✳ PRIORITY CONCEPT EXEMPLARS

ACID-BASE BALANCE

Acidosis, 190

CELLULAR REGULATION

Breast Cancer, 1440
Cirrhosis, 1169
Colorectal Cancer, 1126
Head and Neck Cancer, 547
Hypothyroidism, 1270
Osteoporosis, 1015
Prostate Cancer, 1481

CLOTTING

Venous Thromboembolism, 742

COGNITION

Alzheimer's Disease, 857
Traumatic Brain Injury, 940

COMFORT

End of Life, 104
Pain, 45

ELIMINATION

Benign Prostatic Hyperplasia, 1474
Chronic Kidney Disease, 1398
Intestinal Obstruction, 1121
Pyelonephritis, 1372
Ulcerative Colitis, 1150
Urinary Incontinence, 1343

FLUID AND ELECTROLYTE BALANCE

Dehydration, 167
Hypercortisolism (Cushing's Disease), 1255

GAS EXCHANGE

Chronic Obstructive Pulmonary Disease, 572
Pneumonia, 598
Pulmonary Embolism, 616
Tracheostomy, 537

GLUCOSE REGULATION

Diabetes Mellitus, 1280

IMMUNITY

Acute Pancreatitis, 1197
Angioedema, 361
Guillain-Barré Syndrome, 912
Hepatitis, 1180
HIV Infection and AIDS, 337
Infection, 413
Leukemia, 817
Multiple Sclerosis, 888
Peptic Ulcer Disease (PUD), 1107
Peritonitis, 1144
Pulmonary Tuberculosis, 605
Rheumatoid Arthritis, 318
Sepsis and Septic Shock, 760

MOBILITY

Fractures, 1032
Osteoarthritis, 305
Parkinson Disease, 868
Spinal Cord Injury, 894

NUTRITION

Cholecystitis, 1191
Esophageal Tumors, 1095
Gastroesophageal Reflux Disease (GERD), 1087
Malnutrition, 1215
Obesity, 1225

PERFUSION

Acute Coronary Syndrome, 769
Amputations, 1050
Atrial Fibrillation, 678
Heart Failure, 691
Hypertension, 720
Hypovolemic Shock, 754
Sickle Cell Disease, 808
Stroke (Brain Attack), 928

SENSORY PERCEPTION

Cataract, 968
Glaucoma, 972
Hearing Loss, 996
Otitis Media, 991

SEXUALITY

Pelvic Inflammatory Disease, 1514
Uterine Leiomyoma, 1459

TISSUE INTEGRITY

Pressure Injuries, 447
Stomatitis, 1076

ACID-BASE BALANCE

Acidosis, 196

CELLULAR REGULATION

Breast Cancer, 1440
Cirrhosis, 1104
Colorectal Cancer, 1123
Head and Neck Cancer, 531
Thrombocytopenia, 776
Osteoporosis, 1011
Prostate Cancer, 1561

CLOTTING

Venous Thromboembolism, 712

COGNITION

Alzheimer's Disease, 855
Traumatic Brain Injury, 938

COMFORT

End Of Life, 106
Pain, 30

ELIMINATION

Benign Prostatic Hyperplasia, 1479
Chronic Kidney Disease, 1366
Intestinal Obstruction, 1131
Pyelonephritis, 1378
Ulcerative Colitis, 1156
Urinary Incontinence, 1367

FLUID AND ELECTROLYTE BALANCE

Dehydration, 167
Hypertension/Fluid Overload, 1985

GAS EXCHANGE

Chronic Obstructive Pulmonary Disease, 577
Pneumonia, 578
Pulmonary Embolism, 696
Atelectasis, 277

GLUCOSE REGULATION

Diabetes Mellitus, 1280

IMMUNITY

Acute Pancreatitis, 1197
Anaphylaxis, 361
Guillain-Barre Syndrome, 915
Hepatitis, 1150
HIV Infection and AIDS, 297
Infection, 354
Leukemia, 812
Multiple Sclerosis, 884
Sickle Cell Disease, 808
Peritonitis, 144
Pulmonary Tuberculosis, 605
Rheumatoid Arthritis, 314
Sepsis and Septic Shock, 740

MOBILITY

Fractures, 1042
Osteoarthritis, 309
Parkinson Disease, 868
Spinal Cord Injury, 894

NUTRITION

Cholecystitis, 1191
Esophageal Tumors, 1085
Gastroesophageal Reflux Disease (GERD), 1079
Malnutrition, 1213
Obesity, 1227

PERFUSION

Acute Coronary Syndrome, 760
Amputation, 1050
Atrial Fibrillation, 678
Heart Failure, 691
Hypertension, 720
Hypovolemic Shock, 754
Sickle Cell Disease, 808
Stroke (Brain Attack), 928

SENSORY PERCEPTION

Cataract, 968
Glaucoma, 972
Hearing Loss, 990
Otitis Media, 991

SEXUALITY

Pelvic Inflammatory Disease, 1514
Uterine Leiomyoma, 1529

TISSUE INTEGRITY

Pressure Injuries, 447
Melanoma, 1024

9th EDITION

Medical-Surgical Nursing

CONCEPTS FOR INTERPROFESSIONAL COLLABORATIVE CARE

Donna D. Ignatavicius, MS, RN, CNE, ANEF
Speaker and Curriculum Consultant for Academic Nursing
 Programs;
Founder, Boot Camp for Nurse Educators;
President, DI Associates, Inc.
Littleton, Colorado

M. Linda Workman, PhD, RN, FAAN
Author and Consultant
Cincinnati, Ohio

Cherie R. Rebar, PhD, MBA, RN, COI
Professor of Nursing
Wittenberg University
Springfield, Ohio

Section Editor:
Nicole M. Heimgartner, MSN, RN, COI
Former Associate Professor of Nursing
Kettering College;
Subject Matter Expert, Author, and Consultant
Louisville, Kentucky

ELSEVIER

ELSEVIER

3251 Riverport Lane
St. Louis, Missouri 63043

Executive Content Strategist: Lee Henderson
Senior Content Development Manager: Laurie Gower
Senior Content Development Specialist: Laura Goodrich
Publishing Services Manager: Jeff Patterson
Senior Project Manager: Jodi M. Willard
Design Direction: Brian Salisbury

Printed in Canada

Last digit is the print number: 9 8 7 6 5 4

CONSULTANTS

Deanne A. Blach, MSN, RN
President
DB Productions of NW AR, Inc.
Green Forest, Arkansas

Richard Lintner, RT (R), (CV), (MR), (CT)
Program Director, School of Interventional
    Radiology
The University of Kansas Health System
Kansas City, Kansas

CONTRIBUTORS

Jeanette Spain Adams, PhD, RN, CRNI, ACNS, BC
Consultant
University of Phoenix
Coconut Grove, Florida

Meg Blair, PhD, MSN, RN, CEN
Professor
Nursing Division
Nebraska Methodist College
Omaha, Nebraska

Andrea A. Borchers, PhD, RN
Assistant Professor
Northern Arizona University
Flagstaff, Arizona

Samuel A. Borchers, OD
Optometrist
Vision Clinic
Northern Arizona VA Healthcare System
Prescott, Arizona

Katherine L. Byar, MSN, APN, BC, BMTCN®
Nurse Practitioner
Nebraska Medicine
Omaha, Nebraska

Michelle Camicia, PhD(c), MSN, CRRN, CCM, FAHA
Director of Operations
Kaiser Foundation Rehabilitation Center
Kaiser Permanente
Vallejo, California;
PhD Candidate
The Betty Irene Moore School of Nursing
University of California, Davis
Davis, California

Lara Carver, PhD, RN, CNE
Professor
Department of Nursing
National University
Las Vegas, Nevada

Tammy Coffee, MSN, RN, ACNP
Nurse
MetroHealth Medical Center
Cleveland, Ohio

Keelin Cromar, MSN, RN
Adjunct Faculty
Mississippi Gulf Coast Community College
Perkinston, Mississippi

Janice Cuzzell, MSN, RN, CWS
Corstrata, Inc.
Savannah, Georgia

Cynthia Danko, DNP, RN
Instructor
Frances Payne Bolton School of Nursing
Case Western Reserve University
Cleveland, Ohio

Laura M. Dechant, DNP, APRN, CCRN, CCNS
Adjunct Clinical Instructor
School of Nursing
Widener University
Chester, Pennsylvania;
Clinical Nurse Specialist
Heart, Vascular and Interventional Services
Christiana Care Health System
Newark, Delaware

Stephanie M. Fox, PsyD
Clinical Psychologist
Littleton, Colorado

Roberta Goff, MSN-Ed, RN-BC, ACNS-BC, ONC
Senior Clinical Analyst
Information Systems
Munson Medical Center
Traverse City, Michigan

Saundra Hendricks, FNP, BC-ADM
Nurse Practitioner
Houston Methodist Hospital
Houston, Texas

Amy Jauch, MSN, RN
Clinical Instructor of Practice
College of Nursing
The Ohio State University
Columbus, Ohio

Gail B. Johnson, MSN, RN, AOCN, CNS
CNS, Midlevel Provider
Division of Surgical Oncology
UC/UCP—University of Cincinnati/
    University of Cincinnati Physicians, Inc.
UCMC—Barrett Cancer Center
Cincinnati, Ohio

Mary K. Kazanowski, PhD, APRN, ACHPN
Palliative Care Nurse Practitioner
Elliot Hospital;
VNA Hospice of Manchester and Southern
    New Hampshire
Manchester, New Hampshire

Harriet Kumar, MSN, ANP-BC
Nurse Practitioner
Division of Hematology/Oncology and Bone
    Marrow Transplantation
University of Cincinnati College of Medicine
Cincinnati, Ohio

Linda Laskowski-Jones, MS, APRN, ACNS-BC, CEN, FAWM, FAAN
Vice President Emergency & Trauma
    Services
Christiana Care Health System
Wilmington, Delaware

Kristin Oneail, MSN, RN
OK! Nurse Consultants
Walbridge, Ohio

Rebecca M. Patton, DNP, RN, CNOR, FAAN
Atkinson Scholar in Perioperative Nursing
Frances Payne Bolton School of Nursing
Case Western Reserve University
Cleveland, Ohio

Julie Ponto, PhD, APRN, CNS, AGCNS-BC, AOCNS®
Professor, Graduate Programs in Nursing
Winona State University—Rochester
Rochester, Minnesota

Jennifer Powers, MSN, RN, FNP-BC
Adjunct Faculty
Department of Nursing
National University
Henderson, Nevada

Harry Rees III, MSN, ACNP-BC
Acute Care Nurse Practitioner
Surgical Intensive Care
Ohio State University Wexner Medical
   Center
Columbus, Ohio

James G. Sampson, DNP, NP-C
Adjunct Assistant Professor
College of Nursing
University of Colorado
Aurora, Colorado;
Clinical Supervisor, Adult Nurse Practitioner
Department of Internal Medicine
Denver Health Medical Center
Denver, Colorado

Melanie H. Simpson, PhD, RN-BC, OCN, CHPN, CPE
Pain Team Coordinator
Department of Nursing
The University of Kansas Health System
Kansas City, Kansas

Tracy Taylor, MSN, RN
Clinical Instructor of Practice
College of Nursing
The Ohio State University
Columbus, Ohio

Karen L. Toulson, MSN, MBA, RN, CEN, NE-BC
Director, Emergency Department Clinical
   Operations
Christiana Care Health System
Newark, Delaware

Kathy Vanderbeck, ARNP, OCNS-C®, CNRN
Joint Center Program Coordinator
Baptist Health
Jacksonville, Florida

Constance G. Visovsky, PhD, RN, ACNP-BC
Associate Dean, Faculty Affairs &
   Partnerships
Director of Diversity
Associate Professor, School of Nursing
University of South Florida
Tampa, Florida

Laura M. Willis, DNP, APRN, FNP-C
Family Nurse Practitioner
Urbana Family Medicine and Pediatrics
Urbana, Ohio

Chris Winkelman, PhD, RN, CNS, CCRN, ACNP, FAANP, FCCM
Associate Professor
Frances Payne Bolton School of Nursing
Case Western Reserve Univesity;
Clinical Support
Trauma/Critical Care Nursing
MetroHealth Medical Center
Cleveland, Ohio

CONTRIBUTORS TO TEACHING/LEARNING RESOURCES

PowerPoint Slides

Nicole M. Heimgartner, MSN, RN, COI
Former Associate Professor of Nursing
Kettering College;
Subject Matter Expert, Author, and Consultant
Louisville, Kentucky

Cherie R. Rebar, PhD, MBA, RN, COI
Professor of Nursing
Wittenberg University
Springfield, Ohio

TEACH for Nurses Lesson Plans

Carolyn Gersch, PhD, MSN, RN, CNE
Director of Nursing Education
Ohio Institute of Allied Health
Dayton, Ohio

Nicole M. Heimgartner, MSN, RN, COI
Former Associate Professor of Nursing
Kettering College;
Subject Matter Expert, Author, and Consultant
Louisville, Kentucky

Cherie R. Rebar, PhD, MBA, RN, COI
Professor of Nursing
Wittenberg University
Springfield, Ohio

Test Bank

Meg Blair, PhD, MSN, RN, CEN
Professor
Nursing Division
Nebraska Methodist College
Omaha, Nebraska

Tami Kathleen Little, RN, DNP, CNE
Dean of Nursing
Brookline College
Albuquerque, New Mexico

Marla Kniewel, EdD, MSN, RN
Associate Professor
Nursing Division
Nebraska Methodist College
Omaha, Nebraska

Case Studies

Candice Kumagai, MSN, RN
Former Clinical Instructor
University of Texas at Austin
Austin, Texas

Linda A. LaCharity, PhD, MN, BSN, RN
Adjunct Faculty
Former Accelerated Program Director and
   Assistant Professor
College of Nursing
University of Cincinnati
Cincinnati, Ohio

Concept Maps

Deanne A. Blach, MSN, RN
President, Nursing Education
DB Productions of NW AR, Inc.
Green Forest, Arkansas

Key Points

Deanne A. Blach, MSN, RN
President, Nursing Education
DB Productions of NW AR, Inc.
Green Forest, Arkansas

Review Questions for the NCLEX Examination

Lisa A. Hollett, MA, BSN, RN, MICN, Certified Forensic Nurse
Stroke Coordinator
Hillcrest Medical Center
Tulsa, Oklahoma

Andrea R. Mann, MSN, RN, CNE
Interim Dean, Third Level Chair
Aria Health School of Nursing
Trevose, Pennsylvania

Molly McClelland, PhD, MSN, BSN, ACNS-BC, CMSRN
Associate Professor
College of Health Professions
University of Detroit Mercy
Detroit, Michigan

Tara McMillan-Queen, MSN, BSN, AA, ANP, GNP
Faculty II, NP
Mercy School of Nursing
Charlotte, North Carolina

Heidi Monroe, MSN
Assistant Professor
Nursing
Bellin College
Green Bay, Wisconsin

Denise Robinson, MS, RN, CNE
Assistant Professor of Nursing
Monroe County Community College
Monroe, Michigan

Kathryn Schartz, MSN, RN, PPCPNP-BC
Assistant Professor of Nursing
School of Nursing
Baker University
Topeka, Kansas

Bethany Sykes, EdD, MSN, BSN, RN, CEN
Emergency Department
St. Luke's Hospital;
CCRN
Critical Care Unit
St. Luke's Hospital
New Bedford, Massachusetts;
Adjunct Faculty
Department of Nursing
Salve Regina University
Newport, Rhode Island;
RN Refresher Course Coordinator
College of Nursing
University of Massachusetts
North Dartmouth, Massachusetts

REVIEWERS

Ramona Bartlow, DNP, MSN, RN
Assistant Professor, Course/Clinical
    Coordinator
Northwestern Oklahoma State University
College of Nursing
Enid, Oklahoma

**Marylee Bressie, DNP, RN, CCNS, CCRN-K,
    CEN**
Core Faculty/MSN Specialization Lead for
    Leadership & Administration
Capella University
School of Nursing & Health Sciences
Department of Nursing
Minneapolis, Minnesota

Ashley Leak Bryant, PhD, RN-BC, OCN
Assistant Professor
The University of North Carolina at Chapel
    Hill
School of Nursing
Chapel Hill, North Carolina

**Margaret-Ann Carno, PhD, MBA, MJ,
    CPNP, ABSM, FAAN**
Professor of Clinical Nursing and Pediatrics
University of Rochester
School of Nursing
Rochester, New York

Mary Cox
Professor
Clemson University
Clemson, South Carolina

**Diane Daddario, ANP-C, ACNS-BC,
    RN-BC, CMSRN**
Hospitalist CRNP in Behavioral Health Unit
Holy Spirit Hospital—A Geisinger Affiliate
Camp Hill, Pennsylvania;
Adjunct Nursing Faculty
Pennsylvania State University
University Park, Pennsylvania

Shirlee Proctor Davidson, MSN, RN
Independent Practitioner and Consultant,
Psychiatric Mental Health Nursing Clinical
    Specialist
Liaison Consultation and Education
Santa Fe, New Mexico

**Laura M. Dechant, APRN, MSN, CCRN,
    CCNS**
Clinical Nurse Specialist
Heart, Vascular and Interventional Services
Christiana Care Health System
Newark, Delaware

**Julie Eggert, NP, PhD, GNP-BC, AGN-BC,
    AOCN, FAAN**
Genetic Risk Consultant
Cancer Risk Screening Program
Bon Secours Hematology & Oncology
Greenville, South Carolina

Selena A. Gilles, DNP, ANP-BC, CCRN
Clinical Assistant Professor
New York University
New York, New York;
Nurse Practitioner
Garden State Pain Management
Clifton, New Jersey

Ruth Gladen, MS, RN
Associate Professor
North Dakota State College of Science
Nursing Department
Wahpeton, North Dakota

Cathy Glennon, RN, MHS, OCN, NE-BC
Director, Brandmeyer Resource Center
University of Kansas Hospital
Cancer Center
Kansas City, Kansas

**Roberta L. Goff, MSN, Ed, RN-BC,
    ACNS-BC, ONC**
Clinical Nurse Specialist
Orthopedics
Munson Medical Center
Traverse City, Michigan

Kathleen Griffith, MSN, RN
Full-Time Lecturer
California State University, Fullerton
School of Nursing
Fullerton, California

Linda Johanson, RN, MS, EdD, CNE
Associate Professor
Appalachian State University
Nursing Department, College of Health
    Sciences
Boone, North Carolina

Janie Lynn Jones, MSN, RN, CNE
Assistant Professor
University of Arkansas at Little Rock
Department of Nursing
Little Rock, Arkansas

**Deanna Jung, DNP, APRN, AGACNP-BC,
    ACCNS-AG**
Assistant Professor
California State University, Fullerton;
Bayside Medical Center
School of Nursing
Fullerton, California

**Marylyn Kajs-Wyllie, MSN, RN, CNS,
    CNRN, CCRN-K, SCRN**
Clinical Associate Professor
Texas State University
St. David's School of Nursing
Round Rock, Texas

Tamara M. Kear, PhD, RN, CNS, CNN
Assistant Professor of Nursing
Villanova University
College of Nursing
Villanova, Pennsylvania

Cheryl Kent, DNP, MS, RN, CNE
Assistant Professor of Nursing
Northwestern Oklahoma State University
Division of Nursing
Enid, Oklahoma

Kari Ksar, RN, MS, CPNP
Pediatric Nurse Practitioner
Lucile Packard Children's Hospital
Pediatric Gastroenterology, Hepatology and
    Nutrition
Palo Alto, California

**Martha E. Langhorne, MSN, RN, FNP,
    AOCN**
Nurse Practitioner
Binghamton Gastroenterology
Binghamton, New York

Shawn M. Mason, MEd, BSN, RN
Nursing Faculty
Kwantlen Polytechnic University, Langley
    Campus
Faculty of Health
Surrey, British Columbia, Canada

Maureen McDonald, MS, RN
Professor, Department Chair
Massasoit Community College
Brockton, Massachusetts

Predrag Miskin, DHSc, RN, PHN, CMSRN
Instructor
De Anza College
Department of Nursing
Cupertino, California

PREFACE

The first edition of this textbook, entitled *Medical-Surgical Nursing: A Nursing Process Approach,* was a groundbreaking work in many ways. The following eight editions built on that achievement and further solidified the book's position as a major trendsetter for the practice of adult health nursing. Now, in its ninth edition, "Iggy" charts the cutting-edge approach for the future of adult nursing practice—an approach reflected in its current title: *Medical-Surgical Nursing: Concepts for Inter-professional Collaborative Care.* The focus of this new edition continues to help students learn how to provide safe, quality nursing care that is patient-centered, evidence-based, and interprofessionally collaborative. In addition to print formats as single- and two-volume texts, this edition is now available in a variety of electronic formats.

The subtitle for this ninth edition was carefully chosen to emphasize the interprofessional nature of today's care, in which the nurse serves as a central role in collaboration with the patient, family, and members of the interprofessional health care team in acute care, community-based, and home settings. This approach reflects the National Academy of Medicine, The Joint Commission, the Quality and Safety Education for Nurses (QSEN) Institute, and the 2010 *Future of Nursing* report that unanimously have called for all health professionals to coordinate and deliver safe, evidence-based, patient-centered care as a collaborative team.

KEY THEMES FOR THE 9TH EDITION

The key themes for this edition strengthen this text's conceptual focus on safety, quality care, patient-centeredness, and clinical judgment to best prepare the student for interprofessional practice in medical-surgical health settings. Each theme is outlined and described below.

- **Enhanced Focus on Professional Nursing and Health Concepts.** This edition uniquely balances a focus on concepts, and a conceptual approach to teaching and learning, with important underpinnings of content. Prelicensure programs that embrace concept-based nursing curriculum, system-focused curriculum, or a hybrid approach will find this edition easy to use. To help students connect previously learned concepts with new information in the text, Chapters 1 and 2 addresses the main concepts used in this edition, giving a working definition upon which the students will reflect and build as they learn new material. These unique features build on basic concepts learned in nursing fundamentals courses, such as gas exchange and safety, to help students make connections between foundational concepts and interprofessional patient care for medical-surgical conditions. For continuity and reinforcement, a list of specific Priority and Interrelated Nursing Concepts is highlighted at the beginning of each chapter. This placement is specifically designed to help students better understand the priority and associated needs that the nurse will address when providing safe, evidence-based, patient-centered care for individuals with selected health problems. When these concepts are discussed in the body of each chapter, they are presented in small capital letters (e.g.,

IMMUNITY) to help students relate and apply essential concepts to provide more focused nursing care.

- **Emphasis on Key Exemplars.** For each priority concept listed in selected chapters, the authors have identified key exemplars. The nursing and interprofesional collaborative care for patients experiencing these exemplar diseases and illnesses is discussed through the lens of the priority and interrelated concepts. In addition, patient problems are presented as a collaborative problem list rather than merely presenting nursing diagnoses.

- **Prioritized Focus on the Core Body of Knowledge and QSEN Competencies.** This edition not only continues to emphasize need-to-know content for the RN level of practice but also includes a continuing emphasis on Quality and Safety Education for Nurses (QSEN) Institute core competencies. Clinical practice settings emphasize the critical need for safe practices and quality improvement to provide interprofessional patient-centered care that is evidence-based. Many hospitals and other health care agencies have formally adopted these QSEN competencies as core values and goals for patient care, and many nursing programs have used these same competencies to build prelicensure nursing curriculum. To help prepare students for the work environment as new graduates, as well as to highlight the foundational underpinning of safety and quality into all nursing actions, this edition prioritizes a focus on these competencies.

- **Emphasis on Patient Safety.** Patient safety is emphasized throughout this edition, not only in the narrative but also in **Nursing Safety Priority boxes** that enable students to immediately identify the most important care needed for patients with specific health problems. These highlighted features are further classified as an Action Alert, Drug Alert, or Critical Rescue. We also continue to include our leading-edge Best Practice for Patient Safety & Quality Care charts to emphasize the most important nursing care. **Highlighted yellow text** also demonstrates the application of The Joint Commission's National Patient Safety Goals initiatives (http://www.jointcommission.org/standards_information/npsgs.aspx) and Core Measures content into everyday nursing practice. The Joint Commission's National Patient Safety Goals initiatives are also set in **boldface type** for further emphasis.

- **Focus on Patient-Centered Care.** Patient-centered care is enhanced in the ninth edition in several ways. The ninth edition continues to use the term "patient" instead of "client" throughout. Although the use of these terms remains a subject of discussion among nursing educators and health care organizations, we have not defined the patient as a dependent person. Rather, the patient can be an individual, a family, or a group—all of whom have rights that are respected in a mutually trusting nurse-patient relationship. Most health care agencies and professional organizations use "patient" in their practice and publications, and most professional nursing organizations support the term.

- **Focus on Gender Considerations.** To increase our emphasis on patient-centered care, **Gender Health Considerations** focus on important gender-associated information that impacts nursing care. Differences in patient values, preferences, and beliefs are addressed in **Chapter 73, Care of Transgender Patients**. Along with other individuals in the LGBTQ population, the health needs of transgender patients have gained national attention through their inclusion in *Healthy People 2020* and The Joint Commission's standards. This chapter, first introduced in the eighth edition, continues to provide tools to help prepare students and faculty to provide safe, evidence-based, patient-centered care for transgender patients who are considering or who have undergone the gender transition process.

- **Emphasis on Evidence-Based Practice.** The ninth edition focuses again on the importance of *using best current evidence in nursing practice* and how to locate and use this evidence to improve patient care. **Evidence-Based Practice boxes** offer a solid foundation in this essential component of nursing practice. Each box summarizes a useful research article and explains the implications of its findings for practice and further research, as well as a rating of the level of evidence based on a well-respected scale.

- **Focus on Quality Improvement.** The QSEN Institute emphasizes, and clinical practice agencies require, that all nurses have *quality improvement* knowledge, skills, and attitudes. To help prepare students for that role, this edition includes unique **Quality Improvement boxes.** Each box summarizes a quality improvement project published in the literature and discusses the implications of the project's success in improving nursing care. The inclusion of these boxes disseminates information and research and helps students understand that quality improvement begins at the bedside as the nurse identifies potential evidence-based solutions to practice problems.

- **Emphasis on Clinical Judgment.** Stressing the importance of clinical judgment skills via prioritization and delegation helps to best prepare students for practice and the NCLEX® Examination. As in the eighth edition, the ninth edition emphasizes the importance of nursing clinical judgment to make timely and appropriate decisions and prioritize care. To help achieve that focus, all-new case-based **Clinical Judgment Challenges** based primarily on QSEN core competencies are integrated throughout the text. Selected Clinical Judgment Challenges highlight ethical dilemmas, as well as delegation and supervision issues. These exercises provide clinical situations in which students can use evolving nursing clinical judgment to help prepare them for the fast-paced world of medical-surgical nursing. Suggested answer guidelines for these Clinical Judgment Challenges are provided on the companion Evolve website (http://evolve.elsevier.com/Iggy/).

Dr. Christine Tanner's clinical judgment framework (Tanner, 2006) is integrated more deeply in this edition to help students apply selected concepts in the Disorders chapters. The components of this model match Tanner's terminology to each nursing process heading, thereby helping students use nursing judgment to provide safe, quality care by:

- Assessment: Noticing
- Analysis: Interpreting
- Planning: Implementation and Responding
- Evaluation: Reflecting

- **Emphasis on Preparation for the NCLEX® Examination.** An enhanced emphasis on the NCLEX Examination and consistency with the 2016 NCLEX-RN® test plan has been refined in this edition. The ninth edition emphasizes "readiness"—readiness for the NCLEX Examination, readiness for disaster and mass casualty events, readiness for safe drug administration, and readiness for the continually evolving world of genetics and genomics. An increased number of new **NCLEX Examination Challenges** are interspersed throughout the text to allow students the opportunity to practice test-taking and decision making. Answers to these Challenges are provided in the back of the book, and their rationales are provided on the Evolve website (http://evolve.elsevier.com/Iggy). In a world that needs more nurses than ever before, it is more critical than ever that students be ready to pass the licensure examination on the first try. To help students and faculty achieve that outcome, **Learning Outcomes** at the beginning of each chapter continue to be consistent with the competencies outlined in the detailed 2016 NCLEX-RN® Test Plan. The ninth edition continues to include an innovative end-of-chapter feature called **Get Ready for the NCLEX® Examination!** This unique and effective learning aid consists of a list of **Key Points** *organized by Client Needs Category* as found in the NCLEX-RN Test Plan. Relevant QSEN and Nurse of the Future competency categories are identified for selected Key Points.

- **New Focus on Care Coordination and Transition Management.** This edition includes a priority focus on continuity of care via a Care Coordination and Transition Management section in each Disorders chapter. Literature continues to emphasize the importance of care coordination and transition management between acute care and community-based care (Lattavo, 2014). To help students prepare for this role, the ninth edition of our text provides coverage focusing on Home Care Management, Self-Management Education, and Health Care Resources.

CLINICAL CURRENCY AND ACCURACY

To ensure currency and accuracy, we listened to students and faculty who have used the previous editions, focusing on their impressions of and experiences with the book. A thorough literature search of current best evidence regarding nursing education and clinical practice helped us validate best practices and national health care trends to shape the focus of the ninth edition.

In-depth reviews of every chapter were commissioned and conducted by a dedicated panel of instructors and clinicians across the United States and Canada. A well-respected interventional radiologist ensured the accuracy of diagnostic testing procedures and associated patient care. The input from these experts guided us in revising chapters into their final format.

The results of these efforts are reflected in the ninth edition's:

- Strong, consistent focus on NCLEX-RN® Examination preparation, clinical judgment, safe patient-centered interprofessional care, pathophysiology, drug therapy, quality improvement, evidence-based clinical practice, and care coordination and transition management
- Foundation of relevant research and best practice guidelines
- Emphasis on critical "need to know" information that entry-level nurses must master to provide safe patient care

With the amount of information that continues to evolve in health care practice and education, it is easy for a book to become larger with each new edition. The reality is that today's nursing students have a limited time to absorb and begin to apply essential information to provide safe medical-surgical nursing care. Materials in this edition were carefully scrutinized to determine what the essential information was that students will actively *use* when providing safe, patient-centered, interprofessional, quality nursing care for adults.

OUTSTANDING READABILITY

Today's students must maximize their study time to read information and quickly understand it. The average reading level of today's learner is 10th to 11th grade. To achieve this level of readability without reducing the quality or depth of material that students need to know, this text uses a direct-address style (where appropriate) that speaks directly to the reader, and sentences are as short as possible without sacrificing essential content. The new edition has improved consistency of difficulty level from chapter to chapter. The result of our efforts is a medical-surgical text of consistently outstanding readability in which content is clear, focused, and accessible.

EASE OF ACCESS

To make this text as easy to use as possible, we have maintained our approach of having smaller chapters of more uniform length. Consistent with our focus on "need to know" material, we chose exemplars to illustrate concepts of care versus detailing every health disorder. The focused ninth edition contains 74 chapters.

The overall presentation of the ninth edition has been updated, including more current, high-quality photographs for realism, as well as design changes to improve accessibility of material. The design of the ninth edition includes appropriate placement of display elements (e.g., figures, tables, and charts) for a chapter flow that enhances text reading without splintering content or confusing the reader. Additional ease-of-access features for this edition include tabbed markings for the answer key, glossary, and index for quick reference. To increase the smoothness of flow and reader concentration, side-turned tables and charts or tables and charts that span multiple pages are infrequently used. Drug tables have been reformatted for consistency and ease of use.

We have maintained the unit structure of previous editions, with vital body systems (cardiovascular, respiratory, and neurologic) appearing earlier in the book. In these three units we continue to provide complex care content in separate chapters that discuss managing critically ill patients with coronary artery disease, respiratory health problems, and neurologic health problems.

To break up long blocks of text and highlight key information, we continue to include streamlined yet eye-catching headings, bulleted lists, tables, charts, and in-text highlights. Key terms are in boldface color type and are defined in the text to foster the learning of need-to-know vocabulary. A glossary is located in the back of the book. Current bibliographic resources at the end of each chapter include research articles, nationally accepted clinical guidelines, and other sources of evidence when available for each chapter. Classic sources from before 2011 are noted with an asterisk (*).

A PATIENT-CENTERED, INTERPROFESSIONAL COLLABORATIVE CARE APPROACH

As in previous editions, we maintain in this edition a collaborative, interprofessional care approach to patient care. In the real world of health care, nurses, patients, and all other providers who are part of the interprofessional team *share* responsibility for the management of patient problems. Thus we present information in a collaborative framework with an increased emphasis on the interprofessional nature of care. In this framework we make no *artificial* distinctions between medical treatment and nursing care. Instead, under each Interprofessional Collaborative Care heading we discuss how the nurse coordinates care and transition management while interacting with members of the interprofessional team.

This edition includes newly redesigned patient-centered Concept Maps that underscore the interprofessional care approach. Each Concept Map contains a case scenario. It then shows how a selected complex health problem is addressed. Each Concept Map spells out the steps of the nursing process and related concepts to illustrate the relationships among disease processes, priority patient problems, collaborative management, and more.

Although our approach has a focus on interprofessional care, the text is first and foremost a *nursing* text. We therefore use a nursing process approach as a tool to organize discussions of patient health problems and their management. Discussions of *major* health problems follow a full nursing process format using this structure:

[Health problem]
Pathophysiology
    Etiology (and Genetic Risk when appropriate)
    Incidence and Prevalence
Health Promotion and Maintenance (when appropriate)
Interprofessional Collaborative Care
    Assessment: Noticing
    Analysis: Interpreting
    Planning and Implementation: Responding
        [Collaborative Intervention Statement (based on priority patient problems)]
        Planning: Expected Outcomes
        Interventions
    Care Coordination and Transition Management
        Home Care Management
        Self-Management Education
        Health Care Resources
    Evaluation: Reflecting

The Analysis sections list the priority patient problems associated with major health problems and disorders. The ninth edition identifies priority collaborative patient problems or needs as the basis for the interprofessional plan of care. These collaborative patient problems pair more clearly with the title's focus than the previous use of NANDA-I language, which addresses primarily nursing-oriented patient problems. With its concentration on collaborative patient problems or needs, the ninth edition aligns with the language of clinical practice.

Discussions of less common or less complex disorders follow a similar, yet abbreviated, format: a discussion of the problem itself (including pertinent information on pathophysiology) followed by a section on interprofessional collaborative care of patients with the disorder. To demonstrate our commitment to providing the content foundational to nursing education, and consistent with the recommendations of Benner and colleagues through the Carnegie Foundation for the Future of Nursing Education, we highlight essential pathophysiologic concepts that are key to understanding the basis for collaborative management.

Integral to the interprofessional care approach is a narrative of who on the health care team is involved in the care of the patient. When a responsibility is primarily the nurse's, the text says so. When a decision must be made jointly by various members of the team (e.g., by the patient, nurse, health care provider, and physical therapist), this is clearly stated. When health care practitioners in different care settings are involved in the patient's care, this is stated.

ORGANIZATION

The 74 chapters of *Medical-Surgical Nursing: Concepts for Interprofessional Collaborative Care* are grouped into 16 units. Unit 1, Foundations for Medical-Surgical Nursing, provides fundamental information for the health care concepts incorporated throughout the text. Unit 2 consists of three chapters on concepts of emergency and trauma care and disaster preparedness.

Unit 3 consists of three chapters on the management of patients with fluid, electrolyte, and acid-base imbalances. Chapters 11 and 12 review key assessments associated with fluid and electrolyte balance, acid-base balance, and related patient care in a clear, concise discussion. The chapter on infusion therapy (Chapter 13) is supplemented with an online Fluids & Electrolytes Tutorial on the companion Evolve website.

Unit 4 presents the perioperative nursing content that medical-surgical nurses need to know. This content provides a solid foundation to help the student better understand the interprofessional care required for the surgical patient regardless of setting. Emphasis is placed on continuous assessment during the perioperative period to prevent complications and improve outcomes as we continue to see an increase in ambulatory care.

Unit 5 provides core content on health problems related to immunity. This material includes information on inflammation and the immune response, altered cell growth and cancer development, and interventions for patients with connective tissue disease, HIV infection, and other immunologic disorders, cancers, and infections.

The remaining 11 units cover medical-surgical content by body system. Each of these units begins with an Assessment chapter and continues with one or more Nursing Care chapters for patients with selected health problems, highlighted via exemplars, in that body system. This framework is familiar to students who learn the body systems in preclinical foundational science courses such as anatomy and physiology.

MULTINATIONAL, MULTICULTURAL, MULTIGENERATIONAL FOCUS

To reflect the increasing diversity of our society, *Medical-Surgical Nursing: Concepts for Interprofessional Collaborative Care* takes a multinational, multicultural, and multigenerational focus. Addressing the needs of both U.S. and Canadian readers, we have included examples of trade names of drugs available in the United States and in Canada. Drugs that are available only in Canada are designated with the Canadian maple leaf symbol(🍁). When appropriate, we identify specific Canadian health care resources, including their websites. In many areas, Canadian health statistics are combined with those of the United States to provide an accurate "North American" picture.

To help nurses provide quality care for patients whose preferences, beliefs, and values may differ from their own, numerous **Cultural/Spiritual Considerations** and **Gender Health Considerations boxes** highlight important aspects of culturally competent care. Chapter 73 is dedicated to the special health care needs of transgender patients.

Increases in life expectancy and aging of the baby-boom generation contribute to a steadily increasing older adult population. To help nurses care for this population, the ninth edition continues to provide thorough coverage of the care of older adults. Chapter 3 offers content on the role of the nurse and interprofessional team in promoting health for older adults, with coverage of common health problems that older adults may experience, such as falls and inadequate nutrition. The text includes many **Nursing Focus on the Older Adult** charts. Laboratory values and drug considerations for older patients are also included throughout the book. Charts specifying normal physiologic changes to expect in the older population are found in each Assessment chapter, and **Considerations for Older Adults boxes** emphasize key points for the student to consider when caring for these patients. A new feature for the ninth edition is **Veterans' Health Considerations**. An increasing number of veterans of wars have multiple physical and mental health problems and require special attention in today's health care environment.

ADDITIONAL LEARNING AIDS

The ninth edition continues to include a rich array of learning aids geared toward adult learners that help students quickly identify and understand key information while serving as study aids.

- Written in "patient-friendly" language, **Patient and Family Education: Preparing for Self-Management charts** provide teaching information that nurses must know to safely transition patients and their families back to the community environment of care.
- **Laboratory Profile charts** summarize important laboratory test information commonly used to evaluate health status. Information typically includes the normal ranges of laboratory values (including differences for older adults, when appropriate) and the significance of abnormal findings.
- The streamlined **Common Examples of Drug Therapy charts** summarize important information about commonly used drugs. Charts include U.S. and Canadian trade names for typically used drugs along with nursing implications and rationales (rationales are indicated by italic type).
- **Key Features charts** highlight the clinical signs and symptoms of important health problems based on pathophysiologic concepts.
- **Evidence-Based Practice boxes**, provided in many chapters, give synopses of recent nursing research articles and other scientific articles applicable to nursing. Each box provides a summary of the research, its level of evidence (LOE), and a brief commentary with implications for nursing practice and future research. This feature helps students identify strengths and weaknesses of evidence while seeing how research guides nursing practice.

- **Quality Improvement boxes** offer anecdotes of recent nursing articles that focus on this important QSEN competency and how nurses at the bedside have an active hand in shaping best practice. Similar to the Evidence-Based Practice boxes, these features provide a brief summary of the research with commentary on the implications for practice.
- As in the previous editions, **Home Care Assessment charts** serve as a convenient summary of essential assessment points for patients who need follow-up home health nursing care.
- Subtypes of **Clinical Judgment Challenges** (CJCs) emphasize the six QSEN core competencies: Patient-Centered Care, Teamwork and Collaboration, Evidence-Based Practice, Quality Improvement, Safety, and Informatics.

AN INTEGRATED MULTIMEDIA RESOURCE BASED ON PROVEN STRATEGIES FOR STUDENT ENGAGEMENT AND LEARNING

Medical-Surgical Nursing: Concepts for Interprofessional Collaborative Care, 9th edition, is the centerpiece of a comprehensive package of electronic and print learning resources that break new ground in the application of proven strategies for student engagement, learning, and evidence-based educational practice. This integrated multimedia resource actively engages the student in problem solving and practicing clinical decision-making skills.

Resources for Instructors

For the convenience of faculty, all Instructor Resources are available on a streamlined, secure instructor area of the Evolve website (http://evolve.elsevier.com/Iggy/). Included among these Instructor Resources are the *TEACH for Nurses* **Lesson Plans.** These Lesson Plans focus on the most important content from each chapter and provide innovative strategies for student engagement and learning. This ninth edition *TEACH for Nurses* product incorporates numerous interprofessional activities that give students an opportunity to practice as an integral part of the health care team. Lesson Plans are provided for each chapter and are categorized into several parts:

Learning Outcomes
Teaching Focus
Key Terms
Nursing Curriculum Standards
    QSEN
    Concepts
    BSN Essentials
Student Chapter Resources
Instructor Chapter Resources
Teaching Strategies

Additional Instructor Resources provided on the Evolve website include:

- A completely revised, updated, high-quality **Test Bank** consisting of more than 1750 items, both traditional multiple-choice and NCLEX-RN® "alternate-item" types. Each question is coded for correct answer, rationale, cognitive level, NCLEX Integrated Process, NCLEX Client Needs Category, and new key words to facilitate question searches. Page references are provided for Remembering (Knowledge)-level and Understanding (Comprehension)-level questions. (Questions at the Applying [Application] and above cognitive level require the student to draw on understanding of multiple or broader concepts not limited to a single textbook page, so page cross references are not provided for these higher-level critical thinking questions.) The Test Bank is provided in the Evolve Assessment Manager and in ExamView and ParTest formats.
- An electronic **Image Collection** containing all images from the book (approximately 550 images), delivered in a format that makes incorporation into lectures, presentations, and online courses easier than ever.
- **PowerPoint Presentations**—a completely revised collection of more than 2000 slides corresponding to each chapter in the text and highlighting key materials with integrated images and Unfolding Case Studies. Audience Response System Questions (three discussion-oriented questions per chapter for use with iClicker and other audience response systems) are included in these slide presentations. Answers and rationales to the Audience Response System Questions and Unfolding Case Studies are found in the "Notes" section of each slide.

Also available for adoption and separate purchase:

- Corresponding chapter-by-chapter to the textbook, *Elsevier Adaptive Quizzing (EAQ)* integrates seamlessly into your course to help students of all skill levels focus their study time and effectively prepare for class, course exams, and the NCLEX® certification exam. *EAQ* is comprised of a bank of high-quality practice questions that allows students to advance at their own pace—based on their performance—through multiple mastery levels for each chapter. A comprehensive dashboard allows students to view their progress and stay motivated. The educator dashboard, grade book, and reporting capabilities enable faculty to monitor the activity of individual students, assess overall class performance, and identify areas of strength and weakness, ultimately helping to achieve improved learning outcomes.
- *Simulation Learning System (SLS) for Medical-Surgical Nursing* is an online toolkit designed to help you effectively incorporate simulation into your nursing curriculum, with scenarios that promote and enhance the clinical decision-making skills of students at all levels. It offers detailed instructions for preparation and implementation of the simulation experience, debriefing questions that encourage critical thinking, and learning resources to reinforce student comprehension. Modularized simulation scenarios correspond to Elsevier's leading medical-surgical nursing texts, reinforcing students' classroom knowledge base, synthesizing lecture and clinicals, and offering the remediation content that is critical to debriefing.

Resources for Students

Resources for students include a revised, updated, and retitled Study Guide, a Clinical Companion, Elsevier Adaptive Learning (EAL), Virtual Clinical Excursions (VCE), and Evolve Learning Resources.

The *Study Guide* has been completely revised and updated and features a fresh emphasis on clinical decision making, priorities of delegation, management of care, and pharmacology.

The pocket-sized *Clinical Companion* is a handy clinical resource that retains its easy-to-use alphabetical organization and streamlined format. It includes "Critical Rescue," "Drug Alert," and "Action Alert" highlights throughout based on the Nursing Safety Priority features in the textbook. National Patient Safety Goals highlights have been expanded as a QSEN feature, focusing on one of six QSEN core competencies while still underscoring the importance of observing vital patient safety standards. This "pocket-sized Iggy" has been tailored to the special needs of students preparing for clinicals and clinical practice.

Corresponding chapter-by-chapter to the textbook, *Elsevier Adaptive Learning (EAL)* combines the power of brain science with sophisticated, patented Cerego algorithms to help students to learn faster and remember longer. It's fun, it's engaging, and it constantly tracks and adapts to student performance to deliver content precisely when it's needed to ensure core information is transformed into lasting knowledge.

Virtual Clinical Excursions, featuring an updated and easy-to-navigate "virtual" clinical setting, is once again available for the eighth edition. This unique learning tool guides students through a virtual clinical environment and helps them "learn by doing" in the safety of a "virtual" hospital.

Also available for students is a dynamic collection of Evolve Student Resources, available at http://evolve.elsevier.com/Iggy/. The Evolve Student Resources include the following:

- Review Questions for the NCLEX® Examination
- Answer Guidelines for NCLEX® Examination and Clinical Judgment Challenges

- Interactive Case Studies
- Concept Maps (digital versions of the 12 Concept Maps from the text)
- Concept Map Creator (a handy tool for creating customized Concept Maps)
- Fluid & Electrolyte Tutorial (a complete self-paced tutorial on this perennially difficult content)
- Key Points (downloadable expanded chapter reviews for each chapter)
- Audio Glossary
- Audio Clips and Video Clips
- Content Updates

In summary, *Medical-Surgical Nursing: Concepts for Interprofessional Collaborative Care,* 9th edition, together with its fully integrated multimedia ancillary package, provides the tools you will need to equip nursing students to meet the opportunities and challenges of nursing practice both now and in an evolving health care environment. The only elements that remain to be added to this package are those that you uniquely provide—your passion, your commitment, your innovation, *your nursing expertise.*

Donna D. Ignatavicius
M. Linda Workman
Cherie R. Rebar

To all the nursing educators who are passionate about teaching, and to all the
nursing students who are passionate about learning.
To my husband, Charles, who has endured countless hours of loneliness while
I've worked on this project, and to Stephanie, my daughter, who has educated me
about the special needs of the LGBTQ community. Thank you!

DONNA

To students everywhere.
To John, still my one.

LINDA

To Michael…you are my everything.
To Gillian…all I do is for you, my beautiful girl.
To Mom and Dad…thank you for roots and wings.
To Donna and Linda…thank you for believing in me!
To our Elsevier team….thank you for your dedication!
To Carolyn, Laura, Nicole, Tracy, and Tracie…my kindred spirits.
To all who study, teach, and practice nursing….you are my heroes.

CHERIE

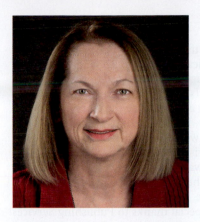

Donna D. Ignatavicius received her diploma in nursing from the Peninsula General School of Nursing in Salisbury, Maryland. After working as a charge nurse in medical-surgical nursing, she became an instructor in staff development at the University of Maryland Medical Center. She then received her BSN from the University of Maryland School of Nursing. For 5 years she taught in several schools of nursing while working toward her MS in Nursing, which she received in 1981. Donna then taught in the BSN program at the University of Maryland, after which she continued to pursue her interest in gerontology and accepted the position of Director of Nursing of a major skilled-nursing facility in her home state of Maryland. Since that time, she has served as an instructor in several associate degree nursing programs. Through her consulting activities, faculty development workshops, and international nursing education conferences (such as Boot Camp for Nurse Educators®),Donna is nationally recognized as an expert in nursing education. She is currently the President of DI Associates, Inc. (http://www.diassociates.com/), a company dedicated to improving health care through education and consultation for faculty. In recognition of her contributions to the field, she was inducted as a charter Fellow of the prestigious Academy of Nursing Education in 2007 and received her Certified Nurse Educator credential in 2016.

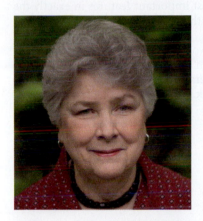

M. Linda Workman, a native of Canada, received her BSN from the University of Cincinnati College of Nursing and Health. After serving in the U.S. Army Nurse Corps and working as an Assistant Head Nurse and Head Nurse in civilian hospitals, Linda earned her MSN from the University of Cincinnati College of Nursing and a PhD in Developmental Biology from the University of Cincinnati College of Arts and Sciences. Linda's 30-plus years of academic experience include teaching at the diploma, associate degree, baccalaureate, master's, and doctoral levels. Her areas of teaching expertise include medical-surgical nursing, physiology, pathophysiology, genetics, oncology, and immunology. Linda has been recognized nationally for her teaching expertise and was inducted as a Fellow into the American Academy of Nursing in 1992. She received Excellence in Teaching awards at the University of Cincinnati and at Case Western Reserve University. She is a former American Cancer Society Professor of Oncology Nursing and held an endowed chair in oncology for 5 years. She has authored several additional textbooks and serves a consultant for major universities.

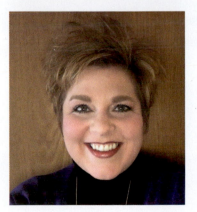

Cherie R. Rebar earned her first degree in education from Morehead State University in Morehead, Kentucky. She returned to school shortly thereafter to earn an Associate of Science degree in Nursing from Kettering College. Cherie's years of clinical practice includes medical-surgical, acute care, ear/nose/throat surgery and allergy, community, and psychiatric-mental health nursing. After earning her MSN and MBA from the University of Phoenix, Cherie combined her love of nursing and education and began teaching Associate and Baccalaureate Completion nursing students at Kettering College while pursuing her Family Nurse Practitioner post-Masters certificate from the University of Massachusetts Boston. Over a decade, Cherie served in numerous leadership positions at Kettering College, including Chair of AS, BSN Completion, and BSN Prelicensure Nursing Programs, as well as Director of the Division of Nursing. She currently is a Professor of Nursing at Wittenberg University, an Affiliate Faculty Member at Indiana Wesleyan University, a Psychiatric–Mental Health Nurse Practitioner Intern through the University of Cincinnati College of Nursing, and a frequent presenter at national nursing conferences. Cherie serves as a consultant with nursing programs and faculty, contributes regularly to professional publications, and holds student success at the heart of all she does.

ACKNOWLEDGMENTS

Publishing a textbook and ancillary package of this magnitude would not be possible without the combined efforts of many people. With that in mind, we would like to extend our deepest gratitude to many people who were such an integral part of this journey.

For the ninth edition, we welcomed section editor Nicole M. Heimgartner to assist in our revision process. Nicole has worked with our team in contributor and ancillary roles over the past editions. Within this edition, she updated and reviewed selected chapters of the text to provide her expertise.

Our contributing authors once again provided excellent manuscripts to underscore the clinical relevancy of this publication. We give special gratitude to Deanne Blach, who revised our Concept Maps, and to Dr. Richard Lintner, who provided expertise in interventional radiologic procedures and associated care. Our reviewers—expert clinicians and instructors from around the United States and Canada—provided invaluable suggestions and encouragement throughout the development of book.

The staff of Elsevier has, as always, provided us with meaningful guidance and support throughout every step of the planning, writing, revision, and production of the ninth edition. Executive Content Strategist Lee Henderson worked closely with us from the early stages of this edition to help us hone and focus our revision plan while coordinating the project from start to finish. Senior Content Development Specialist Laura Goodrich then worked with us to bring the logistics of the ninth edition from vision to publication. Laura also held the reins of our complex ancillary package and worked with a gifted group of writers and content experts to provide an outstanding library of resources to complement and enhance the text.

Senior Project Manager Jodi Willard was, as always, an absolute joy with whom to work. If the mark of a good editor is that his or her work is invisible to the reader, then Jodi is the consummate editor. Her unwavering attention to detail, flexibility, and conscientiousness helped to make the ninth edition consistently readable, while making the production process incredibly smooth. Also, a special thanks to Publishing Services Manager Jeff Patterson.

Designer Brian Salisbury is responsible for the beautiful cover and the new interior design of the ninth edition. Brian's work on this edition has cast important features in exactly the right light, contributing to the readability and colorful beauty of this edition.

Our acknowledgments would not be complete without recognizing our dedicated team of Educational Solutions Consultants and other key members of the Sales and Marketing staff who helped to put this book into your hands.

Donna D. Ignatavicius
M. Linda Workman
Cherie R. Rebar

CONTENTS

UNIT I Foundations for Medical-Surgical Nursing

1 **Overview of Professional Nursing Concepts for Medical-Surgical Nursing**, 1
Donna D. Ignatavicius
   Quality and Safety Education for Nurses Core
      Competencies, 2
   Patient-Centered Care, 2
   Safety, 3
   Teamwork and Interprofessional Collaboration, 5
   Evidence-Based Practice, 6
   Quality Improvement, 7
   Informatics and Technology, 7
   Clinical Judgment, 8
   Ethics, 8
   Health Care Organizations, 9
   Health Care Disparities, 10

2 **Overview of Health Concepts for Medical-Surgical Nursing**, 13
Donna D. Ignatavicius and Kristin Oneail
   Acid-Base Balance, 13
   Cellular Regulation, 14
   Clotting, 15
   Cognition, 16
   Comfort, 17
   Elimination, 18
   Fluid and Electrolyte Balance, 19
   Glucose Regulation, 20
   Gas Exchange, 20
   Immunity, 21
   Mobility, 23
   Nutrition, 24
   Perfusion, 25
   Sensory Perception, 26
   Sexuality, 27
   Tissue Integrity, 27

3 **Common Health Problems of Older Adults**, 29
Donna D. Ignatavicius
   Overview, 30
   Health Issues for Older Adults in Community-Based
      Settings, 30
      Decreased Nutrition and Hydration, 30
      Decreased Mobility, 31
      Stress, Loss, and Coping, 32
      Accidents, 33
      Drug Use and Misuse, 34
      Inadequate Cognition, 35
      Substance Use, 38
      Elder Neglect and Abuse, 39
   Health Issues for Older Adults in Hospitals and
      Long-Term Care Settings, 39
      Problems of Sleep, Nutrition, and Continence, 40
      Confusion, Falls, and Skin Breakdown, 40

      Care Coordination and Transition
         Management, 42

4 **Assessment and Care of Patients With Pain**, 45
Melanie H. Simpson and Donna D. Ignatavicius
   *Pain, 45
      Scope of the Problem, 45
      Definitions of Pain, 46
      Categorization of Pain by Duration, 46
      *Categorization of Pain by Underlying
         Mechanisms, 47*
   Interprofessional Collaborative Care, 48

5 **Principles of Genetics and Genomics for Medical-Surgical Nursing**, 71
M. Linda Workman
   Genetic Biology Review, 72
      DNA, 72
      Gene Structure and Function, 74
      Gene Expression, 76
      Protein Synthesis, 76
      Mutations and Variations, 76
      Microbiome, 77
   Patterns of Inheritance, 77
      Pedigree, 77
      *Autosomal Dominant Pattern of
         Inheritance, 78*
      *Autosomal Recessive Pattern of
         Inheritance, 79*
      *Sex-Linked Recessive Pattern of
         Inheritance, 79*
      *Complex Inheritance and Familial
         Clustering, 80*
   Genetic Testing, 80
      Purpose of Genetic Testing, 80
      Benefits and Risks of Genetic Testing, 80
      Genetic Counseling, 81
      Ethical Issues, 81
   The Role of the Medical-Surgical Nurse in Genetic
      Counseling, 82
      Communication, 82
      Privacy and Confidentiality, 83
      Information Accuracy, 83
      Patient Advocacy and Support, 83

6 **Rehabilitation Concepts for Chronic and Disabling Health Problems**, 86
Michelle Camicia and Donna D. Ignatavicius
   Overview, 87
      Chronic and Disabling Health Conditions, 87
      Rehabilitation Settings, 87
      The Rehabilitation Interprofessional Team, 88

7 **End-of-Life Care Concepts**, 103
Mary K. Kazanowski
   Overview of Death, Dying, and End of Life, 103
   Pathophysiology of Dying, 104
   *End of Life, 104
      Hospice and Palliative Care, 106
   Postmortem Care, 114
   Ethics and Dying, 114

Asterisk (*) denotes a Concept Exemplar.

UNIT II Principles of Emergency Care and Disaster Preparedness

8 Principles of Emergency and Trauma Nursing, 117
Linda Laskowski-Jones and Karen L. Toulson
The Emergency Department Environment of Care, 118
Demographic Data and Vulnerable Populations, 118
Special Nursing Teams—Members of the Interprofessional Team, 118
Interprofessional Team Collaboration, 119
Staff and Patient Safety Considerations, 120
Staff Safety, 120
Patient Safety, 121
Scope of Emergency Nursing Practice, 122
Core Competencies, 122
Training and Certification, 123
Emergency Nursing Principles, 123
Triage, 123
Disposition, 124
The Impact of Homelessness, 127
Trauma Nursing Principles, 127
Trauma Centers and Trauma Systems, 127
Mechanism of Injury, 128
Primary Survey and Resuscitation Interventions, 129
The Secondary Survey and Resuscitation Interventions, 130
Disposition, 130

9 Care of Patients With Common Environmental Emergencies, 133
Linda Laskowski-Jones
Heat-Related Illnesses, 133
Heat Exhaustion, 133
Heat Stroke, 134
Snakebites and Arthropod Bites and Stings, 135
Lightning Injuries, 141
Cold-Related Injuries, 142
Hypothermia, 142
Frostbite, 144
Altitude-Related Illnesses, 145
Drowning, 147

10 Principles of Emergency and Disaster Preparedness, 149
Linda Laskowski-Jones
Types of Disasters, 149
Impact of External Disasters, 150
Emergency Preparedness and Response, 151
Mass Casualty Triage, 151
Notification and Activation of Emergency Preparedness/Management Plans, 153
Hospital Emergency Preparedness: Personnel Roles and Responsibilities, 153
Event Resolution and Debriefing, 156
Critical Incident Stress Debriefing, 156
Administrative Review, 157
Role of Nursing in Community Emergency Preparedness and Response, 157
Psychosocial Response of Survivors to Mass Casualty Events, 157

UNIT III Interprofessional Collaboration for Patients With Problems of Fluid, Electrolyte, and Acid-Base Balance

11 Assessment and Care of Patients With Problems of Fluid and Electrolyte Balance, 160
M. Linda Workman
Anatomy and Physiology Review, 160
Filtration, 161
Diffusion, 162
Osmosis, 163
Fluid Balance, 164
Body Fluids, 164
Hormonal Regulation of Fluid Balance, 165
Significance of Fluid Balance, 166
Disturbances of Fluid and Electrolyte Balance, 167
*Dehydration, 167
Fluid Overload, 171
Electrolyte Balance and Imbalances, 172
Sodium, 173
Potassium, 175
Calcium, 179
Magnesium, 181

12 Assessment and Care of Patients With Problems of Acid-Base Balance, 185
M. Linda Workman
Maintaining Acid-Base Balance, 185
Acid-Base Chemistry, 186
Body Fluid Chemistry, 187
Acid-Base Regulatory Actions and Mechanisms, 188
Acid-Base Imbalances, 190
*Acidosis, 190
Alkalosis, 195

13 Concepts of Infusion Therapy, 199
Jeanette Spain Adams
Overview, 199
Types of Infusion Therapy Fluids, 200
Prescribing Infusion Therapy, 201
Vascular Access Devices, 201
Peripheral Intravenous Therapy, 202
Short Peripheral Catheters, 202
Midline Catheters, 204
Central Intravenous Therapy, 205
Peripherally Inserted Central Catheters, 205
Nontunneled Percutaneous Central Venous Catheters, 206
Tunneled Central Venous Catheters, 207
Implanted Ports, 207
Hemodialysis Catheters, 208
Infusion Systems, 208
Containers, 208
Administration Sets, 209
Rate-Controlling Infusion Devices, 211
Nursing Care for Patients Receiving Intravenous Therapy, 211
Educating the Patient, 211
Performing the Nursing Assessment, 212
Securing and Dressing the Catheter, 212
Changing Administration Sets and Needleless Connectors, 214

Controlling Infusion Pressure, 214
Flushing the Catheter, 214
Obtaining Blood Samples from Central Venous Catheters, 215
Removing the Vascular Access Device, 215
Documenting Intravenous Therapy, 216
Complications of Intravenous Therapy, 216
Catheter-Related Bloodstream Infection, 216
Other Complications of Intravenous Therapy, 216
Intravenous Therapy and Care of the Older Adult, 216
Skin Care, 216
Vein and Catheter Selection, 222
Cardiac and Renal Changes, 222
Subcutaneous Infusion Therapy, 223
Intraosseous Infusion Therapy, 223
Intra-Arterial Infusion Therapy, 224
Intraperitoneal Infusion Therapy, 225
Intraspinal Infusion Therapy, 225

UNIT IV Interprofessional Collaboration for Perioperative Patients

14 Care of Preoperative Patients, 228
Cynthia L. Danko and Rebecca M. Patton
Overview, 229
Categories and Purposes of Surgery, 229
Surgical Settings, 229
15 Care of Intraoperative Patients, 251
Cynthia L. Danko and Rebecca M. Patton
Overview, 251
Members of the Surgical Team, 252
The Surgical Suite—Patient and Team Safety, 252
Anesthesia, 256
16 Care of Postoperative Patients, 270
Rebecca M. Patton and Cynthia Danko
Overview, 270

UNIT V Interprofessional Collaboration for Patients With Problems of Immunity

17 Principles of Inflammation and Immunity, 289
M. Linda Workman
Overview, 289
Self Versus Non-Self, 289
Organization of the Immune System, 290
General Immunity: Inflammation, 291
Infection, 292
Cell Types Involved in Inflammation, 292
Phagocytosis, 294
Sequence of Inflammation, 294
Specific Immunity, 295
Antibody-Mediated Immunity, 295
Cell-Mediated Immunity, 299
Age-Related Changes in Immunity, 300
Transplant Rejection, 300
Hyperacute Rejection, 301
Acute Rejection, 301
Chronic Rejection, 301
Management of Transplant Rejection, 301

18 Care of Patients With Arthritis and Other Connective Tissue Diseases, 304
Roberta Goff and Kathy Vanderbeck
*Osteoarthritis, 305
*Rheumatoid Arthritis, 318
Lupus Erythematosus, 326
Systemic Sclerosis, 329
Gout, 330
Lyme Disease, 332
Disease-Associated Arthritis, 332
Fibromyalgia Syndrome, 333
19 Care of Patients With Problems of HIV Disease, 337
James G. Sampson and M. Linda Workman
*HIV Infection and AIDS, 337
20 Care of Patients With Hypersensitivity (Allergy) and Autoimmunity, 360
M. Linda Workman
HYPERSENSITIVITIES/ALLERGIES, 360
Type I: Rapid Hypersensitivity Reactions, 360
*Angioedema, 361
Allergic Rhinosinusitis, 365
Type II: Cytotoxic Reactions, 366
Type III: Immune Complex Reactions, 366
Type IV: Delayed Hypersensitivity Reactions, 367
AUTOIMMUNITY, 367
21 Principles of Cancer Development, 372
M. Linda Workman
Pathophysiology, 372
Biology of Normal Cells, 372
Biology of Abnormal Cells, 373
Cancer Development, 375
Carcinogenesis/Oncogenesis, 375
Cancer Classification, 375
Cancer Grading, Ploidy, and Staging, 376
Cancer Etiology and Genetic Risk, 377
Cancer Prevention, 381
Primary Prevention, 381
Secondary Prevention, 382
22 Care of Patients With Cancer, 384
Constance G. Visovsky and Julie Ponto
Impact of Cancer on Physical Function, 384
Impaired Immunity and Clotting, 385
Altered GI Function, 385
Altered Peripheral Nerve Function, 385
Motor and Sensory Deficits, 385
Cancer Pain, 385
Altered Respiratory and Cardiac Function, 386
Cancer Management, 386
Surgery, 386
Radiation Therapy, 387
Cytotoxic Systemic Therapy, 390
Oncologic Emergencies, 407
Sepsis and Disseminated Intravascular Coagulation, 407
Syndrome of Inappropriate Antidiuretic Hormone, 407
Spinal Cord Compression, 408
Hypercalcemia, 408
Superior Vena Cava Syndrome, 408
Tumor Lysis Syndrome, 409

23 **Care of Patients With Infection**, 413
    Donna D. Ignatavicius
    *Infection, 413
        Transmission of Infectious Agents, 414
        Physiologic Defenses for Infection, 416
        Health Promotion and Maintenance, 417
        Infection Control in Health Care Settings, 417
        Methods of Infection Control and
            Prevention, 417
    Multidrug-Resistant Organism Infections and
        Colonizations, 421
        Methicillin-Resistant Staphylococcus aureus
            (MRSA), 422
        Vancomycin-Resistant Enterococcus (VRE), 422
        Carbapenem-Resistant Enterobacteriaceae
            (CRE), 422
    Occupational and Environmental Exposure to
        Sources of Infection, 423
    Problems Resulting From Inadequate Antimicrobial
        Therapy, 423
    Critical Issues: Emerging Infections and Global
        Bioterrorism, 427

UNIT VI Interprofessional Collaboration for
         Patients With Problems of the Skin,
         Hair, and Nails

24 **Assessment of the Skin, Hair, and Nails**, 431
    Janice Cuzzell
    Anatomy and Physiology Review, 431
        Structure of the Skin, 431
        Structure of the Skin Appendages, 432
        Functions of the Skin, 433
        Skin Changes Associated With Aging, 433
    Assessment: Noticing and Interpreting, 433
        Patient History, 433
        Nutrition Status, 436
        Family History and Genetic Risk, 436
        Current Health Problems, 436
        Skin Assessment, 436
        Hair Assessment, 441
        Nail Assessment, 441
        Skin Assessment Techniques for Patients With Darker
            Skin, 443
        Psychosocial Assessment, 444
        Diagnostic Assessment, 444
25 **Care of Patients With Skin Problems**, 447
    Janice Cuzzell
    *Pressure Injuries, 447
    Minor Skin Irritations, 461
        Pruritis, 461
        Urticaria, 462
    Common Inflammations, 462
    Psoriasis, 463
    Skin Infections, 466
    Parasitic Disorders, 470
        Pediculosis, 470
        Scabies, 470
        Bedbugs, 471
    Trauma, 471
    Skin Cancer, 474

    Other Skin Disorders, 478
        Toxic Epidermal Necrolysis and Stevens-Johnson
            Syndrome, 478
26 **Care of Patients With Burns**, 481
    Tammy Coffee
    Introduction to Burn Injury, 481
    Health Promotion and Maintenance, 488
    Resuscitation Phase of Burn Injury, 489
    Acute Phase of Burn Injury, 497
    Rehabilitative Phase of Burn Injury, 504

UNIT VII Interprofessional Collaboration for
          Patients With Problems of the
          Respiratory System

27 **Assessment of the Respiratory System**, 508
    Harry Rees
    Anatomy and Physiology Review, 508
        Upper Respiratory Tract, 509
        Lower Respiratory Tract, 510
        Oxygen Delivery and the Oxygen-Hemoglobin
            Dissociation Curve, 512
        Respiratory Changes Associated With Aging, 512
        Health Promotion and Maintenance, 512
    Assessment: Noticing and Interpreting, 515
        Patient History, 515
        Physical Assessment, 517
        Psychosocial Assessment, 521
        Diagnostic Assessment, 521
28 **Care of Patients Requiring Oxygen Therapy or**
    Tracheostomy, 529
    Harry Rees
    Oxygen Therapy, 529
    *Tracheostomy, 537
29 **Care of Patients With Noninfectious Upper Respiratory**
    Problems, 547
    M. Linda Workman
    *Head and Neck Cancer, 547
    Cancer of the Nose and Sinuses, 556
    Fractures of the Nose, 556
    Epistaxis, 557
    Facial Trauma, 558
    Obstructive Sleep Apnea, 559
    Laryngeal Trauma, 559
    Upper Airway Obstruction, 560
30 **Care of Patients With Noninfectious Lower Respiratory**
    Problems, 563
    M. Linda Workman
    Asthma, 563
    *Chronic Obstructive Pulmonary Disease, 572
    Cystic Fibrosis, 581
    Pulmonary Arterial Hypertension, 584
    Idiopathic Pulmonary Fibrosis, 585
    Lung Cancer, 586
31 **Care of Patients With Infectious Respiratory**
    Problems, 596
    Meg Blair
    Seasonal Influenza, 596
    Pandemic Influenza, 597
    Middle East Respiratory Syndrome
        (MERS), 598

*Pneumonia, 598
*Pulmonary Tuberculosis, 605
Rhinosinusitis, 610
Peritonsillar Abscess, 611
Inhalation Anthrax, 611
Pertussis, 613
Coccidioidomycosis, 613

32 Care of Critically Ill Patients With Respiratory Problems, 616
Harry Rees
*Pulmonary Embolism, 616
Acute Respiratory Failure, 624
Acute Respiratory Distress Syndrome, 626
The Patient Requiring Intubation and
  Ventilation, 628
Chest Trauma, 636
  Pulmonary Contusion, 636
  Rib Fracture, 636
  Flail Chest, 637
  Pneumothorax and Hemothorax, 637

UNIT VIII Interprofessional Collaboration for Patients With Problems of the Cardiovascular System

33 Assessment of the Cardiovascular System, 641
Laura M. Dechant
Anatomy and Physiology Review, 642
  Heart, 642
  Vascular System, 645
  Cardiovascular Changes Associated With Aging, 646
Assessment: Noticing and
  Interpreting, 646
  Patient History, 646
  Physical Assessment, 651
  Psychosocial Assessment, 655
  Diagnostic Assessment, 655

34 Care of Patients With Dysrhythmias, 664
Laura M. Dechant and Nicole M. Heimgartner
Review of Cardiac Conduction System, 664
Electrocardiography, 665
  Lead Systems, 666
  Continuous Electrocardiographic
    Monitoring, 667
  Electrocardiographic Complexes, Segments, and
    Intervals, 667
  Electrocardiographic Rhythm Analysis, 670
Overview of Normal Cardiac Rhythms, 671
Common Dysrhythmias, 671
Sinus Dysrhythmias, 672
  Sinus Tachycardia, 673
  Sinus Bradycardia, 674
Atrial Dysrhythmias, 675
  Premature Atrial Complex, 676
  Supraventricular Tachycardia, 676
*Atrial Fibrillation, 678
Ventricular Dysrhythmias, 683
  Premature Ventricular Complex, 683
  Ventricular Tachycardia, 684
  Ventricular Fibrillation, 684
  Ventricular Asystole, 686

35 Care of Patients With Cardiac Problems, 691
Laura M. Dechant
*Heart Failure, 691
Valvular Heart Disease, 705
Inflammations and Infections, 711
  Infective Endocarditis, 711
  Pericarditis, 712
  Rheumatic Carditis, 714
  Cardiomyopathy, 714

36 Care of Patients With Vascular Problems, 720
Nicole M. Heimgartner
*Hypertension, 720
Arteriosclerosis and Atherosclerosis, 728
Peripheral Arterial Disease, 731
Acute Peripheral Arterial Occlusion, 737
Aneurysms of the Central Arteries, 738
Aneurysms of the Peripheral Arteries, 740
Aortic Dissection, 740
Other Arterial Health Problems, 741
Peripheral Venous Disease, 741
*Venous Thromboembolism, 742
Venous Insufficiency, 746
Varicose Veins, 748

37 Care of Patients With Shock, 751
Nicole M. Heimgartner
Overview, 751
  Review of Gas Exchange and Tissue
    Perfusion, 752
  Types of Shock, 752
*Hypovolemic Shock, 754
*Sepsis and Septic Shock, 760

38 Care of Patients With Acute Coronary Syndromes, 768
Laura M. Dechant
Chronic Stable Angina Pectoris, 768
*Acute Coronary Syndrome, 769

UNIT IX Interprofessional Collaboration for Patients With Problems of the Hematologic System

39 Assessment of the Hematologic System, 795
M. Linda Workman
Anatomy and Physiology Review, 795
  Bone Marrow, 795
  Blood Components, 796
  Accessory Organs of Blood
    Formation, 797
  Hemostasis and Blood Clotting, 798
  Anti-Clotting Forces, 799
  Hematologic Changes Associated
    With Aging, 800
Assessment: Noticing and
  Interpreting, 800
  Patient History, 800
  Nutrition Status, 802
  Family History and Genetic Risk, 802
  Current Health Problems, 802
  Physical Assessment, 802
  Psychosocial Assessment, 803
  Diagnostic Assessment, 803

40 **Care of Patients With Hematologic Problems,** 808
Katherine L. Byar
  *Sickle Cell Disease, 808
  Anemia, 813
  Polycythemia Vera, 816
  Hereditary Hemochromatosis, 817
  Myelodysplastic Syndromes, 817
  *Leukemia, 817
  Malignant Lymphomas, 828
  Multiple Myeloma, 829
  Autoimmune Thrombocytopenic
    Purpura, 830
  Thrombotic Thrombocytopenic Purpura, 831
  Hemophilia, 831
  Heparin-Induced Thrombocytopenia, 832
  Transfusion Therapy, 832
    Pretransfusion Responsibilities, 832
    Transfusion Responsibilities, 833
    Types of Transfusions, 834
    Acute Transfusion Reactions, 835
    Autologous Blood Transfusions, 836

**UNIT X   Interprofessional Collaboration
        for Patients With Problems of
        the Nervous System**

41 **Assessment of the Nervous System,** 839
Donna D. Ignatavicius
  Anatomy and Physiology Review, 839
    *Nervous System Cells: Structure and
      Function, 839*
    *Central Nervous System: Structure and
      Function, 840*
    *Peripheral Nervous System: Structure and
      Function, 842*
    *Autonomic Nervous System: Structure and
      Function, 842*
    Neurologic Changes Associated With Aging, 844
    Health Promotion and Maintenance, 845
  Assessment: Noticing and Interpreting, 846
    Patient History, 846
    Physical Assessment, 846
    Psychosocial Assessment, 850
    Diagnostic Assessment, 851

42 **Care of Patients With Problems of the Central Nervous
      System: The Brain,** 857
Donna D. Ignatavicius
  *Alzheimer's Disease, 857
  *Parkinson Disease, 868
  Migraine Headache, 873
  Seizures and Epilepsy, 876
  Meningitis, 880
  Encephalitis, 883

43 **Care of Patients With Problems of the Central Nervous
      System: The Spinal Cord,** 887
Laura M. Willis and Donna D. Ignatavicius
  *Multiple Sclerosis, 888
  *Spinal Cord Injury, 894
  Back Pain, 903
    Low Back Pain (Lumbosacral Back Pain), 903
    Cervical Neck Pain, 909

44 **Care of Patients With Problems of the Peripheral
      Nervous System,** 912
Donna D. Ignatavicius
  *Guillain-Barré Syndrome, 912
  Myasthenia Gravis, 917
  Restless Legs Syndrome, 922
  Trigeminal Neuralgia, 923
  Facial Paralysis, 924

45 **Care of Critically Ill Patients With Neurologic
      Problems,** 927
Laura M. Willis
  Transient Ischemic Attack, 927
  *Stroke (Brain Attack), 928
  *Traumatic Brain Injury, 940
  Brain Tumors, 950

**UNIT XI   Interprofessional Collaboration
        for Patients With Problems of
        the Sensory System**

46 **Assessment of the Eye and Vision,** 957
Samuel A. Borchers and Andrea A. Borchers
  Anatomy and Physiology Review, 957
    Structure, 957
    Function, 960
    Eye Changes Associated With Aging, 961
    Health Promotion and Maintenance, 961
  Assessment: Noticing and Interpreting, 962
    Patient History, 962
    Physical Assessment, 963
    Psychosocial Assessment, 964
    Diagnostic Assessment, 965

47 **Care of Patients With Eye and Vision Problems,** 968
Samuel A. Borchers and Andrea A. Borchers
  *Cataract, 968
  *Glaucoma, 972
  Corneal Disorders, 977
    Corneal Abrasion, Ulceration, and Infection, 977
    Keratoconus and Corneal Opacities, 977
  Retinal Disorders, 979
    Macular Degeneration, 979
    Retinal Holes, Tears, and Detachments, 979
    Retinitis Pigmentosa, 980
  Refractive Errors, 980
  Trauma, 981
    Foreign Bodies, 981
    Lacerations, 981
    Penetrating Injuries, 982

48 **Assessment and Care of Patients With Ear and Hearing
      Problems,** 984
Samuel A. Borchers and Andrea A. Borchers
  Anatomy and Physiology Review, 984
    Structure, 984
    Function, 986
  Assessment: Noticing and Interpreting, 986
    Patient History, 986
    Physical Assessment, 988
    General Hearing Assessment, 989
    Psychosocial Assessment, 990
    Diagnostic Assessment, 990
  *Otitis Media, 991

External Otitis, 993
Cerumen or Foreign Bodies, 994
Mastoiditis, 995
Trauma, 995
Tinnitus, 995
Ménière's Disease, 995
Acoustic Neuroma, 996
*Hearing Loss, 996

UNIT XII Interprofessional Collaboration for Patients With Problems of the Musculoskeletal System

49 Assessment of the Musculoskeletal System, 1004
Donna D. Ignatavicius
   Anatomy and Physiology Review, 1005
      Skeletal System, 1005
      Muscular System, 1007
      Musculoskeletal Changes Associated
         With Aging, 1007
      Health Promotion and Maintenance, 1007
   Assessment: Noticing and Interpreting, 1008
      Patient History, 1008
      Assessment of the Skeletal System, 1009
      Assessment of the Muscular System, 1011
      Psychosocial Assessment, 1011
      Diagnostic Assessment, 1011

50 Care of Patients With Musculoskeletal Problems, 1015
Donna D. Ignatavicius
   *Osteoporosis, 1015
   Osteomyelitis, 1022
   Bone Tumors, 1024
   Disorders of the Hand, 1028
   Disorders of the Foot, 1028
      Common Foot Deformities, 1028
      Plantar Fasciitis, 1029
      Other Problems of the Foot, 1029

51 Care of Patients With Musculoskeletal Trauma, 1031
Roberta Goff and Donna D. Ignatavicius
   *Fractures, 1032
   Selected Fractures of Specific Sites, 1046
      Upper-Extremity Fractures, 1046
      Lower-Extremity Fractures, 1047
      Fractures of the Chest and Pelvis, 1049
      Compression Fractures of the Spine, 1050
   *Amputations, 1050
   Knee Injuries, 1056
   Carpal Tunnel Syndrome, 1057
   Rotator Cuff Injuries, 1059

UNIT XIII Interprofessional Collaboration for Patients With Problems of the Gastrointestinal System

52 Assessment of the Gastrointestinal System, 1061
Amy Jauch
   Anatomy and Physiology Review, 1061
      Structure, 1061
      Function, 1062
      Gastrointestinal Changes Associated With Aging, 1064

   Assessment: Noticing and Interpreting, 1065
      Patient History, 1065
      Physical Assessment, 1066
      Psychosocial Assessment, 1068
      Diagnostic Assessment, 1068

53 Care of Patients With Oral Cavity Problems, 1075
Tracy Taylor
   *Stomatitis, 1076
   Oral Cavity Disorders, 1078
      Oral Tumors: Premalignant Lesions, 1078
      Oral Cancer, 1079
   Disorders of the Salivary Glands, 1084
      Acute Sialadenitis, 1084
      Post-Irradiation Sialadenitis, 1085

54 Care of Patients With Esophageal Problems, 1087
Tracy Taylor
   *Gastroesophageal Reflux Disease (GERD), 1087
   Hiatal Hernias, 1092
   *Esophageal Tumors, 1095
   Esophageal Diverticula, 1101
   Esophageal Trauma, 1101

55 Care of Patients With Stomach Disorders, 1103
Lara Carver
   Gastritis, 1103
   *Peptic Ulcer Disease (PUD), 1107
   Gastric Cancer, 1115

56 Care of Patients With Noninflammatory Intestinal Disorders, 1121
Keelin Cromar
   *Intestinal Obstruction, 1121
   Polyps, 1126
   *Colorectal Cancer, 1126
   Irritable Bowel Syndrome, 1135
   Herniation, 1137
   Hemorrhoids, 1139
   Malabsorption Syndrome, 1141

57 Care of Patients With Inflammatory Intestinal Disorders, 1144
Keelin Cromar
   Acute Inflammatory Bowel Disorders, 1144
      *Peritonitis, 1144
      Appendicitis, 1147
      Gastroenteritis, 1148
   Chronic Inflammatory Bowel Disease, 1150
      *Ulcerative Colitis, 1150
      Crohn's Disease, 1157
      Diverticular Disease, 1162
      Celiac Disease, 1164
   Anal Disorders, 1164
      Anorectal Abscess, 1164
      Anal Fissure, 1165
      Anal Fistula, 1165
   Parasitic Infection, 1165

58 Care of Patients With Liver Problems, 1169
Lara Carver and Jennifer Powers
   *Cirrhosis, 1169
   *Hepatitis, 1180
   Fatty Liver (Steatosis), 1185
   Liver Trauma, 1186
   Cancer of the Liver, 1186
   Liver Transplantation, 1187

59 **Care of Patients With Problems of the Biliary System and Pancreas,** 1191
Lara Carver and Jennifer Powers
   *Cholecystitis, 1191
   *Acute Pancreatitis, 1197
   Chronic Pancreatitis, 1202
   Pancreatic Abscess, 1205
   Pancreatic Pseudocyst, 1205
   Pancreatic Cancer, 1205

60 **Care of Patients With Malnutrition: Undernutrition and Obesity,** 1211
Laura M. Willis and Cherie Rebar
   Nutrition Standards for Health Promotion and Maintenance, 1211
   Nutrition Assessment, 1212
    Initial Nutrition Screening, 1212
    Anthropometric Measurements, 1213
   *Malnutrition, 1215
   *Obesity, 1225

UNIT XIV Interprofessional Collaboration for Patients With Problems of the Endocrine System

61 **Assessment of the Endocrine System,** 1234
M. Linda Workman
   Anatomy and Physiology Review, 1235
    Hypothalamus and Pituitary Glands, 1236
    Gonads, 1237
    Adrenal Glands, 1237
    Thyroid Gland, 1238
    Parathyroid Glands, 1239
    Pancreas, 1239
    Endocrine Changes Associated With Aging, 1240
   Assessment: Noticing and Interpreting, 1240
    Patient History, 1240
    Physical Assessment, 1241
    Psychosocial Assessment, 1242
    Diagnostic Assessment, 1242

62 **Care of Patients With Pituitary and Adrenal Gland Problems,** 1245
M. Linda Workman
   Disorders of the Anterior Pituitary Gland, 1245
    Hypopituitarism, 1245
    Hyperpituitarism, 1247
   Disorders of the Posterior Pituitary Gland, 1250
    Diabetes Insipidus, 1250
    Syndrome of Inappropriate Antidiuretic Hormone, 1251
   Disorders of the Adrenal Gland, 1253
    Adrenal Gland Hypofunction, 1253
    Hypercortisolism (Cushing's Disease), 1255
    Hyperaldosteronism, 1260
    Pheochromocytoma, 1261

63 **Care of Patients With Problems of the Thyroid and Parathyroid Glands,** 1264
M. Linda Workman
   Thyroid Disorders, 1264
    Hyperthyroidism, 1264
    Hypothyroidism, 1270
    Thyroiditis, 1275
    Thyroid Cancer, 1275

   Parathyroid Disorders, 1275
    Hyperparathyroidism, 1275
    Hypoparathyroidism, 1277

64 **Care of Patients With Diabetes Mellitus,** 1280
Saundra Hendricks
   *Diabetes Mellitus, 1280

UNIT XV Interprofessional Collaboration for Patients With Problems of the Renal/Urinary System

65 **Assessment of the Renal/Urinary System,** 1321
Chris Winkelman
   Anatomy and Physiology Review, 1322
    Kidneys, 1322
    Ureters, 1327
    Urinary Bladder, 1327
    Urethra, 1327
    Kidney and Urinary Changes Associated With Aging, 1328
   Assessment: Noticing and Interpreting, 1329
    Patient History, 1329
    Physical Assessment, 1330
    Psychosocial Assessment, 1331
    Diagnostic Assessment, 1331

66 **Care of Patients With Urinary Problems,** 1343
Chris Winkelman
   *Urinary Incontinence, 1343
   Cystitis, 1354
   Urethritis, 1359
   Urolithiasis, 1361
   Urothelial Cancer, 1366
   Bladder Trauma, 1369

67 **Care of Patients With Kidney Disorders,** 1372
Chris Winkelman
   *Pyelonephritis, 1372
   Acute Glomerulonephritis, 1376
   Chronic Glomerulonephritis, 1378
   Nephrotic Syndrome, 1378
   Nephrosclerosis, 1379
   Polycystic Kidney Disease, 1379
   Hydronephrosis and Hydroureter, 1382
   Renovascular Disease, 1384
   Diabetic Nephropathy, 1384
   Renal Cell Carcinoma, 1385
   Kidney Trauma, 1387

68 **Care of Patients With Acute Kidney Injury and Chronic Kidney Disease,** 1390
Chris Winkelman
   Acute Kidney Injury, 1391
   *Chronic Kidney Disease, 1398

UNIT XVI Interprofessional Collaboration for Patients With Problems of the Reproductive System

69 **Assessment of the Reproductive System,** 1428
Donna D. Ignatavicius
   Anatomy and Physiology Review, 1428
    Structure and Function of the Female Reproductive System, 1428

Structure and Function of the Male Reproductive System, 1430
Reproductive Changes Associated With Aging, 1431
Health Promotion and Maintenance, 1431
Assessment: Noticing and Interpreting, 1431
Patient History, 1431
Physical Assessment, 1433
Psychosocial Assessment, 1433
Diagnostic Assessment, 1433

70 Care of Patients With Breast Disorders, 1440
Gail B. Johnson and Harriet Kumar
*Breast Cancer, 1440
Benign Breast Disorders, 1455
Fibroadenoma, 1455
Fibrocystic Breast Condition, 1455
Issues of Large-Breasted Women, 1456
Issues of Small-Breasted Women, 1456

71 Care of Patients With Gynecologic Problems, 1459
Donna D. Ignatavicius
*Uterine Leiomyoma, 1459
Pelvic Organ Prolapse, 1464
Endometrial (Uterine) Cancer, 1465
Ovarian Cancer, 1467
Cervical Cancer, 1469
Vulvovaginitis, 1470
Toxic Shock Syndrome, 1471

72 Care of Patients With Male Reproductive Problems, 1473
Donna D. Ignatavicius
*Benign Prostatic Hyperplasia, 1474
*Prostate Cancer, 1481
Testicular Cancer, 1486
Erectile Dysfunction, 1489

73 Care of Transgender Patients, 1492
Donna D. Ignatavicius and Stephanie M. Fox
Patient-Centered Terminology, 1493
Transgender Health Issues, 1494
Stress and Transgender Health, 1494
The Need to Improve Transgender Health Care, 1494

74 Care of Patients With Sexually Transmitted Infections, 1504
Donna D. Ignatavicius
Overview, 1504
Health Promotion and Maintenance, 1505
Genital Herpes, 1506
Syphilis, 1508
Condylomata Acuminata (Genital Warts), 1510
Chlamydia Infection, 1511
Gonorrhea, 1512
*Pelvic Inflammatory Disease, 1514

Glossary, G-1
NCLEX® Examination Challenges Answer Key, AK-1

GUIDE TO SPECIAL FEATURES

BEST PRACTICE FOR PATIENT SAFETY AND QUALITY CARE

Acute Adrenal Insufficiency, 1253

AIDS, Infection Control for Home Care, 357

Alteplase, Nursing Interventions During and After Administration, 936

Altitude-Related Illnesses, 146

Alzheimer's Disease, Promoting Communication, 863

Anaphylaxis, 365

Anesthesia, Spinal and Epidural, Recognizing Serious Complications, 275

Anticoagulant Therapy, 744

Anticoagulant, Fibrinolytic, or Antiplatelet Therapy and Prevention of Injury, 623

Arteriovenous Fistula or Arteriovenous Graft, 1415

Artificial Airway Suctioning, 541

Aspiration Prevention During Swallowing, 543

Autologous Blood Salvage and Transfusion, Intraoperative, 264

Autonomic Dysreflexia: Immediate Interventions, 898

Benzodiazepine Overdose, 281

Breast Mass Assessment, 1445

Breast Reconstruction, Postoperative Care, 1451

Breast Self-Examination, 1444

Burn Patient and Fluid Resuscitation, 495

Burns, Emergency Management, 489

Cancer Pain Management with Intrathecal Pump, 62

Carpal Tunnel Syndrome Prevention, 1058

Catheter-Associated Urinary Tract Infections (CAUTI), 1356

Cervical Diskectomy and Fusion, 910

Chest Discomfort, 775

Chest Tube Drainage System Management, 592

Chronic Diarrhea, Special Skin Care, 1142

Cognition Assessment, 847

Colonoscopy, 1073

Colorectal Cancer Screening Recommendations, 1128

Communicating With Patients Unable To Speak, 550

Continuous Passive Motion (CPM) Machine, 316

Contractures, Positioning to Prevent, 503

Dark Skin, Assessing Changes, 444

Death Pronouncement, 114

Dehydration, 169

Diagnostic Testing, Precautions for Use of Iodine-Based or Gadolinium Contrast, 852

Diarrhea, 19

Driver Safety Improvement in Older Adults, 34

Dysrhythmias, 672

Ear Irrigation, 994

Eardrops Instillation, 993

Emergency Department and Patient and Staff Safety, 120

Endocrine Testing, 1243

Energy Conservation, 826

Esophageal Surgery and Nasogastric Tube, 1100

Extremity Fracture, 1038

Eyedrops Instillation, 966

Fall Prevention in Older Adults, 41

Feeding Tube Maintenance, 1222

Fires in Health Care Facility, 150

Fluid Volume Management, 1405

Fundoplication Procedures and Postoperative Complications, 1094

Gait Training, 95

Gastrointestinal Health History, 1065

Genetic Testing and Counseling, 82

Genital Herpes, Self-Management, 1507

Gynecologic Cancer, Brachytherapy and Health Teaching, 1466

Hand Hygiene, 418

Hearing Impairment and Communication, 998

Heart Transplant, Signs and Symptoms of Rejection, 716

Heat Stroke, 135

Hemodialysis, 1416

HIV, Recommendations for Preventing Transmission by Health Care Workers, 345

Hypertensive Urgency or Crisis, 727

Hypokalemia, 177

Hypophysectomy, 1249

Hypovolemic Shock, 759

Immunity, Reduced, Care of Hospitalized Patients, 351

Infection, Nursing Interventions for the Patient at Risk, 417

Inflammatory Bowel Disease, Pain Control and Skin Care, 1156

Intestinal Obstruction, 1124

Intraoperative Positioning, Prevention of Complications, 267

Kidney Test or Procedure Using Contrast Medium, 1338

LGBTQ Patients, TJC Recommendations for Creating Safe Environment, 1495

Lumbar Spinal Surgery, Assessment and Management of Complications, 907

Magnetic Resonance Imaging Preparation, 1013

Malignant Hyperthermia, 260

Mechanical Ventilation Care, 630

Meningitis, 882

Minimally Invasive Inguinal Hernia Repair (MIIHR), 1139

Musculoskeletal Injury Prevention, 908

Musculoskeletal Injury, Neurovascular Status Assessment, 1037

Myasthenia Gravis, Improving Nutrition, 921

Myelosuppression and Neutropenia, 397

Myxedema Coma, 1274

Nosebleed, Anterior, 557

Nutrition Screening Assessment, 1213

Ocular Irrigation, 981

Ophthalmic Ointment Instillation, 970

Opioid Overdose, 285

Oral Cavity Problems, 1077

Oxygen Therapy, 530

Pain, Reducing Postoperative and Promoting Comfort, 285

Paracentesis, 1177

Parkinson Disease, 870

Pericarditis, 713

Peritoneal Dialysis Catheter, 1420

Phlebostatic Axis Identification, 780

Plasmapheresis, Preventing and Managing Complications, 915
Postmortem Care, 114
Postoperative Hand-off Report, 271
Post-Traumatic Stress Disorder Prevention in Staff Following a Mass Casualty Event, 156
Pressure Injuries and Wound Management, 457
Pressure Injury Prevention, 449
Primary Osteoporosis, Risk Assessment, 1017
Prostatectomy, Open Radical, 1484
Pulmonary Embolism Prevention, 617
Pulmonary Embolism, 619
Radioactive Sealed Implants, 389
Relocation Stress in Older Adults, 33
Reproductive Health Problem Assessment, 1432
Restraint Alternatives, 42
Seizures, Tonic-Clonic or Complete Partial, 878
Sickle Cell Crisis, 811
Skin Problem, Nursing History, 435
Sports-Related Injuries, 1056
Surgical Wound Evisceration, 283
Systemic Sclerosis and Esophagitis, 330
Thrombocytopenia and Prevention of Injury, 398
Thrombocytopenia, 825
Thyroid Storm, 1270
Total Parenteral Nutrition, Care and Maintenance, 1224
Tracheostomy Care, 542
Transfusion in Older Adults, 834
Transfusion Therapy, 833
Transurethral Resection of the Prostate, 1480
Tube-Feeding Care and Maintenance, 1221
Urinary Incontinence, Bladder Training and Habit Training to Reduce, 1351
Venous Catheters, Placement of Short Peripheral, 203
Vertebroplasty and Kyphoplasty, 1050
Viral Hepatitis Prevention in Health Care Workers, 1182
Vision Reduction, 975
Wandering, Prevention in Hospitalized Patients, 864
Wound Care, Perineal, 1133
Wound Monitoring, 460

COMMON EXAMPLES OF DRUG THERAPY

Acute Coronary Syndrome (Nitrates, Beta Blockers, Antiplatelets), 776
Adrenal Gland Hypofunction, 1255
Antidysrhythmic Medication, 677
Asthma, 569
Biologic Disease-Modifying Antirheumatic Drugs (DMARDs), 370
Biological Response Modifiers for Rheumatoid Arthritis and Other Connective Tissue Diseases, 323
Burn Wounds, 501
Diabetes Mellitus, 1292
Glaucoma, 976
HIV Infection, 351
Hypertension Management, 725
Hyperthyroidism, 1268
Hypovolemic Shock, 759
Inhalation Anthrax, Prophylaxis and Treatment, 612
Intravenous Vasodilators and Inotropes, 783
Kidney Disease, 1410
Nausea and Vomiting, Chemotherapy-Induced, 399

Osteoporosis, 1021
Pain, Postoperative, 284
Peptic Ulcer Disease, 1106
Plaque Psoriasis, 466
Pulmonary Embolism, 621
Transplant Rejection, 302
Tuberculosis, First-Line Treatment, 608
Urinary Incontinence, 1350
Urinary Tract Infections, 1360

CONCEPT MAP

Benign Prostatic Hyperplasia, 1478
Chronic Kidney Disease, 1406
Chronic Obstructive Pulmonary Disease, 575
Cirrhosis, 1176
Community-Acquired Pneumonia (CAP), 602
Diabetes Mellitus Type 2, 1290
Hypertension, 724
Hypovolemic Shock, 757
Multiple Sclerosis, 893
Pressure Injury, 456
Primary Open-Angle Glaucoma, 973

KEY FEATURES

Acidosis, 193
Acute Leukemia, 819
Adrenal Insufficiency, 1254
AIDS, 346
Alkalosis, 196
Alzheimer's Disease, 860
Anaphylaxis, 364
Anemia, 814
Angina and Myocardial Infarction, 773
Asthma Control Levels, 566
Asthma Control, Step System for Medication Use, 566
Autonomic Dysreflexia, 896
Bowel Obstructions, Small and Large, 1123
Brain Tumors, Common, 951
Celiac Disease, 1164
Cervical Diskectomy and Fusion Complications, 910
Cholecystitis, 1193
Compartment Syndrome, 1034
Cor Pulmonale, 574
Diabetes Insipidus, 1250
Esophageal Tumors, 1096
Fluid Overload, 172
Gastric Cancer, Early Versus Advanced, 1116
Gastritis, 1105
Gastroesophageal Reflux Disease, 1088
Gastrointestinal Bleeding, Upper, 1109
Guillain-Barré Syndrome, 914
Heat Stroke, 134
Hiatal Hernias, 1093
Hypercortisolism (Cushing's Disease/Syndrome), 1257
Hyperthyroidism, 1265
Hypothermia, 143
Hypothyroidism, 1271
Infective Endocarditis, 711
Inhalation Anthrax, 612
Intracranial Pressure (ICP), Increased, 936

Kidney Disease, Severe Chronic and End-Stage, 1403
Liver Trauma, 1186
Meningitis, 881
Migraine Headaches, 874
Multiple Sclerosis, 889
Myasthenia Gravis, 917
Nephrotic Syndrome, 1379
Oral Cancer, 1080
Osteomyelitis, Acute and Chronic, 1023
Pancreatic Cancer, 1206
Pancreatitis, Chronic, 1203
Peripheral Arterial Disease, Chronic, 732
Peritonitis, 1145
Pituitary Hyperfunction, 1248
Pituitary Hypofunction, 1246
Polycystic Kidney Disease, 1381
Pressure Injuries, 452
Pulmonary Edema, 702
Pulmonary Emboli: Fat Embolism Versus Blood Clot
    Embolism, 1034
Pulmonary Embolism, 618
Pyelonephritis, Acute, 1374
Pyelonephritis, Chronic, 1374
Renovascular Disease, 1384
Rheumatoid Arthritis, 318
Shock, 752
Skin Conditions, Inflammatory, 463
Skin Infections, Common, 467
Stroke Syndromes, 933
Strokes, Left and Right Hemisphere, 933
Sustained Tachydysrhythmias and Bradydysrhythmias, 672
Systemic Lupus Erythematosus (SLE) and Systemic
    Sclerosis (SSc), 326
Transient Ischemic Attack, 928
Traumatic Brain Injury, Mild, 945
Ulcers, Lower-Extremity, 734
Uremia, 1398
Urinary Tract Infection, 1358
Valvular Heart Disease, 706
Ventricular Failure, Left, 695
Ventricular Failure, Right, 696

EVIDENCE-BASED PRACTICE

Ambulation and Ambulation Protocol Effectiveness, 24
Benign Prostatic Hyperplasia Surgery and
    Quality of Life, 1481
Bone Loss, Risk Factors in Men, 1017
Central Venous Access Device, Best Method for Securing, 213
Chronic Pain Management in Older Adults, 56
Dementia Caregivers and Telephone Support, 867
End-of-Life Care for Prisoners, 106
Hearing Loss in Combat, 997
Heat Stroke and On-Site Treatment, 135
Hepatitis C, Care of Military Veterans, 1183
Hip Fracture, Resources for Caregivers, 1049
HIV Self-Management and mHealth Technology Among
    African-American Women, 345
Hysterectomy and Sexuality, 1462
Noninvasive Ventilation (NIV) Effectiveness, 535
Opioid Usage, 279
Oral Care, Preoperative and Postsurgical Outcomes, 1082

Preoperative Assessment, 239
Pressure Injury Reduction Using Skin Integrity
    Care Bundle, 449
Sickle Cell Disease and Self-Care in Young Adults, 813
Traumatic Brain Injury (TBI) and Mannitol to Reduce
    Mortality, 948
Veterans with Dementia, Reducing Hospital Admissions and
    Emergency Department Visits, 126

FOCUSED ASSESSMENT

AIDS, 356
Diabetic Foot, 1306
Diabetic Patient, Home or Clinic Visit, 1318
Hearing, 998
Hypophysectomy for Hyperpituitarism, 1249
Infection Risk, 821
Kidney Transplant, 1425
Oral Cancer and the Postoperative Older Adult, 1082
Pneumonia Recovery, 605
Postanesthesia Care Unit Discharge to
    Medical-Surgical Unit, 272
Preoperative Patient, 238
Pressure Injuries, 461
Seizures, Nursing Observations and Documentation, 878
Sexually Transmitted Infection, 1507
Thyroid Dysfunction, 1274
Total Abdominal Hysterectomy, Postoperative Care, 1462
Tracheostomy, 542
Urinary Incontinence, 1346

HOME CARE ASSESSMENT

Amputation, Lower-Extremity, 1056
Breast Cancer Surgery Recovery, 1453
Cataract Surgery, 971
Chronic Obstructive Pulmonary Disease, 581
Colostomy, 1134
Heart Failure, 704
Inflammatory Bowel Disease, 1158
Laryngectomy, 554
Myocardial Infarction, 790
Peripheral Vascular Disease, 737
Pulmonary Embolism, 624
Sepsis Risk, 766
Ulcer Disease, 1115

LABORATORY PROFILE

Acid-Base Assessment, 188
Acid-Base Imbalances (Uncompensated), 193
Adrenal Gland Assessment, 1255
Anticoagulation Therapy and Monitoring With
    Blood Tests, 622
Blood Glucose Values, 1288
Burn Assessment During the Resuscitation Phase, 493
Cardiovascular Assessment, 656
Connective Tissue Disease, 320
Gastrointestinal Assessment, 1069
Hematologic Assessment, 804
Hypovolemic Shock, 758
Kidney Disease, 1395

Kidney Function Blood Studies, 1332
Musculoskeletal Assessment, 1012
Parathyroid Function, 1276
Reproductive Assessment, 1434
Respiratory Assessment, 522
Thyroid Function for Adults, 1267
Urinalysis, 1333
Urine Collections, 24-Hour, 1336

NURSING FOCUS ON THE OLDER ADULT

Acid-Base Imbalance, 191
Burn Injury Complications, 490
Cancer Assessment, 380
Cardiovascular System, 647
Cerumen Impaction, 995
Coronary Artery Bypass Graft Surgery, 790
Coronary Artery Disease, 779
Diverticulitis, 1163
Dysrhythmias, 682
Ear and Hearing Changes, 987
Electrolyte Values, 165
Endocrine System Changes, 1241
Eye and Vision Changes, 961
Fecal Impaction Prevention, 1126
Fluid Balance, 165
Gastrointestinal System Changes, 1064
Heat-Related Illness Prevention, 134
Hematologic Assessment, 800
Immune Function, 291
Infection, Factors That May Increase Risk, 415
Integumentary System, 434
Intraoperative Nursing Interventions, 264
Low Back Pain, 904
Malnutrition Risk Assessment, 1216
Musculoskeletal System Changes, 1007
Nervous System, 845
Nutrition Intake Promotion, 1219
Pain, 59
Preoperative Considerations for Care Planning, 236
Renal System Changes, 1328
Reproductive System Changes, 1431
Respiratory Disorder, Chronic, 564
Respiratory System, 513
Shock, Risk Factors, 764
Skin Care, Postoperative, 281
Spinal Cord Injury, 902
Surgical Risk Factors, 234
Thyroid Problems, 1274
Total Hip Arthroplasty, 311
Traumatic Brain Injury, 944
Urinary Incontinence, Contributing Factors, 1346
Vision Impairment, Promoting Independent Living, 974

PATIENT AND FAMILY EDUCATION: PREPARING FOR SELF-MANAGEMENT

Arthritis and Energy Conservation, 324
Arthropod Bite/Sting Prevention, 137
Asthma Management, 568
Bariatric Surgery, Discharge Teaching, 1231
Beta Blocker/Digoxin Therapy, 705
Bleeding Risk, 827
Brain Injury, Mild, 949
Breast Cancer Surgery Recovery, 1453
Breathing Exercises, 578
Cancer Risk, Dietary Habits to Reduce, 379
Cardioverter/Defibrillator, 688
Caregiver Stress Reduction, 866
Cast Removal and Extremity Care, 1045
Central Venous Catheter Home Care, 826
Cerumen Removal and Self–Ear Irrigation, 987
Cervical Ablation Therapies, 1470
Cervical Biopsy Recovery, 1437
Chest Pain Management at Home, 792
Cirrhosis, 1179
Condom Use, 1508
Coronary Artery Disease and Activity, 791
Coronary Artery Disease Prevention, 771
Cortisol Replacement Therapy, 1260
Death, Emotional Signs of Approaching, 108
Death, Physical Manifestations, 113
Death, Physical Signs and Symptoms of Approaching, 107
Dry Powder Inhaler (DPI) Use, 571
Dry Skin Prevention, 462
Dysrhythmias Prevention, 682
Ear Infection or Trauma Prevention, 1000
Ear Surgery Recovery, 993
Epilepsy and Health Teaching, 880
Epinephrine Injectors, Care and Use of Automatic, 364
Exercise, 1301
Eyedrops Use, 962
Foot Care Instructions, 1307
Gastritis Prevention, 1104
Gastroenteritis, Preventing Transmission, 1150
Glucosamine Supplements, 309
Halo Device, 899
Hearing Aid Care, 999
HIV Testing and One-Time Screening, CDC Recommendations, 341
Hyperkalemia, Nutritional Management, 179
Hypoglycemia, Home Management, 1310
Hysterectomy, Total Vaginal or Abdominal, 1463
Ileostomy Care, 1157
Infection Prevention, 351
Infection Prevention, 397
Infection Prevention, 827
Inhaler, Correct Use, 570
Injury and Bleeding Prevention, 398
Injury and Bleeding Prevention, 623
Insulin Administration, Subcutaneous, 1297
Joint Protection Instructions, 317
Kidney and Genitourinary Trauma Prevention, 1387
Kidney and Urinary Problem Prevention, 1402
Laparoscopic Nissen Fundoplication (LNF) and Paraesophageal Repair via Laparoscope, Postoperative Instructions, 1094
Laryngectomy Home Care, 554
Leg Exercises, Postoperative, 245
Lightning Strike Prevention, 141
Low Back Pain and Injury Prevention, 904
Low Back Pain Exercises, 906
Lupus Erythematosus and Skin Protection, 328
Lyme Disease Prevention and Early Detection, 333

Migraine Attack Triggers, 876
MRSA, Preventing Spread, 469
Mucositis and Mouth Care, 400
Myasthenia Gravis and Drug Therapy, 922
Oral Cancer and Home Care, 1083
Oral Cavity Maintenance, 1076
Osteoarthritis and Rheumatoid Arthritis Exercises, 317
Pacemakers, Permanent, 676
Pancreatitis, Chronic, Enzyme Replacement, 1203
Pancreatitis, Chronic, Prevention of Exacerbations, 1204
Peak Flow Meter Use, 568
Pelvic Muscle Exercises, 1347
Peripheral Neuropathy, Chemotherapy-Induced, 401
Peripheral Vascular Disease and Foot Care, 737
Pneumonia Prevention, 600
Polycystic Kidney Disease, 1382
Polycythemia Vera, 817
Post-Mastectomy Exercises, 1449
Radiation Therapy and Skin Protection, 390
Radioactive Isotope Safety Precautions, 1269
Reflux Control, 1090
Respiratory Care, Perioperative, 244
Sexually Transmitted Infections and Oral
 Antibiotic Therapy, 1516
Sick-Day Rules, 1314
Sickle Cell Crisis Prevention, 812
Skin Cancer Prevention, 476
Smoking Cessation, 515
Snakebite Prevention, 136
Sperm Banking, 1488
Stretta Procedure, Postoperative Instructions, 1091
Stroke and Modifiable Risk Factors, 930
Supraglottic Method of Swallowing, 553
Testicular Self-Examination, 1486
Total Hip Arthroplasty, 312

Toxic Shock Syndrome Prevention, 1471
Urinary Calculi, 1366
Urinary Catheter Care at Home, 1486
Urinary Incontinence, 1353
Urinary Tract Infection Prevention, 1357
Valvular Heart Disease, 710
Venous Insufficiency, 747
Viral Hepatitis, 1185
Viral Hepatitis, Health Practices to Prevent, 1182
Vulvovaginitis Prevention, 1471
Warfarin (Coumadin) and Interference of
 Food and Drugs, 746
Wellness Promotion Through Lifestyles and Practices, 30
West Nile Virus Protection, 884

QUALITY IMPROVEMENT

Core Measure and Interprofessional Collaboration, 601
Diabetes and Increasing Blood Glucose Control and
 Insulin-Mealtime Match, 1310
Electrode Placement and Proper Skin Preparation, 668
Improving Medication Reconciliation With a Nurse-Led
 Protocol, 4
Joint Replacement and Shortening Hospital
 Length of Stay, 314
Opioid-Induced Respiratory Depression, Reducing with
 Capnography, 524
Oral Anticancer Agents, Text Message Reminders Improve
 Adherence, 394
Safe Handling Practices and Protection of
 Health Care Staff, 93
Sepsis, Early Recognition and Intervention, 763
Surgical Site Infection Prevention, 786
Tracheostomies and Reducing Caregiver Anxiety, 555
Urinary Tract Infections, Reducing Catheter-Associated, 415

CHAPTER 33

Assessment of the Cardiovascular System

Laura M. Dechant

PRIORITY AND INTERRELATED CONCEPTS

The priority concept for this chapter is PERFUSION.

The interrelated concept for this chapter is FLUID AND
ELECTROLYTE BALANCE.

LEARNING OUTCOMES

Safe and Effective Care Environment

1. Collaborate with the interprofessional team to perform a complete cardiovascular (CV) assessment, including PERFUSION status and FLUID AND ELECTROLYTE BALANCE.
2. Prioritize evidence-based care for patients having invasive CV diagnostic testing affecting PERFUSION.

Health Promotion and Maintenance

3. Teach evidence-based ways for adults to decrease their risk for CV health problems.
4. Explain how physiologic aging changes of the CV system affect PERFUSION and associated care of older adults.

Psychosocial Integrity

5. Implement nursing interventions to decrease the psychosocial impact caused by a CV health problem.

Physiological Integrity

6. Apply knowledge of anatomy and physiology to perform a patient-centered assessment for the patient with a CV health problem, including cultural and spiritual considerations.
7. Use clinical judgment to document the cardiovascular assessment in the electronic health record.
8. Interpret assessment findings for patients with a suspected or actual CV health problem.
9. Identify the CV assessment components that contribute to disparities in certain populations.

The cardiovascular (CV) system is responsible for supplying oxygen to body organs and other tissues (PERFUSION). It is made up of the heart and blood vessels (both arteries and veins).

The heart muscle, called the myocardium, must receive sufficient oxygen to pump blood to other parts of the body. The arteries must be patent so the pumped blood can reach the rest of the body. Oxygen in the blood is required for cells to live and

function properly. When diseases or other problems of the CV systems occur, gas exchange and PERFUSION decrease, often resulting in life-threatening events or a risk for these events.

The CV system works with the respiratory and hematologic systems to meet the human need for gas exchange and tissue PERFUSION. Any problem in these systems requires the CV system to work harder to meet gas exchange and tissue perfusion needs.

Cardiovascular disease (CVD) continues to be the number-one cause of death in the United States. An average of one death in the United States occurs every 40 seconds from CVD (Mozaffarian et al., 2016). The disease kills more people than the next four causes of death combined, including cancer, chronic lower respiratory diseases, accidents, and diabetes. Of particular concern is that CVD is the leading cause of death for women. In addition, the American Heart Association (AHA) estimates that more than one in three adults are living with some form of the disease. About 20% of people who experience a myocardial infarction will die within 1 year from the initial cardiac event (Mozaffarian et al., 2016).

ANATOMY AND PHYSIOLOGY REVIEW

Heart

Structure

The human heart is a fist-sized, muscular organ located in the mediastinum between the lungs (Fig. 33-1). Each beat of the heart pumps about 60 mL of blood, or 5 L/min. During strenuous physical activity, the amount of blood pumped can double to meet the body's increased gas exchange needs. A covering called the *pericardium* protects the heart. A muscular wall (septum) separates the heart into two halves: right and left. Each half has an atrium and a ventricle (Fig. 33-2).

The *right atrium (RA)* receives *deoxygenated* venous blood, which is returned from the body through the superior and inferior vena cava. It also receives blood from the heart muscle through the coronary sinus. Most of this venous return flows passively from the RA, through the opened tricuspid valve, and to the right ventricle during ventricular diastole, or filling. The RA actively propels the remaining venous return into the right ventricle during atrial systole, or contraction.

The *right ventricle (RV)* is a muscular pump located behind the sternum. It generates enough pressure to close the tricuspid valve, open the pulmonic valve, and propel blood into the pulmonary artery and the lungs.

After blood is *reoxygenated* in the lungs, it flows freely from the four pulmonary veins into the left atrium. Blood then flows through an opened mitral valve into the left ventricle during ventricular diastole. When the left ventricle is almost full, the *left atrium (LA)* contracts, pumping the remaining blood volume into the left ventricle. With systolic contraction, the *left ventricle (LV)* generates enough pressure to close the mitral valve and open the aortic valve. Blood is propelled into the aorta and the systemic arterial circulation. Blood flow through the heart is shown in Fig. 33-2.

Blood moves from the aorta throughout the systemic circulation to the various tissues of the body. The pressure of blood in the aorta of a young adult averages about 100 to 120 mm Hg, whereas the pressure of blood in the RA averages about 0 to 5 mm Hg. These differences in pressure produce a pressure gradient, with blood flowing from an area of higher pressure to an area of lower pressure. The heart and vascular structures are responsible for maintaining these pressures.

The four *cardiac valves* are responsible for maintaining the forward flow of blood through the chambers of the heart (see Fig. 33-2). These valves open and close when pressure and volume change within the heart's chambers. The cardiac valves are classified into two types: atrioventricular (AV) valves and semilunar valves.

The *AV valves* separate the atria from the ventricles. The *tricuspid valve* separates the RA from the RV. The *mitral*

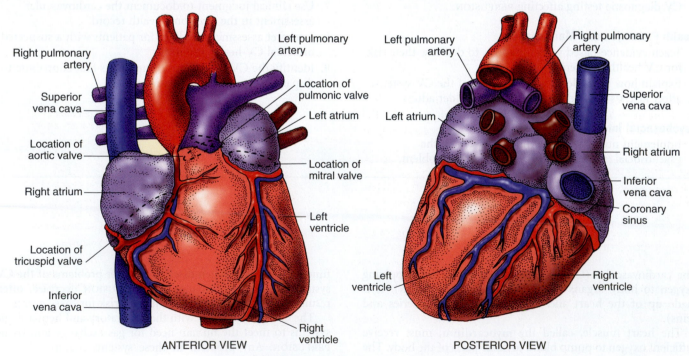

FIG. 33-1 Surface anatomy of the heart.

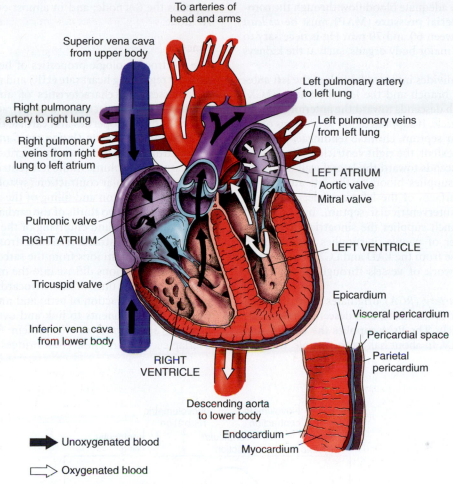

FIG. 33-2 Blood flow through the heart.

(bicuspid) valve separates the LA from the LV. During ventricular diastole, these valves act as funnels and help move the flow of blood from the atria to the ventricles. During systole, the valves close to prevent the backflow (valvular regurgitation) of blood into the atria.

The *semilunar valves* are the pulmonic valve and the aortic valve, which prevent blood from flowing back into the ventricles during diastole. The *pulmonic valve* separates the right ventricle from the pulmonary artery. The *aortic valve* separates the left ventricle from the aorta.

The heart muscle receives blood to meet its metabolic needs through the coronary arterial system (Fig. 33-3). The coronary arteries originate from an area on the aorta just beyond the aortic valve. All of the coronary arteries feeding the left heart originate from the left main coronary artery (LMCA). The right coronary artery (RCA) branches from the aorta to perfuse the right side of the heart and inferior wall of the left side of the heart.

Coronary artery blood flow to the myocardium occurs primarily during diastole, when coronary vascular resistance is

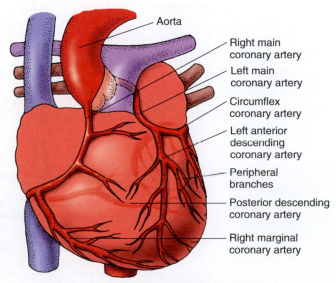

FIG. 33-3 Coronary arterial system.

minimized. To maintain adequate blood flow through the coronary arteries, **mean arterial pressure (MAP)** must be *at least 60 mm Hg*. A MAP between 60 and 70 mm Hg is necessary to maintain PERFUSION of major body organs, such as the kidneys and brain.

The *left main artery* divides into two branches: the left anterior descending (LAD) branch and the left circumflex (LCX) branch. The LAD branch descends toward the anterior wall and the apex of the left ventricle. It supplies blood to portions of the left ventricle, ventricular septum, chordae tendineae, papillary muscle, and, to a lesser extent, the right ventricle.

The LCX branch descends toward the lateral wall of the left ventricle and apex. It supplies blood to the left atrium, the lateral and posterior surfaces of the left ventricle, and sometimes portions of the interventricular septum. In about half of people, the LCX branch supplies the sinoatrial (SA) node. In a very small number of people, it supplies the AV node. Peripheral branches arise from the LAD and LCX branches and form an abundant network of vessels throughout the entire myocardium.

The *right coronary artery (RCA)* originates from the right sinus of Valsalva, encircles the heart, and descends toward the apex of the right ventricle. The RCA supplies the RA, RV, and inferior portion of the LV. In about half of the people, the RCA

supplies the SA node; and in almost everyone, it supplies the AV node.

Function

The electrophysiologic properties of heart muscle are responsible for regulating heart rate (HR) and rhythm. Cardiac muscle cells possess the characteristics of automaticity, excitability, conductivity, contractility, and refractoriness. Chapter 34 describes these properties and cardiac conduction in detail.

Sequence of Events During the Cardiac Cycle. The phases of the cardiac cycle are generally described in relation to changes in pressure and volume in the left ventricle during filling (diastole) and ventricular contraction (systole) (Fig. 33-4). **Diastole** consists of relaxation and filling of the atria and ventricles and comprises about two thirds of the cardiac cycle. **Systole** consists of the contraction and emptying of the atria and ventricles.

Myocardial contraction results from the release of large numbers of calcium ions from the sarcoplasmic reticulum and the blood. These ions diffuse into the myofibril sarcomere (the basic contractile unit of the myocardial cell). Calcium ions promote the interaction of actin and myosin protein filaments, causing these filaments to link and overlap. Cross-bridges, or linkages, are formed as the protein filaments slide over or overlap each other. These cross-bridges act as force-generating

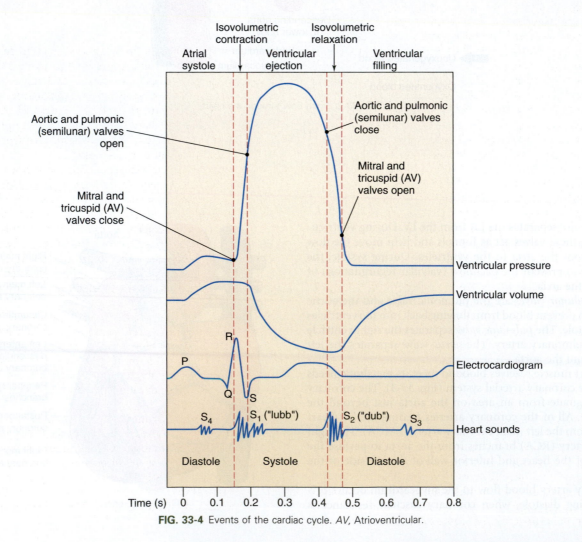

FIG. 33-4 Events of the cardiac cycle. *AV,* Atrioventricular.

sites. The sliding of these protein filaments shortens the sarcomeres, producing myocardial contraction.

Cardiac muscle relaxes when calcium ions are pumped back into the sarcoplasmic reticulum, causing a decrease in the number of calcium ions around the myofibrils. This reduced number of ions causes the protein filaments to disengage, the sarcomere to lengthen, and the muscle to relax.

Mechanical Properties of the Heart. The electrical and mechanical properties of cardiac muscle determine the function of the cardiovascular system. The healthy heart can adapt to various pathophysiologic conditions (e.g., stress, infections, hemorrhage) to maintain PERFUSION to the various body tissues. Blood flow from the heart into the systemic arterial circulation is measured clinically as **cardiac output (CO)**, the amount of blood pumped from the left ventricle each minute. CO depends on the relationship between heart rate (HR) and stroke volume (SV); it is the product of these two variables:

$$\text{Cardiac output} = \text{Heart rate} \times \text{Stroke volume}$$

In adults the CO ranges from 4 to 7 L/min. Because CO requirements vary according to body size, the cardiac index is calculated to adjust for differences in body size. The **cardiac index** can be determined by dividing the CO by the body surface area. The normal range is 2.8 to 4.2 L/min/m^2 (Pagana et al., 2017).

Heart rate (HR) refers to the number of times the ventricles contract each minute. The normal resting HR for an adult is between 60 and 100 beats/min. Increases in rate increase myocardial oxygen demand. The HR is extrinsically controlled by the autonomic nervous system (ANS), which adjusts rapidly when necessary to regulate cardiac output. The parasympathetic (vagus nerve) system *slows* the HR, whereas sympathetic stimulation *increases* the heart rate. An increase in circulating catecholamines (e.g., epinephrine and norepinephrine) usually causes an increase in HR and contractility. Many cardiovascular drugs, particularly beta blockers, block this sympathetic (fight or flight) pattern by decreasing the HR.

Stroke volume (SV) is the amount of blood ejected by the left ventricle during each contraction. Several variables influence SV and, ultimately, CO. These variables include HR, preload, afterload, and contractility.

Preload refers to the degree of myocardial fiber stretch at the end of diastole and just before contraction. The stretch imposed on the muscle fibers results from the volume contained within the ventricle at the end of diastole. Preload is determined by the amount of blood returning to the heart from both the venous system (right heart) and the pulmonary system (left heart) (left ventricular end-diastolic [LVED] volume).

An increase in ventricular volume increases muscle-fiber length and tension, thereby enhancing contraction and improving stroke volume. This statement is derived from Starling's law of the heart: The more the heart is filled during diastole (within limits), the more forcefully it contracts. However, excessive filling of the ventricles results in excessive LVED volume and pressure and may result in decreased cardiac output.

Another factor affecting stroke volume, **afterload,** is the pressure or resistance that the ventricles must overcome to eject blood through the semilunar valves and into the peripheral blood vessels. The amount of resistance is directly related to arterial blood pressure and the diameter of the blood vessels.

Impedance, the peripheral component of afterload, is the pressure that the heart must overcome to open the aortic valve.

The amount of impedance depends on aortic compliance and total systemic vascular resistance, a combination of blood viscosity (thickness) and arteriolar constriction. A decrease in stroke volume can result from an increase in afterload without the benefit of compensatory mechanisms, thus leading to a decrease in cardiac output.

Myocardial contractility affects stroke volume and CO and is the force of cardiac contraction independent of preload. Contractility is increased by factors such as sympathetic stimulation, calcium release, and positive inotropic drugs. It is decreased by factors such as hypoxia and acidemia.

Vascular System

The vascular system serves several purposes:
- Provides a route for blood to travel from the heart to nourish the various tissues of the body
- Carries cellular wastes to the excretory organs
- Allows lymphatic flow to drain tissue fluid back into the circulation
- Returns blood to the heart for recirculation

The vascular system is divided into the arterial system and the venous system. In the arterial system, blood moves from the larger arteries to a network of smaller blood vessels, called *arterioles*, which meet the capillary bed. In the venous system, blood travels from the capillaries to the venules and to the larger system of veins, eventually returning in the vena cava to the heart for recirculation.

Arterial System

The primary function of the arterial system is to deliver oxygen and nutrients to various tissues in the body. Nutrients are carried through arteries to arterioles, then branch into smaller terminal arterioles, and finally join with capillaries and venules to form a capillary network. Within this network, nutrients are exchanged across capillary membranes by three primary processes: osmosis, filtration, and diffusion. (See Chapter 11 for detailed discussions of these processes.)

The arterial system delivers blood to various tissues for oxygen and nourishment. At the tissue level, nutrients, chemicals, and body defense substances are distributed and exchanged for cellular waste products, depending on the needs of the particular tissue. The arteries transport the cellular wastes to the excretory organs (e.g., kidneys and lungs) to be reprocessed or removed. These vessels also contribute to temperature regulation in the tissues. Blood can be either directed toward the skin to promote heat loss or diverted away from it to conserve heat.

Blood pressure (BP) is the *force* of blood exerted against the vessel walls. Pressure in the larger arterial blood vessels is greater (about 80 to 100 mm Hg) and decreases as blood flow reaches the capillaries (about 25 mm Hg). By the time blood enters the right atrium, the BP is about 0 to 5 mm Hg. Volume, ventricular contraction, and vascular tone are necessary to maintain blood pressure.

BP is determined primarily by the quantity of blood flow or cardiac output (CO) and by the resistance in the arterioles.

Any factor that increases CO or total peripheral vascular resistance increases the BP. In general, BP is maintained at a relatively constant level. Therefore an increase or decrease in total peripheral vascular resistance is associated with a decrease or an increase in CO, respectively. Three mechanisms mediate and regulate BP:

- The autonomic nervous system (ANS), which excites or inhibits sympathetic nervous system activity in response to impulses from chemoreceptors and baroreceptors
- The kidneys, which sense a change in blood flow and activate the renin-angiotensin-aldosterone mechanism
- The endocrine system, which releases various hormones (e.g., catecholamine, kinins, serotonin, histamine) to stimulate the sympathetic nervous system at the tissue level

Systolic BP is the amount of pressure/force generated by the left ventricle to distribute blood into the aorta with each contraction of the heart. It is a measure of how effectively the heart pumps and is an indicator of vascular tone. **Diastolic BP** is the amount of pressure/force against the arterial walls during the relaxation phase of the heart.

BP is regulated by balancing the sympathetic and parasympathetic nervous systems of the autonomic nervous system. Changes in autonomic activity are responses to messages sent by the sensory receptors in the various tissues of the body. These receptors, including the baroreceptors, chemoreceptors, and stretch receptors, respond differently to the biochemical and physiologic changes of the body.

Baroreceptors in the arch of the aorta and at the origin of the internal carotid arteries are stimulated when the arterial walls are stretched by an increased BP. Impulses from these baroreceptors inhibit the vasomotor center, which is located in the pons and the medulla. Inhibition of this center results in a drop in BP.

Several 1- to 2-mm collections of tissue have been identified in the carotid arteries and along the aortic arch known as **peripheral chemoreceptors**. These receptors are sensitive primarily to hypoxemia (a decrease in the partial pressure of arterial oxygen [Pao_2]). When stimulated, these chemoreceptors send impulses along the vagus nerves to activate a vasoconstrictor response and raise BP.

The central chemoreceptors in the respiratory center of the brain are also stimulated by **hypercapnia** (an increase in partial pressure of arterial carbon dioxide [$Paco_2$]) and acidosis. However, the direct effect of carbon dioxide on the central nervous system (CNS) is 10 times stronger than the effect of hypoxia on the peripheral chemoreceptors.

Stretch receptors in the vena cava and the right atrium are sensitive to pressure or volume changes. When a patient is hypovolemic, stretch receptors in the blood vessels sense a reduced volume or pressure and send fewer impulses to the CNS. This reaction stimulates the sympathetic nervous system to increase the heart rate (HR) and constrict the peripheral blood vessels.

The kidneys also help regulate cardiovascular activity. When renal blood flow or pressure decreases, the kidneys retain sodium and water. BP tends to rise because of fluid retention and activation of the renin-angiotensin-aldosterone mechanism (see Fig. 11-6). This mechanism results in vasoconstriction and sodium retention (and thus fluid retention). Vascular volume is also regulated by the release of antidiuretic hormone (vasopressin) from the posterior pituitary gland (see Chapter 11).

Other factors can also influence the activity of the cardiovascular system. Emotional behaviors (e.g., excitement, pain, anger) stimulate the sympathetic nervous system to increase BP and HR. Increased physical activity such as exercise also increases BP and HR during the activity. Body temperature can affect the metabolic needs of the tissues, thereby influencing the delivery of blood. In hypothermia, tissues require fewer nutrients, and BP falls. In hyperthermia, the metabolic requirement of the tissues is greater, and BP and HR rise.

Venous System

The primary function of the venous system is to complete the circulation of blood by returning blood from the capillaries to the right side of the heart. It is composed of a series of veins that are located next to the arterial system. A second superficial venous circulation runs parallel to the subcutaneous tissue of the extremity. These two venous systems are connected by communicating veins that provide a means for blood to travel from the superficial veins to the deep veins. Blood flow is directed toward the deep venous circulation.

Veins have the ability to accommodate large shifts in volume with minimal changes in venous pressure. This flexibility allows the venous system to accommodate the administration of IV fluids and blood transfusions and to maintain pressure during blood loss and dehydration. Veins in the superficial and deep venous systems (except the smallest and the largest veins) have valves that direct blood flow back to the heart and prevent backflow. Skeletal muscles in the extremities provide a force that helps push the venous blood forward. The superior vena cava and inferior vena cava are valveless and large enough to allow blood flow to return easily to the heart.

Gravity exerts an increase in **hydrostatic pressure** in the capillaries when the patient is in an upright position, delaying venous return. Hydrostatic pressure is decreased in dependent areas such as the legs when the patient is lying down; thus there is less hindrance of venous return to the heart.

Cardiovascular Changes Associated With Aging

A number of physiologic changes in the cardiovascular system occur with advancing age (Chart 33-1). Many of these changes result in a loss of cardiac reserve. These changes are usually not evident when the older adult is resting. They become apparent only when the person is physically or emotionally stressed and the heart cannot meet the increased metabolic demands of the body.

ASSESSMENT: NOTICING AND INTERPRETING

Patient History

The focus of the patient history is on obtaining information about risk factors and symptoms of cardiovascular disease. Assess *nonmodifiable* (uncontrollable) risk factors, including the patient's age, gender, ethnic origin and a family history of cardiovascular disease. Ask about any chronic disease or illness that the patient may have. The incidence of conditions such as coronary artery disease (CAD) and valvular disease increases with age. The incidence of CAD also varies with the patient's gender. Men have a higher risk for CAD than women of all ages except in the oldest age-group of 75 years and older (Mozaffarian et al., 2016).

Heart disease is the leading cause of diabetes-related death for both men and women. Adults with diabetes have heart disease death rates two to four times higher than those without diabetes. The risk for stroke is also two to four times higher among people with diabetes.

Modifiable (controllable) risk factors should also be assessed. *Modifiable* risk factors are personal lifestyle habits, including cigarette use, physical inactivity, obesity, and psychological

CHART 33-1 Nursing Focus on the Older Adult

Changes in the Cardiovascular System Related to Aging

CHANGE	NURSING INTERVENTIONS	RATIONALES
Cardiac Valves		
Calcification and mucoid degeneration occur, especially in mitral and aortic valves.	Assess heart rate and rhythm and heart sounds for murmurs. Question patients about dyspnea.	Murmurs may be detected before other symptoms. Valvular abnormalities may result in rhythm changes.
Conduction System		
Pacemaker cells decrease in number. Fibrous tissue and fat in the sinoatrial node increase. Few muscle fibers remain in the atrial myocardium and bundle of His. Conduction time increases.	Assess the electrocardiogram (ECG) and heart rhythm for dysrhythmias or a heart rate less than 60 beats/min.	The sinoatrial (SA) node may lose its inherent rhythm. Atrial dysrhythmias occur in many older adults; 80% of older adults experience premature ventricular contractions (PVCs).
Left Ventricle		
The size of the left ventricle increases. The left ventricle becomes stiff and less distensible. Fibrotic changes in the left ventricle decrease the speed of early diastolic filling by about 50%.	Assess the ECG for a widening QRS complex and a longer QT interval. Assess the heart rate at rest and with activity. Assess for activity intolerance.	Ventricular changes result in decreased stroke volume, ejection fraction, and cardiac output during exercise; the heart is less able to meet increased oxygen demands. Maximum heart rate with exercise is decreased. The heart is less able to meet increased oxygen demands.
Aorta and Other Large Arteries		
The aorta and other large arteries thicken and become stiffer and less distensible. Systolic blood pressure increases to compensate for the stiff arteries. Systemic vascular resistance increases as a result of less distensible arteries; therefore the left ventricle pumps against greater resistance, contributing to left ventricular hypertrophy.	Assess blood pressure. Note increases in systolic, diastolic, and pulse pressures. Assess for activity intolerance and shortness of breath. Assess the peripheral pulses.	Hypertension may occur and must be treated to avoid target organ damage.
Baroreceptors		
Baroreceptors become less sensitive.	Assess the patient's blood pressure with the patient lying and then sitting or standing. Assess for dizziness when the patient changes from a lying to a sitting or standing position. Teach the patient to change positions slowly.	Orthostatic (postural) and postprandial changes occur because of ineffective baroreceptors. Changes may include blood pressure decreases of 10 mm Hg or more, dizziness, and fainting.

GENDER HEALTH CONSIDERATIONS

Patient-Centered Care QSEN

Postmenopausal women are two to three times more likely than premenopausal women to have CAD. The incidence for the disease in women is about 10 years later than in men and 20 years later for myocardial infarction (MI) and death to occur. After an acute MI, women tend to have a higher mortality rate and suffer more complications when compared with men (Mozaffarian et al., 2016).

Women with waist and abdominal obesity (greater waist-hip ratio) are more likely to experience cardiovascular disease (CVD) than are women with excess fat in their buttocks, hips, and thighs.

variables. Ask the patient about each of these common risk factors.

Cigarette smoking is a major risk factor for CVD, specifically coronary artery disease (CAD) and peripheral vascular disease (PVD). Three compounds in cigarette smoke have been implicated in the development of CAD: tar, nicotine, and carbon monoxide. The smoking history should include the number of cigarettes smoked daily, the duration of the smoking habit, and the age of the patient when smoking started. Record the smoking history in **pack-years,** which is the number of packs per day multiplied by the number of years the patient has smoked.

Ask about the patient's desire to quit, past attempts to quit, and the methods used. Determine nicotine dependence by asking questions such as:

- How soon after you wake up in the morning do you smoke?
- Do you wake up in the middle of your sleep time to smoke?
- Do you find it difficult not to smoke in places where smoking is prohibited?
- Do you smoke when you're ill?

Three to four years after a patient has stopped smoking, his or her CVD risk appears to be similar to that of a person who has never smoked. Be sure to ask those who do not currently smoke whether they have ever smoked and when they quit. Passive smoke significantly reduces blood flow in healthy young adults' coronary arteries, and the risk for dying increases among those who are exposed to secondhand smoke (American Heart Association [AHA], 2015b).

A *sedentary lifestyle* is also a major risk factor for heart disease. Regular physical activity promotes cardiovascular fitness and produces beneficial changes in blood pressure and levels of blood lipids and clotting factors. Unfortunately, few people in the United States follow the recommended exercise guidelines: 150 minutes of moderate exercise or 75 minutes of vigorous exercise per week (or a combination of the two) plus completing muscle-strengthening exercises at least 2 days per week (Mozaffarian et al., 2016). According to the AHA (2015b), only 20.9% of people in the United States meet the guidelines for physical activity. Encourage increased physical exercise as part of a lifestyle change to reduce the risk for CAD. Ask patients about the type of exercise they perform, how long a period they have participated in the exercise, and the frequency and intensity of the exercise.

About two thirds of American adults are overweight as defined by a body mass index (BMI) of 25 to 30. Obesity, defined as a BMI greater than 30, is particularly a problem for African-American women and Mexican Americans; however, the exact cause of this cultural difference is unknown (Mozaffarian et al., 2016). Asian Americans, with the exception of Filipino adults, have the lowest prevalence of obesity. Obesity is also associated with hypertension, hyperlipidemia, and diabetes; all are known contributors to CVD.

The American Heart Association provides guidelines to combat obesity and improve cardiac health, including ingesting more nutrient-rich foods that have vitamins, minerals, fiber, and other nutrients but are low in calories. To get the necessary nutrients, teach patients to choose foods such as vegetables, fruits, unrefined whole-grain products, and fat-free dairy products most often. Also teach patients to not eat more calories than they can burn every day (AHA, 2015a).

A variety of *psychological factors* make people more vulnerable to the development of heart disease. Those who are highly competitive, overly concerned about meeting deadlines, and often hostile or angry are at higher risk for heart disease. Psychological stress, anger, depression, and hostility are all closely associated with risk for developing heart disease.

You might ask the patient, "How do you respond when you have to wait for an appointment?" Chronic anger and hostility appear to be closely associated with CVD. The constant arousal of the sympathetic nervous system as a result of anger may influence BP, serum fatty acids and lipids, and clotting mechanisms. Observe the patient and assess his or her response to stressful situations.

Review the patient's medical history, noting any major illnesses such as diabetes mellitus, renal disease, anemia, high BP, stroke, bleeding disorders, connective tissue diseases, chronic pulmonary diseases, heart disease, and thrombophlebitis. These conditions can influence the patient's cardiovascular status.

Ask about previous treatment for CVD, identify previous diagnostic procedures (e.g., ECG, cardiac catheterization), and request information about any medical or invasive treatment of CVD. Ask specifically about recurrent tonsillitis, streptococcal infections, and rheumatic fever, because these conditions may lead to valvular abnormalities of the heart. In addition, inquire about any known congenital heart defects. Many patients with congenital heart problems live into adulthood because of improved treatment and surgeries.

Ask patients about their drug history, beginning with any current or recent use of prescription or over-the-counter (OTC) medications or herbal/natural products. Inquire about known sensitivities to any drug and the nature of the reaction (e.g., nausea, rash). Patients should be asked whether they have recently used cocaine or any IV "street" drugs, because these substances are often associated with heart disease.

🧩 GENDER HEALTH CONSIDERATIONS
Patient-Centered Care **QSEN**

Research is clear that women frequently present with CAD differently than men. Assess women for nonspecific cardiovascular symptoms, such as fatigue, malaise, anxiety, and shortness of breath. Although knowledge of presentation in women is increasing, educational needs remain, because heart disease remains the leading cause of death in women (Froedge, 2015).

The *social history* includes information about the patient's living situation, including having a domestic partner, other household members, environment, and occupation. Identification of support systems is especially important in exploring the possibility that the patient might have difficulty paying for medications or treatment. Ask about occupation, including the type of work performed and the requirements of the specific job. For instance, does the job involve physical exertion such as lifting heavy objects? Is the job emotionally stressful? What does a day's work entail? Does the patient's job require him or her to be outside in extreme weather conditions?

♥ VETERANS' HEALTH CONSIDERATIONS
Patient-Centered Care **QSEN**

The risk of heart disease in the veteran population has been assumed as increased as a result of increased incidence of poor physical and mental health. This assumption was based on the number of veterans facing mental health issues such as depression and post-traumatic stress disorder (PTSD) and the increased incidence of health-compromising behaviors such as smoking. However, recent research suggests that veterans are at a higher risk of having new-onset heart disease, and this link may be independent of health behaviors and chronic medical conditions (Assari, 2014). Research suggests that targeted teaching interventions should be considered in veterans before the development of heart disease to decrease their risk for heart disease (Assari, 2014).

Nutrition History

A nutrition history includes the patient's recall of food and fluid intake during a 24-hour period, self-imposed or medically prescribed dietary restrictions or supplementations, and the amount and type of alcohol consumption. If needed, the dietitian may review the type of foods selected by the patient for the amount of sodium, sugar, cholesterol, fiber, and fat. Cultural beliefs and economic status can influence the choice of food items and therefore are seriously considered. Family members or significant others who are responsible for shopping and cooking should be included in this screening.

 NCLEX EXAMINATION CHALLENGE 33-2

Health Promotion and Maintenance

The nurse is teaching a client with a newly diagnosed cardiovascular disorder. Which statement made by the client demonstrates health promotion?

A. "My heart disease will go away when I cut down to one cigarette a day."

B. "I'm glad I don't have to change my diet and can continue to eat whatever I want."

C. "I need to get at least 150 minutes of moderate exercise a week."

D. "I finally have my blood pressure to a normal level of 150/85."

Family History and Genetic Risk

Review the family history and obtain information about the age, health status, and cause of death of immediate family members. A positive family history for CAD in a first-degree relative (parent, sibling, or child) is a major risk factor. It is *more* important than other factors such as hypertension, obesity, diabetes, or sudden cardiac death.

 GENETIC/GENOMIC CONSIDERATIONS

Patient-Centered Care QSEN

Cardiovascular disease has many contributory factors, including a genetic tendency. A significant association between familial cardiac history and CVD is consistently demonstrated in the evidence of multiple large-scale prospective epidemiology studies (Mozaffarian et al., 2016). Although several genes have been reported to be associated with heart disease, stroke, and hypertension, the impact of each individual gene is not fully understood. Genetic association studies are under way to determine more specific genetic variants that may underlie the family history (Roberts, 2014). Additional discussions about genetic factors related to specific CVDs are found in other chapters in this unit.

Current Health Problems

Ask the patient to describe his or her health concerns. Expand on the description of these concerns by obtaining information about their onset, duration, sequence, frequency, location, quality, intensity, associated symptoms, and precipitating, aggravating, and relieving factors. Major symptoms usually identified by patients with CVD include chest pain or discomfort, dyspnea, fatigue, palpitations, weight gain, syncope, and extremity pain.

Pain or discomfort, considered a traditional symptom of heart disease, can result from ischemic heart disease, pericarditis, and aortic dissection. Chest pain can also be caused by noncardiac conditions such as pleurisy, pulmonary embolus, hiatal hernia, gastroesophageal reflux disease, neuromuscular abnormalities, and anxiety.

Ask the patient to identify when the symptoms were first noticed (onset):

- Did the symptoms begin suddenly or develop gradually (manner of onset)?
- How long did the symptoms last (duration)?

If he or she has repeated painful episodes, assess how often the symptoms occur (frequency). If pain is present, ask whether it

! NURSING SAFETY PRIORITY QSEN

Action Alert

Thoroughly evaluate the nature and characteristics of the chest pain. Because pain resulting from myocardial ischemia is life threatening and can lead to serious complications, its cause should be considered ischemic (reduced or obstructed blood flow to the myocardium) until proven otherwise. When assessing for symptoms, ask the patient if he or she has "discomfort," "heaviness," "pressure," and/or "indigestion." It is important to note that chest pain can occur in any setting. Proper assessment of the pain can decrease the potential for serious complications.

GENDER HEALTH CONSIDERATIONS

Patient-Centered Care QSEN

Some patients, especially women, do not experience pain in the chest but, instead, feel discomfort or indigestion. Women often present with a "triad" of symptoms. In addition to indigestion or a feeling of abdominal fullness, chronic fatigue despite adequate rest and feelings of an "inability to catch my breath" (dyspnea) are also common in heart disease. The patient may also describe the sensation as aching, choking, strangling, tingling, squeezing, constricting, or viselike. Others with severe neuropathy may experience few or no traditional symptoms except shortness of breath, despite major ischemia. Be aware that CVD affects younger people as well. According to the American Heart Association (2015b), 31% to 48% of women over the age of 20 have cardiovascular disease.

is different from any other episodes of pain. Ask the patient to describe which activities he or she was doing when it first occurred, such as sleeping, arguing, or running (precipitating factors). If possible, the patient should point to the area where the chest pain occurred (location) and describe if and how the pain radiated (spread).

In addition, ask how the pain feels and whether it is sharp, dull, or crushing (quality of pain). To understand the severity of the pain, ask the patient to grade it from 0 to 10, with 10 indicating severe pain (intensity). He or she may also report other signs and symptoms that occur at the same time (associated symptoms), such as dyspnea, diaphoresis (excessive sweating), nausea, and vomiting. Other factors that need to be addressed are those that may have made the chest pain worse (aggravating factors) or less intense (relieving factors). Chest pain can arise from a variety of sources (Table 33-1). By obtaining the appropriate information, you can help identify the source of the discomfort.

Dyspnea (difficult or labored breathing) can occur as a result of both cardiac and pulmonary disease. It is experienced by the patient as uncomfortable breathing or shortness of breath. When obtaining the history, ask which factors precipitate and relieve dyspnea, what level of activity produces dyspnea, and what the patient's body position was when dyspnea occurred.

Dyspnea that is associated with activity, such as climbing stairs, is referred to as **dyspnea on exertion (DOE)**. This is usually an early symptom of heart failure and may be the *only* symptom experienced by women.

The patient with advanced heart disease may experience **orthopnea** (dyspnea that appears when he or she lies flat). Several pillows may be needed to elevate the head and chest, or a recliner to prevent breathlessness may be used. The number of pillows or the amount of head elevation needed to provide

TABLE 33-1 Assessment of Chest Discomfort: How Various Types of Chest Pain Differ

ONSET	QUALITY AND SEVERITY	LOCATION AND RADIATION	DURATION AND RELIEVING FACTORS
Angina			
Sudden, usually in response to exertion, emotion, or extremes in temperature	Squeezing, viselike pain	Usually the left side of chest without radiation Substernal; may spread across the chest and the back and/or down the arms	Usually lasts less than 15 min; relieved with rest, nitrate administration, or oxygen therapy
Myocardial Infarction			
Sudden, without precipitating factors, often in early morning	Intense stabbing, viselike pain or pressure, severe	Substernal; may spread throughout the anterior chest and to the arms, jaw, back, or neck	Continuous or no chest discomfort; relieved with morphine, cardiac drugs, and oxygen therapy
Pericarditis			
Sudden	Sharp, stabbing, moderate to severe	Substernal; usually spreads to the left side or the back	Intermittent; relieved with sitting upright, analgesia, or administration of anti-inflammatory agents
Pleuropulmonary			
Variable	Moderate ache, worse on inspiration	Lung fields	Continuous until the underlying condition is treated or the patient has rested
Esophageal-Gastric			
Variable	Squeezing, heartburn, variable severity	Substernal; may spread to the shoulders or the abdomen	Variable; may be relieved with antacid administration, food intake, or taking a sitting position
Anxiety			
Variable, may be in response to stress or fatigue	Dull ache to sharp stabbing; may be associated with numbness in fingers	Not well located and usually does not radiate to other parts of the body as pain	Usually lasts a few minutes

restful sleep often measures the severity of orthopnea. This symptom is usually relieved within a matter of minutes by sitting up or standing.

Paroxysmal nocturnal dyspnea (PND) develops after the patient has been lying down for several hours. In this position, blood from the lower extremities is redistributed to the venous system, which increases venous return to the heart. A diseased heart cannot compensate for the increased volume and is ineffective in pumping the additional fluid into the circulatory system. Pulmonary congestion results, and the patient awakens abruptly, often with a feeling of suffocation and panic. He or she sits upright and dangles the legs over the side of the bed to relieve the dyspnea. This sensation may last for 20 minutes.

Fatigue may be described as a feeling of tiredness or weariness resulting from activity. The patient may report that an activity takes longer to complete or that he or she tires easily after activity. Although fatigue in itself is not diagnostic of heart disease, many people with heart failure are limited by leg fatigue during exercise. Fatigue that occurs after mild activity and exertion usually indicates inadequate cardiac output (due to low stroke volume) and anaerobic metabolism in skeletal muscle. It can also accompany other symptoms or may be an early indication of heart disease in women.

Ask about the time of day the patient experiences fatigue and the activities that he or she can perform. Fatigue resulting from decreased cardiac output is often worse in the evening. Ask whether the patient can perform the same activities as he or she

could perform a year ago or the same activities as others of the same age. Often he or she limits activities in response to fatigue and, unless questioned, is unaware how much less active he or she has become.

A feeling of fluttering or an unpleasant feeling in the chest caused by an irregular heartbeat is referred to as **palpitations**. They may result from a change in heart rate or rhythm or from an increase in the force of heart contractions. Rhythm disturbances that may cause palpitations include paroxysmal supraventricular tachycardia, premature contractions, and sinus tachycardia. Those that occur during or after strenuous physical activity, such as running and swimming, may indicate overexertion or possibly heart disease. Noncardiac factors that may precipitate palpitations include anxiety; stress; fatigue; insomnia; hyperthyroidism; and the ingestion of caffeine, nicotine, or alcohol. Ask the patient about specific factors that cause his or her palpitations.

A sudden weight increase of 2.2 lb (1 kg) can result from excess fluid (1 L) in the interstitial spaces. The *best indicator* of fluid balance is weight. Excess fluid accumulation is commonly known as **edema**. It is possible for weight gains of up to 10 to 15 lb (4.5 to 6.8 kg, or 4 to 7 L of fluid) to occur before edema is apparent. Ask whether the patient has noticed a tightness of shoes, indentations from socks, or tightness of rings.

Syncope refers to a brief loss of consciousness. The most common cause is decreased perfusion to the brain. Any condition that suddenly reduces cardiac output, resulting in decreased cerebral blood flow, can lead to a syncopal episode. Conditions such as cardiac rhythm disturbances, especially ventricular dysrhythmias, and valvular disorders such as aortic stenosis may trigger this symptom. Near-syncope refers to dizziness with an inability to remain in an upright position. Explore the circumstances that lead to dizziness or syncope.

CONSIDERATIONS FOR OLDER ADULTS
Patient-Centered Care QSEN

Syncope in the aging person may result from hypersensitivity of the carotid sinus bodies in the carotid arteries. Pressure applied to these arteries while turning the head, shrugging the shoulders, or performing a Valsalva maneuver (bearing down during defecation) may stimulate a vagal response. A decrease in blood pressure and heart rate can result, which can produce syncope. This type of syncopal episode may also result from postural (orthostatic) or postprandial (after eating) hypotension.

Extremity pain may be caused by two conditions: ischemia from atherosclerosis and venous insufficiency of the peripheral blood vessels. Patients who report a moderate-to-severe cramping sensation in their legs or buttocks associated with an activity such as walking have intermittent claudication related to decreased arterial tissue PERFUSION. Resting or lowering the affected extremity to decrease tissue demands or to enhance arterial blood flow usually relieves claudication pain. Leg pain that results from prolonged standing or sitting is related to venous insufficiency from either incompetent valves or venous obstruction. Elevating the extremity may relieve this pain.

Functional History
After the history of the patient's cardiovascular status is obtained, he or she may be classified according to the New York Heart Association Functional Classification (Table 33-2) or other system. The four classifications (I, II, III, and IV) depend on the degree to which ordinary physical activities (routine ADLs) are affected by heart disease. The Killip Classification provides a more objective description of the hemodynamics of heart failure and is described in Chapter 38.

Physical Assessment
A thorough physical assessment is the foundation for the nursing database and the patient's priority problems. Any changes noted during the course of illness can be compared with this initial database. Evaluate the patient's vital signs on admission to the hospital or during the initial visit to the clinic or primary care provider's office.

General Appearance
Physical assessment begins with the patient's general appearance. Assess general build and appearance, skin color, distress level, level of consciousness, shortness of breath, position, and verbal responses.

Patients can have left- or right-sided heart failure, or both. They can also be diagnosed with systolic and/or diastolic heart failure. As a result, poor cardiac output and decreased cerebral PERFUSION may cause confusion, memory loss, and slowed verbal responses, especially in older adults. Patients with chronic heart failure may also appear malnourished, thin, and cachectic. Late signs of severe right-sided heart failure are ascites, jaundice, and anasarca (generalized edema) as a result of prolonged congestion of the liver. Heart failure may also cause fluid

---

TABLE 33-2   New York Heart Association Functional Classification of Cardiovascular Disability

Class I
- Patients with cardiac disease but without resulting limitations of physical activity
- Ordinary physical activity does not cause undue fatigue, palpitation, dyspnea, or anginal pain

Class II
- Patients with cardiac disease resulting in slight limitation of physical activity
- Comfortable at rest
- Ordinary physical activity results in fatigue, palpitation, dyspnea, or anginal pain

Class III
- Patients with cardiac disease resulting in marked limitation of physical activity
- Comfortable at rest
- Less than ordinary physical activity causes fatigue, palpitation, dyspnea, or anginal pain

Class IV
- Patients with cardiac disease resulting in inability to carry on any physical activity without discomfort
- Symptoms of cardiac insufficiency or of the anginal syndrome may be present, even at rest
- If any physical activity is undertaken, discomfort is increased

Excerpted from The New York Heart Association. (1964). *Diseases of the heart and blood vessels: Nomenclature and criteria for diagnosis* (6th ed.). Boston: Little, Brown.

---

retention and may be manifested by obvious generalized dependent edema. Chapter 35 differentiates right and left failure and systolic from diastolic heart failure in detail.

Skin
Skin assessment includes color and temperature. The best areas in which to assess circulation include the nail beds, mucous membranes, and conjunctival mucosa, because small blood vessels are located near the surface of the skin in those areas.

If there is normal blood flow or adequate perfusion to a given area in light-colored skin, it appears pink, perhaps rosy, and is warm. Decreased PERFUSION is manifested as cool, pale, and moist skin. Pallor is characteristic of anemia and can be seen in areas such as the nail beds, palms, and conjunctival mucous membranes in any patient.

A bluish or darkened discoloration of the skin and mucous membranes in *light-skinned* adults is referred to as cyanosis. This condition results from an increased amount of deoxygenated hemoglobin. It is not an early sign of decreased perfusion but occurs later with other symptoms. *Dark-skinned* adults may experience cyanosis as a graying of the same tissues.

Central cyanosis involves decreased oxygenation of the arterial blood in the lungs and appears as a bluish tinge of the conjunctivae and the mucous membranes of the mouth and tongue. Central cyanosis may indicate impaired lung function or a right-to-left shunt found in congenital heart conditions. Because of impaired circulation, there is marked desaturation of hemoglobin in the peripheral tissues, which produces a bluish or darkened discoloration of the nail beds, earlobes, lips, and toes.

Peripheral cyanosis occurs when blood flow to the peripheral vessels is decreased by peripheral vasoconstriction. Constriction results from a low cardiac output or an increased extraction of oxygen from the peripheral tissues. Peripheral cyanosis localized in an extremity is usually a result of arterial or venous insufficiency. Rubor (dusky redness) that replaces pallor in a dependent foot suggests arterial insufficiency.

Skin *temperature* can be assessed for symmetry by touching different areas of the body with the dorsal (back) surface of the hand or fingers. Decreased blood flow results in decreased skin temperature. It is lowered in several clinical conditions, including heart failure, peripheral vascular disease, and shock.

Extremities

Assess the patient's hands, arms, feet, and legs for skin changes, vascular changes, clubbing, and edema. Skin mobility and turgor are affected by fluid status. Dehydration and aging reduce skin turgor, and edema decreases skin elasticity. Vascular changes in an affected extremity may include paresthesia, muscle fatigue and discomfort, numbness, pain, coolness, and loss of hair distribution from a reduced blood supply.

Clubbing of the fingers and toes is caused by *chronic* oxygen deprivation in body tissues. It is common in patients with advanced chronic pulmonary disease, congenital heart defects, and cor pulmonale (right-sided heart failure). The angle of the normal nail bed is 160 degrees. With clubbing, the nail straightens out to an angle of 180 degrees and the base of the nail becomes spongy. Fig. 30-10 shows late clubbing.

Peripheral edema (fluid accumulation in the legs and feet) is a common finding in patients with cardiovascular problems. The location of edema helps determine its potential cause. Bilateral edema of the legs may be seen in those with heart failure or chronic venous insufficiency. Abdominal and leg edema can be seen in patients with heart disease and cirrhosis of the liver. Localized edema in one extremity may be the result of venous obstruction (thrombosis) or lymphatic blockage of the extremity (lymphedema). Edema may also be noted in dependent areas, such as the sacrum, when a patient is confined to bed. In other patients, edema results from third spacing when plasma proteins decrease. Dependent foot and ankle edema is also a common side effect of certain antihypertensive drugs, such as amlodipine (Norvasc).

Document the location of edema as precisely as possible (e.g., midtibial or sacral) and the number of centimeters from an anatomic landmark. The extent of edema can be assessed as mild, moderate, or severe (or 1+, 2+, 3+, or 4+). However, these values are not precise and are very unreliable. Determine whether the edema is pitting (the skin can be indented) (Fig. 33-5) or nonpitting.

The finger is typically used for pulse oximetry as a noninvasive method for assessing oxygenation and PERFUSION of many medical-surgical nursing patients. Correct placement of the pulse oximetry sensor is essential for accurate readings. Oxygen saturation levels of above 90% are considered normal, depending on the patient's age. Detailed information about this assessment method can be found in Chapter 27.

Blood Pressure

Arterial blood pressure is measured *indirectly* by sphygmomanometry. This technique of measurement is described in detail in nursing skills textbooks.

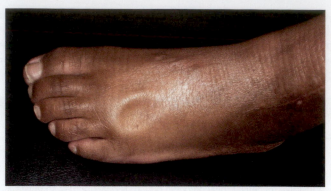

FIG. 33-5 Peripheral pitting edema. (From Sahrmann, S. (2011). Movement system impairment syndromes of the extremities, cervical and thoracic spines. St. Louis: Mosby.)

The Eighth National High Blood Pressure Education Program National Committee (JNC) on Prevention, Detection, Evaluation, and Treatment of High Blood Pressure (James et al., 2014) defines hypertension as a systolic pressure of 140 mm Hg or higher or a diastolic pressure of 90 mm Hg or higher or taking drugs to control blood pressure. Specific treatment goals were outlined for patients based on age and comorbidities. Chapter 36 describes hypertension in detail.

A BP less than 90/60 mm Hg (hypotension) may not be adequate for providing enough oxygen and sufficient nutrition to body cells. In certain circumstances such as shock, the Korotkoff sounds are less audible or are absent. In these cases palpate the BP, use an ultrasonic device (Doppler device), or obtain a direct measurement by arterial catheter in the critical care setting. When BP is palpated, only the systolic pressure can be determined. Patients may report dizziness or light-headedness when they move from a flat, supine position to a sitting or a standing position at the edge of the bed. Normally these symptoms are transient and pass quickly; pronounced symptoms may be due to postural hypotension. Postural (orthostatic) hypotension occurs when the BP is not adequately maintained while moving from a lying to a sitting or standing position. It is defined as a decrease of more than 20 mm Hg of the systolic pressure or more than 10 mm Hg of the diastolic pressure and a 10% to 20% increase in heart rate. The causes of postural hypotension include cardiovascular drugs, blood volume decrease, prolonged bedrest, age-related changes, or disorders of the nervous system.

To detect orthostatic changes in BP, first measure the BP when the patient is supine. After remaining supine for at least 3 minutes, the patient changes position to sitting or standing. Normally systolic pressure drops slightly or remains unchanged as the patient rises, whereas diastolic pressure rises slightly. After the position change, wait for at least 1 minute before auscultating BP and counting the radial pulse. The cuff should remain in the proper position on the patient's arm. Observe and record any signs or symptoms of dizziness. If the patient cannot tolerate the position change, return him or her to the previous position of comfort.

Paradoxical blood pressure is an exaggerated decrease in systolic pressure by more than 10 mm Hg during the inspiratory phase of the respiratory cycle (normal is 3 to 10 mm Hg). Certain clinical conditions that potentially alter the filling pressures in the right and left ventricles may produce a paradoxical BP. Such conditions include pericardial tamponade, constrictive pericarditis, and pulmonary hypertension. During inspiration, the filling pressures normally decrease slightly. However, decreased fluid volume in the ventricles resulting from these pathologic conditions produces a marked reduction in cardiac output. The difference between the systolic and diastolic values is referred to as **pulse pressure**. This value can be used as an indirect measure of cardiac output. Narrowed pulse pressure is rarely normal and results from increased peripheral vascular resistance or decreased stroke volume in patients with heart failure, hypovolemia, or shock. It can also be seen in those with mitral stenosis or regurgitation. An increased pulse pressure may occur in patients with slow heart rates, aortic regurgitation, atherosclerosis, hypertension, and aging.

The **ankle-brachial index (ABI)** can be used to assess the vascular status of the lower extremities. A BP cuff is applied to the lower extremity just above the malleolus. The systolic pressure is measured by Doppler ultrasound at both the dorsalis pedis and posterior tibial pulses. The higher of these two pressures is then divided by the higher of the two brachial pulses to obtain the ABI.

Normal values for the ABI are 1.00 or higher because BP in the legs is usually higher than BP in the arms. ABI values less than 0.90 usually indicate moderate vascular disease, whereas values less than 0.50 indicate severe vascular compromise. Although used primarily to help identify peripheral vascular disease, the ABI may be effective as a risk factor in predicting other CVD. An ABI of ≤0.90 and ≥1.40 suggests an increased risk of CVD and mortality; a result between 0.91 and 1.0 indicates moderate risk (Aboyans et al., 2012).

A **toe brachial pressure index (TBPI)** may be performed instead of or in addition to the ABI to determine arterial perfusion in the feet and toes. TBPI is the toe systolic pressure divided by the brachial (arm) systolic pressure.

Venous and Arterial Pulses

Observe the venous pulsations in the neck to assess the adequacy of blood volume and central venous pressure (CVP). Specially educated or critical care nurses can assess jugular venous pressure (JVP) to estimate the filling volume and pressure on the right side of the heart. An increase in JVP causes **jugular venous distention (JVD)**.

Normally the JVP is 3 to 10 cm H_2O. Increases are usually caused by right ventricular failure. Other causes include tricuspid regurgitation or stenosis, pulmonary hypertension, cardiac tamponade, constrictive pericarditis, hypervolemia, and superior vena cava obstruction.

Assessment of *arterial pulses* provides information about vascular integrity and circulation. For patients with suspected or actual vascular disease, major peripheral pulses should be assessed for presence or absence, amplitude, contour, rhythm, rate, and equality. Palpate the peripheral arteries in a head-to-toe approach with a side-to-side comparison (Fig. 33-6).

A *hypokinetic* pulse is a weak pulse indicative of a narrow pulse pressure. It is seen in patients with hypovolemia, aortic stenosis, and decreased cardiac output. A *hyperkinetic* pulse is a large, "bounding" pulse caused by an increased ejection of blood. It occurs in patients with a high cardiac output (with exercise, sepsis, or thyrotoxicosis) and in those with increased sympathetic system activity (with pain, fever, or anxiety).

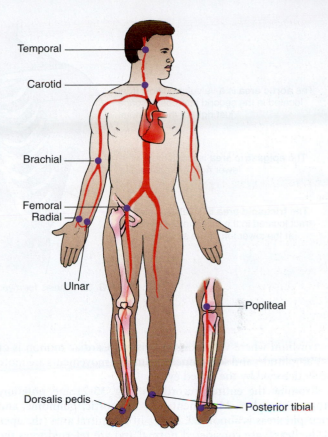

FIG. 33-6 Pulse points for assessment of arterial pulses.

Auscultation of the major arteries (e.g., carotid and aorta) is necessary to assess for bruits. **Bruits** are swishing sounds that may occur from turbulent blood flow in narrowed or atherosclerotic arteries. Assess for the absence or presence of bruits by placing the bell of the stethoscope on the neck over the carotid artery while the patient holds his or her breath. Normally there are no sounds if the artery has uninterrupted blood flow. A bruit may develop when the internal diameter of the vessel is narrowed by 50% or more, but this does not indicate the severity of disease in the arteries. Once the vessel is blocked 90% or greater, the bruit often cannot be heard.

Precordium

Assessment of the precordium (the area over the heart) involves inspection, palpation, percussion, and auscultation. In most settings, the medical-surgical nurse seldom performs precordial palpation and percussion. Critical care nurses and advanced practice nurses are qualified to perform the complete assessment. Therefore only inspection and auscultation are described here. Begin by placing the patient in a supine position, with the head of the bed slightly elevated for comfort. Some patients may require elevation of the head of the bed to 45 degrees for ease and comfort in breathing.

Inspection

A cardiac examination is usually performed in a systematic order, beginning with inspection. Inspect the chest from the side, at a right angle, and downward over areas of the

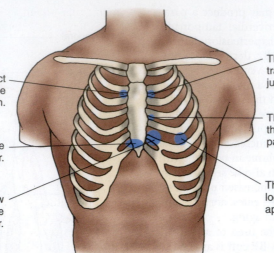

The **aortic area** is a valvular outflow tract located in the second intercostal space just right of the sternum.

The **epigastric area** is located over the lower right sternal border.

The **tricuspid area** is a valvular outflow tract located in the fifth intercostal space at the lower left of the sternal border.

The **pulmonic area** is a valvular outflow tract located in the second intercostal space just left of the sternum.

The **right ventricular area** is located over the lower half of the sternum and the left parasternal area.

The **mitral area** is a valvular outflow tract located in the fifth intercostal space at the apex of the heart.

FIG. 33-7 Areas for myocardial inspection and auscultation.

precordium where vibrations are visible. Cardiac motion is of low amplitude, and sometimes the inward movements are more easily detected by the naked eye.

Examine the entire precordium (Fig. 33-7) and note any prominent pulses. Movement over the aortic, pulmonic, and tricuspid areas is abnormal. Pulses in the mitral area (the apex of the heart) are considered normal and are referred to as the **apical impulse,** or the **point of maximal impulse (PMI).** The PMI should be located at the left fifth intercostal space (ICS) in the midclavicular line. If it appears in more than one ICS and has shifted lateral to the midclavicular line, the patient may have left ventricular hypertrophy.

Auscultation

Auscultation evaluates heart rate and rhythm, cardiac cycle (systole and diastole), and valvular function. The technique of auscultation requires a good-quality stethoscope and extensive clinical practice. Identifying specific abnormal heart sounds is most important in critical care and telemetry.

Listen to heart sounds in a systematic order. Examination usually begins at the aortic area and progresses slowly to the apex of the heart. The diaphragm of the stethoscope is pressed tightly against the chest to listen for high-frequency sounds and is useful in listening to the first and second heart sounds and high-frequency murmurs. Repeat the progression from the base to the apex of the heart using the bell of the stethoscope, which is held lightly against the chest. The bell can screen out high-frequency sounds and is useful in listening for low-frequency gallops (diastolic filling sounds) and murmurs.

Normal Heart Sounds. The **first heart sound (S1)** is created by the closure of the mitral and tricuspid valves (atrioventricular valves) (see Fig. 33-4). When auscultated, S_1 is softer and longer; it is of a low pitch and is best heard at the lower left sternal border or the apex of the heart. Palpating the carotid pulse while listening may help to identify S_1. S_1 marks the beginning of ventricular systole and occurs right after the QRS complex on the ECG.

S_1 can be accentuated or intensified in conditions such as exercise, hyperthyroidism, and mitral stenosis. A decrease in sound intensity occurs in patients with mitral regurgitation and

heart failure. If you have difficulty hearing heart sounds, have the patient lean forward or roll to his or her left side.

The *second heart sound (S_2)* is created by the closing of the aortic and pulmonic valves (semilunar valves) (see Fig. 33-4). S_2 is characteristically shorter. It is higher pitched and is heard best at the base of the heart at the end of ventricular systole.

The splitting of heart sounds is often difficult to differentiate from diastolic filling sounds (gallops). A splitting of S_1 (closure of the mitral valve followed by closure of the tricuspid valve) occurs physiologically because left ventricular contraction occurs slightly before right ventricular contraction. However, closure of the mitral valve is louder than closure of the tricuspid valve, so splitting is often not heard. Normal splitting of S_2 occurs because of the longer systolic phase of the right ventricle. Splitting of S_1 and S_2 can be accentuated by inspiration (due to increased venous return), and it narrows during expiration.

Abnormal Heart Sounds. Abnormal splitting of S_2 is referred to as **paradoxical splitting** and has a wider split heard on expiration. Paradoxical splitting of S_2 is heard in patients with severe myocardial depression that causes early closure of the pulmonic valve or a delay in aortic valve closure. Such conditions include myocardial infarction (MI), left bundle-branch block, aortic stenosis, aortic regurgitation, and right ventricular pacing.

Gallops and murmurs are common abnormal heart sounds that may occur with heart disease, but they can occur in some healthy people. Diastolic filling sounds (S_3 and S_4) are produced when blood enters a noncompliant chamber during rapid ventricular filling. The third heart sound (S_3) is produced during the rapid passive filling phase of ventricular diastole when blood flows from the atrium to a noncompliant ventricle. The sound arises from vibrations of the valves and supporting structures. The fourth heart sound (S_4) occurs as blood enters the ventricles during the active filling phase at the end of ventricular diastole.

S_3 is called a **ventricular gallop,** and S_4 is referred to as **atrial gallop.** These sounds can be caused by decreased compliance of either or both ventricles. Left ventricular diastolic filling sounds are best heard with the patient on his or her left side. The bell of the stethoscope is placed at the apex and at the left lower sternal border during expiration.

An S_3 heart sound is most likely to be a normal finding in those younger than 35 years. An S_3 gallop in patients older than 35 years is considered abnormal and represents a decrease in left ventricular compliance. It can be detected as an early sign of heart failure or as a ventricular septal defect.

An atrial gallop (S_4) may be heard in patients with hypertension, anemia, ventricular hypertrophy, MI, aortic or pulmonic stenosis, and pulmonary emboli. It may also be heard with advancing age because of a stiffened ventricle.

Murmurs reflect turbulent blood flow through normal or abnormal valves. They are classified according to their timing in the cardiac cycle: *systolic* murmurs (e.g., aortic stenosis and mitral regurgitation) occur between S_1 and S_2, whereas *diastolic* murmurs (e.g., mitral stenosis and aortic regurgitation) occur between S_2 and S_1. Murmurs can occur during presystole, midsystole, or late systole or diastole or can last throughout both phases of the cardiac cycle. They are also graded by the primary care provider according to their intensity, depending on their level of loudness (Table 33-3).

Although you are not expected to grade murmurs as a medical-surgical nurse, describe their location based on where they are best heard. Some murmurs transmit or radiate from their loudest point to other areas, including the neck, the back, and the axilla. The configuration is described as *crescendo* (increases in intensity) or *decrescendo* (decreases in intensity). The quality of murmurs can be further characterized as harsh, blowing, whistling, rumbling, or squeaking. They are also described by pitch—usually *high* or *low*.

A **pericardial friction rub** originates from the pericardial sac and occurs with the movements of the heart during the cardiac cycle. Rubs are usually transient and are a sign of inflammation, infection, or infiltration. They may be heard in patients with pericarditis resulting from MI, cardiac tamponade, or post-thoracotomy.

Psychosocial Assessment

To most people, the heart is a symbol of their ability to exist, survive, and love. A patient with a heart-related illness, whether acute or chronic, usually perceives it as a major life crisis. The patient and family confront not only the possibility of death but also fears about pain, disability, lack of self-esteem, physical dependence, and changes in family dynamics. Assess the meaning of the illness to the patient and family by asking, "What do you understand about what happened to you (or the patient)?" and "What does that mean to you?" When they perceive the stressor as overwhelming, formerly adequate support

systems may no longer be effective. In these circumstances, the patient and family members attempt to cope to regain a sense or feeling of control.

Coping behaviors vary among patients and their families. Those who feel helpless to meet the demands of the situation may exhibit behaviors such as disorganization, fear, and anxiety. Ask them, "Have you ever encountered such a situation before?" "How did you manage that situation?" and "To whom can you turn for help?" The answers to these questions often reassure the patient and family that they have encountered difficult situations in the past and have the ability and resources to cope with them.

A common and normal response is *denial,* which is a defense mechanism that enables the patient to cope with threatening circumstances. He or she may deny the current cardiovascular condition, may state that it was present but is now absent, or may be excessively cheerful. Denial becomes maladaptive when the patient is noncompliant or does not adhere to the interdisciplinary plan of care.

Family members and significant others may be more anxious than the patient. Often they recall all events of the illness, are unprotected by denial, and are afraid of recurrence. Disagreements may occur between the patient and family members over adherence to appropriate follow-up care.

> ### ❓ CLINICAL JUDGMENT CHALLENGE 33-1
> #### *Safety; Teamwork and Collaboration* **QSEN**
>
> A middle-age man presents to the emergency department (ED) with reports of chest pain and indigestion. He reports some minor discomfort in his jaw. The patient is alert and oriented; BP 90/50; HR/80. You are the RN assigned to his care. There is an unlicensed assistive personnel (UAP) working with you.
> 1. Which assessment data will you perform on his arrival to the ED? Why?
> 2. The provider orders labs, 12-lead ECG, IV fluids, blood pressure checks, medication for chest pain, and oxygen at 2 L per nasal cannula. What part of the patient's care will you delegate to the UAP? Which information will you communicate on delegation?
> 3. Which interventions will you implement to ensure this patient's safety?
> 4. Which priority information will you document in the patient's electronic health record?
> 5. The patient's wife is very concerned about her husband returning to work as owner of a roofing company. What education will you provide the patient and his wife at this time? With which health care team members will you collaborate to ensure positive patient outcomes?

Diagnostic Assessment
Laboratory Assessment

Assessment of the patient with cardiovascular dysfunction includes examination of the blood for abnormalities. The examination is performed to help establish a diagnosis, detect concurrent disease, assess risk factors, and monitor response to treatment. Normal values for serum cardiac enzymes and serum lipids are listed in Chart 33-2.

Serum Markers of Myocardial Damage. Events leading to cellular injury cause a release of enzymes from intracellular storage, and circulating levels of these enzymes are dramatically elevated. Acute myocardial infarction (MI), also known as **acute coronary syndrome,** can be confirmed by abnormally high levels of certain proteins or isoenzymes.

TABLE 33-3	**Grading of Heart Murmurs**
Grade I	Very faint
Grade II	Faint but recognizable
Grade III	Loud but moderate in intensity
Grade IV	Loud; accompanied by a palpable thrill
Grade V	Very loud; accompanied by a palpable thrill; audible with the stethoscope partially off the patient's chest
Grade VI	Extremely loud; may be heard with the stethoscope slightly above the patient's chest; accompanied by a palpable thrill

CHART 33-2   Laboratory Profile

Cardiovascular Assessment

NORMAL RANGE	SIGNIFICANCE OF ABNORMAL FINDINGS
Serum Lipids	
Total lipids 400-1000 mg/dL	Elevation indicates increased risk for coronary artery disease (CAD).
Cholesterol Less than 200 mg/dL	Elevation indicates increased risk for CAD.
Triglycerides Females: 35-135 mg/dL Males: 40-160 mg/dL	Elevation indicates increased risk for CAD.
Plasma high-density lipoproteins (HDLs) Females: >55 mg/dL Males: >45 mg/dL Older adults: range increases with age	Elevations protect against CAD.
Plasma low-density lipoproteins (LDLs) <130 mg/dL	Elevation indicates increased risk for CAD.
HDL:LDL ratio 3:1	Elevated ratios may protect against CAD.
VLDL 7-32 ng/dL	Elevated level indicates risk for CAD.
C-reactive protein (CRP) <1.0 mg/dL	Elevation may indicate tissue infarction or damage.
Serum Markers	
Troponins Cardiac troponin T <0.10 ng/mL Cardiac troponin I <0.03 ng/mL	Elevations indicate myocardial injury or infarction.

VLDL, Very-low-density lipoproteins.

Troponin is a myocardial muscle protein released into the bloodstream with injury to myocardial muscle. Troponins T and I are not found in healthy patients, so any rise in values indicates cardiac necrosis or acute MI. Specific markers of myocardial injury, troponins T and I, have a wide diagnostic time frame, making them useful for patients who present several hours after the onset of chest pain. Even low levels of troponin T are treated aggressively because of increased risk for death from cardiovascular disease (CVD). Obtaining cardiac markers at the bedside in the emergency department can be done as "point-of-care" (POC) testing for patients experiencing or at risk for acute MI, with results available within 15 to 20 minutes. These markers are evaluated in addition to clinical signs and symptoms and electrocardiogram (ECG) changes when identifying at-risk patients. Following initial troponin assessment, levels should be assessed again in 3 to 6 hours. Before the development of highly sensitive troponin levels, providers relied on creatinine kinase (CK), its isoenzyme (CK-MB), and myoglobin to assist with diagnosis of acute myocardial infarction. Use of these cardiac markers is no longer recommended (Amsterdam et al., 2014; Jaffe & Morrow, 2015).

Serum Lipids. Elevated lipid levels are considered a risk factor for coronary artery disease (CAD). **Cholesterol, triglycerides**, and the protein components of **high-density lipoproteins (HDLs)** and **low-density lipoproteins (LDLs)** are evaluated to assess the risk for CAD. The desired ranges for lipids are (Pagana et al., 2017):
- Total cholesterol less than 200 mg/dL
- Triglycerides between 40 and 160 mg/dL for men and between 35 and 135 mg/dL for women
- HDL more than 45 mg/dL for men; more than 55 mg/dL for women ("good" cholesterol)
- LDL less than 130 mg/dL

Each of the lipoproteins contains varying proportions of cholesterol, triglyceride, protein, and phospholipid. HDL contains mainly protein and 20% cholesterol, whereas LDL is mainly cholesterol. Elevated LDL levels are positively correlated with CAD, whereas elevated HDL levels are negatively correlated and appear to be protective for heart disease. LDL pattern size is of significant importance in determining risk for CVD. LDL pattern A is associated with non–insulin resistance; normal glucose, insulin, and HDL levels; and normal blood pressure. LDL pattern B is associated with insulin resistance; increased glucose, insulin, and triglyceride levels; and hypertension.

A fasting blood sample for the measurement of serum cholesterol levels is preferable to a nonfasting sample. If triglycerides are to be evaluated with cholesterol, the health care provider requests the specimen after a 12-hour fast.

Lipoprotein-a, or Lp(a), is a modified form of LDL, the most common familial lipoprotein disorder in patients with premature coronary artery disease. Lp(a) is atherogenic (increases atherosclerotic plaques) and prothrombotic (increases clots). Therefore the desired outcome is a value less than 30 mg/dL. The patient should be fasting and avoid smoking before the test (Pagana et al., 2017).

Other Laboratory Tests. **Homocysteine** is an amino acid that is produced when proteins break down. A certain amount of homocysteine is present in the blood, but elevated values may be an independent risk factor for the development of CVD. Although the relationship between homocysteine and CVD remains controversial, elevated levels of homocysteine may increase the risk for disease as much as smoking and hyperlipemia, especially in women. High-risk patients who have a personal or family history of premature heart disease should be screened. A level less than 14 mmol/dL is considered optimal, but this level increases as one ages (Pagana et al., 2017).

Inflammation is a common and critical component to the development of atherothrombosis. **Highly sensitive C-reactive protein (hsCRP)** has been the most studied marker of inflammation. Any inflammatory process can produce CRP in the blood. Elevations also are seen with hypertension, infection, and smoking. A level less than 1 mg/dL is considered low risk; a level over 3 mg/dL places the patient at high risk for heart disease. The CRP is very helpful in determining treatment outcomes in patients at risk for coronary disease and in managing statin therapy after an acute myocardial infarction. The most useful time to measure CRP appears to be for risk assessment in middle-age or older persons.

Microalbuminuria, or small amounts of protein in the urine, has been shown to be a clear marker of widespread endothelial dysfunction in cardiovascular disease (along with elevated CRP). It should be screened annually in all patients with hypertension, metabolic syndrome, or diabetes mellitus. Microalbuminuria has also been used as a marker for renal disease, particularly in patients with hypertension and diabetes.

Blood coagulation studies evaluate the ability of the blood to clot. They are important in patients with a greater tendency to form thrombi (e.g., those with atrial fibrillation, prosthetic valves, or infective endocarditis). These tests are also essential for monitoring patients receiving anticoagulant therapy (e.g., during cardiac surgery, during treatment of an established thrombus).

Prothrombin time (PT) and *international normalized ratio (INR)* are used when initiating and maintaining therapy with oral anticoagulants, such as sodium warfarin (Coumadin, Warfilone). They measure the activity of prothrombin, fibrinogen, and factors V, VII, and X. INR is the most reliable way to monitor anticoagulant status in warfarin therapy. The therapeutic ranges vary significantly based on the reason for the anticoagulation and the patient's history. The normal INR is 1.

Partial thromboplastin time (PTT) is assessed in patients who are receiving heparin (Hepalean). It measures deficiencies in all coagulation factors except VII and XIII.

Arterial blood gas (ABG) determinations are often obtained in patients with CVD. Determination of tissue oxygenation, carbon dioxide removal, and acid-base status is essential to appropriate treatment. (See Chapter 12 for a complete discussion of ABGs.)

FLUID AND ELECTROLYTE BALANCE is essential for normal cardiovascular performance. Cardiac manifestations often occur when there is an imbalance in either fluids or electrolytes in the body. For example, the cardiac effects of hypokalemia (low serum potassium level) include increased electrical instability, ventricular dysrhythmias, and an increased risk for digitalis toxicity. The effects of hyperkalemia on the myocardium include slowed ventricular conduction, peaked T waves on the ECG, and contraction followed by asystole (cardiac standstill).

Cardiac manifestations of hypocalcemia are ventricular dysrhythmias, a prolonged QT interval, and cardiac arrest. Hypercalcemia shortens the QT interval and causes atrioventricular block, digitalis hypersensitivity, and cardiac arrest. Serum sodium values reflect fluid balance and may be decreased, indicating fluid excess in patients with heart failure (dilutional hyponatremia).

Because magnesium regulates some aspects of myocardial electrical activity, hypomagnesemia has been implicated in some forms of ventricular dysrhythmias known as *torsades de pointes*. Hypomagnesemia prolongs the QT interval, causing this specific type of ventricular tachycardia. Chapter 11 describes these electrolytes in more detail.

The *erythrocyte (red blood cell [RBC]) count* is usually decreased in rheumatic fever and infective endocarditis. It is increased in heart diseases as needed to compensate for decreased available oxygen.

Decreased *hematocrit and hemoglobin* levels (e.g., caused by hemorrhage or hemolysis from prosthetic valves) indicate anemia and can lead to angina or aggravate heart failure. Vascular volume depletion with hemoconcentration (e.g., hypovolemic shock and excessive diuresis) results in an elevated hematocrit.

The *leukocyte (white blood cell [WBC]) count* typically is elevated after an MI and in various infectious and inflammatory diseases of the heart (e.g., infective endocarditis and pericarditis).

Other Diagnostic Assessment

Posteroanterior (PA) and left lateral *x-ray* views of the chest are routinely obtained to determine the size, silhouette, and position of the heart. In acutely ill patients, a simple anteroposterior (AP) view may be obtained at the bedside. Cardiac enlargement, pulmonary congestion, cardiac calcifications, and placement of central venous catheters, endotracheal tubes, and hemodynamic monitoring devices are assessed by x-ray.

Angiography of the arterial vessels, or **arteriography**, is an invasive diagnostic procedure that involves fluoroscopy and the use of contrast media. This procedure is performed when an arterial obstruction, narrowing, or aneurysm is suspected. The interventional radiologist performs selective arteriography to evaluate specific areas of the arterial system. For example, a coronary arteriography, which is performed during left-sided cardiac catheterization, assesses arterial circulation within the heart. It can also be performed on arteries in the extremities, mesentery, and cerebrum. Angiography is discussed under the appropriate associated diseases elsewhere in this text.

Cardiac Catheterization. The most definitive but most invasive test in the diagnosis of heart disease is cardiac catheterization. **Cardiac catheterization** may include studies of the right or left side of the heart and the coronary arteries. Some of the most common indications for cardiac catheterization are listed in Table 33-4.

Patient Preparation. Assess the patient's physical and psychosocial readiness and knowledge level about the procedure because many patients have anxiety and fear about cardiac catheterization. Review the purpose of the procedure, inform the patient about the length of the procedure, state who will be present, and describe the appearance of the catheterization laboratory. Tell the patient about the sensations that he or she may experience during the procedure, such as palpitations (as the catheter is passed up to the left ventricle), a feeling of heat or a hot flash (as the medium is injected into either side of the heart), and a desire to cough (as the medium is injected into the right side of the heart). Written, electronic, or illustrated materials or DVDs may be used to assist in understanding.

The cardiologist explains the risks of cardiac catheterization. The risks vary with the procedures to be performed and the patient's physical status (Table 33-5). Although not common, several serious complications may follow coronary arteriography, such as:

- Myocardial infarction (MI)
- Stroke

TABLE 33-4 Indications for Cardiac Catheterization

- To confirm suspected heart disorders, including congenital abnormalities, coronary artery disease, myocardial disease, valvular disease, and valvular dysfunction
- To determine the location and extent of the disease process
- To assess:
  - Stable, severe angina unresponsive to medical management
  - Unstable angina pectoris
  - Uncontrolled heart failure, ventricular dysrhythmias, or cardiogenic shock associated with acute myocardial infarction, papillary muscle dysfunction, ventricular aneurysm, or septal perforation
- To determine best therapeutic option (percutaneous transluminal coronary angioplasty, stents, coronary artery bypass graft, valvulotomy versus valve replacement)
- To evaluate effects of medical or invasive treatment on cardiovascular function, percutaneous transluminal coronary angioplasty, or coronary artery bypass graft patency

TABLE 33-5 Complications of Cardiac Catheterization

Right-Sided Heart Catheterization
- Thrombophlebitis
- Pulmonary embolism
- Vagal response

Left-Sided Heart Catheterization and Coronary Arteriography
- Myocardial infarction
- Stroke
- Arterial bleeding or thromboembolism
- Dysrhythmias

Right-Sided or Left-Sided Heart Catheterization*
- Cardiac tamponade
- Hypovolemia
- Pulmonary edema
- Hematoma or blood loss at insertion site
- Reaction to contrast medium

*In addition to those cited for each procedure.

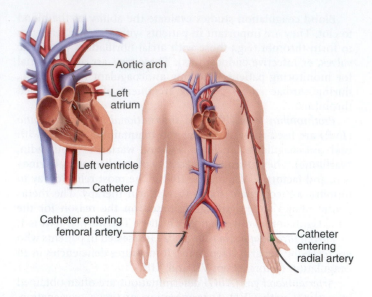

FIG. 33-8 Left-sided cardiac catheterization.

- Arterial bleeding
- Thromboembolism
- Lethal dysrhythmias
- Arterial dissection
- Death

The cardiologist or interventional radiologist obtains a written informed consent from the patient or responsible party before the procedure.

The patient is admitted to the hospital on the day of the catheterization procedure. He or she may be admitted earlier if there is renal dysfunction. Fluids may be given 12 to 24 hours before the procedure for renal protection. Contrast-induced renal dysfunction can result from vasoconstriction and the direct toxic effect of the contrast agent on the renal tubules. Hydration pre- and post-study helps eliminate or minimize contrast-induced renal toxicity.

Standard preoperative tests are performed, which usually include a chest x-ray, complete blood count, coagulation studies, and 12-lead ECG. Patients may ingest clear liquids up to 2 hours prior; solids and other liquids are held 6 hours before the procedure. The catheterization site is antiseptically prepared with hairs clipped according to agency policy.

Before the procedure, take the patient's vital signs, auscultate the heart and the lungs, and assess the peripheral pulses. Question him or her about any history of allergy to iodine-based contrast agents. An antihistamine or steroid may be given to a patient with a positive history or to prevent a reaction. **Be sure that the signed informed consent is completed, as required by The Joint Commission's National Patient Safety Goals (NPSGs).** A mild sedative is usually administered before the procedure. Certain medications, such as diuretics, may be held before the procedure. In addition, warfarin and other oral anticoagulants are held if it is anticipated that the femoral artery will be used for access. Analysis of electrolytes, blood urea nitrogen (BUN), creatinine, coagulation profile, and complete blood count (CBC) is essential before and after the procedure; and abnormalities are discussed with the health care provider.

Procedure. The patient is taken to the cardiac catheterization laboratory (sometimes referred to as the *cath lab*), placed in the supine position on the x-ray table, and securely strapped to the table. The physician injects a local anesthetic at the insertion site. During the procedure, the patient is instructed to report any chest pain, pressure, or other symptoms to the staff.

The *right side of the heart* is catheterized first and may be the only side examined. The cardiologist inserts a catheter through the femoral vein to the inferior vena cava or through the basilic vein to the superior vena cava. The catheter is advanced through either the inferior or the superior vena cava and, guided by fluoroscopy, is advanced through the right atrium, through the right ventricle, and, at times, into the pulmonary artery. Intracardiac pressures (right atrial, right ventricular, pulmonary artery, and pulmonary artery wedge pressures) and blood samples are obtained. A contrast medium is usually injected to detect any cardiac shunts or regurgitation from the pulmonic or tricuspid valves.

In a *left-sided heart catheterization,* the cardiologist advances the catheter against the blood flow from the femoral, brachial, or radial artery up the aorta, across the aortic valve, and into the left ventricle (Fig. 33-8). Radial artery access has recently become the most common access site for diagnostic heart catheterization examinations. Because of the size of stent delivery catheters, radial artery access is not possible for all patients. Alternatively, the catheter may be passed from the right side of the heart through the atrial septum, using a special needle to puncture the septum. Intracardiac pressures and blood samples are obtained. The pressures of the left atrium, left ventricle, and aorta and mitral and aortic valve status are evaluated. The cardiologist injects contrast dye into the ventricle; digital subtraction angiography evaluates left ventricular motion. Calculations are made regarding end-systolic volume, end-diastolic volume, stroke volume, and ejection fraction.

The technique for *coronary arteriography* is the same as for left-sided heart catheterization. The catheter is advanced into the aortic arch and positioned selectively in the right or left coronary artery. Injection of a contrast medium permits viewing the coronary arteries. By assessing the flow of the medium through the coronary arteries, information about the site and severity of coronary lesions is obtained.

An alternative to injecting a medium into the coronary arteries is **intravascular ultrasonography (IVUS)**, which introduces a flexible catheter with a miniature transducer at the distal tip to view the coronary arteries. The transducer emits sound waves, which reflect off the plaque and the arterial wall to create an image of the blood vessel. IVUS can be used in vessels as small as 2 mm to assess the nature of plaques or vessel condition following an intervention.

Fractional flow reserve (FFR) can also be assessed to determine if a blockage needs to be revascularized. FFR is an objective method to measure the flow across the stenosis in the coronary artery. A special pressure wire is passed through the area of stenosis, and measurements are taken proximal and distal to the area of stenosis. These two measurements are used to calculate the FFR. A measure of 0.8 or less indicates that the stenosis is clinically significant and the artery should be revascularized.

Follow-Up Care. The patient recovers in a specialty area equipped with monitored beds. After cardiac catheterization, restrict him or her to bedrest and keep the insertion site extremity straight. A soft knee brace can be applied to prevent bending of the affected extremity. Some cardiologists allow the head of the bed to be elevated up to 30 degrees during the period of bedrest, whereas others prefer that the patient remain supine. Current practice is for patients to remain in bed for 2 to 6 hours depending on the type of vascular closure device used. Various types of vascular closure devices are used to eliminate the need for manual compression after the catheterization. Examples include arteriotomy sutures and collagen plugs to seal the insertion site. Radial artery access is growing in popularity because it allows for a faster discharge (when compared with femoral access) and has fewer post-discharge restrictions on the patient than femoral or brachial artery access.

Monitor the patient's vital signs every 15 minutes for 1 hour, then every 30 minutes for 2 hours or until vital signs are stable, and then every 4 hours or according to agency policy. Assess the insertion site for bloody drainage or hematoma formation. Complications with vascular closure devices are not common but can be very serious. Assess peripheral pulses in the affected extremity and skin temperature and color with every vital sign check. Observe for complications of cardiac catheterization (see Table 33-5).

> **! NURSING SAFETY PRIORITY** **QSEN**
> ### Critical Rescue
>
> If the patient experiences symptoms of cardiac ischemia such as chest pain, dysrhythmias, bleeding, hematoma formation, or a dramatic change in peripheral pulses in the affected extremity, contact the Rapid Response Team or provider immediately to provide prompt intervention! Remain with the patient and obtain a 12-lead ECG for patients experiencing chest pain or dysrhythmias. For bleeding or hematoma formation, hold steady, firm pressure to the access site until the Rapid Response Team arrives. Neurologic changes indicating a possible stroke, such as visual disturbances, slurred speech, swallowing difficulties, and extremity weakness, should also be reported immediately.

Because the contrast medium acts as an osmotic diuretic, monitor urine output and ensure that the patient receives sufficient oral and IV fluids for adequate excretion of the medium. Pain medication for insertion site or back discomfort may be given as prescribed.

Review home instructions and risk factor modification with the patient before discharge. Remind the patient to:

- Limit activity for several days, including avoiding lifting and exercise
- Leave the dressing in place for at least the first day at home
- Observe the insertion site over the next few weeks for increased swelling, redness, warmth, and pain. (Bruising or a small hematoma is expected.)

> ### ? NCLEX EXAMINATION CHALLENGE 33-3
> #### Physiological Integrity
>
> Which statement made by the client on the way to the catheterization laboratory requires an **immediate** action by the nurse?
> A. "My allergies are bothering me, so I took some Benadryl last night before bed."
> B. "I was nervous last night, but I still remembered to take my warfarin."
> C. "I sure am hungry. I haven't had anything to eat since I went to bed last night."
> D. "I don't know what I will do if they find a blockage in my heart."

Electrocardiography. The electrocardiogram (ECG) is a routine part of every cardiovascular evaluation and is one of the most valuable diagnostic tests. Various forms are available: resting ECG, continuous ambulatory ECG (Holter monitoring), exercise ECG (stress test), signal-averaged ECG, and 30-day event monitoring. The resting ECG provides information about cardiac dysrhythmias, myocardial ischemia, the site and extent of MI, cardiac hypertrophy, electrolyte imbalances, and the effectiveness of cardiac drugs. The normal ECG pattern and a detailed discussion of the interpretation of abnormal patterns are discussed in Chapter 34.

Electrophysiologic Studies. An **electrophysiologic study (EPS)** is an invasive procedure during which programmed electrical stimulation of the heart is used to cause and evaluate lethal dysrhythmias and conduction abnormalities. Patients who have survived cardiac arrest, have recurrent tachydysrhythmias, or experience unexplained syncopal episodes may be referred for EPS. Induction of the dysrhythmia during EPS helps find an accurate diagnosis and aids in effective treatment. These procedures have risks similar to those for cardiac catheterization and are performed in a special catheterization laboratory, where conditions are strictly controlled and immediate treatment is available for any adverse effects.

Exercise Electrocardiography (Stress Test). The **exercise electrocardiography** test (also known as **exercise tolerance**, or **stress test**) assesses cardiovascular response to an increased workload. The stress test helps determine the functional capacity of the heart and screens for asymptomatic coronary artery disease. Dysrhythmias that develop during exercise may be identified, and the effectiveness of antidysrhythmic drugs can be evaluated.

Patient Preparation. Because risks are associated with exercising, the patient must be adequately informed about the purpose of the test, the procedure, and the risks involved. Written consent must be obtained. Anxiety and fear are common before stress testing. Therefore assure the patient that the procedure is performed in a controlled environment in which prompt nursing and medical attention are available.

Instruct the patient to get plenty of rest the night before the procedure. He or she may have a light meal 2 hours before the test but should avoid smoking or drinking alcohol or caffeine-containing beverages on the day of the test. The cardiologist decides whether the patient should stop taking any cardiac medications. Usually cardiovascular drugs such as beta blockers or calcium channel blockers are withheld on the day of the test to allow the heart rate to increase during the stress portion of the test. Patients are advised to wear comfortable, loose clothing and rubber-soled, supportive shoes. Remind them to tell the provider if symptoms such as chest pain, dizziness, shortness of breath, and an irregular heartbeat are experienced during the test.

Before the stress test, a resting 12-lead ECG, cardiovascular history, and physical examination are performed to check for any ECG abnormalities or medical factors that might interfere with the test. Check to see that all emergency supplies such as cardiac drugs, a defibrillator, and other necessary resuscitation equipment are available in the room in which the stress test is performed. It is important to be proficient in the use of resuscitation equipment when assisting the provider because chest pain, dysrhythmias, and other ECG changes may occur.

Procedure. The technician places electrodes on the patient's chest and attaches them to a multilead monitoring system. Note baseline blood pressure (BP), heart rate (HR), and respiratory rate. The two major modes of exercise available for stress testing are pedaling a bicycle ergometer and walking on a treadmill. A bicycle ergometer has a wheel operated by pedals that can be adjusted to increase the resistance to pedaling. The treadmill is a motorized device with an adjustable conveyor belt. It can reach speeds of 1 to 10 miles/hr and can also be adjusted from a flat position to a 22-degree incline.

After the patient is shown how to use the bicycle or walk on the treadmill, he or she begins to exercise. During the test, the BP and ECG are closely monitored as the resistance to cycling or the speed and incline of the treadmill are increased (Fig. 33-9). The patient exercises until one of these findings occurs:

- A predetermined HR is reached and maintained.
- Signs and symptoms such as chest pain, fatigue, extreme dyspnea, vertigo, hypotension, and ventricular dysrhythmias appear.
- Significant ST-segment depression or T-wave inversion occurs.
- The 20-minute protocol is completed.

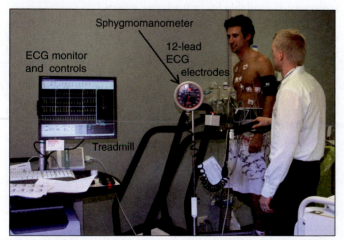

FIG. 33-9 Patient using a treadmill for a stress test. (From Baker, T., Nikolic, G., & O'Connor, S. (2008). *Practical cardiology,* (2nd ed.). Sydney: Churchill Livingstone Australia.)

Follow-Up Care. After the test, the nurse or other qualified health care team member monitors the ECG and BP until the patient has completely recovered. After recovery, he or she can return home if the test was performed on an ambulatory basis. Advise him or her to avoid a hot shower for 1 to 2 hours after the test because this may cause hypotension. If he or she does not recover but continues to have pain or ventricular dysrhythmias or appears medically unstable, admission to a telemetry unit for observation is needed.

For patients who cannot exercise because of conditions such as peripheral vascular disease or arthritis, pharmacologic stress testing with inotropes such as dobutamine and a vasodilator such as adenosine, dipyridamole, or regadenoson may be indicated. The nursing considerations are similar to those for the patient who has undergone an exercise ECG.

Echocardiography. As a noninvasive, risk-free test, echocardiography is easily performed at the bedside or on an ambulatory care basis. Echocardiography uses ultrasound waves to assess cardiac structure and mobility, particularly of the valves. It helps assess and diagnose cardiomyopathy, valvular disorders, pericardial effusion, left ventricular function, ventricular aneurysms, and cardiac tumors.

There is no special *preparation* for echocardiography. Inform the patient that the test is painless and takes 30 to 60 minutes to complete. The patient is instructed to lie quietly during the test and on his or her left side with the head elevated 15 to 20 degrees.

During an echocardiogram, a small transducer lubricated with gel to facilitate movement and conduction is placed on the patient's chest at the level of the third or fourth intercostal space near the left sternal border. The transducer transmits high-frequency sound waves and receives them as they are reflected from different structures. These echoes are usually videotaped simultaneously with the echocardiogram and can be recorded on graph paper for a permanent record.

After the images are taped, cardiac measurements that require several images can be obtained. Routine measurements include chamber size, ejection fraction, and flow gradient across the valves. There is no specific *follow-up care* for a patient who has undergone an echocardiogram.

A slightly more aggressive form of echocardiogram is a pharmacologic stress echocardiogram using either dobutamine or dipyridamole. This test is usually used when patients cannot tolerate exercise. Dobutamine (Dobutrex) increases the heart's contractility; dipyridamole (Persantine, Apo-Dipyridamole) is a coronary artery dilator. Patients are required to be NPO for 3 to 6 hours before the test, except for sips of water with medications. The technician ensures that IV access is present before the procedure and monitors BP and pulse continuously throughout the procedure. After the procedure, vital signs are monitored until BP returns to baseline and the pulse rate slows to less than 100 beats/min.

Transesophageal Echocardiography. Echocardiograms may also be performed transesophageally (through the esophagus). Transesophageal echocardiography (TEE) examines cardiac structure and function with an ultrasound transducer placed immediately behind the heart in the esophagus or stomach. The transducer provides especially detailed views of posterior cardiac structures such as the left atrium, mitral valve, and aortic arch. Preparation and follow-up are similar to that for an upper GI endoscopic examination (see Chapter 52).

Myocardial Nuclear Perfusion Imaging. The use of radionuclide techniques in cardiovascular assessment is called **myocardial nuclear perfusion imaging (MNPI)**. Cardiovascular abnormalities can be viewed, recorded, and evaluated using radioactive tracer substances. These studies are useful for detecting myocardial infarction (MI) and decreased myocardial blood flow and for evaluating left ventricular ejection. Conducting myocardial nuclear imaging tests, in conjunction with exercise or the administration of vasodilating agents, allows clearer identification of how the heart responds to stress.

Inform the patient that these tests are noninvasive. Because the amount of radioisotope is small, radiation exposure risks are minimal. If a dilating agent is to be used, advise the patient to avoid cigarettes and caffeinated food or drinks for 4 hours before administration of the vasodilator.

Common tests in nuclear cardiology include technetium (^{99m}Tc) pyrophosphate scanning, thallium imaging, and multigated cardiac blood pool imaging. Each test requires the injection of different types of radioactive isotopes into the antecubital vein. After the cells and tissues have time to take up the radioactive substances, usually 10 minutes to 2 hours, nuclear imaging can detect the difference between healthy and unhealthy tissue.

During the *technetium scan*, radioisotopes (^{99m}Tc pyrophosphate) accumulate in damaged myocardial tissue, which appears as a "hot spot" during the scan. This test helps detect the location and size of acute myocardial infarctions.

Alternatively, during the *thallium imaging scan*, necrotic or ischemic tissue does not absorb the radioisotope (thallium-201) and appears as "cold spots" on the scan. Thallium imaging is used to assess myocardial scarring and perfusion, to detect the location and extent of an acute or chronic myocardial infarction, to evaluate graft patency after coronary bypass surgery, and to evaluate antianginal therapy, thrombolytic therapy, or balloon angioplasty.

Thallium imaging may be performed during an exercise test or with the patient at rest. Thallium imaging performed during an exercise test may demonstrate perfusion deficits not apparent at rest. First the stress test procedure is performed. After the patient reaches maximum activity level, a small dose of thallium-201 is injected IV. The patient continues to exercise for about 1 to 2 minutes, after which the scanning is performed. Nuclear cardiologists often compare the resting and stress images to differentiate between fixed and reversible defects in the myocardium.

If a patient cannot exercise on a bike or treadmill, dipyridamole (Persantine, Apo-Dipyridamole) or dobutamine hydrochloride (Dobutrex) is administered to simulate the effects of exercise. Tell the patient that these vasodilators may cause flushing, headache, dyspnea, and chest tightness for a few moments after injection.

Cardiac blood pool imaging is a noninvasive test for evaluating cardiac motion and calculating ejection fraction. It uses a computer to synchronize the patient's ECG with pictures taken by a special camera. The technician attaches the patient to an ECG and injects a small amount of ^{99m}Tc IV. The radioisotope is not taken up by tissue but remains "tagged" to red blood cells in the circulation. The camera may take pictures of the radioactive material as it makes its first pass through the heart.

During **multigated blood pool scanning**, the computer breaks the time between R waves on the ECG into fractions of a second, called *gates*. The camera records blood flow through the heart during each of these gates. By analyzing the information from multiple gates, the computer can evaluate the ventricular wall motion and calculate ejection fraction (percentage of the left ventricular volume that is ejected with each contraction) and ejection velocity. Areas of decreased, absent, or paradoxical movement of the left ventricle may also be identified.

Positron emission tomography (PET) scans are used to compare cardiac perfusion and metabolic function and differentiate normal from diseased myocardium. The technician administers the first radioisotope (nitrogen-13-ammonia) and then begins a 20-minute scan to detect myocardial perfusion. Next the technician administers a second radioisotope (fluoro-18-deoxyglucose). After a pause, a second scan is performed to detect the metabolically active myocardium, which is using glucose.

The two scans are compared. In a normal heart, performance and metabolic function will match. In an ischemic heart, there will be a mismatch (i.e., a reduction in perfusion and increased glucose uptake by the ischemic myocardium). The scanning procedure takes 2 to 3 hours, and the patient may be asked to use a treadmill or exercise bicycle in conjunction with the scan.

Depending on which test is performed, the patient may report fatigue or discomfort at the antecubital injection site. If a stress test was paired with the study, he or she will need follow-up care for the stress test.

Computed Tomography Imaging. Cardiac computed tomography (CT) imaging is a noninvasive option to evaluate calcium formation in the coronary arteries. This modality requires a low resting heart rate as images are taken during end systole and mid-diastole. Beta blockers or calcium channel blockers may be given to assist with slowing the heart rate. Coronary artery calcium (CAC) calculation is often performed during the CT and may help identify patients at risk for coronary artery disease. To identify areas of stenosis, ionated contrast may be administered IV to visualize the coronary arteries. This is referred to as *CT angiography (CTA)*. Presence of coronary stents can make this test less reliable. Use of IV ionated contrast puts the patient at risk for contrast-induced nephropathy (CIN) or renal damage. Assess renal function before and after the test and ensure adequate hydration by administering IV fluids as ordered. Encourage oral fluids after testing.

Magnetic Resonance Imaging. Magnetic resonance imaging (MRI) is a noninvasive diagnostic option. An image of the heart or great vessels is produced through the interaction of magnetic fields, radio waves, and atomic nuclei showing hydrogen density. Simply put, the radio waves "bounce off" the body tissue being examined. Because each tissue has its own density, the computer image clearly differentiates between various types of tissues. MRI permits determination of cardiac wall thickness, chamber dilation, valve and ventricular function, and blood movement in the great vessels. Improved MRI techniques allow coronary artery blood flow to be mapped with nearly the accuracy of a cardiac catheterization.

Before an MRI, ensure that the patient has removed all metallic objects, including watches, jewelry, clothing with metal fasteners, and hair clips. Patients with pacemakers or implanted defibrillators may not be able to have an MRI because the magnetic fields can deactivate them. However, some newer MRI machines have eliminated this complication. A few patients may experience claustrophobia during the 15 to 60 minutes required to complete the scan.

GET READY FOR THE NCLEX® EXAMINATION!

KEY POINTS

Review these Key Points for each NCLEX Examination Client Needs Category.

Safe and Effective Care Environment

- Assess patients for allergy to iodine-based contrast media before having invasive diagnostic tests requiring an iodine-based contrast agent. **QSEN: Safety**
- After invasive cardiovascular diagnostic testing, such as angiography and cardiac catheterization, monitor the insertion site for bleeding and hematoma formation. **QSEN: Safety**
- Assess vital signs carefully in patients having invasive cardiovascular testing; report and document any new dysrhythmias after testing. **QSEN: Informatics**

Health Promotion and Maintenance

- Identify patients at risk for cardiovascular disease, especially those with hyperlipidemia, hypertension, excess weight, physical inactivity, smoking, psychological stress, a positive family history, and diabetes. **QSEN: Evidence-Based Practice**
- Teach patients how to reduce the risk for heart disease through modifiable factors such as exercise, diet modification, smoking cessation, and medications, as needed. **QSEN: Patient-Centered Care**
- Inform patients that genetics and other nonmodifiable risk factors, such as family history and gender, contribute to the development of coronary artery disease (CAD). **QSEN: Evidence-Based Practice**
- Assess the older adult for cardiovascular changes associated with aging as described in Chart 33-1. **QSEN: Safety**

Psychosocial Integrity

- Discuss with the patient any feelings or concerns that he or she might have about the stress of cardiac illness, diagnostic testing, or other issues and use therapeutic measures to decrease anxiety. **QSEN: Patient-Centered Care**
- Recognize that denial is a common and normal response to help patients cope with threatening circumstances. **QSEN: Patient-Centered Care**

- Be aware that coping behaviors of those who have cardiovascular problems vary from patient to patient. **QSEN: Patient-Centered Care**
- Allow the patient to express feelings about an actual or perceived loss of health or social status related to cardiovascular disease. **QSEN: Patient-Centered Care**

Physiological Integrity

- Be aware of the importance of recalling the anatomy and physiology of the cardiovascular (CV) system to best understand how to care for patients with CV health problems. **Clinical Judgment**
- Assess the patient's report of pain to differentiate the pain of angina and myocardial infarction (MI) from other noncardiac causes; *discomfort, indigestion, squeezing, heaviness,* and *viselike* are common terms used to describe chest pain of cardiac origin. **Clinical Judgment**
- Be aware that gender differences in CVD exist; with women often experiencing more vague symptoms such as fatigue, indigestion, and shortness of breath. **Health Care Disparities**
- Recall that syncope is a transient loss of consciousness and is common in older adults.
- Be aware that the veteran population has increased risk for development of cardiovascular disease. **Health Care Disparities**
- Assess for bruits, which are swishing sounds that develop in narrowed arteries. **QSEN: Patient-Centered Care**
- Auscultate the heart for normal first and second sounds and for abnormalities such as an S_3, S_4, murmur, or gallop. **QSEN: Patient-Centered Care**
- Monitor serum markers of myocardial damage and other cardiac-related laboratory tests as listed in Chart 33-2. **QSEN: Patient-Centered Care**
- Prepare patients having a cardiac catheterization for expectations of the procedure and postprocedure care. **QSEN: Patient-Centered Care**
- Assess patients having cardiac catheterizations for potential complications as listed in Table 33-5. **QSEN: Safety**
- Include all relevant findings of the patient's CV assessment in the electronic health record. **QSEN: Informatics**

SELECTED BIBLIOGRAPHY

Asterisk indicates a classic or definitive work on this subject.

*Aboyans, V., Criqui, M., Abraham, P., Allison, M., Creager, M., Diehm, C., et al. (2012). Measurement and interpretation of the ankle-brachial index: A scientific statement from the American Heart Association. *Circulation, 126,* 2890–2909.

American Heart Association (AHA). (2015a). *Diet and lifestyle recommendations* (updated August 12, 2015). www.heart.org/HEARTORG/GettingHealthy/Diet-and-Lifestyle-Recommendations_UCM_305855_Article.jsp.

American Heart Association. (2015b). *Statistical Fact Sheet.* 2015 Update. https://www.heart.org/idc/groups/heart-public/@wcm/@sop/@smd/documents/downloadable/ucm_462014.pdf.

Amsterdam, E. A., Wenger, N. K., Brindis, R. G., Casey, D. E., Ganiats, T. G., Holmes, D. R., et al. (2014). AHA/ACCC guideline for the management of patients with non-ST-elevation acute coronary syndrome: A report of the American college of cardiology/American heart association task force on practice guidelines. *Journal of the American College of Cardiology, 64,* e139–e228.

Assari, S. (2014). Veterans and risk of heart disease in the United States: A cohort with 20 years of follow up. *International Journal of Preventative Medicine., 5*(6), 703–709.

*Bashore, T., Balter, S., Barac, A., Byrne, J., Cavendish, J., Chambers, C., et al. (2012). 2012 American College of Cardiology Foundation/Society for Cardiovascular Angiography and Interventions expert consensus document on cardiac catheterization laboratory standards update. *Journal of the American College of Cardiology, 59*(24), 2221–2305.

Froedge, W. (2015). Coronary artery disease in women. *Nursing 2015 Critical Care, 10*(3), 17–20. doi:10.1097/01.CCN.0000464302 .64634.9d.

Hannibal, G. (2013). Interpretation of serum troponin elevation. *AACN Advanced Critical Care, 24*(2), 224–228.

James, P. A., Oparil, S., Carter, B. L., Cushman, W. C., Dennison-Himmelfarb, C., Handler, J., et al. (2014). 2014 evidence-based guidelines for the management of high blood pressure in adults: Report from the panel members appointed to the Eighth Joint National Committee (JNC 8). *The Journal of the American Medical Association, 311*(5), 507–520.

Jaffe, A., & Morrow, D. (2015). *Troponins as biomarkers of cardiac injury.* https://www.uptodate.com/contents/troponin-testing -clinical-use.

King, J., & Magdic, K. (2014). Chest pain: A time for concern? *AACN Advanced Critical Care, 25*(3), 279–283.

*Landgraf, J., Wishner, S. H., & Kloner, R. A. (2010). Comparison of automatic oscillometric versus auscultatory blood pressure measurement. *American Journal of Cardiology, 106*(3), 386–388.

McCance, K., Huether, S., Brashers, V., & Rote, N. (2014). *Pathophysiology: The biologic basis for disease in adults and children* (7th ed.). St. Louis: Mosby.

Mozaffarian, D., Benjamin, E., Go, A., Arnett, D., Blaha, M., Cushman, M., et al. (2016). Heart disease and stroke statistics—2016 update. *Circulation, 131.* doi:10.1161/CIR0000000000000152.

Pagana, K., Pagana, T., & Pagana, T. (2017). *Mosby's diagnostic and laboratory test reference* (13th ed.). St. Louis: Elsevier.

Ramos, L. (2014). Cardiac diagnostic testing: What bedside nurses need to know. *Critical Care Nurse, 34*(3), 16–28.

Roberts, R. (2014). Genetics of coronary artery disease. *Circulation Research, 114*, 1890–1903.

Tebaldi, M., Campo, G., & Biscaglia, S. (2015). Fractional flow reserve: Current applications and overview of the available data. *World Journal of Clinical Cases, 3*(8), 678–681.

*The New York Heart Association. (1964). *Diseases of the heart and blood vessels: Nomenclature and criteria for diagnosis* (6th ed.). Boston: Little, Brown.

Wray, W. (2014). Preventing cardiovascular disease in women. *Canadian Nurse, 110*(3), 24–29. https://www.canadian-nurse.com/en/ articles/issues/2014/april-2014/preventing-cardiovascular-disease -in-women.

Care of Patients With Dysrhythmias

Laura M. Dechant and Nicole M. Heimgartner

ⓔ http://evolve.elsevier.com/Iggy/

PRIORITY AND INTERRELATED CONCEPTS

The priority concept for this chapter is PERFUSION.

✳ The PERFUSION concept exemplar for this chapter is Atrial Fibrillation, p. 678.

The interrelated concepts for this chapter are:
- FLUID AND ELECTROLYTE BALANCE
- CLOTTING

LEARNING OUTCOMES

Safe and Effective Care Environment

1. Collaborate with the interprofessional team to coordinate high-quality care to promote PERFUSION in patients with dysrhythmias.
2. Provide a safe environment for patients and staff when using a cardiac defibrillator.

Health Promotion and Maintenance

3. Teach the patient and caregiver(s) about drug therapy used for common dysrhythmias.
4. Teach the patient with a pacemaker or implantable cardioverter/defibrillator about self-management when in the community.

Psychosocial Integrity

5. Implement patient and family-centered nursing interventions to decrease the psychosocial impact caused by life-threatening dysrhythmias and emergency care procedures.

Physiological Integrity

6. Apply knowledge of pathophysiology to assess patients with common dysrhythmias.
7. Analyze an ECG rhythm strip to identify normal sinus rhythm and common or life-threatening dysrhythmias.
8. Use clinical judgment to plan care coordination and transition management for patients experiencing common dysrhythmias.
9. Plan evidence-based nursing care to promote PERFUSION to prevent complications in patients experiencing dysrhythmias.
10. Explain the need to perform evidence-based emergency care procedures, such as cardiopulmonary resuscitation (CPR) and automated external defibrillation.

The heart is an intricate pump that works to perfuse the body. When the heart does not work effectively as a pump, PERFUSION to vital organs and peripheral tissues can be impaired, resulting in organ dysfunction or failure. Cardiac dysrhythmias are abnormal rhythms of the heart's electrical system that can affect its ability to effectively pump *oxygenated* blood throughout the body. Some dysrhythmias are life threatening, and others are not. They are the result of disturbances in cardiac electrical impulse formation, conduction, or both.

Many health problems, especially coronary artery disease (CAD), electrolyte imbalances, impaired gas exchange, and drug toxicity (both legal and illicit drugs), can cause abnormal heart rhythms. Dysrhythmias can occur in people of any age but occur most often in older adults. To provide collaborative patient-centered care using best practices, a *basic* understanding of cardiac electrophysiology, the conduction system of the heart, and the principles of electrocardiography is needed as a medical-surgical nurse. Specialty nurses and advanced practice nurses have a more in-depth knowledge because they manage patients with these cardiac problems in critical care and ambulatory care settings.

REVIEW OF CARDIAC CONDUCTION SYSTEM

Conduction begins with the sinoatrial (SA) node (also called the *sinus node*), located close to the surface of the right atrium near its junction with the superior vena cava. *The SA node is the heart's primary pacemaker.* It can spontaneously and rhythmically generate electrical impulses at a rate of 60 to 100 beats/min and therefore has the greatest degree of automaticity (pacing function). The SA node is richly supplied by the sympathetic and parasympathetic nervous systems, which increase and decrease the rate of discharge of the sinus node, respectively. This process results in changes in the heart rate.

Impulses from the sinus node move directly through atrial muscle and lead to atrial depolarization, which is *reflected in a P wave on the electrocardiogram (ECG)*. Atrial muscle contraction should follow. Within the atrial muscle are slow and fast conduction pathways leading to the atrioventricular (AV) node.

The **atrioventricular (AV) junctional** area consists of a transitional cell zone, the AV node itself, and the bundle of His. The AV node lies just beneath the right atrial endocardium, between the tricuspid valve and the ostium of the coronary sinus. Here T-cells (transitional cells) cause impulses to slow down or be delayed in the AV node before proceeding to the ventricles. This delay is reflected in the *PR segment* on the ECG. This slow conduction provides a short delay, allowing the atria to contract and the ventricles to fill. The contraction is known as *atrial kick* and contributes additional blood volume for a greater cardiac output. The AV node is also controlled by both the sympathetic and the parasympathetic nervous systems. The bundle of His connects with the distal portion of the AV node and continues through the interventricular septum.

The *bundle of His* extends as a right bundle branch down the right side of the interventricular septum to the apex of the right ventricle. On the left side, it extends as a left bundle branch, which further divides.

At the ends of both the right and the left bundle branch systems are the Purkinje fibers. These fibers are an interweaving network located on the endocardial surface of both ventricles, from apex to base. The fibers then partially penetrate into the myocardium. **Purkinje cells** make up the bundle of His, bundle branches, and terminal Purkinje fibers. These cells are responsible for the rapid conduction of electrical impulses throughout the ventricles, leading to ventricular depolarization and the subsequent ventricular muscle contraction. A few nodal cells in the ventricles also occasionally demonstrate automaticity, giving rise to ventricular beats or rhythms.

The cardiac conduction system consists of specialized myocardial cells (Fig. 34-1). The electrophysiologic properties of these cells regulate heart rate and rhythm and possess unique properties: automaticity, excitability, conductivity, and contractility.

Automaticity (pacing function) is the ability of cardiac cells to generate an electrical impulse spontaneously and repetitively. Normally only the sinoatrial (SA) node can generate an electrical impulse. However, under certain conditions, such as myocardial ischemia (decreased blood flow), electrolyte imbalance, hypoxia, drug toxicity, and infarction (cell death), any cardiac cell may produce electrical impulses independently and create dysrhythmias. Disturbances in automaticity may involve either an increase or a decrease in pacing function.

Excitability is the ability of nonpacemaker heart cells to respond to an electrical impulse that begins in pacemaker cells. **Depolarization** occurs when the normally negatively charged cells within the heart muscle develop a positive charge.

Conductivity is the ability to send an electrical stimulus from cell membrane to cell membrane. As a result, excitable cells depolarize in rapid succession from cell to cell until all cells have depolarized. The wave of depolarization causes the deflections in the ECG waveforms that are recognized as the P wave and the QRS complex. Disturbances in conduction result when conduction is too rapid or too slow, when the pathway is totally blocked, or when the electrical impulse travels an abnormal pathway.

Contractility is the ability of atrial and ventricular muscle cells to shorten their fiber length in response to electrical stimulation, causing sufficient pressure to push blood forward through the heart. In other words, *contractility is the mechanical activity of the heart.*

ELECTROCARDIOGRAPHY

The **electrocardiogram (ECG)** provides a graphic representation, or picture, of cardiac electrical activity. The cardiac electrical currents are transmitted to the body surface. Electrodes, consisting of a conductive gel on an adhesive pad, are placed on specific sites on the body and attached to cables connected to an ECG machine or to a monitor. The cardiac electrical current

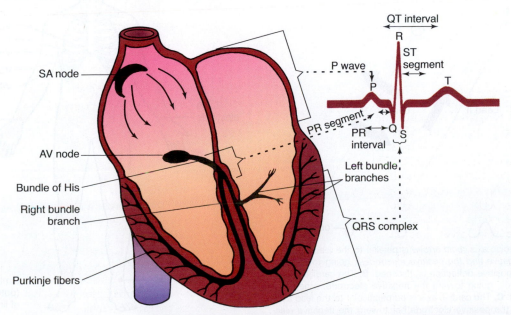

FIG. 34-1 The cardiac conduction system.

is transmitted via the electrodes and through the lead wires to the machine or monitor, which displays the cardiac electrical activity. A **lead** provides one view of the heart's electrical activity. Multiple leads, or views, can be obtained. Electrode placement is the same for male and female patients.

Lead systems are made up of a positive pole and a negative pole. An imaginary line joining these two poles is called the **lead axis**. The direction of electrical current flow in the heart is the **cardiac axis**. The relationship between the cardiac axis and the lead axis is responsible for the deflections seen on the ECG pattern:

- The baseline is the **isoelectric** line. It occurs when there is no current flow in the heart after complete depolarization and also after complete repolarization. Positive deflections occur above this line, and negative deflections occur below it. Deflections represent depolarization and repolarization of cells.
- If the direction of electrical current flow in the heart (cardiac axis) is toward the positive pole, a **positive deflection** (above the baseline) is viewed (Fig. 34-2A).
- If the direction of electrical current flow in the heart (cardiac axis) is moving away from the positive pole toward the negative pole, a **negative deflection** (below the baseline) is viewed (Fig. 34-2B).
- If the cardiac axis is moving neither toward nor away from the positive pole, a biphasic complex (both above and below baseline) will result (Fig. 34-2C).

Lead Systems

The standard 12-lead ECG consists of 12 leads (or views) of the heart's electrical activity. Six of the leads are called *limb leads* because the electrodes are placed on the four extremities in the frontal plane. The remaining six leads are called *chest (precordial) leads* because the electrodes are placed on the chest in the horizontal plane.

Standard bipolar *limb leads* consist of three leads (I, II, and III) that each measure the electrical activity between two points and a fourth lead (right leg) that acts as a ground electrode. Of the three measuring leads, the right arm is always negative, the left leg is always positive, and the left arm can be either positive or negative.

Other lead systems include the 18-lead ECG, which adds six leads placed on the horizontal plane on the right side of the chest to view the right side of the heart. This is sometimes referred to as a *right-sided ECG*. The extra leads are sometimes placed on the back. Unipolar limb leads consist of a positive electrode only. The unipolar limb leads are aVR, aVL, and aVF, with *a* meaning augmented; *V* is a designation for a unipolar lead. The third letter denotes the positive electrode placement: *R* for right arm, *L* for left arm, and *F* for foot (left leg). The positive electrode is at one end of the lead axis. The other end is the center of the electrical field, at about the center of the heart.

There are six unipolar (or V) *chest leads,* determined by the placement of the chest electrode. The four limb electrodes are placed on the extremities, as designated on each electrode (right arm, left arm, right leg, and left leg). The fifth (chest) electrode on a monitor system is the positive, or exploring, electrode and is placed in one of six designated positions to obtain the desired chest lead. With a 12-lead ECG, four leads are placed on the limbs, and six are placed on the chest, eliminating the need to move any electrodes about the chest (Fig. 34-3).

Positioning of the electrodes is crucial in obtaining an accurate ECG. Comparisons of ECGs taken at different times will be valid only when electrode placement is accurate and identical at each test. Positioning is particularly important when working with patients with chest deformities or large breasts. Patients may be asked to move the breasts to ensure proper electrode placement. For serial ECGs, a surgical marker may be used to mark the electrode placement site to allow for accurate placement. It is important to remove the electrodes following the ECG because skin breakdown can occur.

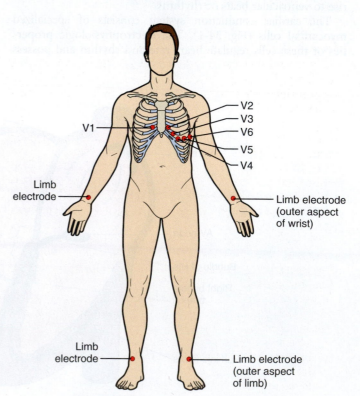

FIG. 34-2 A, The cardiac axis *(bold arrow)* is parallel to the lead axis *(the line between the negative and the positive electrodes),* going toward the positive electrode; a positive deflection is inscribed. **B,** The cardiac axis is parallel to the lead axis, going toward the negative electrode; a negative deflection is inscribed. **C,** The cardiac axis is perpendicular to the lead axis, going neither toward the positive electrode nor toward the negative electrode; a biphasic deflection is inscribed.

FIG. 34-3 Electrode positions for 12-lead ECG.

While obtaining a 12-lead ECG, remind the patient to be as still as possible in a semi-reclined position, breathing normally. Any repetitive movement will cause artifact and could lead to inaccurate interpretation of the ECG.

Nurses are sometimes responsible for obtaining 12-lead ECGs; but more commonly, technicians are trained to perform this skill. Remind the technician to notify the nurse or physician of any suspected abnormality. A nurse may direct a technician to take a 12-lead ECG on a patient experiencing chest pain to observe for diagnostic changes, but it is ultimately the primary health care provider's responsibility to definitively interpret the ECG.

Continuous Electrocardiographic Monitoring

For continuous ECG monitoring, the electrodes are not placed on the limbs because movement of the extremities causes "noise," or motion artifact, on the ECG signal. Place the electrodes on the trunk, a more stable area, to minimize such artifacts and to obtain a clearer signal. If the monitoring system provides five electrode cables, place the electrodes as follows:

- Right arm electrode just below the right clavicle
- Left arm electrode just below the left clavicle
- Right leg electrode on the lowest palpable rib, on the right midclavicular line
- Left leg electrode on the lowest palpable rib, on the left midclavicular line
- Fifth electrode placed to obtain one of the six chest leads

With this placement, the monitor lead-select control may be changed to provide lead I, II, III, aVR, aVL, aVF, or one chest lead. The monitor automatically alters the polarity of the electrodes to provide the lead selected.

The clarity of continuous ECG monitor recordings is affected by skin preparation and electrode quality. To ensure the best signal transmission and decrease skin impedance, clean the skin and clip hairs if needed. Make sure that the area for electrode placement is dry. The gel on each electrode must be moist and fresh. Attach the electrode to the lead cable and then to the contact site. The contact site should be free of any lotion, tincture, or other substance that increases skin impedance. Electrodes cannot be placed on irritated skin or over scar tissue. Electrodes may be applied by unlicensed assistive personnel (UAP), but the nurse determines which lead to select and checks for correct electrode placement. Assess the quality of the ECG rhythm transmission to the monitoring system.

The ECG cables can be attached directly to a wall-mounted monitor (a hard-wired system) if the patient's activity is restricted to bedrest and sitting in a chair, as in a critical care unit. For an ambulatory patient, the ECG cable is attached to a battery-operated transmitter (a **telemetry** system) held in a pouch. The ECG is transmitted to a remote monitor via antennae located in strategic places, usually in the ceiling. Telemetry allows freedom of movement within a certain area without losing transmission of the ECG.

Most acute care facilities have monitor technicians (monitor "techs") who are educated in ECG rhythm interpretation and are responsible for:

- Watching a bank of monitors on a unit
- Printing ECG rhythm strips routinely and as needed
- Interpreting rhythms
- Reporting the patient's rhythm and significant changes to the nurse

The technical support is particularly helpful on a telemetry unit that does not have monitors at the bedside. The nurse is responsible for accurate patient assessment and management.

Some units have full-disclosure monitors, which continuously store ECG rhythms in memory up to a certain amount of time. This system allows nurses and health care providers to access and print rhythm strips for more thorough patient assessment. Routine strips and any changes in rhythm are printed and documented in the patient's record.

The health care provider is responsible for determining when monitoring can be suspended, such as during showering. He or she also determines whether monitoring is needed during off-unit testing procedures and for transportation to other facilities. Clinical alarms, such as those associated with continuous ECG monitoring, have been identified as one of the top ten technology hazards. The Joint Commission has responded to this hazard with a National Patient Safety Goal to improve the safety of clinical alarms. As part of implementation, hospitals are asked to implement specific policy and procedure regarding clinical alarm safety. Lukasewicz & Mattox (2015) suggest that the best method for reduction of alarm hazards is through proactive alarm management. *Think carefully before suspending an alarm or adjusting alarm parameters* and be informed regarding organizational policy regarding alarm management. (See the Quality Improvement box for proactive alarm management.)

Prehospital personnel, such as paramedics and emergency medical technicians (EMTs) with advanced training, frequently monitor ECG rhythms at the scene and on the way to a health care facility. They function under medical direction and protocols but may also be communicating with a nurse in the emergency department.

The ECG strip is printed on graph paper (Fig. 34-4), with each small block measuring 1 mm in height and width. ECG recorders and monitors are standardized at a speed of 25 mm/sec. Time is measured on the horizontal axis. At this speed, each small block represents 0.04 second. Five small blocks make up one large block, defined by darker bold lines and representing 0.20 second. Five large blocks represent 1 second, and 30 large blocks represent 6 seconds. Vertical lines in the top margin of the graph paper are usually 15 large blocks apart, representing 3-second segments (Fig. 34-5).

Electrocardiographic Complexes, Segments, and Intervals

Complexes that make up a normal ECG consist of a P wave, a QRS complex, a T wave, and possibly a U wave. Segments include the PR segment, the ST segment, and the TP segment. Intervals include the PR interval, the QRS duration, and the QT interval (Fig. 34-6).

The **P wave** is a deflection representing atrial depolarization. The shape of the P wave may be a positive, negative, or biphasic (both positive and negative) deflection, depending on the lead selected. When the electrical impulse is consistently generated from the sinoatrial (SA) node, the P waves have a consistent shape in a given lead. If an impulse is then generated from a different (ectopic) focus, such as atrial tissue, the shape of the P wave changes in that lead, indicating that an ectopic focus has fired.

The **PR segment** is the isoelectric line from the end of the P wave to the beginning of the QRS complex, when the electrical impulse is traveling through the atrioventricular (AV) node,

QUALITY IMPROVEMENT (QSEN)

Proper Skin Preparation and Electrode Placement to Decrease Clinical Alarms

Walsh-Irwin, C., & Jurgens, C. (2015). Proper skin preparation and electrode placement decreases alarms on a telemetry unit. *Dimensions of Critical Care Nursing. 34*(3). doi: 10.1097.

For patients who have cardiovascular disease, electrocardiogram (ECG) monitoring is common practice and an integral part of safe care within the hospital setting. However, with ECG monitoring comes the responsibility of alarm management. Walsh-Irwin & Jurgens (2015) estimate that 85% to 99% of ECG alarms are false. Repeated response leads to alarm fatigue, which is the desensitization of nurses to clinical alarms as a result of an overload of alarms. Alarm fatigue has resulted in sentinel events creating national concern. Current studies indicate that nurses do not properly prepare the skin for electrode placement before monitoring.

As a result of existing research, a quality improvement project was initiated at Veterans' Hospital to test the effect of proper skin preparation and ECG electrode placement on the number of alarms on a telemetry unit. This study was an application of current evidence on a standard of care. Telemetry alarms were measured for 24 hours.

Following the baseline assessment, electrodes were replaced using proper skin preparation. The following steps were used: (1) clip hair; (2) wash skin with soap and water; (3) dry skin with washcloth; (4) attach electrodes to leads; and (5) place electrodes in correct anatomical position. Following the change in electrodes, alarms were monitored again for a 24-hour period with mean results showing a 44% decrease in alarms.

Commentary: Implications for Practice and Research

The Joint Commission's (TJC's) National Patient Safety Goal specific to alarm management requires alarm management strategies. These strategies include educating staff about alarms and developing policy and procedure for alarm management. This quality improvement study provides additional evidence that proper skin preparation and correct electrode placement will decrease clinical alarms. In addition, this project clearly demonstrates implementation of TJC's National Patient Safety Goal. Although these steps may take additional time, the safety benefits are clear. Additional research to address parameters for alarms is needed to determine best practice.

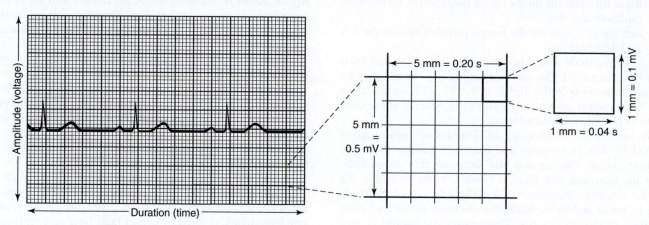

FIG. 34-4 Electrocardiographic waveforms are measured in amplitude (voltage) and duration (time).

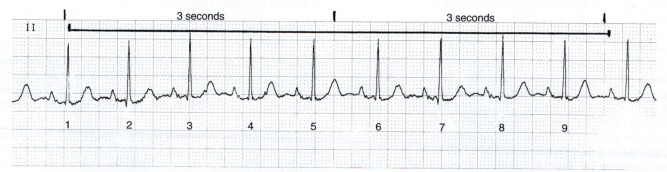

FIG. 34-5 Each segment between the dark lines *(above the monitor strip)* represents 3 seconds when the monitor is set at a speed of 25 mm per second. To estimate the ventricular rate, count the QRS complexes in a 6-second strip and multiply that number by 10 to estimate the rate for 1 minute. In this example, there are 9 QRS complexes in 6 seconds. Therefore the heart rate can be estimated to be 90 beats/min.

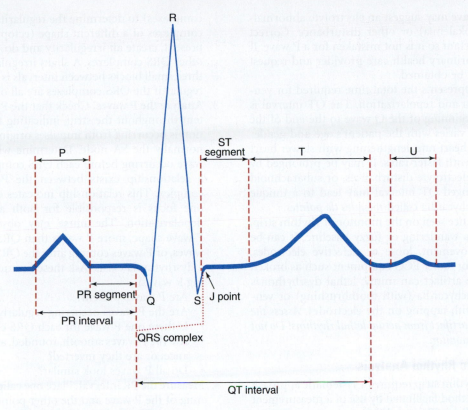

FIG. 34-6 The components of a normal electrocardiogram.

P wave:	Represents atrial depolarization.
PR segment:	Represents the time required for the impulse to travel through the AV node, where it is delayed, and through the bundle of His, bundle branches, and Purkinje fiber network, just before ventricular depolarization.
PR interval:	Represents the time required for atrial depolarization as well as impulse travel through the conduction system and Purkinje fiber network, inclusive of the P wave and PR segment. It is measured from the beginning of the P wave to the end of the PR segment.
QRS complex:	Represents ventricular depolarization and is measured from the beginning of the Q (or R) wave to the end of the S wave.
J point:	Represents the junction where the QRS complex ends and the ST segment begins.
ST segment:	Represents early ventricular repolarization.
T wave:	Represents ventricular repolarization.
U wave:	Represents late ventricular repolarization.
QT interval:	Represents the total time required for ventricular depolarization and repolarization and is measured from the beginning of the QRS complex to the end of the T wave.

where it is delayed. It then travels through the ventricular conduction system to the Purkinje fibers.

The **PR interval** is measured from the beginning of the P wave to the end of the PR segment. It represents the time required for atrial depolarization, the impulse delay in the AV node, and the travel time to the Purkinje fibers. It normally measures from 0.12 to 0.20 second (five small blocks).

The **QRS complex** represents ventricular depolarization. The shape of the QRS complex depends on the lead selected. The Q wave is the first negative deflection and is not present in all leads. When present, it is small and represents initial ventricular septal depolarization. When the Q wave is abnormally present in a lead, it represents myocardial necrosis (cell death). The R wave is the first positive deflection. It may be small, large, or absent, depending on the lead. The S wave is a negative deflection following the R wave and is not present in all leads.

The **QRS duration** represents the time required for depolarization of both ventricles. It is measured from the beginning of

the QRS complex to the J point (the junction where the QRS complex ends and the ST segment begins). It normally measures from 0.04 to 0.12 second (up to three small blocks).

The **ST segment** is normally an isoelectric line and represents early ventricular repolarization. It occurs from the J point to the beginning of the T wave. Its length varies with changes in the heart rate, the administration of medications, and electrolyte disturbances.

The **T wave** follows the ST segment and represents ventricular repolarization. It is usually positive, rounded, and slightly asymmetric. T waves may become tall and peaked; inverted (negative); or flat as a result of myocardial ischemia, potassium or calcium imbalances, medications, or autonomic nervous system effects.

The **U wave,** when present, follows the T wave and may result from slow repolarization of ventricular Purkinje fibers. It is of the same polarity as the T wave, although generally it is smaller. It is not normally seen in all leads and is more common in lead

V₃. An abnormal U wave may suggest an electrolyte abnormality (particularly hypokalemia) or other disturbance. Correct identification is important so it is not mistaken for a P wave. If in doubt, notify the primary health care provider and request that a potassium level be obtained.

The QT interval represents the total time required for ventricular depolarization and repolarization. The QT interval is measured from the beginning of the Q wave to the end of the T wave. This interval varies with the patient's age and gender and changes with the heart rate, lengthening with slower heart rates and shortening with faster rates. It may be prolonged by certain medications, electrolyte disturbances, or subarachnoid hemorrhage. A prolonged QT interval may lead to a unique type of ventricular tachycardia called *torsades de pointes*.

Artifact is interference seen on the monitor or rhythm strip, which may look like a wandering or fuzzy baseline. It can be caused by patient movement, loose or defective electrodes, improper grounding, or faulty ECG equipment such as broken wires or cables. Some artifact can mimic lethal dysrhythmias such as ventricular tachycardia (with toothbrushing) or ventricular fibrillation (with tapping on the electrode). *Assess the patient to differentiate artifact from actual lethal rhythms! Do not rely only on the ECG monitor.*

Electrocardiographic Rhythm Analysis

Analysis of an ECG rhythm strip requires a systematic approach using an eight-step method facilitated by use of a measurement tool called an ECG caliper (Palmer, 2011):

1. **Determine the heart rate.** The most common method is to count the number of QRS complexes in 6 seconds and multiply that number by 10 to calculate the rate for a full minute. This is called the *6-second strip method* and is a quick method to determine the mean or *average* heart rate. Normal heart rates fall between 60 and 100 beats/min. A rate less than 60 beats/min is called bradycardia. A rate greater than 100 beats/min is called tachycardia. Current monitoring systems will display a continuous heart rate and print it on the ECG strip. *Use caution and confirm that the rate is correct by assessing the patient's heart rate directly.* Many factors can incorrectly alter the rate displayed by the monitor.

2. **Determine the heart rhythm.** Assess for atrial and/or ventricular regularity. Heart rhythms can be either regular or irregular. Irregular rhythms can be regularly irregular, occasionally irregular, or irregularly irregular. Check the regularity of the atrial rhythm by assessing the PP intervals, placing one caliper point on a P wave and the other point on the precise spot on the next P wave. Then move the caliper from P wave to P wave along the entire strip ("walking out" the P waves) to determine the regularity of the rhythm. P waves of a different shape (ectopic waves), if present, create an irregularity and do not walk out with the other P waves. A slight irregularity in the PP intervals, varying no more than three small blocks, is considered essentially regular if the P waves are all of the same shape. This alteration is caused by changes in intrathoracic pressure during the respiratory cycle.

   Check the regularity of the ventricular rhythm by assessing the RR intervals, placing one caliper point on a portion of the QRS complex (usually the most prominent portion of the deflection) and the other point on the precise spot of the next QRS complex. Move the caliper from QRS complex to QRS complex along the entire strip (walking out the QRS

complexes) to determine the regularity of the rhythm. QRS complexes of a different shape (ectopic QRS complexes), if present, create an irregularity and do not walk out with the other QRS complexes. A slight irregularity of no more than three small blocks between intervals is considered essentially regular if the QRS complexes are all of the same shape.

3. **Analyze the P waves.** Check that the P-wave shape is consistent throughout the strip, indicating that atrial depolarization is occurring from impulses originating from one focus, normally the SA node. Determine whether there is one P wave occurring before each QRS complex, establishing that a relationship exists between the P wave and the QRS complex. This relationship indicates that an impulse from one focus is responsible for both atrial and ventricular depolarization. The nurse may observe more than one P-wave shape, more P waves than QRS complexes, absent P waves, or P waves coming after the QRS, each indicating that a dysrhythmia exists. Ask these five questions when analyzing P waves:
   - Are P waves present?
   - Are the P waves occurring regularly?
   - Is there one P wave for each QRS complex?
   - Are the P waves smooth, rounded, and upright in appearance; or are they inverted?
   - Do all P waves look similar?

4. **Measure the PR interval.** Place one caliper point at the beginning of the P wave and the other point at the end of the PR segment. The PR interval normally measures between 0.12 and 0.20 second. The measurement should be constant throughout the strip. The PR interval cannot be determined if there are no P waves or if P waves occur after the QRS complex. Ask these three questions about the PR interval:
   - Are PR intervals greater than 0.20 second?
   - Are PR intervals less than 0.12 second?
   - Are PR intervals constant across the ECG strip?

5. **Measure the QRS duration.** Place one caliper point at the beginning of the QRS complex and the other at the J point, where the QRS complex ends and the ST segment begins. The QRS duration normally measures between 0.04 and 0.10 second. The measurement should be constant throughout the entire strip. Check that the QRS complexes are consistent throughout the strip. When the QRS is narrow (0.10 second or less), it indicates that the impulse was not formed in the ventricles and is referred to as *supraventricular* or *above the ventricles*. When the QRS complex is wide (greater than 0.10 second), it indicates that the impulse is either of ventricular origin or of supraventricular origin with aberrant conduction, meaning deviating from the normal course or pattern. More than one QRS complex pattern or occasionally missing QRS complexes may be observed, indicating a dysrhythmia. Ask these questions to evaluate QRS intervals:
   - Are QRS intervals less than or greater than 0.12 second?
   - Are the QRS complexes similar in appearance across the ECG paper?

6. **Examine the ST segment.** The normal ST segment begins at the isoelectric line. ST elevation or depression is significant if displacement is 1 mm (one small box) or more above or below the line and is seen in two or more leads. ST *elevation* may indicate problems such as myocardial infarction, pericarditis, and hyperkalemia. ST *depression* is associated with hypokalemia, myocardial infarction, or ventricular hypertrophy.

7. **Assess the T wave.** Note the shape and height of the T wave for peaking or inversion. Abnormal T waves may indicate problems such as myocardial infarction and ventricular hypertrophy.

8. **Measure the QT interval.** A normal QT interval should be equal to or less than one-half the distance of the RR interval.

Using steps 1 through 8, you can interpret the cardiac rhythm and differentiate normal and abnormal cardiac rhythms (dysrhythmias).

OVERVIEW OF NORMAL CARDIAC RHYTHMS

Normal sinus rhythm (NSR) is the rhythm originating from the sinoatrial (SA) node (dominant pacemaker) that meets these ECG criteria (Fig. 34-7):

- *Rate:* Atrial and ventricular rates of 60 to 100 beats/min
- *Rhythm:* Atrial and ventricular rhythms regular
- *P waves:* Present, consistent configuration, one P wave before each QRS complex
- *PR interval:* 0.12 to 0.20 second and constant
- *QRS duration:* 0.04 to 0.10 second and constant

Sinus arrhythmia is a variant of NSR. It results from changes in intrathoracic pressure during breathing. In this context, the term *arrhythmia* does not mean an absence of rhythm, as the term suggests. Instead, the heart rate increases slightly during inspiration and decreases slightly during exhalation. This irregular rhythm is frequently observed in healthy adults.

Sinus arrhythmia has all the characteristics of NSR except for its irregularity. The PP and RR intervals vary, with the difference between the shortest and the longest intervals being greater than 0.12 second (three small blocks):

- *Rate:* Atrial and ventricular rates between 60 and 100 beats/min
- *Rhythm:* Atrial and ventricular rhythms irregular, with the shortest PP or RR interval varying at least 0.12 second from the longest PP or RR interval
- *P waves:* One P wave before each QRS complex; consistent configuration
- *PR interval:* Normal, constant
- *QRS duration:* Normal, constant

Sinus arrhythmias occasionally are due to nonrespiratory causes such as digitalis or morphine. These drugs enhance vagal tone and cause decreased heart rate and irregularity unrelated to the respiratory cycle.

COMMON DYSRHYTHMIAS

Any disorder of the heartbeat is called a **dysrhythmia**. Historically the term *arrhythmia* has been used in the literature. Although the terms often are used interchangeably, *dysrhythmia* is more accurate. Although many dysrhythmias have no signs and symptoms, many others have serious consequences if not treated.

❖ PATHOPHYSIOLOGY

Dysrhythmias are classified in several ways. As broad categories, they include premature complexes, bradydysrhythmias (bradycardias), and tachydysrhythmias (tachycardias).

Premature Complexes

Premature complexes are early rhythm complexes. They occur when a cardiac cell or cell group, other than the sinoatrial (SA) node, becomes irritable and fires an impulse before the next sinus impulse is produced. The abnormal focus is called an *ectopic focus* and may be generated by atrial, junctional, or ventricular tissue. After the premature complex, there is a pause before the next normal complex, creating an irregularity in the rhythm. The patient with premature complexes may be unaware of them or may feel **palpitations** or a "skipping" of the heartbeat. If premature complexes, especially those that are ventricular, become more frequent, the patient may experience symptoms of decreased cardiac output.

Premature complexes may occur *repetitively in a rhythmic fashion:*

- **Bigeminy** exists when normal complexes and premature complexes occur alternately in a repetitive two-beat pattern, with a pause occurring after each premature complex so complexes occur in pairs.
- **Trigeminy** is a repeated three-beat pattern, usually occurring as two sequential normal complexes followed by a premature complex and a pause, with the same pattern repeating itself in triplets.
- **Quadrigeminy** is a repeated four-beat pattern, usually occurring as three sequential normal complexes followed by a premature complex and a pause, with the same pattern repeating itself in a four-beat pattern.

Bradydysrhythmias

Bradydysrhythmias occur when the heart rate is less than 60 beats/min. These rhythms can also be significant because:

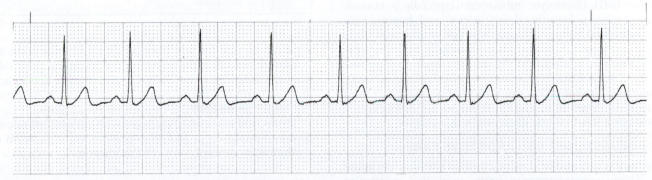

FIG. 34-7 Normal sinus rhythm. Both atrial and ventricular rhythms are essentially regular (a slight variation in rhythm is normal). Atrial and ventricular rates are both 87 beats/min. There is one P wave before each QRS complex, and all the P waves are of a consistent morphology, or shape. The PR interval measures 0.18 second and is constant; the QRS complex measures 0.06 second and is constant.

- Myocardial oxygen demand is reduced from the slow heart rate, which can be beneficial.
- Coronary PERFUSION time may be adequate because of a prolonged diastole, which is desirable.
- Coronary perfusion pressure may decrease if the heart rate is too slow to provide adequate cardiac output and blood pressure; this is a serious consequence.

Therefore the patient may tolerate the bradydysrhythmia well if the blood pressure is adequate. If the blood pressure is not adequate, symptomatic bradydysrhythmias may lead to myocardial ischemia or infarction, dysrhythmias, hypotension, and heart failure.

Tachydysrhythmias

Tachydysrhythmias are heart rates greater than 100 beats/min. They are a major concern in the adult patient with coronary artery disease (CAD). Coronary artery blood flow occurs mostly during diastole when the aortic valve is closed and is determined by diastolic time and blood pressure in the root of the aorta. Tachydysrhythmias are serious because they:

- Shorten the diastolic time and therefore the coronary PERFUSION time (the amount of time available for blood to flow through the coronary arteries to the myocardium)
- Initially increase cardiac output and blood pressure (However, a continued rise in heart rate decreases the ventricular filling time because of a shortened diastole, decreasing the stroke volume. Consequently, cardiac output and blood pressure will begin to decrease, reducing aortic pressure and therefore coronary PERFUSION pressure.)
- Increase the work of the heart, increasing myocardial oxygen demand

The patient with a tachydysrhythmia may have:

- Palpitations
- Chest discomfort (pressure or pain from myocardial ischemia or infarction)
- Restlessness and anxiety
- Pale, cool skin
- Syncope ("blackout") from hypotension

Tachydysrhythmias may also lead to heart failure. Presenting symptoms of heart failure may include dyspnea, lung crackles, distended neck veins, fatigue, and weakness (see Chapter 35). Chart 34-1 summarizes key features of sustained bradydysrhythmias and tachydysrhythmias.

Etiology

Dysrhythmias occur for many reasons, including myocardial infarction (MI), electrolyte imbalances (especially potassium and magnesium), hypoxia, drug toxicity, and hypovolemia (decreased blood volume). People who use cocaine and illicit inhalants are particularly at risk for potentially fatal dysrhythmias. Stress, fear, anxiety, and caffeine can cause an increased heart rate (tachycardia or premature ventricular contractions). Nicotine and alcohol excess can lead to abnormal heart rates such as atrial fibrillation. Specific etiologies are described for each common dysrhythmia discussed in this chapter.

❖ INTERPROFESSIONAL COLLABORATIVE CARE

Dysrhythmias may also be classified by their site of origin in the heart. These include common sinus, atrial, and ventricular dysrhythmias. Although many specific dysrhythmias can occur, general assessment and interventions for patient care may be similar (Chart 34-2). Assess the patient's apical and radial pulses

---

⏵⏵ CHART 34-1   Key Features
Sustained Tachydysrhythmias and Bradydysrhythmias

- Chest discomfort, pressure, or pain, which may radiate to the jaw, the back, or the arm
- Restlessness, anxiety, nervousness, confusion
- Dizziness, syncope
- Palpitations (in tachydysrhythmias)
- Change in pulse strength, rate, and rhythm
- Pulse deficit
- Shortness of breath, dyspnea
- Tachypnea
- Pulmonary crackles
- Orthopnea
- S_3 or S_4 heart sounds
- Jugular venous distention
- Weakness, fatigue
- Pale, cool, skin; diaphoresis
- Nausea, vomiting
- Decreased urine output
- Delayed capillary refill
- Hypotension

◎ CHART 34-2   Best Practice for Patient Safety & Quality Care QSEN
Care of the Patient With Dysrhythmias

- Assess vital signs at least every 4 hours and as needed.
- Monitor patient for cardiac dysrhythmias.
- Evaluate and document the patient's response to dysrhythmias.
- Encourage the patient to notify the nurse when chest pain occurs.
- Assess chest pain (e.g., location, intensity, duration, radiation, and precipitating and alleviating factors).
- Assess peripheral circulation (e.g., palpate for presence of peripheral pulses, edema, capillary refill, color, and temperature of extremity).
- Provide antidysrhythmic therapy according to unit policy (e.g., antidysrhythmic medication, cardioversion, or defibrillation), as appropriate.
- Monitor and document patient's response to antidysrhythmic medications or interventions.
- Monitor appropriate laboratory values (e.g., cardiac enzymes, electrolyte levels).
- Monitor the patient's activity tolerance and schedule exercise/rest periods to avoid fatigue.
- Observe for respiratory difficulty (e.g., shortness of breath, rapid breathing, labored respirations).
- Promote stress reduction.
- Offer spiritual support to the patient and/or family (e.g., contact clergy), as appropriate.

---

for a full minute for any irregularity, which may occur with premature beats or atrial fibrillation. If the apical pulse differs from the radial pulse rate, a pulse deficit exists and indicates that the heart is not pumping adequately to achieve optimal PERFUSION to the body.

Dysrhythmias are often managed with antidysrhythmic drug therapy. Specific drugs and other treatments for common dysrhythmias are discussed later in this chapter.

SINUS DYSRHYTHMIAS

The sinoatrial (SA) node in the right atrium is the pacemaker in all sinus dysrhythmias. Innervation from sympathetic and parasympathetic nerves is normally in balance to ensure a normal sinus rhythm (NSR). An imbalance increases or decreases the rate of SA node discharge either as a normal response to activity or physiologic changes or as a pathologic response to disease. Sinus tachycardia and sinus bradycardia are the two most common types of sinus dysrhythmias.

SINUS TACHYCARDIA

❖ PATHOPHYSIOLOGY

Sympathetic nervous system stimulation or vagal (parasympathetic) inhibition results in an increased rate of SA node discharge, which increases the heart rate. When the rate of SA node discharge is more than 100 beats/min, the rhythm is called **sinus tachycardia** (Fig. 34-8A). From age 10 years to adulthood, the heart rate normally does not exceed 100 beats/min except in response to activity and then usually does not exceed 160 beats/min. Rarely does the heart rate reach 180 beats/min.

Sinus tachycardia initially increases cardiac output and blood pressure. However, continued increases in heart rate decrease coronary PERFUSION time, diastolic filling time, and coronary PERFUSION pressure while increasing myocardial oxygen demand.

Increased sympathetic stimulation is a normal response to physical activity but may also be caused by anxiety, pain, stress, fever, anemia, hypoxemia, and hyperthyroidism. Drugs such as epinephrine, atropine, caffeine, alcohol, nicotine, cocaine, aminophylline, and thyroid medications may also increase the heart rate. In some cases, sinus tachycardia is a compensatory response to decreased cardiac output or blood pressure, as

occurs in dehydration, hypovolemic shock, myocardial infarction (MI), infection, and heart failure. Assess patients for signs and symptoms of hypovolemia and dehydration, including increased pulse rate, decreased urinary output, decreased blood pressure, and dry skin and mucous membranes.

❖ INTERPROFESSIONAL COLLABORATIVE CARE

The patient may be asymptomatic except for an increased pulse rate. However, if the rhythm is not well tolerated, he or she may have symptoms of instability.

> **⚠ NURSING SAFETY PRIORITY** **QSEN**
> **Action Alert**
>
> For patients with sinus tachycardia, assess for fatigue, weakness, shortness of breath, orthopnea, decreased oxygen saturation, increased pulse rate, and decreased blood pressure. Also assess for restlessness and anxiety from decreased cerebral perfusion and for decreased urine output from impaired renal perfusion. The patient may also have anginal pain and palpitations. The ECG pattern may show T-wave inversion or ST-segment elevation or depression in response to myocardial ischemia.

The desired outcome is to decrease the heart rate to normal levels by treating the underlying cause. Remind the patient to remain on bedrest if the tachycardia is causing hypotension or weakness. Teach the patient to avoid substances that increase cardiac rate, including caffeine, alcohol, and nicotine. Help patients develop stress-management strategies or refer the patient to a mental health professional.

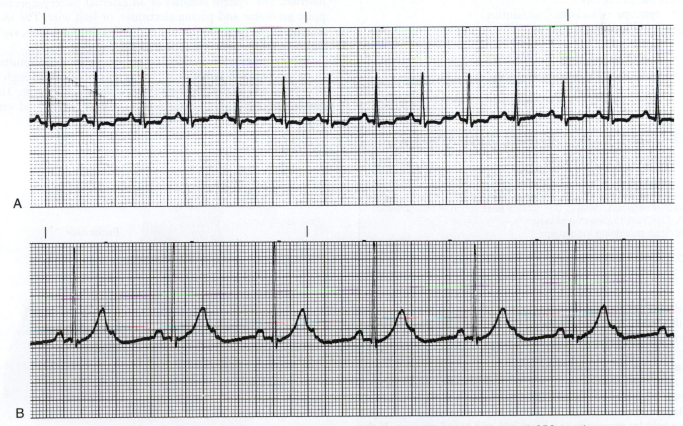

FIG. 34-8 Sinus rhythms. **A,** Sinus tachycardia (heart rate, 115 beats/min; PR interval, 0.12 second; QRS complex, 0.08 second). **B,** Sinus bradycardia (heart rate, 52 beats/min; PR interval, 0.18 second; QRS complex, 0.08 second).

SINUS BRADYCARDIA

❖ PATHOPHYSIOLOGY

Excessive vagal (parasympathetic) stimulation to the heart causes a decreased rate of sinus node discharge. It may result from carotid sinus massage, vomiting, suctioning, Valsalva maneuvers (e.g., bearing down for a bowel movement or gagging), ocular pressure, or pain. Increased parasympathetic stimuli may also result from hypoxia, inferior wall MI, and the administration of drugs such as beta-adrenergic blocking agents, calcium channel blockers, and digitalis. Lyme disease, ELECTROLYTE disturbances, neurologic disorders, and hypothyroidism may also cause bradycardia.

The stimuli slow the heart rate and decrease the speed of conduction through the heart. When the sinus node discharge rate is less than 60 beats/min, the rhythm is called sinus bradycardia (Fig. 34-8B). Sinus bradycardia increases coronary PERFUSION time, but it may decrease coronary perfusion pressure. However, myocardial oxygen demand is *decreased*. Well-conditioned athletes with bradycardia have a hypereffective heart in which the strong heart muscle provides an adequate stroke volume and a low heart rate to achieve a normal cardiac output.

❖ INTERPROFESSIONAL COLLABORATIVE CARE

◆ Assessment: Noticing

The patient with sinus bradycardia may be asymptomatic except for the decreased pulse rate. In many cases, the cause of sinus bradycardia is unknown. Assess the medication administration record (MAR) to determine if the patient is receiving medications that slow the conduction through the SA or AV node. Assess the patient for:

- Syncope ("blackouts" or fainting)
- Dizziness and weakness
- Confusion
- Hypotension
- Diaphoresis (excessive sweating)
- Shortness of breath
- Chest pain

❓ NCLEX EXAMINATION CHALLENGE 34-1

Physiological Integrity

During routine suctioning of a client with a tracheostomy, the client becomes diaphoretic and nauseous, and the heart rate decreases to 39 beats/min. What is the nurse's **best** action at this time?
A. Continue to clear the airway.
B. Stop suctioning the patient.
C. Administer atropine.
D. Call the health care provider immediately.

◆ Interventions: Responding

If the patient is stable, treatment includes identification and treatment of the underlying cause. If the patient has any of these symptoms and the underlying cause cannot be determined, the treatment is to administer drug therapy with atropine 0.5 mg IV, increase intravascular volume via IV fluids, and apply oxygen. Drugs suspected of causing the bradycardia are discontinued. If beta-blocker overdose is suspected, administration of glucagon may help by increasing the heart rate and blood pressure. If the heart rate does not increase sufficiently, prepare for transcutaneous

or transvenous pacing to increase the heart rate. If treatment of the underlying cause does not restore normal sinus rhythm, the patient will require permanent pacemaker implantation.

Temporary Pacing. Temporary pacing is a nonsurgical intervention that provides a timed electrical stimulus to the heart when either the impulse initiation or the conduction system of the heart is defective. The electrical stimulus then spreads throughout the heart to depolarize the cells, which should be followed by contraction and cardiac output. Electrical stimuli may be delivered to the right atrium or right ventricle (single-chamber pacemakers) or to both (dual-chamber pacemakers).

Temporary pacing is used for patients with symptomatic bradydysrhythmias who do not respond to atropine or for patients with asystole. There are two types of temporary pacing: transcutaneous and transvenous.

Transcutaneous pacing is accomplished through the application of two large external electrodes. The electrodes are attached to an external pulse generator. The generator emits electrical pulses, which are transmitted through the electrodes and then transcutaneously to stimulate ventricular depolarization when the patient's heart rate is slower than the rate set on the pacemaker. Transcutaneous pacing is used as an *emergency* measure to provide demand ventricular pacing in a profoundly bradycardic or asystolic patient until invasive pacing can be used or the patient's heart rate returns to normal. This method of pacing is painful and may require administration of pain and sedative medications for the patient to tolerate the therapy. Transcutaneous pacing is used only as a temporary measure to maintain heart rate and PERFUSION until a more permanent method of pacing is used.

A temporary transvenous system can be inserted in an emergency as a bridge until a permanent pacemaker can be inserted. This system consists of an external battery-operated pulse generator and pacing electrodes, or lead wire. The wire attaches to the generator on one end and is threaded to the right ventricle via the subclavian or femoral vein (Fig. 34-9).

In pacemaker systems, electrical pulses, or stimuli, are emitted from the negative terminal of the generator, flow through a lead wire, and stimulate the cardiac cells to depolarize. The current seeks ground by returning through the other lead wire

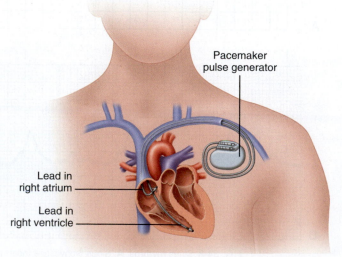

Pacemaker
pulse generator

Lead in
right atrium

Lead in
right ventricle

FIG. 34-9 Placement of pacemaker in chest and heart leads.

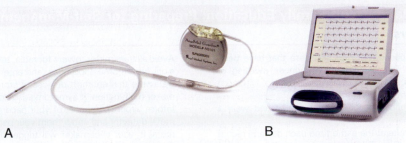

FIG. 34-10 Permanent pacemaker **(A)** and programmer **(B)**. (From Fischell, T. A., et al. [2010]. Initial clinical results using intracardiac electrogram monitoring to detect and alert patients during coronary plaque rupture and ischemia, *Journal of the American College of Cardiology, 56*(14), 1089-1098.)

to the positive terminal of the generator, thus completing a circuit. The intensity of electrical current is set by selecting the appropriate current output, measured in milliamperes.

The two major modes of pacing are synchronous (demand) pacing and asynchronous (fixed-rate) pacing. Temporary pacing is *usually* done in the synchronous (demand) pacing mode. The pacemaker's sensitivity is set to sense the patient's own beats. When the patient's heart rate is above the rate set on the pulse generator, the pacemaker does not fire (inhibits itself). When the patient's heart rate is less than the generator setting, the pacemaker provides electrical impulses (paces).

When a pacing stimulus is delivered to the heart, a spike (or pacemaker artifact) is seen on the monitor or ECG strip. The spike should be followed by evidence of depolarization (i.e., a P wave, indicating atrial depolarization, or a QRS complex, indicating ventricular depolarization). This pattern is referred to as *capture*, indicating that the pacemaker has successfully depolarized, or captured, the chamber.

Permanent Pacemaker. Permanent pacemaker insertion is performed to treat conduction disorders that are not temporary, including complete heart block. These pacemakers are usually powered by a lithium battery and have an average life span of 10 years. After the battery power is depleted, the generator must be replaced by a procedure done with the patient under local anesthesia. Some pacemakers are nuclear powered and have a life span of 20 years or longer. Other pacemakers can be recharged externally. Combination pacemaker/defibrillator devices are also available.

A biventricular pacemaker may be used to coordinate contractions between the right and left ventricles. In addition to pacing used in the right side of the heart, an additional lead is placed in the left lateral wall of the left ventricle through the coronary sinus. This procedure allows synchronized depolarization of the ventricles and is used in patients with moderate-to-severe heart failure to improve functional ability.

The electrophysiologist implants the pulse generator in a surgically made subcutaneous pocket at the shoulder in the right or left subclavicular area, which may create a visible bulge (see Fig. 34-9). The leads are introduced transvenously via the cephalic or the subclavian vein to the endocardium on the right side of the heart. After the procedure, monitor the ECG rhythm to check that the pacemaker is working correctly. Assess the implantation site for bleeding, swelling, redness, tenderness, and infection. The dressing over the site should remain clean and dry. The patient should be afebrile and have stable vital signs. The health care provider prescribes initial activity restrictions, which are then gradually increased. Complications of permanent pacemakers are similar to those of temporary

invasive pacing and include development of pericardial effusion, pericardial tamponade, and diaphragmatic pacing. In diaphragmatic pacing, the patient may report pain at the level of the diaphragm. Observe for muscle contractions over the diaphragm that are synchronous with the heart rate.

Pacemaker checks are done on an ambulatory-care basis at regular intervals. Reprogramming may be needed if pacemaker problems develop. The pulse generator is interrogated using an electronic device to determine the pacemaker settings and battery life (Fig. 34-10). In addition, most pacemaker manufacturers offer wireless home transmitter devices. Data are then sent via landline telephone to a database, which is then accessed by the device clinic or primary health care provider. Stress the need to keep follow-up appointments for more detailed pacemaker checks and reprogramming, if necessary, and for assessment.

Give written and verbal information to patients who have a *permanent pacemaker* about the type and settings of their pacemaker. Teach the patient to report any pulse rate lower than that set on the pacemaker. Review the proper care of the pacemaker insertion site and the importance of reporting any fever or any redness, swelling, or drainage at the pacemaker insertion site. If the surgical incision is near either shoulder, advise the patient to avoid lifting the arm over the head or lifting more than 10 lb for the next 4 weeks because this could dislodge the pacemaker wire. Encourage the patient that usual arm movement is encouraged to prevent shoulder stiffness.

> ⚠ **NURSING SAFETY PRIORITY** QSEN
>
> **Action Alert**
>
> Teach patients who have permanent pacemakers to:
> - Keep handheld cellular phones at least 6 inches away from the generator, with the handset on the ear opposite the side of the generator
> - Avoid sources of strong electromagnetic fields, such as magnets and telecommunications transmitters (These may cause interference and could change the pacemaker settings, causing a malfunction. Magnetic resonance imaging (MRI) is usually contraindicated, depending on the machine's technology.)
> - Carry a pacemaker identification card provided by the manufacturer and wear a medical alert bracelet at all times

Chart 34-3 outlines the major points for patient and family teaching after the insertion of a permanent pacemaker.

ATRIAL DYSRHYTHMIAS

In patients with atrial dysrhythmias, the focus of impulse generation shifts away from the sinus node to the atrial tissues.

CHART 34-3   Patient and Family Education: Preparing for Self-Management

Permanent Pacemakers

- Follow the instructions for pacemaker site skin care that have been specifically prepared for you. Report any fever or redness, swelling, or drainage from the incision site to your physician.
- Do not manipulate the pacemaker generator site.
- Keep your pacemaker identification card in your wallet and wear a medical alert bracelet.
- Take your pulse for 1 full minute at the same time each day and record the rate in your pacemaker diary. Take your pulse any time you feel symptoms of a possible pacemaker failure and report your heart rate and symptoms to your primary health care provider.
- Know the rate at which your pacemaker is set and the basic functioning of your pacemaker. Know which rate changes to report to your primary health care provider.
- Do not apply pressure over your generator. Avoid tight clothing or belts.
- You may take baths or showers without concern for your pacemaker.
- Inform all health care providers that you have a pacemaker. Certain tests that they may wish to perform (e.g., magnetic resonance imaging) could affect or damage it.
- Know the indications of battery failure for your pacemaker as you were instructed and report these findings to your primary health care provider if they occur.
- Do not operate electrical appliances directly over your pacemaker site because this may cause your pacemaker to malfunction.
- Do not lean over electrical or gasoline engines or motors. Be sure that electrical appliances or motors are properly grounded.

- Avoid all transmitter towers for radio, television, and radar. Radio, television, other home appliances, and antennas do not pose a hazard.
- Be aware that antitheft devices in stores may cause temporary pacemaker malfunction. If symptoms develop, move away from the device.
- Inform airport personnel of your pacemaker before passing through a metal detector and show them your pacemaker identification card. The metal in your pacemaker will trigger the alarm in the metal detector device.
- Stay away from any arc welding equipment.
- Be aware that it is safe to operate a microwave oven unless it does not have proper shielding (old microwave ovens) or is defective.
- Report any of these symptoms to your primary health care provider if you experience them: difficulty breathing, dizziness, fainting, chest pain, weight gain, and prolonged hiccupping. If you have any of these symptoms, check your pulse rate and call your primary health care provider.
- If you feel symptoms when near any device, move 5 to 10 feet away from it and check your pulse. Your pulse rate should return to normal.
- Keep all of your health care provider and pacemaker clinic appointments.
- Take all medications prescribed for you as instructed.
- Follow your prescribed diet.
- Follow instructions about restrictions on physical activity, such as no sudden, jerky movement, for 8 weeks to allow the pacemaker to settle in place.

The shift changes the axis (direction) of atrial depolarization, resulting in a P-wave shape that differs from normal P waves. The most common atrial dysrhythmias are:

- Premature atrial complexes
- Supraventricular tachycardia
- Atrial fibrillation

PREMATURE ATRIAL COMPLEXES

A **premature atrial complex (contraction) (PAC)** occurs when atrial tissue becomes irritable. This ectopic focus fires an impulse before the next sinus impulse is due. The premature P wave may not always be clearly visible because it can be hidden in the preceding T wave. Examine the T wave closely for any change in shape and compare with other T waves. A PAC is usually followed by a pause.

- The causes of atrial irritability include:
- Stress
- Fatigue
- Anxiety
- Inflammation
- Infection
- Caffeine, nicotine, or alcohol
- Drugs such as epinephrine, sympathomimetics, amphetamines, digitalis, or anesthetic agents

PACs may also result from myocardial ischemia, hypermetabolic states, electrolyte imbalance, or atrial stretch. Atrial stretch can result from congestive heart failure, valvular disease, and pulmonary hypertension with cor pulmonale.

The patient usually has no symptoms except for possible heart palpitations. No intervention is needed except to treat causes such as heart failure. If PACs occur frequently, they may lead to more serious atrial tachydysrhythmias and therefore may need treatment. Administration of prescribed antidysrhythmic drugs may be necessary (Chart 34-4). Teach the patient measures to

manage stress and substances to avoid, such as caffeine and alcohol, that are known to increase atrial irritability.

SUPRAVENTRICULAR TACHYCARDIA

❖ PATHOPHYSIOLOGY

Supraventricular tachycardia (SVT) involves the rapid stimulation of atrial tissue at a rate of 100 to 280 beats/min in adults. During SVT, P waves may not be visible, especially if there is a 1:1 conduction with rapid rates, because the P waves are embedded in the preceding T wave. *SVT may occur in healthy young people, especially women.*

SVT is usually caused by a re-entry mechanism in which one impulse circulates repeatedly throughout the atrial pathway, re-stimulating the atrial tissue at a rapid rate. The term **paroxysmal supraventricular tachycardia (PSVT)** is used when the rhythm is intermittent. It is initiated suddenly by a premature complex such as a PAC and terminated suddenly with or without intervention.

❖ INTERPROFESSIONAL COLLABORATIVE CARE

Signs and symptoms depend on the duration of the SVT and the rate of the ventricular response. In patients with a *sustained* rapid ventricular response, assess for palpitations, chest pain, weakness, fatigue, shortness of breath, nervousness, anxiety, hypotension, and syncope. Cardiovascular deterioration may occur if the rate does not sustain adequate blood pressure. In that case, SVT can result in angina, heart failure, and cardiogenic shock. With a *nonsustained* or slower ventricular response, the patient may be asymptomatic except for occasional palpitations.

If SVT occurs in a healthy person and stops on its own, no intervention may be needed other than eliminating identified causes. If it continues, the patient should be studied in the electrophysiology study (EPS) laboratory. The preferred

CHART 34-4 Common Examples of Drug Therapy

Antidysrhythmic Medication

DRUG CATEGORY	SELECTED NURSING IMPLICATIONS

Class I: Sodium Channel Blockers—There are three subgroups of Class I drugs.

Common examples of sodium channel blockers:

Type IA
- Disopyramide phosphate (Norpace)

Type IB
- Lidocaine (Xylocaine, Xylocard ✦)
- Mexiletine hydrochloride (Mexitil)
- Tocainide hydrochloride (Tonocard)

Type IC
- Flecainide acetate (Tambocor)
- Propafenone hydrochloride (Rythmol)

Monitor BP and HR; *hypotension and bradycardia can occur.*
Monitor for arrhythmias; *these agents affect conduction patterns, sometimes increasing the frequency or severity of dysrhythmias.*
Monitor for CNS side effects such as dizziness, anxiety, ataxia, insomnia, confusion, seizures, and GI distress; *these side effects may require dose reduction or discontinuation of the drug.*
Monitor for signs of heart failure; *many Class I agents can also cause HF.*

Class II: Beta Blockers—Only four beta blockers are approved for the treatment of dysrhythmias.

Common examples of beta blockers:
- Propanolol (Inderal, Apo-Propanolol ✦)
- Acebutolol (Sectral)
- Esmolol (Brevibloc)
- Sotalol (Betapace)
  - Sotalol is a Class II dysrhythmic and a Class III drug because of effect on the QT interval and delay of repolarization.
  - Assess ventricular arrhythmias because this drug can have proarrhythmic effects.

Monitor HR and BP; *bradycardia and decreased BP are expected effects.*
Assess for wheezing or shortness of breath; *beta₂-blocking effects on the lungs can cause bronchospasm.*
Assess for insomnia, fatigue, and dizziness; *side effects may require a decrease in dosage or discontinuation of the drug.*

Class III: Potassium Channel Blockers—There are currently five Class III agents. Each drug works to delay repolarization and prolongs the QT interval. Although their effects are similar, the side effects and mechanism of action vary greatly. **Selected examples** of drug-specific side effects with associated rationales are listed.

- Sotalol (Betapace)
  - Used for atrial and ventricular dysrhythmias.
- Amiodarone (Cordarone)
  - Used for atrial and ventricular dysrhythmias.
  - Continually monitor ECG rhythm during infusion; *bradycardia and AV block can occur.*
  - This drug can cause serious toxicities (lung damage, visual impairment). As a result, *approval is limited to use for life-threatening dysrhythmias. However, because of efficacy, use remains very common* (Burchum & Rosenthal, 2016).
  - Corneal pigmentation occurs in most patients, but it generally does not interfere with vision.
- Dronedarone (Multaq)
  - Used for AF and atrial flutter.
  - Teach patient to take with meals and to avoid grapefruit juice; *this drug is better absorbed with food and grapefruit juice alters the effect of the drug.*
  - Teach patient to notify provider with signs of HF; *this drug is contraindicated for patient with HF.*
- Ibutilide (Corvert)
  - Used for AF and atrial flutter.
  - Stop infusion as soon as the dysrhythmia is terminated or in the event of VT; *this drug may cause potentially fatal dysrhythmias.*
  - Assess potassium and magnesium levels before infusion.
- Dofetilide (Tikosyn)
  - Used for AF and atrial flutter.
  - Teach patient to change positions slowly; *orthostatic hypotension is a common side effect.*

For all Class III potassium channel blockers:
- Monitor BP and HR; *hypotension and bradycardia can occur.*
- Monitor for arrhythmias; *these agents affect conduction patterns, sometimes increasing the frequency or severity of dysrhythmias.*

Class IV: Calcium Channel Blockers—Only two calcium channel blockers are approved for use in the treatment of dysrhythmias.

- Verapamil (Calan, Isoptin)
- Diltiazem (Cardizem, Tiazac XC ✦)

For all Class IV calcium channel blockers:
- Monitor HR and BP; *bradycardia and hypotension are common side effects.*
- Teach patients to change position slowly when receiving oral therapy; *orthostatic hypotension can occur until tolerance develops.*
- Used for AF and atrial flutter.
- Teach patients to report dyspnea, orthopnea, distended neck veins, or swelling of the extremities; *HF can occur, necessitating a decrease in dosage or discontinuation of drug.*

Continued

CHART 34-4   Common Examples of Drug Therapy—cont'd

Antidysrhythmic Medication

DRUG CATEGORY	SELECTED NURSING IMPLICATIONS

Class: Other—Other drugs used in the treatment of dysrhythmias fall outside of the previous categories. They are unclassified drugs for dysrhythmia treatment.

Common examples of other dysrhythmia medications:
- Digoxin (Lanoxin, Toloxin ✦)
  - Used for AF and atrial flutter.
  - Assess apical HR before administration; *decreased HR is an expected response.*
  - Teach patient to report nausea, vomiting, diarrhea, paresthesias, confusion, or visual disturbance; *these can indicate digoxin toxicity.*
- Atropine sulfate
  - Used for bradycardia.
  - Monitor HR and rhythm after administration; *increased heart rate is expected.*
- Adenosine (Adenocard)
  - Used for paroxysmal SVT.
  - Have emergency equipment available *because a short period of asystole is common after administration; bradycardia and hypotension may occur.*
  - Facial flushing, shortness of breath, and chest pain are common side effects.

AF, Atrial fibrillation; *AV,* atrioventricular; *BP,* blood pressure; *BUN,* blood urea nitrogen; *CAD,* coronary artery disease; *CHF,* congestive heart failure; *CNS,* central nervous system; *ECG,* electrocardiogram; *HF,* heart failure; *HR,* heart rate; *SVT,* supraventricular tachycardia.

---

treatment for recurrent SVT is radiofrequency catheter ablation, described later in this chapter with treatment of atrial fibrillation. In sustained SVT with a rapid ventricular response, the desired outcomes of treatment are to decrease the ventricular response, convert the dysrhythmia to a sinus rhythm, and treat the cause.

Vagal maneuvers induce vagal stimulation of the cardiac conduction system, specifically the SA and AV nodes. Although not as common today, vagal maneuvers may be attempted to treat supraventricular tachydysrhythmias and include carotid sinus massage and Valsalva maneuvers. However, the results of these interventions are often temporary and may cause "rebound" tachycardia or severe bradycardia. Further therapy must be initiated.

In *carotid sinus massage,* the health care provider massages over one carotid artery for a few seconds, observing for a change in cardiac rhythm. This intervention causes vagal stimulation, slowing SA and AV nodal conduction. Prepare the patient for the procedure. Instruct him or her to turn the head slightly away from the side to be massaged and observe the cardiac monitor for a change in rhythm. An ECG rhythm strip is recorded before, during, and after the procedure. After the procedure, assess vital signs and the level of consciousness. Complications include bradydysrhythmias, asystole, ventricular fibrillation (VF), and cerebral damage. Because of these risks, carotid massage is not commonly performed. *A defibrillator and resuscitative equipment must be immediately available during the procedure.*

To stimulate a *vagal reflex,* the health care provider instructs the patient to bear down as if straining to have a bowel movement. Assess the patient's heart rate, heart rhythm, and blood pressure. Observe the cardiac monitor and record an ECG rhythm strip before, during, and after the procedure to determine the effect of therapy.

Drug therapy is prescribed for some patients to convert SVT to a normal sinus rhythm (NSR). Adenosine (Adenocard) is used to terminate the acute episode and given rapidly (over several seconds) followed by a normal saline bolus.

> **! NURSING SAFETY PRIORITY** QSEN
>
> **Drug Alert**
>
> Side effects of adenosine include significant bradycardia with pauses, nausea, and vomiting. When administering adenosine, be sure to have emergency equipment readily available!

AV nodal blocking agents, such as beta and calcium channel blockers, are also given to treat SVT. Chart 34-4 lists medications that may be used for SVT.

If symptoms of poor PERFUSION are severe and persistent, the patient may require synchronized cardioversion to immediately terminate the SVT. For long-term treatment, patients are referred to an electrophysiologist for radiofrequency catheter ablation. Synchronized cardioversion and catheter ablation are discussed later in this chapter with treatment of atrial fibrillation.

✳ PERFUSION CONCEPT EXEMPLAR
Atrial Fibrillation

Atrial fibrillation (AF) is the most common dysrhythmia seen in clinical practice. AF can be encountered and treated in the ambulatory and acute care settings. It can impair quality of life and cause considerable morbidity and mortality, largely related to CLOTTING concerns such as embolic stroke, deep venous thrombosis (DVT) or pulmonary embolism (PE).

❖ PATHOPHYSIOLOGY

In patients with AF, multiple rapid impulses from many atrial foci depolarize the atria in a totally disorganized manner at a rate of 350 to 600 times per minute; ventricular response is usually 120 to 200 beats/min. The result is a chaotic rhythm with no clear P waves, no atrial contractions, loss of atrial kick, and an irregular ventricular response (Fig. 34-11). The atria merely quiver in fibrillation (commonly called *A fib*). Often the ventricles beat with a rapid rate in response to the numerous

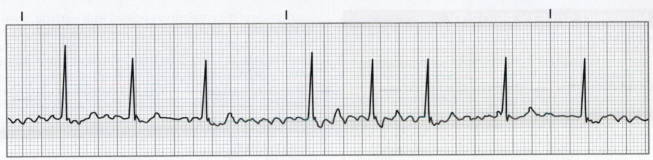

FIG. 34-11 Atrial fibrillation. Note wavy baseline with atrial electrical activity and irregular ventricular rhythm.

atrial impulses. The rapid and irregular ventricular rate decreases ventricular filling and reduces cardiac output. This alteration in cardiac function allows for blood to pool, placing the patient at risk for CLOTTING concerns such as DVT or PE. AF is frequently associated with underlying cardiovascular disease (Urden et al., 2016).

Etiology and Genetic Risk

AF is associated with atrial fibrosis and loss of muscle mass. These structural changes are common in heart diseases such as hypertension, heart failure, and coronary artery disease. For those without an underlying disorder leading to the development of AF, as many as 30 genetic mutations have been identified as the potential cause (Palatinus & Das, 2015). Investigation continues in the development of genetic testing to identify patients at risk and targeted treatment (Palatinus & Das, 2015). As AF progresses, cardiac output decreases by as much as 20% to 30%.

Incidence and Prevalence

Currently, about 2.7 to 6.1 million people in the United States are diagnosed with AF; it occurs more often in those of European ancestry and African Americans (January et al., 2014). The incidence of AF increases with age; it causes serious problems in older people, leading to stroke and/or heart failure. Risk factors include hypertension (HTN), previous ischemic stroke, transient ischemic attack (TIA) or other thromboembolic event, coronary heart disease, diabetes mellitus, heart failure, obesity, hyperthyroidism, chronic kidney disease, excessive alcohol use, and mitral valve disease.

❖ INTERPROFESSIONAL COLLABORATIVE CARE

◆ Assessment: Noticing

History. When obtaining a history, assess for prior history of AF or other dysrhythmias. Recurrence of AF is common, and assessment of previous conduction issues can be helpful in developing the plan of care. Assess for history of cardiovascular disease. The risk of AF is much higher in patients with a history of hypertension, heart failure, obesity, or acute coronary syndrome (Urden, Stacy & Lough, 2016).

Physical Assessment/Signs and Symptoms. On physical examination, the apical pulse may be irregular. Symptoms depend on the ventricular rate. Because of the loss of atrial kick, the patient in uncontrolled AF is at greater risk for inadequate cardiac output. Signs of poor PERFUSION may be seen. Assess the patient for fatigue, weakness, shortness of breath, dizziness, anxiety, syncope, palpitations, chest discomfort or pain, and hypotension. Some patients may be asymptomatic.

Psychosocial Assessment. Patients with AF, especially those with a high ventricular rate, can feel very anxious. With increased heart rate, cardiac output decreases, which can create dyspnea, contributing to feelings of anxiety. Assess patients who have chronic atrial fibrillation for methods of coping with a long-term conduction issue. Patients with chronic AF may have anxiety related to anticoagulation medications and the potential for emboli development.

Other Diagnostic Assessment. Definitive diagnosis occurs by obtaining a 12-lead ECG. AF is classified into five categories based on length of time in the rhythm: paroxysmal, persistent, long-standing persistent, permanent, and nonvalvular. AF is termed *paroxysmal* when the patient experiences an episode within 7 days that converts back to sinus rhythm. Episode lengths vary but do not continue beyond a week. *Persistent AF* is experienced as episodes that occur for longer than 7 days. AF sustained for more than 12 months is categorized as *long-standing persistent*. *Permanent AF* is defined as patients who remain in AF, and a decision is made not to restore or maintain sinus rhythm by either medical or surgical intervention. *Nonvalvular AF* occurs in the absence of mitral valve disease or repair.

◆ Analysis: Interpreting

The priority collaborative problems for most patients with atrial fibrillation are:
1. Potential for embolus formation due to irregular cardiac rhythm
2. Potential for heart failure due to altered conduction pattern

◆ Planning and Implementation: Responding

Interventions for AF depend on the severity of the problem and the patient's response. Be sure to individualize care based on the patient's values and preferences, your clinical expertise, and best current evidence. Drug therapy is often effective for treating AF.

Preventing Embolus Formation

Planning: Expected Outcomes. The expected outcome is that the patient will remain free of embolus formation by restoring regular cardiac conduction.

Interventions. The purpose of collaborative care is to restore regular blood flow through the atrium when possible. Correcting the rhythm and controlling the rate of the rhythm restore blood flow, which helps prevent embolus formation and increases cardiac output. Drug therapy is often effective for treating AF.

Traditional interventions for AF include antidysrhythmic drugs to slow the ventricular conduction or to convert the

Action Alert

The loss of coordinated atrial contractions in AF can lead to pooling of blood, resulting in CLOTTING. *The patient is at high risk for pulmonary embolism!* Thrombi may form within the right atrium and then move through the right ventricle to the lungs. If pulmonary embolism is suspected, remain with the patient and monitor for shortness of breath, chest pain, and/or hypotension. Initiate the Rapid Response Team and notify the provider.

In addition, the patient is at risk for systemic emboli, particularly an embolic stroke, which may cause severe neurologic impairment or death. Monitor patients carefully for signs of stroke. Initiate Rapid Response Team if stroke is suspected to facilitate timely diagnosis.

Patients with AF who have valvular disease are particularly at risk for venous thromboembolism (VTE). In VTE, the patient may complain of lower extremity pain and swelling. Anticipate ultrasound of vasculature and initiation of systemic anticoagulation.

AF to normal sinus rhythm (NSR). Examples of drugs to slow conduction are calcium channel blockers such as diltiazem (Cardizem, Tiazac XC ♦) or, for more difficult-to-control AF, amiodarone (Cordarone). Dronedarone (Multaq) is a medication similar to amiodarone, yet better tolerated by patients, for maintenance of sinus rhythm after cardioversion. However, dronedarone should not be used in patients with heart failure because it can cause an exacerbation of cardiac symptoms or with permanent AF because it increases the risk of stroke, myocardial infarction, or cardiovascular death.

Beta blockers, such as metoprolol (Toprol, Betaloc ♦) and esmolol (Brevibloc), may also be used to slow ventricular response. Digoxin (Lanoxin, Toloxin ♦) is given for patients with heart failure and AF. It is useful in controlling the rate of ventricular response. However, it does not convert AF to sinus rhythm. Carefully monitor the pulse rate of patients taking these drugs.

Medications used for rhythm control of AF include flecainide (Tambocor), dofetilide (Tikosyn), propafenone (Rythmol), and ibutilide (Corvert). These medications are usually started within the acute care setting because of the risk of developing prolonged QT intervals and bradycardia. Continuous cardiac monitoring and frequent 12-lead ECGs are needed. Amiodarone is also used but does not require an acute care stay. If permanent AF is present, rhythm control antiarrhythmic medications should not be used. The medications used for rate and rhythm control are further discussed in Chart 34-4.

The primary health care provider weighs the benefit of anticoagulant use versus risk of bleeding to determine the treatment path. The patient should be made aware of the risk of stroke development verses the risk of bleeding, and his or her preferences should also be a part of the decision-making process.

Because of the unpredictable drug response and many food-drug interactions, laboratory test monitoring (e.g., international normalized ratio [INR]) is required when a patient is taking warfarin. Teach patients the importance of avoiding foods high in vitamin K and to avoid herbs such as ginger, ginseng, goldenseal, *Ginkgo biloba*, and St. John's wort, which could interfere with the drug's action. Chapter 36 describes care of patients receiving anticoagulant therapy.

Because of the problems associated with warfarin, novel oral anticoagulants (NOACs) such as dabigatran (Pradaxa), rivaroxaban (Xarelto), apixaban (Eliquis), or edoxaban (Savaysa) may be given on a long-term basis to prevent strokes associated with nonvalvular AF. Because these drugs achieve a steady state, there is no need for laboratory test monitoring. Prothrombin time (PT) and INR are not accurate predictors of bleeding time when NOACs are used. However, if the patient does experience severe bleeding, the only NOAC with a reversal agent is dabigatran (Pradaxa).

For those taking dabigatran (Pradaxa), a reversal agent has been approved by the U.S. Food and Drug Administration (FDA). Idarucizumab (Praxbind), an intravenous monoclonal antibody, binds to dabigatran, thereby preventing dabigatran from inhibiting thrombin. Side effects of idarucizumab (Praxbind) include hypokalemia, confusion, constipation, fever, and pneumonia. Use of idarucizumab (Praxbind) increases the risk of CLOTTING and stroke and should only be used in the event of life-threatening bleeding.

Drug Alert

Teach patients taking any type of anticoagulant drug to report bruising, bleeding nose or gums, and other signs of bleeding to their primary health care provider immediately.

? NCLEX EXAMINATION CHALLENGE 34-2
Physiological Integrity

The primary health care provider prescribes warfarin (Coumadin) for a client with atrial fibrillation. Which statement made by the client indicates that additional education is needed?
A. "I need to go to the clinic once a week to have my blood level checked."
B. "If my stools turn black, I will be sure to call my primary health care provider"
C. "I'm glad I don't need to change my diet. Salads are my favorite food."
D. "I need to stop taking my herbal supplement."

Preventing Heart Failure

Planning: Expected Outcomes. The expected outcome is that the patient will remain free of heart failure by restoration of normal conduction with a controlled ventricular rate.

Interventions. Collaborative care to prevent heart failure and improve cardiac output generally begins with drug therapy; however, the patient may require other nonsurgical or surgical interventions if medication is not successful in meeting optimal outcomes.

Nonsurgical Interventions. Nonsurgical interventions most commonly include electrical cardioversion, left atrial appendage closure, radiofrequency catheter ablation, and pacing.

Electrical Cardioversion. Electrical cardioversion is a *synchronized* countershock that may be performed to restore normal conduction in a hospitalized patient with *new-onset* AF. A cardioversion can also be scheduled electively for stable AF that is resistant to medical therapy. When the onset of AF is greater than 48 hours, the patient must take anticoagulants for 4 to 6 weeks before the procedure to prevent clots from moving from the heart to the brain or lungs. If the onset of AF is uncertain, a transesophageal echocardiogram (TEE) may be performed to assess for clot formation in the left atrium.

The shock depolarizes a large amount of myocardium during the cardiac depolarization. It is intended to stop the re-entry circuit and allow the sinus node to regain control of the heart. Emergency equipment must be available during the procedure. The physician, advanced practice nurse, or other qualified nurse explains the procedure to the patient and family. Help the patient sign a consent form unless the procedure is an emergency for a life-threatening dysrhythmia. Because he or she is usually conscious, a short-acting anesthetic agent is administered for sedation.

One electrode is placed to the left of the precordium, and the other is placed on the right next to the sternum and below the clavicle. The defibrillator should be set in the synchronized mode. A dot or line will be indicated over each QRS complex, confirming the synchronized mode. This avoids discharging the shock during the T wave, which may increase ventricular irritability, causing ventricular fibrillation (VF). Charge the defibrillator to the energy level requested, usually starting at a low rate of 120 to 200 joules for biphasic machines.

! NURSING SAFETY PRIORITY QSEN

Critical Rescue

For safety before cardioversion, turn oxygen off and away from patient; fire could result. Shout "CLEAR" before shock delivery for electrical safety!

After cardioversion, assess the patient's response and heart rhythm. Therapy is repeated, if necessary, until the desired result is obtained or alternative therapies are considered. If the patient's condition deteriorates into VF after cardioversion, check to see that the synchronizer is turned off so immediate defibrillation can be administered.

Nursing care after cardioversion includes:

- Maintaining a patent airway
- Administering oxygen
- Assessing vital signs and the level of consciousness
- Administering antidysrhythmic drug therapy, as prescribed
- Monitoring for dysrhythmias
- Assessing for chest burns from electrodes
- Providing emotional support
- Documenting the results of cardioversion

Left Atrial Appendage Closure. For patients who are high risk for stroke and who are not candidates for anticoagulation, the left atrial appendage (LAA) occlusion device may be an option (Cheng & Hijazi, 2015). The LAA is a small sac in the wall of the left atrium. For those with nonvalvular AF, the LAA is the most common site of blood clot development leading to the risk of stroke. Inserted percutaneously via the femoral vein, a device to occlude the LAA is delivered via a transseptal puncture. In the United States, the Watchman, (nitinol frame with fenestrated fabric) is the only device approved for use in atrial fibrillation patients. After insertion, anticoagulation

with aspirin and warfarin is required. A repeat TEE is performed approximately 45 days after insertion to assess for leaks around the device. If no leak is detected, the warfarin is stopped, and antiplatelet therapy is continued. Complications are similar to those for undergoing cardiac ablation procedure.

Radiofrequency Catheter Ablation. Radiofrequency catheter ablation (RCA) is an invasive procedure that may be used to destroy an irritable focus in atrial or ventricular conduction. The patient must first undergo electrophysiologic studies and mapping procedures to locate the focus. Then radiofrequency waves are delivered to abolish the irritable focus. When ablation is performed in the AV nodal or His bundle area, damage may also occur to the normal conduction system, causing heart blocks and requiring implantation of a permanent pacemaker.

In AF, pulmonary vein isolation and ablation create scar tissue that blocks impulses and disconnects the pathway of the abnormal rhythm. Patients with AF with a rapid ventricular rate not responsive to drug therapy may have AV nodal ablation performed to totally disconnect the conduction from the atria to the ventricles, which requires implantation of a permanent pacemaker. AF ablation should not be performed if long-term anticoagulation is contraindicated.

Biventricular Pacing. This type of pacing may be another alternative for patients with heart failure and conduction disorders. Biatrial pacing, anti-tachycardia pacing, and implantable atrial defibrillators are other methods used to suppress or resolve AF. (See full pacing discussion earlier in this chapter.)

Surgical Interventions. Patients in AF with heart failure (discussed in Chapter 35) may benefit from the *surgical* **maze procedure**, an open-chest surgical technique often performed with coronary artery bypass grafting (CABG). Before this procedure, electrophysiologic mapping studies are done to confirm the diagnosis of AF. The surgeon places a maze of sutures in strategic places in the atrial myocardium, pulmonary artery, and possibly the superior vena cava to prevent electrical circuits from developing and continuing AF. Sinus impulses can then depolarize the atria before reaching the AV node and preserve the atrial kick. Postoperative care is similar to that after other open-heart surgical procedures (see Chapter 38).

The surgical MAZE procedure is being replaced by catheter procedures using a minimally invasive form. The *catheter* maze procedure is done by inserting a catheter through a leg vein into the atria and dragging a heated ablating catheter along the atria to create lines (scars) of conduction block. Patients having this minimally invasive form of the procedure have fewer complications, less pain, and a quicker recovery than those with the open, surgical maze procedure.

Care Coordination and Transition Management

Home Care. Patients discharged from the hospital may have considerable needs, often more related to their underlying chronic diseases than to their dysrhythmia. A case manager or care coordinator can assess the need for health care resources and coordinate access to services.

The focus of the home care nurse's interventions is assessment and health teaching. The community-based nurse provides the patient and family members with an opportunity to verbalize their concerns and fears. Provide emotional support and

CONSIDERATIONS FOR OLDER ADULTS
Patient-Centered Care **QSEN**

Older adults are at increased risk for dysrhythmias because of normal physiologic changes in their cardiac conduction system. The sinoatrial node has fewer pacemaker cells. There is a loss of fibers in the bundle branch system. Therefore older adults are at risk for sinus node dysfunction and may require pacemaker therapy. The most common dysrhythmias are premature atrial contractions, premature ventricular contractions, and atrial fibrillation. Dysrhythmias tend to be more serious in older patients because of underlying heart disease, causing cardiac decompensation. Consequently, blood flow to organs that may already be decreased because of the aging process may be further compromised, leading to multisystem organ dysfunction. Chart 34-5 highlights special considerations for older adults receiving antidysrhythmic therapy.

CHART 34-5   Nursing Focus on the Older Adult

Dysrhythmias

Special nursing considerations for the older patient with dysrhythmias are:
- Evaluate the patient with dysrhythmias immediately for the presence of a life-threatening dysrhythmia or hemodynamic deterioration.
- Assess the patient with a dysrhythmia for angina, hypotension, heart failure, and decreased cerebral and renal perfusion.
- Consider these causes of dysrhythmias when taking the patient's history: hypoxia, drug toxicity, electrolyte imbalances, heart failure, and myocardial ischemia or infarction.
- Assess the patient's level of education, hearing, learning style, and ability to understand and recall instructions to determine the best approaches for teaching.
- Assess the patient's ability to read written instructions.
- Teach the patient the generic and trade names of prescribed antidysrhythmic drugs and their purposes, dosage, side effects, and special instructions for use.
- Provide clear written instructions in basic language and easy-to-read print.
- Provide a written drug dosage schedule for the patient, considering all the drugs the patient is taking and possible drug interactions.
- Assess the patient for possible side effects or adverse reactions to drugs, considering age and health status.
- Teach the patient to take his or her pulse and to report significant changes in heart rate or rhythm to the primary health care provider.
- Inform the patient of available resources for blood pressure and pulse checks, such as blood pressure clinics, home health agencies, and cardiac rehabilitation programs.
- Instruct the patient about the importance of keeping follow-up appointments with the primary health care provider and reporting symptoms promptly.
- Include the patient's family members or significant other in all teaching whenever possible.
- Teach the patient to avoid drinking caffeinated beverages, stop smoking, drink alcohol only in moderation, and follow his or her prescribed diet.

 CHART 34-6   Patient and Family Education: Preparing for Self-Management

How to Prevent or Decrease Dysrhythmias

For Patients at Risk for Vasovagal Attacks Causing Bradydysrhythmias
- Avoid doing things that stimulate the vagus nerve, such as raising your arms above your head, applying pressure over your carotid artery, applying pressure on your eyes, bearing down or straining during a bowel movement, and stimulating a gag reflex when brushing your teeth or putting objects in your mouth.

For Patients With Premature Beats and Ectopic Rhythms
- Take the medications that have been prescribed for you and report any adverse effects to your physician.
- Stop smoking, avoid caffeinated beverages and energy drinks as much as possible, and drink alcohol only in moderation.
- Learn ways to manage stress and avoid getting too tired.

For Patients With Ischemic Heart Disease
- If you have an angina attack, treat it promptly with rest and nitroglycerin administration as prescribed by your physician. This decreases your chances of experiencing a dysrhythmia.
- If chest pain is not relieved after taking the amount of nitroglycerin that has been prescribed for you, seek medical attention promptly. Also seek prompt medical attention if the pain becomes more severe or you experience other symptoms, such as sweating, nausea, weakness, and palpitations.

For Patients at Risk for Potassium Imbalance
- Know the symptoms of decreased potassium levels, such as muscle weakness and cardiac irregularity.
- Eat foods high in potassium, such as tomatoes, beans, prunes, avocados, bananas, strawberries, and lettuce.
- Take the potassium supplements that have been prescribed for you.

---

referrals for ongoing care in the community. Assess the patient for possible side effects of antidysrhythmic agents or anticoagulation therapy.

Self-Management Education. Patients and their families must have a thorough understanding of the prescribed *medication therapy*, including antidysrhythmic and anticoagulant agents. Pharmacies provide written instructions with filled prescriptions. Teach patients and families the generic and trade names of their drugs and the drugs' purposes, using basic terms that are easily understood. Clear instructions regarding dosage schedules and common side effects are important (see Chart 34-4). Emphasize the importance of reporting these side effects and any dizziness, nausea, vomiting, chest discomfort, or shortness of breath to the primary care provider. Be sure to include education that medication should not be stopped abruptly unless instructed by the primary health care provider. Teach the patient the signs and symptoms of bleeding. Advise patients to call the provider if any signs of bleeding are identified.

Teach all patients and their family members how to take a pulse and blood pressure. Some patients may want to use technology to calculate and record their pulse rate. Several applications (apps) for handheld mobile devices (such as the iPhone) are available, but their accuracy varies. "Instant Health Rate" and "Quick Heart Rate" are examples of apps used to calculate pulse rate.

Remind patients to report any signs of a change in heart rhythm, such as a significant decrease in pulse rate, a rate more than 100 beats/min, or increased rhythm irregularity. Smart Blood Pressure (SmartBP) is a blood pressure and pulse-management system that records, tracks, and analyzes data to share via an iPhone or iPad. The patient can send these readings to his or her primary health care provider as needed to maintain frequent vital sign monitoring (Chart 34-6).

Health Care Resources. The cardiac rehabilitation nurse typically provides written and oral information about dysrhythmias, antidysrhythmic drugs, and anticoagulant drugs. In addition, information about cardiac exercise programs, educational programs, and support groups is provided. The office or ambulatory care nurse may also provide information about resources. Teach the patient how to contact the local chapter of the American Heart Association (www.americanheart.org) or the provincial chapter of the Heart and Stroke Foundation in Canada (www.heartandstroke.ca) for information about dysrhythmias, pacemakers, and CPR training.

◆ Evaluation: Reflecting

Evaluate the care of the patient with AF on the basis of the identified patient problems. The expected outcomes include that the patient will:

- Remain free of embolus formation associated with AF
- Remain free of heart failure with regular heart rate and rhythm

VENTRICULAR DYSRHYTHMIAS

Ventricular dysrhythmias are potentially more life threatening than atrial dysrhythmias because the left ventricle pumps oxygenated blood throughout the body to perfuse vital organs and other tissues. The most common or life-threatening ventricular dysrhythmias include:

- Premature ventricular complexes
- Ventricular tachycardia
- Ventricular fibrillation
- Ventricular asystole

PREMATURE VENTRICULAR COMPLEXES

❖ PATHOPHYSIOLOGY

Premature ventricular complexes (PVCs), also called *premature ventricular contractions*, result from increased irritability of ventricular cells and are seen as early ventricular complexes followed by a pause. When multiple PVCs are present, the QRS complexes may be unifocal or uniform, meaning that they are of the same shape (Fig. 34-12A), or multifocal or multiform, meaning that they are of different shapes (Fig. 34-12B). PVCs frequently occur in repetitive rhythms, such as bigeminy (two), trigeminy (three), and quadrigeminy (four). Two sequential PVCs are a pair, or couplet. Three or more successive PVCs are usually called **nonsustained ventricular tachycardia (NSVT)**.

Premature ventricular contractions are common, and their frequency increases with age. They may be insignificant or may occur with problems such as myocardial infarction, chronic heart failure, chronic obstructive pulmonary disease (COPD), and anemia. PVCs may also be present in patients with hypokalemia or hypomagnesemia. Sympathomimetic agents, anesthesia drugs, stress, nicotine, caffeine, alcohol, infection, or surgery can also cause PVCs, especially in older adults. Postmenopausal women often find that caffeine causes palpitations and PVCs.

❖ INTERPROFESSIONAL COLLABORATIVE CARE

The patient may be asymptomatic or experience palpitations or chest discomfort caused by increased stroke volume of the normal beat after the pause. Peripheral pulses may be

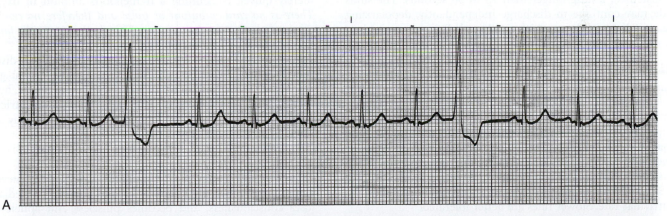

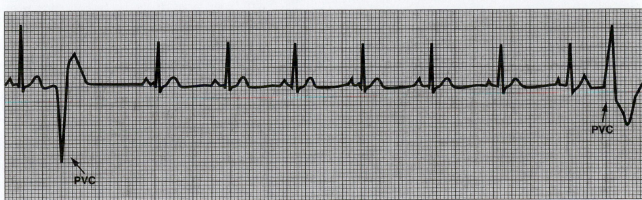

FIG. 34-12 Premature ventricular contractions. **A,** Normal sinus rhythm with unifocal premature ventricular complexes (PVCs). **B,** Normal sinus rhythm with multifocal PVCs (one negative and the other positive).

diminished or absent with the PVCs themselves because the decreased stroke volume of the premature beats may *decrease peripheral* PERFUSION.

> ### ❗ NURSING SAFETY PRIORITY QSEN
> **Action Alert**
>
> Because other dysrhythmias can cause widened QRS complexes, assess whether the premature complexes perfuse to the extremities. Palpate the carotid, brachial, or femoral arteries while observing the monitor for widened complexes or auscultating apical heart sounds. With acute MI, PVCs may be considered as a warning, possibly triggering life-threatening ventricular tachycardia (VT) or ventricular fibrillation (VF).

If there is no underlying heart disease, PVCs are not usually treated other than by eliminating or managing any contributing cause (e.g., caffeine, stress). Potassium or magnesium is given for replacement therapy if hypokalemia or hypomagnesemia is the cause. If the number of PVCs in a 24-hour period is excessive, the patient may be placed on beta-adrenergic blocking agents (beta blockers) (see Chart 34-4).

VENTRICULAR TACHYCARDIA

❖ PATHOPHYSIOLOGY

Ventricular tachycardia (VT), sometimes referred to as *V tach*, occurs with repetitive firing of an irritable ventricular ectopic focus, usually at a rate of 140 to 180 beats/min or more (Fig. 34-13). VT may result from increased automaticity or a re-entry mechanism. It may be intermittent (nonsustained VT) or sustained, lasting longer than 15 to 30 seconds. The sinus node may continue to discharge independently, depolarizing the atria but not the ventricles, although P waves are seldom seen in sustained VT.

❖ INTERPROFESSIONAL COLLABORATIVE CARE

Ventricular tachycardia may occur in patients with ischemic heart disease, MI, cardiomyopathy, hypokalemia, hypomagnesemia, valvular heart disease, heart failure, drug toxicity (e.g., steroids), or hypotension. Patients who use cocaine or illicit inhalants are at a high risk for VT. *In patients who go into cardiac arrest, VT is commonly the initial rhythm before deterioration into ventricular fibrillation (VF) as the terminal rhythm!*

Signs and symptoms of sustained VT partially depend on the ventricular rate. Slower rates are better tolerated.

> ### ❗ NURSING SAFETY PRIORITY QSEN
> **Critical Rescue**
>
> In some patients, VT causes cardiac arrest. Assess the patient's circulation and airway, breathing, level of consciousness, and oxygenation level. For the *stable* patient with sustained VT, administer oxygen and confirm the rhythm via a 12-lead ECG. Amiodarone (Cordarone), lidocaine, or magnesium sulfate may be given.

Current Advanced Cardiac Life Support (ACLS) guidelines state that elective cardioversion is highly recommended for stable VT. The primary health care provider may prescribe an oral antidysrhythmic agent, such as mexiletine (Mexitil) or sotalol (Betapace, Rylosol ✦), to prevent further occurrences. If the patient has been taking digoxin, the drug is withheld for up to 48 hours before an elective cardioversion. Digoxin increases ventricular irritability and puts the patient at risk for VF after the countershock. Patients who persist with episodes of stable VT may require radiofrequency catheter ablation. *Unstable* VT without a pulse is treated the same way as ventricular fibrillation as described in the following paragraphs.

VENTRICULAR FIBRILLATION

❖ PATHOPHYSIOLOGY

Ventricular fibrillation (VF), sometimes called *V fib*, is the result of electrical chaos in the ventricles and is *life threatening!* Impulses from many irritable foci fire in a totally disorganized manner so ventricular contraction cannot occur. There are no recognizable ECG deflections (Fig. 34-14A). The ventricles merely quiver, consuming a tremendous amount of oxygen. *There is no cardiac output or pulse and therefore no cerebral, myocardial, or systemic perfusion. This rhythm is rapidly fatal if not successfully ended within 3 to 5 minutes.*

VF may be the first manifestation of coronary artery disease (CAD). Patients with myocardial infarction (MI) are at great risk for VF. It may also occur in those with hypokalemia, hypomagnesemia, hemorrhage, drug therapy, rapid supraventricular tachycardia (SVT), or shock. Surgery or trauma may also cause VF.

❖ INTERPROFESSIONAL COLLABORATIVE CARE

Emergency care for ventricular fibrillation is critical for survival. When VF begins, the patient becomes faint, immediately loses consciousness, and becomes pulseless and apneic (no

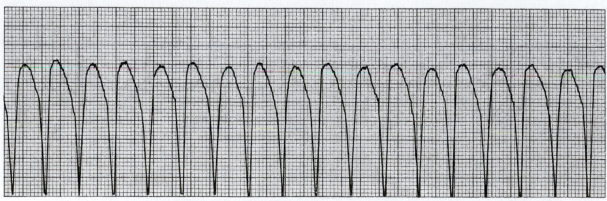

FIG. 34-13 Sustained ventricular tachycardia at a rate of 166 beats/min.

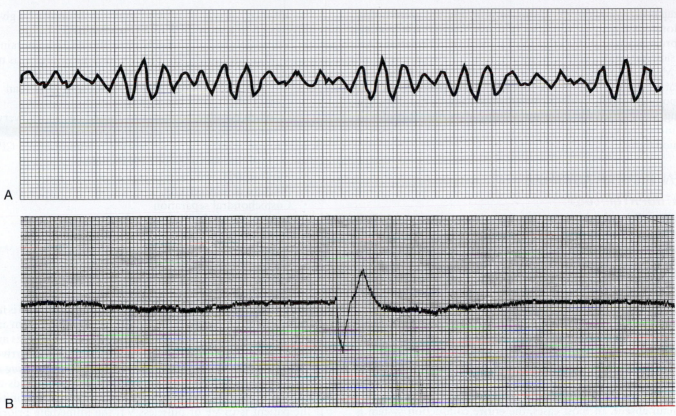

FIG. 34-14 Ventricular dysrhythmias. **A,** Coarse ventricular fibrillation. **B,** Ventricular asystole with one idioventricular complex.

breathing). There is no blood pressure, and heart sounds are absent. Respiratory and metabolic acidosis develop. Seizures may occur. Within minutes, the pupils become fixed and dilated, and the skin becomes cold and mottled. *Death results without prompt intervention.*

The desired outcomes of collaborative care are to resolve VF promptly and convert it to an organized rhythm. *Therefore the priority is to defibrillate the patient immediately according to ACLS protocol.* If a defibrillator is not readily available, high-quality CPR must be initiated and continued until the defibrillator arrives. An automated external defibrillator (AED) is frequently used because it is simple for both medical and lay personnel. Defibrillation is discussed with cardiopulmonary resuscitation later in this chapter.

Drug therapy is used when dysrhythmias are sustained and/or life threatening. Drug therapy from one or more classes of antidysrhythmic agents is often used (see Chart 34-4). The Vaughn-Williams classification is commonly used to categorize drugs according to their effects on the action potential of cardiac cells (Classes I through IV). Other drugs also have antidysrhythmic effects but do not fit the Vaughn-Williams classification.

Class I antidysrhythmics are membrane-stabilizing agents used to decrease automaticity. The three subclassifications in this group include type IA drugs, which moderately slow conduction and prolong repolarization, prolonging the QT interval. These drugs are used to treat or prevent supraventricular and ventricular premature beats and tachydysrhythmias, but they are not as commonly used as other drugs. An example is procainamide hydrochloride (Pronestyl). Type IB drugs shorten repolarization. These drugs are used to treat or prevent

ventricular premature beats, ventricular tachycardia (VT), and ventricular fibrillation (VF). Examples include lidocaine and mexiletine hydrochloride (Mexitil). Type IC drugs markedly slow conduction and widen the QRS complex. These agents are used primarily to treat or to prevent recurrent, life-threatening ventricular premature beats, VT, and VF. Examples include flecainide acetate (Tambocor) and propafenone hydrochloride (Rythmol).

Class II antidysrhythmics control dysrhythmias associated with excessive beta-adrenergic stimulation by competing for receptor sites, thereby decreasing heart rate and conduction velocity. Beta-adrenergic blocking agents, such as propranolol (Inderal) and esmolol hydrochloride (Brevibloc), are Class II drugs. They are used to treat or prevent supraventricular and ventricular premature beats and tachydysrhythmias. Sotalol hydrochloride (Betapace, Sotacor) is an antidysrhythmic agent with both noncardioselective beta-adrenergic blocking effects (Class II) and action potential duration prolongation properties (Class III). It is an oral agent that may be used for the treatment of documented ventricular dysrhythmias such as VT that are life threatening.

Class III antidysrhythmics lengthen the absolute refractory period and prolong repolarization and the action potential duration of ischemic cells. Class III drugs include amiodarone (Cordarone) and ibutilide (Corvert) and are used to treat or prevent ventricular premature beats, VT, and VF.

Class IV antidysrhythmics slow the flow of calcium into the cell during depolarization, thereby depressing the automaticity of the sinoatrial (SA) and atrioventricular (AV) nodes, decreasing the heart rate, and prolonging the AV nodal refractory period and conduction. Calcium channel blockers, such as verapamil hydrochloride (Calan, Isoptin, and diltiazem hydrochloride [Cardizem]), are Class IV drugs. They are used to treat supraventricular tachycardia (SVT) and atrial fibrillation (AF) to slow the ventricular response.

Magnesium sulfate is an electrolyte administered to treat refractory VT or VF because these patients may be hypomagnesemic, with increased ventricular irritability. The drug is also used for a life-threatening VT called torsades de pointes that can result from certain antidysrhythmics such as amiodarone.

VENTRICULAR ASYSTOLE

❖ *PATHOPHYSIOLOGY*

Ventricular asystole, sometimes called *ventricular standstill,* is the complete absence of any ventricular rhythm (Fig. 34-14B). There are no electrical impulses in the ventricles and therefore *no* ventricular depolarization, no QRS complex, no contraction, no cardiac output, and no PERFUSION to the rest of the body.

❖ *INTERPROFESSIONAL COLLABORATIVE CARE*

◆ *Assessment: Noticing*

The patient in ventricular asystole has no pulse, respirations, or blood pressure. *The patient is in full cardiac arrest.* In some cases, the sinoatrial (SA) node may continue to fire and depolarize the atria, with only P waves seen on the ECG. However, the sinus impulses do not conduct to the ventricles, and QRS complexes remain absent. In most cases, the entire conduction system is electrically silent, with no P waves seen on the ECG.

Ventricular asystole usually results from myocardial hypoxia, which may be a consequence of advanced heart failure. It may also be caused by severe hyperkalemia and acidosis. If P waves are seen, asystole is likely because of severe ventricular conduction blocks.

◆ *Interventions: Responding*

When cardiac arrest occurs, cardiac output stops. The underlying rhythm is usually ventricular tachycardia (VT), ventricular fibrillation (VF), or asystole. Without cardiac output, the patient is pulseless and becomes unconscious because of inadequate cerebral PERFUSION and gas exchange. Shortly after cardiac arrest, respiratory arrest occurs. Therefore cardiopulmonary resuscitation is essential to prevent brain damage and death.

Cardiopulmonary Resuscitation and Defibrillation. Cardiopulmonary resuscitation (CPR), also known as Basic Cardiac Life Support (BCLS), must be initiated immediately when asystole occurs. When finding an unresponsive patient, confirm unresponsiveness and call 911 (in community or long-term care setting) or the emergency response team (in the hospital). Gather the AED or defibrillator *before initiating CPR.* Guidelines for CPR have changed from an ABC (airway-breathing-compressions) approach to the initial priorities of CAB (compressions-airway-breathing) (AHA, 2015).

- Check for a carotid pulse for 5 to 10 seconds.
- *If carotid pulse is absent,* start chest **c**ompressions of 100 to 120 **c**ompressions per minute and a compression depth of at least 2 inches with no more than 2.4 inches. Push hard and fast! Avoid leaning into the chest after each compression to allow for full chest wall recoil.
- Maintain a patent **a**irway.
- Ventilate (**b**reathing) with a mouth-to-mask device. Give rescue breaths at a rate of 10 to 12 breaths/min. If an advanced airway is in place, one breath should be given every 6 to 8 seconds (8 to 10 breaths/min).
- Ventilation-to-compression ratio should be maintained at 30 compressions to 2 breaths if advanced airway is not in place.
  - Limit interruptions to compressions to less than 10 seconds.
  - When possible, compressors should be rotated every 2 minutes to maintain effective compressions.

Be sure to use Standard Precautions when administering CPR. Be aware that complications of CPR include:
- Rib fractures
- Fracture of the sternum
- Costochondral separation
- Lacerations of the liver and spleen
- Pneumothorax
- Hemothorax
- Cardiac tamponade
- Lung contusions
- Fat emboli

As soon as help arrives, place a board under the patient who is not on a firm surface. To make room for the resuscitation team and the crash cart, ask that the area be cleared of movable items and unnecessary personnel. When the AED or defibrillator arrives, *do not stop chest compressions while the defibrillator is being set up.* If trained to use the AED or defibrillator, apply hands-off defibrillator pads to the patient's chest and turn on the monitor. If the patient is in VF or pulseless VT, the immediate priority is to defibrillate! Defibrillation, an *asynchronous* countershock, depolarizes a critical mass of myocardium simultaneously to stop the re-entry circuit, allowing the sinus node to regain control of the heart. After defibrillation, CPR is resumed. CPR must continue at all times except during defibrillation.

> **! NURSING SAFETY PRIORITY** **QSEN**
> ### *Critical Rescue*
>
> Early defibrillation is critical in resolving pulseless ventricular tachycardia (VT) or ventricular fibrillation (VF). It must not be delayed for any reason after the equipment and skilled personnel are present. The earlier defibrillation is performed, the greater the chance of survival! *Do not defibrillate ventricular asystole.* The purpose of defibrillation is disruption of the chaotic rhythm. allowing the SA node signals to restart. In ventricular asystole, no electrical impulses are present to disrupt.
>
> Before defibrillation, loudly and clearly command all personnel to clear contact with the patient and the bed and check to see they are clear before the shock is delivered. Deliver shock and immediately resume CPR for 5 cycles or about 2 minutes. Reassess the rhythm every 2 minutes and if indicated. Charge the defibrillator to deliver an additional shock at the same energy level previously used. During the 2-minute intervals while high-quality CPR is being delivered, the Advanced Cardiac Life Support (ACLS) team administers medications and performs interventions to try and restore an organized cardiac rhythm. *Discussion of ACLS protocol is beyond the scope of this text.*

After the ACLS team initiates interventions, the role of the medical-surgical nurse is to provide information about the patient. Specific nursing responsibilities include providing a brief summary of the patient's medical condition and the events that occurred up until the time of cardiac arrest. Report the patient's initial cardiac rhythm. Remain in the room to answer questions, document the event, and assist with compressions. If family is present, provide emotional support and explanation of events in the room.

An emerging clinical practice is allowing or encouraging family presence at resuscitation attempts. This can be a positive experience for family members and significant others because it promotes closure after the death of a loved one. Although there may be staff resistance and some limits to family presence, overall it is a beneficial practice that should be considered in all resuscitation attempts.

When spontaneous circulation resumes, the patient is transported to the intensive care unit. Be ready to give hand-off report to the ICU nurse using SBAR communication or other agency system and assist with patient transport.

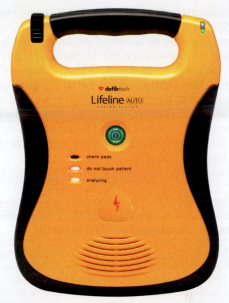

FIG. 34-15 Automated external defibrillator. (Courtesy Defibtech LLC, Guilford, CT).

🔆 NCLEX EXAMINATION CHALLENGE 34-3

Safe and Effective Care Environment

A client in the telemetry unit is on a cardiac monitor. The monitor technician notices that there are no ECG complexes, and the alarm sounds. What is the **first** action by the nurse?

A. Suspend the alarm.
B. Call the emergency response team.
C. Press the record button to get an ECG strip.
D. Assess the client and check lead placement.

👤 CLINICAL JUDGMENT CHALLENGE 34-1

Teamwork and Collaboration; Evidence-Based Practice; Safety QSEN

A 48-year-old male was found unresponsive in the stands at a basketball game. An AED was used on site and delivered a shock to the patient. He was admitted to the hospital following the event. Currently the patient is in sinus rhythm with frequent PVCs and reports intermittent chest pain. HR is 112, BP 92/48, and the patient is dyspneic.

1. What is the initial treatment for this patient at this time?
2. What drugs should you anticipate administering to this patient? Why are they indicated?
3. What evidence-based precautions must be taken to promote safety?
4. If this rhythm deteriorates to ventricular fibrillation or VT without a pulse, what steps should you take? Why?

Automated External Defibrillation. The American Heart Association promotes the use of automated external defibrillators (AEDs) for use by laypersons and health care professionals responding to cardiac arrest emergencies (Fig. 34-15). These devices are found in many public places such as malls, airports, and commercial jets. The patient in cardiac arrest must be on a firm, dry surface. The rescuer places two large adhesive-patch electrodes on the patient's chest in the same positions as for defibrillator electrodes. The rescuer stops CPR and commands anyone present to move away, ensuring that no one is touching the patient. This measure eliminates motion artifact when the machine analyzes the rhythm. The rescuer presses the "analyze" button on the machine. After rhythm analysis, which may take up to 30 seconds, the machine advises either that a shock is necessary or that a shock is not indicated. *Shocks are recommended for VF or pulseless VT only.*

If a shock is indicated, issue a command to clear all contact with the patient and press the charge button. Once the AED is charged, press the shock button, and the shock will be delivered. The shock is delivered through the patches; so it is hands-off

defibrillation, which is safer for the rescuer. The rescuer then resumes CPR until the AED instructs to "stop CPR" to analyze the rhythm. If the rhythm is VF or VT and another shock is indicated, the AED will instruct the rescuer to charge and deliver another shock. Newer AEDs perform rhythm analysis and defibrillation without the need for a rescuer to press a button to analyze or shock the victim. It is essential that Advanced Cardiac Life Support (ACLS) be provided as soon as possible. Use of AEDs allows for earlier defibrillation. Therefore there is a greater chance of successful rhythm conversion and patient survival.

Implantable Cardioverter/Defibrillator. The implantable cardioverter/defibrillator (ICD) is indicated for patients who have experienced one or more episodes of spontaneous sustained ventricular tachycardia (VT) or ventricular fibrillation (VF) not caused by a myocardial infarction (MI). Collaborate with the physician and the electrophysiology nurse to prepare the patient for this procedure. A psychological profile is done to determine whether the patient can cope with the discomfort and fear associated with internal defibrillation from the ICD. Many patients report anxiety, depression, and decreased quality of life, which improves for the majority of patients after 12 months.

Two types of lead systems are available: transvenous and subcutaneous. In the traditional transvenous system, the leads are introduced via the subclavian vein, and the generator is implanted in the left pectoral area, similar to a permanent pacemaker insertion. In the subcutaneous ICD, the leads are tunneled underneath the skin and placed to the left of the sternum to form a right angle just below the xiphoid, where they attach to the generator. The generator is implanted in the left midaxillary chest wall. The subcutaneous ICD is recommended for younger patients (<40 years), patients without venous access, and patients who do not require concomitant pacemaker therapy. This procedure is performed in the electrophysiology laboratory. If the patient experiences a VT or VF episode after ICD placement and the ICD therapies are not successful, the qualified nurse or health care provider promptly externally defibrillates and initiates high-quality CPR.

The generator may be activated or deactivated by the provider placing a magnet over the implantation site for a few moments. The patient requires close monitoring in the postoperative period for dysrhythmias and complications such as bleeding and cardiac tamponade. The nurse must know whether the ICD is activated or deactivated. Care of the patient is similar to that after implantation of a permanent pacemaker, discussed earlier in this chapter. Chart 34-7 highlights the important points for health teaching.

Some patients use a lightweight, automated wearable cardioverter/defibrillator (WCD). This external vestlike device is worn 24 hours a day except when the patient showers or bathes. One popular brand is the Zoll Lifecore LifeVest, which is programmed to monitor for VT and VF. A family member must be present to call 911 and initiate CPR if the patient experiences pulseless VT or VF while in the shower. If the patient is conscious while experiencing VT, he or she can press a button to prevent a shock. This precaution is an advantage over implantable devices because ICDs are programmed to always deliver a shock when VT or VF occurs.

CHART 34-7   Patient and Family Education: Preparing for Self-Management

Implantable Cardioverter/Defibrillator

- Follow the instructions for implantable cardioverter/defibrillator (ICD) site skin care that have been specifically prepared for you.
- Report to your primary health care provider any fever or redness, swelling, soreness, or drainage from your incision site.
- Do not wear tight clothing or belts that could cause irritation over the ICD generator.
- Do not manipulate your generator site.
- Avoid activities that involve rough contact with the ICD implantation site.
- Keep your ICD identification card in your wallet and consider wearing a medical alert bracelet.
- Know the basic functioning of your ICD device, its rate cutoff, and the number of consecutive shocks it can deliver.
- Avoid magnets directly over your ICD because they can inactivate the device. If beeping tones are coming from the ICD, move away from the electromagnetic field immediately (within 30 seconds) before the inactivation sequence is completed and notify your primary health care provider.
- Inform all health care providers caring for you that you have an ICD implanted, because certain diagnostic tests and procedures must be avoided to prevent ICD malfunction. These include diathermy, electrocautery, and nuclear magnetic resonance tests.
- Avoid other sources of electromagnetic interference, such as devices emitting microwaves (not microwave ovens); transformers; radio, television, and radar transmitters; large electrical generators; metal detectors, including handheld security devices at airports; antitheft devices; arc welding equipment; and sources of 60-cycle (Hz) interference.

- Also avoid leaning directly over the alternator of a running motor of a car or boat.
- Report to your primary health care provider symptoms such as fainting, nausea, weakness, blackout, and rapid pulse rates.
- Take all medications prescribed for you as instructed.
- Follow instructions on restrictions on physical activity, such as not swimming, driving motor vehicles, or operating dangerous equipment.
- Keep all health care provider and ICD clinic appointments.
- Sit or lie down immediately if you feel dizzy or faint to avoid falling if the ICD discharges.
- Know how to contact the local emergency medical services (EMS) systems in your community. Inform them in advance that you have an ICD so they can be prepared if they need to respond to an emergency call for you.
- Encourage family members to learn how to perform CPR. Family members should know that, if they are touching you when the device discharges, they may feel a slight shock but this is not harmful to them.
- Follow instructions on what to do if the ICD successfully discharges, after which you feel well. This may include maintaining a diary of the date, the time, activity preceding the shock, symptoms, the number of shocks delivered, and how you feel after the shock. The physician may wish to be notified each time the device discharges.
- Avoid strenuous activities that may cause your heart rate to meet or exceed the rate cutoff of your ICD because this causes the device to discharge inappropriately.
- Notify your primary health care provider for information regarding access to health care if you are leaving town or relocating.

GET READY FOR THE NCLEX® EXAMINATION!

KEY POINTS

Review these Key Points for each NCLEX Examination Client Needs Category.

Safe and Effective Care Environment

- Be very careful to protect patients and staff to prevent electrical injury when assisting with invasive pacemakers, cardioversion, and defibrillation. **QSEN: Safety**
- For safety during cardioversion, turn oxygen off and away from the patient to prevent a fire. Shout "CLEAR" before shock delivery for electrical safety. **QSEN: Safety**
- Teach patients who have permanent pacemakers to keep cell phones at least 6 inches away from the generator, avoid electromagnetic fields such as telecommunication transmitters, wear a medical alert bracelet at all times, and carry a pacemaker identification card. **QSEN: Safety**

Health Promotion and Maintenance

- Teach patients with dysrhythmias the correct drug, dose, route, time, and side effects of prescribed drugs and teach them to notify their primary care provider if adverse effects occur (see Chart 34-4).
- Teach patients taking anticoagulant therapy to report any signs of bruising or unusual bleeding immediately to their primary health care provider.
- Teach family members where to learn cardiopulmonary resuscitation (CPR) to decrease their anxiety while living with a patient with dysrhythmias or ICD/pacemaker. **QSEN: Patient-Centered Care**
- Teach patients the importance of adhering to their prescribed cardiac regimen, such as checking their pulse to ascertain pacemaker function.

Physiological Integrity

- Assess patients with dysrhythmias for a decrease in cardiac output resulting in inadequate gas exchange and perfusion to vital organs (see Chart 34-2); typical assessment findings include shortness of breath, dizziness or syncope, weakness and fatigue, and irregular pulse. **Clinical Judgment**
- Monitor patients with dysrhythmias, including conducting a physical assessment and health history and interpreting ECG rhythm strips. Report significant changes to the primary health care provider. **Clinical Judgment**
- Interpret common dysrhythmias, especially bradycardia, tachycardia, atrial fibrillation (AF) and ventricular fibrillation (VF), premature ventricular contractions (PVCs), and asystole, using the steps of ECG analysis.
- Use special considerations when caring for older adults with dysrhythmias, as described in Chart 34-5. **QSEN: Patient-Centered Care**

- Recognize that noninvasive pacing is an emergency measure to provide demand ventricular pacing in patients with profound bradycardia or asystole. Teach patients to expect possible discomfort.
- Identify and intervene in life-threatening situations by providing cardiopulmonary resuscitation, electrical therapy, or drug administration. **QSEN: Evidence-Based Practice**
- Be aware that automated external defibrillators (AEDs) are used by medical and lay personnel as an essential intervention for VF.
- Do not perform CPR while the patient is being defibrillated. **QSEN: Safety**
- Educate patients who have permanent pacemakers or ICDs about self-management (see Charts 34-3 and 34-7).

SELECTED BIBLIOGRAPHY

Asterisk indicates a classic or definitive work on this subject.

Akintade, B., Chapa, D., Friedmann, E., & Thomas, S. (2015). The influence of depression and anxiety symptoms on health-related quality of life in patients with atrial fibrillation and atrial flutter. *Journal of Cardiovascular Nursing, 30*(1), 66–73.

American Heart Association (AHA). (2015). 2015 guidelines highlights. <https://eccguidelines.heart.org/index.php/guidelines-highlights/>.

Aziz, S., Leon, A., & El-Chami, M. (2014). The subcutaneous defibrillator: A review of the literature. *Journal of the American College of Cardiology, 63*(15), 1473–1479.

Borak, M., Francisco, M., Stokas, M., Maroney, M., Bednar, V., Miller, M., et al. (2014). Every second counts: Innovations to increase timely defibrillation rates. *Journal of Nursing Care Quality, 29*(4), 311–317.

Burchum, J., & Rosenthal, L. (2016). Lehne's pharmacology for nursing care (9th ed.). St. Louis: Elsevier.

*Calkins, H., Kuck, K., Cappato, R., Brugada, J., Camm, A., Chen, S., et al. (2012). 2012 HRS/EHRA/ECAS expert consensus statement on catheter and surgical ablation of atrial fibrillation: Recommendations for patient selection, procedural techniques, patient management and follow-up, definitions, endpoints and research trial design. *Heart Rhythm, 9*(4), 632–696.

Cheng, A., & Hijazi, Z. (2015). Nonpharmacologic therapy to prevent embolization in patients with AF. Up to Date. Retrieved from <www.uptodate.com>.

Copley, D., & Hill, K. (2016). Atrial fibrillation: A review of treatments and current guidelines. *AACN Advanced Critical Care, 27*(1), 120–128.

*Cronin, E., & Varma, N. (2012). Remote monitoring of cardiovascular implanted electronic devices: A paradigm shift for the 21st century. *Expert Reviews, 9*(4), 367–376.

Cutugno, C. (2015). Atrial fibrillation: Updated management guidelines and nursing implications. *American Journal of Nursing, 115*(5), 26–38.

Epstein, A., Abraham, W., Bianco, N., Kern, K., Mirro, M., Rao, S., et al. (2013). Wearable cardioverter-defibrillator use in patients perceived to be at high risk early post-myocardial infarction. *Journal of the American College of Cardiology, 62*(21), 2000–2007.

Food and Drug Administration (FDA). (2015). FDA approves Praxbind, the first reversal agent for the anticoagulant Pradaxa. <www.fda.gov.NewsEvents/Newsroom/PressAnnouncements/ucm467300.htm>.

Frankel, D., Parker, S., Rosenfeld, L., & Gorelick, P. (2014). NRS/NSA 2014 survey of atrial fibrillation and stroke: Gaps in knowledge and perspective, opportunities for improvement. *Heart Rhythm, 12*(8), e105–e113.

Hoke, L., & Streletsky, Y. (2015). Catheter ablation of atrial fibrillation. *American Journal of Nursing, 115*(10), 32–42.

January, C., Wann, S., Alpert, J., Calkins, H., Cigarroa, J., Cleveland, J., et al. (2014). 2014 AHA/ACC/HRS Guideline for the management of patients with atrial fibrillation: Executive Summary. *Journal of the American College of Cardiology, 64*(21), 2246–2280.

*Keseg, D. P. (2010). Reducing interruptions: Continuous compression CPR & minimally interrupted CPR result in improved survival. A *Journal of Emergency Medical Services, 35*(1), 14–17.

*Kireyev, D., Fernandez, S., Gupta, V., Arkhipow, M., & Paris, J. (2012). Targeting tachycardia: Diagnostic tips and tools. *Journal of Family Practice, 61*(5), 258–263.

Klein, H., Goldenberg, I., & Moss, A. (2013). Risk stratification for implantable cardioverter defibrillator therapy: the role of the wearable cardioverter-defibrillator. *European Heart Journal, 34*, 2230–2242.

Lukasewicz, C., & Mattox, E. (2015). Understanding clinical alarm safety. *Critical Care Nurse, 34*(4), 45–55.

Masoudi, F., Caulkins, H., Kavinsky, C., Drozda, J., Gainsley, P., Slotwiner, D., et al. (2015). 2015 ACC/HRS/SCAI left atrial appendage occlusion device societal overview: A professional society overview from the American College of Cardiology, Heart Rhythm Society and Society for Cardiovascular Angiography and Interventions. *Journal of the American College of Cardiology, 66*, 1497–1513.

Mooney, T. (2013). Use of dabigatran to prevent stroke in patients with atrial fibrillation. *Nursing Standard, 27*(27), 35–41.

Nair, V., & Barkley, T. (2015). Percutaneous closure of the left atrial appendage for stroke prevention in atrial fibrillation: An alternative to long-term anticoagulation. *Critical Care Nursing Quarterly, 38*(4), 371–384.

Page, R., Joglar, J., Al-Khatib, S., Caldwell, M., Caulkins, H., Conti, J., et al. (2015). 2015 ACC/AHA/HRS guideline for the management of adult patients with supraventricular tachycardia: Executive summary: a report of the American College of Cardiology/American Heart Association Task Force on clinical practice guidelines and Heart Rhythm Society. *Circulation, 132*, doi:10.1161/CIR0000000000000310.

Palatinus, J., & Das, S. (2015). Your father and grandfather's atrial fibrillation: A review of the genetics of the most common pathological cardiac dysrhythmia. *Current Genomics, 16*(2), 75–81.

*Palmer, B. (2011). Systematic cardiac rhythm strip analysis. *Medsurg Nursing, 20*(2), 96–97.

Pedersen, C., Kay, G. N., Kalman, J., Borggrefe, M., Della-Bella, P., Dickfeld, T., et al. (2014). EHRA/HRS/APHRS expert consensus on ventricular arrhythmias. *Heart Rhythm Society*, 11(10), e166–e196.

Poulidakis, E., & Manolis, A. (2014). Transvenous temporary cardiac pacing. *Hospital Chronicles*, 9(3), 190–198.

*Sellers, M. B., & Newby, L. K. (2011). Atrial fibrillation, anticoagulants, fall risk, and outcomes in elderly patients. *American Heart Journal*, 161(2), 241–246.

Slotwiner, D., Varma, N., Akar, J., Annas, G., Beardsall, M., Fogel, R., et al. (2015). HRS expert consensus statement on remote interrogation and monitoring for cardiovascular implantable electronic devices. *Heart Rhythm*, 12(7), e69–e100.

Spivak, I. (2015). Oral anticoagulants and atrial fibrillation: An update for the clinical nurse. *Medsurg Nursing*, 24(2), 95–100.

Swift, J. (2013). Assessment and treatment of patients with acute unstable bradycardia. *Nursing Standard*, 27(22), 48–56.

*Tracy, C., Epstein, A., Darbar, D., DiMarco, J., Dunbar, S., Estes, M., et al. (2012). 2012 ACCF/AHA/HRS focused update of the 2008 guidelines for device-based therapy of cardiac rhythm abnormalities. *Journal of the American College of Cardiology*, 60(14), 1247–1313. doi:10.1016/j.jacc2012.08.009.

Urden, L., Stacy, K., & Lough, M. (2016). Priorities in critical care nursing (7th ed.). St. Louis: Elsevier.

Vallerand, A., & Sanoski, C. (2017). Davis's Canadian drug guide for nurses (15th ed.). Philadelphia, PA: F.A. Davis.

Walsh-Irwin, C., & Jurgens, C. (2015). Proper skin preparation and electrode placement decreases alarms on a telemetry unit. *Dimensions of Critical Care Nursing*, 34(3), 134–139.

*Wann, L. S., Curtis, A. B., Ellenbogen, K. A., Estes, N. A., III, Ezekowitz, M. D., Jackman, W. M., et al. (2011). 2011 ACCF/AHA/HRS focused update on the management of patients with atrial fibrillation (update on dabigatran): A report of the American College of Cardiology Foundation/American Heart Association Task Force on Practice Guidelines. *Journal of the American College of Cardiology*, 57(11), 1330–1337.

Zarraga, I., & Kron, I. (2013). Oral anticoagulation in elderly adults with atrial fibrillation: Integrating new options with old concepts. *Journal of the American Geriatrics Society*, 61, 143–150. doi:10.1111/jgs.12042.

CHAPTER 35

Care of Patients With Cardiac Problems

Laura M. Dechant

(e) http://evolve.elsevier.com/Iggy/

PRIORITY AND INTERRELATED CONCEPTS

The priority concept for this chapter is PERFUSION.

✳ The PERFUSION concept exemplar for this chapter is Heart Failure, below.

The interrelated concepts for this chapter are:
- GAS EXCHANGE
- COMFORT
- IMMUNITY

LEARNING OUTCOMES

Safe and Effective Care Environment

1. Collaborate with the interprofessional team to provide high-quality care for patients with cardiac problems that impact PERFUSION and GAS EXCHANGE.
2. Teach the patient and caregiver(s) about home safety affected by cardiac problems.
3. Prioritize evidence-based care for patients with common cardiac problems affecting PERFUSION.

Health Promotion and Maintenance

4. Plan care coordination and transition management for patients and caregiver(s) with cardiac problems.
5. Teach the patient and caregiver(s) about drug therapy used for cardiac problems.

Psychosocial Integrity

6. Implement patient and family-centered nursing interventions to decrease the psychosocial impact of living with chronic cardiac problems.

Physiological Integrity

7. Apply knowledge of anatomy and physiology to perform an evidence-based assessment for the patient with a cardiovascular problem.
8. Explain how common drug therapies improve cardiac output, enhance peripheral perfusion, and prevent worsening cardiovascular problems.
9. Plan nursing care to promote PERFUSION and prevent complications such as altered GAS EXCHANGE, altered COMFORT, and altered IMMUNITY in patients with cardiovascular problems.
10. Use clinical judgment to assess laboratory data and signs and symptoms to prioritize nursing care for patients with a cardiovascular problem.
11. Plan postoperative care for patients requiring cardiovascular surgery.
12. Provide emergency care for patients experiencing life-threatening complications, such as cardiac tamponade and pulmonary edema.

Heart failure is the most common reason for hospital stays in patients over 65 years of age in the United States. When the heart is diseased, it cannot effectively pump an adequate amount of arterial blood to the rest of the body. Arterial blood carries *oxygen* and nutrients to vital organs, such as the kidneys and brain, and to peripheral tissues. When these organs and other body tissues are not adequately *perfused*, they may not function properly. This chapter focuses on heart failure and its common causes in the adult population; coronary artery disease is discussed in Chapter 38.

✳ PERFUSION CONCEPT EXEMPLAR Heart Failure

Heart failure, also called *pump failure,* is a general term for the inability of the heart to work effectively as a pump. It results from a number of acute and chronic cardiovascular problems that are discussed in this chapter and within the cardiovascular unit.

❖ PATHOPHYSIOLOGY

Heart failure (HF) is a common *chronic* health problem, with acute episodes often causing hospitalization. Acute coronary disease and other structural or functional problems of the heart can lead to *acute* HF. Both acute and chronic HF can be life threatening if they are not adequately treated or if the patient does not respond to treatment.

Types of Heart Failure

The major types of heart failure are:

- Left-sided heart failure
- Right-sided heart failure
- High-output failure

Because the two ventricles of the heart represent two separate pumping systems, it is possible for one to fail by itself for a short period. *Most heart failure begins with failure of the left ventricle and progresses to failure of both ventricles.* Typical causes of left-sided heart (ventricular) failure include hypertension, coronary artery disease, and valvular disease. Decreased tissue PERFUSION from poor cardiac output and pulmonary congestion from increased pressure in the pulmonary vessels indicate left ventricular failure (LVF).

Left-sided heart failure was formerly referred to as congestive heart failure (CHF); however, not all cases of LVF involve fluid accumulation. In the clinical setting, though, the term *CHF* is still commonly used. Left-sided failure may be acute or chronic and mild to severe. It can be further divided into two subtypes: systolic heart failure and diastolic heart failure.

Systolic heart failure (heart failure with reduced ejection fraction [HFrEF]) results when the heart cannot contract forcefully enough during systole to eject adequate amounts of blood into the circulation. Preload increases with decreased contractility, and afterload increases as a result of increased peripheral resistance (e.g., hypertension) (McCance et al., 2014). The ejection fraction (the percentage of blood ejected from the heart during systole) drops from a normal of 50% to 70% to below 40% with ventricular dilation. As it decreases, tissue PERFUSION diminishes and blood accumulates in the pulmonary vessels. Manifestations of systolic dysfunction may include symptoms of inadequate tissue PERFUSION or pulmonary and systemic congestion. Systolic heart failure is often called *forward failure* because cardiac output is decreased and fluid backs up into the pulmonary system. Because these patients are at high risk for sudden cardiac death, patients with an ejection fraction of less than 30% are considered candidates for an implantable cardioverter/defibrillator (ICD) (see Chapter 34).

In contrast, diastolic heart failure (heart failure with preserved left ventricular function [HFpEF]) occurs when the left ventricle cannot relax adequately during diastole. Inadequate relaxation or "stiffening" prevents the ventricle from filling with sufficient blood to ensure an adequate cardiac output. Although ejection fraction is more than 40%, the ventricle becomes less compliant over time because more pressure is needed to move the same amount of volume compared with a healthy heart. Diastolic failure represents about 20% to 40% of all heart failure, primarily in older adults and in women who have chronic hypertension and undetected coronary artery disease. Signs and symptoms and management of diastolic failure are similar to those of systolic dysfunction (McCance et al., 2014).

Right-sided heart (ventricular) failure may be caused by left ventricular failure, right ventricular myocardial infarction (MI), or pulmonary hypertension. In this type of heart failure (HF), the right ventricle cannot empty completely. Increased volume and pressure develop in the venous system, and peripheral edema results.

High-output heart failure can occur when cardiac output remains normal or above normal, unlike left- and right-sided heart failure, which are typically low-output states. High-output failure is caused by increased metabolic needs or hyperkinetic conditions, such as septicemia, high fever, anemia, and hyperthyroidism. This type of heart failure is not as common as other types.

Classification and Staging of Heart Failure

The American College of Cardiology (ACC) and American Heart Association (AHA) have developed evidence-based guidelines for staging and managing heart failure as a chronic, progressive disease. These guidelines do not replace the New York Heart Association (NYHA) functional classification system, which is used to describe symptoms that a patient may exhibit (see Table 33-2 in Chapter 33).

The ACC/AHA staging system when compared with the NYHA system categorizes patients as:

A. Patients at high risk for developing heart failure (Class I NYHA)

B. Patients with cardiac structural abnormalities or remodeling who have not developed HF symptoms (Class I NYHA)

C. Patients with current or prior symptoms of heart failure (Class II or III NYHA)

D. Patients with refractory end-stage heart failure (Class IV NYHA)

Another method for staging heart failure is the Killip classification system, which is based on the heart's hemodynamic ability. Table 38-3 outlines this system.

Compensatory Mechanisms

When cardiac output is insufficient to meet the demands of the body, compensatory mechanisms work to improve it (Fig. 35-1). Although these mechanisms may initially increase cardiac output, they eventually have a damaging effect on pump function. Major compensatory mechanisms include:

- Sympathetic nervous system stimulation
- Renin-angiotensin system (RAS) activation (also called *renin-angiotensin-aldosterone [RAAS] activation*)
- Other chemical responses
- Myocardial hypertrophy

In heart failure (HF), *stimulation of the sympathetic nervous system* (i.e., increasing catecholamines) as a result of tissue hypoxia represents the most immediate compensatory mechanism. Stimulation of the adrenergic receptors causes an increase in heart rate (beta adrenergic) and blood pressure from vasoconstriction (alpha adrenergic).

Because cardiac output (CO) is the product of heart rate (HR) and stroke volume (SV), an increase in HR results in an immediate *increase in CO*. The HR is limited, though, in its ability to compensate for decreased CO. If it becomes too rapid, diastolic filling time is limited, and CO may start to decline. An increase in HR also significantly increases oxygen demand by the myocardium. If the heart is poorly perfused because of arteriosclerosis, HF may worsen.

Stroke volume (SV) is also *improved* by sympathetic stimulation. Sympathetic stimulation increases venous return to the heart, which further stretches the myocardial fibers causing dilation. According to Starling's law, increased myocardial stretch results in more forceful contraction. More forceful contractions increase SV and CO. After a critical point is reached

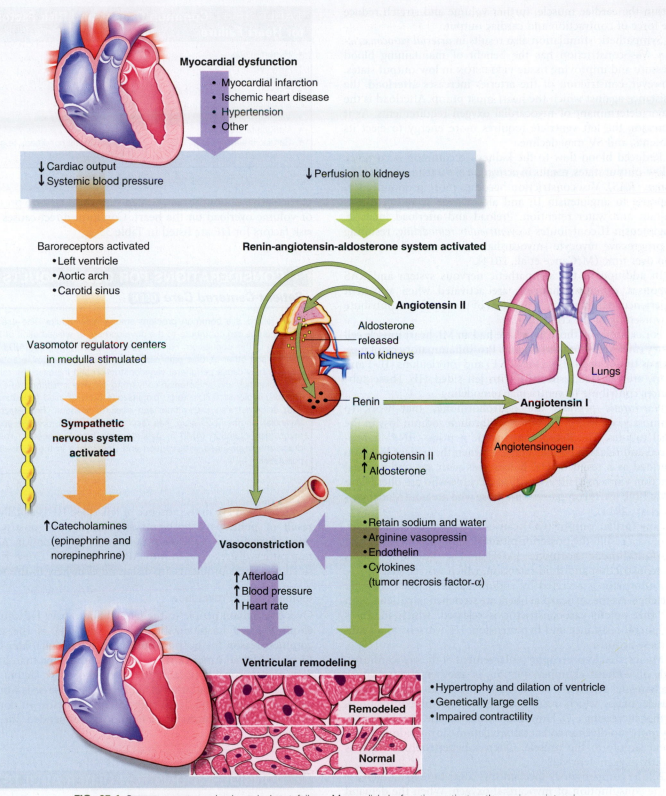

FIG. 35-1 Compensatory mechanisms in heart failure. Myocardial dysfunction activates the renin-angiotensin-aldosterone and sympathetic nervous systems, releasing neurohormones (angiotensin II, aldosterone, catecholamines, and cytokines). (From McCance, K. L., Huether S. E., Brashers, V., & Rote, N. [2014]. *Pathophysiology: The biologic basis for disease in adults and children* [7th ed.]. St. Louis: Mosby. Redrawn from Carelock, J., Clark, A. P. [2001]. *The American Journal of Nursing 101*[12], 27.)

within the cardiac muscle, further volume and stretch reduce the force of contraction and cardiac output.

Sympathetic stimulation also results in *arterial vasoconstriction*. Vasoconstriction has the benefit of maintaining blood pressure and improving tissue PERFUSION in low-output states. However, constriction of the arteries increases afterload, the resistance against which the heart must pump. Afterload is the major determinant of myocardial oxygen requirements. As it increases, the left ventricle requires more energy to eject its contents, and SV may decline.

Reduced blood flow to the kidneys, a common occurrence in low-output states, results in *activation of the renin-angiotensin system (RAS)*. Vasoconstriction becomes more pronounced in response to angiotensin II, and aldosterone secretion causes sodium and water retention. Preload and afterload increase. Angiotensin II contributes to *ventricular remodeling*, resulting in progressive myocyte (myocardial cell) contractile dysfunction over time (McCance et al., 2014).

In addition to the sympathetic nervous system and RAS responses, other mechanisms are activated when a patient experiences heart failure (HF). Most of these actions contribute to worsening of the condition.

For example, in those who have had an MI, heart muscle cell injury causes an *immune response*. Pro-inflammatory cytokines, such as tumor necrosis factor (TNF) and interleukins (IL-1 and IL-6), are released, especially with left-sided HF. These substances contribute to ventricular remodeling.

Natriuretic peptides are neurohormones that work to promote vasodilation and diuresis through sodium loss in the renal tubules. The B-type natriuretic peptide (BNP) is produced and released by the ventricles when the patient has fluid overload as a result of HF. It increases with age and as renal function worsens (Hill et al., 2014). People who are obese have lower BNP levels compared with those who are not (Madamanchi et al., 2014).

Low cardiac output (CO) causes decreased cerebral perfusion. As a result, the posterior pituitary gland secretes *vasopressin* (antidiuretic hormone [ADH]). The hormone causes vasoconstriction and fluid retention, which worsen HF.

Endothelin is secreted by endothelial cells when they are stretched. As the myocardial fibers are stretched in patients with HF, this potent vasoconstrictor is released, which increases peripheral resistance and hypertension. HF worsens as a result of these actions.

Myocardial hypertrophy (enlargement of the myocardium), with or without chamber dilation, is another compensatory mechanism. The walls of the heart thicken to provide more muscle mass, which results in more forceful contractions, further increasing CO. However, cardiac muscle may hypertrophy more rapidly than collateral circulation can provide adequate blood supply to the muscle. Often a hypertrophied heart is slightly oxygen deprived.

All the compensatory mechanisms contribute to an increase in the consumption of myocardial oxygen. When the demand for oxygen increases and the myocardial reserve has been exhausted, signs and symptoms of HF develop.

Etiology

Heart failure (HF) is caused by systemic hypertension in most cases. Some patients experiencing myocardial infarction (MI, "heart attack") also develop HF. The next most common cause is structural heart changes, such as valvular dysfunction,

TABLE 35-1 Common Causes and Risk Factors for Heart Failure

- Hypertension
- Coronary artery disease
- Cardiomyopathy
- Substance abuse (alcohol and illicit/prescribed drugs)
- Valvular disease
- Congenital defects
- Cardiac infections and inflammations
- Dysrhythmias
- Diabetes mellitus
- Smoking/tobacco use
- Family history
- Obesity
- Severe lung disease
- Sleep apnea
- Hyperkinetic conditions (e.g., hyperthyroidism)

particularly pulmonic or aortic stenosis, which leads to pressure or volume overload on the heart. Common direct causes and risk factors for HF are listed in Table 35-1.

CONSIDERATIONS FOR OLDER ADULTS
Patient-Centered Care QSEN

Heart failure is a common problem among older adults. The use of certain drugs can contribute to the development or exacerbation of the problem in this population. For example, long-term use of NSAIDs for arthritis and other chronic pain can cause fluid and sodium retention. NSAIDs may cause peripheral vasoconstriction and increase the toxicity of diuretics and angiotensin-converting enzyme inhibitors (ACEIs). Thiazolidinediones (TZDs) (e.g., pioglitazone [Actos]) used for patients with diabetes) also cause fluid and sodium retention. Rosiglitazone (Avandia), another TZD drug, has recently been found to cause acute myocardial infarction (AMI) in patients with type 2 diabetes. These drugs should be used with caution and restrictions in the older-adult population.

Right-sided HF in the absence of left-sided HF is usually the result of pulmonary problems such as chronic obstructive pulmonary disease (COPD) or pulmonary hypertension. Acute respiratory distress syndrome (ARDS) may also cause right-sided HF. These problems are discussed elsewhere in this text.

Incidence and Prevalence

Over five million people in the United States have HF, causing about 875,000 hospitalizations each year. HF is the most common reason for hospital admission for people older than 65 years. African Americans are affected more often than Euro-Americans, probably because they have more risk factors that can lead to HF (Mozaffarian et al., 2015). The disease is a major cause of disability and death after MI, often because of nonadherence to the treatment plan and recommended lifestyle changes.

CONSIDERATIONS FOR OLDER ADULTS
Patient-Centered Care QSEN

Heart failure has been referred to as a U.S. epidemic, although it is a major problem worldwide. One of the U.S. *Healthy People 2020* objectives is to reduce the number of hospitalizations of older adults with HF as the principal diagnosis. Patient and family education can help meet this objective (Table 35-2). As the "baby boomer" population reaches 65 years of age, the numbers of hospital stays and deaths from HF are likely to increase dramatically.

TABLE 35-2 Meeting *Healthy People* 2020 Objectives

Cardiac Disease

To reduce hospitalizations of older adults with heart failure as the principal diagnosis:

- For patients hospitalized for heart failure, collaborate with the case manager for discharge planning, including adequate support in the community.
- Provide a continuing plan of care for patients and their families or other caregivers when the patient is discharged from the hospital.
- If the patient is discharged to home, call to check that he or she has no impending signs and symptoms of heart failure (the case manager may make calls).
- Teach the patient and family or other caregiver about when to call the health care provider for health changes so the patient can be treated at home.
- Ensure that the interprofessional team provides the patient with follow-up care in the home or nursing home.

❖ **INTERPROFESSIONAL COLLABORATIVE CARE**

◆ **Assessment: Noticing**

History. When obtaining a history, keep in mind the many conditions that can lead to HF. Carefully question the patient about his or her medical history, including hypertension, angina (cardiac pain), MI, rheumatic heart disease, valvular disorders, endocarditis, and pericarditis. Ask about the patient's perception of his or her activity tolerance, breathing pattern, sleeping pattern, urinary pattern, and fluid volume status and his or her knowledge about HF.

Left-Sided Heart Failure. With left ventricular systolic dysfunction, cardiac output (CO) is diminished, leading to impaired tissue PERFUSION, anaerobic metabolism, and unusual fatigue. Assess activity tolerance by asking whether the patient can perform normal ADLs or climb flights of stairs without fatigue or dyspnea. Many patients with heart failure (HF) experience weakness or fatigue with activity or have a feeling of heaviness in their arms or legs. Ask about their ability to perform simultaneous arm and leg work (e.g., walking while carrying a bag of groceries). Such activity may place an unacceptable demand on the failing heart. Ask the patient to identify his or her most strenuous activity in the past week. Many people unconsciously limit their activities in response to fatigue or dyspnea and may not realize how limited they have become.

Perfusion to the myocardium is often impaired as a result of left ventricular failure, especially with cardiac hypertrophy. The patient may report *chest discomfort* or may describe palpitations, skipped beats, or a fast heartbeat.

As the amount of blood ejected from the left ventricle diminishes, hydrostatic pressure builds in the pulmonary venous system and results in fluid-filled alveoli and pulmonary congestion, which results in a *cough*. The patient in early HF describes the cough as irritating, nocturnal (at night), and usually nonproductive. *As HF becomes very severe, he or she may begin expectorating frothy, pink-tinged sputum—a sign of life-threatening pulmonary edema.*

Dyspnea also results from increasing pulmonary venous pressure and pulmonary congestion. Carefully question about the presence of dyspnea and when and how it developed. The patient may refer to dyspnea as "trouble catching my breath," "breathlessness," or "difficulty breathing."

▷▷ **CHART 35-1 Key Features**

Left Ventricular Failure

Decreased Cardiac Output	Pulmonary Congestion
• Fatigue	• Hacking cough, worse at night
• Weakness	• Dyspnea/breathlessness
• Oliguria during the day (nocturia at night)	• Crackles or wheezes in lungs
• Angina	• Frothy, pink-tinged sputum
• Confusion, restlessness	• Tachypnea
• Dizziness	• S_3/S_4 summation gallop
• Tachycardia, palpitations	
• Pallor	
• Weak peripheral pulses	
• Cool extremities	

As **exertional dyspnea** develops (also called *dyspnea upon* or *on exertion [DUE/DOE]*), the patient often stops previously tolerated levels of activity because of shortness of breath. Dyspnea at rest in the recumbent (lying flat) position is known as **orthopnea**. Ask how many pillows are used to sleep or whether the patient sleeps in an upright position in a bed, recliner, or other type of chair.

Patients who describe sudden awakening with a feeling of breathlessness 2 to 5 hours after falling asleep have **paroxysmal nocturnal dyspnea (PND)**. Sitting upright, dangling the feet, or walking usually relieves this condition.

Right-Sided Heart Failure. Signs of systemic congestion occur as the right ventricle fails, fluid is retained, and pressure builds in the venous system. Edema develops in the lower legs and may progress to the thighs and abdominal wall. Patients may notice that their shoes fit more tightly, or their shoes or socks may leave indentations on their swollen feet. They may have removed their rings because of swelling in their fingers and hands. Ask about weight gain. An adult may retain 4 to 7 liters of fluid (10 to 15 lb [4.5 to 6.8 kg]) before pitting edema occurs.

Reports of *nausea and anorexia* may be a direct consequence of liver engorgement (congestion) resulting from fluid retention. In *advanced* heart failure (HF), *ascites* and an increased abdominal girth may develop from severe liver congestion. Another common finding related to fluid retention is *diuresis at rest*. At rest, fluid in the peripheral tissue is mobilized and excreted, and the patient describes frequent awakening at night to urinate.

Obtain a careful nutritional history, questioning about the use of salt and the types of food consumed. Ask about daily fluid intake. Patients with HF may experience increased thirst and drink excessive fluid (4000 to 5000 mL/day) because of sodium retention.

Physical Assessment/Signs and Symptoms. Signs and symptoms of HF depend on the type of failure, the ventricle involved, and the underlying cause. Impaired tissue PERFUSION and pulmonary congestion are associated with *left* ventricular failure (Chart 35-1). Conversely, systemic venous congestion and peripheral edema are associated with *right* ventricular failure (Chart 35-2).

Left-Sided Heart Failure. Left ventricular failure is associated with decreased cardiac output and elevated pulmonary venous pressure. It may appear clinically as:

- Weakness
- Fatigue

CHART 35-2   Key Features

Right Ventricular Failure

Systemic Congestion
- Jugular (neck vein) distention
- Enlarged liver and spleen
- Anorexia and nausea
- Dependent edema (legs and sacrum)
- Distended abdomen
- Swollen hands and fingers
- Polyuria at night
- Weight gain
- Increased blood pressure (from excess volume) or decreased blood pressure (from failure)

- Dizziness
- Acute confusion
- Pulmonary congestion
- Breathlessness
- Oliguria (scant urine output)

Decreased blood flow to the major body organs can cause dysfunction, especially renal failure. Nocturia may occur when the patient is at rest.

The pulse may be tachycardic, or it may alternate in strength (**pulsus alternans**). Take the apical pulse for a full minute, noting any irregularity in heart rhythm. *An irregular heart rhythm resulting from premature atrial contractions (PACs), premature ventricular contractions (PVCs), or atrial fibrillation (AF) is common in HF* (see Chapter 34). The sudden development of an irregular rhythm may further compromise CO. Carefully monitor the patient's respiratory rate, rhythm, and character, as well as oxygen saturation. The respiratory rate typically exceeds 20 breaths/min.

Assess whether the patient is oriented to person, place, and time. A short mental status examination may be used if there are concerns about orientation. Objective assessment is important because many people are skillful at covering up memory loss. Older adults are frequently disoriented or confused when the heart fails as a result of brain hypoxia (decreased oxygen).

Increased heart size is common with a displacement of the apical impulse to the left. A third heart sound, S_3 **gallop**, is an early diastolic filling sound indicating an increase in left ventricular pressure. This sound is often the first sign of HF. A fourth heart sound (S_4) also can occur; it is not a sign of failure but is a reflection of decreased ventricular compliance.

Auscultate for crackles and wheezes of the lungs. Late inspiratory crackles and fine profuse crackles that repeat themselves from breath to breath and do not diminish with coughing indicate HF. *Crackles are produced by intra-alveolar fluid and are often noted first in the bases of the lungs and spread upward as the condition worsens.* Wheezes indicate a narrowing of the bronchial lumen caused by engorged pulmonary vessels. Identify the precise location of crackles and wheezes and whether the wheezes are heard on inspiration, expiration, or both.

Right-Sided Heart Failure. Right ventricular failure is associated with increased systemic venous pressures and congestion. On inspection, assess the neck veins for distention and measure abdominal girth. Hepatomegaly (liver engorgement), hepatojugular reflux, and ascites may also be assessed. Abdominal fluid can reach volumes of more than 10 liters. When the fluid accumulates in the abdomen, pressure is placed on the stomach and intestines. This pressure can lead to early satiety and malnutrition.

Assess for dependent edema. In ambulatory patients, edema commonly presents in the ankles and legs. When patients are restricted to bedrest, the sacrum is dependent, and fluid accumulates there.

 ! NURSING SAFETY PRIORITY QSEN

Action Alert

Edema is an extremely unreliable sign of HF. Be sure that accurate daily weights are taken to document fluid retention. Assessing weight at the same time of the morning using the same scale is important. *Weight is the most reliable indicator of fluid gain and loss!*

? NCLEX EXAMINATION CHALLENGE 35-1

Physiological Integrity

A client is diagnosed with right-sided heart failure. Which assessment findings will the nurse expect the client to have? **Select all that apply.**
A. Peripheral edema
B. Crackles in both lungs
C. Increased abdominal girth
D. Ascites
E. Tachypnea

Psychosocial Assessment. Chronic heart failure (HF) typically is a slow, debilitating disease. Anxiety and frustration are common. Symptoms such as dyspnea increase the patient's anxiety level.

Patients with HF, especially those with advanced disease, are at high risk for depression. It is not certain whether the functional impairments contribute to the depression or depression affects functional ability. Older hospitalized patients may be depressed, particularly those who have been re-admitted for an acute episode of HF. Lifestyle changes and quality-of-life issues can also cause depression many months after the initial diagnosis of HF.

Assess patients and their families for anxiety and depression. Ask them about their usual methods of coping and any history of depression. If anxiety or depression is present, notify the primary health care provider for further assessment. Social workers, certified clinical chaplains, or psychologists may administer specific assessment tools to determine the extent of the problem. Some patients need drug therapy and nonpharmacologic modalities, such as cognitive behavior therapy, biofeedback, or relaxation training.

Hope is a major indicator of well-being for patients with HF. Those who are hopeful tend to feel better and are more socially involved. Ask patients about their daily activities and how often they interact with the significant people in their life to help determine patient and family coping strategies.

Laboratory Assessment. Electrolyte imbalance may occur from complications of HF or as side effects of drug therapy, especially diuretic therapy. Regular evaluations of a patient's serum electrolytes, including sodium, potassium, magnesium, calcium, and chloride, are essential. Any impairment of renal function resulting from inadequate perfusion causes elevated blood urea nitrogen and serum creatinine and decreased creatinine clearance levels. Hemoglobin and hematocrit tests should be performed to identify HF resulting from anemia. If the patient has fluid volume excess, the hematocrit levels may be low as a result of hemodilution.

B-type natriuretic peptide (BNP) is used for diagnosing HF (in particular, diastolic HF) in patients with acute dyspnea. As discussed earlier, it is part of the body's response to decreased cardiac output (CO) from either left or right ventricular dysfunction. An absence of elevation in BNP, in conjunction with history and physical, rules out HF as the cause of acute dyspnea and points to a primary lung dysfunction (Hill et al., 2014). Patients with renal disease may have elevated BNP levels (Hill et al., 2014). In the ambulatory care setting, BNP trends may be used over time to guide ambulatory care treatment (Traughton et al., 2014). As therapy is optimized, BNP levels decrease. If BNP levels increase, alternate causes such as ischemia are considered before intensifying treatment.

Urinalysis may reveal proteinuria and high specific gravity. *Microalbuminuria* is an early indicator of decreased compliance of the heart and occurs before the BNP rises. It serves as an "early warning detector" that lets the primary health care provider know that the heart is experiencing early signs of decreased compliance long before symptoms occur.

⚙ CONSIDERATIONS FOR OLDER ADULTS
Patient-Centered Care QSEN

> Thyroxine (T_4) and thyroid-stimulating hormone (TSH) levels should be assessed in patients who are older than 65 years, have atrial fibrillation, or have evidence of thyroid disease. Heart failure (HF) may be caused or aggravated by hypothyroidism or hyperthyroidism.

Arterial blood gas (ABG) values often reveal hypoxemia (low blood oxygen level) because oxygen does not diffuse easily through fluid-filled alveoli. Respiratory alkalosis may occur because of hyperventilation; respiratory acidosis may occur because of carbon dioxide retention. Metabolic acidosis may indicate an accumulation of lactic acid.

Imaging Assessment. Chest x-rays can be helpful in diagnosing left ventricular failure. Typically the heart is enlarged (cardiomegaly), representing hypertrophy or dilation. Pleural effusions develop less often and generally reflect biventricular failure. *Echocardiography is considered the best tool in diagnosing heart failure.* Cardiac valvular changes, pericardial effusion, chamber enlargement, and ventricular hypertrophy can be diagnosed with this noninvasive technique. The test can also be used to determine ejection fraction.

Radionuclide studies (thallium imaging or technetium pyrophosphate scanning) can also indicate the presence and cause of HF. Multigated acquisition (MUGA) scans, also called *multigated blood pool scans,* provide information about left ventricular ejection fraction and velocity, which are typically low in patients with HF. These tests are discussed in Chapter 33.

Other Diagnostic Assessment. An *electrocardiogram* (ECG) is also performed. It may show ventricular hypertrophy; dysrhythmias; and any degree of myocardial ischemia, injury, or infarction. However, it is *not* helpful in determining the presence or extent of HF.

Invasive hemodynamic monitoring allows the direct assessment of cardiac function and volume status in acutely ill patients. Although medical-surgical nurses do not manage these systems on general hospital units, they should be familiar with the interpretation of some of the major hemodynamic pressures as they relate to patient assessment. These measurements can confirm the diagnosis and guide the management of HF. For example, right atrial pressure is either normal or elevated in left ventricular failure and elevated in right ventricular failure. Pulmonary artery pressure (PAP) and pulmonary artery wedge pressure (PAWP) are elevated in left-sided HF because volumes and pressures are increased in the left ventricle. Hemodynamic monitoring is described in Chapter 38.

◆ *Analysis: Interpreting*

The priority collaborative problems for most patients with heart failure (HF) include:

1. Decreased gas exchange due to ventilation/perfusion imbalance
2. Potential for decreased PERFUSION due to inadequate cardiac output
3. Fatigue due to hypoxemia
4. Potential for pulmonary edema due to left-sided HF

◆ *Planning and Implementation: Responding*

The patient-centered collaborative care that patients with HF need depends on their disease stage and severity of signs and symptoms. Be sure to individualize care based on the patient's values and preferences, your clinical expertise, and best current evidence.

Increasing Gas Exchange

Planning: Expected Outcomes. The expected outcome is that the patient will have an optimal spontaneous breathing pattern that increases GAS EXCHANGE and maintains a serum carbon dioxide level that is within normal limits.

Interventions. The purpose of collaborative care is to help promote GAS EXCHANGE. *Ventilation assistance* may be needed because the oxygen content of the blood is often decreased in patients who have pulmonary congestion. Monitor the patient's respiratory rate, rhythm, and quality every 1 to 4 hours. Auscultate breath sounds every 4 to 8 hours.

❗ NURSING SAFETY PRIORITY QSEN
Action Alert

> Provide the necessary amount of supplemental oxygen within a range prescribed by the health care provider *to maintain oxygen saturation at 90% or greater.* If the patient has dyspnea, place in a high-Fowler's position with pillows under each arm to maximize chest expansion and improve gas exchange. Repositioning and performing coughing and deep-breathing exercises every 2 hours helps to improve gas exchange and prevents atelectasis. Interprofessional collaboration with the respiratory therapist is important to plan the most effective methods for assisting with ventilation.

Increasing Perfusion

Planning: Expected Outcomes. The expected outcome is that the patient will have increased perfusion with adequate cardiac output.

Interventions. Collaborative care begins with nonsurgical interventions, but the patient may need surgery if these are not successful in meeting optimal outcomes.

Nonsurgical Management. Nonsurgical management relies primarily on a variety of drugs (Table 35-3). If drug therapy is ineffective, other nonsurgical options are available. Drugs to

TABLE 35-3 Commonly Used Drug Classifications for Patients With Systolic Heart Failure

Angiotensin-converting enzyme (ACE) inhibitors or angiotensin-receptor blockers (ARBs)

Diuretics:
- High-ceiling
- Potassium-sparing

Human B-type natriuretic peptides

Nitrates

Inotropics:
- Beta-adrenergic agonists
- Phosphodiesterase inhibitors
- Calcium sensitizers
- Digoxin (Lanoxin)

Beta-adrenergic blockers

Angiotensin receptor neprilysin inhibitor (ARNI):
- Sacubitril/valsartan (Entresto)

Aldosterone antagonist

HCN Channel blocker
- Ivabradine (Corlanor)

HCN, Hyperpolarization-activated cyclic nucleotide-gated.

improve stroke volume include those that reduce afterload, reduce preload, and improve cardiac muscle contractility. A major role of the nurse is to give medications as prescribed, monitor for their therapeutic and adverse effects, and teach the patient and family about drug therapy.

Drugs That Reduce Afterload. By relaxing the arterioles, arterial vasodilators can reduce the resistance to left ventricular ejection (afterload) and improve cardiac output (CO). These drugs do not cause excessive vasodilation but reverse some of the inappropriate or excessive vasoconstriction common in HF.

Angiotensin-Converting Enzyme Inhibitors and Angiotensin-Receptor Blockers. Patients with even mild heart failure (HF) resulting from left ventricular dysfunction are given a trial of angiotensin-converting enzyme (ACE) inhibitors or angiotensin-receptor blockers (ARBs). Both ACE inhibitors (e.g., enalapril [Vasotec] and fosinopril [Monopril]) and ARBs (e.g., valsartan [Diovan], irbesartan [Avapro], and losartan [Cozaar]) improve function and quality of life for patients with HF. ACE inhibitors are the first-line drug of choice, but some health care providers prefer to start the patient on an ARB because ACE inhibitors can cause a nagging, dry cough. For patients with *acute* HF, the health care provider may prescribe an IV-push ACE inhibitor such as Vasotec IV.

The ACE inhibitors and ARBs suppress the renin-angiotensin system (RAS), which is activated in response to decreased renal blood flow. ACE inhibitors prevent conversion of angiotensin I to angiotensin II, resulting in arterial dilation and increased stroke volume. ARBs block the effect of angiotensin II receptors and thus decrease arterial resistance and arterial dilation. In addition, these drugs block aldosterone, which prevents sodium and water retention, thus decreasing fluid overload. *Both ACEIs and ARBs work more effectively for Euro-Americans than for African-American populations.* Volume-depleted patients should receive a low starting dose, or the fluid volume should be restored before beginning the prescribed drug. Monitor for hyperkalemia, a potential adverse drug effect in patients who have renal dysfunction.

A new combination medication, sacubitril/valsartan (Entresto), has demonstrated a reduction in death and hospitalization in patients with Class II-IV HF with a decreased ejection fraction. Entresto is a first-in-class medication as an angiotensin receptor neprilysin inhibitor (ARNI). It is used in place of an ACE inhibitor or ARB and should not be given in patients with a history of angioedema. Other side effects are similar to those of ACE inhibitors and include hypotension, hyperkalemia, cough, dizziness, and renal failure. Monitor potassium and creatinine levels while on therapy.

> ! **NURSING SAFETY PRIORITY** QSEN
> ### Drug Alert
>
> ACEIs and ARBs are started slowly and cautiously. The first dose may be associated with a rapid drop in blood pressure (BP). Patients at risk for hypotension usually have an initial systolic BP less than 100 mm Hg, are older than 75 years, have a serum sodium level less than 135 mEq/L, or are volume depleted. Monitor BP every hour for several hours after the initial dose and each time the dose is increased. Immediately report to the health care provider and document a systolic blood pressure of less than 90 mm Hg (or designated protocol level). If this problem occurs, place the patient flat and elevate legs to increase cerebral perfusion and promote venous return.

Assess for orthostatic hypotension, acute confusion, poor peripheral perfusion, and reduced urine output in patients with low systolic blood pressure. Monitor serum potassium and creatinine levels to determine renal dysfunction.

Human B-Type Natriuretic Peptides. Human B-type natriuretic peptides (hBNPs) such as nesiritide (Natrecor) are often used to treat *acute* HF. Endogenous BNP is released in response to decreased CO and causes *natriuresis,* or loss of sodium in the renal tubules, and vasodilation. Natrecor lowers pulmonary capillary wedge pressure (PCWP) and improves renal glomerular filtration. It is given as an IV bolus over 60 seconds followed with a continuous infusion for up to 48 hours.

> ! **NURSING SAFETY PRIORITY** QSEN
> ### Drug Alert
>
> When giving Natrecor, monitor BP and pulse carefully because significant decreases in BP may occur. Although the patient's systolic BP may be between 90 and 100 mm Hg, he or she is usually asymptomatic. *Give Natrecor through a separate infusion line because it is incompatible with heparin and most other parenteral medications.* Expect an increase in the serum BNP after drug administration.

Interventions That Reduce Preload. Ventricular fibers contract less forcefully when they are overstretched, such as in a failing heart. Interventions aimed at reducing preload attempt to decrease volume and pressure in the left ventricle, increasing ventricular muscle stretch and contraction. Preload reduction is appropriate for HF accompanied by congestion with total body sodium and water overload.

Nutrition Therapy. In HF, nutrition therapy is aimed at reducing sodium and water retention to decrease the workload of the heart. The primary care provider may restrict sodium intake in an attempt to decrease fluid retention. Many patients need to omit table salt (no added salt) from their diet, thus reducing sodium intake to about 3 g daily.

If salt intake must be reduced further, the patient may need to eliminate high-sodium foods (e.g., ham, bacon, pickles) and all salt in cooking, thus reducing sodium intake to 2 g daily. If needed, collaborate with the dietitian to help the patient select foods that meet such a restricted therapeutic diet. There is no current evidence to suggest that less than 2 g of sodium daily is helpful; in fact, it may be harmful (Reilly et al., 2015)

Few patients are placed on severe fluid restrictions. However, patients with excessive aldosterone secretion may experience thirst and drink 3 to 5 liters of fluid each day. As a result, their fluid intake may be limited to a more normal 2 liters daily. *Supervise unlicensed assistive personnel (UAP) to ensure that they limit the prescribed intake and accurately record intake and output.*

Weigh the patient daily or delegate this activity to UAP and supervise that it is done. Keep in mind that *1 kg of weight gain or loss equals 1 liter of retained or lost fluid.* The same scale should be used every morning before breakfast for the most accurate assessment of weight. Monitor for an expected *decrease* in weight because excess fluid is excreted from the body.

Drug Therapy. Common drugs prescribed to reduce preload are diuretics and venous vasodilators. *Morphine sulfate* is also given for patients in *acute* HF to reduce anxiety, decrease preload and afterload, slow respirations, and reduce pain associated with a myocardial infarction (MI).

The primary health care provider adds *diuretics* to the regimen when diet and fluid restrictions have not been effective in managing the symptoms of HF. Diuretics are the first-line drug of choice in older adults with HF and fluid overload. These drugs enhance the renal excretion of sodium and water by reducing circulating blood volume, decreasing preload, and reducing systemic and pulmonary congestion.

The type and dosage of diuretic prescribed depend on the severity of HF and renal function. Loop diuretics such as furosemide (Lasix), torsemide (Demadex), and bumetanide (Burinex ♣) are most effective for treating fluid volume overload.

🌐 CONSIDERATIONS FOR OLDER ADULTS

Patient-Centered Care **QSEN**

> Loop diuretics continue to work even after excess fluid is removed. As a result, some patients, especially older adults, can become dehydrated. Observe for signs of dehydration in the older adult, especially acute confusion, decreased urinary output, and dizziness. Provide evidence-based interventions to reduce the risk for falls, as discussed in Chapter 3.

For patients with *acute* HF, furosemide (Lasix) or bumetanide (Burinex ♣) can be administered by IV push (IVP). Lasix can be given in doses of 20 to 40 mg IVP and increased by 20 mg every 2 hours until the desired diuresis is obtained. The usual IVP initial dose for bumetanide is 1 to 2 mg once or twice daily, but it is more often given in a continuous infusion of 10 mg over 24 hours.

The health care provider may initially prescribe a thiazide diuretic, such as hydrochlorothiazide (HCTZ) (Microzide, Urozide ♣) and metolazone (Zaroxolyn), for *older adults* with *mild* volume overload. Zaroxolyn is a long-acting agent and therefore is often given every second, third, or fourth day, depending on patient need and tolerance.

Unlike loop diuretics, the action of thiazides is self-limiting (i.e., diuresis decreases after edema fluid is lost). Therefore the dehydration that may occur with loop diuretics is not common

with these drugs. Patients also prefer thiazides because of the gradual onset of diuresis.

As HF progresses, many patients develop diuretic resistance with refractory edema. The health care provider may choose to manage this problem by prescribing both types of diuretics. Other strategies include IV continuous infusion of furosemide or bumetanide or rotating loop diuretics.

Monitor for and prevent potassium deficiency (hypokalemia) from diuretic therapy. The primary signs of hypokalemia are nonspecific neurologic and muscular symptoms, such as generalized weakness, depressed reflexes, and irregular heart rate. A potassium supplement may be prescribed for some patients. Other practitioners prescribe a potassium-sparing diuretic, such as spironolactone (Aldactone), for patients at risk for dysrhythmias from hypokalemia. Although not as effective as other diuretics, spironolactone helps retain potassium, which decreases the risk for ventricular dysrhythmias, and is usually used in stage III/IV heart failure. Monitor for hyperkalemia and renal failure and anticipate stopping the medication if potassium or creatinine levels rise.

Patients being managed with ACE inhibitors or ARBs and diuretics at the same time may not experience hypokalemia. However, if their kidneys are not functioning well, they may develop hyperkalemia (elevated serum potassium level). Review the patient's serum creatinine level. *If the creatinine is greater than 1.8 mg/dL, notify the health care provider before administering supplemental potassium.*

The health care provider may prescribe *venous vasodilators* (e.g., nitrates) for the patient with HF who has persistent dyspnea. Significant constriction of venous and arterial blood vessels occurs to compensate for reduced CO. Constriction reduces the volume of fluid that the vascular bed can hold and increases preload. Venous vasodilators may benefit by:

- Returning venous vasculature to a more normal capacity
- Decreasing the volume of blood returning to the heart
- Improving left ventricular function

Nitrates may be administered IV, orally, or topically. IV nitrates are used most often for *acute* HF. These drugs cause primarily venous vasodilation but also a significant amount of arteriolar vasodilation. Monitor the patient's blood pressure when starting nitrate therapy or increasing the dosage. Patients may initially report headache, but assure them that they will develop a tolerance to this effect and that the headache will cease or diminish. Acetaminophen (Tylenol, Exdol) can be given to help relieve discomfort.

Unfortunately, tolerance to the vasodilating effects develops when nitrates are given around-the-clock. To prevent this tolerance, the health care provider may prescribe at least one 12-hour nitrate-free period out of every 24 hours (usually overnight). Nitrates such as isosorbide (Imdur, ISMO) are prescribed to provide nitrate-free periods and reduce the problem of tolerance. Chapter 38 discusses nitrates in more detail.

Drugs That Enhance Contractility. Contractility of the heart can also be enhanced with drug therapy. Positive inotropic drugs are most commonly used, but vasodilators and beta-adrenergic blockers may also be administered. For *chronic* HF, low-dose beta blockers are most commonly used. Digoxin (Lanoxin) may be prescribed to improve symptoms, thereby decreasing dyspnea and improving functional activity. This older and long-used drug is not expensive. In some settings, nesiritide (Natrecor) may be administered for end-stage HF, although this drug is very expensive (see discussion of nesiritide [Natrecor] for acute HF later in this chapter).

Digoxin. Although not as commonly used today, digoxin (Lanoxin, Novo-digoxin), a cardiac glycoside, has been demonstrated to provide symptomatic benefits for patients in *chronic heart failure (HF)* with sinus rhythm and atrial fibrillation. Digoxin (sometimes called *dig*) therapy reduces exacerbations of HF and hospitalizations when added to a regimen of ACE inhibitors or ARBs, beta blockers, and diuretics. However, it may increase mortality as a result of drug toxicity, especially in older adults.

The potential benefits of digoxin include:

- Increased contractility
- Reduced heart rate (HR)
- Slowing of conduction through the atrioventricular node
- Inhibition of sympathetic activity while enhancing parasympathetic activity

Digoxin is absorbed from the GI tract erratically. Many drugs, especially antacids, interfere with its absorption. It is eliminated primarily by renal excretion. Older patients should be maintained on lower doses of the drug than younger patients.

❓ NCLEX EXAMINATION CHALLENGE 35-2

Physiological Integrity

An 84-year-old client with heart failure presents to the emergency department (ED) with confusion, blurry vision, and an upset stomach. Which assessment data are **most** concerning to the nurse?

A. Digoxin (Lanoxin) therapy daily
B. Daily metoprolol (Lopressor)
C. Furosemide (Lasix) twice daily
D. Currently taking an antacid for upset stomach

⚠ NURSING SAFETY PRIORITY QSEN

Drug Alert

Increased cardiac automaticity occurs with toxic digoxin levels or in the presence of hypokalemia, resulting in ectopic beats (e.g., premature ventricular contractions [PVCs]). Changes in potassium level, especially a decrease, cause patients to be more sensitive to the drug and cause toxicity.

The signs and symptoms of digoxin toxicity are often vague and nonspecific and include anorexia, fatigue, blurred vision, and changes in mental status, especially in older adults. Toxicity may cause nearly any dysrhythmia, but PVCs are most commonly noted. Assess for early signs of toxicity such as bradycardia and loss of the P wave on the ECG. Carefully monitor the apical pulse rate and heart rhythm of patients receiving digoxin.

The health care provider determines the desirable heart rate (HR) to achieve. Some health care providers prefer a rate between 50 and 60 beats/min. Report the development of either an irregular rhythm in a patient with a previously regular rhythm or a regular rhythm in a patient with a previously irregular one. Monitor serum digoxin and potassium levels (hypokalemia potentiates digoxin toxicity) to identify toxicity. Older adults are more likely than other patients to become toxic because of decreased renal excretion.

Any drug that increases the workload of the failing heart also increases its oxygen requirement. Be alert for the possibility that the patient may experience angina (chest pain) in response to digoxin.

Other Inotropic Drugs. Patients experiencing *acute* heart failure are candidates for IV drugs that increase contractility. For example, *beta-adrenergic agonists,* such as dobutamine (Dobutrex), are used for short-term treatment of *acute* episodes of HF. Dobutamine improves cardiac contractility and thus cardiac output and myocardial-systemic perfusion.

A more potent drug used for *acute* HF, milrinone (Primacor), functions as a vasodilator/inotropic agent with phosphodiesterase activity. Also known as a *phosphodiesterase inhibitor,* this drug increases cyclic adenosine monophosphate (cAMP), which enhances the entry of calcium into myocardial cells to increase contractile function. Like the beta-adrenergic agonists, Primacor is given IV.

Levosimendan (Simdax) is a calcium-sensitizing medication and a positive inotropic drug. It appears to bind to troponin C in the heart muscle and therefore increases the contraction of the heart. Simdax is used most often in patients who have had or are at high risk for myocardial infarction. Chapter 38 discusses inotropic drugs in more detail.

Beta-Adrenergic Blockers. Beta-adrenergic blockers (commonly referred to as *beta blockers*) improve the condition of some patients in HF. Prolonged exposure to increased levels of sympathetic stimulation and catecholamines worsens cardiac function. Beta-adrenergic blockade reverses this effect, improving morbidity, mortality, and quality of life for patients in HF.

Beta blockers must be started slowly for HF. *Patients in acute HF should not be started on these drugs.* Carvedilol (Coreg), metoprolol succinate (Toprol XL, Betaloc ✦), and bisoprolol (Zebeta) are approved for treatment of *chronic* HF. **Do not confuse metoprolol tartrate with metoprolol succinate.** Current guidelines only recommend the sustained-release formulation of metoprolol for chronic HF treatment. The first dose is extremely low. Monitor the patient either in the hospital or in the primary health care provider's office to assess for bradycardia or hypotension after the first dose is given.

Instruct the patient to weigh daily and report any signs of worsening HF immediately. The primary health care provider gradually increases the drug dose if HF worsens. The patient is evaluated at least weekly for changes in BP, pulse, activity tolerance, and orthopnea. A modest drop in BP is acceptable if he or she remains asymptomatic and can stand without experiencing dizziness or a further drop in BP. The resting heart rate (HR) should remain between 55 and 60 and increase slightly with exercise. Activity tolerance improves, and less orthopnea is experienced. Most patients with mild and moderate HF demonstrate improved ejection fraction, decreased hospital admissions, and improvement in symptoms when beta blockers are added to their treatment regimens. The benefits of this therapy are seen over a long period rather than immediately.

Aldosterone Antagonists. Those with Class II-IV HF with EF <35% or history of diabetes should be prescribed aldosterone antagonists (spironolactone [Aldactone] or eplerenone [Inspra]). As a potassium-sparing diuretic, aldosterone antagonists decrease the risk for dysrhythmias from hypokalemia. Aldosterone antagonists also block the effect of aldosterone, which decreases the amount of water and sodium retained. Monitor the patient for hyperkalemia and renal failure and anticipate stopping the medication if potassium or creatinine levels rise. Every-other-day dosing is an alternative for patients at risk of developing hyperkalemia.

HCN Channel Blocker. Ivabradine (Corlanor) is a new medication, approved by the Food and Drug Administration (FDA) in 2015, for the treatment of stabilized chronic heart failure. This medication is a first-in-class, hyperpolarization-activated cyclic nucleotide-gated (HCN) channel blocker, which slows the heart rate by inhibiting a specific channel in the sinus node. It has been shown to reduce the risk of hospitalization rate in HF patients. Ivabradine is used for HF patients who have an ejection fraction (EF) <35% who are in sinus rhythm with a resting heart rate ≥70 beats/min. This medication is used for patients who are either on the maximally tolerated dose of beta-blocker therapy or have a contraindication to it.

Ivabradine is contraindicated with hypotension, sick sinus syndrome, third-degree heart block, pacemaker dependence, severe hepatic impairment, and use of cytochrome P4503A4 inhibitors. Side effects include bradycardia, hypertension, atrial fibrillation, and luminous phenomena (visual brightness).

Advise the patient to take this medication with meals but to avoid taking St. John's wort or drinking grapefruit juice while on it. Teach the patient how to check radial pulse and to report low heart rate or irregularity to provider. Advise him or her that visual changes associated with light may occur with initial treatment. These visual changes are usually transient and will disappear with time (Aschenbrenner, 2015). Patients should use caution when driving or using machines in situations where light intensity may change abruptly.

💡 NCLEX EXAMINATION CHALLENGE 35-3

Physiological Integrity

A client with chronic heart failure presents to the ED with a new onset of atrial fibrillation. Which of the following medications would the nurse question?
A. Lasix (furosemide)
B. Toprol XL (metoprolol succinate)
C. Cardizem (diltiazem)
D. Corlanor (ivabradine)

For patients with *diastolic* HF, drug therapy has not been as effective. Calcium channel blockers, ACE inhibitors, and beta blockers have been used with various degrees of success.

Other Nonsurgical Options. In addition to drug therapy, other nonsurgical options, both noninvasive and invasive, may be used and include:

- Continuous positive airway pressure (CPAP)
- Cardiac resynchronization therapy (CRT)
- CardioMEMS™ implantable monitoring system
- Investigative gene therapy

Continuous positive airway pressure (CPAP) is a respiratory treatment that improves obstructive sleep apnea in patients with HF. It also improves cardiac output (CO) and ejection fraction (EF) by decreasing afterload and preload, blood pressure (BP), and dysrhythmias. Sleep apnea is directly correlated with coronary artery disease as a result of diminished oxygen supply to the heart during apneic episodes. This respiratory problem is discussed in detail in Chapter 29.

Cardiac resynchronization therapy (CRT), also called *biventricular pacing*, uses a permanent pacemaker alone or is combined with an implantable cardioverter/defibrillator. Electrical stimulation causes more synchronous ventricular contractions to improve EF, CO, and mean arterial pressure. This

modality is indicated for patients with Class III or IV HF, an EF of less than 35%, and presence of a left bundle branch block. CRT improves the patient's ability to perform ADLs. Chapter 34 discusses pacing in more detail.

CardioMEMS™ implantable monitoring system is inserted into the pulmonary artery and allows the patient to take a daily reading of the pulmonary artery pressure. These data are transmitted to the provider's office and allow for management and adjustment of medications. The device, about the size of the quarter, is implanted during a right heart catheterization and is permanent. The patient is provided a special pillow with an antenna and portable electronic unit. He or she turns the system on, places the pillow on the bed, and lies on top of the pillow. The device will advise if the position needs to be changed and when reading is complete. The CardioMEMS™ device can detect increases in pulmonary pressures, indicating fluid retention before the patient demonstrates symptoms. Therapy can be adjusted before symptoms, which may prevent readmission to the hospital and improve quality of life.

Gene therapy may be indicated for patients in end-stage HF who are not candidates for heart transplantation. This therapy replaces damaged genes with normal or modified genes by a series of injections of growth factor into the left ventricle. Although still investigative, this therapy may result in improved exercise tolerance and regrowth of cardiac cells.

Surgical Management. Heart transplantation is still the ultimate choice for end-stage HF (see the Heart Transplantation section). Several surgical procedures are available to improve CO in patients who are *not* candidates for a transplant or are awaiting transplant.

Ventricular Assist Devices. Patients with debilitating end-stage heart failure are often sent home on drug therapy and referred to hospice. However, ventricular assist devices (VADs) can dramatically improve the lives of many patients. In this procedure, a mechanical pump is implanted to work with the patient's own heart (Fig. 35-2). Both left and right VADs are available, depending on the type of HF the patient has. Those with end-stage kidney disease, severe chronic lung disease, clotting disorders, and infections that do not respond to antibiotics are not candidates for this surgery. Postoperative complications include

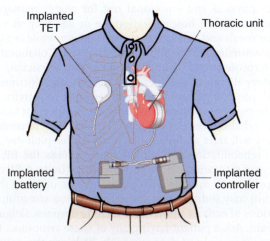

FIG. 35-2 The AbioCor Implantable Replacement Heart has four main parts that are placed inside the body. *TET,* Transtelephonic electrocardiographic transmission device. (Courtesy Abiomed, Inc., Danvers, MA.)

bleeding, infective endocarditis, ventricular dysrhythmias, and stroke. Nursing care is similar to that described for cardiac surgery in Chapter 38.

VADs can be used short-term while awaiting heart transplantation (a "bridge-to-transplant" procedure) or long-term (destination therapy). Most patients survive with a VAD until a transplant is available.

Other Surgical Therapies. HF causes ventricular remodeling, or dilation, which worsens as the disease progresses. Several new therapies are used to reshape the left ventricle in patients with HF. Perioperative care is similar to that for the patient having a coronary artery bypass graft (CABG) (see Chapter 38). The most common ventricular reconstructive procedures include:

- Partial left ventriculectomy (PLV)
- Endoventricular circular patch cardioplasty
- Acorn cardiac support device
- Myosplint

Also known as *heart reduction surgery*, PLV (sometimes referred to as the *Batista procedure)* involves removing a triangle-shaped section of the weakened heart in the left lateral ventricle to reduce the ventricle's diameter and decrease wall tension. In *endoventricular circular patch cardioplasty,* the surgeon removes portions of the cardiac septum and left ventricular wall and grafts a circular patch (synthetic or autologous) into the opening. This procedure provides a more normal shape to the left ventricle to improve the heart's ejection fraction (EF) and cardiac output (CO).

The Acorn cardiac support device is a polyester mesh jacket that is placed over the ventricles to provide support and avoid overstretching the myocardial muscle. The material for the jacket has been used for other procedures, such as vascular grafts. The jacket appears to reduce hypertrophy of the heart muscle and assists with improvement of the EF.

The Myosplint has recently been approved for use in the United States. Electrical stimulation of several tension pads (splints) on the outside of the ventricle changes it to a more normal shape to improve function.

Decreasing Fatigue

Planning: Expected Outcomes. The expected outcomes are that the patient will have decreased fatigue and gain energy as HF improves.

Interventions. The patient in severe heart failure initially requires physical and emotional rest for *energy management.* On the first day of hospitalization, he or she may sit up in a chair for meals and perform basic leg exercises while out of bed. Organize nursing care to allow periods of rest. Collaborate with the interprofessional team, including the physician, nurse, respiratory therapist, and clergy, to observe and document the patient's physiologic and emotional response to activity.

As the patient's condition improves, it is important to consult cardiac rehabilitation specialists. The cardiac rehabilitation specialist will start ambulation, usually on hospital day 2. The cardiac rehabilitation specialist or nurse checks the BP, pulse, and oxygen saturation before and after the activity. A BP change of more than 20 mm Hg or a pulse increase of more than 20 beats/min may indicate that the activity is too stressful. Other indications of activity intolerance include dyspnea, fatigue, and chest pain. Ask a patient having any of these symptoms to rate exertion on a scale of 1 to 20, with 20 being the maximum perceived exertion. If the patient rates the exertion more than 12, remind him or her to slow down. If activity is tolerated, the cardiac rehabilitation specialist steadily increases the activity

level until the patient is ambulating 200 to 400 feet several times per day.

If the patient is able, the cardiac rehabilitation specialist (or assistive nursing or physical therapy personnel) might time him or her for 6 minutes while walking at a comfortable pace. The distance the patient can walk can be used to determine his or her functional level and activity plan. At discharge, encourage the patient to continue with cardiac rehabilitation. In addition to exercise programs, cardiac rehabilitation provides education on risk factor modification, medication adherence, and diet and weight management.

Preventing or Managing Pulmonary Edema

Planning: Expected Outcomes. The most desirable outcome is that the patient will not develop pulmonary edema as a result of heart failure (HF). However, if the patient progresses to pulmonary edema, the expected outcome is that he or she will recover from this complication without other problems.

Interventions. Monitor for signs of acute pulmonary edema, a life-threatening event that can result from severe HF (with fluid overload), acute myocardial infarction (MI), mitral valve disease, and possibly dysrhythmias. In pulmonary edema, the left ventricle fails to eject sufficient blood, and pressure increases in the lungs as a result. The increased pressure causes fluid to leak across the pulmonary capillaries and into the lung airways and tissues.

> ! **NURSING SAFETY PRIORITY** QSEN
>
> ### *Critical Rescue*
>
> Assess for and report early symptoms, such as crackles in the lung bases, dyspnea at rest, disorientation, and confusion, especially in older patients. Document the precise location of the crackles because the level of the fluid progresses from the bases to higher levels in the lungs as the condition worsens. The patient in acute pulmonary edema is typically extremely anxious, tachycardic, and struggling for air. As pulmonary edema becomes more severe, he or she may have a moist cough productive of frothy, blood-tinged sputum; and his or her skin may be cold, clammy, or cyanotic. Chart 35-3 lists the major signs and symptoms of this complication.

The patient diagnosed with pulmonary edema is admitted to the acute care hospital, often in a critical care unit. Reassure the patient and family that his or her distress will decrease with proper management.

If the patient's systolic blood pressure is above 100, give sublingual nitroglycerin (NTG) to decrease afterload and

---

> ►► **CHART 35-3** **Key Features**
>
> ### *Pulmonary Edema*
>
> - Crackles
> - Dyspnea at rest
> - Disorientation or acute confusion (especially in older adults as early symptom)
> - Tachycardia
> - Hypertension or hypotension
> - Reduced urinary output
> - Cough with frothy, pink-tinged sputum
> - Premature ventricular contractions and other dysrhythmias
> - Anxiety
> - Restlessness
> - Lethargy

Critical Rescue

If the patient is not hypotensive, place in a sitting (high-Fowler's) position with the legs down to decrease venous return to the heart. The *priority nursing action* is to administer oxygen therapy at 5 to 12 L/min by simple facemask or at 6 to 10 L/min by nonrebreathing mask with reservoir (which may deliver up to 100% oxygen) to promote GAS EXCHANGE and PERFUSION (Urden et al., 2016). Apply a pulse oximeter and titrate the oxygen flow to keep the patient's oxygen saturation above 90%. If supplemental oxygen does not resolve the patient's respiratory distress, collaborate with the respiratory therapist, physician, advanced practice nurse, or physician assistant for more aggressive therapy, such as continuous positive airway pressure (CPAP) or bi-level positive airway pressure (BiPAP) ventilation. Intubation and mechanical ventilation may be needed for some patients.

preload every 5 minutes for three doses while establishing IV access for additional drug therapy. The health care provider prescribes rapid-acting diuretics, such as furosemide (Lasix) or bumetanide (Bumex). Give furosemide (Lasix) IV push (IVP) over 1 to 2 minutes, usually at a starting dose of 20 to 40 mg for diuretic-naive patients and another 40 mg if needed in 30 minutes. Patients already on oral diuretic therapy should be given an amount that is the same or doubled in milligrams as initial IV diuretic therapy. Administer each increment of 40 mg of Lasix over 1 to 2 minutes to avoid ototoxicity. Bumetanide (Bumex) may be administered 1 to 2 mg IVP or as a continuous infusion to provide consistent fluid removal over 24 hours. Monitor vital signs frequently, at least every 30 to 60 minutes.

If the patient's blood pressure is adequate, IV morphine sulfate may be prescribed, 1 to 2 mg at a time, to reduce venous return (preload), decrease anxiety, and reduce the work of breathing. Monitor respiratory rate and BP closely. Other drugs, such as IV NTG and drugs to treat HF, may be administered. Monitor the patient's vital signs closely (especially BP) while these drugs are being given.

In severe cases of fluid overload and renal dysfunction or diuretic resistance, ultrafiltration may be used. Ultrafiltration can remove up to 500 mL/hr and uses a blood flow rate of 10 to 40 mL/hr. Peripheral lines are used for IV access. See Chapter 68 for a complete discussion of this procedure and nursing implications.

The benefits of ultrafiltration include:
- Decrease in cardiac filling pressures
- Decrease in pulmonary arterial pressure
- Increase in cardiac index
- Reduction in norepinephrine, rennin, and aldosterone

Care Coordination and Transition Management

Patients who are not adequately prepared for discharge or do not have adequate community support and follow-up for self-management are at high risk for repeated hospital admissions for heart failure (HF). Collaborate with the case manager or care coordinator to assess the patient's needs for health care resources.

The Heart Failure Core Measure Set must be determined for hospitals accredited by The Joint Commission. These measures include that the patient with HF has:
- Discharge instructions (including information on diet, activity, medications, weight monitoring, and planning for worsening symptoms)

Safety; Patient-Centered Care; Evidence-Based Practice; Informatics QSEN

A 73-year-old woman is admitted to the telemetry unit with right-sided heart failure, type 2 diabetes mellitus, hypertension, and chronic obstructive pulmonary disease (COPD). When the patient arrives to the unit, you observe that her color is pale, she is becoming increasingly dyspneic, and she reports a new onset of chest discomfort. The patient's husband is very concerned because he thinks his wife is slightly disoriented. Her oxygen saturation levels are 88% on oxygen 2 liters per nasal cannula.
1. Using clinical judgment, what should you assess first?
2. What evidence-based actions will you plan to implement at this time based on your assessment? What is the source of the evidence?
3. The patient's health care provider prescribes an initial dose of furosemide (Lasix) 40 mg IVP. What assessments will you perform to determine if the drug was effective?
4. The patient's husband remains very anxious and asks to stay at her bedside. What will you tell him about her condition at this time? Should the patient's husband be present during her emergency treatment? Why or why not?
5. After two doses of furosemide, the patient's condition improves. What data will you document in the electronic medical record (EMR)?

- Evaluation of left ventricular systolic function
- An ACEI or ARB for left ventricular systolic dysfunction
- Adult smoking-cessation advice/counseling (if appropriate)
- Posthospitalization visit with the primary health care provider within 7 days of discharge

An inability to obtain help in activities such as food shopping and obtaining medications is a major contributor to hospital readmission. If home support is available, the patient may be discharged home in the care of a family member or other caregiver. Home care nurses may direct the care and assess for adherence to the discharge plan; home health aides may provide assistance with ADLs for a short time. If the patient has multiple health problems or has been severely compromised by heart disease, he or she may require admission to a skilled unit for either transitional or long-term care.

Home Care Management. The home care nurse's interventions focus on assessment and health teaching, which are reimbursable by Medicare and other third-party payers. Chart 35-4 lists the major areas of home health assessment.

Patients with chronic HF need to make many adjustments in their lifestyles. They must adhere to the collaborative plan of care that includes dietary restrictions, activity, prescriptions, and drug therapy. They need careful, concise explanations of the self-management plan. The community-based nurse in any setting encourages the patient to verbalize fears and concerns about his or her illness and helps to explore coping skills. Patient participation in self-management can help alleviate and control symptoms.

Self-Management Education. Health teaching is essential for promoting self-management (also called *self-care*). Many patients are re-admitted to hospitals because they do not maintain their prescribed treatment plan, including lifestyle changes. Because of the need for extensive discharge instructions, most hospitals are using teaching packets with videos, CDs, and easy-to-read information about the importance of adhering to specific self-management strategies at home. One standardized and

CHART 35-4 Home Care Assessment
The Patient With Heart Failure

Assess for signs of heart failure, including:
- Changes in vital signs (heart rate >100 beats/min at rest, new atrial fibrillation, blood pressure <90 or >150 systolic)
- Indications of poor tissue perfusion:
  - Fatigue
  - Angina
  - Activity intolerance
  - Changes in mental status
  - Pallor or cyanosis
  - Cool extremities
- Indications of congestion:
  - Presence of cough or dyspnea
  - Weight gain
  - Jugular venous distention and peripheral edema

Assess functional ability, including:
- Performance of ADLs
- Mobility and ambulation (review frequency and duration of walking, development of symptoms, and pulse rate)
- Cognitive ability

Assess nutritional status, including:
- Food and fluid intake
- Intake of sodium-rich foods
- Alcohol consumption
- Skin turgor

Assess home environment, including:
- Safety hazards, especially related to oxygen therapy
- Structural barriers affecting functional ability
- Social support (family, home health services)

Assess the patient's adherence and understanding of illness and its treatment, including:
- Signs and symptoms to report to primary health care provider
- Dosages, effects, and side or toxic effects of medications
- When to report for laboratory and health care provider visits
- Ability to accurately weigh self on scale
- Presence of advance directive
- Use of home oxygen, if appropriate

Assess patient and caregiver coping skills.

TABLE 35-4 Heart Failure Self-Management Health Teaching (MAWDS)

Medications:
- Take medications as prescribed and do not run out.
- Know the purpose and side effects of each drug.
- Avoid NSAIDs to prevent sodium and fluid retention.

Activity:
- Stay as active as possible but don't overdo it.
- Know your limits.
- Be able to carry on a conversation while exercising.

Weight:
- Weigh each day at the same time on the same scale to monitor for fluid retention.

Diet:
- Limit daily sodium intake to 2 to 3 grams as prescribed.
- Limit daily fluid intake to 2 liters.

Symptoms:
- Note any new or worsening symptoms and notify the health care provider immediately.

commonly used self-management plan called *MAWDS* is outlined in Table 35-4. Medication reconciliation is also important to be sure that similar drugs are not being prescribed and that patients meet the Core Measure requirements for HF. It is important to perform a learning needs assessment and tailor

education to the patient's particular need to see changes in behavior and improved outcomes.

Ambulatory care clinics for HF patients are also becoming increasingly common. Their purpose is to offer assessments, drug therapy, and health teaching. Some nurses specialize in caring for patients with health failure.

Activity Schedule. Encourage patients with HF to stay as active as possible and to develop a regular exercise regimen (e.g., home walking program). However, teach the patient not to overdo it. Patients should be referred to cardiac rehabilitation programs. Medicare and third-party payers are now reimbursing for this service, but patients may need to wait 6 weeks to fully participate in the program.

Remind patients with persistent crackles and uncontrolled edema to begin exercise after their condition stabilizes. When exercise is indicated, teach the patient to begin walking 200 to 400 feet per day. At home the patient should try to walk at least 3 times a week and should slowly increase the amount of time walked over several months. If chest pain or severe dyspnea occurs while exercising or the patient has fatigue the next day, he or she is probably advancing the activity too quickly and should slow down. Encourage him or her to keep a diary that documents the time and duration of each exercise session, heart rate, and any symptoms that occur with exercise.

Indications of Worsening or Recurrent Heart Failure. Many patients who are re-admitted to hospitals for treatment of HF fail to seek medical attention promptly when symptoms recur.

! NURSING SAFETY PRIORITY QSEN
Action Alert

Per the HF Core Measure for discharge instructions, teach the patient and caregiver to immediately report to the primary health care provider the occurrence of *any* of these symptoms, which could indicate worsening or recurrent heart failure:
- Rapid weight gain (3 lb in a week or 1 to 2 lb overnight)
- Decrease in exercise tolerance lasting 2 to 3 days
- Cold symptoms (cough) lasting more than 3 to 5 days
- Excessive awakening at night to urinate
- Development of dyspnea or angina at rest or worsening angina
- Increased swelling in the feet, ankles, or hands

Drug Therapy. Provide oral, written, and video instructions about the drug regimen. Teach the caregiver and patient how to count a pulse rate, especially if the patient is taking digoxin, beta blockers, or ivabradine (Corlanor). Chart 35-5 lists instructions for the patient taking beta blockers and digoxin.

Advise the patient taking diuretics to take them in the morning to avoid waking during the night for voiding. After determining whether he or she has a weight scale and can use it, emphasize the importance of weighing each morning at the same time. Daily weights indicate whether the patient is losing or retaining fluid. Some patients are taught to use a sliding scale to adjust their daily diuretic dose, depending on their daily weight, similar to the way a patient with diabetes adjusts an insulin dose based on the capillary glucose level.

Teach patients taking ACEIs, ARBs, or sacubitril/valsartan (Entresto) to move slowly when changing positions, especially from a lying to a sitting position. Remind them to report

CHART 35-5 Patient and Family Education: Preparing for Self-Management

Beta Blocker/Digoxin Therapy

- Establish same time of day to take this medication every day.
- Continue taking this medication unless your health care provider tells you to stop.
- Do not take digoxin at the same time as antacids or cathartics (laxatives).
- Take your pulse rate before taking each dose of digoxin. Notify your health care provider of a change in pulse rate (60 to 100 beats/min is typically normal, depending on your baseline pulse rate) or rhythm and increasing fatigue, muscle weakness, confusion, or loss of appetite (signs of digoxin toxicity).
- If you forget to take a dose, it may be delayed a few hours. However, if you do not remember it until the next day, you should take only your usual daily dose.
- Report for scheduled laboratory tests (e.g., potassium and digoxin levels).
- If potassium supplements are prescribed, continue the dose until told to stop by your health care provider.

dizziness, light-headedness, and cough to the health care provider.

Serum potassium level and renal function are monitored at least every few months for patients taking diuretics and ACE inhibitors, ARBs or sacubitril/valsartan (Entresto). Diuretics, especially loop diuretics such as furosemide (Lasix) and bumetanide (Burinex ✦), deplete potassium and often cause hypokalemia. Conversely, ACE inhibitors, ARBs, sacubitril/valsartan (Entresto), or potassium-sparing diuretics may result in potassium retention. If serum potassium levels drop below 4 mEq/L, the health care provider may prescribe potassium supplements or add a potassium-sparing diuretic such as spironolactone (Aldactone) or eplerenone (Inspra). Provide information about potassium-rich foods to include in the diet for patients at risk for hypokalemia (see Chapter 11).

Nutrition Therapy. Remind patients with chronic HF to restrict their dietary sodium. In collaboration with the home care nurse or dietitian, provide written instructions on low- or restricted-sodium diets. A 3-g sodium diet is recommended for *mild-to-moderate* disease. Remind the patient to avoid salty foods and table salt. Patients usually find this diet acceptable and fairly easy to follow. Teach patients how to read food labels, specifically ingredients that include sodium.

A 2-g sodium diet may be needed for patients with *severe* HF. They should not add salt during or after meal preparation, avoid milk and milk products, use few canned or prepared foods, and read food labels to determine sodium content. This diet is not easily tolerated for many patients, and the cost of low-sodium foods can be a financial burden.

Commercial salt substitutes typically contain potassium. Teach patients that their renal status and serum potassium level must be evaluated while using these products. Suggest that patients try lemon, spices, and herbs to enhance the flavor of low-salt foods.

Advance Directives. HF is a chronic, progressive debilitating disease. The only potential cure is transplantation. Early in the diagnosis stage, patients and families should be made aware of the progressive nature of this disease process. About 50% of deaths from HF are sudden—many without any warning or worsening of symptoms. Assess whether the patient has written

advance directives. If not, provide information about them during the hospital stay. Because most of these deaths occur at home, it is important for the primary health care provider or home care nurse to discuss advance directives with the patient and family. The family should be prepared to act in agreement with the patient's wishes in the event of cardiac arrest. If resuscitation is desired, be sure that the family knows how to activate the emergency medical system (EMS) and how to provide cardiopulmonary resuscitation (CPR) until an ambulance arrives. If CPR is not desired, the patient, family, and nurse plan how the family will respond. Palliative consultation can provide support to the patient and the family as condition progresses and the patient's conditions declines. Goals of palliative care are to improve the quality of life, manage symptoms, and provide support. As the patient approaches end of life, hospice consultation would be appropriate. Chapter 7 discusses hospice and end-of-life care in detail.

Health Care Resources. A home care nurse, ambulatory care clinic, or nurse-led follow-up program may be needed to assess the patient's adherence to drug and nutrition therapy and to monitor for worsening or recurrent HF. Many large hospitals use follow-up telephone calls or teleconferencing/videoconferencing devices to monitor patients at home. Teleconferencing can also assess the patient's heart and lung sounds. These follow-up processes have been very successful in decreasing repeated hospital stays for chronic HF patients.

In addition to home care support, other resources are available for patient education and family support. The American Heart Association is an excellent community resource for print and electronic pamphlets, books, newsletters, and videotapes or DVDs related to HF and heart disease. The organization also provides referrals to various local support groups for patients and their caregivers.

For equipment needs (e.g., home oxygen therapy, hospital bed), medical supply companies provide setup and maintenance services. Chapter 28 provides a detailed description of home oxygen therapy.

◆ Evaluation: Reflecting

Evaluate the care of the patient with HF on the basis of the identified patient problems. The expected outcomes include that the patient will:

- Have adequate pulmonary tissue PERFUSION
- Have increased cardiac pump effectiveness
- Take actions to manage energy
- Be free of pulmonary edema

VALVULAR HEART DISEASE

❖ PATHOPHYSIOLOGY

Acquired valvular dysfunctions include mitral stenosis, mitral regurgitation, mitral valve prolapse, aortic stenosis, and aortic regurgitation (Chart 35-6). The tricuspid valve is not affected often and may occur following endocarditis in IV drug abusers.

Mitral Stenosis

Mitral stenosis usually results from rheumatic carditis, which can cause valve thickening by fibrosis and calcification. Rheumatic fever is the most common cause of the problem. In mitral stenosis, the valve leaflets fuse and become stiff, and the chordae tendineae contract and shorten. The valve opening narrows, preventing normal blood flow from the left atrium to the left

>> **CHART 35-6** **Key Features**

Valvular Heart Disease

MITRAL STENOSIS	MITRAL REGURGITATION	MITRAL VALVE PROLAPSE	AORTIC STENOSIS	AORTIC REGURGITATION
Fatigue	Fatigue	Atypical chest pain	Dyspnea on exertion	Palpitations
Dyspnea on exertion	Dyspnea on exertion	Dizziness, syncope	Angina	Dyspnea
Orthopnea	Orthopnea	Palpitations	Syncope on exertion	Orthopnea
Paroxysmal nocturnal dyspnea	Palpitations	Atrial tachycardia	Fatigue	Paroxysmal nocturnal dyspnea
Hemoptysis	Atrial fibrillation	Ventricular tachycardia	Orthopnea	Fatigue
Hepatomegaly	Neck vein distention	Systolic click	Paroxysmal nocturnal dyspnea	Angina
Neck vein distention	Pitting edema		Harsh, systolic crescendo-decrescendo murmur	Sinus tachycardia
Pitting edema	High-pitched holosystolic murmur			Blowing, decrescendo diastolic murmur
Atrial fibrillation				
Rumbling, apical diastolic murmur				

ventricle. As a result of these changes, left atrial pressure rises, the left atrium dilates, pulmonary artery pressures increase, and the right ventricle hypertrophies.

Pulmonary congestion and right-sided heart failure occur first. Later, when the left ventricle receives insufficient blood volume, preload is decreased and cardiac output (CO) falls.

People with mild mitral stenosis are usually asymptomatic. As the valvular orifice narrows and pressure in the lungs increases, the patient experiences dyspnea on exertion, orthopnea, paroxysmal nocturnal dyspnea (sudden dyspnea at night), palpitations, and dry cough. Hemoptysis (coughing up blood) and pulmonary edema occur as pulmonary hypertension and congestion progress. Right-sided HF can cause hepatomegaly (enlarged liver), neck vein distention, and pitting dependent edema late in the disorder.

On palpation, the pulse may be normal, rapid, or irregularly irregular (as in atrial fibrillation). Because the development of atrial fibrillation indicates that the patient may decompensate, the health care provider should be notified immediately of the development of an irregularly irregular rhythm. A rumbling, apical diastolic murmur is noted on auscultation.

Mitral Regurgitation (Insufficiency)

The fibrotic and calcific changes occurring in **mitral regurgitation** (insufficiency) prevent the mitral valve from closing completely during *systole*. Incomplete closure of the valve allows the backflow of blood into the left atrium when the left ventricle contracts. During *diastole*, regurgitant output again flows from the left atrium to the left ventricle along with the normal blood flow. The increased volume must be ejected during the next systole. To compensate for the increased volume and pressure, the left atrium and ventricle dilate and hypertrophy.

The primary causes of mitral regurgitation are mitral valve prolapse and rheumatic heart disease (McCance et al., 2014). Other causes include infective endocarditis, papillary muscle dysfunction, or rupture resulting from ischemic heart disease or congenital anomalies. Rheumatic heart disease is the number-one cause in developing nations. When it results from rheumatic heart disease, it usually coexists with some degree of mitral stenosis; it affects women more often than men.

Mitral regurgitation usually progresses slowly; patients may remain symptom-free for decades. Symptoms begin to occur when the left ventricle fails in response to chronic blood volume overload. They include fatigue and chronic weakness as a result of reduced CO. Dyspnea on exertion and orthopnea develop later. A significant number of patients report anxiety, atypical chest pains, and palpitations. Assessment may reveal normal BP, atrial fibrillation, or changes in respirations characteristic of left ventricular failure.

When right-sided HF develops, the neck veins become distended, the liver enlarges (hepatomegaly), and pitting edema develops. A high-pitched systolic murmur at the apex, with radiation to the left axilla, is heard on auscultation. Severe regurgitation often exhibits a third heart sound (S_3).

Mitral Valve Prolapse

Mitral valve prolapse (MVP) occurs because the valvular leaflets enlarge and prolapse into the left atrium during systole. This abnormality is usually benign but may progress to pronounced mitral regurgitation in some patients.

The etiology of MVP is variable and has been associated with conditions such as Marfan syndrome and other congenital cardiac defects. MVP also has a familial tendency. Usually, however, no other cardiac abnormality is found.

Most patients with MVP are asymptomatic. However, some may report chest pain, palpitations, or exercise intolerance. Chest pain is usually atypical, with patients describing a sharp pain localized to the left side of the chest. Dizziness, **syncope** ("blackouts"), and palpitations may be associated with atrial or ventricular dysrhythmias.

A normal heart rate and BP are usually found on physical examination. A midsystolic click and a late systolic murmur may be heard at the apex of the heart. The intensity of the murmur is not related to the severity of the prolapse.

Aortic Stenosis

Aortic stenosis is the most common cardiac valve dysfunction in the United States and is often considered a disease of "wear and tear." In **aortic stenosis,** the aortic valve orifice narrows and obstructs left ventricular outflow during systole. This increased resistance to ejection or afterload results in ventricular hypertrophy. As stenosis worsens, cardiac output becomes fixed and cannot increase to meet the demands of the body during exertion. Symptoms then develop. Eventually the left ventricle fails, blood backs up in the left atrium, and the pulmonary system becomes congested. Right-sided HF can occur late in the disease. *When the surface area of the valve becomes 1 cm or less, surgery is indicated on an urgent basis!*

Congenital bicuspid or unicuspid aortic valves are the primary causes for aortic stenosis in many patients. Rheumatic aortic stenosis occurs with rheumatic disease of the mitral valve and develops in young and middle-age adults. Atherosclerosis and degenerative calcification of the aortic valve are the major causative factors in older adults. *Aortic stenosis has become the most common valvular disorder in all countries with aging populations.*

The classic symptoms of aortic stenosis result from fixed cardiac output: dyspnea, angina, and syncope occurring on exertion. When cardiac output falls in the late stages of the disease, the patient experiences marked fatigue, debilitation, and peripheral cyanosis. A narrow pulse pressure is noted when the BP is measured. A diamond-shaped, systolic crescendo-decrescendo murmur is usually noted on auscultation.

Aortic Regurgitation (Insufficiency)

In patients with **aortic regurgitation**, the aortic valve leaflets do not close properly during diastole; and the *annulus* (the valve ring that attaches to the leaflets) may be dilated, loose, or deformed. This allows flow of blood from the aorta back into the left ventricle during diastole. The left ventricle, in compensation, dilates to accommodate the greater blood volume and eventually hypertrophies.

Aortic insufficiency usually results from nonrheumatic conditions such as infective endocarditis, congenital anatomic aortic valvular abnormalities, hypertension, and Marfan syndrome (a rare, generalized, systemic disease of connective tissue).

Patients with aortic regurgitation remain asymptomatic for many years because of the compensatory mechanisms of the left ventricle. As the disease progresses and left ventricular failure occurs, the major symptoms are exertional dyspnea, orthopnea, and paroxysmal nocturnal dyspnea. Palpitations may be noted with severe disease, especially when the patient lies on the left side. Nocturnal angina with diaphoresis often occurs.

On palpation, the nurse notes a "bounding" arterial pulse. The pulse pressure is usually widened, with an elevated systolic pressure and diminished diastolic pressure. The classic auscultatory finding is a high-pitched, blowing, decrescendo diastolic murmur.

❖ INTERPROFESSIONAL COLLABORATIVE CARE

◆ Assessment: Noticing

A patient with valvular disease may suddenly become ill or slowly develop symptoms over many years. Collect information about the patient's family health history, including valvular or other forms of heart disease to which he or she may be genetically predisposed. Ask about attacks of rheumatic fever and infective endocarditis, the specific dates when these occurred, and the use of antibiotics to prevent recurrence of these diseases. Also ask the patient about a history of IV drug abuse, a common cause of infective endocarditis. Discuss his or her fatigue and tolerated activity levels, the presence of angina or dyspnea, and the occurrence of palpitations, if present.

As part of the physical assessment, obtain vital signs, inspect for signs of edema, palpate and auscultate the heart and lungs, and palpate the peripheral pulses. Assessment findings are summarized in Chart 35-6.

Echocardiography is the noninvasive diagnostic procedure of choice to visualize the structure and movement of the heart. The more invasive transesophageal echocardiography (TEE) or transthoracic echocardiography (TTE) is also performed to assess most valve problems. Exercise tolerance testing (ETT) and stress echocardiography are sometimes done to evaluate symptomatic response and assess functional capacity. With either mitral or aortic stenosis, cardiac catheterization may be indicated to assess the severity of the stenosis and its other effects on the heart.

In patients with mitral stenosis, the chest x-ray shows left atrial enlargement, prominent pulmonary arteries, and an enlarged right ventricle. In those with mitral regurgitation (insufficiency), the chest x-ray reveals an increased cardiac shadow, indicating left ventricular and left atrial enlargement.

In the later stages of aortic stenosis, the chest x-ray may show left ventricular enlargement and pulmonary congestion. Left atrial and left ventricular dilation appear on the chest x-ray of patients with aortic regurgitation (insufficiency). If HF is present, pulmonary venous congestion is also evident.

The health care provider also requests an ECG to assess abnormalities such as left ventricular hypertrophy, as seen with mitral regurgitation and aortic regurgitation, or right ventricular hypertrophy, as seen in severe mitral stenosis. Atrial fibrillation is a common finding in both mitral stenosis and mitral regurgitation and may develop in aortic stenosis because of left atrial dilation.

◆ Interventions: Responding

Management of valvular heart disease depends on which valve is affected and the degree of valve impairment. Some patients can be managed with annual monitoring and drug therapy, whereas others require invasive procedures or heart surgery.

Nonsurgical Management. Nonsurgical management focuses on drug therapy and rest. During the course of valvular disease, left ventricular failure with pulmonary or systemic congestion may develop.

Drug Therapy. Diuretics, beta blockers, ACE inhibitors, digoxin, and oxygen are often administered to improve the symptoms of HF. Nitrates are administered cautiously to patients with aortic stenosis because of the potential for syncope associated with a reduction in left ventricular volume (preload). Vasodilators such as calcium channel blockers may be used to reduce the regurgitant flow for patients with aortic or mitral stenosis.

! NURSING SAFETY PRIORITY **QSEN**

Drug Alert

Teach patients with valve disease the importance of prophylactic antibiotic therapy before any invasive dental or oral procedure. This includes patients with a previous history of endocarditis and cardiac transplant or valve recipients. Have patients demonstrate appropriate oral hygiene because optimal oral health is the best intervention to prevent endocarditis.

Prophylactic antibiotics are *not* recommended before GI procedures such as upper GI endoscopy, colonoscopy, or procedures requiring genitourinary instrumentation.

A major concern in valvular heart disease is maintaining cardiac output (CO) if atrial fibrillation develops. With mitral valvular disease, left ventricular filling is especially dependent on atrial contraction. When atrial fibrillation develops, there is no longer a single coordinated atrial contraction. CO can decrease, and HF may occur. Ineffective atrial contraction may also lead to the stasis of blood and thrombi in the left atrium. Monitor the patient for the development of an irregular rhythm and notify the primary care provider if it develops. (See Chapter 34 for a detailed explanation of atrial fibrillation.)

The primary care provider usually starts drug therapy first to control the heart rate (HR) and maintain CO (HR < 100 is considered a controlled ventricular response). After these outcomes are met, drugs are used in an attempt to restore normal sinus rhythm (NSR). In some cases, the provider elects to convert a patient from atrial fibrillation to sinus rhythm using IV diltiazem (Cardizem, Apo-Diltiaz) or amiodarone (Cordarone, Pacerone). Monitor the patient on a unit where both cardiac rhythm and BP can be watched closely. Synchronized countershock (cardioversion) may be attempted if atrial fibrillation is rapid, the patient's condition worsens, and the rhythm is unresponsive to medical treatment (see Chapter 34).

If the patient remains in atrial fibrillation, low-dose amiodarone (Cordarone) is often prescribed to slow ventricular rate. Procainamide hydrochloride (Procan ♣) may be added to the regimen. A beta-blocking agent (e.g., metoprolol) may also be considered to slow the ventricular response.

For valvular heart disease and chronic atrial fibrillation, anticoagulation with sodium warfarin (Coumadin, Warfilone) is usually a part of the plan of care to prevent thrombus formation. Thrombi (clots) may form in the atria or on defective valve segments, resulting in systemic emboli. If a portion breaks off and travels to the brain, one or more strokes may occur. Assess the patient's baseline neurologic status and monitor for changes. A transesophageal echocardiography (TEE) is often done before synchronized cardioversion to ensure that thrombi that could embolize when this therapy is administered are not present. The novel oral anticoagulants (NOACs) *rivaroxaban* (Xarelto), *dabigatran* (Pradaxa), *apixaban* (Eliquis), and *edoxaban* (Savaysa) are *not recommended* to anticoagulate patients with atrial fibrillation related to valvular disease.

Rest is often an important part of treatment. Activity may be limited because CO cannot meet increased metabolic demands and angina or HF can result. A balance of rest and exercise is needed to prevent skeletal muscle atrophy and fatigue.

Noninvasive Heart Valve Reparative Procedures. Reparative procedures are becoming more popular because of continuing problems with thrombi, endocarditis, and left ventricular dysfunction after valve replacement. Reparative procedures do not result in a normal valve, but they usually "turn back the clock," resulting in a more functional valve and an improvement in CO. Turbulent blood flow through the valve may persist, and degeneration of the repaired valve is possible.

Balloon valvuloplasty, an invasive nonsurgical procedure, is possible for stenotic mitral and aortic valves; however, careful selection of patients is needed. It may be the initial treatment of choice for people with noncalcified, mobile mitral valves. Patients selected for *aortic* valvuloplasty are usually older and are at high risk for surgical complications or have refused operative treatment. The benefits of this procedure for aortic stenosis tend to be short lived, rarely lasting longer than 6 months.

When performing *mitral* valvuloplasty, the physician passes a balloon catheter from the femoral vein, through the atrial septum, and to the mitral valve. The balloon is inflated to enlarge the mitral orifice. For *aortic* valvuloplasty, the physician inserts the catheter through the femoral artery and advances it to the aortic valve, where it is inflated to enlarge the orifice. The procedure usually offers immediate relief of symptoms because the balloon has dilated the orifice and improved leaflet mobility. The results are comparable with those of surgical commissurotomy for appropriately selected patients.

Minimally invasive techniques have expanded. For patients who are not surgical candidates, *transcatheter aortic valve replacement (TAVR)* is an alternate option for treatment of aortic stenosis (Fig. 35-3). A bioprosthetic valve is placed percutaneously via either the transfemoral or transapical route under general anesthesia in a hybrid operating room (a combination of a catheterization laboratory and cardiovascular operating room). After initial balloon aortic valvuloplasty, the new valve, which is wrapped around a balloon on a large catheter, is inserted via the femoral artery (see Fig. 35-3A-B). The patient is transvenously paced at a rate of about 200 beats/min to mimic ventricular standstill. The balloon is then inflated, and the valve deployed (see Fig. 35-3C-D). In the transapical approach, a small incision is made at the apex of the heart. The

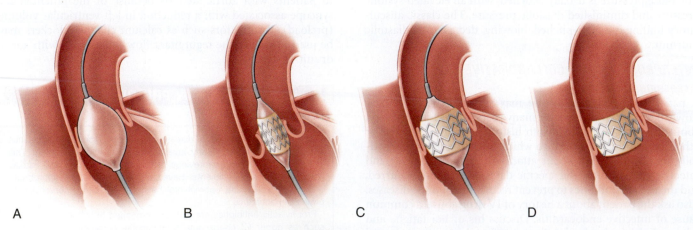

A   B   C   D

FIG. 35-3 Transcatheter aortic valve replacement (TAVR) procedure. **A,** Balloon aortic valvuloplasty. **B,** New valve placed around balloon. **C,** Balloon inflated, deploying valve. **D,** Catheter removed, valve in place.

catheter is then threaded through the incision and the left ventricle to gain access to the aortic valve. As in the transvenous approach, the balloon and catheter are deployed during rapid transvenous pacing. This procedure is performed by a health care team consisting of interventional cardiologists and cardiovascular surgeons. The team must be prepared to convert to an open or traditional aortic valve replacement (AVR) if necessary. Care of the patient is similar to that of the patient undergoing coronary artery bypass graft (CABG) (see Chapter 38); however, this patient population only needs anticoagulation with aspirin and clopidogrel (Plavix) after the procedure.

The pulmonary valve can also be replaced percutaneously by a device using a similar procedure to the TAVR. The Mitraclip is used to repair the mitral valve in patients with mitral regurgitation. Under general anesthesia, access is gained percutaneously via the femoral vein, and the catheter and Mitraclip are advanced in the left atria and then the left ventricle. The Mitraclip is then retracted and deployed to hold the leaflets of the valve together. Care is similar to that of the patient undergoing CABG (see Chapter 38).

> ### ⚠ NURSING SAFETY PRIORITY QSEN
>
> #### *Action Alert*
>
> After valvuloplasty, observe the patient closely for bleeding from the catheter insertion site and institute post-angiogram precautions. Bleeding is likely because of the large size of the catheter. Assess for signs of a regurgitant valve by closely monitoring heart sounds, CO, and heart rhythm. Because vegetations (thrombi) may have been dislodged from the valve, observe for any indication of systemic emboli (see the Infective Endocarditis section in this chapter).

Surgical Management. Surgeries for patients with valvular heart disease include invasive reparative procedures and replacement. These procedures are performed after symptoms of left ventricular failure have developed but before irreversible dysfunction occurs. Surgical therapy is the *only* definitive treatment of *aortic stenosis* and is recommended when angina, syncope, or dyspnea on exertion develops.

Invasive Heart Valve Reparative Procedures. *Direct (open) commissurotomy* is accomplished with cardiopulmonary bypass during open-heart surgery. The surgeon visualizes the valve, removes thrombi from the atria, incises the fused commissures (leaflets), and débrides calcium from the leaflets, widening the orifice.

Mitral valve annuloplasty (reconstruction) is the reparative procedure of choice for most patients with acquired mitral insufficiency. To make the annulus (the valve ring that attaches to and supports the leaflets) smaller, the surgeon may suture the leaflets to an annuloplasty ring or take tucks in the patient's annulus. Leaflet repair is often performed at the same time. Elongated leaflets may be shortened, and shortened leaflets may be repaired by lengthening the chordae that bind them in place. Perforated leaflets may be patched with synthetic grafts.

Annuloplasty and leaflet repair result in an annulus of the appropriate size and leaflets that can close completely. Thus regurgitation is eliminated or markedly reduced.

Heart Valve Replacement Procedures. The development of a wide variety of *prosthetic* (synthetic) and *biologic* (tissue) valves has improved the surgical therapy and prognosis of valvular heart disease. Each type has advantages and disadvantages. An aortic valve can be replaced only with a prosthetic valve for symptomatic adults with aortic stenosis and aortic insufficiency. A biologic valve cannot be used because of the high pressure within the aorta.

Biologic valve replacements may be **xenograft** (from other species), such as a porcine valve (from a pig) (Fig. 35-4) or a bovine valve (from a cow). Because tissue valves are associated with little risk for clot formation, long-term anticoagulation is *not* indicated. Xenografts are not as durable as prosthetic valves and usually must be replaced every 7 to 10 years. The durability of the graft is related to the age of the recipient. Calcium in the blood, which is present in larger quantities in younger patients, breaks down the valves. The older the patient, the longer the xenograft will last. Valves donated from human cadavers and **pulmonary autographs** (relocation of the patient's own pulmonary valve to the aortic position [Ross procedure]) are also used for valve replacement.

Patients having a valve replacement have open-heart surgery similar to the procedure for a CABG (see Chapter 38). Ideally surgery is an elective and planned procedure. Patients need to have a preoperative dental examination. If dental caries or periodontal disease is present, these problems must be resolved before valve replacement. Teach patients receiving oral anticoagulants to stop taking them before surgery, usually at least 72

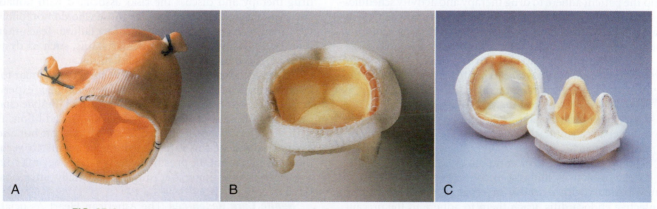

FIG. 35-4 Examples of biologic (tissue) heart valves. **A,** Freestyle, a stentless pig valve with no frame. **B,** Hancock II, a stented pig valve. **C,** Carpentier-Edwards pericardial bioprosthesis. (**A** and **B** courtesy Medtronic, Inc., Minneapolis, MN; **C** courtesy Baxter Healthcare Corporation, Edwards CVS Division, Santa Ana, CA.)

hours before the procedure. Inform the patient and family about the management of postoperative pain, incision care, and strategies to prevent infection and respiratory complications. Postoperative nursing interventions for patients with valve replacement are similar to those for a CABG (see Chapter 38).

! **NURSING SAFETY PRIORITY** QSEN

Critical Rescue

Patients with mitral stenosis often have pulmonary hypertension and stiff lungs. Therefore monitor respiratory status closely during weaning from the ventilator. Be especially alert for bleeding in those with aortic valve replacements because of a higher risk for postoperative hemorrhage. If heart rate or blood pressure decreases, call the Rapid Response Team or other health care provider immediately!

Patients with valve replacements are also more likely to have significant reductions in cardiac output (CO) after surgery, especially those with aortic stenosis or left ventricular failure from mitral valve disease. Carefully monitor CO and assess for indications of heart failure. Report any indications of HF to the surgeon immediately, and prepare for collaborative management (see earlier discussion on HF in this chapter).

When a patient has a mechanical valve, lifelong anticoagulant therapy with warfarin (Coumadin) is required. Teach the patient that the international normalized ratio (INR) will need to be monitored frequently. The therapeutic goal for patients with mechanical heart valves is 3.0 to 4.0 (Pagana et al., 2017). However, therapy must be individualized to each patient. Low-dose aspirin (75 to 100 mg) is also recommended. Novel oral anticoagulants (NOACs) *are not recommended* in patients with valve replacement. Teach patient the signs and symptoms of bleeding and to report these symptoms to the primary health care provider.

Care Coordination and Transition Management

The patient with valvular heart disease may be discharged home on medical therapy or after valve repair or replacement surgery. Because fatigue is a common problem, ensure that the home environment can provide rest while moving the patient toward increased activity levels. Some older adults with aortic stenosis live in long-term care settings.

Home Care Management. A home care nurse may be needed to help the patient adhere to drug therapy and activity schedules and to detect any problems, particularly with anticoagulant therapy. Patients who have undergone surgery may require a nurse for help with incision care. A home care aide may assist with ADLs if the patient lives alone or is older.

Self-Management Education. The teaching plan for the patient with valvular heart disease includes:
- The disease process and the possibility of HF
- Drug therapy, including diuretics, vasodilators, beta blockers, calcium channel blockers, antibiotics, and anticoagulants
- The prophylactic use of antibiotics
- A plan of activity and rest to conserve energy

Because patients with defective or repaired valves are at risk for infective endocarditis, teach them to adhere to the precautions described for endocarditis. Remind them to inform all health care providers of the valvular heart disease history. Tell

---

👤 **CHART 35-7** **Patient and Family Education: Preparing for Self-Management**

Valvular Heart Disease

- Notify all your health care providers that you have a defective heart valve.
- Remind the health care provider of your valvular problem when you have any invasive dental work (e.g., extraction).
- Request antibiotic prophylaxis before and after these procedures if the health care provider does not offer it.
- Clean all wounds and apply antibiotic ointment to prevent infection.
- Notify your primary health care provider immediately if you experience fever, petechiae (pinpoint red dots on your skin), or shortness of breath.

---

providers that they require antibiotic administration before all invasive dental procedures. Health teaching for the patient is summarized in Chart 35-7.

Patients who have had valve replacements with prosthetic valves require lifetime prophylactic anticoagulation therapy to prevent thrombus formation. Teach patients taking anticoagulants how to manage their drug therapy successfully, including nutritional considerations (if taking warfarin) and the prevention of bleeding. For example, the patient should be taught to avoid foods high in vitamin K, especially dark green leafy vegetables, and to use an electric razor to avoid skin cuts. In addition, teach him or her to report any bleeding or excessive bruising to the primary health care provider.

For patients who have surgery, reinforce how to care for the sternal incision and instruct them to watch for and report any fever, drainage, or redness at the site. Most patients can usually return to normal activity after 6 weeks but should avoid heavy physical activity involving their upper extremities for 3 to 6 months to allow the incision to heal. Those who have had valvular surgery should also avoid invasive dental procedures for 6 months because of the potential for endocarditis. Those with prosthetic valves need to avoid any procedure using magnetic resonance unless the newest technology is available. Remind patients to obtain a medical alert bracelet, card, or necklace to indicate that they have a valve replacement and are taking anticoagulants.

Patients with valvular heart disease may have complicated medication schedules that can potentially lead to inadequate self-management. Provide clear, concise instructions about drug therapy and discuss the risks associated with nonadherence. Patients with a failed valve or those who do not follow the treatment plan are at high risk for heart failure. Teach them to report any changes in cardiovascular status, such as dyspnea, syncope, dizziness, edema, and palpitations.

The psychological response to valve surgery is similar to that after coronary artery bypass surgery. Patients may experience an altered self-image as a result of the required lifestyle changes or the visible medial sternotomy incision. In addition, those with prosthetic valves may need to adjust to a soft but audible clicking sound of the valve. Encourage patients to verbalize their feelings about the prosthetic heart valve. They may display a variety of emotions after surgery, especially after hospital discharge.

Health Care Resources. The American Heart Association's *Mended Hearts, Inc.* (www.mendedhearts.org) is a community resource that provides information about valvular heart disease.

CHART 35-8 **Key Features**
Infective Endocarditis

- Fever associated with chills, night sweats, malaise, and fatigue
- Anorexia and weight loss
- Cardiac murmur (newly developed or change in existing)
- Development of heart failure
- Evidence of systemic embolization
- Petechiae
- Splinter hemorrhages
- Osler's nodes (on palms of hands and soles of feet)
- Janeway's lesions (flat, reddened maculae on hands and feet)
- Positive blood cultures

A wallet-size card can be obtained to identify the patient as needing prophylactic antibiotics. An identification bracelet or necklace that states the name of the drugs the patient is taking should also be worn.

INFLAMMATIONS AND INFECTIONS
INFECTIVE ENDOCARDITIS
❖ PATHOPHYSIOLOGY

Infective endocarditis (previously called *bacterial endocarditis*) is a microbial infection (e.g., viruses, bacteria, fungi) of the endocardium. The most common infective organism is *Streptococcus viridans* or *Staphylococcus aureus.*

Infective endocarditis occurs primarily in patients who abuse IV drugs, have had valve replacements, have experienced systemic alterations in IMMUNITY, or have structural cardiac defects. With a cardiac defect, blood may flow rapidly from a high-pressure area to a low-pressure zone, eroding a section of endocardium. Platelets and fibrin adhere to the denuded endocardium, forming a vegetative lesion. During bacteremia, bacteria become trapped in the low-pressure "sinkhole" and are deposited in the vegetation. Additional platelets and fibrin are deposited, which cause the vegetative lesion to grow. The endocardium and valve are destroyed. Valvular insufficiency may result when the lesion interferes with normal alignment of the valve. If vegetations become so large that blood flow through the valve is obstructed, the valve appears stenotic and then is very likely to *embolize* (i.e., cause emboli to be released into the systemic circulation) (McCance et al., 2014).

Possible ports of entry for infecting organisms include:

- The oral cavity (especially if dental procedures have been performed)
- Skin rashes, lesions, or abscesses
- Infections (cutaneous, genitourinary, GI, systemic)
- Surgery or invasive procedures, including IV line placement

❖ INTERPROFESSIONAL COLLABORATIVE CARE
◆ Assessment: Noticing

Because the mortality rate remains high, early detection of infective endocarditis is essential. Unfortunately, many patients (especially older adults) are misdiagnosed. Signs and symptoms typically occur within 2 weeks of a bacteremia (Chart 35-8).

Most patients have recurrent fevers from 99° to 103° F (37.2° to 39.4° C). However, as a result of physiologic changes associated with aging, older adults may be afebrile. The severity of symptoms may depend on the virulence of the infecting organism.

Physical Assessment/Signs and Symptoms. Assess the patient's *cardiovascular status.* Almost all patients with infective endocarditis develop murmurs. Carefully auscultate the precordium, noting and documenting any new murmurs (usually regurgitant in nature) or any changes in the intensity or quality of an old murmur. An S_3 or S_4 heart sound also may be heard.

HF is the most common complication of infective endocarditis. Assess for right-sided HF (as evidenced by peripheral edema, weight gain, and anorexia) and left-sided HF (as evidenced by fatigue, shortness of breath, and crackles on auscultation of breath sounds). See the discussion of HF earlier in this chapter.

Arterial embolization is a major complication in up to half of patients with infective endocarditis. Fragments of vegetation (clots) break loose and travel randomly through the circulation. When the left side of the heart is involved, vegetation fragments are carried to the spleen, kidneys, GI tract, brain, and extremities. When the right side of the heart is involved, emboli enter the pulmonary circulation.

Splenic infarction with sudden abdominal pain and radiation to the left shoulder can also occur. When performing an *abdominal assessment,* note rebound tenderness on palpation. The classic alteration in COMFORT described with renal infarction is flank pain that radiates to the groin and is accompanied by hematuria (red blood cells in the urine) or pyuria (white blood cells in the urine). Mesenteric emboli cause diffuse abdominal pain, often after eating, and abdominal distention.

About a third of patients have *neurologic changes;* others have signs and symptoms of pulmonary problems. Emboli to the central nervous system cause either transient ischemic attacks (TIAs) or a stroke. Confusion, reduced concentration, and aphasia or dysphagia may occur. Pleuritic chest pain, dyspnea, and cough are symptoms of pulmonary infarction related to embolization.

Petechiae (pinpoint red spots) occur in many patients with endocarditis. Examine the mucous membranes, the palate, the conjunctivae, and the skin above the clavicles for small, red, flat lesions. Assess the distal third of the nail bed for splinter hemorrhages, which appear as black longitudinal lines or small red streaks.

Diagnostic Assessment. The most reliable criteria for diagnosing endocarditis include positive blood cultures, a new regurgitant murmur, and evidence of endocardial involvement by echocardiography.

A positive *blood culture* is a prime diagnostic test. Both aerobic and anaerobic specimens are obtained for culture. Some slow-growing organisms may take 3 weeks and require a specialized medium to isolate. Low hemoglobin and hematocrit levels may also be present.

Echocardiography has improved the ability to diagnose infective endocarditis accurately. Transesophageal echocardiography (TEE) allows visualization of cardiac structures that are difficult to see with transthoracic echocardiography (TTE) (see Chapter 33).

◆ Interventions: Responding

Care of the patient with endocarditis usually includes antimicrobials, rest balanced with activity, and supportive therapy for HF. If these interventions are successful, surgery is usually not required.

Nonsurgical Management. The major component of treatment for endocarditis is drug therapy. Other interventions help prevent the life-threatening complications of the disease.

Antimicrobials are the main treatment, with the choice of drug depending on the specific organism involved. Because vegetations surround and protect the offending microorganism, an appropriate drug must be given in a sufficiently high dose to ensure its destruction. Antimicrobials are usually given IV, with the course of treatment lasting 4 to 6 weeks. For most bacterial cases, the ideal antibiotic is one of the penicillins or cephalosporins.

Patients may be hospitalized for several days to institute IV therapy and then are discharged for continued IV therapy at home. After hospitalization, most patients who respond to therapy may continue it at home when they become afebrile, have negative blood cultures, and have no signs of HF or embolization.

Anticoagulants do not prevent embolization from vegetations. Because they may result in bleeding, these drugs are avoided unless they are required to prevent thrombus formation (clotting) on a prosthetic valve.

The patient's activities are balanced with *adequate rest.* Consistently use appropriate aseptic technique to protect the patient from contact with potentially infective organisms. Continue to assess for signs of HF (e.g., rapid pulse, fatigue, cough, dyspnea) throughout the antimicrobial regimen and report significant changes.

Surgical Management. The cardiac surgeon may be consulted if antibiotic therapy is ineffective in sterilizing a valve, if refractory HF develops secondary to a defective valve, if large valvular vegetations are present, or if multiple embolic events occur. Current surgical interventions for infective endocarditis include:

- Removing the infected valve (either biologic or prosthetic)
- Repairing or removing congenital shunts
- Repairing injured valves and chordae tendineae
- Draining abscesses in the heart

Preoperative and postoperative care of patients having surgery involving the valves is similar to that described earlier in this chapter for valve replacement.

Care Coordination and Transition Management

Community-based care for patients with infective endocarditis is essential to resolve the problem, prevent relapse, and avoid complications. Patients and families need to be willing and have the knowledge, physical ability, and resources to administer IV antibiotics at home. **Collaborate with the home care nurse to complete health teaching started in the hospital and to monitor patient adherence and health status as directed by The Joint Commission's National Patient Safety Goals.**

In collaboration with the case manager, the home care nurse and pharmacist arrange for appropriate supplies to be available to the patient at home. Supplies include the prepared antibiotic, IV pump with tubing, alcohol wipes, IV access device, normal saline solution, and a saline flush solution drawn up in syringes. A saline lock, peripherally inserted central catheter (PICC) line, or central catheter is positioned at a venous site that is easily accessible to the patient or a family member.

Teach the patient and family how to administer the antibiotic and care for the infusion site while maintaining aseptic technique. The patient or family member should demonstrate this technique before the patient is discharged from the hospital. Emphasize the importance of maintaining a blood level of the antibiotic by administering the antibiotics as scheduled. After stabilization at home, the case manager or other nurse contacts the patient every week to determine whether he or she is adhering to the antibiotic therapy and whether any problems have been encountered.

Encourage proper oral hygiene. Advise patients to use a soft toothbrush, to brush their teeth at least twice per day, and to rinse the mouth with water after brushing. They should not use irrigation devices or floss the teeth because bacteremia may result. Teach them to clean any open skin areas well and apply an antibiotic ointment.

> **! NURSING SAFETY PRIORITY QSEN**
> **Action Alert**
>
> Patients must remind health care providers (including their dentists) of their endocarditis. Guidelines for antibiotic prophylaxis have been revised and are recommended only if the patient with a prosthetic valve, a history of infective endocarditis, or an unrepaired cyanotic congenital heart disease undergoes an invasive dental or oral procedure.
>
> Instruct patients to note any indications of recurring endocarditis such as fever. Remind them to monitor and record their temperature daily for up to 6 weeks. Teach them to report fever, chills, malaise, weight loss, increased fatigue, sudden weight gain, or dyspnea to their primary care provider.

PERICARDITIS

❖ PATHOPHYSIOLOGY

Acute pericarditis is an inflammation or alteration of the pericardium (the membranous sac that encloses the heart). The problem may be fibrous, serous, hemorrhagic, purulent, or neoplastic. Acute pericarditis is most commonly associated with:

- Infective organisms (bacteria, viruses, or fungi) (usually respiratory)
- Post–myocardial infarction (MI) syndrome (Dressler's syndrome)
- Post-pericardiotomy syndrome
- Acute exacerbations of systemic connective tissue disease

Chronic constrictive pericarditis occurs when chronic pericardial inflammation causes a fibrous thickening of the pericardium. It is caused by tuberculosis, radiation therapy, trauma, renal failure, or metastatic cancer. In chronic constrictive pericarditis, the pericardium becomes rigid, preventing adequate filling of the ventricles and eventually resulting in cardiac failure.

❖ INTERPROFESSIONAL COLLABORATIVE CARE

◆ Assessment: Noticing

Assessment findings for patients with *acute pericarditis* include substernal precordial pain that radiates to the left side of the neck, the shoulder, or the back. The alteration in COMFORT is classically grating and oppressive and is aggravated by breathing (mainly on inspiration), coughing, and swallowing. The pain is worse when the patient is in the supine position and may be relieved by sitting up and leaning forward. Ask specific questions to evaluate chest discomfort to differentiate it from the pain associated with an acute MI (see Chapter 38).

A pericardial friction rub may be heard with the diaphragm of the stethoscope positioned at the left lower sternal border. This scratchy, high-pitched sound is produced when the inflamed, roughened pericardial layers create friction as their surfaces rub together.

Patients with acute pericarditis may have an elevated white blood cell count and usually have a fever. Therefore blood culture and sensitivity may be analyzed in the laboratory. The ECG usually shows ST elevation in all leads, which returns to baseline with treatment. Atrial fibrillation is also common. Echocardiograms may be used to determine a pericardial effusion.

The proposed diagnostic criteria for acute pericarditis are presence of two of the following:

- Pericardial chest pain
- Presence of pericardial rub
- New ST elevation in all ECG leads or PR-segment depression
- New or worsening pericardial effusion

Patients with *chronic constrictive pericarditis* (lasting longer than 3 months) have signs of right-sided HF, elevated systemic venous pressure with jugular distention, hepatic engorgement, and dependent edema. Exertional fatigue and dyspnea are common complications. Thickening of the pericardium is seen on echocardiography or a computed tomography (CT) scan.

◆ Interventions: Responding

The focus of collaborative management is to promote COMFORT and treat the cause of pericarditis before severe complications occur.

Promoting Comfort. The health care provider usually prescribes NSAIDs for pain associated with pericarditis. Patients who do not obtain pain relief and who do not have bacterial pericarditis may receive corticosteroid therapy. Help the patient assume positions of COMFORT—usually sitting upright and leaning slightly forward. If the pain is not relieved within 24 to 48 hours, notify the primary health care provider. Colchicine 0.5 mg orally twice a day for 3 months has been shown to prevent pericarditis recurrence.

The various causes of pericarditis require specific therapies. For example, bacterial pericarditis (acute) usually requires antibiotics and pericardial drainage. The usual clinical course of acute pericarditis is short term (2 to 6 weeks), but episodes may recur. Chronic pericarditis caused by malignant disease may be treated with radiation or chemotherapy, whereas uremic pericarditis is treated by hemodialysis. The definitive treatment for chronic constrictive pericarditis is surgical excision of the pericardium (**pericardiectomy**).

Monitor all patients for **pericardial effusion**, which occurs when the space between the parietal and visceral layers of the pericardium fills with fluid. This complication puts the patient at risk for **cardiac tamponade**, or excessive fluid within the pericardial cavity.

Emergency Care: Acute Cardiac Tamponade. Acute cardiac tamponade may occur when small volumes (20 to 50 mL) of fluid accumulate rapidly in the pericardium and cause a sudden decrease in cardiac output (CO). If the fluid accumulates slowly, the pericardium may stretch to accommodate several hundred milliliters of fluid. Report any suspicion of this complication to the health care provider immediately. Findings of cardiac tamponade include:

- Jugular venous distention
- **Paradoxical pulse**, also known as *pulsus paradoxus* (systolic blood pressure 10 mm Hg or more higher on expiration than on inspiration) (Chart 35-9)
- Decreased heart rate, dyspnea, and fatigue
- Muffled heart sounds
- Hypotension

Cardiac tamponade is an emergency! The health care provider may initially manage the decreased CO with increased fluid volume administration while awaiting an echocardiogram or x-ray to confirm the diagnosis. Unfortunately, these tests are not always helpful because the fluid volume around the heart may be too small to visualize. Hemodynamic monitoring in a specialized critical care unit usually demonstrates compression of the heart, with all pressures (right atrial, pulmonary artery, and wedge) being similar and elevated (plateau pressures).

The health care provider may elect to perform a **pericardiocentesis** to remove fluid and relieve the pressure on the heart. Under echocardiographic or fluoroscopic and hemodynamic monitoring, the cardiologist inserts an 8-inch (20.3-cm), 16- or 18-gauge pericardial needle into the pericardial space. When the

---

 CHART 35-9   Best Practice for Patient Safety & Quality Care QSEN

Care of the Patient With Pericarditis

- Assess the nature of the patient's chest discomfort. (Pericardial pain is typically substernal. It is worse on inspiration and decreases when the patient leans forward.)
- Auscultate for a pericardial friction rub.
- Assist the patient to a position of comfort.
- Provide anti-inflammatory agents as prescribed.
- Explain that anti-inflammatory agents usually increase COMFORT within 48 hours.
- Avoid the administration of aspirin and anticoagulants because these may increase the possibility of tamponade.
- Auscultate the blood pressure carefully to detect paradoxical blood pressure (pulsus paradoxus), a sign of tamponade:
  - Palpate the blood pressure and inflate the cuff above the systolic pressure.
  - Deflate the cuff gradually and note when sounds are first audible on expiration.
  - Identify when sounds are also audible on inspiration.
  - Subtract the inspiratory pressure from the expiratory pressure to determine the amount of pulsus paradoxus (>10 mm Hg is an indication of tamponade).
- Inspect for other indications of tamponade, including jugular venous distention with clear lungs, muffled heart sounds, and decreased cardiac output.
- Notify the health care provider if tamponade is suspected.

needle is positioned properly, a catheter is inserted, and all available pericardial fluid is withdrawn. A pericardial drain may be placed temporarily. Monitor the pulmonary artery, wedge, and right atrial pressures during the procedure. The pressures should return to normal as the fluid compressing the heart is removed, and the signs and symptoms of tamponade should resolve. In situations in which the cause of the tamponade is unknown, pericardial fluid specimens may be sent to the laboratory for culture and sensitivity tests and cytology.

> **! NURSING SAFETY PRIORITY** **QSEN**
>
> **Action Alert**
>
> After the pericardiocentesis, closely monitor the patient for the recurrence of tamponade. Pericardiocentesis alone often does not resolve acute tamponade. Be prepared to provide adequate fluid volumes to increase CO and to prepare the patient for emergency sternotomy if tamponade recurs.

If the patient has a recurrence of tamponade or recurrent effusions or adhesions from chronic pericarditis, a portion or all of the pericardium may need to be removed to allow adequate ventricular filling and contraction. The surgeon may create a pericardial window, which involves removing a portion of the pericardium to permit excessive pericardial fluid to drain into the pleural space. In more severe cases, removal of the toughened encasing pericardium (pericardiectomy) may be necessary.

RHEUMATIC CARDITIS

❖ PATHOPHYSIOLOGY

Rheumatic carditis, also called *rheumatic endocarditis,* is a sensitivity response that develops after an upper respiratory tract infection with group A beta-hemolytic *Streptococci*. It occurs in almost half of patients with rheumatic fever. The precise mechanism by which the infection causes inflammatory lesions in the heart is not established; however, inflammation is evident in all layers of the heart. The inflammation results in impaired contractile function of the myocardium, thickening of the pericardium, and valvular damage.

Rheumatic carditis is characterized by the formation of Aschoff bodies (small nodules in the myocardium that are replaced by scar tissue). A diffuse cellular infiltrate also develops and may be responsible for the resulting heart failure (HF). The pericardium becomes thickened and covered with exudate, and a serosanguineous pleural effusion may develop. The most serious damage occurs to the endocardium, with inflammation of the valve leaflets developing. Hemorrhagic and fibrous lesions form along the inflamed surfaces of the valves, resulting in stenosis or regurgitation of the mitral and aortic valves (McCance et al., 2014).

❖ INTERPROFESSIONAL COLLABORATIVE CARE

Rheumatic carditis is one of the major indicators of rheumatic fever. The common signs and symptoms are:

- Tachycardia
- **Cardiomegaly** (enlarged heart)
- Development of a new murmur or a change in an existing murmur
- Pericardial friction rub

- Precordial pain
- Electrocardiogram (ECG) changes (prolonged P-R interval)
- Indications of HF
- Evidence of an existing streptococcal infection

Primary prevention is extremely important. Teach all patients to remind their primary health care providers to provide appropriate antibiotic therapy if they develop the indications of streptococcal pharyngitis:

- Moderate-to-high fever
- Abrupt onset of a sore throat
- Reddened throat with exudate
- Enlarged and tender lymph nodes

Penicillin is the antibiotic of choice for treatment. Erythromycin (Eryc, Erythromid) is the alternative for penicillin-sensitive patients.

Once a diagnosis of rheumatic fever is made, antibiotic therapy is started immediately. Teach the patient to continue the antibiotic administration for the full 10 days to prevent re-infection. Suggest ways to manage fever, such as maintaining hydration and taking antipyretics. Encourage the patient to get adequate rest.

Explain to the patient and family that a recurrence of rheumatic carditis is most likely the result of reinfection by *Streptococcus*. Antibiotic prophylaxis is necessary for the rest of the patient's life to prevent infective endocarditis discussed earlier in this chapter (see Infective Endocarditis).

CARDIOMYOPATHY

❖ PATHOPHYSIOLOGY

Cardiomyopathy is a subacute or chronic disease of cardiac muscle, and the cause may be unknown. Cardiomyopathies are classified into four categories on the basis of abnormalities in structure and function: dilated cardiomyopathy, hypertrophic cardiomyopathy, restrictive cardiomyopathy, and arrhythmogenic right ventricular cardiomyopathy (Table 35-5). **Dilated cardiomyopathy (DCM)** is the structural abnormality most commonly seen. DCM involves extensive damage to the myofibrils and interference with myocardial metabolism. Ventricular wall thickness is normal, but both ventricles are dilated (left ventricle is usually worse) and systolic function is impaired. Causes may include alcohol abuse, chemotherapy, infection, inflammation, and poor nutrition. Decreased CO from inadequate pumping of the heart causes the patient to experience dyspnea on exertion (DOE), decreased exercise capacity, fatigue, and palpitations.

The cardinal features of **hypertrophic cardiomyopathy (HCM)** are asymmetric ventricular hypertrophy and disarray of the myocardial fibers. Left ventricular hypertrophy leads to a stiff left ventricle, which results in diastolic filling abnormalities. Obstruction in the left ventricular outflow tract is seen in most patients with HCM. In about half of patients, HCM is transmitted as a single-gene autosomal-dominant trait (McCance et al., 2014). Some patients die without any symptoms; whereas others have DOE, syncope, dizziness, and palpitations. Many athletes who die suddenly probably had hypertrophic cardiomyopathy.

Restrictive cardiomyopathy, the rarest of the cardiomyopathies, is characterized by stiff ventricles that restrict filling during diastole. Symptoms are similar to those of left or right HF or both. The disease can be primary or caused by endocardial

TABLE 35-5 Pathophysiology, Signs and Symptoms, and Treatment of Common Cardiomyopathies

DILATED CARDIOMYOPATHY	HYPERTROPHIC CARDIOMYOPATHY	
	NONOBSTRUCTED	OBSTRUCTED
Pathophysiology		
Fibrosis of myocardium and endocardium Dilated chambers Mural wall thrombi prevalent	Hypertrophy of all walls Hypertrophied septum Relatively small chamber size	Same as for nonobstructed except for obstruction of left ventricular outflow tract associated with the hypertrophied septum and mitral valve incompetence
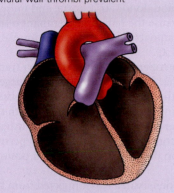	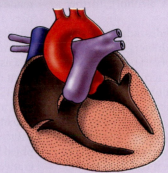	
Signs and Symptoms		
Fatigue and weakness Heart failure (left side) Dysrhythmias or heart block Systemic or pulmonary emboli S_3 and S_4 gallops Moderate to severe cardiomegaly	Dyspnea Angina Fatigue, syncope, palpitations Mild cardiomegaly S_4 gallop Ventricular dysrhythmias Sudden death common Heart failure	Same as for nonobstructed except with mitral regurgitation murmur Atrial fibrillation
Treatment		
Symptomatic treatment of heart failure Vasodilators Control of dysrhythmias Surgery: heart transplant	For both: Symptomatic treatment Beta blockers Conversion of atrial fibrillation Surgery: ventriculomyotomy or muscle resection with mitral valve replacement Nitrates and other vasodilators *contraindicated* with the obstructed form	

or myocardial disease such as sarcoidosis or amyloidosis. The prognosis for this type of cardiomyopathy is poor.

Arrhythmogenic right ventricular cardiomyopathy (dysplasia) results from replacement of myocardial tissue with fibrous and fatty tissue. Although the name implies right ventricle disease, about a third of patients also have left ventricle (LV) involvement. This disease has a familial association and most often affects young adults. Some patients have symptoms, and others do not.

❖ INTERPROFESSIONAL COLLABORATIVE CARE

◆ Assessment: Noticing

Findings in cardiomyopathy depend on the structural and functional abnormalities. For example, left ventricular or biventricular failure is characteristic of *dilated* cardiomyopathy (DCM). Some patients with DCM are asymptomatic for months to years and have left and/or right ventricular dilation confirmed on x-ray examination or echocardiography. Others experience sudden, pronounced symptoms of left ventricular failure, such as progressive dyspnea on exertion, orthopnea, palpitations, and activity intolerance. Right-sided HF develops late in the disease and is associated with a poor prognosis.

Atrial fibrillation occurs in some patients and is associated with embolism.

The clinical picture of *hypertrophic cardiomyopathy* (HCM) results from the hypertrophied septum causing a reduced stroke volume (SV) and cardiac output (CO). Most patients are asymptomatic until late adolescence or early adulthood. The primary symptoms of HCM are exertional dyspnea, angina, and syncope. The chest pain is atypical in that it usually occurs at rest, is prolonged, has no relation to exertion, and is not relieved by the administration of nitrates. A high incidence of ventricular dysrhythmias is associated with HCM. Sudden death occurs and may be the first manifestation of the disease.

Echocardiography, radionuclide imaging, and angiocardiography during cardiac catheterization are performed to diagnose and differentiate cardiomyopathies.

◆ Interventions: Responding

The treatment of choice for the patient with cardiomyopathy varies with the type of cardiomyopathy and may include both medical and surgical interventions.

Nonsurgical Management. The care of patients with dilated or restrictive cardiomyopathy is initially the same as that for HF.

Drug therapy includes the use of diuretics, vasodilating agents, and cardiac glycosides to increase CO. Because patients are at risk for sudden death, teach them to report any palpitations, dizziness, or fainting, which might indicate a dysrhythmia. Antidysrhythmic drugs or implantable cardiac defibrillators may be used to control life-threatening dysrhythmias. To block inappropriate sympathetic stimulation and tachycardia, beta blockers (e.g., metoprolol) are used. If cardiomyopathy has developed in response to a toxin (such as alcohol), further exposure to that toxin must be avoided.

Management of obstructive HCM includes administering negative inotropic agents such as beta-adrenergic blocking agents (carvedilol) and calcium antagonists (verapamil). These drugs decrease the outflow obstruction that accompanies exercise. They also decrease heart rate (HR), resulting in less angina, dyspnea, and syncope. Vasodilators, diuretics, nitrates, and cardiac glycosides are contraindicated in patients with obstructive HCM because vasodilation and positive inotropic effects may worsen the obstruction (Sherrid & Arabadjian, 2012). Strenuous exercise is also prohibited because it can increase the risk for sudden death. Excess alcohol intake and dehydration should also be avoided. Depending on risk stratification, an implantable cardioverter defibrillator (ICD) may be recommended to prevent sudden cardiac death. Patients with HCM are encouraged to seek genetic counseling. First-degree relatives should be screened for the presence of HCM, and echocardiography should be offered starting at age 12.

Surgical Management

Myomectomy and Ablation. The type of surgery performed depends on the type of cardiomyopathy. The most commonly used surgical treatment for obstructive HCM involves excising a portion of the hypertrophied ventricular septum to create a wider outflow tract (ventriculomyomectomy; also called *ventricular septal myectomy*). This procedure results in long-term improvement in activity tolerance for most patients.

Percutaneous alcohol septal ablation is another option for patients with HCM. Absolute alcohol is injected into a target septal branch of the left anterior descending coronary artery to produce a small septal infarction.

The patient with arrhythmogenic right ventricular cardiomyopathy who does not respond to drug therapy may have a radiofrequency catheter ablation or placement of an implantable defibrillator (see Chapter 34 for discussion of these procedures).

Heart Transplantation. Heart transplantation (surgical replacement with a donor heart) is the treatment of choice for patients with severe DCM and may be considered for patients with restrictive cardiomyopathy. The procedure may be done also for end-stage heart disease caused by coronary artery disease, valvular disease, or congenital heart disease.

Preoperative Care. Criteria for candidate selection for heart transplantation include:

- Life expectancy less than 1 year
- Age generally less than 65 years
- New York Heart Association (NYHA) Class III or IV
- Normal or only slightly increased pulmonary vascular resistance
- Absence of active infection
- Stable psychosocial status
- No evidence of current drug or alcohol abuse

Once the candidate is eligible and a heart is available, provide preoperative care as described in Chapter 14.

Operative Procedures. The surgeon transplants a heart from a donor with a comparable body weight and ABO compatibility into a recipient less than 6 hours after procurement. In the most common procedure (bicaval technique), the intact right atrium of the donor heart is preserved by anastomoses at the patient's (recipient's) superior and inferior venae cavae. In the more traditional orthotopic technique, cuffs of the patient's right and left atria are attached to the donor's atria. Anastomoses are made between the recipient and donor atria, aorta, and pulmonary arteries (Fig. 35-5). Because the remaining remnant of the recipient's atria contains the sinoatrial (SA) node, two unrelated P waves are visible on the ECG.

Postoperative Care. The postoperative care of the heart transplant recipient is similar to that for conventional cardiac surgery (see Chapter 38). However, the nurse must be especially observant to identify occult bleeding into the pericardial sac with the potential for tamponade. The patient's pericardium has usually stretched considerably to accommodate the diseased, hypertrophied heart, predisposing him or her to have concealed postoperative bleeding.

The transplanted heart is denervated (disconnected from the body's autonomic nervous system) and unresponsive to vagal stimulation. In the early postoperative phase, isoproterenol (Isuprel) may be titrated to support the heart rate and maintain cardiac output. Atropine, digoxin, and carotid sinus pressure are not used because they do not have their usual effects on the new heart. Denervation of the heart may cause pronounced orthostatic hypotension in the immediate postoperative phase. Caution the patient to change position slowly to help prevent this complication. Some patients also require a permanent pacemaker that is rate responsive to his or her activity level. The purpose is to increase CO and improve activity tolerance.

To suppress natural defense mechanisms (especially T- and B-cell function) and prevent transplant rejection, patients require a combination of immunosuppressants for the rest of their lives. Chapter 17 describes transplant rejection and prevention in detail.

! NURSING SAFETY PRIORITY QSEN

Critical Rescue

After surgery, perform comprehensive cardiovascular and respiratory assessments frequently according to agency or heart transplant surgical protocol. Chart 35-10 lists the signs and symptoms of rejection that are specific to heart transplant. Report any of these manifestations to the surgeon immediately! To detect rejection, the surgeon performs right endomyocardial biopsies at regularly scheduled intervals and whenever symptoms occur.

◎ CHART 35-10   Best Practice for Patient Safety & Quality Care QSEN

Assessing for Signs and Symptoms of Heart Transplant Rejection

- Shortness of breath
- Fatigue
- Fluid gain (edema, increased weight)
- Abdominal bloating
- New bradycardia
- Hypotension
- Atrial fibrillation or flutter
- Decreased activity tolerance
- Decreased ejection fraction (late sign)

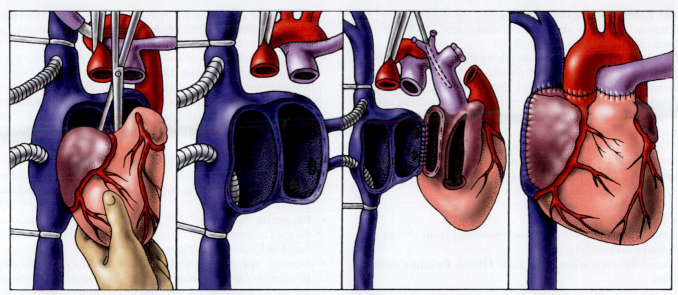

1. After the recipient is placed on cardiopulmonary bypass, the heart is removed.

2. The posterior walls of the recipient's left and right atria are left intact.

3. The left atrium of the donor heart is anastomosed to the recipient's residual posterior atrial walls, and the other atrial walls, the atrial septum, and the great vessels are joined.

POSTOPERATIVE RESULT

FIG. 35-5 One technique for heart transplantation.

Be very careful about handwashing and aseptic technique because patients are immunosuppressed from drug therapy. *Infection is the major cause of death* and usually develops in the immediate post-transplant period or during treatment for acute rejection.

About 50% of patients survive 10 years after transplantation (Gustafsson, 2016). Many of the surviving patients have a form of coronary artery disease (CAD) called **coronary artery vasculopathy (CAV)**, which presents as diffuse plaque in the arteries of the donor heart. The cause is thought to involve a combination of immunologic and nonimmunologic processes that result in vascular endothelial injury and an inflammatory response (Gustafsson, 2016). Because the heart is denervated, patients do not usually experience angina. Regularly scheduled exercise tolerance tests and angiography are required to identify CAV. Only a small percentage of patients with CAV benefit from revascularization procedures such as balloon angioplasty or coronary artery bypass surgery. Stents are beginning to show some promise in managing these patients. Retransplantation may be done in select patients.

To delay the development of CAV, encourage patients to follow lifestyle changes similar to those with primary CAD (see Chapter 38). The provider may prescribe a calcium channel blocker such as diltiazem (Cardizem) to prevent coronary spasm and closure. Stress the importance of strict adherence to nutritional modifications and drug regimens. Teach the patient the importance of participating in a regular exercise program. Collaborate with the physical therapist and the cardiac rehabilitation specialist to plan the most appropriate exercise plan for the patient.

Discharge planning involves a collaborative, interdisciplinary approach. Patients require extensive health teaching for self-management and community resources for support. Counseling and support groups can help patients cope with their fear of organ rejection. Drug therapy adherence is crucial to prevent this problem. Continuing community-based care for patients with a heart transplant is similar to that for heart failure discussed earlier in this chapter.

GET READY FOR THE NCLEX® EXAMINATION!

KEY POINTS

Review these Key Points for each NCLEX Examination Client Needs Category.

Safe and Effective Care Environment

- Provide information about continuing care for patients with heart failure (HF) after discharge to the community.

- Assess whether patients with end-stage HF have advance directives. If not, provide information about them.
- Collaborate with members of the health care team when developing and implementing a plan of care for patients with HF. **QSEN: Teamwork and Collaboration**
- Teach patients about community support groups and resources such as the American Heart Association.

Health Promotion and Maintenance

- Provide teaching about self-management at home for patients with HF (see Table 35-4).
- Monitor older adults who are taking digoxin for manifestations of toxicity. Monitor potassium levels to check for hypokalemia (see Chart 35-5). **QSEN: Safety**
- Teach patients taking ACE inhibitors, ARBs, or sacubitril/valsartan (Entresto) to change positions slowly to avoid orthostatic hypotension, especially older adults. **QSEN: Safety**
- Teach the patient with valvular dysfunction, cardiac infection, or cardiomyopathy the necessity of taking preventive antibiotic therapy before any invasive dental procedure. **QSEN: Evidence-Based Practice**

Psychosocial Integrity

- Assess the patient for depression resulting from altered self-concept and anxiety.
- Assess the patient's coping skills. **QSEN: Patient-Centered Care**

Physiological Integrity

- Assess the patient for manifestations of right- and left-sided HF (see Charts 35-1 and 35-2).
- Weigh daily and record intake and output of patients with HF.
- Assess for early signs and symptoms of pulmonary edema (e.g., crackles in the lung bases, dyspnea at rest, disorientation, confusion), especially in older adults. **QSEN: Safety**
- Assess for symptoms of worsening HF: rapid weight gain (3 lb in a week), a decrease in exercise tolerance lasting 2 to 3 days, cold symptoms (cough) lasting more than 3 to 5 days, nocturia, development of dyspnea or angina at rest, or unstable angina. **QSEN: Safety**
- Monitor the HF patient on beta blockers carefully for hypotension and bradycardia. **QSEN: Safety**
- Monitor the pulse of patients taking digoxin before administration and report to the health care provider a pulse that is not within the desired parameters.
- Monitor for manifestations of pulmonary edema as listed in Chart 35-3.
- Place the patient in a sitting position and provide oxygen therapy at a high flow rate (unless otherwise contraindicated) if pulmonary edema is suspected. **QSEN: Evidence-Based Practice**
- Recognize that home care nurses perform and document focused physical assessments for cardiac patients as delineated in Chart 35-4. **QSEN: Informatics**
- Monitor the patient with valvular dysfunction for atrial fibrillation, which may lead to hemostasis and mural thrombi. Monitor for an irregular cardiac rhythm and administer warfarin as indicated.
- Document neurovascular status frequently because emboli from valvular disease may cause strokes. **QSEN: Informatics**
- Differentiate major types of cardiomyopathy as described in Table 35-5.
- Observe for symptoms of heart transplant rejection as listed in Chart 35-10.
- Provide care for patients with pericarditis as outlined in Chart 35-9.

SELECTED BIBLIOGRAPHY

Asterisk indicates a classic or definitive work on this subject.

Adler, Y., Charron, P., Imazio, M., Badano, L., Baron-Esquivias, G., et al. (2015). 2015 ESC guidelines for the diagnosis and management of pericardial disease. *European Heart Journal*, *36*(42), 2921–2964.

*Albert, N. M. (2012). Fluid management strategies in heart failure. *Critical Care Nurse*, *32*(2), 20–32.

Amgen. (2015). *Highlights of prescribing information*. pi.amgen.com/united_states/corlanor/corlanor_pi_hcp.pdf.

Aschenbrenner, D. (2015). Drug Watch: New drug for chronic heart failure. *American Journal of Nursing*, *115*(8), 48–49.

Baddour, L., Wilson, W., Bayer, A., Fowler, V., Tleyjeh, I., Rybak, M., et al. (2015). Infective endocarditis in adults: Diagnosis, antimicrobial therapy, and management of complications: A scientific statement for healthcare professionals from the American Heart Association. *Circulation*, *132*, 1435–1486.

Boekstegers, P., Hausleiter, J., Baldus, S., von Bardeleben, R. S., Beucher, H., Butter, C., et al. (2014). Percutaneous interventional mitral regurgitation treatment using the Mitra-Clip system. *Clinical Research Cardiology*, *103*, 85–96.

Bonacchi, M., Harmelin, G., & Sani, G. (2014). The actual role of cardiocirculatory assistance in heart-failure treatment as destination therapy and bridge to life. *Heart Failure Clinic*, *10*, S13–S25.

Broglio, K., Eichholz-Heller, F., & Nakagawa, S. (2015). Left ventricular assist devices: When bridge to transplantation becomes destination. *Journal of Hospice & Palliative Nursing*, *17*(5), 374–379.

Buonocore, D., & Wallace, E. (2014). Comprehensive guideline for care of patients with heart failure. *AACN Advanced Critical Care*, *25*(2), 151–162.

Caboral-Stevens, M. (2014). A snapshot of the latest heart failure guidelines. *The Nurse Practitioner*, *39*(7), 49–54.

*Chen, W., Tran, K., & Maisel, A. (2010). Biomarkers in heart failure. *Heart (British Cardiac Society)*, *96*, 314–320.

Clark, A., McDougall, G., Riegel, B., Joiner-Rogers, G., Innerarity, S., Meraviglia, M., et al. (2015). Health status and self-care outcomes after an education-support intervention for people with chronic heart failure. *Journal of Cardiovascular Nursing*, *30*(4S), S3–S13.

Colin-Ramirez, E., McAlister, F., Zheng, Y., Sharma, S., Armstrong, P., & Ezekowitz, J. (2015). The long-term effect of dietary sodium restriction on clinical outcomes in patients with heart failure. The SODIUM-HF (Study of dietary intervention under 100 mmol in heart failure): A pilot study. *American Heart Journal*, *169*(2), 274–281.

*Cooper, K. L. (2011). Care of the lower extremities in patients with acute decompensated heart failure. *Critical Care Nurse*, *31*(4), 21–29.

Cooper, K. (2015). Biventricular pacemakers in patients with heart failure. *Critical Care Nurse*, *35*(2), 20–27.

Elliott, P., Anastasaki, A., Borger, M., Borggrefe, M., Cecchi, F., Charron, P., et al. (2014). 2014 ESC guidelines on diagnosis and management of hypertrophic cardiomyopathy. *European Heart Journal*, *35*, 2733–2779.

Eun, J., & Smith, A. (2015). Safety and efficacy of colchicine therapy in the prevention of recurrent pericarditis. *American Journal of Health-System Pharmacy*, *71*, 1277–1281.

*Fard, A., Taub, P., Iqbal, N., & Maisel, A. (2012). Natriuretic peptides in the hospital: Risk stratification and treatment titration. In A. Maisel (Ed.), *Cardiac biomarkers: Expert advice for clinicians* (pp. 128–139). London: JP Medical Publishers.

Fergenbaum, J., Bermingham, S., Krahn, M., Alter, D., & Demers, C. (2015). Care in the home for the management of chronic heart failure: Systematic review and cost-effectiveness analysis. *Journal of Cardiovascular Nursing, 30*(4S), S44–S51.

Grodanz, E. (2015). Robotic mitral valve repair. *Journal of Cardiovascular Nursing, 30*(4), 325–331.

Gustafsson, F. (2016). *Diagnosis and prognosis of cardiac allograft vasculopathy. Up to Date.* https://www.uptodate.com/contents/diagnosis-and-prognosis-of-cardiac-allograft-vasculopathy?source=see_link.

Habib, G., Lancellotti, P., Antunes, M., Bongiorni, M., Casalta, J., Del Zotti, F., et al. (2015). 2015 ESC guidelines for the management of infective endocarditis. *European Heart Journal, 36*(44), 3075–3128.

*Hannibal, G. (2012). ECG characteristics of acute pericarditis. *AACN Advanced Critical Care, 23*(3), 341–344.

Hill, S., Booth, R., Santaguida, L., Don-Wauchope, A., Brown, J., Oremus, M., et al. (2014). Use of BNP and NT-proBNP for the diagnosis of heart failure in the emergency department: A systematic review of the evidence. *Heart Failure Review, 19*, 421–438.

Hjelm, C., Bostrom, A., Riegel, B., Arestedt, K., & Stromberg, A. (2014). The association between cognitive function and self-care in patients with chronic heart failure. *Heart and Lung: The Journal of Critical Care, 44*, 113–119.

Huntsinger, M., Rabara, R., Peralta, I., & Doshi, R. (2015). Current technology to maximize cardiac resynchronization therapy benefit for patients with symptomatic heart failure. *AACN Advanced Critical Care, 26*(4), 329–340.

Imazio, M., & Adler, Y. (2015). Pharmacological therapy of pericardial disease. *Current Pharmaceutical Design, 21*, 525–530.

Imazio, M., Gaita, F., & LeWinter, M. (2015). Evaluation and treatment of pericarditis: A systematic review. *Journal of the American Medical Association, 314*(14), 1498–1506.

Kalowes, P. (2015). Improving end-of-life-care prognostic discussions: Role of the advance practice nurse. *AACN Advanced Critical Care, 26*(2), 151–166.

Keteyian, S., Squires, R., Ades, P., & Thomas, R. (2014). Incorporating patients with chronic heart failure into outpatient cardiac rehabilitation: Practical recommendations for exercise and self-care counseling—a clinical review. *Journal of Cardiopulmonary Rehabilitation and Prevention, 34*, 223–232.

Kuhn, D., & Brown, C. (2015). Exploration of factors associated with hospital readmissions in patients with chronic heart failure: A pilot study. *Professional Case Management, 20*(2), 106–109.

Lachell, A., & Henry, L. (2015). Transcatheter aortic valve replacement options for severe aortic stenosis in high-risk patients. *Journal of Cardiovascular Nursing, 30*(3), 242–247.

Laing, C. (2014). Left ventricular assist device for end-stage heart failure. *The Nurse Practitioner, 39*(2), 42–47.

Madamanchi, C., Alhosainti, H., Sumida, A., & Runge, M. (2014). Obesity and natriuretic peptides, BNP and NT-proBNP: Mechanisms and diagnostic implications for heart failure. *International Journal of Cardiology, 176*(3), 611–617.

Marron, B., Ommen, S., Semsarian, C., Spirito, P., Olivotto, I., & Maron, M. (2015). Hypertrophic cardiomyopathy: Present and future, with translation into contemporary cardiovascular medicine. *Journal of the American College of Cardiology, 64*(1), 83–99.

McCance, K., Huether, S., Brashers, V., & Rote, N. (2014). *Pathophysiology: The biologic basis for disease in adults and children* (7th ed.). St. Louis: Mosby.

McMurray, J., Packer, M., Desai, A., Gong, J., Lefkowitz, M., Rizkala, A., et al. (2014). Angiotensin-neprilysin inhibition versus enalapril in heart failure. *The New England Journal of Medicine, 371*(11), 993–1004.

Mozaffarian, D., Benjamin, E., Go, A., Arnett, D., Blaha, M., Cushman, M., et al. (2015). Heart disease and stroke statistics—2015 update. *Circulation, 131*, e29–e322. doi:10.1161/CIR0000000000000152.

Nishimura, R., Otto, C., Bonow, R. W., Barabello, B. A., Erwin, J. P., Guyton, R. A., et al. (2014). 2014 AHA/ACC guideline for the management of patients with valvular heart disease: A report of the American College of Cardiology/American Heart Association task

force on practice guidelines. *Journal of the American College of Cardiology, 63*(22), e57–e185.

O'Neill, B., & Kazer, M. (2014). Destination to nowhere: A new look at aggressive treatment for heart failure—a case study. *Critical Care Nurse, 34*(2), 47–56.

Orso, F., Fabbri, G., Baldasseroni, S., & Maggioni, A. (2014). Newest additions to heart failure treatment. *Expert Opinion on Pharmacotherapy, 15*(13), 1849–1861.

Pagana, K., Pagana, T., & Pagana, T. (2017). *Mosby's diagnostic and laboratory test reference* (13th ed.). St. Louis: Mosby.

Panos, A., & George, E. (2014). Transcatheter aortic valve implantation options for treating severe aortic stenosis in the elderly. *Dimensions in Critical Care Nurse, 33*(2), 49–56.

Paul, S., & Hice, A. (2014). Role of the acute care nurse in managing patients with heart failure using evidence-based care. *Critical Care Nursing Quarterly, 37*(4), 357–376.

Prasun, M. (2015). New heart failure treatment and nursing care. *Heart and Lung: The Journal of Critical Care, 44*, 367.

Reilly, C., Anderson, K., Baas, L., Johnson, E., Lennie, T., Lewis, C., et al. (2015). American Association of Heart Failure Nurses Best Practices paper: Literature synthesis and guideline review for dietary sodium restriction. *Heart and Lung: The Journal of Critical Care, 44*, 289–298. doi:10.1016/j.hrtlng.2015.03.003.

Schell, W. (2014). A review: Discharge navigation and its effect on heart failure readmissions. *Professional Case Management, 19*(5), 224–234.

Schwier, N., Coons, J., & Rao, S. (2015). Pharmacotherapy update of acute idiopathic pericarditis. *Pharmacotherapy, 35*(1), 99–111.

Sherrid, M., & Arabadjian, M. (2012). A primer of disopyramide treatment of obstructive hypertrophic cardiomyopathy. *Progress in Cardiovascular Diseases, 54*(6), 483–492.

Sterne, P., Grossman, S., Migliardi, J., & Swallow, A. (2014). Nurses' knowledge of heart failure: Implications for decreasing 30-day readmission rates. *Medical Surgical Nursing, 23*(5), 321–329.

Suter, P., Gorski, L., Hennessey, B., & Suter, W. (2012). Best practices for heart failure: A focused review. *Home Healthcare Nurse, 30*(7), 394–405.

*Swedberg, K., Komajda, M., Bohm, M., Borer, J., Ford, I., Dubost-Brama, A., et al. (2010). Ivabradine and outcomes in chronic heart failure (SHIFT): A randomized placebo-controlled study. *The Lancet, 376*(9744), 875–885.

Townsend, T. (2015). Aortic stenosis. *Nursing Critical Care, 10*(1), 15–17.

Traughton, R., Frampton, C., Brunner-LaRocca, H., Pfisterer, M., Eurlings, L., Erntell, H., et al. (2014). Effect of B-type natriuretic peptide-guided treatment of chronic heart failure on total mortality and hospitalization: An individual patient meta-analysis. *European Heart Journal, 35*, 1559–1567.

Urden, L., Stacy, K., & Lough, M. (2016). *Priorities in critical care nursing* (7th ed.). St. Louis: Elsevier.

Xin, W., Lin, Z., & Mi, S. (2015). Does B-type natriuretic peptide-guided therapy improve outcomes in patients with chronic heart failure? A systematic review and meta-analysis of randomized controlled trials. *Heart Failure Review, 20*, 69–80.

*Yancy, C., Jessup, M., Bozkurt, B., Butler, J., Casey, D., Drazner, M., et al. (2013). 2013 ACCF/AHA Guideline for the management of heart failure: Executive Summary: A report of the American College of Cardiology Foundation/American Heart Association Task Force on Practice Guidelines. *Journal of the American College of Cardiology, 62*(16), 1495–1539.

Yancy, C., Jessup, M., Bozkurt, B., Butler, J., Casey, D., Colvin, M., et al. (2016). 2016 ACC/AHA/HFSA focused update on new pharmacological therapy for heart failure: An Update of the 2013 ACCF/AHA guideline for the management of heart failure. *Circulation, 134*, e282–e293. doi:10.1161/CIR.0000000000000435.

Zhang, P., & Melander, S. (2014). Transcatheter aortic valve replacement for severe aortic stenosis. *Critical Care Nursing Quarterly, 37*(4), 346–356.

Care of Patients With Vascular Problems

Nicole M. Heimgartner

 http://evolve.elsevier.com/Iggy/

PRIORITY AND INTERRELATED CONCEPTS

The priority concepts for this chapter are:
- PERFUSION
- CLOTTING

✳ The PERFUSION concept exemplar for this chapter is Hypertension, below.

✳ The CLOTTING concept exemplar for this chapter is Venous Thromboembolism, p. 742.

The interrelated concept for this chapter is IMMUNITY.

LEARNING OUTCOMES

Safe and Effective Care Environment

1. Collaborate with the interprofessional team to provide high-quality care for patients with vascular problems that impact PERFUSION and CLOTTING.
2. Prioritize evidence-based care for patients with vascular problems affecting PERFUSION and CLOTTING.

Health Promotion and Maintenance

3. Teach patients about lifestyle modifications to reduce the risk for vascular problems.
4. Teach patient and caregiver(s) about common drugs used for vascular problems, including anticoagulants to prevent CLOTTING.

Psychosocial Integrity

5. Implement nursing interventions to decrease the psychosocial impact of living with chronic vascular disease.

Physiological Integrity

6. Apply knowledge of anatomy and physiology to perform an evidence-based assessment for the patient with a vascular problem.
7. Plan nursing care to promote PERFUSION and prevent complications such as CLOTTING or altered IMMUNITY.
8. Use clinical judgment to assess laboratory data and signs and symptoms to prioritize care for patients with vascular problems.

✳ PERFUSION CONCEPT EXEMPLAR Hypertension

Hypertension, or high blood pressure (BP), is the most common health problem seen in primary care settings and can cause stroke, myocardial infarction (heart attack), kidney failure, and death if not treated early and effectively. The Eighth Joint National Committee (JNC 8) on Prevention, Detection, Evaluation, and Treatment of High Blood Pressure recently published *Evidence-Based Guidelines for the Management of High Blood Pressure in Adults* (James et al., 2014).

According to JNC 8, in the general population ages 60 years and older, the desired BP is below 150/90. For people younger than 60 years, the desired BP is below 140/90. Patients whose BPs are above these desired goals should be treated with drug therapy (James et al., 2014). Adult patients with specific risk factors for developing hypertension should be treated at any age, as described later under Drug Therapy.

❖ PATHOPHYSIOLOGY

To best understand the pathophysiology of hypertension, a review of normal BP and how it is normally maintained is essential.

Mechanisms That Influence Blood Pressure

The systemic arterial BP is a product of cardiac output (CO) and total peripheral vascular resistance (PVR). Cardiac output is determined by the stroke volume (SV) multiplied by heart rate (HR) ($CO = SV \times HR$). Control of peripheral vascular resistance (i.e., vessel constriction or dilation) is maintained by the autonomic nervous system and circulating hormones, such as norepinephrine and epinephrine. Consequently, any factor that increases peripheral vascular resistance, heart rate, or stroke volume increases the systemic arterial pressure. Conversely, any factor that decreases peripheral vascular resistance, heart rate, or stroke volume decreases the systemic arterial pressure and can cause decreased PERFUSION to body tissues.

Stabilizing mechanisms exist in the body to exert an overall regulation of systemic arterial pressure and to prevent circulatory collapse. Four control systems play a major role in maintaining blood pressure:

- The arterial baroreceptor system
- Regulation of body fluid volume
- The renin-angiotensin-aldosterone system
- Vascular autoregulation

Arterial baroreceptors are found primarily in the carotid sinus, aorta, and wall of the left ventricle. They monitor the level of arterial pressure and counteract a rise in arterial pressure through vagally mediated cardiac slowing and vasodilation with decreased sympathetic tone. Therefore reflex control of circulation elevates the systemic arterial pressure when it falls and lowers it when it rises. Why baroreceptor control fails in hypertension is not clear (McCance et al., 2014).

Changes *in fluid volume* also affect the systemic arterial pressure. For example, if there is an excess of sodium and/or water in a person's body, the BP rises through complex physiologic mechanisms that change the venous return to the heart, producing a rise in cardiac output. If the kidneys are functioning adequately, a rise in systemic arterial pressure produces diuresis (excessive voiding) and a fall in pressure. Pathologic conditions change the pressure threshold at which the kidneys excrete sodium and water, thereby altering the systemic arterial pressure.

The *renin-angiotensin-aldosterone* system also regulates BP (see discussion in Chapter 11). The kidney produces renin, an enzyme that acts on angiotensinogen to split off angiotensin I, which is converted by an enzyme in the lung to form angiotensin II. Angiotensin II has strong vasoconstrictor action on blood vessels and is the controlling mechanism for aldosterone release. Aldosterone then works on the collecting tubules in the kidneys to reabsorb sodium. Sodium retention inhibits fluid loss, thus increasing blood volume and subsequent BP.

Inappropriate secretion of renin may cause increased peripheral vascular resistance in patients with hypertension. When the BP is high, renin levels should decrease because the increased renal arteriolar pressure usually inhibits renin secretion. However, for most people with essential hypertension, renin levels remain normal.

The process of *vascular autoregulation*, which keeps PERFUSION of tissues in the body relatively constant, appears to be important in causing hypertension. However, the exact mechanism of how this system works is poorly understood.

Classifications of Hypertension

Hypertension can be essential (primary) or secondary. **Essential hypertension** is the most common type and is not caused by an existing health problem. However, a number of risk factors can increase a person's likelihood of becoming hypertensive. Continuous BP elevation in patients with essential hypertension results in damage to vital organs by causing medial hyperplasia (thickening) of the arterioles. As the blood vessels thicken and PERFUSION decreases, body organs are damaged. These changes can result in myocardial infarctions, strokes, peripheral vascular disease (PVD), or kidney failure.

Specific disease states and drugs can increase a person's susceptibility to hypertension. A person with this type of elevation in BP has **secondary hypertension**.

Malignant hypertension is a severe type of elevated BP that rapidly progresses. A person with this health problem usually has symptoms such as morning headaches, blurred vision, and dyspnea and/or symptoms of uremia (accumulation in the blood of substances ordinarily eliminated in the urine). Patients are often in their 30s, 40s, or 50s with their systolic BP greater than 200 mm Hg. The diastolic BP is greater than 150 mm Hg or greater than 130 mm Hg when there are pre-existing complications. Unless intervention occurs promptly, a patient with malignant hypertension may experience kidney failure, left ventricular heart failure, or stroke.

Etiology and Genetic Risk

Essential hypertension can develop when a patient has any one or more of the risk factors listed in Table 36-1.

Kidney disease is one of the most common causes of *secondary* hypertension. Hypertension can develop when there is any sudden damage to the kidneys. Renovascular hypertension is associated with narrowing of one or more of the main arteries carrying blood directly to the kidneys, known as *renal artery stenosis (RAS)*. Many patients have been able to reduce the use of their antihypertensive drugs when the narrowed arteries are dilated through angioplasty with stent placement.

Dysfunction of the adrenal medulla or the adrenal cortex can also cause secondary hypertension. *Adrenal-mediated hypertension* is caused by primary excesses of aldosterone, cortisol, and catecholamines. In *primary aldosteronism,* excessive aldosterone causes hypertension and hypokalemia (low potassium levels). It usually arises from benign adenomas of the adrenal cortex. *Pheochromocytomas* are tumors that originate most commonly in the adrenal medulla and result in excessive secretion of catecholamines, resulting in life-threatening high blood pressure. In *Cushing's syndrome,* excessive glucocorticoids are excreted from the adrenal cortex. The most common cause of Cushing's syndrome is either adrenocortical hyperplasia or adrenocortical adenoma (tumor).

Drugs that can cause secondary hypertension include estrogen, glucocorticoids, mineralocorticoids, sympathomimetics, cyclosporine, and erythropoietin. The use of estrogen-containing oral contraceptives is likely the most common cause of secondary hypertension in women. Drugs that cause hypertension are discontinued to reverse this problem.

TABLE 36-1 **Etiology of Hypertension**	
ESSENTIAL (PRIMARY)	**SECONDARY**
• Family history of hypertension	• Kidney disease
• African-American ethnicity	• Primary aldosteronism
• Hyperlipidemia	• Pheochromocytoma
• Smoking	• Cushing's disease
• Older than 60 years or postmenopausal	• Coarctation of the aorta
• Excessive sodium and caffeine intake	• Brain tumors
• Overweight/obesity	• Encephalitis
• Physical inactivity	• Pregnancy
• Excessive alcohol intake	• Drugs:
• Low potassium, calcium, or magnesium intake	• Estrogen (e.g., oral contraceptives)
• Excessive and continuous stress	• Glucocorticoids
	• Mineralocorticoids
	• Sympathomimetics

Incidence and Prevalence

Hypertension is a worldwide epidemic. In the United States, it is estimated that 80 million adults have high blood pressure (Mozaffarian et al., 2016). The disease can shorten life expectancy.

GENDER HEALTH CONSIDERATIONS
Patient-Centered Care QSEN

A higher percentage of men than women have hypertension until 45 years of age. From ages 45 to 64, the percentages of men and women with hypertension are similar. After age 64, women have a higher percentage of the disease (Mozaffarian et al., 2016). The causes for these differences are not known.

CULTURAL/SPIRITUAL CONSIDERATIONS
Patient-Centered Care QSEN

The prevalence of hypertension in African Americans in the United States is among the highest in the world and is constantly increasing. When compared with Euro-Americans, they develop high blood pressure earlier in life, making them much more likely to die from strokes, heart disease, and kidney disease (Mozaffarian et al., 2016). The exact reasons for these differences are not known. Raising awareness of hypertension through education within African-American communities, including the importance of receiving treatment and controlling blood pressure, has been somewhat successful (Mozaffarian et al., 2016). Because of the prevalence in the African-American population, the JNC-8 Guideline differentiates first-line therapy based on race (Davis, 2015).

Health Promotion and Maintenance

Control of hypertension has resulted in major decreases in cardiovascular morbidity and mortality. The U.S. *Healthy People 2020* campaign includes a number of objectives related to hypertension to decrease cardiovascular mortality (Table 36-2).

The *2013* American College of Cardiology (ACC) and American Heart Association (AHA) *Guidelines on Lifestyle Management to Reduce Cardiovascular Risk* outlines evidence-based dietary and exercise practices to help lower blood pressure (Eckel et al., 2014). These guidelines are similar to the Dietary Approaches to Stop Hypertension (DASH) and include:

- Consume a dietary pattern that emphasizes intake of vegetables, fruits, and whole grains.
- Consume low-fat dairy products, poultry, fish, legumes, nontropical vegetable oils, and nuts.
- Limit intake of sweets, sugar-sweetened beverages, and red meats.
- Lower sodium intake to no more than 2400 mg per day; a limit of 1500 mg of sodium per day is preferred.
- Engage in aerobic physical activity three or four times a week. Each session should last for 40 minutes on average and involve moderate-to-vigorous physical activity.

In addition to following specific dietary and physical activity guidelines, teach patients ways to decrease other modifiable risk factors for hypertension, such as smoking and excessive alcohol intake. Risk factor prevention and lifestyle changes are discussed in more detail in Chapter 38.

TABLE 36-2 Meeting *Healthy People 2020* Objectives

Heart Disease and Stroke

Selected objectives retained from *Healthy People 2010:*
- Increase the proportion of adults with high blood pressure who are taking action to help control their blood pressure.
- Increase the proportion of adults who have had their blood pressure measured within the preceding 2 years and can state whether their blood pressure was normal or high.

Selected objectives retained but modified from *Healthy People 2010:*
- Reduce the proportion of people in the population with hypertension.
- Increase the proportion of adults with prehypertension who meet the recommended guidelines for:
  a. Body mass index (BMI)
  b. Saturated fat consumption
  c. Sodium intake
  d. Physical activity
  e. Moderate alcohol consumption
- Increase the proportion of adults with hypertension who meet the [above] recommended guidelines.

New objectives for Healthy People 2020:
- Increase the proportion of adults with hypertension who are taking the recommended medications to decrease their blood pressure.

Data from www.healthypeople.gov/2020.

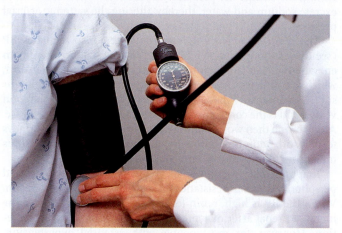

FIG. 36-1 Blood pressure screening during history and physical examination. (From Wilson S. F., Giddens J.F. [2017]. *Health assessment for nursing practice* [ed. 6.]. St. Louis: Mosby.)

❖ INTERPROFESSIONAL COLLABORATIVE CARE
◆ Assessment: Noticing

History. Review the patient's risk factors for hypertension. Collect data on the patient's age; ethnic origin or race; family history of hypertension; average dietary intake of calories, sodium- and potassium-containing foods and alcohol; and exercise habits. Also assess any past or present history of kidney or cardiovascular disease and current use of drug therapy or illicit drugs.

Physical Assessment/Signs and Symptoms. When a diagnosis of hypertension is made, most people have no symptoms. However, some patients experience headaches, facial flushing (redness), dizziness, or fainting as a result of the elevated blood pressure. Obtain blood pressure readings in both arms. Two or more readings may be taken at each visit (Fig. 36-1). Some patients have high blood pressure due to anxiety associated with visiting a health care provider. Be sure to take an accurate blood pressure by using an appropriate-size cuff.

To detect postural (orthostatic) changes, take readings with the patient in the supine (lying) or sitting position and at least 2 minutes later when standing. **Orthostatic hypotension** is a decrease in blood pressure (20 mm Hg systolic and/or 10 mm Hg diastolic) when the patient changes position from lying to sitting.

Funduscopic examination of the eyes to observe vascular changes in the retina is done by a skilled health care practitioner. The appearance of the retina can be a reliable index of the severity and prognosis of hypertension. Physical assessment is also helpful in diagnosing several conditions that produce secondary hypertension. The presence of abdominal bruits is typical of patients with renal artery stenosis. Tachycardia, sweating, and pallor may suggest a pheochromocytoma (adrenal medulla tumor). Coarctation of the aorta is evidenced by elevation of blood pressure in the arms, with normal or low blood pressure in the lower extremities.

Psychosocial Assessment. Assess for psychosocial stressors that can worsen hypertension and affect the patient's ability to adhere to treatment. Evaluate job-related, economic, and other life stressors and the patient's response to these stressors. Some patients may have difficulty coping with the lifestyle changes needed to control hypertension. Be sure to assess past coping strategies.

Diagnostic Assessment. Although no laboratory tests are diagnostic of essential hypertension, several laboratory tests can assess possible causes of secondary hypertension. Kidney disease can be diagnosed by the presence of protein and red blood cells in the urine, elevated levels of blood urea nitrogen (BUN), and elevated serum creatinine levels. The creatinine clearance test directly indicates the glomerular filtration ability of the kidneys. The normal value is 107 to 139 mL/min for men and 87 to 107 mL/min for women (Pagana et al., 2017). Decreased levels indicate acute or chronic kidney disease.

Urinary test results are positive for the presence of catecholamines in patients with a pheochromocytoma (tumor of the adrenal medulla). An elevation in levels of serum corticoids and 17-ketosteroids in the urine is diagnostic of Cushing's disease.

No specific x-ray studies can diagnose hypertension. Routine chest radiography may help recognize cardiomegaly (heart enlargement). An electrocardiogram (ECG) determines the degree of cardiac involvement. Left atrial and ventricular hypertrophy is the first ECG sign of heart disease resulting from hypertension. Left ventricular remodeling can be detected on the 12-lead ECG (see Chapter 38 for discussion of remodeling).

◆ *Analysis: Interpreting*

The priority collaborative problems for most patients with hypertension are:

1. Need for health teaching due to the plan of care for hypertension management
2. Potential for decreased adherence due to side effects of drug therapy and necessary changes in lifestyle

◆ *Planning and Implementation: Responding*

Health Teaching

Planning: Expected Outcomes. The patient with hypertension is expected to verbalize his or her individualized plan of care for hypertension (see the Concept Map on Hypertension).

Interventions. Lifestyle changes are considered the foundation of hypertension control. If these changes are unsuccessful, the primary care provider considers the use of antihypertensive drugs. There is no surgical treatment for essential hypertension. However, surgery may be indicated for certain causes of secondary hypertension, such as kidney disease, coarctation of the aorta, and pheochromocytoma.

Lifestyle Changes. In collaboration with the health care team, teach the patient to (Scordo & Pickett, 2015):

- Restrict sodium intake in the diet per the ACC/AHA guidelines
- Reduce weight, if overweight or obese
- Use alcohol sparingly (no more than one drink a day for women and two drinks a day for men)
- Exercise 3 or 4 days a week for 40 minutes each day per the ACC/AHA guidelines
- Use relaxation techniques to decrease stress
- Stop smoking and tobacco use

Strategies to help patients make these changes are discussed in Chapter 38.

Complementary and Integrative Health. Garlic and coenzyme Q_{10} have been used for a number of health problems, but evidence to support their use to prevent hypertension is controversial. Evidence by consensus and case reports does support garlic's cholesterol-lowering ability and its ability to decrease blood pressure in patients with hypertension (National Center for Complementary and Alternative Medicine, 2015). Teach patients to check with their primary health care provider before starting garlic or any herbal therapy because of possible side effects and interactions with other herbs, foods, or drugs. Garlic can damage the liver and cause bleeding in some patients, especially if they have invasive procedures such as surgery.

Some patients have also had success with biofeedback, meditation, and acupuncture as part of their overall management plan. These methods may be most useful as adjuncts for patients who experience continuous and severe stress.

Drug Therapy. Drug therapy is individualized for each patient, with consideration given to culture, age, other existing illness, severity of blood pressure elevation, and cost of drugs and follow-up. Once-a-day drug therapy is best, especially for the older adult, because the more doses required each day, the higher the risk that a patient will not follow the treatment regimen. However, many patients with hypertension need two or more drugs to adequately control blood pressure.

In the largest hypertensive trial done to date, Antihypertensive and Lipid-Lowering Treatment to Prevent Heart Attack Trial (ALLHAT), the use of diuretics has been practically unmatched in preventing the cardiovascular complications of hypertension. The *2014 Evidence-Based Guidelines for the Management of High Blood Pressure in Adults* presented by JNC 8 recommends the use of one or more of these four classes of drugs: thiazide-type diuretics, calcium channel blockers (CCBs), angiotensin-converting enzyme inhibitors (ACEIs), and angiotensin II receptor blockers (ARBs). Patients who do not respond to these first-line drugs may be placed on an aldosterone receptor antagonist (blocker), beta-adrenergic blocker, or renin inhibitor. Examples of commonly used drug classes for hypertension are listed in Chart 36-1. JNC 8 recommendations for pharmacologic management are summarized in Table 36-3.

CONCEPT MAP

PERFUSION · IMMUNITY · HYPERTENSION

INTERVENTIONS—RESPONDING

1 | Data Collection

Assess risk factors: age, ethnicity, family history, diet history, alcohol consumption, drug use, history of renal or CV disease. Reviews modifiable and nonmodifiable risk factors that decrease PERFUSION and provides a foundation for teaching lifestyle changes.

2 | Physical Assessment: Pattern of Responses—Noticing

- Assess BP in both arms with accurately sized BP cuff. Determines orthostatic changes; increased incidence of hypertension in patients with atherosclerosis.
- Palpate all pulses and note differences; palpate each carotid artery separately. Prevents blocking PERFUSION to the brain.
- Check temperature differences in lower extremities; check capillary filling. Indicator of poor PERFUSION that is often present in patients with DM.

3 | Foundation of Control—Lifestyle Modifications

- Teach the patient to follow the DASH dietary guidelines, restrict sodium, identify potassium-rich foods, control weight, consume alcohol sparingly, increase exercise, use relaxation techniques, and avoid tobacco and caffeine. Educates about decreasing modifiable risk factors to control hypertension and stresses the importance of lifestyle choices.
- Identify ways to encourage drug adherence. Encourages the patient without physical symptoms, economic restraints, or forgetfulness, the importance of taking medications as prescribed to prevent decreased PERFUSION.

4 | Psychosocial Assessment: Pattern of Responses—Noticing

Evaluate economic and other life stressors as well as patient's response to stressors. Assess past coping strategies. Determines the patient's coping ability and gauges probability of treatment compliance; stressors can worsen hypertension and affect the patient's ability to follow treatment.

5 | Interpreting Laboratory Values

Notice and respond for abnormal lab values: total cholesterol, HDL-C, LDL-C, triglycerides, blood sugar. Monitors lipid levels; patients with DM can have increased lipid levels leading to early severe atherosclerosis, arterial damage, and CAD.

6 | Drug Therapy

- Administer antihypertensive and lipid lowering treatment as prescribed. Controls hypertension and lipid levels; medications are instituted if lifestyle changes prove unsuccessful.
- Notice for signs of orthostatic hypotension. Promotes safety in the older patient who is at greatest risk for postural hypotension because of perfusion changes associated with aging.

7 | Nursing Safety Priority: Drug Alert!

Interpret and respond to K^+ levels, irregular pulse and muscle weakness, which may indicate decreased K^+. Patients taking potassium-depleting diuretics should eat foods high in K^+; supplements may be needed. Helps prevent electrolyte imbalance which can cause cardiac dysrhythmias.

8 | Complementary and Integrative Therapies

Help the patient explore complementary and alternative therapies. Gives the patient alternatives to replace or supplement conventional therapies. Garlic and Q_{10} may prevent/treat hypertension and have short-term lipid-lowering abilities; biofeedback, meditation, and acupuncture may help with continuous and severe stress.

Concept Map by Deanne A. Blach, MSN, RN

NOTICE IN THE HISTORY

Mike Jones is an older adult admitted for control of his blood pressure. He has a history of hypertension and type 2 diabetes. He takes captopril (Capoten) 50 mg BID, metformin (Glucaphage) 850 mg daily, gemfibrozil (Lopid) 600 mg BID, and hydrochlorothiazide (HCTZ) 20 mg daily.

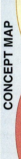

NOTICING—Physical Assessment

- BP 170/86 mm Hg; HR 80; Chol - 240; LDL-C 150; HDL-C 40; triglycerides - 400; HgA,C 7%; BS 170
- Face is flushed, patient is dizzy
- Recently divorced, consumes lots of canned goods, lives alone on fixed income

Data Synthesis

Identifying Risk Factors HTN

- Family history of CV and PVD; African-American male
- Type 2 diabetes, alcoholism
- Postoperative pain
- 45 lbs overweight
- Divorced, shares custody of 2 teenagers with ex-wife

Data Synthesis

PATIENT PROBLEMS

- Need for health teaching due to the plan of care for hypertension management
- Potential for nonadherence due to side effects of drug therapy and necessary changes in lifestyle

Planning

EXPECTED OUTCOMES

- Verbalize plan to change lifestyle to reduce modifiable factors of hypertension
- Patient with diabetes will target BP of <130/90 mm Hg; patient without diabetes will target BP of <120/80 mm Hg
- Lab goals:
  Cholesterol: <200 mg/dL
  LDL-C <70 mg/dL with CVD or DM
  HDL-C >40 mg/dL
  Triglycerides <150 mg/dL
  HgA1C: 6%
  BS <130 mg/dL

CHART 36-1   Common Examples of Drug Therapy

Hypertension Management

DRUG CATEGORY	NURSING IMPLICATIONS
Diuretics	
Common examples of diuretics: • Potassium-sparing: Spironolactone (Aldactone) • Loop: Furosemide (Lasix); bumetanide (Bumex, Burinex 🍁) • Thiazide: Hydrochlorothiazide (Microzide, Urozide 🍁); chlorothiazide (Diuril)	Assess for weakness, dizziness, or a new onset of confusion *because these drugs can cause hypovolemia and dehydration.* Teach older adults to rise slowly *because the medication can cause orthostatic hypotension associated with diuresis.* For potassium-sparing agents: • Teach the patient to decrease intake of foods that are high in potassium and have follow-up laboratory tests for electrolyte levels *because these agents cause retention of K⁺ in the body.* • Teach the patient to report weakness and irregular pulse to the primary health care provider *because these symptoms may indicate hyperkalemia.* For loop and thiazide agents: • Teach the patient to eat foods high in K⁺ and to have follow-up laboratory tests to monitor electrolyte levels *because these agents cause K⁺ and Mg²⁺ excretion.* • Use with caution in patients with diabetes *because glucose control can be affected.* • Use with caution in patients with gout *because uric acid retention can occur.*
Beta Blockers	
Common examples of beta blockers: • Atenolol (Tenormin, Apo-Atenol) • Metoprolol (Lopressor, Toprol XL, Betaloc)	Assess heart rate (HR) and blood pressure (BP) before administration *because beta blockers cause a decrease in HR and cardiac output and suppress renin activity.* • Do not administer if HR is <50-60 beats/min. • Hold for systolic <90-100 mm HG and contact the health care provider. • Monitor for orthostatic hypotension *because this is a common adverse effect that can contribute to falls and confusion, especially in older adults.* Use with caution in patients with diabetes *because glucose production may be affected.* Teach the patient that these agents can cause fatigue, depression, and sexual dysfunction. These adverse effects should be reported to the primary health care provider.
Calcium Channel Blockers	
Common examples of calcium channel blockers: • Verapamil (Calan, Isoptin, Nu-Verap 🍁) • Amlodipine (Norvasc) • Diltiazem (Cardizem)	Monitor pulse and BP before taking each day *because the drug slows SA and AV conduction, which decreases HR and vasodilation and causes decreased BP.* Teach patients to avoid grapefruit juice and grapefruit while taking calcium channel blockers *because grapefruit and its juice can enhance the action of the drug, causing organ dysfunction or death.*
Angiotensin-Converting Enzyme (ACE) Inhibitors	
Common examples of ACE inhibitors: • Lisinopril (Prinivil, Zestril) • Enalapril (Vasotec) • Captopril (Capoten, Apo-Capto 🍁)	Report persistent, dry cough to the primary health care provider *because this is a common and annoying side effect and another type of antihypertensive medication may be necessary.* Monitor BP carefully, especially orthostatic pressures, *because these agents result in vasodilation and decreased BP.* • Do not give the drug without checking with the health care provider if systolic BP is below 100. Assess for hyperkalemia *because ACE inhibitors reduce the excretion of potassium.*
Angiotensin II Receptor Blockers (ARBs)	
Common examples of ARBs: • Valsartan (Diovan) • Losartan (Cozaar)	Teach patients to avoid foods high in potassium *because ARBs can cause hyperkalemia, especially when combined with other hypertensive agents.* Monitor BP carefully, especially orthostatic pressures, *because these agents result in vasodilation and decreased BP.* • Do not give the drug without checking with the health care provider if systolic BP is below 100.

AV, Atrioventricular; *SA,* sinoatrial.

! NURSING SAFETY PRIORITY QSEN
Drug Alert

Teach men that they may experience decreased libido (desire for sex) and decreased sexual performance when taking thiazide diuretics. Thiazide diuretics should be used with caution in patients with diabetes mellitus because they can interfere with serum glucose control. Caution is also indicated for patients with gout or a history of significant hyponatremia (decreased serum sodium level) because these problems can worsen when thiazides are taken.

! NURSING SAFETY PRIORITY QSEN
Drug Alert

The most frequent side effect associated with *thiazide and loop diuretics* is hypokalemia (low potassium level). Monitor serum potassium levels and assess for irregular pulse, dysrhythmias, and muscle weakness, which may indicate hypokalemia. Teach patients taking potassium-depleting diuretics to eat foods high in potassium, such as bananas, potatoes, and orange juice. Most people also need a potassium supplement to maintain adequate serum potassium levels.

Assess for hyperkalemia (high potassium level) for patients taking potassium-sparing diuretics such as spironolactone. Like hypokalemia, an increased potassium level can also cause weakness, irregular pulse, and cardiac dysrhythmias. In some cases, patients may have painful muscle spasms (cramping) in their legs. These electrolyte imbalances are described in detail in Chapter 11.

Diuretics. Diuretics are the first type of drugs for managing hypertension. Three basic types of diuretics are used to decrease blood volume and lower blood pressure in the order of how commonly they are typically prescribed:

- Thiazide (low-ceiling) diuretics, such as hydrochlorothiazide (Microzide, Urozide ✤), inhibit sodium, chloride, and water reabsorption in the distal tubules while promoting potassium, bicarbonate, and magnesium excretion. However, they decrease calcium excretion, which helps prevent kidney stones and bone loss. Because of the low cost and high effectiveness of thiazide-type diuretics, they are usually the drugs of choice for patients with uncomplicated hypertension. These drugs can be prescribed as a single agent or in combination with other classes of drugs.
- Loop (high-ceiling) diuretics, such as furosemide (Lasix, Apo-Furosemide ✤) and torsemide (Demadex), inhibit sodium, chloride, and water reabsorption in the ascending loop of Henle and promote potassium excretion.

🌐 CONSIDERATIONS FOR OLDER ADULTS
Patient-Centered Care QSEN

Loop diuretics are not used commonly for older adults because they can cause dehydration and orthostatic hypotension. These complications increase the patient's risk for falls. Teach families to monitor for and report patient dizziness, falls, or confusion to the primary health care provider as soon as possible and discontinue the drug.

- Potassium-sparing diuretics, such as spironolactone (Aldactone), triamterene (Dyrenium), and amiloride (Midamor ✤), act on the distal renal tubule to inhibit reabsorption of sodium ions in exchange for potassium, thereby *retaining* potassium in the body. When used, they are typically in combination with another diuretic or antihypertensive drug to *conserve* potassium.

Frequent voiding caused by any type of diuretic may interfere with daily activities. Teach patients to take their diuretic in the morning rather than at night to prevent nocturia (voiding during the night).

Other Antihypertensive Drugs. Calcium channel blockers, such as verapamil hydrochloride (Calan, Nu-Verap SR ✤) and amlodipine (Norvasc), lower blood pressure by interfering with the transmembrane flux of calcium ions. This results in vasodilation, which *decreases* blood pressure. These drugs also block sinoatrial (SA) and atrioventricular (AV) node conduction, resulting in a decreased heart rate. Calcium channel blockers are most effective in older adults and African Americans (Mozaffarian et al., 2016).

Some calcium channel blockers (CCBs), especially felodipine (Plendil, Renedil) and nifedipine (Adalat, Apo-Nifed), react with grapefruit and grapefruit juice. Teach the patient to avoid grapefruit juice to prevent complications such as kidney failure, heart failure, GI bleeding, or even death. A newer CCB, clevidipine butyrate (Cleviprex), is available only in IV form and must be administered using an infusion pump. This drug is indicated when oral therapy is not possible and is used for severe hypertension. The most common side effects are headache and nausea. Monitor the patient's blood pressure frequently to check for hypotension (Burchum & Rosenthal, 2016).

Angiotensin-converting enzyme inhibitors (ACE inhibitors or ACEIs), known as the "-pril" drugs, are also used as single or combination agents in the treatment of hypertension. These

TABLE 36-3 Select 2014 Evidence-Based Recommendations for the Management of High Blood Pressure in Adults (JNC 8)

- In the general population ages 60 years and older, start drug therapy to lower blood pressure (BP) at systolic blood pressure (SBP) equal to or greater than 150 mm Hg or diastolic blood pressure (DBP) equal to or greater than 90 mm Hg. The goal is to decrease BP to below 150/90.
- In the general population younger than 60 years, start drug therapy to lower BP at SBP equal to or greater than 140 mm Hg or DBP equal to or greater than 90 mm Hg. The goal is to decrease BP to below 140/90.
- In people ages 18 years and older with chronic kidney disease (CKD), start drug therapy to lower BP to less than 140/90.
- In the general *nonblack* population, including those with diabetes mellitus, initial drug therapy should include a thiazide-type diuretic, calcium channel blocker (CCB), angiotensin-converting enzyme inhibitor (ACEI), or angiotensin receptor blocker (ARB).
- In the general *black* population, including those with diabetes mellitus, initial drug therapy should include a thiazide-type diuretic or CCB.
- If the goal BP is not reached within a month of treatment, increase drug dosage or add a second drug from one of the recommended classes.

Data from James, P.A., Oparil, S., Carter, B.L., Cushman, W.C., Dennison-Himmelfarb, C., Handler, J., et al. (2014). 2014 evidence-based guidelines for the management of high blood pressure in adults: Report from the panel members appointed to the Eighth National Committee (JNC 8). *Journal of the American Medical Association, 311*(5), 507-520. Retrieved from http://jama.jamanetwork.com/article.aspx?articleid=1791497.

drugs block the action of the ACE as it attempts to convert angiotensin I to angiotensin II, one of the most powerful vasoconstrictors in the body. This action also decreases sodium and water retention and lowers peripheral vascular resistance, both of which lower blood pressure. ACE inhibitors include capto*pril* (Capoten), lisino*pril* (Prinivil, Zestril), and enala*pril* (Vasotec). *The most common side effect of this group of drugs is a nagging, dry cough.* Teach patients to report this problem to their primary health care provider as soon as possible. If a cough develops, the drug is discontinued.

❗ NURSING SAFETY PRIORITY QSEN
Drug Alert

Instruct the patient receiving an ACE inhibitor for the first time to get out of bed slowly to avoid the severe hypotensive effect that can occur with initial use. Orthostatic hypotension may occur with subsequent doses, but it is usually less severe. If dizziness continues or there is a significant decrease in the systolic blood pressure (more than a change of 20 mm Hg), notify the health care provider or teach the patient to notify the health care provider. *The older patient is at the greatest risk for postural hypotension because of the cardiovascular changes associated with aging.*

Angiotensin II receptor antagonists, also called *angiotensin II receptor blockers (ARBs)* or the *-sartan drugs,* make up a group of drugs that selectively block the binding of angiotensin II to receptor sites in the vascular smooth muscle and adrenal tissues by competing directly with angiotensin II but not inhibiting ACE. Examples of drugs in this group are cande*sartan* (Atacand), val*sartan* (Diovan), lo*sartan* (Cozaar), and azil*sartan* (Edarbi). ARBs can be used alone or in combination with other antihypertensive drugs. These drugs are excellent options for patients who report a nagging cough associated with ACE inhibitors. In addition, they do not require initial adjustment of the dose for older adults or for any patient with renal impairment. Like the ACEs, the ARBs are not as effective in African Americans unless they are taken with diuretics or another category such as a beta blocker or calcium channel blocker (Mozaffarian et al., 2016).

Beta-adrenergic blockers, identified by the ending -olol, are categorized as cardioselective (working only on the cardiovascular system) and noncardioselective. Cardioselective beta blockers, affecting only beta$_1$ receptors, may be prescribed to lower blood pressure by blocking beta receptors in the heart and peripheral vessels. By blocking these receptors, the drug decreases heart rate and myocardial contractility. Teach patients about common side effects of beta blockers, including fatigue, weakness, depression, and sexual dysfunction. The potential for side effects depends on the "selective" blocking effects of the drug. Aten*olol* (Tenormin, Apo-Atenol), bisopr*olol* (Zebeta), and metopr*olol* (Lopressor, Toprol, Toprol-XL, Betaloc) are cardioselective beta blockers given for hypertension.

Patients with diabetes who take beta blockers may not have the usual manifestations of hypoglycemia because the sympathetic nervous system is blocked. The body's responses to hypoglycemia such as gluconeogenesis may also be inhibited by certain beta blockers.

Beta blockers are often the drug of choice for hypertensive patients with ischemic heart disease (IHD) because the heart is the most common target of end-organ damage with hypertension. If this drug is not tolerated, a long-acting calcium channel blocker can be used. In patients with unstable angina or myocardial infarction (MI), beta blockers or calcium channel blockers should be used initially in combination with ACE inhibitors or ARBs, with addition of other drugs if needed to control the blood pressure (see Chapter 38).

tailor the therapeutic regimen to his or her lifestyle and daily schedule.

Patients who do not adhere to antihypertensive treatment are at a high risk for target organ damage and **hypertensive crisis**, a severe elevation in blood pressure (greater than 180/120), which can cause organ damage in the kidneys or heart (target organs) (Chart 36-2). Patients in hypertensive crisis are admitted to critical care units, where they receive IV antihypertensive therapy such as nitroprusside (Nipride), nicardipine (Cardene IV), fenoldopam (Corlopam), or labetalol (Trandate). These drugs act quickly as vasodilators to decrease blood pressure by no more than 25% within 2 to 6 hours. A gradual reduction in blood pressure is preferred because rapid reduction can cause cerebral ischemia, MI, and renal failure. Provide oxygen to the patient and monitor oxygen saturation levels. When the patient's blood pressure stabilizes, oral antihypertensive drugs are given (Burchum & Rosenthal, 2016).

Care Coordination and Transition Management

Home Care Management. Hypertension is a chronic illness. Allow patients to verbalize feelings about the disease and its treatment. Emphasize that their involvement in the collaborative plan of care can lead to control of the disease and can prevent complications.

Some patients do not adhere to their drug therapy regimen at home because they have no symptoms or they simply forget to take their drugs. Others may think they are not sick enough to need medication. Some patients may assume that, once their blood pressure (BP) returns to normal levels, they no longer need treatment. They may also stop taking their drugs because of side effects or cost. Develop a plan with the patient and family and identify ways to encourage adherence to the plan of care.

Promoting Adherence to the Plan of Care

Planning: Expected Outcomes. The patient with hypertension is expected to adhere to the plan of care, including making necessary lifestyle changes.

Interventions. Patients who require medications to control essential hypertension usually need to take them for the rest of their lives. Some patients stop taking them because they have no symptoms and have troublesome side effects.

In the hospital setting, interprofessional collaboration with the pharmacist to discuss the outcomes of therapy with the patient, including potential side effects can help the patient

---

◎ CHART 36-2 Best Practice for Patient Safety & Quality Care QSEN

Emergency Care of Patients With Hypertensive Urgency or Crisis

Assess
- Severe headache
- Extremely high blood pressure (BP)
- Dizziness
- Blurred vision
- Shortness of breath
- Epistaxis (nosebleed)
- Severe anxiety

Intervene
- Place patient in a semi-Fowler's position.
- Administer oxygen.
- Start IV of 0.9% normal saline (NS) solution slowly to prevent fluid overload (which would increase BP).
- Administer IV beta blocker or nicardipine (Cardene IV) or other infusion drug as prescribed; when stable, switch to oral antihypertensive drug.
- Monitor BP every 5 to 15 minutes until the diastolic pressure is below 90 and not less than 75; then monitor BP every 30 minutes to ensure that BP is not lowered too quickly.
- Observe for neurologic or cardiovascular complications, such as seizures; numbness, weakness, or tingling of extremities; dysrhythmias; or chest pain (possible indicators of target organ damage).

Self-Management Education. Health teaching is essential to help patients become successful in managing their BP. Provide oral and written information about the indications, dosage, times of administration, side effects, and drug interactions for antihypertensives. Stress that medication must be taken as prescribed; when all of it has been consumed, the prescription must be renewed on a continual basis. Suddenly stopping drugs such as beta blockers can result in angina (chest pain), myocardial infarction (MI), or rebound hypertension. Urge patients to report unpleasant side effects such as excessive fatigue, cough, or sexual dysfunction. In many instances, an alternative drug can be prescribed to minimize certain side effects.

Teach the patient to obtain an ambulatory BP monitoring (ABPM) device for use at home so the pressure can be checked. Evaluate the patient's and family's ability to use this device. If weight reduction is a desired outcome, suggest having a scale in the home for weight monitoring. For patients who do not want to self-monitor, are not able to self-monitor, or have "white-coat" syndrome when they go to their primary health care provider (causing elevated BP), continuous ABPM may be used. The monitor is worn for 24 hours or longer while patients perform their normal daily activities. BP is automatically taken every 15 to 30 minutes and recorded for review later. The advantage of this technique is that the primary health care provider can view the changes in BP readings throughout the 24-hour period to get a picture of a true BP value. Research strongly supports 24-hour ambulatory BP monitoring as a first-line procedure to determine the need for antihypertensive therapy (Kaplan & Townsend, 2015).

Instruct the patient about sodium restriction, weight maintenance or reduction, alcohol restriction, stress management, and exercise. If necessary, also explain about the need to stop using tobacco, especially smoking.

Health Care Resources. A home care nurse may be needed for follow-up to monitor the BP. Evaluate patient or family ability to obtain accurate BP measurements and assess adherence with treatment. The American Heart Association (www.aha.org), the Red Cross, or a local pharmacy may be used for free BP checks if patients cannot buy equipment to monitor their BP. Health fairs and BP screening programs located in faith-based centers are also available in most locations.

◆ Evaluation: Reflecting

Evaluate the care of the patient with hypertension on the basis of the identified patient problems. The expected outcomes are that the patient will:

- Verbalize understanding of the plan of care, including drug therapy and any necessary lifestyle changes
- Report adverse drug effects, such as coughing, dizziness, or sexual dysfunction, to the primary health care provider immediately
- Consistently adhere to the plan of care, including regular follow-up with the primary health care provider

ARTERIOSCLEROSIS AND ATHEROSCLEROSIS

❖ PATHOPHYSIOLOGY

Arteriosclerosis is a thickening, or hardening, of the arterial wall that is often associated with aging. **Atherosclerosis,** a type of arteriosclerosis, involves the formation of plaque within the arterial wall and is the leading risk factor for cardiovascular disease. Usually the disease affects the larger arteries, such as

---

⑦ CLINICAL JUDGMENT CHALLENGE 36-1

Patient-Centered Care; Teamwork and Collaboration; Evidence-Based Practice QSEN

A 43 year old African-American male finance executive presents to the primary health care provider for a routine checkup. The patient reports a history of smoking and has a body mass index (BMI) of 31.

Both of his parents have hypertension. Initial nursing assessment reveals a heart rate of 88 beats/min, blood pressure of 190/110, and respiratory rate of 24 breaths/min.

1. What physical assessment data will you collect from the patient? What laboratory data or relevant testing do you anticipate given the patient's clinical presentation?
2. What risk factors for hypertension are present? Are they modifiable or nonmodifiable?
3. What health teaching will you provide for the patient? What evidence do you have to support your answer?
4. What type of drug therapy may be prescribed for this patient? What are your nursing responsibilities when giving these drugs?
5. What members of the interprofessional health care team may be involved in this patient's care?
6. What community resources are available to help this patient self-manage his hypertension?

---

coronary artery beds; aorta; carotid and vertebral arteries; renal, iliac, and femoral arteries; or any combination of these.

The exact pathophysiology of atherosclerosis is not known, but the condition is thought to occur from blood vessel damage that causes inflammation, which is an alteration in IMMUNITY (see the discussion of inflammation in Chapter 17) (Fig. 36-2). After the vessel becomes inflamed, a fatty streak appears on the intimal surface (inner lining) of the artery. Through the process of cellular proliferation, collagen migrates over the fatty streak, forming a fibrous plaque. The fibrous plaque is often elevated and protrudes into the vessel lumen, partially or completely obstructing blood flow through the artery. Plaques are either stable or unstable. Unstable plaques are prone to rupture and are often clinically silent until they rupture (McCance et al., 2014).

In the final stage, the fibrous plaques become calcified, hemorrhagic, ulcerated, or thrombosed and affect all layers of the vessel. The rate of progression of the process may be influenced by genetic factors; certain chronic diseases (e.g., diabetes mellitus); and lifestyle habits, including smoking, eating habits, and level of exercise.

When *stable* plaque ruptures, thrombosis (blood clot) and constriction obstruct the vessel lumen, causing inadequate PERFUSION and oxygenation to distal tissues. *Unstable* plaque rupture causes more severe damage. After the rupture occurs, the exposed underlying tissue causes platelet adhesion and rapid thrombus formation. The thrombus may suddenly block a blood vessel, resulting in ischemia and infarction (e.g., myocardial infarction).

Endothelial (intimal) injury of the major arteries of the body can be caused by many factors. Elevated levels of **lipids** (fats) such as low-density lipoprotein cholesterol (LDL-C) and decreased levels of high-density lipoprotein cholesterol (HDL-C) can cause chemical injuries to the vessel wall. (Chapter 33 discusses lipids in detail.) Chemical injury can also be caused by elevated levels of toxins in the bloodstream, which may occur with renal failure or by carbon monoxide circulating in the bloodstream from cigarette smoking. The vessel wall can be

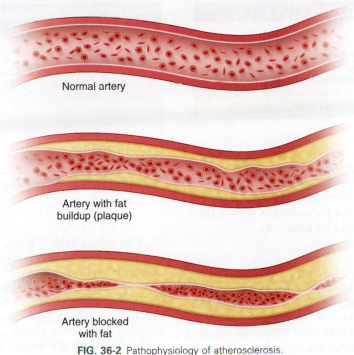

Normal artery

Artery with fat
buildup (plaque)

Artery blocked
with fat

FIG. 36-2 Pathophysiology of atherosclerosis.

TABLE 36-4	**Risk Factors for Atherosclerosis**
• Low HDL-C	• Sedentary lifestyle
• High LDL-C	• Smoking
• Increased triglycerides	• Stress
• Genetic predisposition	• African-American or Hispanic ethnicity
• Diabetes mellitus	• Older adult
• Obesity	

HDL-C, High-density lipoprotein cholesterol; *LDL-C,* low-density lipoprotein cholesterol.

weakened by the natural process of aging or by diseases such as hypertension.

Genetic predisposition and diabetes have a major effect on the development of atherosclerosis. Some patients have familial **hyperlipidemia,** an elevation of serum lipid levels. In these people, the liver makes excessive cholesterol and other fats. However, some people with hereditary atherosclerosis have a normal blood cholesterol level. The reason for the development and progression of plaque in these patients is not understood (McCance et al., 2014).

Adult patients of any age with severe diabetes mellitus frequently have premature and severe atherosclerosis from microvascular damage. The premature atherosclerosis occurs because diabetes promotes an increase in LDL-C and triglycerides (lipids) in plasma. In addition, arterial damage may result from the effect of hyperglycemia.

Other factors are indirectly related to atherosclerosis development. A list of risk factors is found in Table 36-4.

It is not known exactly how many people have atherosclerosis, but small plaques are almost always present in the arteries of young adults. The incidence can be better quantified by assessing the number of cardiovascular diseases (CVDs) that result from atherosclerosis. An estimated 85.6 million U.S.

adults have one or more types of CVD (Mozaffarian et al., 2016). About half of those with CVD are older than 60 years, and many more are middle-age. The number of people affected by atherosclerosis is likely to increase as the population ages.

❖ **INTERPROFESSIONAL COLLABORATIVE CARE**
◆ **Assessment: Noticing**

The assessment of a patient with atherosclerosis includes a complete cardiovascular assessment because associated heart disease is often present. Because of the high incidence of hypertension in patients with atherosclerosis, assess the blood pressure in both arms.

Palpate pulses at all of the major sites on the body and note any differences. *Palpate each carotid artery separately to prevent blocking blood flow to the brain!* Also feel for temperature differences in the lower extremities and check capillary filling. Prolonged capillary filling (>3 seconds in young-to–middle-age adults; >5 seconds in older adults) generally indicates poor circulation, *although this is not the most reliable indicator of* PERFUSION. With severe atherosclerotic disease, the extremity may be cool or cold with a diminished or absent pulse.

Many patients with vascular disease have a bruit in the larger arteries, which can be heard with a stethoscope or Doppler probe. A **bruit** is a turbulent, swishing sound, which can be soft or loud in pitch. It is heard as a result of blood trying to pass through a narrowed artery. A bruit is considered abnormal, but it does not indicate the severity of disease. Bruits often occur in the carotid, aortic, femoral, and popliteal arteries.

Patients with atherosclerosis often have elevated lipids, including cholesterol and triglycerides. Elevated cholesterol levels are confirmed by HDL and LDL measurements. Increased low-density lipoprotein cholesterol (LDL-C) ("bad" cholesterol) levels and low high-density lipoprotein cholesterol (HDL-C) ("good" cholesterol) indicate that a person is at an increased

TABLE 36-5 Commonly Used Drugs for Lowering LDL-C Levels

HMG-CoA REDUCTASE INHIBITORS (STATINS)	COMBINATION DRUGS
• Lovastatin (Mevacor) • Atorvastatin (Lipitor) • Simvastatin (Zocor) • Fluvastatin (Lescol) • Rosuvastatin (Crestor) • Pravastatin (Pravachol) • Pitavastatin (Livalo)	• Ezetimibe and simvastatin (Vytorin) • Amlodipine and atorvastatin (Caduet) • Niacin and lovastatin (Advicor)

HMG-CoA, 3-hydroxy-3-methylglutaryl coenzyme A.

risk for atherosclerosis. The *triglyceride* level may also be elevated with atherosclerosis. Elevated triglycerides are considered a marker for other lipoproteins. They also suggest metabolic syndrome, which increases the risk for coronary disease (see Chapter 33 for in-depth serum lipid information).

◆ **Interventions: Responding**

Atherosclerosis progresses for years before signs and symptoms occur. Adults who are at risk for the disease can often be identified through cholesterol screening and history. Because of the high incidence in the United States, low-risk people 20 years of age and older are advised to have their total serum cholesterol level evaluated at least once every 5 years. More frequent measurements are suggested for people with multiple risk factors and those older than 40 years of age.

People with multiple risk factors are grouped into high-risk patient categories.

Interventions for patients with atherosclerosis or those at high risk for the disease focus on lifestyle changes. Teach patients about the need to make daily changes by avoiding or minimizing modifiable risk factors. *Modifiable risk factors* are those that can be changed or controlled by the patient, such as smoking, weight management, and exercise. Nutrition is one of the most important parts of the risk-reduction plan. Chapter 38 describes how to manage modifiable risk factors. If lipoprotein levels do not improve after lifestyle changes, the primary health care provider may prescribe drug therapy to lower cholesterol and/or triglycerides.

Nutrition Therapy. The ACC and AHA publish dietary recommendations for lowering LDL-C levels (Eckel et al., 2014). These recommendations are based on the best current evidence from randomized controlled trials and include:

- Consume a dietary pattern that emphasizes intake of vegetables, fruits, and whole grains.
- Consume low-fat dairy products, poultry, fish, legumes, nontropical (e.g., canola) vegetable oils, and nuts.
- Limit intake of sweets, sugar-sweetened beverages, and red meats.
- Aim for a dietary pattern that includes 5% to 6% of calories from saturated fat.
- Reduce percent of calories from *trans* fat.

These guidelines are similar to the Dietary Approaches to Stop Hypertension (DASH), which also recommend daily sodium, potassium, and fiber amounts (National Heart, Lung, and Blood Institute, 2015). Interprofessional collaboration with the dietitian to teach the patient about the types of fat content in food is encouraged. Meats and eggs contain mostly saturated fats and are high in cholesterol. Instruct patients about increasing dietary fiber to 30 g each day, which is consistent with DASH guidelines.

Physical Activity. The ACC/AHA also recommends that adults engage in aerobic physical activity three or four times a week to reduce LDL-C levels. Each session should last for 40 minutes on average and involve moderate-to-vigorous physical activity (Eckel et al., 2014).

Drug Therapy. For patients with elevated total and LDL-C levels that do not respond adequately to dietary intervention, the primary health care provider prescribes a cholesterol-lowering agent. Drug choice and dosing depend on the serum cholesterol level, the degree to which the level needs to be decreased, and the patient's age (Stone et al., 2014). Because most of these drugs can produce side effects, they are generally given only when nonpharmacologic management has been unsuccessful.

A class of drugs known as *3-hydroxy-3-methylglutaryl coenzyme A (HMG-CoA) reductase inhibitors (statins)* successfully reduces total cholesterol in most patients when used for an extended period. Examples include lovastatin (Mevacor), simvastatin (Zocor), and pitavastatin (Livalo), which lower both LDL-C and triglyceride levels (Table 36-5).

The American College of Cardiology (ACC)/American Heart Association (AHA) publishes recommendations for treatment of high cholesterol to reduce atherosclerotic cardiovascular disease (ASCVD) in adults (Stone et al., 2014). These evidence-based recommendations are highlighted in Table 36-6. It is important to note that, although these guidelines support regular monitoring of laboratory data, the focus of care is on risk modification versus just reduction of the laboratory value. Statin therapy should be used as an adjunct therapy for risk reduction versus simply a medication to modify cholesterol levels (Sherrod et al., 2015).

A different type of lipid-lowering agent, ezetimibe (Zetia), may be used in place of or in combination with statin-type drugs. This drug inhibits the absorption of cholesterol through the small intestine. Vytorin is a combination drug containing ezetimibe and simvastatin. This drug works two ways—by reducing the absorption of cholesterol and by decreasing the amount of cholesterol synthesis in the liver. Other statin combinations have been developed to improve lipid levels, such as Advicor—a combination of niacin and lovastatin. Aspirin and pravastatin are combined as Pravigard. Amlodipine (Norvasc) and atorvastatin are combined as Caduet to decrease blood pressure while decreasing triglycerides (TGs), increasing HDL, and lowering LDL. Combining drugs may improve adherence for the patient who is often taking multiple drugs.

The Food and Drug Administration (FDA) recently approved a new drug class, PCSK9 inhibitors, for use in patients with familial hypercholesterolemia or for those who are unable to reduce LDLs with existing therapies. These potent drugs inhibit

TABLE 36-6   Selected 2013 ACC/AHA Recommendations for the Treatment of Serum Cholesterol to Reduce Atherosclerotic Cardiovascular Disease Risk in Adults

Primary Prevention

- All people with LDL-C equal to or greater than 190 mg/dL should be evaluated for secondary causes of hyperlipidemia and treated with statin therapy.
- Adults with diabetes mellitus who are 40 to 75 years of age should be treated with high-intensity statin therapy.
- Adults 40 to 75 years of age with LDL-C of 70 to 189 mg/dL without clinical signs of ASCVD or diabetes should be treated with moderate- to high-intensity statin therapy.

Secondary Prevention

- High-intensity statin therapy should be initiated or continued as first-line treatment in adults 75 years of age or younger who have signs and symptoms of ASCVD, unless contraindicated.
- In people older than 75 years, the potential for ASCVD risk-reduction benefits, adverse drug effects, and drug-drug interactions should be evaluated.

ASCVD, Atherosclerotic cardiovascular disease; *LDL-C*, low-density lipoprotein cholesterol.
Data from Stone, N. J., Robinson, J., Lichtenstein, A. H., Merz, N. B., Blum, C. B., Eckel, R. H., et al. (2014). 2013 ACC/AHA guidelines on the treatment of blood cholesterol to reduce atherosclerotic cardiovascular risk in adults: A report of the American College of Cardiology/American Heart Association Task Force on Practice Guidelines. *Circulation, 129*(25 Suppl 2), S1-S45.

! NURSING SAFETY PRIORITY QSEN

Drug Alert

Statins reduce cholesterol synthesis in the liver and increase clearance of LDL-C from the blood. Therefore they are contraindicated in patients with active liver disease or during pregnancy because they can cause muscle myopathies and marked decreases in liver function. Statins also have the potential for interactions with other drugs, such as warfarin, cyclosporine, and selected antibiotics. They are discontinued if the patient has muscle cramping or elevated liver enzyme levels. Some patients also report abdominal bloating, flatulence, diarrhea, and/or constipation as side effects of these drugs. Remind patients to have laboratory testing follow-up as prescribed by their primary health care provider.

Teach patients taking statin drugs, especially those taking atorvastatin, lovastatin, and simvastatin, to *avoid grapefruit and grapefruit juice in their diet*. Grapefruit contains a group of chemicals called *furanocoumarins* that bind to and inactivate the enzyme *CYP3A4*. This enzyme is important for metabolism of many drugs, including statins. If it is inactivated, too much of the statin drug can remain in the patient's bloodstream, causing possible kidney failure, heart failure, GI bleeding, or even death (Bailey et al., 2013).

PCSK9, which is a protease produced primarily in the liver that can cause elevations in LDLs. Alirocumab (Praluent) and evolocumab (Repatha) are administered by subcutaneous injection on a monthly or bimonthly basis for patients who are on maximally tolerated doses of statins.

Complementary and Integrative Health. Nicotinic acid or niacin (Niaspan), a B vitamin, may lower LDL-C and very-low-density lipoprotein (VLDL) cholesterol levels and increase HDL-C levels in some patients, although the evidence supporting its use is lacking. It is used as a single agent or in combination with an acid-binding resin drug or a statin. Low doses are recommended because many patients experience flushing and a very warm feeling all over. Higher doses can result in an elevation of hepatic enzymes.

Lovaza (omega-3 ethyl esters) is approved by the FDA as an adjunct to diet to reduce TGs that are greater than 500 mg/dL. This drug also decreases plaque growth and inflammation and reduces CLOTTING.

? NCLEX EXAMINATION CHALLENGE 36-2

Health Promotion and Maintenance

A client diagnosed with atherosclerosis and hypertension has been newly prescribed a combination drug of amlodipine and atorvastatin (Caduet). Which statement by the client indicates a need for further teaching?
A. "I'll continue to take my amlodipine with the new medication."
B. "I'll follow up with my nurse practitioner on a regular basis."
C. "I need to quit smoking as soon as I possibly can."
D. "I shouldn't drink grapefruit juice while on this drug."

PERIPHERAL ARTERIAL DISEASE

❖ PATHOPHYSIOLOGY

Peripheral vascular disease (PVD) includes disorders that change the natural flow of blood through the arteries and veins of the peripheral circulation, causing decreased PERFUSION to body tissues. It affects the legs much more frequently than the arms. Generally, a diagnosis of PVD implies arterial disease (peripheral arterial disease [PAD]) rather than venous involvement. Some patients have both arterial and venous disease. The cost of the disease is very high and is expected to increase as baby boomers age and obesity in the United States continues to be a major health problem.

PAD is a result of systemic atherosclerosis. It is a chronic condition in which partial or total arterial occlusion (blockage) decreases PERFUSION to the extremities. The tissues below the narrowed or obstructed arteries cannot live without an adequate *oxygen* and nutrient supply. PAD in the legs is sometimes referred to as *lower-extremity arterial disease (LEAD)*.

Obstructions are classified as inflow or outflow, according to the arteries involved and their relationship to the inguinal ligament (Fig. 36-3). *Inflow* obstructions involve the distal end of the aorta and the common, internal, and external iliac arteries. They are located above the inguinal ligament. *Outflow* obstructions involve the femoral, popliteal, and tibial arteries and are below the superficial femoral artery (SFA). Gradual inflow occlusions may not cause significant tissue damage. Gradual outflow occlusions typically do.

Atherosclerosis is the most common cause of chronic arterial obstruction; therefore the risk factors for atherosclerosis apply to PAD as well (see Table 36-4). Advancing age also increases the risk for disease related to atherosclerosis. Patients with PAD have an increased risk for developing chronic angina, MI, or stroke and are much more likely to die within 10 years than those who do not have the disease (Mozaffarian et al., 2016). About 8.5 million people in the United States, age 40 and older, have PAD. African Americans are affected more often than any other group, most likely because they have many risk factors such as diabetes and hypertension (Mozaffarian et al., 2016).

❖ INTERPROFESSIONAL COLLABORATIVE CARE
◆ Assessment: Noticing

The clinical course of chronic PAD can be divided into four stages (Chart 36-3). Patients do not experience symptoms in the early stages of disease. Most patients are not diagnosed until they develop leg pain.

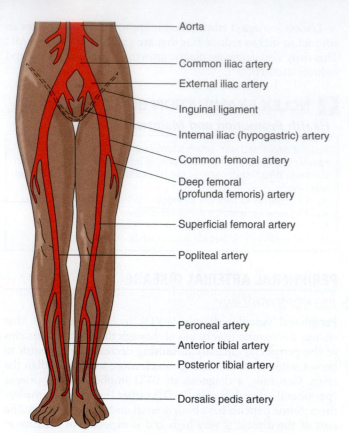

- Aorta
- Common iliac artery
- External iliac artery
- Inguinal ligament
- Internal iliac (hypogastric) artery
- Common femoral artery
- Deep femoral (profunda femoris) artery
- Superficial femoral artery
- Popliteal artery
- Peroneal artery
- Anterior tibial artery
- Posterior tibial artery
- Dorsalis pedis artery

FIG. 36-3 Common locations of inflow and outflow lesions.

▶ **CHART 36-3 Key Features**

Chronic Peripheral Arterial Disease

Stage I: Asymptomatic
- No claudication is present.
- Bruit or aneurysm may be present.
- Pedal pulses are decreased or absent.

Stage II: Claudication
- Muscle pain, cramping, or burning occurs with exercise and is relieved with rest.
- Symptoms are reproducible with exercise.

Stage III: Rest Pain
- Pain while resting commonly awakens the patient at night.
- Pain is described as numbness, burning, toothache-type pain.
- Pain usually occurs in the distal part of the extremity (toes, arch, forefoot, or heel), rarely in the calf or the ankle.
- Pain is relieved by placing the extremity in a dependent position.

Stage IV: Necrosis/Gangrene
- Ulcers and blackened tissue occur on the toes, forefoot, and heel.
- Distinctive gangrenous odor is present.

Most patients initially seek medical attention for a classic leg pain known as **intermittent claudication** (a term derived from a word meaning "to limp"). Usually they can walk only a certain distance before discomfort, such as cramping or burning muscular pain, forces them to stop. The pain stops with rest. When patients resume walking, they can walk the same distance before it returns. Thus the pain is considered reproducible. As

the disease progresses, they can walk only shorter and shorter distances before pain recurs. Ultimately it may occur even while at rest.

Rest pain, which may begin while the disease is still in the stage of intermittent claudication, is a numb or burning sensation, often described as feeling like a toothache that is severe enough to awaken patients at night. It is usually located in the toes, the foot arches, the forefeet, the heels, and, rarely, in the calves or ankles. Patients can sometimes alleviate pain by keeping the limb in a dependent position (below the heart). Those with rest pain often have advanced disease that may result in limb loss.

Patients with **inflow disease** have discomfort in the lower back, buttocks, or thighs. Patients with *mild* inflow disease have discomfort after walking about two blocks. This discomfort is not severe but causes them to stop walking. It is relieved with rest. Patients with *moderate* inflow disease experience pain in these areas after walking about one or two blocks. The discomfort is described as being more like pain, but it eases with rest most of the time. *Severe* inflow disease causes severe pain after walking less than one block. These patients usually have rest pain.

Patients with **outflow disease** describe burning or cramping in the calves, ankles, feet, and toes. Instep or foot discomfort indicates an obstruction below the popliteal artery. Those with *mild* outflow disease experience discomfort after walking about five blocks. Rest relieves this discomfort. Patients with *moderate* outflow disease have pain after walking about two blocks. Intermittent rest pain may be present. Those with *severe* outflow disease usually cannot walk more than one-half block. They may hang their feet off the bed at night for comfort and report more frequent rest pain than patients with inflow disease.

Specific findings for PAD depend on the severity of the disease. Observe for loss of hair on the lower calf, ankle, and foot; dry, scaly, dusky, pale, or mottled skin; and thickened toenails. With severe arterial disease, the extremity is cold and gray-blue (cyanotic) or darkened. Pallor may occur when the extremity is elevated. Dependent **rubor** (redness) may occur when the extremity is lowered (Fig. 36-4). Muscle atrophy can result from prolonged chronic arterial disease.

▣ **CULTURAL/SPIRITUAL CONSIDERATIONS**

Patient-Centered Care **QSEN**

Only severe cyanosis is evident in the skin of dark-skinned patients. To detect cyanosis, assess the skin and nail beds for a dull, lifeless color. The soles of the feet and the toenails are less pigmented and allow detection of cyanosis or duskiness in the lower extremities.

Palpate all pulses in both legs. The most sensitive and specific indicator of arterial function is the quality of the posterior tibial pulse because the pedal pulse is not palpable in a small percentage of people. The strength of each pulse should be compared bilaterally.

Note early signs of ulcer formation or complete ulcer formation, a complication of PAD. Arterial and venous stasis ulcers differ from diabetic ulcers (Chart 36-4). Initially, **arterial ulcers** are painful and develop on the toes (often the great toe), between the toes, or on the upper aspect of the foot. With prolonged occlusion, the toes can become gangrenous.

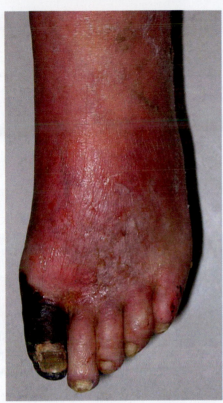

FIG. 36-4 Dependent rubor in the left leg of a patient with peripheral arterial disease. (From Brooks, M., & Jenkins, M. P. (2008). Acute and chronic ischaemia of the limb. *Surgery 26*(1), 17-20.)

Typically, the ulcer is small and round with a "punched out" appearance and well-defined borders. Skin lesions are discussed in further detail in Chapter 25.

Magnetic resonance angiography (MRA) is commonly used to assess blood flow in the peripheral arteries. A contrast medium is used to help visualize blood flow through these arteries. This test is often the only one used to diagnose PAD, although a computed tomography angiography (CTA) may also be performed.

Using a Doppler probe, *segmental systolic blood pressure measurements* of the lower extremities at the thigh, calf, and ankle are an inexpensive, noninvasive method of assessing PAD. Normally, blood pressure readings in the thigh and calf are higher than those in the upper extremities. With the presence of arterial disease, these pressures are lower than the brachial pressure.

With *inflow* disease, pressures taken at the thigh level indicate the severity of disease. Mild inflow disease may cause a difference of only 10 to 30 mm Hg in pressure on the affected side compared with the brachial pressure. Severe inflow disease can cause a pressure difference of more than 40 to 50 mm Hg. The ankle pressure is normally equal to or more than the brachial pressure.

To evaluate *outflow* disease, compare ankle pressure with the brachial pressure, which provides a ratio known as the **ankle-brachial index (ABI)**. The value can be derived by dividing the ankle blood pressure by the brachial blood pressure. *An ABI of less than 0.90 in either leg is diagnostic of PAD. Patients with diabetes are known to have a falsely elevated ABI.*

Exercise tolerance testing (by chemical stress test or treadmill) may give valuable information about claudication (muscle pain). The technician obtains resting pulse volume recordings

and asks the patient to walk on a treadmill until the symptoms are reproduced. At the time of symptom onset or after about 5 minutes, the technician obtains another pulse volume recording. Normally, there may be an increased waveform with minimal, if any, drop in the ankle pressure. In patients with arterial disease, the waveforms are decreased (dampened), and there is a decrease in the ankle pressure of 40 to 60 mm Hg for 20 to 30 seconds in the affected limb. If the return to normal pressure is delayed (longer than 10 minutes), the results suggest abnormal arterial flow in the affected limb.

Plethysmography can also be performed to evaluate arterial flow in the lower extremities. The measurement provides graphs or tracings of arterial flow in the limb. If an occlusion is present, the waveforms are decreased to flattened, depending on the degree of occlusion.

◆ Interventions: Responding

Collaborative management of PAD may include nonsurgical interventions and/or surgery. The patient must first be assessed to determine if the altered tissue PERFUSION is caused by arterial disease, venous disease, or both.

Nonsurgical Management. Exercise, positioning, promoting vasodilation, drug therapy, and invasive nonsurgical procedures are used to increase *arterial* flow to the affected leg(s).

Using Exercise and Positioning. *Exercise* may improve arterial blood flow to the affected leg through buildup of the collateral circulation. **Collateral circulation** provides blood to the affected area through smaller vessels that develop and compensate for the occluded vessels. Exercise is individualized for each patient, but people with severe rest pain, venous ulcers, or gangrene should not participate. Others with PAD can benefit from exercise that is started gradually and slowly increased. Instruct the patient to walk until the point of claudication, stop and rest, and then walk a little farther. Eventually, he or she can walk longer distances as collateral circulation develops. Collaborate with the primary health care provider and physical therapist in determining an appropriate exercise program. Exercise rehabilitation has been used to relieve symptoms but requires a motivated patient. Supervised sessions generally are not reimbursed by health care insurance.

Positioning to promote circulation has been somewhat controversial. Some patients have swelling in their extremities. Teach them to avoid raising their legs above the heart level because extreme elevation slows arterial blood flow to the feet. In severe cases, patients with PAD and swelling may sleep with the affected leg hanging from the bed or sit upright in a chair for comfort.

> **! NURSING SAFETY PRIORITY** QSEN
>
> **Action Alert**
>
> Instruct all patients with the disease to avoid crossing their legs and avoid wearing restrictive clothing (e.g., garters to hold up nylon stockings, particularly common among older women), which interfere with blood flow. Teach them the importance of inspecting their feet daily for color or other changes.

Promoting Vasodilation. Vasodilation can be achieved by providing warmth to the affected extremity and preventing long periods of exposure to cold. Encourage the patient to maintain a warm environment at home and to wear socks or insulated

CHART 36-4   Key Features

Lower-Extremity Ulcers

FEATURE	ARTERIAL ULCERS	VENOUS ULCERS	DIABETIC ULCERS
History	Patient reports claudication after walking about 1-2 blocks Rest pain usually present Pain at ulcer site Two or three risk factors present	Chronic nonhealing ulcer No claudication or rest pain Moderate ulcer discomfort Patient reports of ankle or leg swelling	Diabetes Peripheral neuropathy No reports of claudication
Ulcer location and appearance	End of the toes Between the toes Deep Ulcer bed pale, with even edges Little granulation tissue	Ankle area Brown pigmentation Ulcer bed pink Usually superficial, with uneven edges Granulation tissue present	Plantar area of foot Metatarsal heads Pressure points on feet Deep Pale, with even edges Little granulation tissue
Other assessment findings	Cool or cold foot Decreased or absent pulses Atrophy of skin Hair loss Pallor with elevation Dependent rubor Possible gangrene When acute, neurologic deficits noted	Ankle discoloration and edema Full veins when leg slightly dependent No neurologic deficit Pulses present May have scarring from previous ulcers	Pulses usually present Cool or warm foot Painless
Treatment	Treat underlying cause (surgical, revascularization) Prevent trauma and infection Patient education, stressing foot care	Long-term wound care (Unna boot, damp-to-dry dressings) Elevate extremity Patient education Prevent infection	Rule out major arterial disease Control diabetes Patient education regarding foot care Prevent infection

Photograph of arterial ulcer from Bonow, R.O., Mann, D.L., Zipes, D.P., & Libby, P. (2011). *Braunwald's heart disease: A textbook of cardiovascular medicine* (9th ed.). Philadelphia: Saunders. Photograph of venous ulcer from Bryant, R., & Nix, D. (2012). *Acute and chronic wounds: Current management concepts* (4th ed.). Philadelphia: Saunders. Photograph of diabetic ulcer from Bryant, R., & Nix, D. (2007). *Acute and chronic wounds: Current management concepts* (3rd ed.). Philadelphia: Saunders.

shoes at all times. *Caution the patient to avoid the application of direct heat to the limb with heating pads or extremely hot water. Sensitivity is decreased in the affected limb. Burns may result.*

Encourage patients to prevent exposure of the affected limb to the cold because cold temperatures cause vasoconstriction (decreasing of the diameter of the blood vessels) and therefore decrease arterial PERFUSION.

Emotional stress, caffeine, and nicotine also can cause vasoconstriction. *Emphasize that complete abstinence from smoking or chewing tobacco is essential to prevent vasoconstriction.* The vasoconstrictive effects of each cigarette may last up to 1 hour after the cigarette is smoked.

Drug Therapy. For patients with chronic PAD, prescribed drugs include hemorheologic and antiplatelet agents. Pentoxifylline (Trental) is a hemorheologic agent that increases the flexibility of red blood cells. It decreases blood viscosity by inhibiting platelet aggregation and decreasing fibrinogen and thus increases blood flow in the extremities. Many patients report limited improvement in their daily lives after taking pentoxifylline. However, those with extremely limited endurance

for walking have reported improvement to the point that they can perform some activities (e.g., walk to the mailbox or dining room) that were previously impossible.

Antiplatelet agents, such as aspirin (acetylsalicylic acid, Asaphen ♣) and clopidogrel (Plavix), are commonly used. Aspirin 325 or 81 mg daily may be recommended for patients with chronic PAD. However, evidence suggests that clopidogrel is better than aspirin for reducing the risk for myocardial infarction (MI), ischemic stroke, and vascular death (Rose, 2015). Patients with PAD and no contraindications to antiplatelet therapy should receive either aspirin or clopidogrel. Some patients receive both drugs (dual antiplatelet therapy), although recent trials indicate no additional benefit of using both (Rose, 2015). Patients who are taking clopidogrel should not eat grapefruit or drink grapefruit juice because of risk of kidney failure, GI bleeding, heart failure, or even death.

Patients who experience disabling intermittent claudication may also benefit from phosphodiesterase inhibitors such as cilostazol (Pletal). This drug can also increase HDL-C levels. Teach patients taking the drug that it may cause headaches and GI disturbances, especially flatulence (gas) and diarrhea.

Controlling hypertension can improve tissue PERFUSION by maintaining pressures that are adequate to perfuse the periphery but not constrict the vessels. Teach about the effect of blood pressure on the circulation and instruct in methods of control. For example, patients taking beta blockers may have drug-related claudication or a worsening of symptoms. The primary health care provider closely monitors those who are receiving beta blockers. If the patient has high serum lipids, lipid-lowering drugs such as statins are used (see discussion of statins earlier in this chapter).

Invasive Nonsurgical Procedures. A nonsurgical but invasive approach for improving arterial flow is the use of **percutaneous vascular intervention**. This procedure requires an arterial puncture in the patient's groin. One or more arteries are dilated with a balloon catheter advanced through a cannula, which is inserted into or above an occluded or stenosed artery. When the procedure is successful, it opens the vessel and improves arterial blood flow. Patients who are candidates for percutaneous procedures must have occlusions or stenoses that are accessible to the catheter. Reocclusion may occur, and the procedure may be repeated. Some patients are occlusion-free for up to 3 to 5 years, whereas others may experience reocclusion within a year.

During percutaneous vascular intervention, intravascular stents (wire meshlike devices) are usually inserted to ensure adequate blood flow in a stenosed vessel. Candidates for stents are patients with stenosis of the common or external iliac arteries. Stents are also available to effectively treat superficial femoral artery disease. Patients have these procedures in same-day surgery or ambulatory care centers.

Another arterial technique to improve blood flow to ischemic legs in people with PAD is mechanical rotational abrasive **atherectomy**. The Rotablator device is designed to scrape plaque from inside the artery while minimizing damage to the vessel surface and is useful at the popliteal artery and below.

> **! NURSING SAFETY PRIORITY** QSEN
>
> **Critical Rescue**
>
> The priority for nursing care following a percutaneous vascular intervention or atherectomy is to observe for bleeding at the arterial puncture site, which is sealed with a special collagen plug. Monitor for manifestations of impending hypovolemic shock, including a decrease in blood pressure, increased pulse rate, and decreased urinary output. Perform frequent checks of the distal pulses in both legs to ensure adequate PERFUSION.

Most patients receive anticoagulant or antiplatelet therapy, such as heparin or clopidogrel (Plavix), before and/or during the procedure. An antiplatelet drug may also be prescribed for 1 to 3 months or longer after the procedure to prevent arterial CLOTTING.

Surgical Management. Patients with severe rest pain or claudication that interferes with the ability to work or threatens loss of a limb become surgical candidates. **Arterial revascularization** is the surgical procedure most commonly used to increase arterial blood flow in an affected limb.

Surgical procedures are classified as *inflow* or *outflow*. Inflow procedures involve bypassing arterial occlusions above the superficial femoral arteries (SFAs). Outflow procedures involve surgical bypassing of arterial occlusions at or below the SFAs. For those who have both inflow and outflow problems, the inflow procedure (for larger arteries) is done before the outflow repair.

Inflow procedures include aortoiliac, aortofemoral, and axillofemoral bypasses. Outflow procedures include femoropopliteal and femorotibial bypasses. Inflow procedures are more successful, with less chance of reocclusion or postoperative ischemia. Outflow procedures are less successful in relieving ischemic pain and are associated with a higher incidence of reocclusion.

Graft materials for bypasses are selected on an individual basis. For outflow procedures, the preferred graft material is the patient's own (**autogenous**) saphenous vein. However, some patients experience coronary artery disease and may need this vein for coronary artery bypass. When the saphenous vein is not usable, the cephalic or basilic arm veins may be used. Grafts made of synthetic materials have also been used when autogenous veins were not available.

Preoperative Care. Preparing the patient for surgery is similar to procedures described for general or epidural anesthesia (see Chapter 14). Documentation of vital signs and peripheral pulses provides a baseline of information for comparison during the postoperative phase. Depending on the surgical procedure, the patient may have one or more IV lines, urinary catheter, central venous catheter, and/or arterial line. To prevent postoperative infection, antibiotic therapy is typically given before the procedure.

Operative Procedures. The anesthesia provider places the patient under general, epidural, or spinal anesthesia. Epidural or spinal induction is preferred for older adults to decrease the risk for cardiopulmonary complications in this age-group. If arterial bypass is to be accomplished by autogenous grafts, the surgeon removes the veins through an incision. The blocked artery is then exposed through an incision, and the replacement vein or synthetic graft material is sutured above and below the occlusion to increase blood flow around the occlusion.

For conventional open *aortoiliac* and *aortofemoral* bypass (AFB) surgery, the surgeon makes a midline incision into the abdominal cavity to expose the abdominal aorta, with additional incisions in each groin (Fig. 36-5). Graft material is tunneled from the aorta to the groin incisions, where it is sutured in place.

In an open *axillofemoral* bypass (Fig. 36-6), the surgeon makes an incision beneath the clavicle and tunnels graft material subcutaneously with a catheter from the chest to the iliac crest, into a groin incision, where it is sutured in place. Neither the thoracic nor the abdominal cavity is entered. For that

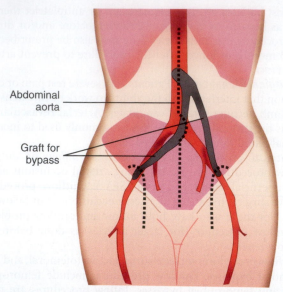

Abdominal aorta

Graft for bypass

FIG. 36-5 In aortoiliac and aortofemoral bypass surgery, a midline incision into the abdominal cavity is required, with an additional incision in each groin.

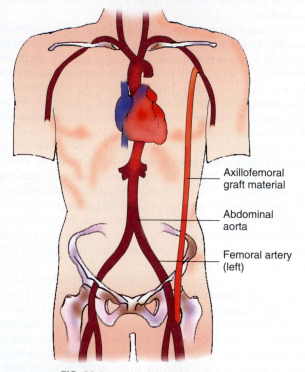

Axillofemoral graft material

Abdominal aorta

Femoral artery (left)

FIG. 36-6 An axillofemoral bypass graft.

reason, the axillofemoral bypass is used for high-risk patients who cannot tolerate a procedure requiring abdominal surgery.

Minimally invasive surgical techniques are beginning to be performed by vascular surgeons using robotic-assisted laparoscopic procedures. These newer surgical techniques require extensive training and further research data to determine their utility.

Postoperative Care. Thorough and ongoing nursing assessment for postoperative arterial revascularization patients is crucial to detect complications. Deep breathing every 1 to 2 hours and using an incentive spirometer are essential to prevent respiratory complications.

Patients who have undergone conventional aortoiliac or aortofemoral bypass are NPO status for at least 1 day after surgery to prevent nausea and vomiting, which could increase intra-abdominal pressure. Those who have undergone bypass surgery of the lower extremities not involving the aorta or abdominal wall (femoropopliteal or femorotibial bypass) may remain NPO until the first postoperative day, when they are allowed clear liquids.

Warmth, redness, and edema of the affected extremity are often expected outcomes of surgery as a result of increased arterial PERFUSION. **Immediately after surgery, the operating suite or postanesthesia care unit (PACU) nurse marks the site where the distal (dorsalis pedis or posterior tibial) pulse is best palpated or heard by Doppler ultrasonography. This information is communicated to the nursing staff on the critical care unit where the patient will be sent. "Hand-off" reporting is essential to promote safety and quality care (as required by The Joint Commission's National Patient Safety Goals).**

To promote graft patency, monitor the patient's blood pressure and notify the surgeon if the pressure increases or decreases beyond the patient's baseline. Hypotension may indicate hypovolemia, which can increase the risk for CLOTTING. Range of motion of the operative leg is usually limited, with no bending of the hip and knee. Consult with the surgeon on a case-by-case basis regarding limitations of movement, including turning. Patients having open procedures may be restricted to bedrest for 24 hours or longer after surgery to prevent disruption of the suture lines. Patients having minimally invasive surgical (MIS) procedures may be ambulatory and eat within the day of surgery. Pain and surgical complications tend to occur less often in patients who have MIS procedures.

❗ NURSING SAFETY PRIORITY QSEN

Critical Rescue

Graft occlusion (blockage) is a postoperative emergency that can occur within the first 24 hours after arterial revascularization. Monitor the patient for and report severe continuous and aching pain, which may be the first indicator of postoperative graft occlusion and ischemia. Many people experience a throbbing pain caused by the increased blood flow to the extremity. Because this alteration in comfort is different from that of ischemic pain, be sure to assess the type of pain that is experienced. Pain from occlusion may be masked by patient-controlled analgesia (PCA). Some patients have ischemic pain that is not relieved by PCA.

Monitor the patency of the graft by checking the extremity every 15 minutes for the first hour and then hourly for changes in color, temperature, and pulse intensity. Compare the operative leg with the unaffected one. *If the operative leg feels cold; becomes pale, ashen, or cyanotic; or has a decreased or absent pulse, contact the surgeon immediately!*

Emergency **thrombectomy** (removal of the clot), which the surgeon may perform at the bedside, is the most common treatment for acute graft occlusion. Thrombectomy is associated with excellent results in prosthetic grafts. Results of thrombectomy in autogenous vein grafts are not as successful and often necessitate graft revision and even replacement.

Local intra-arterial thrombolytic (clot-dissolving) therapy with an agent such as tissue plasminogen activator (t-PA) or an infusion of a platelet inhibitor such as abciximab (ReoPro) may be used for acute graft occlusions. This therapy is provided in select settings in which health care providers are experts in its

CHART 36-5   Home Care Assessment

The Patient With Peripheral Vascular Disease

Assess tissue perfusion to affected extremity(ies), including:
- Distal circulation, sensation, and motion
- Presence of pain, pallor, paresthesias, pulselessness, paralysis, poikilothermy (coolness)
- Ankle-brachial index

Assess adherence to therapeutic regimen, including:
- Following foot care instructions
- Quitting smoking
- Maintaining dietary restrictions
- Participating in exercise regimen
- Avoiding exposure to cold and constrictive clothing

Assess ability to manage wound care and prevent further injury, including:
- Use of compression stockings or compression pumps as directed
- Use of various dressing materials
- Signs and symptoms to report to nurse

Assess coping ability of patient and family members.

Assess home environment, including:
- Safety hazards, especially related to falls

CHART 36-6   Patient and Family Education: Preparing for Self-Management

Foot Care for the Patient With Peripheral Vascular Disease

- Keep your feet clean by washing them with a mild soap in room-temperature water.
- Keep your feet dry, especially the ankles and between the toes.
- Avoid injury to your feet and ankles. Wear comfortable, well-fitting shoes. Never go without shoes.
- Keep your toenails clean and filed. Have someone cut them if you cannot see them clearly. Cut your toenails straight across.
- To prevent dry, cracked skin, apply a lubricating lotion to your feet.
- Prevent exposure to extreme heat or cold. Never use a heating pad on your feet.
- Avoid constricting garments.
- If a problem develops, see a podiatrist or health care provider.
- Avoid extended pressure on your feet or ankles, such as occurs when you lean against something.

use. Other antiplatelet drugs such as the glycoprotein IIb/IIIa inhibitors *tirofiban (Aggrastat)* and *eptifibatide (Integrilin)* may be used as alternatives. The health care provider considers these therapies when the surgical alternative (e.g., thrombectomy with or without graft revision or replacement) carries high morbidity or mortality rates or when surgery for this type of occlusion has traditionally yielded poor results. Closely assess the patient for manifestations of bleeding if thrombolytics are used.

Graft or wound infections can be life threatening. Use sterile technique when providing incisional care and observe for symptoms of infection. Assess the area for induration, erythema, tenderness, warmth, edema, or drainage. Also monitor for fever and leukocytosis (increased serum white blood cell count). Notify the surgeon promptly if any of these symptoms occur. Patients having conventional open bypass procedures are usually hospitalized for 5 to 7 days. Those having MIS procedures usually have shorter stays of 2 or 3 days.

Peripheral arterial disease (PAD) is a chronic, long-term problem with frequent complications. Patients may benefit from a case manager who can follow them across the continuum of care. The desired outcome is that the patient can be maintained in the home.

Management at home often requires an interprofessional team approach, including several home care visits. Chart 36-5 outlines the assessment highlights for home care patients with peripheral vascular disease (PVD).

Instruct patients on methods to promote vasodilation. Teach them to avoid raising their legs above the level of the heart unless venous stasis is also present. Provide written and oral instructions on foot care and methods to prevent injury and ulcer development (Chart 36-6).

Patients who have had surgery require additional instruction on incision care (see Chapter 16). Encourage all patients to avoid smoking and to limit dietary fat intake to 5% to 6% of the total daily calories (Eckel et al., 2014). Remind them to drink adequate fluids to prevent dehydration.

Patients with chronic arterial obstruction may fear recurrent occlusion or further narrowing of the artery. They often fear that they might lose a limb or become debilitated in other ways. Indeed, chronic PAD may worsen, especially in those with diabetes mellitus. Reassure them that participation in prescribed exercise, nutrition therapy, and drug therapy, along with cessation of smoking, can limit further formation of atherosclerotic plaques.

Patients with arterial compromise may need assistance with ADLs if activity is limited by pain. They may need to limit or avoid stair climbing, depending on the severity of disease. Patients who have undergone surgery or need to limit activity usually need temporary help with ADLs by the family or other caregiver. Patients who must limit activity because of PAD may benefit from the assistance of a home care aide. Those who have undergone surgery may require a home care nurse to help with incision care. In collaboration with the case manager, arrange for home care resources before discharge.

ACUTE PERIPHERAL ARTERIAL OCCLUSION

❖ PATHOPHYSIOLOGY

Although chronic peripheral arterial disease (PAD) progresses slowly, the onset of acute arterial occlusions is sudden and dramatic. An embolus (piece of a clot that travels and lodges in a new area) is the most common cause of peripheral occlusions, although a local thrombus may be the cause. Occlusion may affect the upper extremities, but it is more common in the lower extremities. Emboli originating from the heart are the most common cause of acute arterial occlusions. Most patients with an embolic occlusion have had an acute myocardial infarction (MI) and/or atrial fibrillation within the previous weeks.

❖ INTERPROFESSIONAL COLLABORATIVE CARE

Patients with an acute arterial occlusion describe severe pain below the level of the occlusion that occurs even at rest. The affected extremity is cool or cold, pulseless, and mottled. Small areas on the toes may be blackened or gangrenous due to lack of PERFUSION. *Those with acute arterial insufficiency often present with the "six P's" of ischemia:*

- Pain
- Pallor
- Pulselessness
- Paresthesia
- Paralysis
- Poikilothermy (coolness)

The primary health care provider must initiate treatment promptly to avoid permanent damage or loss of an extremity. Anticoagulant therapy with unfractionated heparin (UFH, Hepalean) is usually the first intervention to prevent further clot formation. The patient may undergo angiography.

A surgical *thrombectomy* or *embolectomy* with local anesthesia may be performed to remove the occlusion. The health care provider makes a small incision, which is followed by an **arteriotomy** (a surgical opening into an artery). A catheter is inserted into the artery to retrieve the embolus. It may be necessary to close the artery with a synthetic or autologous (patient's own blood vessel) patch graft.

! NURSING SAFETY PRIORITY QSEN

Critical Rescue

After an arterial thrombectomy, observe the affected extremity for improvement in color, temperature, and pulse every hour for the first 24 hours or according to the postoperative surgical protocol. Monitor patients for manifestations of new thrombi or emboli, especially pulmonary emboli (PE). Chest pain, dyspnea, and acute confusion (older adults) typically occur in patients with PE. Notify the health care provider or Rapid Response Team immediately if these symptoms occur.

Alterations in comfort should significantly diminish after the surgical procedure, although mild incisional pain remains. Watch closely for complications caused by reperfusing the artery after thrombectomy or embolectomy, either of which includes spasms and swelling of the skeletal muscles. Swelling of the skeletal muscles can result in compartment syndrome.

Compartment syndrome occurs when tissue pressure within a confined body space becomes elevated and restricts blood flow. The resulting ischemia can lead to tissue damage and eventually tissue death. Assess the motor and sensory function of the affected extremity. Monitor for increasing pain, swelling, and tenseness. Report any of these symptoms to the health care provider immediately. **Fasciotomy** (surgical opening into the tissues) may be necessary to prevent further injury and save the limb.

The use of *systemic thrombolytic therapy* for acute arterial occlusions has been disappointing because bleeding complications often outweigh the benefits obtained. Catheter-directed intra-arterial thrombolytic therapy with *fibrinolytics*, such as alteplase (Activase) or t-PA, has emerged as an alternative to surgical treatment in selected settings. A catheter is placed percutaneously (through the skin) into the artery with or without ultrasound guidance by the vascular surgeon or interventional radiologist. The tip of the catheter is embedded in the clot to directly deliver the thrombolytic infusion for 24 to 36 hours until the clot dissolves.

During infusion, monitor the patient for complications such as bleeding and hemorrhagic stroke. Maintaining a normal blood pressure is essential in preventing a potential stroke. As the clot dissolves, the patient typically experiences severe pain due to reperfusion that requires patient-controlled analgesia (PCA).

! NURSING SAFETY PRIORITY QSEN

Drug Alert

When *fibrinolytics* are given, assess for signs of bleeding, bruising, or hematoma. For patients receiving any *platelet inhibitor*, monitor platelet counts for the first 3, 6, and 12 hours after the start of the infusion or per agency protocol. If the platelet count decreases to below 100,000/mm^3, the infusion needs to be readjusted or discontinued. If any of these complications occur, notify the health care provider or Rapid Response Team immediately.

ANEURYSMS OF THE CENTRAL ARTERIES

❖ PATHOPHYSIOLOGY

An **aneurysm** is a permanent localized dilation of an artery, which enlarges the artery to at least two times its normal diameter. It may be described as *fusiform* (a diffuse dilation affecting the entire circumference of the artery) or *saccular* (an outpouching affecting only a distinct portion of the artery). Aneurysms may also be described as *true* or *false*. In true aneurysms, the arterial wall is weakened by congenital or acquired problems. False aneurysms occur as a result of vessel injury or trauma to all three layers of the arterial wall. *Dissecting aneurysms* differ from aneurysms in that they are formed when blood accumulates in the wall of an artery.

Aneurysms tend to occur at specific anatomic sites (Fig. 36-7), most commonly in the abdominal aorta. They often occur at a point where the artery is not supported by skeletal muscles or on the lines of curves or flexion in the arterial tree. This chapter discusses aneurysms of the central arteries. Brain aneurysms are discussed in Chapter 45.

An aneurysm forms when the middle layer (media) of the artery is weakened, producing a stretching effect in the inner layer (intima) and outer layers of the artery. As the artery widens, tension in the wall increases; and further widening occurs, thus enlarging the aneurysm and increasing the risk for arterial rupture. Elevated blood pressure can also increase the rate of aneurysmal enlargement and risk for early rupture. When *dissecting* aneurysms occur, the aneurysm enlarges, blood is lost, and blood flow to organs is diminished.

Abdominal aortic aneurysms (AAAs) account for most aneurysms, are commonly asymptomatic, and frequently rupture. Most of these are located between the renal arteries and the aortic bifurcation (dividing area).

Thoracic aortic aneurysms (TAAs) are not quite as common and are frequently misdiagnosed. They are typically discovered when advanced imaging is used to assess other conditions. TAAs commonly develop between the origin of the left subclavian artery and the diaphragm. They are located in the descending, ascending, and transverse sections of the aorta. They can also occur in the aortic arch and are very difficult to manage surgically.

Aneurysms can cause symptoms by exerting pressure on surrounding structures or by rupturing. *Rupture is the most frequent complication and is life threatening because abrupt and massive hemorrhagic shock results.* Thrombi within the wall of an aneurysm can also be the source of emboli in distal arteries below the aneurysm.

Atherosclerosis is the most common cause of aneurysms, with hypertension, hyperlipidemia, and cigarette smoking being

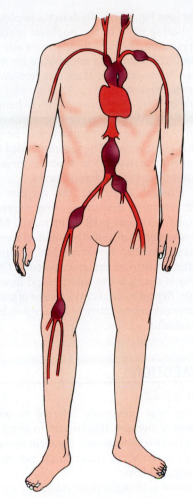

FIG. 36-7 Common anatomic sites of arterial aneurysms.

contributing factors. Age, gender, and family history also play a role (McCance et al., 2014).

❖ INTERPROFESSIONAL COLLABORATIVE CARE

◆ Assessment: Noticing

Most patients with abdominal or thoracic aneurysms are asymptomatic when their aneurysms are first discovered by routine examination or during an imaging study performed for another reason. However, a few patients do have symptoms that bring them to their primary health care provider or the emergency department.

Assess patients with a known or suspected *abdominal aortic aneurysm (AAA)* for abdominal, flank, or back pain. Pain is usually described as steady with a gnawing quality, unaffected by movement, and lasting for hours or days.

A pulsation in the upper abdomen slightly to the left of the midline between the xiphoid process and the umbilicus may be present. A detectable aneurysm is at least 5 cm in diameter. *Auscultate for a bruit over the mass, but avoid palpating the mass because it may be tender and there is risk for rupture!* If expansion and impending rupture of an AAA are suspected, assess for severe pain of sudden onset in the back or lower abdomen, which may radiate to the groin, buttocks, or legs.

Patients with a rupturing AAA are *critically ill* and are at risk for hypovolemic shock caused by hemorrhage. Signs and symptoms include hypotension, diaphoresis, decreased level of consciousness, oliguria (scant urine output), loss of pulses distal to the rupture, and dysrhythmias. Retroperitoneal hemorrhage is manifested by hematomas in the flanks (lower back). Rupture into the abdominal cavity causes abdominal distention.

When a *thoracic aortic aneurysm* is suspected, assess for back pain and manifestations of compression of the aneurysm on adjacent structures. Signs include shortness of breath, hoarseness, and difficulty swallowing. TAAs are not often detected by physical assessment, but occasionally a mass may be visible above the suprasternal notch. Assess the patient with suspected rupture of a thoracic aneurysm for sudden and excruciating back or chest pain. Hypovolemic shock also occurs with TAA.

Computed tomography (CT) scanning with contrast is the standard tool for assessing the size and location of an abdominal or thoracic aneurysm. *Ultrasonography* is also used.

◆ Interventions: Responding

The size of the aneurysm and the presence of symptoms determine patient management. The nurse's role is to perform frequent patient assessments, including blood pressure, pulse, and peripheral circulation checks.

Nonsurgical Management. The desired outcome of nonsurgical management is to monitor the growth of the aneurysm and maintain the blood pressure at a normal level to decrease the risk for rupture. Patients with hypertension are treated with antihypertensive drugs to decrease the rate of enlargement and the risk for early rupture.

For those with small or asymptomatic aneurysms, frequent ultrasound or CT scans are necessary to monitor the growth of the aneurysm. Emphasize the importance of following through with scheduled tests to monitor the growth. Also explain the signs and symptoms of aneurysms that need to be promptly reported.

Surgical Management. Surgical management of an aneurysm may be an elective or an emergency procedure. *For patients with a rupturing abdominal aortic or a thoracic aneurysm, emergency surgery is performed.* Patients with smaller aneurysms that are producing symptoms are advised to have elective surgery. Those with smaller aneurysms that are not causing symptoms are treated nonsurgically until symptoms occur or the aneurysm enlarges.

The most common surgical procedure for AAA has traditionally been a resection or repair (**aneurysmectomy**). However, the mortality rate for elective resection is high and markedly increases for emergency surgery. Endovascular stent grafts have improved mortality rates and shortened the hospital stay for select patients who need AAA repair.

The repair of AAAs with **endovascular stent grafts** is the procedure of choice for almost all patients on an elective or emergent basis. Stents (wirelike devices) are inserted percutaneously (through the skin), avoiding abdominal incisions and therefore decreasing the risk for a prolonged postoperative recovery. Postoperative care is similar to care required after an arteriogram (angiogram).

Different designs of endovascular stent grafts are used, depending on the anatomic involvement of the aneurysm. The stent graft is flexible with either Dacron or polytetrafluoroethylene (PTFE) material. It is inserted through a skin incision into the femoral artery by way of a catheter-based system. The catheter is advanced to a level above the aneurysm away from the renal arteries. The graft is released from the catheter, and the stent graft is placed with a series of hooks. This procedure is done in collaboration with the vascular surgeon, interventional radiologist, operating suite team, and, at some centers, the vascular medicine physician.

Complications of stent repair include:
- Conversion to open surgical repair
- Bleeding
- Aneurysm rupture
- Peripheral embolization
- Misplacement of the stent graft
- Endoleak

The endovascular repair of AAAs has decreased the length of hospital stay for patients requiring repair of abdominal aneurysms. However, the patient needs to be closely monitored, in the hospital and at home, for the development of complications after the procedure. Expert nursing care is required to allow for early identification of problems, and complications require timely surgical intervention. In addition, coordination and interprofessional collaboration with the health care team are required for discharge planning and follow-up ca\re for patients at home.

Most patients are discharged to home after aneurysm repair. However, in the absence of family or other support systems, the postoperative patient may be discharged to a transitional care or long-term care facility for rehabilitation.

If discharged to home, the patient must follow instructions regarding activity level and incisional care. Because stair climbing may be restricted initially, he or she may need a bedside commode if the bathroom is inaccessible. Teach the patient who has undergone surgical repair about activity restrictions, wound care, and pain management. Patients may not perform activities that involve lifting heavy objects (usually more than 15 to 20 lb [6.8 to 9.1 kg]) for 6 to 12 weeks after surgery. Advise them to use caution for activities that involve pulling, pushing, or straining. Most patients are restricted from driving a car for several weeks after discharge.

For patients who have not undergone surgical aneurysm repair, the teaching plan emphasizes the importance of compliance with the schedule of frequent ultrasound scanning to monitor the size of the aneurysm.

> ### ! NURSING SAFETY PRIORITY QSEN
> #### *Action Alert*
>
> Teach patients receiving treatment for hypertension about the importance of continuing to take prescribed drugs. Instruct them about the signs and symptoms that must be reported promptly to the primary health care provider, which include:
> - Abdominal fullness or pain or back pain
> - Chest or back pain
> - Shortness of breath
> - Difficulty swallowing or hoarseness

In collaboration with the case manager or social worker, assess the availability of transportation to and from appointments for patients needing ultrasound monitoring. Those who have undergone surgery may require the services of a home care nurse for initial assistance with dressing changes. A home care aide may be needed to assist with ADLs, depending on the patient's support system.

ANEURYSMS OF THE PERIPHERAL ARTERIES

Although femoral and popliteal aneurysms are not common, they may be associated with an aneurysm in another location of the arterial tree (see Fig. 36-7). To detect a popliteal aneurysm, assess for a pulsating mass in the popliteal space. To detect a femoral aneurysm, observe a pulsatile mass over the femoral artery. *To prevent its rupture, do not palpate the mass!* Evaluate both extremities because more than one femoral or popliteal aneurysm may be present.

The patient may have symptoms of limb ischemia (decreased PERFUSION), including diminished or absent pulses, cool to cold skin, and pain. Alterations in comfort may be present if an adjacent nerve is compressed. The recommended treatment for either type of aneurysm, regardless of size, is surgery because of the risk for thromboembolic complications.

To treat a femoral aneurysm, the surgeon removes the aneurysm and restores circulation using a synthetic or an autogenous saphenous vein graft-stent repair. Most surgeons prefer to bypass rather than resect a popliteal aneurysm.

After surgery, monitor for lower-limb ischemia. Palpate pulses below the graft to assess graft patency. Often Doppler ultrasonography is necessary to assess blood flow when pulses are not palpable. *Report sudden development of pain or discoloration of the extremity immediately to the surgeon because it may indicate graft occlusion.*

AORTIC DISSECTION

❖ *PATHOPHYSIOLOGY*

Aortic dissection was previously referred to as a *dissecting aneurysm.* However, because this condition is more accurately described as a *dissecting hematoma,* the term *aortic dissection* is more commonly used. Aortic dissection is not common but is a life-threatening problem.

Aortic dissection is thought to be caused by a sudden tear in the aortic intima, allowing blood to enter the aortic wall. Degeneration of the aortic media may be the primary cause for this condition, with hypertension being an important contributing factor. It is often associated with genetic connective tissue disorders such as Marfan syndrome. It occurs also in middle-age and older people, peaking in adults in their 50s and 60s. Men are more commonly affected than women.

The circulation of any major artery arising from the aorta can be impaired in patients with aortic dissection; therefore this condition is highly lethal and represents an emergency situation. Although the ascending aorta and descending thoracic aorta are the most common sites, dissections can also occur in the abdominal aorta and other arteries.

❖ *INTERPROFESSIONAL COLLABORATIVE CARE*
◆ *Assessment: Noticing*

The most common symptom is pain. It is described as "sharp," "tearing," "ripping," and "stabbing" and tends to move from its point of origin. Depending on the site of dissection, the patient may feel pain in the anterior chest, back, neck, throat, jaw, or teeth at a level of 10 on a 0-to-10 pain intensity scale.

Diaphoresis (excessive sweating), nausea, vomiting, faintness, and apprehension are also common. Blood pressure is usually elevated unless complications such as cardiac tamponade or rupture have occurred. In these cases, the patient becomes rapidly hypotensive. A decrease or absence of peripheral pulses is common, as is aortic regurgitation, which is characterized by a musical murmur best heard along the right sternal border. Neurologic deficits such as an altered level of consciousness, paraparesis, and strokes also can occur.

If the patient is medically stable, a thoracic MRI is the test of choice to confirm diagnosis. However, the patient is often too unstable to be transported, and a transesophageal echocardiography (TEE) may be performed at the bedside to confirm diagnosis (Manning, 2015)

◆ *Interventions: Responding*

The expected outcomes for emergency care for a patient with an aortic dissection are increased comfort and reduction of systolic blood pressure to 100 to 120 mm Hg. Make sure that the patient has two large-bore IV catheters to infuse 0.9% sodium chloride and give medication. Insert an indwelling urinary catheter. The health care provider prescribes IV morphine sulfate to relieve pain and an IV beta blocker, such as esmolol (Brevibloc), to lower heart rate and blood pressure (Manning, 2015). If this regimen is not effective, nicardipine hydrochloride (Cardene) or other antihypertensive may be used.

Subsequent treatment depends on the location of the dissection. Patients receive continued medical treatment for uncomplicated distal dissections and surgical treatment for proximal dissections. For long-term medical treatment, the systolic blood pressure must be maintained at or below 130 to 140 mm Hg. Beta blockers (e.g., propranolol) and calcium channel antagonists (e.g., amlodipine) are prescribed to assist with blood pressure maintenance once the patient is stabilized. Patients having surgical intervention for a proximal dissection typically require cardiopulmonary bypass (CPB) (see Chapter 38). The surgeon removes the intimal tear and sutures edges of the dissected aorta. Usually a synthetic graft is used.

OTHER ARTERIAL HEALTH PROBLEMS

Less common health problems affecting peripheral and central arteries are summarized in Table 36-7.

PERIPHERAL VENOUS DISEASE

To function properly, veins must be patent (open) with competent valves. Vein function also requires the assistance of the surrounding muscle beds to help pump blood toward the heart. If one or more veins are not operating properly, they become distended, and signs and symptoms occur.

Three health problems alter the blood flow in veins:

- Thrombus formation (*venous thrombosis*) can lead to pulmonary embolism (PE), a life-threatening complication. Venous thromboembolism (VTE) is the current term that includes both deep vein thrombosis and PE.
- Defective valves lead to *venous insufficiency* and *varicose veins*, which are not life threatening but are problematic.
- Skeletal muscles do not contract to help pump blood in the veins. This problem can occur when weight bearing is limited or muscle tone decreases.

TABLE 36-7	Interprofessional Collaborative Care for Other Arterial Health Problems	
Assessment: Noticing	**Interventions: Responding**	**Nursing Implications**
Buerger's Disease		
Claudication in feet and lower extremities worse at night; causes ischemia and fibrosis of vessels in extremities with increased sensitivity to cold; ulcerations and gangrene on digits; cause unknown but is associated with smoking	Vasodilating drugs, such as nifedipine (Procardia); management of ulceration and gangrene; chronic pain management modalities	Teach patient about smoking cessation, avoiding cold by wearing gloves and warm clothes, managing stress, avoiding caffeine; teach patient taking nifedipine to avoid grapefruit and grapefruit juice to prevent severe adverse effects, including possible death; teach patients on vasodilators about side effects such as facial flushing, hypotension, headaches.
Raynaud's Phenomenon/Disease		
Painful vasospasms of arteries and arterioles in extremities, especially digits; causes red-white-blue skin color changes on exposure to cold or stress; cause unknown, occurs more in women, and may be autoimmune because it is associated with many rheumatic diseases such as systemic lupus erythematosus	Same as for Buerger's disease	Same as for Buerger's disease
Subclavian Steal		
Occurs in upper extremities as result of subclavian artery occlusion or stenosis causing ischemia in the arm and pain; paresthesias and dizziness are also common; blood pressure difference in arms and presence of subclavian bruit on the affected side	Surgical interventions for cyanosis or unrelenting pain, such as endarterectomy, bypass, or dilation of subclavian artery	Monitor patient closely for new signs and symptoms; postoperative, check pulses and observe for ischemic changes, including severe pain or color changes (e.g., cyanosis).
Thoracic Outlet Syndrome		
Compression of subclavian artery by rib or muscle that is more common in women and those who have to keep arms moving or above their heads (e.g., golfers, swimmers); also present with trauma; causes neck, arm, and shoulder pain with numbness and possible cyanosis	Physical therapy for exercise program; avoiding aggravating positions; surgery as last resort for severe pain	Health teaching about avoiding activities and positions that aggravate pain; monitor for new signs and symptoms; neurovascular assessments; postoperative care if needed.

✳ CLOTTING CONCEPT EXEMPLAR Venous Thromboembolism

❖ PATHOPHYSIOLOGY

Venous thromboembolism (VTE) is one of health care's greatest challenges and includes both thrombus and embolus complications. A thrombus (also called a *thrombosis*) is a blood clot believed to result from an endothelial injury, venous stasis, or hypercoagulability. The thrombosis may be specifically attributable to one element, or it may involve all three elements. It is often associated with an inflammatory process. When a thrombus develops, IMMUNITY is altered, causing inflammation to occur around the clot, thickening of the vein wall, and possible embolization (the formation of an embolus). Pulmonary embolism (PE) is the most common type of embolus and is discussed in detail in Chapter 32.

Phlebothrombosis is a thrombus without inflammation. Thrombophlebitis refers to a thrombus that is associated with inflammation. Thrombophlebitis can occur in superficial veins. However, it most frequently occurs in the deep veins of the lower extremities.

Deep vein thrombophlebitis, commonly referred to as deep vein thrombosis (DVT), is the most common type of thrombophlebitis. It is more serious than superficial thrombophlebitis because it presents a greater risk for PE. With PE, a dislodged blood clot travels to the pulmonary artery—a medical emergency! DVT develops most often in the legs but can also occur in the upper arms as a result of increased use of central venous devices.

Etiology

Thrombus formation has been associated with stasis of blood flow, endothelial injury, and/or hypercoagulability, known as Virchow's triad. The precise cause of these events remains unknown; however, a few predisposing factors have been identified.

The highest incidence of clot formation occurs in patients who have undergone hip surgery, total knee replacement, or open prostate surgery. Other conditions that seem to promote thrombus formation are ulcerative colitis, heart failure, cancer, oral contraceptives, and immobility. Complications of immobility occur during prolonged bedrest such as when a patient is confined to bed for an extensive illness. People who sit for long periods (e.g., on an airplane or at a computer) are also at risk. Phlebitis (vein inflammation) associated with invasive procedures such as IV therapy can also predispose patients to thrombosis.

Incidence and Prevalence

Millions of people in the United States are affected by DVT each year, and many die from pulmonary embolism. The largest number of deaths occurs in older adults. Among patients who have a DVT, over half will have long-term complications, and one third will have a recurrence within 10 years (Mozaffarian et al., 2016).

❖ INTERPROFESSIONAL COLLABORATIVE CARE

◆ Assessment: Noticing

History. Assess the patient for a history of any type of VTE. In addition, assess him or her for risks that may be associated with the development of VTE such as prolonged periods of sitting or bedrest, recent surgical procedures, or any factors that may affect coagulation.

The Joint Commission's VTE Core Measure Set requires that hospitals report data on six areas related to VTE prophylaxis and management (Table 36-8). If VTE is not prevented or adequately managed, the hospital may not be paid by the third-party payer (e.g., Medicare) for the patient's care. In the *inpatient setting*, all patients must be assessed for risk for VTE on admission. A systematic literature review by Anthony (2013) found a valid and reliable model for placing patients in high- and low-risk groups for DVT. This model is highly predictive of DVT development. During the nursing assessment, one point is given for each of nine characteristics, which include:

- Active cancer, paralysis, or casting of an extremity
- Bedridden for more than 3 days
- Major surgery with general anesthesia during the previous 3 months
- Localized tenderness along the deep venous system
- Swelling of the entire leg
- Calf swelling of greater than 3 cm larger when compared with the other leg
- Pitting edema in one leg
- Dilated superficial veins in one leg
- Previously documented DVT

A score of 2 or more indicates that a DVT is likely to occur.

Physical Assessment/Signs and Symptoms. People with DVT may have symptoms or may be asymptomatic. *The classic signs and symptoms of DVT are calf or groin tenderness and pain*

TABLE 36-8	Venous Thromboembolism (VTE) Core Measure Set
CORE MEASURE	**ASSESSMENT OF MEASURE**
VTE-1	**VTE Prophylaxis:** Number of patients who received VTE prophylaxis or have documented why no VTE prophylaxis was given the day of or the day after hospital admission or surgery
VTE-2	**ICU VTE:** Number of patients who received VTE prophylaxis on ICU admission or have documented why no VTE prophylaxis was given the day of admission, transfer, or surgery
VTE-3	**VTE Patients With Anticoagulant Overlap Therapy:** Number of patients diagnosed with confirmed VTE who received overlap of parenteral anticoagulant and warfarin
VTE-4	**VTE Patients Receiving Unfractionated Heparin:** Number of patients receiving heparin with dosages/platelet count monitoring by protocol or nomogram
VTE-5	**VTE Warfarin Therapy Discharge Instructions:** Number of patients who received written instructions that address these four criteria: • Compliance issues • Dietary advice • Follow-up monitoring • Information about potential for adverse drug reactions/interactions
VTE-6	**Hospital-Acquired Potentially Preventable VTE:** Number of patients who developed VTE while hospitalized

ICU, Intensive care unit.
Data from www.jointcommission.org/venous_thromboembolism/.

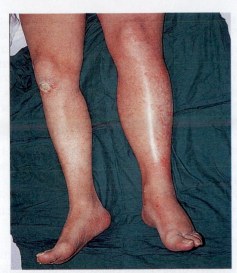

FIG. 36-8 Deep vein thrombosis (DVT) of lower left leg. (From Forbes, C. D., & Jackson, W. F. [2003]. *Colour atlas and text of clinical medicine* [3rd ed.]. London: Mosby.)

and sudden onset of unilateral swelling of the leg. Pain in the calf on dorsiflexion of the foot (positive Homans' sign) appears in only a small percentage of patients with DVT, and false-positive findings are common. *Therefore checking a Homans' sign is not advised because it is an unreliable tool!* Examine the area described as painful, comparing this site with the other limb. *Gently* palpate the site, observing for **induration** (hardening) along the blood vessel and for warmth and edema. Redness may also be present (Fig. 36-8).

Other Diagnostic Assessments. If a definitive diagnosis is lacking from physical assessment findings alone, diagnostic tests may be performed. The preferred diagnostic test for DVT is *venous duplex ultrasonography,* a noninvasive ultrasound that assesses the flow of blood through the veins of the arms and legs. *Doppler flow studies* may also be useful in the diagnosis, but they are more sensitive in detecting proximal rather than distal DVT. Normal venous circulation creates audible signals, whereas thrombosed veins produce little or no sound. The accuracy of the scanning depends on the technical skill of the health care professional performing the test. If the test is negative but a DVT is still suspected, a venogram may be needed to make an accurate diagnosis.

Impedance plethysmography assesses venous outflow and can detect most DVTs that are located above the popliteal vein. It is not helpful in locating clots in the calf and is less sensitive than Doppler studies.

Magnetic resonance direct thrombus imaging (MRI), another noninvasive test, is useful in finding a DVT in the proximal deep veins and is better than traditional venography in finding DVT in the inferior vena cava or pelvic veins.

A D-dimer test is a global marker of coagulation activation and measures fibrin degradation products produced from fibrinolysis (clot breakdown). The test is used for the diagnosis of DVT when the patient has few clinical signs and stratifies patients into a high-risk category for recurrence. Useful as an adjunct to noninvasive testing, a negative D-dimer test can exclude a DVT without an ultrasound.

Physical and diagnostic assessment of patients with pulmonary embolism is described in Chapter 32.

◆ **Analysis: Interpreting**

The priority collaborative problem for most patients with venous thromboembolism (VTE) is:

1. Potential for injury due to complications of VTE and anticoagulation therapy.

◆ **Planning and Implementation: Responding**

Preventing Injury

Planning: Expected Outcomes. The patient with VTE is expected to remain free of injury from VTE complications and the use of anticoagulant therapy.

Interventions. The focus of managing thrombophlebitis is to prevent complications such as pulmonary emboli, further thrombus formation, and an increase in size of the thrombus. Patients with deep vein thrombosis (DVT) may be hospitalized for treatment, although this practice is changing as a result of the use of newer drugs.

Nonsurgical Management. DVT is usually treated medically with a combination of rest and drug therapy. Prevention of DVT and other types of VTE is crucial for patients at risk. For those at moderate-to-high risk, initiate these interventions to prevent VTE:

- Patient education
- Leg exercises
- Early ambulation
- Adequate hydration
- Graduated compression stockings
- Intermittent pneumatic compression, such as sequential compression devices (SCDs)
- Venous plexus foot pump
- Anticoagulant therapy

Supportive therapy for DVT has typically included bedrest and elevation of the extremity. However, research shows that ambulation does not increase the risk for pulmonary embolus (Lip & Hull, 2015). The risk of pulmonary embolism (PE) associated with more aggressive activity is unknown. The accepted approach is a gradual increase in ambulation as tolerated by the patient. Allowing patients to ambulate may decrease their fear and anxiety about dislodging the clot and life-threatening complications.

Teach the patient to elevate his or her legs when in the bed and chair. To help prevent chronic venous insufficiency, instruct patients with active and resolving DVT to wear knee- or thigh-high sequential or graduated compression stockings for an extended period. Be sure to select the correct stocking size for the patient according to the sizing chart provided.

Some health care providers prescribe intermittent or continuous warm, moist soaks to the affected area. *To prevent the thrombus from dislodging and becoming an embolus, do not massage the affected extremity.* Monitor all patients for signs and symptoms of PE, which include shortness of breath, chest pain, and acute confusion (in older adults). Emboli may also travel to the brain or heart, but these complications are not as common as PE. Chapter 32 describes PE manifestations in detail.

Drug Therapy. Anticoagulants are the drugs of choice for actual DVT and for patients at risk for DVT. However, these drugs are known to cause medical complications and even death. **Therefore The Joint Commission's National Patient Safety Goals (NPSGs) include elements of performance to reduce the likelihood of patient harm associated with the use of anticoagulant therapy.**

The conventional treatment has been IV unfractionated heparin followed by oral anticoagulation with warfarin (Coumadin). However, unfractionated heparin can be problematic because each patient's response to the drug is unpredictable and hospital admission is usually required for laboratory monitoring and dose adjustments. The use of low–molecular-weight heparin (LMWH) and the development of novel oral anticoagulants (NOACs, also referred to as *direct oral anticoagulants [DOACs]*) has changed the management of both DVT and PE.

Unfractionated Heparin Therapy. Some patients with a confirmed diagnosis of an existing blood clot are started on a regimen of IV unfractionated heparin (UFH, Hepalean) therapy. The health care provider prescribes UFH to prevent further CLOT-TING, which often develops in the presence of an existing clot, and to prevent enlargement of the existing clot. Over a long period of time, the body slowly absorbs the existing clot.

Before UFH administration, a baseline prothrombin time (PT), activated partial thromboplastin time (APTT or aPTT), international normalized ratio (INR), complete blood count (CBC) with platelet count, urinalysis, stool for occult blood, and creatinine level are required. Notify the primary health care provider if the platelet count is below 100,000 to 120,000/mm³, depending on agency protocol.

UFH is initially given in a bolus IV dose of about 80 to 100 units/kg of body weight in a prefilled syringe or 5000 units followed by continuous infusion via an infusion pump. The infusion is regulated by a reliable electronic pump that protects against accidental free flow of solution. The health care provider or clinical pharmacist prescribes concentrations of UFH (in 5% dextrose in water) and the number of units or milliliters per hour needed to maintain a therapeutic aPTT (usually 18 to 20 units/kg/hr or at least 30,000 units over 24 hours). aPTT is measured at least daily, and results are reported to the health care provider as soon as they are available to allow adjustment of heparin dosage. Therapeutic levels of aPTT are usually $1\frac{1}{2}$ to 2 times normal control levels.

> **! NURSING SAFETY PRIORITY** QSEN
>
> **Critical Rescue**
>
> Notify the health care provider if the aPTT value is greater than 70 seconds or follow hospital protocol for reporting critical laboratory values. Assess patient for signs and symptoms of bleeding, which include hematuria, frank or occult blood in the stool, ecchymosis (bruising), petechiae, an altered level of consciousness, or pain. If bleeding occurs, stop the anticoagulant immediately and call the health care provider or Rapid Response Team!

UFH can also decrease platelet counts. Mild reductions are common and are resolved with continued heparin therapy. Severe platelet reductions, although rare, result from the development of antiplatelet bodies within 6 to 14 days after the beginning of treatment. Platelets aggregate into "white clots" that can cause thrombosis, usually in the form of an acute arterial occlusion. The health care provider discontinues heparin administration if severe **heparin-induced thrombocytopenia (HIT)** (platelet count <150,000), or "white clot syndrome," occurs. Low–molecular-weight heparin is used more commonly today because of the complications involved with unfractionated heparin.

Bivalirudin (Angiomax) and argatroban injection are *highly selective direct thrombin inhibitors* that may be used as alternatives to heparin or for patients who have had HIT. Like heparin, these drugs increase the risk for bleeding. Monitor hemoglobin, hematocrit, aPTT, platelet count, urinalysis, fecal occult blood test, and blood pressure for indications of this complication. An oral anticoagulant such as warfarin (Coumadin) may also be substituted for heparin if necessary.

Ensure that protamine sulfate, the antidote for heparin, is available if needed for excessive bleeding. Chart 36-7 highlights information important to nursing care and patient education associated with anticoagulant therapy.

To *prevent* DVT, unfractionated heparin may be given in low doses subcutaneously for high-risk patients, especially after orthopedic surgery.

Alternatives to unfractionated heparin include:
- Low–molecular-weight heparin (e.g., enoxaparin [Lovenox]) (drug class of choice after orthopedic surgery)
- Novel oral anticoagulants (dabigatran [Pradaxa], rivaroxaban [Xarelto], apixaban, [Eliquis], edoxaban [Savaysa])
- Warfarin (Coumadin, Warfilone)

Low-Molecular-Weight Heparin. Subcutaneous low-molecular-weight heparins (LMWHs) such as enoxaparin (Lovenox) or dalteparin (Fragmin) have a consistent action and are preferred for prevention and treatment of DVT. LMWHs bind less to plasma proteins, blood cells, and vessel walls, resulting in a longer half-life and more predictable response. These drugs inhibit thrombin formation because of reduced factor IIa activity and enhanced inhibition of factor Xa and thrombin.

Some patients taking LMWH may be safely managed at home with visits from a home care nurse. Candidates for home

> **◎ CHART 36-7 Best Practice for Patient Safety & Quality Care** QSEN
>
> **The Patient Receiving Anticoagulant Therapy**
>
> - Carefully check the dosage of anticoagulant to be administered, even if the pharmacy prepared the drug.
> - Monitor the patient for signs and symptoms of bleeding, including hematuria, frank or occult blood in the stool, ecchymosis, petechiae, altered mental status (indicating possible cranial bleeding), or pain (especially abdominal pain, which could indicate abdominal bleeding).
> - Monitor vital signs frequently for decreased blood pressure and increased pulse (indicating possible internal bleeding).
> - Have antidotes available as needed (e.g., protamine sulfate for heparin; vitamin K for warfarin [Coumadin, Warfilone]).
> - Monitor activated partial thromboplastin time (aPTT) for patients receiving unfractionated heparin. Monitor prothrombin time (PT)/international normalized ratio (INR) for patients receiving warfarin or low–molecular-weight heparin (LMWH).
> - Apply prolonged pressure over venipuncture and injection sites.
> - When administering *subcutaneous* heparin, apply pressure over the site and do not massage.
> - Teach the patient going home while taking an anticoagulant to:
>   - Use only an electric razor
>   - Take precautions to avoid injury (e.g., do not use tools such as hammers or saws where accidents commonly occur)
>   - Report signs and symptoms of bleeding, such as blood in the urine or stool, nosebleeds, ecchymosis, or altered mental status
>   - Take the prescribed dosage of drug at the precise time that it was prescribed to be taken
>   - Do not stop taking the drug abruptly; the health care provider usually tapers the anticoagulant gradually

therapy must have stable DVT or PE, low risk for bleeding, adequate renal function, and normal vital signs. They must be willing to learn self-injection or have a family member, friend, or home care nurse administer the subcutaneous injections.

Some health care providers place the patient on a regimen of IV unfractionated heparin (UFH) for several days and then follow up with an LMWH. In this case, the UFH is discontinued at least 30 minutes before the first LMWH injection. The usual dose of enoxaparin is 1 mg/kg of body weight, not to exceed 90 mg, and is repeated every 12 hours. If the patient's creatinine level is greater than 2 mg/dL (indicating renal insufficiency), the health care provider lowers the dose. Dalteparin can be given once daily at 200 units/kg of body weight and does not require dose adjustment for renal insufficiency. Assess all stools for occult blood. The aPTTs are not checked on an ongoing basis because the doses of LMWH are not adjusted.

Warfarin Therapy. If the patient is receiving continuous UFH, warfarin (Coumadin), an oral anticoagulant, may be *added*. This anticoagulant drug overlap is necessary for a period of at least 5 days because heparin and warfarin work differently. Warfarin works in the liver to inhibit synthesis of the four vitamin K–dependent clotting factors and takes 3 to 4 days before it can exert therapeutic anticoagulation. The heparin continues to provide therapeutic anticoagulation until this effect is achieved. IV heparin is then discontinued. Patients receiving LMWH are placed on the oral drug after the first dose.

According to the National Patient Safety Goals, therapeutic levels of warfarin must be monitored by measuring the international normalized ratio (INR) at frequent intervals. Because prothrombin times are often inconsistent and misleading, the INR was developed. Most laboratories report both results. Most patients receiving warfarin should have an INR between 1.5 and 2.0 to prevent future DVT and to minimize the risk for stroke or hemorrhage (Pagana et al., 2017). For patients with additional cardiovascular problems or pulmonary embolus, the desired INR is higher, up to 3.5 or 4.0. The health care provider specifies the desired INR level to obtain. Be aware of the critical value for INR according to agency policy (ranges between 4.5 and 6.0). Notify the health care provider immediately if your patient's INR is at a critical value.

After obtaining the patient's baseline INR, warfarin therapy should be started with low doses, at least 5 mg, and gradually titrated up according to the INR. Patients usually receive this drug for 3 to 6 months or longer after an episode of DVT if no precipitating factors were discovered, with recurrence, or if there are continuing risk factors.

> ! **NURSING SAFETY PRIORITY** QSEN
>
> *Drug Alert*
>
> For patients taking warfarin, assess for any bleeding, such as hematuria or blood in the stool. *Ensure that vitamin K, the antidote for warfarin, is available in case of excessive bleeding* (see Chart 36-7). Report any bleeding to the health care provider and document in the patient's health record. Teach patients to avoid foods with high concentrations of vitamin K, especially dark green leafy vegetables. These foods interfere with the action of warfarin, which is a vitamin K synthesis inhibitor.

Novel Oral Anticoagulants (NOACs). The latest development in anticoagulation is the use of NOACs (also referred to as direct oral anticoagulants [DOACs]). These medications (dabigatran [Pradaxa], rivaroxaban [Xarelto], apixaban [Eliquis], edoxaban

[Savaysa]) were developed to have fewer drug interactions and a wide therapeutic index to allow for fixed dosing without the need for frequent laboratory monitoring (Goldstein, 2015). Current research suggests that efficacy with NOACs is similar to that of warfarin therapy in the treatment of VTE (Mookadam et al., 2015). Prothrombin time (PT) and INR are not accurate predictors of bleeding time when NOACs are used. If the patient does experience severe bleeding, the only NOAC with a reversal agent is dabigatran.

The FDA has approved the use of idarucizumab (Praxbind) as an antidote or reversal agent for dabigatran. Idarucizumab binds to dabigatran, which prevents dabigatran from inhibiting thrombin. Side effects of idarucizumab include hypokalemia, confusion, constipation, fever, and pneumonia. Use of idarucizumab increases the risk of CLOTTING and should only be used in the event of life-threatening bleeding.

Expect to see an increase in the use of NOACs, specifically dabigatran, given the recent FDA approval of the reversal agent idarucizumab (Leung, 2015). Patients should be informed that this medication should not be stopped prematurely because of a significant risk of CLOTTING. Initial laboratory values, including PT and aPTT, are suggested. However, recurrent laboratory monitoring is not required with this medication. Dosage is decreased when renal insufficiency is present. The same teaching specific to all anticoagulants, with the exception of repeat laboratory testing, applies to patients taking NOACs.

Thrombolytic Therapy. Thrombolytic therapy using a catheter-directed approach can be used. However, anticoagulant therapy is preferred for most patients with an uncomplicated DVT, reserving thrombolytic therapy for extensive DVT.

> ? **NCLEX EXAMINATION CHALLENGE 36-4**
>
> *Physiological Integrity*
>
> A client is being discharged home following 5 days of acute care for treatment of a deep vein thrombosis. Which statement made by the client indicates a need for further teaching?
> A. "I will be going home on oral Heparin and warfarin."
> B. "I have an appointment for follow-up care with my primary care provider."
> C. "I will avoid dark green leafy vegetables while taking warfarin."
> D. "I will report any signs of bleeding to my primary health care provider."

Surgical Management. A deep vein thrombus is rarely removed surgically unless there is a massive occlusion that does not respond to medical treatment and the thrombus is of recent (1 to 2 days) onset. **Thrombectomy** is a surgical procedure for clot removal. Preoperative and postoperative care of patients undergoing thrombectomy is similar to the care for those undergoing arterial surgery (see the Peripheral Arterial Disease section).

For patients with recurrent deep vein thrombosis (DVT) or pulmonary emboli that do not respond to medical treatment and for patients who cannot tolerate anticoagulation, **inferior vena cava filtration** may be indicated. The surgeon or interventional radiologist inserts a filter device into the femoral vein or jugular vein. The device is meant to trap emboli in the inferior vena cava before they progress to the lungs. Holes in the device allow blood to pass through, without interfering with the return of blood to the heart. Several new filter brands are available that are designed for removal if and when DVT risks diminish.

Preoperative care is similar to that provided for patients receiving local anesthesia (see Chapter 14). If they have recently been taking anticoagulants, collaborate with the health care provider about interrupting this therapy in the preoperative period to avoid hemorrhage.

After surgery, inspect the groin insertion site for bleeding and signs or symptoms of infection. Other postoperative nursing care is similar to that for any patient undergoing local anesthesia (see Chapter 16).

Care Coordination and Transition Management

Home Care. Patients recovering from thrombophlebitis or DVT are ambulatory when they are discharged from the hospital. The primary focus of planning for discharge is to educate the patient and family about anticoagulation therapy. Patients who have experienced DVT may fear recurrence of a thrombus. They may also be concerned about treatment with warfarin and the risk for bleeding. Assure them that the prescribed treatment will help resolve this problem and that ongoing assessment of prothrombin times and INR values decreases the risks for bleeding.

Self-Management Education. Teach patients recovering from DVT to stop smoking and avoid the use of oral contraceptives to decrease the risk for recurrence. Alternative forms of birth control may be used. Most patients are discharged on a regimen of warfarin (Coumadin) or low–molecular-weight heparin (LMWH). Patients receiving subcutaneous LMWH injections at home need instruction on self-injection. Teach the appropriate caregiver and family members or friends, if necessary, to administer the injections. The VTE Core Measures and the Joint Commission's National Patient Safety Goals require that patients be given written discharge instructions about anticoagulant therapy that address:

- Drug compliance issues (need to take drug as prescribed)
- Dietary advice (e.g., foods to avoid)
- Follow-up monitoring (e.g., Coumadin clinic, INR testing)
- Information about potential for adverse drug reactions/ interactions (e.g., bleeding, bruising)

Instruct patients and their families to avoid potentially traumatic situations, such as participation in contact sports. Provide written and oral information about the signs and symptoms of bleeding (see Chart 36-7). Reinforce the need to report any of these manifestations to the primary health care provider immediately. The anticoagulant effect of warfarin may be reversed by omitting one or two doses of the drug or by the administration of vitamin K. In case of injury, teach patients to apply pressure to bleeding wounds and to seek medical assistance immediately. Encourage them to carry an identification card or wear a medical alert bracelet that states that they are taking warfarin or any other anticoagulant.

Instruct patients to tell their dentist and other health care providers that they are taking warfarin before receiving treatment or prescriptions. Prothrombin times are affected by many prescription and over-the-counter drugs such as NSAIDs. Teach patients to avoid high-fat and vitamin K–rich foods (Chart 36-8). Remind them to drink adequate fluids to stay well hydrated, avoid alcohol (which can cause dehydration), and avoid sitting for prolonged periods.

Health Care Resources. Collaborate with the case manager (CM) or office nurse to arrange for the patient to obtain a device to self-monitor INR at home. Some insurance companies do not pay for the INR monitoring device. Clinical studies show

---

CHART 36-8   Patient and Family Education: Preparing for Self-Management

Foods and Drugs That Interfere With Warfarin (Coumadin)

Eat only small amounts of foods rich in vitamin K each day, including any of these:	If possible, avoid:
• Broccoli • Cauliflower • Spinach • Kale • Other green leafy vegetables • Brussels sprouts • Cabbage • Liver	• Allopurinol • NSAIDs • Acetaminophen • Vitamin E • Histamine blockers • Cholesterol-reducing drugs • Antibiotics • Oral contraceptives • Antidepressants • Thyroid drugs • Antifungal agents • Other anticoagulants • Corticosteroids • Herbs, such as St. John's wort, garlic, ginseng, *Ginkgo biloba*

---

that self-monitoring the INR and self-adjusting anticoagulation therapy result in better anticoagulation control, improve patient satisfaction, and improve quality of life (Michaels & Regan, 2013). The device used to self-monitor is similar to a glucometer for glucose testing and requires a finger stick blood sample. If the patient cannot use a monitoring device, teach a family member or other caregiver how to perform the procedure. If the patient lives alone, collaborate with the CM to arrange for follow-up laboratory appointments to have blood drawn at frequent intervals—usually every week until the patient's values are stabilized. Communication with the primary health care provider is essential while patients are receiving warfarin.

◆ Evaluation: Reflecting

Evaluate the care of the patient with VTE on the basis of the identified priority problem. The expected outcome is that he or she:

- Remains free of injury associated with VTE complications such as pulmonary embolism and bleeding associated with anticoagulation therapy.

VENOUS INSUFFICIENCY

❖ PATHOPHYSIOLOGY

Venous insufficiency occurs as a result of prolonged venous hypertension that stretches the veins and damages the valves. Valvular damage can lead to a backup of blood and further venous hypertension, resulting in edema and decreased tissue perfusion. With time, this stasis (stoppage) results in venous stasis ulcers, swelling, and cellulitis.

The veins cannot function properly when thrombosis occurs or when valves are not working correctly. Venous hypertension can occur in people who stand or sit in one position for long periods (e.g., teachers, office personnel). Obesity can also cause chronically distended veins, which lead to damaged valves. Thrombus formation can contribute to valve destruction. Chronic venous insufficiency also often occurs in patients who have had thrombophlebitis. In severe cases, venous ulcers develop.

Venous leg ulcers are a major cause of pain, death, and health care costs. Most venous ulcer care is delivered in the community setting by home care nurses or through self-management.

❖ INTERPROFESSIONAL COLLABORATIVE CARE

◆ Assessment: Noticing

Venous insufficiency may result in edema of both legs. There may be stasis dermatitis or reddish-brown discoloration along the ankles, extending up to the calf. In people with long-term venous insufficiency, stasis ulcers often form. They can result from the edema or from minor injury to the limb. Ulcers typically occur over the malleolus, more often medially (inner ankle) than laterally (outer ankle). The ulcer usually has irregular borders. In general, these ulcers are chronic and difficult to heal (see Chart 36-4). Many people live with ulcers for years, and recurrence is common. Some may lose one or both legs if ulcers are not controlled.

◆ Interventions: Responding

The focus of treating venous insufficiency is to decrease edema and promote venous return from the affected leg. Patients are not usually hospitalized for venous insufficiency alone unless it is complicated by an ulcer or another disorder is occurring at the same time.

Treatment of chronic venous insufficiency is nonsurgical unless it is complicated by a venous stasis ulcer that requires surgical débridement. The desired outcomes of managing venous stasis ulcers are to heal the ulcer, prevent infection, and prevent stasis with recurrence of ulcer formation. Interprofessional collaboration with the wound care nurse or wound, ostomy, and continence nurse (WOCN) is essential in providing ulcer care. A dietitian can suggest dietary supplements such as zinc and vitamins A and C, as well as high-protein foods, to promote wound healing.

Patients with chronic venous insufficiency wear graduated compression stockings, which fit from the middle of the foot to just below the knee or to the thigh. Stockings should be worn during the day and evening. Explain the purpose and importance of wearing the compression stockings. Be sure to use the sizing chart that comes with the stockings to select the best fit. Teach patients to not roll them down and to report if they become too tight or uncomfortable.

Teach the patient to elevate his or her legs for at least 20 minutes four or five times per day. When the patient is in bed, remind him or her to elevate the legs above the level of the heart (Chart 36-9).

Coordinate with the health care provider about the use of intermittent sequential pneumatic compression or foot plexus pumps for patients with past or present venous stasis ulcers. If an open venous ulcer is present, the device may be applied over a dressing such as an Unna boot. Instruct the patient to apply the pump as directed during the period of healing. Because of the high incidence of venous ulcer recurrence, encourage patients with chronic venous insufficiency whose ulcers have healed to continue compression therapy for life.

Venous stasis ulcers are slightly more manageable than ulcers resulting from arterial disease. They are chronic in nature, with some patients having the same ulcer for years. Ulcers often heal, only to recur in the same area several years later.

Two types of occlusive dressings are used for venous stasis ulcers: oxygen-permeable dressings and oxygen-impermeable dressings. Because the role of atmospheric oxygen in wound

---

👤 CHART 36-9 Patient and Family Education: Preparing for Self-Management

Venous Insufficiency

Graduated Compression Stockings (GCSs)
- Wear stockings as prescribed, usually during the day and evening.
- Put the stockings on upon awakening and before getting out of bed.
- When applying the stockings, do not "bunch up" and apply like socks. Instead, place your hand inside the stocking and pull out the heel. Then place the foot of the stocking over your foot and slide the rest of the stocking up. Be sure that rough seams on the stocking are on the outside, not next to your skin.
- Do not push stockings down for comfort because they may function like a tourniquet and further impair venous return.
- Put on a clean pair of stockings each day. Wash them by hand (not in a washing machine) in a gentle detergent and warm water.
- If the stockings seem to be "stretched out," replace them with a new pair.
- Be sure to assess sizing if the patient has gained or lost weight.

Dos and Don'ts
- Elevate your legs for at least 20 minutes 4 or 5 times a day. When in bed, elevate your legs above the level of your heart.
- Avoid prolonged sitting or standing.
- Do not cross your legs. Crossing at the ankles is acceptable for short periods.
- Do not wear tight, restrictive pants. Avoid girdles and garters.

---

healing is controversial, opinions vary with regard to which type of dressing is preferred. An oxygen-permeable polyethylene film and an oxygen-impermeable hydrocolloid dressing (e.g., DuoDERM) are common. Hydrocolloid dressings are left in place for a minimum of 3 to 5 days for best effect. Use medical aseptic technique when changing dressings. If the wound is infected, use Contact Precautions in addition to Standard Precautions.

Artificial skin products can be used for difficult-to-heal venous leg ulcers. These first-generation products are very expensive but are laying the foundation in the field, with costs anticipated to come down in the future. Except for cultured epithelial autografts, artificial skins are only temporary. Artificial skin serves as a biologic cover to secrete growth factors to promote more growth factor secretion from the patient's own skin to speed the wound healing process.

If the patient is ambulatory, an Unna boot may be used. An Unna boot dressing is constructed of gauze that has been moistened with zinc oxide. Apply the boot to the affected limb, from the toes to the knee, after the ulcer has been cleaned with normal saline solution. It is then covered with an elastic wrap and hardens like a cast. This promotes venous return and prevents stasis. The Unna boot also forms a sterile environment for the ulcer. The health care provider changes the boot about once a week. Instruct the patient to report increased pain, which indicates that the boot may be too tight.

The primary health care provider may prescribe topical agents, such as Accuzyme, to chemically débride the ulcer, eliminating necrotic tissue and promoting healing. Remind patients that they may temporarily feel a burning sensation when the agent is applied. If an infection or cellulitis develops, systemic antibiotics are necessary.

Surgery for chronic venous insufficiency is not usually performed because it is not successful. Attempts at transplanting vein valves have had limited success. Surgical débridement of venous ulcers is similar to that performed for arterial ulcers.

The desired outcome for the patient with chronic venous insufficiency is to be managed in the home. For patients with frequent acute complications and repeated hospital admissions, case management can help meet appropriate clinical and cost outcomes. Help patients plan for opportunities and facilities that allow for elevation of the lower extremities in and outside the home. In addition, collaborate with the wound specialist to plan care of the ulcers at home.

If the primary health care provider prescribes graduated compression stockings, teach patients to apply these stockings before they get out of bed in the morning and to remove them just before going to bed at night (see Chart 36-9). Also advise them that they will probably need to wear these stockings for the rest of their lives.

To improve circulation and aid in weight reduction, collaborate with the physical therapist to prescribe an exercise program on an individual basis. Encourage all patients to maintain an optimal weight and consult with the dietitian to plan a weight-reduction diet.

Patients with venous stasis disease, especially those with venous stasis ulcers, may require long-term emotional support to help them meet long-term needs. They may also need help to cope with necessary lifestyle adjustments, such as possible changes in occupation. Patients with venous stasis ulcers may need the assistance of a home care nurse to perform dressing changes. Those with Unna boots need weekly transportation to their primary health care provider for dressing changes. Collaborate with the case manager to arrange for a sequential compression device in the home if the primary health care provider prescribes one.

VARICOSE VEINS

❖ PATHOPHYSIOLOGY

Varicose veins are distended, protruding veins that appear darkened and tortuous. They can occur in anyone, but they are common in adults older than 30 years whose occupations require prolonged standing or heavy physical activity. Varicose veins are also frequently seen in patients with systemic problems (e.g., heart disease), obesity, high estrogen states, and a family history of varicose veins.

As the vein wall weakens and dilates, venous pressure increases, and the valves become incompetent (defective), causing venous reflux. The incompetent valves enhance the vessel dilation, and the veins become tortuous and distended. The severity of the disease depends on the extent of the distention and reflux. **Telangiectasias** (spider veins) are dilated *intradermal* veins less than 1 to 3 mm in diameter that are visible on the skin surface. Most patients are not bothered by them but may consider them unattractive. Most telangiectasias do not develop into the more severe varicose vein disease.

More advanced disease causes venous distention (bulging), edema, a feeling of fullness in the legs, and pruritus (itching). As a result, signs and symptoms of venous insufficiency may occur, including venous stasis ulcers, brown pigmentation from extravasated red blood cells (also called *skin staining*), and pain. Varicose veins and reflux are diagnosed by simple or duplex ultrasonography.

❖ INTERPROFESSIONAL COLLABORATIVE CARE

The overall purpose of management for patients with varicose veins is to improve and maintain optimal venous return to the heart and prevent disease progression. Conservative measures are the treatment of choice, including the three Es: **e**lastic compression hose, **e**xercise, and **e**levation. Graduated compression stockings (GCSs) rely on graduated external pressure to improve venous return by applying pressure to the muscles. They are available in many grades or strengths, ranging from 8 to 50 mm Hg pressure. Exercise increases venous return by helping the muscles pump blood back to the heart. Teach patients to avoid high-impact exercises such as horseback riding and running. Daily walks and ankle flexion exercises while sitting are common exercises that are helpful in promoting circulation. Elevating the extremities as much as possible allows gravity to work with the valves in promoting venous return and prevent reflux.

Patients who continue to have pain or unsightly veins despite using the three Es may opt for more invasive approaches. Surgical ligation and/or removal of veins ("stripping") were the procedures of choice for many years. Sclerotherapy to occlude the affected vessel is also an option.

However, newer, less-invasive treatments are more common today. They are less painful and have a shorter recovery time. A common procedure is an endovenous ablation, which occludes the varicose vein, most commonly the saphenous vein. Using ultrasound guidance, the clinician advances a catheter into the vein and injects an anesthetic agent. Then the vessel is ablated (occluded) while the catheter is slowly removed.

After the procedure, teach the patient the importance of using a GCS or other form of compression (such as elastic compression bandages) for 24 hours a day, except for showers, for at least the first week. Follow-up ultrasonography ensures that the treated vein is closed. The patient is monitored carefully for the first 6 to 8 weeks to determine how healing has progressed. Some patients require continued use of the three Es for many years, depending on the severity of their disease.

Assess the affected limb for vascular status, including any changes in color or temperature of the leg. Monitor for pain, edema, and paresthesias that could indicate complications such as DVT or nerve damage. Nerve damage is usually temporary and minimal; it usually resolves within a few months (Armstrong, 2013).

GET READY FOR THE NCLEX® EXAMINATION!

KEY POINTS

Review these Key Points for each NCLEX Examination Client Needs Category.

Safe and Effective Care Environment

- Plan care for the patient with atherosclerosis and hypertension, in collaboration with the health care team, including the dietitian, pharmacist, and primary health care provider, as needed. **QSEN: Teamwork and Collaboration**
- To reduce the risk for injury, caution patients about orthostatic hypotension when taking antihypertensive drugs. **QSEN: Safety**
- Monitor blood pressure carefully in patients who have hypertension; be aware that they may develop a hypertensive crisis, a life-threatening medical emergency (see Chart 36-2). **QSEN: Safety**

Health Promotion and Maintenance

- In collaboration with the dietitian, help the patient incorporate healthy eating behaviors to lower cholesterol and saturated fats and increase fresh fruits, vegetables, and fiber in the diet. For overweight patients, assist in a weight-reduction plan. **QSEN: Teamwork and Collaboration**
- Teach patients to engage in 40 minutes of moderate-to-vigorous physical activity three or four times a week to lower blood pressure and LDL-C levels.
- Assess the patient for modifiable and nonmodifiable risk factors for vascular disease and teach health promotion behaviors to the patient and family. Pay particular attention to the patient with a family history of cardiovascular disease (see Table 36-4). **QSEN: Patient-Centered Care**

Physiological Integrity

- Remember that risk factors such as smoking increase the pathophysiologic process of atherosclerosis (see Table 36-4).
- Remember that atherosclerosis occurs when fatty plaques occlude arteries and prevent adequate PERFUSION to vital body tissues.
- Monitor total cholesterol, HDL-C, and LDL-C levels to assess patient risk for atherosclerosis.
- Teach patients taking any of the statins in Table 36-5 to report any adverse effects, including muscle cramping, to their primary health care provider. Monitor the patient's liver enzymes carefully.
- Teach patients to decrease saturated and *trans* fats in their diet; instruct them to consume a diet rich in fruits, vegetables, and whole grains; and instruct them to include legumes, poultry, fish, and low-fat dairy products. **QSEN: Evidence-Based Practice**

- Hypertension is categorized as either essential or secondary; the risk factors and causes for each type are described in Table 36-1.
- Closely observe the patient receiving anticoagulants or fibrinolytics for signs of bleeding and monitor appropriate laboratory values for desired outcome values (see Chart 36-7). **QSEN: Safety**
- Monitor for decreased serum potassium levels when patients are taking thiazide or loop diuretics; hypokalemia could cause life-threatening cardiac dysrhythmias (see Chart 36-1). **QSEN: Safety**
- Teach patients to move slowly when changing position if taking any of the antihypertensive drugs listed in Chart 36-1. **QSEN: Safety**
- Recognize that signs and symptoms of peripheral vascular disease (PVD) depend on whether it affects the arteries or veins. In addition to pallor, rubor, or cyanosis, key features of chronic peripheral arterial disease are listed in Chart 36-3.
- Vasodilating drugs or surgery can be used for arterial vascular diseases.
- Deep vein thrombosis (DVT) is the most common type of peripheral vascular problem. When symptoms are present, they include swelling, redness, localized pain, and warmth.
- Be aware that DVT can lead to pulmonary embolism, a life-threatening emergency! **Clinical Judgment**
- Teach patients to prevent VTE by leg exercises, early ambulation, adequate hydration, graduated compression stockings (GCSs), sequential compression devices (SCDs), and anticoagulant therapy.
- Monitor aPTT values for patients receiving unfractionated heparin; monitor INR for patients receiving warfarin (Coumadin). **QSEN: Safety**
- Assess for venous and arterial ulcers as described in Chart 36-4.
- Teach foot care for patients with PVD as outlined in Chart 36-6.
- Teach patients about precautions for anticoagulant therapy as described in Chart 36-7.
- Teach about food and drugs that interfere with warfarin (Coumadin) as listed in Chart 36-8. **QSEN: Evidence-Based Practice**
- Monitor for indications of aneurysm rupture: diaphoresis, nausea, vomiting, pallor, hypotension, tachycardia, severe pain, and decreased level of consciousness. **QSEN: Safety**
- Varicose veins can cause severe pain and reflux requiring the three Es: **e**lastic compression hose, **e**xercise, and **e**levation.

SELECTED BIBLIOGRAPHY

Asterisk indicates a classic or definitive work on this subject.
*ALLHAT Officers and Coordinators for the ALLHAT Collaborative Research Group. (2002). Major outcomes in high-risk hypertensive patients randomized to angiotensin-converting enzyme inhibitor or calcium channel blocker vs diuretic. The Antihypertensive and Lipid-Lowering Treatment to Prevent Heart Attack Trial (ALLHAT). *Journal of the American Medical Association, 288*(23), 2981-2997.

American Heart Association. (2016). *American Heart Association recommendations for physical activity in adults.* http://www.heart.org/HEARTORG/GettingHealthy/PhysicalActivity/FitnessBasics/

American-Heart-Association-Recommendations-for-Physical-Activity-in-Adults_UCM_307976_Article.jsp#.Vp5JhVMrKCQ.

*Anthony, M. (2013). Nursing assessment of deep vein thrombosis. *Medsurg Nursing, 22*(2), 95-98.

Armstrong, K. E. (2013). Stop the reflux: An update on treatment for symptomatic varicose veins. *Nursing, 43*(2), 27-34.

*Bailey, D. G., Dresser, D., & Arnold, J. M. O. (2013). Grapefruit-medication interactions: Forbidden fruit or avoidable consequences. *CMAJ: Canadian Medical Association Journal, 185*, 309-316.

Burchum, J., & Rosenthal, L. (2016). *Lehne's pharmacology for nursing care.* (9th ed.). St. Louis: Elsevier.

Davis, L. (2015). Hypertension: Evidence-based treatments for maintaining blood pressure control. *The Nurse Practitioner 40*(6), 32-37.

Eckel, R. H., Jakicic, J. M., Ard, J. D., Hubbard, V. S., de Jesus, J. M., Lee, I. M., et al. (2014). 2013 AHA/ACC guideline on lifestyle management to reduce cardiovascular risk: A report of the American College of Cardiology/American Heart Association Task Force on Practice Guidelines. *Circulation, 129*(25 Suppl. 2), S76–S99.

Elisha, S., Heiner, J., Nagelhout, J., & Gabot, M. (2015). Venous thromboembolism: New concepts in perioperative management. *AANA Journal, 83*(3), 211-221.

Felicilda-Reynaldo, R., & Kenneally, M. (2015a). A review of antihypertensive medications: Part 1. *Medsurg Nursing, 24*(3), 177-181.

Felicilda-Reynaldo, R., & Kenneally, M. (2015b). A review of antihypertensive medications: Part 2. *Medsurg Nursing, 24*(5), 331-335.

*Gay, V., Hamilton, R., Heiskell, S., & Sparks, A. M. (2009). Influence of bedrest or ambulation in the clinical treatment of acute deep vein thrombosis on patient outcomes: A review and synthesis of the literature. *Medsurg Nursing, 18*(5), 293-299.

Goldstein, P. (2015). Drug update: Venous thromboembolic (VTE) prophylaxis: Part II. *MedSurg Matters, 24*(4), 9-13.

*Hiratzka, L. F., Bakris, G. L., Beckman, J. A., Bersin, R. M., Carr, V. F., Casey, D. E., et al. (2010). *Guidelines for the diagnosis and management of patients with thoracic aortic disease.* Philadelphia: Lippincott Williams & Wilkins.

James, P. A., Oparil, S., Carter, B. L., Cushman, W. C., Dennison-Himmelfarb, C., Handler, J., et al. (2014). 2014 evidence-based guidelines for the management of high blood pressure in adults: Report from the panel members appointed to the Eighth National Committee (JNC 8). *Journal of the American Medical Association, 311*(5), 507–520. http://jama.jamanetwork.com/article.aspx?articleid=1791497.

Kaplan, N., & Townsend, R. (2015). *Ambulatory and home blood pressure monitoring and white coat syndrome in adults.* www.uptodate.com.

Leung, L. (2015). *Anticoagulation with direct thrombin inhibitors and direct factor Xa inhibitors.* www.uptodate.com.

Lip, G., & Hull, R. (2015). *Overview of the treatment of lower extremity deep venous thrombosis.* www.uptodate.com.

McCance, K., Huether, S., Brashers, V., & Rote, N. (2014). *Pathophysiology: The biologic basis for disease in adults and children* (7th ed.). St. Louis: Mosby.

Manning, W. (2015). *Management of aortic dissection.* www.uptodate.com.

*Michaels, K., & Regan, N. (2013). Teaching patients INR self-management. *Nursing, 43*(5), 67-69.

Mookadam, M., Shamoun, F., Ramakrishna, H., Obeid, H., Rife, R., Mookadam, F. (2015). Perioperative venous thromboembolic disease and the emerging role of the novel oral anticoagulants: An analysis of the implications for perioperative management. *Annals of Cardiac Anaesthesia, 18*(4), 517-527.

Mozaffarian, D., Benjamin, E., Go, A., Arnett, D., Blaha, M., Cushman, M., et al. (2016). Heart disease and stroke statistics—2016 update. *Circulation* doi:10.1161/CIR0000000000000350.

National Center for Complementary and Alternative Medicine. (2015). *Herbs at a glance: Garlic.* https://nccih.nih.gov/health/garlic/ataglance.htm.

*National Cholesterol Education Program. (2002). *Third Report of the Expert Panel on Detection, Evaluation, and Treatment of High Blood Cholesterol in Adults (Adult Treatment Panel III).* NIH Publication No. 02-5215. Bethesda, MD: National Heart, Lung, and Blood Institute.

National Heart, Lung, and Blood Institute. (2015). *Description of the DASH eating plan.* https://www.nhlbi.nih.gov/health/health-topics/topics/dash.

Pagana, K., Pagana, T. J., & Pagana, T. N. (2017). *Mosby's diagnostic and laboratory test reference* (13th ed.). St. Louis: Mosby.

Rose, M. (2015). A review of peripheral arterial disease (PAD). *British Journal of Cardiac Nursing, 10*(6), 277-282.

Scordo, K., & Pickett, K. (2015). Managing hypertension: Piecing together the guidelines. *Nursing2015, January,* 28-33.

Simmons, S. (2015). Understanding Raynaud phenomenon. *Nursing 2015, July,* 43-45. doi:10.1097/01.NURSE.0000461849.16529.30.

*Stone, N. J., Robinson, J., Lichtenstein, A. H., Merz, N. B., Blum, C. B., Eckel, R. H., et al. (2014). 2013 ACC/AHA guidelines on the treatment of blood cholesterol to reduce atherosclerotic cardiovascular risk in adults: A report of the American College of Cardiology/American Heart Association Task Force on Practice Guidelines. *Circulation, 129*(25 Suppl. 2), S1-S45.

Sherrod, M., Sherrod, N., & Cheek, D. (2015). Follow the guideline for reducing cardiovascular risk with statins. *Nursing 2015,* 41-46.

CHAPTER 37

Care of Patients With Shock

Nicole M. Heimgartner

http://evolve.elsevier.com/Iggy/

PRIORITY AND INTERRELATED CONCEPTS

The priority concepts for this chapter are:
- PERFUSION
- IMMUNITY

✳ The PERFUSION concept exemplar for this chapter is Hypovolemic Shock, p. 754.

✳ The IMMUNITY concept exemplar for this chapter is Sepsis and Septic Shock, p. 760.

The interrelated concepts for this chapter are:
- CLOTTING
- GAS EXCHANGE

LEARNING OUTCOMES

Safe and Effective Care Environment

1. Collaborate with the interprofessional team to coordinate high-quality care and promote PERFUSION in patients who are experiencing shock.

Health Promotion and Maintenance

2. Teach adults how to decrease the risk for sepsis and shock.

Psychosocial Integrity

3. Implement nursing interventions to help the patient and family cope with the psychosocial impact caused by shock or its complications.

Physiological Integrity

4. Apply knowledge of anatomy and physiology to assess critically ill patients with respiratory problems affecting PERFUSION or IMMUNITY.

5. Implement evidence-based nursing interventions to prevent complications of sepsis and shock.

OVERVIEW

All organs, tissues, and cells need a continuous supply of oxygen to function properly. The lungs first bring oxygen into the body through ventilation and GAS EXCHANGE, and the cardiovascular system (heart, blood, and blood vessels) delivers oxygen by PERFUSION to all tissues and removes cellular wastes. **Shock** is widespread abnormal cellular metabolism that occurs when gas exchange with oxygenation and tissue perfusion needs are not met sufficiently to maintain cell function (McCance et al., 2014). It is a condition rather than a disease and is the "whole-body" response that occurs when too little oxygen is delivered to the tissues. All body organs are affected by shock and either work harder to adapt and compensate for reduced gas exchange or perfusion or fail to function because of hypoxia. Shock is a "syndrome" because the problems resulting from it occur in a predictable sequence.

Any problem that impairs PERFUSION and GAS EXCHANGE to tissues and organs can start the syndrome of shock and lead to a life-threatening emergency. Shock is often a result of cardiovascular problems. Patients in acute care settings are at higher risk, but shock can occur in any setting. For example, older patients in long-term care settings are at risk for sepsis and shock related to urinary tract infections. When the body's adaptive adjustments (compensation) or health care interventions are not effective and shock progresses, it can lead to cell loss, multiple organ dysfunction syndrome (MODS), and death.

Shock is classified by the type of impairment causing it into the categories of hypovolemic shock, cardiogenic shock, distributive shock (which includes septic shock, neurogenic shock, and anaphylactic shock), and obstructive shock. Table 37-1 describes this classification and common causes of shock.

Most signs and symptoms of shock are similar regardless of what starts the process or which tissues are affected first. Symptoms result from physiologic adjustments (*compensatory mechanisms*) that the body makes in the attempt to ensure continued PERFUSION of vital organs. Compensatory actions are triggered by the sympathetic nervous system's stress response activating

TABLE 37-1   Causes and Types of Shock by Functional Impairment

Hypovolemic Shock

Overall Cause

Total body fluid decreased (in all fluid compartments).

Specific Cause or Risk Factors

- Hemorrhage
- Trauma
- GI ulcer
- Surgery
- Inadequate CLOTTING
- Hemophilia
- Liver disease
- Cancer therapy
- Anticoagulation therapy
- Dehydration
- Vomiting
- Diarrhea
- Heavy diaphoresis
- Diuretic therapy
- Nasogastric suction
- Diabetes insipidus

Cardiogenic Shock

Overall Cause

Direct pump failure (fluid volume not affected).

Specific Cause or Risk Factors

- Myocardial infarction
- Cardiac arrest
- Ventricular dysrhythmias
- Cardiac amyloidosis
- Cardiomyopathies
- Myocardial degeneration

Distributive Shock

Overall Cause

Fluid shifted from central vascular space (total body fluid volume normal or increased).

Specific Cause or Risk Factors

- Neural-induced
- Pain
- Anesthesia
- Stress
- Spinal cord injury
- Head trauma
- Chemical-induced
- Anaphylaxis
- Sepsis
- Capillary leak
- Burns
- Extensive trauma
- Liver impairment
- Hypoproteinemia

Obstructive Shock

Overall Cause

Cardiac function decreased by noncardiac factor (indirect pump failure). Total body fluid is not affected, although central volume is decreased.

Specific Cause or Risk Factors

- Cardiac tamponade
- Arterial stenosis
- Pulmonary embolus
- Pulmonary hypertension
- Constrictive pericarditis
- Thoracic tumors
- Tension pneumothorax

CHART 37-1   Key Features

Shock

Cardiovascular Symptoms

- Decreased cardiac output
- Increased pulse rate
- Thready pulse
- Decreased blood pressure
- Narrowed pulse pressure
- Postural hypotension
- Low central venous pressure
- Flat neck and hand veins in dependent positions
- Slow capillary refill in nail beds
- Diminished peripheral pulses

Respiratory Symptoms

- Increased respiratory rate
- Shallow depth of respirations
- Increased $PaCO_2$
- Decreased PaO_2
- Cyanosis, especially around lips and nail beds

Gastrointestinal Symptoms

- Decreased motility
- Diminished or absent bowel sounds
- Nausea and vomiting
- Constipation

Neuromuscular Symptoms

Early

- Anxiety
- Restlessness
- Increased thirst

Late

- Decreased central nervous system activity (lethargy to coma)
- Generalized muscle weakness
- Diminished or absent deep tendon reflexes
- Sluggish pupillary response to light

Kidney Symptoms

- Decreased urine output
- Increased specific gravity
- Sugar and acetone present in urine

Integumentary Symptoms

- Cool to cold
- Pale to mottled to cyanotic
- Moist, clammy
- Mouth dry; pastelike coating present

$PaCO_2$, Partial pressure of arterial carbon dioxide; PaO_2, partial pressure of arterial oxygen.

the endocrine and cardiovascular systems. Symptoms unique to any one type of shock result from specific tissue dysfunction. The common features of shock are listed in Chart 37-1.

Review of Gas Exchange and Tissue Perfusion

GAS EXCHANGE and PERFUSION depend on how much oxygen from arterial blood perfuses the tissue. Perfusion is related to mean arterial pressure (MAP). The factors that influence MAP include:

- Total blood volume
- Cardiac output
- Size and integrity of the vascular bed, especially capillaries

Total blood volume and cardiac output are directly related to MAP, so increases in either total blood volume or cardiac output *raise* MAP. Decreases in either total blood volume or cardiac output *lower* MAP.

The size of the vascular bed is inversely (negatively) related to MAP. This means that increases in the size of the vascular bed *lower* MAP and decreases *raise* MAP (Fig. 37-1). The small arteries and veins connected to capillaries can increase in diameter by relaxing the smooth muscle in vessel walls (dilation) or decrease in diameter by contracting the muscle (vasoconstriction). When

blood vessels dilate and total blood volume remains the same, blood pressure decreases and blood flow is slower. When blood vessels constrict and total blood volume remains the same, blood pressure increases and blood flow is faster.

Blood vessels are innervated by the sympathetic nervous system. Some nerves continuously stimulate vascular smooth muscle so the blood vessels are normally partially constricted, a condition called sympathetic tone. Increases in sympathetic stimulation constrict smooth muscle even more, raising MAP. Decreases in sympathetic tone relax smooth muscle, dilating blood vessels and lowering MAP.

PERFUSION (blood flow) to organs adjusts to changes in tissue oxygen needs. The body can selectively increase blood flow to some areas while reducing flow to others. The skin and skeletal muscles can tolerate low levels of oxygen for hours without dying or being damaged. Other organs (e.g., heart, brain, liver, pancreas) do not tolerate hypoxia (low levels of tissue oxygen), and a few minutes without oxygen results in serious damage and cell death.

Types of Shock

Types of shock vary because shock is a problem caused by a pathologic condition rather than a disease state (see Table 37-1). *More than one type of shock can be present at the same time.* For example, trauma caused by a car crash may trigger hemorrhage (leading to hypovolemic shock) and a myocardial infarction (leading to cardiogenic shock).

Hypovolemic shock occurs when too little circulating blood volume decreases MAP, resulting in inadequate total body PERFUSION and GAS EXCHANGE. Common problems leading to

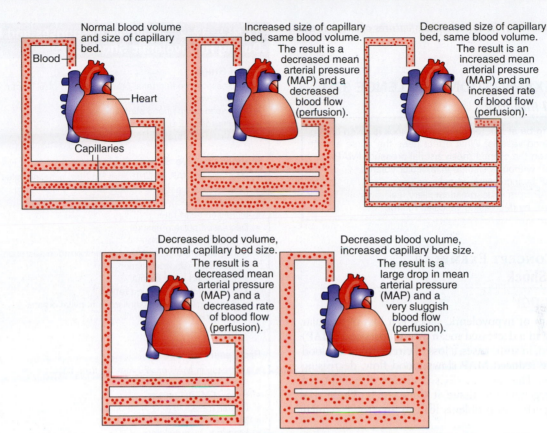

FIG. 37-1 Interaction of blood volume and the size of the capillary bed affecting mean arterial pressure (MAP).

hypovolemic shock are dehydration and poor CLOTTING with hemorrhage. A complete discussion of the pathophysiology and management of hypovolemic shock begins with the PERFUSION concept exemplar.

Cardiogenic shock occurs when the heart muscle is unhealthy and pumping is impaired. Myocardial infarction is the most common cause of direct pump failure (Warise, 2015). Other causes are listed in Table 37-1. Any type of pump failure decreases cardiac output and MAP. Chapter 38 discusses the pathophysiology and care for the adult with shock from myocardial infarction.

Distributive shock occurs when blood volume is not lost from the body but is distributed to the interstitial tissues where it cannot perfuse organs. It can be caused by blood vessel dilation, pooling of blood in venous and capillary beds, and increased capillary leak. All these factors decrease MAP and may be started either by nerve changes *(neural-induced)* or by the presence of some chemicals *(chemical-induced)*.

Neural-induced distributive shock is a loss of MAP that occurs when sympathetic nerve impulses are decreased and blood vessel smooth muscles relax, causing vasodilation and poor PERFUSION. Shock results when vasodilation is widespread. Problems leading to loss of sympathetic tone are listed in Table 37-1.

Chemical-induced distributive shock has three common origins: anaphylaxis, sepsis, and capillary leak syndrome. It occurs when certain body chemicals or foreign substances in the blood and vessels start widespread changes in blood vessel walls. The chemicals are usually **exogenous** (originate outside the body), but this type of shock also can be induced by substances normally found in the body, such as excessive amounts of histamine.

Anaphylaxis is an extreme type of allergic reaction. It begins within seconds to minutes after exposure to a specific allergen in a susceptible adult. The result is widespread loss of blood vessel tone, with decreased blood pressure and cardiac output. Chapter 20 describes the pathophysiology, prevention, and care of the patient with anaphylactic shock.

Sepsis is a widespread infection that triggers whole-body inflammation. It leads to distributive shock when infectious microorganisms are present in the blood and is most commonly called **septic shock**. A complete discussion of the pathophysiology, prevention, and care for the patient with sepsis and septic shock begins with the IMMUNITY concept exemplar.

Capillary leak syndrome is the response of capillaries to the presence of histamine and other chemicals that enlarge capillary pores and allow fluid to shift from the capillaries into the interstitial tissues. These fluids are stagnant, and no GAS EXCHANGE occurs. Problems causing fluid shifts include severe burns, liver disorders, ascites, peritonitis, large wounds, kidney disease, hypoproteinemia, and trauma.

Obstructive shock is caused by problems that impair the ability of the normal heart to pump effectively. The heart itself remains normal, but conditions outside the heart prevent either adequate filling of the heart or adequate contraction of the healthy heart muscle. The most common cause of obstructive shock is cardiac tamponade (see Table 37-1). Care of the adult with cardiac tamponade is presented in Chapter 35 (pericarditis) and Chapter 38.

Although the causes and initial signs and symptoms associated with the different types of shock vary, eventually the effects of hypotension and **anaerobic cellular metabolism** *(metabolism* *without oxygen) result in the common key features of shock listed in Chart 37-1.*

✴ PERFUSION CONCEPT EXEMPLAR
Hypovolemic Shock

❖ PATHOPHYSIOLOGY

The basic problem of hypovolemic shock is a loss of vascular volume, resulting in a decreased mean arterial pressure (MAP) (see Fig. 37-1) and, in some cases, a loss of circulating red blood cells (RBCs). The reduced MAP slows blood flow, decreasing tissue PERFUSION. The loss of RBCs decreases the ability of the blood to oxygenate the tissue it does reach. These GAS EXCHANGE and perfusion problems lead to anaerobic cellular metabolism.

The main trigger leading to hypovolemic shock is a sustained decrease in MAP from decreased circulating blood volume. A decrease in MAP of 5 to 10 mm Hg below the patient's normal baseline value is detected by pressure-sensitive nerve receptors *(baroreceptors)* in the aortic arch and carotid sinus. This information is transmitted to brain centers, which stimulate compensatory mechanisms to help ensure continued blood flow and oxygen delivery to vital organs while limiting blood flow to less vital areas. The movement of blood into selected areas while bypassing others ("shunting") results in some shock symptoms.

If the events that caused the initial decrease in MAP are halted now, compensatory mechanisms provide adequate GAS EXCHANGE and PERFUSION without intervention. If events continue and MAP decreases further, some tissues function under anaerobic conditions. This condition increases lactic acid levels and other harmful metabolites (e.g., protein-destroying enzymes, oxygen free radicals) (McCance et al., 2014). These substances cause acidosis with tissue-damaging effects and depressed heart muscle activity. The effects are temporary and reversible if the cause of shock is corrected within 1 to 2 hours after onset. When shock conditions continue for longer periods without help, the resulting increased metabolites cause so much cell damage in vital organs that they are unable to perform their critical functions. When this problem, known as *multiple organ dysfunction syndrome (MODS),* occurs to the extent that vital organs die, recovery from shock is no longer possible (see the section on Refractory Stage of Shock. Table 37-2 summarizes the progression of shock.

Stages of Shock

The syndrome of shock progresses in four stages when the conditions that cause shock remain uncorrected and poor cellular oxygenation continues. These stages are:

TABLE 37-2 Adaptive Responses and Events During Hypovolemic Shock

Initial Stage
- Decrease in mean arterial pressure (MAP) of 5-10 mm Hg from baseline value
- Increased sympathetic stimulation
- Mild vasoconstriction
- Increased heart rate

Nonprogressive Stage
- Decrease in MAP of 10-15 mm Hg from baseline value
- Continued sympathetic stimulation
- Moderate vasoconstriction
- Increased heart rate
- Decreased pulse pressure
- Chemical compensation
- Renin, aldosterone, and antidiuretic hormone secretion
  - Increased vasoconstriction
  - Decreased urine output
  - Stimulation of the thirst reflex
  - Some anaerobic metabolism in nonvital organs
- Mild acidosis
- Mild hyperkalemia

Progressive Stage
- Decrease in MAP of >20 mm Hg from baseline value
- Anoxia of nonvital organs
- Hypoxia of vital organs
- Overall metabolism is anaerobic
- Moderate acidosis
- Moderate hyperkalemia
- Tissue ischemia

Refractory Stage
- Severe tissue hypoxia with ischemia and necrosis
- Release of myocardial depressant factor from the pancreas
- Buildup of toxic metabolites
- Multiple organ dysfunction syndrome (MODS)
- Death

1. Initial stage
2. Nonprogressive stage
3. Progressive stage
4. Refractory stage

Initial Stage. The initial stage is present when the patient's baseline MAP is decreased by less than 10 mm Hg. Compensatory mechanisms are effective at returning systolic pressure to normal at this stage; thus oxygen PERFUSION to vital organs is maintained. Cellular changes include increased anaerobic metabolism in some tissues with production of lactic acid, although overall metabolism is still aerobic. The compensation responses of vascular constriction and increased heart rate are effective, and both cardiac output and MAP are maintained within the normal range. Because vital organ function is not disrupted, the indicators of shock are difficult to detect at this stage.

❗ NURSING SAFETY PRIORITY QSEN

Action Alert

Be aware that increased heart and respiratory rates or a slight *increase* in diastolic blood pressure may be the only sign of this stage of shock.

Nonprogressive Stage. The nonprogressive stage of shock occurs when MAP decreases by 10 to 15 mm Hg from baseline. Kidney and hormonal compensatory mechanisms are activated because cardiovascular responses alone are not enough to maintain MAP and supply oxygen to vital organs.

The ongoing decrease in MAP triggers the release of renin, antidiuretic hormone (ADH), aldosterone, epinephrine, and norepinephrine to start kidney compensation. Urine output decreases, sodium reabsorption increases, and widespread blood vessel constriction occurs. ADH increases water reabsorption in the kidney, further reducing urine output, and increases blood vessel constriction in the skin and other less vital tissue areas. Together these actions compensate for shock by maintaining the fluid volume within the central blood vessels.

Tissue hypoxia occurs in nonvital organs (e.g., skin, GI tract) and in the kidney, but it is not great enough to cause permanent damage. Buildup of metabolites from anaerobic metabolism causes acidosis (low blood pH) and increased blood potassium levels.

Signs and symptoms of this stage include changes resulting from decreased tissue PERFUSION. Subjective changes include thirst and anxiety. Objective changes include restlessness, tachycardia, increased respiratory rate, decreased urine output, falling systolic blood pressure, rising diastolic blood pressure, narrowing pulse pressure, cool extremities, and a 2% to 5% decrease in oxygen saturation. *Comparing these changes with the values and observations obtained earlier is critical to identifying this stage of shock.*

If the patient is stable and compensatory mechanisms are supported by interventions, he or she can remain in this stage for hours without having permanent damage. *Stopping the conditions that started shock and providing supportive interventions can prevent the shock from progressing.* The effects of this stage are reversible when nurses recognize the problem and coordinate the interprofessional health care team to start appropriate interventions.

Progressive Stage. The progressive stage of shock occurs when there is a sustained decrease in MAP of more than 20 mm Hg from baseline. Compensatory mechanisms are functioning but can no longer deliver sufficient oxygen, even to vital organs. Vital organs develop hypoxia, and less vital organs become **anoxic** (no oxygen) and **ischemic** (cell dysfunction or death from lack of oxygen). As a result of poor PERFUSION and a buildup of metabolites, some tissues die.

Indications of the progressive stage include a *worsening* of changes resulting from decreased tissue PERFUSION. The patient may express a sense of "something bad" (impending doom) about to happen. He or she may be confused, and thirst increases. Objective changes are a rapid, weak pulse; low blood pressure; pallor to cyanosis of oral mucosa and nail beds; cool and moist skin; anuria; and a 5% to 20% decrease in oxygen saturation. Laboratory data may show a low blood pH, along with rising lactic acid and potassium levels.

Refractory Stage and Multiple Organ Dysfunction Syndrome. The refractory stage of shock occurs when too much cell death and tissue damage result from too little oxygen reaching the tissues. Vital organs have extensive damage and cannot respond effectively to interventions, and shock continues. So much damage has occurred with release of metabolites and enzymes that damage to vital organs continues despite interventions.

The sequence of cell damage caused by the massive release of toxic metabolites and enzymes is termed **multiple organ**

? NCLEX EXAMINATION CHALLENGE 37-2

Safe and Effective Care Environment

A client who is in the progressive stage of hypovolemic shock has all of the following signs, symptoms, or changes. Which ones does the nurse attribute to ongoing compensatory mechanisms? **Select all that apply.**
A. Increasing pallor
B. Increasing thirst
C. Increasing confusion
D. Increasing heart rate
E. Increasing respiratory rate
F. Decreasing systolic blood pressure
G. Decreasing blood pH
H. Decreasing urine output

---

dysfunction syndrome (MODS). Once the damage has started, the sequence becomes a vicious cycle as more dead cells open and release metabolites. These trigger small clots (*microthrombi*) to form, which block tissue PERFUSION and damage more cells, continuing the devastating cycle. Liver, heart, brain, and kidney functions are lost first. The most profound change is damage to the heart muscle.

Signs are a rapid loss of consciousness; nonpalpable pulse; cold, dusky extremities; slow, shallow respirations; and unmeasurable oxygen saturation. *Therapy, including fluid replacement, is not effective in saving the patient's life, even if the cause of shock is corrected and MAP temporarily returns to normal.*

Etiology

Hypovolemic shock occurs when too little circulating blood volume causes a MAP decrease that prevents total body PERFUSION and adequate GAS EXCHANGE. Problems leading to hypovolemic shock are listed in Table 37-1.

Hypovolemic shock from hemorrhage is common after trauma or surgery; and internal hemorrhage occurs with blunt trauma, GI ulcers, and poor control of surgical bleeding. Hemorrhage leading to hypovolemia also can be caused by any problem that reduces the levels of CLOTTING factors (see Table 37-1). Hypovolemia from dehydration can be caused by any problem that decreases fluid intake or increases fluid loss (see Table 37-1).

Incidence and Prevalence

The exact incidence of hypovolemic shock is not known because it is a response rather than a disease. It is a common complication among hospitalized patients in emergency departments and after surgery or invasive procedures.

Health Promotion and Maintenance

Recognizing hypovolemic shock is a major nursing responsibility. Keep in mind that just being a patient in the acute care setting is a risk factor. Also identify patients at risk for dehydration and assess for early signs and symptoms. This is especially important for those who have reduced cognition or mobility or who are on NPO status.

Assess all patients with invasive procedures or trauma for obvious or occult bleeding from impaired CLOTTING. Compare pulse quality and rate with baseline. Compare urine output with fluid intake. Check vital signs of patients who have persistent thirst. Assess for shock in any patient who develops a change in mental status, an increase in pain, or an increase in anxiety.

Teach patients who have invasive procedures about the signs and symptoms of shock. Stress the importance of seeking immediate help for obvious heavy bleeding, persistent thirst, decreased urine output, light-headedness, or a sense of impending doom.

❖ INTERPROFESSIONAL COLLABORATIVE CARE

Hypovolemic shock is an emergent problem that is usually managed in an acute care setting. If complications from the problem or its treatment are ongoing, patients may be cared for in a variety of community settings. The Concept Map addresses assessment and nursing care issues related to hypovolemic shock.

◆ Assessment: Noticing

History. Ask about risk factors related to hypovolemic shock. If the patient is alert, question him or her directly. If the patient is not alert, collect information from family members. Ask about recent illness, trauma, procedures, or chronic health problems that may lead to shock (e.g., GI ulcers, general surgery, hemophilia, liver disorders, prolonged vomiting or diarrhea). Ask about the use of drugs such as aspirin, other NSAIDs, and diuretics that may cause changes leading to hypovolemic shock.

Ask about fluid intake and output during the previous 24 hours. *Information about urine output is especially important because urine output is reduced during the first stages of shock, even when fluid intake is normal.*

Assess the patient for factors that can lead to shock. Areas to examine for poor CLOTTING and hemorrhage include the gums, wounds, and sites of dressings, drains, and vascular accesses. Also check *under* the patient for blood. Observe for any swelling or skin discoloration that may indicate an internal hemorrhage.

Physical Assessment/Signs and Symptoms. Most signs and symptoms of hypovolemic shock are caused by the changes resulting from compensatory efforts. Shock may first be evident as changes in cardiovascular function. As shock progresses, changes in the renal, respiratory, integumentary, musculoskeletal, and central nervous systems become evident. Ensure that vital sign measurements are accurate and monitor them for trends indicating shock.

Cardiovascular changes that occur with hypovolemic shock start with decreased mean arterial pressure (MAP) leading to compensatory responses. Assess the central and peripheral pulses for rate and quality. In the initial stage of shock, the pulse rate increases above the patient's baseline to keep cardiac output and MAP at normal levels, even though the actual [stroke volume](#) (amount of blood pumped out from the heart) per beat

is decreased. *Increased heart rate is the first sign of shock.* Because stroke volume is decreased, the peripheral pulses are difficult to palpate and easily blocked. As shock progresses, peripheral pulses may not be palpable, and a Doppler may be needed.

With vasoconstriction, diastolic pressure increases, but systolic pressure remains the same. As a result, the difference between the systolic and diastolic pressures *(pulse pressure)* is smaller or "narrower." Monitor blood pressure for changes from baseline levels and for changes from the previous measurement. For accuracy, use the same equipment on the same extremity. Validate an abnormal electronic BP reading with a manual BP reading.

Systolic pressure decreases as shock progresses and cardiac output decreases. A reduced systolic pressure narrows the pulse pressure even further. When shock continues and interventions are not adequate, compensation fails, both systolic and diastolic pressures decrease, and blood pressure is difficult to hear. Palpation or a Doppler device may be needed to detect the systolic blood pressure.

Oxygen saturation is assessed through pulse oximetry. Pulse oximetry values between 90% and 95% occur with the nonprogressive stage of shock, and values between 75% and 80% occur with the progressive stage of shock. *Any value below 70% is considered a life-threatening emergency and may signal the refractory stage of shock.*

Respiratory changes with shock are an adaptive response to help maintain GAS EXCHANGE when tissue PERFUSION is decreased. Assess the rate and depth of respiration. Respiratory rate increases during shock to ensure that oxygen intake is increased so it can be delivered to critical tissues.

Kidney and urinary changes occur with shock to compensate for decreased mean arterial pressure (MAP) by saving body water through decreased filtration and increased water reabsorption. Assess urine for volume, color, specific gravity, and the presence of blood or protein. *Decreased urine output is a sensitive indicator of early shock. Measure urine output at least every hour. In severe shock, urine output may be absent.* When hypoxia or anoxia persists beyond about an hour, patients are at risk for acute kidney injury (AKI) and kidney failure.

Skin changes occur because of reduced blood flow in the skin. An early compensatory mechanism is skin blood vessel constriction, which reduces skin PERFUSION. This allows more

CONCEPT MAP

PERFUSION

GAS EXCHANGE

HYPOVOLEMIC SHOCK

CLOTTING

IMMUNITY

NOTICE IN THE HISTORY

A 59-year-old involved in a motor vehicle crash comes to the ED in a confused and restless state with HR 120 (weak and thready), RR 24, BP 100/60 mm Hg. No open wounds, abdomen distended, hypoactive bowel sounds.

NOTICING—
Physical Assessment

Subjective signs: Thirst, anxiety

Objective signs: Restlessness, rapid, weak pulse, ↑ RR, ↓ diastolic BP, ↓ systolic BP (narrowing pulse pressure), ↓ U/O, ↓ O₂ sat, cool extremities, ↓ pH, cyanosis, pallor, ↑ lactic acid, ↑ K⁺

Data Synthesis

PATIENT PROBLEMS

- Decreased GAS EXCHANGE due to hypovolemia
- Inadequate PERFUSION due to active fluid volume loss and hypotension
- Anxiety related to potential for death and decreased cerebral PERFUSION
- Decreased cognition due to decreased cerebral PERFUSION

Notice and Interpret Risk Factors

Data Synthesis

- Hemorrhage after blunt trauma
- Insufficient clotting factors

Planning

EXPECTED OUTCOMES

Maintain normal aerobic cellular metabolism as evidenced by:
- Clear thought processes
- MAP <10 mm Hg from baseline
- BP, HR, RR, ABGs, O₂ saturation return to baseline
- U/O significantly >30 mL/hr
- No development of complications with supportive and drug therapies

INTERVENTIONS—RESPONDING

1
Nursing Priority – Ensuring a Patent Airway
- Administer oxygen; monitor and respond to: ↑ RR, shallow depth; ↓ PaCO₂; ↓ PaO₂; cyanosis, especially around lips and nail beds. *Monitors for progression of shock and inadequate PERFUSION and GAS EXCHANGE.*
- Assess oxygen saturation through pulse oximetry. *Indicates life-threatening emergency when O₂ saturation is below 70%.*

2
Nursing Safety Priority: Critical Rescue!
Do not leave the patient. RN (not LPN or UAP) must assess vital signs. *An unstable patient requires the assessment skills of an RN.*

3
Interpreting Vital Signs in Shock
Monitor vital signs at least every 15 minutes until shock is controlled and patient's condition improves. Assess pulse (rate, regularity, quality), blood pressure, pulse pressure, central venous pressure, respiratory rate, skin and mucosal color, oxygen saturation, cognition, and urine output. *Determines the patient's condition and the effectiveness of therapy.*

4
Nursing Safety Priority: Action Alert!
Interpret and respond to changes in heart and respiratory rates or a slight increase in diastolic blood pressure as the only sign of early shock. *Changes in systolic blood pressure are not always present in the initial stage of shock.*

5
Minimizing Bleeding
- Apply direct pressure for overt bleeding. Check under the patient for blood. Observe for swelling or skin discoloration. *Discoloration may indicate internal hemorrhage.*
- Prepare the patient for surgical intervention. *Corrects internal bleeding for the patient's survival.*

6
Fluid Replacement Therapy
Increase the rate of IV fluid delivery: crystalloids, colloids, and/or blood products. *Restores fluid volume and improves perfusion to vital organs, which is the primary intervention for hypovolemic shock.*

7
Nursing Safety Priority: Action Alert!
Use only normal saline for infusion with blood or blood products. *Calcium in Ringer's lactate induces CLOTTING of the infusing blood.*

8
Drug Therapy
Administer drugs for shock, vasoconstrictors, inotropic agents, and/or drugs that enhance cardiac PERFUSION when volume loss is severe and the patient does not respond sufficiently to fluid replacement and blood products. *Increases likelihood to recover from shock by increasing venous return, improving cardiac contractility, or improving cardiac PERFUSION by dilating the coronary vessels.*

9
Nursing Safety Priority: Drug Alert!
Monitor the patient closely. *Drugs that dilate coronary blood vessels, such as nitroprusside, can cause systemic vasodilation and increase shock if the patient is volume depleted. Drugs that increase heart muscle contraction increase heart oxygen consumption and can cause angina or infarction.*

Concept Map by Deanne A. Blach, MSN, RN

blood to perfuse the vital organs, which cannot tolerate low oxygen levels.

Assess the skin for temperature, color, and moisture. With shock, it feels cool or cold to the touch and is moist. Color changes appear first in oral mucous membranes and in the skin around the mouth. In dark-skinned patients, pallor or cyanosis is best assessed in the oral mucous membranes. Other color changes are noted first in the skin of the extremities and then in the central trunk area. The skin feels clammy or moist to the touch, not because sweating increases but because the normal fluid lost through the skin does not evaporate well on cool skin. As shock progresses, skin becomes mottled. Lighter-skinned patients have an overall grayish-blue color; and darker-skinned patients appear darker, without an underlying reddish glow.

Evaluate capillary refill time by pressing on the patient's fingernail until it blanches and then observing how fast the nail bed resumes color when pressure is released. Normally capillaries resume color as soon as pressure is released. With shock, capillary refill is slow or may be absent. Capillary refill is not a reliable indicator for peripheral blood flow in older patients or those with anemia, diabetes, or peripheral vascular disease.

Central nervous system (CNS) changes with shock first manifest as thirst. Thirst is caused by stimulation of the thirst centers in the brain in response to decreased blood volume.

Assess the patient's level of consciousness (LOC) and orientation, which are sensitive to cerebral hypoxia. In the initial and nonprogressive stages, patients may be restless or agitated and may be anxious or have a feeling of impending doom. As hypoxia progresses, confusion and lethargy occur, which progress to loss of consciousness as cerebral hypoxia worsens.

Skeletal muscle changes during shock include weakness and pain in response to tissue hypoxia and anaerobic metabolism, which are later indications. Weakness is generalized and has no specific pattern. Deep tendon reflexes are decreased or absent.

Psychosocial Assessment. *Changes in mental status and behavior occur early in shock.* Assess mental status by evaluating LOC and noting whether the patient is asleep or awake. If the patient is asleep, attempt to awaken him or her and document how easily he or she is aroused. If the patient is awake, determine whether he or she is oriented to person, place, and time. Avoid asking questions that can be answered with a "yes" or a "no" response. Consider these points during assessment:

- Is it necessary to repeat questions to obtain a response?
- Does the response answer the question asked?
- Does the patient have difficulty making word choices?
- Is the patient irritated or upset by the questions?
- Can the patient concentrate on a question long enough to answer, or is the attention span limited?

Talk with the family to determine whether the patient's behavior and cognition are typical or represent a change.

Laboratory Assessment. Although no single test confirms or rules out shock, changes in laboratory data may support the diagnosis. Chart 37-2 lists laboratory changes occurring with hypovolemic shock. As shock progresses, arterial blood gas values become abnormal. The pH decreases, the partial pressure of arterial oxygen (Pao_2) decreases, and the partial pressure of arterial carbon dioxide ($Paco_2$) increases. Other laboratory changes occur with specific causes of hypovolemic shock.

Hematocrit and hemoglobin levels decrease if shock is caused by hemorrhage from poor CLOTTING. When shock is caused by dehydration or a fluid shift, hematocrit and hemoglobin levels are elevated.

CHART 37-2   Laboratory Profile

Hypovolemic Shock

TEST	NORMAL RANGE FOR ADULTS	SIGNIFICANCE OF ABNORMAL FINDINGS
pH (arterial)	7.35-7.45	Decreased: insufficient tissue oxygenation causing anaerobic metabolism and acidosis
Pao_2	80-100 mm Hg	Decreased: anaerobic metabolism
$Paco_2$	35-45 mm Hg	Increased: anaerobic metabolism
Lactic acid (lactate) (arterial)	3-7 mg/dL 0.3-0.8 mmol/L	Increased: anaerobic metabolism with buildup of metabolites
Hematocrit	*Females:* 37%-47% (0.37-0.47 volume fraction) *Males:* 42%-52% (0.42-0.52 volume fraction)	Increased: fluid shift, dehydration Decreased: hemorrhage
Hemoglobin	*Females:* 12-16 g/dL (120-160 g/L) *Males:* 14-18 g/dL (140-180 g/L)	Increased: fluid shift, dehydration Decreased: hemorrhage
Potassium	3.5-5.0 mEq/L or mmol/L	Increased: dehydration, acidosis

$Paco_2$, Partial pressure of arterial carbon dioxide; *Pao_2,* partial pressure of arterial oxygen.
Data from Pagana, K., Pagana, T. J., & Pagana, T. N. (2017). *Mosby's diagnostic and laboratory test reference* (13th ed.). St. Louis: Mosby; and Pagana, K., Pagana, T., & Pike-MacDonald, S. (2013). *Mosby's Canadian manual of diagnostic and laboratory tests.* St. Louis: Mosby.

◆ Analysis: Interpreting

The priority collaborative problems for patients with hypovolemic shock are:

- Hypoxia due to hypovolemia
- Inadequate PERFUSION due to active fluid volume loss and hypotension
- Anxiety due to potential for death and decreased cerebral PERFUSION
- Decreased cognition due to decreased cerebral PERFUSION

◆ Planning and Implementation: Responding

Interventions for patients in hypovolemic shock focus on reversing the shock, restoring fluid volume to the normal range, and preventing complications. Monitoring is critical to determine whether the patient is responding to therapy or whether shock is progressing and a change in intervention is needed. Surgery may be needed to correct some causes of shock. Chart 37-3 lists best practices for patients in hypovolemic shock.

Nonsurgical Management. The purposes of shock management are to maintain tissue GAS EXCHANGE, increase vascular volume, and support compensatory mechanisms. Oxygen therapy, fluid replacement therapy, and drug therapy are useful.

Oxygen therapy is used at any stage of shock and is delivered by mask, hood, nasal cannula, endotracheal tube, or tracheostomy tube. Chapter 28 describes oxygen-delivery methods.

IV therapy for fluid resuscitation is a primary intervention for hypovolemic shock. Crystalloids and colloids are often used for volume replacement. Crystalloid solutions contain nonprotein substances (e.g., minerals, salts, sugars). Colloid solutions contain large molecules of proteins or starches (see Chapter 11).

Crystalloid fluids help maintain an adequate fluid and electrolyte balance. Two common solutions are normal saline and Ringer's lactate. Normal saline (0.9% sodium chloride in water) is a replacement solution used to increase plasma volume and can be infused with any blood product. Ringer's lactate contains sodium, chloride, calcium, potassium, and lactate. This isotonic solution expands volume, and the lactate buffers acidosis. To date, no research has shown one type of crystalloid solution to be better than another overall. Selection of specific fluid is based on the patient's fluid and electrolyte status, acid-base status, and organ function (Pavlik et al., 2015).

! NURSING SAFETY PRIORITY QSEN

Action Alert

Use only normal saline for infusion with blood or blood products because the calcium in Ringer's lactate induces CLOTTING of the infusing blood.

 CHART 37-3   Best Practice for Patient Safety & Quality Care QSEN

The Patient in Hypovolemic Shock

- Ensure a patent airway.
- Insert an IV catheter or maintain an established catheter.
- Administer oxygen.
- Elevate the patient's feet, keeping his or her head flat or elevated to no more than a 30-degree angle.
- Examine the patient for overt bleeding.
- If overt bleeding is present, apply direct pressure to the site.
- Administer drugs as prescribed.
- Increase the rate of IV fluid delivery.
- Do not leave the patient.

Protein-containing colloid fluids help restore osmotic pressure and fluid volume. Blood products are used when shock is caused by blood loss. These fluids most often include packed red blood cells (PRBCs) and plasma.

PRBCs increase hematocrit and hemoglobin levels along with some fluid volume. Massive transfusion therapy, defined as 10 units of PRBCs given within the first 6 hours of severe hemorrhage, can improve outcomes and prevent death from acute traumatic coagulopathy (Day et al., 2013). See Chapter 40 for nursing care during transfusion therapy.

Plasma, an acellular blood product containing clotting factors, is given to restore osmotic pressure when hematocrit and hemoglobin levels are normal. Plasma protein fractions (e.g., Plasmanate) and synthetic plasma expanders (e.g., hetastarch [hydroxyethyl starch, Hespan]) increase volume and are used for hypovolemic shock before a cause is identified. Newer "supra-plasma expanders" that also include substances to carry oxygen are in development (Tsai et al., 2015).

Drug therapy is used in addition to fluid therapy when volume loss is severe and the patient does not respond sufficiently to fluid replacement and blood products. Drugs for shock increase venous return, improve cardiac contractility, or improve cardiac PERFUSION by dilating the coronary vessels. Chart 37-4 lists common drugs used to treat shock.

! NURSING SAFETY PRIORITY QSEN

Drug Alert

Monitor the patient closely because drugs that dilate coronary blood vessels, such as nitroprusside, can cause systemic vasodilation and increase shock if the patient is volume depleted. Drugs that increase heart muscle contraction increase heart oxygen consumption and can cause angina or infarction.

 CHART 37-4   Common Examples of Drug Therapy

Hypovolemic Shock

DRUG CATEGORY	NURSING IMPLICATIONS
Vasoconstrictors—Improve mean arterial pressure by increasing peripheral resistance, increasing venous return, and increasing myocardial contractility.	
Dopamine (Intropin, Revimine) Norepinephrine (Levophed) Phenylephrine HCl	Assess patient for chest pain *because these drugs increase myocardial consumption and can cause angina or ischemia.* Monitor urine output hourly *because higher doses decrease kidney perfusion and urine output.* Assess blood pressure every 15 min *because hypertension is a symptom of overdose.* Assess patient for headache *because headache is an early symptom of drug excess.* Assess every 30 min for extravasation; check extremities for color and perfusion *because if the drug gets into the tissues, it can cause severe vasoconstriction, tissue ischemia, and tissue necrosis.* Assess for chest pain *because the drug can cause rapid onset of vasoconstriction in the myocardium and impair cardiac oxygenation.*
Inotropic Agents—Directly stimulate beta-adrenergic receptors on the heart muscle, improving contractility	
Dobutamine (Dobutrex) Milrinone (Primacor)	Assess for chest pain *because these drugs increase myocardial oxygen consumption and can cause angina or infarction.* Assess blood pressure every 15 min *because hypertension is a symptom of overdose.*
Agents Enhancing Myocardial Perfusion—Improve myocardial perfusion by dilating coronary arteries rapidly for a short time.	
Sodium nitroprusside (Nitropress, Nipride)	Protect drug container from light *because light degrades the drug quickly.* Assess blood pressure at least every 15 min *because the drug can cause systemic vasodilation and hypotension, especially in older adults.*

Monitoring vital signs and level of consciousness is a major nursing action to determine the patient's condition and the effectiveness of therapy. Monitor these patient responses:

- Pulse (rate, regularity, and quality)
- Blood pressure
- Pulse pressure
- Central venous pressure (CVP)
- Respiratory rate
- Skin and mucosal color
- Oxygen saturation
- Cognition
- Urine output

Assess these parameters at least every 15 minutes until the shock is controlled and the patient's condition improves. Hemodynamic monitoring in critical care settings includes intra-arterial monitoring, mixed venous oxygen saturation (Svo_2), pulmonary artery monitoring, and pulmonary capillary wedge pressures.

Insertion of a CVP catheter allows pressure to be monitored in the patient's right atrium or superior vena cava while providing venous access. A decrease in CVP from baseline levels reflects hypovolemic shock with reduced venous return to the right atrium.

Intra-arterial catheters allow continuous blood pressure monitoring and are an access for arterial blood sampling. They are inserted into an artery (radial, brachial, femoral, or dorsalis pedis). The catheter is attached to pressure tubing and a transducer, which converts arterial pressure into an electrical signal seen as a waveform on an oscilloscope and as a numeric value.

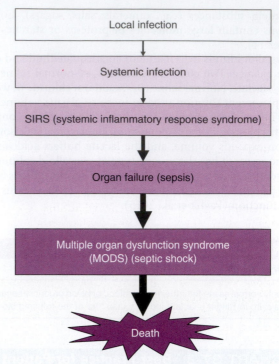

FIG. 37-2 Common progression of events leading to septic shock.

❋ IMMUNITY CONCEPT EXEMPLAR
Sepsis and Septic Shock

❖ *PATHOPHYSIOLOGY*

Sepsis leading to septic shock is a complex type of distributive shock that usually begins as a bacterial or fungal infection and progresses to a critical emergency over a period of days. The progression of sepsis to septic shock is outlined in Fig. 37-2. *As progression occurs, the pathologic problems occur faster and to a greater degree. Thus control of sepsis and prevention of severe sepsis and septic shock are easier to achieve early in the process. Failure to recognize and intervene in early sepsis is a major factor for progression to septic shock and death.*

Infection

When infection is confined to a local area, it should not lead to sepsis and shock. In the adult whose IMMUNITY and inflammatory responses are effective, the presence of organism invasion first starts a helpful, local response of inflammation to confine and eliminate the organism and prevent the infection from becoming worse or widespread.

The white blood cells (WBCs) in the area of invasion secrete cytokines to trigger local inflammation and bring more WBCs to kill the invading organisms. The results of this response constrict the small veins and dilate the arterioles in the area, which increases PERFUSION to locally infected tissues.

Capillary leak occurs, allowing plasma to leak into the tissues. This response causes swelling (edema). The duration of inflammation depends on the size and severity of the infection, but usually it subsides within a few days, when the infection has been managed by these responses. A benefit of inflammation is that it is limited only to the area of infection and stops as soon as it is no longer needed. The patient does not have fever,

Surgical Management. Surgical intervention in addition to nonsurgical management may be needed to correct the cause of shock. Such procedures include vascular repair, surgical hemostasis of major wounds, closure of bleeding ulcers, and chemical scarring (chemosclerosis) of varicosities.

Care Coordination and Transition Management

Hypovolemic shock is a complication of another condition and is resolved before patients are discharged from the acute care setting. Because surgery and many other invasive procedures now occur on an ambulatory care basis, more patients at home are at increased risk for hypovolemic shock. Teach patients and family members the early indicators of shock (increased thirst, decreased urine output, light-headedness, sense of apprehension) and to seek immediate medical attention if they appear.

tachycardia, decreased oxygen saturation, or reduced urine output.

Sepsis and Systemic Inflammatory Response Syndrome

The most recent definition of sepsis is a life-threatening organ dysfunction resulting from a dysregulated host response to infection (Kleinpell et al., 2016). It occurs as the presence of infection with systemic signs and symptoms (Chong et al., 2015). Infectious organisms have entered the bloodstream. As their numbers increase, widespread inflammation, known as *systemic inflammatory response syndrome (SIRS)*, is triggered as a result of infection escaping local control. With the organisms and their toxins in the bloodstream and entering other body areas, inflammation becomes an enemy, leading to extensive hormonal, tissue, and vascular changes and oxidative stress that further impair GAS EXCHANGE and tissue PERFUSION. The WBCs produce many pro-inflammatory cytokines, especially interleukin-1 (IL-1), interleukin-6 (IL-6), and tumor necrosis factor-alpha (Abbas et al., 2015). (See Chapter 17 for a discussion of cytokines.) As a result, there is widespread vasodilation and blood pooling, allowing stasis (Schell-Chaple & Lee, 2014). The patient has mild hypotension, a low urine output, and an increased respiratory rate. These responses result in a hypodynamic state with decreased cardiac output. Body temperature varies depending on the duration of the sepsis and on WBC function. Some patients have a low-grade fever and others have a high fever. Still others may have a below-normal body temperature. Fever and hypotension result from SIRS. The reduced urine output and increased respiratory rate are the compensatory responses to impaired GAS EXCHANGE and PERFUSION. Often the patient has the elevated WBC count expected with a systemic infection.

Inappropriate CLOTTING with microthrombi forming in some organ capillaries causes hypoxia and reduces organ function. This problem is hard to detect but, if sepsis is stopped at this point, the organ damage is reversible. The microthrombi increase hypoxic conditions, which then generate more toxic metabolites. These damage more cells and increase the production of pro-inflammatory cytokines, leading to an amplification of SIRS and a vicious repeating cycle of poor GAS EXCHANGE and PERFUSION (Fig. 37-3). Although these signs are subtle, they indicate sepsis and SIRS and will progress unless intervention begins immediately.

Unfortunately, this early hypodynamic state has a relatively short duration, and indicators are so subtle that the condition is often missed or misdiagnosed. When early sepsis and SIRS are identified and treated aggressively at this stage, the cycle of progression is stopped, and the outcome is good. When sepsis and SIRS are not identified and treated at this stage, they progress and become much harder to control. Nurses and all other health care professionals have a responsibility to identify cues that indicate sepsis before it becomes severe (Kleinpell et al., 2016). Identifying criteria have been established (Table 37-3) and must be used to ensure that interventions are instituted at this stage.

> **! NURSING SAFETY PRIORITY** **QSEN**
> *Critical Rescue*
>
> Monitor the patient at risk for sepsis to recognize symptoms that meet the criteria for sepsis and SIRS. If *any* of these are present, respond by notifying the health care provider or the Rapid Response Team.

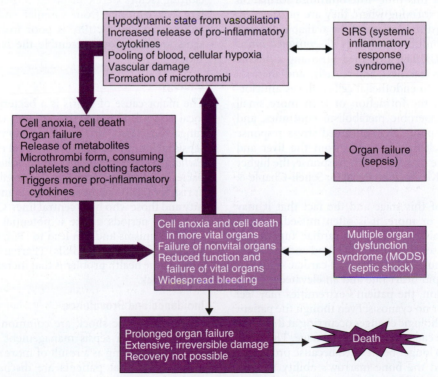

FIG. 37-3 Vicious cycle of systemic inflammatory response syndrome (SIRS) and multiple organ dysfunction syndrome (MODS) in septic shock.

TABLE 37-3 Sepsis With Systemic Inflammatory Response Syndrome (SIRS) Criteria

Suspected or identified infection with some of the following:

- Temperature of more than 101°F (38.3°C) or less than 96.8°F (36°C)
- Heart rate of more than 90 beats/min
- Respiratory rate of more than 20 breaths/min
- Abnormal WBC count (>12,000/mm³ or <4000/mm³)
- Normal WBC count with >10% bands
- Plasma C-reactive protein >2 standard deviations above normal
- Plasma prolactin >2 standard deviations above normal
- Arterial hypotension (SBP <90 mm Hg; MAP <70 mm Hg)
- Arterial hypoxemia (PaO₂/FiO₂ <300)
- Urine output <0.5 mL/kg/hr for 2 hours despite adequate fluid resuscitation
- Creatinine increase >0.5 mg/dL
- INR >1.5 or aPTT >60
- Absent bowel sounds
- Platelet count <100,000/mm³
- Total bilirubin >4 mg/dL
- Elevated lactic acid (lactate) levels
- Decreased capillary refill or presence of mottling
- Hyperglycemia (plasma glucose >140 mg/dL or 7.7 mmol/L) in absence of diabetes
- Unexplained change in mental status
- Significant edema or positive fluid balance

aPTT, Activated partial thromboplastin time; *FiO₂,* fraction of inspired oxygen; *INR,* international normalized ratio; *MAP,* mean arterial pressure; *PaO₂,* partial pressure of arterial oxygen; *SBP,* systolic blood pressure; *WBC,* white blood cell.
Data from Dellinger, R. P., Levy, M., Rhodes, A., Annane, D., Gerlach, H., Opal, S. M., et al. (2013). Surviving Sepsis Campaign. (2015). Updated bundles in response to new evidence. http://www.survivingsepsis.org/SiteCollectionDocuments/SSC_Bundle.pdf.

TABLE 37-4 Conditions Predisposing to Sepsis and Septic Shock

- Malnutrition
- Immunosuppression
- Large, open wounds
- Mucous membrane fissures in prolonged contact with bloody or drainage-soaked packing
- GI ischemia
- Exposure to invasive procedures
- Cancer
- Older than 80 years
- Infection with resistant microorganisms
- Receiving cancer chemotherapy
- Alcoholism
- Diabetes mellitus
- Chronic kidney disease
- Transplantation recipient
- Hepatitis
- HIV/AIDS

AIDS, Acquired immune deficiency syndrome; *HIV,* human immune deficiency virus.

When SIRS becomes amplified, all tissues are involved and are hypoxic to some degree. Some organs are experiencing cell death and dysfunction at this time. Microthrombi formation is widespread, with clots forming where they are not needed. This process uses up (consumes) many of the available platelets and clotting factors, a condition known as *disseminated intravascular coagulation (DIC)*. The amplified SIRS and cytokine release increase capillary leakiness, injure cells, and increase cell metabolism. Damage to endothelial cells reduces anticlotting actions and triggers the formation of even more small clots, increasing DIC. Anaerobic metabolism continues, and cell uptake of oxygen is poor. The continued stress response triggers the continued release of glucose from the liver and causes hyperglycemia. The more severe the response, the higher the blood glucose level (Kleinpell et al., 2016; Schell-Chaple & Lee, 2014).

Despite the severity of this stage and the fact that it may be present for 24 hours or more, it is often missed. One of the reasons it may be missed is that the cardiac function is hyperdynamic in this phase. The pooling of blood and the widespread capillary leak stimulate the heart, and cardiac output is *increased* with a more rapid heart rate and an elevated systolic blood pressure. In addition, the patient's extremities may feel warm, and there is little or no cyanosis. Even though the patient may "look" better, the pathologic changes occurring at the tissue level are serious and have caused significant damage. The WBC count at this time may no longer be elevated because prolonged sepsis may have exceeded the bone marrow's ability to keep producing and releasing new mature neutrophils and other WBCs. The WBC count may be extremely low, especially the segmented neutrophils (segs).

Signs and symptoms include a lower oxygen saturation, rapid respiratory rate, decreased-to-absent urine output, and a change in the patient's cognition and affect. Appropriate and aggressive interventions at this stage can still prevent septic shock, although mortality after a patient reaches this stage is much higher than for sepsis and SIRS. *At this point, the downhill course leading to septic shock is extremely rapid.*

Septic Shock

Septic shock is sepsis-induced hypotension persisting despite adequate fluid resuscitation. It is the stage of sepsis and SIRS when multiple organ dysfunction syndrome (MODS) with organ failure is evident and poor CLOTTING with uncontrolled bleeding occurs (see Fig. 37-3). *Even with appropriate intervention, the death rate among patients in this stage of sepsis is very high* (Dellinger et al., 2013). Severe hypovolemic shock and hypodynamic cardiac function are present as a result of an inability of the blood to clot because the platelets and clotting factors were consumed earlier. Vasodilation and capillary leak continue from vascular endothelial cell disruption, and cardiac contractility is poor from cellular ischemia. The signs and symptoms resemble the late stage of hypovolemic shock.

Etiology

The major cause of sepsis is a bacterial infection that escapes local control, although in patients with reduced IMMUNITY, fungal infections also cause it. Common organisms causing sepsis include gram-negative bacteria (*Pseudomonas aeruginosa, Escherichia coli,* and *Klebsiella pneumoniae*) and gram-positive bacteria (*Staphylococcus* and *Streptococcus*). Patients especially at risk for sepsis are those who have any type of reduced immunity and those who have central lines. Central lines in place even for short periods create a potential direct access point for microorganisms and can lead to central line–associated bloodstream infections (CLABSIs) (Earhart, 2013). Table 37-4 lists some of the health problems that increase the risk for sepsis and septic shock.

Incidence and Prevalence

Sepsis and septic shock are common events (Dellinger et al., 2013). Although sepsis management has improved, the incidence is increasing as a result of more drug-resistant organisms and the fact that patients are discharged from the hospital "quicker and sicker" (Lopez-Bushnell et al., 2014). Sepsis takes time to develop, and the patient may be discharged before signs and symptoms are obvious.

Health Promotion and Maintenance

Prevention is the best management strategy for sepsis and septic shock. Evaluate all patients for their risk for sepsis, especially older adults, because the death rate from sepsis in adults older than 65 years is nearly twice that of younger adults. Table 37-4 lists health problems that increase the risk for septic shock. Use aseptic technique during invasive procedures and when working with nonintact skin and mucous membranes in patients with reduced IMMUNITY. Remove indwelling urinary catheters and IV access lines as soon as they are no longer needed. Ensure that patients receiving mechanical ventilation are weaned from the ventilator as soon as possible (Kleinpell et al., 2016).

Because sepsis can be a complication of many conditions found in acute care settings, always consider its possibility. *Early detection of sepsis before progression to septic shock is a major nursing responsibility.* The nurse is the health care professional most in contact with the patient and is in a unique position to detect subtle changes in appearance and behavior that can indicate sepsis. Use the assessment techniques described earlier for changes in vital signs, laboratory findings, appearance, and behavior to identify early any characteristics of sepsis and sepsis progression at least every shift for potentially infected seriously ill patients (Kleinpell & Schorr, 2014; Kurczewski et al., 2015). Using an evidence-based electronic alert system in acute care settings to identify patients who may be in early sepsis can improve the timing of implementing an appropriate sepsis bundle intervention (see the Quality Improvement box).

Early detection can be made by patients and families, as well as health care personnel. This is especially important for patients discharged to home after invasive procedures or surgery. Teach patients and families the signs and symptoms of local infection (local redness, pain, swelling, purulent drainage, loss of function) and early sepsis (fever, urine output less than intake, light-headedness). Teach them how to use a thermometer and to take the temperature twice a day and whenever they are not feeling well. Urge those with symptoms of early sepsis to immediately contact their health care provider. Teach them that, if antibiotics are prescribed, to take these drugs as prescribed and to complete the entire course.

❖ INTERPROFESSIONAL COLLABORATIVE CARE

Sepsis and septic shock may occur in any setting. Successful outcomes from management usually require intensive interventions in an acute care setting.

◆ Assessment: Noticing

Sepsis and septic shock differ from other types of shock in many ways. The entire syndrome may occur over many hours to days, and the signs and symptoms are less obvious. The chance for recovery is good when the patient is recognized as having sepsis with SIRS and appropriate interventions are started within 6 hours. Septic shock, on the other hand, has a rapid downhill course, and chances for recovery are relatively poor. Identifying patients in the earlier stages of sepsis can make the greatest difference in survival.

History. Age is important because sepsis develops more easily among older, debilitated patients who have reduced IMMUNITY (Abbas et al., 2015; Englert & Ross, 2015; Umberger et al., 2015). Chart 37-5 lists factors that increase the older adult's risk for shock. Ask about the patient's medical history, including recent illness, trauma, invasive procedures, or chronic conditions that

QUALITY IMPROVEMENT QSEN

Using Electronic Alerts for Early Sepsis Recognition and Intervention

Kurczewski, L., Sweet, M., McKnight, R., & Halbritter, K. (2015). Reduction in time to first action as a result of electronic alerts for early sepsis recognition. *Critical Care Nurse Quarterly, 38*(2), 182–187.

The Surviving Sepsis Campaign promotes early recognition of systemic inflammatory response syndrome (SIRS), or sepsis. After prevention, the greatest positive factor for surviving sepsis is early recognition of the condition, which leads to implementation of evidence-based interventions through early goal-directed therapy (EGDT). The SSC has identified care bundles that have shown a decrease in mortality rates. However, success with intervention is contingent on early recognition and swift intervention.

One hospital implemented hospital-wide sepsis alerts. These alerts were generated through the electronic medical records using predetermined SIRS criteria (temperature, heart rate, respiratory rate, white blood cell count). Real time patient data were used to trigger an alert that prompted the provider to consider sepsis potential and intervene based on standards of care. This study showed significant potential in decreasing the time of recognition to sepsis-related intervention. This was attributed to the real-time data as well as to the inability of the provider to "ignore" the warning because action regarding the data was required. In addition, the alerts were not physician specific but rather were for all caregivers.

Commentary: Implications for Practice and Research

Evidence-based practice has demonstrated that early recognition of patients with SIRS or sepsis is the first step in improving survival from this devastating condition. The implementation of a hospital-wide alert system using the electronic medical record has decreased the time associated with the first sepsis-related intervention. Although this alert system was proven effective within this health care system, more research is needed to determine its applicability to other health care systems and settings.

may lead to sepsis. Check which drugs the patient has used in the past week. Some drugs may directly cause changes leading to shock. A drug regimen may also indicate a disorder or problem that can contribute to sepsis (e.g., drugs that include aspirin, corticosteroids, antibiotics, and cancer drugs).

Physical Assessment/Signs and Symptoms. Signs and symptoms of sepsis and septic shock occur over many hours, and some change during the progression. See Table 37-3 for a listing of specific symptoms and laboratory changes that often occur with sepsis and septic shock.

Cardiovascular changes differ in the stages of sepsis and septic shock. Cardiac output and blood pressure are low in early sepsis and very low in septic shock. In severe sepsis, cardiac output is higher as are heart rate and blood pressure, although this is an indication of a worsening condition rather than an improvement. Increased cardiac output is reflected by tachycardia, increased stroke volume, a normal systolic blood pressure, and a normal central venous pressure (CVP). Increased cardiac output and vasodilation make the skin color appear normal with pink mucous membranes and the skin is warm to the touch. This situation is temporary, and eventually the cardiac output is greatly reduced.

With progression, disseminated intravascular coagulation (DIC) occurs as a result of excessive CLOTTING, with formation of thousands of small clots in the tiny capillaries of the liver, kidney, brain, spleen, and heart. DIC reduces PERFUSION and

---

CHART 37-5   Nursing Focus on the Older Adult

Risk Factors for Shock

Hypovolemic Shock
- Diuretic therapy
- Diminished thirst reflex
- Immobility
- Use of aspirin-containing products
- Use of complementary therapies such as *Ginkgo biloba*
- Anticoagulant therapy

Cardiogenic Shock
- Diabetes mellitus
- Presence of cardiomyopathies

Distributive Shock
- Diminished immune response
- Reduced skin integrity
- Presence of cancer
- Peripheral neuropathy
- Strokes
- Being in a hospital or extended-care facility
- Malnutrition
- Anemia

Obstructive Shock
- Pulmonary hypertension
- Presence of cancer

GAS EXCHANGE and decreases oxygen saturation, causing widespread hypoxia and ischemia.

The huge number of small clots uses clotting factors and fibrinogen faster than they can be produced, which eventually leads to poor CLOTTING. This leads to hemorrhage, which occurs in the septic shock stage. Coupled with continued capillary leak, bleeding causes hypovolemia and a dramatic decrease in cardiac output, blood pressure, and pulse pressure. The signs and symptoms of this phase are the same as those of the later stages of hypovolemic shock.

Respiratory changes are first caused by compensatory mechanisms that try to maintain oxygenation with a rate increase. The lungs are susceptible to damage, and the complication of acute respiratory distress syndrome (ARDS) may occur in septic shock. ARDS in septic shock is caused by the continued systemic inflammatory response syndrome (SIRS) increasing the formation of oxygen free radicals, which damage lung cells. *ARDS in a patient with septic shock has a high mortality rate.*

Skin changes differ at different stages of sepsis. In the hyperdynamic stage, the skin is warm and no cyanosis is evident. With progression to septic shock and compromised circulation, it is cool and clammy with pallor, mottling, or cyanosis. In DIC, petechiae and ecchymoses can occur anywhere. Blood may ooze from the gums, other mucous membranes, and venipuncture sites and around IV catheters.

A *kidney/urinary change* of low urine output compared with fluid intake indicates shock. When a patient who has no known kidney problems suddenly starts having a low urine output, be suspicious of severe sepsis or septic shock. Reduced output is caused by low circulating volume and hormonal changes. Kidney function decreases, and serum creatinine levels rise.

Psychosocial Assessment. An indicator that patients may be in the beginning of severe sepsis is often a change in affect or behavior. Compare the patient's current behavior, verbal responses, and general affect with those assessed earlier in the day or the day before. They may seem just slightly different in their reactions to greetings, comments, or jokes. They may be less patient than usual or act restless or fidgety. Patients may make statements such as, "I feel as if something is wrong, but I don't know what." If behavior is changed from prior assessments, consider the possibility of severe sepsis and shock.

Laboratory Assessment. No single laboratory test confirms the presence of sepsis and septic shock, although hallmarks of sepsis are a rising serum procalcitonin level, an increasing serum lactate level, a normal or low total white blood cell (WBC) count, and a decreasing segmented neutrophil level with a rising band neutrophil level (left shift, see Chapter 17). The presence of bacteria in the blood supports the diagnosis of sepsis, although this finding may not be present. Obtain specimens of urine, blood, sputum, and any drainage for culture to identify the causative organisms. Blood cultures should be taken before antibiotic therapy is started, provided that this action does not delay antibiotic therapy by more than 45 minutes (Dellinger et al., 2013). Other abnormal laboratory findings that occur with septic shock include changes in the white blood cell (WBC) count; the differential leukocyte count may show a left shift. Hematocrit and hemoglobin levels usually do not change until late in septic shock. At that point, the hematocrit and hemoglobin levels, fibrinogen levels, and platelet count are low from disseminated intravascular coagulation (DIC). The serum lactate level is above normal, and the serum bicarbonate levels are lower than normal. Unfortunately these parameters may take time to change and cannot be relied on as sensitive indicators of the patient's worsening condition.

Another indicator of sepsis and septic shock is a low blood level of activated protein C. Protein C is an enzyme that prevents inappropriate clot formation. It is activated when it binds to healthy vascular endothelial cells. In severe sepsis, the injured endothelial cells cannot activate protein C, and thousands of small clots form in the capillaries of vascular organs. Decreasing levels of activated protein C indicate the beginning of severe sepsis even before other symptoms are evident.

Other biologic indicators of severe sepsis and septic shock are changes in plasma D-dimer levels, cytokine, and interleukin levels. These indicators have a lag time, and changes may not be present soon enough to identify sepsis with SIRS before severe sepsis or septic shock develops.

Because the results of blood cultures may not be available until the patient's condition has progressed to severe sepsis or septic shock, other biomarkers for sepsis and SIRS are needed to help identify the condition when it can be managed and cured. Two such markers are increasing lactic acid levels and increasing procalcitonin levels (Sullivan & Von Rueden, 2016; Walker, 2015).

The actual diagnosis of sepsis is difficult to make, yet the best outcome depends on an early diagnosis and the implementation of appropriate aggressive interventions within 6 hours. In general, sepsis is considered to exist when an infection is present along with some of the additional established criteria listed in Table 37-3.

? NCLEX EXAMINATION CHALLENGE 37-4

Safe and Effective Care Environment

With which client should the nurse remain alert for the possibility of sepsis and septic shock?

A. 41-year-old man who sustained closed depression fractures of the face when hit with a baseball

B. 53-year-old woman who had an open abdominal hysterectomy 3 days ago to remove several large fibroid tumors.

C. 67-year-old woman on chronic corticosteroid therapy who had several teeth extracted 2 days ago.

D. 72-year-old man with severe allergies who is undergoing radiation therapy for early-stage prostate cancer.

◆ **Analysis: Interpreting**

The priority collaborative problems for patients with sepsis and septic shock are:

1. Widespread infection due to inadequate IMMUNITY
2. Potential for myocardial dysfunction due to inappropriate CLOTTING, poor PERFUSION, and poor GAS EXCHANGE from widespread infection and inflammation

◆ **Planning and Implementation: Responding**

The priority problem for patients with septic shock is potential for multiple organ dysfunction syndrome (MODS).

Planning: Expected Outcomes. With appropriate interventions, the patient with sepsis or septic shock is expected to have normal aerobic cellular metabolism. Indicators include:

- Arterial blood gases (pH, Pao₂, and Paco₂) within the normal range
- Maintenance of a urine output of at least 20 mL/hr
- Maintenance of mean arterial blood pressure within 10 mm Hg of baseline
- Absence of multiple organ dysfunction syndrome (MODS)

Interventions. Interventions for sepsis and septic shock focus on identifying the problem as early as possible, correcting the conditions causing it, and preventing complications. The use of a sepsis resuscitation bundle for treatment of sepsis within 6 hours is the standard of practice. A *bundle* is a group of two or more specific interventions that have been shown to be effective when applied together or in sequence. The Surviving Sepsis Campaign (SSC) is a national initiative that was started to standardize sepsis care and promote early recognition of patients with sepsis and septic shock. In 2004, SSC care "bundle" guidelines were developed to reduce sepsis-related deaths. These bundles were updated based on practice evidence, most recently in 2015, and are reflective of goal-directed therapy for prevention of sepsis-related mortality (Lehman & Thiessen, 2015; Surviving Sepsis Campaign, 2015). Table 37-5 details the bundles updated by the SSC.

Oxygen therapy is useful whenever poor tissue PERFUSION and poor GAS EXCHANGE are present. The patient with septic shock is more likely to be mechanically ventilated. Care of the patient being mechanically ventilated is discussed in detail in Chapter 32.

Drug therapy to enhance cardiac output and restore vascular volume is essentially the same as that used in hypovolemic shock (see Chart 37-4). In addition, drug therapy is needed to combat sepsis, adrenal insufficiency, hyperglycemia, and clotting problems.

Although septic shock can be caused by any organism, the most common agents are gram-negative bacteria. In accordance with the recommendations of The Joint Commission's National Patient Safety Goals (NPSGs), IV antibiotics with known activity against gram-negative bacteria are given before organisms are identified, preferably within 1 hour of a sepsis diagnosis. Multiple antibiotics with broad-spectrum activity are prescribed, based on the site of infection and the most common geographic infections, until the actual causative organism is known (Droege et al., 2016).

The stress of severe sepsis can cause adrenal insufficiency. Adrenal support may involve providing the patient with low-dose corticosteroids during the treatment period. Drugs used for this purpose are IV hydrocortisone and oral fludrocortisone (Florinef).

Patients with sepsis or septic shock usually have elevated blood glucose levels (>180 mg/dL or >10 mmol/L), which is associated with a poor outcome. Insulin therapy is used to maintain blood glucose levels between 110 mg/dL (6.2 mmol/L) and 150 mg/dL (8.4 mmol/L). Keeping the blood glucose level below 110 mg/dL (6.2 mmol/L) is associated with increased mortality.

During severe sepsis, patients have microvascular abnormalities and form many small clots. Heparin therapy with fractionated heparin is used to limit inappropriate CLOTTING and prevent the excessive consumption of clotting factors.

Blood replacement therapy is used when poor CLOTTING with hemorrhage occurs and may include clotting factors, platelets, fresh frozen plasma (FFP), or packed red blood cells. Chapter 40 discusses in detail the care of the patient during blood replacement. The use of platelet transfusion is recommended ahead of other blood products for patients with septic shock to improve CLOTTING (Dellinger et al., 2013).

Care Coordination and Transition Management

Identified sepsis should be resolved before patients are discharged from the acute care setting. Because more patients are receiving treatment on an ambulatory care basis and are being discharged earlier from acute care settings, more patients at home are at increased risk for sepsis.

TABLE 37-5 Bundles for Resuscitation and Management of Severe Sepsis

Surviving Sepsis Care Bundle

Within the first 3 hours of suspecting severe sepsis:
1. Measure serum lactate levels.
2. Obtain blood cultures *before* administering antibiotics.
3. Administer broad-spectrum antibiotics.
4. Administer 30 mL/kg crystalloids intravenously for hypotension or lactate ≥4 mmol/L.

Within 6 hours of initial indications of suspected septic shock:
5. Administer prescribed vasopressors for hypotension that does not respond to initial fluid resuscitation measures to maintain MAP ≥65 mm Hg.
6. If arterial hypotension persists despite initial fluid volume resuscitation or lactate remains ≥4 mmol/L (36 mg/dL), reassess volume status and tissue perfusion and document findings (reassessment of volume status and tissue perfusion as outlined below).
7. Remeasure lactate level if initial value was elevated.

Document reassessment of volume status and tissue perfusion with EITHER:
- Repeat focused examination (after initial fluid resuscitation), including vital signs, cardiopulmonary, capillary refill, pulse, and skin findings

OR TWO OF THE THREE FOLLOWING:
- Measure of central venous pressure
- Measure of central venous oxygen saturation
- Bedside cardiovascular ultrasound
- Dynamic assessment of fluid responsiveness with passive leg raise or fluid challenge

Data from *Surviving Sepsis Campaign* http://www.survivingsepsis.org/bundles/Pages/default.aspx; Kleinpell, R., Schorr, C., Balk, R. (2016). The new sepsis definitions: Implications for critical care practitioners. *American Journal of Critical Care, 25*(53), 457-464; *Surviving Sepsis Campaign.* (2015). Updated bundles in response to new evidence. http://www.survivingsepsis.org/SiteCollectionDocuments/SSC_Bundle.pdf. *MAP,* Mean arterial pressure.

CLINICAL JUDGMENT CHALLENGE 37-1

Safety; Patient-Centered Care; Teamwork and Collaboration QSEN

A 47-year-old obese woman with a history of type 2 diabetes and previous deep vein thrombosis of the right leg comes to the emergency department with an enlarged abdomen, nausea, and a high blood glucose level of 278 mg/dL (15.4 mmol/L). She says she has felt tired for 2 days and has not eaten or taken any of her usual drugs (rivaroxaban [Xarelto] 20 mg, losartan [Cozaar] 50 mg, and metformin [Glucophage] 850 mg). Your initial assessment findings include pale skin and mucous membranes, abdominal tenderness, an irregular pulse of 118, an oral temperature of 96.4°F (35.8°C), a blood pressure of 102/40, and a pulse oximetry reading of 89%. Immediate orders are to draw blood for a complete blood count with differential, serum electrolytes, and serum lactate; start an IV of D5% in 0.45% sodium chloride at 200 mL/hr; and apply oxygen by nasal cannula at 4 L/min.

1. Which action should you perform first? Provide a rationale for your choice.
2. What signs or symptoms of shock are present?
3. What risk factors does this patient have for sepsis or septic shock?
4. What other assessment data would be helpful in determining whether sepsis or septic shock is present?
5. How frequently should this patient be assessed? Provide a rationale for your answer.

Home Care Management. Evaluate the home environment for safety regarding infection hazards. Note the general cleanliness, especially in the kitchen and bathrooms. Chart 37-6 lists focused patient and environmental assessment data to obtain during a home visit.

Self-Management Education. Protecting frail patients from infection and sepsis at home is an important nursing function. Teach about the importance of self-care strategies, such as good

CHART 37-6 Home Care Assessment

The Patient at Risk for Sepsis

Assess the patient for any signs and symptoms of infection, including:
* Temperature, pulse, respiration, and blood pressure
* Color of skin and mucous membranes
* The mouth and perianal area for fissures or lesions
* Any nonintact skin area for the presence of exudates, redness, increased warmth, swelling
* Any pain, tenderness, or other discomfort anywhere
* Cough or any other symptoms of a cold or the flu
* Urine; or ask patient whether urine is dark or cloudy, has an odor, or causes pain or burning during urination

Assess patient's and caregiver's adherence to and understanding of infection prevention techniques.

Assess home environment, including:
* General cleanliness
* Kitchen and bathroom facilities, including refrigeration
* Availability and type of soap for handwashing
* Presence of pets, especially cats, rodents, or reptiles

hygiene, handwashing, balanced diet, rest and exercise, skin care, and mouth care. If patients or family members do not know how to take a temperature or read a thermometer, teach them and obtain a return demonstration. Teach patients and families to notify the primary health care provider immediately if fever or other signs of infection appear. General recommendations for Infection Precautions for patients at risk for sepsis are listed in Chart 22-4.

◆ **Evaluation: Reflecting**

Evaluate the care of the patient with sepsis or septic shock. The expected outcome is that the patient will maintain normal aerobic cellular metabolism.

GET READY FOR THE NCLEX® EXAMINATION!

KEY POINTS

Review these Key Points for each NCLEX Examination Client Needs Category.

Safe and Effective Care Environment

* Ensure that vital sign measurements are accurate and monitor them for changes indicating the presence of shock. **QSEN: Safety**
* Identify patients at high risk for infection caused by age, disease, or the environment. **QSEN: Safety**
* Use the recommended criteria to assess for the presence of sepsis (see Table 37-3). **QSEN: Evidence-Based Practice**
* Use strict aseptic techniques when performing invasive procedures, administering IV drugs, changing dressings, and handling nonintact skin. **QSEN: Safety**
* Use good handwashing techniques before providing any care to a patient who has impaired IMMUNITY. **QSEN: Safety**
* Assign a registered nurse rather than a licensed practical nurse/licensed vocational nurse (LPN/LVN) or unlicensed assistive personnel (UAP) to assess the vital signs of a patient who is suspected of having hypovolemic shock. **QSEN: Safety**

Health Promotion and Maintenance

* Teach all adults how to avoid dehydration. **QSEN: Patient-Centered Care**
* Teach all adults to use safety devices to avoid trauma. **QSEN: Patient-Centered Care**
* Instruct all patients going home after surgery or invasive procedures to seek immediate attention for persistent signs of early shock. **QSEN: Patient-Centered Care**
* Teach all patients who have a local infection to seek medical attention when signs of systemic infection appear. **QSEN: Patient-Centered Care**

Psychosocial Integrity

* Assess all patients at risk for shock for a change in affect, reduced cognition, altered level of consciousness, and increased anxiety. **QSEN: Patient-Centered Care**
* Stay with the patient in shock. **QSEN: Patient-Centered Care**
* Reassure patients who are in shock that the appropriate interventions are being instituted. **QSEN: Patient-Centered Care**

Physiological Integrity

- Be aware of the role of the systemic inflammatory response syndrome (SIRS) in the signs, symptoms, and progression of sepsis and septic shock. **QSEN: Safety**
- Assess the immunocompromised patient every shift for infection. **QSEN: Safety**
- Assess the skin integrity of the patient with reduced IMMUNITY at least every shift. **QSEN: Patient-Centered Care**
- Immediately assess vital signs of patients who have a change in level of consciousness, increased thirst, or anxiety. **QSEN: Evidence-Based Practice**
- Assess for changes in pulse rate and quality or a decrease in urine output rather than blood pressure as an indicator of shock. **QSEN: Evidence-Based Practice**

- Give oxygen to any patient in shock. **QSEN: Evidence-Based Practice**
- Assess hourly urine output to evaluate the adequacy of treatment for hypovolemic shock. **QSEN: Evidence-Based Practice**
- Before administering prescribed antibiotics, obtain blood cultures and cultures of urine, wound drainage, and sputum for any patient suspected to have sepsis. **QSEN: Evidence-Based Practice**
- Administer prescribed antibiotics within 1 hour of a diagnosis of sepsis. **QSEN: Evidence-Based Practice**

SELECTED BIBLIOGRAPHY

Abbas, A., Lichtman, A., & Pillai, S. (2015). *Cellular and molecular immunology* (8th ed.). Philadelphia: Saunders.

Bernstein, M., & Lynn, S. (2013). Helping patients survive sepsis. *American Nurse Today*, 8(1), 24–28.

Chen, L. (2015). A study in scarlet: Restrictive red blood cell transfusion strategy. *Critical Care Nursing Quarterly*, 38(2), 217–219.

Chong, J., Dumant, T., Francis-Frank, L., & Balaan, M. (2015). Sepsis and septic shock: A review. *Critical Care Nursing Quarterly*, 38(2), 111–120.

Day, D., Matsumoto, K., & Passion, C. (2013). Acute traumatic coagulopathy: The latest intervention strategies. *American Nurse Today*, 8(11), 8–11.

Dellinger, R. P., Levy, M., Rhodes, A., Annane, D., Gerlach, H., Opal, S. M., et al. (2013). Surviving sepsis campaign: International guidelines for management of severe sepsis and septic shock: 2012. *Critical Care Medicine*, 41(2), 580–637.

Droege, M., Van Fleet, S., & Mueller, E. (2016). Application of pharmacodynamics and dosing principles in patients with sepsis. *Critical Care Nurse*, 36(2), 22–32.

Earhart, A. (2013). Recognizing, preventing, and troubleshooting central line complications. *American Nurse Today*, 8(11), 18–22.

Englert, N., & Ross, C. (2015). The older adult experiencing sepsis. *Critical Care Nursing Quarterly*, 38(2), 175–181.

Kleinpell, R., & Schorr, C. (2014). Targeting sepsis as a performance improvement metric: Role of the nurse. *AACN Advanced Critical Care*, 25(2), 179–180.

Kleinpell, R., Schorr, C., & Balk, R. (2016). The new sepsis definitions: Implications for critical care practitioners. *American Journal of Critical Care*, 25(5), 457–464.

Kurczewski, L., Sweet, M., McKnight, R., & Halbritter, K. (2015). Reduction in time to first action as a result of electronic alerts for early sepsis recognition. *Critical Care Nursing Quarterly*, 38(2), 182–187.

Lehman, K., & Thiessen, K. (2015). Sepsis guidelines: Clinical practice implications. *The Nurse Practitioner*, 40(6), 1–6.

Lopez-Bushnell, K., Demaray, W., & Jaco, C. (2014). Reducing sepsis mortality. *Medsurg Nursing*, 23(1), 9–14.

McCance, K., Huether, S., Brashers, V., & Rote, N. (2014). *Pathophysiology: The biologic basis for disease in adults and children* (7th ed.). St. Louis: Mosby.

Pagana, K., Pagana, T. J., & Pagana, T. N. (2017). *Mosby's diagnostic and laboratory test reference* (13th ed.). St. Louis: Mosby.

Pagana, K., Pagana, T., & Pike-MacDonald, S. (2013). *Mosby's Canadian manual of diagnostic and laboratory tests*. St. Louis: Mosby.

Pavlik, D., Simpson, R., Horn, E., King, L., & Finoli, L. (2015). Pharmacology of sepsis. *Critical Care Nursing Quarterly*, 38(2), 121–126.

Schell-Chaple, H. (2015). Connecting the dots leads to suspicion of sepsis. *American Nurse Today*, 10(3), 24.

Schell-Chaple, H., & Lee, M. (2014). Reducing sepsis deaths: A systems approach to early detection and management. *American Nurse Today*, 9(7), 26–30.

Sullivan, S., & Von Rueden, K. (2016). Using procalcitonin in septic shock to guide antibacterial therapy. *Dimensions of Critical Care Nursing*, 35(2), 66–73.

Surviving Sepsis Campaign. (2015). *Updated bundles in response to new evidence*. http://www.survivingsepsis.org/SiteCollectionDocuments/SSC_Bundle.pdf.

Thibeault, A. (2015). Massive transfusion for hemorrhagic shock: What every critical care nurse needs to know. *Critical Care Nursing Clinics of North America*, 27(1), 47–53.

Touhy, T., & Jett, K. (2016). *Ebersole and Hess' toward healthy aging: Human needs and nursing response* (9th ed.). St. Louis: Mosby.

Tsai, A., Vazquez, B., Hofmann, A., Acharya, S., & Intaglietta, M. (2015). Supra-plasma expanders: The future of treating blood loss and anemia without red cell transfusions? *Journal of Infusion Nursing*, 38(3), 217–222.

Umberger, R., Callen, B., & Brown, M. (2015). Severe sepsis in older adults. *Critical Care Nursing Quarterly*, 38(3), 259–270.

Walker, C. (2015). Procalcitonin-guided antibiotic therapy duration in critically ill adults. *AACN Advanced Critical Care*, 26(2), 99–106.

Warise, L. (2015). Understanding cardiogenic shock. *Dimensions of Critical Care Nursing*, 34(2), 67–78.

38 | CHAPTER

Care of Patients With Acute Coronary Syndromes

Laura M. Dechant

 http://evolve.elsevier.com/Iggy/

PRIORITY AND INTERRELATED CONCEPTS

The priority concept for this chapter is PERFUSION.

❋ The PERFUSION concept exemplar for this chapter is Acute Coronary Syndrome, p. 769.

The interrelated concept for this chapter is COMFORT.

LEARNING OUTCOMES

Safe and Effective Care Environment

1. Collaborate with the interprofessional team to provide high-quality care for patients with acute coronary syndromes that impact PERFUSION and COMFORT.
2. Prioritize evidence-based care for patients with acute coronary syndromes affecting PERFUSION and COMFORT.

Health Promotion and Maintenance

3. Teach patients about lifestyle modifications to reduce modifiable and nonmodifiable risk factors for acute coronary syndromes.
4. Teach the patient and caregiver(s) about common drugs used for acute coronary syndromes.

Psychosocial Integrity

5. Implement nursing interventions to decrease the psychosocial impact of acute coronary events, especially myocardial infarction (MI).

Physiological Integrity

6. Apply knowledge of anatomy and physiology to provide evidence-based nursing care for patients with stable angina, unstable angina, and MI.
7. Use clinical judgment to prioritize nursing care to promote PERFUSION and prevent complications in patients with chest pain.
8. Use laboratory data and signs and symptoms to prioritize care for the patient with acute coronary syndrome.
9. Develop a plan of care using quality improvement measures for the patient who requires percutaneous or surgical coronary intervention to promote PERFUSION.

Coronary artery disease (CAD) is a broad term that includes chronic stable angina and acute coronary syndromes. It affects the arteries that provide blood, oxygen, and nutrients to the myocardium. When blood flow through the coronary arteries is partially or completely blocked, ischemia and infarction of the myocardium may result. **Ischemia** occurs when *insufficient oxygen* is supplied to meet the requirements of the myocardium. **Infarction** (necrosis, or cell death) occurs when severe ischemia is prolonged and decreased PERFUSION causes irreversible damage to tissue.

Coronary artery disease (CAD), also called *coronary heart disease (CHD)* or simply *heart disease,* is the single largest killer of American men and women in all ethnic groups. When the arteries that supply the **myocardium** (heart muscle) are diseased, the heart cannot pump blood effectively to adequately perfuse vital organs and peripheral tissues. The organs and

tissues need oxygen in arterial blood for survival. When PERFUSION is impaired, the patient can have life-threatening signs and symptoms and possibly death.

The death rate from CAD has declined over the past decade (Mozaffarian et al., 2016). This decline is due to many factors, including increasingly effective treatment and an increased awareness and emphasis on reducing major cardiovascular risk factors (e.g., hypertension, smoking, high cholesterol). However, some coronary events occur in patients without common risk factors.

CHRONIC STABLE ANGINA PECTORIS

Angina pectoris is chest pain caused by a temporary imbalance between the coronary arteries' ability to supply oxygen and the cardiac muscle's demand for oxygen. **Ischemia** (lack of oxygen) that occurs with angina is limited in duration and does not cause permanent damage of myocardial tissue.

Angina may be of two main types: stable angina and unstable angina. **Chronic stable angina (CSA)** is chest discomfort that occurs with moderate to prolonged exertion in a pattern that is familiar to the patient. The frequency, duration, and intensity of symptoms remain the same over several months. CSA results in only slight limitation of activity and is usually associated with a *fixed* atherosclerotic plaque. It is usually relieved by nitroglycerin or rest and often is managed with drug therapy. Rarely does CSA require aggressive treatment. *Unstable* angina is discussed in the following Acute Coronary Syndrome section.

✳ PERFUSION CONCEPT EXEMPLAR
Acute Coronary Syndrome

❖ PATHOPHYSIOLOGY

The term **acute coronary syndrome (ACS)** is used to describe patients who have either *unstable* angina or an acute myocardial infarction. In ACS, it is believed that the atherosclerotic plaque in the coronary artery *ruptures*, resulting in platelet aggregation ("clumping"), thrombus (clot) formation, and vasoconstriction (Fig. 38-1). The amount of disruption of the atherosclerotic plaque determines the degree of coronary artery obstruction (blockage) and the specific disease process. The artery has to

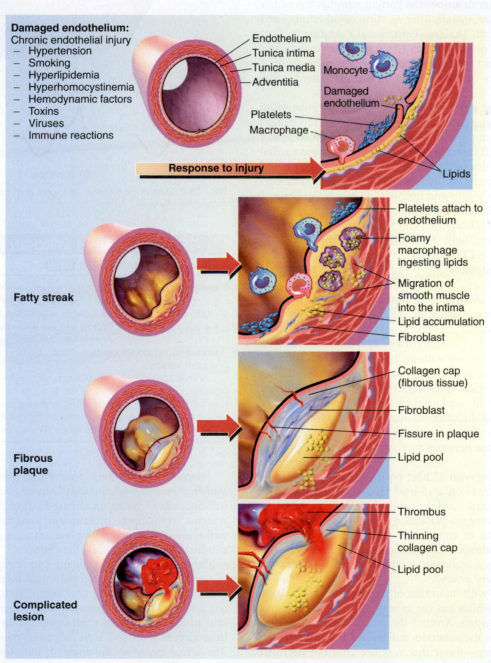

Damaged endothelium:
Chronic endothelial injury
- Hypertension
- Smoking
- Hyperlipidemia
- Hyperhomocystinemia
- Hemodynamic factors
- Toxins
- Viruses
- Immune reactions

Endothelium
Tunica intima
Tunica media
Adventitia
Monocyte
Damaged endothelium
Platelets
Macrophage

Response to injury

Lipids

Fatty streak

Platelets attach to endothelium
Foamy macrophage ingesting lipids
Migration of smooth muscle into the intima
Lipid accumulation
Fibroblast

Fibrous plaque

Collagen cap (fibrous tissue)
Fibroblast
Fissure in plaque
Lipid pool

Complicated lesion

Thrombus
Thinning collagen cap
Lipid pool

FIG. 38-1 A cross-section of an atherosclerotic coronary artery. (From Huether S. E., McCance, K. L., Brashers, V. L., & Rote, N. S. [2014]. *Understanding pathophysiology* [6th ed.]. St. Louis: Mosby.)

have at least 40% plaque accumulation before it starts to block blood flow (McCance et al., 2014).

Unstable angina (UA) is chest pain or discomfort that occurs at rest or with exertion and causes severe activity limitation. An increase in the number of attacks and in the intensity of the pressure indicates UA. The pressure may last longer than 15 minutes or may be poorly relieved by rest or nitroglycerin. Unstable angina describes a variety of disorders, including *new-onset angina*, *variant (Prinzmetal's) angina*, and *pre-infarction angina*. *Patients with unstable angina may present with ST changes on a 12-lead ECG but do not have changes in troponin levels.* Ischemia is present but is not severe enough to cause detectable myocardial damage or cell death. As the assays for troponins become more sensitive, the diagnosis of UA is decreasing.

New-onset angina describes the patient who has his or her first angina symptoms, usually after exertion or other increased demands on the heart. Variant (Prinzmetal's) angina is chest pain or discomfort resulting from coronary artery spasm and typically occurs after rest. Pre-infarction angina refers to chest pain that occurs in the days or weeks before a myocardial infarction.

The most serious acute coronary syndrome is myocardial infarction (MI), often referred to as *acute MI* or *AMI*. Undiagnosed or untreated angina can lead to this very serious health problem. Myocardial infarction (MI) occurs when myocardial tissue is abruptly and severely deprived of oxygen. When blood flow is quickly reduced by 80% to 90%, ischemia develops. Ischemia can lead to injury and necrosis of myocardial tissue if blood flow is not restored. There are two types of MI: non–ST-segment elevation MI (NSTEMI) and ST elevation MI (STEMI).

Patients presenting with NSTEMI typically have ST and T-wave changes on a 12-lead ECG. This indicates myocardial ischemia. Initially troponin may be normal, but it elevates over the next 3 to 12 hours. The combination of changes on the ECG and elevation in cardiac troponin indicates myocardial cell death or necrosis. Causes of NSTEMI include coronary vasospasm, spontaneous dissection, and sluggish blood flow due to narrowing of the coronary artery. It is important to note that changes in ECG along with elevation of troponin should always be assessed in conjunction with the clinical presentation and history of the patient. Patients with elevated troponin and ECG changes without typical symptoms of acute coronary syndrome (i.e., chest discomfort, shortness of breath, nausea) typically have a condition other than CAD (such as sepsis), causing the imbalance between myocardial oxygen supply and demand.

Patients presenting with STEMI typically have ST elevation in two contiguous leads on a 12-lead ECG. This indicates MI/necrosis. STEMI is attributable to rupture of the fibrous atherosclerotic plaque leading to platelet aggregation and thrombus formation at the site of rupture (McCance et al., 2014). *The thrombus causes an abrupt 100% occlusion to the coronary artery, is a medical emergency, and requires immediate revascularization of the blocked coronary artery.*

Often MIs begin with infarction of the subendocardial layer of cardiac muscle, which has the *greatest* oxygen *demand* and the *poorest* oxygen *supply*. Around the initial area of infarction (zone of necrosis) in the subendocardium are two other zones: (1) the zone of injury—tissue that is injured but not necrotic; and (2) the zone of ischemia—tissue that is oxygen deprived. This pattern is illustrated in Fig. 38-2.

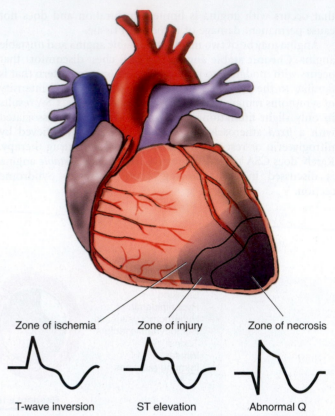

Zone of ischemia | Zone of injury | Zone of necrosis

T-wave inversion | ST elevation | Abnormal Q

FIG. 38-2 Electrocardiographic changes and patterns associated with myocardial infarction.

GENDER HEALTH CONSIDERATIONS
Patient-Centered Care QSEN

Many women with symptomatic ischemic heart disease or abnormal stress testing do not have abnormal coronary angiography. Studies implicate microvascular disease or endothelial dysfunction or both as the causes for risk for CAD in women. Endothelial dysfunction is the inability of the arteries and arterioles to dilate due to lack of nitric oxide production by the endothelium. Nitric oxide is a relaxant of vascular smooth muscle.

Women typically have smaller coronary arteries and frequently have plaque that breaks off and travels into the small vessels to form an embolus (clot). Positive remodeling, or outward remodeling (lesions that protrude outward), is more common in women (McCance et al., 2014). This outpouching may be missed on coronary angiography.

Infarction is a dynamic process that does not occur instantly. Rather, it evolves over a period of several hours. Hypoxemia from ischemia may lead to local vasodilation of blood vessels and acidosis. Potassium, calcium, and magnesium imbalances, as well as acidosis at the cellular level, may cause changes in normal conduction and contractile functions.

Catecholamines (epinephrine and norepinephrine) released in response to hypoxia and pain may increase the heart's rate, contractility, and afterload. These factors increase *oxygen* requirements in tissue that is already oxygen deprived. This may lead to life-threatening ventricular dysrhythmias. The area of infarction may extend into the zones of injury and ischemia. The actual extent of the zone of infarction depends on three factors: collateral circulation, anaerobic metabolism, and workload demands on the myocardium.

Obvious physical changes do not occur in the heart until 6 hours after the infarction, when the infarcted region appears blue and swollen. *These changes explain the need for intervention within the first 4 to 6 hours of symptom onset!* After 48 hours, the infarcted area turns gray with yellow streaks as neutrophils invade the tissue and begin to remove the necrotic cells. By 8 to 10 days after infarction, granulation tissue forms at the edges of the necrotic tissue. Over a 2- to 3-month period, the necrotic area eventually develops into a shrunken, thin, firm scar. Scar tissue permanently changes the size and shape of the entire left ventricle, called ventricular remodeling. Remodeling may decrease left ventricular function, cause heart failure, and increase morbidity and mortality. The scarred tissue does not contract, nor does it conduct electrically. Thus this area is often the cause of chronic ventricular dysrhythmias surrounding the infarcted zone (McCance et al., 2014).

The patient's response to an MI also depends on which coronary artery or arteries were obstructed and which part of the left ventricle wall was damaged: anterior, septal, lateral, inferior, or posterior. Fig. 33-3 shows the location of the major coronary arteries.

Obstruction of the left anterior descending (LAD) artery causes *anterior* or *septal* MIs because it perfuses the anterior wall and most of the septum of the left ventricle. Patients with anterior wall MIs (AWMIs) have the highest mortality rate because they are most likely to have left ventricular failure and dysrhythmias from damage to the left ventricle.

The circumflex artery supplies the lateral wall of the left ventricle and possibly portions of the posterior wall or the sinoatrial (SA) and atrioventricular (AV) nodes. Patients with obstruction of the circumflex artery may experience a *posterior* wall MI (PWMI) or a *lateral* wall MI (LWMI) and sinus dysrhythmias.

In most people, the right coronary artery (RCA) supplies most of the SA and AV nodes, as well as the right ventricle and inferior or diaphragmatic portion of the left ventricle. Patients with obstruction of the RCA often have inferior wall MIs (IWMIs). About half of all inferior wall MIs are associated with an occlusion of the RCA, causing significant damage to the right ventricle. *Thus it is important to obtain a "right-sided" ECG to assess for right ventricular involvement.*

Etiology and Genetic Risk

Atherosclerosis is the primary factor in the development of CAD. Numerous risk factors, both nonmodifiable and modifiable, contribute to atherosclerosis and subsequently to CAD. Atherosclerosis is described in Chapter 36. Nonmodifiable and modifiable risk factors are described in detail in Chapter 33. Chart 38-1 also discusses risk factors for CAD.

Metabolic syndrome, also called *syndrome X,* has been recognized as a risk factor for cardiovascular (CV) disease and is being researched aggressively. Patients who have three of the factors in Table 38-1 are diagnosed with metabolic syndrome. This health problem increases the risk for developing diabetes and CAD. About 22.9% of adults older than 20 years in the United States have metabolic syndrome (Mozaffarian et al., 2016). Prevalence is higher in Mexican Americans, American Indians, and Alaska Native people living in the southwestern United States. This increase is likely a result of physical inactivity and the current obesity epidemic. Management is aimed at reducing risks, managing hypertension, and preventing complications.

CHART 38-1 Patient and Family Education: Preparing for Self-Management

Prevention of Coronary Artery Disease

Smoking/Tobacco Use
- If you smoke or use tobacco, quit.
- If you don't smoke or use tobacco, don't start.

Diet
- Consume sufficient calories for your body to include:
  - 5% to 6% from saturated fats
  - Avoiding *trans* fatty acids
- Limit your cholesterol intake to less than 200 mg/day.
- Limit your sodium intake as specified by your health care provider, or under 1500 mg/day, if possible.

Cholesterol
- Have your lipid levels checked regularly.
- If your cholesterol and LDL-C levels are elevated, follow your health care provider's advice, including taking statin medications as indicated.

Physical Activity
- If you are middle-age or older or have a history of medical problems, check with your health care provider before starting an exercise program.
- Exercise periods should be at least 40 minutes long with 10-minute warm-up and 5-minute cool-down periods.
- If you cannot exercise moderately 3 to 4 times each week, walk daily for 30 minutes at a comfortable pace.
- If you cannot walk 30 minutes daily, walk any distance you can (e.g., park farther away from a site than necessary; use the stairs, not the elevator, to go one floor up or two floors down).

Diabetes Mellitus
- Manage your diabetes with your health care provider.

Hypertension
- Have your blood pressure checked regularly.
- If your blood pressure is elevated, follow your health care provider's advice.
- Continue to monitor your blood pressure at regular intervals.

Obesity
- Avoid severely restrictive or fad diets.
- Restrict intake of saturated fats, sweets, sweetened beverages, and cholesterol-rich foods.
- Increase your physical activity.

LDL-C, Low-density lipoprotein–cholesterol.

CULTURAL/SPIRITUAL CONSIDERATIONS

Patient-Centered Care QSEN

Several groups have a higher genetic risk for CAD than others. For example, African-American and Hispanic women have higher CAD risk factors than white women of the same socioeconomic status. Of American Indians and Alaskan Natives 18 years of age and older, about 46.7% have one or more CAD risk factors (hypertension [HTN], smoking, high cholesterol, excess weight, or diabetes mellitus). The leading cause of death for both men and women in the Euro-American population is cardiovascular disease, even though they may not have genetic predispositions to developing cardiovascular risk factors (Mozaffarian et al., 2016).

TABLE 38-1 Indicators of Risk Factors for Metabolic Syndrome

RISK FACTOR	INDICATOR
Hypertension	Either blood pressure of 130/85 mm Hg or higher OR taking antihypertensive drug(s)
Decreased HDL-C (usually with high LDL-C) level	Either HDL-C <45 mg/dL for men or <55 mg/dL for women OR taking an anticholesterol drug
Increased level of triglycerides	Either 160 mg/dL or higher for men or 135 mg/dL or higher for women OR taking an anticholesterol drug
Increased fasting blood glucose (caused by diabetes, glucose intolerance, or insulin resistance)	Either 100 mg/dL or higher OR taking antidiabetic drug(s)
Large waist size (excessive abdominal fat causing central obesity)	40 inches (102 cm) or greater for men or 35 inches (89 cm) or greater for women

HDL-C, High-density lipoprotein–cholesterol; *LDL-C,* low-density lipoprotein–cholesterol.

GENDER HEALTH CONSIDERATIONS
Patient-Centered Care QSEN

Age is the most important risk factor for developing CAD in women. The older a woman is, the more likely it is that she will have the disease. When compared with men, women are usually 10 years older when they have CAD. Only 56% of women are aware that heart disease is the leading cause of death in women, and even fewer can identify the symptoms of a heart attack (Mozaffarian et al., 2016). Women who have MIs have a greater risk for dying during hospitalization. When they are older than 40 years, women are more likely than men to die within 1 year after their MI. If women do survive, they are less likely to participate in cardiac rehabilitation programs (Mozaffarian et al., 2016).

Incidence and Prevalence

The average age of a person having a first MI is 65.1 years for men and 72 years for women (Mozaffarian et al., 2016). Every 34 seconds, a person in the United States has a major coronary event, and every 84 seconds, an American will die from CAD (Mozaffarian et al., 2016). Many people die from CAD without being hospitalized. Most of these are sudden deaths caused by cardiac arrest.

GENDER HEALTH CONSIDERATION QSEN
Patient-Centered Care

Premenopausal women have a lower incidence of MI than men. However, for postmenopausal women in their 70s or older, the incidence of MI equals that of men. Family history is also a risk factor for women; those whose parents had CAD are more susceptible to the disease. Women with abdominal obesity (androidal shape) and metabolic syndrome are also at increased risk for CAD. Because lesbian and bisexual women have a higher incidence of obesity and smoking than women who are not lesbian or bisexual, they should be considered an especially high-risk group for CAD. The reasons for these trends are not known (Roberts, 2015).

Many patients who survive MIs are not able to return to work. CAD is the leading cause of premature, permanent disability in the United States and the world.

Health Promotion and Maintenance

Ninety-five percent of sudden cardiac arrest victims die before reaching the hospital, largely because of ventricular fibrillation ("v fib"). To help combat this problem, automatic external defibrillators (AEDs) are found in many public places, such as in shopping centers and on airplanes. Employees are taught how to use these devices if a sudden cardiac arrest occurs. Some patients with diagnosed CAD have AEDs in their homes or at work. The procedure for using this device is described in Chapter 34.

Health promotion efforts are directed toward controlling or altering modifiable risk factors for CAD. For patients at risk for coronary artery disease (CAD), especially MI, assess specific risk factors and implement an individualized health teaching plan. Teach people who have one or more of these risk factors the importance of modifying or eliminating them to decrease their chances of CAD (see Chart 38-1). Chapter 36 describes health teaching and evidence-based interventions for preventing and managing atherosclerosis and hypertension. Smoking cessation is discussed in Chapter 27.

❓ NCLEX EXAMINATION CHALLENGE 38-1
Health Promotion and Maintenance

A 48-year-old female client having an annual physical asks the nurse about her risk for developing a myocardial infarction (MI). The nurse discusses risk factors with the client.
  Which modifiable risk factors will the nurse assess to guide the client's teaching plan? **Select all that apply.**
A. Older age
B. Tobacco use
C. Female
D. High-fat diet
E. Family history
F. Obesity

❖ INTERPROFESSIONAL COLLABORATIVE CARE
◆ Assessment: Noticing

History. If symptoms of CAD are present at the time of the interview, delay collecting data until interventions for symptom relief, vital sign instability, and dysrhythmias are started and discomfort resolves. If the patient had pain, ask about how he or she has managed the discomfort and other symptoms and which drugs he or she may be taking. When the patient is pain free, obtain information about family history and modifiable risk factors, including eating habits, lifestyle, and physical activity levels. Ask about a history of smoking and how much alcohol is consumed each day. Collaborate with the dietitian to assess current body mass index (BMI) and weight as needed.

Physical Assessment/Signs and Symptoms. Rapid assessment of the patient with chest pain or other presenting symptoms is crucial. It is important to differentiate among the types of chest pain and identify the source. Question the patient to determine the characteristics of the alterations in COMFORT. However, patients may deny pain and report that they feel "pressure." Appropriate questions to ask concerning the discomfort include onset, location, radiation, intensity, duration, and precipitating and relieving factors.

If pain is present, ask the patient if the pain is in the chest, epigastric area, jaw, back, shoulder, or arm. Ask the patient to rate the pain on a scale of 0 to 10, with 10 being the highest level of discomfort. Some patients describe the discomfort as tightness, a burning sensation, pressure, or indigestion. A complete pain assessment is described in Chapter 4.

GENDER HEALTH CONSIDERATIONS

Patient-Centered Care QSEN

> *Many women of any age experience atypical angina.* **Atypical angina** manifests as indigestion, pain between the shoulders, an aching jaw, or a choking sensation that occurs with exertion. These symptoms typically manifest during stressful circumstances or ADLs. Women may curtail activity as a result of angina, and health care providers need to ask about changes in routine. Symptoms in women typically include chest discomfort, unusual fatigue, and dyspnea (McSweeney et al., 2014).

Chart 38-2 provides a comparison of angina and infarction pain. Because angina pain is ischemic pain, it usually improves when the imbalance between oxygen supply and demand is resolved. For example, rest reduces tissue demands, and nitroglycerin improves oxygen supply. Discomfort from a myocardial infarction (MI) does not usually resolve with these measures. Ask about any associated symptoms, including *nausea, vomiting, diaphoresis, dizziness, weakness, palpitations,* and *shortness of breath.*

Assess *blood pressure* and *heart rate.* Interpret the patient's cardiac rhythm and presence of *dysrhythmias.* Sinus tachycardia with premature ventricular contractions (PVCs) frequently occurs in the first few hours after an MI.

Next assess *distal peripheral pulses* and *skin temperature.* The skin should be warm with all pulses palpable. In the patient with

CHART 38-2 Key Features

Angina and Myocardial Infarction

ANGINA	MYOCARDIAL INFARCTION
• Substernal chest discomfort:	• Pain or discomfort:
• Radiating to the left arm	• Substernal chest pain/pressure radiating to the left arm
• Precipitated by exertion or stress (or rest in variant angina)	• Pain or discomfort in jaw, back, shoulder, or abdomen
• Relieved by nitroglycerin or rest	• Occurring without cause, usually in the morning
• Lasting less than 15 minutes	• Relieved only by opioids
• Few, if any, associated symptoms	• Lasting 30 minutes or more
	• Frequent associated symptoms:
	• Nausea/vomiting
	• Diaphoresis
	• Dyspnea
	• Feelings of fear and anxiety
	• Dysrhythmias
	• Fatigue
	• Palpitations
	• Epigastric distress
	• Anxiety
	• Dizziness
	• Disorientation/acute confusion
	• Feeling "short of breath"

CONSIDERATIONS FOR OLDER ADULTS

Patient-Centered Care QSEN

> The presence of associated symptoms without chest discomfort is significant. In up to 40% of all patients with MI, primarily older women and patients with diabetes, chest pain, or discomfort may be mild or absent. Instead they have associated symptoms. Some older patients may think they are having indigestion and therefore not recognize that they are having an MI. Others report shortness of breath as the only symptom. Because of the ambiguity of symptoms, the older adult is more likely to wait before seeking treatment. The major manifestation of MI in people older than 80 years may be disorientation or acute confusion because of poor cardiac output and inadequate coronary perfusion.
>
> In some older adults with MI, absence of chest pain may be caused by cognitive impairment or inability to verbalize pain sensation. However, in most cases it is probably the result of increased collateral circulation. Silent myocardial ischemia increases the incidence of new coronary events and should be treated aggressively.

unstable angina or MI, poor cardiac output may be manifested by cool, diaphoretic ("sweaty") skin and diminished or absent pulses. *Auscultate for an S_3 gallop, which often indicates heart failure—a serious and common complication of MI.* In adults, the S_3 heart sound is heard with the bell of the stethoscope over the apex of the heart (Jarvis, 2016).

Assess the *respiratory rate* and breath sounds for signs of heart failure. An increased respiratory rate is common because of anxiety and pain, but *crackles or wheezes* may indicate *left-sided* heart failure. Assess for the presence of jugular venous distention and peripheral edema.

The patient with MI may experience a *temperature elevation* for several days after infarction. Temperatures as high as 102°F (38.9°C) may occur in response to myocardial necrosis, indicating the inflammatory response.

Psychosocial Assessment. Denial is a common early reaction to chest discomfort associated with angina or MI. On average, the patient with an acute MI waits more than 2 hours before seeking medical attention. Often he or she rationalizes that symptoms are caused by indigestion or overexertion. In some situations, denial is a normal part of adapting to a stressful event. However, denial that interferes with identifying a symptom such as chest discomfort can be harmful. Explain the importance of reporting any discomfort to the health care provider.

Fear, depression, anxiety, and anger are other common reactions of many patients and their families. Assist in identifying these feelings. Encourage them to explain their understanding of the event and clarify any misconceptions.

Laboratory Assessment. Although there is no single test to diagnose MI, the most common laboratory tests include troponins T and I. Troponin is specific for MI and cardiac necrosis. Troponins T and I rise quickly. These tests are described in more detail in Chapter 33. If serial troponins are negative, the patient has a nuclear medicine test such as those described in the next section.

Imaging Assessment. Unless there is associated cardiac dysfunction (e.g., valve disease) or heart failure, a chest x-ray is not diagnostic for angina or MI. A chest x-ray may be performed to help rule out aortic dissection, which may mimic an MI. If the x-ray demonstrates a widened mediastinum, further testing for aortic dissection with either transesophageal echography (TEE) or CT scan is needed.

Thallium scans use radioisotope imaging to assess for ischemia or necrotic muscle tissue related to angina or MI. Areas of decreased or absent PERFUSION, referred to as *cold spots,* identify ischemia or infarction. Thallium may be used with the exercise tolerance test. Dipyridamole (Persantine) thallium scanning (DTS) may also be used.

Contrast-enhanced cardiovascular magnetic resonance (CMR) imaging may also be done as a noninvasive approach to detect CAD. *Echocardiography* may be used to visualize the structures of the heart.

Use of the 64-slice computed tomography coronary angiography (CTCA) has been found to be helpful in diagnosing CAD in symptomatic patients identified as having a "low- or intermediate-pretest probability" risk for CAD. This new generation of high-speed CT scanners is becoming a highly reliable, noninvasive way to evaluate CAD.

Other Diagnostic Assessment. Twelve-lead ECGs allow the health care provider to examine the heart from varying perspectives. By identifying the lead(s) in which ECG changes are occurring, the health care provider can identify both the occurrence and the location of ischemia (angina) or necrosis (infarction). In addition to the traditional 12-lead ECG, the health care provider may request a "right-sided" or 18-lead ECG to determine whether ischemia or infarction has occurred in the right ventricle. *The ECG should be obtained within 10 minutes of patient presentation with chest discomfort!*

An ischemic myocardium does not repolarize normally. Thus 12-lead ECGs obtained during an angina episode reveal ST depression, T-wave inversion, or both. Variant angina, caused by coronary vasospasm (vessel spasm), usually causes elevation of the ST segment during angina attacks. These ST and T-wave changes usually subside when the ischemia is resolved and pain is relieved. However, the T wave may remain flat or inverted for a period of time. If the patient is not experiencing angina at the moment of the test, the ECG is usually normal unless he or she has evidence of an old MI.

When infarction occurs, one of two ECG changes is usually observed: ST-elevation MI (STEMI), or non–ST-elevation MI (NSTEMI). An abnormal Q wave (wider than 0.04 seconds or more than one third the height of the QRS complex) may develop, depending on the amount of myocardium that has necrosed. Women having an MI often present with an NSTEMI.

The Q wave may develop because necrotic cells do not conduct electrical stimuli. Hours to days after the MI, the ST-segment and T-wave changes return to normal. However, when the Q wave exists, it may become permanent. The Q waves may disappear after a number of years, but their absence does not necessarily mean that the patient has not had an MI.

After the acute stages of an unstable angina episode, the health care provider often requests an *exercise tolerance test (stress test)* on a treadmill to assess for ECG changes consistent with ischemia, evaluate medical therapy, and identify those who might benefit from invasive therapy. Pharmacologic stress-testing agents such as dobutamine (Dobutrex) may be used instead of the treadmill. Treadmill exercise testing is only moderately accurate for women when compared with men. The results are also not as reliable in tall, obese men when compared with short, thinner men. In women with suspected CAD, stress echocardiography or single photon emission CT (SPECT) should be performed.

Cardiac catheterization may be performed to determine the extent and exact location of coronary artery obstructions. It allows the cardiologist and cardiac surgeon to identify patients who might benefit from percutaneous coronary intervention (PCI) or from coronary artery bypass grafting (CABG). Each of these diagnostic tests is described in detail in Chapter 33.

◆ Analysis: Interpreting

The patient with coronary artery disease (CAD) may have either stable angina or acute coronary syndrome (ACS). If ACS is suspected or cannot be completely ruled out, the patient is admitted to a telemetry unit for continuous monitoring or to a critical care unit if hemodynamically unstable.

The priority collaborative problems for most patients with ACS include:

1. Acute Pain due to an imbalance between myocardial oxygen supply and demand
2. Decreased myocardial tissue perfusion due to interruption of arterial blood flow
3. Decreased functional ability due to fatigue caused by the imbalance between oxygen supply and demand
4. Decreased ability to cope due to the effects of acute illness and major changes in lifestyle
5. Potential for dysrhythmias due to ischemia and ventricular irritability
6. Potential for heart failure due to left ventricular dysfunction

◆ Planning and Implementation: Responding

Astute assessment skills, timely analysis of troponin, and analysis of the 12-lead ECG (or 18-lead ECG for a suspected right ventricular infarction) are essential to ensure appropriate patient care management. This is particularly important since the average time a patient waits before seeking treatment is over 2 hours. This delay lessens the 4- to 6-hour window of opportunity for the most advantageous treatment with percutaneous intervention.

Managing Acute Pain. Patients with *diabetes mellitus* and CAD may not experience chest pain or pressure because of diabetic neuropathy. In this patient population, the onset of ACS may be signaled by new onset of atrial fibrillation. With new-onset atrial fibrillation, a cardiac workup should be done to rule out ACS.

Planning: Expected Outcomes. The expected outcome is that the patient will verbalize increased COMFORT as a result of prompt collaborative interventions to increase PERFUSION.

Interventions. The purpose of interprofessional collaborative care is to promote COMFORT, decrease myocardial oxygen demand, and increase PERFUSION (myocardial oxygen supply).

Emergency Care: Myocardial Infarction. Evaluate any report of pain, obtain vital signs, ensure an IV access, and notify the health care provider of the patient's condition. Chart 38-3 summarizes the emergency interventions for the patient with symptoms of CAD.

Pain relief helps increase the oxygen supply and decrease myocardial oxygen demand. The American Heart Association (AHA) recommends several pain management strategies, including nitroglycerin, morphine sulfate, and oxygen.

Drug Therapy. At home or in the hospital, the patient may take nitroglycerin to relieve episodic anginal pain. Aspirin 325 mg, an antiplatelet drug, may also be taken daily to prevent clots that further block coronary arteries.

Nitroglycerin (NTG), a nitrate often referred to as *nitro,* increases collateral blood flow, redistributes blood flow toward the subendocardium, and dilates the coronary arteries. In addition, it decreases myocardial oxygen demand by peripheral vasodilation, which decreases both preload and afterload.

Emergency Care of the Patient With Chest Discomfort

- Assess airway, breathing, and circulation (ABCs). Defibrillate as needed.
- Provide continuous ECG monitoring.
- Obtain the patient's description of pain or discomfort.
- Obtain the patient's vital signs (blood pressure, pulse, respiration).
- Assess/provide vascular access.
- Consult chest pain protocol or notify the health care provider or Rapid Response Team for specific intervention.
- Obtain a 12-lead ECG within 10 minutes of report of chest pain.
- Provide pain relief medication and aspirin (non–enteric coated) as prescribed.
- Administer oxygen therapy to maintain oxygen saturation ≥90%.
- Remain calm. Stay with the patient if possible.
- Assess the patient's vital signs and intensity of pain 5 minutes after administration of medication.
- Remedicate with prescribed drugs (if vital signs remain stable) and check the patient every 5 minutes.
- Notify the provider if vital signs deteriorate.

! **NURSING SAFETY PRIORITY** QSEN

Drug Alert

Before administering NTG, ensure that the patient has not taken any phosphodiesterase inhibitors for erectile dysfunction such as sildenafil (Viagra, Revatio), tadalafil (Cialis), or vardenafil (Levitra) within the past 24 to 48 hours. Concomitant use of NTG with these inhibitors can cause profound hypotension. Remind patients not to take these medications within 24 to 48 hours of one another.

Some phosphodiesterase inhibitors are also used in the treatment of pulmonary arterial hypertension (PAH). Patients with PAH cannot stop taking the phosphodiesterase inhibitor. As a result, NTG is contraindicated in this patient population.

Teach the patient to hold the NTG tablet under the tongue and drink 5 mL (1 teaspoon) of water, if necessary, to allow the tablet to dissolve. NTG spray is also available and is more quickly absorbed. Pain relief should begin within 1 to 2 minutes and should be clearly evident in 3 to 5 minutes. After 5 minutes, recheck the patient's pain intensity and vital signs. If the blood pressure (BP) is less than 100 mm Hg systolic or 25 mm Hg lower than the previous reading, lower the head of the bed and notify the health care provider.

If the patient is experiencing some but not complete relief and vital signs remain stable, another NTG tablet or spray may be used. In 5-minute increments, a total of three doses may be administered in an attempt to relieve angina pain. If the patient uses NTG spray instead of the tablet, teach him or her to sit upright and spray the dose under the tongue. NTG topical patches should be placed below the nipple line to decrease discomfort.

Angina usually responds to NTG. The patient typically states that the pain is relieved or markedly diminished. When simple measures, such as taking three sublingual nitroglycerin tablets, in timed increments, one after the other, do not relieve chest discomfort, the patient may be experiencing an MI.

When ischemia persists, the health care provider may prescribe IV NTG for management of the chest pain. Begin the drug infusion slowly, checking the blood pressure (BP) and pain level every 3 to 5 minutes. The NTG dose is increased until the pain is relieved, the BP falls excessively, or the maximum prescribed dose is reached (Chart 38-4).

! **NURSING SAFETY PRIORITY** QSEN

Critical Rescue

If the patient is experiencing an MI, prepare him or her for transfer to a specialized unit where close monitoring and appropriate management can be provided. If the patient is at home or in the community, call 911 for transfer to the closest emergency department.

When the pain or other symptoms have subsided and the patient is stabilized, the health care provider may change the drug to an oral or topical nitrate. During administration of long-term oral and topical nitrates, an 8- to 12-hour nitrate-free period should be maintained to prevent tolerance. The patient may initially report a headache. Give acetaminophen (Tylenol, Abenol ♣) before the nitrate to ease some of this discomfort.

The health care provider may prescribe *morphine sulfate (MS)* to relieve discomfort that is unresponsive to nitroglycerin. Morphine promotes COMFORT, decreases myocardial oxygen demand, relaxes smooth muscle, and reduces circulating catecholamines. It is usually administered in 1- to 5-mg doses IV every 5 to 30 minutes until the maximum prescribed dose is reached or the patient experiences relief or signs of toxicity. Monitor for adverse effects of morphine, which include respiratory depression, hypotension, bradycardia, and severe vomiting. Treatment for morphine toxicity is naloxone (Narcan) 0.2 to 0.8 mg IV, vasopressor drugs, IV fluids, and oxygen therapy.

If hypoxemia is present, the health care provider may prescribe oxygen at a flow of 2 to 4 L/min to maintain an arterial oxygen saturation of 90% or higher. The use of oxygen in the absence of hypoxemia has been shown to increase coronary vascular resistance, decrease coronary blood flow, and increase mortality. Monitor the patient's vital signs and cardiac rhythm every few minutes. If the BP is stable, help the patient assume any position of comfort. Placing the patient in semi-Fowler's position often enhances comfort and tissue oxygenation. A quiet, calm environment and explanations of interventions often reduce anxiety and help relieve chest pain. If needed, remind the patient to take several deep breaths to increase oxygenation.

These strategies are often enough to relieve the pain. If they are not adequate, additional interventions identified in the Increasing Myocardial Tissue Perfusion section may be attempted.

⚙ **CLINICAL JUDGMENT CHALLENGE 38-1**

Patient-Centered Care; Evidence-Based Practice; Clinical Judgment; Informatics QSEN

A 70-year-old man has been having periods of chest pain and pressure that have been ignored until he became short of breath and diaphoretic with the episode of chest pain. The patient called 911 and was taken via ambulance to the emergency department (ED).

1. As his ED nurse, what is your first action in response to his report of chest pain? What evidence supports this decision?
2. The provider prescribes nitroglycerin for pain. What assessment will you perform before administering this drug and why? What administration route do you anticipate?
3. What other drugs might the provider prescribe at this time and why?
4. The patient's ECG indicated ST elevation and elevated troponins. What does the nurse anticipate in the care of this patient?
5. What will you document in the electronic health record about this patient's care?

CHART 38-4 **Common Examples of Drug Therapy**

Acute Coronary Syndrome (Nitrates, Beta Blockers, Antiplatelets)

DRUG CATEGORY	NURSING IMPLICATIONS
Nitrates Common examples of nitrates: • Sublingual tablets: Nitrostat, Nitroquick • Sublingual spray: Nitrolingual • Transdermal nitroglycerin: Minitran, Nitro Dur, Nitrek • Isosorbide dinitrate (Isordil, Iso-Bid) • Isosorbide mononitrate (Imdur)	Monitor blood pressure (BP) and pay close attention to orthostatic changes *because a decrease in BP occurs with vasodilation.* • Dizziness can occur with drop in BP. Monitor for headache *because vasodilation is generalized.* **Do not administer to patients taking drugs used to treat sexual dysfunction (e.g., sildenafil, tadalafil, vardenafil)** *because very serious, possibly fatal interactions can occur.* Always assess for pain relief *because additional medication may be required.* With sublingual tablets or spray: • Instruct patient to lie down when taking *because the hypotensive response can be dramatic.* • Tablets can be taken every 5 minutes *for pain relief,* up to 3 tablets. • Be sure to allow the tablet to dissolve *because it is absorbed through the mucous membranes.* • Check expiration date *because the efficacy decreases over time and should be replaced every 3-5 months.* With transdermal nitroglycerin: • Apply the patch to a clean, dry, hairless area *because the medication will be better absorbed.* • Rotate application sites *to prevent skin irritation.* • Remove the patch before defibrillation *to prevent burns.* • Remove patch after 12-14 hours each day *to prevent drug tolerance.*
Beta Blockers Common examples of beta blockers: • Carvedilol (Coreg, Coreg CR) • Metoprolol (Lopressor, Toprol XL, Betaloc ✦), a cardioselective beta-adrenergic blocker	Assess HR and BP before administration *because beta blockers cause a decrease in HR and cardiac output and suppress renin activity.* • Do not administer if heart rate is <50-60 beats/min. • Hold for systolic <90-100 mm Hg. Observe for signs of heart failure such as cough, edema, shortness of breath, and weight gain *because this can occur with a decrease in cardiac output.* Assess for wheezing and shortness of breath *because beta₂-blocking effects in the lungs can cause bronchoconstriction.*

Antiplatelets
Common examples of antiplatelets:
• Aspirin (Ecotrin, Asaphen ✦)
• P2Y12 Inhibitors
  • Clopidogrel (Plavix)
  • Prasugrel (Effient)
  • Ticagrelor (Brilinta)
  • Cangrelor (Kengreal)
• PAR-1 Inhibitor
  • Vorapaxar sulfate (Zontivity)
	Inform patients to report any unusual bleeding or bruising *because bleeding is a side effect for all medications in this category.*
	Avoid over-the-counter pain medications that contain additional aspirin.
	With aspirin therapy:
	• Take with food *because gastric irritation may occur.*
	• Assess for ringing in ears *because this can be a sign of aspirin toxicity.*
	• Teach patient that aspirin is an important cardiac medication that should not be stopped unless indicated by the provider *as studies indicate better survival rates for patients with CAD receiving aspirin.*
	With P2Y12 platelet inhibitors:
	• Take with food *because drug can cause diarrhea and GI upset.*
	• **Do not confuse Plavix with Paxil.**

Increasing Myocardial Tissue Perfusion

Planning: Expected Outcomes. The primary outcome is that the patient will have increased myocardial PERFUSION as evidenced by an adequate cardiac output, normal sinus rhythm, and vital signs within normal limits.

Interventions. Because myocardial infarction (MI) is a dynamic process, restoring PERFUSION to the injured area (usually within 4 to 6 hours for NSTEMI and 60 to 90 minutes for STEMI) often limits the amount of extension and improves left ventricular function. Complete, sustained reperfusion of coronary arteries after an acute coronary syndrome (ACS) has decreased mortality rates.

Drug Therapy. *Aspirin (ASA)* therapy is recommended by the American College of Cardiology (ACC) and the American Heart Association (AHA). It inhibits both platelet aggregation and vasoconstriction, thereby decreasing the likelihood of thrombosis. *If the patient has new-onset angina at home, teach him or her*

to chew aspirin 325 mg (4 "baby aspirins" that are 81 mg each) immediately and call 911! The antiplatelet effect of ASA begins within 1 hour of use and continues for several days. In the hospital setting, aspirin should be given on arrival to the emergency department or when an MI occurs in the hospital. Administer 81 to 325 mg non–enteric-coated aspirin every day to all patients with suspected CAD unless absolutely contraindicated. Instruct the patient to chew and swallow the drug and continue taking it as prescribed unless adverse effects occur.

Glycoprotein (GP) IIb/IIIa inhibitors such as abciximab (ReoPro), eptifibatide (Integrilin), or tirofiban (Aggrastat) may be administered IV to prevent fibrinogen from attaching to activated platelets at the site of a thrombus. These medications are used in unstable angina and NSTEMI. They are also given before and during percutaneous coronary intervention (PCI) to maintain patency of an artery with a large clot and are given with fibrinolytic agents after STEMI.

Antiplatelets, such as clopidogrel (Plavix) or ticagrelor (Brilinta), also known as P2Y12 platelet inhibitors, may be given with an initial loading dose followed by a daily dose for up to 12 months after diagnosis. Prasugrel (Effient) is only recommended in those undergoing primary coronary intervention, discussed later in this chapter. These oral agents work to prevent platelets from aggregating (clumping) together to form clots. A newly approved antiplatelet agent (also known as a protease-activated receptor inhibitor PAR-1), vorapaxar (Zontivity), is shown to decrease the risk of recurrent MI when added to the regimen of aspirin and clopidogrel. The main side effect is bleeding, including an increased risk of intracranial hemorrhage.

In addition to antiplatelet therapy, *anticoagulation therapy* may also be used to prevent clot formation. Choice of anticoagulant is determined by provider preference because national guidelines do not currently recommend one agent over another. Anticoagulation is stopped before cardiac catheterization and is usually not continued following coronary intervention unless a high risk for clot reformation exists following the intervention. See Chapter 36 for full discussion of anticoagulation therapy.

Once-a-day *beta-adrenergic blocking agents* (e.g., metoprolol XL [Toprol XL], carvedilol CR [Coreg CR]), sometimes just called *beta blockers (BBs),* decrease the size of the infarct, the occurrence of ventricular dysrhythmias, and mortality rates in patients with MI. The provider usually prescribes a cardioselective beta-blocking agent within the first 1 to 2 hours after an MI if the patient is hemodynamically stable. Beta blockers slow the heart rate and decrease the force of cardiac contraction (see Chart 38-4). Thus these agents prolong the period of diastole and increase myocardial PERFUSION while reducing the force of myocardial contraction. With beta blockade, the heart can perform more work without ischemia. During beta-blocking therapy, monitor for:

- Bradycardia
- Hypotension
- Decreased level of consciousness (LOC)
- Chest discomfort

Assess the lungs for crackles (indicative of heart failure) and wheezes (indicative of bronchospasm). Hypoglycemia, depression, nightmares, and forgetfulness are also problems with beta blockade, especially in older patients. Many of these side effects decrease with time. Unless contraindicated, all patients experiencing NSTEMI and STEMI should be discharged on beta-blocker therapy. If the patient has a history or new onset of heart failure, metoprolol succinate, carvedilol, or bisoprolol should be used because these agents have been shown to reduce mortality in patients with heart failure.

Health care providers frequently prescribe *angiotensin-converting enzyme inhibitors (ACEIs)* or *angiotensin receptor blockers (ARBs)* within 48 hours of ACS if the ejection fraction is equal to or less than 40% in those with hypertension, diabetes mellitus, or stable chronic kidney disease to prevent ventricular remodeling and the development of heart failure. Both ACEIs and ARBs increase survival after an MI. Monitor the patient for decreased urine output, hypotension, and cough. Check for changes in serum potassium, creatinine, and blood urea nitrogen. If ACEIs or ARBs are initiated, they should be continued on discharge indefinitely. Chapter 36 provides a more detailed discussion of ACEIs and ARBs.

For patients with angina, the health care provider may prescribe *calcium channel blockers* (CCBs) to promote vasodilation and myocardial PERFUSION. These drugs are indicated for patients with variant angina or for those who are hypertensive and continue to have angina despite therapy with beta blockers (unstable angina). They are *not* indicated after an acute MI unless beta blockade is contraindicated. Monitor the patient for hypotension and peripheral edema and review the frequency of angina episodes.

Calcium channel blockers are also used for chronic stable angina (CSA). When they are not successful in managing CSA, *ranolazine (Ranexa)* may be added to the drug regimen. This drug has anti-angina and anti-ischemic properties and is often effective in relieving the pain associated with CSA.

Statin therapy reduces the risk of developing recurrent MI, mortality, and stroke. Before discharge, all diagnosed with ACS should be started on high-intensity statin therapy despite results of lipid panel testing. High-intensity statins lower the LDL-C by ≥50% and include atorvastatin (Lipitor) 80 mg and rosuvastatin (Crestor) 20 mg daily.

Reperfusion Therapy. As time passes, myocardial tissue can become increasingly ischemic and necrotic. Therefore, based on the location and skill set within the health care institution, one of two reperfusion strategies are used to open a blocked artery in a patient experiencing acute MI: thrombolytic therapy or percutaneous coronary intervention (PCI).

Thrombolytic Therapy. Thrombolytic therapy using fibrinolytics dissolves thrombi in the coronary arteries and restores myocardial blood flow. Examples of these agents, which target the fibrin component of the coronary thrombosis, include:

- Tissue plasminogen activator (t-PA, alteplase [Activase]) (IV or intracoronary)

- Reteplase (Retavase) (IV or intracoronary)
- Tenecteplase (TNKase) (IV push [IVP])

Intracoronary fibrinolytics may be delivered during cardiac catheterization. Thrombolytic agents are most effective when administered within the first 6 hours of a coronary event. They are used in men and women, young and old.

Thrombolytic therapy is given in a unit where the patient can be monitored continuously. It is indicated for chest pain of longer than 30 minutes' duration that is unrelieved by nitroglycerin, with *indications of STEMI by the ECG*. It is *not* indicated for the NSTEMI patient population. The Joint Commission Acute Myocardial Infarction Core Measure Set requires that fibrinolytic therapy begin within 30 minutes of ED arrival. Contraindications include recent abdominal surgery or stroke, because bleeding may occur when fresh clots are lysed (broken down or dissolved). Table 38-2 lists the current contraindications to thrombolytic therapy.

! NURSING SAFETY PRIORITY QSEN

Drug Alert

During and after thrombolytic administration, immediately report any indications of bleeding to the health care provider or Rapid Response Team. Observe for signs of bleeding by:
- Documenting the patient's neurologic status (in case of intracranial bleeding)
- Observing all IV sites for bleeding and patency
- Monitoring clotting studies
- Observing for signs of internal bleeding (Monitor hemoglobin, hematocrit, and blood pressure.)
- Testing stools, urine, and emesis for occult blood

TABLE 38-2 Contraindications to Thrombolytic Therapy

Absolute
- Any prior intracranial hemorrhage
- Known structural cerebral vascular lesion (e.g., arteriovenous malformations)
- Known malignant intracranial neoplasm (primary or metastatic)
- Ischemic stroke within 3 months EXCEPT acute ischemic stroke within 3 hours
- Suspected aortic dissection
- Active bleeding or bleeding diathesis (excluding menses)
- Significant closed-head or facial trauma within 3 months

Relative
- History of chronic, severe, poorly controlled hypertension
- Severe uncontrolled hypertension on presentation (SBP >180 mm Hg or DBP >110 mm Hg)*
- History of prior ischemic stroke within 3 months, dementia, or known intracranial pathology not covered in contraindications
- Traumatic or prolonged (≥10 minutes) CPR or major surgery (within 3 weeks)
- Recent (within 2-4 weeks) internal bleeding
- Noncompressible vascular punctures
- For streptokinase/anistreplase: prior exposure (>5 days ago) or prior allergic reaction to these agents
- Pregnancy
- Active peptic ulcer
- Current use of anticoagulants; the higher the INR, the higher risk for bleeding

CPR, Cardiopulmonary resuscitation; *DBP,* diastolic blood pressure; *INR,* international normalized ratio; *MI,* myocardial infarction; *SBP,* systolic blood pressure.
*Could be an absolute contraindication in low-risk patients with MI.

Patients who receive fibrinolytics require percutaneous coronary intervention (PCI) for more definitive treatment such as stent placement. Therefore, if criteria for PCI are met, it is more advantageous to go directly to the catheterization laboratory where definitive treatment, not just clot resolution, can be performed.

Monitor the patient for indications that the clot has been lysed (dissolved) and the artery reperfused. These indications include:
- Abrupt cessation of pain or discomfort
- Sudden onset of ventricular dysrhythmias
- Resolution of ST-segment depression/elevation or T-wave inversion
- A peak at 12 hours of markers of myocardial damage

After clot lysis with thrombolytics, large amounts of thrombin are released into the system, increasing the risk for vessel reocclusion. To maintain the patency of the coronary artery after thrombolytic therapy, the health care provider usually prescribes aspirin and IV heparin, a *high-alert drug*. Maintain the heparin infusion via pump for 3 to 5 days as prescribed and monitor the activated partial thromboplastin time (aPTT). The target aPTT range is usually $1\frac{1}{2}$ to $2\frac{1}{2}$ times the control sample. The heparin antifactor Xa assay (heparin assay) test may be used instead of the aPTT in some clinical facilities. Low–molecular-weight heparin (LMWH) (enoxaparin [Lovenox]) may be substituted for IV heparin. Therapeutic dosing of LMWH in this patient population should be based on weight (1 mg/kg). Chapter 36 describes care of the patient receiving heparin or LMWH in detail.

? NCLEX EXAMINATION CHALLENGE 38-2

Physiological Integrity

The nurse is assessing a client with chest pain. Which symptoms assessed by the nurse would be **most** indicative of myocardial infarction? **Select all that apply.**
A. Substernal chest discomfort associated with exertion
B. Chest pain that is relieved with rest.
C. Chest pain associated with ECG changes
D. Chest pain relieved with nitroglycerin
E. Chest pain relieved only by opioids
F. Chest pain associated with shortness of breath
G. Chest pain that lasts less than 10 minutes

Percutaneous Coronary Intervention. For some patients experiencing ACS, primary percutaneous coronary intervention (PCI) may be used to reopen the clotted coronary artery and restore PERFUSION. Percutaneous intervention has been associated with excellent return of blood flow through the coronary artery when an interventional cardiologist can perform it within 2 to 3 hours of the onset of symptoms. Many community hospitals can now perform emergent PCI. When primary PCI is not available, patients should receive immediate thrombolytic agents if they are appropriate candidates and then be transferred to a facility that can perform PCI. After PCI with stent placement, the patient requires dual antiplatelet therapy, explained in this chapter.

Increasing Functional Ability

Planning: Expected Outcomes. The patient is expected to increase functional ability without chest pain and the need for supplemental oxygen as a result of a collaborative cardiac rehabilitation program.

Interventions. A planned program of cardiac rehabilitation increases functional ability and tolerance to activity. Cardiac rehabilitation is implemented primarily by the nurse and cardiac rehabilitation specialist and is continued after discharge.

Cardiac rehabilitation is the process of actively assisting the patient with cardiac disease in achieving and maintaining a vital and productive life while remaining within the limits of the heart's ability to respond to increases in activity and stress. It can be divided into three phases. *Phase 1* begins with the acute illness and ends with discharge from the hospital. *Phase 2* begins after discharge and continues through convalescence at home. *Phase 3* refers to long-term conditioning.

In the acute phase (phase 1), promote rest and ensure limited mobility. Assistance may be needed for some ADLs, such as ambulation to the bathroom. Patients progress at their own rate to increasing levels of activity, depending on their clinical status, age, and physical capabilities.

The next step in phase 1 is independent ambulation of the patient in the room and to the bathroom. Encourage progressive ambulation in the hallway, usually 50, 100, and then 200 feet three times a day. In addition, the patient may begin showering for 5 or 10 minutes with warm water. A chair should be available to facilitate rest and maintain balance.

! NURSING SAFETY PRIORITY QSEN

Action Alert

During cardiac rehabilitation, assess the patient's heart rate, blood pressure (BP), respiratory rate, and level of fatigue with each higher level of activity. Decreases greater than 20 mm Hg in the systolic BP, changes of 20 beats/min in the pulse rate, and/or reports of dyspnea or chest pain indicate intolerance of activity. If these manifestations develop, notify the health care provider and do not advance the patient to the next level. Older adults with CAD often have needs and concerns different from those of younger adults, as described in Chart 38-5.

CHART 38-5 Nursing Focus on the Older Adult

Coronary Artery Disease

- Recognize that chest pain may not be evident in the older patient. Examples of associated symptoms are unexplained dyspnea, confusion, or GI symptoms.
- Although older adults have a greater reduction in mortality rate from myocardial infarction (MI) with the use of thrombolytics, they also have the most severe side effects. Monitor older patients receiving thrombolytics extremely carefully.
- Dysrhythmia may be a normal age-related change rather than a complication of MI. Determine whether the dysrhythmia is causing significant symptoms. Then notify the health care provider.
- If beta blockers are used, assess the patient carefully for the development of side effects. Exacerbation of the depression some older adults have is a significant problem with beta blockade.
- Plan slow, steady increases in activity. Older adults with minimal previous exercise show particular benefit from a gradual increase in activity.
- Older adults should plan longer warm-up and cool-down periods when participating in an exercise program. Their pulse rates may not return to baseline until 30 minutes or longer after exercise.

All patients with ACS should be referred to a phase 2 cardiac rehabilitation program on discharge from the hospital. Interprofessional collaboration with the case manager to plan for the patient's continuing care is important.

Increasing Ability to Cope

Planning: Expected Outcomes. The patient is expected to learn to cope with the cardiac event and identify effective coping strategies with the help of support systems.

Interventions. Assess the patient's level of anxiety while allowing expression of any apprehension and attempt to define its origin. Simple, repeated explanations of therapies, expectations, and surroundings, as well as patient progress, may help relieve anxiety.

Identify the patient's current *coping* mechanisms. The most common are denial, anger, and depression. Denial allows the patient to decrease a threat and use problem-focused coping mechanisms. The patient may avoid discussing what has happened and yet comply with treatment regimens. This type of denial decreases anxiety and should not be discouraged. *However, denial that results in a patient who refuses to follow treatment regimens can be harmful.* Because this behavior is usually caused by extreme anxiety or fear, threats only worsen the behavior. Remain calm and avoid confronting the patient. Clearly indicate when a behavior is not acceptable and is potentially harmful as a result of nonadherence to the plan of care.

Anger may represent an attempt to regain control of life. Encourage the patient to verbalize the source of frustration and provide opportunities for decision making and control. Collaborate with the certified spiritual chaplain or social worker in the hospital to help the patient cope with the situation based on his or her preferences, values, and beliefs. Help the patient identify support systems such as family, friends, church, or social group.

Depression may be a response to grief and loss of function. Listen as the patient verbalizes feelings of loss, being careful not to offer false or general reassurances. Acknowledge depression, but encourage the patient to perform ADLs and other activities within restrictions.

Identifying and Managing Dysrhythmias

Planning: Expected Outcomes. The most desired outcome for the patient is that he or she will be free of dysrhythmias. If dysrhythmias occur, they will be identified and managed early to prevent complications or death.

Interventions. *Dysrhythmias are the leading cause of prehospital death in most patients with ACS.* Even in the early period of hospitalization, most patients with ACS experience some abnormal cardiac rhythm. When a dysrhythmia develops:

- Identify the dysrhythmia.
- Assess hemodynamic status.
- Evaluate for discomfort.

Dysrhythmias are treated when they cause hemodynamic compromise, increase myocardial oxygen requirements, or predispose the patient to lethal ventricular dysrhythmias.

Typical dysrhythmias for the patient with an *inferior* ACS are bradycardias and second-degree atrioventricular (AV) blocks resulting from ischemia of the AV node. These rhythms tend to be intermittent. Monitor the cardiac rhythm and rate and the hemodynamic status. If the patient becomes hemodynamically unstable, a temporary pacemaker may be necessary.

The patient with an *anterior* ACS is likely to exhibit premature ventricular contractions (PVCs) caused by ventricular irritability. Third-degree or bundle branch block is a serious complication in this patient because it indicates that a large portion of the left ventricle is involved. The health care provider may insert a pacemaker. Observe the patient closely to detect the development of heart failure. Appropriate interventions for dysrhythmias are described in Chapter 34.

Monitoring for and Managing Heart Failure

Planning: Expected Outcomes. The most desired outcome for the patient is that he or she will be free of heart failure. However, if it occurs, the outcome is that the heart failure will be identified and treated early to prevent further complications.

Interventions. Decreased cardiac output due to heart failure is a relatively common complication after an MI resulting from left ventricular dysfunction, rupture of the intraventricular septum, papillary muscle rupture with valvular dysfunction, or right ventricular infarction. The most severe form of acute heart failure, *cardiogenic shock,* discussed later in this chapter, causes most in-hospital deaths after an ACS. The type of management used to increase cardiac output depends on the location of the ACS and the type of heart failure that resulted from the infarction.

Managing Left Ventricular Failure. When a patient with ACS experiences damage to the left ventricle, rupture of the intraventricular septum, or tear of a papillary muscle, the amount of blood that the heart can eject is reduced. When volume and pressure are markedly increased in the pulmonary vasculature, pulmonary complications can develop.

Assess for manifestations of left ventricular failure and pulmonary edema by listening for crackles and identifying their location in the lung fields. Wheezing, tachypnea, and frothy sputum may also occur with pulmonary edema. Auscultate the heart, paying particular attention to the presence of an S_3 heart sound.

⚠ NURSING SAFETY PRIORITY QSEN

Critical Rescue

Monitor for, report, and document these signs of inadequate organ PERFUSION that may result from decreased cardiac output:
- A change in orientation or mental status
- Urine output less than 0.5-1 mL/kg/hr
- Cool, clammy extremities with decreased or absent pulses
- Unusual fatigue
- Recurrent chest pain

Hemodynamic Monitoring. Hemodynamic monitoring is an invasive system used in critical care areas to provide quantitative information about vascular capacity, blood volume, pump effectiveness, and tissue PERFUSION. It directly measures pressures in the heart and great vessels. These procedures are usually performed for more seriously ill patients and can provide more accurate measurements of blood pressure, heart function, and volume status. Although medical-surgical nurses do not manage these systems on general hospital units, they should be familiar with the interpretation of some of the major hemodynamic pressures as they relate to patient assessment.

Hemodynamic monitoring does involve significant risks, although complications are uncommon. Therefore informed consent is required. After obtaining consent, the critical care nurse prepares a pressure-monitoring system. The components of this system are a catheter with an infusion system, a transducer, and a monitor. The catheter receives the pressure waves

---

◎ CHART 38-6 Best Practice for Patient Safety & Quality Care QSEN

Identification of the Phlebostatic Axis

1. Position the patient supine.
2. Palpate the fourth intercostal space at the sternum.
3. Follow the fourth intercostal space to the side of the patient's chest.
4. Determine the midway point between anterior and posterior.
5. Find the intersection between the midway point and the line from the fourth intercostal space and mark it with an X in indelible ink. This is the phlebostatic axis.

(mechanical energy) from the heart or the great vessels. The transducer converts the mechanical energy into electrical energy, which is displayed as waveforms or numbers on the monitor. Patency of the catheter is maintained with a slow continuous flush of normal saline, usually infused at 3 to 4 mL/hr under pressure to prevent the backup of blood and occlusion of the catheter.

To prepare the transducer, balance and calibrate it according to hospital policy and the manufacturer's specifications. Finally, identify the phlebostatic axis (Chart 38-6) and level the transducer to it. The physician inserts a balloon-tipped catheter percutaneously through a large vein, usually the internal jugular or subclavian, and directs it to the right atrium (RA). When the catheter tip reaches the RA, the balloon is inflated. The catheter advances with the flow of blood through the tricuspid valve, into the right ventricle, past the pulmonic valve, and into a branch of the pulmonary artery. The balloon is deflated after the catheter tip reaches the pulmonary artery. Waveforms are viewed on the monitor as the pulmonary artery catheter is advanced (Fig. 38-3). A chest x-ray is used to check the location of the catheter.

A pulmonary artery catheter is a multi-lumen catheter with the capacity to measure right atrial and indirect left atrial pressures or pulmonary artery wedge pressure (PAWP), also known as the **pulmonary artery occlusive pressure (PAOP)**. A cardiac output measurement, cardiac index, and systemic and pulmonary vascular resistance may also be obtained.

Right atrial (RA) pressure is measured by a pressure sensor on the catheter inside the RA. Normal RA pressure ranges from 2 to 6 mm Hg. *Increased RA pressures may occur with right ventricular failure, whereas low RA pressures usually indicate hypovolemia.*

Normal pulmonary artery pressure (PAP) ranges from 15 to 26 mm Hg systolic/5 to 15 mm Hg diastolic (mean, 15) and is constantly visible on the monitor. When the balloon at the catheter tip is inflated, the catheter advances and wedges in a branch of the pulmonary artery. The tip of the catheter can sense pressures transmitted from the left atrium, which reflect left ventricular end-diastolic pressure (LVEDP). The pressure measured during balloon inflation is called the **pulmonary artery wedge pressure (PAWP)**. PAWP closely reflects left atrial pressure and LVEDP in patients with normal left ventricular function, normal heart rates, and no mitral valve disease. The PAWP is a mean pressure and normally ranges between 4 and 12 mm Hg.

Elevated PAWP measurements may indicate left ventricular failure, hypervolemia, mitral regurgitation, or intracardiac shunt. A decreased PAWP is seen with hypovolemia or afterload

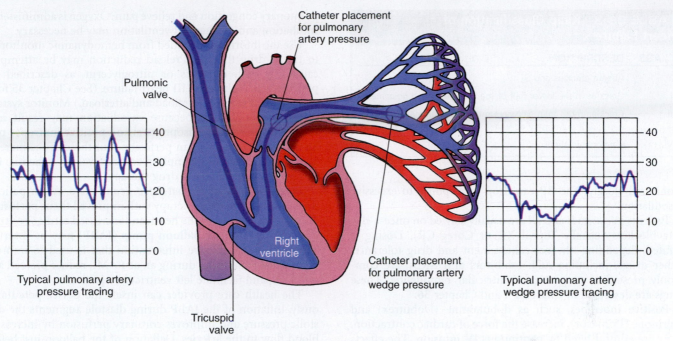

Pulmonic valve

Catheter placement for pulmonary artery pressure

Right ventricle

Tricuspid valve

Catheter placement for pulmonary artery wedge pressure

Typical pulmonary artery pressure tracing

Typical pulmonary artery wedge pressure tracing

FIG. 38-3 Cardiac pressure waveforms can be seen on the monitor.

reduction. Individual values may be less important than the trend in values.

The critical care nurse obtains and records RA pressure, PAP, and PAWP at appropriate intervals (usually every 1 to 4 hours). Single values of these measurements are less significant than the trend of values combined with the patient's signs and symptoms. They help health care providers identify heart failure and guide the administration of fluids and vasoactive drugs. During pressure recording, it is important that the transducer be at the level of the phlebostatic axis. The patient is usually supine with the head elevated up to 45 degrees during hemodynamic readings, although the position may not affect results. If the balloon remains in the wedge position after PAWP measurement, try to change the catheter's position by asking the patient to cough or by changing his or her position. *If these methods are not successful, notify the health care provider immediately.*

Change the occlusive sterile dressing over the catheter according to hospital policy. Inspect the insertion site for redness, induration, swelling, drainage, and intactness of the sutures. Detailed discussion of the management and care of patients with pulmonary artery catheters can be found in textbooks on critical care nursing.

Be sure to assess for a number of complications associated with pulmonary artery catheters. For example, pulmonary infarction or pulmonary rupture may occur if the catheter remains in the wedge position. Air embolism is possible if the balloon has ruptured and repeated attempts are made to inflate it. Ventricular dysrhythmias may occur during insertion or if the catheter tip slips back into the right ventricle and irritates the myocardium. Thrombus and embolus formation may occur at the catheter site. Infection may result, and bleeding may be pronounced if the infusion system becomes disconnected.

Direct measurement of *arterial BP* is done by invasive arterial catheter in critically ill patients. The physician or specially trained health care professional inserts an intra-arterial catheter into the radial or femoral artery. After the catheter is inserted,

it is attached to pressure tubing. A normal saline flush solution is infused constantly under pressure to maintain the integrity of the system. A transducer attached to the tubing allows continuous direct monitoring of the arterial BP. Direct measurements of BP are usually 10 to 15 mm Hg greater than indirect (cuff) measurements. The arterial catheter may also be used to obtain blood samples for arterial blood gas values and other blood tests.

Because the arterial vasculature is a high-pressure system, frequent assessment of the arterial site and infusion system is essential. *Note any bleeding around the intra-arterial catheter or any loose connections and correct the situation immediately.* Collateral circulation must be assessed by Doppler before and while the arterial catheter is in place. Carefully monitor color, pulse, and temperature distal to the insertion site for any early signs of circulatory compromise. Complications of systemic intra-arterial monitoring include pain, infection, arteriospasm, or obstruction at the site with the potential for distal infarction, air embolism, and hemorrhage.

Classification of Post–Myocardial Infarction Heart Failure. Several classification systems may be used to categorize heart failure after an MI. For example, the classic Killip system identifies four classes based on prognosis (Table 38-3). This system complements the ACC/AHA heart failure classification of function assessment discussed in Chapter 35.

Patients with *class I* heart failure often respond well to reduction in preload with IV nitrates and diuretics. Monitor the urine output hourly, check vital signs hourly, continue to assess for signs of heart failure, and review the serum potassium level.

Patients with *class II* and *class III* heart failure may require diuresis and more aggressive medical intervention, such as afterload reduction and/or enhancement of contractility. IV nitroprusside or nitroglycerin may be used to decrease both preload and afterload. These drugs are given as continuous infusions in specialized units where the PAWP and BP can be

TABLE 38-3 Killip Classification of Heart Failure

CLASS	DESCRIPTION
I	Absent crackles and S_3
II	Crackles in the lower half of the lung fields and possible S_3
III	Crackles more than halfway up the lung fields and frequent pulmonary edema
IV	Cardiogenic shock

monitored closely. The BP can drop in response to excessive vasodilation.

Patients in *classes II and III* are usually started on once-a-day beta blockers (usually Toprol XR or Coreg CR). Dosing is titrated, depending on goal achievement and drug tolerance. Other drugs, including ACE inhibitors and ARBs, are commonly prescribed to promote ventricular remodeling. These drugs are described in Chart 38-4 and Chapter 36.

Positive inotropes, such as dobutamine (Dobutrex) and milrinone (Primacor), increase the force of cardiac contraction. They are administered by continuous IV infusion. The effects of these drugs on the blood vessels and heart rate vary and may be dose dependent. The infusions are titrated to promote cardiac output.

> **! NURSING SAFETY PRIORITY** QSEN
>
> **Drug Alert**
>
> Use caution when giving positive inotropes because of the potential risk for increasing myocardial oxygen consumption and further decreasing cardiac output. Monitor the patient frequently, paying particular attention to the development of chest pain.

Class IV heart failure is cardiogenic shock. In **cardiogenic shock**, necrosis of more than 40% of the left ventricle occurs. Most patients have a stuttering pattern of chest pain, resulting in piecemeal extension of the ACS.

> **! NURSING SAFETY PRIORITY** QSEN
>
> **Critical Rescue**
>
> Monitor for, report, and document manifestations of cardiogenic shock immediately. These signs and symptoms include:
> - Tachycardia
> - Hypotension
> - Systolic BP less than 90 mm Hg or 30 mm Hg less than the patient's baseline
> - Urine output less than 0.5-1 mL/kg/hr
> - Cold, clammy skin with poor peripheral pulses
> - Agitation, restlessness, or confusion
> - Pulmonary congestion
> - Tachypnea
> - Continuing chest discomfort
>
> *Early detection is essential because undiagnosed cardiogenic shock has a high mortality rate!*

Drug Therapy. Medical interventions aim to relieve pain and decrease myocardial oxygen requirements through preload and afterload reduction (see Chart 38-4; Chart 38-7). The health care provider prescribes IV morphine, which is used to decrease pulmonary congestion and relieve pain. Oxygen is administered. Intubation and mechanical ventilation may be necessary.

Use the information gained from hemodynamic monitoring to titrate drug therapy. Preload reduction may be attempted cautiously with diuretics or nitroglycerin, as described for patients with Killip class III heart failure. (See Chapter 35 for a complete discussion of preload and afterload.) Monitor systolic pressure continuously because vasodilation may result in a further decline in BP. Vasopressors and positive inotropes may be used to maintain organ perfusion, but these drugs increase myocardial oxygen consumption and can worsen ischemia. Use extreme caution in giving drug therapy.

Other Interventions for Left-Sided Heart Failure. When patients do not respond to drug therapy with improved tissue perfusion, decreased workload of the heart, and increased cardiac contractility, an **intra-aortic balloon pump (IABP)** may be inserted. The IABP is an invasive intervention that is used to improve myocardial PERFUSION during an acute MI, reduce preload and afterload, and facilitate left ventricular ejection.

The health care provider can insert the device percutaneously. Inflation of the IABP during diastole augments the diastolic pressure and improves coronary perfusion by increasing blood flow to the arteries. Deflation of the balloon just before systole reduces afterload at the time of systolic contraction. This action facilitates emptying of the left ventricle and improves cardiac output. The balloon catheter is attached to a pump console, which is triggered by an ECG tracing and arterial waveform.

In patients undergoing high-risk percutaneous coronary intervention (PCI) or those at risk for cardiogenic shock, a *percutaneous ventricular assist device* may be used. These devices are temporary to decrease the myocardial workload and oxygen consumption of the heart and increase cardiac output and peripheral perfusion.

Immediate reperfusion is an invasive intervention that shows some promise for managing cardiogenic shock. The patient is taken to the cardiac catheterization laboratory, and an emergency left-sided heart catheterization is performed. If he or she has a treatable occlusion or occlusions, the interventional cardiologist performs a PCI in the catheterization laboratory, or the patient is transferred to the operating suite for a coronary artery bypass graft (CABG).

Managing Right Ventricular Failure. Conditions other than left ventricular failure may result in decreased cardiac output after an ACS. In about a third of patients with inferior MIs, right ventricular infarction and failure develop. In this instance, the right ventricle fails independently of the left. Decreased cardiac output with a paradoxical pulse, clear lungs, and jugular venous distention occurs when the patient is in semi-Fowler's position.

The desired outcome of management is to improve right ventricular stroke volume by increasing right ventricular fiber stretch or preload. To enhance right ventricular preload, give sufficient fluids (as much as 200 mL/hr) to increase right atrial pressure to 20 mm Hg. In the critical care unit, *monitor the pulmonary artery wedge pressure (PAWP)—attempting to maintain below 15 to 20 mm Hg—and auscultate the lungs to assess for left-sided heart failure. If symptoms of this complication occur, notify the health care provider immediately.*

Monitoring for and Managing Recurrent Symptoms and Extension of Injury

Planning: Expected Outcomes. The most desired outcome is that the patient will not have recurrent symptoms or an extension of myocardial injury. If these problems occur, they

CHART 38-7 Common Examples of Drug Therapy

Commonly Used Intravenous Vasodilators and Inotropes

DRUG CATEGORY	NURSING IMPLICATIONS
Nitrates	
Nitroprusside sodium (Nipride, Nitropress)	This agent is a potent, rapidly reversible vasodilator acting on both peripheral venous and arterial musculature. • Monitor BP every 2-5 minutes when initiating therapy. • Monitor PAWP, SVR, BP, heart rate, urine output frequently. Titrate medication to obtain the desired effect. Protect from light *because this medication is light sensitive.* Administered in mcg/kg/min. Higher doses are associated with thiocyanate or cyanide toxicity. • Monitor for metabolic acidosis, confusion, and hyperreflexia, *which are symptoms of toxicity.*
Nitroglycerin (Tridil)	This agent produces systemic vasodilation and dilates coronary arteries rapidly. • Monitor BP every 1-3 minutes when initiating therapy *because BP may drop in 1 minute.* • Monitor RAP, PAWP, SVR, BP, HR, and urine output frequently. • Assess for headache *because this is a frequent side effect of initial therapy.* • Tolerance to this agent can develop with continued administration.
Milrinone (Primacor) Fenoldopam (Corlopam)	Assess BP and HR every 5 minutes *because hypotension is a common adverse effect.* • If systolic BP drops 30 mm Hg, stop infusion and call the health care provider. Monitor I&O and weight *because this drug causes diuresis.*
Sympathomimetics	
Dopamine (Intropin)	This agent is a dose-dependent activator of alpha, beta, and dopaminergic receptors. • Assess reason for use and expected result. • Observe HR, BP, PAWP, SVR, cardiac output, and urine output every 5 minutes to 1 hour. • Titrate dosage to maintain dose range and obtain the desired effect. • Infuse through central line *because extravasation can cause tissue necrosis and sloughing.* • Monitor for ectopy and angina.
Dobutamine (Dobutrex)	Observe patients continuously during administration *because this agent is a very strong beta₁-receptor activator and a moderately strong beta₂-receptor activator.* • Titrate the drug on the basis of adequate tissue perfusion: mentation, skin temperature, peripheral pulses, PAWP, cardiac output, SVR, and urine output. Monitor for atrial and ventricular ectopy *because dysrhythmias are an adverse effect.*

BP, Blood pressure; *ECG,* electrocardiogram; *I&O,* input and output; *PAWP,* pulmonary artery wedge pressure; *RAP,* right atrial pressure; *SVR,* systemic vascular resistance.

will be identified and treated early to prevent further complications or death.

Interventions. *Recurrent discomfort despite medical therapy is one of the major indications for surgical management of CAD.* Patients who continue to have chest discomfort despite medical therapy or who have ischemia during a stress test may require invasive correction by PCI or CABG to resolve angina or prevent MI. Before invasive treatment, a left-sided cardiac catheterization with coronary angiogram is performed to document that the lesions are correctable and that left ventricular pump function is adequate.

Percutaneous Coronary Intervention. **Percutaneous coronary intervention (PCI)** is an invasive but nonsurgical technique that is performed within 90 minutes of an acute MI (AMI) diagnosis. It is performed to reduce the frequency and severity of discomfort for patients with angina and to bridge patients to CABG surgery. It combines clot retrieval, coronary angioplasty, and stent placement. Under fluoroscopic guidance, the cardiologist performs initial coronary angiography. In the STEMI patient, if a clot is seen, a clot retrieval device is inserted over the guidewire, and the clot is removed. Once the clot is removed in the STEMI patient or area of narrowing is identified in the NSTEMI patient, a balloon-tipped catheter is introduced through a guidewire to the coronary artery occlusion. The physician activates a compressor that inflates the balloon (angioplasty) to force the plaque against the vessel wall, thus dilating the wall, and reduces or eliminates the occluding clot. Balloon inflation may be repeated until angiography indicates a decrease in the stenosis (narrowing) to less than 50% of the vessel's diameter (Fig. 38-4). The balloon catheter is then withdrawn, and a balloon catheter with stent is introduced. Once the stent and balloon are in position, the stent is deployed by the balloon inflation. The balloon is deflated and the stent stays in place, acting as scaffolding to hold the diseased artery open. **Stents** are expandable metal mesh devices that are used to maintain the patent lumen created by angioplasty or atherectomy. Bare metal or drug-eluting stents (DESs) (drug-coated) may be used. By providing a supportive scaffold, these devices prevent closure of the vessel from arterial dissection or vasospasm. Fig. 38-5 shows a stent positioned in a coronary artery.

Patients who are most likely to benefit from PCI have single- or double-vessel disease with discrete, proximal, noncalcified lesions or clots. This procedure often does not work for complex clots. When identifying which lesions are treatable with PCI, the cardiologist considers the clot's complexity and location and the amount of myocardium at risk. Although treating lesions located in the left main artery places a large amount of myocardial tissue at risk if the vessel closes quickly, these lesions are now being treated more with PCI. In the past, CABG was the intervention used for these patients. PCI may also be used for the patient with an evolving acute MI, either alone or with thrombolytic therapy or glycoprotein (GP) IIb/IIIa inhibitor, to reperfuse the damaged myocardium.

Without stent placement, the artery often reoccludes because of its normal elasticity and memory. Patients who undergo PCI are required to take dual antiplatelet therapy (DAT) consisting of aspirin and a platelet inhibitor (see Chart 38-4). Before the procedure, the patient receives an initial dose of a platelet

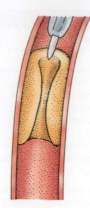
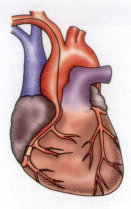
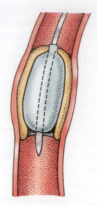
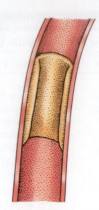

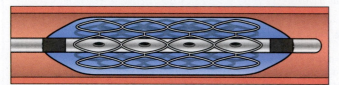

1. The balloon-tipped catheter is positioned in the artery.

2. The uninflated balloon is centered in the obstruction.

3. The balloon is inflated, which flattens plaque against the artery wall.

4. The balloon is removed, and the artery is left unoccluded.

FIG. 38-4 Percutaneous coronary intervention.

FIG. 38-5 A coronary stent open after balloon inflation.

inhibitor (clopidogrel [Plavix]) or ticagrelor [Brilinta]) and aspirin. If prasugrel (Effient) is the preferred platelet inhibitor, it is given immediately after PCI. Cangrelor (Kengreal) is a newly Food and Drug Administration (FDA)–approved IV alternative. Infusion is started before PCI and continued for at least 2 hours or the entire duration of the procedure. Administration of an oral platelet inhibitor is required after the infusion. If there are any concerns that the patient may require CABG, the platelet inhibitor may be held until after the procedure. The inhibition of the platelets is permanent and increases the risk for postoperative bleeding. Patients should wait 5 (clopidogrel and ticagrelor) to 7 (prasugrel) days before undergoing CABG. If the patient has received thrombolytic therapy, clopidogrel (Plavix) is the preferred drug. Use of cangrelor infusion as an antiplatelet bridge to CABG is currently under investigation. Early studies suggest that cangrelor provides antiplatelet protection and less risk of bleeding when the infusion is stopped the day of surgery. Further research is necessary to determine best use.

During the procedure, the patient may receive boluses of IV heparin or a continuous infusion of bivalirudin (Angiomax). Heparin is used to maintain an elevated activated clotting time and prevent clotting on wires and catheters during the procedure. It is discontinued before removal of the catheters. Bivalirudin (Angiomax) is a direct thrombin inhibitor and is frequently used as an alternative to glycoprotein IIb/IIIa platelet inhibitors and heparin. It has a short half-life (25 minutes) and is less dependent on renal function. IV or intracoronary nitroglycerin or diltiazem (Cardizem) is given to prevent coronary vasospasm. PCI initially reopens the vessel in most patients. However, within the first 24 hours, a small percentage of patients have re-stenosis. At 6 months, a larger number have one or more blockages.

The health care provider also prescribes a long-term nitrate and beta blocker, and an ACE inhibitor or ARB is added for patients who have had primary angioplasty after an MI. Some patients may experience hypokalemia after the procedure and require careful monitoring and potassium supplements. The nursing interventions for patients receiving these drugs are described in Chart 38-4. Provide careful explanations of drug therapy and any recommended lifestyle changes.

> **! NURSING SAFETY PRIORITY** **QSEN**
>
> ***Critical Rescue***
>
> After PCI, monitor for potential problems, including acute closure of the vessel (causes chest pain and potential ST elevation on 12-lead ECG), bleeding from the insertion site, and reaction to the contrast medium used in angiography. Also monitor for and document hypotension, hypokalemia, and dysrhythmias. Document and report any of these findings to the health care provider or Rapid Response Team immediately!

Other Procedures. Other techniques being used to ensure continued patency of the vessel are laser angioplasty (the laser breaks up the clot) and atherectomy. **Atherectomy** devices can either excise and retrieve plaque or emulsify it. One of the advantages of this procedure is that it creates a less bulky vessel with better elastic recoil. Another procedure that may be performed is rheolytic thrombectomy (e.g., AngioJet, Vortex), which uses low-pressure, high-speed saline jets to break up the clot. The EndiCOR X-SIZER lances and aspirates a clot simultaneously.

Injecting vascular endothelial growth factor (VEGF) during angioplasty has increased PERFUSION to the wall of the heart. Also, VEGF helps initiate new blood vessel growth and development, which results in increased blood supply to cardiac muscle.

Traditional Coronary Artery Bypass Graft Surgery. Over 390,000 traditional open **coronary artery bypass graft (CABG)** surgeries are performed in the United States each year (Mozaffarian et al., 2016). It is the most common type of cardiac surgery and the most common procedure for older adults. Almost half of all CABGs are done for patients older than 65 years. The occluded coronary arteries are bypassed with the patient's own venous or arterial blood vessels or synthetic grafts. The internal mammary artery (IMA) is the current graft of choice because it has an excellent patency rate many years after the procedure.

CABG is indicated when patients do not respond to medical management of CAD or when disease progression is evident. Because of the development of drug-eluting stents (DESs), patients who previously had no option other than CABG have been able to have their vessels revascularized without surgery. The decision for surgery is based on the patient's symptoms and the results of cardiac catheterization. Candidates for surgery are patients who have:

- Angina with greater than 50% occlusion of the left main coronary artery that cannot be stented
- Unstable angina with severe two-vessel disease, moderate three-vessel disease, or small-vessel disease in which stents could not be introduced
- Ischemia with heart failure
- Acute MI with cardiogenic shock
- Signs of ischemia or impending MI after angiography or percutaneous transluminal coronary angioplasty (PTCA)
- Valvular disease
- Coronary vessels unsuitable for PCI

The vessels to be bypassed should have proximal clots blocking more than 70% of the vessel's diameter but with good distal runoff. Bypass of less occluded vessels may result in poor PERFUSION through the graft and early obstruction. CABG is most effective when adequate ventricular function remains and the ejection fraction is close to or greater than 50%. Patients with lower ejection fractions are subject to develop more complications.

For most patients, the risk is low, and the benefits of bypass surgery are clear. Surgical treatment of CAD does not appear to affect the life span. Left ventricular function is the most important long-term indicator of survival. CABG improves the quality of life for most patients. Most are pain free 1 year after surgery and remain so 5 years after the procedure. The percentage of patients experiencing some pain increases sharply after 5 years.

Preoperative Care. CABG surgery may be planned as an elective procedure or performed as an emergency. It may be done as a *traditional* operative technique or performed as a *minimally invasive surgical (MIS)* technique, discussed later in this chapter. Patients undergoing elective surgery are admitted on the morning of surgery. Preoperative preparations and teaching are completed during prehospitalization interviews. Teach patients that their drugs will be changed after surgery. Ensure that the necessary drugs have been administered before surgery.

One potential complication of CABG is sternal wound infection. To decrease risk, have the patient shower with 4% chlorhexidine gluconate (CHG). This decreases the number of microorganisms on the skin. Surgical sites are prepared by clipping hair and applying CHG with isopropyl alcohol (either 0.5% or 2%). In addition, IV antibiotics are administered 1 hour before the surgical procedure.

Familiarize the patient and family with the cardiac surgical–critical care unit (sometimes referred to as the *open heart unit*) and prepare them for postoperative care. If the procedure is elective, demonstrate and have the patient return a demonstration of how to splint the chest incision, cough, deep breathe, and perform arm and leg exercises. Stress that:

- The patient should report any pain to the nursing staff.
- Most of the pain will be in the site where the vessel was harvested. (With the use of endovascular vessel harvesting [EVH] and one or two small incisions, the pain and edema are less than for previously performed procedures.)
- Analgesics will be given to promote COMFORT.

- Coughing and deep breathing are essential to prevent pulmonary complications.
- Early ambulation is important to decrease the risk for venous thrombosis and possible embolism.

For the traditional surgical procedure, explain that the patient will have a sternal incision; possibly a large leg incision; one, two, or three chest tubes; an indwelling urinary catheter; pacemaker wires; and hemodynamic monitoring. An endotracheal tube will be connected to a ventilator for several hours after surgery. Tell the patient and family that the patient will not be able to talk while the endotracheal tube is in place. When describing the postoperative course, emphasize that close monitoring and the use of sophisticated equipment are standard treatment. (See the Quality Improvement box regarding prevention of surgical site infections.)

Preoperative anxiety is common and can negatively affect postoperative outcomes. An appropriate nursing assessment should identify the level of anxiety and the coping methods that patients have used successfully in the past. Some patients may find it helpful to define their fears. Common sources of fear include fear of the unknown, fear of bodily harm, and fear of death.

In elective procedures, patients may benefit from detailed information about the surgery, depending on individual preferences and cultural practices. Others may feel overwhelmed by so much material. Some patients need to discuss their feelings in detail or describe the experiences of people they know who have undergone CABG. Assess patients' anxiety level and help them cope.

Operative Procedures. Coronary artery bypass surgery is performed with the patient under general anesthesia for both cardiopulmonary bypass and off-pump surgery. For the *traditional operative procedure,* the cardiac surgical team begins the procedure with a median sternotomy incision and visualization of the heart and great vessels. Another surgical team may begin harvesting the vein if it is to be used for the graft. Synthetic grafts may be used instead.

Cardiopulmonary bypass (CPB) is used to provide oxygenation, circulation, and hypothermia during induced cardiac arrest. Blood is diverted from the heart to the bypass machine, where it is heparinized, oxygenated, and returned to the circulation through a cannula placed in the ascending aortic arch or femoral artery (Fig. 38-6). During bypass, the patient's core temperature remains between 95°F (35°C) (cold cardioplegia) and normal temperature (warm cardioplegia). Although cooling decreases the rate of metabolism and demand for oxygen, keeping the heart "warm" decreases postoperative complications that were more common when cold cardioplegia was used. The heart is perfused with a potassium solution, which decreases myocardial oxygen consumption and causes the heart to stop during diastole. This process ensures a motionless operative field and prevents myocardial ischemia.

Once the heart is arrested, the grafting procedure can begin. The surgeon uses the internal mammary artery (IMA), a saphenous vein, and/or a radial artery to bypass blockages in the coronary arteries (Fig. 38-7). The distal end of the vessel graft is dissected and attached below the clot in the coronary artery. If the surgeon uses a venous graft or the radial artery, it is anastomosed (sutured) proximally to the aorta and distally to the coronary artery just beyond the occlusion, thus improving myocardial perfusion. After flow rates through the grafts are measured, the heart is rewarmed slowly. The cardioplegic

QUALITY IMPROVEMENT QSEN

Achieving and Sustaining Zero: Preventing Surgical Site Infections

Kles, C., Murrah, P., Smith, K., Baugus-Welmeir, E., Hurry, T., & Morris. C. (2015). Achieving and sustaining zero: Preventing surgical site infections after isolated coronary artery bypass with saphenous vein harvest through implementation of a staff-driven quality improvement process. *Dimensions of Critical Care Nursing, 34*(5), 265-272.

Surgical site infections (SSIs) associated with coronary artery bypass grafting can create significant complications for patients. SSIs increase morbidity and mortality, hospital cost, and overall length of stay following surgery. Deep sternal wound infections create an even larger burden because of the need for long-term antibiotic therapy, advanced wound care, and additional surgeries. Kles et al. (2015) estimate that the cost for one deep sternal wound infection is $17,944, with an average length of hospital stay of 25.7 days.

One hospital, joining with the Centers for Medicare and Medicaid Services initiative "Partnerships for Patients," launched a quality improvement process with a goal of 40% reduction in SSIs for CABG patients over a 1-year period. The hospital used a Six Sigma approach, which is based on a five-step, systematic methodology: define, measure, analyze, improve, and control. An interprofessional team was developed, including frontline staff to help identify potential variables and examine practice associated with SSIs. During observation, inconsistencies in process showing a variance from evidence-based guidelines were discovered. These variances were associated with hair removal, MRSA prevention strategies, and glycemic control.

As a result of following the quality improvement process, the hospital was able to identify gaps in practice and make changes to decrease the SSIs surpassing their targeted goal, with zero SSIs since May 2012. Changes included hair removal in preoperative short stay without exception, topical nasal mupirocin for MRSA prevention for a course of 5 days before surgery, and glycemic maintenance of 180 mg/dL before surgery. In addition, new best practices were implemented such as antibiotic-coated sutures, midsternal dressing care impregnated with silver, disposable pacer wires and electrocardiogram leads, preoperative chlorohexidine gluconate bath, and chlorohexidine gluconate mouthwash until discharge. Each new policy was incorporated into preprinted orders, and staff education was completed to ensure that all shifts were operating with the same prevention measures. As of December 2014, the estimated cost avoidance for this hospital was $606,498.

Commentary: Implications for Practice and Research

Quality improvement initiatives can make a significant difference in patient outcomes and overall cost associated with care. As indicated in this study, a bundled approach with multiple interventions was effective in decreasing SSIs. It is important to note that these interventions for improvement are interdisciplinary, which emphasized the importance of interprofessional collaboration in the quest for quality improvement. Assessing current practice and involving all staff encouraged ownership of the outcomes, which was a huge step toward change in practice. Further research is indicated to isolate which interventions made the most significant impact to the decrease in SSIs.

CABG, Coronary artery bypass graft; *MRSA,* methicillin-resistant *Staphylococcus aureus.*

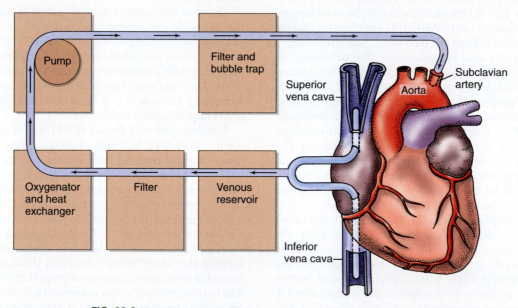

FIG. 38-6 Heart-lung bypass circuitry used during cardiopulmonary bypass.

solution is flushed from the heart. The heart regains its rate and rhythm, or it may be defibrillated to return it to a normal rhythm. When the procedure is completed, the patient may be rewarmed (if cold cardioplegia was used) and weaned from the bypass machine while the grafts are observed for patency and leakage. The surgeon may place atrial and ventricular pacemaker wires and mediastinal and pleural chest tubes. Finally the surgeon closes the sternum with wire sutures.

Postoperative Care. After traditional surgery, the patient is transported to a post–open heart surgery unit and undergoes mechanical ventilation for 3 to 6 hours. He or she requires highly skilled nursing care from a nurse qualified to provide post–cardiac surgery care, including routine postoperative care described in Chapter 16. *Be sure to use sterile technique when changing sternal or donor-site dressings.*

Connect the mediastinal tubes to water-seal drainage systems and ground the epicardial pacer wires by connecting them to the pacemaker generator. Monitor pulmonary artery and arterial pressures, as well as the heart rate and rhythm, which are displayed on a monitor.

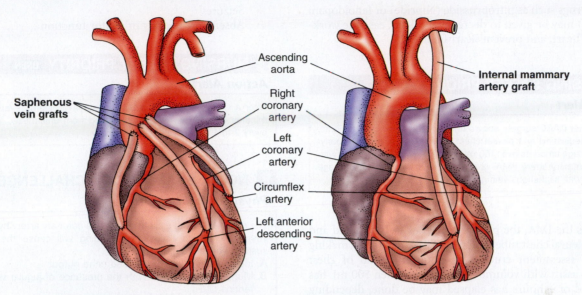

Ascending
aorta

Right
coronary
artery

Left
coronary
artery

Circumflex
artery

Left anterior
descending
artery

**Internal mammary
artery graft**

**Saphenous
vein grafts**

FIG. 38-7 Two methods of coronary artery bypass grafting. The procedure used depends on the nature of the coronary artery disease, the condition of the vessels available for grafting, and the patient's health status.

Closely assess the patient for dysrhythmias, such as brady-dysrhythmias, atrial fibrillation, or heart block. Manage symptomatic dysrhythmias according to unit protocol or the health care provider's prescription. Hypoxemia and hypokalemia are frequent causes of ventricular dysrhythmias. If the patient has symptomatic bradydysrhythmias or heart block, turn on the pacemaker and adjust the pacemaker settings as prescribed. Monitor for, report, and document other complications of CABG, including:

- Fluid and electrolyte imbalance
- Hypotension
- Hypothermia
- Hypertension
- Bleeding
- Cardiac tamponade
- Decreased level of consciousness
- Anginal pain

Managing Fluid and Electrolyte Imbalance. Assessing fluid and electrolyte balance is a high priority in the early postoperative period. Edema is common. However, decisions concerning fluid administration are made on the basis of BP, pulmonary artery wedge pressure (PAWP), right atrial pressure, cardiac output, cardiac index, systemic vascular resistance, blood loss, and urine output. An experienced specialized nurse interprets the assessment findings and adjusts fluid administration on the basis of standing unit policies or specific prescription from the health care provider.

Serum electrolytes (especially calcium, magnesium, and potassium) may be decreased after surgery and are monitored carefully. Because the serum potassium level can fluctuate dramatically, electrolyte levels are checked frequently, since imbalances can cause dysrhythmias. Potassium and magnesium depletions are common and may result from hemodilution or diuretic therapy. Calcium replacement is based on the *ionized* serum calcium. The desired potassium level is 4.0 mEq/L, and the magnesium level should be 2.2 mEq/L.

If the serum potassium level is decreased, the health care provider may prescribe IV potassium replacement. The dose of

potassium given often exceeds the usual recommended level of no more than 20 mEq of potassium per hour. The drug must be given through a central catheter and controlled by an infusion pump. The patient is placed on a cardiac monitor for intense, focused nursing observation.

Managing Other Complications. Hypotension (systolic BP <90 mm Hg) is a major problem because it may result in the collapse of the coronary graft. Decreased preload (decreased PAWP) can result from hypovolemia or vasodilation. If the patient is hypovolemic, it might be appropriate to increase fluid administration or administer blood. The health care provider may manage the patient with volume replacement followed by vasopressor therapy to increase the BP. However, if hypotension is the result of left ventricular failure (increased PAWP), IV inotropes might be needed.

Hypothermia is a common problem after surgery. Although warm cardioplegia is now the usual operative procedure used, it is not uncommon for the body temperature to drift downward after the patient leaves the surgical suite. Monitor the body temperature and institute rewarming procedures if the temperature drops below 96.8° F (36° C). Rewarming may be accomplished with warm blankets, lights, or thermal blankets. The danger of rewarming patients too quickly is that they may begin shivering, resulting in metabolic acidosis, increased myocardial oxygen consumption, and hypoxia. To prevent shivering, rewarming should proceed at a rate no faster than 1.8° F (1° C) per hour. Discontinue the procedure when the body temperature approaches 98.6° F (37° C) and the patient's extremities feel warm.

Hypothermia is a significant risk for the patient after CABG surgery because it promotes vasoconstriction and *hypertension.* Other factors contributing to hypertension in the CABG patient include CPB, drug therapy, and increased sympathetic nervous system activity.

After surgery, many patients experience *hypertension* (hypertension is defined as a systolic BP greater than 140 to 150 mm Hg). Hypertension is dangerous because increased pressure promotes leakage from suture lines and may cause bleeding. Drugs such as nitroprusside (Nipride) or fenoldopam (Corlopam) may be given to decrease afterload, ease the workload of the heart, and prevent heart failure.

> **! NURSING SAFETY PRIORITY** **QSEN**
>
> **Action Alert**
>
> Bleeding after CABG surgery occurs to a limited extent in all patients. Measure mediastinal and pleural chest tube drainage at least hourly. Report drainage amounts over 150 mL/hr to the surgeon. Patients with internal mammary artery (IMA) grafts may have more chest drainage than those with saphenous vein grafts (from the leg).

To access the IMA, the pleural space has to be entered and requires a pleural chest tube with the mediastinal tubes, making pulmonary assessment crucial. An autotransfusion of chest drainage to assist with volume management when 500 mL has accumulated or 4 hours has elapsed may be done, depending on the clinical pathway or the health care provider's protocol. Maintain the patency of the mediastinal and pleural chest tubes. One effective way of promoting chest tube drainage is to prevent a dependent loop from forming in the tubing.

If the patient is bleeding and the mediastinal tubes are not kept patent, fluid (blood) may accumulate around the heart. The myocardium is then compressed, and cardiac tamponade results. The fluid compresses the atria and ventricles, preventing them from filling adequately and thus reducing cardiac output.

> **! NURSING SAFETY PRIORITY** **QSEN**
>
> **Critical Rescue**
>
> Assess for, document, and report manifestations of cardiac tamponade immediately, including:
> - Sudden cessation of previously heavy mediastinal drainage
> - Beck's Triad:
>   - Jugular venous distention but clear lung sounds
>   - Distant, muffled heart sounds
>   - Hypotension
> - Pulsus paradoxus (BP more than 10 mm Hg higher on expiration than on inspiration)
> - An equalizing of PAWP and right atrial pressure
> - Cardiovascular collapse

Prepare the patient for echocardiogram or chest x-ray to confirm the diagnosis. Pericardiocentesis (withdrawal of fluid from the pericardium via a large needle) may not be appropriate for tamponade after CABG because the blood in the pericardium may have clotted. Volume expansion and emergency sternotomy with drainage are the treatments of choice.

The patient may also demonstrate *changes in level of consciousness*, which may be permanent or transient (temporary, short term). Transient changes related to anesthesia, cardiopulmonary bypass (CPB), air emboli, or hypothermia occur in many patients. Assess for neurologic deficits, which may include slowness to arouse, memory loss, and new-onset confusion.

Patients with transient neurologic deficits usually return to baseline neurologic status within 4 to 8 hours. *Permanent* deficits associated with an intraoperative stroke may be manifested by:
- Abnormal pupillary response
- Failure to awaken from anesthesia

- Seizures
- Absence of sensory or motor function

> **! NURSING SAFETY PRIORITY** **QSEN**
>
> **Action Alert**
>
> After a CABG, check the patient's neurologic status every 30 to 60 minutes until he or she has awakened from anesthesia. Then check every 2 to 4 hours or per agency policy.

> **? NCLEX EXAMINATION CHALLENGE 38-3**
>
> **Physiological Integrity**
>
> The nurse assesses a client who had a coronary artery bypass graft yesterday. Which assessment finding will cause the nurse to suspect cardiac tamponade?
> A. Incisional pain with decreased urine output
> B. Muffled heart sounds with the presence of jugular venous distention (JVD)
> C. Sternal wound drainage with nausea
> D. Increased blood pressure and decreased heart rate

Managing Pain. Differentiate between *sternotomy pain*, which is expected after CABG, and *anginal pain*, which might indicate graft failure. Typical sternotomy pain is localized, does not radiate, and often becomes worse when the patient coughs or breathes deeply. He or she may describe the pain as sharp, aching, or burning. Pain may stimulate the sympathetic nervous system, which increases the heart rate and vascular resistance while decreasing cardiac output. Administer enough of the prescribed analgesic in adequate doses to control pain. However, during the process of weaning the patient from mechanical ventilation, it may be necessary to use short-acting analgesics and limit pain medication because of the respiratory depressant effects of analgesia.

Transfer from the Special Care Unit. Mechanical ventilation is usually provided for 3 to 6 hours after surgery until the patient is breathing adequately and is hemodynamically stable. During the first day, the patient usually has pacemaker wires, hemodynamic monitoring lines, and mediastinal tubes removed. He or she is then transferred to an intermediate care unit. *All CABG patients, especially those with IMA grafts, are at high risk for atelectasis, the number-one complication.* Encourage them to splint, cough, turn, and deep breathe to expectorate secretions. Early ambulation after surgery is essential. Two hours after extubation (removal of the endotracheal tube), patients should be dangled as tolerated and turned side to side. Within 4 to 8 hours after extubation, help patients out of bed into a chair. By the first day after surgery, they should be out of bed in a chair and ambulating 25 to 100 feet three times a day as tolerated. Continue to monitor for decreased cardiac output, pain, dysrhythmias, decreased oxygen saturation, and infection during these activities.

Many patients have supraventricular dysrhythmias (especially atrial fibrillation) during the postoperative period, usually on the second or third postoperative day. Examine the monitor pattern for atrial fibrillation. When auscultating the heart, listen for an irregular rhythm.

Sternal wound infections develop between 5 days and several weeks after surgery in a small number of patients and

Action Alert

Monitor the neurovascular status of the donor arm of patients whose radial artery was used as a graft in CABG. Assess the hand color, temperature, pulse (both ulnar and radial), and capillary refill every hour initially. In addition, check the fingertips, hand, and arm for sensation and mobility at least every 4 hours. IV nitroglycerin is often given for the first 24 hours after surgery to promote vasodilation in the donor arm and therefore maintain circulation.

are responsible for increased costs and longer hospital stays. Be alert for **mediastinitis** (infection of the mediastinum) by observing for:

- Fever continuing beyond the first 4 days after CABG
- Instability (bogginess) of the sternum
- Redness, induration, swelling, or drainage from suture sites
- An increased white blood cell count

The health care provider may perform a needle biopsy to confirm a sternal infection. Surgical débridement, antibiotic wound irrigation, and IV antibiotics are usually indicated. If sternal osteomyelitis has developed, 4 to 6 weeks of IV antibiotics are required. Prophylactic use of mupirocin (Bactroban) intranasally may be prescribed to decrease the incidence of sternal wound infection.

Postpericardiotomy syndrome is a source of chest discomfort for some post–cardiac surgery patients. The syndrome is characterized by pericardial and pleural pain, pericarditis, a friction rub, elevated temperature and white blood cell count, and dysrhythmias. Postpericardiotomy syndrome may occur days to weeks after surgery and seems to be associated with blood remaining in the pericardial sac. Observe for the development of pericardial or pleural pain. For most patients, the syndrome is mild and self-limiting. However, they may require treatment similar to that for pericarditis. Be prepared to detect acute cardiac (pericardial) tamponade.

Minimally Invasive Direct Coronary Artery Bypass. The **minimally invasive direct coronary artery bypass (MIDCAB)** (also known as *keyhole surgery*) may be indicated for patients with a lesion of the left anterior descending (LAD) artery. In one of the most common MIDCAB procedures, a 2-inch left thoracotomy incision is made, and the fourth rib is removed. Then the left internal mammary artery (IMA) is dissected and attached to the still-beating heart below the level of the lesion. Cardiopulmonary bypass (CPB) is not required.

After surgery, assess for chest pain and ECG changes (Q waves and ST-segment and T-wave changes in leads V_2 to V_6) because occlusion of the IMA graft occurs acutely in only a small percentage of patients. *If there is any question of acute graft closure, immediately notify the health care provider.* Patients tend to have more incisional pain after MIDCAB than after traditional CABG surgery, but usually it can be managed with oxycodone or codeine. Because they have a thoracotomy incision and a chest tube or smaller-lumen vacuum chest device, patients are encouraged to cough, deep breathe, and use an incentive spirometer for a week after surgery. Most patients spend less than 6 hours in a critical care unit and are discharged in 2 or 3 days.

Endovascular (Endoscopic) Vessel Harvesting. Regardless of whether the traditional CABG or the MIDCAB is performed,

the donor vessel may be obtained using an endoscope rather than a large surgical incision. The radial artery or a vein in the leg may be taken with this method. Instead of a large, painful incision, the patient has one or two very small incisions in the leg or arm. This procedure has decreased hospital length of stay, postoperative complications, and pain.

Transmyocardial Laser Revascularization. **Transmyocardial laser revascularization** is a procedure for patients with unstable angina and inoperable CAD with areas of reversible myocardial ischemia. After a single-lung intubation, a left anterior thoracotomy is performed and the heart is visualized. A laser is used to create 20 to 24 long, narrow channels through the left ventricular muscle to the left ventricle. These channels will eventually allow oxygenated blood to flow during diastole from the left ventricle to nourish the muscle. After surgery, the patient is transported to a critical care unit, where hemodynamic monitoring is used to assess for anginal episodes and bleeding disturbances.

Off-Pump Coronary Artery Bypass. Off-pump coronary artery bypass (OPCAB) is a procedure in which open-heart surgery is performed without the use of a heart-lung bypass machine. Advantages include shorter hospital stays and decreased mortality rate, risk for infection, and cost. The disadvantage of OPCAB is that it requires cardiac surgeons to have increased skill to master the technique.

Robotic Heart Surgery. Robotic heart surgery is a new step toward less invasive open-heart surgery. Surgeons operate endoscopically through very small incisions in the chest wall. Use of robotics provides surgeons with capabilities that simplify the surgical process, eliminate tremors that can exist with human hands, increase the ability to reach otherwise inaccessible sites, and improve depth perception and visual acuity.

Other advantages of robotic procedures include shorter hospital stays (average stay is 2 to 3 days), less pain because of smaller incisions, no need for heart-lung bypass machine, less anxiety for the patient, and greater patient acceptance. The use of robotics also allows surgeons to perform telesurgery, performing heart procedures over long distances.

Disadvantages include computer failure, limited numbers of surgeons skilled in these techniques, and the length of surgery time (the time is about 50 minutes longer than the conventional surgery).

Care Coordination and Transition Management

Home Care Management. Case management is most appropriate for patients who meet high-cost, high-volume, and high-risk criteria. Patients with coronary artery disease (CAD) clearly meet all these criteria. Clinical pathways and case-management programs for those with CAD are used in most U.S. hospitals. By focusing on cardiovascular risk reduction and improving the continuity of care, health care professionals have reduced the length and cost of hospital stays. Posthospital case management should reduce hospital readmission rates and improve patient health.

Patients who have experienced a myocardial infarction (MI), angina, or coronary artery bypass graft (CABG) surgery are usually discharged to home or to a transitional care setting with drug therapy and specific activity prescriptions. Depending on the procedure, hospital stays may be 3 to 5 days for patients with MI or those undergoing CABG and only 1 to 2 days for those undergoing percutaneous coronary intervention (PCI) or newer surgeries. Therefore patients are still recovering when they are discharged from the hospital and need continuing care.

Patients should not be discharged to home alone. Assess whether the patient has family or friends to provide assistance. In some cases, a home care nurse may be needed (Chart 38-8). Older adults are often living alone when coronary events occur and may have a greater need for home assistance after CABG surgery (Chart 38-9). A patient who was a resident in a long-term care facility may be returned there after hospitalization for unstable angina, MI, or CABG surgery.

CHART 38-8   Home Care Assessment

The Patient Who Has Had a Myocardial Infarction

Assess cardiovascular function, including:
- Current vital signs (compare with previous to identify changes)
- Recurrence of discomfort (characteristics, frequency, onset)
- Indications of heart failure (weight gain, crackles, cough, dyspnea)
- Adequacy of tissue perfusion (mentation, skin temperature, peripheral pulses, urine output)
- Indications of serious dysrhythmia (very irregular pulse, palpitations with fainting or near fainting)

Assess coping skills, including:
- Is patient displaying denial, anger, or fear?
- Is caregiver providing adequate support?
- Are patient and caregiver disagreeing about treatment?

Assess functional ability, including:
- Activity tolerance (examine the patient's activity diary: review distance, duration, frequency, and symptoms occurring during exercise)
- ADLs (is any assistance needed?)
- Household chores (who performs them?)
- Does patient plan to return to work? When?

Assess nutritional status, including:
- Food intake (review patient's intake of fats and cholesterol)

Assess patient's understanding of illness and treatment, including:
- How to treat chest discomfort
- Signs and symptoms to report to health care provider
- Dosage, effects, and side effects of medications
- How to advance and when to limit activity
- Modification of risk factors for coronary artery disease

CHART 38-9   Nursing Focus on the Older Adult

Coronary Artery Bypass Graft Surgery

- Be aware that perioperative mortality rates are higher for the older patient than for the patient younger than 60 years.
- Monitor neurologic and mental status carefully because older adults are more likely to have transient neurologic deficits after coronary artery bypass graft (CABG) surgery than younger adults are.
- Observe for side effects of cardiac drugs because older patients are more likely to develop toxic effects from positive inotropes (dobutamine) and potent antihypertensives (nitroglycerin or nitroprusside).
- Monitor the patient closely for dysrhythmias because older adults are more likely to have dysrhythmias such as atrial fibrillation or supraventricular tachycardia after CABG surgery.
- Be aware that recuperation after CABG surgery is slower for older patients and that their average hospital stay is longer.
- Teach the patient and family that, during the first 2 to 5 weeks after discharge, fatigue, chest discomfort, and lack of appetite may be particularly bothersome for older adults.
- Teach the patient to let someone know where he or she is walking outside.

Cardiac rehabilitation is available in most communities for patients after an MI or CABG surgery, but only a small percentage participate in structured rehabilitation programs. The most frequently cited reasons for nonparticipation are lack of insurance coverage, a health care provider's decision that it is unnecessary, and the patient's decision that it is not necessary. Those who participate in these programs report greater improvement in exercise tolerance and improved ability to control stress. However, no difference in their return to work has been seen.

Self-Management Education. The need for health teaching depends in part on the treatment plan or type of procedure that the patient received. Because hospital stays are short and patients are quite ill during hospitalization, most in-hospital education programs concentrate on the skills essential for self-care after discharge.

As part of home visits or a cardiac rehabilitation program, identify the additional educational needs of the patient and family and their readiness to learn. Develop a teaching plan, which usually includes education about the normal anatomy and physiology of the heart, the pathophysiology of angina and MI, risk factor modification, activity and exercise protocols, cardiac drugs, and when to seek medical assistance. Teach patients that myocardial healing after an MI begins early and is usually complete in 6 to 8 weeks. Remind those who have undergone traditional CABG that the sternotomy should heal in about 6 to 8 weeks, but upper body exercise needs to be limited for several months.

Patients who have undergone CABG require instruction on incision care for the sternum and the graft site. Teach them to inspect the incisions daily for any redness, swelling, or drainage. The leg of a saphenous vein donor site is often edematous. Instruct patients to avoid crossing legs, to wear elastic stockings until the edema subsides, and to elevate the surgical limb when sitting in a chair. Teach patients who have had a radial artery graft to open and close the hand vigorously 10 times every 2 hours.

Risk Factor Modification. Modification of risk factors is a necessary part of a patient's management and involves changing his or her health maintenance patterns. Such modifications may include tobacco cessation, altered dietary patterns, regular exercise, BP control, and blood glucose control.

For patients who use tobacco, explain its negative effects, especially cigarette smoking. Many patients choose to quit smoking soon after an MI. Chart 27-1 also provides information on this lifestyle change.

The mainstays of cholesterol control are nutritional therapy and antihyperlipidemic agents, as described in Chapter 36. Teach patients to avoid adding salt when beginning a meal. A reduction of 80 mg/day of sodium can reduce the systolic blood pressure (SBP) by 5 mm Hg and 3 mm Hg for the diastolic blood pressure (DBP). Maintain adequate dietary potassium, calcium, and magnesium intake. Increasing potassium may reduce the SBP by 8 mm Hg. Booklets and cookbooks that can help the patient learn to cook with reduced fats, oils, and salt are available from the American Heart Association (AHA).

Collaborate with the cardiac rehabilitation specialist to establish an activity and exercise schedule as part of rehabilitation, depending on the cardiac procedure that was performed. Instruct the patient to remain near home during the first week after discharge and to continue a walking program. Patients may engage in light housework or any activity done while

CHART 38-10 Patient and Family Education: Preparing for Self-Management

Activity for the Patient With Coronary Artery Disease

- Begin by walking the same distance at home as in the hospital (usually 400 feet) 3 times each day.
- Carry nitroglycerin with you.
- Check your pulse before, during, and after the exercise.
- Stop the activity for a pulse increase of more than 20 beats/min, shortness of breath, angina, or dizziness. Make gradual increases in walking distance.
- Exercise outdoors when the weather is good.
- After an exercise tolerance test and with your health care provider's approval, walk at least 3 times each week, increasing the distance every other week, until the total distance is 1 mile.
- Avoid straining (lifting, push-ups, pull-ups, and straining at bowel movements).

sitting and that does not precipitate angina. During the second week, they are encouraged to increase social activities and possibly to return to work part time. By the third week, they may begin to lift objects as heavy as 15 lb (e.g., 2 gallons of milk) but should avoid lifting or pulling heavier objects for the first 6 to 8 weeks. Chart 38-10 lists suggested instructions for activity level.

Patients may begin a simple walking program by walking 400 feet twice a day at the rate of 1 mile/hr the first week after discharge and increasing the distance and rate as tolerated, usually weekly, until can walk 2 miles at 3 to 4 miles/hr. Teach them to take their pulse reading before, halfway through, and after exercise. Teach the patient to stop exercising if the target pulse rate is exceeded or if dyspnea or angina develops.

After a limited exercise tolerance test, the cardiac rehabilitation specialist or nurse encourages the patient to join a formal exercise program, ideally one that helps him or her monitor cardiovascular progress. The program should include 5- to 7-minute warm-up and cool-down periods and 30 minutes of aerobic exercise. The patient should engage in aerobic exercise a minimum of 3 (and preferably 5) times a week.

Complementary and Integrative Health. Additional therapies can aid in reducing the patient's anxiety about progressive activity both in the immediate postoperative period and during the rehabilitation phase. Many patients who have had cardiac surgery or other invasive procedures use complementary and integrative therapy practices. However, they often do not share with their health care providers that they use these practices. Techniques such as progressive muscle relaxation, guided imagery, music therapy, pet therapy, and therapeutic touch may decrease anxiety, reduce depression, and increase compliance with activity and exercise regimens after heart surgery.

Teach patients that adding omega-3 fatty acids from fish and plant sources has been effective for some patients in reducing lipid levels, stabilizing atherosclerotic plaques, and reducing sudden death from an MI. The preferred source of omega-3 acids is from fish two times a week or a daily fish oil nutritional supplement (1-2 g/day) (American Heart Association [AHA], 2016). Patients often take a number of other supplements, such as vitamin E, coenzyme Q_{10}, Pantesin, and vitamin B complex to decrease the risk for heart disease. However, studies do not show that these substances are helpful in reducing coronary artery disease.

Sexual Activity. Sexual activity is often a subject of great concern to patients and their partners. Inform the patient and his or her partner that engaging in their usual sexual activity is unlikely to damage the heart. Patients can resume sexual intercourse on the advice of the health care provider, usually after an exercise-tolerance assessment. In general, those who can walk one block or climb two flights of stairs without symptoms can usually safely resume sexual activity.

Suggest that initially these patients have intercourse after a period of rest. They might try having intercourse in the morning when they are well rested or wait $1\frac{1}{2}$ hours after exercise or a heavy meal. The position selected should be comfortable for both the patient and his or her partner so no undue stress is placed on the heart or suture line.

Drug Therapy. Assess patients with diabetes mellitus for their ability to control hyperglycemia. Review the prescribed dosage of insulin or oral antidiabetic drugs with the patient and family. The patient and/or family should demonstrate accurate testing of blood for glucose levels and the technique for insulin administration, if used.

Teach the patient about the type of prescribed cardiac drugs, the benefit of each drug, potential side effects, and the correct dosage and time of day to take each drug. Drug regimens vary considerably. Many patients with angina are discharged while taking aspirin, a beta blocker, a calcium channel blocker, a statin agent, and a nitrate. Those who have experienced an MI may require dual antiplatelet therapy with aspirin and a P2Y12 inhibitor, a beta blocker, a statin drug, and, if the ejection fraction is <40%, an ACEI and/or an ARB. It is recommended that all patients with cardiovascular disease receive an annual influenza vaccine and that patients over age 56 should also receive the pneumococcal vaccine. Determine whether the patient can comply with the instructions.

! NURSING SAFETY PRIORITY QSEN
Drug Alert

The FDA has strengthened the warnings associated with NSAIDs and cardiovascular risk. Use of nonaspirin NSAIDs can increase the chance of heart attack or stroke. This risk of heart attack or stroke can occur early in treatment and may increase with length of treatment. Those with CVD have the greatest risk for adverse cardiovascular events. Teach the patient that NSAIDs are commonly available over the counter so it is very important to read box labels. Acetaminophen products provide an alternative for pain relief and fever reduction.

! NURSING SAFETY PRIORITY QSEN
Drug Alert

Use of sublingual or spray nitroglycerin (NTG) deserves special attention. *Teach the patient to carry NTG at all times.* Keep the tablets in a glass, light-resistant container. The drug should be replaced every 3 to 5 months before it loses its potency or stops producing a tingling sensation when placed under the tongue. Chart 38-11 gives instructions for management of chest discomfort at home.

Seeking Medical Assistance. Teach patients to notify their health care provider if they have:

- Heart rate remaining less than 50 after arising
- Wheezing or difficulty breathing
- Weight gain of 3 lb in 1 week or 1 to 2 lb overnight
- Persistent increase in NTG use
- Dizziness, faintness, or shortness of breath with activity

CHART 38-11 Patient and Family Education: Preparing for Self-Management

Management of Chest Pain at Home

- Keep fresh nitroglycerin available for immediate use.
- At the first indication of chest discomfort, cease activity and sit or lie down.
- Place one nitroglycerin tablet or spray under your tongue, allowing the tablet to dissolve.
- Wait 5 minutes for relief.
- If no relief results, call 911 for transportation to a health care facility.
- While waiting for emergency medical services (EMS), repeat the nitroglycerin and wait 5 more minutes.
- If there is no relief, repeat and wait 5 more minutes.
- Carry a medical identification card or wear a bracelet or necklace that identifies a history of heart problems.

Remind them to always call 911 for transportation to the hospital if they have:

- Chest discomfort that does not improve after 5 minutes or one sublingual NTG tablet or spray
- Extremely severe chest or epigastric discomfort with weakness, nausea, or fainting
- Other associated symptoms that are particular to them, such as fatigue and nausea

Health Care Resources. The American Heart Association (AHA) is an excellent source for booklets, films, CDs, DVDs, cookbooks, and professional service referrals for the patient with coronary artery disease (CAD). Many local chapters have their own cardiac rehabilitation programs. Specifically for women, the AHA has established the Go Red Heart Match.

This online program matches women with similar conditions and experience, which provides a connection and support system.

Within the community, cardiac rehabilitation programs may be affiliated with local hospitals, community centers, or other facilities such as clinics. Many shopping malls open before shopping hours to allow a measured walking program indoors.

This opportunity is particularly popular with older patients because it provides a good support group and allows for an appropriate place to exercise in inclement weather.

Mended Hearts is a nationwide program with local chapters that provides education and support to coronary artery bypass graft (CABG) patients and their families. Smoking-cessation programs and clinics and weight-reduction programs are located within the community. Many hospitals and places of worship also sponsor health fairs, BP screening, and risk-factor modification programs.

CLINICAL JUDGMENT CHALLENGE 38-2

Teamwork and Collaboration; Safety QSEN

A 55-year-old woman had a CABG surgical procedure and is scheduled for discharge from the hospital tomorrow. The patient lives with her daughter and is anxious to resume her active lifestyle.
1. What elements are essential to address for home care management of the patient?
2. What members of the interprofessional health care team should the nurse collaborate to ensure the patient's continuity of care?
3. What are the expected outcomes for this patient as a result of cardiac rehabilitation?
4. What community resources might this patient use after the completion of her cardiac rehabilitation program?
5. For what surgical complications is she still at risk?

◆ **Evaluation: Reflecting**

Evaluate the care of the patient with CAD based on the identified priority patient problems. The expected outcomes are that the patient will:

- State that discomfort or other symptoms are alleviated
- Have adequate blood flow through the coronary vasculature to ensure heart function
- Walk 200 feet four times a day without discomfort, shortness of breath, or other symptoms of CAD
- Identify support systems and other sources to assist in effective coping with the cardiac event
- Be free of complications such as dysrhythmias and heart failure

GET READY FOR THE NCLEX® EXAMINATION!

KEY POINTS

Review these Key Points for each NCLEX Examination Client Needs Category.

Safe and Effective Care Environment
- Collaborate with members of the interprofessional health care team (e.g., cardiac rehabilitation specialist, case manager, home care providers) when caring for patients participating in cardiac rehabilitation. **QSEN: Teamwork and Collaboration**

Health Promotion and Maintenance
- Assess the patient for risk factors for coronary artery disease (CAD). Examples of modifiable risk factors that can be managed or controlled include obesity, smoking, high serum

lipids, and hypertension; examples of nonmodifiable risk factors that cannot be altered include older age, being African American, and having a family history of CAD.
- Teach patients about the importance of decreasing their risk for CAD (see Chart 38-1). **QSEN: Safety**

Psychosocial Integrity
- Allow patients to verbalize and express feelings of fear, anxiety, anger, denial, and grief regarding their CAD. **QSEN: Patient-Centered Care**
- Address the needs of the family and significant others and provide teaching and information regarding the disease process. Clarify any misconceptions.

Physiological Integrity

- Teach patients that angina is the pain associated with decreased blood flow to the heart muscle. An MI indicates necrosis of heart muscle tissue (see Chart 38-2).
- Identify and interpret diagnostic values for cardiac markers, such as troponins and myoglobin, and other indicators of CAD. **Clinical Judgment**
- Monitor patients receiving thrombolytics and anticoagulants, such as heparin, for bleeding and bruising. **QSEN: Safety**
- For patients undergoing invasive cardiac procedures, assess for signs and symptoms of active bleeding. **QSEN: Safety**
- Interpret and assess the patient with CAD for dysrhythmias.
- Evaluate the patient for pain characteristics (e.g., type, location, duration, cause, intensity, and measures taken to relieve symptoms).
- Teach patients and their families about drug therapy, including how to use nitroglycerin if they have chest or other cardiac-related pain (see Chart 38-4).

- After percutaneous cardiac intervention, monitor the patient for potential complications such as chest pain, bleeding from the insertion site, hypotension, hypokalemia, and dysrhythmias. Document and report any of these findings immediately. **QSEN: Safety**
- Identify and assess for complications for post–cardiac surgery patients, especially fluid and electrolyte imbalance, bleeding, hypothermia, hypertension, and angina pain.
- Provide emergency care for the patient with chest pain as described in Chart 38-3.
- For patients having coronary artery bypass graft (CABG) surgery, be sure to manage pain adequately, assess fluid and electrolyte balance, and monitor for potential complications. Examples of complications include fluid and electrolyte imbalances (especially hypokalemia), hypothermia, hypertension, bleeding, sternal wound infections, and neurologic deficits. **Clinical Judgment; QSEN: Evidence-Based Practice, Quality Improvement**

SELECTED BIBLIOGRAPHY

Asterisk indicates a classic or definitive work on this subject.

American Heart Association (AHA). (2016). *The American Heart Association's diet and lifestyle recommendations* (updated: October 2016). www.heart.org/HEARTORG/GettingHealthy/Diet-and-Lifestyle-Recommendations_UCM_305855_Article.jsp.

Amsterdam, E., Wenger, N., Brindis, R., Casey, D., Ganiats, T., Holmes, D., et al. (2014). 2014 AHA/ACC guideline for the management of patients with non–ST-elevation acute coronary syndromes. *Journal of the American College of Cardiology, 64*(4), e139–e228.

Beckie, T., & McCabe, P. (2015). Depression among patients with acute coronary syndrome. *Journal of Cardiovascular Nursing, 29*(4), 288–290.

Bhandari, B., & Mehta, B. (2014). Vorapaxar, a protease-activated receptor-1 antagonist, a double-edged sword! *Recent Advances in Cardiovascular Drug Discovery, 9*(2), 1–5.

Casey, A., Itrakjy, A., Birkett, C., Clethro, A., Bonser, R., Graham, T., et al. (2015). A comparison of the efficacy of 70% v/v isopropyl alcohol with either 0.5% w/v or 2% w/v chlorhexidine gluconate for skin preparation before harvest of the long saphenous vein used in coronary artery bypass grafting. *American Journal of Infection Control, 43*, 816–820.

Clark, M., Beavers, C., & Osborne, J. (2015). Managing the acute coronary syndrome patient: Evidence-based recommendations for anti-platelet therapy. *Heart and Lung: The Journal of Critical Care, 44*, 141–149.

Frazer, C. (2015). Metabolic syndrome. *Medical Surgical Nursing, 42*(2), 125–126.

*Gara, P., Kushner, F., Ascheim, D., Casey, D., Chung, M., de Lemos, J., et al. (2013). 2013 ACCF/AHA guideline for the management of ST-elevation myocardial infarction. *Circulation, 127*, e362–e425.

Gibson, J., & Raphael, B. (2014). Understanding beta blockers. *Nursing, 44*(6), 55–59.

Gillis, N., Arslanian-Engoren, C., & Struble, L. (2014). Acute coronary syndromes in older adults: A review of the literature. *Journal of Emergency Nursing, 40*(3), 270–275.

*Grundy, S. M., Cleeman, J. I., Daniels, S. R., Donato, K. A., Eckel, R. H., Franklin, B. A., et al. (2005). Diagnosis and management of the metabolic syndrome: An American Heart Association/National Heart, Lung, and Blood Institute scientific statement. *Circulation, 112*(17), 2735–2752.

*Hillis, D., Smith, P., Anderson, J., Bittl, J., Bridges, C., Byrne, J., et al. (2011). 2011 ACCF/AHA guideline for coronary artery bypass graft surgery: Executive summary: A report of the American College of

Cardiology Foundation/American Heart Association Task Force on Practice Guidelines. *Circulation, 124*, 2610–2642.

Huber, K., Bates, E., Valgimigli, M., Wallentin, L., Kristensen, S., Anderson, J., et al. (2014). Antiplatelet and anticoagulation agents in acute coronary syndromes: What is the current status and what does the future hold? *American Heart Journal, 168*, 611–621.

Hussar, D. (2015). New drugs 2015. *Nursing 2015*, part 2, *45*(7), 34–41.

Injean, P., McKinnell, J., Hsiue, P., Vangala, S., Miller, L., Benharash, P., et al. (2014). Survey of preoperative infection prevention for coronary bypass graft procedures. *Infection Control and Hospital Epidemiology, 35*(6), 736–737.

Jarvis, C. (2016). *Physical examination & health assessment* (7th ed.). St. Louis: Saunders.

Joseph, H., Whitcomb, J., & Taylor, W. (2015). Effect of anxiety on individuals and caregivers after coronary artery bypass grafting surgery: A review of the literature. *Dimensions of Critical Care Nursing, 34*(5), 285–288.

King, J., & Magdic, K. (2014). Chest pain: A time for concern. *AACN Advanced Critical Care, 25*(3), 279–283.

Kles, C., Murrah, C., Smith, K., Baugus-Wellmeier, E., Hurry, T., & Morris, C. (2015). Achieving and sustaining zero: Preventing surgical site infections after isolated coronary artery bypass with saphenous vein harvest site through implementation of a staff-driven quality improvement process. *Dimensions of Critical Care Nursing, 34*(5), 265–272.

Le, R., Kosowksy, J., Landman, A., Bixho, I., Melanson, S., & Tanasijevic, M. (2015). Clinical and financial impact of removing creatine kinase-MB from the routine testing menu in the emergency setting. *American Journal of Emergency Medicine, 33*, 72–75.

Levine, G., O'Gara, P., Bates, E., Blankenship, J., Kushner, F., Bailey, S., et al. (2015). 2015 ACC/AHA/SCAI Focused Update on primary percutaneous coronary intervention for patients with ST-elevation myocardial infarction: An update of the 2011 ACCF/AHA/SCAI guideline for percutaneous coronary intervention and the 2013 ACF/AHA guideline for the management of ST-elevation myocardial infarction. *Journal of the American College of Cardiology*, doi:10.1016/.jacc.2015.10.005.

*Lindholm, D., Varenhorst, C., Cannon, C., Harrington, R., Himmelmann, A., Maya, J., et al. (2013). Ticagrelor versus clopidogrel in patients with non-ST-elevation acute coronary syndrome: Results from the PLATO trial. *Journal of the American College of Cardiology, 61*(10), doi:http://dx.doi.org/10.1016/S0735-1097(13)60002-9.

McCance, K., Huether, S., Brashers, V., & Rote, N. (2014). *Pathophysiology: The biologic basis for disease in adults and children* (7th ed.). St. Louis: Mosby.

McSweeney, J., Cleves, M., Fischer, E., Moser, D., Wei, J., Pettey, C., et al. (2014). Predicting coronary heart disease events in women: A longitudinal cohort study. *Journal of Cardiovascular Nursing, 29*(6), 482–492.

Mozaffarian, D., Benjamin, E., Go, A., Arnett, D., Blaha, M., Cushman, M., et al. (2016). Heart disease and stroke statistics—2016 update. *Circulation*, doi:10.1161/CIR0000000000000350.

O'Keefe-McCarthy, S., McGillion, M., Clarke, S., & McFetridge-Durdle, J. (2015). Pain and anxiety in rural acute coronary syndrome patients awaiting diagnostic cardiac catheterization. *Journal of Cardiovascular Nursing, 30*(6), 546–557.

Roberts, S. (2015). Primary care of women who have sex with women recommendations from the research. *The Nurse Practitioner, 40*(12), 24–32. doi:10.1097/01.NPR.0000431883.32986.81.

Sherrod, M. M., Sherrod, N. M., Spitzer, M. T., & Cheek, D. J. (2013). AHA recommendations for preventing heart disease in women. *Nursing, 43*(5), 61–66.

Stone, N., Robinson, J., Lichtenstein, A., Bairey, N., Blum, C., Eckel, R., et al. (2013). 2013 ACC/AHA guideline on the treatment of blood cholesterol to reduce atherosclerotic cardiovascular risk in adults: A report of the American College of Cardiology/American Heart Association task force on practice guidelines. *Circulation, 129*(Suppl. 2), S1–S45.

*Thygesen, K., Alpert, J., Jaffe, A., Simoons, M., Chaitman, B., White, H., et al. (2012). Third universal definition of myocardial infarction. *Circulation, 126*, 2020–2035.

U.S. Food and Drug Administration. (May, 2014). *FDA approves Zontivity to reduce the risk of heart attacks and stroke in high-risk patients.* [News Release]. www.fda.gov/NewsEvents/Newsroom/PressAnnouncements/ucm396585.htm.

U.S. Food and Drug Administration. (July, 2015). *FDA strengthens warning of heart attack and stroke risk for non-steroidal anti-inflammatory drugs.* http://www.fda.gov/ForConsumers/ConsumerUpdates/ucm453610.htm.

Waite, L., Phan, Y., & Spinler, S. (2014). Cangrelor: A novel intravenous antiplatelet agent with a questionable future. *Pharmacotherapy, 34*(10), 1061–1076.

CHAPTER **39**

Assessment of the Hematologic System

M. Linda Workman

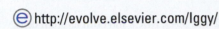
http://evolve.elsevier.com/Iggy/

PRIORITY AND INTERRELATED CONCEPTS

The priority concepts for this chapter are:
- CLOTTING
- PERFUSION

LEARNING OUTCOMES

Safe and Effective Care Environment

1. Collaborate with the interprofessional team to perform a complete hematologic assessment, including CLOTTING and PERFUSION.

Health Promotion and Maintenance

2. Explain how physiologic aging changes the hematologic functions of CLOTTING and PERFUSION and how these changes affect the associated care of older adults.
3. Teach all adults how to protect the hematologic system.

Psychosocial Integrity

4. Implement patient-centered nursing interventions to help the patient and family cope with the psychosocial impact of a possible hematologic health problem.

Physiological Integrity

5. Apply knowledge of anatomy and physiology, including information about genetic risk, to perform an evidence-based assessment for the patient with a possible hematologic problem.
6. Interpret assessment findings for the patient undergoing hematologic assessment.
7. Teach the patient and caregivers about diagnostic procedures associated with hematologic assessment.
8. Explain the effects of anticoagulants, fibrinolytics, and inhibitors of platelet activity on CLOTTING and PERFUSION.
9. Prioritize nursing care for the patient after bone marrow aspiration or biopsy.

The blood, blood cells, lymph, and organs involved with blood formation or blood storage compose the hematologic system. The concepts of peripheral and central tissue PERFUSION and gas exchange (oxygenation) rely on the hematologic system, because the blood is the oxygen delivery system (Fig. 39-1). Perfusion is the total arterial blood flow through the tissues (peripheral perfusion) and blood that is pumped by the heart (central perfusion). All systems depend on the blood for oxygen perfusion, and any problem of the hematologic system affects total body health. In addition, the concept of CLOTTING is a function of this system. Clotting is a complex, multi-step process by which blood forms a protein-based structure (clot) in an appropriate area of tissue injury to prevent excessive bleeding while maintaining whole-body blood flow (perfusion).

Chapter 2 further explains these concepts. This chapter, together with Chapter 17, reviews the normal physiology of the hematologic system and assessment of hematologic status.

ANATOMY AND PHYSIOLOGY REVIEW

Bone Marrow

Bone marrow is responsible for blood formation by producing red blood cells (RBCs, erythrocytes), white blood cells (WBCs, leukocytes), and platelets. Bone marrow also is involved in the immune responses (see Chapter 17).

Each day the bone marrow normally releases about 2.5 billion RBCs, 2.5 billion platelets, and 1 billion WBCs per kilogram of body weight. In adults, cell-producing marrow is present only in flat bones (sternum, skull, pelvic and shoulder girdles) and the ends of long bones. With aging, fatty tissue replaces active bone marrow, and only a small portion of the remaining marrow continues to produce blood in older adults (Touhy & Jett, 2016).

The bone marrow first produces **blood stem cells**, which are immature, unspecialized (undifferentiated) cells that are capable of becoming any type of blood cell, depending on the body's needs (Fig. 39-2) (McCance et al., 2014).

The next stage in blood cell production is the *committed stem cell* (or *precursor* cell). A committed stem cell enters one growth pathway and can at that point specialize (differentiate) into only one cell type. Committed stem cells actively divide but require the presence of a specific growth factor for specialization. For example, erythropoietin is a growth factor specific for the RBC. Other growth factors control WBC and platelet growth (see Chapters 17, 22, and 40 for discussion of growth factors and cytokines).

Blood Components

Blood is composed of plasma and cells. Plasma is an extracellular fluid similar to the interstitial fluid found between tissue cells, but containing much more protein. The three major types of plasma proteins are albumin, globulins, and fibrinogen.

Albumin maintains the osmotic pressure of the blood, preventing the plasma from leaking into the tissues (see Chapter 11). *Globulins* have many functions, such as transporting other substances and, as antibodies, protecting the body against infection. *Fibrinogen* is activated to form fibrin, which is critical in the blood CLOTTING process.

The blood cells include RBCs, WBCs, and platelets. These cells differ in structure, site of maturation, and function.

Red blood cells (**erythrocytes**) are the largest proportion of blood cells. Mature RBCs have a biconcave disk shape and no nucleus. Together with a flexible membrane, this feature allows RBCs to change their shape without breaking as they pass through narrow, winding capillaries. The number of RBCs an adult has varies with gender, age, and general health, but the normal range is from 4,200,000 to 6,100,000/mm³ (4.2 to 6.1 × 10^{12}/L).

As shown in Figs. 39-2 and 39-3, RBCs start out as stem cells, enter the myeloid pathway, and progress in stages to mature erythrocytes. Healthy, mature, circulating RBCs have a life span of about 120 days. As RBCs age, their membranes become more fragile. These old cells are trapped and destroyed in the tissues, spleen, and liver. Some parts of destroyed RBCs (e.g., iron, hemoglobin) are recycled and used to make new RBCs.

The RBCs produce hemoglobin (Hgb). Each normal mature RBC contains hundreds of thousands of hemoglobin molecules. Each hemoglobin molecule needs iron to be able to transport up to four molecules of oxygen. *Therefore iron is an essential part of hemoglobin.* Hemoglobin also carries carbon dioxide. RBCs also help maintain acid-base balance.

The most important feature of hemoglobin is its ability to combine loosely with oxygen. Only a small drop in tissue oxygen levels increases the transfer of oxygen from hemoglobin to

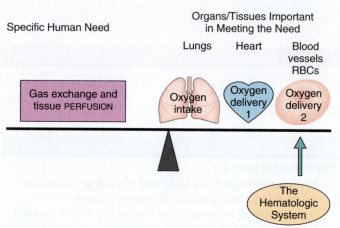

FIG. 39-1 Role of the hematologic system in gas exchange and tissue PERFUSION. *RBCs,* Red blood cells.

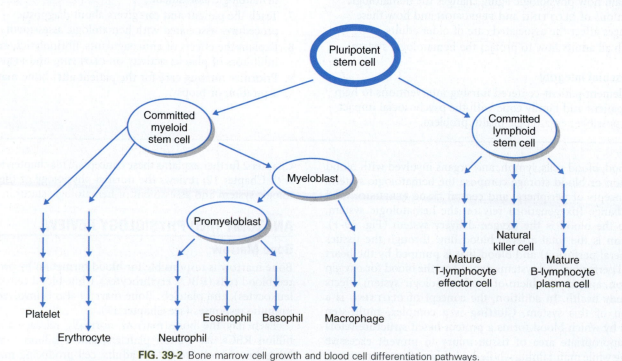

FIG. 39-2 Bone marrow cell growth and blood cell differentiation pathways.

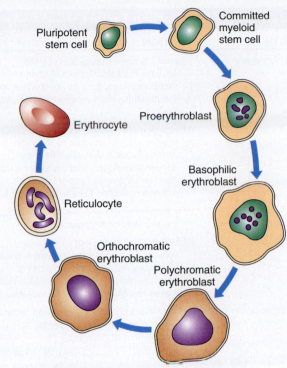

FIG. 39-3 Erythrocyte (red blood cell) growth pathway.

TABLE 39-1	Functions of Specific Leukocytes
LEUKOCYTE	**FUNCTION**
Inflammation	
Neutrophil	Nonspecific ingestion and phagocytosis of microorganisms and foreign protein
Macrophage	Nonspecific recognition of foreign proteins and microorganisms; ingestion and phagocytosis
Monocyte	Destruction of bacteria and cellular debris; matures into macrophage
Eosinophil	Weak phagocytic action; releases vasoactive amines during allergic reactions
Basophil	Releases histamine and heparin in areas of tissue damage
Antibody-Mediated Immunity	
B-lymphocyte	Becomes sensitized to foreign cells and proteins
Plasma cell	Secretes immunoglobulins in response to the presence of a specific antigen
Memory cell	Remains sensitized to a specific antigen and can secrete increased amounts of immunoglobulins specific to the antigen on re-exposure
Cell-Mediated Immunity	
T-lymphocyte helper/inducer T-cell	Enhances immune activity through the secretion of various factors, cytokines, and lymphokines
Cytotoxic-cytolytic T-cell	Selectively attacks and destroys non-self cells, including virally infected cells, grafts, and transplanted organs
Natural killer cell	Nonselectively attacks non-self cells, especially body cells that have undergone mutation and become malignant; also attacks grafts and transplanted organs

tissues, known as **oxygen dissociation**. See Chapter 27 for a discussion of oxygen dissociation.

An adult's total number of RBCs is carefully controlled to ensure that enough are present for good PERFUSION with oxygen and for CLOTTING without having too many cells that could "thicken" the blood and slow its flow. RBC production or **erythropoiesis** (selective growth of stem cells into mature erythrocytes) must be properly balanced with RBC destruction or loss. When balanced, this process helps tissue perfusion by ensuring adequate delivery of oxygen. The trigger for RBC production is an increase in the tissue need for oxygen. The kidney produces the RBC growth factor erythropoietin at the same rate as RBC destruction or loss occurs to maintain a constant normal level of circulating RBCs. When tissue oxygen is less than normal (**hypoxia**), the kidney releases more erythropoietin, which then increases RBC production in the bone marrow. When tissue oxygen is normal or high, erythropoietin levels fall, slowing RBC production. Synthetic erythrocyte-stimulating agents (ESAs) such as Procrit, Epogen, and EPO have the same effect on bone marrow as the naturally occurring erythropoietin.

Many substances are needed to form hemoglobin and RBCs, including iron, vitamin B_{12}, folic acid, copper, pyridoxine, cobalt, and nickel. A lack of any of these substances can lead to anemia, which results in unmet tissue oxygen needs because of a reduction in the number or function of RBCs.

White blood cells (WBCs, leukocytes) also are formed in the bone marrow. The many types of WBCs all have specialized functions that provide protection through inflammation and immunity (Table 39-1). WBC function is presented in Chapter 17.

Platelets are the third type of blood cells. They are the smallest blood cells, formed in the bone marrow from megakaryocyte precursor cells. When activated, platelets stick to injured blood vessel walls and form platelet plugs that can stop the flow of blood at the injured site. They also produce substances important to blood CLOTTING and *aggregate* (clump together) to perform most of their functions. Platelets help keep small blood vessels intact by initiating repair after damage.

Production of platelets is controlled by the growth factor thrombopoietin. After platelets leave the bone marrow, they are stored in the spleen and then released slowly to meet the body's needs. Normally 80% of platelets circulate and 20% are stored in the spleen.

Accessory Organs of Blood Formation

The spleen and liver are important accessory organs for blood production. They help regulate the growth of blood cells and form factors that ensure proper CLOTTING.

The spleen contains three types of tissue: white pulp, red pulp, and marginal pulp. These tissues help balance blood cell production with blood cell destruction and assist with immunity. White pulp is filled with white blood cells (WBCs) and is a major site of antibody production. As whole blood filters through the white pulp, bacteria and old RBCs are removed. Red pulp is the storage site for RBCs and platelets. Marginal pulp contains the ends of many blood vessels.

The spleen destroys old or imperfect RBCs, breaks down the hemoglobin released from these destroyed cells, stores platelets, and filters antigens. Anyone who has had a splenectomy has reduced immune functions and an increased risk for infection and sepsis.

The liver produces prothrombin and other blood CLOTTING factors. Also, proper liver function is important in forming vitamin K in the intestinal tract. (Vitamin K is needed to produce clotting factors VII, IX, and X and prothrombin.) Large amounts of whole blood and blood cells can be stored in the liver. The liver also stores extra iron within the protein *ferritin*.

Hemostasis and Blood Clotting

Hemostasis is the multi-stepped process of controlled blood CLOTTING. It results in localized blood clotting in damaged blood vessels to prevent excessive blood loss while continuing blood PERFUSION to all other areas. This complex function balances blood clotting actions with anti-clotting actions. When injury occurs, hemostasis starts the formation of a platelet plug and continues with a series of steps that eventually cause the formation of a fibrin clot. Three sequential processes result in blood clotting: platelet aggregation with platelet plug formation, the blood clotting cascade, and the formation of a complete fibrin clot.

Platelet aggregation begins forming a platelet plug by having platelets clump together, a process essential for blood CLOTTING. Platelets normally circulate as individual small cells that do not clump together until activated. Activation causes platelet membranes to become sticky, allowing them to clump together. When platelets clump, they form large, semi-solid plugs in blood vessels, disrupting local blood flow. *These platelet plugs are **not** clots and last only a few hours. Thus they cannot provide complete hemostasis but only start the hemostatic process.*

Substances that activate platelets and cause clumping include adenosine diphosphate (ADP), calcium, thromboxane A_2 (TXA_2), and collagen. Platelets secrete some of these substances, and other activating substances are external to the platelet. Platelet plugs start the cascade action that ends with local blood CLOTTING and are important at most steps within the cascade. When too few platelets are present, clotting is impaired, increasing the risk for excessive bleeding.

Blood clotting is a cascade triggered by the formation of a platelet plug, which then rapidly amplifies the cascade. The final result is much larger than the triggering event. Thus the cascade works like a landslide—a few stones rolling down a steep hill can eventually dislodge large rocks, trees, and soil, causing an enormous movement of earth. Just like landslides, cascade reactions are hard to stop once set into motion.

Intrinsic factors are conditions, such as circulating debris or venous stasis, within the blood itself that can activate platelets and trigger the blood CLOTTING cascade (Fig. 39-4). Continuing the cascade to blood clotting requires sufficient amounts of all the clotting factors and cofactors (Table 39-2).

Extrinsic factors outside of the blood can also activate platelets. The most common extrinsic event is trauma that damages blood vessels and exposes the collagen in vessel walls. Collagen then activates platelets to form a platelet plug within seconds. The blood clotting cascade is started sooner by this pathway because some intrinsic pathway steps are bypassed. Other blood vessel changes that can activate platelets include inflammation, bacterial toxins, or foreign proteins.

Whether the platelet plugs are formed because of abnormal blood (intrinsic factors) or by exposure to inflamed or damaged blood vessels (extrinsic factors), the end result of the cascade is the same: *formation of a fibrin clot and local blood CLOTTING (coagulation).* The cascade, from the formation of a platelet plug to the formation of a fibrin clot, depends on the presence

TABLE 39-2	The Clotting Factors
FACTOR	**ACTION**
I: Fibrinogen	Factor I is converted to fibrin by the enzyme *thrombin*. Individual fibrin molecules form fibrin threads, which are the mesh for clot formation and wound healing.
II: Prothrombin	Factor II is the inactive thrombin. Prothrombin is activated to thrombin by clotting factor X. Activated thrombin converts fibrinogen (clotting factor I) into fibrin and activates factors V and VIII. Synthesis is vitamin K–dependent.
III: Tissue thromboplastin	Factor III interacts with factor VII to initiate the extrinsic clotting cascade.
IV: Calcium	Calcium (Ca^{2+}), a divalent cation, is a cofactor for most of the enzyme-activated processes required in blood clotting. Calcium enhances platelet aggregation and makes red blood cells clump together.
V: Proaccelerin	Factor V is a cofactor for activated factor X, which is essential for converting prothrombin to thrombin.
VI: Is an artifact	No factor VI is involved in blood clotting.
VII: Proconvertin	Factor VII activates factors IX and X, which are essential in converting prothrombin to thrombin. Synthesis is vitamin K–dependent.
VIII: Antihemophilic factor	Factor VIII together with activated factor IX activates factor X. Factor VIII combines with von Willebrand's factor to help platelets adhere to capillary walls in areas of tissue injury. A lack of factor VIII results in classic hemophilia (hemophilia A).
IX: Plasma thromboplastin component (Christmas factor)	Factor IX, when activated, activates factor X to convert prothrombin to thrombin. A lack of factor IX causes hemophilia B. Synthesis is vitamin K–dependent.
X: Stuart-Prower factor	Factor X, when activated, converts prothrombin into thrombin. Synthesis is vitamin K–dependent.
XI: Plasma thromboplastin antecedent	Factor XI, when activated, assists in the activation of factor IX. However, a similar factor must exist in tissues. People who are deficient in factor XI have mild bleeding problems.
XII: Hageman factor	Factor XII is critically important in the intrinsic pathway for the activation of factor XI.
XIII: Fibrin-stabilizing factor	Factor XIII assists in forming cross-links among the fibrin threads to form a strong fibrin clot.

of specific clotting factors, calcium, and more platelets at every step.

Clotting factors (see Table 39-2) are inactive enzymes that become activated in a sequence. At each step, the activated enzyme from the previous step activates the next enzyme. The last two steps in the cascade are the activation of thrombin from prothrombin and the conversion (by thrombin) of fibrinogen

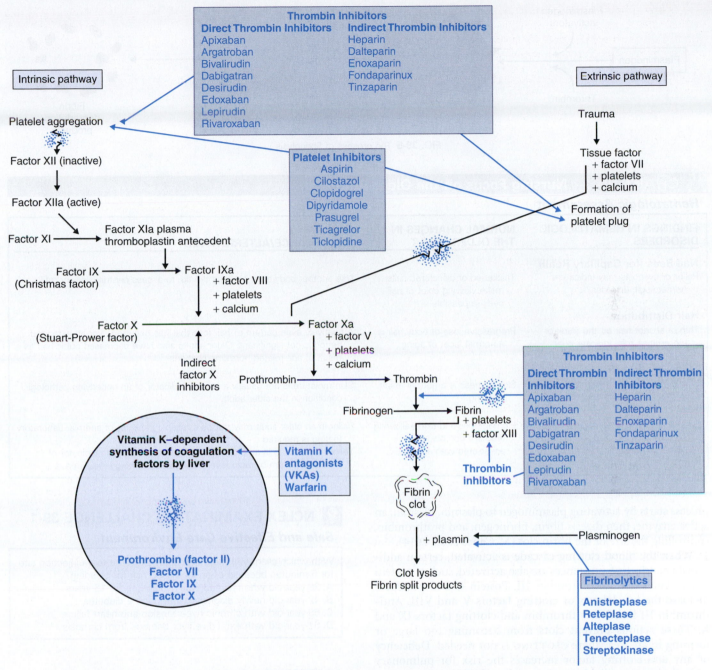

FIG. 39-4 Summary of the blood clotting cascade.

into fibrin. Only fibrin molecules can begin the formation of a true clot.

Fibrin clot formation is the last phase of blood CLOTTING. Fibrinogen is an inactive protein made in the liver. The activated enzyme *thrombin* removes the end portions of fibrinogen, converting it to active fibrin that can link together to form fibrin threads. Fibrin threads make a meshlike base to form a blood clot.

After the fibrin mesh is formed, clotting factor XIII tightens up the mesh, making it more dense and stable. More platelets stick to the threads of the mesh and attract other blood cells and proteins to form an actual blood clot. As this clot tightens (retracts), the serum is squeezed out, and clot formation is complete.

Anti-Clotting Forces

Because blood CLOTTING occurs through a rapid cascade process, in theory it keeps forming fibrin clots whenever the cascade is set into motion until all blood throughout the entire body has coagulated and PERFUSION stops. Therefore, whenever the clotting cascade is started, anti-clotting forces are also started to limit clot formation only to damaged areas so normal perfusion is maintained everywhere else. When blood clotting and anti-clotting actions are balanced, clotting occurs only where it is needed, and normal perfusion is maintained. The anti-clotting forces both ensure that activated clotting factors are present only in limited amounts and also cause fibrinolysis to prevent overenlargement of the fibrin clot. **Fibrinolysis** is the process that dissolves fibrin clot edges with special enzymes (Fig. 39-5). The

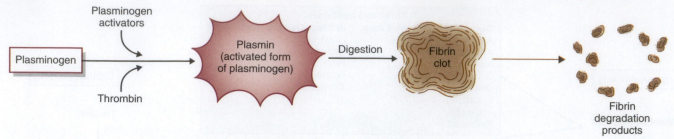

FIG. 39-5 The process of fibrinolysis.

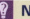 **CHART 39-1   Nursing Focus on the Older-Adult**

Hematologic Assessment

FINDINGS IN HEMATOLOGIC DISORDERS	NORMAL CHANGES IN THE OLDER ADULT	SIGNIFICANCE/ALTERNATIVES
Nail Beds (for Capillary Refill) Pallor or cyanosis may indicate a hematologic disorder.	Thickened or discolored nails make viewing color of nail beds impossible.	Use another body area, such as the lip, to assess central capillary refill.
Hair Distribution Thin or absent hair on the trunk or extremities may indicate poor PERFUSION to a particular area.	Progressive loss of body hair is a normal facet of aging.	A relatively even pattern of hair loss that has occurred over an extended period is not significant. Older adults also have decreased pubic hair as a result of age-related hormone changes.
Skin Moisture Skin dryness may indicate any of a number of hematologic disorders.	Skin dryness is a normal result of aging.	Skin moisture is not usually a reliable indicator of an underlying pathologic condition in the older adult.
Skin Color Skin color changes, especially pallor and jaundice, are associated with some hematologic disorders.	Pigment loss and skin yellowing are common changes associated with aging.	Pallor in an older adult may not be a reliable indicator of anemia. Laboratory testing is required. Yellow-tinged skin in an older adult may not be a reliable indicator of increased serum bilirubin levels. Laboratory testing is required.

process starts by activating plasminogen to plasmin. Plasmin, an active enzyme, then digests fibrin, fibrinogen, and prothrombin, controlling the size of the fibrin clot (McCance et al., 2014).

When the blood clotting cascade is activated, certain additional anti-clotting substances are also activated, such as protein C, protein S, and antithrombin III. Protein C and protein S increase the breakdown of clotting factors V and VIII. Antithrombin III inactivates thrombin and clotting factors IX and X. These actions prevent clots from becoming too large or forming in an area where CLOTTING is not needed. Deficiency of any anti-clotting factor increases the risk for pulmonary embolism, myocardial infarction, and strokes.

Hematologic Changes Associated With Aging

Aging changes the blood components (Touhy & Jett, 2016). The older adult has a decreased blood volume with lower levels of plasma proteins. The lower plasma protein level may be related to a low dietary intake of proteins and to reduced protein production by the older liver. Chart 39-1 lists assessment tips for older adults.

As bone marrow ages, it produces fewer blood cells. Total red blood cell (RBC) and white blood cell (WBC) counts are lower among older adults, although platelet counts do not change. Lymphocytes become less reactive to antigens and lose immune function. Antibody levels and responses are lower and slower in older adults. The WBC count does not rise as high in response to infection in older adults as it does in younger adults.

Hemoglobin levels in men and women fall after middle age. Iron-deficient diets may play a role in this reduction.

 NCLEX EXAMINATION CHALLENGE 39-1

Safe and Effective Care Environment

With which client will the nurse apply pressure to an injection site for 5 minutes because of an increased risk for bleeding?
A. 28-year-old who has had type 1 diabetes for 15 years
B. 42-year-old newly diagnosed with type 2 diabetes
C. 58-year-old with chronic hypertension and heart failure
D. 62-year-old with extensive liver damage from cirrhosis

ASSESSMENT: NOTICING AND INTERPRETING

Patient History

Age and gender are important to consider when assessing the patient's hematologic status. Bone marrow function and immune activity decrease with age.

GENDER HEALTH CONSIDERATIONS

Patient-Centered Care **QSEN**

At all ages, women have lower red blood cell counts than do men. This difference is greater during menstrual years because menstrual blood loss may occur faster than blood cell production. This difference also is related to blood dilution caused by fluid retention from female hormones. Always assess for RBC adequacy in a woman hospitalized for any reason.

TABLE 39-3 Drugs Impairing the Hematologic System

DRUGS CAUSING BONE MARROW SUPPRESSION	DRUGS CAUSING HEMOLYSIS	DRUGS DISRUPTING PLATELET ACTION
• Altretamine	• Acetohydroxamic acid	• Aspirin
• Amphotericin B	• Amoxicillin	• Carbenicillin
• Azathioprine	• Chlorpropamide	• Carindacillin
• Chemotherapeutic agents	• Doxapram	• Dipyridamole
• Chloramphenicol	• Glyburide	• Ibuprofen
• Chromic phosphate	• Mefenamic acid	• Meloxicam
• Colchicine	• Menadiol diphosphate	• Naproxen
• Didanosine	• Methyldopa	• Oxaprozin
• Eflornithine	• Nitrofurantoin	• Pentoxifylline
• Foscarnet sodium	• Penicillin G benzathine	• Sulfinpyrazone
• Ganciclovir	• Penicillin V	• Ticarcillin
• Interferon alfa	• Primaquine	• Ticlopidine
• Pentamidine	• Procainamide hydrochloride	• Valproic acid
• Sodium iodide	• Quinidine polygalacturonate	
• Zalcitabine	• Quinine	
• Zidovudine	• Sulfonamides	
	• Tolbutamide	
	• Vitamin K	

Liver function, the presence of known immunologic or hematologic disorders, current drug use, dietary patterns, and socioeconomic status are important to assess. Because the liver makes CLOTTING factors, ask about symptoms that may indicate liver problems, such as jaundice, anemia, and gallstones. Previous radiation therapy for cancer may impair hematologic function if marrow-forming bones were in the radiation path.

Ask about the patient's occupation and hobbies and whether the home is located near an industrial setting. This information may identify exposure to agents that affect bone marrow and hematologic function.

Check all drugs that the patient is using or has used in the past 3 weeks. Ask about the use of drugs listed in Table 39-3 that are known to change hematologic function. Check a drug handbook to determine whether other drugs the patient takes can affect hematologic function.

Ask the patient about use of blood "thinners" and NSAIDs, which change blood CLOTTING activity. Such drugs include anticoagulants and platelet inhibitors. Many patients refer to these drugs as *blood thinners,* although they do not change blood thickness (viscosity). Fig. 39-4 shows where in the blood clotting cascade these agents work.

Anticoagulant drugs work by interfering with one or more steps involved in the blood CLOTTING cascade. Thus these agents *prevent* new clots from forming and limit or prevent extension of formed clots. *Anticoagulants do not break down existing clots.* These drugs are classified as direct thrombin inhibitors, indirect thrombin inhibitors, and vitamin K antagonists.

Direct thrombin inhibitors (DTIs) can be given by the parenteral route and orally. The parenteral drugs include lepirudin (Refludan), desirudin (Iprivask), bivalirudin (Angiomax), and argatroban (ARGATROBAN, Novastin ✦). Oral agents include apixaban (Eliquis), dabigatran (Pradaxa, Pradax ✦), edoxaban

(Savaysa), and rivaroxaban (Xarelto). These drugs prevent the conversion of prothrombin (factor X) to its active form, thrombin (factor Xa). Less thrombin disrupts the CLOTTING cascade by reducing the amount of fibrinogen that is converted to active fibrin (Burchum & Rosenthal, 2016).

A clinical problem with the DTIs has been a lack of an antidote to administer when excessive bleeding is present as a result of DTI therapy. A recently approved IV antidote for dabigatran is idarucizumab (Praxbind), which is a monoclonal antibody that specifically binds to the structure of dabigatran (O'Malley, 2015; Siegal, et al., 2015). It is not effective against other thrombin inhibitors. Two other drugs under current study for reversal of bleeding related to other thrombin inhibitors are andexanet alfa and ciraparantag (Aripazine).

Indirect thrombin inhibitors include the heparins and heparinoids. These drugs include enoxaparin (Lovenox), dalteparin (Fragmin), tinzaparin (Innohep), and fondaparinux (Arixtra). All are given parenterally. Lower molecular weight drugs are preferred for home use. The drugs cause anticoagulation by binding to and increasing the activity of antithrombin III (AT III). By activating ATIII, coagulation factor Xa (thrombin) is indirectly inhibited.

Vitamin K antagonists (VKAs) decrease vitamin K synthesis in the intestinal tract, which then reduces the production of vitamin K–dependent CLOTTING factors II, VII, IX, and X. When clotting factor synthesis is reduced, anticoagulation results. The most commonly used VKA is warfarin (Coumadin, Jantoven), an oral agent.

Fibrinolytic drugs (also known as *thrombolytic drugs* or "clot busters") selectively break down fibrin threads present in formed blood clots. The mechanism starts with activation of the inactive tissue protein *plasminogen* to its active form, *plasmin.* Plasmin directly attacks and degrades the fibrin molecule. Fibrinolytic drugs include alteplase (Activase), reteplase (Retavase), tenecteplase (TNKase), and urokinase (Abbokinase, Kinlytic). All are IV agents. Urokinase is approved for use only in patients who have a massive pulmonary embolism.

The use of fibrinolytic drugs results in the best clot breakdown with less disruption of blood CLOTTING. These drugs are the first-line therapy for problems caused by small, localized formed clots such as myocardial infarction (MI), limited arterial thrombosis, and thrombotic strokes. For some problems such as MI, these drugs are usually given only within the first 6 hours after the onset of symptoms. This time limitation is not related to drug activity because fibrinolytic agents can break down clots older than 6 hours. Rather, the tissue that has been anoxic for more than 6 hours as a result of an acute event is not likely to benefit from this therapy, making the risks to the patient greater than the advantages.

Platelet inhibitors or antiplatelet drugs prevent either platelet activation or aggregation (clumping). The most widely used drug for this effect is aspirin, which irreversibly inhibits the production of substances that activate platelets, such as thromboxane. Other drugs change the platelet membrane, reducing its "stickiness," or prevent activators from binding to platelet receptors by inhibiting a variety of enzymes important to platelet activation. These drugs include cilostazol (Pletal), clopidogrel (Plavix), dipyridamole (Persantine), prasugrel (Effient), ticagrelor (Brilinta), and ticlopidine (Ticlid). Another group of drugs that inhibits platelets by binding to certain membrane proteins includes abciximab (ReoPro), eptifibatide (Integrilin), and tirofiban (Aggrastat), which are all administered parenterally.

The complementary therapy agents St. John's wort and Ginkgo biloba also inhibit platelet activity.

Nutrition Status

Diet can alter cell quality and affect CLOTTING. Ask patients to recall what they have eaten during the past week. Use this information to assess possible iron, protein, mineral, or vitamin deficiencies. Diets high in fat and carbohydrates and low in protein, iron, and vitamins can cause many types of anemia and decrease the functions of all blood cells. Diets high in vitamin K, found in leafy green vegetables, may increase the rate of blood clotting. Assess the amount of salads and other raw vegetables that the patient eats and whether supplemental vitamins and calcium are used. Ask about alcohol consumption because chronic alcoholism causes nutrition deficiencies and impairs the liver, both of which reduce blood CLOTTING.

Ask about personal resources, such as finances and social support. An adult with a low income may have a diet deficient in iron and protein because foods containing these substances are more expensive.

Family History and Genetic Risk

Assess family history because many disorders affecting blood and blood CLOTTING are inherited. Ask whether anyone in the family has had hemophilia, frequent nosebleeds, postpartum hemorrhages, excessive bleeding after tooth extractions, or heavy bruising after mild trauma. Ask whether any family member has sickle cell disease or sickle cell trait. Although sickle cell disease is seen most often among African Americans, anyone can have the trait.

Current Health Problems

Ask about lymph nodes swelling, excessive bruising or bleeding, and whether the bleeding was spontaneous or induced by trauma. Ask about the amount and duration of bleeding after routine dental work. Ask women to estimate the number of pads or tampons used during the most recent menstrual cycle and whether this amount represents a change from the usual pattern of flow. Ask whether clots are present in menstrual blood. If menstrual clots occur, ask women to estimate clot size using coins or fruit for comparison.

Assess and record whether the patient has shortness of breath on exertion, palpitations, frequent infections, fevers, recent weight loss, headaches, or paresthesias. Any or all of these symptoms may occur with hematologic disease.

The most common symptom of anemia is fatigue as a result of decreased oxygen delivery to cells. Cells use oxygen to produce the high-energy chemical *adenosine triphosphate (ATP)* needed to perform most cellular work. When oxygen delivery to cells is reduced, cellular work decreases, and fatigue increases. Ask patients about feeling tired, needing more rest, or losing endurance during normal activities. Ask them to compare their activities during the past month with those of the same month a year ago. Determine whether other symptoms of anemia, such as vertigo, tinnitus, and a sore tongue, are present.

Physical Assessment

Assess the whole body because blood problems may reduce oxygen delivery and tissue PERFUSION to all systems (Jarvis, 2016). Some assessment findings associated with hematologic problems are less reliable when seen in the older adult (see Chart 39-1). Equipment needed for hematologic assessment includes gloves, a stethoscope, a blood pressure cuff, and a penlight. Remember to gently handle the patient suspected of having a hematologic problem or reduced CLOTTING to avoid causing bruising, petechiae, or excessive bleeding.

Skin Assessment

Inspect the skin and mucous membranes for pallor or jaundice. Assess nail beds for pallor or cyanosis. Pallor of the gums, conjunctivae, and palmar creases (when the palm is stretched) indicates decreased hemoglobin levels and poor tissue oxygenation. Assess the gums for active bleeding in response to light pressure or brushing the teeth with a soft-bristled brush and assess any lesions or draining areas. Inspect for petechiae and large bruises *(ecchymoses)*. Petechiae are pinpoint hemorrhagic lesions in the skin. Bruises may cluster together. For hospitalized patients, determine whether there is bleeding around nasogastric tubes, endotracheal tubes, central lines, peripheral IV sites, or Foley catheters. Check the skin turgor and ask about itching because dry skin from poor perfusion itches. Assess body hair patterns. Areas with poor circulation, especially the lower legs and toes, may have sparse or absent hair, although this may be a normal finding in an older adult.

🌐 CULTURAL/SPIRITUAL CONSIDERATIONS
Patient-Centered Care QSEN

Pallor and cyanosis are more easily detected in adults with darker skin by examining the oral mucous membranes and the conjunctiva of the eye. Jaundice can be seen more easily on the roof of the mouth. Petechiae may be visible only on the palms of the hands or the soles of the feet. Bruises can be seen as darker areas of skin and palpated as slight swellings or irregular skin surfaces. Ask the patient about pain when skin surfaces are touched lightly or palpated. (Chapter 24 provides tips for assessing darker skin.)

Head and Neck Assessment

Check for pallor or ulceration of the oral mucosa. The tongue is smooth in pernicious anemia and iron deficiency anemia or smooth and beefy red in other nutrition deficiencies. These symptoms may occur with fissures at the corners of the mouth. Assess for scleral jaundice.

Inspect and palpate all lymph node areas. Document any lymph node enlargement, including whether palpation of the enlarged node causes pain and whether the enlarged node moves or remains fixed with palpation.

Respiratory Assessment

When blood problems reduce oxygen delivery, the lungs work harder to maintain tissue PERFUSION. Assess the rate and depth of respiration while the patient is at rest and during and after mild physical activity (e.g., walking 20 steps in 10 seconds). Note whether the patient can complete a 10-word sentence without stopping for a breath. Assess whether he or she is fatigued easily, has shortness of breath at rest or on exertion, or needs extra pillows to breathe well at night. Anemia can cause these problems as a result of respiratory changes made as adjustments to the reduced tissue oxygen levels.

Cardiovascular Assessment

When blood problems reduce oxygen delivery, the heart works harder to help maintain tissue PERFUSION. Pulses may become weak and thready. Observe for distended neck veins, edema, or indications of phlebitis. Use a stethoscope to listen for abnormal heart sounds and irregular rhythms. Assess blood pressure (BP). Systolic BP tends to be lower than normal in patients with anemia and higher than normal when the patient has excessive red blood cells.

Kidney and Urinary Assessment

The kidneys have many blood vessels, and bleeding problems may cause *hematuria* (blood in the urine). Inspect urine for color. Hematuria may be seen as grossly bloody red or dark-brownish gold urine. Test the urine for proteins with a urine test dipstick because blood contains protein and blood in the urine increases its protein content. Keep in mind that the adult with chronic kidney disease (CKD) produces less natural erythropoietin and often is anemic.

Musculoskeletal Assessment

Rib or sternal tenderness may occur with leukemia (blood cancer) when the bone marrow overproduces cells, increasing the pressure in the bones. Examine the skin over superficial bones, including the ribs and sternum, by applying firm pressure with the fingertips. Assess the range of joint motion and document any swelling or joint pain.

Abdominal Assessment

The normal adult spleen is usually *not* palpable, but an enlarged spleen occurs with many hematologic problems. An enlarged spleen may be detected by palpation, but this is usually performed by the primary health care provider because an enlarged spleen is tender and ruptures easily.

> **! NURSING SAFETY PRIORITY** QSEN
>
> ### Action Alert
>
> Do not palpate the splenic area of the abdomen for any patient with a suspected hematologic problem. An enlarged spleen ruptures easily and can lead to hemorrhage and death.

Palpating the edge of the liver in the right upper quadrant of the abdomen can detect enlargement, which often occurs with hematologic problems. The normal liver may be palpable as much as 4 to 5 cm below the right costal margin but is usually not palpable in the epigastrium.

A common cause of anemia among older adults is a chronically bleeding GI ulcer or intestinal polyp. If the ulcer is located in the stomach or the small intestine, obvious blood may not be visible in the stool, or such a small amount is passed each day that the patient is not aware of it. Obtain a stool specimen for occult blood testing.

Central Nervous System Assessment

Assessing cranial nerves and testing neurologic function are important in hematologic assessment because some problems cause specific changes. Vitamin B_{12} deficiency impairs nerve function, and severe chronic deficiency may cause permanent neurologic degeneration. Many neurologic problems can develop in patients who have leukemia because leukemia can cause bleeding, infection, or tumor spread within the brain. When the patient with a suspected bleeding disorder has any head trauma, expand the assessment to include frequent neurologic checks and checks of cognitive function (see Chapter 41).

Psychosocial Assessment

Regardless of the type of hematologic problem, each patient brings his or her own coping style to the illness. Develop a rapport with the patient and learn which coping mechanisms he or she has used successfully in the past.

Ask the patient and family members about social support networks and financial resources. A problem in these areas can interfere with the patient's adherence to therapy.

Diagnostic Assessment
Laboratory Tests

Laboratory test results provide definitive information about hematologic problems. Chart 39-2 lists laboratory data used to assess hematologic function. When a venipuncture is necessary, apply pressure to the site for at least 5 minutes on a patient suspected of having a hematologic problem to prevent bleeding and hematoma formation.

Tests of Cell Number and Function. A peripheral blood smear is made by taking a drop of blood and spreading it over a slide. It can be read by an automated calculator or a technologist with a microscope. This rapid test provides information on the sizes, shapes, and proportions of different blood cell types within the peripheral blood.

A complete blood count (CBC) includes a number of studies: red blood cell (RBC) count, white blood cell (WBC) count, hematocrit, and hemoglobin level. The RBC count measures circulating RBCs in 1 mm^3 (or 1 L) of blood. The WBC count measures all leukocytes present in 1 mm^3 (or 1 L) of blood. To determine the percentages of different types of leukocytes circulating in the blood, a WBC count with differential leukocyte count is performed (see Chapter 17). The hematocrit (Hct) is the percentage of RBCs in the total blood volume (also known as *volume fraction*). The hemoglobin (Hgb) level is the total amount of hemoglobin in blood and is measured as g/dL (or g/L).

The CBC can measure other features of the RBCs. The mean corpuscular volume (MCV) measures the average volume or size of individual RBCs and is useful for classifying anemias. When the MCV is elevated, the cell is larger than normal (*macrocytic*), as seen in megaloblastic anemias. When the MCV is decreased, the cell is smaller than normal (*microcytic*), as seen in iron deficiency anemia. The mean corpuscular hemoglobin (MCH) is the average amount of hemoglobin by weight in a single RBC. The mean corpuscular hemoglobin concentration (MCHC) measures the average amount of hemoglobin by percentage in a single RBC. When the MCHC is decreased, the cell has a hemoglobin deficiency and is *hypochromic* (a lighter

CHART 39-2 Laboratory Profile

Hematologic Assessment

TEST	REFERENCE RANGE	CANADIAN REFERENCE UNITS	SIGNIFICANCE OF ABNORMAL FINDINGS
Red blood cell (RBC) count	*Females:* 4.2-5.4 million/μL *Males:* 4.7-6.1 million/μL	$4.2\text{-}5.4 \times 10^{12}$ cells/L $4.7\text{-}6.1 \times 10^{12}$ cells/L	*Decreased levels* indicate possible anemia or hemorrhage. *Increased levels* indicate possible chronic hypoxia or polycythemia vera.
Hemoglobin (Hgb)	*Females:* 12-16 g/dL *Males:* 14-18 g/dL	120-160 g/L 140-180 g/L	Same as for RBC.
Hematocrit (Hct)	*Females:* 37%-47% *Males:* 42%-52%	0.37-0.47 volume fraction 0.42-0.52 volume fraction	Same as for RBC.
Mean corpuscular volume (MCV)	80-95 fL	Same as reference range	*Increased levels* indicate macrocytic cells, possible anemia. *Decreased levels* indicate microcytic cells, possible iron deficiency anemia.
Mean corpuscular hemoglobin (MCH)	27-31 pg	Same as reference range	Same as for MCV.
Mean corpuscular hemoglobin concentration (MCHC)	32-36 g/dL or 32%-36%	Same as reference range	*Increased levels* may indicate spherocytosis or anemia. *Decreased levels* may indicate iron deficiency anemia or a hemoglobinopathy.
White blood cell (WBC) count	5000-10,000/mm³	$5.0\text{-}10.0 \times 10^{9}$ cells/L	*Increased levels* are associated with infection, inflammation, autoimmune disorders, and leukemia. *Decreased levels* may indicate prolonged infection or bone marrow suppression.
Reticulocyte count	0.5%-2.0% of RBCs	Same as reference range	*Increased levels* may indicate chronic blood loss. *Decreased levels* indicate possible inadequate RBC production.
Total iron-binding capacity (TIBC)	250-460 mcg/dL	45-82 mcmol/L	*Increased levels* indicate iron deficiency. *Decreased levels* may indicate anemia, hemorrhage, hemolysis.
Iron (Fe)	*Females:* 60-160 mcg/dL *Males:* 80-180 mcg/dL	11-29 mcmol/L 14-32 mcmol/L	*Increased levels* indicate iron excess, liver disorders, hemochromatosis, megaloblastic anemia. *Decreased levels* indicate possible iron deficiency anemia, hemorrhage.
Serum ferritin	*Females:* 10-150 ng/mL *Males:* 12-300 ng/mL	10-150 mcg/L 12-300 mcg/L	Same as for iron.
Platelet count	150,000-400,000/mm³	$150\text{-}400 \times 10^{9}$/L	*Increased levels* may indicate polycythemia vera or malignancy. *Decreased levels* may indicate bone marrow suppression, autoimmune disease, hypersplenism.
Hemoglobin electrophoresis	Hgb A_1: 95%-98% Hgb A_2: 2%-3% Hgb F: 0.8%-2% Hgb S: 0% Hgb C: 0% Hgb E: 0%	Same as reference range	*Variations* indicate hemoglobinopathies.
Direct and indirect Coombs' test	Negative	Negative	*Positive findings* indicate antibodies to RBCs.
International normalized ratio (INR)	0.8-1.1 times the control value	Same as reference range	*Increased values* indicate longer clotting times. This is desirable for anticoagulation therapy with warfarin. *Decreased values* indicate hypercoagulation and increased risk for venous thromboembolic events.
Prothrombin time (PT)	11-12.5 sec 85%-100%	Same as reference range	*Increased time* indicates possible deficiency of clotting factors V and VII. *Decreased time* may indicate vitamin K excess.

Data from Pagana, K., Pagana, T., & Pike-MacDonald, S. (2013). *Mosby's Canadian manual of diagnostic and laboratory tests.* St. Louis: Mosby; Pagana, K., Pagana, T. J., & Pagana, T. N. (2017). *Mosby's diagnostic and laboratory test reference* (13th ed.). St. Louis: Mosby.

fL, Femtoliter; *pg,* picograms.

color), as in iron deficiency anemia. These three tests can help determine possible causes of low RBC counts that are not related to blood loss.

Reticulocyte count is helpful in determining bone marrow function. A reticulocyte is an immature RBC that still has its nucleus. An elevated reticulocyte count indicates that RBCs are being produced and released by the bone marrow before they mature. Normally only about 2% of circulating RBCs are reticulocytes. An elevated reticulocyte count is desirable in an anemic patient or after hemorrhage because this indicates that the bone marrow is responding to a decrease in the total RBC level. An elevated reticulocyte count without a precipitating cause usually indicates health problems, such as polycythemia vera (a malignant condition in which the bone marrow overproduces RBCs).

A platelet count, also known as a thrombocyte count, reflects the number of platelets in circulation. The normal range is 150,000 to 400,000/mm³ (150 to 400×10^9/L). When this value is low *(thrombocytopenia),* the patient is at greater risk for bleeding because platelets are critical for blood clotting. Patients who have values between 40,000/mm³ (40×10^9/L) and 80,000/mm³ (800×10^9/L) may have prolonged bleeding from trauma, dental work, and surgery. With platelet values below 20,000/mm³ (20×10^9/L), the patient may have spontaneous bleeding that is very difficult to stop.

Hemoglobin electrophoresis detects abnormal forms of hemoglobin, such as hemoglobin S in sickle cell disease. Hemoglobin A is the major type of hemoglobin in an adult.

Leukocyte alkaline phosphatase (LAP) is an enzyme produced by normal mature neutrophils. Elevated LAP levels occur during episodes of infection or stress. An elevated neutrophil count without an elevation in LAP level occurs with some types of leukemia.

Coombs' tests, both direct and indirect, are used for blood typing. The direct test detects antibodies against RBCs that may be attached to a patient's RBCs. Although healthy adults can make these antibodies, in certain diseases (e.g., systemic lupus erythematosus, mononucleosis) these antibodies are directed against the patient's own RBCs. Excessive amounts of these antibodies can cause hemolytic anemia (Pagana et al., 2017).

The indirect Coombs' test detects the presence of circulating antiglobulins. The test is used to determine whether the patient has serum antibodies to the type of RBCs that he or she is about to receive by blood transfusion (Pagana et al., 2017).

Serum ferritin, transferrin, and the total iron-binding capacity (TIBC) tests measure iron levels. Abnormal levels of iron and TIBC occur with problems such as iron deficiency anemia.

The serum ferritin test measures the amount of free iron present in the plasma, which represents 1% of the total body iron stores. Therefore the serum ferritin level provides a means to assess total iron stores. Adults with serum ferritin levels at least 10 ng/100 mL have adequate iron stores; adults with levels less than 10 ng/100 mL have inadequate iron stores and have difficulty recovering from any blood loss.

Transferrin is a protein that transports dietary iron from the intestines to cell storage sites. Measuring the amount of iron that can be bound to serum transferrin indirectly determines whether an adequate amount of transferrin is present. This test is the total iron-binding capacity (TIBC) test. Normally only about 30% of the transferrin is bound to iron in the blood. TIBC increases when a patient is deficient in serum iron and stored iron levels. Such a value indicates that an adequate amount of transferrin is present but less than 30% of it is bound to serum iron.

Tests Measuring Bleeding and Coagulation. Tests that measure bleeding and coagulation provide information that reflects the effectiveness of different aspects of blood CLOTTING. These tests are used to diagnose specific hematologic health problems, determine drug therapy effectiveness, and identify risk for excessive bleeding or clotting.

Prothrombin time (PT) measures how long blood takes to clot, reflecting the level of clotting factors II, V, VII, and X and how well they are functioning. When enough of these clotting factors are present and functioning, the PT shows blood CLOTTING between 11 and 12.5 seconds or within 85% to 100% of the time needed for a control sample of blood to clot. PT is prolonged when one or more of these clotting factors are deficient.

The PT test is now used less often to assess how fast blood clots, because control blood is taken from different adults and may not be the same even in one laboratory from one day to the next. To reduce PT errors as a result of control blood variation or in some of the chemicals used in the test, the international normalized ratio is used to assess clotting time.

International normalized ratio (INR) measures the same process as the PT by establishing a normal mean or standard for PT. The INR is calculated by dividing the patient's PT by the established standard PT. A normal INR ranges between 0.8 and 1.1 (Pagana et al., 2013; Pagana et al., 2017). When using the INR to monitor warfarin therapy, the desired outcome is usually to maintain the patient's INR between 2.0 and 3.0, regardless of the actual PT in seconds. However, the desired INR range for any patient is individualized for specific patient factors and medical conditions.

The partial thromboplastin time (PTT) assesses the intrinsic CLOTTING cascade and the action of factors II, V, VIII, IX, XI, and XII. PTT is prolonged whenever any of these factors is deficient, such as in hemophilia or disseminated intravascular coagulation (DIC). Because factors II, IX, and X are vitamin K–dependent and are produced in the liver, liver disease can prolong the PTT. Desired therapeutic ranges for anticoagulation are usually between 1.5 and 2.0 times normal values but can be greater depending on the reason the adult is receiving anticoagulation therapy.

The anti-factor Xa test measures the amount of anti-activated factor X (anti-Xa) in blood, which is affected by heparin. It is used mainly to monitor heparin levels in patients treated with either standard unfractionated heparin or low-molecular-weight heparin. For adults not receiving heparin in any form, the reference range is less than 0.1 IU/mL. The usual therapeutic range for patients receiving standard heparin is 0.5 to 1.0 IU/mL, and the usual therapeutic range for patients receiving low-molecular-weight heparin is 0.3 to 0.7 IU/mL. Test results are affected by age, gender, health history, and the specific laboratory technique used for the test.

Platelet aggregation, or the ability to clump, is tested by mixing the patient's plasma with an agonist substance that should cause clumping. The degree of clumping is noted. Aggregation can be impaired in von Willebrand's disease and during the use of drugs such as aspirin, anti-inflammatory agents, psychotropic agents, and platelet inhibitors.

NCLEX EXAMINATION CHALLENGE 39-3

Health Promotion and Maintenance

What is the **most important** precaution for the nurse to teach a client whose platelet counts usually range between 50,000 to 60,000/mm³ (50×10^9/L to 60×10^9/L)?
A. "Drink at least 3 liters of fluid daily."
B. "Take a multiple vitamin that contains iron."
C. "Avoid aspirin and aspirin-containing drugs."
D. "Increase your intake of dark green, leafy vegetables."

Imaging Assessment

Assessment of the patient with a suspected hematologic problem can include radioisotopic imaging. Isotopes are used to evaluate the bone marrow for sites of active blood cell formation and iron storage. Radioactive colloids are used to determine organ size and liver and spleen function.

The patient is given an IV radioactive isotope by about 3 hours before the procedure. Once in the nuclear medicine department, he or she must lie still for about an hour during the scan. No special patient preparation or follow-up care is needed for these tests.

Standard x-rays may be used to diagnose some hematologic problems. For example, multiple myeloma causes classic bone destruction, with a "Swiss cheese" appearance on x-ray.

Bone Marrow Aspiration and Biopsy

Bone marrow aspiration and biopsy, which are similar invasive procedures, help evaluate the patient's hematologic status when other tests show abnormal findings that indicate a possible problem in blood cell production or maturation. Results provide information about bone marrow function, including the production of all blood cells and platelets. In a bone marrow aspiration, cells and fluids are suctioned from the bone marrow. In a bone marrow biopsy, solid tissue and cells are obtained by coring out an area of bone marrow with a large-bore needle.

A hematologic health care provider's prescription and a signed informed consent are obtained before either procedure is performed. Bone marrow aspiration may be performed by a physician, an advanced practice nurse, or a physician assistant, depending on the agency's policy and regional law. The procedure may be performed at the patient's bedside, in an examination room, or in a laboratory.

After learning which specific tests will be performed on the marrow, check with the hematology laboratory to determine how to handle the specimen. Some tests require that heparin or other solutions be added to the specimen.

Patient Preparation. Most patients are anxious before a bone marrow aspiration, even those who have had one in the past. You can help reduce anxiety and allay fears by providing accurate information and emotional support. Some patients like to have their hand held during the procedure.

Explain the procedure and reassure the patient that you will stay during the entire procedure. Tell the patient that the local anesthetic injection will feel like a stinging or burning sensation. Tell him or her to expect a heavy sensation of pressure and pushing while the needle is being inserted. Sometimes a crunching sound can be heard or scraping sensation felt as the needle punctures the bone. Explain that a brief sensation of painful pulling will be experienced as the marrow is being aspirated by mild suction in the syringe. If a biopsy is performed, the patient may feel more discomfort as the needle is rotated into the bone.

Assist the patient onto an examining table and expose the site (usually the iliac crest). If this site is not available or if more marrow is needed, the sternum may be used. If the iliac crest is the site, place the patient in the prone or side-lying position. Depending on the tests to be performed on the specimen, a laboratory technician may also be present to ensure its proper handling.

Procedure. The procedure usually lasts from 5 to 15 minutes. The type and amount of anesthesia or sedation depend on the clinician's preference, the patient's preference and previous experience with bone marrow aspiration and biopsy, and the setting.

A local anesthetic agent is injected into the skin around the site. The patient may also receive a mild tranquilizer or a rapid-acting sedative, such as midazolam (Versed), lorazepam (Ativan, Apo-Lorazepam ✚, Novo-Lorazem ✚), or etomidate (Amidate). Some patients do well with guided imagery or autohypnosis.

> ### ! NURSING SAFETY PRIORITY QSEN
> #### Action Alert
>
> Aspiration or biopsy procedures are invasive, and sterile technique must be observed.

The skin over the site is cleaned. For an aspiration, the needle is inserted with a twisting motion, and the marrow is aspirated by pulling back on the plunger of the syringe. When sufficient marrow has been aspirated to ensure accurate analysis, the needle is withdrawn rapidly while the tissues are supported. For a biopsy, a small skin incision is made, and the biopsy needle is inserted. Pressure and several twisting motions are needed to ensure coring and loosening of an adequate amount of marrow tissue. Apply external pressure to the site until hemostasis is ensured. A pressure dressing or sandbags may be applied to reduce bleeding at the site.

Follow-Up Care. The nursing priority after a bone marrow aspiration or biopsy is prevention of excessive bleeding. Cover the site with a dressing after bleeding is controlled, and closely observe it for 24 hours for signs of bleeding and infection. A mild analgesic (aspirin-free) may be given for discomfort, and ice packs can be placed over the site to limit bruising. If the patient goes home the same day as the procedure, instruct him or her to inspect the site every 2 hours for the first 24 hours to assess for active bleeding or bruising. Advise the patient to avoid any activity that might result in trauma to the site for 48 hours.

Information obtained from bone marrow aspiration or biopsy reflects the degree and quality of bone marrow activity present. The counts made on a marrow specimen can indicate whether different cell types are present in the expected quantities and proportions. In addition, bone marrow aspiration or biopsy can confirm the spread of cancer cells from other tumor sites.

> ### ? CLINICAL JUDGMENT CHALLENGE 39-1
> #### Ethics, Patient-Centered Care, Teamwork and Collaboration QSEN
>
> The patient is Joe, a 28-year-old man with Down syndrome who lives at home with his parents. His blood cell counts are all abnormal, and the next diagnostic test scheduled is a bone marrow aspiration. Joe can read at a fourth grade level and is very friendly; however, he is afraid of needles and had to be restrained during the venipuncture for blood testing.
>
> 1. From whom should informed consent be obtained for the procedure, Joe or his parents?
> 2. Should anyone explain to Joe what the procedure entails? Why or why not?
> 3. Who is responsible for obtaining the informed consent?
> 4. If Joe says he does not want the test but his parents insist that he have it, what if any, ethical principles may be violated? (If necessary, review the ethical principles in Chapter 1.)
> 5. What members of the interprofessional team could provide guidance in this situation?

GET READY FOR THE NCLEX® EXAMINATION!

KEY POINTS

Review the following Key Points for each NCLEX Examination Client Needs Category.

Safe and Effective Care Environment

- Verify that a patient having a bone marrow aspiration or biopsy has signed an informed consent statement. **QSEN: Safety**
- Handle patients with suspected hematologic problems gently to avoid bleeding or bruising. **QSEN: Safety**
- Do not palpate the splenic area of any patient suspected of having a hematologic problem. **QSEN: Safety**
- Maintain pressure over a venipuncture site for at least 5 minutes to prevent excessive bleeding. **QSEN: Safety**

Health Promotion and Maintenance

- Teach adults to avoid unnecessary contact with environmental chemicals or toxins. If contact cannot be avoided, teach them to use safety precautions.
- Instruct patients about the importance of eating a diet with adequate amounts of foods that are good sources of iron, folic acid, and vitamin B_{12}. **QSEN: Patient-Centered Care**

Psychosocial Integrity

- Support the patient during a bone marrow aspiration or biopsy. **QSEN: Patient-Centered Care**

Physiological Integrity

- Interpret blood cell counts and clotting tests to assess hematologic status. **QSEN: Evidence-Based Practice**
- Be aware that:
  - Tissue oxygenation and perfusion rely on normal hematologic function for oxygen delivery.

- The most common symptom of a hematologic problem is fatigue.
- A platelet plug and a fibrin clot are not the same.
- Both clotting forces and anticlotting forces are needed to maintain adequate perfusion.
- Use the lip rather than nail beds to assess capillary refill on older adults. **QSEN: Evidence-Based Practice**
- Rely on laboratory tests rather than skin color changes in older adults to assess anemia or jaundice. **QSEN: Evidence-Based Practice**
- Assess the patient's endurance in performing ADLs.
- Teach patients and family members about what to expect during procedures to assess hematologic function, including restrictions, drugs, and follow-up care. **QSEN: Patient-Centered Care**
- Ask patients about their activity level and whether they are satisfied with the energy they have for activities. **QSEN: Patient-Centered Care**
- Apply an ice pack to the needle site after a bone marrow aspiration or biopsy. **QSEN: Patient-Centered Care**
- Check the needle insertion site at least every 2 hours after a bone marrow aspiration or biopsy. If the patient is going home, teach the patient and family how to assess the site for bleeding and when to seek help. **QSEN: Patient-Centered Care**
- Instruct patients to avoid activities that may traumatize the site after a bone marrow aspiration or biopsy. **QSEN: Evidence-Based Practice**

SELECTED BIBLIOGRAPHY

Burchum, J., & Rosenthal, L. (2016). *Lehne's pharmacology for nursing care* (9th ed.). St. Louis: Elsevier.

Drug News. (2014). Edoxaban compares well to warfarin. *Nursing 2014, 44*(2), 10.

Jarvis, C. (2016). *Physical examination & health assessment* (7th ed.). St. Louis: Saunders.

McCance, K., Huether, S., Brashers, V., & Rote, N. (2014). *Pathophysiology: The biologic basis for disease in adults and children* (7th ed.). St. Louis: Mosby.

O'Malley, P. (2015). Waiting for the antidote. *Clinical Nurse Specialist, 29*(5), 262–264.

Pagana, K., Pagana, T. J., & Pagana, T. N. (2017). *Mosby's diagnostic and laboratory test reference* (13th ed.). St. Louis: Mosby.

Pagana, K., Pagana, T., & Pike-MacDonald, S. (2013). *Mosby's Canadian manual of diagnostic and laboratory tests*. St. Louis: Mosby.

Rauen, C. (2012). Beyond the bloody mess: Hematologic assessment. *Critical Care Nurse, 32*(5), 42–46.

Sendir, M., Buyukylmaz, F., Celik, Z., & Taskopru, I. (2015). Comparison of 3 methods to prevent pain and bruising after subcutaneous heparin administration. *Clinical Nurse Specialist, 29*(3), 174–180.

Siegal, D., Curnutte, J., Connolly, S., Lu, G., Conley, P., Wiens, B., et al. (2015). Adexanel alfa for reversal of factor Xa inhibitor activity. *New England Journal of Medicine, 373*(25), 2413–2414.

Straznitskas, A., & Giarratano, M. (2014). Emergent reversal of oral anticoagulation: Review of current treatment strategies. *AACN Advanced Clinical Care, 25*(1), 5–12.

Touhy, T., & Jett, K. (2016). *Ebersole and Hess' toward healthy aging* (9th ed.). St. Louis: Mosby.

Care of Patients With Hematologic Problems

Katherine L. Byar

(e) http://evolve.elsevier.com/Iggy/

PRIORITY AND INTERRELATED CONCEPTS

The priority concepts for this chapter are:
- PERFUSION
- IMMUNITY

✳ The PERFUSION concept exemplar for this chapter is Sickle Cell Disease, below.

✳ The IMMUNITY concept exemplar for this chapter is Leukemia, p. 817.

The interrelated concepts for this chapter are:
- CELLULAR REGULATION
- GAS EXCHANGE
- CLOTTING

LEARNING OUTCOMES

Safe and Effective Care Environment

1. Collaborate with the interprofessional team to coordinate high-quality care to patients who have a hematologic problem affecting CLOTTING, IMMUNITY, PERFUSION, or GAS EXCHANGE.
2. Teach the patient and caregiver(s) about home safety related to impaired IMMUNITY, impaired CLOTTING, and other changes caused by hematologic problems or their management.

Health Promotion and Maintenance

3. Identify community resources for patients with a chronic hematologic problem.
4. Teach adults undergoing therapy for a hematologic problem how to reduce the risk for infection and bleeding related to impaired IMMUNITY and impaired CLOTTING.

Psychosocial Integrity

5. Implement nursing interventions to help the patient and family cope with the psychosocial impact caused by chronic or life-threatening hematologic problems and their therapies.

Physiological Integrity

6. Apply knowledge of pathophysiology to assess patients with common complications caused by hematologic problems and their therapies.
7. Teach the patient and caregiver(s) about common drugs used as therapy for hematologic problems and their complications, including pain, impaired IMMUNITY, and impaired CLOTTING.
8. Prioritize nursing responsibilities during transfusion therapy.

The hematologic system is responsible for the production and function of blood cells, which are critical for PERFUSION, IMMUNITY, CLOTTING, and GAS EXCHANGE. These vital activities can be impaired by any hematologic problem that interferes with the production, function, and maintenance of blood cells. The type and severity of the problem determine the impact on health. This chapter discusses mild hematologic disorders and those that are potentially life threatening, such as sickle cell disease and hematologic malignancies.

✳ **PERFUSION CONCEPT EXEMPLAR**
Sickle Cell Disease

❖ **PATHOPHYSIOLOGY**

Sickle cell disease (SCD), formerly called *sickle cell anemia*, is one of several related genetic hemoglobin disorders that

result in chronic anemia, pain, disability, organ damage, increased risk for infection, and early death as a result of poor blood perfusion. Other similar disorders in this category include hemoglobin C disease and the thalassemias. SCD overall is more severe than the other hemoglobin disorders, although there is great variation in disease severity and when complications start. **PERFUSION** is adequate arterial blood flow through the tissues (peripheral perfusion) and blood that is pumped by the heart (central perfusion) to oxygenate body tissues. Chapter 2 provides a summary discussion of issues about the concept.

SCD results in the formation of abnormal hemoglobin chains. In healthy adults, the normal hemoglobin (hemoglobin A [HbA]) molecule has two alpha chains and two beta chains of amino acids. Normal adult red blood cells usually contain 98% to 99% HbA, with a small percentage of a fetal form of hemoglobin (HbF).

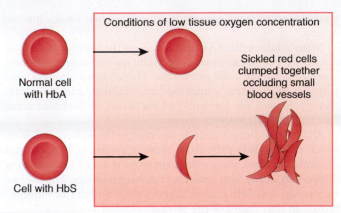

FIG. 40-1 Red blood cell actions under conditions of low tissue oxygenation. (*HbA*, Hemoglobin A; *HbS*, hemoglobin S.)

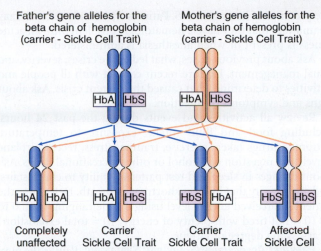

FIG. 40-2 Possible transmission of sickle cell disease and sickle cell trait when both parents are carriers. (*HbA*, Hemoglobin A; *HbS*, hemoglobin S.)

In SCD, at least 40% (and often much more) of the total hemoglobin is composed of an abnormal beta chain (**hemoglobin S [(HbS]**). HbS is sensitive to low oxygen content of the red blood cells (RBCs). When RBCs with large amounts of HbS are exposed to decreased oxygen conditions, the abnormal beta chains contract and pile together within the cell, distorting the cell into a sickle shape. Sickled cells become rigid and clump together, causing the RBCs to become "sticky" and fragile. The clumped masses of sickled RBCs block blood flow and PERFUSION (Fig. 40-1), known as a *vaso-occlusive event (VOE)*. VOE leads to further tissue **hypoxia** (reduced oxygen supply) and more sickle-shaped cells, which then leads to more blood vessel obstruction, inadequate perfusion, and ischemia in the affected tissues. Conditions that cause sickling include hypoxia, dehydration, infection, venous stasis, pregnancy, alcohol consumption, high altitudes, low or high environmental or body temperatures, acidosis, strenuous exercise, emotional stress, and anesthesia.

Usually sickled cells go back to normal shape when the precipitating condition is removed and the blood oxygen level is normalized, which allows tissue PERFUSION to resume. Although the cells then appear normal, some of the hemoglobin remains twisted, decreasing cell flexibility. The cell membranes are damaged over time, and cells are permanently sickled. The membranes of cells with HbS are more fragile and more easily broken. The average life span of an RBC containing 40% or more of HbS is about 10 to 20 days, much less than the 120-day life span of normal RBCs (McCance et al., 2014). This reduced RBC life span causes **hemolytic** (blood cell–destroying) anemia in patients with SCD.

The patient with SCD has periodic episodes of extensive cellular sickling, called **crises**. The crises have a sudden onset and can occur as often as weekly or as seldom as once a year. Many patients are in good health much of the time, with crises occurring only in response to conditions that cause local or systemic **hypoxemia** (deficient oxygen in the blood).

Repeated VOEs and impaired PERFUSION in large blood vessels cause long-term damage to tissues and organs. Most damage results from tissue hypoxia, anoxia, ischemia, and cell death. Organs develop small infarcted areas and scar tissue formation, and eventually organ failure results. The spleen, liver, heart, kidney, brain, joints, bones, and retina are affected most often.

Etiology and Genetic Risk

Sickle cell disease (SCD) is a genetic disorder with an autosomal-recessive pattern of inheritance (see Chapter 5). A specific mutation in the hemoglobin gene alleles on chromosome 11 leads to the formation of HbS instead of HbA. In SCD, the patient has two HbS gene alleles, one inherited from each parent, usually resulting in 80% to 100% of the hemoglobin being HbS. Because both hemoglobin alleles are S, SCD is sometimes abbreviated "SS." Patients with SCD often have severe symptoms and greatly impaired PERFUSION, even when triggering conditions are mild. If a patient with SCD has children, each child will inherit one of the two abnormal gene alleles and at least have sickle cell trait.

Sickle cell trait occurs when one normal gene allele and one abnormal gene allele for hemoglobin are inherited and only about half of the hemoglobin chains are abnormal. Sickle cell trait is abbreviated "AS." The patient is a carrier of the HbS gene allele (Fig. 40-2) and can pass the trait on to his or her children. However, the patient has only mild symptoms of the disease when precipitating conditions are present because less hemoglobin is abnormal.

Incidence and Prevalence

Sickle cell trait and different forms of SCD occur in people of all races and ethnicities but is most common among African Americans in the United States. About 90,000 to 100,000 people have SCD, occurring in 1 in 500 African Americans. About 1 in 12 to 1 in 15 (8%) African Americans are carriers of one sickle cell gene allele and have AS (Centers for Disease Control and Prevention [CDC], 2015).

❖ INTERPROFESSIONAL COLLABORATIVE CARE

Sickle cell disease (SCD) is a chronic disease that reduces PERFUSION, and complications become worse over time, especially in adults. Patients must self-manage continually at home or other residential settings. When crises or other acute complications occur, patients are cared for in an acute care environment, usually in a medical-surgical setting.

◆ Assessment: Noticing

History. An adult with SCD usually has a long-standing diagnosis of the disorder. Those with sickle cell trait usually have no symptoms or abnormal laboratory findings other than the presence of hemoglobin S. Patients with sickle cell trait may be unaware that they have a hematologic problem until an acute illness is present or when anesthesia is administered.

Ask about previous crises, what led to the crises, severity, and usual management. Explore recent contact with ill people and activities to determine what caused the current crisis. Ask about signs and symptoms of infection.

Review all activities and events during the past 24 hours, including food and fluid intake, exposure to temperature extremes, drugs taken, exercise, trauma, stress, recent airplane travel, and ingestion of alcohol or other recreational drugs. Ask about changes in sleep and rest patterns, ability to climb stairs, and any activity that induces shortness of breath. Determine the patient's perceived energy level using a scale ranging from 0 to 10 (0 = not tired with plenty of energy; 10 = total exhaustion) to assess the degree of fatigue.

Physical Assessment/Signs and Symptoms. *Pain is the most common symptom of SCD crisis* (Matthie & Jenerette, 2015). Others vary with the site of reduced PERFUSION and the tissue damaged.

Cardiovascular changes, including the risk for high-output heart failure, occur because of the anemia. Assess the patient for shortness of breath and general fatigue or weakness. Other problems may include murmurs, the presence of an S_3 heart sound, and increased jugular-venous pulsation or distention. Assess the cardiovascular status by comparing peripheral pulses, temperature, and capillary refill in all extremities. Extremities distal to blood vessel occlusion are cool to the touch with slow capillary refill and may have reduced or absent pulses, which indicate reduced PERFUSION. Heart rate may be rapid, and blood pressure may be low to normal with anemia.

Respiratory system changes occur over time. Many patients with SCD develop pulmonary hypertension, and all are at risk for recurrent pneumonia. Further assessment with pulmonary function testing of the adult with SCD who has symptoms of pulmonary disease is recommended (U.S. Department of Health and Human Services [USDHHS], 2014). (See Chapter 27 for a discussion of pulmonary function testing.)

Acute chest syndrome is a common reason for hospitalization and is the most common cause of death (USDHHS, 2014). This life-threatening condition is usually associated with respiratory infection and can also be caused by fat embolism and pulmonary debris from sickled cells. Symptoms are similar to pneumonia with cough, shortness of breath, abnormal breath sounds, and an infiltrate on chest x-ray. Fever may or may not be present. Without intervention, this complication can lead to respiratory failure and failure of all other organ systems.

Priapism is a prolonged penile erection that can occur in men who have SCD. The cause is excessive vascular engorgement in erectile tissue. The condition is very painful and can last for hours. During the priapism episode, the patient usually cannot urinate.

Skin changes include pallor or cyanosis because of poor GAS EXCHANGE from decreased PERFUSION and anemia. Examine the lips, tongue, nail beds, conjunctivae, palms, and soles of the feet at least every 8 hours for subtle color changes. With cyanosis, the lips and tongue are gray; and the palms, soles, conjunctivae, and nail beds have a bluish tinge.

Another skin sign of SCD is jaundice. Jaundice results from RBC destruction and release of bilirubin. To assess for jaundice in patients with darker skin, inspect the roof of the mouth for a yellow appearance. Examine the sclera closest to the cornea to assess jaundice more accurately. Jaundice often causes intense itching.

Many adults with SCD have ulcers on the lower legs that are caused by poor PERFUSION, especially on the outer sides and inner aspect of the ankle or the shin. These lesions often become necrotic or infected, requiring débridement and antibiotic therapy. Inspect the legs and feet for ulcers or darkened areas that may indicate necrotic tissue.

Abdominal changes include damage to the spleen and liver, which often occurs early from many episodes of hypoxia and ischemia. In crisis, abdominal pain from reduced PERFUSION is diffuse and steady, also involving the back and legs. The liver or spleen may feel firm and enlarged with a nodular or "lumpy" texture in later stages of the disease.

Kidney and urinary changes are common as a result of poor PERFUSION and decreased tissue GAS EXCHANGE. Chronic kidney disease occurs as a result of anoxic damage to the kidney nephrons (USDHHS, 2014). Early damage makes the kidneys less effective at filtration and reabsorption. The urine contains protein, and the patient may not concentrate urine. Eventually the kidneys fail, resulting in little or no urine output.

Musculoskeletal changes occur because arms and legs are often sites of blood vessel occlusion. Joints may be damaged from hypoxic episodes and have necrotic degeneration. Inspect the arms and legs and record any areas of swelling, temperature, or color difference. Ask patients to move all joints. Record the range of motion and any pain with movement.

Central nervous system (CNS) changes may occur in SCD. During crises, patients may have a low-grade fever. Long-term effects of reduced PERFUSION to the CNS may result in infarcts with repeated episodes of hypoxia, causing the patient to have seizures or symptoms of a stroke (USDHHS, 2014). Assess for the presence of "pronator drift," bilateral hand grasp strength, gait, and coordination. See Chapter 41 for details of neurologic assessment.

Psychosocial Assessment. Often cognitive and behavioral changes are early indications of cerebral hypoxia from poor PERFUSION. Assess the patient and document mental status examination results. Ask family members whether the current behavior and mental status are usual for the patient. Assess the patient and family for knowledge and understanding of SCD and how to live with the disease to the highest level of wellness possible.

SCD is a painful, life-limiting disorder that can be passed on to one's children. When assessing psychosocial needs, keep in mind new factors that might contribute to a crisis. Also assess established support systems, use of coping patterns, disease progression, and the impact that all of these have on the patient and family.

Laboratory Assessment. The diagnosis of SCD is based on the percentage of hemoglobin S (HbS) on electrophoresis. A person who has AS usually has less than 40% HbS, and the patient with SCD may have 80% to 100% HbS. This percentage does not change during crises. Another indicator of SCD is the number of RBCs with permanent sickling. This value is less than 1% among people with no hemoglobin disease, 5% to 50% among people with AS, and up to 90% among patients with SCD.

Other laboratory tests can indicate complications of the disease, especially during crises. The hematocrit of patients with SCD is low (between 20% and 30% [0.2 and 0.3 volume fraction]) because of RBC shortened life span and destruction. This value decreases even more during crises or stress (aplastic crisis). The reticulocyte count is high, indicating anemia of long duration. The total bilirubin level may be high because damaged RBCs release iron and bilirubin.

The total white blood cell (WBC) count is usually high in patients with SCD. This elevation is related to chronic inflammation caused by tissue hypoxia and ischemia.

Imaging Assessment. Bone changes occur as a result of chronically stimulated marrow and low bone oxygen levels. The skull may show changes on x-ray as a result of bone surface cell destruction and new growth, giving the skull a "crew cut" appearance on x-ray. X-rays of joints may show necrosis and destruction. Ultrasonography, CT, positron emission tomography (PET), and MRI may show soft-tissue and organ changes from poor PERFUSION and chronic inflammation.

Other Diagnostic Assessment. ECG changes document cardiac infarcts and tissue damage. Specific ECG changes are related to the area of the heart damaged. Echocardiograms may show cardiomyopathy and decreased cardiac output (low ejection fraction).

◆ Analysis: Interpreting

The priority collaborative problems for the patient with sickle cell disease include:

1. Pain due to poor tissue oxygenation and joint destruction
2. Potential for infection, sepsis, multiple organ dysfunction, and death

◆ Planning and Implementation: Responding

Managing Pain

Planning: Expected Outcomes. The pain associated with sickle cell disease may be acute during crises and chronic as a result of complications (Matthie & Jenerette, 2015). Acute pain episodes have a sudden onset, usually involving the chest, back, abdomen, and extremities. Complications of SCD can cause severe, chronic pain, requiring large doses of opioid analgesics. Regardless of the pain type, expected outcomes include that the patient's pain is controlled to a level acceptable to him or her (e.g., a 3 or less on a pain intensity rating scale of 0 to 10) and can participate in self-care or other activities to the degree he or she wishes (Lentz & Krautz, 2017).

Interventions. The pain with sickle cell crisis is the result of tissue injury caused by poor PERFUSION and tissue GAS EXCHANGE from obstructed blood flow. Mild pain can be managed at home. However, pain is often severe enough to require hospitalization and opioid analgesics.

Ask whether the pain is typical of past pain episodes. If not, other pain causes or disease complications must be explored. Ask the patient to rate pain on a scale ranging from 0 to 10 and evaluate the effectiveness of interventions based on the ratings.

Concerns about substance abuse can lead to inadequate pain treatment in these patients. Opioid addiction is rare in patients with SCD (Matthie & Jenerette, 2015). Because the pain of crisis has no objective signs, pain management is based on past pain history, previous drug use, disease complications, and current pain assessment. Many patients have had negative interactions with nurses and other members of the interprofessional team who suggest that the pain is not a problem and that patients with SCD may be "drug seekers" (O'Connor et al., 2014). Health care professionals need to be aware of their own attitudes when caring for this population. If substance abuse occurs, management of addiction is incorporated into the overall

---

◎ CHART 40-1 Best Practice for Patient Safety & Quality Care

Care of the Patient in Sickle Cell Crisis

- Administer oxygen.
- Administer prescribed pain medication.
- Hydrate the patient with normal saline IV and with beverages of choice (without caffeine) orally.
- Remove any constrictive clothing.
- Encourage the patient to keep extremities extended to promote venous return.
- Do not raise the knee position of the bed.
- Elevate the head of the bed no more than 30 degrees.
- Keep room temperature at or above 72°F (22.2°C).
- Avoid taking blood pressure with external cuff.
- Check circulation in extremities every hour:
  - Pulse oximetry of fingers and toes
  - Capillary refill
  - Peripheral pulses
  - Toe temperature

---

treatment plan. *Addicted patients in acute pain crisis still need opioids.*

Drug therapy for patients in acute sickle cell crisis often starts with at least 48 hours of IV analgesics. (Chart 40-1 lists best practices for nursing care of the patient in sickle cell crisis.) Morphine and hydromorphone (Dilaudid) are given IV on a routine schedule or by infusion pump using patient-controlled analgesia (PCA). Once relief is obtained, the IV dose can be tapered and the drug given orally. Avoid "as needed" (PRN) schedules because they do not provide adequate relief. Moderate pain may be managed with oral doses of opioids or NSAIDs. (See Chapter 4 for more information on pain management.)

Hydroxyurea (Droxia) may reduce the number of sickling and pain episodes by stimulating fetal hemoglobin (HbF) production. Increasing the level of HbF reduces sickling of red blood cells in some but not all patients with sickle cell disease (Vacce & Blank, 2017). However, this drug increases the risk for leukemia. Long-term complications should be discussed with the patient before this therapy is started. Hydroxyurea also suppresses bone marrow function, including IMMUNITY, and regular follow-up to monitor complete blood counts (CBCs) for drug toxicity is important.

! NURSING SAFETY PRIORITY QSEN

Action Alert

Hydroxyurea is **teratogenic** (can cause birth defects). Teach sexually active women of childbearing age using hydroxyurea to adhere to strict contraceptive measures while taking it and for 1 month after it is discontinued.

Hydration by the oral or IV route helps reduce the duration of pain episodes. Urge the patient to drink water or juices. Because the patient is often dehydrated and his or her blood is hypertonic, hypotonic fluids are usually infused at 250 mL/hr for 4 hours. Once the patient's blood osmolarity is reduced to the normal range of 270 to 300 mOsm, the IV rate is reduced to 125 mL/hr if more hydration is needed.

Complementary and integrative therapies and other measures, such as keeping the room warm, using distraction and relaxation techniques, positioning with support for painful areas, aroma therapy, therapeutic touch, and warm soaks or compresses, all help reduce pain perception.

NCLEX EXAMINATION CHALLENGE 40-1
Physiological Integrity

Which change in laboratory test results of a client with sickle cell disease who was started on therapy with hydroxyurea 4 weeks ago indicates to the nurse that the therapy is effective?

A. Increased HbF from 2% to 10%
B. Decreased HbA from 3% to 2.5%
C. Increased platelets from 250,000/mm³ (250 × 10⁹/L) to 300,000/mm³ (300 × 10⁹/L)
D. Decreased white blood cells from 8200/mm³ (8.2 × 10⁹/L) to 7700/mm³ (7 × 10⁹/L)

Preventing Sepsis, Multiple Organ Dysfunction Syndrome, and Death

Planning: Expected Outcomes. The patient with SCD is expected to remain free from infection and sepsis. Indicators include:

- Absence of fever and foul-smelling or purulent drainage
- Absence of cough, chest pain, and dyspnea
- Absence of pain, burning on urination

Interventions. The patient with SCD is at greater risk for bacterial infection because of reduced IMMUNITY from anoxic damage to the spleen. Interventions focus on preventing infection, controlling infection, and starting drug therapy early when infection is present. The patient with a fever should have diagnostic testing for sepsis, including complete blood count (CBC) with differential, blood cultures, reticulocyte count, urine culture, and a chest x-ray. Usually these patients are started on prophylactic antibiotics.

Prevention and early detection strategies are used to protect the patient in sickle cell crisis from infection. Frequent, thorough handwashing is of the utmost importance. Any person with an upper respiratory tract infection who enters the patient's room must wear a mask. Strict aseptic technique is used for all invasive procedures.

Continually assess the patient for infection and monitor the daily CBC with differential WBC count. Inspect the mouth every 8 hours for lesions indicating fungal or viral infection. Listen to the lungs every 8 hours for crackles, wheezes, or reduced breath sounds. Inspect voided urine for odor and cloudiness and ask about urgency, burning, or pain on urination. Take vital signs at least every 4 hours to assess for fever or supervise this action when performed by others.

Drug therapy by prophylaxis with twice-daily oral penicillin reduces the number of pneumonia and other streptococcal infections. Urge the patient to receive a pneumonia vaccination and annual influenza vaccinations. Drug therapy for an actual infection depends on the sensitivity of the specific organism and the extent of the infection.

Continued blood vessel occlusion by clumping of sickled cells increases the risk for multiple organ dysfunction. Acute chest syndrome, in which a vaso-occlusive event (VOE) causes infiltration and damage to the pulmonary system, is a major cause of death in adults with SCD. Thus preventing heart and lung damage is a priority. Management focuses on prevention of VOEs and promotion of PERFUSION.

Assess the patient admitted in sickle cell crisis for adequate PERFUSION to all body areas. Remove restrictive clothing and instruct the patient to avoid flexing the knees and hips.

Hydration is needed because dehydration increases cell sickling and must be avoided. Help the patient maintain adequate hydration. The patient in acute crisis needs an oral or IV fluid intake of at least 200 mL/hr.

Oxygen is given during crises because lack of oxygen is the main cause of sickling. Ensure that oxygen therapy is nebulized to prevent dehydration. Monitor oxygen saturation. If saturation is low, evaluation of arterial blood gases (ABGs) and a chest x-ray may be needed.

Transfusion with RBCs can be helpful to increase HbA levels and dilute HbS levels, although they must be prescribed cautiously to prevent iron overload from repeated transfusions (Martin & Haines, 2016). Transfusion therapy in some centers is a mainstay of SCD management to reduce the risk for stroke. Monitor the patient for transfusion complications (discussed in the Acute Transfusion Reactions section).

Hematopoietic stem cell transplantation (HSCT) may correct abnormal hemoglobin permanently during childhood. However, HSCT is expensive and may result in life-threatening complications. At this time, HSCT is not approved as therapy for SCD in adults (Vacce & Blank, 2017).

Care Coordination and Transition Management

Care focuses on teaching the patient and family how to prevent crises and complications (Chart 40-2). The patient with SCD may receive care in acute care, subacute care, extended or assistive care, and home care settings.

Self-Management Education. Having the patient and family be partners in the life-long management of SCD is critical for improved outcomes. Thus self-management education is extensive and should be reinforced at every health care encounter with a patient who has SCD. Both income level and education level have a positive correlation with the patient's ability to be successful in the performance of self-care (Matthie et al.,

CHART 40-2 Patient and Family Education: Preparing for Self-Management
Prevention of Sickle Cell Crisis

- Drink at least 3 to 4 liters of liquids every day.
- Avoid alcoholic beverages.
- Avoid smoking cigarettes or using tobacco in any form.
- Contact your primary health care provider at the first sign of illness or infection.
- Be sure to get a "flu shot" every year.
- Ask your primary health care provider about taking the pneumonia vaccine.
- Avoid temperature extremes of hot or cold.
- Be sure to wear socks and gloves when going outside on cold days.
- Avoid planes with unpressurized passenger cabins.
- Avoid travel to high altitudes (e.g., cities such as Denver and Santa Fe).
- Ensure that any health care professional who takes care of you knows that you have sickle cell disease, especially the anesthesia provider and radiologist.
- Consider genetic counseling.
- Avoid strenuous physical activities.
- Engage in mild, low-impact exercise at least 3 times a week when you are not in crisis.

EVIDENCE-BASED PRACTICE (QSEN)

Which Factors Positively Influence Self-Care in Young Adults With Sickle Cell Disease?

Matthie, N., Jenerette, C., & McMillan, S. (2015). Role of self-care in sickle cell disease. *Pain Management Nursing, 16*(3), 257–266.

Sickle cell disease (SCD) is a serious, lifelong condition with complications that impair physical function and shorten life span. Consistent practice of recommended self-care activities can result in fewer or less severe complications and a longer life span. Once considered a childhood problem, more patients with SCD are living to adulthood and transitioning from a pediatric hematologic or SCD management setting to adult hematologic management. As young adults, these patients are expected to assume more responsibility for self-care in the management of SCD.

The study reported here, which was a descriptive cross-sectional design using secondary analysis of existing data, sought to identify the personal and sociodemographic factors that positively influenced self-care in an SCD population. Self-care was defined as "One's perceived ability to participate in general therapeutic activities aimed at improving health status and quality of life, as well as the actual performance of those activities." Self-care actions included maintaining adequate hydration, avoiding temperature extremes, eating a healthy diet, obtaining regular checkups, and ensuring adequate rest. Data from 103 adults with SCD ranging in age from 18 to 30 years were examined for demographic information, SCD self-care efficacy, perceived social support, self-care, and the annual number of hospital visits for pain crises.

Several factors demonstrated importance in promoting self-care management. Patients who had more education and more social support had overall higher scores for SCD self-efficacy, which included self-care management, perceived self-care ability, and participation in self-care actions. Social support in particular had the most significant effect on self-care. There was a negative association between income level and number of hospital visits for pain crises. The interpretation of this finding was that adult SCD patients with health insurance and/or higher incomes were able to access and obtain primary care, which reduce the number of pain crises experienced.

Level of Evidence: 3

The study reanalyzed data from a much larger, multisite study and had adequate power to generate statistically significant results for the guiding research hypotheses. The instruments used to measure the concepts of SCD self-efficacy, perceived social support, perceived self-care ability, and self-care actions were all well established with appropriate validity and reliability.

Commentary: Implications for Practice and Research

The finding that social support was most positively associated with SCD self-care is consistent with the findings of other studies regarding self-care in chronic disease management. Nurses can have an impact in promoting social support by working to help SCD patients, family, and friends have an adequate understanding of the disease, complication-avoiding activities, and performance of self-care activities. Although the availability of such information and professional support is a critical component of pediatric SCD management centers, it may not be nearly as well developed in the adult hematologic care setting. This lack becomes more significant as the SCD population ages and more adults with the disease are managed in nonpediatric settings. The authors conclude that more knowledge on the part of nursing students and practicing nurses in the adult setting about the care and education needs of SCD patients and families could have a positive effect on increasing social support.

2015b). See the Evidence-Based Practice box for a discussion of the role of self-care in SCD management.

Teach the patient to avoid specific activities that lead to reduced GAS EXCHANGE from hypoxia and hypoxemia. Stress the recognition of the early symptoms of crisis or infection so interventions can be started early to prevent pain, complications, and permanent tissue damage. Teach the patient and family the correct use of opioid analgesics at home.

Health Care Resources. Some adults are unfamiliar with the hereditary aspects of SCD. For those who need it, refer patients to genetic counselors. These professionals can provide information about birth control methods and pregnancy options.

Many patients and family members can be helped by local support groups. Provide information about the closest local chapter of the Sickle Cell Foundation. Often local children's hospitals have sickle cell support groups that include adults with the disease.

GENDER HEALTH CONSIDERATIONS

Patient-Centered Care (QSEN)

Pregnancy in women with SCD may be life threatening. Barrier methods of contraception (cervical cap, diaphragm, or condoms with or without spermicides) are often recommended for women with SCD who are sexually active. The use of combination hormone drugs for contraception may increase CLOTTING, especially among smokers, predisposing them to impaired PERFUSION and crises. The use of progestin-only hormonal contraception is recommended to reduce the risk for venous thrombotic events (VTEs) (USDHHS, 2014). Urge women using hormone-based contraceptives not to smoke.

◆ Evaluation: Reflecting

Evaluate the care of the patient with SCD based on the identified priority patient problems. The expected outcomes include that the patient will:

- Report pain to be maintained at an acceptable level
- Maintain PERFUSION and GAS EXCHANGE to extremities and vital organs
- Remain free of infection and sepsis

CLINICAL JUDGMENT CHALLENGE 40-1

Safety; Patient-Centered Care (QSEN)

A young woman who has sickle cell disease comes to the emergency department with severe joint and back pain, a cough, a temperature of 102.2°F (39°C), and shortness of breath. She appears anxious and states, "I have never felt this way before." The primary health care provider prescribes 3 mg of morphine IV and a stat chest x-ray.

1. What additional assessment data are most important to obtain? Provide a rationale for your selection.
2. Should you be concerned about the morphine causing respiratory depression? Why or why not?
3. Should oxygen be started even though it has not yet been prescribed? Why or why not?
4. What can you do to reduce her anxiety?

ANEMIA

Anemia is a reduction in the number of RBCs, the amount of hemoglobin, or the hematocrit (percentage of packed RBCs per deciliter of blood). It is a clinical indicator, not a specific disease,

TABLE 40-1   Common Causes of Anemia

TYPE OF ANEMIA	COMMON CAUSES
Sickle cell disease	Autosomal-recessive inheritance of two defective gene alleles for hemoglobin synthesis
Glucose-6-phosphate dehydrogenase (G6PD) deficiency anemia	X-linked recessive deficiency of the enzyme G6PD
Autoimmune hemolytic anemia	Abnormal immune function in which a person's immune reactive cells fail to recognize his or her own red blood cells as self-cells
Iron deficiency anemia	Inadequate iron intake caused by: • Iron-deficient diet • Chronic alcoholism • Malabsorption syndromes • Partial gastrectomy Rapid metabolic (anabolic) activity caused by: • Pregnancy • Adolescence • Infection
Vitamin B$_{12}$ deficiency anemia	Dietary deficiency Failure to absorb vitamin B$_{12}$ from intestinal tract as a result of: • Partial gastrectomy • Pernicious anemia • Malabsorption syndromes
Folic acid deficiency anemia	Dietary deficiency Malabsorption syndromes Drugs: • Oral contraceptives • Anticonvulsants • Methotrexate
Aplastic anemia	Exposure to myelotoxic agents: • Radiation • Benzene • Chloramphenicol • Alkylating agents • Antimetabolites • Sulfonamides • Insecticides Viral infection (unproven): • Epstein-Barr virus • Hepatitis B • Cytomegalovirus

because it occurs with many health problems. Anemia can result from dietary problems, genetic disorders, bone marrow disease, or excessive bleeding. GI bleeding is the most common reason for anemia in adults.

There are many types and causes of anemia (Table 40-1). Some are caused by a deficiency in one of the components needed to make fully functional RBCs. Others are caused by decreased RBC production, increased RBC destruction, or chronic RBC loss. Despite the many causes, the symptoms (Chart 40-3) and the nursing interventions are similar for all types of anemia.

❖ PATHOPHYSIOLOGY

Iron deficiency anemia is the most common anemia worldwide, especially among women, older adults, and people with poor diets (Touhy & Jett, 2016). It can result from blood loss, poor

CHART 40-3   Key Features

Anemia

Integumentary Signs and Symptoms
• Pallor, especially of the ears, the nail beds, the palmar creases, the conjunctivae, and around the mouth
• Cool to the touch
• Intolerance of cold temperatures
• Nails become brittle and become concave over time

Cardiovascular Signs and Symptoms
• Tachycardia at basal activity levels, increasing with activity and during and immediately after meals
• Murmurs and gallops heard on auscultation when anemia is severe
• Orthostatic hypotension

Respiratory Signs and Symptoms
• Dyspnea on exertion
• Decreased oxygen saturation levels

Neurologic Signs and Symptoms
• Increased somnolence and fatigue
• Headache

GI absorption of iron, and an inadequate diet (McCance et al., 2014). The problem is a decreased iron supply for the developing RBC. Any adult with iron deficiency should be evaluated for abnormal bleeding, especially from the GI tract.

Adults usually have between 2 and 6 total-body grams of iron, depending on the size of the person and the amount of hemoglobin in the cells. With chronic iron deficiency, RBCs are small (**microcytic**); and the patient has mild symptoms of anemia, including weakness and pallor. Other symptoms include fatigue, reduced exercise tolerance, and fissures at the corners of the mouth. Serum ferritin values are less than 10 ng/mL (normal range is 12 to 300 ng/mL [12 to 300 mcg/L]).

Vitamin B$_{12}$ deficiency anemia results in failure to activate enzymes that move folic acid into precursor RBCs cells so cell division and growth into functional RBCs can occur. These precursor cells then undergo improper DNA synthesis and increase in size. This type of anemia is called *megaloblastic* or **macrocytic anemia** because of the large size of these abnormal cells.

Causes of vitamin B$_{12}$ deficiency include vegan diets or diets lacking dairy products, small bowel resection, chronic diarrhea, diverticula, tapeworm, or overgrowth of intestinal bacteria. Anemia resulting from failure to absorb vitamin B$_{12}$ (**pernicious anemia**) is caused by a deficiency of **intrinsic factor** (a substance normally secreted by the gastric mucosa), which is needed for intestinal absorption of vitamin B$_{12}$.

Vitamin B$_{12}$ deficiency anemia may be mild or severe and usually develops slowly. Indications of this type of anemia include pallor and jaundice, **glossitis** (a smooth, beefy-red tongue) (Fig. 40-3), fatigue, and weight loss. Patients with pernicious anemia may also have **paresthesias** (abnormal sensations) in the feet and hands and poor balance.

Folic acid deficiency anemia may have symptoms similar to those of vitamin B$_{12}$ deficiency. However, nervous system functions remain normal because folic acid deficiency does not affect nerve function and does not result in paresthesias. The disease develops slowly.

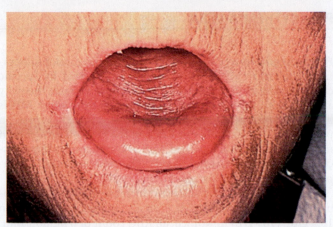

FIG. 40-3 Glossitis, a smooth tongue as a result of vitamin B₁₂ deficiency anemia. (From Feldman, M., Friedman, L., & Brandt, L. [2010]. *Sleisenger and Fordtran's gastrointestinal and liver disease* [9th ed.]. Philadelphia: Saunders.)

Common causes of folic acid deficiency are poor nutrition, malabsorption, and drugs. Poor nutrition, especially a diet lacking green leafy vegetables, liver, yeast, citrus fruits, dried beans, and nuts, is the most common cause. Malabsorption syndromes, such as Crohn's disease, are the second most common cause. Anticonvulsants and oral contraceptives can contribute to folic acid deficiency and anemia.

CONSIDERATIONS FOR OLDER ADULTS

Patient-Centered Care (QSEN)

Older patients often have restricted diets and may be unable to eat meat because of tooth loss or economic reasons and thus are at risk for iron deficiency anemia. Ask about a family history of anemia. B₁₂ deficiency anemia often occurs in patients 50 to 80 years of age and may result from an inherited genetic mutation (Touhy & Jett, 2016). Because symptoms are vague, the disorder can easily be overlooked.

Aplastic anemia is a deficiency of circulating red blood cells (RBCs) because of impaired CELLULAR REGULATION of the bone marrow, which then fails to produce these cells. It is caused by an injury to the immature precursor cell for RBCs. Although aplastic anemia sometimes occurs alone, it usually occurs with **leukopenia** (a reduction in white blood cells [WBCs]) and **thrombocytopenia** (a reduction in platelets), a condition known as **pancytopenia**. Disease onset may be slow or rapid.

The most common type of the disease is caused by long-term exposure to toxic agents, drugs (see Table 39-3), ionizing radiation, or infection; but often the cause is unknown. The disease also may follow viral infection. The most common hereditary form of the disease is Fanconi's anemia. These problems all result in loss of normal CELLULAR REGULATION.

The patient has symptoms of severe anemia. A complete blood count (CBC) shows severe macrocytic anemia, leukopenia, and thrombocytopenia. A bone marrow biopsy may show replacement of cell-forming marrow with fat. Infection is common.

Glucose-6-phosphate dehydrogenase (G6PD) deficiency anemia is caused by a genetic problem in which there is a deficiency of the enzyme G6PD. This disease is inherited as an X-linked recessive disorder, with more severe expression in males and mild partial expression in carrier females. It affects about 10% of all African Americans and also is more common in adults from the Middle East and Asia (McCance et al., 2014).

G6PD stimulates reactions in glucose metabolism important for energy in RBCs because they contain no other way to produce adenosine triphosphate (ATP). Cells with reduced amounts of G6PD break more easily during exposure to some drugs (e.g., sulfonamides, aspirin, quinine derivatives, chloramphenicol, dapsone, high doses of vitamin C, and thiazide diuretics), benzene, and other toxins.

New RBCs have some G6PD, but the enzyme diminishes as the cells age. The patient usually does not have symptoms until exposed to triggering agents or until a severe infection develops. After exposure to a precipitating cause, acute RBC breakage begins and lasts 7 to 12 days. During this acute phase, anemia and jaundice develop. The hemolytic reaction is limited because only older RBCs, containing less G6PD, are destroyed.

Immunohemolytic anemia, also referred to as *autoimmune hemolytic anemia* (McCance et al., 2014) is caused by abnormal IMMUNITY that results in the excessive destruction of RBC membranes (*lysis*) followed by accelerated RBC production. Immune system products (e.g., antibodies) attack a person's own RBCs for unknown reasons. Regardless of the cause, RBCs are viewed as non-self by the immune system and are attacked and destroyed.

The two types of immunohemolytic anemia are warm antibody anemia and cold antibody anemia. **Warm antibody anemia** occurs with immunoglobulin G (IgG) antibody excess. These antibodies are most active at 98.6°F (37°C) and may be triggered by drugs, chemicals, or other autoimmune problems. **Cold antibody anemia** has complement protein fixation on immunoglobulin M (IgM) and occurs most at body temperatures around 86°F (30°C). This problem often occurs with a Raynaud's-like response in which the arteries in the hands and feet constrict profoundly in response to cold temperatures or stress.

NCLEX EXAMINATION CHALLENGE 40-2

Physiological Integrity

Which signs and symptoms does the nurse expect to find in clients with any type of anemia? **Select all that apply.**
A. Exercise intolerance
B. Fatigue
C. Glossitis
D. Jaundice
E. Leukopenia
F. Microcytic red blood cells
G. Paresthesias of the hands and feet
H. Tachycardia

❖ INTERPROFESSIONAL COLLABORATIVE CARE

Iron deficiency anemia management involves increasing the oral intake of iron from food sources (e.g., red meat, organ meat, egg yolks, kidney beans, leafy green vegetables, and raisins). If iron losses are mild, oral iron supplements are started until the hemoglobin level returns to normal. If the supplements cause GI distress, the preparations can be taken with meals. When iron deficiency anemia is severe, iron solutions (iron dextran [Dexferrum, INFeD, Pri-Dextra]; ferumoxytol [Feraheme]) can be given parenterally. Ferumoxytol now carries a black box warning of an increased risk for life-threatening anaphylaxis that can occur during or within 5 minutes after receiving the infusion (Aschenbrenner, 2015).

Vitamin B$_{12}$ deficiency anemia is managed by teaching the patient to increase his or her intake of foods rich in vitamin B$_{12}$ (animal proteins, fish, eggs, nuts, dairy products, dried beans, citrus fruit, and leafy green vegetables). Vitamin supplements may be prescribed when anemia is severe. Patients who have pernicious anemia are given vitamin B$_{12}$ injections weekly at first and then monthly for the rest of their lives. Oral B$_{12}$ preparations and nasal spray or sublingual cobalamin preparations may be used to maintain vitamin levels after the patient's deficiency has first been corrected by the traditional injection method.

Folic acid deficiency anemia is best managed by identifying adults at risk and preventing the deficiency. High-risk adults include older, debilitated patients with alcoholism; patients at risk for malnutrition; and those with increased folic acid requirements. A diet rich in foods containing folic acid and vitamin B$_{12}$ prevents a deficiency. This type of anemia is managed with scheduled folic acid replacement therapy.

Aplastic anemia is managed differently depending on the absolute cause. For transient or drug-induced aplastic anemia, short-term management may include blood transfusions along with discontinuing the offending drug. Blood transfusions are used when the anemia causes disability or when bleeding is life threatening because of low platelet counts. Unnecessary transfusion increases the chances for developing immune reactions to platelets and shortens the life span of the transfused cell. This therapy is discontinued as soon as the bone marrow begins to produce RBCs if the problem is transient.

Immunosuppressive therapy helps patients who have the types of aplastic anemia with a disease course similar to that of autoimmune problems. Drugs such as prednisone, antithymocyte globulin (ATG), and cyclosporine A (Sandimmune) have resulted in partial or complete remissions. For moderate aplastic anemia, daclizumab (Zenapax) has improved both blood counts and transfusion requirements. Splenectomy may be needed for patients with an enlarged spleen that is either destroying normal RBCs or suppressing their development.

Hematopoietic stem cell transplantation with donor cells is the most successful method of treatment for aplastic anemia that does not respond to other therapies. Cost, availability, and complications limit this treatment. For patients who are unable to undergo such treatment or lack a suitable donor, immunosuppressive therapy remains the treatment of choice.

Glucose-6-phosphate dehydrogenase deficiency anemia management has prevention as the most important therapeutic measure. Men who belong to the high-risk groups should be tested for this problem before being given drugs that can cause the hemolytic reaction.

Hydration is important during an episode of hemolysis to prevent debris and hemoglobin from collecting in the kidney tubules, which can lead to acute kidney injury (AKI). Osmotic diuretics, such as mannitol (Osmitrol), help prevent this complication. Transfusions are needed when anemia is present and kidney function is normal (see the Transfusion Therapy section).

Immunohemolytic anemia management depends on disease severity. Steroid therapy to suppress IMMUNITY is temporarily effective in most patients. Splenectomy and more intense immunosuppressive therapy with chemotherapy drugs may be used if steroid therapy fails. Plasma exchange therapy with antibody removal is effective for patients who do not respond to chemotherapy drugs.

POLYCYTHEMIA VERA

❖ PATHOPHYSIOLOGY

Polycythemia vera (PV) is one of the chronic myeloproliferative neoplasms (MPNs), which are characterized by specific clonal proliferation of myeloid cells that have variable maturity and function. PV is distinguished clinically from other MPNs by the presence of an elevated red blood cell (RBC) mass. In polycythemia, the number of RBCs in the blood is *greater* than normal. The blood of a patient with polycythemia is hyperviscous (thicker than normal blood). The problem may be temporary (because of other conditions) or chronic.

PV is a disease with a sustained increase in blood hemoglobin levels greater than 18 g/dL (180 g/L) in men or greater than 16.5 g/dL (165 g/L) in women, an RBC count of 6 million/mm^3 (6×10^{12}), or a hematocrit of 55% (0.55 volume fraction) or greater. PV is a cancer of the RBCs with three major hallmarks: massive production of RBCs, excessive leukocyte production, and excessive production of platelets. More than 90% of patients with PV show a mutation of the *JAK2* kinase gene in the affected cell; this mutation causes a loss of CELLULAR REGULATION over blood cells (McCance et al., 2014). Extreme hypercellularity (cell excess) of the peripheral blood occurs in people with PV.

The patient's facial skin and mucous membranes have a dark, purple or cyanotic, flushed (plethoric) appearance with distended veins. Intense itching caused by dilated blood vessels and poor PERFUSION is common. The thick blood moves more slowly and places increased demands on the heart, resulting in hypertension. In some areas, blood flow may be so slow that stasis occurs. Vascular stasis causes thrombosis (CLOTTING) within the smaller vessels, occluding them, which leads to tissue hypoxia, anoxia and, later, to infarction and necrosis. Tissues most at risk for this problem are the heart, spleen, and kidneys, although damage can occur in any organ.

Because the actual number of cells in the blood is greatly increased and the cells are not completely normal, cell life spans are shorter. The shorter life spans and increased cell production cause a rapid turnover of circulating blood cells. This rapid turnover increases the amount of cell debris (released when cells die) in the blood, adding to the general "sludging" of the blood. This debris includes uric acid and potassium, which cause the symptoms of gout and hyperkalemia (elevated serum potassium level).

Even though the number of RBCs is greatly increased, their oxygen-carrying capacity is impaired, and patients have poor GAS EXCHANGE with severe hypoxia. Bleeding problems are common because of platelet impairment with poor CLOTTING.

❖ INTERPROFESSIONAL COLLABORATIVE CARE

PV is a malignant disease that progresses in severity over time. If left untreated, few people with PV live longer than 2 years after diagnosis. With management by repeated phlebotomy with apheresis (two to five times per week), the patient may live 10 to 15 years or longer. (Apheresis is the withdrawal of whole blood and removal of some of the patient's blood components, in this case RBCs. The plasma is then reinfused back into the patient.) Increasing hydration and promoting venous return help prevent clot formation. Therapy for PV also includes the use of anticoagulants. Chart 40-4 lists health tips for patients with PV.

Aggressive IV chemotherapy is no longer recommended because of its increased risk for inducing leukemia. Aspirin

CHART 40-4 Patient and Family Education: Preparing for Self-Management

Polycythemia Vera

- Drink at least 3 liters of liquids each day.
- Avoid tight or constrictive clothing, especially garters and girdles.
- Wear gloves when outdoors in temperatures lower than 50°F (10°C).
- Keep all health care–related appointments.
- Contact your primary health care provider at the first sign of infection.
- Take anticoagulants as prescribed.
- Wear support hose or stockings while you are awake and up.
- Elevate your feet whenever you are seated.
- Exercise slowly and only on the advice of your primary health care provider.
- Stop activity at the first sign of chest pain.
- Use an electric shaver.
- Use a soft-bristled toothbrush to brush your teeth.
- Do not floss between your teeth.
- If you are a smoker, strongly consider smoking cessation.

therapy may be used to decrease CLOTTING but increases the risk for GI bleeding. Hydroxyurea, an oral chemotherapy drug, may be prescribed for severe disease symptoms. Pegylated interferon has also shown some benefit in controlling RBC production.

HEREDITARY HEMOCHROMATOSIS

Hereditary hemochromatosis is an autosomal-recessive disorder in which a mutation in both alleles of the *HFE* gene causes increased intestinal absorption of dietary iron (Online Mendelian Inheritance in Man [OMIM], 2016a). The excess iron is deposited in a variety of tissues and organs, including the liver, spleen, heart, joints, skin, and pancreas. Iron deposits can damage the organs, leading to organ failure. Usually the disease is more common in men, and symptoms appear in men during their 40s. Women have symptoms later because the loss of menstrual blood before menopause helps remove excess iron. Common signs and symptoms are abdominal pain, liver enlargement, hyperglycemia, and a gradual darkening of the skin. Later problems include diabetes, liver cirrhosis, endocrine gland failure, heart disease, and death.

The disorder is diagnosed on the basis of symptoms and altered iron levels. Genetic testing is available to determine carrier status. When the disorder is identified early before organ damage, management is simple and can prevent severe organ damage and early death (Quigley, 2016). Phlebotomy and removal of 500 mL of blood at a time, occurring as often as twice weekly at first, is performed to reduce the overall iron load of the blood. The desired outcome is to reduce blood ferritin levels to less than 9 to 50 micrograms per liter (9 to 50 mcg/L). Once this level is achieved, phlebotomy frequency can be reduced to once every 2 to 4 months for maintenance.

MYELODYSPLASTIC SYNDROMES

❖ PATHOPHYSIOLOGY

Myelodysplastic syndromes (MDS) are a group of disorders caused by the formation of abnormal cells in the bone marrow. These abnormal cells are usually destroyed shortly after they are released into the blood. As a result, patients with MDS have a decrease in all blood cell types. Anemia is the most common problem with MDS, although neutropenia (low white blood cell count [WBC]) and thrombocytopenia (low platelets) are also often present.

MDS most often occurs in people ages 65 years or older. It has cancer-like features and is considered to be a *precancerous* state. Like cancer, it arises from a single population of abnormal cells that have lost normal CELLULAR REGULATION. About 30% of all patients with MDS eventually develop acute leukemia (McCance et al., 2014). The subtypes of MDS have different prognoses and responses to therapy. Patients are categorized into risk groups (i.e., low, intermediate [1 and 2], high) based on the severity of pancytopenia (low counts of all blood cell types), cytogenetic abnormalities, and numbers of blast cells (immature WBC cells) found in the bone marrow.

The exact cause of MDS is not clear. Risk factors include normal physiologic changes associated with aging, chemical exposures (pesticides, benzene), tobacco smoke, and exposure to radiation or chemotherapy drugs. Diagnosis is made by examination of the chromosomes and the genes within the chromosomes (cytogenetic testing) of the bone marrow cells. Peripheral blood smears are used to assess the level of cell maturation and the proportion of abnormal cells.

❖ INTERPROFESSIONAL COLLABORATIVE CARE

The only potentially curative treatment for MDS is allogeneic hematopoietic stem cell transplantation, which is often not an option because of the advanced age of many patients. Several alternate management strategies have demonstrated some promise. For low-risk and intermediate-1-risk MDS, the anti-tumor immunomodulatory agent lenalidomide (Revlimid) is approved for patients whose dysplastic cells have the chromosome abnormality of a deleted 5q. Two other agents approved for intermediate-2-risk and high-risk MDS are azacitidine (Vidaza) and decitabine (Dacogen). These drugs often require at least 3 to 6 months to achieve a clinical response; therefore supportive care is necessary.

Supportive care includes blood transfusions for anemia and platelet transfusions when platelet levels are very low. Erythrocyte stimulating agents (ESAs) such as epoetin alfa (Epogen, Procrit) or darbepoetin alfa (Aranesp) may be given in addition to transfusions.

✳ IMMUNITY CONCEPT EXEMPLAR Leukemia

As discussed in Chapter 17, white blood cells (WBCs), or leukocytes, provide protection from infection and cancer development. This protection depends on maintaining normal numbers and ratios of the different mature circulating WBCs. When any one type of WBC is present in either abnormal amounts (too high or too low), IMMUNITY, GAS EXCHANGE, and CLOTTING are altered to some degree, placing patients at risk for many complications.

❖ PATHOPHYSIOLOGY

Leukemia is cancer that results from a loss of normal CELLULAR REGULATION, leading to uncontrolled production of immature WBCs ("blast" cells) in the bone marrow. As a result, the bone marrow becomes overcrowded with immature, nonfunctional cells, and production of normal blood cells is greatly decreased. Leukemia may be acute, with a sudden onset, or chronic, with a slow onset and symptoms that persist for years.

Leukemia is classified by cell type. Leukemic cells coming from the lymphoid pathways (see Fig. 17-3) are classified as **lymphocytic** or **lymphoblastic**. Leukemic cells coming from the myeloid pathways are classified as **myelocytic** or **myelogenous**. Several subtypes exist for each of these diseases, which are classified according to the degree of maturity of the abnormal cell and the specific cell type involved. These are identified as M0 through M8. M3 is a subtype (referred to as acute promyelocytic leukemia [APL]) that has a specific treatment different from other AMLs. It is identified by a translocation of chromosomes 15 and 17. *Biphenotypic leukemia* is acute leukemia that shows both lymphocytic and myelocytic features.

With leukemia, cancer most often occurs in the stem cells or early precursor leukocyte cells, causing excessive growth of a specific type of immature leukocyte. In some chronic leukemias, the cancerous cells may be more mature. These cells are abnormal, and their excessive production in the bone marrow stops normal bone marrow production, leading to anemia, thrombocytopenia, and leukopenia. Often the number of immature, abnormal WBCs ("blasts") in the blood is greatly elevated, but these cells do not provide infection protection. Leukemic cells may also be in the spleen, liver, lymph nodes, and central nervous system. With acute leukemia, these changes occur rapidly and, without intervention, progress to death from infection or hemorrhage. Chronic leukemia may be present for years before changes appear.

Etiology and Genetic Risk

The exact cause of leukemia is unknown, although many genetic and environmental factors are involved in its development. The basic problem involves damage to genes controlling cell growth, resulting in a loss of normal CELLULAR REGULATION. This damage then changes cells from normal to **malignant** (cancer). Bone marrow analysis shows abnormal chromosomes about 50% of the time (McCance et al., 2014). Possible risk factors for leukemia development include ionizing radiation, viral infection, exposure to chemicals and drugs, disorders such as myelodysplastic syndrome or Fanconi's anemia, genetic factors, IMMUNITY factors, environmental factors, and the interaction of these factors.

Ionizing radiation exposures such as radiation therapy for cancer treatment or heavy accidental exposures increase the risk for leukemia development, particularly acute myelogenous leukemia (AML). Chemicals and drugs have been linked to leukemia development because of their ability to damage DNA and disrupt normal CELLULAR REGULATION. Previous treatment for cancer with some chemotherapy drugs (e.g., melphalan, doxorubicin, etoposide, and cyclophosphamide) poses risks for leukemia development about 5 to 8 years after treatment. Table 39-3 lists chemicals and drugs that damage the hematologic system.

Genetic and IMMUNITY factors influence leukemia development. There is an increased incidence of the disease among patients with genetic conditions such as Down syndrome, Bloom syndrome, Klinefelter syndrome, and Fanconi's anemia. Immune deficiencies may promote the development of leukemia. Chronic lymphocytic leukemia often has a familial predisposition.

Incidence and Prevalence

Leukemia accounts for 3% to 4% of all new cases of cancer and 4% to 5% of all deaths from cancer (American Cancer Society

[ACS], 2017). In Canada, leukemia accounts for 6.3% of new cancer cases and 6.9% of all deaths from cancer (Canadian Cancer Society [CCS], 2016). The incidence depends on many factors, including the type of WBC affected, age, gender, race, and geographic locale.

About 60,140 new cases of leukemia occur each year in the United States, and about 6200 new cases occur in Canada (ACS, 2017; CCS, 2016). Leukemia is classified into five different types based on the cell type and how fast the disease progresses (Table 40-2)

❖ INTERPROFESSIONAL COLLABORATIVE CARE

Leukemia can be cured; but the acute phase of treatment is long, affects every aspect of a patient's life, and is best managed by an interprofessional team. In addition to hematology oncologists and oncology nurses, other professionals important to ensuring optimal management include registered dieticians, pharmacists, occupational therapists, social workers, patient navigators, community health workers, mental health practitioners, and spiritual care advisors. Like many disorders, leukemia management is most effective when the patient and family are full partners with the health care team.

Initial care usually occurs in an inpatient setting, as does care for treatment complications such as infection. Some therapy is provided on an outpatient basis; even stem cell transplant recipients may be managed as outpatients in some health centers. Care coordination is extensive, and patient and family education is an ongoing process.

◆ Assessment: Noticing

History. Ask the patient about exposure to risk factors and related genetic factors. Age is important because the risk for

TABLE 40-2 Classification of Leukemia Types

LEUKEMIA TYPE	FEATURES
Acute myelogenous leukemia (AML)	Most common in adults Has eight subtypes
Acute promyelocytic leukemia (APL)	Subtype of AML Most curable of adult leukemias
Acute lymphocytic leukemia (ALL)	Forms about 10% of adult-onset leukemias Often is Philadelphia chromosome–positive
Chronic myelogenous leukemia (CML)	Forms about 20% of adult-onset leukemias Occurs most often after age 50 years Usually is Philadelphia chromosome–positive Has three phases: • *Chronic:* slow growing with mild manifestations that respond to therapy • *Accelerated:* more rapid growing with more severe manifestations, increased blast cells, and failure to respond to therapy • *Blast:* very aggressive leukemia with high percentage of blast and promyelocytes that spread to other organs
Chronic lymphocytic leukemia (CLL)	Most common chronic leukemia in adults; occurs most often after age 50 years Is associated with a genetic predisposition Survival time can extend to 10 years or more in patients diagnosed with early-stage disease

adult-onset leukemia increases with age. Occupation and hobbies may reveal exposure to agents that increase the risk for leukemia. Previous illnesses and the medical history may reveal exposure to ionizing radiation or drugs that increase risk.

Changes in IMMUNITY increase the risk for infection in the patient with leukemia. Even when the blood count shows a normal or high level of WBCs, these cells are immature and cannot protect the patient from infection. Ask about the frequency and severity of infections, such as colds, influenza, pneumonia, bronchitis, or unexplained fevers, during the past 6 months.

Platelet function is reduced with leukemia, interfering with CLOTTING. Ask about any excessive bleeding episodes, such as:

- A tendency to bruise easily or longer after minor trauma
- Nosebleeds
- Increased menstrual flow
- Bleeding from the gums
- Rectal bleeding
- Hematuria (blood in the urine)

If the patient has experienced such an episode, ask whether this type and extent of bleeding is his or her usual response to injury or represents a change.

The patient with leukemia often has weakness and fatigue from anemia and from the increased metabolism of the leukemic cells. Ask whether any of these problems have occurred:

- Headaches
- Behavior changes
- Increased somnolence; decreased alertness; fatigue
- Decreased attention span
- Muscle weakness
- Loss of appetite
- Weight loss

A 24-hour activity history may reveal activity intolerance, changes in behavior, and unexplained fatigue. Assess how long the patient has had any of these debilitating problems.

Physical Assessment/Signs and Symptoms. Leukemia affects all blood cells, which then influence the health and function of all organs and systems. Thus many body areas and systems may be affected (Chart 40-5). The following problems occur with acute leukemia and chronic leukemia in the blast phase.

Cardiovascular changes often are related to adjustments needed when PERFUSION and GAS EXCHANGE are reduced from anemia. The heart rate is increased, and blood pressure is decreased. Murmurs (abnormal blood flow sounds in the heart) and bruits (abnormal blood flow sounds over arteries) may be heard. Capillary refill is slow. When the WBC count is greatly elevated and blood is highly viscous, blood pressure is elevated with a bounding pulse.

Respiratory changes are related to reduced GAS EXCHANGE from anemia and to infection. Respiratory rate increases as anemia becomes more severe. If a respiratory infection is present, the patient may have coughing and dyspnea. Abnormal breath sounds are heard on auscultation.

Skin changes include pallor and coolness to the touch as a result of reduced PERFUSION from anemia. Pallor is most evident on the face, around the mouth, and in the nail beds. The conjunctiva of the eye also is pale, as are the creases on the palm of the hand. Petechiae may be present on any area of skin surface, especially the legs and feet. The petechiae may be unrelated to any obvious trauma. Inspect for skin infections or injured areas that have failed to heal. Inspect the mouth

> ## CHART 40-5 Key Features
> ### Acute Leukemia
>
> **Integumentary Signs and Symptoms**
> - Ecchymoses
> - Petechiae
> - Open infected lesions
> - Pallor of the conjunctivae, the nail beds, the palmar creases, and around the mouth
>
> **Gastrointestinal Signs and Symptoms**
> - Bleeding gums
> - Anorexia
> - Weight loss
> - Enlarged liver and spleen
>
> **Renal Signs and Symptoms**
> - Hematuria
>
> **Musculoskeletal Signs and Symptoms**
> - Bone pain
> - Joint swelling and pain
>
> **Cardiovascular Signs and Symptoms**
> - Tachycardia at basal activity levels
> - Orthostatic hypotension
> - Palpitations
>
> **Respiratory Signs and Symptoms**
> - Dyspnea on exertion
>
> **Neurologic Signs and Symptoms**
> - Fatigue
> - Headache
> - Fever

for gum bleeding and any sore or lesion that may indicate infection.

Intestinal changes may be related to an increased bleeding tendency and fatigue. Weight loss, nausea, and anorexia are common. Examine the rectal area for fissures, and test stool for occult blood. Many patients with leukemia have reduced bowel sounds and are constipated because reduced blood flow to intestinal tissue leads to decreased peristalsis. Enlargement of the liver and spleen and abdominal tenderness also may be present from leukemic cells trapped in these organs.

Central nervous system (CNS) changes include cranial nerve problems, headache, and papilledema from leukemic invasion of the CNS. Seizures and coma also may occur.

Miscellaneous changes can include bone and joint tenderness as the marrow is damaged and the bone reabsorbs. Leukemic cells invade lymph nodes, causing enlargement.

Psychosocial Assessment. The patient and family with newly diagnosed leukemia may be very anxious and fearful of the disease outcome. Assess what the diagnosis means to the patient and family and what they expect in the future (Albrecht, 2014).

A diagnosis of leukemia has serious consequences for the patient's lifestyle. Hospitalization for initial treatment often lasts weeks and may result in boredom, loneliness, isolation, and financial stress. Assess coping patterns, including activities that the patient finds enjoyable and methods that help him or her relax. After initial therapy, the patient may resume work, depending on the occupation. Often the patient must make adjustments for changes in functional status. He or she may be hospitalized repeatedly for complications.

Laboratory Assessment. The patient with acute leukemia usually has decreased hemoglobin and hematocrit levels, a low platelet count, and an abnormal white blood cell (WBC) count. The WBC count may be low, normal, or elevated. The patient with a high WBC count consisting of mostly blast cells at diagnosis has a poorer prognosis.

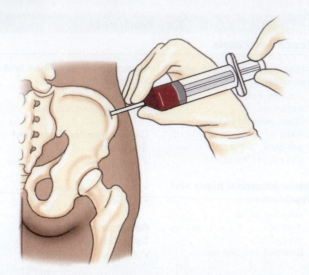

FIG. 40-4 Bone marrow aspiration from the posterior iliac crest. (From Leonard, P. C. [2012]. *Building a medical vocabulary: With Spanish translations* [8th ed.]. St. Louis: Saunders.)

The definitive test for leukemia is an examination of cells obtained from bone marrow aspiration and biopsy (Fig. 40-4). The bone marrow is full of leukemic **blast phase cells** (immature cells that are dividing). The proteins (**antigens**) on the surfaces of the leukemic cells are "markers" that help diagnose the type of leukemia and may indicate prognosis. These include the T11 protein, terminal deoxynucleotidyl transferase (TDT), the common acute lymphoblastic leukemia antigen (CALLA), and the CD33 antigen.

Blood CLOTTING times and factors are usually abnormal with acute leukemia. Reduced levels of fibrinogen and other clotting factors are common. Whole-blood clotting time is prolonged, as is the activated partial thromboplastin time (aPTT).

Chromosome analysis (cytogenetic studies) of the leukemic cells may identify marker chromosomes to help diagnose the type of leukemia, predict the prognosis, and determine therapy effectiveness. An example is the Philadelphia chromosome, which is important in the diagnosis and treatment of some types of chronic myelogenous leukemia (CML) and adult acute lymphocytic leukemia (ALL). The Philadelphia chromosome is an abnormal chromosome caused by a translocation of the *ABL* gene from chromosome 9 onto the *BCR* gene of chromosome 22. The new protein produced by this mutation causes loss of normal CELLULAR REGULATION by inhibiting cell apoptosis and DNA repair (Jorde et al., 2016).

Imaging Assessment. Specific signs and symptoms determine the need for specific tests. In a patient with dyspnea, a chest x-ray is needed to determine whether leukemic infiltrates are present in the lung. Skeletal x-rays may help determine whether loss of bone minerals and bone density is present.

◆ **Analysis: Interpreting**

The priority collaborative problems for patients with acute myelogenous leukemia (AML), the most common type of acute leukemia seen in adults, include:

1. Potential for infection due to decreased IMMUNITY and chemotherapy

2. Potential for injury due to poor CLOTTING from thrombocytopenia and chemotherapy

3. Fatigue due to decreased GAS EXCHANGE and increased energy demands

◆ **Planning and Implementation: Responding**

Preventing Infection

Planning: Expected Outcomes. The patient with leukemia is expected to remain free from infection. Indicators include:

• Absence of fever and foul-smelling or purulent drainage
• Absence of cough, chest pain, and dyspnea
• Absence of urinary frequency, urgency, or pain and burning
• Intact skin and mucous membranes

Interventions. *Infection is a major cause of death in the patient with leukemia* because the white blood cells (WBCs) are immature and cannot function or WBCs are depleted from chemotherapy, leading to sepsis. Infection occurs through both **auto-contamination** (normal flora overgrows and penetrates the internal environment) and **cross-contamination** (organisms from another person or the environment are transmitted to the patient). The most common sources of infection are the skin, respiratory tract, and intestinal tract.

Gram-negative bacteria are the most common cause of infection, although infections from other causes do occur. Interventions aim to halt infection and control infections early. Chart 40-6 lists areas to assess for the patient at risk for infection.

Drug Therapy for Acute Leukemia. Drug therapy for patients with AML is divided into three distinctive phases: induction, consolidation, and maintenance.

Induction therapy is intense combination chemotherapy started at the time of diagnosis. The purpose of this therapy is to achieve a rapid, complete remission of all disease symptoms. Agencies and oncologists differ in drug combinations used and the treatment schedule. One example of aggressive induction therapy is continuous IV cytosine arabinoside for 7 days together with an anthracycline for the first 3 days, sometimes referred to as a *7 plus 3 regimen*. This therapy results in severe bone marrow suppression with neutropenia and reduced IMMUNITY, making the patient even more at risk for infection. For acute promyelocytic leukemia (APL), the agent tretinoin (Vesanoid) is added to the chemotherapy regimen.

Prolonged hospitalizations are common while the patient is neutropenic. Recovery of bone marrow function requires at least 2 to 3 weeks, during which the patient must be protected from life-threatening infection. Other side effects of drugs used for induction therapy include nausea, vomiting, diarrhea, **alopecia** (hair loss), **stomatitis** (mouth sores), kidney toxicity, liver toxicity, and cardiac toxicity. (See Chapter 22 for information on effects of anticancer agents.) Older patients have a greater infection-related death rate during this phase than do younger patients. Patients with APL are at greater risk for sepsis with disseminated intravascular coagulation (DIC) during induction therapy than are patients with other subtypes of AML.

Consolidation therapy consists of another course of either the same drugs used for induction at a different dosage or a different combination of chemotherapy drugs. This treatment occurs early in remission, and its intent is to cure. Consolidation therapy may be either a single course of chemotherapy or repeated courses. Hematopoietic stem cell transplantation also

CHART 40-6 Focused Assessment

Patients at Risk for Infection

General Condition
- Age
- History of allergies
- History of chemotherapy, radiation therapy, or other immunosuppressive therapies such as steroid use
- Chronic diseases
- History of febrile neutropenia and associated symptoms
- Nutrition status
- Functional status—problems with immobility
- Tobacco use—cigarettes, pipe, cigars, oral
- Recreational drug use
- Alcohol use
- Prescribed and over-the-counter drug use
- Baseline and ongoing vital signs—blood pressure, heart rate, respiratory rate, and temperature

Skin and Mucous Membranes
- Thorough inspection of all skin surfaces with attention to axillae, anorectal area, and under breasts; inspection of skin for color, vascularity, bleeding, lesions, edema, moist areas, excoriation, irritation, erythema; general condition of hair and nails, pressure areas, swelling, pain, tenderness, biopsy or surgical sites, wounds, enlarged lymph nodes, catheters, or other devices
- Inspection of oral cavity, including lips, tongue, mucous membranes, gingiva, teeth, and throat—color, moisture, bleeding, ulcerations, lesions, exudate, mucositis, stomatitis, plaque, swelling, pain, tenderness, taste changes, amount and character of saliva, ability to swallow, changes in voice, dental caries, patient's oral hygiene routine
- History of current skin or mucous membrane problems

Head, Eyes, Ears, Nose
- Pain, tenderness, exudate, crusting, enlarged lymph nodes

Cardiopulmonary
- Respiratory rate and pattern, breath sounds (presence/absence, adventitious sounds), quantity and characteristics of sputum, shortness of breath, use of accessory muscles, dysphagia, diminished gag reflex, tachycardia, blood pressure

Gastrointestinal
- Pain, diarrhea, bowel sounds, character and frequency of bowel movements, constipation, rectal bleeding, hemorrhoids, change in bowel habits, sexual practices, erythema, ulceration

Genitourinary
- Dysuria, frequency, urgency, hematuria, pruritus, pain, vaginal or penile discharge, vaginal bleeding, burning, lesions, ulcerations, characteristics of urine

Central Nervous System
- Cognition, level of consciousness, personality, behavior

Musculoskeletal
- Tenderness, pain, loss of function

---

may be considered, depending on the disease subtype and the patient's response to induction therapy.

Maintenance therapy may be prescribed for months to years after successful induction and consolidation therapies for acute lymphocytic leukemia (ALL) and acute promyelocytic leukemia (APL). The purpose is to maintain the remission achieved through induction and consolidation. Not all types of leukemia respond to maintenance therapy.

Drug Therapy for Chronic Leukemia. Imatinib mesylate (Gleevec) is a common first-line drug therapy for CML that is Philadelphia chromosome positive. This oral drug is well tolerated and has been effective at inducing remission for early stages of CML. Other drugs approved for first-line therapy or for patients whose disease is resistant or intolerant to imatinib are dasatinib (Sprycel), nilotinib (Tasigna), or bosutinib (Bosulif). Other drugs used to treat CML include interferon-alfa, which slows the growth of leukemic cells. Patient responses to therapy are evaluated on the basis of hematologic, cytogenetic, and molecular criteria.

Chronic lymphocytic leukemia (CLL) is the most prevalent form of leukemia in adults, affecting women more often than men. Cytogenetic testing is important in the prognosis. Partial deletion of chromosome 13 is associated with a favorable prognosis, whereas a deletion of chromosome 11 or in chromosome 17 (*Tp53* mutation) is associated with a poor prognosis. Treatment of CLL with standard chemotherapy can cause remissions but does not cure the disease. The decision to initiate therapy is based on disease stage, symptoms, and disease activity. Rituximab (Rituxan) is often combined with standard chemotherapy

drugs or used as a single agent. Another drug approved for CLL is bendamustine (Treanda), which may be used alone or along with rituximab. Other monoclonal antibodies approved for CLL are ofatumumab (Arzerra), alemtuzumab (Campath), and obinutuzumab (Gazyva). Current investigational therapies for CLL include ibrutinib (Imbruvica), idelalisib (Zydelig), lenalidomide (Revlimid), and venetoclax (ABT-199).

Hematopoietic stem cell transplantation in patients with CLL is an option that offers curative potential or prolonged disease-free survival. However, it comes with considerable risk for mortality and is not an appropriate alternative for all patients.

Drug Therapy for Infection. Drug therapy is the main defense against infections that develop in patients undergoing therapy for AML. Drugs used depend on the sensitivity of the organism causing the infection, as well as on infection severity. Drugs for infection include antibacterial, antiviral, and antifungal agents.

Infection Protection. A major focus in caring for the patient with leukemia and reduced IMMUNITY is protection from infection. All personnel must use extreme care during all nursing procedures. Frequent, thorough handwashing is of the utmost importance. Anyone with an upper respiratory tract infection who enters the patient's room must wear a mask. Observe strict asepsis when changing dressings or accessing a central venous catheter. Maintain strict aseptic technique in the care of these catheters at all times.

If possible, ensure that the patient is in a private room to reduce cross-contamination. Other precautions are used, such as not allowing standing water in vases, denture cups, or humidifiers in the patient's room, because they are breeding grounds for organisms.

Some facilities place the immunosuppressed patient in a room with a high-efficiency particulate air (HEPA) filtration or laminar airflow system. These systems decrease the number of airborne pathogens. It is not known whether they benefit patients.

Continually assess the patient for the presence of infection. This task is difficult because symptoms are not obvious in the patient with leukopenia. He or she may have a severe infection without pus and with only a low-grade fever.

Monitor the patient's daily complete blood count (CBC) with differential WBC count and absolute neutrophil count (ANC). Inspect the mouth during every shift for lesions and mucosa breakdown. Assess the lungs every 8 hours for crackles, wheezes, and reduced breath sounds that indicate impaired GAS EXCHANGE. Assess urine for odor and cloudiness. Ask about any urgency, burning, or pain on urination. Take vital signs at least every 4 hours to assess for fever.

⚠ NURSING SAFETY PRIORITY (QSEN)

Critical Rescue

A temperature elevation of even 1°F (or 0.5°C) above baseline is significant for a patient with leukopenia and indicates infection until it has been proven otherwise. Monitor patients with reduced IMMUNITY closely to recognize indications of infection. When any temperature elevation is present in a patient with leukemia, respond by reporting it to the primary health care provider immediately and implement standard infection protocols.

Many hospital units that specialize in the care of patients with neutropenia have specific protocols for antibiotic therapy if infection is suspected. Usually the hematology oncologist is notified immediately, and specific specimens are obtained for culture. Obtain blood for bacterial and fungal cultures from peripheral IV sites and the central venous catheter. Obtain urine specimens, sputum specimens, and specimens from open lesions for culture. Chest x-rays are taken. After the specimens are obtained, the patient begins IV antibiotics.

Skin care is important for preventing infection in the patient with leukemia and reduced IMMUNITY because the skin may be the only intact defense. Teach him or her about hygiene and urge daily bathing. If the patient is immobile, turn him or her every hour and apply skin lubricants.

Perform pulmonary hygiene every 2 to 4 hours. Listen to the lungs for crackles, wheezes, and reduced breath sounds. Urge the patient to cough and deep breathe or to use an incentive spirometer every hour while awake to promote GAS EXCHANGE.

Hematopoietic Stem Cell Transplantation. Hematopoietic stem cell transplantation (HSCT), sometimes called *bone marrow transplantation (BMT)*, is standard treatment for the patient with leukemia who has a closely matched donor and who is in temporary remission after induction therapy. It is used also for lymphoma, multiple myeloma, aplastic anemia, sickle cell disease, and many solid tumors.

The bone marrow is the actual site of production of leukemic cells. It can be difficult to ensure that all leukemic cells have been eradicated during induction therapy. Therefore before HSCT, additional chemotherapy with or without total body irradiation is given to purge (condition or clean) the marrow of leukemic cells. *These treatments are lethal to the bone marrow; and, without replacement of stem cells by transplantation, the patient would die of infection or hemorrhage.*

After conditioning, new healthy stem cells are given to the patient. The new cells go to the marrow and then begin the process of hematopoiesis, which results in normal, properly functioning blood cells and, ideally, a permanent cure.

Many hospitals have transplant units. With long-term survival increasing after HSCT, nurses can expect to be caring for these people—if not during the actual transplantation or recovery period, then after the recovery period—in a variety of health care settings.

HSCT started with the use of allogeneic bone marrow transplantation (transplantation of bone marrow from a sibling or matched unrelated donor) and has advanced to the use of human leukocyte antigen (HLA)–matched stem cells from the umbilical cords of unrelated donors. Transplants are classified by the source of stem cells (Table 40-3). Stem cells for transplantation may be obtained by bone marrow harvest, peripheral stem cell apheresis, or umbilical cord blood stem cell banking. Transplantation has five phases: stem cell obtainment, conditioning regimen, transplantation, engraftment, and post-transplantation recovery.

Obtaining the Stem Cells. Stem cells are taken from the patient directly (*autologous stem cells*), an HLA-identical twin (*syngeneic stem cells*), or an HLA-matched person (*allogeneic stem cells*). For allogeneic HSCT, best results occur when the donor is an HLA-identical sibling; however, transplant also can be successful between closely but not perfectly matched HLA types. The chance of matching with any given sibling is 25%. Donor registries keep records of potential donors who can provide stem cells for patients who do not have a family member HLA match. The chance of matching with an unrelated donor is 1 in 5000.

Patients often believe that a donor's blood type must be a match to theirs. Although the tissue type must be a close match for a successful stem cell transplant, the blood type is not related to tissue type, and its compatibility is not needed for donor criteria.

TABLE 40-3 Classification of Transplants

TYPE OF TRANSPLANT	SOURCES OF STEM CELLS
Autologous	
Self-donation	Bone marrow harvest Peripheral stem cell apheresis Umbilical cord blood
Syngeneic	
Patient's HLA identical twin or other identical sibling	Bone marrow harvest Peripheral stem cell apheresis
Allogeneic	
HLA-matched relative	Bone marrow harvest
Unrelated HLA-matched donor	Peripheral stem cell apheresis
Mismatched or partially HLA-matched family member or unrelated donor (donor registries)	Umbilical cord blood

HLA, Human leukocyte antigen.

💡 NCLEX EXAMINATION CHALLENGE 40-3

Health Promotion and Maintenance

A client diagnosed with acute leukemia tells the nurse that his brother cannot donate stem cells for a transplant because the brother has type O blood and he has type A blood. How will the nurse respond?

A. "Don't worry about it. You may not need a stem cell transplant."

B. "Because you are of Asian descent, finding an unrelated donor will be easy."

C. "Blood type and tissue type are not connected. If your brother's tissue type matches yours, you can receive his stem cells."

D. "Because type O blood is considered to be a universal donor and you have type A blood, you can receive your brother's stem cells."

Bone marrow harvesting occurs after a suitable donor is identified by tissue typing. The procedure occurs in the operating room, where marrow is removed through multiple aspirations from the iliac crests, although this technique is used less often today. About 500 to 1000 mL of marrow is aspirated, and the donor's marrow regrows within a few weeks. The marrow is then filtered and, if autologous, is treated to rid the marrow of any remaining cancer cells. Allogeneic marrow is transfused into the recipient immediately. Autologous marrow is frozen for later use.

Monitor the donor for fluid loss, assess for complications of anesthesia, and manage pain. During surgery, donors may lose a large amount of fluid in addition to the volume of marrow taken. Donors are hydrated with saline infusions before and immediately after surgery. Assess the harvest sites to ensure that the dressings are dry and intact and that bleeding is not excess.

Marrow donation is usually a same-day surgical procedure. Teach the donor to inspect the harvest sites for bleeding and take analgesics for pain. Pain at the harvest sites (hips) is common and is managed with oral non–aspirin-containing analgesics. Some donors may require opioid analgesics for pain control.

Peripheral blood stem cell (PBSC) harvesting requires three phases: mobilization, collection by apheresis, and reinfusion. PBSCs are stem cells that have been released from the bone marrow and circulate within the blood. Although there are fewer stem cells in peripheral blood than in bone marrow, their numbers can be increased artificially. During the mobilization phase, chemotherapy or hematopoietic growth factors are given to the patient for an autologous collection, depending on the cancer type; and hematopoietic growth factors alone are given to the donor for an allogeneic or syngeneic collection. These agents increase the numbers of stem cells and WBCs in the peripheral blood. An agent used for some other types of hematologic cancers to mobilize stem cells before harvesting in combination with hematopoietic growth factors is plerixafor (Mozobil). This drug decreases the number of apheresis collections needed.

After mobilization, stem cells are collected by apheresis (withdrawing whole blood, filtering out the cells, and returning the plasma to the patient). One to five apheresis procedures, each lasting 2 to 4 hours, are needed to obtain enough stem cells for transplantation. The cells are frozen and stored for reinfusion after the patient's conditioning regimen is completed.

Monitor the patient or donor closely during apheresis. Complications include catheter clotting and hypocalcemia (caused by anticoagulants). Low calcium levels may cause numbness or tingling in the fingers and toes, abdominal or muscle cramping, or chest pain. Oral calcium supplements may be used to manage these symptoms. Monitor vital signs at least every hour during apheresis. The patient may become hypotensive from fluid loss during the procedure.

Cord blood harvesting obtains stem cells from umbilical cord blood of newborns. This blood has a high concentration of stem cells. These cells are obtained through a simple blood draw from the placenta after birth and before the placenta detaches. The blood is sent to the Cord Blood Registry for processing and storage. The stem cells may be used later for an unrelated recipient or stored in case the infant develops a serious illness later in life and needs them.

Conditioning Regimen. Fig. 40-5 outlines the timing and steps involved in transplantation. The day the patient receives the stem cells is day T-0. Before transplantation, the conditioning

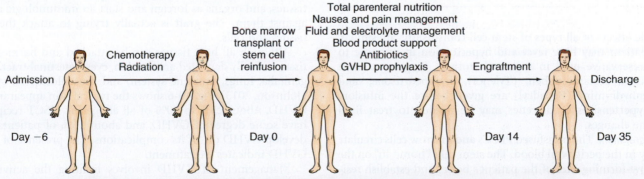

Total parenteral nutrition
Nausea and pain management
Fluid and electrolyte management
Blood product support
Antibiotics
GVHD prophylaxis

Chemotherapy
Radiation

Bone marrow
transplant or
stem cell
reinfusion

Engraftment

Admission

Day −6

Day 0

Day 14

Discharge

Day 35

FIG. 40-5 Timing and steps of allogeneic bone marrow transplantation. *GVHD*, Graft-versus-host disease.

days are counted in reverse order from T-0, just like a rocket countdown. After transplantation, days are counted in order from the day of transplantation.

The patient first undergoes a conditioning regimen, which varies with the diagnosis and type of transplant to be received. The conditioning regimen serves two purposes: (1) to "wipe out" the patient's own bone marrow, thus preparing him or her for optimal graft take; and (2) to give higher-than-normal doses of chemotherapy and/or radiotherapy to rid the person of cancer cells (*myeloablation*). Usually a period of 5 to 10 days is required. The regimen usually includes high-dose chemotherapy and, less commonly, total-body irradiation (TBI). Each conditioning regimen is tailored to the patient's specific disease, overall health, and previous treatment.

Because of the problems and risk for death associated with this conditioning regimen, a nonmyeloablative approach may be used instead. Nonmyeloablative regimens use lower doses of chemotherapy and/or a lower dose of TBI that allows for recovery of a recipient's own immune system. The use of nonmyeloablative conditioning regimens decreases the chemotherapy side effects but relies on the development of graft-versus-host disease (GVHD) for the control of the cancer. In contrast, myeloablative conditioning regimens use high doses of chemotherapy with or without radiation therapy to completely destroy a recipient's bone marrow, allowing for replacement by a new immune system.

During conditioning, bone marrow and normal tissues respond immediately to the chemotherapy and radiation. The patient has all of the expected side effects associated with both therapies (see Chapter 22). When chemotherapy is given in high doses, these side effects are more intense than those seen with standard doses.

Late effects from the conditioning regimen may occur as long as 3 to 10 years later. These effects include veno-occlusive disease (VOD), skin problems, cataracts, lung fibrosis, second cancers, cardiomyopathy, endocrine complications, and neurologic changes.

Transplantation. Day T-0 is the day of transplantation. The transplantation itself is very simple. Frozen marrow, PBSCs, or umbilical cord blood cells are thawed and infused through the patient's central catheter like an ordinary blood transfusion.

> ### ⚠ NURSING SAFETY PRIORITY **QSEN**
> #### Action Alert
>
> Do not use blood administration tubing to infuse stems cells because the cells could get caught in the filter, resulting in the patient receiving fewer stem cells. Usually standard, larger-bore, IV administration tubing is used.

Side effects of all types of stem cell transfusions are similar. The patient may have fever and hypertension in response to the preservative used in stem cell storage. To prevent these reactions, acetaminophen (Tylenol), hydrocortisone, and diphenhydramine (Benadryl) are given before the infusion. Antihypertensives or diuretics may be needed to treat fluid volume changes.

Engraftment. The transfused PBSCs and marrow cells circulate briefly in the peripheral blood. The stem cells "home-in" on the marrow-forming sites of the patient's bones and establish residency there.

Engraftment, the successful "take" of the transplanted cells in the patient's bone marrow, is key to the whole transplantation process. For the stem cells to "rescue" the patient after his or her own bone marrow has been "wiped out," the stem cells must survive and grow in the patient's bone marrow sites. The average time to engraftment ranges from 14 to 21 days. To aid engraftment, growth factors, such as granulocyte colony-stimulating factor or granulocyte-macrophage colony-stimulating factor, may be given. When engraftment occurs, the patient's WBC, RBC, and platelet counts begin to rise. Engraftment syndrome (ES) with fever and weight gain may occur at this time (Thoele, 2014).

Monitoring engraftment involves checking the patient's blood for *"chimerism,"* which is the presence of blood cells that show a genetic profile or marker different from those of the patient. Mixed chimerism is the presence of both the patient's cells and those from the donor. Progressive chimerism with increasing percentages of donor cells indicates engraftment. Regressive chimerism with increasing percentages of the patient's cells indicates graft failure. When engraftment is successful, only the donor's cells are present.

Prevention of Complications. The period after transplantation is difficult. Infection and poor CLOTTING with bleeding are severe problems because the patient remains without any IMMUNITY until the transfused cells grow and engraft. Care for this patient is the same as that for the patient during induction therapy for AML. Helping the patient maintain hope through this long recovery period is challenging. Complications are often severe and life threatening. Help the patient have a positive attitude and be involved in his or her own recovery. Encourage the patient to express his or her feelings and concerns while maintaining a supportive presence and trusting nurse-patient relationship.

In addition to the problems related to the period of **pancytopenia** (low levels of all circulating blood cells), other complications of HSCT include failure to engraft, development of graft-versus-host disease (GVHD), and veno-occlusive disease (VOD).

Failure to engraft occurs when the donated stem cells fail to grow and function in the bone marrow. This issue is discussed in advance with the patient and donor. Failure to engraft occurs more often with allogeneic HSCT than with autologous HSCT. The causes include too few cells transplanted, attack or rejection of donor cells by the recipient's remaining immune system cells, infection of transplanted cells, and unknown biologic factors. *If the transplanted cells fail to engraft, the patient will die unless another stem cell transplant is successful.*

GVHD occurs mostly in allogeneic transplants but also can occur in autologous transplants. The immunocompetent cells of the donated marrow recognize the patient's (recipient) cells, tissues, and organs as foreign and start an immunologic attack against them. The graft is actually trying to attack the host tissues and cells.

Although all host tissues can be attacked and harmed, the tissues usually damaged are the skin, eyes, intestinal tract, liver, genitalia, lungs, immune system, and musculoskeletal system (Johnson, 2013). Fig. 40-6 shows the typical skin appearance of GVHD. About 25% to 50% of all allogeneic HSCT recipients have some degree of GVHD, and about 15% of patients who develop GVHD die of its complications. The presence of some GVHD indicates engraftment.

Management of GVHD involves limiting the activity of donor T-cells by using drugs to suppress IMMUNITY such as

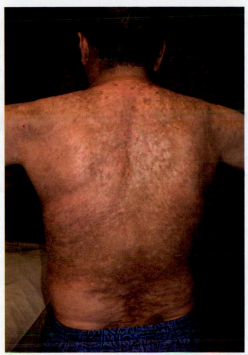

FIG. 40-6 Typical skin manifestations of graft-versus-host disease.

cyclosporine, tacrolimus, methotrexate, corticosteroids, mycophenolate mofetil (Cellcept, MMF), and antithymocyte globulin (ATG). Care is taken to avoid suppressing the new immune system to the extent that either infection risk increases or the new cells stop engrafting.

Veno-occlusive disease (VOD) is the blockage of liver blood vessels by CLOTTING and inflammation (phlebitis) and occurs in about one fifth of patients with HSCT. Problems usually begin within the first 30 days after transplantation. Patients who received high-dose chemotherapy with alkylating agents are at risk for life-threatening liver problems. Symptoms include jaundice, pain in the right upper quadrant, ascites, weight gain, and liver enlargement.

Because there is no way of opening the liver vessels, treatment is supportive. Early detection improves the chance for survival. Fluid management is also crucial. Assess the patient daily for weight gain, fluid retention, ascites, and hepatomegaly.

Minimizing Injury. Bone marrow production of platelets is severely limited with acute myelogenous leukemia (AML), leading to thrombocytopenia. The patient is at great risk for poor CLOTTING with excessive bleeding in response to minimal trauma. Thrombocytopenia can also be caused by induction therapy for AML or high-dose chemotherapy for transplantation.

Planning: Expected Outcomes. The patient with leukemia is expected to remain free from bleeding. Indicators include:

- Maintenance of hematocrit and hemoglobin within normal limits
- Absence of visible bleeding, petechiae, or ecchymosis
- Absence of evidence of occult bleeding (e.g., abdominal swelling, tarry stools)

Interventions. The platelet count is decreased as a side effect of chemotherapy. During the period of greatest bone marrow suppression (the **nadir**), the platelet count may be less than 10,000/mm³ (10×10^9/L). The patient is at extreme risk for bleeding once the platelet count falls below 50,000/mm³ (50 ×

10^9/L), and spontaneous bleeding may occur when the count is lower than 20,000/mm³ (20×10^9/L).

Bleeding Precautions are used to protect the patient at increased risk for injury from impaired CLOTTING (Chart 40-7). Assess at least every 4 hours for evidence of bleeding: oozing, enlarging bruises, petechiae, or purpura. Inspect all stools, urine, drainage, and vomit for blood and test for occult blood. Measure any blood loss as accurately as possible and measure the abdominal girth daily. Increases in abdominal girth can indicate internal hemorrhage. Institute the Bleeding Precautions listed in Chart 40-7. Platelet levels return to normal more slowly than do either WBCs or RBCs, and the patient remains at bleeding risk for weeks after discharge.

Monitor laboratory values daily, especially CBC results, to assess bleeding risk and actual blood loss. The patient with a platelet count below 10,000/mm³ (10×10^9/L) may need a platelet transfusion. For the patient with severe blood loss, packed RBCs may be prescribed (see the Red Blood Cell Transfusions section).

Conserving Energy. Production of RBCs is limited in leukemia, causing anemia and fatigue. In addition, leukemic cells have high rates of metabolism, increasing fatigue in the anemic patient. Anemia may also occur as a side effect of chemotherapy.

Planning: Expected Outcomes. The patient with leukemia is expected to have no increase in fatigue. Indicators include that the patient consistently demonstrates these behaviors:

- Participates in self-care
- Recognizes indicators of fatigue
- Changes activity level to match energy level

Interventions. Interventions to reduce fatigue focus on conserving energy and improving RBC counts.

Nutrition therapy is needed to help the patient eat enough calories to meet at least basal energy requirements. However, increasing food intake can be difficult with fatigue. Collaborate with a dietitian to provide small, frequent meals high in protein and carbohydrates.

Blood transfusions are sometimes indicated for the patient with fatigue. Transfusions with packed RBCs increase the blood's oxygen-carrying capacity and replace missing RBCs. (See Chart 40-12 for nursing care during transfusions.)

Drug therapy with colony-stimulating growth factors may reduce the severity and duration of anemia and neutropenia after intensive chemotherapy. For anemia, erythropoiesis-stimulating agents (ESAs) that boost production of RBCs may be used. These agents now carry a warning for causing hypertension and increasing the risk for myocardial infarction. ESAs must be given with care and should be avoided in patients with myeloid malignancies. They are not used unless the hemoglobin level is lower than 10 mg/dL (100 g/L) and are stopped when this level is reached. Assess for side effects such as hypertension, headaches, fever, myalgia (muscle aches), and rashes. (See Chapter 22 for information on hematopoietic growth factors.)

Activity management helps conserve the patient's energy (Chart 40-8). Examine the patient's schedule of prescribed and routine activities. Assess activities that do not have a direct positive effect on the patient's condition in terms of their usefulness. If the benefit of an activity is less than its worsening of fatigue, coordinate with other interprofessional team members about eliminating or postponing it. Activities that may be postponed include physical therapy and invasive diagnostic tests not needed for assessment or treatment of current problems.

Care Coordination and Transition Management

The patient with leukemia is discharged after induction chemotherapy and recovery of blood cell production. Follow-up care continues on an ambulatory care basis. Although many transplant centers discharge patients after engraftment, some centers give high-dose chemotherapy and stem cell infusion on an ambulatory care basis. This plan involves daily clinic visits and frequent follow-up by nurses in the home care setting.

Home Care Management. Planning for home care for the patient with leukemia begins as soon as remission is achieved. Assess the available support systems. Many patients need a visiting nurse to assist with dressing changes for central venous catheters, infusions, and to answer questions. Home transfusion therapy for blood components may be needed.

Coordination of the home care team is critical for the patient receiving stem cell transplantation in the home setting. Potential candidates are evaluated in advance. Criteria include a knowledgeable caregiver, a clean home environment, location near the hospital, telephone access, and emotional stability of the patient and caregiver.

Home care nurses give chemotherapy and monitor for complications. Nurses visit the patient once or twice per day and spend between 4 and 8 hours per day in the home. The patient receives the stem cell transplant infusion in the ambulatory care clinic. Nursing care is similar to that provided in the hospital. If complications such as sepsis or veno-occlusive disease (VOD) occur, the patient is admitted to the inpatient facility.

Self-Management Education. Instruct the patient and family about the importance of continuing therapy and medical follow-up. Many patients go home with a central venous catheter in place and need instructions about its care. Chart 40-9 lists guidelines for central venous catheter care at home. These guidelines may be altered, depending on the home setting, assistance available, and agency policy.

Protecting the patient from infection at home is just as important as it was during hospitalization. (See Chart 40-6 for focused assessment for the patient at risk for infection.) Teach

---

⊚ CHART 40-8 Best Practice for Patient Safety & Quality Care

Conserving Energy

- Reassure the patient that fatigue is temporary and energy levels will improve over a period of weeks to months. Stress that a return to previous energy levels may take as long as a year.
- Teach the patient that shortness of breath and palpitations are symptoms of over-activity.
- Instruct the patient to stop activity when shortness of breath or palpitations are present.
- Space care activities at least an hour apart and avoid the time right before or right after meals.
- Schedule care activities at times when the patient has more energy (e.g., immediately after naps).
- Perform complete bed bath only every other day. Between complete baths, ensure cleansing of face, hands, axillae, and perineum.
- In collaboration with other members of the health care team, cancel or reschedule nonessential tests and activities.
- Provide four to six small, easy-to-eat meals instead of three larger ones.
- Urge the patient to drink small amounts of protein shakes or other nutritional supplements.
- During periods of extreme fatigue, encourage the patient to allow others to perform personal care.
- Help the patient identify one or two lead visitors (those designated as allowed to visit at any time and who do not disturb the patient).
- Selectively limit nonlead visitors when the patient is resting or sleeping.
- Remind families that, although independence is important, independence in ADLs during extreme fatigue can be detrimental to the patient's health.
- Monitor oxygen saturation and respiratory rate during any activity to determine patient responses and activity tolerance.

👤 CHART 40-9 Patient and Family Education: Preparing for Self-Management

Home Care of the Central Venous Catheter

- To maintain patency, flush the catheter briskly with saline once a day and after completing infusions.
- Change the Luer-Lok cap on each catheter lumen weekly.
- Change the dressing as often as prescribed:
  - Use clean technique with thorough handwashing.
  - Clean the exit site with alcohol and povidone-iodine (Betadine) or with chlorhexidine.
  - Apply antibacterial ointment to the site, if prescribed.
  - Cover the site with dry sterile gauze dressing, taped securely, or with transparent adherent dressing.
- To prevent tension, always tape the catheter to yourself.
- Look for and report any signs of infection (redness, swelling, or drainage at the exit site).
- In case of a break or puncture in the catheter lumen, immediately clamp the catheter between yourself and the opening. *Notify your primary health care provider immediately.*

CHART 40-10 Patient and Family Education: Preparing for Self-Management

Prevention of Infection

- Avoid crowds and other gatherings of people who might be ill.
- Do not share personal toilet articles, such as toothbrushes, toothpaste, washcloths, or deodorant sticks, with others.
- If possible, bathe daily.
- Wash the armpits, groin, genitals, and anal area at least twice a day with an antimicrobial soap.
- Clean your toothbrush daily by either running it through the dishwasher or rinsing it in liquid laundry bleach and then rinsing it with running water.
- Wash your hands thoroughly with an antimicrobial soap before you eat or drink, after touching a pet, after shaking hands with anyone, as soon as you come home from any outing, and after using the toilet.
- Eat a low-bacteria diet and avoid salads, raw fruits and vegetables, and undercooked meat.
- Wash dishes between uses with hot, sudsy water or use a dishwasher.
- Do not drink water that has been standing for longer than 15 minutes.
- Do not reuse cups and glasses without washing.
- Avoid changing pet litter boxes. If unavoidable, use gloves or wash hands immediately.
- Avoid keeping turtles and reptiles as pets.
- Do not feed pets raw or undercooked meat.
- Take your temperature at least twice a day.
- Report any of these indications of infection to your primary health care provider immediately:
  - Temperature greater than 100°F (38°C)
  - Persistent cough (with or without sputum)
  - Pus or foul-smelling drainage from any open skin area or normal body opening
  - Presence of a boil or abscess
  - Urine that is cloudy, foul smelling, or burning on urination
- Take all drugs as prescribed.
- Do not dig in the garden or work with houseplants.
- Avoid travel to areas of the world with poor sanitation or inadequate health care facilities.

CHART 40-11 Patient and Family Education: Preparing for Self-Management

The Patient at Risk for Bleeding

- Use an electric shaver.
- Use a soft-bristled toothbrush and do not floss.
- Do not have dental work done without consulting your primary health care provider.
- Do not take aspirin or any aspirin-containing products. Read the label to be sure that the products do not contain aspirin or salicylates.
- Wear shoes or slippers with a sole to avoid foot injury.
- Do not participate in contact sports or any activity likely to result in your being bumped, scratched, or scraped.
- If you are bumped, apply ice to the site for at least 1 hour.
- Notify your primary health care provider if you:
  - Experience an injury and persistent bleeding results
  - Have excessive menstrual bleeding
  - See blood in your urine or bowel movement
  - Have a headache that does not respond to acetaminophen
- Avoid anal intercourse.
- Take a stool softener to prevent straining during a bowel movement.
- Do not use enemas or rectal suppositories.
- Avoid bending over at the waist.
- Do not wear clothing or shoes that are tight or that rub.
- Avoid blowing your nose or placing objects in your nose. If you must blow your nose, do so gently without blocking either nasal passage.

about proper hygiene and the need to avoid crowds or others with infections. Neither the patient nor any household member should receive live virus immunization (poliomyelitis, measles, or rubella) for 2 years after transplantation. In general, the patient receives no vaccinations for the first year after transplantation because his or her immune function has not returned sufficiently to generate antibodies in response to vaccination. Instruct the patient to continue mouth care regimens at home. Stress to the patient that he or she should immediately notify the primary health care provider if a fever or any other indications of infection develop. Chart 40-10 lists guidelines for infection prevention among patients with reduced IMMUNITY.

Many patients return home still at risk for bleeding because platelet recovery is slower than recovery of other cells and CLOTTING remains slow. Reinforce safety and bleeding precautions and emphasize that these precautions must be followed until the platelet count remains above 50,000/mm^3 (50 × 10^9/L). Teach the patient and family to assess for petechiae, avoid trauma and sharp objects, apply pressure to wounds for 10 minutes, and report blood in the stool or urine or headache that does not respond to acetaminophen. Chart 40-11 lists guidelines for patients with reduced CLOTTING.

Psychosocial Preparation. A diagnosis of leukemia may threaten the patient's sense of self and his or her role within the family. The patient faces the possibility of death, and treatment may cause major changes in self-image. Changes occur in body image, level of independence, and lifestyle. Some feel threatened by the environment, seeing everything as infectious. Patients who are cared for in protective isolation may feel lonely and isolated. Help the patient and family define priorities, understand the illness and its treatment, and find hope. Make referrals and encourage patients and their families to attend support groups sponsored by organizations such as the American Cancer Society or the Leukemia and Lymphoma Society of America.

One problem that lasts for a long period of time after transplantation is severe fatigue. Although the acute period after transplantation requires energy conservation with reduced activity, in the later recovery period, exercise provides benefits and fatigue reduction (Albrecht, 2014). Help the patient and family understand the benefits of low-impact exercise and encourage them to organize their day with exercise included.

Health Care Resources. The patient with limited social support may need help at home until strength and energy return. A home care aide may suffice for some patients, whereas for others a visiting nurse may be needed. The patient may also need equipment for ADLs and ambulation. Assess financial resources. Cancer treatment is expensive, and coordination with the social services department is needed to ensure that insurance is adequate. If the patient is uninsured, other sources, such as drug company–sponsored compassionate aid programs and local cancer center foundations, are explored. The Leukemia and Lymphoma Society of America also offers limited financial help.

Prolonged outpatient contact and follow-up are necessary, and patients need transportation to the outpatient facility. Many local units of the American Cancer Society and the Canadian Cancer Society offer free transportation to patients with cancer or leukemia.

◆ *Evaluation: Reflecting*

Evaluate the care of the patient with leukemia based on the identified priority patient problems. The expected outcomes include that the patient will:

- Remain free of infection and sepsis
- Not experience episodes of bleeding
- Be able to balance activity and rest
- Use energy conservation techniques

? NCLEX EXAMINATION CHALLENGE 40-4

Health Promotion and Maintenance

The family of a client who had a successful stem cell transplant for leukemia 3 months ago asks the nurse whether they should obtain influenza vaccinations now. How will the nurse respond?

A. "No. You need to wait at least 2 years before receiving any vaccination."

B. "Yes. Obtain the vaccination now to protect your family member from influenza."

C. "If you have no small children in the household, influenza vaccinations are not needed for anyone."

D. "Yes. If you and the client are older than 50, you should all receive influenza vaccinations immediately."

MALIGNANT LYMPHOMAS

Lymphomas are cancers of the lymphoid tissues with abnormal overgrowth of lymphocytes. They are cancers of committed lymphocytes rather than stem cell precursors (as in leukemia). This growth occurs as solid tumors in lymphoid tissues scattered throughout the body, especially the lymph nodes and spleen, rather than in the bone marrow. The two major adult forms of lymphoma are Hodgkin's lymphoma (HL) and non-Hodgkin's lymphoma (NHL).

❖ PATHOPHYSIOLOGY

Hodgkin's lymphoma (HL) is a cancer that can affect any age-group. However, it appears to peak in two different age-groups: (1) teens and young adults, and (2) adults in their 50s and 60s (McCance et al., 2014). HL affects younger men and women equally, but the disease is more prevalent in men in the older group. About 8500 cases are diagnosed in the United States each year, and another 1000 are diagnosed in Canada (ACS, 2017; CCS, 2016).

The exact cause of HL is uncertain. Possible causes include viral infections (i.e., Epstein-Barr virus [EBV], human T-cell leukemia/lymphoma virus [HTLV], human immune deficiency virus [HIV]), and exposure to chemicals. However, most cases of the disease occur in people without known risk factors.

This cancer usually starts in a single lymph node or a single chain of nodes. These nodes contain a specific cancer cell type, the Reed-Sternberg cell, a marker for HL. HL often spreads predictably from one group of lymph nodes to the next, unlike non-Hodgkin's lymphoma.

Non-Hodgkin's lymphoma (NHL) includes all lymphoid cancers that do not have the Reed-Sternberg cell. There are over 60 subtypes of NHL divided into either indolent or aggressive lymphomas. NHL generally spreads through the lymphatic system in a less orderly fashion than HL. About 72,500 new cases are diagnosed each year in the United States (ACS, 2017),

and 8200 are diagnosed in Canada (CCS, 2016). The disease is more common in men and older adults.

The exact cause of NHL is unknown, although the incidence is higher among patients with solid organ transplantation, immunosuppressive drug therapy, and HIV disease. Chronic infection from *Helicobacter pylori* is associated with a type of NHL called *mucosa-associated lymphoid tissue (MALT) lymphoma,* and Epstein-Barr viral infection has been associated with Burkitt's lymphoma. There is an increased incidence of NHL among people exposed to pesticides, insecticides, and dust.

NHL is not a single disease but, rather, a group of diseases. The specific subtype of lymphoma must be classified because management varies with the subtype. Classification is based on histology, immunophenotyping by flow cytometry, and genetic (chromosomal changes and molecular rearrangements) and clinical features. NHLs are broadly classified as B-cell or T-cell lymphomas, depending on the lymphocyte type that gave rise to the cancer. B-cell lymphomas are most common.

Patients with indolent (slow-growing) lymphomas usually have painless lymph node swelling at diagnosis. Those with more aggressive B-cell lymphomas may have large masses at diagnosis and symptoms. Constitutional symptoms, as seen in Hodgkin's lymphoma, occur in about one third of patients with aggressive lymphomas and rarely in indolent lymphomas. Bone marrow involvement in indolent lymphomas is common.

❖ INTERPROFESSIONAL COLLABORATIVE CARE
◆ Assessment: Noticing

The most common assessment finding for any lymphoma is a large but painless lymph node or nodes. The patient may also have constitutional symptoms ("B symptoms") that include fevers (>101.5°F [>38.6°C]), drenching night sweats, and unplanned weight loss (>10% of normal body weight). The presence of these symptoms often means a poorer prognosis. Many patients have no symptoms at time of diagnosis, and specific symptoms often depend on the site and extent of disease.

Diagnosis and subtype of HL are established when biopsy reveals Reed-Sternberg cells (McCance et al., 2014). HL is then classified into one of several different subtypes. The diagnosis of NHL is made only after the biopsy of an involved lymph node is reviewed by a hematopathologist.

After diagnosis of HL, staging is performed to determine the extent of disease. This process is detailed and must be accurate because the treatment regimen is determined by the extent of disease. Staging usually includes a history and physical examination; CBC; electrolyte panel; kidney and liver function tests; erythrocyte sedimentation rate (ESR); bone marrow aspiration and biopsy; and CT of the neck, chest, abdomen, and pelvis. Positron emission tomography (PET) is used to stage the disease and monitor response to therapy. After staging procedures are complete, the stage of the disease is determined by the Lugano Modification of the Ann Arbor Staging System for primary nodal lymphoma (Table 40-4).

Classification of NHL is complicated and is based on the World Health Organization (WHO) classification system. In addition, lactate dehydrogenase (LDH) levels and beta$_2$-microglobulin levels are also evaluated to measure tumor growth rates and calculate prognosis. (High LDH levels and high beta$_2$-microglobulin levels are associated with a poorer prognosis.) Cerebrospinal fluid is evaluated when lymphoma is

TABLE 40-4 Lugano Modification of Ann Arbor Staging System* (for Primary Nodal Lymphomas)

STAGE	INVOLVEMENT	EXTRANODAL STATUS
Limited		
Stage I	One node or group of adjacent nodes	Single extranodal lesions without nodal involvement
Stage II	Two or more nodal groups on the same side of the diaphragm	Stage I or II by nodal extent with limited, contiguous extranodal involvement
Bulky stage II†	Stage II as with "bulky" disease >7.5 cm	N/A
Advanced		
Stage III	Nodes on both sides of the diaphragm Nodes above the diaphragm with spleen involvement	N/A
Stage IV	Additional noncontiguous extranodal involvement	N/A

N/A, Not applicable.
*Extent of disease is determined by PET-CT for avid lymphomas and CT for non-avid histologies.
NOTE: Tonsils, Waldeyer's ring, and spleen are considered nodal tissue.
†Whether II bulky is treated as limited or advanced disease may be determined by histology and a number of prognostic factors.
Categorization of A versus B has been removed from the Lugano Modification of Ann Arbor Staging and is only used for Hodgkin's lymphoma.

present in the CNS, around the spinal cord, brain, or testes and when HIV-related lymphoma is diagnosed.

◆ Interventions: Responding

HL is one of the most treatable types of cancer. For stages I and II disease, the treatment is external radiation of involved lymph node regions. With more extensive disease, radiation and combination chemotherapy are used to achieve remission. (See Chapter 22 on general care of patients receiving radiation and chemotherapy.) An important issue is that, when the disease is in the inguinal area, radiation therapy usually results in permanently reduced fertility and, most often, sterility in men. Sperm banking before therapy begins is an option to assist in future reproductive plans.

Treatment options for patients with NHL vary based on the subtype of the tumor, international prognostic index (IPI) score, stage of the disease, performance status, and overall tumor burden. Special consideration for patients with additional health problems is important, especially among older-adult patients. Many new therapies have evolved over the past decade for various subtypes of NHL. These therapies include combinations of chemotherapy drugs alone or in combination with other therapies, depending on the stage of the disease. Therapies include monoclonal antibodies (e.g., rituximab and alemtuzumab); localized radiation therapy; radiolabeled antibodies (^{131}I tositumomab and ^{90}Y ibritumomab tiuxetan); targeted or novel therapies of lenalidomide (Revlimid), ibrutinib (Imbruvica), and bortezomib (Velcade); hematopoietic stem cell transplantation; and investigational agents.

Nursing management of the patient undergoing treatment for HL or NHL focuses on the acute side effects of therapy, especially:
- Drug-induced pancytopenia with increased risk for infection, anemia, and bleeding from impaired IMMUNITY and CLOTTING
- Severe nausea and vomiting
- Skin problems at the site of radiation
- Constipation or diarrhea
- Permanent sterility for male patients receiving radiation to the lower abdomen or pelvic region in combination with specific chemotherapy drugs (The patient is informed and given the option to store sperm in a sperm bank *before* treatment.)
- Secondary cancer development from drug-induced impaired CELLULAR REGULATION and the need for long-term follow-up

With the use of biotherapy for NHL, close monitoring for infusion-related reactions is needed during and after the delivery of monoclonal antibodies. (See Chapter 22 for general care of patients undergoing treatment with biotherapy).

? CLINICAL JUDGMENT CHALLENGE 40-2

Patient-Centered Care; Evidence-Based Practice QSEN

The patient is a 20-year-old male full-time college student who comes to the student health clinic with an enlarged lymph node in his left axillary, drenching night sweats, and fevers (>101.5° F [>38.6° C]. A lymph node biopsy reveals Hodgkin's lymphoma. He is then referred to an oncologist who completes staging and determines the disease to be stage IIIb with some involvement in his inguinal nodes. He is scheduled to start on combination chemotherapy drugs and radiation therapy. The patient tells you that he is worried because he is adopted and has no biologic siblings who could donate stem cells for a lifesaving transplant. He is very afraid that he will die from the disease. He also asks whether he will lose his hair.
1. Is his fear of death justified? Why or why not?
2. What will you tell him about stem cell transplantation?
3. Is there anything specific he should do to prepare himself for the prescribed therapy?
4. What will you tell him about possible hair loss? (You may need to refer to Chapter 22 for more guidance on this issue.)

MULTIPLE MYELOMA

❖ PATHOPHYSIOLOGY

Multiple myeloma is a white blood cell (WBC) cancer that involves a mature B-lymphocyte called a *plasma cell,* which secretes antibodies. These cells are overgrown in the bone marrow. When they become cancerous, they produce excessive antibodies (gamma globulins). Thus the disorder is called a *gammopathy.* When myeloma cells are overproduced, fewer red blood cells (RBCs), WBCs, and platelets are produced, leading to anemia and increased risk for infection and bleeding.

In addition to the excess antibodies, multiple myeloma cells also produce excess cytokines (see Chapter 17) that increase cancer cell growth and destroy bone. The excess antibodies are in the blood, increasing the serum protein levels and clogging blood vessels in the kidney and other organs. Without treatment, the disease causes progressive bone destruction, bleeding problems, kidney failure, reduced IMMUNITY, and death.

Multiple myeloma accounts for about 11,000 deaths per year in the United States and 1400 in Canada (ACS, 2017; CCS, 2016). The disease is most common in people older than 65 years. The incidence is higher in American blacks than in whites, with a much higher incidence in men.

The cause of multiple myeloma is unknown. Possible risk factors include radiation exposure, chemical exposure, and infection with human herpes virus-8 (HHV-8). This cancer can be distinguished by changes in immunoglobulin structure that begin within a single clone of cells even before transformation to cancer occurs. When the specifically altered immunoglobulin is present in a high enough quantity, the type can be recognized as a unique "spike" pattern on a serum electrophoresis test of plasma proteins. Because one clone of cells develops into cancer cells, the abnormal immunoglobulin produced by these cells is a *monoclonal* paraprotein.

❖ INTERPROFESSIONAL COLLABORATIVE CARE

◆ Assessment: Noticing

Some patients have no symptoms at time of the diagnosis. An elevation of serum total protein or a detection of a monoclonal protein (also known as *paraprotein*) in the blood or urine may be the only finding. Other common symptoms include fatigue, anemia, bone pain, pathologic fractures, recurrent bacterial infections, and kidney dysfunction.

A positive finding of a serum monoclonal protein is not sufficient to make a diagnosis of multiple myeloma. About 1% of the population produces a monoclonal protein in the blood but does not have multiple myeloma. This condition is labeled **m**onoclonal **g**ammopathy of **u**ndetermined **s**ignificance or MGUS, which is a premalignant condition. Follow-up of patients with MGUS is important because a small percentage eventually will develop multiple myeloma. Multiple myeloma is distinguished from MGUS by having more than 10% of the bone marrow infiltrated with plasma cells, the presence of a monoclonal protein in the serum or urine, and the presence of osteolytic bone lesions.

The staging system for multiple myeloma divides patients into stages and prognostic groups on the basis of the serum beta₂-microglobulin and albumin levels. Other factors that help determine prognosis include age, performance status, serum creatinine, serum albumin, serum calcium, lactate dehydrogenase (LDH) level, C-reactive protein, hemoglobin level, platelet count, quantitative immunoglobulins, beta₂-microglobulin, serum-free light chains, serum protein electrophoresis (SPEP) with immunofixation, 24-hour urine for SPEP, and cytogenetic abnormalities found in the bone marrow biopsy (Kurtin & Faiman, 2013).

The patient usually first notices fatigue, easy bruising, and bone pain. Bone fractures, hypertension, infection, hypercalcemia, and fluid imbalance may occur as the disease progresses. Diagnosis is made by x-ray findings of bone thinning with areas of bone loss that resemble Swiss cheese, high immunoglobulin and plasma protein levels, and the presence of Bence-Jones protein (protein composed of incomplete antibodies) in the urine. A bone marrow biopsy is performed to diagnose the disease and determine chromosome changes. An abnormality of chromosome 11 predicts a longer survival, and absence of chromosome 13 is a poor prognostic factor.

◆ Interventions: Responding

Treatment options vary. For minimal disease, watchful waiting may be an option instead of chemotherapy. Standard treatment for multiple myeloma is the use of proteasome inhibitors, such as bortezomib (Velcade) or carfilzomib (Kyprolis), and immunomodulating drugs such as thalidomide (Thalomid) or lenalidomide (Revlimid). All these agents, which are types of targeted cancer therapy (see Chapter 22), may be used alone or in combination with steroids such as dexamethasone (Decadron). Drug selection is based on whether the patient is eligible for an autologous stem cell transplant. If eligible, drug therapy is used to reduce tumor burden before transplantation. For patients who are not eligible for autologous stem cell transplantation, standard chemotherapy drugs such as melphalan, prednisone, vincristine, cyclophosphamide, doxorubicin, and carmustine are usually effective in controlling but not curing the disease.

Side effects and severe toxicities can occur with these agents. Myelosuppression is an expected side effect of many myeloma therapies. A nursing priority is to teach the patient about the symptoms. The risk for thromboembolic events is increased with the use of thalidomide and lenalidomide. Peripheral neuropathy can be challenging, causing pain and poor quality of life. GI side effects, such as nausea, vomiting, diarrhea, and constipation, are severe and can be life threatening if not managed properly.

Despite therapy, multiple myeloma remains largely incurable (Kurtin & Faiman, 2013). Best outcomes are seen with autologous hematopoietic stem cell transplantation, although few patients can pursue this option (Mangan et al., 2013). Because most patients with multiple myeloma have bone pain, analgesics and alternative approaches for pain management, such as relaxation techniques, aromatherapy, or hypnosis, are used. The bone disease of multiple myeloma is treated with bisphosphonates (pamidronate [Aredia], zoledronic acid [Zometa], denosumab [Xgeva]), which inhibit bone resorption and can help reduce the skeletal complications.

AUTOIMMUNE THROMBOCYTOPENIC PURPURA

Pathophysiology

Autoimmune thrombocytopenic purpura is also called *idiopathic thrombocytopenic purpura (ITP)*. The number of circulating platelets is greatly reduced in ITP, even though platelet production is normal.

Patients with this disorder make an antibody against the surface of their own platelets (an antiplatelet antibody). This antibody coats the platelet surfaces, making destruction by macrophages easier (see Chapter 17). The spleen has many macrophages, and the blood vessels of the spleen are long and twisted. These conditions increase destruction of antibody-coated platelets in the spleen. When platelet destruction exceeds platelet production, the number of circulating platelets decreases, and CLOTTING is impaired.

The trigger for the production of autoantibodies is unknown, but viral infection is suspected. ITP is most common among women between the ages of 20 and 50 years and among people who have other autoimmune disorders (McCance et al., 2014).

❖ INTERPROFESSIONAL COLLABORATIVE CARE

◆ Assessment: Noticing

Symptoms of ITP are at first seen in the skin and mucous membranes: large ecchymoses (bruises) or a petechial rash on the arms, legs, upper chest, and neck; mucosal bleeding occurs easily. If the patient has had significant blood loss, anemia may also be present.

A rare complication is intracranial bleeding–induced stroke. Assess for neurologic function and mental status (see Chapter 41).

ITP is diagnosed by a low platelet count and increased megakaryocytes in the bone marrow. Antiplatelet antibodies may be detected in the blood. If the patient has any episodes of bleeding, hematocrit and hemoglobin levels may be low.

◆ **Interventions: Responding**

As a result of the decreased platelet count, the patient is at great risk for poor CLOTTING and increased bleeding. Interventions include therapy for the underlying condition and protection from bleeding episodes. Management is often limited to patients with platelet counts lower than 50,000/mm³ (50×10^9/L), those who are bleeding, and those at high risk for bleeding.

Drug therapy to control ITP includes drugs that suppress immune function. Drugs such as corticosteroids, azathioprine (Imuran), eltrombopag, rituximab (Rituxan), and romiplostim are used to inhibit production of antiplatelet autoantibodies. IV immunoglobulin and IV anti-Rho can help prevent the destruction of antibody-coated platelets, although anti-Rho carries a black box warning for increased risk for intravascular hemolysis and death. Aggressive therapy involves low doses of chemotherapy drugs.

Platelet transfusions are used when platelet counts are less than 10,000/mm³ (10×10^9/L) or the patient has an acute life-threatening bleeding episode. Transfusions are not performed routinely because the donated platelets are destroyed by the spleen just as rapidly as the patient's own platelets. (See the discussion in the Platelet Transfusions section.)

Maintaining a safe environment helps protect the patient from bleeding. Closely monitor the amount of bleeding that is occurring. (For nursing care actions, see the discussion of Minimizing Injury in the Leukemia section.)

Surgical management with a splenectomy may be needed for the patient who does not respond to drug therapy (Greenberg, 2017). (The spleen is the site of excessive platelet destruction.)

Depending on the size of the spleen and the risk for bleeding, splenectomy may be performed as an open abdominal surgery or as minimally invasive surgery by laparoscopy. Nursing care after surgery is the same as for any other abdominal surgery (see Chapter 16). After splenectomy, the patient is at increased risk for infection because the spleen performs many protective immune functions, especially antibody generation. For this reason, vaccinations against pneumococcal and meningococcal disorders and *Haemophilus influenzae* are recommended either 2 weeks before a planned splenectomy or 2 weeks after the surgery. Teaching patients about their increased risk for infection, avoiding crowds and people who are ill, and consulting with the primary health care provider is a nursing priority.

THROMBOTIC THROMBOCYTOPENIC PURPURA

In thrombotic thrombocytopenic purpura (TTP), platelets clump together abnormally in the capillaries, and too few platelets remain in circulation. The patient has inappropriate CLOTTING, yet the blood fails to clot when trauma occurs. The cause of TTP appears to be an autoimmune reaction in small blood vessel cells (endothelial cells) that starts platelet aggregation and clotting there. Tissues become ischemic, leading to kidney failure, myocardial infarction, and stroke. Untreated, this disorder is often fatal within 3 months.

Management of the patient with TTP focuses on preventing platelet clumping and stopping the autoimmune process.

Plasma removal and the infusion of fresh frozen plasma reduce the clumping caused by elements in the patient's blood. Drugs that inhibit platelet clumping, such as aspirin, alprostadil (Prostin), and plicamycin, also may be helpful. Immunosuppressive therapy reduces the intensity of this disorder.

HEMOPHILIA

❖ PATHOPHYSIOLOGY

Hemophilia is a hereditary bleeding disorder with two forms resulting from different CLOTTING factor deficiencies. Hemophilia A (classic hemophilia) is a deficiency of factor VIII and accounts for 80% of cases of hemophilia. Hemophilia B (Christmas disease) is a deficiency of factor IX and accounts for 20% of cases. The incidence of both disorders is 1 in 10,000 (McCance et al., 2014; National Hemophilia Foundation, 2017).

GENETIC/GENOMIC CONSIDERATIONS

Patient-Centered Care QSEN

Hemophilia is an X-linked recessive trait. Women who are **carriers** (can pass on the gene without expressing bleeding problems) have a 50% chance of passing the hemophilia gene to their daughters (who then are carriers) and to their sons (who then have hemophilia). Hemophilia A affects mostly males, none of whose sons will have the gene for hemophilia and all of whose daughters will be carriers. About 30% of patients with hemophilia have no family history, and their disease may be the result of a new gene mutation (OMIM, 2016b). Ensure that the family is referred to the appropriate level of genetic counseling.

The clinical pictures of hemophilias A and B are identical. The patient has abnormal bleeding in response to any trauma because of a deficiency of the specific CLOTTING factor. Hemophiliacs form platelet plugs at the bleeding site, but the clotting factor deficiency impairs the formation of stable fibrin clots. This allows excessive bleeding, which may be mild, moderate, or severe, depending on the degree of factor deficiency.

❖ INTERPROFESSIONAL COLLABORATIVE CARE

Assessment of the patient with hemophilia shows:

- Excessive bleeding from minor cuts, bruises, or abrasions (from abnormal platelet function)
- Joint and muscle hemorrhages that lead to disabling long-term problems and may require joint replacement
- A tendency to bruise easily
- Prolonged and potentially fatal hemorrhage after surgery

The laboratory test results for a patient with hemophilia show a prolonged activated partial thromboplastin time (aPTT), a normal bleeding time, and a normal prothrombin time (PT). The most common problem that occurs with hemophilia is degenerating joint function as a result of chronic bleeding into the joints, especially the hips and knees.

The bleeding problems of hemophilia A are managed by either regularly scheduled infusions of synthetic factor VIII or the infusion of this substance only when injury or bleeding occurs. The cost of factor VIII replacement is prohibitive for many people with hemophilia. The source of factor VIII varies (Table 40-5); and the traditional sources, derived from pooled human serum, are no longer recommended because of the risk for transfusion-related infections (National Hemophilia Foundation, 2017).

HEPARIN-INDUCED THROMBOCYTOPENIA

Heparin-induced thrombocytopenia (HIT) is a serious IMMUNITY-mediated CLOTTING disorder with an unexplained drop in platelet count after heparin treatment. The occurrence is increasing because of the increased use of heparin. Unlike other clotting disorders, HIT is an immune-mediated drug reaction that is caused by heparin-dependent platelet-activating immunoglobulin G (IgG) antibodies in which heparin binds with platelet factor 4 (PF4). This drug binding leads to the development of a highly reactive immune complex that activates the platelets. Once activated, platelets release procoagulants and PF4, which neutralizes heparin and increases thrombin generation from prothrombin.

HIT can occur in patients receiving any type of heparin, although it is more common after exposure to unfractionated heparin. The incidence is higher among patients with risk factors of (1) duration of heparin use longer than 1 week, (2) exposure to unfractionated heparin, (3) postsurgical thrombo-prophylaxis, and (4) being female.

Symptoms of HIT include venous thromboembolism (VTE) such as deep vein thrombosis and pulmonary embolism. The diagnosis is based on the patient's exposure to heparin, which can be up to 100 days before the event. Thrombocytopenia after heparin exposure is the hallmark sign of HIT. Clinical and laboratory findings are needed to diagnose this disorder.

Once HIT is diagnosed, anticoagulation therapy is started. Drug management for HIT management is with a direct thrombin inhibitor such as argatroban (Acova) and lepirudin (Refludan) (Greenberg, 2017).

TRANSFUSION THERAPY

Any blood component may be removed from a donor and transfused into a recipient. Blood components may be transfused individually or collectively, with varying degrees of benefit to the recipient. Table 40-6 lists indications for transfusion therapy.

Pretransfusion Responsibilities

Nursing actions during transfusions focus on prevention or early recognition of adverse transfusion reactions. Preparation of the patient for transfusion is critical, and blood product administration procedures must be followed carefully. Before infusing any blood product, review agency policies and procedures. Chart 40-12 lists best practices for transfusion therapy.

A primary health care provider's prescription is needed to administer blood components. The prescription specifies the type of component, the volume, and any special conditions. In many hospitals, a separate consent form is obtained from the patient before a transfusion is performed.

A blood specimen is obtained for type and crossmatch (testing of the donor's blood and the recipient's blood for compatibility). The procedures for obtaining this specimen are specified by hospital policy. Usually a new type- and crossmatch-specimen is required every 72 hours.

Both Y-tubing and straight tubing sets are used for blood component infusion (Fig. 40-7). A blood filter (about 170 microns) to remove sediment from the stored blood products is included with blood administration sets and must be used to transfuse most, but not all, blood products.

TABLE 40-5 Antihemophilic Drugs

DRUG TYPES	SOURCES
High purity antihemophilic factor • Alphanate • Humate-P • Koate-DIV	Pooled human serum
Monoclonal antibody purified antihemophilic factor • Hemofil-M • Monarc-M • Monoclate-P	Pooled human serum
Recombinant antihemophilic factor • Helixate FS • Kogenate FS • Recombinate	Recombinant DNA technology
B-domain deleted (BDD) recombinant antihemophilic factor • ReFacto	Recombinant DNA technology
Recombinant antihemophilic factor plasma/protein-free method (rAHF-PFM) • Advate	Recombinant DNA technology
Recombinant antihemophilic factor plasma/albumin-free method • Xyntha	Recombinant DNA technology
Porcine factor VIII • Hyate: C	Animal serum

TABLE 40-6 Indications for Treatment With Blood Components

COMPONENT	VOLUME	INFUSION TIME	INDICATIONS
Packed red blood cells (PRBCs)	200-250 mL	2-4 hr	Anemia; hemoglobin <6 g/dL (<60 g/L), 6-10 g/dL (60-100 g/L), depending on symptoms
Washed red blood cells (WBC-poor PRBCs)	200 mL	2-4 hr	History of allergic transfusion reactions Hematopoietic stem cell transplant patients
Platelets			
Pooled	About 300 mL	15-30 min	Thrombocytopenia, platelet count <20,000 (<20 × 10^9/L) Patients who are actively bleeding with a platelet count <50,000 (<50 × 10^9/L)
Single donor	200 mL	30 min	History of febrile or allergic reactions
Fresh frozen plasma	200 mL	15-30 min	Deficiency in plasma coagulation factors Prothrombin or partial thromboplastin time 1.5 times normal
White blood cells (WBCs)	400 mL	1 hr	Sepsis, neutropenic infection not responding to antibiotic therapy

CHART 40-12 Best Practice for Patient Safety & Quality Care

Transfusion Therapy

NURSING ACTIONS	RATIONALES
Before Infusion	
1. Assess laboratory values.	Many institutions have specific guidelines for blood product transfusions (e.g., platelet count <20,000 [<20 × 10^9/L] or hemoglobin <6 g/dL [<60 g/L]).
2. Verify the medical prescription.	Legally a primary health care provider's prescription is required for transfusions. The prescription should state the type of product, dose, and transfusion time.
3. Assess the patient's vital signs, urine output, skin color, and history of transfusion reactions.	Determine whether the patient can tolerate infusion. Baseline information may be needed to help identify transfusion reactions.
4. Obtain venous access. Use a central catheter or at least a 19-gauge needle if possible.	The larger-bore needle allows cells to flow more easily without occluding the lumen of the catheter.
5. Obtain blood products from a blood bank. Transfuse as soon as possible after first performing **all the required safety checks.**	Once a blood product has been released from the blood bank, the product should be transfused as soon as possible (e.g., red blood cell transfusions should be completed within 4 hours of removal from refrigeration).
6. With another registered nurse, verify the patient by name and number, check blood compatibility, and note expiration time.	Human error is the most common cause of ABO incompatibility reactions.
During Infusion	
7. Administer the blood product using the appropriate filtered tubing.	Filters are needed to remove aggregates and possible contaminants.
8. Dilute blood products with only normal saline solution.	Hemolysis occurs if some other IV solution is used.
9. Remain with the patient during the first 15 to 30 minutes of the infusion.	Hemolytic reactions occur most often within the first 50 mL of the infusion.
10. Infuse the blood product at the prescribed rate.	Fluid overload is a potential complication of rapid infusion.
11. Monitor vital signs.	Vital sign changes often indicate transfusion reactions.
After Infusion	
12. When the transfusion is completed, discontinue infusion and dispose of the bag and tubing properly.	Bloodborne pathogens may be spread inadvertently through improper disposal.
13. Document.	The patient record should indicate the type of product infused, product number, volume infused, time of infusion, and any adverse reactions.

Use normal saline as the solution to administer with blood products, although this practice is not evidence-based (Kessler, 2013). Ringer's lactate and dextrose in water are not used for infusion with blood products because they may cause CLOT-TING or hemolysis of blood cells, although there is not sufficient evidence of hemolysis when using hypotonic fluids (Kessler, 2013; Tolich et al., 2013).

! NURSING SAFETY PRIORITY QSEN

Action Alert

Never add to or infuse other drugs with blood products because they may clot the blood during transfusion.

In compliance with recommendations by The Joint Commission's National Patient Safety Goals (NPSG) and before the transfusion, the priority actions are to determine that the blood component delivered is correct and that identification of the patient is correct. Check the primary health care provider's prescription together with another registered nurse to determine the patient's identity and whether the hospital identification band name and number are identical to those on the blood component tag. According to The Joint Commission's National Patient Safety Goals, *the patient's room number is not an acceptable form of identification.* Some facilities use a bar code—point of care (BC-POC) system, similar to drug-dispensing systems, in an attempt to improve patient safety and reduce identification errors.

! NURSING SAFETY PRIORITY QSEN

Action Alert

The nurse who will actually infuse the blood products must be one of the two professionals comparing the patient's identification with the information on the blood component bag.

Examine the blood bag label, the attached tag, and the requisition slip to ensure that the ABO and Rh types are compatible with those of the patient. Check the expiration date and inspect the product for discoloration, gas bubbles, or cloudiness, which are all indicators of bacterial growth or hemolysis.

Transfusion Responsibilities

Before starting the transfusion, explain the procedure to the patient. Assess vital signs and temperature immediately before starting the infusion. Begin the infusion slowly. *Remain with the patient for the first 15 to 30 minutes.* Any severe reaction usually occurs with infusion of the first 50 mL of blood. Ask the patient

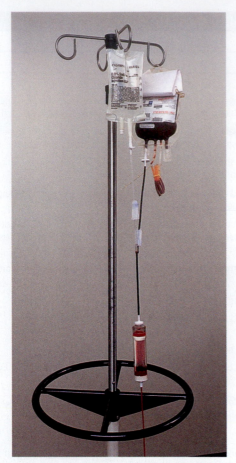

FIG. 40-7 Blood administration setup. (From deWit, S. C., & O'Neill, P. [2014]. *Fundamental concepts and skills for nursing* [4th ed.]. St. Louis: Saunders.)

TABLE 40-7   Compatibility Chart for Red Blood Cell Transfusions

	RECIPIENT			
DONOR	**A**	**B**	**AB**	**O**
A	X		X	
B		X	X	
AB			X	
O	X	X	X	X

to report unusual sensations such as chills, shortness of breath, hives, itching, or back pain. Assess vital signs 15 minutes after starting the infusion for indications of a reaction. If there are none, the rate can be increased to transfuse 1 unit in 2 hours (depending on the patient's cardiac status and facility policy for rate of administration). Take vital signs every hour during the transfusion or as specified by agency policy. Some facilities continuously monitor patients during transfusions using a wireless remote monitoring device.

Blood components without large amounts of red blood cells (RBCs) can be infused more quickly. The identification checks are the same as for RBC transfusions. It may be necessary to infuse blood products at a slower rate for older patients. Best practices related to the nursing care needs of older patients during transfusion therapy are listed in Chart 40-13.

Electrolyte imbalances are possible as a result of transfusions, especially with packed red blood cells (PRBCs). During transfusions, some cells are damaged, releasing potassium and raising the patient's serum potassium level above normal (hyperkalemia). This problem is more likely when the blood being transfused has been frozen or is several weeks old.

Types of Transfusions

At one time, transfusion with whole blood was a common form of transfusion therapy. Today whole blood transfusions are extremely rare (AABB, 2014). When a whole blood donation is made, it is centrifuged on arrival at the blood-banking facility and separated into various components. The individual components are transfused according to patients' specific needs.

Red Blood Cell Transfusions

RBCs are given to replace cells lost from trauma or surgery. Patients with problems that destroy RBCs or impair RBC maturation also may receive RBC transfusions. PRBCs, supplied in 250-mL bags, are a concentrated source of RBCs and are the most common component given to RBC-deficient patients.

Blood transfusions are transplantations of tissue from one person to another. Therefore the donor and recipient blood must be checked carefully for compatibility to prevent lethal reactions (Table 40-7). Compatibility is determined by two different antigen systems (cell surface proteins): the ABO system antigens and the Rh antigen, present on the membranes of RBCs.

RBC antigens are inherited. For the ABO system, a person inherits one of these:

- A antigen (type A blood)
- B antigen (type B blood)
- Both A and B antigens (type AB blood)
- Neither A nor B antigens (type O blood)

People develop circulating antibodies against the blood type antigens they did not inherit. For example, a person with type

A blood forms antibodies against type B blood. A person with type O blood has not inherited either A or B antigens and will form antibodies against RBCs with either A or B antigens. If RBCs that have an antigen are infused into a recipient who does not share that antigen, the infused blood is recognized by the recipient's antibodies as non-self, and the recipient then has a reaction to the transfused products.

The Rh antigen system is slightly different. An Rh-negative person is born without the Rh-antigen on his or her RBCs and does not form antibodies unless specifically sensitized to it. Sensitization can occur with RBC transfusions from an Rh-positive person or from exposure during pregnancy and birth. Once an Rh-negative person has been sensitized and antibodies develop, any exposure to Rh-positive blood can cause a transfusion reaction. Antibody development can be prevented by giving anti-Rh–immunoglobulin as soon as exposure to the Rh antigen is suspected. *Adults who have Rh-positive blood can receive an RBC transfusion from an Rh-negative donor, but Rh-negative adults must not receive Rh-positive blood.*

Platelet Transfusions

Platelets are given to patients with platelet counts below 10,000/mm³ (10×10^9/L) and to patients with thrombocytopenia who are actively bleeding or are scheduled for an invasive procedure. Platelet transfusions are pooled from as many as 10 donors and do not have to be of the same blood type as the patient has. For patients who are having hematopoietic stem cell transplantation (HSCT) or who need multiple platelet transfusions, platelets from a single donor may be prescribed, which reduces the chances of allergic reactions.

Platelet infusion bags contain about 300 mL for pooled platelets and 200 mL for single-donor platelets. Platelets are fragile and must be infused immediately after being brought to the patient's room, usually over a 15- to 30-minute period. A special transfusion set with a smaller filter and shorter tubing is used. Platelet filters help remove WBCs from the platelets for patients who have a history of febrile reactions or who need multiple platelet transfusions.

> **! NURSING SAFETY PRIORITY** QSEN
>
> *Action Alert*
>
> When infusing platelets, do not use the standard blood administration set because the longer tubing increases platelet adherence to the lumen.

Take the vital signs before the infusion, 15 minutes after the infusion starts, and at its completion. A patient who has had a transfusion reaction in the past may be given diphenhydramine (Benadryl) and acetaminophen (Tylenol) before the transfusion to reduce the fever and severe chills (rigors) that often occur during platelet transfusions.

Plasma Transfusions

Plasma infusions may be given fresh to replace blood volume and CLOTTING factors. More often, plasma is frozen immediately after donation, forming **fresh frozen plasma (FFP)**. Infuse FFP immediately after thawing while the clotting factors are still active.

ABO compatibility is required for transfusion of plasma products because the plasma contains the donor's ABO antibodies that could react with the recipient's RBC antigens. The infusion bag contains about 200 mL. Infuse FFP as rapidly as the patient can tolerate, generally over a 30- to 60-minute period, through a regular Y-set or straight filtered tubing.

Granulocyte (White Blood Cell) Transfusions

Rarely, neutropenic patients with infections receive white blood cell (WBC) replacement transfusions. WBC surfaces have many antigens that can cause severe reactions when infused into a patient whose immune system recognizes these antigens as non-self.

WBCs are suspended in 400 mL of plasma and should be infused slowly, usually over a 45- to 60-minute period, depending on the concentration of cells being infused. Agency policies often require stricter monitoring during WBC infusions because reactions are more common. A physician may need to be present in the hospital unit, and vital signs may need to be taken every 15 minutes throughout the transfusion. Amphotericin B infusion should be separated from WBC transfusions by 4 to 6 hours because this drug can hemolyze the blood cells. In addition, amphotericin B has so many side effects that these may mask a transfusion reaction.

Acute Transfusion Reactions

Patients can develop any of these transfusion reactions: febrile, hemolytic, allergic, or bacterial reactions; circulatory overload; or transfusion-associated graft-versus-host disease (TA-GVHD). To prevent complications, remain alert during transfusions to detect early reactions and initiate appropriate management. Instructing the patient to immediately report any change in physical or emotional status such as new-onset joint, back, chest, or abdominal pain; chills; nausea; feeling unwell; or feeling uneasy, which may help identify a possible transfusion reaction (Menendez & Edwards, 2016).

Febrile transfusion reactions occur most often in the patient with anti-WBC antibodies, which can develop after multiple transfusions, WBC transfusions, and platelet transfusions. The patient develops chills, tachycardia, fever, hypotension, and tachypnea. Giving leukocyte-reduced blood or single-donor HLA-matched platelets reduces the risk for this type of reaction. WBC filters may be used to trap WBCs and prevent their infusion into the patient.

Hemolytic transfusion reactions are caused by blood type or Rh incompatibility. When blood containing antigens different from the patient's own antigens is infused, antigen-antibody complexes are formed in his or her blood. These complexes destroy the transfused cells and start inflammatory responses in the blood vessel walls and organs. The reaction may be mild, with fever and chills, or life threatening, with disseminated intravascular coagulation (DIC) and circulatory collapse (McCance et al., 2014). Other symptoms include:

- Apprehension
- Headache
- Chest pain
- Low back pain
- Tachycardia
- Tachypnea
- Hypotension
- Hemoglobinuria
- A sense of impending doom

The onset of a hemolytic reaction may be immediate or may not occur until subsequent units have been transfused.

Allergic transfusion reactions (anaphylactic transfusion reactions) are most often seen in patients with other allergies. They may have urticaria, itching, bronchospasm, or anaphylaxis. Onset usually occurs during or up to 24 hours after the transfusion. Patients with an allergy history can be given leukocyte-reduced or washed RBCs, in which the WBCs, plasma, and immunoglobulin A have been removed, reducing the risk for an allergic reaction.

Bacterial transfusion reactions occur from infusion of contaminated blood products, especially those contaminated with a gram-negative organism. Symptoms include tachycardia, hypotension, fever, chills, and shock. The onset of a bacterial transfusion reaction is rapid. (See Chapter 37 for care of the patient with septic shock.)

Transfusion-related acute lung injury (TRALI) is a life-threatening event that occurs most often when donor blood contains antibodies against the recipient's neutrophil antigens, HLA, or both. Common symptoms are a rapid onset of dyspnea and hypoxia within 6 hours of the transfusion. Early recognition is key to survival. Most patients require intubation and mechanical ventilation for respiratory support.

Transfusion-associated circulatory overload (TACO) can occur when a blood product is infused too quickly, especially in an older adult (Touhy & Jett, 2016). It is a pulmonary reaction that may be difficult at first to differentiate from TRALI (Bockhold & Crumpler, 2015). This is most common with whole-blood transfusions or when the patient receives multiple packed RBC transfusions. Symptoms include:

- Hypertension
- Bounding pulse
- Distended jugular veins
- Dyspnea
- Restlessness
- Confusion

Manage and prevent this complication by monitoring intake and output, infusing blood products more slowly, and giving diuretics. (See Chapter 11 for management of fluid overload.)

Transfusion-associated graft-versus-host disease (TA-GVHD) is a rare but life-threatening problem that occurs more often in an immunosuppressed patient. Its cause in immunosuppressed patients is similar to that of GVHD that occurs with allogeneic stem cell transplantation, (discussed in the interventions section under Acute Leukemia), in which donor T-cell lymphocytes attack host tissues.

Symptoms usually occur within 1 to 2 weeks and include thrombocytopenia, anorexia, nausea, vomiting, chronic hepatitis, weight loss, and recurrent infection. TA-GVHD has an 80% to 90% mortality rate but can be prevented by using irradiated blood products. Irradiation destroys most T-cells and their cytokine products.

Acute pain transfusion reaction or APTR is a rare event that can occur during or shortly after transfusion of any blood product. Its cause is not known. Symptoms are severe chest pain, back pain, joint pain, hypertension, anxiety, and redness of the head and neck (Hardwick et al., 2013). The reaction does not appear to be life threatening, and most patients respond well with drugs for pain and rigors. Although symptoms are general, diagnosis can be supported with a positive direct antibody test

(DAT), indicating that some degree of hemolysis has occurred but is not widespread. APTR management focuses on patient support and drugs to control or reduce symptoms.

Interventions for transfusion reactions occurring during transfusion (hemolytic reactions, allergic reactions, and bacterial reactions) begin with stopping the transfusion and removing the blood tubing. (For hemolytic and suspected bacterial reactions, return the component bag, labels, and all tubing to the blood bank or laboratory.) Notify the Rapid Response Team. If the patient has no other IV access, keep the access and flush with normal saline. *Do not flush the contents of the blood transfusion tubing, which would allow more of the reaction-causing blood to enter the patient.* Usually oxygen is applied, and diphenhydramine (Benadryl) is administered by IV push. If indications of shock are present, fluid resuscitation and hemodynamic monitoring are needed. Blood pressure support with vasopressors may be needed (see Chapter 37). Other drug therapy is supportive, such as antipyretics for fever, antibiotics for suspected bacterial contamination, and meperidine for rigors.

Autologous Blood Transfusions

Autologous blood transfusions involve collection and infusion of the patient's own blood. This type of transfusion eliminates compatibility problems and reduces the risk for transmitting bloodborne diseases. The four types of autologous blood transfusions are preoperative autologous blood donation, acute normovolemic hemodilution, intraoperative autologous transfusion, and postoperative blood salvage.

Autologous blood donation before surgery is the most common type of autologous blood transfusion. It involves collecting whole blood from a qualified patient, dividing it into components, and storing it for later use. As long as hematocrit and hemoglobin levels are within a safe range, the patient can donate blood on a weekly basis until the prescribed amount of blood is obtained. Fresh packed RBCs may be stored for 40 days. For patients with rare blood types, blood may be frozen for up to 10 years.

Acute normovolemic hemodilution involves withdrawal of a patient's RBCs and volume replacement just before a surgical procedure. The goal is to decrease RBC loss during surgery. The blood is stored at room temperature for up to 6 hours and reinfused after surgery. This type of autologous transfusion is not used with anemic patients or those with poor kidney function.

Intraoperative autologous transfusion and blood salvage after surgery are the recovery and reinfusion of a patient's own blood from an operative field or from a bleeding wound. Special devices collect, filter, and drain the blood into a transfusion bag. This blood is used for trauma or surgical patients with severe blood loss. The salvaged blood must be reinfused within 6 hours.

Transfuse autologous blood products using the guidelines previously described. Although the patient receiving autologous blood is not at risk for some types of transfusion reactions, circulatory overload or bacterial transfusion reactions can still occur and are managed in the same way that these complications are managed in transfusions derived from donors.

GET READY FOR THE NCLEX® EXAMINATION!

KEY POINTS

Review these Key Points for each NCLEX Examination Client Needs Category.

Safe and Effective Care Environment

- Use aseptic technique during all central line dressing changes or any invasive procedure. **QSEN: Safety**
- Use good handwashing techniques before providing any care to a patient who is either immunocompromised or has reduced IMMUNITY. **QSEN: Safety**
- Modify the environment to protect patients who have thrombocytopenia. **QSEN: Safety**
- Use Bleeding Precautions for any patient with thrombocytopenia or pancytopenia (see Chart 40-7). **QSEN: Safety**
- Ensure that informed consent is obtained before any invasive procedure or transfusion. **QSEN: Safety**
- Verify with another registered nurse prescriptions for transfusion of blood products. **QSEN: Safety**
- Use at least two forms of identification for the patient who is to receive a blood product transfusion (e.g., name, birthdate, identification number). **QSEN: Safety**
- Teach patients with sickle cell disease to avoid conditions that are known to trigger crises. **QSEN: Patient-Centered Care**
- Teach the patient and family about the symptoms of infection and when to seek medical advice. **QSEN: Patient-Centered Care**
- Instruct patients who have anemia as a result of dietary deficiency which foods are good sources of iron, folic acid, and vitamin B_{12}. **QSEN: Patient-Centered Care**
- Teach precautions to take to avoid injury (see Chart 40-11) to patients at risk for poor CLOTTING and increased bleeding. **QSEN: Patient-Centered Care**
- Report any temperature over $100°F$ ($37.8°C$) in a patient with neutropenia. **QSEN: Evidence-Based Practice**

Health Promotion and Maintenance

- Make referrals to support groups sponsored by organizations such as the Sickle Cell Foundation Support Group, American Cancer Society, Leukemia and Lymphoma Society of America, and National Hemophilia Foundation. **QSEN: Teamwork and Collaboration**

- Teach people to avoid unnecessary contact with environmental chemicals or toxins. If contact cannot be avoided, teach people to use safety precautions. **QSEN: Evidence-Based Practice**
- Identify patients at high risk for infection because of disease or therapy. **QSEN: Patient-Centered Care**

Psychosocial Integrity

- Allow the patient and family the opportunity to express their feelings regarding the diagnosis of leukemia or lymphoma or the treatment regimen. **QSEN: Patient-Centered Care**
- Explain all procedures, restrictions, drugs, and follow-up care to the patient and family. **QSEN: Patient-Centered Care**
- Reassure patients having pain that using opioid analgesics for needed pain relief is not drug abuse. **QSEN: Patient-Centered Care**

Physiological Integrity

- Pace nonurgent health care activities to reduce the risk for fatigue among patients with anemia or pancytopenia. **QSEN: Patient-Centered Care**
- Assess patients in the induction phase of chemotherapy, those after HSCT, and anyone with neutropenia every 8 hours for indicators of infection. **QSEN: Evidence-Based Practice**
- Assess the skin integrity of the perianal region of a patient with leukemia or profound neutropenia after every bowel movement. **QSEN: Patient-Centered Care**
- Administer analgesics on a schedule rather than PRN. **QSEN: Evidence-Based Practice**
- Use normal saline as the solution infusing with blood products. **QSEN: Safety**
- Transfuse blood products more slowly to older patients or those who have a cardiac problem. **QSEN: Patient-Centered Care**
- Remain with the patient during the first 15 minutes of infusion of any blood product. **QSEN: Safety**
- Do not administer any drugs in the same line with infusing blood products. **QSEN: Evidence-Based Practice**

SELECTED BIBLIOGRAPHY

AABB. (2014). *Circular information for the use of human blood and blood components.* www.aabb.org/tm/coi/Documents/coi1113.pdf.

Albrecht, T. (2014). Physiologic and psychological symptoms experienced by adults with acute leukemia: An integrative literature review. *Oncology Nursing Forum, 41*(3), 286–295.

Al-Eidan, F. A. S. (2015). Pharmacotherapy of heparin-induced thrombocytopenia: Therapeutic options and challenges in the clinical practices. *Journal of Vascular Nursing, 33*(1), 10–20.

American Cancer Society (ACS). (2017). *Cancer facts and figures 2017.* Report No. 01-300M–No. 500817. Atlanta: Author.

Aschenbrenner, D. (2015). Drug watch: Antianemia drug receives boxed warning. *The American Journal of Nursing, 115*(8), 48.

Betcher, J., Van Ryan, V., & Mikhael, J. (2015). Chronic anemia and the role of the infusion therapy nurse. *Journal of Infusion Nursing, 38*(5), 341–348.

Blix, A. (2014). Personalized medicine, genomics, and pharmacogenomics: A primer for nurses. *Clinical Journal of Oncology Nursing, 18*(4), 437–441.

Bockhold, C., & Crumpler, S. (2015). Responding to pulmonary-related blood transfusion reactions. *Nursing, 45*(9), 37–41.

Burchum, J., & Rosenthal, L. (2016). *Lehne's pharmacology for nursing care* (9th ed.). St. Louis: Elsevier.

Cadogan, S., & Miller, S. (2014). Aspergillus pneumonia in adult patients with acute leukemia. *Clinical Journal of Oncology Nursing, 18*(2), 243–246.

Canadian Cancer Society (CCS), Statistics Canada. (2016). *Canadian cancer statistics, 2016.* Toronto: Canadian Cancer Society. http://www.cancer.ca/~/media/cancer.ca/CW/cancer%20information/cancer%20101/Canadian%20cancer%20statistics/Canadian-Cancer-Statistics-2016-EN.pdf.

Centers for Disease Control and Prevention (CDC). (2015). *Sickle cell disease: Data & statistics.* www.cdc.gov/ncbddd/sicklecell/data.html.

Crookston, K., Hoenig, S., & Reyes, M. (2015). Transfusion reaction identification and management at the bedside. *Journal of Infusion Nursing, 38*(2), 104–113.

Divers, J., & O'Shaughnessy, J. (2015). Stomatitis associated with use of mTOR inhibitors: Implications for patients with invasive breast cancer. *Clinical Journal of Oncology Nursing, 19*(4), 468–474.

Gonella, S., & Giulio, P. (2015). Delayed chemotherapy-induced nausea and vomiting in the hematologic population: A review of the literature. *Clinical Journal of Oncology Nursing, 19*(4), 438–443.

Greenberg, E. (2017). Thrombocytopenia: A destruction of platelets. *Journal of Infusion Nursing, 40*(1), 41–50.

Guerrero, M., & Swenson, K. (2014). Herpes simplex virus-related mucositis in patients with lymphoma. *Oncology Nursing Forum, 41*(3), 327–330.

Hardwick, J., Osswald, M., & Walker, D. (2013). Acute pain transfusion reaction. *Oncology Nursing Forum, 40*(6), 543–545.

Hitch, D. (2013). What every nurse should know about hemophilia. *American Nurse Today, 8*(3), 22–26.

Jarvis, C. (2016). *Physical examination & health assessment* (7th ed.). St. Louis: Elsevier.

Johnson, N. (2013). Ocular graft-versus-host disease after allogeneic transplantation. *Clinical Journal of Oncology Nursing, 17*(6), 621–626.

Jorde, L., Carey, J., & Bamshad, M. (2016). *Medical genetics* (5th ed.). Philadelphia: Elsevier.

Kannan, R., Madden, K., & Andrews, S. (2014). Primer on immune-oncology and immune response. *Clinical Journal of Oncology Nursing, 18*(3), 311–317.

Katrancha, E., & Gonzalez, L. (2014). Trauma-induced coagulopathy. *Critical Care Nurse, 34*(4), 54–63.

Kelly, D., Lyon, D., Ameringer, S., Elswick, R., & McCarty, J. (2015). Symptoms, cytokines, and quality of life in patients diagnosed with chronic graft-versus-host disease following allogeneic hematopoietic stem cell transplantation. *Oncology Nursing Forum, 42*(3), 265–275.

Kessler, C. (2013). Priming blood transfusion tubing: A critical review of the blood transfusion process. *Critical Care Nurse, 33*(3), 80–83.

Kurtin, S., & Faiman, B. (2013). The changing landscape of multiple myeloma: Implications for oncology nurses. *Clinical Journal of Oncology Nursing, S17*(6), S2, S7-S11.

Lassiter, M., & Schneider, S. (2015). A pilot study comparing the neutropenic diet to a non-neutropenic diet in the allogeneic hematopoietic stem cell transplantation population. *Clinical Journal of Oncology Nursing, 19*(3), 273–278.

Lentz, M., & Kautz, D. (2017). Acute vaso-occlusive crisis in patients with sickle cell disease. *Nursing, 47*(1), 67–68.

Mangan, P., Gleason, C., & Miceli, T. (2013). Autologous hematopoietic stem cell transplantation for multiple myeloma. *Clinical Journal of Oncology Nursing, 17*(6), 43–47.

Martin, M., & Haines, D. (2016). Clinical management of patients with thalassemia syndromes. *Clinical Journal of Oncology Nursing, 20*(3), 310–317.

Matthie, N., & Jenerette, C. (2015). Sickle cell disease in adults: Developing an appropriate care plan. *Clinical Journal of Oncology Nursing, 19*(5), 562–568.

Matthie, N., Brewer, C., Moura, V., & Jenerette, C. (2015a). Breathing exercises for inpatients with sickle cell disease. *Medsurg Nursing, 24*(1), 35–38.

Matthie, N., Jenerette, C., & McMillan, S. (2015b). Role of self-care in sickle cell disease. *Pain Management Nursing, 16*(3), 257–266.

McCance, K., Huether, S., Brashers, V., & Rote, N. (2014). *Pathophysiology: The biologic basis for disease in adults and children* (6th ed.). St. Louis: Mosby.

Menendez, J., & Edwards, B. (2016). Early identification of acute hemolytic transfusion reactions: Realistic implications for best practice in patient monitoring. *Medsurg Nursing, 25*(2), 88–90, 109.

National Hemophilia Foundation. (2017). *Bleeding disorders: Hemophilia A.* Retrieved from https://www.hemophilia.org/Bleeding-Disorders/Types-of-Bleeding-Disorders/Hemophilia-A.

O'Connor, S., Hanes, D., Lindsey, A., Weiss, M., Petty, L., & Overcash, J. (2014). Attitudes among healthcare providers and patients diagnosed with sickle cell disease: Frequent hospitalizations and stressors. *Clinical Journal of Oncology Nursing, 18*(6), 675–680.

Online Mendelian Inheritance in Man (OMIM). (2016a). *Hemochromatosis, type1; HFE1.* https://www.omim.org/entry/235200.

Online Mendelian Inheritance in Man (OMIM). (2016b). *Hemophilia A; HEMA.* https://www.omim.org/entry/306700.

Online Mendelian Inheritance in Man (OMIM). (2016c). *Sickle cell anemia.* https://www.omim.org/entry/603903.

Pagana, K., Pagana, T. J., & Pagana, T. N. (2017). *Mosby's diagnostic and laboratory test reference* (13th ed.). St. Louis: Mosby.

Quigley, P. (2016). Hereditary hemochromatosis: Dealing with iron overload. *Nursing, 46*(5), 36–43.

Smithson, C., & Schneider, S. (2015). Ibrutinib: A new targeted therapy for hematologic cancers. *Clinical Journal of Oncology Nursing, 19*(3), E47–E51.

Stupnyckyj, C., Smolarek, S., Reeves, C., McKeith, J., & Magnan, M. (2014). Changing blood transfusion policy and practice. *The American Journal of Nursing, 114*(12), 50–59.

Sullivan, K., Vu, T., Richardson, G., Castillo, E., & Martinez, F. (2015). Evaluating the frequency of vital sign monitoring during blood transfusion: An evidence-based practice initiative. *Clinical Journal of Oncology Nursing, 19*(5), 516–520.

The Joint Commission (TJC). (2014). *Implementation guide for The Joint Commission patient blood management performance measures.* www.jointcommission.org/patient_blood_management_performance_measures_project/.

Thoele, K. (2014). Engraftment syndrome in hematopoietic stem cell transplantations. *Clinical Journal of Oncology Nursing, 18*(3), 349–354.

Thomson, B., Gorospe, G., Cooke, L., Giesie, P., & Johnson, S. (2015). Transitions of care: A hematopoietic stem cell transplantation nursing education project across the trajectory. *Clinical Journal of Oncology Nursing, 19*(4), E74–E79.

Tolich, D., Blackmur, S., Stahorsky, K., & Wabeke, D. (2013). Blood management: Best practice transfusion strategies. *Nursing, 43*(1), 40–47.

Touhy, T., & Jett, K. (2016). *Ebersole and Hess' toward healthy aging* (9th ed.). St. Louis: Mosby.

U.S. Department of Health and Human Services (USDHHS). (2014). National Institutes of Health: *Evidence-based management of sickle cell disease-Expert panel report, 2014.* https://www.nhlbi.nih.gov/sites/www.nhlbi.nih.gov/files/sickle-cell-disease-report.pdf.

U.S. Department of Health and Human Services (USDHHS). (2015). *Why minority donors are needed.* www.organdonor.gov/whydonate/minorities.html.

Vacce, V., & Blank, L. (2017). Sickle cell disease: Where are we now? *Nursing, 47*(4), 26–34.

CHAPTER **41**

Assessment of the Nervous System

Donna D. Ignatavicius

http://evolve.elsevier.com/Iggy/

PRIORITY AND INTERRELATED CONCEPTS

The priority concepts for this chapter are:
- COGNITION
- MOBILITY
- SENSORY PERCEPTION

The interrelated concept for this chapter is PERFUSION.

LEARNING OUTCOMES

Safe and Effective Care Environment
1. Coordinate with the interprofessional health care team to perform a complete neurologic assessment based on the patient's history and presenting signs and symptoms.

Health Promotion and Maintenance
2. Identify factors such as risky behaviors or lifestyle choices that place patients at risk for neurologic health problems.
3. Provide patient-centered health teaching for preparation and follow-up care for selected neurologic diagnostic testing.
4. Apply knowledge of common physiologic changes associated with aging to accurately interpret neurologic assessment findings and plan interventions to ensure patient safety.

Psychosocial Integrity
5. Identify possible psychological responses to neurologic health problems, including the influence of cultural and spiritual factors.

Physiological Integrity
6. Document findings from the neurologic nursing assessment to identify changes in MOBILITY and SENSORY PERCEPTION.
7. Perform a focused neurologic assessment to identify changes in COGNITION, especially level of consciousness and memory, to ensure patient safety.
8. Use clinical judgment to interpret assessment findings based on the Glasgow Coma Scale.
9. Describe evidence-based precautions for the use of iodine-based or gadolinium contrast for diagnostic testing to ensure patient safety.
10. Monitor for signs of early complications from selected invasive neurologic diagnostic testing.

The major divisions of the nervous system are the central nervous system (CNS) (brain and spinal cord) and peripheral nervous system (PNS). The divisions of the nervous system work together to control COGNITION, MOBILITY, and SENSORY PERCEPTION. See Chapter 2 for review of these health concepts.

ANATOMY AND PHYSIOLOGY REVIEW

Nervous System Cells: Structure and Function

The basic unit of the nervous system, the **neuron**, transmits impulses, or "messages." Some neurons are **motor** (causing purposeful physical movement or MOBILITY), and some are sensory (resulting in the ability to perceive stimulation through one's sensory organs or SENSORY PERCEPTION). Some process information, and some retain information (COGNITION). When a neuron receives an impulse from another neuron, the effect may be excitation (increasing action) or inhibition (decreasing action). Each neuron has a *cell body,* or *soma;* short, branching processes called *dendrites;* and a single *axon* (Fig. 41-1).

Afferent neurons, also known as *sensory neurons,* are specialized to send impulses toward the CNS, away from the PNS. *Efferent* neurons are motor nerve cells that carry signals away from the CNS to the cells in the PNS. Each dendrite synapses with another cell body, axon, or dendrite and sends impulses along the efferent and afferent neuron pathways.

Many axons are covered by a myelin sheath—a white, lipid covering. Myelinated axons appear whitish and therefore are also called white matter. Nonmyelinated axons have a grayish cast and are called gray matter. Myelinated axons have gaps in the myelin called *nodes of Ranvier.* The nodes of Ranvier play a major role in impulse conduction (see Fig. 41-1). When the myelin is impaired, the impulses cannot travel from the brain to the rest of the body, such as in patients with multiple sclerosis.

The enlarged distal end of each axon is called the *synaptic* or *terminal knob.* Within the synaptic knobs are the mechanisms for manufacturing, storing, and releasing a transmitter substance. Each neuron produces a specific neurotransmitter chemical (e.g., acetylcholine and serotonin) that can either enhance or inhibit the impulse, but cannot do both.

Impulses are transmitted to their eventual destination through synapses, or spaces between neurons. There are two distinct types of synapses: *neuron to neuron* and *neuron to muscle* (or gland). Between the terminal knob and the next cell is a small space called the *synaptic cleft.* The knob, the cleft, and the portion of the cell to which the impulse is being transmitted make up the synapse.

Neuroglia cells, which vary in size and shape, provide protection, structure, and nutrition for the neurons. They are classified into four types: astroglial cells, ependymal cells, oligodendrocytes, and microglial cells. These cells are also part of the blood-brain barrier and help regulate cerebrospinal fluid (CSF) (McCance et al., 2014).

Central Nervous System: Structure and Function

The central nervous system (CNS) is composed of the *brain,* which directs the regulation and function of the nervous system and all other systems of the body, and the *spinal cord,* which starts reflex activity and transmits impulses to and from the brain.

Brain

The meninges form the protective covering of the brain and the spinal cord. The outside layer is the *dura mater.* The subdural space is located between the dura mater and the middle layer, the *arachnoid.* The *pia mater* is the most inner layer. Situated between the arachnoid and pia mater is the subarachnoid space, where CSF circulates. A potential space, referred to as the epidural space, is located between the skull and the outer layer of the dura mater. This area also extends down the spinal cord and is used for the delivery of epidural analgesia and anesthesia.

The dura mater also lies between the cerebral hemispheres and the cerebellum and is called the *tentorium.* It helps decrease or prevents the transmission of force from one hemisphere to another and protects the lower brainstem when head trauma occurs. Clinical references may be made to a lesion (e.g., a tumor) as being supratentorial (above the tentorium) or infratentorial (below the tentorium).

Major Parts of the Brain. The brain consists of three main areas—the forebrain, the cerebellum, and the brainstem. The *forebrain* lies above the brainstem and cerebellum and is the most advanced in function complexity. This area of the brain is further divided into three areas—the diencephalon, the cerebrum, and the cerebral cortex.

The *diencephalon,* which lies below the cerebrum, includes the thalamus, hypothalamus, and epithalamus (Fig. 41-2). The *thalamus* is the major "relay station," or "central switchboard," for the CNS. The *hypothalamus* plays a major role in autonomic nervous system control (controlling temperature and other functions) and COGNITION. The *epithalamus* connects the pathways to regulate emotion and contribute to smooth voluntary motor function.

The *cerebrum* is the largest part of the brain and controls intelligence, creativity, and memory. The "gray matter" of the cerebrum is the central cortex—the center that receives information from the thalamus and all the lower areas of the brain. The cerebrum consists of two halves, referred to as the *right hemisphere* and the *left hemisphere,* which are joined by the corpus callosum. The *left* hemisphere is the dominant hemisphere in most people (even in many left-handed people). Within the deeper structures of the cerebrum are the right and

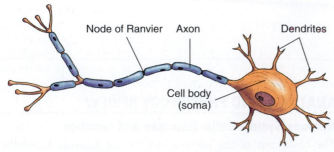

FIG. 41-1 Structure of a typical neuron.

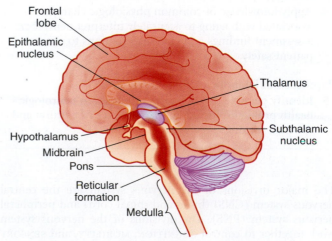

FIG. 41-2 Structures of the brainstem and diencephalon.

TABLE 41-1 Cerebral Lobe Main Functions

Frontal Lobe

- Primary motor area (also known as the *motor "strip"* or *cortex*)
- Broca's speech center on the dominant side
- Voluntary eye movement
- Access to current sensory data
- Access to past information or experience
- Affective response to a situation
- Behavior regulation
- Judgment
- Ability to develop long-term goals
- Reasoning, concentration, abstraction

Parietal Lobe

- Understanding sensory input such as texture, size, shape, and spatial relationships
- Three-dimensional (spatial) perception
- Needed for singing, playing musical instruments, and processing nonverbal visual experiences
- Perception of body parts and body position awareness
- Taste impulses for interpretation

Temporal Lobe

- Auditory center for sound interpretation
- Complicated memory patterns
- Wernicke's area for speech

Occipital Lobe

- Primary visual center

TABLE 41-2 Brainstem Functions

Medulla

- Cardiac-slowing center
- Respiratory center
- Cranial nerve nuclei IX (glossopharyngeal), X (vagus), XI (accessory), and XII (hypoglossal) and parts of cranial nerves VII (facial) and VIII (vestibulocochlear)

Pons

- Cardiac acceleration and vasoconstriction centers
- Pneumotaxic center that helps control respiratory pattern and rate
- Cranial nerve nuclei V (trigeminal), VI (abducens), VII (facial), and VIII (vestibulocochlear)

Midbrain

- Contains the cerebral aqueduct or aqueduct of Sylvius
- Location of periaqueductal gray, which may abolish pain when stimulated
- Cranial nerve nuclei III (oculomotor) and IV (trochlear)

left lateral ventricles. At the base of the cerebrum near the ventricles is a group of neurons called the *basal ganglia,* which help regulate motor function.

The *cerebral cortex* is part of the cerebrum and is involved with almost all of the higher functions of the brain. This part of the brain processes and communicates all information coming from the peripheral nervous system (PNS). It also translates the impulses into understandable feelings and thoughts. The cerebral cortex is so complex that it is further divided into four lobes: the frontal lobe, parietal lobe, temporal lobe, and occipital lobe. Table 41-1 summarizes the major functions of each lobe.

The *cerebellum* receives immediate and continuous information about the condition of the muscles, joints, and tendons. Cerebellar function enables a person to:

- Keep an extremity from overshooting an intended target
- Move from one skilled movement to another in an orderly sequence
- Predict distance or gauge the speed with which one is approaching an object
- Control voluntary movement
- Maintain equilibrium

Unlike the motor cortex, cerebellar control of the body is *ipsilateral* (situated on the same side). The right side of the cerebellum controls the right side of the body, and the left cerebellum controls the left side of the body.

The *brainstem* includes the midbrain, pons, and medulla. The functions of these structures are presented in Table 41-2. Throughout the brainstem are special cells that constitute the reticular activating system (RAS), which controls awareness and alertness. For example, this tissue awakens a person from sleep when presented with a stimulus such as loud noise or pain

or when it is time to awaken. The reticular formation area has many connections with the cerebrum, the rest of the brainstem, and the cerebellum.

Circulation in the Brain. Circulation in the brain originates from the carotid and vertebral arteries (Fig. 41-3). The internal carotid arteries branch into the anterior cerebral artery (ACA) and middle cerebral artery (MCA), the largest ones. The two posterior vertebral arteries become the basilar artery, which then divides into two posterior cerebral arteries. The anterior, middle, and posterior cerebral arteries are joined together by small communicating arteries to form a ring at the base of the brain known as the circle of Willis.

The *middle* cerebral artery supplies the lateral surface of the cerebrum from about the mid-temporal lobe upward (i.e., the area for hearing and upper body motor and sensory neurons). The *anterior* cerebral artery supplies the midline, or medial, aspect of the same area (i.e., the lower body motor and sensory neurons). The *posterior* cerebral arteries supply the area from the mid-temporal region down and back (occipital lobe), as well as much of the brainstem. When blood flow is interrupted in any of these arteries (e.g., by a clot), the area of the brain being supplied is affected and may not function as it should.

The *blood-brain barrier (BBB)* seems to exist because the endothelial cells of the cerebral capillaries are joined tightly together. This barrier keeps some substances in the bloodstream out of the cerebrospinal circulation and out of brain tissue. Substances that can pass through the BBB include oxygen, glucose, carbon dioxide, alcohol, anesthetics, and water. Large molecules such as albumin, any substance bound to albumin, and many antibiotics are prevented from crossing the barrier.

Cerebrospinal fluid (CSF) also circulates, surrounds, and cushions the brain and spinal cord. While moving through the subarachnoid space, the fluid is continuously produced by the choroid plexus, reabsorbed by the arachnoid villi, and then channeled into the superior sagittal sinus. Expanded areas of subarachnoid space, where there are large amounts of CSF, are called *cisterns.* The largest one is the lumbar cistern, the site of lumbar puncture, from the level of the second lumbar vertebra to the second sacral vertebra (L2-S2) (Jarvis, 2014).

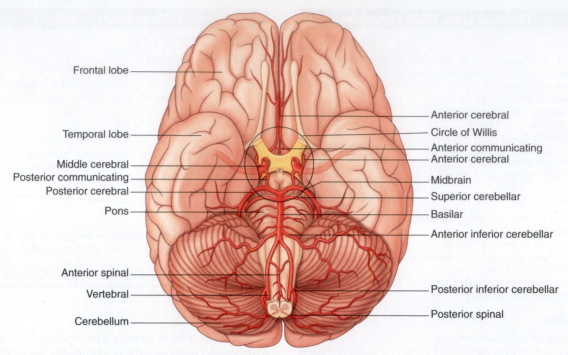

FIG. 41-3 Cerebral circulation and the circle of Willis at the base of the brain. (Modified from Patton, K. T. & Thibodeau, G. A. [2016]. *Anatomy and physiology* [9th ed.]. St. Louis: Mosby.)

Spinal Cord

The spinal cord controls MOBILITY; regulates organ function; processes SENSORY PERCEPTION information from the extremities, trunk, and many internal organs; and transmits information to and from the brain. It contains H-shaped *gray matter* (neuron cell bodies) that is surrounded by *white matter* (myelinated axons). Groups of cells in the white matter (ascending and descending tracts) have been fairly well identified. These tracts carry impulses from the spinal cord to the brain (ascending tracts, such as the spinothalamic tract) or from the brain to the spinal cord (descending tracts, such as the corticospinal tract).

Peripheral Nervous System: Structure and Function

The peripheral nervous system (PNS) is composed of the spinal nerves, cranial nerves, and autonomic nervous system.

There are 31 pairs of spinal nerves (8 cervical, 12 thoracic, 5 lumbar, 5 sacral, and 1 coccygeal) exiting from the spinal cord. Each of the nerves has a posterior and an anterior branch. The posterior branch carries SENSORY PERCEPTION information to the cord *(afferent pathway)*. The anterior branch transmits motor impulses to the muscles of the body to allow MOBILITY *(efferent pathway)*.

Each spinal nerve is responsible for the muscle innervation and sensory reception of a given area of the body. The cervical and thoracic spinal nerves are relatively close to their areas of responsibility, whereas the lumbar and sacral spinal nerves are some distance from theirs. Because the spinal cord ends between L1 and L2, the axons of the lumbar and sacral cord extend downward before exiting at the appropriate intervertebral foramen. The area controlled by each spinal nerve is roughly reflected in the dermatomes. **Dermatomes** represent sensory input from spinal nerves to specific areas of the skin (Fig. 41-4). For example, the patient with an injury to cervical spinal nerves

C6 and C7 has sensory changes in the thumb, index finger, middle finger, middle of the palm, and back of the hand.

Sensory receptors throughout the body monitor and transmit impulses of pain, temperature, touch, vibration, pressure, visceral sensation, and proprioception. Sensory receptors also monitor and transmit the sensory perceptions of the special senses (i.e., vision, taste, smell, and hearing).

The cell bodies of the anterior spinal nerves are located in the anterior gray matter (anterior horn) of each level in the spinal cord. The anterior motor neurons are also referred to as *lower motor neurons*. As each nerve axon leaves the spinal cord, it joins other spinal nerves to form **plexuses** (clusters of nerves). Plexuses continue as trunks, divisions, and cords and finally branch into individual peripheral nerves.

The **reflex arc** is a closed circuit of spinal and peripheral nerves and therefore requires no control by the brain (Fig. 41-5).

Reflexes consist of sensory input from:
- Skeletal muscles, tendons, skin, organs, and special senses
- Small cells in the spinal cord lying between the posterior and anterior gray matter (interneurons)
- Anterior motor neurons, along with the muscles they innervate

There are 12 *cranial nerves*. Their number, name, origin, type, and function are summarized in Table 41-3. Cranial nerve function is an important part of the complete neurologic assessment (Jarvis, 2014).

Autonomic Nervous System: Structure and Function

The **autonomic nervous system (ANS)** is composed of two parts: the sympathetic nervous system (SNS) and the parasympathetic nervous system. ANS functions are not usually under conscious control but may be altered in some people by using biofeedback and other methods.

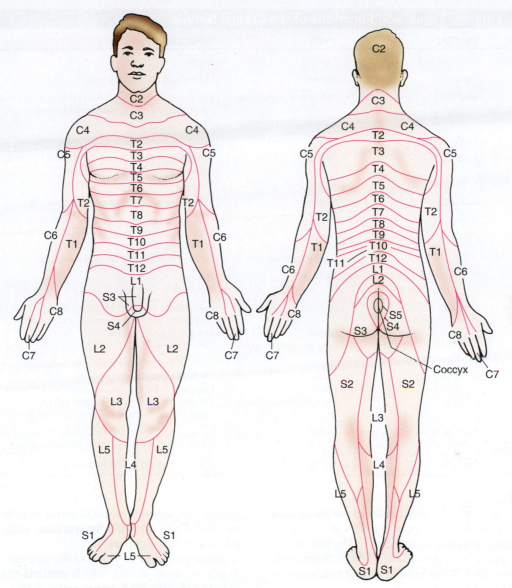

FIG. 41-4 Dermatomes (cutaneous innervation of spinal nerves). *C*, Cervical; *L*, lumbar; *S*, sacral; *T*, thoracic.

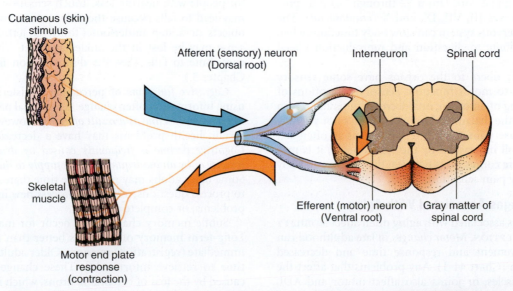

FIG. 41-5 An example of reflex activity. Stimulation of skin results in involuntary muscle contraction (reflex arc).

TABLE 41-3 Origins, Types, and Functions of the Cranial Nerves

CRANIAL NERVE	ORIGIN	TYPE	FUNCTION
I: Olfactory	Olfactory bulb	Sensory	Smell
II: Optic	Midbrain	Sensory	Central and peripheral vision
III: Oculomotor	Midbrain	Motor to eye muscles	Eye movement via medial and lateral rectus and inferior oblique and superior rectus muscles; lid elevation via the levator muscle
		Parasympathetic-motor	Pupil constriction; ciliary muscles
IV: Trochlear	Lower midbrain	Motor	Eye movement via superior oblique muscles
V: Trigeminal	Pons	Sensory	Sensory perception from skin of face and scalp and mucous membranes of mouth and nose
		Motor	Muscles of mastication (chewing)
VI: Abducens	Inferior pons	Motor	Eye movement via lateral rectus muscles
VII: Facial	Inferior pons	Sensory	Pain and temperature from ear area; deep sensations from the face; taste from anterior two thirds of the tongue
		Motor	Muscles of the face and scalp
		Parasympathetic-motor	Lacrimal, submandibular, and sublingual salivary glands
VIII: Vestibulocochlear	Pons-medulla junction	Sensory	Hearing Equilibrium
IX: Glossopharyngeal	Medulla	Sensory	Pain and temperature from ear; taste and sensations from posterior one third of tongue and pharynx
		Motor	Skeletal muscles of the throat
		Parasympathetic-motor	Parotid glands
X: Vagus	Medulla	Sensory	Pain and temperature from ear; sensations from pharynx, larynx, thoracic and abdominal viscera
		Motor	Muscles of the soft palate, larynx, and pharynx
		Parasympathetic-motor	Thoracic and abdominal viscera; cells of secretory glands; cardiac and smooth muscle innervation to the level of the splenic flexure
XI: Accessory	Medulla (anterior gray horn of the cervical spine)	Motor	Skeletal muscles of the pharynx and larynx and sternocleidomastoid and trapezius muscles
XII: Hypoglossal	Medulla	Motor	Skeletal muscles of the tongue

The SNS cells originate in the gray matter of the spinal cord from T1 through L2 or L3. This part of the ANS is considered *thoracolumbar* because of its anatomic location. The SNS stimulates the functions of the body needed for "fight or flight" (e.g., heart and respiratory rate). It also inhibits certain functions not needed in urgent and stressful situations.

The parasympathetic cells originate in the gray matter of the sacral area of the spinal cord (from S2 through S4) plus portions of cranial nerves III, VII, IX, and X *(craniosacral)*. The parasympathetic nervous system can slow body functions when needed and contribute to digestion and reproduction ("feed and breed").

Parasympathetic fibers to the organs have some sensory ability in addition to motor function. Sensory perceptions of irritation, stretching of an organ, or a decrease in tissue oxygen are transmitted to the thalamus through pathways not yet fully understood. Because pain from internal organs is often felt below the body wall innervated by the spinal nerve, it is presumed that there are connections between the viscera and body structure that relay pain sensation.

Neurologic Changes Associated With Aging

Neurologic changes associated with aging often affect MOBILITY and SENSORY PERCEPTION. *Motor changes* in late adulthood can cause slower movement and response time and decreased sensory perception (Chart 41-1). Any problems that affect the nerves, bones, muscles, or joints also affect motor and ADL ability. Determining functional status (i.e., a combination of COGNITION, MOBILITY, and SENSORY PERCEPTION) is a recommended Core Measure for patients with complex chronic conditions (www.cms.gov).

Sensory changes in older adults can also affect their ADLs. Pupils decrease in size, which restricts the amount of light entering the eye, and adapt more slowly. Older adults need increased lighting to see. Chapter 48 describes collaborative care for people with hearing loss. Touch sensation decreases, which may lead to falls because the older person may not feel small objects or a step underfoot (Touhy & Jett, 2014). Vibration sense may be lost in the ankles and feet. These changes can contribute to falls. (See the discussion on fall prevention in Chapter 3.)

Cognitive functions of perceiving, registering, storing, and using information often change as a normal part of aging. *Intellect does not decline as a result of aging.* However, a person with certain health problems may have a decrease in COGNITION. *Cognitive decline is frequently caused by drug interactions or toxicity or by an inadequate oxygen supply to the brain (hypoxia).* Some older adults may need more time than a younger person to process questions, learn and process new information, solve problems, or complete analogies.

Subtle memory changes can occur for many older people. Long-term memory often seems better than recall (recent) or immediate (registration) memory. Older adults may need more time to retrieve information. These changes may be partly caused by the loss of cerebral neurons, which is associated with the aging process.

CHART 41-1 Nursing Focus on the Older Adult

Changes in the Nervous System Related to Aging

PHYSIOLOGIC CHANGES	NURSING IMPLICATIONS	RATIONALES
Slower processing time	Provide sufficient time for the affected older adult to respond to questions and/or direction.	Allowing adequate time for processing helps differentiate normal findings from neurologic deterioration.
Recent memory loss	Reinforce teaching by repetition, using written teaching and memory aids such as electronic alarms or applications for electronic devices that provide recurrent alerts.	Greatest loss of brain weight is in the white matter of the frontal lobe. Intellect is not impaired, but the learning process is slowed. Repetition helps the patient learn new information and recall it when needed.
Decreased sensory perception of touch	Remind the patient to look where his or her feet are placed when walking. Instruct the patient to wear shoes that provide good support when walking. If the patient is unable, change his or her position frequently (every hour) while he or she is in the bed or chair.	Decreased sensory perception may cause the patient to fall.
Change in perception of pain	Ask the patient to describe the nature and specific characteristics of pain. Monitor additional assessment variables to detect possible health problems.	Accurate and complete nursing assessment ensures that the interventions will be appropriate for the older adult (see Chapter 4).
Change in sleep patterns	Ascertain sleep patterns and preferences. Ask if sleep pattern interferes with ADLs. Adjust the patient's daily schedule to his or her sleep pattern and preference as much as possible (e.g., evening versus morning bath).	Older adults require as much sleep as younger adults. It is more common for older adults to fall asleep early and arise early.
Altered balance and/or decreased coordination	Instruct the patient to move slowly when changing positions. If needed, advise the patient to hold on to handrails when ambulating. Assess the need for an ambulatory aid, such as a cane.	The patient may fall if moving too quickly. Assistive and adaptive aids provide support and prevent falls.
Increased risk for infection	Monitor carefully for infection.	Older adults often have structural deterioration of microglia, the cells responsible for cell-mediated immune response in the central nervous system (CNS).
Changes in sleep patterns	Assess sleep habits. Provide usual bedtime routines. Decrease noise and light at night.	Age-related changes include more time in bed spent awake before falling asleep, reduced sleep time, daytime napping, and changes in circadian rhythm leading to "early to bed and early to rise."

Biorhythms vary among people. Circadian responses are reduced in older adults, and the sleep-wake cycle may become less responsive to stimuli that signal patterns of sleep. Older adults may experience changes in sleep habits and sleeping patterns (Touhy & Jett, 2014). For example, older adults are more likely to go bed earlier and experience an earlier awakening compared with younger adults. They are also more likely to experience more periods of wakefulness lasting 30 or more minutes during the night. On average, an older person needs as much sleep as a younger person but is more likely to nap in the afternoon.

Sleep deprivation, common in many inpatient settings, is related to both the earlier onset and greater severity of delirium (acute confusion) in older adults. Lack of sleep can worsen symptoms of mild dementia (chronic confusion). Sleep deprivation can also interfere with normal immune function and wound healing.

Mental status may be impaired as a result of infection, hypoxia, and hypoglycemia or hyperglycemia in the older adult. These conditions are usually easily assessed and managed. During an acute change in mental status, assess the adult for peripheral oxygenation saturation (SpO_2), serum glucose (fingerstick), and potential infection (e.g., fever, urine with sediment or odor, sputum production, red or draining wound). *Often a decrease or change in mental status (e.g., acute confusion) is a key early sign of an infectious process in the older patient, such as a urinary tract infection.*

Health Promotion and Maintenance

Prevention of neurologic health problems includes avoiding risky behaviors and practicing a healthy lifestyle. Young adults, especially men, are particularly at risk for engaging in risky physical activities, such as motorcycle or car racing without wearing a helmet or taking other safety precautions, or diving into shallow water. Unfortunately, these activities often lead to serious spinal cord or traumatic brain injuries and should be avoided. Remind adults of any age to avoid excessive alcohol or other substances that can impair judgment and cause an accident.

Active military men and women who are in or near combat areas are also at risk for neurologic problems, especially traumatic brain injury (TBI). The most common cause of TBI in this population is a blast from an improvised explosive device (IED). Continued improvements in IED detection and protective headgear may help decrease these injuries. TBI in veterans is discussed later in Chapter 45.

Practicing a healthy lifestyle can help promote nervous system health. For example, smoking constricts blood vessels and can lead to decreased PERFUSION to the brain, resulting in a brain attack or stroke. Teach these patients the importance of smoking cessation as discussed elsewhere in this text.

Sleep deprivation at any age can lead to significant changes in COGNITION. Interrupted sleep and sleep deprivation can also impair physical function and self-management. Sleep and rest are both necessary to promote health. Teach patients that proper nutrition and regular exercise are also important to prevent neurologic impairment. For example, the brain requires adequate glucose to function properly. Decreased blood glucose can cause light-headedness and dizziness, leading to falls, especially among older adults. Skipping meals or poor nutrition can affect the function of the body's neurons.

NCLEX EXAMINATION CHALLENGE 41-1

Health Promotion and Maintenance

The nurse performs an initial assessment on an older client. Which assessment findings would the nurse expect to be the result of normal physiologic aging? **Select all that apply.**
A. Confusion
B. Hearing loss
C. Decerebrate positioning
D. Slurred speech
E. Constipation
F. Urinary incontinence

ASSESSMENT: NOTICING AND INTERPRETING

Patient History

Obtain information from the patient about health problems, drug therapy history, smoking and substance abuse history, occupation, and current lifestyle. During your introduction, note the patient's appearance and assess his or her speech, affect, and movement. If he or she seems to have COGNITION deficits or has trouble speaking or hearing, ask a family member or significant other to stay during the interview to help obtain an accurate history. Be sure that glasses, contact lenses, and hearing aids are available if the patient wears any of these devices.

Ask the patient about his or her medical history to determine its association with the current health problem. Inquire about the ability to perform ADLs. Knowing the level of daily activity helps establish a baseline for later comparison as the patient improves or worsens. Ask whether the patient is right handed or left handed. This information is important for several reasons:

- The patient may be somewhat stronger on the dominant side, which is expected.
- The effects of cerebral injury or disease are more pronounced if the dominant hemisphere is involved.

Ask about family neurologic history such as stroke. Some diseases occur more often in certain groups of people and may be caused by a genetic influence or other reason. A number of neurologic diseases have a genetic basis, such as neurodegenerative disorders, migraine headaches, and epilepsy. These genetic risks are described with specific neurologic health problems found later in this unit.

Physical Assessment

Compare each assessment with the patient's baseline, between right and left sides, and between upper and lower extremities. *Two types of neurologic assessments may be performed: a complete assessment and a focused assessment.* Some focused assessments are specifically designed to be rapid to ease repetition when recurrent neurologic assessments are needed to monitor the patient's condition over time. The type chosen depends on the information needed, the time available with the patient, and your clinical skill level. Advanced practice registered nurses (APRNs) and other primary health care providers usually perform the *complete* assessment, with selected parts done by the nurse generalist or staff nurse. Collaborate with the interprofessional health care team to determine which components each member will perform. It is important to understand each component of the assessment and what the results might indicate.

Complete Neurologic Assessment

A complete neurologic assessment includes a history and evaluation of mental status, cranial nerves (see Table 41-3), MOBILITY and motor system function, deep tendon reflexes, SENSORY PERCEPTION, and cerebellar function. Although not all components of a complete assessment are performed by the nurse generalist or staff nurse, noting abnormalities at baseline or with disease progression is important. During any neurologic assessment, look for asymmetry, such as subtle unequal movement in the facial muscles.

The complete neurologic assessment is performed by the primary health care provider (PHCP) to consider whether a single lesion or more than one site in the nervous system may be contributing to abnormal physical assessment findings. If the lesion or injury is in the CNS, the assessment can further help the health care provider determine if abnormalities are in the cortex, below the cortex, or multifocal. These findings, along with patient history, help determine the urgency of treatment. For example, a sudden unilateral (one side of the body) loss in motor function and sensation is an emergency requiring a stroke center and staff with expertise to diagnose and intervene during a "brain attack." A gradual unilateral loss or a variable loss (with waxing and waning symptoms) may be less urgent and not require stroke center expertise. Generally, the nurse completes a *focused* or *rapid assessment* to detect major changes in signs and symptoms.

Assessment of Mental Status. Mental status assessment is generally divided into assessment of *consciousness* and *cognition.* Consciousness is the ability to be aware of the environment, an object, and oneself; it is often documented as one's level of consciousness. **Level of consciousness (LOC)** usually refers to the degree of alertness or amount of stimulation needed to engage a patient's attention and can range from *alert* to *coma.*

The patient who is described as *alert* is awake, engaged, and responsive. A patient may be alert but not oriented to person, place, or time. Patients who are less than alert are labeled *lethargic, stuporous,* or *comatose.* A **lethargic** patient is drowsy but is easily awakened. One who is arousable only with vigorous or painful stimulation is **stuporous**. The **comatose** patient is unconscious and cannot be aroused despite vigorous or noxious simulation.

After determining alertness, the next step is to evaluate *orientation.* Once the patient's attention is engaged, ask questions to determine orientation. Varying the sequence of questioning on repeated assessments prevents the patient from memorizing

Critical Rescue

Be aware that a change in level of consciousness and orientation is the earliest and most reliable indication that central neurologic function has declined! If a decline occurs, contact the Rapid Response Team or PHCP immediately. Perform a focused neurologic assessment as described later in this chapter to determine if additional changes are present.

the answers. Responses that indicate orientation include ability to answer questions about person, place, and time such as:

- The patient's ability to relate the onset of symptoms
- The name of the PHCP or nurse
- The year and month
- Home address
- The name of the health care agency

Time of day, drug therapy, and the need for sleep, glucose, or oxygen may affect these responses. Be sure to link any changes in orientation with respiratory status, changes in drug regimens or use of intermittent drugs, time of day/sleep deprivation, or current serum glucose values. Education, occupation, interest, culture, anxiety, and depression affect performance during assessment of mental status. What is considered "normal" may not be so for a particular patient, so adaptation of questions suggested for mental status assessment may be necessary. Be alert to both *sudden* and *subtle* changes, particularly when changes are noted by family members or others who know the patient.

NCLEX EXAMINATION CHALLENGE 41-2

Physiological Integrity

During a client's neurologic assessment, the nurse finds that the client continues to be drowsy but is easily awakened. How does the nurse document this client's level of consciousness?
A. Stuporous
B. Lethargic
C. Comatose
D. Alert

COGNITION typically is evaluated in a rapid or focused manner using tests of memory and attention that require verbal or written ability (Chart 41-2). *Loss of memory, especially recent memory, tends to be an early sign of neurologic problems.* Three types of memory can be tested: long-term (remote) memory, recall (recent) memory, and immediate memory.

Many *speech and language* skills can be assessed during the initial interview. Language skills include understanding the spoken or written word and being able to speak or write. The patient demonstrates understanding by following directions on admission (e.g., getting undressed). If he or she hesitates, it may be that he or she does not understand the vocabulary or word. When speech hesitation or performance hesitation occurs, point to objects and ask the patient to name them, such as the door or bed. Speech is assessed as being normal, slow, garbled, difficult to find words, or other impairments. If the change in speech is new and represents a deterioration from a previous ability to communicate, this change must be urgently reported to the primary health care provider because it may indicate a stroke, new onset of confusion, or other serious neurologic condition. The speech-language pathologist

CHART 41-2 Best Practice for Patient Safety & Quality Care

Assessment of Cognition

Perform assessment at the following care interactions:
- On admission to and discharge from an institutional care setting
- On transfer from one care setting to another
- Every 8 to 12 hours throughout hospitalization
- Following major changes in pharmacotherapy
- With behavior that is unusual for the person and/or inappropriate to the situation

Assess and document (noting "sometimes," "frequently," or "always" as observed):
- Does the patient respond to voice; require being shaken awake to communicate; doze off during a conversation or when no activities occur; or not respond to voice or touch?
- Is speech clear and understandable; disoriented to person, place, or time; inappropriate; or incomprehensible/garbled?
- Can the patient name the place, reason for admission or visit, month, and age?
- Can the patient follow one-step commands: open/close eyes; make fist/let go?
- Can the patient switch to a different topic or activity versus loses the thread of the conversation or is easily distracted (inattention)?
- Can the patient recognize a familiar object and its purpose or a familiar person and name relationship?
- Can the patient respond relevantly and quickly?
- Does the patient have unrealistic thoughts or act distrustful of others (e.g., does not dare to take his/her medicine; says that people are "listening")?
- Is the patient cooperative, euphoric, hostile, anxious, withdrawn, or guarded?
- Is the patient's appearance, behavior, or facial expression appropriate for the situation?

(SLP) completes additional language tests such as reading comprehension.

CULTURAL/SPIRITUAL CONSIDERATIONS

Patient-Centered Care QSEN

Remember that some patients cannot read or write or may speak a language different from that of the clinician. In this case, modify the examination accordingly such as having the patient copy something that has been drawn (e.g., a cross, circle, diamond, or square). In some cases, an interpreter may be needed.

Several COGNITION screening tests are used by nurses in clinical settings to assess for delirium (acute confusion) or dementia (chronic confusion). Chapter 3 describes common tests for assessing delirium; Chapter 42 describes tests for dementia in the Alzheimer's disease section.

Assessment of Cranial Nerves. Cranial nerves are typically tested to establish a baseline from which to compare progress or deterioration. However, they are not routinely tested unless the patient has a suspected problem affecting one or more of them (see Table 41-3). Adding the specific cranial nerves to be tested to the documentation record of a patient with a problem affecting them helps to ensure continued comparison and assessment.

Testing pupils is a common cranial nerve test performed by nurses. Pupil constriction is a function of cranial nerve III, the oculomotor nerve. **P**upils should be **e**qual in size, **r**ound and **r**egular in shape, and react to **l**ight and **a**ccommodation

(PERRLA). Estimate the size of both pupils using a millimeter ruler or a pupillometer. Patients who have had eye surgery for cataracts or glaucoma often have irregularly shaped pupils. Those using eyedrops for either cataracts or glaucoma may have unequal pupils if only one eye is being treated, and the pupillary response may be altered.

To test for pupil constriction, ask the patient to close his or her eyes and dim the room lights. Bring a penlight in from the side of the patient's head and shine the light in the eye being tested as soon as the patient opens his or her eyes. The pupil being tested should constrict (direct response). The other pupil should also constrict slightly (consensual response). To test accommodation, relight the room and ask the patient to focus on a distant object and then immediately look at an object 4 to 5 inches from the nose. The eyes should converge, and the pupils should constrict. Pinpoint or severely dilated nonreactive pupils are usually late signs of neurologic deterioration (Jarvis, 2014).

Assessment of Motor Function. Throughout the physical assessment, observe the patient for involuntary tremors or movements. Describe these movements as accurately as possible, such as "pill-rolling with the thumbs and fingers at rest" or "intention tremors of both hands" (tremors that occur when the patient tries to do something). These abnormalities can indicate certain diseases, such as multiple sclerosis, or the effects of selected psychotropic drugs. In addition, assess the patient for motor movements that indicate irritability, hyperactivity, or slowed movements. Measure the patient's hand *strength* by asking him or her to grasp and squeeze two fingers of each of your hands. Then compare the grasps for equality of strength. As another means of evaluating strength, try to withdraw the fingers from the patient's grasp and compare the ease or difficulty. He or she should release the grasps on command—another assessment of consciousness and the ability to follow commands.

Collaborate with the physical therapist to test the patient's strength. To test strength against resistance, ask the patient to resist the examiner's bending or straightening of the arm, hand, leg, or foot being tested (Fig. 41-6). A five-point rating scale is commonly used (see Chapter 49). Always evaluate and compare strength on each side. Compare previous results with current findings and report all decreases to the primary health care provider.

Cerebral motor or *brainstem* integrity may also be assessed. Ask the patient to close his or her eyes and hold the arms perpendicular to the body with the palms up for 15 to 30 seconds.

If there is a cerebral or brainstem reason for muscle weakness, the arm on the weak side will start to fall, or "drift," with the palm pronating (turning inward). This is called a pronator drift. The same can be done for the lower extremities, with the patient lying on his or her stomach with the legs bent upward at the knees. However, it is easier for most patients to sit on the side of the bed and extend the legs outward.

Decortication is abnormal motor movement seen in the patient with lesions that interrupt the corticospinal pathways (Fig. 41-7A). The patient's arms, wrists, and fingers are flexed with internal rotation and plantar flexion of the legs. Decerebration is abnormal movement with rigidity characterized by extension of the arms and legs, pronation of the arms, plantar flexion, and opisthotonos (body spasm in which the body is bowed forward) (Fig. 41-7B). Decerebration is usually associated with dysfunction in the brainstem area.

Assessment of Reflex Activity. The primary health care provider, including the APRN, may assess deep tendon reflexes (DTRs) and superficial (cutaneous) reflexes. The deep tendon reflexes of the biceps, triceps, brachioradialis, and quadriceps muscles and of the Achilles tendon can be tested as part of the complete neurologic assessment (Jarvis, 2014). Striking the tendon with the reflex hammer should cause contraction of the muscle. The appropriate muscle contraction indicates an intact reflex arc.

The cutaneous (superficial) reflexes usually tested are the plantar reflexes and sometimes the abdominal reflexes. The plantar reflex is tested with a pointed (but not sharp) object, such as the handle end of the reflex hammer or the rounded end of bandage scissors. The normal response is plantar flexion of all toes. Babinski's sign, a dorsiflexion of the great toe and fanning of the other toes, is abnormal in anyone older than 2 years and represents the presence of central nervous system (CNS) disease. The terms *positive Babinski's sign* (abnormal response) and *negative Babinski's sign* (normal response) are clinically used terms but are not technically accurate. Health care team members may also use the terms *upgoing* or *downgoing* to refer to the toes of the stimulated foot. Upgoing toes are an abnormal response that indicates the presence of pathology in the CNS. Babinski's sign can occur with drug and alcohol intoxication, after a seizure, or in patients with multiple sclerosis or severe liver disease.

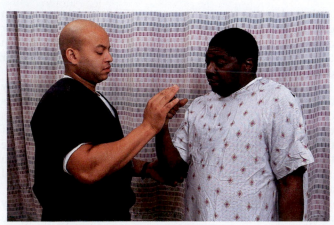

FIG. 41-6 Testing for strength against resistance.

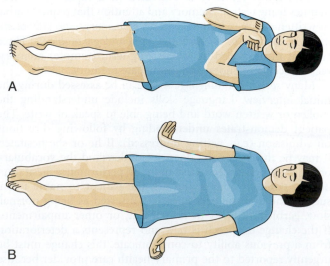

FIG. 41-7 Posturing. **A,** Decorticate posturing. **B,** Decerebrate posturing.

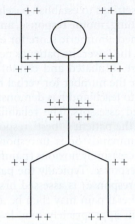

0	Absent, no response
1 (+)	Weaker than normal, hypoactive
2 (++)	Normal
3 (+++)	Stronger or more brisk than normal
4 (++++)	Hyperactive
	(Note: 1 and 3 may be normal for some individuals.)

FIG. 41-8 Stick figure and scale for recording reflex activity.

Hyperactive reflexes indicate possible upper motor neuron disease (damage to the brain or upper spinal cord). *Hypoactive* reflexes may result from lower motor neuron disease (damage to the lower spinal cord) or neuromuscular diseases.

Asymmetry of reflexes is an important finding because it probably indicates a disease process or injury. The results of reflex testing are recorded by the use of a stick figure and a scale of 0 to 4 (Fig. 41-8). A score of 2 is considered normal, although scores of 1 (hypoactive) or 3 (stronger than normal) may be normal for a particular patient. Clonus (also called *myoclonus*) is the sudden, brief, jerking contraction of a muscle or muscle group often seen in seizures.

Assessment of Sensory Function. The acuity level of the patient determines how often the sensory assessment is done. For example, patients with acute spinal cord trauma or ascending Guillain-Barré syndrome (GBS) are assessed every hour until stable and then every 4 hours. As the condition improves, sensory assessment may be needed only once each shift. Findings are documented according to agency protocol. A special spinal cord assessment flow sheet may be used to document sensory and/or motor findings for the patient with a spinal cord injury.

Pain and temperature sensation are transmitted by the same nerve endings. Therefore if one sensation is tested and found to be intact, it can safely be assumed that the other is intact. Testing temperature sensation can usually be accomplished using a cold reflex hammer and the warm touch of the hand for patients with known or suspected spinal problems.

Assess for *pain perception* with any sharp or dull object, such as the tips of a cotton-tipped applicator. While the patient's eyes are open, demonstrate what will be done. Then ask him or her to keep eyes closed and to indicate whether the touch is sharp or dull. The sharp and dull ends should be changed at random so he or she does not anticipate the next type of stimulus for SENSORY PERCEPTION. Not all areas need to be tested unless a spinal cord injury has occurred. If testing begins on the hands and feet, there is no need to test the other parts of the extremities because the tracts transmitting pain and

temperature sensations are intact. Compare reactions on each side. A sensation reported as dull when the stimulus was actually sharp requires further testing. A patient with sensory loss as a result of diabetes mellitus or peripheral vascular disease may or may not be aware of the loss until tested. Some patients with chronic illness may report that they have had sensory losses for a long time. Before testing for pain, the nurse must check to determine whether the patient is on anticoagulant therapy. If the patient is on anticoagulant therapy, avoid any testing with a sharp object because it can cause bleeding.

Light touch discrimination is likely to be normal if pain and temperature sensory tracts are intact. Touch discrimination and two-point discrimination may be assessed as part of a complete neurologic examination by the PHCP.

For testing *touch discrimination*, the patient closes his or her eyes. The practitioner touches the patient with a finger and asks that he or she point to the area touched. This procedure is repeated on each extremity at random rather than at sequential points. Next, the practitioner touches the patient on each side of the body on corresponding sites at the same time. The patient should be able to point to both sites.

The clinician then touches the patient in two places on the same extremity with two objects, such as cotton-tipped applicators. A person can normally identify two points fairly close together, depending on the location of the stimuli. When an area is heavily innervated, the *two-point discrimination will feel closer.*

Abnormal sensory findings may have a CNS or a peripheral nervous system (PNS) cause. The neuropathies of diabetes, malnutrition, and vascular problems have a PNS cause. Damage to a specific spinal nerve may not result in significant sensory loss because the spinal nerves overlap. Injury to several nearby spinal nerves is manifested as decreased or absent SENSORY PERCEPTION in the dermatomes of those nerves.

CNS problems in the brainstem, thalamus, and cortex generally result in loss of sensation on the contralateral (opposite) side of the body. Cerebellar lesions result in sensory deficits on the *same* side of the body.

Assessment of Cerebellar Function. Most of the assessment of cerebellar function can be performed with the patient sitting on the side of the bed or examining table. Fine *coordination* of muscle activity is tested. If cerebellar problems are suspected or diagnosed, ask the patient to perform these tasks with his or her eyes closed:

- Run the heel of one foot down the shin of the other leg and repeat with the other leg (the patient should be able to do this smoothly and keep the heel on the shin).
- Place the hands palm-up and then palm-down on each thigh, repeating as fast as possible (this can normally be done rapidly).
- With arms out at the side, touch the finger to the nose two or three times, with eyes open and then with eyes closed (this can be done with alternating arms or with each arm individually).

For the last part of the cerebellar assessment, the *ambulatory* patient stands for testing of *gait and equilibrium*. Gait and equilibrium are usually tested at the end or beginning of the entire neurologic assessment. Ask the patient to walk across the room, turn, and return. Observe for uneven steps, difficulty walking, and so forth. To evaluate balance, ask him or her to stand on one foot and then on the other. Tiptoe and heel-to-toe walking can also demonstrate gait problems. For patients with sciatic nerve involvement, pain may worsen when they walk on their toes or heels.

To test equilibrium, ask the patient to stand with arms at the sides, feet and knees close together, and eyes open. Check for swaying and then ask him or her to close his or her eyes and maintain position. The examiner should be close enough to prevent falling if the patient cannot stay erect. If he or she sways with the eyes closed but not when the eyes are open (the **Romberg sign**), the problem is probably **proprioceptive** (awareness of body position). If the patient sways with the eyes both open and closed, the neurologic disturbance is probably *cerebellar* in origin (Jarvis, 2014).

If the patient cannot perform any of these activities smoothly, the problem is manifested on the same side as the cerebellar lesion. If both lobes of the cerebellum are involved, the incoordination affects both sides of the body (bilateral).

Rapid/Focused Neurologic Assessment

A rapid/focused neurologic assessment, or "neuro check," is completed when the patient is admitted to a health care facility on an emergent basis. It is also a major part of frequent ongoing patient assessment and performed in the event of a sudden change in neurologic status. The typical record contains data related to alertness, orientation, movement of arms and legs, and pupil size and reaction to light. *Be sure to document all aspects of the rapid neurologic assessment frequently in the designated or standardized part of the electronic record as needed per agency protocol or health care provider request.*

An example of a standard rapid neurologic assessment tool is the **Glasgow Coma Scale (GCS)** (Fig. 41-9). The GCS is used in many acute care settings to establish baseline data in each of these areas: eye opening, motor response, and verbal response. The patient is assigned a numeric score for each of these areas. The lower the score, the lower the patient's neurologic function. For patients who are intubated and cannot talk, record their score with a "t" after the number for verbal response.

The GCS is easy to teach and has demonstrated a consistent score among trained assessors. The reliability of the GCS is based on recording the patient's "best" response. If the patient does not follow commands or is unresponsive to voice, the nurse proceeds to increasingly noxious (painful) stimuli to elicit an eye and motor response. Typically the patient's response to central pain (brain response) is assessed first. On the basis of this response, peripheral pain may then be assessed. Failure to apply painful stimuli appropriately may lead to an incorrect conclusion about the patient's neurologic status. If the patient responds fully to voice or light touch, there is no need to progress to more vigorous or painful stimuli.

Start with the least noxious irritation or pressure and proceed to more painful stimulation if the patient does not respond. Begin each phase of the assessment by speaking in a normal voice. If no response is obtained, use a loud voice. If the patient does not respond, gently shake him or her. The shaking should be similar to that used in attempting to wake up a child. If that is unsuccessful, apply painful stimuli using one of these methods:

- Supraorbital (above eyes) pressure by placing a thumb under the orbital rim in the middle of the eyebrow and pushing upward (Do not use this technique if the patient has orbital or facial fractures.)
- Trapezius muscle squeeze by pinching or squeezing the trapezius muscle located at the angle of the shoulder and neck muscle
- Mandibular (jaw) pressure to the jaw by using your index and middle fingers to pinch the lower jaw
- Sternal (breastbone) rub by making a fist and rubbing/twisting your knuckles against the sternum

The tissue in these areas is tender, and bruising is not unusual. Therefore do not use this technique for older adults or for patients who may experience severe bruising (e.g., recipients of anticoagulant therapy). Peripheral pain is assessed with pressure at the base of the nail on one finger or one toe, both on the right and left.

The patient may respond to painful stimuli in several ways. Although the initial response to pain may be abnormal flexion or extension, continued application of pain for no more than 20 to 30 seconds may demonstrate that he or she can localize or withdraw. If the patient does not respond after 20 to 30 seconds, stop applying the painful stimulus.

Psychosocial Assessment

Patients vary in their responses to a suspected or actual health problem, often depending on whether it is acute or chronic. Response is also influenced by MOBILITY, SENSORY PERCEPTION, and/or COGNITION; these abilities can be temporarily or permanently altered as a result of neurologic disease or injury. For example, patients who have a mild stroke and no lasting neurologic deficits are less likely to be severely depressed than patients who experience a loss of independent movement or impaired communication as a result of a stroke.

Depression can result in cognitive and behavioral changes that are similar to delirium or dementia. Depression is a

---

GLASGOW COMA SCALE*

Eye Opening

Spontaneous	4
To sound	3
To pain	2
Never	1

Motor Response

Obeys commands	6
Localizes pain	5
Normal flexion (withdrawal)	4
Abnormal flexion	3
Extension	2
None	1

Verbal Response

Oriented	5
Confused conversation	4
Inappropriate words	3
Incomprehensible sounds	2
None	1

* The highest possible score is 15.

FIG. 41-9 The Glasgow Coma Scale.

! NURSING SAFETY PRIORITY QSEN

Critical Rescue

A decrease of 2 or more points in the Glasgow Coma Scale total is clinically significant and should be communicated to the primary health care provider (PHCP) immediately. Other findings requiring urgent communication with the health care provider include a new finding of abnormal flexion or extension, particularly of the upper extremities (decerebrate or decorticate posturing); pinpoint or dilated nonreactive pupils; and sudden or subtle changes in mental status. Remember, a change in level of consciousness is the earliest sign of neurologic deterioration. Communicate early recognition of neurologic changes to the Rapid Response Team or primary health care provider for the best opportunity to prevent complications and preserve CNS function.

? NCLEX EXAMINATION CHALLENGE 41-3

Physiological Integrity

The nurse is assessing a client who opens both eyes when spoken to, obeys commands, and seems confused during conversation. Which Glasgow Coma Score (GCS) will the nurse document?

A. 15
B. 14
C. 11
D. 9

common mental health disorder that is often missed in a variety of health care settings, especially in settings that care for older adults (Touhy & Jett, 2014). Consider using a depression screening tool such as the Center for Epidemiological Studies Depression-Revised (CESD-R) or the Geriatric Depression Scale (short form) to identify patients with depressive symptoms. Refer them to the appropriate provider (both primary care and mental health care) if the screening is positive. Chapter 3 discusses depression in older adults. More information on depression can be found in mental/behavioral health resources.

⊕ CULTURAL/SPIRITUAL CONSIDERATIONS

Patient-Centered Care QSEN

Age may also be a factor in how a patient accepts the illness. For instance, a young adult who has a motorcycle crash causing a traumatic brain injury (TBI) may react differently from an older adult who has a spinal injury. In some cases, the patient's emotional responses result from the health problem itself, especially for TBI patients.

Men may feel differently about their illness than women. Male patients who have had strokes are typically depressed more often than women who have had strokes. Discussions of these response differences can be found in the following chapters on specific neurologic health problems.

Regardless of what the health problem is, do not assume that everyone reacts the same way to his or her illness or injury. Consider the cultural and spiritual background of the patient because this will influence his or her reaction. Patients experiencing the grieving process may fluctuate among denial, anger, and depression. Encourage patients to express their feelings and have hope. Refer them to the appropriate support services as needed, including counseling, social work, or clergy, depending on patient preference and service availability. Assess the patient's support systems, including family members and friends, if available. Be sure to document your assessment and interventions.

Diagnostic Assessment

Laboratory Assessment

Fluid, electrolyte, and glucose abnormalities can cause neurologic impairment. The basic metabolic panel (BMP) and serum calcium, phosphorus, and magnesium are evaluated. Both anemia and malnutrition can contribute to neurologic disorders so a complete blood count and serum levels of albumin and minerals/vitamins (particularly B vitamins) are collected. Arterial blood to evaluate pH, oxygen, and carbon dioxide levels may be collected because these three results, when either too high or too low, can alter neurologic status. For patients with a neurologic problem resulting from an infection, cultures are necessary to identify the pathogen. Although the cause of infection must be determined for any patient, this is especially true for those with existing CNS disease. The blood-brain barrier is often not intact in neurologic disease; and the patient is more likely to get an infection of the nervous system, such as meningitis or encephalitis.

Imaging Assessment

In general, for any image that involves being placed in a scanner, the nurse needs to be aware of special circumstances that can either prevent the procedure from taking place or interfere with it. If the patient is alert and claustrophobic, two options are available: one is a mild sedative such as diazepam (Valium) to calm the patient; the other option is an open scanner. The nurse must determine whether the patient has any metal prosthetics, such as heart valves or shrapnel in the part of the body to be scanned. If he or she does have any type of metal object in the body part to be examined, the nurse must notify the radiology department immediately because the procedure may need to be cancelled. If the patient does have a metal prosthetic or device, the nurse should ask the patient or significant other if he or she carries a medical alert card from the manufacturer. Medical device manufacturers issue cards to PHCPs for their patients to carry with the device number and instructions if radiologic diagnostic testing is needed.

Plain X-Rays. Plain *x-rays* of the skull and spine are used to determine bony fractures, curvatures, bone erosion, bone dislocation, and possible calcification of soft tissue, which can damage the nervous system. Several views are taken (i.e., anteroposterior, lateral, oblique, and, when necessary, special views of the facial bones). *In head trauma and multiple injuries, after assessing the ABCs (airway, breathing, and circulation), one of the first priorities is to rule out cervical spine fracture.*

Explain that the x-ray procedure for the skull and spine is similar to that for a chest x-ray. The patient must remain still during the procedure. Remind him or her that the exposure to radiation is minimal. If the patient is in traction and a portable x-ray unit is not available, the nurse may need to accompany him or her to help with positioning. Any patient who cannot walk from a wheelchair to the x-ray table should be transferred to the radiology department on a stretcher. Hospitals may have specific procedures for transferring patients in wheelchairs or on stretchers. Check with your hospital on this procedure. For example, with a patient who is confused or disoriented, the hospital radiology department staff may require two or more hospital personnel to assist with the transfer. The patient is positioned for each of the desired views and is asked to not move just before each x-ray. Follow-up care is not required.

Cerebral Angiography. Cerebral angiography (arteriography) is done to visualize the cerebral circulation to detect blockages in the arteries or veins in the brain, head, or neck that impair PERFUSION. It remains the gold standard for the diagnosis of intracranial vascular disease and is required for any transcatheter therapy or for surgical intervention. Angiography may be used to identify aneurysms, traumatic injuries, strictures/occlusions, tumors, blood vessel displacement from edema, and arteriovenous (AV) malformations.

Patient Preparation. Risk factors for adverse events must be determined before scheduling the test. Patients sensitive to iodine may be sensitive to iodinated contrast agents. Patients with a history of hypersensitivity in general (e.g., multiple food allergies or asthma) are more likely to have an adverse reaction than the general population. Seafood allergies are no longer considered an indicator of iodinated contrast allergy. Patients with known contrast sensitivity are pre-treated with steroids. Chart 41-3 summarizes the precautions that must be taken for patients having any test using contrast agents.

To minimize the risk for aspiration during the procedure, assess for the presence of nausea or recent vomiting and medicate as needed before the test. Ensure that the patient is NPO 4 to 6 hours before the test. Assess and document neurologic signs, vital signs, and neurovascular checks.

Reinforce these important points:

- Your head is immobilized during the procedure.
- Do not move during the procedure.
- Contrast dye is injected through a catheter placed in the femoral artery. You will feel a warm or hot sensation when the dye is injected; this is normal.
- You will be able to talk to the physician; let him or her know if you are in pain or have any concerns.

Procedure. The patient is placed on an examining table and made as comfortable as possible. At this time, dentures and hearing aids must be removed. He or she is then connected to cardiac monitoring throughout the procedure. Deep or moderate sedation is usually not used, although the patient may be given medication for relaxation.

The interventional radiologist or other specially trained physician numbs the area at the groin and inserts a catheter into the femoral artery. Under fluoroscopic guidance, the catheter is advanced into a carotid or vertebral artery. Then the physician injects contrast material into each vessel while recording images from different angles over the head and neck. After all the vessels have been imaged, the radiologist reviews all the images and consults with the referring physician to decide whether the patient could benefit from a therapeutic radiologic procedure or surgery to treat the problem. An arterial closure device is typically used to seal the artery and prevent bleeding.

The x-ray images are stored on a computer. With older equipment, a two-dimensional picture of the vessels is produced. Most radiographic systems now come with software to create three-dimensional images of the blood vessels in the head and/or neck. These systems can also display a "subtracted image" made from two images—one just before the contrast was injected and one with the contrast in the artery.

Follow-Up Care. Follow agency policy regarding care of the injection site, which may include:

- Check the dressing for bleeding and swelling around the site.
- Apply an ice pack to site.
- Keep the extremity straight and immobilized.
- Maintain the pressure dressing for 2 hours.

Check the extremity for adequate circulation to include skin color and temperature, pulses distal to the injection site, and capillary refill. Be sure to monitor for the risks of the procedure, including contrast reaction (usually manifested by hives and flushing), thrombosis (clotting), and bleeding from the entry site. If bleeding is present, maintain manual pressure on the site and notify the physician immediately. Assess vital signs and neurologic status. Increase oral or IV fluid intake

---

◎ **CHART 41-3** **Best Practice for Patient Safety & Quality Care**

Precautions for the Use of Iodine-Based or Gadolinium Contrast for Diagnostic Testing

Special precautions are taken for patients who will receive an iodinated or high-osmolar contrast agent (e.g., gadolinium) as part of their diagnostic test. These measures include:

- Following agency guidelines regarding informed consent.
- Screening patients at risk for developing contrast-induced kidney damage:
  - Ask the patient about all allergies (food, drug, environmental antigens), asthma, and prior reaction to contrast agents.
  - Review for the presence of these conditions:
    - Pre-existing renal disease such as a diagnosis of chronic kidney disease
    - Diabetic nephropathy
    - Heart failure
    - Dehydration
    - Older age
    - Drugs that interfere with renal perfusion such as metformin or NSAIDs
    - Administration of contrast media in the previous 72 hours
- Evaluating current kidney function. Patients with a serum creatinine greater than or equal to 1.5 mg/dL *or* a calculated glomerular filtration rate (GFR) of less than 60 mL/min are at highest risk for kidney damage from contrast media.

- Communicating with the health care provider before diagnostic testing when risk factors and allergic reaction to iodinated contrast are present:
  - Consider including a discussion of the patient's serum creatinine as a component of the "time-out" process before a diagnostic procedure.
  - Document the date, time, and name of the health care provider with whom communication of risk occurred and which actions were prescribed, if any.
  - Hold medications that are associated with kidney damage for 24-48 hours before *and* after the test.
- Providing adequate hydration before and after contrast administration:
  - Collaborate with the health care provider to determine whether hydration before the diagnostic test, typically with IV normal saline, is needed. Bicarbonate with normal saline; or an IV dose of *N*-acetylcysteine may be used in a high-risk patient.
  - Determine the optimal post-diagnostic intake and output. Provide sufficient hydration to flush out the contrast with oral or IV fluids over the 4-5 hours following the test.
- Re-evaluating serum creatinine and glomerular filtration rate (GFR) 24-48 hours after the diagnostic test. Communicate an increase of serum creatinine 0.5 mg/dL above baseline and a decrease in GFR >25% to the health care provider. Document communication and follow-up interventions, if any. Generally the peak creatinine rise is at 48-72 hours after the administration of contrast.

unless contraindicated. Document all nursing assessments and interventions.

Computed Tomography. Computed tomography (CT) scanning is an accurate, quick, easy, noninvasive, painless, and least-expensive method of diagnosing neurologic problems. Using x-rays (i.e., ionizing radiation), pictures are taken at many horizontal levels, or slices, of the brain or spinal cord. A computer then generates three-dimensional detailed anatomic pictures of tissues, typically the brain, spinal cord, or peripheral neuromuscular system in neurologic testing. A contrast medium may be used to enhance the image. CT scans distinguish bone, soft tissue (e.g., the brain, vascular system, and ventricular system), and fluids such as cerebrospinal fluid (CSF) or blood. Tumors, infarctions, hemorrhage, hydrocephalus, and bone malformations can also be identified.

The patient is placed on a movable table in a head-holding device. He or she must remain completely still during the test, which may be difficult. The table is positioned in the machine—a large, donut-shaped structure. Depending on the scan, the patient may be completely enclosed or in a more open situation. A noncontrast series of pictures are taken first. Then, if needed, the patient is withdrawn from the scanner and given an injection of the iodinated contrast medium. The scan is then repeated. Each set of head scans takes less than 5 minutes in newer scanners. Spinal studies take about 10 minutes per body section (cervical, thoracic, lumbar) and are less likely to require contrast injection.

Most patients with new cranial neurologic symptoms have both a precontrast and postcontrast study of the head. Contrast-enhanced CT is especially useful in locating and identifying tumor types and abscesses. For situations in which bleeding is the only concern (e.g., in trauma patients), contrast scans are not usually required.

After a standard CT scan, imaging software digitally removes images of soft tissue so only images of bone remain. Through the use of this technology, bone deformities, trauma, and birth defects are more easily identified.

CT angiography involves administering contrast dye IV before the CT scan. It is used to identify blockages or narrowing of blood vessels, aneurysms, and other blood vessel abnormalities.

A *CT perfusion study* is an important tool in the evaluation of patients with acute stroke-like symptoms. There are several causes of these symptoms, and the cause must be determined as quickly as possible so the correct treatment can begin for optimal outcomes. Perfusion CT is performed using an advanced CT scanner with a special software system. For the patient, though, it will seem like a standard CT examination.

An *intrathecal contrast-enhanced CT* scan is performed to diagnose disorders of the spine and spinal nerve roots. A lumbar puncture is performed so a small amount of spinal fluid can be removed and mixed with contrast dye and injected. The patient is positioned to allow for the contrast medium to move around the spinal cord and nerve roots as needed. He or she may have a headache after the procedure. Follow facility policy regarding patient positioning after the procedure.

Magnetic Resonance Imaging. Magnetic resonance imaging (MRI or MR) has advantages over CT in the diagnostic imaging of the brain, spinal cord, and nerve roots. It does not use ionizing radiation but instead relies on magnetic fields. Multiple sets of images are taken that are used to determine normal and abnormal anatomy. Images may be enhanced with the use of gadolinium, a non–iodine-based contrast medium. MRIs of the

? NCLEX EXAMINATION CHALLENGE 41-4
Physiological Integrity

The nurse is teaching a client about what to expect during a cerebral angiographic examination. Which statement by the client indicates a need for **further** teaching?

A. "I can't have this test because I am allergic to shellfish."
B. "My head will be strapped in place so I don't move."
C. "I'll have to keep my leg very still after the procedure."
D. "I'll have a temporary dressing on my groin."

spine have largely replaced CT scans and myelography for evaluation. Bony structures cannot be viewed with MRI; CT scans are the best way to see bones. Some facilities have a *functional MRI (fMRI)* machine that can assess blood flow to the brain rather than merely show its anatomic structure.

In addition to the traditional MRI, *magnetic resonance angiography (MRA)*, *magnetic resonance spectroscopy (MRS)*, or *diffusion imaging (DI)* may be requested. MRA is used to evaluate PERFUSION and blood vessel abnormalities such as an arterial blockage, intracranial aneurysms, and AV malformations. MRS is used to detect abnormalities in the brain's biochemical processes, such as that which occurs in epilepsy, Alzheimer's disease, and brain attack (stroke). DI uses MRI techniques to evaluate ischemia in the brain to determine the location and severity of a stroke.

Newer, open-sided units ("open MRI") now produce adequate images for patients who are claustrophobic or do not want standard MRI scanners. However, image quality from these scanners is not as good as that from long-bore traditional scanners. Traditional scanners have higher magnetic field strength and provide better resolution, especially for patients with neurologic health problems.

MRI has been contraindicated for patients with cardiac pacemakers, other implanted pumps or devices, and ion-containing metal aneurysm clips. Extensive trials are testing ways to safely scan some patients with pacemakers. Other implanted devices, such as vascular stents, intravascular catheter (IVC) filters, and metal antiembolic devices, may be scanned immediately or after a certain period of time, depending on manufacturer recommendations. MRI may also be contraindicated in patients who are confused or agitated, have unstable vital signs, are on continuous life support, or have older tattoos (which contain lead). New physiologic monitoring systems made specifically for the scanner allow some patients who are unstable to be scanned. A comprehensive online list of medical devices tested for MRI safety and compatibility can be found at *www.mrisafety.com*. Medical personnel must remove any medical devices they are carrying or wearing and ensure that only approved devices are allowed in the MRI room.

Computed Tomography–Positron Emission Tomography. Single PET machines are no longer commonly used or available. Instead, the newest PET machines are combination CT-PET scanners that fuse images together to produce better information about the type and location of neurologic dysfunction. They are particularly useful in staging brain, spinal cord, and other primary cancers.

The physician or nuclear medicine technologist injects the patient with IV deoxyglucose, which is tagged to an isotope. The isotope emits activity in the form of positrons, which are scanned and converted into a color image by computer. The more active a given part of the brain, the greater the glucose uptake. This test is used to evaluate drug metabolism and detect areas of metabolic alteration that occur in dementia, epilepsy, psychiatric and degenerative disorders, neoplasms, and Alzheimer's disease. The level of radiation is equivalent to that of five or six x-rays but much less than exposure during CT.

Teach the patient that he or she will be NPO the night before morning testing and 4 hours before afternoon testing. Patients with diabetes have their test in the morning before taking their antidiabetic drugs. During this 2- to 3-hour procedure, the patient may be blindfolded and have earplugs inserted for all or part of the test. He or she is asked to perform certain mental functions to activate different areas of the brain. Older adults and patients with mental health/behavioral health problems may be too anxious to have a CT-PET scan.

Single-Photon Emission Computed Tomography.

The single-photon emission computed tomography (SPECT) uses a radiopharmaceutical agent that enables radioisotopes to cross the blood-brain barrier. The agent is administered by IV injection. Gamma-emitting radionuclides have longer half-lives, therefore eliminating the need for a cyclotron near the scanner. Although SPECT is less expensive than PET, the resolution of the images is limited. SPECT is particularly useful in studying cerebral blood flow, amnesia, neoplasms, head trauma, or persistent vegetative state. The test is contraindicated in women who are breast-feeding.

The patient is injected with the material about 1 hour before the actual scan by the radiologist, certified nuclear medicine technologist, or specially trained RN. The patient is positioned on an x-ray table in a quiet dark room for the actual scans. Several gamma cameras scan his or her head. When completed, the images are downloaded to a computer.

Magnetoencephalography.

Magnetoencephalography (MEG) is a noninvasive imaging technique used to measure the magnetic fields produced by electrical activity in the brain via extremely sensitive devices such as superconducting quantum interference devices (SQUIDs). MEG is somewhat similar to electroencephalography (EEG). The advantage is greater accuracy because of the minimal distortion of the signal. This allows for more usable and reliable localization of brain function. The brain can be observed "in action" rather than just from viewing a still MRI image. These machines are not widely available because of their extremely high cost.

Other Diagnostic Assessment

Electromyography. Electromyography (EMG) is used to identify nerve and muscle disorders, as well as spinal cord disease. (See Chapter 42 for a description of patient preparation, procedure, and follow-up care.) Electromyography and electroneurography or nerve-conduction velocity studies (NCVSs) are usually used together and are referred to as *electromyoneurography.*

Electroencephalography. Electroencephalography (EEG) records the electrical activity of the cerebral hemispheres. Each graphic recording represents electrical impulses within the brain. The frequency, amplitude, and characteristics of the brain waves are recorded. For example, a cerebral tumor or infarct may have abnormally slow waveforms.

Patient Preparation. Fasting is avoided before EEG testing because hypoglycemia can alter the test results. Ensure that hair is clean and without conditioners, hair creams, lotions, sprays, or styling gels. Teach the patient to avoid the use of sedatives or stimulants in the 12 to 24 hours preceding the EEG. Ensure a quiet room with signage to inform visitors of EEG recording in progress. Instruct the patient or family members about the reasons for periodic or continuous monitoring. The reasons for EEG monitoring include:

- Determining the general activity of the cerebral hemispheres
- Determining the origin of seizure activity (epilepsy)
- Determining cerebral function in epilepsy and other pathologic conditions such as tumors, abscesses, cerebrovascular disease, hematomas, injury, metabolic diseases, degenerative brain disease, and drug intoxication
- Differentiating between organic and hysterical or feigned blindness or deafness
- Monitoring cerebral activity during surgical anesthesia or sedation in the intensive care unit
- Diagnosing sleep disorders (If the EEG is related to a sleep disorder diagnosis, the patient may be asked to sleep less the night before the EEG.)
- Assisting in the determination of brain death

Procedure. The patient is placed on a reclining chair or bed. Multiple electrodes are applied to the scalp with a jellylike substance and connected to the machine. The physician or EEG technician places glue over the electrodes to prevent slippage. The patient must lie still with his or her eyes closed during the initial recording. The rest of the test engages the patient in certain activities: hyperventilation, photic stimulation, and sleep. A portable EEG may be performed at the bedside if necessary, but the preference is for the EEG to be done in a very quiet room.

Hyperventilation produces cerebral vasoconstriction and alkalosis, which increase the likelihood of seizure activity. The patient is asked to breathe deeply 20 times per minute for 3 minutes. In *photic stimulation,* a flashing bright light is placed in front of the patient. Frequencies of 1 to 20 flashes per second are used with the patient's eyes open and then closed. If the patient's seizures are photosensitive in origin, seizure activity may be seen on the EEG. A *sleep* EEG may be performed to aid in the detection of abnormal brain waves that are seen only when the patient is sleeping, such as with frontal lobe epilepsy.

During an EEG test, which takes 45 to 120 minutes, the recording can be stopped about every 5 minutes to allow the patient to move. If he or she moves during the recording, movement creates a change in the brain waves, and the technician will note movements on the graph. Examples of unintentional movement that can affect the recordings are tongue movement, eye blinking, and muscle tensing. The technician may induce or request certain movements or sensory stimulation and record these events on the EEG record to link changes in brain waves with motor activity or sensory stimulation; these intentional movements are also documented on the EEG recording.

Follow-Up Care. The gel and glue used for placing electrodes can be washed out immediately after the test ends. Acetone or witch hazel will dissolve the paste. Advise the patient who has had a sleep-deprived EEG to have someone drive the patient home.

Evoked Potentials. Evoked potentials (also called *evoked response*) measure the electrical signals to the brain generated by sound, touch, or light. These tests are used to assess sensory nerve problems and confirm neurologic conditions, including multiple sclerosis, brain tumor, acoustic neuroma (small tumors of the inner ear), and spinal cord injury. Evoked potentials are also used to monitor brain activity in comatose patients and confirm brain death. During evoked potentials, a second set of electrodes is attached to the part of the body that will experience sensation. A stimulus is applied, and the amount of time it takes for the impulse generated by the stimulus to reach the brain is recorded. Under normal circumstances, the process of signal transmission is instantaneous.

Auditory evoked potentials (also called *brainstem auditory evoked response*) are used to assess high-frequency hearing loss, diagnose any damage to the acoustic nerve and auditory pathways in the brainstem, and detect acoustic neuromas. The patient sits in a soundproof room and wears headphones. Clicking sounds are delivered one at a time to one ear while a masking sound is sent to the other ear.

Visual evoked potentials detect loss of vision from optic nerve damage (in particular, damage caused by multiple sclerosis). The patient sits close to a screen and is asked to focus on the center of a shifting checkerboard pattern. Only one eye is tested at a time. The other eye is either kept closed or covered with a patch.

Somatosensory evoked potentials measure response from stimuli to the peripheral nerves and can detect nerve or spinal cord damage or nerve degeneration from multiple sclerosis and other degenerating diseases. Tiny electrical shocks are delivered by electrode to a nerve in an arm or leg.

Lumbar Puncture. Lumbar puncture (spinal tap) is the insertion of a spinal needle into the subarachnoid space between the third and fourth (sometimes the fourth and fifth) lumbar vertebrae.

A lumbar puncture (LP) is used to:
- Obtain cerebrospinal fluid (CSF) pressure readings with a manometer
- Obtain CSF for analysis
- Check for spinal blockage caused by a spinal cord lesion
- Inject contrast medium or air for diagnostic study
- Inject spinal anesthetics
- Inject selected drugs

Patient Preparation. Because of the danger of sudden release of CSF pressure, a lumbar puncture is not done for patients with symptoms indicating severely increased intracranial pressure (ICP). The procedure is also not performed in patients with skin infections at or near the puncture site because of the danger of introducing infective organisms into the CSF.

! NURSING SAFETY PRIORITY QSEN

Action Alert

It is very important that the patient not move during a lumbar puncture. If the patient is restless or cannot cooperate, two people may need to assist instead of one. The patient may need a sedative to reduce movement. Consider patient needs for additional assistance or sedation before beginning the procedure.

Procedure. In preparation for the procedure, position the patient in a fetal side-lying position to separate the vertebrae and move the spinal nerve roots away from the area to be accessed. The primary health care provider (PHCP) then cleans the skin site thoroughly. The injection site is determined, and a local anesthetic is injected. In a few minutes, a spinal needle is inserted between the third and fourth lumbar vertebrae. Instruct the patient to inform the provider if there is shooting pain or a tingling sensation. After determining proper placement in the subarachnoid space by removing the stylet and seeing CSF, the patient is asked to relax as much as possible so the pressure reading will be accurate. Opening and closing pressure readings are taken and recorded. The normal opening pressure should be no more than 20 cm H_2O; the CSF should be clear and colorless and contain only a few cells. Three to five test tubes of CSF are usually collected and numbered sequentially. After specimen collection, the needle is withdrawn, slight pressure is applied, and an adhesive bandage strip is placed over the insertion site.

Examination of CSF has been a useful diagnostic tool for some time. Recent technical advances are increasing the number of analyses that can be done on CSF. Gram-stain smears can test for particular types of meningitis, such as tubercular meningitis. CSF can be cultured, and sensitivity studies determine the best choice of antibiotic if an infection is diagnosed. A specific test for neurosyphilis is the fluorescent treponemal antibody absorption (FTA-ABS) test. Cytologic studies of CSF can identify tumor cells.

Follow-Up Care. Obtain vital signs and perform frequent neurologic checks as directed by agency protocol. Follow agency policy regarding how long the patient should be on bedrest and remain flat. Encourage the patient to increase fluid intake unless contraindicated. Monitor for complications, especially increased ICP (severe headache, nausea, vomiting, photophobia, and change in level of consciousness). Serious complications of lumbar puncture, although not common, include brainstem herniation (discussed in Chapter 45), infection, CSF leakage, and hematoma formation. Observe the needle insertion site for leakage and notify the physician if it occurs. Provide the prescribed medication for patient report of headache. Be sure to notify the health care provider if the medication does not relieve pain.

Transcranial Doppler Ultrasonography. Intracranial hemodynamics can be evaluated through the use of the transcranial Doppler (TCD), which uses sound waves to measure blood flow through the arteries. The test is particularly valuable in evaluating cerebral vasospasm or narrowing of arteries. TCD is safe, can be used repeatedly for the same patient, and is an inexpensive alternative to angiography.

GET READY FOR THE NCLEX® EXAMINATION!

KEY POINTS

Review these Key Points for each NCLEX Examination Client Needs Category.

Safe and Effective Care Environment
- Coordinate with the health care provider, physical therapist, and speech-language pathologist to establish priorities in neurologic assessment based on the patient's history and

presenting signs and symptoms. **QSEN: Teamwork and Collaboration**

Health Promotion and Maintenance
- Identify risk factors that place patients at risk for neurologic health problems such as behaviors that result in serious harm (e.g., driving recklessly) and lifestyle choices. **QSEN: Patient-Centered Care**

- Teach patients how to prepare for selected neurologic diagnostic tests, including what to expect during and after the test.
- Be sure to be aware of the normal neurologic changes that occur in older adults when interpreting assessment data (see Chart 41-1).
- Recognize that older adults do not normally experience deterioration in COGNITION and memory but do experience physical and physiological changes that affect MOBILITY and SENSORY PERCEPTION (see Chart 41-1). **QSEN: Patient-Centered Care**
- Provide a safe environment when memory loss is part of the older adult's health status by using memory aids and assistive technology to meet teaching or self-care goals. **QSEN: Safety**
- Provide safe opportunities for MOBILITY, including physical activity such as walking, when caring for older adults. **QSEN: Safety**

Psychosocial Integrity

- Assess the reaction of the person to neurologic disease. The psychological responses to neurologic health problems can vary by age, gender, and cultural background. **QSEN: Patient-Centered Care**
- Encourage patients to express their feelings and refer them to appropriate support services as needed.

Physiological Integrity

- Take a patient history before performing a complete neurologic assessment if the situation is not emergent. **QSEN: Patient-Centered Care**
- Detect neurologic changes early with health screening and physical assessment strategies that reflect the prioritized assessment. Recall that a deterioration in level of consciousness (e.g., from alert to lethargic) is the most sensitive and reliable indicator of an adverse neurologic change. **QSEN: Evidence-Based Practice; Clinical Judgment**

- Perform a neurologic examination that may be either comprehensive or focused as determined by patient needs. **QSEN: Patient-Centered Care**
- Use the Glasgow Coma Scale for patients with new traumatic brain injury.
- Include assessment of gait, balance, and coordination to determine risk for falls. **QSEN: Safety**
- Check cranial nerve III by examining pupils for size, shape, and reaction to light. Pupils should be equal in size and round and regular in shape and become smaller in bright light. Changes in eye signs can indicate new neurologic deterioration in nonverbal patients. **QSEN: Evidence-Based Practice**
- Assess for cognition using the guidelines in Chart 41-2.
- Be sure to monitor for potentially life-threatening complications after invasive diagnostic testing. For example, monitor for bleeding in patients who have cerebral angiography. If bleeding is observed, call the radiologist or primary physician immediately. Monitor for cerebrospinal fluid (CSF) leakage after a lumbar puncture. **QSEN: Safety; Clinical Judgment**
- Use serum creatinine or estimated glomerular filtration rate to identify patients with reduced kidney function. Older adults and patients with chronic kidney disease, diabetes, or heart failure are at high risk for kidney damage from iodinated and gadolinium contrast media. Provide adequate fluid intake before and after diagnostic testing to flush contrast after a diagnostic test (see Chart 41-3).
- Before MRI, check for implanted devices such as pacemakers, vascular stents, pumps, and aneurysm clips. **QSEN: Safety**
- Recall that CSF should be clear and colorless with few cells.
- Remember that decerebrate or decorticate posturing and pinpoint or dilated nonreactive pupils are late signs of neurologic deterioration.

SELECTED BIBLIOGRAPHY

Barr, J., Fraser, G. L., Puntillo, K., Ely, E. W., Gélinas, C., Dasta, J. F., et al. (2013). Clinical practice guidelines for the management of pain, agitation, and delirium in adult patients in the intensive care unit. *Critical Care Medicine, 41*(1), 263–306.

Boudreaux, A. (2014). Strengthening your neurologic assessment techniques. *Nursing2014 Critical Care, 9*(3), 32–37.

Centers for Medicare & Medicaid (2016). Recommend Core Measures. http://www.cms.gov/Regulations-and-Guidance/Legislation/EHRIncentivePrograms/Recommended_Core_Set.html.

Faraklas, I., Holt, B., Tran, S., Lin, H., Saffle, J., & Cochran, A. (2013). Impact of a nursing-driven sleep hygiene protocol on sleep quality. *Journal of Burn Care and Research, 34*(2), 249–254.

Hickey, J. V. (2013). The clinical practice of neurological and neurosurgical nursing (7th ed.). Philadelphia: Lippincott Williams & Wilkins.

Iacono, L. A., Wells, C., & Mann-Finnerty, K. (2014). Standardizing neurological assessments. *The Journal of Neuroscience Nursing, 46*(2), 125–132.

Institute for Magnetic Resonance Safety, Education, and Research. (2014). MRI Safety. http://www.mrisafety.com/.

Jarvis, C. (2014). Physical examination & health assessment (7th ed.). St. Louis: Elsevier Saunders.

McCance, K., Huether, S., Brashers, V., & Rote, N. (2014). Pathophysiology: The biologic basis for disease in adults and children (7th ed.). St. Louis: Mosby.

Rank, W. (2013). Performing a focused neurologic assessment. *Nursing, 43*(12), 37–40.

Touhy, T. A., & Jett, K. F. (2014). *Gerontological nursing and healthy aging* (4th ed.). St. Louis: Mosby.

CHAPTER 42

Care of Patients With Problems of the Central Nervous System: The Brain

Donna D. Ignatavicius

 http://evolve.elsevier.com/Iggy/

PRIORITY AND INTERRELATED CONCEPTS

The priority concepts for this chapter are:
- COGNITION
- MOBILITY

✳ The COGNITION concept exemplar for this chapter is Alzheimer's Disease, below.

✳ The MOBILITY concept exemplar for this chapter is Parkinson Disease, p. 868.

The interrelated concept for this chapter is COMFORT.

LEARNING OUTCOMES

Safe and Effective Care Environment

1. Plan with the interprofessional health care team for transitions in care, including discharge to home or other setting for patients with Alzheimer's disease (AD) or Parkinson disease (PD).
2. Prioritize nursing interventions for the patient who has AD to ensure safety needed as a result of impaired COGNITION.

Health Promotion and Maintenance

3. Teach patients with migraine headaches about preventive and management approaches to therapy.
4. Develop a teaching plan about drug therapy for patients with epilepsy.
5. Teach patients about health promotion strategies to prevent meningitis and encephalitis.

Psychosocial Integrity

6. Teach family/informal caregivers about strategies to prevent stress when caring for patients with AD.
7. Plan interventions to promote self-concept in patients experiencing PD.

Physiological Integrity

8. Differentiate the major stages of AD, including the effect of each stage on COGNITION and MOBILITY.
9. Plan nursing care for the patient with AD to promote communication, functional ability, and COMFORT.
10. Identify vulnerable populations at risk for AD and other types of dementia, including war veterans.
11. Plan care for the patient with PD to ensure safety and promote optimum functioning and MOBILITY.
10. Differentiate the common types of seizures, including presenting signs and symptoms.
11. Prioritize evidence-based care for patients with a seizure disorder, including appropriate seizure precaution interventions.
12. Identify nursing priorities for patients with meningitis and encephalitis.
13. Prevent or reduce the risk for common complications that contribute to functional decline and decreased quality of life in adults with AD and PD.

Neurologic disorders can interfere with self-management and functional ability; many of them cause impaired COGNITION, decreased MOBILITY, and chronic impaired COMFORT. Chapter 2 reviews these health concepts. Care of patients with health problems affecting the brain requires coordination by nurses and interprofessional collaboration.

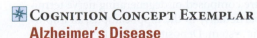 ✳ COGNITION CONCEPT EXEMPLAR
Alzheimer's Disease

❖ PATHOPHYSIOLOGY

Alzheimer's disease (AD) is the most common type of dementia that typically affects people older than 65 years. Dementia,

TABLE 42-1 Comparison of the Two Major Types of Dementia: Alzheimer's Disease and Vascular Dementia

	ALZHEIMER'S DISEASE	VASCULAR DEMENTIA
Cause	Genetic and environmental factors; possibly viral	Strokes or other vascular disorders that decrease blood flow to the brain
Pathophysiologic changes	Chronic, terminal disease that is characterized by formation of neuritic plaques, neurofibrillary tangles, and vascular degeneration in the brain	Impaired blood flow to the brain, causing ischemia or necrosis of brain neurons
Course of dementia	Steady and gradual decline of cognitive, mobility, and ADL function from mild through severe stages; patients usually die from complications of immobility	Stepwise progression of dementia symptoms that get significantly worse after each vascular event, such as a stroke or series of mini-strokes; symptoms may improve as collateral circulation to vital neurons develops
Risk factors	Female Over 65 years of age Down syndrome Traumatic brain injury	Male Over 65 years of age History of diabetes mellitus (DM), high cholesterol, myocardial infarction, atherosclerosis, hypertension, smoking, obesity
Management	Safety measures to prevent injury, wandering, or falls Cholinesterase inhibitors Behavior management ADL and mobility assistance as needed based on stage	Identification of risk factors and management of the risk for or actual vascular event (e.g., antidiabetes drugs for DM, antihypertensive drugs, low-fat diet, smoking cessation, weight loss) Safety measures to prevent injury or falls Behavior management

sometimes referred to as a *chronic* confusional state or syndrome, is a general term for progressive loss of brain function and impaired COGNITION. Other common types of dementia include vascular dementia, Lewy body dementia, and frontotemporal dementia (formerly called *Pick's disease*), which occurs in middle-age adults (Klug, 2014). Table 42-1 compares AD with vascular dementia, the second most common type of dementia. Vascular dementia, sometimes called *multi-infarct dementia*, results from strokes or other vascular disorders that decrease blood flow to the brain.

Any type of dementia affects a person's ability to learn new information and eventually impairs language, judgment, and behavior. As the disease progresses, the patient's functional ability declines, and death occurs as a result of complications of decreased MOBILITY.

The brain of the older adult usually weighs less and occupies less space in the cranium than does the brain of a younger person. Other changes in the brain that occur with aging include widening of the cerebral sulci, narrowing of the gyri, and enlargement of the ventricles. In the presence of AD and other types of dementia, these normal changes are greatly accelerated. Brain weight is reduced further. Marked atrophy of the cerebral cortex and loss of cortical neurons occur.

Microscopic changes of the brain found in people with AD include neurofibrillary tangles, amyloid-rich senile or neuritic plaques, and vascular degeneration. *Neurofibrillary tangles* are composed of fibrous tissue that impairs the ability of impulses from being transmitted from neuron to neuron (McCance et al., 2014).

Neuritic plaques are composed of degenerating nerve terminals and are found particularly in the hippocampus, an important part of the limbic system. Deposited within the plaques are increased amounts of an abnormal protein called *beta amyloid*. These proteins have a tendency to accumulate and form the neurotoxic plaques found in the brain that impair neuronal transmission (Fig. 42-1) (McCance et al., 2014).

Although *vascular degeneration* occurs in the normally aging brain, its presence is significantly increased in patients with dementia. Vascular degeneration accounts for at least partial loss of the ability of nerve cells to function properly. This pathologic change contributes to the cognitive decline and mortality associated with AD.

In addition to the structural changes in the brain associated with this disorder, abnormalities in the neurotransmitters (acetylcholine [ACh], norepinephrine, dopamine, and serotonin) may occur. High levels of beta amyloid can reduce the amount of acetyltransferase in the hippocampus. This loss is important because the decrease in Ach interferes with cholinergic innervation to the cerebral cortex. This change results in impaired COGNITION, recent memory, and the ability to acquire new memories (McCance et al., 2014).

Etiology and Genetic Risk

The exact cause of AD is unknown. It is well established that *age, gender, and genetics are the most important risk factors*. Age is strongly linked to the incidence of AD for people older than 65, and women are more likely to develop the disease than men (McCance et al., 2014). As older adults age further, they become more at risk for the disease. Although not commonly occurring, when AD is diagnosed in people in their 40s and 50s, it is referred to as *early dementia, Alzheimer type*, or *presenile dementia*. Other risk factors for AD have been studied, including chemical imbalances, environmental agents, immunologic changes, excessive stress, and ethnicity/race. Environmental agents, especially certain viruses such as herpes zoster and herpes simplex, and toxic metals such as zinc and copper have also been suggested as causes. Patients who have experienced a traumatic brain injury (TBI) (e.g., war veterans) or repeated head trauma (e.g., boxers) may be more at risk for AD and at an earlier age than others. There is also a high incidence of AD in people who have Down syndrome.

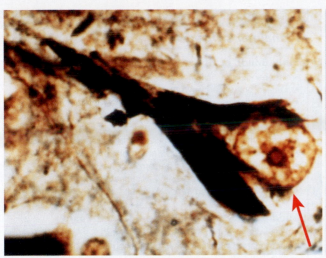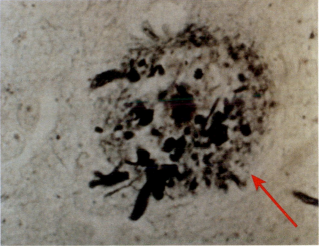

FIG. 42-1 Plaques and neurofibrillary tangles in the brain of a patient with Alzheimer's disease. (Courtesy Armstrong, D. Baylor College of Medicine and Texas Children's Hospital, Houston. In Nussbaum, R. L., et al. [2016]. *Thompson & Thompson Genetics in medicine* [8th ed.]. Philadelphia: Elsevier.)

♥ VETERANS' HEALTH CONSIDERATIONS

Patient-Centered Care QSEN

Studies suggest that war veterans who have a current or past history of post-traumatic stress disorder (PTSD) are at an increased risk of AD and other dementias (Sibener et al., 2014). A factor that further increases the veteran's risk of AD is being a prisoner of war (POW). Many POWs have PTSD as a result of this experience (Meziab et al., 2014).

⚕ GENETIC/GENOMIC CONSIDERATIONS

Patient-Centered Care QSEN

There is little doubt that many patients with AD had a genetic predisposition to the development of the disease. The most well-established genetic factor for AD in Euro-Americans is apolipoprotein E *(APOE)*, a protein that transports cholesterol.

Another set of genes have been identified that are involved in the formation of the plaque and neurofibrillary tangles in AD. These genes include the beta-amyloid precursor *(APP)*, the presenilin 1 *(PSEN1)*, and presenilin 2 *(PRESN2)* genes. A third family of genes associated with AD progression is responsible for processes that help deliver neurotransmitters. These genes are phosphatidylinositol-binding clathrin assembly protein *(PICALM)* and Bridging Integrator 1 *(BIN1)* (Bettens et al., 2013). The genetic studies in AD are an example of how genetics and genomics and proteomics are not only finding genes associated with the condition but also illustrating the mechanisms of pathology in complex conditions among diverse populations.

Incidence and Prevalence

There is a significant increase in both the incidence and prevalence of AD after 65 years of age, although it may affect anyone older than 40 years. The number of people in the United States with AD is estimated at over 5 million and expected to triple in the next three decades as baby boomers age (Barnes & Bennett, 2014). An increasing number of young veterans are at risk for dementia as a result of PTSD and/or TBI. AD has a significant impact on health care costs, including direct (such as drug therapy and health care provider visits) and indirect medical costs (such as home care or nursing home care) worldwide

🌐 CULTURAL/SPIRITUAL CONSIDERATIONS

Patient-Centered Care QSEN

African Americans and Hispanics have a greater risk for developing AD earlier than non-Hispanic whites (Euro-Americans). The APOE gene along with a new gene, ABCA7, is associated with an increased risk of AD among African Americans. The ABCA7 gene is thought to be responsible for transport of beta amyloid in the brain. Other risk factors that may help account for this ethnic difference include increased body mass index (obesity), smoking, and depression, which occur more commonly in these minority groups when compared to non-Hispanic whites (Barnes & Bennett, 2014).

Most AD research has not included the diagnosis, signs and symptoms, or disease progression in minority populations. However, a few studies suggest that African American and Hispanic patients with AD begin their cognitive impairment earlier and live longer with the disease than non-Hispanic whites. The reasons for these differences are unknown and require additional research because the number of minority older adults is expected to rapidly increase in the next few decades (Barnes & Bennett, 2014).

(Schaller et al., 2015). Millions of informal caregivers, most often spouses/partners or other family members, provide care at home for years for most patients with AD. Many of these individuals are at risk for physical and psychosocial problems as a result of the burden of caregiving.

Health Promotion and Maintenance

There are no proven ways to prevent AD; however, research is ongoing. Many patients with AD have other chronic health problems, such as diabetes mellitus, strokes, and atherosclerosis. Maintaining a healthy lifestyle helps to prevent these problems, such as eating a well-balanced diet, using soy products, and consuming sufficient amounts of folate and vitamins B_{12}, C, and E. Walking, swimming, and other exercise not only increase tone and muscle strength but also may decrease cognitive decline. Potentially harmful lifestyle habits that increase the individual's risk of stroke and cardiovascular disease should be avoided, such as smoking and excessive alcohol intake.

❖ INTERPROFESSIONAL COLLABORATIVE CARE
◆ Assessment: Noticing

History. A thorough history and physical assessment are necessary to differentiate AD from other, possibly reversible causes of impaired COGNITION. Some patients experience cognitive impairment as acute confusion (delirium) as discussed in Chapter 3. Table 2-1 compares dementia and delirium. Patients who have dementia are at an increased risk of delirium when hospitalized or admitted to a long-term care (LTC) setting (Struble et al., 2014).

Obtain information from family members or significant others because the patient may be unaware of the problems, denying their existence or covering them up. Some family members often do not recognize or may deny early changes in their loved one as well. Others may recognize subtle changes early in the disease process.

The most important information to be obtained is the onset, duration, progression, and course of the symptoms. Question the patient and the family about changes in memory or increasing forgetfulness and about the ability to perform ADLs. Ask about current employment status; work history; military history; and ability to fulfill household responsibilities, including cleaning, grocery shopping, and preparing meals. Inquire about changes in driving ability, ability to handle routine financial transactions, and language and communication skills. In addition, document any changes in personality and behavior. Assessing functional status for complex chronic conditions such as dementia is a recommended core measure by the Centers for Medicare and Medicaid Services.

There is increasing evidence that an altered sense of smell is associated with the development of AD. Therefore ask about changes in the ability to smell or the sense of smell. The history taking concludes with a review of the patient's medical history. Of particular importance is a history of TBI, viral illness, or exposure to metal or toxic waste and any family history of AD or Down syndrome.

Physical Assessment/Signs and Symptoms

Stages of Alzheimer's Disease. In recent years, the National Institute of Aging in the United States has recognized three phases of AD to include (Barnes & Bennett, 2014):
- Asymptomatic preclinical phase
- Symptomatic pre-dementia phase (mild impaired COGNITION)
- Dementia phase

The signs and symptoms associated with the dementia phase can be grouped into three broad stages based on the progress of the disease (Chart 42-1). The patient does not necessarily progress from one stage to the next in an orderly fashion. A stage may be bypassed, or he or she may exhibit symptoms of one or several stages. Each patient exhibits different disease stages and signs and symptoms. Consequently, most authorities now use broader terms such as *early (mild), middle (moderate),* and *late (severe)* stages, although other staging systems exist.

The primary focus of the nursing assessment of patients with AD is to identify abnormalities in COGNITION, including language, personality, and behavior. Physical manifestations of neurologic impairment (seizures, tremors, or ataxia) tend to occur late in the disease process.

Changes in Cognition. As defined in Chapter 2, **cognition** is the complex integration of mental processes and intellectual

---

⏩ CHART 42-1   Key Features
Alzheimer's Disease

Early (Mild), or Stage I (First Symptoms up to 4 Years)
- Independent in ADLs
- Denies presence of symptoms
- Forgets names; misplaces household items
- Has short-term memory loss and difficulty recalling new information
- Shows subtle changes in personality and behavior
- Loses initiative and is less engaged in social relationships
- Has mild impaired COGNITION and problems with judgment
- Demonstrates decreased performance, especially when stressed
- Unable to travel alone to new destinations
- Often has decreased sense of smell

Middle (Moderate), or Stage II (2 to 3 Years)
- Has impairment of all cognitive functions
- Demonstrates problems with handling or unable to handle money and finances
- Is disoriented to time, place, and event
- Is possibly depressed and/or agitated
- Is increasingly dependent in ADLs
- Has visuospatial deficits: has difficulty driving and gets lost
- Has speech and language deficits: less talkative, decreased use of vocabulary, increasingly nonfluent, and eventually aphasic
- Incontinent
- Has episodes of wandering; trouble sleeping

Late (Severe), or Stage III
- Completely incapacitated; bedridden
- Totally dependent in ADLs
- Has loss of MOBILITY and verbal skills
- Has agnosia (loss of facial recognition)

---

function for the purposes of reasoning, learning, and memory. Therefore assess patient for deficits in these abilities:
- Attention and concentration
- Judgment and perception
- Learning and memory
- Communication and language
- Speed of information processing

One of the first symptoms of AD is short-term memory impairment. New memory and defects in information retrieval result from dysfunction in the hippocampal, frontal, or parietal region. Alterations in communication abilities, such as **apraxia** (inability to use words or objects correctly), **aphasia** (inability to speak or understand), **anomia** (inability to find words), and **agnosia** (loss of sensory comprehension), are due to dysfunction of the temporal and parietal lobes. Frontal lobe impairment causes problems with judgment, an inability to make decisions, decreased attention span, and a decreased ability to concentrate. As the disease progresses to a later stage, the patient loses all cognitive abilities, is totally unable to communicate, and becomes less aware of the environment.

To more clearly identify the nature and extent of the patient's impaired COGNITION, the neurologist or psychologist administers several neuropsychological tests. The tests selected depend on clinician preference and the ability of the patient to participate in testing. All of the tests focus on cognitive ability and may be repeated over time to measure changes. Folstein's Mini-Mental State Examination (MMSE) is an example of a tool used to determine the onset and severity of cognitive impairment. The MMSE is also known as the "mini-mental exam." The MMSE assesses five major areas—orientation, registration, attention and calculation, recall, and speech-language (including reading). The patient performs certain cognitive tasks that are scored and added together for a total score of 0 to 30. The lower the score is, the greater the severity of the dementia. It is not unusual for a patient with advanced AD to score below 5.

Although the MMSE is used frequently by specialists and researchers, it is a copyrighted tool, and the patient must be able to read. For the patient who cannot read or for a quicker screening test, the "set test" can be used. The patient is asked to name 10 items in each of four sets or categories: fruits, animals, colors, and towns (FACT). Other categories can be used, if needed. The patient receives 1 point for each item for a possible maximum score of 40. Patients who score above 25 do not have dementia. Although this assessment is easy to administer, it should not be used for patients with hearing impairments or speech and language problems.

Another brief tool to screen for dementia that has validity and reliability in acute care settings is the Short Blessed Test (www.mybraintest.org) or the Clock Drawing Test (CDT). The CDT does not require that the patient can read and is non-threatening to perform. In LTC settings, the federally required Brief Interview for Mental Status (BIMS) is included as part of the Minimum Data Set 3.0 for Nursing Homes (see Chapter 3).

Changes in Behavior and Personality. One of the most difficult aspects of AD and dementia with which families and caregivers cope is the behavioral changes that can occur in advanced disease. Assess the patient for:

- Aggressiveness, especially verbal and physical abusive tendencies
- Rapid mood swings
- Increased confusion at night or when light is not adequate (sundowning) or in excessively fatigued patients

The patient may wander and become lost or may go into other rooms to rummage through another's belongings. Hoarding or hiding objects is also common. For example, patients may hoard washcloths in the long-term care setting.

For some patients with dementia, emotional and behavioral problems occur with the primary disease. They may experience paranoia (suspicious behaviors), delusions, hallucinations, and depression. Document these behaviors and ensure the patient's safety. (Refer to a mental health/behavior health nursing textbook for a complete discussion of these psychiatric disorders.)

Changes in Self-Management Skills. Observe for changes in the patient's self-management skills that decline over time, such as:

- Decreased interest in personal appearance
- Selection of clothing that is inappropriate for the weather or event
- Loss of bowel and bladder control
- Decreased appetite or ability to eat (often due to forgetting how to chew food and swallow in late dementia)

Over time, the patient becomes less mobile, and complications of impaired MOBILITY develop. These potential complications are listed in Table 2-3. The patient eventually becomes totally immobile and requires total physical care.

Psychosocial Assessment. In people with dementia, the cognitive changes and biochemical and structural dysfunctions affect personality and behavior. In the early stage, patients often recognize that they are experiencing memory or cognitive changes and may attempt to hide the problems. They begin the grieving process because of anticipated loss, experiencing denial, anger, bargaining, and depression at varying times.

Research shows that depression or depressive symptoms in patients with mild cognitive impairment are associated with the progression to AD (Van der Mussele et al., 2014).

When the patient and family receive the diagnosis, one or more family members may desire genetic testing. Support the patient's/family's decisions regarding testing and help them find credible resources for testing and professional genetics counseling.

As the disease progresses, patients begin to display major changes in emotional and behavioral affect. Of particular importance is the need for an assessment of the patients' reactions to changes in routine or environment. For example, a hospital admission is very traumatic for most patients with dementia. It is not unusual for them to exhibit a catastrophic response or overreact to any change by becoming excessively aggressive or abusive. This is referred to as *traumatic relocation syndrome.*

Sexual disinhibition is one of the most challenging symptoms for both family and staff members. Sexually inappropriate behaviors may include masturbating publicly, attempting sexual acts on staff or other patients, disrobing or exposing the genital area, and/or making sexualized comments to staff or other patients (Murphy, 2015). Assess a history of or current manifestation of these behaviors to include into the patient's plan of care.

Neuropsychiatric symptoms are common in patients with AD and increase as the disease progresses and aphasia increases. The patient's emotions are often displayed as nonverbal behaviors, including hitting, yelling, and agitation. Any new hospital procedure may cause anxiety and fear as a trigger for these behaviors. Psychoses, such as delusions and hallucinations, are also common (Struble et al., 2014).

As patients become unaware of their behavior, the focus of the psychosocial assessment shifts to the family or significant others. The interprofessional health care team assesses their ability to cope with the chronicity and progression of the disease and identifies possible support systems.

Laboratory and Imaging Assessment. No laboratory test can confirm the diagnosis of AD. Definitive diagnosis is made on the basis of brain tissue examination at autopsy, which confirms the presence of neurofibrillary tangles and neuritic plaques.

Genetic testing, specifically for *apolipoprotein E4 (APOE 4),* may be helpful as an ancillary test (not a predictive test) for the differential diagnosis of AD. *Amyloid beta protein precursor (soluble)* (sBPP) may be measured for patients to diagnose AD and other types of dementia. A decrease in the patient's sBPP in the cerebrospinal fluid (CSF) supports the diagnosis because the amyloid tends to deposit in the brain and is not circulating in the CSF (Pagana et al., 2017).

A variety of laboratory tests (CT or MRI) may be performed to rule out other treatable causes of dementia or delirium. The CT scan typically shows cerebral atrophy and ventricular enlargement, wide sulci, and shrunken gyri in the later stages of the disease. An MRI scan can also rule out other causes of neurologic disease.

◆ **Analysis: Interpreting**

The priority collaborative problems for patients with Alzheimer's disease (AD) include:

1. Decreased memory and COGNITION due to neuronal degeneration in the brain
2. Potential for injury or accident due to wandering or inability to ambulate independently

? NCLEX EXAMINATION CHALLENGE 42-1
Psychosocial Integrity

The nurse assesses an older adult with a diagnosis of severe, late-stage Alzheimer's disease. Which assessment findings would the nurse expect for this client? **Select all that apply.**
A. Acute confusion
B. Hallucinations
C. Wandering
D. Urinary incontinence
E. Difficulty eating

3. Potential for elder abuse by caregivers due to the patient's prolonged progression of disability and the patient's increasing care needs

◆ Planning and Implementation: Responding

The priority for interprofessional care is safety! Chronic confusion and physical deficits place the patient with AD at a high risk for injury, accidents, and elder abuse.

Managing Memory and Cognitive Dysfunction

Planning: Expected Outcomes. In the very early stages of the disease, the patient with AD is expected to maintain the ability to perform basic mental processes. As the disease progresses, patients cannot meet this outcome. Instead, the desired outcome is to maintain memory and cognitive function for as long as possible to keep patients safe and increase their quality of life.

Interventions. Although drug therapy may be used for patients with AD, nonpharmacologic interventions are the main focus of nursing teamwork and interprofessional collaboration. Teach family members and significant others about the importance of being consistent in following the individualized plan of care.

Nonpharmacologic Management

Behavioral Management in a Structured Environment. The primary health care provider should answer the patient's questions truthfully concerning the diagnosis of AD. In this way, the patient and family can more fully participate in the interprofessional plan of care. Interventions are the same whether he or she is cared for at home, in an adult day-care center, in an assisted-living center, in an LTC facility, or in a hospital. *The patient with memory problems benefits best from a structured and consistent environment.* Training in communication can help nurses and health care team members interact with better affect and compassion.

Many factors, including physical illness and environmental factors, can exacerbate (worsen) the signs and symptoms of AD. The patient with dementia frequently has other health problems such as cardiovascular disease, arthritis, renal insufficiency, and pulmonary disease. Changes in vision and hearing also may be present. Managing these problems often improves the patient's functional ability.

Approaches to managing the patient who has AD include:
- Cognitive stimulation and memory training
- Structuring the environment
- Orientation and validation therapy
- Promoting self-management
- Promoting bowel and bladder continence
- Promoting communication

The purpose of *cognitive stimulation and memory training* is to reinforce or promote desirable cognitive function and facilitate memory. Research has shown that cognitive-stimulation therapy programs and mindfulness provide some benefit for patients (Mapelli et al., 2013). Interactive pet therapy may also help patients with mild-to-moderate impaired cognition to enhance cognitive function (Friedmann et al., 2015).

As the disease progresses, the patient may experience an inability to recognize oneself and other familiar faces. Encourage the family to provide pictures of family members and close friends that are labeled with the person's name on the picture. In addition, advise the family to reminisce with the patient about pleasant experiences from the past. Use *reminiscence therapy* while assisting the patient with ADLs or performing a treatment or assessment. Refer to a personal item in the room to help the patient begin to talk about its meaning in the present and in the past.

It is not unusual for the patient to talk to his or her image in the mirror. This behavior should be allowed as long as it is not harmful. If the patient becomes frightened by the mirror image, remove or cover the mirror. In some long-term care or assisted-living memory care units, a picture of the patient is placed on the room door to help with facial recognition and to help the patient locate his or her room. This picture also helps the staff locate the patient in case of elopement (running away).

Teach the family to keep environmental distractions and noise to a minimum. The patient's home, hospital room, or nursing home room should not have pictures on the wall or other decorations that could be misinterpreted as people or animals that could harm the patient. An abstract painting or wallpaper might look like a fire or an explosion and scare the patient. The room should have adequate, nonglare lighting and no potentially frightening shadows.

In addition to disturbed sleep, other negative effects of high noise levels include decreased nutritional intake, changes in blood pressure and pulse rates, and feelings of increased stress and anxiety. The patient with AD is especially susceptible to these changes and needs to have as much undisturbed sleep at night as possible. Fatigue increases confusion and behavioral manifestations such as agitation and aggressiveness.

! NURSING SAFETY PRIORITY QSEN
Action Alert

When a patient with Alzheimer's disease is in a new setting or environment, collaborate with the staff and admitting department to select a room that is in the quietest area of the unit and away from obvious exits, if possible. A private room may be needed if the patient has a history of agitation or wandering. The television should remain off unless the patient turns it on or requests that it be turned on.

Objects such as furniture, a hairbrush, and eyeglasses should be kept in the same place. Establish a daily routine and follow it as much as possible. Arrange for a communication board or digital handheld device for scheduled activities and other information to promote orientation such as the day of the week, the month, and the year. Pictures of people familiar to the patient can also be placed on this board.

Explain changes in routine to the patient before they occur, repeating the explanation immediately before the changes take place. Clocks and single-date calendars also help the patient maintain day-to-day orientation to the environment in the early stages of the disease process. *For the patient with early disease, reality orientation is usually appropriate.* Teach family members and health care staff to frequently reorient the patient to the environment. Remind the patient what day and time it is, where he or she is, and who you are.

For the patient in the later stages of AD or dementia, reality orientation does not work and often increases agitation. *The interprofessional health care team uses validation therapy for the patient with moderate or severe AD. In* validation therapy, *the staff member recognizes and acknowledges the patient's feelings and concerns.* For example, if the patient is looking for his or her mother, ask him or her to talk about what Mother looks like and what she might be wearing. This response does not argue with the patient but also does not reinforce the patient's belief that Mother is still living.

As the disease progresses, altered thought processes affect the *ability to perform ADLs.* Encourage the patient to perform as much self-care as possible and to maintain independence in daily living skills as long as possible. For example, in the home setting, complete clothing outfits that can be easily placed on a single hanger are preferred for patient selection. When possible, the patient should participate in meal preparation, grocery shopping, and other household routines. Many patients cannot make purposeful movements as the disease progresses.

NCLEX EXAMINATION CHALLENGE 42-2

Psychosocial Integrity

A client with **early** dementia asks the nurse to find her mother, who is deceased. What is the nurse's **most appropriate** response?
A. "We can call her in a little while if you want."
B. " Your mother died over 20 years ago."
C. "What did your mother look like?"
D. "I'll ask your father to find her when he visits."

Collaborate with the occupational and physical therapists to provide a complete evaluation and assistance in helping the patient become more independent. Adaptive devices, such as grab bars in the bathtub or shower area, an elevated commode, and adapted eating utensils, may enable him or her to maintain independence in grooming, toileting, and feeding. The physical therapist prescribes an exercise program to improve physical health and functionality.

The patient may remain continent of bowel and bladder for long periods if taken to the bathroom or given a bedpan or urinal every 2 hours. Toileting may be needed more often during the day and less frequently at night. Unlicensed assistive personnel (UAP) or home caregivers should encourage the patient to drink adequate fluids to promote optimal voiding. A patient may refuse to drink enough fluids because of a fear of incontinence. Assure the patient that he or she will be toileted on a regular schedule to prevent incontinent episodes.

When patients with dementia are in the hospital or other unfamiliar place, avoid the use of restraints, including side rails. Serious injury can occur when a patient with dementia attempts to get out of bed with either limb restraints or side rail use. Use frequent surveillance, toileting every 2 hours, and other strategies to prevent falls. Restraint reduction has been associated with a reduced length of stay and fewer injuries. In some cases,

sitters may be used to help prevent patient injury. Chapter 3 discusses fall prevention in detail.

Maintain a clear path between the bed and bathroom at all times. For patients who are too weak to walk to the bathroom, a bedside commode may be used. Some patients may void in unusual places, such as the sink or a wastebasket. As a reminder of where they should toilet, place a picture of the commode on the bathroom door.

Complementary and Integrative Health. If culturally appropriate and if the patient allows being touched by staff, teach UAP to provide a massage before bedtime to promote sleep or at other times to reduce stress and promote relaxation. Use some type of oil or lotion if the patient does not have allergies to these substances. Slow, rhythmic massage strokes on the upper back, neck, and shoulders can be very relaxing and calming (Westman & Blaisdell, 2016). Essential oils such as lavender and bergamot may also produce a calming effect and promote relaxation (Allard & Katseres, 2016).

Use redirection by attracting the patient's attention to promote communication. Keep the environment as free from distractions as possible. Speak directly to the patient in a distinct manner. Sentences should be clear and short. Remind the patient to perform one task at a time and allow sufficient time for completion. It may be necessary to break each task down into many small steps and limit choices. Chart 42-2 lists other best practices for promoting communication with patients with AD.

As the disease progresses, the patient is unable to perform tasks when asked. Show the patient what needs to be done, or provide cues to remind him or her how to perform the task. When possible, explain and demonstrate the task that the patient is asked to perform.

Patients with dementia disorders typically have specific speech and language problems. Recognize that emotional and physical behaviors may be a form of communication. Interpret the meaning of these behaviors to address them. For example, restlessness may indicate urinary retention, pain, infection, or hypoxia (lack of oxygen to the brain). Collaborate with the speech-language pathologist to assist with communication ability.

Drug Therapy. Few drugs are helpful in treating Alzheimer's disease. Psychotropic drugs may be prescribed to help control the signs and symptoms of associated mental/behavioral health problems (e.g., depression, anxiety, paranoia).

CHART 42-2 Best Practice for Patient Safety & Quality Care QSEN

Promoting Communication With the Patient With Alzheimer's Disease

- Ask simple, direct questions that require only a "yes" or "no" answer if the patient can communicate.
- Provide instructions with pictures in a place that the patient will see if he or she can read them.
- Use simple, short sentences and one-step instructions.
- Use gestures to help the patient understand what is being said.
- Validate the patient's feelings as needed.
- Limit choices; too many choices cause frustration and increased confusion.
- Never assume that the patient is totally confused and cannot understand what is being communicated.
- Try to anticipate the patient's needs and interpret nonverbal communication.

Cholinesterase inhibitors are drugs approved for treating AD symptoms. They work to improve cholinergic neurotransmission in the brain by delaying the destruction of acetylcholine (ACh) by the enzyme *cholinesterase.* This action slows the onset of cognitive decline in some patients, but none of these drugs alters the course of the disease. In some cases, cholinesterase inhibitors can improve functional ADL ability. Examples include donepezil (Aricept), galantamine (Reminyl), and rivastigmine (Exelon) (Burchum & Rosenthal., 2016).

> ⚠ **NURSING SAFETY PRIORITY** **QSEN**
>
> *Drug Alert*
>
> Teach the family to monitor the patient's heart rate and report dizziness or falls because these drugs can cause bradycardia. Therefore they are used cautiously for patients who have a history of heart disease.

Memantine (Namenda) is the first of a new class of drugs that is a low-to-moderate affinity **N-methyl-D-aspartate (NMDA) receptor antagonist.** Overexcitation of NMDA receptors by the neurotransmitter *glutamate* may play a role in AD. This drug blocks excess amounts of glutamate that can damage nerve cells. It is indicated for advanced AD and has been shown to slow the pace of deterioration (Burchum & Rosenthal, 2016). Memantine may help maintain patient function for a few months' longer. Some patients also have improved memory and thinking skills. This drug can be given with donepezil (Aricept), a cholinesterase inhibitor.

Some patients with AD develop depression and may be treated with **antidepressants.** Selective serotonin reuptake inhibitors (SSRIs), such as paroxetine (Paxil) and sertraline (Zoloft), are usually prescribed. Tricyclic antidepressants, such as amitriptyline (Elavil), should not be used because of their anticholinergic effect, especially for older adults. Anticholinergic drugs frequently cause serious side effects, including increased confusion, urinary retention, and constipation.

Psychotropic drugs, also called *antipsychotic* or *neuroleptic drugs,* should be reserved for patients with mental/behavioral health problems that sometimes accompany dementia, such as hallucinations and delusions. However, in clinical practice, these drugs are sometimes incorrectly used for agitation, combativeness, or restlessness. Psychotropic drugs are considered chemical restraints because they decrease MOBILITY and patients' self-management ability. Therefore most geriatricians recommend that they be used as a last resort and with caution in low doses for a specific mental/behavioral health problem. The specific drug prescribed depends on side effects, the condition of the patient, and expected outcomes. Follow agency policy and The Joint Commission standards concerning the use of chemical restraints.

Although not U.S. Food and Drug Administration (FDA)–approved at this time, nasal insulin for patients with mild impaired COGNITION or mild-to-moderate Alzheimer's dementia has proven to improve cognition. Both men and women taking 20 units of insulin benefited, but only men showed improvement with 40 units of insulin, possibly suggesting that gender differences may account for disparities in responses to treatment for AD (Claxton, 2015).

Preventing Injuries or Accidents

Planning: Expected Outcomes. The patient with dementia is expected to remain free from physical harm and not injure anyone else.

Interventions. Many patients with dementia tend to wander and may easily become lost. In later stages of the disease, some patients may become severely agitated and physically or verbally abusive to others. Teach the family the importance of a patient identification badge or bracelet. The badge should include how to contact the primary caregiver. In an inpatient setting, check the patient frequently and place him or her in a room that can be monitored easily. The room should be away from exits and stairs. Some health care agencies place large stop signs or red tape on the floor in front of exits. Others have installed alarm systems to indicate when a patient is opening the door or getting out of a bed or chair.

Restlessness may be decreased if the patient is taken for frequent walks. If the patient begins to wander, redirect him or her. For example, if the patient insists on going shopping for clothes, he or she is redirected to his or her closet to select clothing that will not be recognized as his ·or her own. This type of activity can be repeated a number of times because the patient has lost short-term memory. Best practices for preventing and managing wandering are listed in Chart 42-3.

 CHART 42-3 **Best Practice for Patient Safety & Quality Care** **QSEN**

Approaches to Prevent and Manage Wandering in Hospitalized Patients

- Identify the patients most at risk for wandering through observation and history provided by family.
- Provide appropriate supervision, including frequent checks (especially at shift-change times).
- Place the patient in an area that provides maximum observation but not in the nurses' station.
- Use family members, friends, volunteers, and sitters as needed to monitor the patient.
- Keep the patient away from stairs or elevators.
- Do not change rooms to prevent increasing confusion.
- Avoid physical or chemical restraints.
- Assess and treat pain.
- Use re-orientation methods and validation therapy, as appropriate.
- Provide frequent toileting and incontinence care as needed.
- If possible, prevent overstimulation, such as excessive noise.
- Use soft music and nonglare lighting if possible.

In any setting, keep the patient busy with structured activities. In a health care agency, an activity therapist or volunteer may work with patients as a group or individually to determine the type of activity that is appropriate for the stage of the disease. Puzzles, board games, art supplies, and computer games are often appropriate. Music and art therapy are also helpful activities to keep patients with AD busy while stimulating COGNITION. These activities allow patients to be engaged and promote their creativity (Volland & Fisher, 2014).

> **! NURSING SAFETY PRIORITY** **QSEN**
> *Action Alert*
>
> In inpatient health care agencies, use the least restrictive physical restraints such as waist belts and geri-chairs with lapboards only as a last resort because they often increase patient restlessness and cause agitation. Federal regulations in long-term care facilities in the United States mandate that all residents have the right to be free of both physical and chemical restraints. All health care agencies accredited by The Joint Commission are required to use alternatives to restraints before resorting to any physical or chemical restraint.

Patients with dementia may be injured because they cannot recognize objects or situations as harmful. Remove or secure all potentially dangerous objects (e.g., knives, drugs, cleaning solutions). Patients are often unaware that their driving ability is impaired and usually want to continue this activity even if their driver's license has been suspended or they are unsafe. Automobile keys must be secured, but the patient should be told why they were taken. (See Chapter 3 for more discussion on older-adult driving.)

Late in the disease process, the patient may experience seizure activity. If he or she is cared for at home, teach caregivers what action to take when a seizure occurs to prevent injury. (See the discussion of Interventions in the Seizures and Epilepsy section.)

Talking calmly and softly and attempting to redirect the patient to a more positive behavior or activity are effective strategies when he or she is agitated. For example, some patients refuse to take a bath or are unable to bathe. Bathing disability predicts decline for patients with dementia and combined with safety issues, often leads the family to place them in long-term care (LTC) settings. LTC staff may label these patients as "difficult" when they aggressively refuse to bathe (Wolf & Czekanski, 2015).

Use calm, positive statements and reassure the patient that he or she is safe. Statements such as, "I'm sorry that you are upset," "I know it's hard," and "I will have someone stay with you until you feel better" may help. Actions to *avoid* when the patient is agitated include raising the voice, confronting, arguing, reasoning, taking offense, or explaining. Teach the caregiver to not show alarm or make sudden movements out of the person's view. If the patient remains agitated, ensure his or her safety and leave the room after explaining that you will return later. Frequent visual checks must be done during this time. If the patient is connected to any type of tubing or other device, he or she may try to disconnect it or pull it out. These devices should be used cautiously in the patient with dementia. For example, if IV access is needed, the catheter or cannula is placed in an area that the patient cannot easily see, or it should be covered.

Another way to manage this problem is to provide a diversion. For example, if the patient is doing an activity or holding

TABLE 42-2 Minimizing Behavioral Problems for Patients With Alzheimer's Disease at Home

- Carefully evaluate the patient's environment to ensure it is safe:
  - Remove small area rugs.
  - Consider replacing tile floors with nonslippery floors.
  - Arrange furniture and room decorations to maximize the patient's safety when walking.
  - Minimize clutter in all rooms in and outside of the house.
  - Install nightlights in patient's room, bathroom, and hallway.
  - Install and maintain smoke alarms, fire alarms, and natural gas detectors.
  - Install safety devices in the bathroom such as handles for changing position (sit-to-stand).
  - Install alarm system or bells on outside doors; place safety locks on doors and gates.
  - Ensure that door locks cannot be easily opened by the patient.
- Help the patient with mild-stage disease remain oriented to the extent possible:
  - Place single-date calendars in patient's room and in kitchen.
  - Use large-face clocks with a neutral background.
- Communicate with the patient based on his or her ability to understand:
  - Explain activity immediately before the patient needs to carry it out.
  - Break complex tasks down to simple steps.
- Allow and encourage the patient to be as independent as possible in ADLs:
  - Place complete outfits for the day on hangers; have the patient select one to wear.
  - Develop and maintain a predictable routine (e.g., meals, bedtime, morning routine).
- When a problem behavior occurs, divert patient to another activity; minimize excessive stimulation:
  - Take the patient on outings when crowds are small.
  - If crowds cannot be avoided, minimize the amount of time the patient is present in a crowd. For example, at family gatherings, provide a quiet room for the patient to rest throughout the visit.
- Arrange for a day-care program to maintain interaction and provide respite for home caregiver.
- In the United States (www.alz.org); in Canada, register the patient with the Alzheimer Society of Canada Medic Alert® Safely Home® program (www.alzheimer.ca).

an item such as a stuffed animal or other special item, he or she might be less likely to pay attention to medical devices. Additional strategies to minimize behavioral problems, especially at home, are listed in Table 42-2.

Patients who are cared for at home are at high risk for neglect or abuse. The Joint Commission requires all patients to be assessed for neglect and abuse on admission to a health care facility. Patients with mild dementia may not report these concerns for fear of retaliation. Those with severe dementia may not have the ability to report the abuse. Asking questions such as, "Who cooks for you?" "Do you get help when you need it?" or "Do you wait long for help to the bathroom?" may be less stressful for the patient to answer.

Preventing Elder Abuse

Planning: Expected Outcomes. The family or other caregivers of the patient with dementia are expected to plan time to care for themselves to promote a reasonable quality of life and satisfaction, which should help prevent patient abuse.

Interventions. AD is a chronic, progressive condition that eventually leaves the patient completely dependent on others for all aspects of care. The patient with moderate or severe dementia requires continual 24-hour supervision and

CHART 42-4 Patient and Family Education: Preparing for Self-Management
Reducing Family/Informal Caregiver Stress

- Maintain realistic expectations for the person with Alzheimer's disease (AD).
- Take each day one at a time.
- Try to find the positive aspects of each incident or situation.
- Use humor with the person who has AD.
- Use the resources of the Alzheimer's Association, including attending local support group meetings.
- Explore alternative care settings early in the disease process for possible use later.
- Establish advance directives with the AD patient early in the disease process.
- Set aside time each day for rest or recreation away from the patient, if possible.
- Seek respite care periodically for longer periods of time.
- Take care of yourself by watching your diet, exercising, and getting plenty of rest.
- Be realistic about what you or they can do and accept help from family, friends, and community resources.
- Use relaxation techniques, including meditation and massage.
- Seek out clergy or other spiritual counselor or support.
- Be mindful about what gives meaning to your life.

caregiving. Severe cognitive changes leave the patient unable to manage finances, property, or personal care. The family needs to seek legal counsel regarding the patient's competency and the need to obtain guardianship or a durable medical power of attorney when necessary.

Millions of family caregivers provide direct care for patients with impaired COGNITION. Family caregivers include relatives, significant others, and neighbors who provide the majority of home health care. Teach these informal caregivers to be aware of their own health and stress levels. Signs of stress include anger, social withdrawal, anxiety, depression, lack of concentration, sleepiness, irritability, and physical health problems. When signs of stress and strain occur, the caregiver should be referred to his or her health care provider or seek one on his or her own. It is not unusual for the caregiver to refuse to accept help from others, even for a few brief hours. Initially, the caregiver may be more comfortable accepting help for just a few minutes a day so he or she could shower, enjoy a cup of tea, or take a brief walk. Some caregivers find that eventually they need to place their loved one into a respite setting or unit so they can re-energize and prevent or manage spiritual distress.

CULTURAL/SPIRITUAL CONSIDERATIONS
Patient-Centered Care **QSEN**

Both religion and spirituality can help family caregivers give meaning to the work they provide for patients with AD. Spirituality is considered an important part of holistic patient care; it may or may not include religion. Spirituality and religion may decrease the incidence of caregiver depression and anxiety. Assess the patient's and family caregiver's cultural beliefs and values related to spirituality and religion. Chart 42-4 lists strategies for reducing caregiver stress and includes interventions to promote spirituality and prevent spiritual distress.

As stated earlier, African Americans and Hispanics have a greater risk for developing AD earlier and typically live longer than non-Hispanic whites (Euro-Americans). These ethnic groups are known to be very family centered and tend to care for their family members at home as needed. As a result of these values and beliefs, an increase in family caregivers is expected as the number of older ethnic minority adults increases dramatically within the next 20 to 30 years. More research that focuses on older adults from these populations is needed to better provide essential care and support (Barnes & Bennett, 2014).

Care Coordination and Transition Management
Home Care Management. In the early stages of AD, patients may be cared for at home with little need for outside intervention. Whenever possible, the patient and family should be assigned a case manager who can assess their needs for health care resources and find the best placement throughout the continuum of care.

The patient usually begins to withdraw from friends and social events as memory impairment and personality and behavior changes progress. The family may begin to decrease their own social activities as the demands of the patient's care take more of their time. Emphasize to the family the importance of maintaining their own social contacts and leisure activities (see Chart 42-4). In a randomized controlled study, Canadian nurse researchers determined the effectiveness of telephone support for caregivers (Martindale-Adams et al., 2013) (see the Evidence-Based Practice box).

In most areas of the United States and Canada, respite care is available for families. The patient may be placed in a respite facility or nursing home for the weekend or for several weeks to give the family a rest from the constant care demands. The family may also be able to obtain respite care in the home through a home care agency or assisted-living facility. Remind the family that respite care is for a short period; it is not permanent placement. Some health care agencies have opened adult day-care centers or memory care units for patients with AD. In the day-care center, patients spend all or part of the day at the facility and participate in activities as their condition permits. Although these centers are usually open only on weekdays, this arrangement allows the caregiver to work or participate in other activities. If patients require 24-hour care, they may be placed in a memory-care unit of a long-term care or assisted-living facility.

Teach the family how to be prepared in case the patient becomes restless, agitated, abusive, or combative. In addition, the family can learn how to use reality orientation or validation therapy, depending on the stage of the disease.

Self-Management Education. Usually patients with AD and dementia are cared for in the home until late in the disease process unless they can afford private-pay care. Because health insurance coverage in the United States and family finances may not be sufficient to cover the services of a private duty nurse or home care aide, family members typically provide the care. The patient plan of care developed by the nurse or case manager, in

EVIDENCE-BASED PRACTICE (QSEN)

Does Telephone Support Assist Caregivers of Patients With Dementia?

Martindale-Adams, J., Nichols, L.O., Burns, R., Graney, M.J., & Zuber, J. (2013). A trial of dementia caregiver telephone support. *Canadian Journal of Nursing Research, 45*(4), 30–48.

The researchers designed and implemented a randomized controlled trial to determine if telephone support was more useful than print educational materials on dementia patient caregiver stress, depression, burden, and well-being. Fifteen (15) treatment groups of five or six caregivers (n=77) were provided with telephone support and compared to control groups (n=77) that only had access to the print materials. Groups met 14 times over a year. Data were collected at 6 and 12 months from all 154 caregivers in the study. Caregivers in the treatment group reported improvement in well-being and coping with stress, but there were no statistical significant differences between groups.

Level of Evidence: 2

This research was a randomized controlled trial that compared two types of interventions.

Commentary: Implications for Practice and Research

Telephone support is an efficient and useful way to provide support for caregivers of patients with dementia. The literature reports major caregiver stress because these patients often live for many years and their health worsens over time. Further research is needed to explore the effect of telephone support, depending on the level of care that patients require.

conjunction with the family, must be reasonable and realistic for the family to implement.

Review how to assist with bathing, dressing, toileting, and other self-management activities. The occupational therapist teaches the family and patient how to use adaptive equipment, such as a brace, a sling, a cane, or modified eating utensils. The patient may have difficulty chewing, swallowing, or tasting foods and may not be able to eat without assistance.

The family and the dietitian should develop a diet plan to increase the patient's nutritional intake. In the late stage of AD, the patient's intake often decreases, and he or she loses weight.

Provide information to the family on what to do in the event of a seizure and how to protect the patient from injury. Instruct them to notify the health care provider if the seizure is prolonged or if the patient's seizure pattern changes.

Review with the family or other caregiver the name, time, and route of administration; the dosage; and the side effects of all drugs. Remind the family to check with the health care provider before using any over-the-counter drugs or herbs because they may interact with prescribed drug therapy.

Emphasis is placed on the need for the patient to have an established exercise program to maintain MOBILITY for as long as possible and to prevent complications of immobility. In collaboration with the family, the physical therapist (PT) develops an individualized exercise program. The PT may continue to work with the patient at home until goals are achieved, depending on the payer source.

Remind the family or other caregiver to take special precautions to maintain the patient safely at home. The environment must be uncluttered, consistent, and structured. All hazardous items (e.g., cooking range and oven, power tools) are removed, secured, or "locked out." All electrical sockets not in use should

be covered with safety plugs. Teach families to install handrails and grab bars in the bathroom. Handrails should be along all stairways, and a guardrail should be placed around porches or open stairwells. Because the patient may have a tendency to wander, especially at night, the family may want to install alarms to all outside doors, the basement, and the patient's bedroom. All outside and basement doors should have deadbolt locks to prevent the patient from going outside unsupervised. Remind the family to adjust the temperature of the water to prevent accidental burns. Nightlights should be used in the patient's bedroom, hallway, and bathroom to prevent fear and to help with orientation.

Health Care Resources. Refer all families to their local chapter of the Alzheimer's Association (www.alz.org) in the United States or to the Alzheimer Society of Canada (www.alzheimer.ca). These organizations provide information and support services to patients and their families, including seminars, audiovisual aids, and publications. In some places, caregiver telephone support is available.

Teach the family to enroll the patient in the Safe Return Program, a U.S. government-funded program of the Alzheimer's Association that assists in the identification and safe, timely return of people with dementia. The program includes registration of the patient and a 24-hour hotline to be called to assist in finding a lost patient. If a patient wanders and becomes lost, the family (or health care institution) should immediately notify the police department. An up-to-date picture of the patient makes it easier for local authorities, the public, and neighbors to identify the missing patient. Devices using radio-wave beacons and a global positioning system (GPS) have been developed to help families and law enforcement officials find a lost patient more easily. These devices include shoes with a GPS unit implanted, jewelry that is hard to remove, and bracelets. Caution families that these devices are not foolproof. Just like cell phones, there are some areas where the signal from the patient may not be picked up easily if at all.

When the patient can no longer be cared for at home, referral to an assisted-living or long-term care facility may be needed. Early in the course of the disease, advise the family that placement might be needed in the late stages of the disease or sooner. This allows the family to begin to search for an appropriate facility before a crisis develops and immediate placement is needed. The national office of the Alzheimer's Association publishes an outline of criteria for a memory-care unit. In the advanced stage of the disease, the patient may need referral to palliative and hospice services for total care. (See the discussion of end-of-life and hospice care in Chapter 7.)

♥ VETERANS' HEALTH CONSIDERATIONS

Patient-Centered Care (QSEN)

For veterans who have AD, help families locate the closest Veterans Administration (VA) for support and services. Services may include home-based primary care, homemaker and home health aides, respite care, adult day health care, outpatient clinics, inpatient hospital services, nursing home, or hospice care. Caregiver support is an essential part of all of these services.

◆ *Evaluation: Reflecting*

Evaluate the care of the patient with AD based on the identified priority patient problems. The expected outcomes include that the patient and/or family will:

- Maintain memory and cognitive function for as long as possible and increase their quality of life
- Remain free from injury and accidents and have a safe environment
- Manage caregiver stress and strain to prevent elder abuse

Specific indicators for these outcomes are listed in the Planning and Implementation section (see earlier).

✳ MOBILITY CONCEPT EXEMPLAR
Parkinson Disease

❖ PATHOPHYSIOLOGY

Parkinson disease (PD), also referred to as *Parkinson's disease* and *paralysis agitans*, is a progressive neurodegenerative disease that is the one of the most common neurologic disorders of older adults. It is a debilitating disease affecting MOBILITY and is characterized by four cardinal symptoms: tremor, muscle rigidity, **bradykinesia** or **akinesia** (slow movement/no movement), and postural instability. Young and middle-age adults with these signs and symptoms may be misdiagnosed as having **Huntington disease**, a rare hereditary disorder that is characterized by progressive dementia and **choreiform movements** (uncontrollable rapid, jerky movements) in the limbs, trunk, and facial muscles. Table 42-3 briefly compares Parkinson and Huntington diseases.

Most people have *primary*, or idiopathic, disease. A few patients have *secondary* parkinsonian symptoms from conditions such as brain tumors and certain anti-psychotic drugs.

Normally, motor activity occurs as a result of integrating the actions of the cerebral cortex, basal ganglia, and cerebellum. The **basal ganglia** are a group of neurons located deep within the cerebrum at the base of the brain near the lateral ventricles.

When the basal ganglia are stimulated, muscle tone in the body is inhibited, and voluntary movements are refined. The secretion of two major neurotransmitters accomplishes this process: dopamine and acetylcholine (ACh).

Dopamine is produced in the substantia nigra and the adrenal glands and is transmitted to the basal ganglia along a connecting neural pathway for secretion when needed. *ACh* is produced and secreted by the basal ganglia and in the nerve endings in the periphery of the body. ACh-producing neurons transmit *excitatory* messages throughout the basal ganglia. Dopamine *inhibits* the function of these neurons, allowing control over voluntary movement. This system of checks and balances usually allows for refined, coordinated movement, such as picking up a pencil and writing.

In PD, widespread degeneration of the *substantia nigra* then leads to a decrease in the amount of dopamine in the brain. When dopamine levels are decreased, a person loses the ability to refine voluntary movement. The large numbers of excitatory ACh-secreting neurons remain active, creating an imbalance between excitatory and inhibitory neuronal activity. The resulting excessive excitation of neurons prevents a person from controlling or initiating voluntary movement (McCance et al., 2014).

Not only does PD interfere with movement as a result of dopamine loss in the brain; it also reduces the sympathetic nervous system influence on the heart, blood vessels, and other areas of the body. This loss results in the orthostatic hypotension, drooling, nocturia (voiding at night), and other autonomic symptoms frequently seen in the patient with PD. Some patients also have neuropsychiatric symptoms, including mood changes.

PD is separated into stages according to the symptoms and degree of disability. Stage 1 is mild disease with unilateral limb

TABLE 42-3 Comparison of Parkinson Disease and Huntington Disease

	PARKINSON DISEASE	HUNTINGTON DISEASE
Cause	*Primary disease:* Cause not known, but could be a combination of genetic and environmental factors *Secondary disease:* Caused by anti-psychotic drugs or another condition such as brain tumor or trauma	Hereditary disease transmitted by an autosomal-dominant trait at conception
Pathophysiologic changes	Chronic, terminal disease caused by degeneration of substantia nigra cells in the basal ganglia of the brain causing decreased dopamine, which normally functions to promote voluntary muscle and sympathetic nervous system control	Chronic, terminal disease caused by alterations in amounts of dopamine, gamma-aminobutyric acid (GABA), and glutamate from the basal ganglia
Course of disease	Steady and gradual decline (typically 10-20 years) of cognitive, mobility, and ADL function from mild through severe stages (see Table 42-4); patients usually die from complications of immobility	Gradual decline (typically about 15 years) of cognitive and neuromuscular symptoms; characterized by progressive dementia and choreiform movements (uncontrollable rapid, jerky movements) in the limbs, trunk, and facial muscles; patients usually die from complications of immobility
Risk factors	**Primary:** Male Over 40 years of age Family history (particularly first-degree relatives (e.g., parent, sibling) **Secondary:** Traumatic brain injury Brain tumor or other lesion	Dominant inheritance 30-50 years of age equally in men and women (when symptoms typically begin)
Management	Safety measures to prevent injury or falls Anti-Parkinson drugs Symptom management ADL and mobility assistance as needed based on stage	Safety measures to prevent injury or falls Supportive care Behavior management ADL and mobility assistance as needed based on stage

TABLE 42-4   Stages of Parkinson Disease
Stage 1: Initial Stage • Unilateral limb involvement • Minimal weakness • Hand and arm trembling Stage 2: Mild Stage • Bilateral limb involvement • Masklike face • Slow, shuffling gait Stage 3: Moderate Disease • Postural instability • Increased gait disturbances Stage 4: Severe Disability • Akinesia • Rigidity Stage 5: Complete ADL Dependence

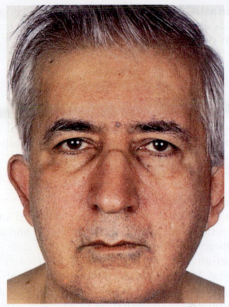

FIG. 42-2 The masklike facial expression typical of patients with Parkinson disease.

involvement, whereas the patient with stage 5 disease is completely dependent in all ADLs. Other classifications refer simply to mild, moderate, and severe disease (Table 42-4).

Etiology and Genetic Risk

Although the exact cause of PD is not known, it is probably the result of environmental and genetic factors. Exposure to pesticides, herbicides, and industrial chemicals and metals and drinking well water, being older than 40 years, and having reduced estrogen levels are known risk factors for the development of PD.

Primary Parkinson disease (PD) often has a familial tendency. The disease is associated with a variety of mitochondrial DNA (mtDNA) variations that often involve deletions in the genetic sequences that are used in central nervous system (CNS) mitochondria, the energy powerhouses of cells. These variations ultimately cause destruction of neurons that produce dopamine in the substantia nigra (McCance et al., 2014).

Incidence and Prevalence

In the United States, about 60,000 new cases of PD are diagnosed each year. As many as 1 million patients live with the disease. As the population ages, the number of people affected by PD is expected to dramatically increase. About 50% more men than women currently have the disease, but the exact reason for this difference is not known (LaRocco, 2015).

❖ INTERPROFESSIONAL COLLABORATIVE CARE

◆ Assessment: Noticing

History. Collect data related to the time and progression of symptoms noticed by the patient or family. The older adult may assume that these behaviors are normal changes associated with aging and therefore ignore early signs and symptoms such as *resting* tremors, bradykinesia (slowed movement), fatigue, and problems with muscular rigidity.

Physical Assessment: Signs and Symptoms. Tremors are usually noticed in the upper extremities first and may increase with stress. Slow voluntary movements and reduced automatic movements may be manifested by a change in the patient's handwriting. Some patients report "freezing" because they feel that they are stuck to the floor. Assess the patient for *rigidity*, or resistance to passive movement of the extremities, which is classified as:

• *Cogwheel,* manifested by a rhythmic interruption of the muscle movement

• *Plastic,* defined as mildly restrictive movement
• *Lead pipe,* or total resistance to movement

Rigidity is present early in the disease process and progresses over time. Observe the patient's ability to relax a muscle or move a selected muscle group. Observe the patient's gait, posture (often unstable), and ability to ambulate with or without ambulatory aids.

Changes in facial expression or a *masklike face* with wide-open, fixed, staring eyes is caused by rigidity of the facial muscles (Fig. 42-2). This rigidity can lead to difficulties in chewing and swallowing, particularly if the pharyngeal muscles are involved. As a result, the patient may have inadequate nutrition. Uncontrolled drooling may occur. Some patients develop dementia later as the disease progresses. In addition to changes in voluntary movement, many patients experience autonomic nervous system symptoms, such as excessive perspiration and orthostatic hypotension. Orthostatic hypotension is likely related to loss of sympathetic innervation in the heart and blood vessel response.

Patients can also develop emotional changes such as depression, irritability, apathy, anxiety, and insecurity (LaRocco, 2015). These symptoms may develop because patients fear that they will not be able to cope with new situations.

Changes in speech pattern are common in PD patients. They may speak very softly, slur or repeat their words, use a monotone voice or a halting speech, hesitate before speaking, or exhibit a rapid speech pattern.

Bowel and bladder problems are commonly seen in PD as a result of malfunction of the autonomic nervous system, which regulates smooth muscle activity. Patients can exhibit symptoms of either urinary incontinence or difficulty urinating. Constipation can occur because of slow motility of the GI tract or because of poor dietary habits and poor fluid intake.

Laboratory and Imaging Assessment. The diagnosis of PD is made based on clinical findings after other neurologic diseases are eliminated as possibilities. There are no specific diagnostic tests. Analysis of cerebrospinal fluid (CSF) may show a decrease in dopamine levels, although the results of other studies are usually normal. Other diagnostic tests may be done such as an MRI or single-photon emission computed tomography (SPECT) to rule out other CNS health problems.

◆ Analysis: Interpreting

The priority collaborative problems for patients with PD include:

1. Decreased mobility (and possible self-care deficit) due to muscle rigidity, tremors, and postural instability
2. Potential for decreased self-esteem due to impaired cognition, tremors, and self-care deficit

◆ Planning and Implementation: Responding

Promoting Mobility

Planning: Expected Outcomes. The expected outcome is that the patient will maintain optimal MOBILITY and not experience complications of impaired mobility.

Interventions

Nonsurgical Management. Care for the patient with PD includes drug therapy, exercise programs or physical therapy, and interprofessional collaboration to promote MOBILITY and self-care and prevent falls or other injuries. Chart 42-5 summarizes best practices for nursing management of the patient with PD.

Drug Therapy. Drugs are prescribed to treat the symptoms of PD with the purpose of increasing the patient's MOBILITY and self-care abilities. An equally important desired outcome is that drugs used for the disease have minimal long-term side effects. Many questions and controversies remain about which drugs to use, when to start therapy, and how to prevent complications. Drug administration is closely monitored, and the health care

provider adjusts the dosage or changes therapy as the patient's condition requires. Teach the patient and family how to monitor for and report adverse effects of drug therapy.

Dopamine agonists mimic dopamine by stimulating dopamine receptors in the brain. They are typically the most effective during the first 3 to 5 years of use. The benefit of these agents is fewer incidents of **dyskinesias** (problems with movement) and "wearing off" phenomenon (loss of response to the drug) when compared with other drugs. This problem is characterized by periods of good mobility ("on") alternating with periods of altered MOBILITY ("off"). Patients report that their most distressing symptom is the "off time."

Examples of dopamine agonists are apomorphine (Apokyn [a morphine derivative]), pramipexole (Mirapex), and ropinirole (Requip). Another drug in this class, rotigotine, is available as a continuous transdermal patch (Neupro) to maintain a consistent level of dopamine.

> ⚠ **NURSING SAFETY PRIORITY** **QSEN**
>
> ### *Drug Alert*
>
> Dopamine agonists are associated with adverse effects such as orthostatic (postural) hypotension, hallucinations, sleepiness, and drowsiness. Remind patients to avoid operating heavy machinery or driving if they have any of these symptoms. Teach them to change from a lying or sitting position to standing by moving slowly. The health care provider should not prescribe drugs in this class to older adults because of their severe adverse drug effects.

Almost all patients are on Sinemet, a combination *levodopa-carbidopa* drug, at some point in their disease. It may be the initial drug of choice if the patient's presenting symptoms are severe or interfere with work or school. Both an immediate-release (IR) and controlled-release (CR) form of Sinemet in varying doses are available. The levodopa agents are less expensive than the dopamine agonists and are better at improving motor function. Long-term use leads to dyskinesia (inability to perform voluntary movement). Teach the patient and family to give the drug before meals to increase absorption and transport across the blood-brain barrier.

Catechol O–methyltransferases (COMTs) are enzymes that inactivate dopamine. Therefore COMT *inhibitors* block this enzyme activity, thus prolonging the action of levodopa. One example is entacapone (Comtan), which is often used in combination with levodopa. Stalevo is a combination of levodopa, carbidopa, and entacapone. The benefit of these combinations is that the disease is treated in several ways with one drug. However, they are not beneficial for patients who need more specific dosages of individual drugs.

Monamine oxidase type B (MAO-B) inhibitors (MAOIs) are more popular for use in patients with early or mild symptoms of PD. Entacapone (Comtan) and selegiline (Deprenyl, Eldepryl) are often given with levodopa for early or mild disease. A newer MAOI-B for PD is rasagiline mesylate (Azilect), which can be given as a single drug or with levodopa. The MAOI-B drugs work by slowing the main type (B) of monamine oxidase in the brain, increasing dopamine concentrations, and helping reduce the signs and symptoms of PD. They may also protect neurons in the brain (Burchum & Rosenthal, 2016).

When other drugs are no longer effective, bromocriptine mesylate (Parlodel), a *dopamine receptor agonist,* may be

---

> ◎ **CHART 42-5   Best Practice for Patient Safety & Quality Care** **QSEN**
>
> ### *Care of the Patient With Parkinson Disease*
>
> - Allow the patient extra time to respond to questions.
> - Administer medications promptly on schedule to maintain continuous therapeutic drug levels.
> - Provide medication for pain and/or tingling in limbs, as needed.
> - Monitor for side effects of medications, especially orthostatic hypotension, hallucinations, and acute confusional state (delirium).
> - Place the patient on Fall Precautions according to agency protocol.
> - Collaborate with physical and occupational therapists to keep the patient as mobile and independent as possible in ADLs.
> - Allow the patient time to perform ADLs and MOBILITY skills; provide assistance only as needed.
> - Implement interventions to prevent complications of impaired MOBILITY, such as constipation, pressure injuries, and contractures.
> - Schedule appointments and activities late in the morning to prevent rushing the patient or schedule them at the time of the patient's optimal level of functioning.
> - Teach the patient to speak slowly and clearly. Use alternative communication methods, such as a communication board or handheld mobile device. Refer to the speech-language pathologist.
> - Monitor the patient's ability to eat and swallow. Monitor actual food and fluid intake.
> - Collaborate with the dietitian to provide high-protein, high-calorie foods or supplements to maintain weight.
> - Recognize that Parkinson disease can affect the patient's self-esteem. Focus on the patient's strengths.
> - Assess for depression and anxiety.
> - Assess for insomnia or sleeplessness.

prescribed to promote the release of dopamine. It may be used alone or in combination with carbidopa/levodopa (Sinemet). Some providers may prescribe Parlodel early in the course of treatment. It is especially useful in the patient who has experienced side effects such as dyskinesias or orthostatic hypotension while receiving Sinemet.

Amantadine (Symmetrel) is an *antiviral drug* that has anti-Parkinson benefits. It may be given early in disease to reduce symptoms. It is also prescribed with Sinemet to reduce dyskinesias. Rivastigmine (Exelon) is a *cholinesterase inhibitor* that is used only when patients with PD have dementia. This drug works to improve the transmission of acetylcholine in the brain by delaying its destruction by the enzyme *acetylcholinesterase.*

For severe motor symptoms such as tremors and rigidity, one of the older *anticholinergic* drugs may be prescribed, but they are rarely used as primary drugs of choice for PD. Examples are benztropine (Cogentin), trihexyphenidyl HCl (Artane), and procyclidine (Kemadrin). *These drugs should be avoided in older adults because they can cause acute confusion, urinary retention, constipation, dry mouth, and blurred vision. Newer and safer drugs are available for this age-group.*

For the patient on any long-term drug therapy regimen, drug tolerance or *drug toxicity* often develops. Drug toxicity may be evidenced by changes in COGNITION such as delirium (acute confusion) or hallucinations and decreased effectiveness of the drug. Delirium may be difficult to assess in the patient who is already suffering from chronic dementia as a result of PD or another disease. If possible, compare the patient's current cognitive and behavioral status with his or her baseline before drug therapy begins.

When drug tolerance is reached, the drug's effects do not last as long as previously. The treatment of PD drug toxicity or tolerance includes:

- A reduction in drug dosage
- A change of drug or in the frequency of administration
- A drug holiday (particularly with levodopa therapy)

During a drug holiday, which typically lasts up to 10 days, the patient receives no drug therapy for PD. Carefully monitor the patient for symptoms of PD during this time and document assessment findings.

Many patients are on additional drugs to help relieve symptoms associated with the disease. For example, muscle spasms may be relieved by baclofen (Kemstro), drooling can be minimized by sublingual atropine sulfate (Atropair), and insomnia may require a sleeping aid such as zolpidem tartrate (Ambien). If patients also become moderately to severely depressed, an antidepressant such as short-acting venlafaxine (Effexor) may be prescribed. This complicated drug regimen may be confusing to patients. Electronic reminders may be effective in helping to educate patients and maintain drug adherence.

Other Interventions. A freezing gait and postural instability are major problems for patients with PD. Nontraditional exercise programs, such as yoga and tai chi, may help elevate mood and improve MOBILITY in the early stage of the disease. Early in the disease process, collaborate with physical and occupational therapists to plan and implement a program to keep the patient flexible, prevent falling, and retain mobility by incorporating active and passive range-of-motion (ROM) exercises, muscle stretching, and out-of-bed activity. Remind the patient to avoid concentrating on his or her feet when walking to prevent falls. *If the patient is hospitalized for any reason, be sure that he or she is placed on Fall Precautions according to agency policy.*

In collaboration with the rehabilitation team, encourage the patient to participate as much as possible in self-management, including ADLs. The team makes the environment conducive to independence in activity and as stress-free and safe as possible. Occupational and physical therapists provide training in ADLs and the use of adaptive devices, as needed, to facilitate independence. The occupational therapist (OT) evaluates the patient for the need for adaptive devices (e.g., special utensils for eating).

Patients with PD tend to not sleep well at night because of drug therapy and the disease itself. Some patients nap for short periods during the day and may not be aware that they have done so. This sleep misperception may put the patient at risk for injury. For example, he or she may fall asleep while driving an automobile. Therefore teach the patient and family to monitor the patient's sleeping pattern and discuss whether he or she can operate machinery or perform other potentially high-risk tasks safely.

Collaborate with the dietitian, if needed, to evaluate the patient's food intake and ability to eat. The patient's intake of calcium, vitamin K, and other nutrients is evaluated, especially in the patient who has difficulty swallowing or is susceptible to injury from falling. The dietitian considers the patient's bowel habits and adjusts the diet if constipation occurs. If the patient has trouble swallowing, collaborate with the speech-language pathologist (SLP) for an extensive swallowing evaluation. Based on these findings and the patient interview, an individualized nutritional plan is developed. Usually a soft diet and thick, cold fluids, such as milk shakes, are tolerated more easily.

Small, frequent meals or a commercial powder, such as Thick-It, added to liquids may assist the patient who has difficulty swallowing. Elevate the patient's head to allow easier swallowing and prevent aspiration. Remind UAP and teach the family to be careful when serving or feeding the patient. The SLP can be very helpful in recommending specific feeding strategies. Be sure that UAP record food intake daily or as needed. The patient loses weight because of altered food intake and the increased number of calories burned secondary to muscle rigidity. Teach the family to weigh the patient once a week so adjustments to the diet can be made as indicated. As the disease progresses and swallowing becomes more of a problem, supplemental feedings become the main source of nutrition to maintain weight, with meals and other foods taken as the patient can tolerate.

Collaborate with the SLP if the patient has speech difficulties. Together with the interprofessional health care team, patient, and family, develop a communication plan. The SLP teaches exercises to strengthen muscles used for breathing, speech, and swallowing. Remind the patient to speak slowly and clearly and to pause and take deep breaths at times during each sentence. Teach the family the importance of avoiding unnecessary environmental noise to increase the listener's ability to hear and understand the patient. Ask the patient to repeat words that the listener does not understand. Have the listener watch the patient's lips and nonverbal expressions for cues to the meaning of conversation. Remind the patient to organize his or her thoughts before speaking and use facial expression and gestures, if possible, to assist with communication. In addition, he or she should exaggerate words to increase the listener's ability to understand. If the patient cannot communicate verbally, he or she can use alternative methods of communication, such as a communication board, mechanical voice synthesizer, computer, or handheld mobile device. The SLP assesses the ability to use these devices before a decision is made about which method to use. Some older patients may not want to use electronic methods to communicate.

❓ NCLEX EXAMINATION CHALLENGE 42-4

Physiological Integrity

The nurse is preparing to administer Sinemet to a client whose highest blood pressure is 88/50 while lying in bed. What is the nurse's **priority** action at this time?
A. Instruct the client to get out of bed slowly.
B. Withhold the drug until contacting the primary health care provider.
C. Ask the client about the presence of hallucinations.
D. Take the client's apical pulse and temperature.

Surgical Management. Several options are available if surgery for the patient with PD is needed. Surgery is a last resort when drugs are not effective in symptom management. The most common surgeries are stereotactic pallidotomy and deep brain stimulation, although newer surgical procedures are being tried. Deep brain stimulation has largely replaced the older thalamotomy procedure.

Stereotactic pallidotomy (opening into the pallidum within the corpus striatum) can be a very effective treatment for controlling the symptoms associated with PD. First, the target area within the pallidum is identified by a CT or MRI scan. Next, the stereotactic head frame is placed on the patient. IV sedation is given, and a burr hole is made into the cranium. An electrode or cylindric rod is inserted into the target area. The target area receives a mild electrical stimulation, and the patient's reaction is assessed for reduction of tremor and rigidity. If this result does not occur or if unexpected visual, motor, or sensory symptoms appear, the probe is repositioned. When the probe is in the ideal location, a permanent lesion (scarring) is made to destroy the tissue. The patient is monitored in the postanesthesia care unit (PACU) for about 1 hour and is then returned to the inpatient unit for continuing observation.

Deep brain stimulation (DBS) is approved as a treatment for PD. In DBS, electrodes are implanted into the brain and connected to a small electrical device called a *pulse generator* that delivers electrical current. The generator is placed under the skin similar to a cardiac pacemaker device. It is externally programmed to deliver an electrical current to decrease involuntary movements known as **dyskinesias**, resulting in a reduced need for levodopa and related drugs. DBS also helps to alleviate fluctuations of symptoms and reduce tremors, slowness of movements, and gait problems (National Institute of Neurological Disorders and Stroke [NINDS], 2017).

Fetal tissue transplantation is an experimental and highly controversial ethical and political treatment. Fetal substantia nigra tissue, either human or pig, is transplanted into the caudate nucleus of the brain. Preliminary reports suggest that patients show clinical improvement in motor symptoms without dyskinesias after receiving the transplanted tissue. Long-term results are yet to be seen or studied (NINDS, 2017).

Promoting Self-Esteem

Planning: Expected Outcomes. The expected outcome is that the patient with PD will not experience altered self-esteem as a result of having strong psychosocial support.

Interventions. Although not all patients with PD have dementia, impaired COGNITION and memory deficits are common. Some patients also experience changes in gait and tremors that are uncontrollable. In the late stages of the disease, they cannot move without assistance, have difficulty talking, have minimal facial expression, and may drool. Patients often state that they are embarrassed and tend to avoid social events or groups of people. They should not be forced into situations in which they feel ashamed of their appearance. Encourage patients to undertake activities that do not require small-muscle dexterity, such as light, modified aerobic exercises.

Teach the family to emphasize the patient's abilities or strengths and provide positive reinforcement when he or she meets expected outcomes. The patient, family or significant other, and rehabilitation team mutually set realistic expected outcomes that can be achieved.

Care Coordination and Transition Management

Home Care Preparation. The long-term management of PD presents a special challenge in the home care setting. A case manager may be required to coordinate interprofessional care and provide support for the patient and family. Impaired MOBILITY can affect the patient's daily lifestyle and self-concept, including sexuality. The case manager or home care nurse uses a holistic approach to ensure that both psychosocial and physical needs are addressed.

Self-Management Education. Teach patients and their families about the need to follow instructions regarding the safe administration of drug therapy. Remind them to immediately report adverse effects of medication such as dizziness, falls, acute confusion (delirium), and hallucinations. For patients who had surgery, review discharge instructions about when to resume activity and contact the surgeon.

Teach family members or other caregivers the importance of maintaining or improving the patient's quality of life by helping to alleviate or manage symptoms. For example, constipation can cause altered COMFORT and can be prevented or managed by encouraging adequate fluids, a high-fiber diet, and a regular bowel-training program with suppositories and bulk-forming laxatives. Sleep disorders may be managed with a good sleep-hygiene program, including avoiding alcohol and caffeine, darkening the bedroom, and bedtime rituals (LaRocco, 2015).

Neuropsychiatric health problems, such as impulse control disorders, altered COGNITION, anxiety, and depression can be very difficult for both the patient and family. Remind families and other caregivers that the patient cannot control these symptoms. Caregiver role strain can be a major problem when caring for patients with PD (see earlier discussion under Alzheimer's disease for caregiver stress management).

Health Care Resources. Collaborate with the social worker or case manager to help the family with financial and health insurance issues, as well as respite care or permanent placement if needed. Refer the patient and family to social and state agencies, support groups, and information as needed. Examples in the United States are the National Parkinson Foundation (www.parkinson.org), American Parkinson Disease Association (www.apdaparkinson.org), and the Parkinson Disease Foundation (www.pdf.org). The Michael J. Fox Foundation for Parkinson's Research (www.michaeljfox.org) provides an extensive list of resources about living with PD. Patients and families in Canada can access Parkinson Canada (www.parkinson.ca) for information about the disease and support groups.

As the disease progresses and drug effectiveness decreases, refer the family to a palliative care organization or hospice. Referral sources can be obtained from the Center to Advance Palliative Care (www.capc.org), which advocates applying the principles of palliative care to chronic disease. Chapter 7 discusses palliative and hospice care in detail.

🧑 CLINICAL JUDGMENT CHALLENGE 42-1

Patient-Centered Care; Safety QSEN

You are assigned to care for a 70-year-old man who was admitted for severe hypotension, dizziness, and frequent falls. The patient has had Parkinson disease (PD) for 5 years and has intentional tremors that are worse in his right hand and arm. He tells you that he served in Vietnam and had a minor head injury from a vehicle accident there. His wife confirms his history but states that the patient has short-term memory loss, which is getting worse. As a result, he sometimes forgets to take his medications. The patient's father also had PD and died of complications of impaired mobility.

1. What safety concerns do you anticipate for this patient?
2. What are the patient's top three priority problems based on the provided information?
3. What additional assessment data do you need to plan this patient's care?
4. What significance might the previous head injury have in planning this patient's care?

◆ Evaluation: Reflecting

Evaluate the care of the patient with PD based on the identified priority patient problems. The expected outcomes include that the patient and/or family will:

- Improve MOBILITY to provide self-care and not experience complications of impaired mobility
- Maintain a positive self-esteem and acceptable quality of life

MIGRAINE HEADACHE

❖ PATHOPHYSIOLOGY

Most individuals experience some type of headache during their lifetime from a variety of causes, such as low blood sugar, sinus infection, alcohol, and stress. These headaches are acute and temporary and often resolve by managing the cause of the headache and/or mild analgesics such as acetaminophen (Tylenol). Some adults have specific types of headache that cause severe, debilitating pain and recur. The most common type is migraine headache. This type of headache is most likely to affect quality of life when compared to other less common types.

A migraine headache is a common clinical syndrome characterized by recurrent episodic attacks of head pain that serve no protective purpose. Migraine headache pain is usually described as throbbing and unilateral. Migraines can be accompanied by associated symptoms such as nausea or sensitivity to light, sound, or head movement and can last 4 to 72 hours. They tend to be familial, and women are affected more commonly than men. Women diagnosed with migraines are more likely to have major depressive disorder (Malone et al., 2015). Migraine sufferers are also at risk for stroke and epilepsy (Malone et al., 2015; McCance et al., 2014).

The cause of migraine headaches is not clear but includes a combination of neuronal hyperexcitability and vascular, genetic, hormonal, and environmental factors. In general, experts suggest that migraines are a neurogenic process with secondary cerebral vasodilation followed by a sterile brain tissue inflammation. Patients may inherit a condition of neuronal hyperexcitability from ion channel variations, particularly calcium and sodium-potassium pump channels, as well as from genetic variations in serotonin and dopamine receptors. Following stimulation of these hyper-excitable neuronal pathways, vascular changes occur. Pain-sensing cells in the blood vessels of the brain initiate the attack. Activation of the trigeminal nerve pathways contributes to the cascade of events that activate nociceptors. Substances that increase sensitivity to pain such as glutamate are synthesized through the trigeminal pathway (McCance et al., 2014). As cerebral arteries dilate, prostaglandins are released (chemicals that cause inflammation and swelling). Vasodilation, in turn, allows prostaglandins and other intravascular molecules to leak (extravasate), contributing to widespread tissue swelling and the sensation of throbbing pain.

Many patients find that certain factors, or *triggers,* such as caffeine, red wine, and monosodium glutamate (MSG), tend to cause migraine headache attacks. Each patient is different regarding which environmental factors trigger headaches. For some patients, stress or a change in weather can lead to an attack. These stimuli are thought to initiate the cascade of events that cause migraines by activating hyper-excitable neurons. Neurons involved in the initiation and propagation of migraines may have an early sensitization to neurotransmitters such that patients become increasingly susceptible to triggers and to the cascade of events that culminate in migraine pain. Thus care includes not only managing pain but also disrupting the migraine cascade to decrease sensitization and recurrent attacks.

❖ INTERPROFESSIONAL COLLABORATIVE CARE
◆ Assessment: Noticing

Migraines fall into three categories: migraines with aura, migraines without aura, and atypical migraines. An aura is a sensation (e.g., visual changes) that signals the onset of a headache or seizure. In a migraine, the aura occurs immediately before the migraine episode. *Most headaches are migraines without aura.* The key features of migraines are listed in Chart 42-6. Atypical migraines are less common and include menstrual and cluster migraines. The stages of migraine may include:

- Prodromal (or prodrome) phase, in which the patient has specific symptoms such as food cravings or mood changes
- Aura phase (if present), which generally involves visual changes, flashing lights, or diplopia (double vision)
- Headache phase, which may last a few hours to a few days
- Termination phase, in which the intensity of the headache decreases

CHART 42-6 **Key Features**

Migraine Headaches

Phases of Migraine With Aura (Classic Migraine)
First, or Prodrome, Phase
- Aura that develops over a period of several minutes and lasts no longer than 1 hour
- Well-defined transient focal neurologic dysfunction exists
- Pain may be preceded by:
  - Visual disturbances
  - Flashing lights
  - Lines or spots
  - Shimmering or zigzag lights
- A variety of neurologic changes, including:
  - Numbness, tingling of the lips or tongue
  - Acute confusional state
  - Aphasia
  - Vertigo
  - Unilateral weakness
  - Drowsiness

Second Phase
- Headache accompanied by nausea and vomiting
- Pain usually beginning in the temple; increases in intensity and becomes throbbing within 1 hour

Third Phase
- Pain changing from throbbing to dull
- Headache, nausea, and vomiting usually lasting from 4 to 72 hours (Older patients may have aura without pain, known as a *visual migraine.*)

Migraine Without Aura (Common Migraine)
- Migraine beginning without an aura before the onset of the headache
- Pain aggravated by performing routine physical activities
- Pain that is unilateral and pulsating
- One of these symptoms is present:
  - Nausea and/or vomiting
  - **Photophobia** (light sensitivity)
  - **Phonophobia** (sound sensitivity)
- Headache lasting for 4 to 72 hours
- Migraine often occurring in the early morning, during periods of stress, or in those with premenstrual tension or fluid retention

Atypical Migraine
- Status migrainous:
  - Headache lasting longer than 72 hours
- Migrainous infarction:
  - Neurologic symptoms not completely reversible within 7 days
  - Ischemic infarct noted on neuroimaging
- Unclassified:
  - Headache not fulfilling all of the criteria to be classified a migraine

- Postprodrome phase, in which the patient is often fatigued, may be irritable, and has muscle pain

The diagnosis of migraine headache is based on the patient's history and on physical, neurologic, and psychological assessment. The typical migraine is described as a unilateral, frontotemporal, *throbbing* pain in the head that is often worse behind one eye or ear. It is often accompanied by a sensitive scalp, anorexia, **photophobia** (sensitivity to light), **phonophobia** (sensitivity to noise), and nausea with or without vomiting. Patients tend to have the same signs and symptoms each time they have a migraine headache. Some may have to refrain from

regular activities for several days if they cannot control or relieve the impaired COMFORT in its early stage.

Some health care providers recommend screening patients with migraines using the Minnesota Multiphasic Personality Inventory–2 to identify personality traits and possible mental health/behavioral health problems such as depression that may contribute to the headache experience (Rausa et al., 2013). Neuroimaging such as MRI may be indicated if the patient has other neurologic findings, a history of seizures, findings not consistent with a migraine, or a change in the severity of the symptoms or frequency of the attacks.

Neuroimaging is also recommended in patients older than 50 years with a new onset of headaches, especially women. Women with a history of migraines with visual symptoms may have an increased risk for stroke, particularly if a migraine with visual symptoms occurred in the past year. Teach women older than 50 years who have migraines about the risk factors for cardiovascular disease. Encourage them to notify their health care provider if they experience symptoms such as facial drooping, arm weakness, or difficulties with speech.

◆ Interventions: Responding

The priority for care of the patient having migraines is pain management. This outcome may be achieved by abortive and preventive therapy. Drug therapy, trigger management, and complementary and integrative therapies are the major approaches to care. Provide detailed patient and family education regarding the collaborative plan of care. Effective health care provider/patient communication is increasingly important in managing the symptoms of migraines.

Abortive Therapy. Abortive therapy is aimed at alleviating pain during the aura phase (if present) or soon after the headache has started. *Drug therapy* is prescribed to manage migraine headaches. Some of the drugs used have major side effects, contraindications, and nursing implications. The health care provider must consider any other medical conditions that the patient has when prescribing drug therapy. In general, the patient is started on a low dose that is increased until the desired clinical effect is obtained. Many new drugs are being investigated for this painful and often debilitating health problem.

Mild migraines may be relieved by acetaminophen (APAP) (Tylenol, Abenol). NSAIDs such as ibuprofen (Motrin) and naproxen (Naprosyn) may also be prescribed. In the United States, the FDA has approved several over-the-counter (OTC) anti-inflammatory drugs for migraines, including Advil migraine capsules, Motrin migraine pain caplets, and Excedrin migraine tablets or caplets (contain APAP, aspirin, and caffeine). Caffeine narrows blood vessels by blocking adenosine, which dilates vessels and increases inflammation. Antiemetics may be prescribed to relieve nausea and vomiting. Metoclopramide (Reglan, Clopra) may be administered with NSAIDs to promote gastric emptying and decrease vomiting.

For more *severe* migraines, drugs such as triptan preparations, ergotamine derivatives, and isometheptene combinations are needed. A potential side effect of these drugs is **rebound headache**, also known as **medication overuse headache**, in which another headache occurs after the drug relieves the initial migraine.

Triptan preparations relieve the headache and associated symptoms by activating the 5-HT (serotonin) receptors on the cranial arteries, the basilar artery, and the blood vessels of the dura mater to produce a vasoconstrictive effect. Examples are sumatriptan (Imitrex), eletriptan (Relpax), naratriptan (Amerge), and almotriptan (Axert). The older drug sumatriptan is available as an oral agent, injection, and nasal spray (Burchum & Rosenthal, 2016). For many patients, these drugs are highly and quickly effective for pain, nausea, vomiting, and light and sound sensitivity with few side effects. However, sumatriptan is most likely to cause chest pain after one or more doses. Therefore most triptans are contraindicated in patients with actual or suspected ischemic heart disease, cerebrovascular ischemia, hypertension, and peripheral vascular disease and in those with Prinzmetal's angina because of the potential for coronary vasospasm. Patients respond differently to drugs, and several types or combinations may be tried before the headache is relieved (Burchum & Rosenthal, 2016).

> ## ! NURSING SAFETY PRIORITY QSEN
> ### Drug Alert
>
> Teach patients taking triptan drugs to take them as soon as migraine symptoms develop. Instruct patients to report angina (chest pain) or chest discomfort to their health care providers immediately to prevent cardiac damage from myocardial ischemia. Remind them to use contraception (birth control) while taking the drugs because the drugs may not be safe for women who are pregnant. Teach them to expect common side effects that include flushing, tingling, and a hot sensation. These annoying sensations tend to subside after the patient's body gets used to the drug. Triptan drugs should not be taken with selective serotonin reuptake inhibitor (SSRI) antidepressants or St. John's wort, an herb used commonly for depression (Burchum & Rosenthal, 2016).

Ergotamine preparations such as Cafergot are taken at the start of the headache. The patient may take up to six tablets in 24 hours or use a rectal suppository. Dihydroergotamine (DHE) may be given IV, IM, or as a nasal spray (Migranal) with an antiemetic if pain control and relief of nausea are not achieved with other drugs. It should not be given within 24 hours of a triptan drug.

Midrin is a combination drug containing APAP, isomeptene, and dichloralphenazone. It is the most common *isomeptene combination* given for treating migraines and is an excellent option when ergotamine preparations are not tolerated or do not work.

Preventive Therapy. Prevention drugs and other strategies are used when a migraine occurs more than twice per week, interferes with ADLs, or is not relieved with acute treatment. Unless otherwise contraindicated, the health care provider may initially prescribe an NSAID, a beta-adrenergic blocker, a calcium channel blocker, or an antiepileptic drug (AED). Propranolol (Inderal, Apo-Propranolol, Novopranol) and timolol (Blocadren, Apo-Timol) are the only *beta blockers* approved for migraine prevention. Verapamil (Calan, Apo-Verap), a *calcium channel blocking agent,* may also be used for some patients. The calcium channel and beta blockers are thought to reduce the activity of hyper-excitable neurons and act on the neurogenic causes of migraine. Both calcium channel blockers and beta blockers interfere with vasodilation, a contributing cause of migraine pain. Both beta-adrenergic blockers and calcium channel blocking drugs can lower blood pressure and decrease pulse rate.

Topiramate (Topamax) is one of the most common *antiepileptic drugs (AEDs)* used for migraines, but it should be used in low doses of 25 to 100 mg daily. The mechanism of action is

> ## ! NURSING SAFETY PRIORITY QSEN
> ### Drug Alert
>
> Teach patients who take beta-adrenergic blockers or calcium channel blockers how to take their pulse. Encourage them to report bradycardia or adverse reactions such as fatigue and shortness of breath to their health care provider as soon as possible.

not clear, but this drug may inhibit the sodium channels, channels that may be hyper-excitable in patients with migraine. Reports of suicides have been associated with this drug when it is used in larger doses of 400 mg daily, most often with patients who have bipolar disorder.

Nortriptyline (Pamelor, Apo-Nortriptyline ♦) is a tricyclic antidepressant that is often effective as a drug to prevent or reduce migraine episodes. The drug is started in a low dose, usually 10 mg, and may be increased to 30 mg or more, depending on the patient's needs. Side effects include dry mouth, urinary retention, and constipation. The drug is not used for older adults because it can also cause delirium or acute confusion.

Encourage patients to keep a headache diary to help identify the type of headache they are experiencing and the response to preventive medication or other intervention. Teach them to notify their health care provider if the quality, intensity, or nature of the headache increases or changes. Encourage them to report whether the headache is associated with new or unusual visual changes and if the prescribed drug is no longer effective.

For chronic migraine, onabotulinumtoxinA (Botox) is the only therapy approved for adults. Doses of 75 to 260 units are administered in seven specific areas of the head and neck by the health care provider. Monthly treatments for up to five treatment cycles are considered safe and effective (Carod-Artel, 2014).

In addition to drug therapy, *trigger avoidance and management* are important interventions for preventing migraine episodes. For example, some patients find that avoiding tyramine-containing products, such as pickled products, caffeine, beer and wine, preservatives; and artificial sweeteners, reduces their headaches. Others have identified specific factors that trigger an attack for them. Help patients identify triggers that could cause migraine episodes and teach them to avoid them once identified (Chart 42-7). For example, at the beginning of a migraine attack, the patient may be able to reduce pain by lying down and darkening the room. He or she may want both eyes covered and a cool cloth on the forehead. If the patient falls asleep, he or she should remain undisturbed until awakening.

External Trigeminal Nerve Stimulator. A new certified medical device called the Cefaly is available in the United States, Europe, and Canada by prescription for the primary health care provider to prevent migraines. This **external trigeminal nerve stimulator (E-TNS)** is a wearable headband that stimulates several branches of the trigeminal nerve that are associated with migraine attacks and pain. Teach the patient to use the device no more than 20 minutes a day as recommended by its manufacturer. For more information, teach the patient to visit either www.cefaly.us or www.cefaly.ca for a video about how to use this nondrug alternative to preventive medications.

Complementary and Integrative Health. Many patients use complementary and integrative therapies as adjuncts to drug

CHART 42-7   Patient and Family Education: Preparing for Self-Management

Factors That May Trigger a Migraine Attack

Teach patients to avoid factors that may trigger a migraine attack, including the following.

Foods Commonly Associated With Migraines

- Alcoholic drinks: beer, wine, and hard liquor
- Aged cheese or other foods with tyramine
- Caffeine found in beverages such as coffee, tea, cola OR caffeine withdrawal
- Chocolate
- Foods with yeast such as pastry and fresh breads
- Monosodium glutamate (MSG)
- Nitrates (meats), pickled or fermented foods
- Nuts
- Artificial sweeteners
- Smoked fish

Drugs Associated With Migraines

- Cimetidine (Tagamet)
- Estrogens
- Nitroglycerin
- Nifedipine (Procardia, Nifed)

Other Factors That Can Trigger a Migraine Attack

- Anger, conflict
- Fatigue
- Hormonal fluctuations, such as menstruation, pregnancy, and menopause
- Light glare
- Missed meals, hypoglycemia
- Psychological stress
- Sleep problems
- Smells, such as tobacco smoke
- Travel to different altitudes

NCLEX EXAMINATION CHALLENGE 42-5

Health Promotion and Maintenance

The nurse is preparing a teaching plan for a client with migraine headaches. Which of these foods or food additives that may trigger a migraine will the nurse include in the teaching? **Select all that apply.**

A. Sugar
B. Salt
C. Monosodium glutamate (MSG)
D. Caffeine
E. Wine
F. Tyramine

Epilepsy is defined by the National Institute of Neurological Disorders and Stroke as two or more seizures experienced by a person. It is a chronic disorder in which repeated unprovoked seizure activity occurs. It may be caused by an abnormality in electrical neuronal activity; an imbalance of neurotransmitters, especially gamma aminobutyric acid (GABA); or a combination of both (McCance et al., 2014).

Types of Seizures

The International Classification of Epileptic Seizures recognizes three broad categories of seizure disorders: generalized seizures, partial seizures, and unclassified seizures.

Five types of **generalized seizures** may occur in adults and involve *both* cerebral hemispheres. The *tonic-clonic seizure* lasting 2 to 5 minutes begins with a **tonic phase** that causes stiffening or rigidity of the muscles, particularly of the arms and legs, and immediate loss of consciousness. **Clonic** or **rhythmic** jerking of all extremities follows. The patient may bite his or her tongue and become incontinent of urine or feces. Fatigue, acute confusion, and lethargy may last up to an hour after the seizure.

Occasionally only tonic or clonic movement may occur. A *tonic seizure* is an abrupt increase in muscle tone, loss of consciousness, and autonomic changes lasting from 30 seconds to several minutes. The *clonic seizure* lasts several minutes and causes muscle contraction and relaxation.

The *myoclonic seizure* causes a brief jerking or stiffening of the extremities that may occur singly or in groups. Lasting for just a few seconds, the contractions may be symmetric (both sides) or asymmetric (one side).

In an *atonic (akinetic) seizure,* the patient has a sudden loss of muscle tone, lasting for seconds, followed by **postictal** (after the seizure) confusion. In most cases, these seizures cause the patient to fall, which may result in injury. This type of seizure tends to be most resistant to drug therapy.

Partial seizures, also called *focal* or *local* seizures, begin in a part of *one* cerebral hemisphere. They are further subdivided into two main classes: complex partial seizures and simple partial seizures. In addition, some partial seizures can become generalized tonic-clonic, tonic, or clonic seizures. Partial seizures are most often seen in adults and generally are less responsive to medical treatment when compared with other types.

Complex partial seizures may cause loss of consciousness (**syncope**), or "blackout," for 1 to 3 minutes. Characteristic automatisms may occur as in absence seizures. The patient is unaware of the environment and may wander at the start of the seizure. In the period after the seizure, he or she may have

therapy. Yoga, meditation, massage, exercise, and biofeedback are helpful in preventing or treating migraines for some patients. Vitamin B_{12} (riboflavin) and magnesium supplements to maintain normal serum values may have a role in migraine prevention (National Center for Complementary and Integrative Health [NCCIH], 2017). A number of herbs are also used for headaches, both for prevention and pain management. Teach patients that all herbs and nutritional remedies should be approved by their health care provider before use because they could interact with prescribed medication.

Acupuncture and acupressure may be effective in relieving pain for some patients (NCCIH, 2017). Some plastic surgeons have resected the trigeminal nerve to relieve chronic migraine pain.

SEIZURES AND EPILEPSY

❖ PATHOPHYSIOLOGY

A **seizure** is an abnormal, sudden, excessive, uncontrolled electrical discharge of neurons within the brain that may result in a change in level of consciousness (LOC), motor or sensory ability, and/or behavior. A single seizure may occur for no known reason. Some seizures are caused by a pathologic condition of the brain, such as a tumor. In this case, once the underlying problem is treated, the patient is often asymptomatic.

amnesia (loss of memory). Because the area of the brain most often involved in this type of epilepsy is the temporal lobe, complex partial seizures are often called *psychomotor* seizures or *temporal lobe* seizures.

CONSIDERATIONS FOR OLDER ADULTS
Patient-Centered Care QSEN

Complex partial seizures are most common among older adults. These seizures are difficult to diagnose because symptoms appear similar to those of dementia, psychosis, or other neurobehavioral disorders, especially in the postictal stage (after the seizure). New-onset seizures in older adults typically are associated with conditions such as hypertension, cardiac disease, diabetes mellitus, stroke, dementia, and recent brain injury (McCance et al., 2014).

The patient with a *simple partial seizure* remains conscious throughout the episode. He or she often reports an aura (unusual sensation) before the seizure takes place. This may consist of a "déjà vu" (already seen) phenomenon, perception of an offensive smell, or sudden onset of pain. During the seizure, the patient may have one-sided movement of an extremity, experience unusual sensations, or have autonomic symptoms. Autonomic changes include a change in heart rate, skin flushing, and epigastric discomfort.

Unclassified or idiopathic seizures account for about half of all seizure activity. They occur for no known reason and do not fit into the generalized or partial classifications.

Etiology and Genetic Risk

Primary or *idiopathic epilepsy* is not associated with any identifiable brain lesion or other specific cause; however, genetic factors most likely play a role in its development. *Secondary seizures* result from an underlying brain lesion, most commonly a tumor or trauma. They may also be caused by:

- Metabolic disorders
- Acute alcohol withdrawal
- Electrolyte disturbances (e.g., hyperkalemia, water intoxication, hypoglycemia)
- High fever
- Stroke
- Head injury
- Substance abuse
- Heart disease

Seizures resulting from these problems are not considered epilepsy. Various risk factors can trigger a seizure, such as increased physical activity, emotional stress, excessive fatigue, alcohol or caffeine consumption, or certain foods or chemicals.

❖ INTERPROFESSIONAL COLLABORATIVE CARE
◆ Assessment: Noticing

Question the patient or family about how many seizures the patient has had, how long they last, and any pattern of occurrence. Ask the patient or family to describe the seizures that the patient has had. Signs and symptoms vary, depending on the type of seizure experienced, as described earlier. Ask about the presence of an aura before seizures begin (preictal phase). Question whether the patient is taking any prescribed drugs or herbs or has had head trauma or high fever. Assess any alcohol and/or illicit drug history. Ask about any other medical condition such as a previous stroke or hypertension.

If the seizure is a new symptom, ask the patient or family if any loss of consciousness or brain injury has occurred, both in the recent and distant past. Often patients may have had a head or brain injury sufficient to cause a loss of consciousness but may not remember this at the time of the seizure, especially if it was during their childhood.

Diagnosis is based on the history and physical examination. A variety of diagnostic tests are performed to rule out other causes of seizure activity and to confirm the diagnosis of epilepsy. Typical diagnostic tests include an electroencephalogram (EEG), CT scan, MRI, or SPECT/PET scan). These tests are described in Chapter 41. Laboratory studies are performed to identify metabolic or other disorders that may cause or contribute to seizure activity.

◆ Interventions: Responding

Removing or treating the underlying condition or cause of the seizure manages *secondary* epilepsy and seizures that are not considered epileptic. In most cases, primary epilepsy is successfully managed through drug therapy.

Nonsurgical Management. Most seizures can be completely or almost completely controlled through the administration of antiepileptic drugs (AEDs), sometimes referred to as *anticonvulsants*, for specific types of seizures.

Drug Therapy. Drug therapy is the major component of management (Table 42-5). The health care provider introduces one antiepileptic drug (AED) at a time to achieve control for the type of seizure that the patient has. If the chosen drug is not effective, the dosage may be increased, or another drug introduced. At times, seizure control is achieved only through a combination of drugs. The dosages are adjusted to achieve therapeutic blood levels without causing major side effects. Because of these potential side effects, teach patients to:

- Follow up on laboratory test appointments to monitor the patient's complete blood count (CBC) and liver enzymes and assess for therapeutic drug levels. Most AEDs can cause leukopenia and liver dysfunction.
- Teach the patient to observe for and report beginning gingival hyperplasia and perform frequent oral care to prevent permanent gingival damage.

Teach patients to take their drugs on time to maintain therapeutic blood levels and maximum effectiveness. Emphasize the importance of taking their AEDs as prescribed. Instruct patients that they can build up sensitivity to the drugs as they age. If sensitivity occurs, tell them they will need to have blood levels

TABLE 42-5 Examples of Drug Therapy
Epilepsy and Seizure Prevention

- Phenytoin (Dilantin, Phenytek) (most widely used)
- Fosphenytoin (Cerbryx)
- Carbamazepine (Tegretol, Tegretol XR, Tegretol-CR ♣, Carbatrol)
- Oxcarbazepine (Oxtellar, Trileptal)
- Lamotrigine (Lamictal)
- Valproic acid (Depakote, Depakoke ER, Epival ♣)
- Primidone (Mysoline)
- Gabapentin (Neurontin)
- Pregabalin (Lyrica)
- Levetiracetam (Keppra)
- Topiramate (Topamax)
- Ezogabine (Potiga) (first approved potassium channel opener drug approved for adjunctive management of partial-onset seizures)

GENDER HEALTH CONSIDERATIONS
Patient-Centered Care QSEN

Management of women with epilepsy is challenging. Hormonal changes from menstrual cycling and the interaction of oral contraceptives with antiepileptic drugs (AEDs) require the primary health care provider and patient to be aware of a variety of guidelines and to more frequently monitor drug effectiveness. AEDs can also contribute to osteoporosis in menopausal women. As a result, coordination between the neurologist, the woman's primary health care provider, and the patient is required for safe, effective care. Nurses can facilitate patient education, communication, and collaboration to promote safe, effective care.

of this drug checked frequently to adjust the dose. In some cases, the antiseizure effects of drugs can decline and lead to an increase in seizures. Because of this potential for "drug decline and sensitivity," patients need to keep their scheduled laboratory appointments to check serum drug levels.

Be aware of drug-drug and drug-food interactions. For instance, warfarin (Coumadin, Warfilone ✦) should not be given with phenytoin (Dilantin). Document side and adverse effects of the prescribed drugs and report to the health care provider. Teach patients that some citrus fruits, such as grapefruit juice, can interfere with the metabolism of these drugs. This interference can raise the blood level of the drug and cause the patient to develop drug toxicity.

Seizure Precautions. Precautions are taken to prevent the patient from injury if a seizure occurs. Specific seizure precautions vary, depending on health care agency policy.

NURSING SAFETY PRIORITY QSEN
Action Alert

Seizure precautions include ensuring that oxygen and suctioning equipment with an airway are readily available. If the patient does not have an IV access, insert a saline lock, especially if he or she is at significant risk for generalized tonic-clonic seizures. The saline lock provides ready access if IV drug therapy must be given to stop the seizure.

Side rails are rarely the source of significant injury, and the effectiveness of the use of padded side rails to maintain safety is debatable. Padded side rails may embarrass the patient and the family. Follow agency policy about the use of side rails because they may be classified as a restraint device. Other methods to protect the patient, such as placing a mattress on the floor, may be used instead of side rails.

Padded tongue blades do not belong at the bedside and should NEVER be inserted into the patient's mouth because the jaw may clench down as soon as the seizure begins! Forcing a tongue blade or airway into the mouth is more likely to chip the teeth and increase the risk for aspirating tooth fragments than prevent the patient from biting the tongue. Furthermore, improper placement of a padded tongue blade can obstruct the airway.

Seizure Management. The actions taken during a seizure should be appropriate for the type of seizure (Chart 42-8). For example, for a simple partial seizure, observe the patient and document the time that the seizure lasted. Redirect the patient's attention away from an activity that could cause injury. Turn the patient on the side during a generalized tonic-clonic or complex partial seizure because he or she may lose consciousness. If possible, turn the patient's head to the side to prevent aspiration

CHART 42-8   Best Practice for Patient Safety & Quality Care QSEN
Care of the Patient During a Tonic-Clonic or Complete Partial Seizure

- Protect the patient from injury.
- Do not force anything into the patient's mouth.
- Turn the patient to the side to prevent aspiration and keep the airway clear.
- Loosen any restrictive clothing the patient is wearing.
- Maintain the patient's airway and suction oral secretions as needed.
- Do not restrain or try to stop the patient's movement; guide movements if necessary.
- Record the time the seizure began and ended.
- At the completion of the seizure:
  - Take the patient's vital signs.
  - Perform neurologic checks.
  - Keep the patient on his or her side.
  - Allow the patient to rest.
  - Document the seizure (see Chart 42-9).

CHART 42-9   Focused Assessment
Seizures: Nursing Observations and Documentation

- How often the seizures occur:
  - Date, time, and duration of the seizure
- Description of each seizure:
  - Tonic, clonic
  - Staring spells, blinking
  - Automatism
- Whether more than one type of seizure occurs
- Sequence of seizure progression:
  - Where the seizure began
  - Body part first involved
- Observations during the seizure:
  - Changes in pupil size and any eye deviation
  - Level of consciousness
  - Presence of apnea, cyanosis, and salivation
  - Incontinence of bowel or bladder during the seizure
  - Eye fluttering
  - Movement and progression of motor activity
  - Lip smacking or other automatism
  - Tongue or lip biting
- How long the seizures last
- When the last seizure took place
- Whether the seizures are preceded by an aura:
  - Dizziness, numbness, or visual disturbances
  - Gustatory (taste) or auditory disturbances
- What the patient does after the seizure:
  - Feels drowsy or weak
  - May resume normal behavior
  - May be unaware that the seizure took place
- How long it takes for the patient to return to pre-seizure status

and allow secretions to drain. Remove any objects that might injure the patient.

It is not unusual for the patient to become cyanotic during a generalized tonic-clonic seizure. The cyanosis is generally self-limiting, and no treatment is needed. Some health care providers prefer to give the high-risk patient (e.g., older adult, critically ill, or debilitated patient) oxygen by nasal cannula or facemask during the postictal phase. For any type of seizure, carefully observe the seizure and document assessment findings (Chart 42-9).

Emergency Care: Acute Seizure and Status Epilepticus Management. Seizures occurring in greater intensity, number, or length than the patient's usual seizures are considered *acute*. They may also appear in clusters that are different from the patient's typical seizure pattern. Treatment with lorazepam (Ativan, Apo-Lorazepam) or diazepam (Valium, Meval, Vivol, Diastat [rectal diazepam gel]) may be given to stop the clusters to prevent the development of status epilepticus. IV phenytoin (Dilantin) or fosphenytoin (Cerebyx) may be added (Burchum & Rosenthal, 2016).

Status epilepticus is a medical emergency and is a prolonged seizure lasting longer than 5 minutes or repeated seizures over the course of 30 minutes. It is a potential complication of all types of seizures. *Seizures lasting longer than 10 minutes can cause death!* Common causes of status epilepticus include:

- Sudden withdrawal from antiepileptic drugs
- Infection
- Acute alcohol or drug withdrawal
- Head trauma
- Cerebral edema
- Metabolic disturbances

! NURSING SAFETY PRIORITY (QSEN)

Critical Rescue

Convulsive status epilepticus must be treated promptly and aggressively! Establish an airway and notify the health care provider or Rapid Response Team immediately if this problem occurs! Establishing an airway is the priority for this patient's care. Intubation by an anesthesia provider or respiratory therapist may be necessary. Administer oxygen as indicated by the patient's condition. If not already in place, establish IV access with a large-bore catheter and start 0.9% sodium chloride. The patient is usually placed in the intensive care unit for continuous monitoring and management.

Blood is drawn to determine arterial blood gas levels and to identify metabolic, toxic, and other causes of the uncontrolled seizure. Brain damage and death may occur in the patient with tonic-clonic status epilepticus. Left untreated, metabolic changes result, leading to hypoxia, hypotension, hypoglycemia, cardiac dysrhythmias, or lactic (metabolic) acidosis. Further harm to the patient occurs when muscle breaks down and myoglobin accumulates in the kidneys, which can lead to renal failure and electrolyte imbalance. *This is especially likely in the older adult.*

The drugs of choice for treating status epilepticus are IV-push lorazepam (Ativan, Apo-Lorazepam) or diazepam (Valium). Diazepam rectal gel (Diastat) may be used instead. Lorazepam is usually given as 4 mg over a 2-minute period. This procedure may be repeated, if necessary, until a total of 8 mg is reached.

! NURSING SAFETY PRIORITY (QSEN)

Drug Alert

To prevent additional tonic-clonic seizures or cardiac arrest, a loading dose of IV phenytoin (Dilantin) is given, and oral doses are administered as a follow-up after the emergency is resolved. Initially give phenytoin at no more than 50 mg/min using an infusion pump. If the drug is piggybacked into an existing IV line, use only normal saline as the primary IV fluid to prevent drug precipitation. Be sure to flush the line with normal saline before and after phenytoin administration (Burchum & Rosenthal, 2016).

An alternative to phenytoin is fosphenytoin (Cerebyx), a water-soluble phenytoin prodrug. It is compatible with most IV solutions. It also causes fewer cardiovascular complications than phenytoin and can be given in an IV dextrose solution. After administration, fosphenytoin converts to phenytoin in the body. Therefore the FDA requires the dosage to be written as a phenytoin equivalent (PE) (e.g., 150 mg of fosphenytoin converts to 100 mg of phenytoin). If given IV, infuse fosphenytoin at a rate of no more than 150 PE/min (Burchum & Rosenthal, 2016).

Teach the patient that serum drug levels are checked every 6 to 12 hours after the loading dose and then 2 weeks after oral phenytoin has started. The desired serum therapeutic range is 10 to 20 mcg/mL (Burchum & Rosenthal, 2016). Drug levels of more than 30 mg/mL are considered an indicator of drug toxicity.

? NCLEX EXAMINATION CHALLENGE 42-6

Safe and Effective Care Environment

A client with a history of seizures is placed on seizure precautions. Which emergency equipment will the nurse provide at the bedside?
Select all that apply.
A. Oropharyngeal airway
B. Oxygen
C. Nasogastric tube
D. Suction setup
E. Padded tongue blade

Surgical Management. Patients who cannot be managed effectively with drug therapy may be candidates for surgery, including vagal nerve stimulation (VNS) and conventional surgical procedures. VNS has been very successful for many patients with epilepsy.

Vagal Nerve Stimulation. VNS may be performed for control of continuous simple or complex partial seizures. Patients with generalized seizures are not candidates for surgery because VNS may result in severe neurologic deficits. The stimulating device (much like a cardiac pacemaker) is surgically implanted in the left chest wall. An electrode lead is attached to the left vagus nerve, tunneled under the skin, and connected to a generator. The procedure usually takes 2 hours with the patient under general anesthesia. The stimulator is activated by the physician either in the operating room or, more commonly, 2 weeks after surgery. Programming is adjusted gradually over a period of time. The pattern of stimulation is individualized to the patient's tolerance. The generator runs continuously, stimulating the vagus nerve according to the programmed schedule.

The patient can activate the VNS with a handheld magnet when experiencing an aura, thus aborting the seizure. Patients experience a change in voice quality, which signifies that the vagus nerve has been stimulated. They usually report a relief in intensity and duration of seizures and an improved quality of life.

Observe for complications after the procedure such as hoarseness (most common), cough, dyspnea, neck pain, or dysphagia (difficulty swallowing). Teach the patient to avoid MRIs, microwaves, shortwave radios, and ultrasound diathermy (a physical therapy heat treatment).

Conventional Surgical Procedures. A small percentage of patients with epilepsy cannot be controlled completely with drug therapy or VNS. When all other options are exhausted, conventional surgery may be needed to improve the patient's quality of life. The largest group of conventional surgical candidates includes those with complex partial seizures in the frontal or temporal lobe.

Before surgery, the patient is admitted to a special inpatient observation unit. While there, he or she has continuous electroencephalogram (EEG) recording, close observation, and in many hospitals, video monitoring at all times except during personal care activities. The patient is taken off all AEDs. After the seizure area is identified, electrodes may be surgically implanted into the brain tissue to identify the extent of the focal area. This step is followed by additional continuous EEG and video monitoring, as well as close observation by the nursing staff. The area is surgically removed if vital areas of brain function will not be affected.

Preoperative care is similar to that described for patients undergoing a craniotomy (see Chapter 45). Preoperative diagnostic tests include MRI and single-photon emission computed tomography (SPECT)/positron emission tomography (PET) scans as described in Chapter 41. An intracarotid amobarbital test (Wada test) and neuropsychological testing are also done. The Wada test assesses hemispheric lateralization of language and memory after injection of amobarbital, a short-acting anesthetic. This procedure establishes the safety of surgery to preserve language memory. Neuropsychological testing evaluates memory, visuospatial function, language function, and intelligence quotient (IQ) to identify deficiencies in the brain that might correspond to areas believed to be the epileptic region. It is also used to compare preoperative and postoperative COGNITION.

Another surgical approach, the *partial corpus callosotomy*, may be used to treat tonic-clonic or atonic seizures in patients who are not candidates for other surgical procedures. The surgeon sections the anterior two thirds of the corpus callosum, preventing neuronal discharges from passing between the two hemispheres of the brain. This surgery usually reduces the number and severity of the seizures, making them more likely to respond to more conventional drug therapy. This procedure is not done as commonly as other surgeries, but it is very successful for some patients.

Care Coordination and Transition Management

Provide self-management education for the patient and family (Chart 42-10). Ask them what they understand about the disorder and correct any misinformation. As new information is presented, be sure that the patient and family can understand it. Refer patients and families to the Epilepsy Foundation of America for more information and community support groups. Encourage patients and their significant others to use information from the Epilepsy Foundation website (www.epilepsy.com).

Emphasize that AEDs must not be stopped even if the seizures have stopped. Discontinuing these drugs can lead to the recurrence of seizures or the life-threatening complication of status epilepticus (discussed earlier). Some patients may stop therapy because they do not have the money to purchase the drugs. Refer limited-income patients to the social services department for assistance or to a case manager to locate other resources.

A balanced diet, proper rest, and stress-reduction techniques usually minimize the risk for breakthrough seizures. Encourage

---

CHART 42-10 Patient and Family Education: Preparing for Self-Management

Health Teaching for the Patient With Epilepsy

- Drug therapy information:
  - Name, dosage, time of administration
  - Actions to take if side effects occur
  - Importance of taking drug as prescribed and not missing a dose
  - What to do if a dose is missed or cannot be taken
  - Importance of having blood drawn for therapeutic or toxic levels as requested by the health care provider
- Do not take any medication, including over-the-counter drugs, without asking your health care provider.
- Wear a medical alert bracelet or necklace or carry an identification card indicating epilepsy.
- Follow up with your neurologist, physician, or other health care provider as directed.
- Be sure that a family member or significant other knows how to help you in the event of a seizure and knows when your health care provider or emergency medical services should be called.
- Investigate and follow state laws concerning driving and operating machinery.
- Avoid alcohol and excessive fatigue.
- Contact the Epilepsy Foundation (www.epilepsy.com) or other organized epilepsy group for additional information. Epilepsy Canada (www.epilepsy.ca) also provides resources and support.

---

the patient to keep a seizure diary to determine whether there are factors that tend to be associated with seizure activity. Patients should follow state law concerning allowances for driving a motor vehicle.

All states prohibit discrimination against people who have epilepsy. Patients who work in occupations in which a seizure might cause serious harm to themselves or others (e.g., construction workers, operators of dangerous equipment, pilots) may need other employment. They may need to decrease or modify strenuous or potentially dangerous physical activity to avoid harm, although this varies with each person. Various local, state, and federal agencies can help with finances, living arrangements, and vocational rehabilitation.

MENINGITIS

❖ PATHOPHYSIOLOGY

Meningitis is an inflammation of the meninges of the brain and spinal cord, specifically the pia mater and arachnoid. Bacterial and viral organisms are most often responsible for meningitis, although fungal and protozoal meningitis also occur. Cancer and some drugs, notably NSAIDs, antibiotics, and IV immunoglobulins, can also cause sterile meningitis. Regardless of cause of meningitis, the symptoms are similar.

The organisms responsible for meningitis enter the central nervous system (CNS) via the bloodstream or are directly introduced into the CNS. Direct routes of entry occur as a result of penetrating trauma, surgical procedures on the brain or spine, or a ruptured brain **abscess**. A basilar skull fracture may lead to meningitis as a result of the direct communication of cerebrospinal fluid (CSF) with the ear or nasal passages, manifested by **otorrhea** (ear discharge) or **rhinorrhea** (nasal discharge, or "runny nose") that is actually CSF. The infecting organisms follow the tract created by skull damage to enter the CNS and circulate in the CSF. The patient with an infection in the head (i.e., eye, ear, nose, mouth) or neck/throat has an increased risk for meningitis because of the proximity of anatomic structures. Infections linked to meningitis include otitis media, acute or chronic sinusitis, and tooth abscess; there are also reports of rare infection from a tongue piercing leading to meningitis. The immunocompromised patient (e.g., one without a spleen receiving treatment for cancer, taking immunosuppressant drugs to manage autoimmune disease or solid organ transplant, and older adults) is also at increased risk for meningitis. The infecting organism may spread to both cranial and spinal nerves, causing irreversible neurologic damage. Increased intracranial pressure (ICP) may occur as a result of blockage of the flow of CSF, change in cerebral blood flow, or thrombus (blood clot) formation (McCance et al., 2014).

Viral meningitis, the most common type, is sometimes referred to as *aseptic meningitis* because no organisms are typically isolated from culture of the CSF. Common viral organisms causing meningitis are enterovirus, herpes simplex virus–2 (HSV-2), varicella zoster virus (VZV) (also causes chickenpox and shingles), mumps virus, and the human immune deficiency virus (HIV) (McCance et al., 2014). The severity of symptoms can vary by the infecting viral agent. For example, the herpes simplex virus alters cellular metabolism, which quickly results in necrosis of the cells. HSV-2 meningitis may be accompanied by genital infections. Other viruses cause an alteration in the production of enzymes or neurotransmitters. Although these alterations result in cell dysfunction, neurologic defects are more likely to be temporary, and a full recovery occurs as the inflammation resolves. Treatment may include the administration of antiviral agents.

Cryptococcus neoformans meningitis is the most common *fungal* infection that affects the CNS of patients with acquired immune deficiency syndrome (AIDS). Fulminant invasive fungal sinusitis is also a recognized cause of fungal meningitis. The signs and symptoms vary because the compromised immune system affects the inflammatory response. For example, some patients have fever, and others do not. Treatment is symptomatic and includes IV antifungal agents.

The most frequently involved organisms responsible for bacterial meningococcal meningitis are *Streptococcus pneumoniae* (pneumococcal disease) and *Neisseria meningitidis*. *N. meningitidis* meningitis is also known as *meningococcal meningitis*. *Meningococcal meningitis is a medical emergency with a fairly high mortality rate, often within 24 hours.* Unlike other types, this disorder is highly contagious. Outbreaks of meningococcal meningitis are most likely to occur in areas of high population density, such as college dormitories, military barracks, and crowded living areas.

❖ INTERPROFESSIONAL COLLABORATIVE CARE
◆ Assessment: Noticing

Perform a complete neurologic and neurovascular assessment to detect signs and symptoms associated with a diagnosis of meningitis or suspected meningitis as outlined in Chart 42-11. These signs and symptoms often include fever, **nuchal rigidity** (neck stiffness), **photophobia** (light sensitivity), **phonophobia** (noise sensitivity), headache, **myalgia** (muscle aches), nausea, and vomiting. Confusion and altered consciousness may be present. A maculopapular rash is seen when the causative organism is an enterovirus. A petechial rash is associated with *N. meningitidis* meningitis. Although the classic nuchal rigidity (stiff neck) and positive Kernig's and Brudzinski's signs have been traditionally used to diagnose meningitis, these findings

---

> **» CHART 42-11   Key Features**
> **Meningitis**
>
> - Decreased (or change in) level of consciousness
> - Disoriented to person, place, and year
> - Pupil reaction and eye movements:
>   - Photophobia
>   - Nystagmus
>   - Abnormal eye movements
> - Motor response:
>   - Normal early in disease process
>   - Hemiparesis, hemiplegia, and decreased muscle tone possible later
>   - Cranial nerve dysfunction, especially CN III, IV, VI, VII, VIII
> - Memory changes:
>   - Attention span (usually short)
>   - Personality and behavior changes
>   - Bewilderment
> - Severe, unrelenting headaches
> - Generalized muscle aches and pain
> - Nausea and vomiting
> - Fever and chills
> - Tachycardia
> - Red macular rash (meningococcal meningitis)

occur in only a small percentage of patients with a definitive diagnosis. Older adults, patients who are immunocompromised, and those who are receiving antibiotics may not have fever. Assess the patient for complications, including increased ICP. Left untreated, increased ICP can lead to herniation of the brain and death (see Chapter 45).

Seizure activity may occur when meningeal inflammation spreads to the cerebral cortex. Inflammation can also result in abnormal stimulation of the hypothalamic area where excessive amounts of antidiuretic hormone (ADH) (vasopressin) are produced. Excess vasopressin results in water retention and dilution of serum sodium caused by increased sodium loss by the kidneys. This syndrome of inappropriate antidiuretic hormone (SIADH, see Chapter 62) may lead to further increases in ICP.

Systemic inflammation (systemic inflammatory response syndrome or **SIRS**), a reaction to either endotoxin produced by infecting bacteria or activation of the immune cells by infecting organisms, can cause a rapidly falling blood pressure and tachycardia. Coagulopathy can occur as a result of systemic inflammation. Assess the patient's vascular status by:

- Observing the color and temperature of the extremities
- Determining the presence of peripheral pulses
- Identifying any indicators of abnormal bleeding

Thrombi may block circulation in the small vessels of the hands and feet, leading to gangrene. Coagulopathy from SIRS may lead to disseminated intravascular coagulation (DIC).

The most significant laboratory test used in the diagnosis of meningitis is the analysis of the *cerebrospinal fluid (CSF)*. Patients older than 60 years, those who are immunocompromised, or those who have signs of increased ICP usually have a CT scan before the lumbar puncture. If there will be a delay in obtaining the CSF, blood is drawn for culture and sensitivity. A broad-spectrum antibiotic should be given before the lumbar puncture. The CSF is analyzed for cell count, differential count, and protein. Glucose concentrations are determined; and culture, sensitivity, and Gram stain studies are performed.

Counterimmunoelectrophoresis (CIE) may be performed to determine the presence of viruses or protozoa in the CSF. CIE is also indicated if the patient has received antibiotics before the CSF was obtained. To identify a bacterial source of infection, specimens for Gram stains and culture are obtained from the urine, throat, and nose when indicated.

A complete blood count (CBC) is performed. The white blood cell (WBC) count is usually elevated well above the normal value. Serum electrolyte values are also assessed to assess and maintain fluid and electrolyte balance.

X-rays of the chest, air sinuses, and mastoids are obtained to determine the presence of infection. A CT or MRI scan may be performed to identify increased ICP, hydrocephalus, or the presence of a brain abscess.

◆ Interventions: Responding

Prevent meningitis by teaching people to obtain vaccination. Vaccines are available to protect against *Haemophilus influenzae* type B (Hib), pneumococcal, mumps, varicella, and meningococcal organisms. Although many of these vaccines were developed to prevent respiratory illness, they have also reduced CNS infections. Mandatory vaccination programs for school enrollment and proof of vaccination as a prerequisite for group home or dormitory experiences have significantly reduced the incidence of meningitis.

Maintain thorough handwashing. Teach visitors to wash hands before and after entering a patient's room. Preventing the transmission of infection through hand cleaning is a National Patient Safety Goal.

The most important nursing interventions for patients with meningitis are accurate monitoring of and documenting their neurologic status. Best practices for nursing care are listed in Chart 42-12.

! NURSING SAFETY PRIORITY QSEN

Action Alert

For the patient with meningitis, assess his or her neurologic status and vital signs at least every 4 hours or more often if clinically indicated. *The priority for care is to monitor for early neurologic changes that may indicate increased ICP, such as decreased level of consciousness (LOC).* The patient is also at risk for seizure activity. Care should be provided as discussed in Interventions in the Seizures and Epilepsy section.

◎ **CHART 42-12** **Best Practice for Patient Safety & Quality Care** QSEN

Care of the Patient With Meningitis

- Prioritize care to maintain airway, breathing, circulation.
- Take vital signs and perform neurologic checks every 2 to 4 hours, as required.
- Perform cranial nerve assessment, with particular attention to cranial nerves III, IV, VI, VII, and VIII, and monitor for changes.
- Manage pain with drug and nondrug methods.
- Perform vascular assessment and monitor for changes.
- Give drugs and IV fluids as prescribed and document the patient's response.
- Record intake and output carefully to maintain fluid balance and prevent fluid overload.
- Monitor body weight to identify fluid retention early.
- Monitor laboratory values closely; report abnormal findings to the physician or nurse practitioner promptly.
- Position carefully to prevent pressure injuries.
- Perform range-of-motion exercises every 4 hours as needed.
- Decrease environmental stimuli:
  - Provide a quiet environment.
  - Minimize exposure to bright lights from windows and overhead lights.
  - Maintain bedrest with head of bed elevated 30 degrees.
- Maintain Transmission-Based Precautions per hospital policy (for bacterial meningitis).
- Monitor for and prevent complications:
  - Increased intracranial pressure
  - Vascular dysfunction
  - Fluid and electrolyte imbalance
  - Seizures
  - Shock

Cranial nerve testing is included as part of the routine neurologic assessment because of possible cranial nerve involvement. Particular attention is given to cranial nerves III, IV, VI, VII, and VIII (i.e., nerves involved in pupillary shape and accommodation to light) (see Chapter 41). *A sixth cranial nerve defect (inability to move the eyes laterally) may indicate the development of* hydrocephalus *(excessive accumulation of CSF within the brain's ventricles).* Other indicators of hydrocephalus include signs of increased ICP and urinary incontinence. Urinary incontinence results from decreasing LOC.

To avoid life-threatening complications, the health care provider prescribes a broad-spectrum antibiotic until the results of the culture and Gram stain are available. After this information is available, the appropriate anti-infective drug to treat the specific type of meningitis is given. Treatment of bacterial meningitis generally requires a 2-week course of IV antibiotics. Drug therapy should begin within 1 to 2 hours after it is prescribed. Monitor and document the patient's response.

Drugs may be used to treat increased ICP or seizures, including mannitol, a hyperosmolar agent for ICP, and antiepileptic drugs (AEDs). Controversy exists as to whether steroids are helpful in the treatment of all adults with meningitis. However, they are recommended for patients with *S. pneumoniae* meningitis.

People who have been in close contact with a patient with *N. meningitidis* should have prophylaxis (preventive) treatment with rifampin (Rifadin, Rofact), ciprofloxacin (Cipro), or ceftriaxone (Rocephin). Preventive treatment with rifampin may be prescribed for those in close contact with a patient with *H. influenzae* meningitis (Burchum & Rosenthal, 2016).

Perform a complete vascular assessment every 4 hours or more often, if indicated, to detect early vascular compromise. Thrombotic or embolic complications are most often seen in circulation to the hand. Assess the patient's temperature, color, pulses, and capillary refill in the fingernails. If vascular compromise is not noticed and left untreated, gangrene can develop quickly, possibly leading to loss of the involved arm. The health care team monitors the patient for other complications, including septic shock, coagulation disorders, acute respiratory distress syndrome, and septic arthritis. These health problems are discussed elsewhere in this textbook.

Standard Precautions are appropriate for all patients with meningitis unless the patient has a bacterial type that is transmitted by droplets, such as *N. meningitides* and *H. influenzae*.

> ### ! NURSING SAFETY PRIORITY QSEN
> #### Action Alert
> Place the patient with bacterial meningitis that is transmitted by droplets on Droplet Precautions *in addition to* Standard Precautions. When possible, place the patient in a private room. Stay at least 3 feet from the patient unless wearing a mask. Patients who are transported outside of the room should wear a mask (see Chapter 23). Teach visitors about the need for these precautions and how to follow them.

ENCEPHALITIS

❖ PATHOPHYSIOLOGY

Encephalitis is an inflammation and infection of the brain tissue and often the surrounding meninges. It affects the cerebrum, the brainstem, and the cerebellum. A viral agent most often causes the disease, although bacteria, fungi, or parasites may also be involved (e.g., malaria). The virus travels to the central nervous system (CNS) via the bloodstream, along peripheral or cranial nerves, or in the meninges (e.g., varicella zoster). Therefore viral encephalitis can be life threatening or lead to persistent neurologic problems such as learning disabilities, epilepsy, memory deficits, or fine motor deficits.

After the virus invades the brain tissue, it begins to reproduce, causing an inflammatory response. Unlike in meningitis, this response does not cause exudate (pus) formation. Inflammation extends over the cerebral cortex, the white matter, and the meninges, causing degeneration of the neurons of the cortex. Demyelination of axons occurs in the involved area because the white matter is destroyed. This destruction leads to hemorrhage, edema, necrosis (cell death), and the development of small lacunae (hollow cavities) within the cerebral hemispheres. Widespread edema can cause compression of blood vessels, leading to a further increase in intracranial pressure (ICP). Death may occur from herniation and increased ICP (McCance et al., 2014).

Arboviruses can be transmitted to humans through the bite of an infected mosquito or tick. The most common types of encephalitis caused by arboviruses are Eastern or Western equine encephalitis, St. Louis encephalitis, California encephalitis, and West Nile virus.

West Nile virus has gained attention in the United States because it has spread rapidly throughout the country and is a potentially serious illness. This infection is typically mild, and usually the patient is asymptomatic. However, a small percentage of patients develop severe disease. The incubation period is 2 to 15 days after being bitten by an infected mosquito. Other possible sources of transmission include blood products, breast milk, or an organ transplant. Diagnostic tests to determine the presence of West Nile virus include enzyme-linked immunosorbent assay and West Nile virus–specific immunoglobulin M (IgM) antibody in the blood or CSF (McCance et al, 2014).

In mild cases of *West Nile virus,* the patient has no symptoms or has mild flu-like symptoms (e.g., fever, body aches, nausea, vomiting). Some people develop serious symptoms that may include high fever, severe headache, decreased level of consciousness, tremors, vision loss, seizures, and muscle weakness or paralysis. These manifestations may last for several weeks, and neurologic deficits may be permanent. A few patients die from the disease, especially those older than 50 years with a weakened immune system.

Echovirus, coxsackievirus, poliovirus, herpes zoster, and viruses that cause mumps and chickenpox are the common *enteroviruses* associated with encephalitis. *Herpes simplex virus type 1 (HSV1)* encephalitis is the most common nonepidemic type of encephalitis in North America. Patients with this disease often have a history of cold sores. The mortality rates for HSV1 encephalitis are very high compared with those for other types of encephalitis.

Amebic meningoencephalitis is caused by the amebae *Naegleria* and *Acanthamoeba.* Both are found in warm freshwater areas and can enter the nasal mucosa of people swimming in ponds or lakes (McCance et al., 2014). The amebae may also be found in soil and decaying vegetation. Although this infection has not often been seen in the past, the incidence in North America is increasing, perhaps because ponds and lakes are becoming more polluted.

❖ INTERPROFESSIONAL COLLABORATIVE CARE

◆ Assessment: Noticing

The typical patient with encephalitis has a high fever and reports nausea, vomiting, and a stiff neck. Assess for other signs and symptoms, including possible:

- Changes in mental status (e.g., agitation)
- Motor dysfunction (e.g., dysphagia [difficulty swallowing])
- Focal (specific) neurologic deficits
- Photophobia (light sensitivity) and phonophobia (noise sensitivity)
- Fatigue
- Symptoms of increased ICP (e.g., decreased LOC)
- Joint pain
- Headache
- Vertigo

Assess LOC using the Glasgow Coma Scale (see Chapter 41) or other agency-approved assessment tool. The patient may be lethargic, stuporous, or comatose. Mental status changes are more extensive in the patient with encephalitis than with meningitis. Changes include acute confusion, irritability, and personality and behavior changes (especially noted in the presence of herpes simplex). Signs of meningeal irritation include the presence of nuchal (neck) rigidity and motor changes that vary from a mild weakness to hemiplegia. The patient may have muscle tremors, spasticity, an ataxic gait (postencephalitic Parkinsonism), myoclonic jerks, and increased deep tendon reflexes. Seizure activity is common (McCance et al., 2014).

Observe for cranial nerve involvement, such as ocular palsies (paralysis), facial weakness, and nystagmus (involuntary lateral eye movements). The herpes zoster lesion affects cranial and spinal nerve root ganglia, which is clinically manifested by a rash, severe pain, itching, burning, or tingling in the areas innervated by these nerves.

! NURSING SAFETY PRIORITY **QSEN**

Critical Rescue

In severe cases of encephalitis, the patient may have increased ICP resulting from cerebral edema, hemorrhage, and necrosis of brain tissue. If the patient is nonverbal or comatose at baseline, monitoring vital signs and pupils becomes essential for detecting worsening neurologic status and increased ICP. Changes in vital signs that require an immediate notification of the health care provider are a widened pulse pressure, new bradycardia, and irregular respiratory effort. Pupils that become increasingly dilated and less responsive to light are also communicated urgently. Left untreated, increased ICP leads to herniation of the brain tissue and possibly death (see Chapter 45).

Lumbar puncture (LP) is done to analyze the CSF for the specific offending organism. A polymerase chain reaction (PCR) test may be used to detect viral DNA or ribonucleic acid (RNA) in the CSF. Specificity and sensitivity in diagnosing encephalitis are excellent, especially with herpes simplex virus (HSV). The test is rapid and noninvasive, replacing the brain biopsy for diagnosis.

An electroencephalogram is done to evaluate brain wave activity to detect seizures. Brain imaging in the form of a CT scan with and without contrast is performed to evaluate elevated intracranial pressure (ICP) or obstructive hydrocephalus.

◆ Interventions: Responding

Teach people who live in mosquito-infested areas to protect themselves and their families from West Nile virus infections. Chart 42-13 lists measures for preventing this infection. There is no curative treatment for West Nile viral encephalitis. Also remind individuals not to swim in lakes and ponds that are not designated for swimming to prevent amebic encephalitis.

Acyclovir (Zovirax) is the antiviral drug of choice for the treatment of herpes encephalitis and is associated with a significantly lower mortality rate than vidarabine (Vira-A) (Burchum & Rosenthal, 2016). Drug therapy is most effective if begun early, before the patient becomes stuporous or comatose. This neurologic decline usually occurs within 4 to 6 days after the initial neurologic symptoms. No specific drug therapy is available for infection by arboviruses or enteroviruses.

👤 CHART 42-13   Patient and Family Education: Preparing for Self-Management

Protecting the Patient and Family From West Nile Virus

- Limit your time outside between dusk and dawn when mosquitoes are out.
- Wear protective clothing, including long sleeves and pants.
- Use an insect repellent containing DEET when outdoors.
- Remove areas of standing water from flower pots, trash cans, and rain gutters.
- Check window and door screens for holes that need repair.
- Keep hot tubs and pools clean and properly chlorinated.

Nursing interventions for encephalitis are similar to those for meningitis with the exception of drug therapy. Supportive nursing care and prompt recognition and treatment of increased ICP are essential components of management. *Maintain a patent airway to prevent the development of atelectasis or pneumonia, which can lead to further brain hypoxia (lack of oxygen).*

Provide supportive nursing care for the patient who is immobile, stuporous, or comatose. Delegate and supervise unlicensed assistive personnel (UAP) to turn, cough, and deep breathe the patient at least every 2 hours. Perform deep tracheal suctioning even in the presence of increased ICP if respiratory status is compromised. Assess vital signs and neurologic signs every 2 hours or more frequently if clinically indicated. Elevate the head of the bed 30 to 45 degrees unless contraindicated (e.g., after lumbar puncture or in the patient with severe hypotension). Keep the patient's room darkened and quiet to promote COMFORT and decrease agitation. Remind UAP to provide safety measures such as keeping the bed in the lowest position.

Provide patient and family support. Families need health teaching to understand how to care for their loved ones. They are often fearful that the patient may not return to his or her baseline. Collaborate with a certified chaplain, social worker, or case manager to provide additional emotional support and counseling.

Patients with encephalitis and permanent neurologic deficits are usually discharged to a rehabilitation setting or a long-term care facility. Those with minimal neurologic problems are discharged to the home setting.

GET READY FOR THE NCLEX® EXAMINATION!

▌KEY POINTS

Review these Key Points for each NCLEX Examination Client Needs Category.

Safe and Effective Care Environment

- Implement best practices for fall prevention and wandering behaviors that are typically seen in patients with impaired COGNITION, such as those with AD (see Chart 42-3). **QSEN: Safety**

- Collaborate with the health care team in discharge planning and health teaching for patients who have chronic seizures or neurodegenerative diseases such as AD and PD. **QSEN: Teamwork and Collaboration**

Health Promotion and Maintenance

- Teach patients with migraine headaches about triggers that could cause an attack, such as tyramine in wine, pickled products, and aged cheeses; nitrates and nitrites in processed and grilled meats; and other dietary or environmental triggers (see Chart 42-7). **QSEN: Patient-Centered Care**

- In addition to prescribed drug therapy, encourage patients with headaches to use complementary and integrative therapies to help relieve altered COMFORT, such as ice, darkened room, and relaxation techniques. **QSEN: Patient-Centered Care**
- Teach the patient with epilepsy to maintain seizure-free health or reduced seizure activity through using prescribed antiepileptic drugs (AEDs) and follow-up medical care.
- Teach the importance of vaccination to prevent some types of infectious meningitis, particularly meningococcal vaccination, to people who are in areas of high population density, such as university residences, military barracks, and crowded living areas. **QSEN: Evidence-Based Practice**
- Teach the importance of strategies to prevent West Nile virus infection that could cause encephalitis as listed in Chart 42-12.

Psychosocial Integrity

- Remind caregivers of patients with chronic neurologic diseases, such as dementia, to find ways to cope with their own stress to remain physically and psychologically healthy, as suggested in Chart 42-4. **QSEN: Patient-Centered Care**
- Teach caregivers of patients with dementia to use validation therapy rather than reality orientation. Acknowledge the patient's feelings and concerns. **QSEN: Patient-Centered Care**
- Emphasize the strengths of patients with PD rather than focus on their limitations; provide positive reinforcement when tasks are completed. Provide encouragement for the patient to promote self-concept. **QSEN: Patient-Centered Care**

Physiological Integrity

- Adults at risk for AD and other dementias include older adults and those who experience a traumatic brain injury (TBI), including war veterans.
- Adapt communication techniques for the patient with dementia as outlined in Chart 42-2.

- Ensure a safe environment for a patient with seizure precautions by ensuring that suction and oxygen are available and that frequent observation occurs to detect seizure activity early. **QSEN: Safety**
- Implement interventions for seizures as listed in Chart 42-8. Patients with status epilepticus have a life-threatening complication. Lorazepam and diazepam are the major drugs used for this emergency. **QSEN: Evidence-Based Practice**
- Assess patients with classic migraine headaches as listed in Chart 42-6.
- Recognize that generalized seizures, such as the tonic-clonic seizure, involve both cerebral hemispheres. Partial seizures, also called *focal* or *local seizures,* usually involve only one hemisphere.
- During a seizure, document the patient's body movements and other assessments as described in Chart 42-9. **QSEN: Informatics**
- Monitor for side and adverse effects of antiepileptic drugs (AEDs) (see Table 42-5 for commonly used drugs). **QSEN: Safety**
- For patients who have had one or more seizures, place on "seizure precautions," which includes having oxygen delivery and suctioning equipment available and starting or maintaining IV access. **QSEN: Safety**
- Assess for signs and symptoms of meningitis as listed in Chart 42-11. For patients with meningitis and encephalitis, carefully monitor neurologic status, including vital signs and neurologic and vascular checks. Observe for signs and symptoms of increased intracranial pressure (ICP) and communicate changes in level of consciousness immediately to the health care provider. **QSEN: Safety**
- Monitor for drug toxicity when patients are taking medications for PD, especially levodopa combinations such as Sinemet. Delirium and decreased drug effectiveness are the most common indicators of toxicity. **QSEN: Safety**
- Document cognitive and functional abilities of the patient with dementia, recognizing that it is a progressive condition (e.g., Alzheimer stages are listed in Chart 42-1).
- For patients with dementia, recall that a few drugs improve function and cognition (cholinesterase inhibitors, such as donepezil [Aricept]) or slow the disease process (Memantine) but do not cure the disease.

SELECTED BIBLIOGRAPHY

Allard, M. E., & Katseres, J. (2016). Using essential oils to enhance nursing practice and for self-care. *American Journal of Nursing, 116*(2), 42–50.

Alzheimer's Disease Education and Referral Center. (2013). *Health disparities and Alzheimer's disease.* https://www.nia.nih.gov/alzheimers/publication/2013-2014-alzheimers-disease-progress-report/health-disparities-and-alzheimers-disease/.

Barnes, L. L., & Bennett, D. A. (2014). *Alzheimer's disease in African Americans: Risk factors and challenges for the future.* http://www.ncbi.nlm.nih.gov.pmc/articles/PMC4084964/.

Bettens, K., Sleegers, K., & Van Broeckhoven, C. (2013). Genetic insights in Alzheimer's disease. *The Lancet. Neurology, 12*(1), 92–104.

Burchum, J. L. R., & Rosenthal, L. D. (2016). *Lehne's pharmacology for nursing care* (9th ed.). St. Louis: Elsevier.

Carod-Artel, F. J. (2014). Tackling chronic migraine: Current perspectives. *Journal of Pain Research, 7,* 185–194.

Claxton, A. (2015). Long-acting intranasal insulin detemir improves cognition for adults with mild cognitive impairment or early-stage Alzheimer's disease dementia. *Journal of Alzheimer's Disease, 42*(3), 897–906.

Deardorff, W. J., & Grossberg, G. T. (2015). The use of cholinesterase inhibitors across all stages of Alzheimer's disease. *Drugs and Aging, 32*(7), 537–547.

Friedmann, E., Galik, E., Thomas, S. A., Hall, P. S., Chung, S. Y., & McCune, S. (2015). Evaluation of a pet-assisted living intervention for improving functional status in assisted-living residents with mild-to-moderate cognitive impairment: A pilot study. *American Journal of Alzheimer's Disease and Other Dementias, 30*(3), 276–289.

Klug, J. R. (2014). Spotlight on frontotemporal dementia. *Nursing, 44*(8), 55–57.

LaRocco, S. A. (2015). Unmasking the nonmotor symptoms of Parkinson disease. *Nursing, 45*(7), 26–32.

Malone, C. D., Bhowmick, A., & Wachholtz, A. B. (2015). Migraine: treatments, comorbidities, and quality of life in the U.S.A. *Journal of Pain Research, 8,* 537–547.

Mapelli, D., Di Rosa, E., Nocita, R., & Sava, D. (2013). Cognitive stimulation in patients with dementia: Randomized controlled trial. *Dementia and Geriatric Cognitive Disorders Extra, 3,* 263–271.

Martindale-Adams, J., Nichols, L. O., Burns, R., Graney, M. J., & Zuber, J. (2013). A trial of dementia caregiver telephone support. *Canadian Journal of Nursing Research, 45*(4), 30–48.

McCance, K., Huether, S., Brashers, V., & Rote, N. (2014). *Pathophysiology: The biologic basis for disease in adults and children* (7th ed.). St. Louis: Mosby.

Meziab, O., Kirby, K. A., Williams, B., Yaffe, K., Byers, A. L., & Barnes, D. E. (2014). Prisoner of war status, posttraumatic stress disorder, and dementia in older veterans. *Alzheimer's & Dementia, 10*(3 Suppl.), S236–S241.

Murphy, K. (2015). What to do about sexually inappropriate behavior in patients with dementia. *Nursing, 45*(9), 53–56.

National Center for Complementary and Integrative Health (NCCIH). (2017). *Headaches: In depth.* https://nccih.nih.gov/health/pain/headachefacts.htm#hed3.

National Institute of Neurological Disorders and Stroke (NINDS). (2017). *Parkinson's disease.* www.ninds.nih.gov/disorders/parkinsons_disease/parkinsons_disease.htm.

Pagana, K. D., Pagana, T. J., & Pagana, T. N. (2017). *Mosby's diagnostic and laboratory test reference* (13th ed.). St. Louis: Elsevier.

Perrar, K. M., Schmidt, H., Eisenmann, Y., Cremer, B., & Voltz, R. (2015). Needs of people with severe dementia at the end-of-life: A systematic review. *Journal of Alzheimer's Disease, 43*(2), 397–413.

Rausa, M., Cevoli, S., Sancisis, E., Grimaldi, D., Pollutru, G., Casoria, M., et al. (2013). Personality traits in chronic daily headache patients with and without psychiatric comorbidity. *Journal of Headache and Pain, 13,* 14–22.

Rovner, B. W., Casten, R. J., & Harris, L. F. (2013). Cultural diversity and views on Alzheimer disease in older African Americans. *Alzheimer Disease and Associated Disorders, 27*(2), 133–137.

Schaller, S., Mauskopf, J., Kriza, C., Wahlster, P., & Kolominsky-Rabas, P. L. (2015). The main cost drivers of dementia: A systematic review. *International Journal of Geriatric Psychiatry, 30*(2), 111–129.

Sibener, L., Zaganjor, I., Snyder, H. M., Bain, L. J., Egge, R., & Carillo, M. C. (2014). Alzheimer's disease prevalence, costs, and prevention for military personnel and veterans. *Alzheimer's & Dementia, 10*(3 Suppl.), S105–S110.

Struble, L. M., Sullivan, B. J., & Hartman, L. S. (2014). Psychiatric disorders impacting critical illness. *Critical Care Nursing Clinics of North America, 26*(1), 115–138.

Van der Mussele, S., Fransend, E., Struyfs, H., Luyckx, J., Marien, P., Saerens, J., et al. (2014). Depression in mild cognitive impairment is associated with progression to Alzheimer's disease: A longitudinal study. *Journal of Alzheimer's Disease, 42*(4), 1239–1250.

Volland, J., & Fisher, A. (2014). Best practices for engaging patients with dementia. *Nursing, 44*(11), 44–50.

Westman, K. F., & Blaisdell, C. (2016). Many benefits, little risk: The use of massage in nursing practice. *American Journal of Nursing, 116*(1), 34–40.

Wolf, Z. R., & Czekanski, K. E. (2015). Bathing disability and bathing persons with dementia. *Medsurg Nursing, 24*(1), 9–22.

CHAPTER 43

Care of Patients With Problems of the Central Nervous System: The Spinal Cord

Laura M. Willis and Donna D. Ignatavicius

PRIORITY AND INTERRELATED CONCEPTS

The priority concepts for this chapter are:

- IMMUNITY
- MOBILITY
- SENSORY PERCEPTION

✳ The IMMUNITY concept exemplar for this chapter is Multiple Sclerosis, p. 888.

✳ The MOBILITY concept exemplar for this chapter is Spinal Cord Injury, p. 894.

The interrelated concepts for this chapter are:

- COMFORT
- COGNITION
- SEXUALITY

LEARNING OUTCOMES

Safe and Effective Care Environment

1. Prioritize nursing care of the patient with an acute spinal cord injury (SCI).
2. Collaborate with interprofessional health care team members to establish outcomes for care and promote optimal functioning for patients with multiple sclerosis (MS) and SCI.

Health Promotion and Maintenance

3. Identify community resources for patients with MS and SCI.
4. Teach adults evidence-based strategies for how to prevent back injury.
5. Teach adults the importance of changing lifestyle practices to prevent SCI.
6. Apply knowledge of adult development to plan health teaching and care for the older adult with an SCI.

Psychosocial Integrity

7. Assess the response of patients to having MS or SCI.
8. Identify resources and strategies for patients with altered SEXUALITY caused by SCI to improve sexual health.

Physiological Integrity

9. Perform a comprehensive assessment of the patient with an SCI.
10. Establish priorities in care for the patient with spinal cord–related problems of MOBILITY, SENSORY PERCEPTION, and COMFORT.
11. Apply knowledge of pathophysiology to promote safety for a patient having autonomic dysreflexia.
12. Apply knowledge of the pathophysiology of MS to identify common assessment findings affecting MOBILITY, SENSORY PERCEPTION, COGNITION, and IMMUNITY.
13. Explain the role of drug therapy in managing patients with MS and associated nursing implications and health teaching.
14. Develop an evidence-based postoperative plan of care for patients having back surgery, including monitoring for complications.

The spinal cord relays messages to and from the brain. Besides injuries, the spinal cord can develop inflammatory and auto-immune diseases, such as multiple sclerosis and tumors, both benign and malignant. The spinal cord itself may be damaged, or the spinal nerves leading from the cord to the extremities may be affected. In some cases, both the spinal cord and the nerves are involved. Signs and symptoms of spinal cord health problems vary, but often include problems with IMMUNITY, MOBILITY, SENSORY PERCEPTION, COMFORT, and SEXUALITY. Interprofessional health care team members with expertise in symptom management collaborate to improve quality of life, promote a safe environment, and prevent complications from impaired mobility and sensory perception. Chapter 2 reviews each of these nursing and health concepts in detail.

✳ **IMMUNITY CONCEPT EXEMPLAR**
Multiple Sclerosis

❖ *PATHOPHYSIOLOGY*

Multiple sclerosis (MS) is a chronic disease caused by immune, genetic, and/or infectious factors that affects the myelin and nerve fibers of the brain and spinal cord. It is one of the leading causes of neurologic disability in young and middle-age adults. MS is characterized by periods of remission and exacerbation (flare), which is commonly referred to as a *relapsing-remitting course*. Patients progress at different rates and over different lengths of time. However, as the severity and duration of the disease progress, the periods of exacerbation become more frequent. Patients with MS can have a normal life expectancy as long as the effects of the disease are managed effectively.

MS is characterized by demyelination and axonal nerve damage. Diffuse random or patchy areas of *plaque* in the white matter of the central nervous system (CNS) are the definitive finding. Initially, remyelination takes place to some degree, and clinical symptoms decrease. However, over time, new lesions develop, and neuronal injury and muscle atrophy occur. Myelin is responsible for the electrochemical transmission of impulses between the brain and spinal cord and the rest of the body; demyelination can result in slowed or stopped impulse transmission. The white fiber tracts that connect the neurons in the brain and spinal cord are also usually involved in MS. The areas particularly affected include optic nerves, pyramidal tracts, posterior columns, brainstem nuclei, and the ventricular region of the brain. Eventually, with repeated exacerbations of the disease, damage to the axons becomes permanent.

The four major types of MS include (McCance et al., 2014):
- Relapsing-remitting
- Primary progressive
- Secondary progressive
- Progressive-relapsing

The classic picture of the relapsing-remitting type of MS (RRMS) occurs in most cases of MS. The course of the disease may be mild or moderate, depending on the degree of disability. Symptoms develop and resolve in a few weeks to months, and the patient returns to baseline. During the relapsing phase, the patient reports loss of function and the continuing development of new symptoms.

Primary progressive MS (PPMS) involves a steady and gradual neurologic deterioration without remission of symptoms. The patient has progressive disability with no acute attacks. Patients with this type of MS tend to be between 40 and 60 years of age at onset of the disease.

Secondary progressive MS (SPMS) begins with a relapsing-remitting course that later becomes steadily progressive. About half of all people with RRMS developed SPMS within 10 years. The current addition of disease-modifying drugs as part of disease management may decrease the development of SPMS.

Progressive-relapsing MS (PRMS) is characterized by frequent relapses with partial recovery but not a return to baseline. This type of MS is seen in only a small percentage of patients. Progressive, cumulative symptoms and deterioration occur over several years.

Etiology

The cause of MS is very complex and involves multiple immune, genetic, and/or infectious factors, although changes in IMMUNITY are the most likely etiology. The environment may also contribute to its development. For example, the disease is seen more often in the colder climates of the northeastern, Great Lakes, and Pacific northwestern states and in Canada. MS is common in areas inhabited by people of northern European ancestry (National Multiple Sclerosis Society, 2017).

🧬 **GENETIC/GENOMIC CONSIDERATIONS**
Patient-Centered Care **QSEN**

Large genome studies of families have helped identify familial patterns of multiple sclerosis (MS). For example, having a first-degree relative such as a parent or sibling with MS increases a person's risk for developing the disease. Research also confirms the association of MS with over 100 gene variants, including interleukin (IL)-7 and IL-2 receptor genes (McCance et al., 2014; National Multiple Sclerosis Society, 2017). These findings have helped guide the development of targeted drug therapies that are important in current disease management.

Incidence/Prevalence

MS usually occurs in people between the ages of 20 and 50 years, but cases may occur at any age. About 400,000 people in the United States have MS. The disease affects over 2.3 million people worldwide (National Multiple Sclerosis Society, 2017). About 100,000 Canadians have it (MS Society of Canada, 2017). Although MS tends to occur more frequently among whites of Northern European ancestry, it affects people of all races and ethnicity.

GENDER HEALTH CONSIDERATIONS
Patient-Centered Care **QSEN**

MS affects women two to three times more often than men, suggesting a possible hormonal role in disease development. Some studies show that the disease occurs up to four times more often in women than men (National Multiple Sclerosis Society, 2017).

❖ *INTERPROFESSIONAL COLLABORATIVE CARE*
◆ *Assessment: Noticing*

History. Multiple sclerosis (MS) often looks like other neurologic diseases, such as amyotrophic lateral sclerosis (ALS), which can make the diagnosis difficult and prolonged. Table 43-1 compares these two neurologic health problems.

Patients often visit many primary health care providers and undergo a variety of diagnostic tests and treatments. Obtaining a thorough history is essential for accurate diagnosis. Ask the patient about a history of vision, MOBILITY, and SENSORY PERCEPTION changes, all of which are early indicators of MS. Symptoms are often vague and nonspecific in the early stages of the disease and may disappear for months or years before returning. Ask about the progression of symptoms. Pay particular attention to whether they are intermittent or are becoming progressively worse. Document the date (month and year) when the patient first noticed these changes.

Next, ask about factors that aggravate the symptoms, such as fatigue, stress, overexertion, temperature extremes, or a hot shower or bath. Ask the patient and the family about any personality or behavioral changes that have occurred (e.g., euphoria [very elated mood], poor judgment, attention loss). In addition, determine whether there is a family history of MS or autoimmune disease.

TABLE 43-1 Comparison of Multiple Sclerosis and Amyotrophic Lateral Sclerosis

	MULTIPLE SCLEROSIS (MS)	AMYOTROPHIC LATERAL SCLEROSIS (ALS)
Pathophysiology/ Etiology	Chronic neurologic disease that affects the brain and spinal cord due to immune-mediated demyelination and nerve injury; characterized by remissions and exacerbations	Chronic neurologic disease of unknown cause (genetic and environmental factors identified) causing progressive muscle weakness and wasting, leading to paralysis of respiratory muscles
Populations Affected	Commonly occurring disease that affects people (women twice as often as men) between the ages of 20 and 50 years; most often affects whites of Northern European ancestry	Uncommon disease that affects people (more men than women) between the ages of 40 and 60 years; incidence increases with each decade of life
Signs and Symptoms	Fatigue Muscle spasticity Blurred or double vision (diplopia) Scotomas Nystagmus Paresthesias Areflexic (flaccid) or spastic bladder Decreased sexual function Intention tremors Gait changes	Fatigue Muscle atrophy (including tongue) Muscle weakness Twitching of face and tongue Dysarthria Dysphagia Stiff and clumsy gait Abnormal reflexes
Interprofessional Collaborative Care	Multiple immunomodulating and antineoplastic drugs available Collaborative care to promote and maintain optimal functioning Symptom management to achieve maximal function Psychosocial support	One approved drug to slow disease (riluzole [Rilutek]) Supportive care to promote optimal function Palliative care for symptom management at end of life Psychosocial support

---

⧉ **CHART 43-1 Key Features**

Multiple Sclerosis

- Muscle weakness and spasticity
- Fatigue
- Intention tremors
- Dysmetria (inability to direct or limit movement)
- Numbness or tingling sensations (paresthesia)
- Hypalgesia (decreased sensitivity to pain)
- Ataxia (decreased motor coordination)
- Dysarthria (slurred speech)
- Dysphagia (difficulty swallowing)
- Diplopia (double vision)
- Nystagmus (involuntary eye movements)
- Scotomas (changes in peripheral vision)
- Decreased visual and hearing acuity
- Tinnitus (ringing in the ears), vertigo (dizziness)
- Bowel and bladder dysfunction
- Alterations in sexual function, such as impotence
- Cognitive changes, such as memory loss, impaired judgment, and decreased ability to solve problems or perform calculations
- Depression

Physical Assessment/Signs and Symptoms. MS produces a wide variety of signs and symptoms (Chart 43-1). Any myelinated fibers of the brain and spinal cord may be affected. The patient often reports increased fatigue and stiffness of the extremities, particularly the legs. Fatigue is one of the most disabling manifestations, affecting almost all patients with MS. Unlike fatigue in other patients, MS fatigue is associated with continuous sensitivity to temperature.

Flexor spasms at night may awaken the patient from sleep. Increased or hyperactive deep tendon reflexes, positive Babinski's reflex, and absent abdominal reflexes may be found. Gait may be unsteady because of leg weakness and spasticity due to cerebral motor strip damage.

Significant *cerebellar* findings include **intention tremor** (tremor when performing an activity), dysmetria (inability to

direct or limit movement), and dysdiadochokinesia (inability to stop one motor impulse and substitute another). Motor movements are often clumsy.

During examination of the *cranial nerves* and brainstem function, the patient may mention episodes of tinnitus (ringing in the ears), vertigo (dizziness), and hearing loss. Speech problems include dysarthria, such as slurred words resulting from weak muscles of the tongue, lips, cheek, or mouth. Scanning is also a type of dysarthria common in MS. Scanning is an abnormal speech pattern with long pauses between words or syllables.

Typical clinical findings from assessment of the patient's visual acuity, visual fields, and pupils include:

- Blurred vision
- **Diplopia** (double vision)
- Decreased visual acuity
- **Scotomas** (changes in peripheral vision)
- **Nystagmus** (involuntary rapid eye movements)

Sensory findings include hypalgesia (diminished sensitivity to pain), paresthesia, facial pain, and decreased temperature perception. The patient may report numbness, tingling, burning, or crawling sensations. Some patients with RRMS report altered COMFORT or pain. Perform a complete pain assessment for all patients with MS as described in Chapter 4.

The patient may have an areflexic (flaccid) bladder or may experience frequency, urgency, or nocturia (spastic bladder). Ask the patient if he or she has constipation or incontinence. Inquire about problems with SEXUALITY, including impotence, difficulty sustaining an erection, and decreased vaginal secretions.

Psychosocial Assessment. A major concern reported by most patients is how long it takes to establish a diagnosis of MS. Many patients go to several primary health care providers, are given varying diagnoses and treatment, and/or are told that their symptoms are related to stress and anxiety. Often, young adults present with weakness, fatigue, or changes in vision and are diagnosed with exhaustion and advised to get more sleep.

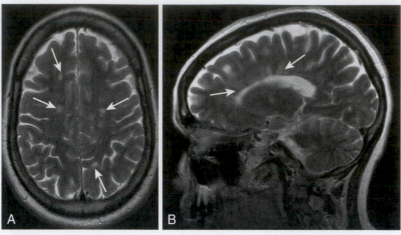

FIG. 43-1 Typical plaques seen in spinal and brain CT of patient with multiple sclerosis. (From Herring W. [2016]. *Learning radiology*, [3rd ed.]. St. Louis: Saunders.)

The patient and family are often relieved to have a definite diagnosis but may express anger and frustration that it took a long time to start appropriate treatment. Therefore establish open and honest communication with the patient and allow him or her to share frustrations, anger, and anxiety.

After the initial diagnosis of MS, the patient is often anxious. Apathy and emotional lability are common problems that occur later. Depression may occur at the time of diagnosis and can also occur later with disease progression. The patient may be euphoric or giddy, either as a result of the disease itself or because of the drugs used to treat it. Assess the patient's previously used coping and stress-management skills in preparing him or her for a chronic, potentially debilitating disease. Secondary depression is the most frequent mental health disorder diagnosed in patients with MS.

Assess the patient for mental status changes. Changes in COGNITION are usually seen late in the course of the disease and can include decreased short-term memory, concentration, and ability to perform calculations; inattentiveness; and impaired judgment.

Assess the impact of bowel and bladder problems. Managing fecal incontinence or constipation can be time-consuming and embarrassing.

SEXUALITY can be affected in people with MS, and sexual dysfunction can have a major impact on quality of life. Assess the patient's fatigue level and pattern, since fatigue contributes to sexual dysfunction. Be sensitive when asking about the patient's sexual practices and orientation. Women often report impaired genital sensation, diminished orgasm, and loss of sexual interest. Men most often report difficulty in achieving and maintaining an erection and delayed ejaculation.

Laboratory Assessment. No single specific laboratory test is definitively diagnostic for MS. However, the collective results of a variety of tests are usually conclusive. Abnormal cerebrospinal fluid (CSF) findings include an elevated protein level and a slight increase in the white blood cell count. CSF electrophoresis reveals an increase in the myelin basic protein and the presence of increased immunoglobulins, especially immunoglobulin G (IgG). IgG bands are seen in most patients with MS (Pagana et al., 2017).

Other Diagnostic Assessment. MRI of the brain and spinal cord demonstrates the presence of plaques and is considered diagnostic for MS. MRI with contrast shows active plaques and reveals older lesions not associated with current symptoms (Fig. 43-1).

A complete history and physical examination are necessary to exclude other disease diagnoses. In general, assessment of cranial nerve function, coordination, strength, reflexes, and sensation are needed to diagnose MS; and a variety of neurologic tests are used to evaluate the many areas in which dysfunction from MS plaques can occur.

◆ *Analysis: Interpreting*

The priority collaborative problems for patients with multiple sclerosis include:

1. Potential for infection/impaired IMMUNITY secondary to disease and drug therapy for disease management
2. Decreased MOBILITY due to spasticity, tremors, and/or fatigue
3. Decreased visual acuity and COGNITION due to dysfunctional central system nerves

◆ *Planning and Implementation: Responding*

The purpose of management is to modify the disease's effects on the immune system, prevent exacerbations, manage symptoms, improve function, and maintain quality of life. As with other spinal cord diseases, care of the patient with MS requires the collaborative efforts of the interprofessional health care team.

Managing Potential for Infection and Impaired Immunity

Planning: Expected Outcomes. The patient with MS is expected to be free from episodes of secondary infection due to impaired IMMUNITY from the disease or from drug therapy used to manage the illness.

Interventions. The patient with MS is treated with a variety of drugs that are used to treat and control the disease progression. Many of these drugs are immunomodulators or anti-inflammatory medications that can alter IMMUNITY and make patients vulnerable to secondary infection. Teach patients receiving drug therapy for MS to avoid crowds and anyone with an infection. If signs and symptoms of an infection occur, remind them to contact their primary health care provider for prompt management and medical observation.

Examples of drugs used for treatment of relapsing types of MS include (Burcham & Rosenthal, 2016):

- Interferon beta-1a (Avonex or Rebif), an immunomodulator that *modifies* the course of the disease and also has antiviral effects
- Interferon beta-1b (Betaseron, Extavia), another immunomodulator with antiviral properties
- Glatiramer acetate (Copaxone), a synthetic protein that is similar to myelin-based protein
- Mitoxantrone (Novantrone), an antineoplastic anti-inflammatory agent used to resolve relapses but with risks for leukemia and cardiotoxicity
- Natalizumab (Tysabri), the first monoclonal antibody approved for MS that binds to white blood cells (WBCs) to prevent further damage to the myelin
- Fingolimod (Gilenya), teriflunomide (Aubagio), and dimethyl fumarate (Tecfidera), newer *oral* immunomodulating drugs
- Corticosteroids (methylprednisolone [Solu-Medrol], dexamethasone, or prednisone), anti-inflammatory and immune-suppressing drugs used short term for acute exacerbation or initial onset

> **! NURSING SAFETY PRIORITY** QSEN
>
> **Drug Alert**
>
> The interferons and glatiramer acetate are subcutaneous injections that patients can self-administer. Teach patients how to give and rotate the site of interferon-beta and glatiramer acetate injections because local injection site (skin) reactions are common. The first dose of these drugs is given under medical supervision to monitor for allergic response, including anaphylactic shock. Teach patients receiving them to avoid crowds and people with infections. Remind them to report any sign or symptom associated with infection immediately to their primary health care provider.

Natalizumab, a humanized monoclonal antibody, is a controversial drug because it can cause many adverse events. It is usually given as an IV infusion in a specialty clinic under careful supervision. The patient is monitored carefully for allergic or anaphylactic reaction when each dose is given because the drug tends to build up in the body. *Patients receiving this drug are at a high risk for* progressive multifocal leukoencephalopathy (PML). This opportunistic viral infection leads to death or severe disability. Monitor for neurologic changes, especially changes in mental state, such as disorientation or acute confusion. PML is confirmed by an MRI and examining the cerebrospinal fluid for the causative pathogen (Burcham & Rosenthal, 2016). Natalizumab also causes damage to hepatic cells. Carefully monitor liver enzymes and teach patients to have frequent laboratory tests to assess for changes.

Mitoxantrone (Novantrone), a chemotherapy drug, has been shown to be effective in reducing neurologic disability. It also decreases the frequency of clinical relapses in patients with secondary progressive, progressive-relapsing, or worsening relapsing-remitting MS.

Fingolimod (Gilenya) was the first oral immunomodulator approved for the management of MS. The capsules may be taken with or without food. Teach patients to monitor their pulse every day because the drug can cause bradycardia, especially within the first 6 hours after taking it. Two other immunomodulating drugs have been approved for MS: teriflunomide (Aubagio) and dimethyl fumarate (Tecfidera). Like fingolimod, these drugs inhibit immune cells and have antioxidant properties

that protect brain and spinal cord cells. Teach the patient that the two most common side effects of all the oral drugs are facial flushing and GI disturbances (Burcham & Rosenthal, 2016). Remind the patient to keep follow-up appointments for laboratory monitoring of the WBC count because the oral drugs can cause a decrease in WBCs, which can predispose the patient to infection.

Immunosuppressive therapy with a combination of cyclophosphamide (Cytoxan) and methylprednisolone (Solu-Medrol) may be used for some patients to stabilize the disease process by decreasing inflammation and the immune response. IV adrenocorticotropic hormone (ACTH) may be given instead of methylprednisolone and tapered gradually over 2 to 4 weeks.

> **? NCLEX EXAMINATION CHALLENGE 43-1**
>
> **Physiological Integrity**
>
> The nurse provides health teaching for a client beginning glatiramer acetate therapy. Which statement by the client indicates a need for **additional** teaching?
> A. "I'll take this drug with food every morning."
> B. "I'll look for signs of skin reaction at the injection site."
> C. "I'll stay away from kids who have colds."
> D. "I'll avoid large crowds so I don't get sick."

Improving Mobility

Planning Expected Outcomes. The patient with MS will have maximal MOBILITY and decreased fatigue as a result of successful interprofessional management and self-care interventions.

Interventions. The symptoms of MS that affect MOBILITY include spasticity, tremor, and fatigue. Referral to rehabilitative services, such as physical and occupational therapy, can help manage functional deficits from MS symptoms. An interprofessional team approach is important to attain patient-centered outcomes for care.

To lessen muscle spasticity, the primary health care provider may prescribe baclofen (Lioresal, Apo-Baclofen ✦), tizanidine (Zanaflex), or dantrolene sodium (Dantrium). Dalfampridine (Ampyra), a potassium channel blocker, is a new oral drug that can be prescribed to improve walking ability and speed. It is not given to patients with a history of seizures or renal disease, and it is not widely prescribed because of side effects (Burcham & Rosenthal, 2016).

Severe muscle spasticity may be treated with intrathecal baclofen (ITB) administered through a surgically implanted pump. Paresthesia may be treated with carbamazepine (Tegretol) or tricyclic antidepressants. Propranolol hydrochloride (Inderal) and clonazepam (Klonopin) have been used to treat cerebellar ataxia.

In collaboration with physical and occupational therapists, plan an exercise program that includes range-of-motion (ROM) exercises and stretching and strengthening exercises to manage spasticity and tremor. If needed as a last resort, neurosurgery (e.g., thalamotomy or deep brain stimulation) may provide some relief from tremors.

Emphasize the importance of avoiding rigorous activities that increase body temperature. Increased body temperature may lead to increased fatigue, diminished motor ability, and decreased visual acuity resulting from changes in the conduction abilities of the injured axons.

In collaboration with the case manager and occupational therapist, assess the patient's home before discharge for any hazards. Any items that might interfere with MOBILITY (e.g., scatter rugs) are removed. In addition, care must be taken to prevent injury resulting from vision problems. Teach the patient and family to keep the home environment as structured and free from clutter as possible. As the disease progresses, the home may need to be adapted for wheelchair accessibility. Adaptation in the kitchen, bedroom, and bathroom may also be needed to promote self-management. Any necessary assistive/adaptive device should be readily available before discharge from the hospital.

The patient with MS is often weak and easily fatigued. The Concept Map highlights the priority problems and interventions for the patient with MS. Teach the patient the importance of planning activities and allowing sufficient time to complete activities. For example, he or she should check that all items needed for work are gathered before leaving the house. Items used on a daily basis should be easily accessible.

If the patient experiences dysarthria (slurred speech) as a result of muscle weakness, refer him or her to the speech-language pathologist (SLP) for evaluation and treatment. It is not unusual for the patient with dysarthria also to have dysphagia (difficulty swallowing). The SLP performs a swallowing evaluation, but further diagnostic testing may be indicated. Monitor the patient to determine if there are problems swallowing at meal time that increase the risk of aspiration. Thickened liquids may be necessary.

Managing Decreased Visual Acuity and Cognition

Planning: Expected Outcomes. The patient with MS will maintain optimal visual acuity and COGNITION with use of available drug treatment and supportive services.

Interventions. Alterations in visual acuity and cognition can occur at any time during the course of the disease process. Areas affected include attention, memory, problem solving, auditory reasoning, handling distractions, and visual perception.

! NURSING SAFETY PRIORITY **QSEN**

Action Alert

For the patient with MS who has cognitive impairment, assist with orientation by using a single-date calendar. Give or encourage the patient to use written lists or recorded messages. To maintain an organized environment, encourage him or her to keep frequently used items in familiar places. Applications for handheld devices such as mobile phones and electronic tablets can also be used for re-orientation, reminders, and behavioral cues.

An eye patch that is alternated from eye to eye every few hours usually relieves diplopia (double vision). For peripheral visual deficits, teach scanning techniques by having the patient move his or her head from side to side. Changes in visual acuity may be helped by corrective lenses.

Complementary and Integrative Health.
Patients with MS often report that complementary therapies are successful in decreasing their symptoms. Some of the CAM therapies used by patients with MS are:

- Reflexology
- Massage
- Yoga
- Relaxation and meditation
- Acupuncture
- Aromatherapy

Marijuana has been used by some patients to relieve muscle spasm pain and is now legal for medical use in many states and in Canada.

Care Coordination and Transition Management

Home Care Management. To help the patient maintain maximum strength, function, and independence, continuity of care by an interprofessional team in the rehabilitation and/or home setting is necessary. Admission to a rehabilitation center may be needed to improve functional ability.

Self-Management Education. The primary health care provider explains to the patient and family the development of MS and the factors that may exacerbate the symptoms. Emphasize the importance of avoiding overexertion, stress, extremes of temperatures (fever, hot baths, use of sauna baths and hot tubs, overheating, and excessive chilling), humidity, and people with infections. Explain all medications to be taken on discharge, including the time and route of administration, dosage, purpose, and side effects. Teach the patient how to differentiate expected side effects from adverse or allergic reactions and provide the name of a resource person to call if questions or problems occur. Provide written instructions as a resource for the patient and caregivers at home.

The physical therapist develops an exercise program appropriate for the patient's tolerance level at home. The patient is instructed in techniques for self-care, daily living skills, and the use of required adaptive equipment such as walkers and electric carts. Include information related to bowel and bladder management, skin care, nutrition, and positioning techniques. Chapter 6 describes in detail these aspects of chronic illness and rehabilitation.

Teach patients about conservation strategies that balance periods of rest and activity, including regular social interactions. Remind them to use assistive devices and modify the environment to avoid fatigue. Explore strategies to manage stress and avoid undue stress. Often patients are anxious and worry about how long the remission will last or when the disease will progress.

MS affects the entire family because of the unpredictability and uncertainty of the course of the disease. Chronic fatigue may also prevent the patient from participating in family and community activities. Assess coping strategies of family members or other caregivers and help them identify support systems that can assist them as they live with the patient with MS.

Because personality changes are not unusual, teach the family or significant others strategies to enable them to cope with these changes. For example, the family may develop a nonverbal signal to alert the patient to potentially inappropriate behavior. This action avoids embarrassment for the patient.

Sexual dysfunction may occur as a result of fatigue, nerve involvement, and/or psychological reasons. Therefore some patients may benefit from counseling. If able, answer the patient's questions or refer him or her to a counselor or urologist with experience in the field of SEXUALITY, intimacy, and disability.

Prostaglandin-5 inhibitors (sildenafil, vardenafil, tadalafil) can be used to help men with erectile dysfunction. Penile prostheses are also used for men. The EROS Clitoral Therapy Device is a U.S. Food and Drug Administration (FDA)–approved therapy for women with impaired sexual response.

INTERVENTIONS—RESPONDING

1

History and Physical Assessment—Noticing

Assess history of onset and severity of signs/symptoms. Ask about their progression and about factors that aggravate or reduce symptoms. Complete a neurological assessment. *A focused history and physical assessment guides effective nursing care.*

2

Nursing Safety Priority: Action Alert!

Assist the cognitively impaired patient with orientation by placing a calendar in the room. Encourage written lists or recorded messages. Suggest keeping frequently used items in familiar places and using mobile device "apps" for re-orientation or reminders. *Cognitive impairment impacts patient safety. Orientation helps the patient to function as safely as possible in the environment.*

3

Responding to Patterns of SENSORY PERCEPTION Management

- Instruct the patient to wear an eye patch, alternating between eyes every few hours. *Relieves diplopia.*
- Teach scanning techniques. *Compensates for peripheral vision loss.*
- Encourage patient to see an ophthalmologist. *Manages changes in visual acuity that may be aided by corrective lenses.*

4

Improving Mobility

Collaborate with a physical/occupational therapist to maintain mobility and promote independence with ADLs. Teach patient to conserve energy and balance activities with periods of rest. Avoid common aggravating factors such as fatigue, stress, overexertion, or temperature extremes. *Maintain mobility by managing MS fatigue, the most disabling symptom. Fatigue level and pattern can contribute to immobility, dysfunction, and depression.*

5

Patterns of Elimination

Assess for urinary hesitancy, dribbling, incontinence, urgency, and constipation. Use a bladder scanner to assess for urinary retention. Implement necessary interventions such as catheterization, bladder pacemaker, or drug therapy. Use best practices to prevent hospital acquired UTIs. *Promotes urinary continence and bowel evacuation. Dysfunction can have a major impact on quality of life.*

6

Drug Management and Altered Immunity

Teach patients receiving medications that are immunomodulators, chemotherapy, or anti-inflammatory medications to avoid crowds and anyone with an infection. *Alters patients' IMMUNITY and makes them vulnerable to secondary infection.*

7

Drug and Complementary Therapies

- Review and provide written instructions of drug therapies for pain, inflammation, and incontinence. *Ensures patient understands drug mechanisms of action for safe administration.*
- Discuss complementary therapies such as massage, yoga, meditation, acupuncture, reflexology, and aromatherapy. *May help the patient to maintain MOBILITY and independence.*

8

Managing Dysarthria and Dysphagia

Collaborate with a speech-language pathologist for evaluation and treatment of slurred speech and swallowing difficulty. *Avoids complications resulting in ineffective airway clearance of secretions and aspiration.*

9

Patterns of Psychosocial Integrity

Assist patient in verbalizing concerns about body image, self-concept, role performance, self-esteem, and SEXUALITY. *Helps patient cope with anxiety and depression over the progression of the disease. Depression is the most frequent mental health disorder diagnosed with MS.*

10

Responding to Sexuality Issues

Assess fatigue level and pattern, being sensitive when asking about sexual practices and orientation. *Contributes to sexual dysfunction SEXUALITY, and sexual dysfunction has a major impact on quality of life.*

Concept Map by Deanne A. Blach, MSN, RN

CONCEPT MAP

COGNITION
MOBILITY
MULTIPLE SCLEROSIS
IMMUNITY
COMFORT
COGNITION
SEXUALITY
COGNITION

EXPECTED OUTCOMES

- Maintain optimal SENSORY PERCEPTION and COGNITION with use of available drug treatment and supportive services.
- Have maximal mobility and decreased fatigue as a result of successful disease management.
- Be free from secondary infection related to decreased IMMUNITY from the disease or from drug therapy.

Analysis: Interpreting of Patient Problems →

PATIENT PROBLEMS

- Potential for infection/decreased IMMUNITY due to disease and drug therapy for disease management
- Decreased MOBILITY due to spasticity, tremors, and/or fatigue
- Decreased visual acuity and COGNITION due to dysfunction of central nerves

← Analysis of Data

Ms. Brown has been diagnosed with PRMS – frequent relapses with partial recovery. Progressive, cumulative symptoms occur over many years from inflammatory damage to myelin in the brain and spinal cord.

↑ Reflect on the Medical Diagnosis

← Data Synthesis

NOTICE IN THE HISTORY

40-year-old Carolyn Brown is admitted with progressive relapsing MS (PRMS) after a fall. She was diagnosed last year after several years of vague and nonspecific symptoms. Married with two school-age children, she is having difficulty managing ADLs. Her marriage is struggling due to these health issues. She is experiencing generalized weakness, muscle spasms, and urinary incontinence.

NOTICING— Physical Assessment →

Subjective Data: "I am so tired, I can hardly get around....and my legs are so stiff, I fall. I just gradually get worse. I sometimes choke when I'm eating." The patient reports weakness, muscle spasms, trouble with balance, and has periods of double vision and vertigo.

Objective Data: Slightly slurred speech. Intention tremor with eating or writing.

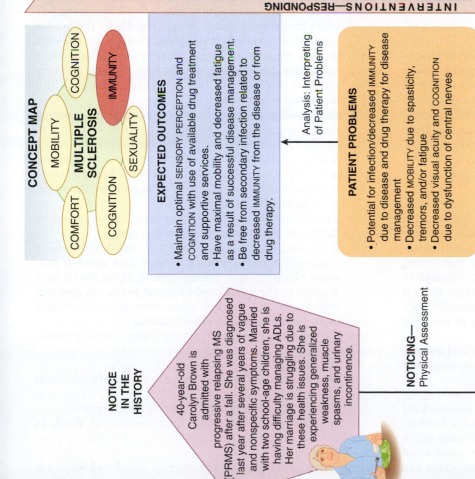

Health Care Resources. Resources required by the patient depend on the course of the disease and the complications that occur. Patients usually are able to live independently, but they may need some assistance. In severe disease, placement in an assisted-living or long-term care facility may be the best alternative. The population of young and middle-age residents in these settings is increasing as people with chronic, disabling diseases live longer. Refer the patient and family members or significant others to the local chapter of the National Multiple Sclerosis Society (www.nationalmssociety.org) or the Multiple Sclerosis Society of Canada (https://mssociety.ca). Other community resources include meal-delivery services (e.g., Meals on Wheels), transportation services for the disabled, and homemaker services.

◆ Evaluation: Reflecting

Evaluate the care of the patient with MS on the basis of the identified priority problems. The expected outcomes are that he or she:

- Remains free of infection as a result of drug therapy affecting IMMUNITY or the disease process
- Maintains maximal MOBILITY and function as a result of managing fatigue and disease progression
- Maintains adequate visual acuity and COGNITION to function independently

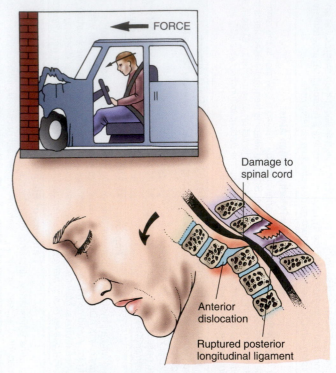

FIG. 43-2 Hyperflexion injury of the cervical spine.

✳ MOBILITY CONCEPT EXEMPLAR
Spinal Cord Injury

❖ PATHOPHYSIOLOGY

Spinal cord injuries (SCIs) are classified as complete or incomplete. A *complete* SCI is one in which the spinal cord has been damaged in a way that eliminates all innervation below the level of the injury. Injuries that allow some function or movement below the level of the injury are described as an *incomplete* SCI. Incomplete injuries are more common than complete SCIs. Loss of or impaired motor function (MOBILITY), SENSORY PERCEPTION, and bowel and bladder control often result from an SCI.

Mechanisms of Injury

When enough force is applied to the spinal cord, the resulting damage causes many neurologic deficits. Sources of force include direct injury to the vertebral column (fracture, dislocation, and subluxation [partial dislocation]) or penetrating injury from violence (gunshot or knife wounds). Although in some cases the cord itself may remain intact, at other times it undergoes a destructive process caused by a contusion (bruise), compression, laceration, or transection (severing of the cord, either complete or incomplete).

The causes of SCI can be divided into primary and secondary mechanisms of injury. Five *primary* mechanisms may result in an SCI:

- **Hyperflexion**: a sudden and forceful acceleration (movement) of the head forward, causing extreme flexion of the neck (Fig. 43-2). This is often the result of a head-on motor vehicle collision or diving accident. Flexion injury to the lower thoracic and lumbar spine may occur when the trunk is suddenly flexed on itself, such as occurs in a fall on the buttocks.

- **Hyperextension** occurs most often in vehicle collisions in which the vehicle is struck from behind or during falls when the patient's chin is struck (Fig. 43-3). The head is suddenly accelerated and then decelerated. This stretches or tears the anterior longitudinal ligament, fractures or subluxates the vertebrae, and perhaps ruptures an intervertebral disk. As with flexion injuries, the spinal cord may easily be damaged.

- **Axial loading or vertical compression** injuries resulting from diving accidents, falls on the buttocks, or a jump in which a person lands on the feet can cause many of the injuries attributable to **axial loading** (vertical compression) (Fig. 43-4). A blow to the top of the head can cause the vertebrae to shatter. Pieces of bone enter the spinal canal and damage the cord.

- **Excessive rotation** results from injuries that are caused by turning the head beyond the normal range.

- **Penetrating trauma** is classified by the speed of the object (e.g., knife, bullet) causing the injury. Low-speed or low-impact injuries cause damage directly at the site or local damage to the spinal cord or spinal nerves. In contrast, high-speed injuries that occur from gunshot wounds cause both direct and indirect damage.

Secondary injury worsens the primary injury. Secondary injuries include:

- Hemorrhage
- Ischemia (lack of oxygen, typically from reduced/absent blood flow)
- Hypovolemia (decreased circulating blood volume)
- Impaired tissue perfusion from neurogenic shock (a *medical emergency*)
- Local edema

Hemorrhage into the spinal cord may be manifested by contusion or petechial leaking into the central gray matter and later

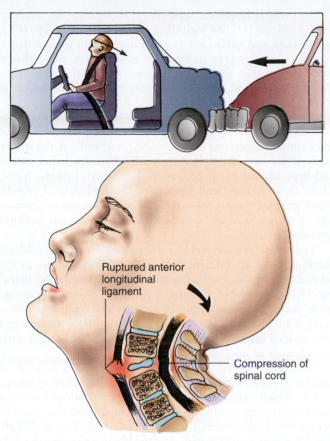

FIG. 43-3 Hyperextension injury of the cervical spine.

Ruptured anterior longitudinal ligament

Compression of spinal cord

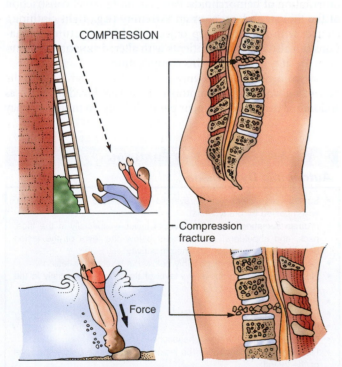

COMPRESSION

Compression fracture

Force

FIG. 43-4 Axial loading (vertical compression) injury of the cervical spine and the lumbar spine.

into the white matter. Systemic hemorrhage can result in shock and decrease perfusion to the spinal cord. Edema occurs with both primary and secondary injuries, contributing to capillary compression and cord ischemia. In neurogenic shock, loss of blood vessel tone (dilation) after *severe* cord injury may result in hypoperfusion (McCance et al., 2014).

Etiology

Trauma is the leading cause of spinal cord injuries (SCIs), with more than a third resulting from vehicle crashes. Other leading causes are falls, acts of violence (usually gunshot wounds [GSWs]), and sport-related accidents (National Spinal Cord Injury Statistical Center, 2016). SCIs from falls are particularly likely among older adults. Spinal cord damage in adults can also result from nontraumatic vertebral fracture and diseases such as benign or malignant tumors.

♥ VETERANS' HEALTH CONSIDERATIONS

Patient-Centered Care QSEN

Be aware that veterans who experience an SCI typically have other major injuries, including traumatic brain injury and amputation of one or more limbs. These additional injuries may take priority over attending to the problems related to the SCI.

Incidence/Prevalence

According to the National Spinal Cord Injury Statistical Center (2016), about 12,500 new SCIs occur every year in the United States. Almost 80% of all SCIs occur in young males, with the majority being Euro-American. Cervical cord injuries are more common than thoracic or lumbar cord injuries. The most common neurologic level of injury is C5. In paraplegia, T12 and L1 are the most common levels (National Spinal Cord Injury Statistical Center, 2016).

❖ INTERPROFESSIONAL COLLABORATIVE CARE

◆ Assessment: Noticing

History. When obtaining a history from a patient with an acute SCI, gather as much data as possible about how the accident occurred and the probable mechanism of injury once the patient is stabilized. Questions include:

- Location and position of the patient immediately after the injury
- Symptoms that occurred immediately with the injury
- Changes that have occurred subsequently
- Type of immobilization devices used and whether any problems occurred during stabilization and transport to the hospital
- Treatment given at the scene of injury or in the emergency department (ED) (e.g., medications, IV fluids)
- Medical history, including osteoporosis or arthritis of the spine, congenital deformities, cancer, and previous injury or surgery of the neck or back
- History of any respiratory problems, especially if the patient has experienced a cervical SCI

Communicate with the ED nurse as he or she "hands off" the patient. Use the situation, background, assessment, recommendation (SBAR) communication technique to collect valuable information for continuing patient care per The Joint Commission's National Patient Safety Goals. (See Chapter 1 for SBAR discussion.)

Physical Assessment/Signs and Symptoms

Initial Assessment. *The initial and priority assessment focuses on the patient's ABCs (**a**irway, **b**reathing, and **c**irculation).* After an airway is established, assess the patient's breathing pattern. The patient with a cervical SCI is at high risk for respiratory compromise because the cervical spinal nerves (C3-5) innervate the phrenic nerve controlling the diaphragm.

Evaluate pulse, blood pressure, and peripheral perfusion such as pulse strength and capillary refill. Multiple injuries may contribute to circulatory compromise from hemorrhagic hypovolemic shock. Assess for indications of *hemorrhage.* All symptoms of circulatory compromise or shock must be treated aggressively to preserve tissue perfusion to the spinal cord. Shock is discussed in detail in Chapter 37.

Use the Glasgow Coma Scale (see Chapter 41) or other agency-approved assessment tool to assess the patient's *level of consciousness (LOC).* Cognitive impairment as a result of an associated traumatic brain injury (TBI) or substance use disorder can occur in patients with traumatic SCIs.

Spinal shock, also called **spinal shock syndrome**, occurs immediately as the cord's response to the injury. The patient has complete but temporary loss of motor, sensory, reflex, and autonomic function that often lasts less than 48 hours but may continue for several weeks (McCance et al., 2014). Spinal shock is NOT the same as neurogenic shock.

Sensory Perception and Mobility Assessment. Perform a detailed assessment of the patient's MOBILITY and SENSORY PERCEPTION status to determine the level of injury and establish baseline data for future comparison. The level of injury is the lowest neurologic segment with intact or normal motor and sensory function. **Tetraplegia** (also called *quadriplegia)* (paralysis) and **quadriparesis** (weakness) involve all four extremities, as seen with cervical cord and upper thoracic injury. **Paraplegia** (paralysis) and **paraparesis** (weakness) involve only the lower extremities, as seen in lower thoracic and lumbosacral injuries or lesions.

Neurologic level defined by the American Spinal Injury Association (ASIA) refers to the highest neurologic level of normal function and is not the same as the *anatomic* level of injury. The neurologic level is determined by evaluation of the zones of sensory and motor function, known as *dermatomes* and *myotomes.* Follow the sensory distribution of the skin dermatomes (see Fig. 41-4), with the examination beginning in the area of reported loss of SENSORY PERCEPTION and ending where sensory perception becomes normal. For example, sensation of the top of the foot and calf of the leg is spinal skin segment (dermatome) levels L3, L4, and L5. The area at the level of the umbilicus is T10, the clavicle (collarbone) is C3 or C4, and finger sensation is C7 and C8. The patient may report a complete sensory loss, **hypoesthesia** (decreased sensation), or **hyperesthesia** (increased sensation).

⚠ NURSING SAFETY PRIORITY QSEN

Critical Rescue

In *acute* SCI, monitor for a decrease in SENSORY PERCEPTION from baseline, especially in a proximal (upward) dermatome and/or new loss of motor function and MOBILITY. The presence of these changes is considered an emergency and requires immediate communication with the primary health care provider using SBAR or other agency-approved protocol for notification. Document these assessment findings in the electronic health record.

The primary health care provider (PHCP) may also test deep tendon reflexes (DTRs), including the biceps (C5), triceps (C7), patella (L3), and ankle (S1). It is not unusual for these reflexes, as well as all MOBILITY or SENSORY PERCEPTION, to be absent immediately after the injury because of spinal shock. After shock has resolved, the reflexes may return if the lesion is incomplete.

Cardiovascular and Respiratory Assessment. *Cardiovascular* dysfunction results from disruption of sympathetic fibers of the autonomic nervous system (ANS), especially if the injury is above the sixth thoracic vertebra. Bradycardia, hypotension, and hypothermia occur because of loss of sympathetic input. These changes may lead to cardiac dysrhythmias. *A systolic blood pressure below 90 mm Hg requires treatment because lack of perfusion to the spinal cord could worsen the patient's condition.*

A patient with a cervical SCI is at risk for *breathing* problems resulting from an interruption of spinal innervation to the respiratory muscles. In collaboration with the respiratory therapist (RT), if available, perform a complete respiratory assessment, including pulse oximetry for arterial oxygen saturation, every 8 to 12 hours. An oxygen saturation 92% or less and adventitious breath sounds may indicate a complication such as atelectasis or pneumonia.

Autonomic dysreflexia (AD), sometimes referred to as *autonomic hyperreflexia,* is a potentially life-threatening condition in which noxious visceral or cutaneous stimuli cause a sudden, massive, uninhibited reflex sympathetic discharge in people with high-level SCI. The signs and symptoms of AD are listed in Chart 43-2. Severely elevated blood pressure can cause a hemorrhagic stroke, discussed in Chapter 45.

The causes of AD are typically GI, gynecologic-urologic (GU), and vascular stimulation. Specific risk factors are bladder distention, urinary tract infection, epididymitis or scrotal compression, bowel distention or impaction from constipation, or irritation of hemorrhoids. Pain; circumferential constriction of the thorax, abdomen, or an extremity (e.g., tight clothing); contact with hard or sharp objects; and temperature fluctuations can also cause AD. Patients with altered SENSORY PERCEPTION are at great risk for this complication.

Gastrointestinal and Genitourinary Assessment. Assess the patient's *abdomen* for symptoms of internal bleeding, such as abdominal distention, pain, or paralytic ileus. Hemorrhage may

---

▶▶ CHART 43-2   Key Features

Autonomic Dysreflexia

- Sudden, significant rise in systolic and diastolic blood pressure, accompanied by bradycardia
- Profuse sweating above the level of lesion—especially in the face, neck, and shoulders; rarely occurs below the level of the lesion because of sympathetic cholinergic activity
- Goose bumps above or possibly below the level of the lesion
- Flushing of the skin above the level of the lesion—especially in the face, neck, and shoulders
- Blurred vision
- Spots in the patient's visual field
- Nasal congestion
- Onset of severe, throbbing headache
- Flushing about the level of the lesion with pale skin below the level of the lesion
- Feeling of apprehension

result from the trauma, or it may occur later from a stress ulcer or the administration of steroids. Monitor for abdominal pain and changes in bowel sounds. Paralytic ileus may develop within 72 hours of hospital admission. During the period of spinal shock, peristalsis decreases, leading to a loss of bowel sounds and to gastric distention. This disruption of the autonomic nervous system may lead to a hypotonic bowel.

After the first few days, when edema subsides, the spinal reflexes that innervate the bowel and bladder usually begin to establish function, depending on the level of the injury. Patients with cervical or high thoracic SCIs have upper motor neuron damage that spares lower spinal reflexes, causing a *spastic* bowel and bladder. Patients with lower thoracic and lumbosacral injuries usually have damage to their lower spinal nerves and therefore have a *flaccid* bowel and bladder.

Assessment of Patients for Long-Term Complications. Patients with complete SCI are at a high risk for complications that result from prolonged immobility, including *skin break-down* and *venous thromboembolism (VTE)*. Assess skin integrity with each turn or repositioning. Monitor for signs of VTE with vital signs, including lower-extremity deep vein thrombosis (DVT). Monitor intake, output, and weight to assess hydration and nutrition status. Assess glycemic and nutritional status, including intake of protein, vitamins, and iron.

Bones can become *osteopenic* and *osteoporotic* without weight-bearing exercise, placing the long-term SCI patient at risk for fractures. Another complication of prolonged immobility is **heterotopic ossification (HO)** (bony overgrowth, often into muscle). Assess for swelling, redness, warmth, and decreased range of motion (ROM) of the involved extremity. The hip is the most common place where HO occurs (Zychowicz, 2013). Changes in the bony structure are not visible until several weeks after initial symptoms appear.

Chapter 2 and 6 describe additional nursing assessments and interventions to help prevent and monitor for complications of decreased mobility.

Psychosocial Assessment. Patients experiencing an SCI may have significant behavior and emotional reactions as a result of changes in functional ability, body image, role performance, and self-concept. Many of these patients are young men who may feel guilty for engaging in high-risk behaviors such as diving into shallow water or racing a vehicle that caused the injury. Some patients with SCI are war veterans. Assess patients for their reaction to the injury and provide opportunities to listen to their concerns. Be realistic about their abilities and projected function but offer hope and encouragement. Aggressive rehabilitation can help most patients live productive and independent lives.

Laboratory and Imaging Assessment. The health care provider requests laboratory studies for the patient with an SCI to establish baseline data. A spine CT and MRI are performed to determine the degree and extent of damage to the spinal cord and detect the presence of blood and bone within the spinal column. In addition, patients may have a series of x-rays of the spine to identify vertebral fractures, subluxation, or dislocation.

◆ **Analysis: Interpreting**

The priority collaborative problems for patients with an *acute* spinal cord injury (SCI) include:

1. Potential for respiratory distress/failure due to aspiration or decreased diaphragmatic innervation

2. Potential for cardiovascular instability (e.g., shock and autonomic dysreflexia) due to loss or interruption of sympathetic innervation or hemorrhage
3. Potential for secondary spinal cord injury due to hypoperfusion, edema, or delayed spinal column stabilization
4. Decreased MOBILITY and sensation due to spinal cord damage and edema

In addition, the patient with a long-term SCI is at risk for multiple problems caused by prolonged immobility or decreased mobility. These problems are discussed in fundamentals textbooks.

◆ **Planning and Implementation: Responding**

Caring for a patient with an SCI requires both a patient- and family-centered collaborative approach and involves every health care team member to help meet the patient's expected outcomes. Optimally, patients with a new SCI are quickly transported to a model SCI System Center. Because of the complexity of an SCI, discharge planning, including the rehabilitation team, needs to begin the day of admission.

The desired outcomes of patient-centered collaborative care following acute SCI are to stabilize the vertebral column, manage damage to the spinal cord, and prevent secondary injuries.

Managing the Airway and Improving Breathing

Planning: Expected Outcomes. The patient with an SCI is expected to not experience respiratory distress as evidenced by a patent airway and adequate ventilation.

Interventions. *Airway management is the priority for a patient with cervical spinal cord injury!* Patients with injuries at or above T6 are especially at risk for respiratory distress and pulmonary embolus during the first 5 days after injury. These complications are caused by impaired functioning of the intercostal muscles and disruption in the innervation to the diaphragm. Depending on the level of injury, intubation or tracheotomy with mechanical ventilation may be needed.

> **! NURSING SAFETY PRIORITY** **QSEN**
>
> *Action Alert*
>
> Assess breath sounds every 2 to 4 hours during the first few days after SCI and document and report any adventitious or diminished sounds. Monitor vital signs with pulse oximetry. Watch for changes in respiratory pattern or airway obstruction. Intervene per agency or PHCP protocol when there is a decrease in oxygen saturation (SpO_2) to below 95%.

Respiratory secretions are managed with manually assisted coughing, pulmonary hygiene, and suctioning. Implement strategies to prevent ventilator-associated pneumonia (VAP) when the patient needs continuous mechanical ventilation as discussed in Chapter 32. Encourage the non–mechanically ventilated patient to use an incentive spirometer. The nurse and respiratory therapist perform a respiratory assessment at least every 8 hours to determine the effectiveness of these strategies. In some cases, it may be necessary to perform oral or nasal suctioning if the patient cannot clear the airway of secretions effectively.

Teach the patient who is tetraplegic to coordinate his or her cough effort with an assistant. The nurse, or other assistant, places

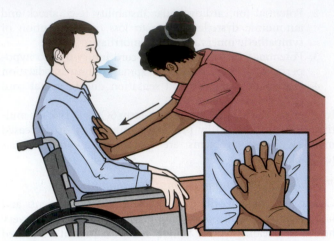

FIG. 43-5 "Cough assist" technique for patient with high spinal cord injury.

his or her hands on the upper abdomen over the diaphragm and below the ribs. Hands are placed one over the other, with fingers interlocked and away from the skin (Fig. 43-5). If the patient is obese, an alternate hand placement is one hand on either side of the rib cage. Have the patient take a breath and cough during expiration. The assistant locks his or her elbows and pushes inward and upward as the patient coughs. This technique is sometimes called *assisted coughing, quad cough,* or **cough assist**. Repeat the coordinated effort, with rest periods as needed, until the airway is clear.

Monitoring for Cardiovascular Instability

Planning: Expected Outcomes. The patient is expected to not develop neurogenic or hypovolemic shock due to hemorrhage; he or she is expected to be free from episodes of autonomic dysreflexia (AD). If any of these potentially life-threatening complications occur, the patient is expected to receive prompt interventions.

Interventions. Maintain adequate hydration through IV therapy and oral fluids as appropriate, depending on the patient's overall condition. Carefully observe for manifestations of **neurogenic shock**, which may occur within 24 hours after injury, most commonly in patients with injuries above T6. This potentially life-threatening problem results from disruption in the communication pathways between upper motor neurons and lower motor neurons.

⚠ NURSING SAFETY PRIORITY QSEN

Critical Rescue

Monitor the patient with acute spinal cord injury at least hourly for:
- Pulse oximetry (SpO$_2$) <95% or symptoms of aspiration (e.g., stridor, garbled speech, or inability to clear airway)
- Symptomatic bradycardia, including reduced level of consciousness and deceased urine output
- Hypotension with systolic blood pressure (SBP) <90 or mean arterial pressure (MAP) <65 mm Hg

Notify the PHCP immediately if these symptoms occur because this problem is an emergency! Respiratory compromise from aspiration may be treated with intubation or bronchial endoscopy. Similar to interventions for any type of shock, neurogenic shock is treated symptomatically by providing fluids to the circulating blood volume, adding vasopressor IV therapy, and providing supportive care to stabilize the patient.

Dextran, a plasma expander, may be used to increase capillary blood flow within the spinal cord and prevent or treat hypotension. *Atropine sulfate* is used to treat bradycardia if the pulse rate falls below 50 to 60 beats/min. Hypotension, if severe, is treated with continuous IV sympathomimetic agents such as *dopamine* or other vasoactive agent. Chapter 37 discusses the care of patients experiencing or at risk for shock in detail.

In addition to observing the patient for shock or hypotension, monitor the patient who has a high SCI injury for the additional risk of autonomic dysreflexia (AD). *AD is a neurologic emergency and must be promptly treated to prevent a hypertensive stroke!* Be sure to reduce potential causes for this complication by preventing bladder and bowel distention, managing pain and room temperature, and monitoring for early vital sign changes.

⚠ NURSING SAFETY PRIORITY QSEN

Critical Rescue

If the patient experiences AD, raise the head of the bed *immediately* to help reduce the blood pressure. Notify the primary health care provider (PHCP) immediately for drug therapy to quickly reduce blood pressure as indicated. Determine the cause of AD and treat it promptly (Chart 43-3). For example, if the bladder is distended, catheterize the patient to relieve the urinary retention. Check the room temperature and bed coverings and adjust as needed for patient COMFORT. Lack of SENSORY PERCEPTION may prevent the patient from noticing temperature variations.

❓ NCLEX EXAMINATION CHALLENGE 43-2

Safe Effective Care Environment

A client who sustained a recent cervical spinal cord injury reports feeling flushed. The client's blood pressure is 180/100. What is the nurse's **best** action at this time?
A. Perform a bladder assessment.
B. Insert an indwelling urinary catheter.
C. Turn on a fan to cool the patient.
D. Place the patient in a sitting position.

◎ CHART 43-3   Best Practice for Patient Safety & Quality Care QSEN

Emergency Care of the Patient Experiencing Autonomic Dysreflexia: Immediate Interventions

- Place patient in a sitting position (first priority!), or return to a previous safe position.
- Notify the primary health care provider or Rapid Response Team.
- Assess for and treat the cause:
  - Check for urinary retention or catheter blockage:
    - Check the urinary catheter tubing (if present) for kinks or obstruction.
  - If a urinary catheter is not present, check for bladder distention and catheterize immediately if indicated:
    - Consider using anesthetic ointment on tip of catheter before catheter insertion to reduce urethral irritation.
- Determine if a urinary tract infection or bladder calculi (stones) are contributing to genitourinary irritation.
- Check the patient for fecal impaction or other colorectal irritation, using anesthetic ointment at rectum. Disimpact if needed.
- Examine skin for new or worsening pressure injury symptoms.
- Monitor blood pressures every 10 to 15 minutes.
- Give nifedipine or nitrate as prescribed to lower blood pressure as needed.
- (Patients with recurrent autonomic dysreflexia may receive an alpha blocker prophylactically.)

Preventing Secondary Spinal Cord Injury

Planning: Expected Outcomes. The patient with an *acute* SCI is expected to have adequate spinal cord stabilization as evidenced by no further deterioration in neurologic status.

Interventions. If the patient has a fractured vertebra, the primary concern of the health care team is to reduce and immobilize the fracture to prevent further damage to the spinal cord from bone fragments. Nonsurgical techniques include external fixation or orthotic devices, but surgery is often needed to stabilize the spine and prevent further spinal cord damage.

Assess the patient's neurologic status, particularly focusing on MOBILITY (motor) and SENSORY PERCEPTION function, vital signs, pulse oximetry, and altered COMFORT, at least every 1 to 4 hours, depending on his or her overall condition. *Document your assessments carefully and in detail, particularly changes in motor or sensory function. Failure to do so may prevent other staff members from quickly recognizing deterioration in neurologic status.*

Regardless of the level of SCI, keep the patient in proper body alignment to prevent further cord injury or irritability. Devices such as traction, orthoses, or collars may be used to keep the spine immobilized during healing and rehabilitation.

Spinal Immobilization and Stabilization. During the immediate care of the patient with a suspected or confirmed cervical spine injury, a hard cervical collar, such as the Miami J or Philadelphia collar, is placed immediately and maintained until a specific order indicates that it can be removed (Fig. 43-6). A daily inspection of skin beneath the collar is recommended while a health care provider helps to maintain neck alignment when the collar is removed. Padding at pressure points beneath and at the edges of the collar, particularly at the occiput, may be necessary to sustain skin integrity. Until the spinal column is stabilized, a jaw-thrust maneuver is preferable to a head-tilt maneuver to open the airway should the patient need an airway intervention. Maintain spinal alignment at all times with log rolling to change position from supine to side-lying.

The patient may be placed in fixed skeletal traction to realign the vertebrae, facilitate bone healing, and prevent further injury,

often after surgical stabilization. The most commonly used device for immobilization of the *cervical spine* is the **halo fixator** device, which is worn for 8 to 12 weeks. This static device is affixed by four pins (or screw) into the outer aspect of the skull (Fig. 43-7). For patients not having surgery, the addition of traction helps reduce the fracture.

! NURSING SAFETY PRIORITY QSEN

Action Alert

Never move or turn the patient by holding or pulling on the halo device. Do not adjust the screws holding it in place. Check the patient's skin frequently to ensure that the jacket is not causing pressure. Pressure is avoided if one finger can be inserted easily between the jacket and the patient's skin. Monitor the patient's neurologic status for changes in movement or decreased strength. A special wrench is needed to loosen the vest in emergencies such as cardiopulmonary arrest. Tape the wrench to the vest for easy and consistent accessibility. Do not use sharp objects (e.g., coat hangers, knitting needles) to relieve itching under the vest; skin damage and infection will slow recovery.

Common complications of the halo device are pin loosening, local infection, and scarring. More serious but less common complications include osteomyelitis (cranial bone infection), subdural abscess, and instability. Hospital policy is followed for pin-site care, which may specify the use of solutions such as saline. Vaseline dressings may also be used. *Monitor vital signs for indications of possible infection (e.g., fever, purulent drainage from the pin sites) and report any changes to the primary health care provider immediately.* Discharge teaching related to halo fixator management is described in Chart 43-4.

Nonsurgical treatment of *thoracic and lumbosacral injuries* is often challenging. Most health care providers choose to refer the patient for surgery and then immobilize the spine with

---

CHART 43-4 **Patient and Family Education: Preparing for Self-Management**

Use of a Halo Device

- Be aware that the weight of the halo device alters balance. Be careful when leaning forward or backward.
- Wear loose clothing, preferably with hook and loop (Velcro) fasteners or large openings for head and arms.
- Bathe in the bathtub or take a sponge bath. (Some primary health care providers [PHCP] allow showers.)
- Wash under the liner of the vest to prevent rashes or sores; use powders or lotions sparingly under the vest.
- Have someone change the liner if it becomes odorous.
- Support the head with a small pillow when sleeping to prevent unnecessary pressure and discomfort.
- Try to resume usual activities to the extent possible; keep as active as possible. (The weight of the device may cause fatigue or weakness.) However, avoid contact sports and swimming.
- Do not drive because vision is impaired with the device.
- Keep straws available for drinking fluids.
- Cut meats and other food into small pieces to facilitate chewing and swallowing.
- Before going outside in cold temperatures, wrap the pins with cloth to prevent the metal from getting cold.
- Have someone clean the pin sites as recommended by the PHCP or hospital protocol.
- Observe the pin sites daily for redness, drainage, or loosening; report changes to the PHCP.
- Increase fluids and fiber in the diet to prevent constipation.
- Use a position of comfort during sexual activity.

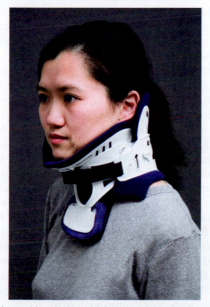

FIG. 43-6 Patient with spinal cord injury wearing a hard cervical (Miami J) collar. (From Browner, B. D., Levine, A. M., Trafton, P. G., Jupiter, J. B., & Krettek, C. [2009]. *Skeletal trauma* [4th ed.]. Philadelphia: Saunders.)

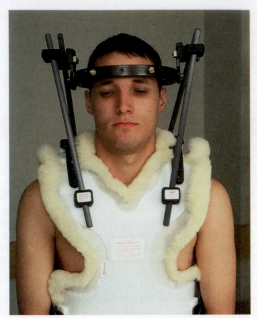

FIG. 43-7 Halo fixation device with jacket.

lightweight, custom-fit thoracic-lumbar sacral orthoses (TLSOs) to prevent prolonged periods of immobility.

? NCLEX EXAMINATION CHALLENGE 43-3

Physiological Integrity

A nurse is caring for a client who has a hard cervical collar for a complete cervical spinal cord injury. Which assessment finding will the nurse report to the primary health care provider?
A. Purulent drainage from the pin sites on the client's forehead
B. Painful pressure injury under the collar
C. Inability to move legs or feet
D. Oxygen saturation of 95% on room air

Drug Therapy. Centrally acting skeletal muscular relaxants, such as tizanidine, may help control severe muscle spasticity. However, these drugs cause severe drowsiness and sedation in most patients and may not be effective in reducing spasticity. As an alternative to these drugs, intrathecal baclofen (ITB) (Lioresal) therapy may be prescribed. This drug is administered through a programmable, implantable infusion pump and intrathecal catheter directly into the cerebrospinal fluid. The pump is surgically placed in a subcutaneous pouch in the lower abdomen. Monitor for common adverse effects, which include sedation, fatigue, dizziness, and changes in mental status. *Seizures and hallucinations may occur if ITB is suddenly withdrawn.*

Other drugs to prevent or treat complications of immobility may be needed *later* during the rehabilitative phase. For example, celecoxib (Celebrex) may be prescribed to prevent or treat heterotopic ossification (bony overgrowth). However, recall that the adverse effects of this drug include an increased risk of myocardial infarction and stroke. Calcium and bisphosphonates may prevent the osteoporosis that results from lack of weight-bearing or resistance activity. Osteoporosis can cause fractures in later years. Early and continued exercise may help decrease the incidence of these complications.

Surgical Management. Surgery within 24 hours of injury to stabilize the vertebral spinal column, particularly if there is evidence of spinal cord compression, results in decreased secondary complications. Emergent surgery also removes bone fragments, hematomas, or penetrating objects such as a bullet. Typical procedures include wiring and spinal fusion for cervical injuries and the insertion of steel or metal rods (e.g., Harrington rods) to stabilize thoracic and lumbar spinal injuries. During a cervical fusion, the surgeon reduces the fracture by placing the bone ends in proper alignment. Metal wiring is then used to secure bone chips taken from the patient's hip or other source of bone grafting. The patient wears a halo vest to immobilize the spine during the healing process. For thoracic and lumbar fusions, metal or steel rods (e.g., Harrington rods) are used to keep the bone ends in alignment after fracture reduction. After surgery, the patient usually wears a molded plastic support (cervical or thoracic-lumbar or both) to keep the injured and operative areas immobilized during recovery. Postoperative care occurs as described in Chapter 16.

! NURSING SAFETY PRIORITY QSEN
Action Alert

After surgical spinal fusion, assess the patient's neurologic status and vital signs at least every hour for the first 4 to 6 hours and then, if the patient is stable, every 4 hours. Assess for complications of surgery, including worsening of motor or sensory function at or above the site of surgery.

Managing Decreased Mobility

Planning: Expected Outcomes. The patient with an SCI is expected to be free from complications of immobility and perform ADLs as independently as possible with or without assistive/adaptive devices.

Interventions. Patients with an SCI are especially at risk for pressure injuries due to altered sensory perception of pressure areas on skin below the level of the injury. They are also at risk for venous thromboembolism (VTE), contractures, orthostatic hypotension (especially in patients with high SCI), and fractures related to osteoporosis. Frequent and therapeutic positioning not only helps prevent complications but also provides alignment to prevent further SCI or irritability. Assess the condition of the patient's skin, especially over pressure points, with each turn or repositioning. Turning may be performed manually, or the patient may be placed on an automatic rotating bed. Reduce pressure on any reddened area and monitor it with the next turn. Reposition patients frequently (every 1 to 2 hours). When sitting in a chair, the patient is repositioned or taught to reposition himself or herself more often than every hour. Paraplegic patients usually perform frequent "wheelchair push-ups" to relieve skin pressure. Use a pressure-reducing mattress and wheelchair or chair pad to help prevent skin breakdown. **Prevent pressure injuries using best practices as described in Chapter 25. Prevent VTE, including using interventions of intermittent pneumatic compression stockings and low–molecular-weight heparin (LMWH). Document pressure injury and VTE prophylaxis in accordance with Core Measures developed by the Centers for Medicare and Medicaid Services and The Joint Commission (www.jointcommision.org).**

Contractures may be prevented or minimized with splints and range-of-motion exercises. Consult with the physical therapist (PT) and occupational therapist (OT) for optimal scheduling for placing/removing splints (typically individually molded to the patient's extremity), applying pressure to trigger points to relieve spasticity, and positioning to maintain joint function. Administer prescribed antispasmodic drugs and monitor the patient's response.

In collaboration with the rehabilitation team, teach or reinforce teaching for bed MOBILITY skills and bed-to-chair transfers. Patients with paraplegia are usually able to transfer from the bed to chair or wheelchair with minimal or no assistance unless balance is a problem (seen in patients with high thoracic injuries). Techniques to improve balance are usually taught by occupational therapists. Tetraplegic patients may learn how to transfer using a slider, also called a *sliding board*. This simple board-like device allows the patient to move from the bed to chair or vice versa by creating a bridge. When using the slider, remind patients to lift his or her buttocks while moving incrementally and slowly across the board. Patients with severe muscle spasticity have more challenges when learning transfer skills.

Patients with cervical cord injuries especially are at high risk for orthostatic (postural) hypotension, but anyone who is immobilized may have this problem. If the patient changes from a lying position to a sitting or standing position too quickly, he or she may experience hypotension, which could result in dizziness and falls. Because of interrupted sympathetic innervation caused by the SCI, the blood vessels do not constrict quickly enough to push blood up into the brain. The resulting vasodilation causes dizziness or light-headedness and possible falls with syncope ("blackout").

All patients with an SCI require bowel and bladder retraining, including adequate fluids and stool softeners to prevent constipation from immobility and the injury itself. Those with *upper* motor neuron lesions (usually cervical and high thoracic injuries) have *spastic* bowel and bladder function with an intact spinal reflex for elimination. However, voiding patterns may be uncontrollable and require long-term indwelling or external catheters. Rectal that suppositories are often successful to promote regular bowel elimination.

The patient with a *lower* motor neuron lesion has a *flaccid* bowel and bladder. Intermittent urinary catheterizations, manual pressure over the bladder area, and bowel impaction on a regular basis help to establish a routine. Chapter 6 describes bowel and bladder training in more detail.

In patients with established or long-term SCI, assess baseline ability and encourage their participation in self-care and management. Encourage family participation in care and support their effort to keep the patient engaged in family life.

Care Coordination and Transition Management

Case managers are ideal care coordinators to act as SCI patient advocates. In some settings, case managers begin working with patients in the emergency department to establish a positive image of SCI rehabilitation. The primary purpose of rehabilitation is to enable patients to function independently in their communities. However, many physical barriers still exist in some communities that prevent the patient in a wheelchair from finding a parking place, using sidewalks, and attending activities or using resources (Fig. 43-8).

Rehabilitation begins in the acute or critical care unit when patients are hemodynamically stable. They are usually transferred from the acute care setting to a rehabilitation setting,

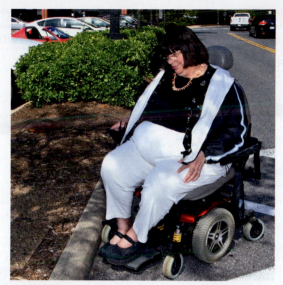

FIG. 43-8 Community physical barrier example: A curb prevents the patient in a wheelchair from getting onto the sidewalk.

where they learn more about self-care, mobility skills, and bladder and bowel retraining.

Psychosocial adaptation is one of the critical factors in determining the success of rehabilitation. The case manager or acute care nurse can help the patient and family members prepare for discharge or transfer to a rehabilitation hospital. Assist in verbalizing feelings and fears about body image, self-concept, role performance, self-esteem, and sexuality. The patient should be told about the expected reactions of those outside the security of the hospital environment. Role playing or anticipating responses to potential problems is helpful. For example, the patient can practice answering questions from children about why he or she is in a wheelchair or cannot move certain parts of the body.

For young men with SCI, sexuality is a major issue. Many patients are concerned about their ability to have sexual intercourse and have children. Most hospitals do not have psychological social workers or counselors to discuss sexuality issues. By contrast, rehabilitation programs often include a sexuality/intimacy counselor as part of the interprofessional team approach to patient care.

Many patients with previous SCIs are admitted to the acute care or long-term care setting for complications of immobility, such as pressure injuries or fractures resulting from osteoporosis. Pressure injuries contribute to local infection, including osteomyelitis and septicemia. Priorities in care may need to be re-evaluated as complications occur and resolve.

Home Care Management. If the patient is discharged home or returns home for a weekend visit from the rehabilitation setting, the environment must be assessed to ensure that it is free from hazards and can accommodate the patient's special needs (e.g., a wheelchair). The occupational or physical therapist, in collaboration with rehabilitation and the home care nurse, usually assesses the patient's temporary or permanent home environment. Ease of accessibility is particularly important at the entrance of the home and in the bathroom, kitchen, and bedroom. The height of the patient's bed may need to be adjusted to allow a smooth transfer into and out of the bed.

CHART 43-5 Nursing Focus on the Older Adult

What Patients Need to Know About Aging With Spinal Cord Injury

NURSING INTERVENTION	RATIONALES
Follow guidelines for adult vaccination, particularly influenza and pneumococcus vaccination recommendations.	Respiratory complications are the most common cause of death after spinal cord injury (SCI).
For women, have Papanicolaou (Pap) smears and mammograms as recommended by the American Cancer Society or your primary health care provider.	Limitations in movement may make breast self-awareness difficult.
Take measures to prevent osteoporosis, such as increasing calcium intake, avoiding caffeine, and not smoking. Exercise against resistance can maintain muscle strength and slow bone loss.	Women older than 50 years often lose bone density, which can result in fractures. Men can also have osteoporotic fractures as a result of immobility.
Practice meticulous skin care, including frequent repositioning, using pressure-reduction surfaces in bed and chairs/wheelchairs, and applying skin protective products.	As a person ages, skin becomes dry and less elastic, predisposing the patient to pressure injuries.
Take measures to prevent constipation, such as drinking adequate fluids, eating a high-fiber diet, adding a stool softener or bowel stimulant daily, and establishing a regular time for bowel elimination.	Constipation is a problem for most patients with SCI, and bowel motility can slow, contributing to constipation later in life.
Modify activities if joint pain occurs; use a powered rather than a manual wheelchair. Ask the health care provider about treatment options.	Arthritis occurs in more than half of people older than 65 years. Patients with SCI are more likely to develop arthritis as a result of added stress on the upper extremities when using a wheelchair.

All adaptive devices that the patient will use at home should be requested and delivered to the rehabilitation facility. This enables the nurse and other therapists to ensure that the items fit correctly and that the patient and family know how to use them correctly.

Self-Management Education. The teaching plan for the patient with an SCI includes:

- MOBILITY skills
- Pressure injury prevention
- ADL skills
- Bowel and bladder program
- Education about SEXUALITY and referral for counseling to promote sexual health
- Prevention of autonomic dysreflexia with appropriate bladder, bowel, and skin-care practices and recognition of early signs or symptoms of autonomic dysreflexia

This information should be reinforced with written handouts, CDs, DVDs, or other patient-education material that the patient and family members can use after discharge to the home. Chart 43-5 provides information about aging for middle-age and older adults with an SCI.

A full-time caregiver or personal assistant is sometimes required if the patient with tetraplegia returns home. The caregiver may be a family member or a nursing assistant employed to help provide care and companionship. A patient who is paraplegic is often able to function without assistance after an appropriate rehabilitation program.

ADL and mobility training for the patient with an SCI includes a structured exercise program to promote strength and endurance. One promising therapy in rehabilitation is functional electrical stimulation (FES). FES uses small electrical pulses to paralyzed muscles to restore or improve their function. It is commonly used for exercise; but it is also used to assist with breathing, grasping, transferring, standing, and walking. The occupational therapist instructs the patient in the correct use of all adaptive equipment and therapies. In collaboration with the therapists, instruct family members or the caregiver in transfer skills, feeding, bathing, dressing, positioning, bowel and bladder training, and skin care as discussed briefly in this chapter and in more detail in Chapter 6.

! NURSING SAFETY PRIORITY QSEN

Drug Alert

Teach the SCI patient and his or her family or other caregiver about the name, purpose, dosage, timing of administration, and side effects of all *drugs*. Make sure they understand the possible interaction of prescribed drugs with over-the-counter drugs or alcohol and illegal drugs.

SEXUALITY is associated with sexual and reproductive function. Sexual function after SCI depends on the level and extent of injury. Incomplete lesions allow some control over SENSORY PERCEPTION and motor ability. Complete lesions disconnect the messages from the brain to the rest of the body and vice versa. However, men with injuries above T6 are often able to have erections by stimulating reflex activity. For example, stroking the penis will cause an erection. Ejaculation is less predictable and may be mixed with urine. However, urine is sterile, so the patient's partner will not get an infection. To prevent autonomic dysreflexia (AD), prophylactic administration of a vasodilator may be needed before intercourse.

Women with an SCI have a different challenge because they have indwelling urinary catheters more commonly than men. However, some women do become pregnant and have full-term children. For others, ovulation stops in response to the injury. In this case, alternate methods for pregnancy, such as *in vitro* fertilization, may be an option. Some women also report vaginal dryness. Recommend a water-soluble lubricant for both partners to promote COMFORT.

For patients who choose not to have intercourse, intimate pleasure can be achieved in other ways, including kissing, hugging, fondling, masturbation, and oral sex. Variations in positioning may be needed to accommodate weak or paralyzed parts of the body. An understanding partner can help the patient adjust to his or her physical changes.

Health Care Resources. Refer the patient and family to local, state or province, and national organizations for more information and support for patients with SCI. These organizations include the National Spinal Cord Injury Association (www.spinalcord.org) in the United States and Spinal Cord Injury Canada (www.sci-can.ca). Many excellent consumer-oriented books, journals, and DVDs are also available. Support groups may help the patient and family adjust to a changed lifestyle and provide solutions to commonly encountered problems.

💜 **VETERANS' HEALTH CONSIDERATIONS**

Patient-Centered Care QSEN

Young male and female veterans may experience an SCI as a result of an explosion or vehicular accident during war or other military operations. In addition to the U.S. Veterans Health Administration services offered in inpatient units and outpatient clinics, the Paralyzed Veterans of America (PVA) (www.pva.org) can assist with educational materials, caregiver services, medical equipment, and support groups. The PVA also sponsors spinal cord research and raises money to help veterans with a variety of needs. It also supports wheelchair-sports teams comprised of veterans with an SCI or diseases that affect the spinal cord.

◆ *Evaluation: Reflecting*

Evaluate the care of the patient with an SCI based on the identified priority patient problems. The expected outcomes are that the patient:

- Exhibits no deterioration in neurologic status
- Maintains a patent airway, a physiologic breathing pattern, and adequate ventilation
- Does not experience a cardiovascular event (e.g., shock, hemorrhage, autonomic dysreflexia) or receives prompt treatment if an event occurs
- Does not experience secondary spinal cord injury, including VTE and heterotopic ossification
- Is free from complications of immobility
- Performs mobility skills and basic ADLs as independently as possible with or without the use of assistive/adaptive devices

BACK PAIN

Back pain affects as many of 80% of adults at some time in their life. It can be recurrent, and subsequent episodes tend to increase in severity. The prevalence of both acute and chronic back pain varies with age; lifestyle factors, including obesity and osteoporosis; and certain types of physical activity such as heavy physical work and lifting. In 2010, back pain was the third most burdensome condition in the United States in terms of mortality or poor health, with only heart disease and chronic obstructive pulmonary disease ranking higher (National Institute of Neurological Disorders and Stroke [NINDS], 2015). Low back pain is the leading cause of work disability and the number one reason why people seek health care from a primary health care provider.

The lumbosacral (lower back) and cervical (neck) vertebrae are most commonly affected because these are the areas where the vertebral column is the most flexible. *Acute* back pain is usually self-limiting and lasts less than 4 weeks. *Subacute* back pain lasts from 4 to 12 weeks. If the alteration in COMFORT continues for 12 weeks (3 months) or more, the patient has *chronic* back pain (Qaseem et al., 2017).

LOW BACK PAIN (LUMBOSACRAL BACK PAIN)

❖ **PATHOPHYSIOLOGY**

Low back pain (LBP) occurs along the lumbosacral area of the vertebral column. Acute pain is caused by muscle strain or spasm, ligament sprain, disk (also spelled "disc") degeneration (osteoarthritis), or herniation of the center of the disk, the nucleus pulposus, past the lateral vertebral border. A **herniated nucleus pulposus (HNP)** in the lumbosacral area can press on the adjacent spinal nerve (usually the sciatic nerve), causing burning or stabbing pain down into the leg or foot which, in some cases, can be severe (Fig. 43-9). Herniated disks occur most often between the fourth and fifth lumbar vertebrae (L4-L5) but may occur at other levels. The specific area of symptoms depends on the level of herniation.

In addition to alterations in the patient's COMFORT, there may be both muscle spasm and numbness and tingling (paresthesia) in the affected leg because spinal nerves have both motor and sensory fibers. The HNP may press on the spinal cord itself,

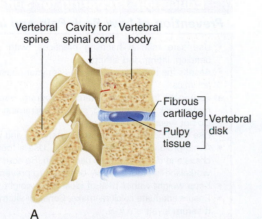

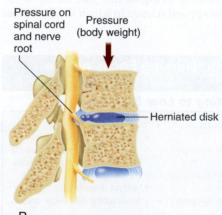

FIG. 43-9 Sagittal section of vertebrae showing a normal disk **(A)** and a herniated disk **(B)**. (From Patton, K. T., & Thibodeau, G. A. [2018]. *The human body in health & disease* [7th ed.]. St. Louis: Mosby.)

causing leg weakness. Bowel and bladder incontinence or retention may occur with motor nerve involvement and because sacral spinal nerves have parasympathetic nerve fibers that help control bowel and bladder function. This can further alter the patient's COMFORT.

Back pain may also be caused by spinal stenosis, which is a narrowing of the spinal canal, nerve root canals, or intervertebral foramina typically seen in people older than 50 years. This narrowing may be caused by infection, trauma, herniated disk, arthritis, and disk degeneration. Most adults older than 50 years have some degree of degenerative disk disease, although they may not be symptomatic.

LBP is most prevalent during the third to sixth decades of life but can occur at any time. *Acute* and *subacute* back pain usually result from injury or trauma such as during a fall, vehicular crash, or lifting a heavy object. The mechanisms of injury include repetitive flexion and/or extension and hyperflexion or hyperextension with or without rotation. Obesity places increased stress on the vertebral column and back muscles, contributing to risk for injury. Smoking has been linked to disk degeneration, possibly caused by constriction of blood vessels that supply the spine. Congenital spinal conditions such as scoliosis can also lead to LBP at any age.

CONSIDERATIONS FOR OLDER ADULTS

Patient-Centered Care QSEN

> Older adults are at high risk for acute, subacute, and chronic LBP. Vertebral fracture from osteoporosis contributes to LBP. Petite, older Euro-American women are at high risk for both bone loss and subsequent vertebral fractures. Chart 43-6 provides a list of specific factors that can cause LBP in the older adult. Vertebral compression fractures are discussed in Chapter 51.

Health Promotion and Maintenance

Many of the problems related to back pain can be prevented by recognizing the factors that contribute to tissue injury and taking appropriate preventive measures to prevent alterations in COMFORT. For example, proper posture and exercise can significantly decrease the incidence of LBP. The U.S. Occupational Safety and Health Administration (OSHA) mandated that all industries develop and implement a plan to decrease musculoskeletal injuries among their workers. One way to meet this requirement is to develop an ergonomic plan for the workplace. Ergonomics is an applied science in which the workplace

CHART 43-6 Nursing Focus on the Older Adult

Factors Contributing to Low Back Pain

- Changes in support structures
  - Spinal stenosis
  - Hypertrophy of the intraspinal ligaments
  - Osteoarthritis
  - Osteoporosis
- Changes in vertebral support and malalignment
  - Scoliosis
  - Lordosis
- Vascular changes
  - Diminished blood supply to the spinal cord or cauda equina caused by arteriosclerosis
  - Blood dyscrasias
- Intervertebral disk degeneration

is designed to increase worker COMFORT (thus reducing injury) while increasing efficiency and productivity. An example is a ceiling lift designed to help nurses assist patients to get out of bed. A variety of equipment can be used to decrease injury related to moving patients. Professional guidelines and legislative rules promote safe patient handling for health care workers (www.nursingworld.org/rnnoharm). Chart 43-7 summarizes various ways to help prevent LBP related to lifting objects and handling patients (ANA, 2013).

❖ INTERPROFESSIONAL COLLABORATIVE CARE

◆ Assessment: Noticing

Physical Assessment/Signs and Symptoms. *The patient's primary concern is continuous pain.* Some patients have so much pain that they walk in a stiff, flexed posture or they may be unable to bend at all. They may walk with a limp, indicating possible sciatic nerve impairment. Walking on the heels or toes often causes severe pain in the affected leg, the back, or both.

Conduct a complete pain assessment as discussed in Chapter 4. Record the patient's current pain score and the worst and best score since the pain began. Ask about precipitating or relieving factors such as symptoms at night or during rest. Determine if a recent injury to the back has occurred. It is not unusual for the patient to say, "I just moved to do something and felt my back go out."

Inspect the patient's back for vertebral alignment and tenderness. Examine the surrounding anatomy and lower extremities for secondary injury. Patients will often describe the altered COMFORT as stabbing, continuous pain in the muscle closest to the affected disk. They often describe a sharp, burning posterior thigh or calf pain that may radiate to the ankle or toes along the path of one or more spinal nerves. Pain usually does not extend the entire length of the limb. Patients may also report the same type of pain in the middle of one buttock or hip. The pain is often aggravated by sneezing, coughing, or straining. Driving a vehicle is particularly painful.

Ask whether paresthesia (tingling sensation) or numbness is present in the involved leg. Both extremities may be checked for SENSORY PERCEPTION by using a cotton ball and a paper clip

CHART 43-7 Patient and Family Education: Preparing for Self-Management

Prevention of Low Back Pain and Injury

- Use safe manual handling practices, with specific attention to bending, lifting, and sitting.
- Assess the need for assistance with your household chores or other activities.
- Participate in a regular exercise program, especially one that promotes back strengthening, such as swimming and walking.
- Do not wear high-heeled shoes.
- Use good posture when sitting, standing, and walking.
- Avoid prolonged sitting or standing. Use a footstool and ergonomic chairs and tables to lessen back strain. Be sure that equipment in the workplace is ergonomically designed to prevent injury.
- Keep weight within 10% of ideal body weight.
- Ensure adequate calcium intake. Consider vitamin D supplementation if serum levels are low.
- Stop smoking. If you are not able to stop, cut down on the number of cigarettes or decrease the use of other forms of tobacco.

for comparison of light or dull and sharp touch. The patient may feel SENSORY PERCEPTION in both legs but may experience a stronger sensation on the unaffected side. Ask about urinary and fecal continence and difficulty with urination or having new-onset constipation.

If the sciatic nerve is compressed, severe pain occurs when the patient's leg is held straight and lifted upward. Foot, ankle, and leg weakness may accompany LBP. To complete the neurologic assessment, evaluate the patient's muscle tone and strength. Muscles in the extremity or lower back can atrophy as a result of severe chronic back pain. The patient has difficulty with movement, and certain movements create more pain than others.

Imaging Assessment. Imaging studies for patients who report mild nonspecific back pain may not be done, depending on the nature of the pain. Patients with severe or progressive motor or SENSORY PERCEPTION deficits or who are thought to have other underlying conditions (e.g., cancer, infection) require complete diagnostic assessment. To determine the exact cause of the pain, a number of diagnostic tests may be used, including:

- Plain x-rays (show general arthritis changes and bony alignment)
- CT scan (shows spinal bones, nerves, disks, and ligaments)
- MRI (provides images of the spinal tissue, bones, spinal cord, nerves, ligaments, musculature, and disks)
- Bone scan (shows bone changes by injecting radioactive tracers, which attach to areas of increased bone production or show increased vascularity associated with tumor or infection)
- Myelogram/post-myelogram CT (evaluates nerve root lesions and any other mass, lesion, or infection of the meninges or spinal cord) (NINDS, 2015).

Electrodiagnostic testing, such as electromyography (EMG) and nerve-conduction studies, may help distinguish motor neuron diseases from peripheral neuropathies and **radiculopathies** (spinal nerve root involvement). These tests are especially useful in chronic diseases of the spinal cord or associated nerves. Chapters 41 and 49 describe these tests in more detail.

◆ Interventions: Responding

Management of patients with low back pain varies with the severity and chronicity of the problem. If acute pain is not treatment or managed effectively, chronic neuropathic pain may occur. Most patients with acute LBP experience a spontaneous resolution of pain and other symptoms over the short term in less than 3 months.

Some patients need only a brief treatment regimen of at-home exercise or physical therapy to manage pain. In general, return to work, if safe, is beneficial for recovery and well-being. Some patients have continuous or intermittent chronic pain that must be managed for an extended period. Referral to an interprofessional team that specializes in pain or back pain can provide expert long-term management.

Nonsurgical Management. A recently published clinical practice guideline recommends interprofessional nonpharmacologic interventions as first-line management for all types of LBP (Qaseem et al., 2017). For *acute* and *subacute* LBP, these interventions may include massage, spinal manipulation, heat, and acupuncture. If these measures are not successful in reducing acute pain, NSAIDs are recommended; acetaminophen is not helpful (Qaseem et al., 2017).

The Williams position is typically more comfortable and therapeutic for the patient with *acute* LBP from a bulging or herniated disk. In this position, the patient lies in the semi-Fowler's position with a pillow under the knees to keep them flexed or sits in a recliner chair. This position relaxes the muscles of the lower back and relieves pressure on the spinal nerve root. Most patients also find that they need to change position frequently. Prolonged standing, sitting, or lying down increases back pain. If the patient must stand for a long time for work or other reason, shoe insoles or special floor pads may help decrease pain. However, bedrest should also be limited, and patients should begin stretching exercises and resume normal daily activities as soon as possible after an injury (NINDS, 2015).

Patients having *chronic* LBP are also initially managed with nonpharmacologic interventions. In addition to the measures described above, patients often benefit from integrative therapies such as stress reduction, mindfulness, progressive muscle relaxation, and yoga. If these measures are not effective in relieving chronic LBP, NSAIDs are prescribed. If NSAIDs do not relieve the pain, tramadol (Ultram), a mild opioid drug, is recommended (Qaseem et al., 2017). The use of stronger opioids is not recommended due to the risk of drug abuse and addiction.

As an adjunct, over-the-counter (OTC) topical creams, sprays, and gels (such as Bio-Freeze) may provide temporary feelings of warmth or cold to dull the sensation of all types of low back pain (NINDS, 2015). Some patients use a transcutaneous electrical nerve stimulator (TENS) unit to help minimize pain. Chapter 4 discusses and includes a photo of this device.

Ziconotide (Prialt) is a drug that can be given for severe chronic back pain. It is given by intrathecal (spinal) infusion with a surgically implanted pump. It is the first available drug in a new class called *N-type calcium channel blockers (NCCBs)*. NCCBs seem to selectively block calcium channels on nerves that usually transmit pain signals to the brain. Ziconotide is also used for patients with cancer, acquired immune deficiency syndrome (AIDS), and unremitting pain from other nervous system disorders.

! NURSING SAFETY PRIORITY QSEN

Drug Alert

Ziconotide can be given with opioid analgesics but should *not* be given to patients with severe mental health/behavioral health problems because it can cause psychosis. *If symptoms such as hallucinations and delusions occur, teach patients to stop the drug immediately and notify their health care provider.*

A physical therapist (PT) works with the patient to develop an individualized exercise program. The type of exercises prescribed depends on the location and nature of the injury and the type of pain. The patient does not begin exercises until acute pain is reduced by other means. Several specific exercises for strengthening muscles to manage LBP are listed in Chart 43-8. Water therapy combined with exercise is helpful for some patients with chronic pain. The water also provides muscle resistance during exercise to prevent atrophy.

Weight reduction may help reduce chronic LBP by decreasing the strain on the vertebrae caused by excess weight. If the

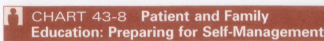

CHART 43-8 Patient and Family Education: Preparing for Self-Management

Typical Exercises for Chronic or Postoperative Low Back Pain

Extension Exercises
- **Stomach lying**: Lie face down with a pillow under your chest; lift legs straight up (alternate legs) (may not be tolerated).
- **Upper trunk extension**: Lie face down with your arms at your sides and lift your head and neck.
- **Prone push-ups**: Lie face down on a mat and, keeping your body stiff, push up to extend your arms.

Flexion Exercises
- **Pelvic tilt**: Lying on your back with your knees bent, tighten your abdominal muscles to push your lower back against the mat.
- **Semi–sit-ups**: Lying on your back with your knees bent, raise your upper body at a 45-degree angle and hold this position for 5 to 10 seconds.
- **Knee to chest**: Lying on your back with your knees bent, tighten your abdominal muscles to push your lower back against the mat. Now bring one or both knees to your chest and hold this position for 5 to 10 seconds.

patient's weight exceeds the ideal by more than 10%, caloric restriction is recommended. Weight reduction can improve patient COMFORT. Health care providers must be sensitive when reinforcing the need for patients to lose weight to prevent or lessen chronic back pain. Behavioral approaches to weight loss and positive reinforcement are important for the nutrition plan.

 NCLEX EXAMINATION CHALLENGE 43-4

Health Promotion and Maintenance

The nurse is teaching a client about self-management measures to help prevent low back pain. Which teaching should be included? **Select all that apply.**

A. "Losing weight can decrease strain on your back."
B. "Avoid twisting at your waist."
C. "Exercise on a regular basis, including walking."
D. "Don't bend at your waist when lifting a heavy object."
E. "Eat foods high in calcium and vitamin D to prevent bone loss."

Surgical Management. Surgery is usually performed if conservative measures fail to relieve unrelenting back pain or if neurologic deficits continue to progress. An orthopedic surgeon and/or neurosurgeon perform these surgeries. Two major types of surgery are used, depending on the severity and exact location of pain: minimally invasive surgery (MIS) and conventional open-surgical procedures. MIS is not done if the disk is pressing into the spinal cord (central cord involvement).

Preoperative Care. Preoperative care for the patient preparing for lumbar surgery is similar to that for any patient undergoing surgery (see Chapter 14). Teach the patient about postoperative expectations, including:
- Techniques to get into and out of bed
- Turning and moving in bed
- Reporting immediately new SENSORY PERCEPTION, such as numbness and tingling, or new motor impairment that may occur in the affected leg or in both legs
- Home care activities and restrictions

Many patients are discharged to home within 23 to 48 hours after surgery. Therefore, before surgery, teach family members or other caregiver how to assist the patient and what restrictions the patient must follow at home.

A bone graft is done if the patient has a *spinal fusion*. The surgeon explains from where the bone for grafting will be obtained. The patient's own bone is used whenever possible, but additional bone from a bone bank may be needed. The surgeon provides verbal and written information about the type and source of bone for surgery. An informed consent is obtained. While the bone graft heals, the patient may wear a back orthotic device for 4 to 6 weeks after surgery. Provide information about the importance of wearing the brace as instructed during the healing process, how to take it off and put it on while maintaining spinal alignment, and how to clean it.

Operative Procedures. *Minimally invasive surgery (MIS)* results in minimal muscle injury, decreased blood loss, and decreased postoperative pain. Therefore the primary advantage of MIS procedures is a shortened hospital stay and the possibility of an ambulatory care (same-day) procedure. Spinal cord and nerve complications are also less likely. Several specific procedures are commonly performed.

A *microdiskectomy* involves microscopic surgery directly through a 1-inch incision using an endoscope. This procedure allows easier identification of anatomic structures, improved precision in removing small fragments, and decreased tissue trauma and pain. A special cutting tool or laser probe is threaded through the cannula for removal or destruction of the *disk pieces* that are compressing the nerve root. This process is also called a **percutaneous endoscopic discectomy (PED)**. A newer procedure combines the PED with *laser thermodiskectomy* to also shrink the herniated disk before removal. Inpatient hospitalization is not necessary for this procedure.

Laser-assisted laparoscopic lumbar diskectomy combines a laser with modified standard disk instruments inserted through the laparoscope using an umbilical ("belly button") incision. The procedure may be used to treat herniated disks that are bulging but do not involve the vertebral canal. The primary risks of this surgery are infection and nerve root injury. The patient is typically discharged in 23 hours but may go home sooner.

The most common *conventional open procedures* are diskectomy, laminectomy, and/or spinal fusion. Artificial disk replacement may also be part of this type of surgery. These procedures involve a surgical incision to expose anatomic landmarks for extensive muscle and soft-tissue dissection.

As the name implies, a *diskectomy* is removal of a herniated disk. A *laminectomy* involves removal of part of the laminae and facet joints to obtain access to the disk space. When repeated laminectomies are performed or the spine is unstable, the surgeon may perform a **spinal fusion (arthrodesis)** to stabilize the affected area. Chips of bone are grafted between the vertebrae for support and to strengthen the back. Metal implants (usually titanium pins, screws, plates, or rods) may be required to ensure the fusion of the spine. In an **interbody cage fusion** surgery, a cagelike device is implanted into the space where the disk was removed. The surgeon may give an **intrathecal** (spinal) or epidural dose of long-acting morphine to decrease postoperative pain.

Postoperative Care. Postoperative care depends on the type of surgery that was performed. In the postanesthesia care unit (PACU), vital signs and level of consciousness are monitored frequently, the same as for any surgery. Best practices for PACU nursing care are discussed in Chapter 16. Patients who have a *minimally invasive spinal surgical procedure* go home the same day or the day after surgery with a Band-Aid or Steri-Strips over the small incision. Those having a microdiskectomy may also have a clear or gauze dressing over the bandage. Most patients notice less pain immediately after surgery, but mild oral analgesics are needed while nerve tissue heals over the next few weeks to promote patient COMFORT. Teach the patient to follow the prescribed exercise program, which begins immediately after discharge. Patients should start walking routinely every day. Complications of MIS are rare.

Early postoperative nursing care focuses on preventing and assessing complications that might occur in the first 24 to 48 hours for patients having conventional open surgery. Major complications include nerve injuries, diskitis (disk inflammation), and dural tears (tears in the dura covering the spinal cord) (Chart 43-9). As for any patient undergoing surgery, take vital signs at least every 4 hours during the first 24 hours to assess for fever, hypotension, or severe pain. Perform a neurologic assessment every 4 hours. Of particular importance are movement, strength, and SENSORY PERCEPTION in the lower extremities.

Carefully check the patient's ability to void. Altered COMFORT and a flat position in bed make voiding difficult, especially for men. An inability to void may indicate damage to the sacral spinal nerves, which control the detrusor muscle in the bladder. The patient with a diskectomy and/or laminectomy typically gets out of bed with assistance on the evening of surgery, which may help with voiding. Altered COMFORT may be relieved with patient-controlled analgesia (PCA) with morphine. The route is changed to oral administration after the patient is able to take fluids.

> ### ! NURSING SAFETY PRIORITY (QSEN)
> #### Action Alert
>
> For the patient after back surgery, inspect the surgical dressing for blood or any other type of drainage. Clear drainage may mean cerebrospinal fluid (CSF) leakage. Blood and CSF may be mixed on the dressing, with the CSF being visible as a "halo" around the outer edges of the dressing. The loss of a large amount of CSF may cause the patient to report having a sudden headache. Report signs of any drainage on the dressing to the surgeon immediately. Bulging at the incision site may be due to a CSF leak or a hematoma, both of which should also be reported to the surgeon.

Empty the surgical drain, usually a Jackson-Pratt or Hemovac, and record the amount of drainage every shift. The surgeon usually removes the drain in 24 to 36 hours.

Correct turning of the patient in bed is especially important. Do not place an overhead trapeze on the bed to assist the patient with MOBILITY skills. This apparatus can cause more back pain and damage the surgical area. Teach the patient to log roll every 2 hours from side to back and vice versa. In log rolling, the patient turns as a unit while his or her back is kept as straight as possible. A turning sheet may be used for obese patients. Either turning method may require additional assistance, depending on how much the patient can assist and on his or

◎ CHART 43-9 Best Practice for Patient Safety & Quality Care (QSEN)

Assessing and Managing the Patient With Major Complications of Open Traditional Lumbar Spinal Surgery

COMPLICATION	ASSESSMENT/INTERVENTIONS
Cerebrospinal fluid (CSF) leakage	Observe for clear fluid on or around the dressing. If leakage occurs, place patient flat. Report CSF leakage immediately to the surgeon. (The patient is usually kept on flat bedrest for several days while the dural tear heals.)
Fluid volume deficit	Monitor intake and output; monitor drain output, which should not be more than 250 mL in 8 hours during the first 24 hours. Monitor vital signs carefully for hypotension and tachycardia.
Acute urinary retention	Assist the patient to the bathroom or a bedside commode as soon as possible after surgery. Help male patients stand at the bedside as soon as possible after surgery.
Paralytic ileus	Monitor for flatus or stool. Assess for abdominal distention, nausea, and vomiting.
Fat embolism syndrome (FES) (more common in people with spinal fusion)	Observe for and report chest pain, dyspnea, anxiety, and mental status changes (more common in older adults). Note petechiae around the neck, upper chest, buccal membrane, and conjunctiva. Monitor arterial blood gas values for decreased PaO_2.
Persistent or progressive lumbar radiculopathy (nerve root pain)	Report pain not responsive to opioids. Document the location and nature of pain. Administer analgesics as prescribed.
Infection (e.g., wound, diskitis, hematoma)	Monitor the patient's temperature carefully (a slight elevation is normal). Increased temperature elevation or a spike after the second postoperative day may indicate infection. Report increased pain or swelling at the wound site or in the legs. Give antibiotics as prescribed if infection is confirmed. Use clean technique for dressing changes.

her weight. Instruct the patient to keep his or her back straight when getting out of bed. He or she should sit in a straight-back chair with the feet resting comfortably on the floor. As with all surgical patients, prevent atelectasis and iatrogenic pneumonia with deep breathing. Follow best practices to avoid venous thromboembolism (VTE) after surgery with early MOBILITY and intermittent sequential compression or pneumatic devices per The Joint Commission's Core Measures.

When a spinal fusion is performed in addition to a laminectomy, more care is taken with MOBILITY and positioning. The nurse or unlicensed assistive personnel (UAP) assist with log rolling the patient every 2 hours. For the conventional fusion, inspect both the iliac and spinal incision dressings for drainage and make sure they are intact. Remind the patient to avoid prolonged sitting or standing. Be sure to check with the surgeon or surgeon's prescription whether to place the orthotic device or brace on the patient before or after getting the patient out of bed.

Care Coordination and Transition Management

The patient with back pain who does not undergo surgery is typically managed at home. If back surgery is performed, the patient is usually discharged to home with support from family or significant others. For older adults without a community support system, a short-term stay in a nursing home or transitional care unit may be needed. Collaborate with the case manager or discharge planner, patient, and family to determine the most appropriate placement.

Home Care Management. Patients having any of the *MIS procedures* may resume normal activities within a few days up to 3 weeks after surgery, depending on the specific procedure and the condition of the patient. He or she may take a shower on the third or fourth day after surgery. Teach the patient to remove the outer clear or gauze dressing, if any is in place, but leave the Steri-Strips in place for removal by the surgeon or until they fall off. Instruct the patient to contact the surgeon immediately if clear drainage seeps from the incision. Clear drainage usually indicates a meningeal tear and that cerebrospinal fluid is leaking.

After *conventional open-back surgery*, the patient may have activity restrictions for the first 4 to 6 weeks, such as:
- Limit daily stair climbing.
- Restrict or limit driving.
- Do not lift objects heavier than 5 lb.
- Restrict pushing and pulling activities (e.g., dog walking).
- Avoid bending and twisting at the waist.
- Take a daily walk.

The duration of home-based recovery depends on the nature of the job and the extent and type of surgery. Most patients return to work after 6 weeks; some patients may not return for 3 to 6 months if their jobs are physically strenuous.

Self-Management Education. The patient with an acute episode of back pain typically returns to his or her usual activities but may fear a recurrence. Remind the patient that he or she may never have another episode if caution is used. However, continuous or repeated altered COMFORT can be frustrating and tiring. Encourage the patient and family members to plan short-term goals and take steps toward recovering each day.

After surgery, in collaboration with the physical therapist, COMFORT can continue to improve. Instruct the patient to:
- Continue with a weight-reduction diet, if needed
- Stop smoking, if applicable
- Perform strengthening exercises as instructed

The physical therapist reviews and demonstrates the principles of body mechanics and muscle-strengthening exercises. The patient is then asked to demonstrate these principles (Chart 43-10). Teach him or her the importance of keeping all appointments and following the prescribed exercise plan.

The health care provider may want the patient to continue taking anti-inflammatory drugs or, if muscle spasm is present, to take muscle relaxants. Remind the patient and family about the possible side effects of drugs and what to do if they occur.

CHART 43-10 Best Practice for Patient Safety & Quality Care QSEN

Prevention of Musculoskeletal Injuries

Use Best Practices to Prevent Back Injury When Moving Objects
- Avoid lifting objects of more than 5-10 lbs without assistance or aid.
- Push objects rather than pull them.
- Do not twist your back during movement.
- Use handles or grips to prevent unintended shifting of the object during movement.
- Avoid prolonged sitting or standing. Use a footstool to lessen back strain.
- Sit in chairs with good support.
- Avoid shoulder stooping; maintain proper posture.
- Do not walk or stand in high-heeled shoes for prolonged periods (for women).

Use Best Practices to Prevent Back Injury When Moving a Person
- Establish an interprofessional team responsible for reviewing and implementing OSHA guidelines for the prevention of musculoskeletal disorders. Originally developed for nursing homes, these guidelines provide guidance for education and practice and programs for health care workers and other stakeholders involved in patient handling, transfers, and movement.
- Build and support a culture of safety in health care settings that protects staff and patients from injury.
- Improve communication among nurses, physical therapists, and family caregivers to facilitate safe patient-handling and movement tasks.
- Develop policies and procedures for the therapeutic use of patient-handling equipment:
  - Select equipment that first provides safety of patients, staff, and family caregivers.
  - Train all staff and family caregivers in the proper and safe operation of all ergonomic-appropriate equipment.
  - Encourage patient participation in the use of assistive equipment such as sit-and-stand lifts that are used as an ambulation aid.
- Develop competency-based assessments that demonstrate proficiency for use of all patient-handling approaches and equipment.
- Encourage quality improvement projects and research that support safe and effective patient handling and movement while maximizing patient-assisted or patient-independent movement. For example, investigate the cost-effectiveness of ergonomic interventions.

OSHA, Occupational Safety and Health Administration.

In a few patients, back surgery is not successful. This situation, referred to as **failed back surgery syndrome (FBSS)**, is a complex combination of organic, psychological, and socioeconomic factors. Repeated surgical procedures often discourage these patients, who must continue aggressive pain management after multiple operations. Nerve blocks, implantable spinal cord stimulators (neurostimulators), and other chronic pain management modalities may be needed on a long-term basis to help with COMFORT.

Spinal cord stimulation is an *invasive* technique that provides COMFORT by applying an electrical field over the spinal cord. A trial with a percutaneous spinal cord stimulator is conducted to determine whether or not permanent placement is appropriate. If the trial is successful, electrodes are surgically placed internally in the epidural space and connected to an external or implanted programmable generator. The patient is taught to program and adjust the device to maximize comfort. Spinal cord stimulation can be extremely effective in select patients, but it is reserved for intractable (unrelenting continuous) neuropathic pain syndromes that have been unresponsive to other treatments.

> **❗ NURSING SAFETY PRIORITY** QSEN
>
> **Critical Rescue**
>
> For patients who have a spinal cord stimulator implanted in the epidural space, assess neurologic status below the level of insertion frequently. Monitor for early changes in SENSORY PERCEPTION, movement, and muscle strength. Ensure that the patient can void without difficulty. *If any changes occur, document and report them immediately to the surgeon!*

Health Care Resources. Help the patient identify support systems (e.g., family, church groups, clubs) after back surgery. For example, a spouse may help the patient with exercises or perform the exercises with the patient. Members of a church group may run errands and do household chores. The patient with back pain may continue physical therapy on an ambulatory basis after discharge. For unresolved comfort alterations, the patient may be referred to pain specialists or clinics. A case manager may be assigned to the patient to help with resource management and utilization.

CERVICAL NECK PAIN
❖ PATHOPHYSIOLOGY

Cervical neck pain most often results from a bulging or herniation of the nucleus pulposus (HNP) in a cervical intervertebral disk, illustrated in Fig. 43-1. The disk tends to herniate laterally where the annulus fibrosus is weakest and the posterior longitudinal ligament is thinned. The result is spinal nerve root compression, with resulting motor and sensory manifestations and altered patient COMFORT, typically in the neck, upper back (over the shoulder), and down the affected arm. The disk between the fifth and sixth cervical vertebrae (C5-C6) is affected most often.

If the disk does not herniate, nerve compression may be caused by osteophyte (bony spur) formation from osteoarthritis. The osteophyte presses on the intervertebral foramen, which results in a narrowing of the disk and pressure on the nerve root. As with sciatic nerve compression, the patient with

> **ⓘ CLINICAL JUDGMENT CHALLENGE 43-1**
>
> **Safety; Clinical Judgment** QSEN
>
> A 52-year-old woman married to a veteran fell down a flight of stairs 10 years ago and sustained an acute herniated disk at the L4-L5 spinal level. A laminectomy and discectomy relieved her pain for about 3 years, when she began having multiple episodes of severe pain and sciatica in her right leg. Two additional surgeries, including a recent spinal fusion, failed to provide pain relief. She is currently taking high-dose gabapentin and ibuprofen to maintain a pain level of 6 on a 0-to-10 pain scale. The patient is admitted to your unit this afternoon; a spinal nerve simulator was implanted as a last resort for pain management. On admission from PACU, she reports that her legs remain "numb" because of her epidural anesthetic. Her vital signs are within her baseline, and her pain level is a 2 on a 0-to-10 pain scale.
>
> 1. Which additional postoperative data will you need to collect and document to ensure patient safety and why?
> 2. For which postoperative complications should you monitor and why?
> 3. The neurosurgeon writes a prescription for the patient to be discharged to home tomorrow morning. Which health teaching will this patient require to ensure her safety?
> 4. The next morning, the patient reports increased lower-extremity numbness and inability to easily move her legs. Her pain is an 8 after you administer her opioid. What is your priority action at this time and why?

cervical nerve compression may have either continuous or intermittent chronic pain. When the disk herniates centrally, pressure on the spinal cord occurs.

Cervical pain—acute or chronic—may also occur from muscle strain, ligament sprain resulting from aging, poor posture, lifting, tumor, rheumatoid arthritis, osteoarthritis, or infection, all of which can affect the patient's COMFORT. The typical history of the patient includes a report of pain when moving the neck, which radiates to the shoulder and down the arm. The pain may interrupt sleep and may be accompanied by a headache or numbness and tingling in the affected arm. To determine the exact cause, imaging studies may be used. Electromyography/nerve conduction studies are used to help differentiate cervical radiculopathy, ulnar or radial neuropathy, carpal tunnel syndrome, or other peripheral nerve problems.

❖ INTERPROFESSIONAL COLLABORATIVE CARE

Conservative treatment for altered COMFORT, specifically acute neck pain, is the same as described for low back pain except that exercises focus on the shoulders and neck. The physical therapist teaches the patient the correct techniques for performing "shoulder shrug," "shoulder squeeze," and "seated rowing." Some primary health care providers prescribe a soft collar to stabilize the neck, especially at night. Using the collar longer than 10 days can lead to decreased muscle strength and range of motion. For that reason, some health care providers do not recommend collars for cervical disk problems. Therapeutic manipulation (chiropractic interventions) alone or in combination with other interventions does not appear to cause harm for most patients but does not consistently reduce pain or disability (Mior et al., 2013).

If conservative treatment is ineffective, surgery may be required, most often using a *conventional open-surgical approach.* A neurosurgeon usually performs this surgery because of the complexity of the nerves and other structures in that area of the spine. Depending on the cause and the location of the herniation, either an anterior or posterior approach is used. An anterior cervical diskectomy and fusion (ACDF) is commonly performed. The patient is fitted with a large neck brace before surgery. Routine preoperative and postoperative care nursing interventions are the same as described in Chapters 14 and 16.

> ## ! NURSING SAFETY PRIORITY QSEN
> ### Critical Rescue
>
> The priority for care in the immediate postoperative period after an ACDF is maintaining an airway and ensuring that the patient has no problem with breathing. Swelling from the surgery can narrow the trachea, causing a partial obstruction. Surgery can also interfere with cranial innervation for swallowing, resulting in a compromised airway or aspiration. If these changes occur, open the patient's airway, sit the patient upright, suction if needed, and provide supplemental oxygen. Promptly notify the surgeon or rapid response team using SBAR and document your assessment and interventions.

Chart 43-11 summarizes best practices for postoperative care and discharge planning. Complications of ACDF can occur from the brace or the surgery itself. The initial brace is worn for 4 to 6 weeks. When it is removed, a soft collar is worn for several more weeks. Potential complications of the anterior surgical approach can be found in Chart 43-12.

Some patients may be candidates for minimally invasive surgery (MIS), such as percutaneous cervical diskectomy (PCD) through an endoscope, with or without laser thermodiskectomy to shrink the herniated portion of the disk. The care for these patients is very similar to that for the patient with low back pain who has MIS (see discussion of surgical management of patients with low back pain earlier in this chapter). Patients may also benefit from the placement of an artificial disk, a surgical option that preserves movement of the vertebrae. Artificial disks are approved by the FDA. Although there is evidence of their safety, the long-term effects on patient health are not yet established.

> ## ◎ CHART 43-11 Best Practice for Patient Safety & Quality Care QSEN
> ### Care of the Patient After an Anterior Cervical Diskectomy and Fusion
>
> **Postoperative Interventions**
> - Assess **a**irway, **b**reathing, and **c**irculation (first priority!).
> - Check for bleeding and drainage at the incision site.
> - Monitor vital signs and neurologic status frequently.
> - Check for swallowing ability.
> - Monitor intake and output.
> - Assess the patient's ability to void (may be a problem secondary to opiates or anesthesia).
> - Manage pain adequately.
> - Assist the patient with ambulation within a few hours of surgery, if he or she is able.
>
> **Discharge Teaching**
> - Be sure that someone stays with the patient for the first few days after surgery.
> - Review drug therapy.
> - Teach care of the incision.
> - Review activity restrictions:
>   - No lifting
>   - No driving until surgeon permission
>   - No strenuous activities
> - Walk every day.
> - Call the surgeon if symptoms of pain, numbness, and tingling worsen or if swallowing becomes difficult.
> - Wear brace or collar per surgeon's prescription.

> ## ⟫ CHART 43-12 Key Features
> ### Postoperative Complications of Anterior Cervical Diskectomy and Fusion
>
> - Hoarseness due to laryngeal injury; may be temporary or permanent
> - Temporary dysphagia; may last few days to several months; usually not severe
> - Esophageal, tracheal, or vertebral artery injury
> - Wound infection
> - Injury to the spinal cord or nerve roots
> - Dura mater tears with associated cerebrospinal fluid leaks
> - Pseudoarthrosis caused by nonunion of fusion
> - Graft and screw loosening if a fusion was performed

GET READY FOR THE NCLEX® EXAMINATION!

▌ KEY POINTS

Review these Key Points for each NCLEX Examination Client Needs Category.

Safe and Effective Care Environment
- Assess airway and breathing *first* for patients with an acute SCI. **QSEN: Evidence-Based Practice; Safety**
- Collaborate with members of the interprofessional health care team when caring for patients with spinal cord problems; assist with transition management to rehabilitation settings and home care. **QSEN: Teamwork and Collaboration**

Health Promotion and Maintenance
- Use safe-object and patient-handling practices to prevent back injury as described in Chart 43-7. **QSEN: Safety**

- Include community resources in discharge planning and teaching for patients with MS and SCI. There are specialty organizations for each of these spinal conditions.
- Apply knowledge of older-adult development to outline special care for older adults with spinal cord injury (see Chart 43-6).

Psychosocial Integrity
- Refer patients to appropriate resources, such as a sexual counselor, for sexual dysfunction resulting from illness or disease. Counsel them as needed about SEXUALITY. **QSEN: Teamwork and Collaboration; Patient-Centered Care**
- Recognize that spinal cord injury and progressive neurologic diseases, such as MS, require the patient and family to make

major adjustments to roles and goals. **QSEN: Patient-Centered Care**
- Determine patient and family coping strategies to help patients adjust to spinal trauma or disease. **QSEN: Patient-Centered Care**

Physiological Integrity
- Assess pain or altered COMFORT level in patients with back injury, including the nature of the pain and location.
- Implement effective drug and nondrug interventions for back pain, including NSAIDs, anticonvulsants, and adjunctives such as heat/cold and exercise.
- Implement interventions to prevent complications associated with immobility, including turning; VTE prophylaxis; early ambulation or transfers out of bed; and airway and breathing management such as bedside suctioning equipment, incentive spirometry, and Aspiration Precautions. **QSEN: Safety**
- Monitor patients with cervical spinal injuries for manifestations of autonomic dysreflexia (see Chart 43-2). Provide a bowel and bladder regimen to prevent retention of stool and urine because these common problems can initiate autonomic dysreflexia. **QSEN: Evidence-Based Practice**
- Provide emergency care for patients who experience autonomic dysreflexia as listed in Chart 43-3. **QSEN: Safety; Clinical Judgment**
- Assess patients with MS for signs and symptoms as listed in Chart 43-1. Fatigue is one of the most common symptoms.
- For patients who have surgery to manage vertebral or spinal cord conditions, observe the incision site for bleeding and cerebrospinal fluid leakage (clear fluid) and document findings (see Charts 43-9 and 43-12). **QSEN: Informatics; Clinical Judgment**
- Log roll during repositioning, especially during acute SCI or following surgical fusion of vertebrae. **QSEN: Safety**
- Reinforce health teaching for exercises for low back pain as described in Chart 43-8; teach principles of body mechanics and lifting to prevent back injury (see Chart 43-10).
- Provide evidence-based postoperative care and discharge teaching for patients having cervical neck surgery as listed in Chart 43-11. **QSEN: Evidence-Based Practice**

SELECTED BIBLIOGRAPHY

Asterisk indicates a classic or definitive work on this subject.

Ahmad, F., Wang, M. Y., & Levi, A. D. (2014). Hypothermia for acute spinal cord injury: A review. *World Neurosurgery, 82*(1–2), 207–214.

American Nurses Association (ANA). (2013). *Safe patient handling and mobility: Interprofessional national standards across the care continuum.* Silver Spring, MD: ANA.

Burcham, J. L. R., & Rosenthal, L. D. (2016). *Lehne's pharmacology for nursing care* (9th ed.). St. Louis: Elsevier.

Jarvis, C. (2014). *Physical examination & health assessment* (7th ed.). St. Louis: Elsevier Saunders.

McCance, K., Huether, S., Brashers, V., & Rote, N. (2014). *Pathophysiology: The biologic basis for disease in adults and children* (7th ed.). St. Louis: Mosby.

Mior, S., Gamble, B., Barnsley, J., Cote, P., & Cote, E. (2013). Changes in primary care physician's management of low back pain in a model of interprofessional collaborative care: An uncontrolled before-after study. *Chiropractic and Manual Therapies, 21*(6), doi:10.1186/2045-709X-21-6.

Multiple Sclerosis Society of Canada. (2017). *What is multiple sclerosis?* https://mssociety.ca/about-ms-what-is-ms.

National Institute of Neurological Disorders and Stroke [NINDS]. (2015). *Back pain fact sheet.* Retrieved from http://www.ninds.nih.gov/disorders/backpain/detail_backpain.htm#3102_3.

National Multiple Sclerosis Society. (2017). *Who gets MS.* www.nationalmssociety.org/about-multiple-sclerosis/what-we-know-about-ms/index.aspx.

National Spinal Cord Injury Statistical Center. (2016). *Spinal cord injury facts and figures at a glance.* www.nscisc.uab.edu/PublicDocuments/fact_figures_docs/Facts2016.pdf.

Pagana, K. D., Pagana, T. J., & Pagana, T. N. (2017). *Mosby's diagnostic and laboratory test reference* (13th ed.). St. Louis: Elsevier.

Parkinson, L., Sibbritt, D., Bolton, P., van Rotterdam, J., & Villadsen, I. (2013). Well-being outcomes of chiropractic intervention for lower back pain: A systematic review. *Clinical Rheumatology, 32*(2), 167–180.

Qaseem, A., Wilt, T. J., McLean, R. M., & Forciea, M. A. (2017). Noninvasive treatments for acute, subacute, and chronic low back pain: A clinical practice guideline from the American College of Physicians. *Annals of Medicine,* annals.org/aim/article/2603228/noninvasive-treatment-acute-subacute-chronic-low-back-pain-clinicalpractice.

Quigley, P. A. (2016). Evidence levels: Applied to select fall and fall injury prevention practices. *Rehabilitation Nursing, 41,* 5–15.

Sezer, N., Akkus, S., & Ugurlu, F. G. (2015). Chronic complications of spinal cord injury. *World journal of orthopedics [electronic resource], 6*(1), 24–30.

*Stahel, P. F., VanderHeiden, T., & Finn, M. A. (2012). Management strategies for acute spinal cord injury: Current options and future perspectives. *Current Opinion in Critical Care, 18*(6), 651–660.

Wegner, I., Widyahening, I. S., van Tulder, M. W., Blomberg, S. E., de Vet, H. C., Brønfort, G., et al. (2013). Traction of low-back pain with or without sciatica. *The Cochrane Database of Systematic Reviews,* online doi:10.1002/14651858.CD003010.pub5.

Zychowicz, M. E. (2013). Pathophysiology of heterotopic ossification. *Orthopaedic Nursing, 32*(3), 173–177.

Care of Patients With Problems of the Peripheral Nervous System

Donna D. Ignatavicius

 http://evolve.elsevier.com/Iggy/

PRIORITY AND INTERRELATED CONCEPTS

The priority concepts for this chapter are:
- MOBILITY
- SENSORY PERCEPTION
- IMMUNITY

✳ The IMMUNITY concept exemplar for this chapter is Guillain-Barré Syndrome, below.

The interrelated concept for this chapter is GAS EXCHANGE.

LEARNING OUTCOMES

Safe and Effective Care Environment
1. Collaborate with interprofessional health care team members when providing care for patients with Guillain-Barré syndrome (GBS) and myasthenia gravis (MG) to promote MOBILITY, GAS EXCHANGE, and self-management.

Health Promotion and Maintenance
2. Identify community resources for peripheral nervous system (PNS) disorders for patients and families as part of care coordination and transition management.

Psychosocial Integrity
3. Plan nursing interventions for patients with GBS and MG for promoting communication based on patient preferences.

Physiological Integrity
4. Describe how to perform focused neurologic assessments for patients with PNS disorders.

5. Compare and contrast the pathophysiology of GBS and MG, including the role of IMMUNITY.
6. Provide information to patients and families on common side effects and administration of drugs for PNS disorders to ensure safety.
7. Prioritize evidence-based nursing interventions for the patient with GBS or MG to maintain adequate MOBILITY and SENSORY PERCEPTION.
8. Differentiate between a myasthenic crisis and a cholinergic crisis.
9. Use clinical nursing judgment to reduce the risk for postoperative complications for patients having a thymectomy.
10. Compare trigeminal neuralgia and facial paralysis assessment findings.

The peripheral nervous system (PNS) is composed of the spinal nerves, cranial nerves, and part of the autonomic nervous system. Its function is to provide communication from the brain and spinal cord to other parts of the body. *Neuropathy* or *peripheral neuropathy (PN)* is a global word that refers to any disease, disorder, or injury to the PNS (Fig. 44-1). These health problems may be acute or chronic. Secondary PN may result from disorders such as peripheral vascular disease and diabetes mellitus. These health problems are discussed elsewhere in this text. PNS health problems can cause impaired or altered MOBILITY, SENSORY PERCEPTION, comfort, and IMMUNITY. A review of each of these health concepts can be found in Chapter 2.

✳ IMMUNITY CONCEPT EXEMPLAR
Guillain-Barré Syndrome

❖ PATHOPHYSIOLOGY

Guillain-Barré syndrome (GBS) is an acute inflammatory disorder that affects the axons and/or myelin of the PNS, causing impaired MOBILITY and SENSORY PERCEPTION as a result of altered IMMUNITY. It is an uncommon disorder, affecting males slightly more than females and peaking after age 55 years (McCance et al., 2014).

GBS may be referred to by a variety of other names, such as acute idiopathic polyneuritis, acute inflammatory demyelinating

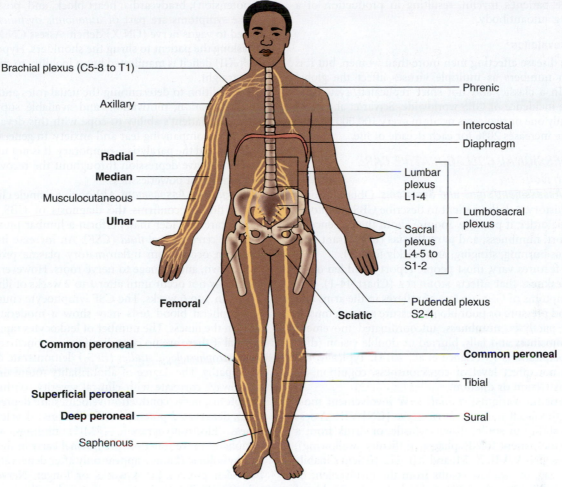

Brachial plexus (C5-8 to T1)
Axillary
Radial
Median
Musculocutaneous
Ulnar

Phrenic
Intercostal
Diaphragm
Lumbar plexus L1-4
Lumbosacral plexus
Sacral plexus L4-5 to S1-2

Femoral
Sciatic

Pudendal plexus S2-4

Common peroneal

Superficial peroneal
Deep peroneal
Saphenous

Common peroneal
Tibial
Sural

FIG. 44-1 Distribution of selected peripheral nerves in the body. The nerves most commonly affected by injury or trauma are highlighted in bold type.

polyneuropathy (AIDP), acute motor axonal neuropathy (AMAN), and acute motor and sensory axonal neuropathy (Arcila-Londono & Lewis, 2012). In some forms of GBS, primarily the axons are affected. In other forms, **demyelination** (destruction of the myelin sheath) of the peripheral nerves occurs. In demyelinating GBS, symptoms typically begin in the legs and spread to the arms and upper body. This is referred to as an ascending paralysis. Paralysis can increase in intensity until the muscles cannot be used at all and the patient is almost totally immobile. As a result, some patients require mechanical ventilation because of a weak or paralyzed diaphragm and accessory muscles for respiration. Healing occurs in reverse; the neurons affected last are the first to recover.

GBS is likely the result of altered IMMUNITY. Antibodies attack the myelin sheath that surrounds the axons of the peripheral nerves. On microscopic examination, groups of lymphocytes are seen at the points of myelin breakdown. In some instances, secondary damage to the cell body, the neurilemma, or the axon occurs. Neurilemma and axonal injury can delay recovery or result in permanent neurologic defects. Segmental demyelination (the destruction of myelin between the nodes of Ranvier) is the major pathologic finding in most variants of GBS. This destruction slows the transmission of impulses from node to node. Damaged motor neurons result in impaired

MOBILITY. Damaged sensory nerves send fewer messages to the brain, affecting the patient's SENSORY PERCEPTION.

Three stages make up the *acute* course of GBS:

- The *acute or initial period* (1 to 4 weeks), which begins with the onset of the first symptoms and ends when no further deterioration occurs
- The *plateau period* (several days to 2 weeks)
- The *recovery phase* (gradually over 4 to 6 months, maybe up to 2 years), which is thought to coincide with remyelination and axonal regeneration (Some patients do not completely recover and have permanent neurologic deficits, referred to as *chronic GBS*.)

Etiology

GBS is often associated with bacterial infection, especially infection with *Campylobacter jejuni*. Influenza, Epstein-Barr, and cytomegalovirus (CMG) viral infections have also been associated with GBS. In countries where the recent Zika virus has emerged, the number of GBS cases has increased, suggesting that the Zika infection can also trigger GBS (Sampathkumar & Sanchez, 2016). There are also reports of some vaccines increasing the risk for GBS slightly, but epidemiologic evidence is weak (Centers for Disease Control and Prevention [CDC], 2017). It is believed that the precipitating infection or event sensitizes the

T-cells to the patient's myelin, resulting in production of a demyelinating autoantibody.

Incidence/Prevalence

GBS is a rare disease affecting men more than women, but it is increasing in numbers as multiple viruses affect the global population. In a classic, and not since replicated, systematic review of the incidence of GBS worldwide, Sejvar et al. (2011) found that only one or two cases occur in every 100,000 people. The incidence increases 20% for each decade of life.

❖ INTERPROFESSIONAL COLLABORATIVE CARE

◆ Assessment: Noticing

Physical Assessment/Signs and Symptoms. Obtain a complete health history. Ask the patient to describe GBS symptoms in chronologic order, if possible. Inquire about the presence of altered comfort, numbness, and paresthesias (unpleasant sensations such as burning, stinging, and prickly feeling).

Although features vary, most people report a sudden onset of muscle weakness that affects MOBILITY (Chart 44-1). The common symptoms of GBS are loss of reflexes in the arms and legs, low blood pressure or poor blood pressure control, muscle weakness or paralysis, numbness, uncoordinated movement leading to clumsiness and falls, blurred or double vision (diplopia), and palpitations (McCance et al., 2014). Typically, the disease does not affect level of consciousness, cognition, or pupillary constriction or dilation.

With any of the variants, *cranial nerve* involvement most often affects the facial nerve (cranial nerve [CN] VII). Assess the patient's ability to smile, frown, whistle, or drink from a straw. Assess the patient for dysphagia (difficulty swallowing), which involves CNs V, VII, X, XI, and XII. The patient's inability to cough, gag, or swallow results from the involvement of CNs IX and X. Monitor the patient closely for varying blood pressure (hypertensive and hypotensive episodes or orthostatic

hypotension), bradycardia, heart block, and, possibly, asystole. These symptoms are part of *autonomic dysfunction*, which is linked to vagus nerve (CN X) deficit. Assess CN XI (accessory) by asking the patient to shrug the shoulders. Hypoglossal nerve (CN XII) deficit is manifested by an inability to stick the tongue out straight.

In addition to determining the usual roles and responsibilities, occupation, motivation, and available support systems, assess the patient's ability to cope with this devastating illness and the accompanying fear and anxiety. In general, GBS is self-limiting, and the paralysis is temporary. It is not unusual for the patient to have depression throughout the recovery period or feel significant powerlessness.

Diagnostic Assessment. Although no single clinical or laboratory finding confirms the diagnosis of GBS, the primary health care provider may perform a lumbar puncture (LP) to evaluate *cerebrospinal fluid (CSF)*. An increase in CSF protein level can occur from inflammatory plasma proteins, myelin breakdown, and damage to nerve roots. However, high protein levels may not occur until after 1 to 2 weeks of illness, reaching a peak in 4 to 6 weeks. The CSF lymphocyte count is normal.

Peripheral blood tests may show a moderate *leukocytosis* early in the illness. The number of leukocytes rapidly returns to normal if there are no complications or concurrent illness.

Electrophysiologic studies (EPSs) demonstrate demyelinating neuropathy. The degree of abnormality found on testing does not always correlate with clinical severity. Within 3 weeks of symptoms, nerve conduction velocities are depressed. In some cases, denervated potentials (fibrillations) develop later in the illness. Electromyographic (EMG) findings, which reflect peripheral nerve function, are normal early in the illness. Electrophysiologic changes appear only after denervation of muscle has been present for 4 weeks or longer. Nerve conduction velocity (NCV) testing is performed with the EMG. Nerve damage or disease may still exist despite normal NCV results. An MRI or CT scan may be requested to rule out other causes of motor weakness. These tests are described in Chapter 41.

Respiratory function manifested by poor GAS EXCHANGE is often compromised in patients with GBS. Therefore vital capacity or tidal volume may be decreased, and respiratory rate increased. Arterial blood gas (ABG) values may be abnormal with a decreased partial pressure of arterial oxygen (Pao_2), increased partial pressure of arterial carbon dioxide ($Paco_2$), or decreased pH.

◆ Analysis: Interpreting

The priority collaborative problems for patients with GBS typically include:

1. Potential for respiratory and/or cardiovascular distress or failure due to thoracic muscle weakness and hypotension
2. Decreased MOBILITY due to skeletal muscle weakness

◆ Planning and Implementation: Responding

Preventing Respiratory and/or Cardiovascular Distress or Failure

Planning: Expected Outcomes. The desired outcome for the patient with GBS is that the patient will not experience cardiopulmonary failure as a result of managing the airway, promoting GAS EXCHANGE, and maintaining normal-range blood pressure.

Interventions. The primary health care provider follows the most recent best practice guidelines from the American

---

> **CHART 44-1** **Key Features**

Guillain-Barré Syndrome

Motor Manifestations Affecting Mobility

- Ascending symmetric muscle weakness → flaccid paralysis without muscle atrophy
- Decreased or absent deep tendon reflexes (DTRs)
- Respiratory compromise (dyspnea, diminished breath sounds, decreased tidal volume, reduced peripheral oxygenation [SpO_2] and vital capacity) and respiratory failure
- Loss of bowel and bladder control (less common)
- Ataxia

Sensory Perception Manifestations

- Paresthesias
- Pain (cramping)

Cranial Nerve Manifestations

- Facial weakness
- Dysphagia
- Diplopia
- Difficulty speaking

Autonomic Manifestations

- Labile blood pressure
- Cardiac dysrhythmias
- Tachycardia

Academy of Neurology for the treatment of GBS. The patient may receive either plasma exchange (also known as *plasmapheresis* or *apheresis*) or IV immunoglobulin (IVIG). Corticosteroids are not used unless medically necessary to treat other associated diseases.

Plasmapheresis removes the circulating antibodies thought to be responsible for the disease. In this procedure, plasma is selectively separated from whole blood. The blood cells are returned to the patient without the plasma. Plasma usually replaces itself, or the patient is transfused with a colloidal substitute such as albumin. Fresh frozen plasma is generally not used because of the associated risk for infection and allergic pulmonary edema. Plasmapheresis should be done within several days after the onset of the illness, although some patients benefit up to 30 days after the onset of symptoms. The patient usually receives three or four treatments, 1 to 2 days apart. Some patients may require a second round of treatment if they deteriorate after the first plasmapheresis.

Nursing interventions for the patient undergoing plasmapheresis include providing information and reassurance, weighing the patient before and after the procedure, caring for the shunt or venous access site, and preventing the complications described in Chart 44-2.

IV Immunoglobulin (IVIG) has been shown to be as effective as plasmapheresis and is immediately available in most settings. Side effects of immunoglobulin therapy range from minor discomforts (e.g., chills, mild fever, myalgia, and headache) to major complications (e.g., anaphylaxis, aseptic meningitis, retinal necrosis, acute renal failure). Infuse IVIG slowly when it

---

! NURSING SAFETY PRIORITY QSEN

Action Alert

If a shunt is used for plasmapheresis, be sure to:
- Check shunt patency by assessing the presence of bruit or thrill every 2 to 4 hours
- Keep double bulldog clamps at the bedside
- Observe the access site for bleeding or ecchymosis (bruising)

---

is started. Observe for and document side and adverse effects and report their occurrence to the health care provider. The rate of administration can be increased based on the patient's tolerance and agency protocol.

Frequent and focused monitoring of both the respiratory and cardiovascular systems can prevent complications from GBS and identify patients in need of critical rescue interventions. Inability to maintain an airway is a high risk and potentially fatal consequence of rapidly ascending GBS. The priority nursing intervention of *airway management* is to promote airway patency and adequate GAS EXCHANGE. Consider implementing Aspiration Precautions that include elevating the head of the bed to 45 degrees or higher and testing for dysphagia before restarting oral drugs or nutrition. Have suctioning equipment available and follow agency procedures for oral or oral-tracheal suctioning if the airway becomes compromised with secretions or food. Monitor the color, consistency, and amount of secretions obtained. Chest physiotherapy, often performed by the respiratory therapist (RT), and frequent

---

◎ CHART 44-2 **Best Practice for Patient Safety & Quality Care** QSEN

Preventing and Managing Complications of Plasmapheresis

COMPLICATION	NURSING INTERVENTIONS
Treatment-Related Complications	
Citrate-induced hypocalcemia	Monitor electrolytes before and after therapy. Communicate abnormal results appropriately to the health care provider. Anticipate calcium replacement therapy (Chapter 11).
Urticarial (skin) reactions from proteins in replacement fluids	Obtain order and administer diphenhydramine (Benadryl) or corticosteroid as premedications when urticaria occurred with previous exchange.
Depletion coagulopathy	Monitor complete blood count and coagulation panel before and after treatment. Communicate abnormal values to the health care provider in an urgent time frame.
Risk for infection from immunoglobulin depletion	Assess and document vital signs, including temperature three times daily. Report symptoms of infection, fever, or abnormal vital signs to the health care provider promptly.
Fluid shift or depletion	Monitor fluid status and vital signs during treatment and at least twice in the first hour following treatment.
Sensitivity reaction (including potential anaphylaxis with incorrect crossmatch or administration) when fresh frozen plasma is used in replacement fluid	Follow institution policy for safe, effective administration of blood products such as fresh frozen plasma.
Site-Related Complications	
Trauma to skin and blood vessels from large-bore needles for access or catheter-related trauma	Teach the patient rationale for and how to monitor access site as follows.
Bleeding, phlebitis, or infection at access site	Anchor tubing securely during treatment. Minimize patient agitation, if present, during treatment. Assess access site immediately following cessation of treatment and at regular intervals (every 4 hours or more often). Assessment includes appearance of site or dressing, palpation of thrill, and auscultation of bruit.
Clotting at access site	Report loss of thrill or bruit, uncontrolled or large-volume bleeding, and presence of redness (particularly along venous pathway), drainage, and swelling to provider immediately.

position changes are combined with breathing exercises (coughing and deep breathing) and the use of an incentive spirometer to prevent pneumonia and atelectasis. Oxygen may be administered by nasal cannula at a flow rate prescribed by the health care provider. Collaborate with the RT to promote GAS EXCHANGE and manage the patient's airway.

⚠ NURSING SAFETY PRIORITY **QSEN**
Action Alert

In the initial phase of Guillain-Barré syndrome, monitor the patient closely for signs of respiratory distress, such as dyspnea, air hunger, adventitious breath sounds, decreased oxygen saturation, and cyanosis. In addition, assess respiratory rate, rhythm, and depth every 1 to 2 hours. In collaboration with the respiratory therapist (RT), check vital capacity every 2 to 4 hours and auscultate the lungs at 4-hour intervals. Monitor the patient's ability to cough and swallow for any change. Assess cognitive status, especially in older adults; a decline in mental status often indicates hypoxia.

Monitor ABG values or end-tidal carbon dioxide ($EtCO_2$) for signs of respiratory failure; pulse oximetry reveals decreasing oxygen saturation. A decrease in vital capacity to less than 15 to 20 mL/kg (or less than two thirds of the patient's normal) and the inability to clear secretions may be indications for elective intubation.

Both the sympathetic and parasympathetic systems may be affected. A patient with acute GBS may require cardiac monitoring because of the risk for dysrhythmias. Monitor trends in vital signs closely. Report significant changes in heart rate and blood pressure to the primary health care provider in an urgent time frame. Hypertension is treated with a beta blocker or nitroprusside (Nitropress). Hypotension is treated with IV fluids and placing the patient in a supine position unless he or she is in extreme respiratory distress. Atropine may be prescribed to treat bradycardia.

Improving Mobility and Preventing Complications of Immobility
Planning: Expected Outcomes. The desired outcome is that the patient will increase MOBILITY to baseline or will not experience any complications of short-term or prolonged immobility.

Interventions. Collaborate with the patient, family, physical and occupational therapists (PTs/OTs), speech-language pathologist (SLP), and dietitian to develop interventions that prevent complications of immobility and to address temporary deficits in self-care. Assess the patient's motor (muscle) strength every 2 to 4 hours as part of the neurologic assessment. The interventions prescribed for MOBILITY and self-management and to prevent complications depend on the degree of motor deficit. The PT and OT can provide assistive devices, as needed, and instructions for their use.

To ensure safety, assist the patient with walking, transfers from bed to chair, position changes, and maintenance of proper body alignment until he or she is able to perform these activities independently. Encourage maximum independence. Perform active or passive range-of-motion (ROM) exercises at least daily or delegate this activity to unlicensed assistive personnel (UAP) with supervision. Teach family members these techniques. See Chapter 6 for detailed discussion of ways to promote self-management and prevent complications of immobility. Monitor the patient's responses, including fatigue level. Provide adequate rest periods between activities.

Muscle weakness can cause dysphagia, which may lead to malnutrition. Collaborate with the dietitian to develop caloric and protein intake goals. The patient may require assistance with feeding. If he or she cannot safely swallow food or liquids, enteral nutrition is prescribed. Weigh the patient three times a week and monitor serum prealbumin each week to evaluate nutritional status.

Immobility and malnutrition place patients at risk for pressure injury. Assess skin integrity at least daily and assist with MOBILITY. While bedbound, ensure that the patient is turned a minimum of every 2 hours. Consider the use of pressure-reducing or pressure-relieving devices, such as a special mattress or overlay. Document the skin assessment daily. Consult with the skin or wound care expert when changes occur that contribute to pressure injury formation (see Chapter 25).

Because venous thromboembolism (VTE) and pulmonary emboli are common complications of immobility, the primary health care provider may prescribe prophylactic anticoagulant therapy, such as subcutaneous low–molecular-weight heparin. Sequential pneumatic compression devices for legs may be used to promote venous return. Ensure documentation of starting and maintaining VTE prophylaxis; this is a Joint Commission Core Measure of high-quality health care delivery in acute and critical care units.

❓ NCLEX EXAMINATION CHALLENGE 44-1
Physiological Integrity

The nurse is caring for a client diagnosed with Guillain-Barré syndrome. Which assessment findings require nursing action? **Select all that apply.**
A. Blood pressure of 80/42
B. Respiratory rate of 24
C. Shallow breathing pattern
D. Peripheral oxygen saturation (SpO_2) of 85%
E. Diminished breath sounds in all lung fields

Care Coordination and Transition Management
Home Care Management. The severity and course of GBS are variable, which makes the prognosis difficult to predict. The most likely residual deficits at discharge from the acute care or rehabilitation setting are related to MOBILITY, self-management, altered SENSORY PERCEPTION, and disturbed self-concept. For patients who have total quadriparesis (weakness in all four extremities) or respiratory paralysis, the course of the rehabilitation phase varies even more and may require weeks to years. The expected outcome of the recovery phase is to move from dependence to independence.

Planning for discharge begins on admission. Include a family member in the education process throughout the patient's hospitalization and in the discharge process. Provide them with both oral and written instructions to improve adherence to the plan of care and promote continuity during care transitions. The patient may transition to home or skilled care. In collaboration with the discharge planner or case manager (CM), the nurse communicates patient status and summarizes the hospital stay to provide safe transitions in care to a rehabilitation or long-term care setting. If the patient is discharged to home, consider referral to a home health care agency or support group. If assistive devices are needed at home, the CM in collaboration with the interprofessional health care team makes certain that the necessary equipment has been delivered after evaluating the home setting. Home care management for patients with GBS is similar to that for those who have had a stroke or spinal cord injury, depending on the nature of the neurologic deficit.

Teach the patient and family about the illness and explain all diagnostic tests and treatments. Assess the patient and family for verbal and nonverbal behaviors that indicate powerlessness, anxiety, fear, and isolation. Encourage the patient to verbalize feelings about the illness and its effects, if possible, while fostering hope. Assess previous decision-making patterns, roles, and responsibilities. To help identify personal factors that influence coping ability, ask the patient and/or family to describe their usual lifestyles and the situations in which they coped effectively. Sleep disturbances related to altered autonomic function may affect the patient's sleep-wake cycle. Allow for regularly scheduled rest periods.

Refer patients who need further psychosocial support to the social worker, certified hospital chaplain or appropriate spiritual resource, and local support groups. If necessary, obtain a psychological consultation for further evaluation and intervention.

Health Care Resources. Self-help and support groups for patients with chronic illness are common. Refer the patient and family to these groups, if indicated. For example, the Guillain-Barré Syndrome Foundation International (www.gbs-cidp.org) provides resources and information for patients and their families. The psychosocial adjustment needed may be minimal or dramatic, depending on the patient's residual deficit, age, gender, usual roles and responsibilities, usual coping strategies, available support systems, and occupation. Help the patient identify other support systems, such as church members, friends, or spiritual resources.

◆ **Evaluation: Reflecting**

Evaluate the care of the patient with GBS on the basis of the identified priority problems. The expected outcomes are that he or she:

- Does not experience respiratory or cardiovascular distress or failure
- Increases mobility to be able to function independently

MYASTHENIA GRAVIS

❖ **PATHOPHYSIOLOGY**

Myasthenia gravis (MG) is an acquired autoimmune disease characterized by muscle weakness. There are two types of MG: ocular and generalized. About two thirds of patients initially present with reports about vision that arise from disturbances of the ocular muscles. MG may take many forms—from mild disturbances of the cranial and peripheral motor neurons to a rapidly developing, generalized weakness that may lead to death from respiratory failure. MG can present at any age, and the incidence is slightly higher among men. It is a progressive disease.

MG is caused by distorted acetylcholine receptors (AChRs) in the muscle motor end plate membranes. Antibodies are attached to the AChRs. As a result, nerve impulses are reduced at the neuromuscular junction; they do not result in muscle contraction. MG and hyperplasia (abnormal growth) of the thymus gland are related because **thymoma** (encapsulated thymus gland tumor) occurs in a few cases.

❖ **INTERPROFESSIONAL COLLABORATIVE CARE**

◆ **Assessment: Noticing**

Physical Assessment/Signs and Symptoms. In addition to the biographic data and history, ask the patient about specific muscle weakness. Although the onset of MG is usually insidious (slow), some instances of fairly rapid development have been caused by infection, pregnancy, or anesthesia. A temporary increase in weakness may be noted after vaccination, menstruation, and exposure to extremes in environmental temperature. The course of the disease may have periods of exacerbation or flares when symptoms worsen. Ask the patient when symptoms worsen, specifically noting the affected muscle groups and any limitation or inability in performing ADLs. Anticipate worsening symptoms with repetitive muscle use. Determine the reason for admission to plan care. Patients with MG are typically hospitalized for myasthenic or cholinergic crisis resulting in respiratory failure or during periods of exacerbation when GAS EXCHANGE is threatened.

Additional areas of inquiry include any history of **ptosis** (drooping eyelids), **diplopia** (double vision), or **dysphagia** (difficulty chewing or swallowing) and the type of diet best tolerated. Assess the patient about a history of respiratory difficulty, choking, or voice weakness. Other areas of assessment include asking about any difficulty holding up the head, brushing teeth, combing hair, or shaving. Assess for the presence of paresthesias or aching in weakened muscles. Finally, ask about a history of thymus gland tumor. The most common symptoms of MG are related to involvement of the levator palpebrae or extraocular muscles (Chart 44-3). These symptoms may last only a few days at the onset and then resolve, only to return weeks or months later. Pupillary responses to light and accommodation are usually normal.

For most patients, the muscles of facial expression, chewing, and speech are affected (**bulbar** involvement) (Fig. 44-2). Note the patient's smile, which may be transformed into a snarl. The jaw may hang so the patient must prop it up with the hand. Chewing and swallowing difficulties, choking, and regurgitation of fluids through the nose may lead to considerable weight loss. Ask about the patient's nutritional intake and any recent weight loss. He or she may have more difficulty eating after talking. After extended conversations, the voice may become

---

> **CHART 44-3** **Key Features**
>
> **Myasthenia Gravis**
>
> **Motor Manifestations Affecting Mobility**
> - Progressive (proximal) muscle weakness that worsens with repetitive use and usually improves with rest
> - Poor posture
> - Ocular palsies
> - Ptosis; incomplete eyelid closure
> - Diplopia
> - Respiratory compromise
> - Loss of bowel and bladder control
> - Fatigue
>
> **Sensory Perception Manifestations**
> - Muscle achiness
> - Paresthesias
> - Decreased sense of smell and taste

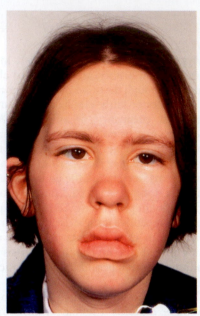

FIG. 44-2 Patient with myasthenia gravis who has changes in facial expression and ptosis. (From Goldman. L., & Schafer, A. I. [2016]. *Goldman-Cecil medicine,* [25th ed.]. St. Louis: Elsevier.)

weaker or exhibit a nasal twang. In some patients, the tongue has fissures (ulcers).

Less often involved are the muscles of the shoulders, the flexors of the neck, and the hip flexors. Because limb weakness is more often *proximal* (closer to the body), the patient may have difficulty climbing stairs, lifting heavy objects, or raising the arms overhead. Neck weakness may be mild or severe enough to cause difficulty in holding the head erect. Among the trunk muscles, the erector spinae are most commonly affected, causing difficulty maintaining a sitting or walking posture.

In the most advanced cases of MG, all muscles are weakened, including those associated with respiratory function and the control of bladder and bowel. In these more severe cases, ask about bowel and bladder function. Assess respiratory rate, depth, pattern, and SpO₂ frequently to ensure adequate GAS EXCHANGE.

Muscle atrophy, although rarely severe, occurs in a small percentage of patients with MG. Some patients report that their weakened muscles ache. If present, paresthesias (painful tingling sensations) affecting the muscles of the face, hands, and thighs are not associated with any loss of sensation.

In Eaton-Lambert syndrome, a form of myasthenia often seen with small cell carcinoma of the lung, the muscles of the trunk and the pelvic and shoulder girdles are most commonly affected. Although weakness increases after exertion, muscle strength may temporarily increase during the first few contractions, followed by rapid decline. Diagnosis is confirmed by electromyography (EMG). Management differs somewhat from that of other types of MG. Treatment includes removing the tumor, managing the cancer, and administering drug therapy to release acetylcholine (ACh). Additional therapies may include plasmapheresis and immunosuppressive therapy (discussed later).

Diagnostic Assessment. Because the incidence of MG is uncommon, diagnosis may be delayed or missed. An experienced clinician can diagnose the disease from the history and physical examination findings. MG may be immediately confirmed by the patient's response to cholinergic drugs. A standard series of laboratory studies is usually performed for patients with known or suspected MG. *Thyroid function* should be tested because thyrotoxicosis (excessive thyroid hormone) is present in a small number of myasthenic patients. *Serum protein electrophoresis* evaluates the patient for immunologic disorders. Immunologic-based diseases, such as rheumatoid arthritis, systemic lupus erythematous, and polymyositis, may be associated with the disease (Pagana et al., 2017).

Several types of antibodies are found in the majority of patients with MG and include forms directed against the acetylcholine receptor (AChR) and the enzyme *muscle-specific kinase* (MuSK). However, although a positive antibody test confirms the diagnosis, a negative finding does not rule out the disease.

Some patients with MG have a thymoma; therefore patients are assessed for this condition. The thymus, an H-shaped gland located in the upper mediastinum beneath the sternum, is where B- and T-cells interact, refining self-recognition of these white blood cells. It is hypothesized that thymic abnormalities cause the breakdown in tolerance that causes the immune-mediated attack on AChR in myasthenia gravis (McCance et al., 2014). A thymoma can be seen on a chest *x-ray* or a *CT scan.*

The most common electrodiagnostic test performed to detect MG is *repetitive nerve stimulation (RNS)* of proximal nerves. Selected nerves are electrically stimulated, which results in progressive decline in the strength of the associated innervated muscle. This test diagnoses most cases of generalized MG but far fewer cases of ocular MG.

During *electromyography* (EMG) to diagnose MG, a recording electrode is placed into skeletal muscle, and the electrical activity of skeletal muscle can be monitored in a manner similar to electrocardiography (ECG) (Pagana et al., 2017). A progressive decrease in the amplitude of the electrical waveform is a classic sign of MG. This study can be combined with nerve conduction studies and may be called an *electromyoneurography*. It can be performed at the bedside by a technician.

Single-fiber EMG (SFEMG) is a newer and most sensitive form of EMG in detecting defects of neuromuscular transmission. This test compares the stability of the firing of one muscle fiber with that of another fiber innervated by the same motor neuron. The time interval between the two firings normally shows a minor degree of variability, called *jitter*. Defective transmission increases jitter or actually blocks successive discharges. This test can diagnose almost all cases of generalized and ocular MG.

Pharmacologic tests with the cholinesterase inhibitor *edrophonium chloride (Enlon, Tensilon)* may be performed. Edrophonium is used most often for testing because of its rapid onset and brief duration of action. This drug inhibits the breakdown of ACh at the postsynaptic membrane, which increases the availability of ACh for excitation of postsynaptic receptors. Within 30 to 60 seconds of the first drug dose, most myasthenic patients show a marked improvement in muscle tone that lasts 4 to 5 minutes. False-positive test results may be caused by increased muscle effort by the patient. False-negative findings may be seen if the tested muscle is extremely weak or refractory to the drug.

Edrophonium may be used also to help determine whether increasing weakness in the previously diagnosed myasthenic patient is due to a cholinergic crisis (too much cholinesterase inhibitor drug) or a myasthenic crisis (too little cholinesterase inhibitor drug). In a cholinergic crisis, muscle tone does not improve after giving the drug. Instead, weakness may actually increase, and **fasciculations** (muscle twitching) may be seen around the eyes and face (Burcham & Rosenthal, 2016).

⚠ NURSING SAFETY PRIORITY QSEN

Drug Alert

Edrophonium can cause cardiac dysrhythmias and cardiac arrest, but these reactions rarely occur. Be sure that the antidote, atropine sulfate, is available in case they occur.

◆ **Interventions: Responding**

MG is one of the most treatable neurologic disorders. The classic presentation of MG is muscle weakness that increases when the patient is fatigued and limits his or her MOBILITY and ability to participate in activities. Management for this disease falls into two categories:

- Treatment that affects the symptoms of MG without influencing the actual course of the disease (anticholinesterases or cholinergic drugs)
- Therapeutic efforts for inducing remission, such as the administration of immunosuppressive drugs or corticosteroids, plasmapheresis, and thymectomy (removal of the thymus gland)

Nonsurgical Management. Although not all patients with MG have respiratory compromise, ongoing assessment and maintenance of respiratory GAS EXCHANGE are nursing care priorities.

Providing Respiratory Support. Both myasthenic and cholinergic crises increase muscle weakness and the patient's risk for respiratory compromise. The diaphragm and intercostal muscles may be affected, which inhibits the patient's ability to maintain adequate GAS EXCHANGE, breathe deeply, and cough effectively. In addition, dysphagia may result in the aspiration of foods, fluids, or saliva, which worsens the respiratory problems. Because of their respiratory muscle involvement, many of these patients have an increased risk for lung infections.

The patient who cannot cough effectively may require oropharyngeal or nasopharyngeal suctioning. If needed, teach the assisted-cough technique, similar to that used by patients who are quadriplegic. Collaborate with the respiratory therapist (RT) to provide chest physiotherapy consisting of postural drainage, percussion, and vibration to mobilize secretions and improve GAS EXCHANGE.

⚠ NURSING SAFETY PRIORITY QSEN

Critical Rescue

Keep a bag-valve-mask setup (e.g., Ambu), equipment for oxygen administration, and suction equipment at the bedside of the patient with myasthenia gravis in case of respiratory distress.

Because breathing difficulty or the inability to breathe easily is frightening, be aware of the patient's mental and emotional status during periods of respiratory compromise. Monitor his or her response to drug therapy for muscle weakness. Monitor for pulmonary congestion that can lead to respiratory complications such as pneumonia and atelectasis.

Noninvasive mechanical ventilation (NIMV) can be used to support patients with acute respiratory failure from MG crisis while awaiting improvement from IV immunoglobulin (IVIG) therapy or plasma exchange. Chapter 32 explains NIMV further.

Promoting Mobility. Assess the patient's muscle strength before and after periods of activity. Provide assistance as necessary to prevent the patient from becoming fatigued. Schedule him or her for tests, treatments, and other activities early in the day or during the energy peaks after giving the prescribed drugs. Assist the patient in planning the periods of rest.

During periods of maximum weakness, provide assistance with positioning and activity. Assess for skin breakdown with each repositioning intervention. Pressure-reducing devices or mattresses are used to help prevent pressure injury. Collaborate with the physical and occupational therapists to develop a program for the patient to assist with MOBILITY, self-care, and energy conservation techniques. Chapter 6 discusses rehabilitation as one strategy to improve functional ability after a period of immobility, and Chapter 25 describes strategies to prevent and manage pressure injuries.

Administering Drug Therapy. Two groups of drugs are typically prescribed for the treatment of myasthenia gravis (MG): anticholinesterases and immunosuppressants. Be sure to *give these drugs on time to maintain blood levels and thus improve muscle strength.* Monitor and document the patient's response to drug therapy. Provide information for the patient and the family about the indications for, effectiveness of, and side effects of the drugs used in the treatment of MG.

Cholinesterase Inhibitor Drugs. *Cholinesterase (ChE) inhibitor drugs are the first-line management of MG.* These drugs are also referred to as *anticholinesterase drugs* or *antimyasthenics.* They enhance neuromuscular impulse transmission by preventing the decrease of ACh by the enzyme *ChE.* This increases the response of the muscles to nerve impulses and improves muscle strength. The ChE inhibitor drug of choice is pyridostigmine (Mestinon, Regonol). Expect a day-to-day variation in dosage, depending on the patient's changing symptoms.

⚠ NURSING SAFETY PRIORITY QSEN

Drug Alert

Instruct the patient to eat meals 45 minutes to 1 hour after taking ChE inhibitors to avoid aspiration. This is especially important if the patient has bulbar involvement. Drugs containing magnesium, morphine or its derivatives, curare, quinine, quinidine, procainamide, or hypnotics or sedatives should be avoided because they may increase the patient's weakness. Antibiotics such as neomycin impair transmitter release and also increase myasthenic symptoms.

A potential adverse effect of ChE inhibitors is cholinergic crisis. Sudden increases in weakness accompanied by hypersalivation, sweating, and increased bronchial secretions help identify this as a cholinergic crisis rather than a myasthenic crisis (Burcham & Rosenthal, 2016).

A cholinergic crisis is also more likely to be associated with nausea, vomiting, and diarrhea *but can cause life-threatening symptoms such as bronchospasm and bradycardia.* Teach the patient and family to monitor for and report these two types of crises immediately:

- Myasthenic crisis—an exacerbation (flare-up or worsening) of the myasthenic symptoms caused by not enough anticholinesterase drugs

TABLE 44-1 Characteristics of Myasthenic and Cholinergic Crises

MYASTHENIC CRISIS	CHOLINERGIC CRISIS	FEATURES COMMON TO BOTH
Increased pulse and respiration	Bradycardia and bronchospasm (life-threatening symptoms!)	Apprehension Restlessness Dyspnea
Rise in blood pressure	Flaccid paralysis	Dysphagia (difficult swallowing)
Bowel and bladder incontinence	Hypersecretion: salivation, tearing, and sweating	Generalized weakness Respiratory failure
Decreased urine output	Nausea/vomiting	
Absence of cough and swallow reflex	Diarrhea	
Improvement of symptoms with edrophonium test*	Abdominal cramps	
	Miosis, blurred vision	
	Worsening of symptoms with edrophonium test	

*Edrophonium (Enlon, Tensilon) is given IV; muscle movement improves immediately in patients with myasthenia or myasthenia crisis.

- Cholinergic crisis—an acute exacerbation of muscle weakness caused by too many anticholinesterase drugs

Because myasthenic and cholinergic crises have many common characteristics, the type of crisis the patient is experiencing must be identified for effective treatment to be provided (Table 44-1). Monitor carefully for early detection of these emergencies if the patient is in a health care setting.

Emergency Care: Myasthenic Crisis. Myasthenic crisis is often caused by some type of infection. For other patients, increasing muscle weakness leads to an overdose of anticholinesterase drugs. As a result, the patient may experience a *mixed* crisis. The edrophonium test described earlier, although not always conclusive, is an important procedure for differentiation because it produces a temporary improvement in myasthenic crisis but worsening or no improvement of symptoms in cholinergic crisis.

The priority for nursing management of the patient in myasthenic crisis is maintaining adequate respiratory function to promote GAS EXCHANGE. The acutely ill patient may need intensive nursing care for monitoring. He or she may require mechanical ventilation or other technologic support. Cholinesterase-inhibiting drugs are withheld because they increase respiratory secretions and are usually ineffective for the first few days after the crisis begins. Drug therapy is restarted gradually and at lower dosages.

Emergency Care: Cholinergic Crisis. In *cholinergic* crisis, do not give anticholinesterase drugs while the patient is maintained with mechanical ventilation. Atropine 1 mg IV may be given and repeated, if necessary. When atropine is prescribed, observe the patient carefully. Secretions can be thickened by the drug, which causes more difficulty with airway clearance and possibly the development of mucus plugs. Unless complications such as pneumonia or aspiration develop, the patient in crisis improves rapidly after the appropriate drugs have been given. Continue to provide assistance as necessary because he or she tires easily after minimal exertion.

Immunosuppressants. Immunosuppression may be accomplished with the use of corticosteroids or other medications (i.e., methotrexate [a chemotherapeutic agent] or rituximab [a biologic agent]) that are effective against B-cells (Burcham & Rosenthal, 2016). B-cells are lymphocytes active in antibody formation (see Chapter 17). For ocular MG, corticosteroid treatment that does not cause significant systemic complications may significantly reduce the prevalence of generalized myasthenia gravis after 2 years on the drug. IV immunoglobulins (IVIGs) may also be used for acute disease management or as a long-term option for disease refractory to other treatment.

Other Interventions. Plasmapheresis is a method by which antibodies are removed from the plasma to decrease symptoms. This is used as short-term management of an exacerbation. Six exchanges occur over a 2-week period, with follow-up exchanges weekly or monthly as needed, usually as an ambulatory care patient. Nursing management of the patient undergoing plasmapheresis is presented in the earlier discussion of Guillain-Barré syndrome and Chart 44-2.

Generalized weakness and fatigue affect the patient's ability to participate in ADLs. Impaired fine-motor control and shoulder weakness, which results in difficulty raising the arms, can compound the problem. Self-care deficits may be complete or partial, depending on the severity of the illness or the patient's response to drugs.

Assess the patient's ability to perform ADLs. Although he or she is encouraged to perform activities as independently as possible, assistance is provided as needed to avoid frustration and fatigue. *For maximizing independence and making attempts at self-management successful, plan activities to follow the administration of medication.* Monitor and document the patient's response to or tolerance of activity, providing periods of rest after an activity. *Rest is critical because repetitive movement can precipitate a crisis.* Occupational and physical therapists evaluate patients for assistive-adaptive devices. In collaboration with the nurse, they also teach the patient and family energy conservation techniques and ideas for making work and self-management easier after discharge from the hospital.

Weakness of the speech and facial muscles often results in dysarthric (slurred) and nasal speech. In collaboration with the speech-language pathologist (SLP), determine the patient's ability to communicate. Instruct him or her to speak slowly while attempting to lip-read. Repeat what the patient says to check that it is correct. Questions that can be answered with "yes" or "no" or by gestures may be used along with other communication systems such as eye blinking, notebook and pencil, computer, handheld mobile devices, and picture, letter, or word boards.

The patient with myasthenia gravis (MG) may have difficulty maintaining an adequate intake of food and fluid because the muscles needed for chewing and swallowing become weakened and tire easily. In collaboration with the dietitian, occupational therapist, and SLP, evaluate the patient's nutritional status and his or her ability to receive adequate oral nutrition. High-calorie snacks are often well tolerated. Monitor the effectiveness of the nutrition program by recording the patient's calorie counts, intake and output, serum prealbumin levels, and daily weights (Chart 44-4). If he or she cannot swallow, a feeding tube may be used.

The patient's inability to completely close the eyes may lead to corneal abrasions and further decrease vision and comfort. During the day, apply artificial tears to keep the corneas moist and free from abrasion. A lubricant gel and shield may be applied to the eyes at bedtime to provide more extensive coverage. To help relieve diplopia, cover the eyes with a patch for 2

CHART 44-4 Best Practice for Patient Safety & Quality Care QSEN

Improving Nutrition in Patients With Myasthenia Gravis

- Assess the patient's gag reflex and ability to chew and swallow.
- Provide frequent oral hygiene as needed.
- Collaborate with the dietitian, speech-language pathologist, and occupational therapist to plan and implement meals that the patient can eat and enjoy.
- Cut food into small bites or request a soft or edentulous diet and encourage the patient to eat slowly.
- Observe the patient for choking, nasal regurgitation, and aspiration.
- Provide high-calorie snacks or supplements (e.g., puddings).
- Keep the head of the bed elevated during meals and for 30 to 60 minutes after the patient eats.
- Consider thickening liquids to avoid choking or aspiration.
- Monitor caloric and food intake.
- Weigh the patient daily.
- Monitor serum prealbumin levels.
- Administer anticholinesterase drugs as prescribed, usually 45 to 60 minutes before meals.

to 3 hours at a time, one eye at a time. At times, patients tape their eyes shut at night.

NCLEX EXAMINATION CHALLENGE 44-2

Physiological Integrity

The nurse is teaching a client about taking a new prescription for pyridostigmine. Which statements by the nurse indicate **correct** information about this drug? **Select all that apply.**

A. "Avoid opioids and other sedating drugs when taking this medication."
B. "Report increased mucous secretions and sweating immediately to the primary health care provider."
C. "Take the prescribed medication after meals to increase intestinal absorption."
D. "Avoid taking antibiotics, especially neomycin, while on this medication."
E. "Maintain the exact same dose of this medication every day."

Surgical Management. For patients with MG, **thymectomy** (removal of the thymus gland) is usually performed early in the disease. The procedure is not always immediately effective. Those who have surgery within 2 years of the onset of myasthenic symptoms show the most improvement, but many patients do not experience a change in status despite thymectomy.

Provide routine preoperative care as discussed in Chapter 14. Because there is no way to predict whether remission or improvement will occur, it is important to avoid making promises but be optimistic. Immediately before surgery, pyridostigmine (Mestinon) may be given with a small amount of water to keep the patient stable during and after surgery. If steroids have been used, they are also given before surgery and are tapered during the postoperative period. Antibiotics are administered immediately before or during the surgery. Plasmapheresis may be used before and after surgery to decrease circulating antibodies.

One of several surgical minimally invasive approaches to remove the thymus or small thymomas is most often used, including the single subxyphoid approach or the trans-subxyphoid

approach with robotic thymectomy (TRT). These surgeries are becoming more popular because they require less surgical time than traditional surgery (i.e., using a sternal incision) and allow more rapid recovery with less discomfort after surgery. Only a small dressing and an IV line are needed after surgery.

The older *sternal split* procedure is preferred when patients have a large thymoma. It allows the surgeon to directly see the mediastinum and areas around the thymus. When a large thymoma is present, all surrounding involved structures (i.e., the pericardium, the innominate vein, a portion of the superior vena cava, and a portion of the lung) are removed. A single chest tube is placed in the anterior mediastinum. The patient is usually admitted to the critical care unit after surgery. Thymoma should be considered as a potentially malignant tumor requiring prolonged follow-up. The presence of myasthenic weakness can still complicate its management.

Although patients with adequate respiratory effort and GAS EXCHANGE may be extubated immediately after surgery, most require a gradual weaning from the ventilator. Prolonged ventilatory assistance is rare. *After the patient is extubated, pay special attention to respiratory status and maintaining a patent airway.* Encourage the patient to turn, breathe deeply three to six times every 15 to 30 minutes in the hours after extubation, and use incentive spirometry.

! NURSING SAFETY PRIORITY QSEN

Critical Rescue

For the patient having a thymectomy, monitor respiratory effort and promote effective GAS EXCHANGE. Observe for signs of pneumothorax or hemothorax, including:
- Chest pain
- Sudden shortness of breath
- Diminished or delayed chest wall expansion
- Diminished or absent breath sounds
- Restlessness or a change in vital signs (decreasing blood pressure or a weak, rapid pulse)

If respiratory distress or symptoms of ineffective gas exchange occur, provide oxygen to the patient and raise the head of the bed to at least 45 degrees. Then report any of these signs and symptoms to the surgeon or Rapid Response Team immediately!

For the sternal surgical technique, provide chest tube care (see Chapter 32). Both surgical approaches require sterile technique for wound care. Observe the patient for signs of infection, such as increasing or purulent drainage; redness, warmth, or swelling around the wound; and elevated temperature. Patient and family teaching about follow-up care is needed before discharge from the hospital.

Care Coordination and Transition Management

The patient with myasthenia gravis (MG) may be cared for in a variety of settings, including the home, long-term acute care facility, rehabilitation setting, or skilled nursing facility. The patient discharged from the hospital may require the assistance of a family member, home care nurse, physical therapist (PT), occupational therapist (OT), and/or home care aide.

Home Care Management. Patients with MG are managed at home. Unless the patient requires new assistive devices, little preparation of the home setting is required. In collaboration with PTs and OTs, the case manager (CM) and nurse make certain that the necessary equipment has been delivered and

TABLE 44-2 Factors Precipitating or Worsening Myasthenia Gravis

- Various drugs, including:
  - Strong cathartics (laxatives)
  - Antidysrhythmics
  - Beta-blocking agents
  - Aminoglycosides and other antibiotics
  - Antirheumatic drugs
  - Antispasmodics, including quinine
  - Antihistamines
  - Opioids
  - Phenytoin (Dilantin)
  - Antidepressants (tricyclics)
- Rheumatoid arthritis
- Alcohol
- Hormonal changes
- Stress
- Infection
- Seasonal temperature changes
- Heat
- Surgery
- Enemas

CHART 44-5 Patient and Family Education: Preparing for Self-Management

Helpful Hints for Teaching Patients With Myasthenia Gravis About Drug Therapy

- Keep prescribed drugs and a glass of water at your bedside if you are weak in the morning.
- Wear a watch with an alarm function (or beeper) to remind you to take your drugs.
- Post your drug schedule so others know it.
- Plan strenuous activities, when possible, when the drug peaks.
- Keep a secure supply of drugs in your car or at work.
- Check with your health care provider before using any over-the-counter drugs.

! NURSING SAFETY PRIORITY QSEN

Action Alert

Because respiratory compromise often occurs in myasthenic patients, encourage family members to learn resuscitation procedures. A manual resuscitation bag, suctioning equipment, and oxygen should be available in the home for patients susceptible to crises. Teach family members the proper use of equipment.

installed properly. Teach the patient and family members how to use the equipment safely. If the patient becomes wheelchair dependent, the discharge planner, CM, or OT checks on any necessary modifications to the home (e.g., the installation of ramps or widening of doorways) that have been completed. Home health care can provide assistance in transitioning from acute to home care.

Self-Management Education. The patient and family need to know about the disease and the drugs used for treatment. Discuss the episodic nature of the disease, including factors that increase the risk for exacerbation, such as infection, stress, surgery, hard physical exercise, sedatives, and enemas or strong cathartics (Table 44-2). Teach the patient the importance of collaborating with the health care team to monitor muscle strength, ability to perform ADLs, and the need to evaluate and adjust drug therapy.

Stress the importance of lifestyle adaptations such as avoiding heat (e.g., sauna, hot tubs, sunbathing), crowds, overeating, erratic changes in sleep habits, or emotional extremes. Teach the signs of exacerbation, such as increased weakness, increased diplopia, ptosis, and problems with chewing or swallowing. Remind the patient to plan activities to allow for rest periods and to conserve energy.

Provide the drug regimen in a written format that includes the names, purposes, dosages, scheduled dosage times, and side effects of the drugs. Explain that the drugs are normally taken before activities such as eating, participating in sports, or working. Stress the importance of maintaining therapeutic blood levels by taking the medications on time and as prescribed and not missing or postponing doses (Chart 44-5). In addition, inform the patient of the side effects of anticholinesterase drugs and drugs that can worsen symptoms, such as corticosteroids, narcotics, antidysrhythmics, and antimalarials. Check with the pharmacist before starting or stopping drugs. In preparing the patient for discharge, explain the signs and symptoms of myasthenic and cholinergic crises and the need to contact the primary health care provider whenever either type of crisis is suspected.

The episodic and progressive nature of MG, the potential or actual loss of independence, and body image changes (e.g., the inability to smile) affect the patient's adjustment. During discharge planning, the CM considers factors such as age, gender, usual roles and responsibilities, available support systems, occupation, and financial status. Because the patient's and family's need for psychosocial adjustment may range from minimal to dramatic, the CM remains sensitive to their needs and provides information and support. Encourage family members or significant others to discuss their feelings with one another.

Health Care Resources. In collaboration with the primary health care provider, patient, and family, the staff nurse or CM may initiate referrals to home care agencies and local self-help groups for people who have chronic illnesses and their families. In the United States, the Myasthenia Gravis Foundation (www.myasthenia.org) provides education and research programs and assistance with financial aid and community resources. Support groups are also available. The Myasthenia Gravis Coalition of Canada (www.mgcc-ccmg.org) is a network of various provincial and local organizations and support groups that are available for patients in Canada with MG. Teach the patient the importance of obtaining and wearing a medical alert (MedicAlert) bracelet or necklace and to carry a medical alert identification card at all times.

RESTLESS LEGS SYNDROME

❖ PATHOPHYSIOLOGY

Restless legs syndrome (RLS) is characterized by leg paresthesias (burning, prickly sensation) associated with an irresistible urge to move. Over 10% of the population in the United States have the problem, and women are affected twice as often as men (National Institute of Neurological Disorders and Stroke [NINDS], n.d.). RLS occurs most often in middle-age and older adults. Stress can exacerbate this condition. RLS is related to a dysfunction in the brain circuits that use the neurotransmitter *dopamine.* Many of those affected with *primary RLS* have a positive family history, indicating a possible genetic basis. The incidence is higher in patients who have diabetes mellitus type

2, chronic kidney disease, iron deficiency, Parkinson disease, and peripheral neuropathy; who use certain medications such as caffeine, calcium channel blockers, lithium, or neuroleptics; or who are withdrawing from sedatives. Although not a cause of hospitalization, RLS may be a comorbidity that complicates recovery from other conditions.

❖ INTERPROFESSIONAL COLLABORATIVE CARE
◆ Assessment: Noticing

The patient reports intense burning or "crawling-type" sensations in the legs and therefore feels the need to move them repeatedly. These symptoms are worse in the evening and at night and when the patient is still for a period of time. Patients feel they need to move to relieve the symptoms. Many move their legs periodically while sleeping. For that reason, they often refer to themselves as "night walkers."

◆ Interventions: Responding

The management of RLS is symptomatic and involves treating the underlying cause or contributing factor, if known. Both nonpharmacologic measures and drug therapy are used. Teach patients to avoid as many risk factors as possible or make lifestyle modifications. Examples are avoiding caffeine and alcohol, quitting smoking, losing weight, and exercising.

Strategies to relieve the symptoms of RLS include walking, stretching, moderate exercise, or a warm bath. In the United States, refer them to The Restless Legs Foundation (www.rls.org) as an excellent resource for information and patient and family support.

Many of the drugs prescribed for RLS are also used for either Parkinson disease (PD) or epilepsy. *Dopamine agonists* such as pramipexole (Mirapex) and ropinirole (Requip) are oral drugs used extensively. Gabapentin enacarbil (Horizant) is an *antiepileptic drug (AED)* that is also approved by the U.S. Food and Drug Administration (FDA) for RLS (Burcham & Rosenthal, 2016).

These agents are usually taken at bedtime because they may cause daytime sleepiness. Teach patients to be cautious of driving or operating heavy equipment when taking them. Correcting iron and magnesium deficiencies can reduce RLS symptoms, and ongoing supplementation of these minerals may be needed.

Some patients have had success with *Sinemet,* a combination of levodopa and carbidopa. This drug is often given with other medications to be more effective in reducing the symptoms of the disease. Other classes of drugs for managing RLS include *benzodiazepines, such as diazepam (Valium), and opioids* as a last resort. Two other AEDs, carbamazepine (Tegretol) and gabapentin (Neurontin), have been particularly effective and are taken in divided doses throughout the day. For insomnia from RLS, *melatonin* may be effective for many people, especially older adults. However, the focus of treatment should be on RLS, not insomnia. Teach patients to inform their health care providers when adding these supplements.

TRIGEMINAL NEURALGIA

❖ PATHOPHYSIOLOGY

Trigeminal neuralgia (TN) is also known as *tic douloureux.* The trigeminal nerve has three branches: the first branch controls sensation in a person's eye, upper eyelid, and forehead; the second branch controls sensation in the lower eyelid, cheek,

nostril, upper lip, and upper gum; and the third branch controls sensations in the jaw, lower lip, lower gum, and some of the muscles used for chewing.

According to the National Institute of Neurological Disorders and Stroke (2013), trigeminal neuralgia has these characteristics:

- Affects the trigeminal (fifth cranial) nerve
- Occurs more often in people older than 50 years and in women more often than men
- Causes a specific type of facial pain, which results in sudden, intense facial spasms
- Is usually provoked by minimal stimulation of a trigger zone (such as dental procedures)
- Is unilateral (one-sided) and confined to the area innervated by the trigeminal nerve, most often the second and third branches (Fig. 44-3)
- Is familial due to an inherited pattern of blood vessel formation

The cause of TN is thought to be related to impaired inhibitory mechanisms in the brainstem caused by excessive firing of irritated fibers in the trigeminal nerve. Trauma and infection of the teeth, jaw, or ear may be contributing factors. Patients younger than 30 years with pain in more than one branch of the trigeminal nerve may be further evaluated to rule out the possibility of a tumor or multiple sclerosis.

❖ INTERPROFESSIONAL COLLABORATIVE CARE
◆ Assessment: Noticing

TN is a chronic syndrome causing impaired comfort, most often severe pain. It can be categorized into two types of pain: classic and atypical. When describing trigeminal pain, patients use terms such as *excruciating, sharp, shooting, piercing, burning,* and *jabbing.* Atypical pain descriptions may include migraine-like headache. Between bursts of pain, which last from seconds to minutes, there is usually no pain. Often no sensory or motor deficits are found on examination. Pain can be initiated by light touch, a change in facial expression (e.g., smiling), or chewing. The fear of precipitating agonizing attacks often causes patients to avoid talking; smiling; eating; or attending to hygienic needs

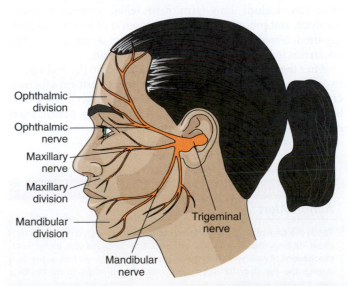

FIG. 44-3 Distribution of the trigeminal nerve and its three divisions: ophthalmic, maxillary, and mandibular.

such as shaving, washing the face, and brushing the teeth. The pain can cause uncontrollable facial twitching. The course of TN involves bouts of classic pain for several weeks or months followed by spontaneous remissions. The length of these remissions may vary from days to years, but attack-free periods tend to become shorter as the patient grows older.

The patient suspected of TN usually has a CT scan and MRI to determine whether there is a reversible cause of trigeminal compression or inflammation. The diagnosis is made based on patient history and the results of these imaging tests.

◆ Interventions: Responding

The priority for care of the patient with TN is pain management. Specific interventions are determined by the amount of pain he or she is experiencing. Drug therapy is the first choice, but surgery can provide satisfactory pain relief in patients who do not respond to drug management or who experience profound adverse drug reactions.

Drug Therapy and Radiosurgery. The first choice for drug therapy is carbamazepine (CBZ, Tegretol), an antiepileptic drug (AED). Other drugs, such as gabapentin (Neurontin), pregabalin (Lyrica), and baclofen (Lioresal, Kemstro), a muscle relaxant, may be used. Some patients also achieve pain relief with complementary therapies, such as acupuncture.

Microvascular decompression, radiosurgery techniques such as a peripheral chemical nerve block with ropivacaine, or stereotactic radiation treatments with the gamma knife are surgical approaches to disrupt trigeminal neuralgia. These minimally invasive procedures prevent the complications of major surgery. Surgical interventions are often combined with drug therapy for pain management of this challenging condition.

In some cases, a **percutaneous stereotactic rhizotomy (PSR)** is performed as an ambulatory care procedure under general anesthesia. The surgeon passes a hollow needle through the inside of the patient's cheek into the trigeminal nerve fibers. A heating current (radiofrequency thermocoagulation) goes through the needle to destroy some of the fibers. As an option to heat, a balloon microcompression of the trigeminal nerve root may be performed. A glycerol injection may also be used as an option, but it is not done as commonly as thermocoagulation.

The entire nerve is not destroyed. The advantages of this procedure include long-term pain relief, absence of facial paralysis, and preservation of the sensation of touch. Puncturing the internal carotid artery is a possible complication. The affected side is permanently insensitive to pain.

After the PSR procedure, apply an ice pack to the PSR operative site on the cheek and jaw for 3 to 4 hours. Perform a focused cranial nerve assessment to assess whether other nerves have been damaged (e.g., facial nerve). Discourage the patient from chewing on the affected side until paresthesias resolve. A soft diet is usually prescribed.

! NURSING SAFETY PRIORITY (QSEN)

Action Alert

Teach the patient who has had percutaneous stereotactic rhizotomy to avoid rubbing the eye on the affected side because the protective mechanism of pain will no longer warn of injury. Instruct him or her to inspect the eye daily for redness or irritation and report to the health care provider any change or blurred vision. Stress the importance of regular dental examinations because the absence of pain may not warn the patient of potential problems.

Surgical Management. In addition to the general preoperative care provided to all patients, the surgeon thoroughly explains the surgical benefits and any expected neurologic deficits. Ensure that the patient understands the procedure to be performed and any risks or complications.

In some patients, a small artery compresses the trigeminal nerve as it enters the pons. Surgical relocation of this artery (**microvascular decompression**) may relieve the pain of TN without compromising facial sensation. This procedure is more invasive, requiring a craniotomy. Though not common, complications include aseptic meningitis, cerebrospinal fluid leak, ataxia, **ipsilateral** (same side) hearing loss, and facial nerve damage. Older adults and patients with other medical problems may not be candidates for this procedure.

In addition to general post-craniotomy care for patients as described in Chapter 45, monitor the patient who has microvascular decompression for signs of complications, including headache, cranial nerve dysfunction, and bleeding. Assess his or her corneal reflex, extraocular muscles, and facial nerve, and report abnormal findings to the surgeon. Document all changes promptly.

Psychosocial considerations for the patient with TN include disappointment with ineffective drug protocols or surgical procedures and fear that the pain may recur with any activity. The patient may fail to move the face in an attempt to prevent pain. This behavior may be misinterpreted by others as withdrawal or depression. Refer patients and their families to the TNA—Facial Pain Association (www.fpa-support.org) for more information and support. TNA of Canada (www.catna.ca) is the national organization in Canada that advocates and informs patients and their families about trigeminal neuralgia.

FACIAL PARALYSIS

❖ PATHOPHYSIOLOGY

Facial paralysis, or **Bell's palsy**, is an acute paralysis of cranial nerve VII but may also affect cranial nerves V (trigeminal) and VIII (vestibulocochlear [auditory]). The condition is also known as *cranial polyneuritis*. Although the incidence may be slightly higher among people with diabetes, Bell's palsy occurs in all ages; however, it is more commonly seen in young adults.

Acute maximum paralysis occurs over 2 to 5 days in almost all patients with this condition. Pain behind the ear or on the face may occur a few hours or even days before paralysis. The disorder involves a drawing sensation and paralysis of all facial muscles on the affected side. The patient cannot close his or her eye, wrinkle the forehead, smile, whistle, or grimace. Tearing may stop or become excessive. The face appears masklike and sags. Taste is usually impaired to some degree, but this symptom seldom persists beyond the second week of paralysis. Tinnitus (ringing in the ears) may also occur. Most patients go into remission within 3 months.

The cause of Bell's palsy is believed to be the result of inflammation triggered by a formerly dormant herpes simplex virus type 1 (HSV-1). Infection, altered IMMUNITY, or exposure to cold may trigger the HSV-1 re-activation. Nurses may encounter patients with Bell's palsy in clinics, office settings, or emergency departments.

❖ INTERPROFESSIONAL COLLABORATIVE CARE

Medical management usually includes corticosteroids, 30 to 60 mg daily, during the first week after the onset of symptoms. Antiviral drugs such as acyclovir (Zovirax), famciclovir

(Famvir), or valacyclovir (Valtrex) may be prescribed for 7 to 10 days after symptoms begin. Mild analgesics may help relieve the altered comfort. Nursing care is directed toward managing the major neurologic deficits and providing psychosocial support. Because the eye does not close, the cornea must be protected from drying and subsequent ulceration or abrasion. Teach the patient to manually close the eyelid at intervals and to instill artificial tears during the day. An ointment to supply moisture can be used at night. The eye may be patched or taped closed at bedtime.

The patient may be unable to chew, sip fluids through a straw, or control drooling on the affected side, creating difficulties at mealtimes. Encourage the patient to eat and drink using the unaffected side of the mouth. High-calorie snacks may supplement meals, and patients may require a soft diet. Explain how to use massage; the application of warm, moist heat; and facial exercises to manage pain and paralysis. In some cases, physical therapy is prescribed. As muscle tone improves, teach the patient to grimace, wrinkle the brow, force the eyes closed, whistle, and blow air out of the cheeks three or four times daily for 5 minutes.

Nerve block to manage pain may be performed, but it is not common. Surgery is reserved for patients with complete, severe Bell's palsy to decompress the facial nerve. In some cases, cosmetic surgery is done.

Although most patients recover fully within a few weeks or months, some may experience permanent neurologic deficits. For chronic pain, gabapentin (Neurontin) may be prescribed. Patients with Bell's palsy may require psychosocial support because body image and self-esteem are affected. Provide both information and psychosocial support. Refer patients and their families to the Bell's Palsy Research Foundation for information (www.angelfire/az/BellsPalsy.com). The Bell's Palsy Association in the United Kingdom is also a good source of Internet-based information (www.bellspalsy.org.uk).

? NCLEX EXAMINATION CHALLENGE 44-3
Safe and Effective Care Environment

The nurse is caring for a client with trigeminal neuralgia. Which patient problem is the **priority** for the nurse?
A. Facial twitching
B. Problems with communication
C. Ptosis and diplopia
D. Severe facial pain

GET READY FOR THE NCLEX® EXAMINATION!

KEY POINTS

Review these Key Points for each NCLEX Examination Client Needs Category.

Safe and Effective Care Environment
- Collaborate with members of the interprofessional health care team, including the primary health care provider, physical and occupational therapists, speech-language pathologist, and dietitian, to establish goals for care and individualized interventions for patients with Guillain-Barré syndrome (GBS) and myasthenia gravis (MG). **QSEN: Teamwork and Collaboration**

Health Promotion and Maintenance
- Refer patients with peripheral nervous system (PNS) disorders to community support groups and health care organizations, such as The Restless Legs Syndrome Foundation and the Myasthenia Gravis Foundation.

Psychosocial Integrity
- Provide alternatives to promote communication for patients with MG, including speaking slowly, lip-reading, and using communication boards or electronic technology. **QSEN: Patient-Centered Care**
- Assess the patient with GBS for altered self-concept and possible depression; assist the patient to identify support resources and other coping strategies. **QSEN: Patient-Centered Care**

Physiological Integrity
- Assess for changes related to GAS EXCHANGE and functional ability for patients with GBS and MG.
- Recall that patients with GBS have ascending paralysis causing impaired MOBILITY, SENSORY PERCEPTION changes, cranial nerve involvement, and autonomic manifestations as a result of demyelination of neurons; the cause of GBS is likely altered IMMUNITY (see Chart 44-1).
- Note that patients with MG have an autoimmune disease in which muscle weakness, including ocular symptoms, is the result of attacks on the acetylcholine receptors at neuromuscular junctions (see Chart 44-3).
- Teach patients about factors that can worsen (exacerbate) MG as listed in Table 44-2. **QSEN: Evidence-Based Practice**
- Remember that the priority for care for patients with GBS and MG is respiratory monitoring and airway management. **QSEN: Safety**
- Prevent complications of immobility for patients with GBS and MG, such as pressure injuries and venous thromboembolic events. **Clinical Judgment**
- Reinforce the need for patients with MG to take their drugs on time. **QSEN: Safety**
- Teach patients on cholinesterase inhibitor drugs and their families about signs and symptoms of cholinergic and myasthenic crises as listed in Table 44-1. **QSEN: Safety**
- For patients having a thymectomy, maintain adequate GAS EXCHANGE and observe for complications such as pneumothorax or hemothorax (e.g., chest pain, shortness of breath). **Clinical Judgment**
- Teach patients with restless legs syndrome to minimize risk factors for the disorder (e.g., exercise, lose weight, and quit smoking). **QSEN: Evidence-Based Practice**
- Recall that trigeminal neuralgia (TN) affects primarily the fifth cranial nerve (although others may be involved) and does not typically involve paralysis or changes in sensation other than excruciating pain along the cranial nerve tract. Facial paralysis (Bell's palsy) affects cranial nerve VII and involves unilateral facial muscle paralysis.
- Prioritize pain management for the care of the patient with TN. **QSEN: Patient-Centered Care**

SELECTED BIBLIOGRAPHY

Asterisk indicates a classic or definitive work on this subject.

*Arcila-Londono, X., & Lewis, R. A. (2012). Guillain-Barré syndrome. *Seminars in Neurology, 32*(3), 179–186.

Burcham, J. L. R., & Rosenthal, L. D. (2016). *Lehne's pharmacology for nursing care* (9th ed.). St. Louis: Elsevier.

Centers for Disease Control and Prevention (CDC). (2017). *Guillain-Barré syndrome.* www.cdc.gov/flu/protect/vaccine/guillainbarre.htm.

*Diaz-Manera, J., Rojas Garcia, R., & Illa, I. (2012). Treatment strategies for myasthenia gravis: An update. *Expert Opinion on Pharmacotherapy, 13*(13), 1873–1883.

*Ibrahim, S. (2012). Trigeminal neuralgia: Diagnostic criteria, clinical aspects and treatment outcomes: A retrospective study. *Gerodontology, 31*(2), 89–94.

Jarvis, C. (2014). *Physical examination & health assessment* (7th ed.). St. Louis: Elsevier Saunders.

*Khan, F., & Amatya, B. (2012). Rehabilitation interventions in patients with acute demyelinating inflammatory polyneuropathy: A systematic review. *European Journal of Physical and Rehabilitation Medicine, 48*(3), 507–522.

Liang, C. L., & Han, S. (2013). Neuromuscular junction disorders. *Physical Medicine and Rehabilitation, 5*(Suppl. 5), S81–S88.

McCance, K., Huether, S., Brashers, V., & Rote, N. (2014). *Pathophysiology: The biologic basis for disease in adults and children* (7th ed.). St. Louis: Mosby.

National Institute of Neurological Disorders and Stroke (NINDS). (n.d.). *Restless leg syndrome.* https://www.ninds.nih.gov/Disorders/All-Disorders/Restless-Legs-Syndrome-Information-Page.

National Institute of Neurological Disorders and Stroke (NINDS). (2013). *Trigeminal neuralgia information page.* www.ninds.nih.gov/disorders/trigeminal_neuralgia/trigeminal_neuralgia.htm.

Pagana, K. D., Pagana, T. J., & Pagana, T. N. (2017). *Mosby's diagnostic and laboratory test reference* (13th ed.). St. Louis: Elsevier.

*Patwa, H. S., Chaudhry, V., Katzerg, H., Rae-Grant, A. D., & So, Y. T. (2012). Evidence-based guideline: Intravenous immunoglobulin in the treatment of neuromuscular disorders. *Neurology, 78*(13), 1009–1015.

Sampathkumar, P., & Sanchez, J. L. (2016). Zika virus in the Americas: A review for clinicians. *Mayo Clinic Proceedings, 91*(4), 514–521.

*Sejvar, J. J., Baughman, A. L., Wise, M., & Morgan, O. W. (2011). Population incidence of Guillain-Barré syndrome: A systematic review and meta-analysis. *Neuroepidemiology, 36*(2), 123–133.

CHAPTER 45

Care of Critically Ill Patients With Neurologic Problems

Laura M. Willis

 http://evolve.elsevier.com/Iggy/

PRIORITY AND INTERRELATED CONCEPTS

The priority concepts for this chapter are:
- PERFUSION
- COGNITION

✳ The PERFUSION concept exemplar for this chapter is Stroke (Brain Attack), p. 928.

✳ The COGNITION concept exemplar for this chapter is Traumatic Brain Injury, p. 940.

The interrelated concepts for this chapter are:
- MOBILITY
- SENSORY PERCEPTION

LEARNING OUTCOMES

Safe and Effective Care Environment

1. Collaborate with members of the interprofessional team to provide safe, effective transitions in care following acute management of patients with a change in PERFUSION and/or COGNITION caused by traumatic brain injury (TBI) and stroke.
2. Prioritize collaborative, evidence-based interventions for patients with a stroke or TBI to ensure optimal functioning and quality of life.

Health Promotion and Maintenance

3. Develop a teaching plan about risk factors for stroke or TBI and prevention of secondary brain injury.
4. Identify community resources to help patients with stroke or TBI achieve or maintain ADL independence.

Psychosocial Integrity

5. Discuss how to support the patient and family coping with life changes that result from stroke, TBI, or brain tumor.

Physiological Integrity

6. Perform a neurologic assessment of patients who are experiencing acute neurologic events of stroke, TBI, or cranial surgery, with a focus on changes in COGNITION.
7. Assess the patient after fibrinolytic therapy for ischemic stroke for potential adverse effects.
8. Apply knowledge of pathophysiology to identify collaborative problems for patients with stroke and TBI, including actual or risk for impaired MOBILITY, SENSORY PERCEPTION, and PERFUSION.
9. Prioritize nursing care for patients having a stroke and TBI, including monitoring for, preventing, and managing increasing intracranial pressure to increase PERFUSION to the brain.
10. Explain the role of chemotherapy, radiation, and surgery in the management of patients with a brain tumor.

Many acute neurologic problems are associated with high mortality and severe morbidity and create significant and enduring impact on patients, their families, and society. Early recognition and comprehensive care of adult patients with acute neurologic compromise by the nurse and interprofessional health care team can reduce mortality and disability. Acute neurologic problems from stroke, brain trauma, and malignancy cause varying degrees of impaired PERFUSION, COGNITION, MOBILITY, and SENSORY PERCEPTION. Chapter 2 reviews each of these health concepts for nursing practice.

TRANSIENT ISCHEMIC ATTACK

Ischemic strokes often follow warning signs such as a **transient ischemic attack (TIA)**. Temporary neurologic dysfunction resulting from a *brief* interruption in cerebral blood flow is easy to ignore or miss, particularly if symptoms resolve by the time the patient reaches the emergency department (ED). Typically, symptoms of a TIA resolve within 30 to 60 minutes (Chart 45-1). TIAs may damage the brain tissue with repeated insults, as seen on MRI or CT scan. Single TIAs indicate a high stroke

CHART 45-1   Key Features

Transient Ischemic Attack

Symptoms resolve typically within 24 hours.

Visual Deficits
- Blurred vision
- Diplopia (double vision)
- Blindness in one eye
- Tunnel vision

Mobility (Motor) Deficits
- Weakness (facial droop, arm or leg drift, hand grasp)
- Ataxia (gait disturbance)

Sensory Perception Deficits
- Numbness (face, hand, arm, or leg)
- Vertigo

Speech Deficits
- Aphasia
- Dysarthria (slurred speech)

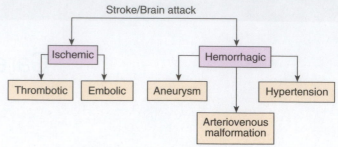

FIG. 45-1 Types of stroke/brain attack.

risk; recurrent and multiple TIAs increase the risk for permanent brain damage.

On admission to the ED, a complete neurologic assessment is performed; and laboratory tests, ECG, and CT scan are performed. If the potential neurologic deficit has resolved, the patient may have further diagnostic testing to evaluate the risk for stroke, including an MRI of carotid and cerebral blood vessels and brain tissue, ultrasound of the carotids, and ECG of the heart. Interprofessional collaborative care focuses on preventing another TIA or possible stroke and may include:

- Reducing high blood pressure (the most common risk factor for stroke) by adding or adjusting drugs to lower blood pressure
- Taking aspirin or other antiplatelet drug (e.g., clopidogrel [Plavix]) to prevent thrombotic or embolic strokes (Amarenco et al., 2014) (see Chapter 36)
- Controlling diabetes (if present) and keeping glucose levels in a target range, typically 100 to 180 mg/dL
- Promoting lifestyle changes, such as smoking cessation, eating more heart-healthy foods, and increasing activity

In collaboration with the interprofessional health team, teach patients about how to achieve a healthier lifestyle to prevent more TIAs or a major stroke. Provide them with information about community resources that can help them meet this desired outcome.

✳ PERFUSION CONCEPT EXEMPLAR
Stroke (Brain Attack)

❖ PATHOPHYSIOLOGY

A stroke is caused by an interruption of PERFUSION to any part of the brain. Chapter 2 reviews the concept of perfusion. The National Stroke Association uses the term brain attack to convey the urgency for acute stroke care similar to that provided for acute myocardial infarction (heart attack). *A stroke is a medical emergency and should be treated immediately to reduce or prevent permanent disability.*

The brain cannot store oxygen or glucose and therefore must receive a constant flow of blood to provide these substances for normal function. In addition, blood flow is important for the removal of metabolic waste (e.g., carbon dioxide, lactic acid). If PERFUSION to any part of the brain is interrupted for more than a few minutes, cerebral tissue dies (infarction). Brain metabolism and blood flow after a stroke can be affected around the infarction and in the contralateral (opposite side) hemisphere. Effects of a stroke on the *nonaffected* side may be the result of brain edema or global changes in PERFUSION in the brain. As a result of brain edema, patients may develop increased intracranial pressure and secondary brain damage.

Types of Strokes

Strokes are generally classified as ischemic (occlusive) or hemorrhagic (Fig. 45-1). Acute ischemic strokes are either thrombotic or embolic in origin (Table 45-1). Most strokes are ischemic.

Ischemic Stroke. An acute ischemic stroke is caused by the occlusion (blockage) of a cerebral or carotid artery by either a thrombus or an embolus. A stroke that is caused by a *thrombus* (clot) is referred to as a thrombotic stroke, whereas a stroke caused by an *embolus* (dislodged clot) is referred to as an embolic stroke.

Thrombotic strokes account for more than half of all strokes and are commonly associated with the development of atherosclerosis in either intracranial or extracranial arteries (usually the carotid arteries). Atherosclerosis is the process by which fatty plaques develop on the inner wall of the affected arterial vessel. Chapter 36 describes this health problem, including its pathophysiology, in detail.

Rupture of one or more atherosclerotic plaques can promote clot formation. When the clot is of sufficient size, it interrupts blood flow to the brain tissue supplied by the vessel, causing an ischemic (occlusive) stroke. The bifurcation (point of division) of the common carotid artery with the internal carotid artery and the vertebral arteries at their junction with the basilar artery are the most common sites involved in atherosclerotic plaque formation because of turbulent blood flow. Because of the gradual nature of clot formation when atherosclerotic plaque is present, thrombotic strokes tend to have a *slow* onset, evolving over minutes to hours.

An *embolic stroke* is caused by a thrombus or a group of thrombi that break off from one area of the body and travel to the cerebral arteries via the carotid artery or vertebrobasilar system. The usual source of emboli is the heart. Emboli can occur in patients with atrial fibrillation, heart valve disease, mural thrombi after a myocardial infarction (MI), a prosthetic heart valve, or endocarditis (infection). Another source of

TABLE 45-1   Differential Features of the Types of Stroke

| FEATURE | ISCHEMIC | | HEMORRHAGIC |
	THROMBOTIC	EMBOLIC	
Evolution	Intermittent or stepwise improvement between episodes of worsening symptoms Completed stroke	Abrupt development of completed stroke Steady progression	Usually abrupt onset
Onset	Gradual (minutes to hours)	Sudden	Sudden; may be gradual if caused by hypertension
Level of consciousness	Preserved (patient is awake)	Preserved (patient is awake)	Deepening lethargy/stupor or coma
Contributing associated factors	Hypertension Atherosclerosis	Cardiac disease	Hypertension Vessel disorders Genetic factors
Prodromal symptoms	Transient ischemic attack (TIA)	TIA	Headache
Neurologic deficits	May be deficits during the first few weeks Slight headache Speech deficits Visual problems Confusion	Maximum deficit at onset Paralysis Expressive aphasia	Focal deficits Severe, frequent
Cerebrospinal fluid	Normal; possible presence of protein	Normal	Bloody
Seizures	No	No	Usually
Duration	Improvements over weeks to months Permanent deficits possible	Usually rapid improvements	Variable Permanent neurologic deficits possible

emboli may be plaque or clot that breaks off from the carotid sinus or internal carotid artery. Emboli tend to become lodged in the smaller cerebral blood vessels at their point of bifurcation or where the lumen narrows.

As the emboli block the vessel, ischemia develops, and the patient experiences the signs and symptoms of the stroke. The occlusion (blockage) may be temporary if the embolus breaks into smaller fragments, enters smaller blood vessels, and is absorbed. For these reasons, embolic strokes are characterized by the *sudden* development and rapid occurrence of neurologic deficits. The symptoms may resolve over a few days. Conversion of an occlusive stroke to a hemorrhagic stroke may occur because the arterial vessel wall is also vulnerable to ischemic damage from blood supply interruption. Sudden hemodynamic stress may result in vessel rupture, causing bleeding directly within the brain tissue.

Hemorrhagic Stroke. The second major classification of stroke is hemorrhagic stroke. In this type of stroke, vessel integrity is interrupted, and bleeding occurs into the brain tissue or into the subarachnoid space.

Intracerebral hemorrhage (ICH) describes bleeding into the brain tissue generally resulting from severe or sustained hypertension. Elevated blood pressure (BP) leads to changes within the arterial wall that leave it likely to rupture. Damage to the brain occurs from bleeding, causing edema, irritation, and displacement, which cause pressure on brain tissue. Cocaine use is one example of a trigger for sudden, dramatic BP elevation leading to hemorrhagic stroke.

Subarachnoid hemorrhage (SAH) is much more common and results from bleeding into the subarachnoid space—the space between the pia mater and arachnoid layers of the meninges covering the brain. This type of bleeding is usually caused by a ruptured aneurysm or arteriovenous malformation.

An aneurysm is an abnormal ballooning or blister along a normal artery commonly developing in a weak spot on the artery wall. Larger aneurysms are more likely to rupture than smaller ones.

An arteriovenous malformation (AVM) is an angled collection of malformed, thin-walled, dilated vessels without a capillary network. This uncommon abnormality occurs during embryonic development. Vasospasm may occur as a result of a sudden and periodic constriction of a cerebral artery, often following an SAH or bleeding from an aneurysm or AVM rupture. This constriction interrupts blood flow to distal areas of the brain. Reduced PERFUSION from vasospasm contributes to secondary cerebral ischemia and further neurologic dysfunction.

Etiology and Genetic Risk

As with many health problems, the causes of stroke are likely a combination of genetic and environmental risk factors. Major risk factors increase the likelihood of strokes and can be divided into those that can be modified and those that cannot (nonmodifiable factors) (see Health Promotion and Maintenance section). Many of these factors have a familial or genetic predisposition and are discussed elsewhere in this text. For example, first-degree (order) relative (mother, father, sister, brother) stroke risk increases with a strong family history of hypertension, atherosclerotic disease, and a diagnosis of aneurysm (McCance et al., 2014). Relatives of a patient with an aneurysm, regardless of vessel location, may be at higher risk for intracranial aneurysms and should consider diagnostic testing and follow-up.

Incidence and Prevalence

Stroke is the fifth leading cause of death in the United States and is considered a major cause of disability worldwide. According to the U.S. Centers for Disease Control and Prevention (CDC), approximately 795,000 people experience new or recurrent stroke; about 130,000 Americans die each year from stroke

(CDC, 2017). About 13,000 Canadians die each year from stroke (Heart and Stroke Foundation, 2017).

Eight southeastern states in the United States are known as the "stroke belt" because they have a mortality rate that is 20% higher than the rest of the nation. The coastal plains of North Carolina, South Carolina, and Georgia have a 40% higher mortality rate. Possible factors influencing these differences include income, education, dietary habits, and access to health care (Bowen, 2016).

It is estimated that there are more than 4.7 million stroke survivors in the United States (CDC, 2017) and 400,000 stroke survivors in Canada living with long-term disability (Heart and Stroke Foundation, 2017). Deaths from stroke have declined over the past 15 years as a result of advances in prompt and effective medical treatment. However, the number of strokes occurring in the younger-adult population is increasing (CDC, 2017). In this group, strokes are associated with illicit drug use because many street drugs cause hypercoagulability, vasospasm, or hypertensive crisis.

Health Promotion and Maintenance

Risk factors that contribute to stroke are divided into three groups: risk factors that can be changed by lifestyle changes (modifiable); those that can be changed with medical management, such as hypertension; and those that cannot be changed, such as family history or race/ethnicity (nonmodifiable).

Lifestyle changes include smoking cessation, if needed; a heart-healthy diet rich in fruits and vegetables and low in saturated fats; and regular activity, including planned exercise. Teach patients that light-to-moderate alcohol consumption may reduce the risk for stroke, but a higher consumption may increase it. Chart 45-2 describes common risk factors that can be changed, often referred to as modifiable risk factors.

Teach patients about the importance of identifying and managing risk factors such as hypertension and diabetes mellitus that contribute to the potential for a major stroke. Remind them to adhere to the plan of care, which may include lifestyle changes, diet therapy, and/or drug therapy to reduce stroke risk.

❖ INTERPROFESSIONAL COLLABORATIVE CARE
◆ Assessment: Noticing

History. Although an accurate history is important in the diagnosis of a stroke, *the first priority is to ensure that the patient is transported to a stroke center.* A stroke center is designated by The Joint Commission (TJC) for its ability to rapidly recognize and effectively treat strokes. TJC designates two distinct levels of stroke-center certification. The *primary certified* stroke center is required to provide diagnostic testing (CT) and stroke therapy

---

CHART 45-2 Patient and Family Education: Preparing for Self-Management

Common Modifiable Risk Factors for Developing a Stroke

- Smoking
- Substance use (particularly cocaine)
- Obesity
- Sedentary lifestyle
- Oral contraceptive use
- Heavy alcohol use
- Use of phenylpropanolamine (PPA), found in antihistamine drugs

---

❓ **NCLEX EXAMINATION CHALLENGE 45-1**
Health Promotion and Maintenance

Which statements about stroke prevention indicate a client's understanding of health teaching by the nurse? **Select all that apply.**
A. "I will take aspirin every day."
B. "I have decided to stop smoking."
C. "I will try to walk at least 30 minutes most days of the week."
D. "I need to cut down a lot on my drinking."
E. "I'm going to decrease salt in my diet."

---

with IV fibrolytic therapy and a stroke team; the *comprehensive* stroke center provides timely and advanced diagnostics and life-saving measures such as endovascular interventions that can prevent long-term disability. Obtaining a history should not delay the patient's arrival to either the stroke center or interventional radiology within the comprehensive stroke center. A focused history to determine if the patient has had a recent bleeding event or is taking an anticoagulant is an important part of the rapid stroke-assessment protocol.

After either receiving fibrinolytic therapy or determining that the patient is not a candidate to receive it, more extensive diagnostic tests and evaluation are done to identify the cause of the stroke and the area of brain involved. Several important parts of the history should be collected:

- What was the patient doing when the stroke began? Hemorrhagic strokes tend to occur during activity.
- How did the symptoms progress? Symptoms of a hemorrhagic stroke tend to occur abruptly, whereas thrombotic strokes generally have a more gradual progression.
- Did the symptoms worsen after the initial onset, or did they begin to improve?
- What is the patient's medical history (with specific attention directed toward a history of head trauma, diabetes, hypertension, heart disease, anemia, and obesity)?
- What are the patient's current medications, including prescribed drugs, over-the-counter (OTC) drugs, herbal and nutritional supplements, and recreational (illicit) drugs?
- What is the patient's social history, including education, employment, travel, leisure activities, and personal habits (e.g., smoking, diet, exercise pattern, drug and alcohol use)?

During the interview, observe the patient's level of consciousness (LOC) and assess for indications of impaired COGNITION and SENSORY PERCEPTION. Question the patient or family member about the presence of SENSORY PERCEPTION deficits or motor changes, visual problems, problems with balance or gait, and changes in reading or writing abilities.

When LOC is suddenly decreased or altered, immediately determine if hypoglycemia or hypoxia is present because these conditions may mimic emergent neurologic disorders. Hypoglycemia and hypoxia are easily treated and reversed, unlike brain injury from inadequate PERFUSION or trauma.

The patient with an SAH, particularly when the hemorrhage is from a ruptured (leaking) aneurysm, often reports the onset of a sudden, severe headache described as "the worst headache of my life." Additional symptoms of SAH or cerebral aneurysmal and AVM bleeding are nausea and vomiting, photophobia, cranial nerve deficits, stiff neck, and change in mental status. There may also be a family history of aneurysms.

Physical Assessment/Signs and Symptoms. First-responder personnel (e.g., paramedics, emergency medical technicians) perform an initial neurologic examination using well-established stroke assessment tools.

> ! **NURSING SAFETY PRIORITY** **QSEN**
> ### *Critical Rescue*
> In the ED, assess the stroke patient within 10 minutes of arrival. This same standard applies to patients already hospitalized for other medical conditions who have a stroke. The priority is assessment of ABCs—**a**irway, **b**reathing, and **c**irculation. Many hospitals have designated stroke teams and centers that are expert in acute stroke assessment and management.

Nurses also perform a complete neurologic assessment on arrival to the ED. The National Institutes of Health Stroke Scale (NIHSS) is a commonly used valid and reliable assessment tool that nurses complete as soon as possible after the patient arrives in the ED and is used as one assessment to determine eligibility for IV fibrinolytics (Table 45-2). The NIHSS includes 11 areas of assessment.

TABLE 45-2 NIH Stroke Scale

CATEGORY AND MEASUREMENT	SCORE*
1a. Level of Consciousness (LOC)	——
0 = Alert; keenly responsive	
1 = Not alert; but arousable by minor stimulation to obey, answer, or respond	
2 = Not alert; requires repeated stimulation to attend or is obtunded and requires strong or painful stimulation to make movements (not stereotyped)	
3 = Responds only with reflex motor or autonomic effects or totally unresponsive, flaccid, and areflexic	
1b. LOC Questions	——
0 = Answers two questions correctly	
1 = Answers one question correctly	
2 = Answers neither question correctly	
1c. LOC Commands	——
0 = Performs two tasks correctly	
1 = Performs one task correctly	
2 = Performs neither task correctly	
2. Best Gaze	——
0 = Normal	
1 = Partial gaze palsy; gaze abnormal in one or both eyes, but forced deviation or total gaze paresis not present	
2 = Forced deviation, or total gaze paresis not overcome by the oculocephalic maneuver	
3. Visual	——
0 = No visual loss	
1 = Partial hemianopia	
2 = Complete hemianopia	
3 = Bilateral hemianopia (blind, including cortical blindness)	
4. Facial Palsy	——
0 = Normal symmetric movements	
1 = Minor paralysis (flattened nasolabial fold, asymmetry on smiling)	
2 = Partial paralysis (total or near-total paralysis of lower face)	
3 = Complete paralysis of one or both sides (absence of facial movement in the upper and lower face)	
5. Motor (Arm)	Right arm:
0 = No drift; limb holds 90 (or 45) degrees for full 10 seconds	——
1 = Drift; limb holds 90 (or 45) degrees, but drifts down before full 10 seconds; does not hit bed or other support	Left arm:
2 = Some effort against gravity; limb cannot get to or maintain (if cued) 90 (or 45) degrees; drifts down to bed but has some effort against gravity	——
3 = No effort against gravity; limb falls	
4 = No movement	
Untestable = Amputation or joint fusion	

Continued

TABLE 45-2 NIH Stroke Scale—cont'd	
CATEGORY AND MEASUREMENT	**SCORE***
6. Motor (Leg)	Right leg: _____
0 = No drift; leg holds 30-degree position for full 5 seconds	Left leg: _____
1 = Drift; leg falls by the end of the 5-second period but does not hit bed	
2 = Some effort against gravity; leg falls to bed by 5 seconds but has some effort against gravity	
3 = No effort against gravity; leg falls to bed immediately	
4 = No movement	
Untestable = Amputation or joint fusion	
7. Limb Ataxia	_____
0 = Absent	
1 = Present in one limb	
2 = Present in two limbs	
Untestable = Amputation or joint fusion	
8. Sensory	_____
0 = Normal; no sensory loss	
1 = Mild-to-moderate sensory loss; patient feels pinprick less sharp or dull on the affected side; or loss of superficial pain with pinprick, but patient aware of being touched	
2 = Severe-to-total sensory loss; patient not aware of being touched in the face, arm, and leg	
9. Best Language	_____
0 = No aphasia; normal	
1 = Mild-to-moderate aphasia; some obvious loss of fluency or facility of comprehension, without significant limitation on ideas expressed or form of expression	
2 = Severe aphasia; all communication is through fragmentary expression; great need for inference, questioning, and guessing by the listener	
3 = Mute, global aphasia; no usable speech or auditory comprehension	
10. Dysarthria	_____
0 = Normal	
1 = Mild-to-moderate dysarthria; patient slurs at least some words and, at worst, can be understood with some difficulty	
2 = Severe dysarthria; patient's speech so slurred as to be unintelligible in the absence of or out of proportion to any dysphasia or is mute/anarthric	
Untestable = Intubated or other physical barrier	
11. Extinction and Inattention (Neglect)	_____
0 = No abnormality	
1 = Visual, tactile, auditory, spatial, or personal inattention or extinction to bilateral simultaneous stimulation in one of the sensory modalities	
2 = Profound hemi-inattention or extinction to more than one modality; does not recognize own hand or orients to only one side of space	

*The patient can have a score of 0 to 40, with 0 having no neurologic deficits and 40 being the most deficits.
Modified from National Institutes of Health (NIH) Stroke Scale, 2013. www.ninds.nih.gov/doctors/NIH_stroke_scale.pdf.

As the patients are transitioned from the ED to other settings, the most important area to assess is the patient's LOC. Use the Glasgow Coma Scale (see Chapter 41) or a modified NIHSS to frequently monitor for changes in LOC throughout the patient's acute care. Specific signs and symptoms of stroke should also be monitored. Stroke symptoms depend on the extent and location of the ischemia and the arteries involved as described in Chart 45-3.

Stroke symptoms can appear at any time of the day or night. The five most common symptoms are (CDC, 2017):

- Sudden confusion or trouble speaking or understanding others
- Sudden numbness or weakness of the face, arm, or leg
- Sudden trouble seeing in one or both eyes
- Sudden dizziness, trouble walking, or loss of balance or coordination
- Sudden severe headache with no known cause

Cognitive Changes. The patient may have impaired COGNITION in addition to changes in LOC. LOC varies, depending on the extent of increased intracranial pressure (ICP) caused by the stroke and the location of the stroke. Assess for:

- Denial of the illness
- Spatial and proprioceptive (awareness of body position in space) dysfunction
- Impairment of memory, judgment, or problem-solving and decision-making abilities
- Decreased ability to concentrate and attend to tasks
- Difficulty in remembering events (past or present)

Dysfunction in one or more of these areas may be severe, depending on the hemisphere involved (Chart 45-4).

The *right* cerebral hemisphere is more involved with visual and spatial awareness and proprioception (sense of body position). A person who has a stroke involving the right cerebral hemisphere is often unaware of any deficits and may

⏩ CHART 45-3 Key Features

Stroke Syndromes

Middle Cerebral Artery Strokes
- Contralateral hemiparesis: arm > leg
- Contralateral sensory perception deficit
- Homonymous hemianopsia
- Unilateral neglect or inattention
- Aphasia, anomia, alexia, agraphia, and acalculia
- Impaired vertical sensation
- Spatial deficit
- Perceptual deficit
- Visual field deficit
- Altered level of consciousness: drowsy to comatose

Posterior Cerebral Artery Strokes
- Perseveration (word or action repetition)
- Aphasia, amnesia, alexia, agraphia, visual agnosia, and ataxia
- Loss of deep sensation
- Decreased touch sensation
- Increased lethargy/stupor, coma

Internal Carotid Artery Strokes
- Contralateral hemiparesis
- Sensory perception deficit
- Hemianopsia, blurred vision, blindness
- Aphasia (dominant side)
- Headache
- Bruit

Anterior Cerebral Artery Strokes
- Contralateral hemiparesis: leg > arm
- Bladder incontinence
- Personality and behavior changes
- Aphasia and amnesia
- Positive grasp and sucking reflex
- Perseveration
- Sensory perception deficit (lower extremity)
- Memory impairment
- Apraxic gait

Vertebrobasilar Artery Strokes
- Headache and vertigo
- Coma
- Memory loss and confusion
- Flaccid paralysis
- Areflexia, ataxia, and vertigo
- Cranial nerve dysfunction
- Dysconjugate gaze
- Visual deficits (uniorbital) and homonymous hemianopsia
- Sensory loss: numbness

⏩ CHART 45-4 Key Features

Left and Right Hemisphere Strokes

FEATURE	LEFT HEMISPHERE*	RIGHT HEMISPHERE
Language	Aphasia Agraphia Alexia	Impaired sense of humor
Memory	Possible deficit	Disorientation to time, place, and person Inability to recognize faces
Vision	Inability to discriminate words and letters Reading problems Deficits in the right visual field Cortical blindness	Visual spatial deficits Neglect of the left visual field Loss of depth perception Cortical blindness
Behavior	Slowness Cautiousness Anxiety when attempting a new task Depression or a catastrophic response to illness Sense of guilt Feeling of worthlessness Worries over future Quick anger and frustration Intellectual impairment	Impulsiveness Lack of awareness of neurologic deficits Confabulation Euphoria Constant smiling Denial of illness Poor judgment Overestimation of abilities (risk for injury)
Hearing	No deficit	Loss of ability to hear tonal variations

*Location for speech in all but 5% to 20% of people.

be disoriented to time and place. Personality changes include impulsivity (poor impulse control) and poor judgment. The *left* cerebral hemisphere, the dominant hemisphere in all but about 15% to 20% of the population, is the center for language, mathematic skills, and analytic thinking. Therefore a left hemisphere stroke may result in:

- **Aphasia**: Inability to speak or comprehend language
- **Alexia** or **dyslexia**: Difficulty reading
- **Agraphia**: Difficulty writing
- **Acalculia**: Difficulty with mathematic calculation

Collaborate with the speech-language pathologist (SLP) who performs the complete assessment of these changes.

Motor (Mobility) Changes. The MOBILITY assessment provides information about which part of the brain is involved. A *right* **hemiplegia** (paralysis on one side of the body) or **hemiparesis** (weakness on one side of the body) indicates a stroke involving the *left* cerebral hemisphere because the motor nerve fibers cross in the medulla before entering the spinal cord and periphery. On the other hand, a *left* hemiplegia or hemiparesis indicates a stroke in the *right* cerebral hemisphere. If the brainstem or cerebellum is affected, the patient may experience hemiparesis or **quadriparesis** (weakness in all extremities), **ataxia** (gait disturbance), and cranial nerve deficits.

In collaboration with the physical therapist (PT) and occupational therapist (OT), assess the patient's muscle tone. The findings may include:

- **Hypotonia,** or **flaccid paralysis**: Inability to overcome the forces of gravity, and the extremities tend to fall to the side when lifted
- **Hypertonia (spastic paralysis)**: Increased muscle activity causing fixed positions or increased tone of the involved extremities.
- **Agnosia**: Inability to use an object correctly

- **Apraxia**: Inability to perform previously learned motor skills or commands (may be verbal or motor)

Sensory Changes. The SENSORY PERCEPTION assessment focuses on the patient's response to touch and painful stimuli. In addition to diminished motor function, decreased sensation typically occurs on the affected side of the body.

Evaluate for sensory changes such as:

- **Unilateral inattention (body neglect) syndrome**: Being unaware of the existence of his or her paralyzed side (particularly common with strokes in the *right* cerebral hemisphere)
- **Ptosis**: Eyelid drooping
- **Hemianopsia**: Blindness in half of the visual field, resulting from damage to the optic tract or occipital lobe
- **Homonymous hemianopsia**: Blindness in the same side of both eyes (Fig. 45-2)
- **Nystagmus**: Involuntary movements of the eyes (can be vertical or horizontal)
- **Paresthesias**: Numbness, tingling, or unusual sensations

Cranial Nerve Function. Assess the patient's ability to chew, which reflects the function of cranial nerve (CN) V. Assessment of the patient's ability to swallow reflects the function of CNs IX and X. In addition, note any facial paralysis or paresis (CN VII), diminished or absent gag reflex (CN IX), or impaired tongue movement (CN XII). The patient who has difficulty chewing or swallowing foods and liquids (**dysphagia**) is at risk for aspiration pneumonia and may become constipated or dehydrated from inadequate fluid intake. Assess for pocketing of food under the tongue or buccal mucosa caused by diminished ability to propel food with the tongue. Also assess the patient's ability to cough, which reflects the function of CN X. If the cough reflex is minimal or absent, the patient is at risk for aspiration.

Cardiovascular Assessment. Patients with embolic strokes may have a heart murmur, dysrhythmias (most often atrial fibrillation), or hypertension. It is not unusual for the patient to be admitted to the hospital with a blood pressure greater than 180 to 200/110 to 120 mm Hg, especially if he or she has a hypertensive bleed. Although a somewhat higher blood pressure of 150/100 mm Hg is needed to maintain cerebral PERFUSION after an acute ischemic stroke, pressures above this reading may lead to extension of the stroke.

Psychosocial Assessment. The typical patient with a stroke is older than 65 years, is hypertensive, and has varying degrees of impaired MOBILITY and level of consciousness. Speech, language, and COGNITION deficits, as well as behavior and memory problems, may also occur.

Assess the patient's reaction to the illness, especially in relation to changes in body image, self-concept, and ability to perform ADLs. In collaboration with the patient's family and friends, identify any problems with coping or personality changes.

Ask about the patient's financial status and occupation, because they may be affected by the residual neurologic deficits of the stroke and the potential long recovery. Patients who do not have disability or health insurance may worry about how their family will cope financially with the disruption in their lives. Early involvement of social services, certified hospital chaplain, or psychological counseling may enhance coping skills.

Assess for **emotional lability** (uncontrollable emotional state) especially if the frontal lobe or right side of the brain has been affected. In such cases, the patient often laughs and then cries unexpectedly for no apparent reason. Explain the cause of uncontrollable emotions to the family or significant others so they do not feel responsible for these reactions.

Laboratory Assessment. Clinical history and presentation are usually enough to identify a stroke once it has occurred. No definitive laboratory tests confirm its diagnosis. Elevated hematocrit and hemoglobin levels are often associated with a severe

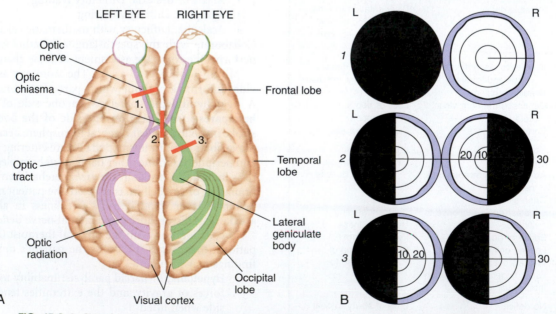

FIG. 45-2 A, Site of lesions causing visual loss. *1,* Total blindness left eye; *2,* Bitemporal hemianopia; *3,* Left homonymous hemianopia. **B,** Visual fields corresponding to lesions shown in **A.** *1,* Total blindness left eye; *2,* Bitemporal hemianopia; *3,* Left homonymous hemianopia. (**A,** From Ball, J. W., Dains, J. E., Flynn, J. A., Solomon, B. S., & Stewart, R. W. [2015]. *Seidel's guide to physical examination* [8th ed.]. St. Louis: Mosby. **B,** modified from Stein, H. A., Slatt, B. J., & Stein, R. M. [1994]. *The ophthalmic assistant* [6th ed.]. St. Louis: Mosby.)

or major stroke as the body attempts to compensate for lack of oxygen to the brain. An elevated white blood cell (WBC) count may indicate the presence of an infection or a response to physiologic stress or inflammation.

The primary health care provider typically requests a prothrombin time (PT) or international normalized ratio (INR) and a partial thromboplastin time (PTT) to establish baseline information before anticoagulation therapy may be started.

Imaging Assessment. For definitive evaluation of a suspected stroke, *CT perfusion scan* is used to assess ischemia of brain tissue (or areas of decreased PERFUSION to or in brain tissue). Cerebral aneurysms or AVM may also be identified. *Magnetic resonance angiography (MRA)* and multimodal techniques such as perfusion-weighted imaging enhance the sensitivity of the MRI to detect early changes in the brain, including confirming blood flow. *Ultrasonography* (carotid duplex scanning) may also be performed.

◆ Analysis: Interpreting

Depending on stroke severity and/or response to immediate management, the priority collaborative problems for patients with a stroke may include:

1. Inadequate PERFUSION to the brain due to interruption of arterial blood flow and a possible increase in ICP
2. Decreased MOBILITY and ability to perform ADLs due to neuromuscular or cognitive impairment
3. Aphasia or dysarthria due to decreased circulation in the brain or facial muscle weakness
4. SENSORY PERCEPTION deficits due to altered neurologic reception and transmission

◆ Planning and Implementation: Responding

Improving Cerebral Perfusion

Planning: Expected Outcomes. The patient with a stroke is expected to have improved cerebral PERFUSION to maintain adequate brain function and prevent further brain injury.

Interventions. Improvements in acute stroke management have helped to decrease deaths from stroke. Most hospitals in the United States have designated stroke centers; however, community and rural acute care settings may not have access to a neurologist or other resources needed to manage an acute stroke. As a result, teleneurology using two-way video technology is a growing strategy to provide acute stroke consultation with a board-certified neurologist (Bowen, 2016).

Interventions for patients experiencing strokes are determined primarily by the type and extent of the stroke. The immediate primary role of the nurse is to manage the patient receiving treatment and continuously assess for increasing intracranial pressure.

Nonsurgical Management. Nursing interventions are initially aimed at monitoring for neurologic changes or complications associated with stroke and its treatment. The two major treatment modalities for patients with acute ischemic stroke are IV fibrinolytic therapy and endovascular interventions. Regardless of the immediate management approach used, once the patient is stable, provide ongoing supportive care. Provide interventions to prevent and/or monitor for early signs of complications, such as hyperglycemia, urinary tract infection, and pneumonia. Implement interventions to prevent patient falls. These health problems are discussed in appropriate chapters in this textbook.

Fibrinolytic Therapy. For select patients with ischemic strokes, early intervention with IV fibrinolytic therapy ("clot-busting drug") is the standard of practice to improve blood flow to viable tissue around the infarct or through the brain. The success of fibrinolytic therapy for a stroke depends on the interval between the time that symptoms begin and treatment is available. IV (systemic) fibrinolytic therapy (also called *thrombolytic therapy*) for an acute ischemic stroke dissolves the cerebral artery occlusion to re-establish blood flow and prevent cerebral infarction. Alteplase (tPA [tissue plasminogen activator], Activase) is the only drug approved at this point for the treatment of acute ischemic stroke. The most important factor in determining whether or not to give alteplase is the time between symptom onset and time seen in the stroke center. Currently, the U.S. Food and Drug Administration (FDA) approves administration of alteplase within 3 hours of stroke onset. The American Stroke Association endorses extension of that time frame to 4.5 hours to administer this fibrinolytic for patients *unless* they fall into one or more of these categories:

- Age older than 80 years
- Anticoagulation regardless of international normalized ratio (INR)
- Imaging evidence of ischemic injury involving more than one third of the brain tissue supplied by the middle cerebral artery
- Baseline National Institutes of Health Stroke Scale score greater than 25
- History of both stroke and diabetes

♥ GENDER HEALTH CONSIDERATIONS

Patient-Centered Care QSEN

> Previous studies have suggested that being a female is a risk factor for delay in recognizing early symptoms of stroke and may contribute to ineligibility for fibrinolytic therapy. Current data show that women have a better understanding of stroke warning signs but may not seek care in an ED at the same speed as men. Women are also less likely to perceive the severity of symptoms, leading to diagnostic or treatment delay (Ramírez-Moreno et al., 2015). A study by Focht et al. (2014) found that women knew more about traditional stroke symptoms than men but did not recognize mild or unusual symptoms.

Fibrinolytic therapy is explained to the patient and/or family member, and informed consent is obtained. The dosage of the drug is based on the patient's actual weight. Each hospital has strict protocols for mixing and administering the fibrinolytic drug and for monitoring the patient before and after fibrinolytic drug administration. In some cases, the patient's blood pressure may be too high to give the medication. In this instance, the patient receives a rapid-acting antihypertensive drug such as labetalol (Normodyne) or nicardipine (Cardene) until the blood pressure is below 185/110 (McKay et al., 2015).

! NURSING SAFETY PRIORITY QSEN

Drug Alert

> In addition to frequent monitoring of vital signs, carefully observe for signs of intracerebral hemorrhage and other signs of bleeding during administration of fibrinolytic drug therapy. Other best practice interventions are listed in Chart 45-5.

CHART 45-5 **Best Practice for Patient Safety & Quality Care** QSEN

Nursing Interventions During and After IV Administration of Alteplase

- Perform a double check of the dose. Use a programmable pump to deliver the initial dose of 0.9 mg/kg (maximum dose 90 mg) over 60 minutes, with 10% of the dose given as a bolus over 1 minute. Do not manually push this drug.
- Admit the patient to a critical care or specialized stroke unit.
- Perform neurologic assessments, including vital signs, every 10 to 15 minutes during infusion and every 30 minutes after that for at least 6 hours; monitor hourly for 24 hours after treatment. Be consistent regarding the device used to obtain blood pressures because blood pressures can vary when switching from a manual to a noninvasive automatic to an intra-arterial device.
- If systolic blood pressure is 180 mm Hg or greater or diastolic is 105 mm Hg or greater during or after tissue plasminogen activator (tPA), give antihypertensive drugs as prescribed (IV is recommended for faster response).
- To prevent bleeding, do not place invasive tubes, such as nasogastric (NG) tubes or indwelling urinary catheters, until the patient is stable (usually for 24 hours).
- Discontinue the infusion if the patient reports severe headache or has severe hypertension, bleeding, nausea, and/or vomiting; notify the health care provider immediately.
- Obtain a follow-up CT scan after treatment before starting antiplatelet or anticoagulant drugs.

NCLEX EXAMINATION CHALLENGE 45-2

Physiological Integrity

The nurse is caring for a patient treated with alteplase following a stroke. Which assessment finding is the **highest priority** for the nurse?

A. Client's blood pressure is 144/90.
B. Client is having epistaxis.
C. Client ate only half of the last meal.
D. Client continues to be drowsy.

Endovascular Interventions. Endovascular procedures to improve PERFUSION include intra-arterial thrombolysis using drug therapy, mechanical embolectomy (clot removal), and carotid stent placement. *Intra-arterial thrombolysis* has the advantage of delivering the fibrinolytic agent directly into the thrombus within 6 hours of the stroke onset. It is particularly beneficial for some patients who have an occlusion of the middle cerebral artery or those who arrive in the ED after the window for IV alteplase. Patients having either fibrinolytic therapy or endovascular interventions are admitted to the critical care setting for intensive collaborative monitoring.

Carotid artery angioplasty with stenting is common to prevent or, in some cases, help manage an acute ischemic stroke. This interventional radiology procedure is usually done under moderate sedation. It may be performed by a cardiovascular surgeon or interventional radiologist. A technique using a distal/embolic protection device has made this procedure very safe. The device is placed beyond the stenosis through a catheter inserted into the femoral artery (groin). The device catches any clot debris that breaks off during the procedure. Placement of a carotid stent is performed to open a blockage in the carotid artery typically at the division of the common carotid artery into the internal and external carotid arteries. Throughout the

---

CHART 45-6 **Key Features**

Increased Intracranial Pressure (ICP)

- Decreased level of consciousness (LOC) (lethargy to coma)
- Behavior changes: restlessness, irritability, and confusion
- Headache
- Nausea and vomiting (may be projectile)
- Change in speech pattern/slurred speech:
  - Aphasia
- Change in sensorimotor status:
  - Pupillary changes: dilated and nonreactive pupils ("blown pupils") or constricted and nonreactive pupils
  - Cranial nerve dysfunction
  - Ataxia
- Seizures (usually within first 24 hours after stroke)
- Cushing's triad:
  - Severe hypertension
  - Widened pulse pressure
  - Bradycardia
- Abnormal posturing:
  - Decerebrate
  - Decorticate

---

procedure, the patient's neurologic and cardiovascular statuses must be carefully assessed.

! **NURSING SAFETY PRIORITY** QSEN

Action Alert

Before discharge after carotid stent placement, teach the patient to report these symptoms to the health care provider as soon as possible:
- Severe headache
- Change in LOC or COGNITION (e.g., drowsiness, new-onset confusion)
- Muscle weakness or motor dysfunction
- Severe neck pain
- Swelling at neck incisional site
- Hoarseness or difficulty swallowing (due to nerve damage)

When the stroke is hemorrhagic and the cause is related to an AVM or cerebral aneurysm, the patient is evaluated for the optimal procedure to stop bleeding. Some procedures can be used to prevent bleeding in an AVM or aneurysm that is discovered *before* symptom onset or SAH. Procedures occur in the interventional radiology suite or operating room.

Following carotid stent placement, *hyperperfusion syndrome* can occur, which has a high morbidity and mortality rate. This syndrome is thought to be the result of an impaired autoregulation of cerebral blood flow that results from long-standing decreased cerebral PERFUSION pressure resulting from carotid artery disease. The signs and symptoms include severe temporal headache, hypertension, seizures, and focal neurologic deficits. This syndrome may be associated with intracranial hemorrhage and may occur within 1 hour after the procedure up to 24 hours or even 1 week later (Orion et al., 2015).

Monitoring for Increased Intracranial Pressure. The patient is most at risk for increased ICP resulting from edema during the first 72 hours after onset of the stroke. Some patients may have worsening of their neurologic status starting within 24 to 48 hours after their endovascular procedure from increased ICP (Chart 45-6). Reassess patients with acute stroke and after endovascular treatment of stroke symptoms every 1 to 4 hours, depending on severity of the condition. Use the approved agency assessment strategy and documentation tools.

Best practices for managing increasing ICP for patients experiencing a stroke include:

- Elevate the head of the bed per agency or primary health care provider (PHCP) protocol to improve PERFUSION pressure.
- Provide oxygen therapy to prevent hypoxia for patients with oxygen saturation less than 94% or per agency or PHCP protocol or prescription.
- Maintain the head in a midline, neutral position to promote venous drainage from the brain.
- Avoid sudden and acute hip or neck flexion during positioning. Extreme hip flexion may increase intrathoracic pressure, leading to decreased cerebral venous outflow and elevated ICP. Extreme neck flexion also interferes with venous drainage from the brain and intracranial dynamics.
- Avoid the clustering of nursing procedures (e.g., giving a bath followed immediately by changing the bed linen). When multiple activities are clustered in a narrow time period, the effect on ICP can be dramatic elevation.
- Hyperoxygenate the patient before and after suctioning to avoid transient hypoxemia and resultant ICP elevation from dilation of cerebral arteries.
- Provide airway management to prevent unnecessary suctioning and coughing that can increase ICP.
- Maintain a quiet environment for the patient experiencing a headache, which is common with a cerebral hemorrhage or increased ICP.
- Keep the room lights low to accommodate any photophobia (sensitivity to light) the patient may have.
- Closely monitor blood pressure, heart rhythm, oxygen saturation, blood glucose, and body temperature to prevent secondary brain injury and promote positive outcomes after stroke.

Although the optimal blood pressure range after stroke is controversial, the primary health care provider often desires that the patient with *acute ischemic stroke* be slightly hypertensive, with a systolic blood pressure (SBP) between 140 and 150 mm Hg to promote cerebral tissue PERFUSION.

Monitoring for Other Complications. Monitor the patient with an aneurysm or arteriovenous malformation (AVM) and patients following repair of these vessel malformations for signs and symptoms of hydrocephalus and vasospasm. Hydrocephalus (increased cerebrospinal fluid [CSF] within the ventricular and subarachnoid spaces) may occur as a result of blood in the CSF. This prevents CSF from being reabsorbed properly by the arachnoid villi because of obstruction by small clots. Cerebral edema, which interferes with the flow of CSF out from the ventricular system, may also develop. Eventually the ventricles become enlarged. If hydrocephalus is left untreated, increased intracranial pressure (ICP) results. Observe for signs and symptoms of hydrocephalus, which are similar to those of ICP elevation, including a change in the LOC. Clinical findings may also include headache, pupil changes, seizures, poor coordination, gait disturbances (if ambulatory), and behavior changes.

If blood is in the subarachnoid space, the patient is at risk for *cerebral vasospasm*. Signs and symptoms of vasospasm may include decreased LOC, motor and reflex changes, and increased neurologic deficits (e.g., cranial nerve dysfunction, motor weakness, and aphasia). The symptoms may fluctuate with the occurrence and degree of vasospasm present. Hemorrhage-related cerebral vasospasm can result in permanent vascular changes and irreversible neurologic impairment.

Rebleeding or rupture is a common complication for the patient with an aneurysm or AVM. Recurrent hemorrhage may occur within 24 hours of the initial bleed or rupture and up to 7 to 10 days later. Assess for severe headache, nausea and vomiting, a decreased LOC, and additional neurologic deficits. Potential consequences of a second cerebral hemorrhagic event may be catastrophic.

Ongoing Drug Therapy. Ongoing drug therapy depends on the type of stroke and the resulting neurologic dysfunction. In general, the purposes of drug therapy are to prevent further thrombotic or embolic episodes (with antithrombotics and anticoagulation) and to protect the neurons from hypoxia.

Antithrombotics include the use of aspirin or other antiplatelet drugs (e.g., clopidogrel [Plavix]) and are the standard of care for treatment following acute ischemic strokes and for preventing future strokes. Sodium heparin and other anticoagulants, such as warfarin (Coumadin, Warfilone), are used in the presence of atrial fibrillation. *Anticoagulants are high-alert drugs that can cause bleeding, including intracerebral hemorrhage.*

An *initial* dose of 325 mg of aspirin (Ecotrin, Ancasal) is recommended within 24 to 48 hours after stroke onset (CDC, 2017). Aspirin should not be given within 24 hours of fibrinolytic administration. Aspirin is an antiplatelet drug that prevents further clot formation by reducing platelet adhesiveness (clumping or "stickiness"). It can cause bruising, hemorrhage, and liver disease over a long-term period. Teach the patient to report any unusual bruising or bleeding to the primary health care provider.

A calcium channel blocking drug that crosses the blood-brain barrier such as nimodipine (Nimotop) may be given to treat or prevent cerebral vasospasm after a subarachnoid hemorrhage. Vasospasm, which usually occurs between 4 and 14 days after the stroke, slows blood flow to the area and causes ischemia. Nimodipine works by relaxing the smooth muscles of the vessel wall and reducing the incidence and severity of the spasm. In addition, this drug dilates collateral vessels to ischemic areas of the brain.

Stool softeners, analgesics for pain, and antianxiety drugs may also be prescribed as needed for symptom management.

Stool softeners also prevent the Valsalva maneuver during defecation to prevent increased ICP.

Promoting Mobility and ADL Ability

Planning: Expected Outcomes. The patient with a stroke is expected to ambulate and provide self-care independently, with or without one or more assistive-adaptive devices.

Interventions. In collaboration with the rehabilitation therapists, assess the patient's functional ability for bed MOBILITY skills, ambulation with or without assistance, and ADL ability, including feeding, bathing, and dressing. Patients who have had a stroke are at risk for aspiration due to impaired swallowing as a result of muscle weakness. Therefore the best practice for all *suspected* and *diagnosed* stroke patients is to maintain NPO status until their swallowing ability is assessed. Follow agency guidelines for screening or use an evidence-based bedside swallowing screening tool to determine if dysphagia is present. Refer the patient to the speech-language pathologist for a swallowing evaluation per stroke protocol as needed. If dysphagia is present, develop a collaborative plan of care to prevent aspiration and support nutrition. A study by Mosselman et al. (2013) found that hospitalized stroke patients become malnourished after 10 days in the acute care setting. Collaborate with the registered dietitian to ensure that nutritional needs are met. Monitor the patient's weight daily and serum pre-albumin levels to notice any decrease from baseline.

Many patients who have an untreated stroke often have flaccid or spastic paralysis. It is not unusual for the patient to eventually have a flaccid arm and spastic leg on the affected side because the affected leg often regains function more quickly than the arm. Be sure to support the affected flaccid arm of the stroke patient, and teach unlicensed assistive personnel (UAP) to avoid pulling on it. Position the arm on a pillow while the patient is sitting to prevent it from hanging freely, which could cause shoulder subluxation. The physical therapist (PT) or occupational therapist (OT) may provide a slinglike device to support the arm during ambulation. Chapter 6 describes interventions for rehabilitation, including improving MOBILITY and promoting self-care.

Patients begin rehabilitation as soon as possible to regain function and prevent complications of immobility, such as pneumonia, atelectasis, and pressure injuries. Another major complication of impaired MOBILITY is the development of venous thromboembolism (VTE), especially deep vein thrombosis (DVT), which can lead to a pulmonary embolism (PE). This risk is highest in older patients and those with a severe stroke. Per The Joint Commission's Core Measures for VTE, provide care to prevent this complication by applying intermittent sequential pneumatic devices, changing the patient's position frequently, and ambulating the patient if possible. Report any indications of DVT to the primary health care provider and document assessments in the patient's record. Chapter 36 discusses VTE prevention in detail.

Promoting Effective Communication

Planning: Expected Outcomes. The patient with a stroke is expected to receive, interpret, and express spoken, written, and nonverbal messages, if possible. However, some patients may need to develop strategies for alternative methods of communication, such as pictures, images, or nonverbal language.

Interventions. Language or speech problems are usually the result of a stroke involving the dominant hemisphere. The left cerebral hemisphere is the speech center in most patients. Speech and language problems may be the result of aphasia or

---

TABLE 45-3	**Types of Aphasia**

Expressive (or Nonfluent)
- Referred to as *Broca's*, or *motor*, *aphasia*
- Difficulty speaking
- Difficulty writing

Receptive
- Referred to as *Wernicke's*, or *sensory*, *aphasia*
- Difficulty understanding spoken words
- Difficulty understanding written words
- Speech often meaningless
- Made-up words

Mixed
- Combination of difficulty understanding words and speech
- Difficulty with reading and writing

Global
- Profound speech and language problems
- Often no speech or sounds that cannot be understood

---

dysarthria. Aphasia is caused by cerebral hemisphere damage; **dysarthria** (slurred speech) is the result of a loss of motor function to the tongue or the muscles of speech, causing facial weakness and slurred speech.

Aphasia can be classified in a number of ways. Most commonly, it is classified as expressive, receptive, or mixed (Table 45-3). **Expressive (Broca's, or motor) aphasia** is the result of damage in Broca's area of the frontal lobe. It is a motor speech problem in which the patient generally understands what is said but cannot speak. He or she also has difficulty writing but may be able to read. Rote speech and automatic speech such as responses to a greeting are often intact. The patient is aware of the deficit and may become frustrated and angry.

Receptive (Wernicke's, or sensory) aphasia is caused by injury involving Wernicke's area in the temporoparietal area. The patient cannot understand the spoken and often the written word. Although he or she may be able to talk, the language is often meaningless.

Usually the patient has some degree of dysfunction in the areas of both expression and reception. This is known as *mixed* or *global aphasia*. Reading and writing ability are equally affected. Few patients have only expressive *or* receptive aphasia. In most cases, though, one type is dominant.

To help communicate with the patient with aphasia, use these guiding principles:

- Present one idea or thought in a sentence (e.g., "I am going to help you get into the chair.").
- Use simple one-step commands rather than ask patients to do multiple tasks.
- Speak slowly but not loudly; use cues or gestures as needed.
- Avoid "yes" and "no" questions for patients with expressive aphasia.
- Use alternative forms of communication if needed, such as a computer, handheld mobile device, communication board, or flash cards (often with pictures).
- Do not rush the patient when speaking.
- For more specific communication strategies for the patient with aphasia or dysarthria, collaborate with the speech-language pathologist.

NCLEX EXAMINATION CHALLENGE 45-3

Physiological Integrity

The nurse is caring for a client with expressive (Broca's) aphasia. Which nursing intervention is **appropriate** for communicating with the client?

A. Refer the client to the speech-language pathologist.
B. Speak loudly to help the client interpret what is being said.
C. Provide pictures to help the client communicate.
D. Ask the client to read messages on a white board.

Managing Changes in Sensory Perception

Planning: Expected Outcomes. The major concern of patients with SENSORY PERCEPTION deficits is adapting to neurologic deficits. Therefore the patient with a stroke is expected to adapt to sensory perception changes in vision, proprioception (position sense), and sensation and to be free from injury.

Interventions. Patients with right hemisphere brain damage typically have difficulty with visual-perceptual or spatial-perceptual tasks. They often have problems with depth and distance perception and with discrimination of right from left or up from down. Because of these problems, patients can have difficulty performing routine ADLs. Caregivers can help the patient adapt to these disabilities by using frequent verbal and tactile cues and by breaking down tasks into discrete steps. *Always approach the patient from the unaffected side, which should face the door of the room!*

Unilateral inattention, or neglect syndrome, occurs most commonly in patients who have had a right cerebral stroke. However, it can occur in any patient who experiences *hemianopsia*, in which the vision of one or both eyes is affected. This problem places the patient at additional risk for injury, especially falls, because of an inability to recognize his or her physical impairment or because of a lack of proprioception (position sense).

- Teach the patient to touch and use both sides of the body.
- When dressing, remind the patient to dress the affected side first.
- If homonymous hemianopsia is present, teach the patient to turn his or her head from side to side to expand the visual field because the same half of each eye is affected. This scanning technique is also useful when the patient is eating or ambulating.

Place objects within the patient's field of vision. A mirror may help visualize more of the environment. If the patient has diplopia (double vision), a patch may be placed over the affected eye and changed every 2 to 4 hours.

The patient with a left hemisphere lesion generally has memory deficits and may show significant changes in the ability to carry out simple tasks, such as eating and grooming. Help with ADLs but encourage the patient to do as much as possible independently. To assist with memory problems, re-orient the patient to the month, year, day of the week, and circumstances surrounding hospital admission. Establish a routine or schedule that is as structured, repetitious, and consistent as possible. Provide information in a simple, concise manner. Apraxia may be present. Typically the patient with apraxia exhibits a slow, cautious, and hesitant behavior style. The physical therapist (PT) helps the patient compensate for loss of position sense.

Care Coordination and Transition Management

The patient with a stroke may be discharged to home, a rehabilitation center, or a skilled nursing facility (SNF). Some patients have no significant neurologic dysfunction and are able to return home and live independently or with minimal support. Other patients are able to return home but require ongoing assistance with ADLs and supervision to prevent accidents or injury. The case or care manager coordinates speech-language, physical, and/or occupational therapy services to continue in the home or on an ambulatory care basis. Patients admitted to an inpatient rehabilitation unit/facility or SNF require continued or more complex nursing care and extensive physical, occupational, recreational, speech-language, or cognitive therapy. The expected outcome for rehabilitation is to maximize the patient's abilities in all aspects of life.

Eight core measures are associated with the care of stroke patients by the interprofessional health care team (The Joint Commission, 2017). Certification as a Primary Stroke Center or a Comprehensive Stroke Center is tied to consistent performance in achieving satisfactory core measures. The core measures may have additional implications in terms of reimbursement in the future. The eight core measures for Ischemic Stroke Care for all patients include:

- Venous thromboembolism (VTE) prophylaxis
- Discharge with antithrombotic therapy
- Discharge with anticoagulation therapy for atrial fibrillation/flutter
- Thrombolytic therapy as indicated
- Antithrombotic therapy re-evaluated by end of hospital day 2
- Discharge on statin medication
- Stroke education provided and documented
- Assessment for rehabilitation

Nurses not only provide direct care to patients with stroke but also contribute to the peer review process to evaluate and monitor the care provided to patients with ischemic stroke who are planning transition from the hospital for continued care.

Home Care Management. Collaborate with the case manager to plan the patient's discharge. Coordinate with rehabilitation therapists to identify needs for assistive or adaptive and safety equipment. The extent of this assessment depends on the patient's disabilities, if any. Teach the patient and family to ensure that the home is free from scatter rugs or other obstacles in the walking pathways. The bathtub and toilet should be equipped with grab bars. Anti-skid patches or strips should be placed in the bathtub to prevent slipping. The PT or OT works with the patient and the family or significant others to obtain all needed assistive devices and home modifications *before* the patient is discharged from the hospital, rehabilitation setting, or SNF. Appointments for ambulatory care speech, physical, and occupational therapy, if needed, are arranged before discharge for seamless transition management and care coordination.

Self-Management Education. As part of the discharge process, teach the family about the signs and symptoms of depression that may occur within 3 months after a stroke. The strongest predictors of post-stroke depression (PSD) are a history of depression, severe stroke, and post-stroke physical or cognitive impairment. Patients may not exhibit typical signs of depression because of their cognitive, physical, and emotional impairments. PSD is associated with increased morbidity and mortality, especially in older men.

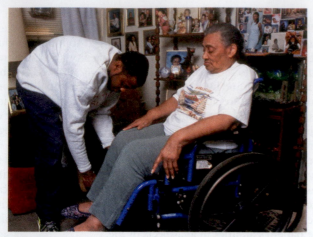

FIG. 45-3 Son adjusting his mother's wheelchair as part of caregiving responsibilities.

The three areas that should be included in patient and family education are disease prevention, disease-specific information, and self-management. The teaching plan may include lifestyle changes, drug therapy, ambulation/transfer skills, communication skills, safety precautions, nutritional management, activity levels, and self-management skills. Health teaching should focus on tasks that must be performed by the patient and the family after hospital discharge. Return demonstrations help to evaluate the family members' competency in tasks required for the patient's care (Fig. 45-3). Provide both written and verbal instruction in all these areas. Pierce & Steiner (2013) described the successful use of an interactive stroke website that was developed in a local community to provide information and support for patients and their families.

Specific teaching for stroke patients (and their families) includes:

- Provide information about prescribed drugs to prevent another stroke and control hypertension. Instruct the patient and the family in the name of each drug, the dosage, the timing of administration, how to take it, and possible side effects.
- Teach the patient how to climb stairs safely, if he or she is able; transfer from the bed to a chair; get into and out of a car; and use any aids for MOBILITY.
- Provide important information regarding what to do in an emergency and who to call for nonemergency questions.

Patients who have had a TIA or stroke are at risk for another stroke. Teach family members to observe for and act on signs of a new stroke using the **F.A.S.T.** pneumonic:

- **F**ace drooping
- **A**rm weakness
- **S**peech or language difficulty
- **T**ime to call 9-1-1

Families may feel overwhelmed by the continuing demands placed on them. Depending on the location of the lesion, the patient may be anxious, slow, cautious, and hesitant and lack initiative (left hemisphere lesions). As a result of right hemisphere lesions, he or she may be impulsive and seemingly unaware of any deficit. Family member caregivers are often uncertain about the progress of the patient and can become depressed the longer they care for him or her (Godwin et al.,

2013; White et al., 2014). Therefore family members need to spend time away from the patient on a routine basis to continue to provide full-time care without sacrificing their own physical and emotional health. Refer the family to social services or other community resources for further support, counseling, and possible respite care.

Health Care Resources. Available resources include a variety of publications from the American Heart Association (www.americanheart.org), including *Stroke: A Guide for Families* and *Stroke: Why Do They Behave That Way?* The National Stroke Association (www.stroke.org) also provides publications and videotapes for caregivers and patients. *Recovering After a Stroke: A Patient and Family Guide* is available from the Agency for Healthcare Research and Quality (www.ahrq.gov). A good resource for stroke information and family support in Canada is the Heart and Stroke Foundation of Canada (www.heartandstroke.com). Refer the patient and family members or significant others to local stroke support groups.

For patients who require symptom management or end-of-life care, refer the family to palliative care or hospice services. Chapter 7 gives a detailed description of end-of-life care and advance directives.

◆ Evaluation: Reflecting

Evaluate the care of the patient with stroke based on the identified priority patient problems. The expected outcomes are that the patient:

- Has adequate cerebral PERFUSION to avoid long-term disability
- Maintains blood pressure and blood sugar within a safe, prescribed range
- Performs self-care and MOBILITY activities independently, with or without assistive devices
- Learns to adapt to SENSORY PERCEPTION changes, if present
- Communicates effectively or develops strategies for effective communication as needed
- Has adequate nutrition and avoids aspiration

✳ COGNITION CONCEPT EXEMPLAR
Traumatic Brain Injury

❖ PATHOPHYSIOLOGY

Traumatic brain injury (TBI) is damage to the brain from an external mechanical force and not caused by neurodegenerative or congenital conditions. TBI can lead to temporary and permanent impairment in COGNITION, MOBILITY, SENSORY PERCEPTION, and/or psychosocial function (see Chapter 2 for review of these concepts).

Various terms are used to describe the brain injuries that occur when a mechanical force is applied either directly or indirectly to the brain. A force produced by a blow to the head is a *direct* injury, whereas a force applied to another body part with a rebound effect to the brain is an *indirect* injury. The brain responds to these forces by movement within the rigid cranial vault. It may also rebound or rotate on the brainstem, causing diffuse nerve axonal injury (shearing injuries). The brain may be contused (bruised) or lacerated (torn) as it moves over the inner surfaces of the cranium, which are irregularly shaped and sharp.

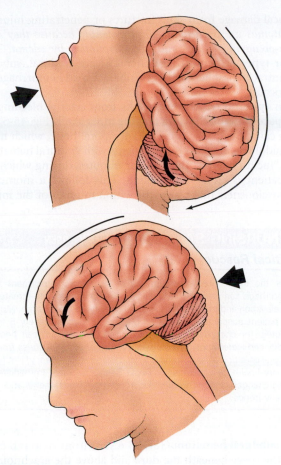

FIG. 45-4 Head movement during acceleration-deceleration injury, which is typically seen in motor vehicle crashes.

Movement or distortion within the cranial cavity is possible because of multiple factors. The first factor is how the brain is supported by cerebrospinal fluid (CSF) within the cranial cavity. When external force is applied to the head, the brain can be injured by the internal surfaces of the skull. The second factor is the consistency of brain tissue, which is very fragile and prone to injury. Brain injury occurs both from initial forces on the cranium and brain and as a result of secondary injury related to mechanical pressure or cerebral edema.

The type of force and the mechanism of injury contribute to TBI. An *acceleration* injury is caused by an external force contacting the head, suddenly placing the head in motion. A *deceleration* injury occurs when the moving head is suddenly stopped or hits a stationary object (Fig. 45-4). These forces may be sufficient to cause the cerebrum to rotate about the brainstem, resulting in shearing, straining, and distortion of the brain tissue, particularly of the axons in the brainstem and cerebellum. Small areas of hemorrhage (contusion, intracranial hemorrhage) may develop around the blood vessels that sustain the impact of these forces (stress), with destruction of adjacent brain tissue. Particularly affected are the basal nuclei and the hypothalamus, which are located deep in the brain.

Primary Brain Injury

Primary brain damage occurs at the time of injury and results from the physical stress (force) within the tissue caused by blunt or penetrating force. A primary brain injury may be categorized as focal or diffuse. A *focal* brain injury is confined to a specific area of the brain and causes localized damage that can often be detected with a CT scan or MRI. *Diffuse* injuries are characterized by damage throughout many areas of the brain. They initially are at a microscopic level and not initially detectable by CT scan. MRI has greater ability to detect microscopic damage, but these areas may not be imaged until necrosis occurs.

Primary brain injuries are also classed as either open or closed. An *open* traumatic brain injury occurs when the skull is fractured or when it is pierced by a penetrating object. The integrity of the brain and the dura is violated, and there is exposure to environmental contaminants. Damage may occur to the underlying vessels, dural sinuses, brain, and cranial nerves. In a *closed* traumatic brain injury, the integrity of the skull is intact, but damage to the brain tissue can still occur as a result of increased intracranial pressure.

TBI is further defined as mild, moderate, or severe. Generally, the determination of severity of TBI is the result of the Glasgow Coma Scale (GCS) score immediately following resuscitation, the presence (or absence) of brain damage imaged by CT or MRI following the trauma, an estimation of the force of the trauma, and symptoms in the injured person.

Secondary Brain Injury

Secondary injury to brain injury includes any processes that occur *after* the initial injury and worsen or negatively influence patient outcomes. Secondary injuries result from physiologic, vascular, and biochemical events that are an extension of the primary injury. The most common secondary injuries result from hypotension and hypoxia, intracranial hypertension, and cerebral edema. Damage to the brain tissue occurs primarily because the delivery of oxygen and glucose to the brain is interrupted from cerebral edema and increasing pressure.

Hypotension and Hypoxia. Both hypotension, defined as a mean arterial pressure less than 70 mm Hg, and hypoxemia, defined as a partial pressure of arterial oxygen (Pao_2) less than 80 mm Hg, restrict the flow of blood to vulnerable brain tissue. Hypotension may be related to shock (see Chapter 37) or other states of reduced PERFUSION to the brain such as clot formation. Hypoxia can be caused by respiratory failure, asphyxiation, or loss of airway and impaired ventilation (see Chapter 32). These problems may occur as a direct result of moderate-to-severe brain injury or secondary to systemic injuries and comorbidities. Low blood flow and hypoxemia contribute to cerebral edema, creating a cycle of deteriorating PERFUSION and hypoxic damage. Patients with hypoxic damage related to moderate or severe brain injury face a poor prognosis and eventually experience decreased COGNITION.

Increased Intracranial Pressure. The cranial contents include brain tissue, blood, and cerebrospinal fluid (CSF). These components are encased in the relatively rigid skull. Within this space, there is little room for any of the components to expand or increase in volume. *A normal level of ICP is 10 to 15 mm Hg.* Periodic increases in pressure occur with straining during defecation, coughing, or sneezing but do not harm the uninjured brain. A sustained ICP of greater than 20 mm Hg is considered detrimental to the brain because neurons begin to die.

As a result of brain injury, the increase in the volume of one component must be compensated for by a decrease in the volume of one of the other components. As a first response to an increase in the volume of any of these components, the CSF is shunted or displaced from the cranial compartment to the spinal subarachnoid space, or the rate of CSF absorption is increased. An additional response, if needed, is a decrease in cerebral blood volume by movement of cerebral venous blood into the sinuses or jugular veins. As long as the brain can compensate for the increase in volume and remain compliant, increases in ICP are minimal.

Increased ICP is the leading cause of death from head trauma in patients who reach the hospital alive. It occurs when compliance no longer takes place and the brain cannot accommodate further volume changes. As ICP increases, cerebral PERFUSION decreases, leading to brain tissue ischemia and edema. If edema remains untreated, the brainstem may herniate downward through the Foramen of Monro or laterally from a unilateral lesion within one cerebral hemisphere, causing irreversible brain damage and possibly death (**brain herniation syndromes**).

Three types of edema may contribute to increased ICP: vasogenic edema, cytotoxic edema, and interstitial edema. *Vasogenic edema* is caused by an abnormal permeability of the walls of the cerebral vessels, which allows protein-rich plasma infiltrate to leak into the extracellular space of the brain. The fluid collects primarily in the white matter. *Cytotoxic edema* may occur as a result of a hypoxic insult, which causes a disturbance in cellular metabolism and active ion transport. The brain is quickly depleted of available oxygen, glucose, and glycogen and converts to anaerobic metabolism. Damage to cell membranes results in cell edema, cell dysfunction, and cell death. Cytotoxic edema may lead to vasogenic edema and a further increase in ICP. *Interstitial edema* occurs with fluid accumulation between the cells of the brain. It is associated with elevated blood pressure or increased CSF pressure. Interstitial edema develops rapidly in the perivascular and periventricular white space and can be controlled through measures to reduce blood pressure or decrease CSF pressures.

Hemorrhage. Hemorrhage, which causes a brain hematoma (collection of blood) or clot, may occur as part of the primary injury and begin at the moment of impact. It may also arise later from vessel damage. Classically, bleeding is caused by vascular damage from the shearing force of the trauma or direct physical damage from skull fractures or penetrating injury. *All hematomas are potentially life threatening because they act as space-occupying lesions and are surrounded by edema.* Three major types of hemorrhage after TBI are epidural, subdural, and intracerebral hemorrhage. Subarachnoid hemorrhage may also occur.

An **epidural hematoma** results from arterial bleeding into the space between the dura and the inner skull (Fig. 45-5). It is often caused by a fracture of the temporal bone, which houses the middle meningeal artery. Patients with epidural hematomas have "lucid intervals" that last for minutes, during which time the patient is awake and talking. This follows a momentary unconsciousness that can occur within minutes of the injury.

> ⚠️ **NURSING SAFETY PRIORITY** QSEN
> ### Critical Rescue
> After the initial interval, symptoms of neurologic impairment from hemorrhage can progress very quickly, with potentially life-threatening ICP elevation and irreversible structural damage to brain tissue. Monitor the patient suspected of epidural bleeding frequently (every 5 to 10 minutes) for changes in neurologic status. The patient can become quickly and increasingly symptomatic. *A loss of consciousness from an epidural or subdural hematoma is a neurosurgical emergency!* Notify the primary health care provider or Rapid Response Team immediately if these changes occur. Carefully document your assessments and identify any trends.

A **subdural hematoma (SDH)** results from venous bleeding into the space beneath the dura and above the arachnoid (see Fig. 45-5). It occurs most often from a tearing of the bridging veins within the cerebral hemispheres or from a laceration of brain tissue. *Bleeding from this injury occurs more slowly than from an epidural hematoma.* SDHs are subdivided into acute, subacute, and chronic. An acute SDH presents within 48 hours after impact; the subacute SDH, between 48 hours and 2 weeks; and the chronic SDH, from 2 weeks to several months after

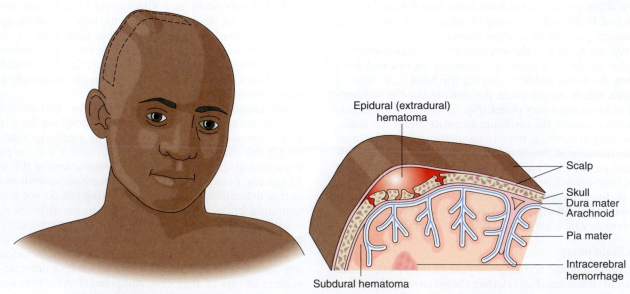

Epidural (extradural) hematoma — Scalp — Skull — Dura mater — Arachnoid — Pia mater — Intracerebral hemorrhage — Subdural hematoma

FIG. 45-5 Epidural hematoma (outside the dura mater of the brain), subdural hematoma (under the dura mater), and intracerebral hemorrhage (within the brain tissue).

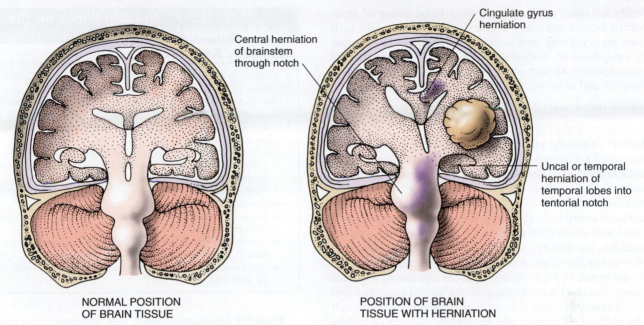

Central herniation of brainstem through notch

Cingulate gyrus herniation

Uncal or temporal herniation of temporal lobes into tentorial notch

NORMAL POSITION OF BRAIN TISSUE

POSITION OF BRAIN TISSUE WITH HERNIATION

FIG. 45-6 Herniation syndromes.

injury. SDHs have the highest mortality rate because they often are unrecognized until the patient presents with severe neurologic compromise.

Traumatic **intracerebral hemorrhage** (ICH) is the accumulation of blood within the brain tissue caused by the tearing of small arteries and veins in the subcortical white matter (see Fig. 45-5). It often acts as a space-occupying lesion (e.g., a tumor) and may be potentially devastating, depending on its location. ICH may also produce significant brain edema and ICP elevations. A traumatic brainstem hemorrhage occurs as a result of a blow to the back of the head, fractures, or torsion injuries to the brainstem. Brainstem injuries have a very poor prognosis.

Hydrocephalus. Hydrocephalus is an abnormal increase in CSF volume. It may be caused by impaired reabsorption of CSF at the arachnoid villi (from subarachnoid hemorrhage or meningitis), called a *communicating hydrocephalus*. It may also be caused by interference or blockage with CSF outflow from the ventricular system (from cerebral edema, tumor, or debris) (called a *noncommunicating hydrocephalus*). The ventricles may dilate from the relative increase in CSF volume. Ultimately, if not treated, this increase may lead to increased ICP.

Brain Herniation. In the presence of increased ICP, the brain tissue may shift and herniate downward. Of the several types of herniation syndromes (Fig. 45-6), *uncal herniation* is one of the most clinically significant because it is life threatening. It is caused by a shift of one or both areas of the temporal lobe, known as the **uncus**. This shift creates pressure on the third cranial nerve. Late findings include dilated and nonreactive pupils, ptosis (drooping eyelids), and a rapidly deteriorating level of consciousness. Central herniation is caused by a downward shift of the brainstem and the diencephalon from a supratentorial lesion. It is clinically manifested by Cheyne-Stokes respirations, pinpoint and nonreactive pupils, and potential hemodynamic instability. All herniation syndromes are potentially life threatening, and the physician must be notified immediately when they are suspected.

Etiology

The most common causes of TBI in the United States are falls and motor vehicle crashes, followed by colliding with a stationary or moving object (CDC, 2017a). Alcohol and drugs are significant contributing factors to the causes of TBI. Summer and spring months, evenings, nights, and weekends are associated with the greatest number of injuries. Young males are more likely than young females to have a TBI. Men tend to play more sports, take more risks when driving, and consume larger amounts of alcohol than women. Falls are the most common cause of TBI in older adults.

♥ VETERANS' HEALTH CONSIDERATIONS
Patient-Centered Care **QSEN**

The United States is seeing increasing numbers of survivors of brain injury from wartime blast injuries. As a result, TBI has become a major health problem among veterans of war and active military personnel.

Incidence and Prevalence

Annually, at least 1.7 million people sustain a TBI in the United States. Of these, about 52,000 die, 275,000 are hospitalized, and 1.4 million are treated and released from an emergency department because of mild TBI (CDC, 2017a). In Canada, statistics are calculated for acquired brain injuries (ABIs), which include both traumatic *and* nontraumatic brain injuries, such as strokes.

Health Promotion and Maintenance

Nurses can educate the public on ways to decrease the incidence of TBI by using safe driving practices such as not driving while impaired and wearing seat belts. Teach people at risk about how alcohol and illicit drug use affect driving ability. Promote the use of helmets for skateboarding and bicycle and motorcycle riding. Help prevent falls by providing a safe environment, especially for older adults. People need to be aware of environmental factors that may increase the likelihood of falls such as inadequate lighting and loose rugs. When possible, install safety equipment in bathtubs and showers. Evaluate balance and coordination as part of a falls prevention strategy inside the hospital and at home.

❖ INTERPROFESSIONAL COLLABORATIVE CARE

◆ Assessment: Noticing

History. Obtaining an accurate history from a patient who has sustained a TBI may be difficult because of changes in the patient's COGNITION. The seriousness of the injury can cause **amnesia** (loss of memory). It is not unusual for the patient to experience amnesia for events before or after the injury. The patient with a serious brain injury may be unconscious or in a confused and combative state. If the patient cannot provide information, the history can be obtained from first responders or witnesses to the injury. Always ask when, where, and how the injury occurred. Did the patient lose consciousness; if so, for how long? Has there been a change in the level of consciousness (LOC)? If trauma is related to drug or alcohol consumption, it may be difficult to differentiate neurologic changes caused by head trauma from those produced by intoxication.

Determine whether the patient had fluctuating consciousness or seizure activity and whether there is a history of a seizure disorder. Obtain precise information about the circumstances of falls, particularly in the older patient (Chart 45-7). Other pertinent information includes hand dominance, any diseases of or injuries to the eyes, and any allergies to drugs or food. Inquire about a history of alcohol or drug use because these substances may interfere with the neurologic baseline assessment. Consider whether the patient is a victim of violence if he or she lives in residential care. The Joint Commission and the Centers for Medicare and Medicaid Services require that all patients be screened for abuse and neglect when they are admitted to any type of health care facility.

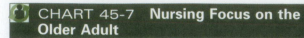

CHART 45-7   Nursing Focus on the Older Adult

Traumatic Brain Injury

- Brain injury is the fifth leading cause of death in older adults (CDC, 2017a).
- The 65- to 75-year age-group has second highest incidence of brain injury of all age-groups (CDC, 2017a).
- Falls and motor vehicle crashes are the most common causes of brain injury (CDC, 2017a).
- Factors that contribute to high mortality are:
  - Falls causing subdural hematomas (closed head injuries), especially chronic subdural hematomas
  - Poorly tolerated systemic stress, which is increased by admission to a high-stimuli environment
  - Medical complications, such as hypotension, hypertension, and cardiac problems
  - Decreased protective mechanisms, which make patients susceptible to infections (especially pneumonia)
  - Decreased immunologic competence, which is further diminished by brain injury

Physical Assessment/Signs and Symptoms. No two brain injuries are alike. The patient with a TBI may have a variety of signs and symptoms depending on the severity of injury and the resulting increase in intracranial pressure (ICP) (Table 45-4). Chart 45-8 lists possible signs and symptoms of mild TBI. For any patient having a TBI, assess for signs of increased ICP, hypotension, hypoxemia (decreased blood level of oxygen), **hypercarbia** ($Paco_2$ greater than 40 to 45 mm Hg or increased partial pressure of carbon dioxide in arterial blood), or **hypocarbia** ($Paco_2$ less than 40 to 45 mm Hg or decreased partial pressure of carbon dioxide in arterial blood). *Hypercarbia* can cause cerebral vasodilation and contribute to elevated ICP. *Hypocarbia* is caused by hyperventilation and can lead to profound vasoconstriction with resulting ischemia. Carbon dioxide levels in an intubated patient can be determined with

TABLE 45-4	Differences Among Mild, Moderate, and Severe Traumatic Brain Injury	
TYPE	**CAUSED BY**	**SYMPTOMS**
Mild traumatic brain injury (MTBI)	Characterized by a blow to the head, transient confusion or feeling dazed or disoriented, and one or more of these conditions: (1) loss of consciousness for up to 30 minutes, (2) loss of memory for events immediately before or after the accident, and (3) focal neurologic deficit(s) that may or not be transient. Loss of consciousness does not have to occur for a person to be diagnosed with MTBI. No evidence of brain damage on a CT or MRI imaging scan.	Includes a wide array of physical and cognitive problems that range from headache and dizziness to changes in behavior listed on Chart 45-7. Symptoms usually resolve within 72 hours. Symptoms may persist and last days, weeks, or months. Persistent symptoms following MTBI are also referred to as *post-concussion syndrome*.
Moderate	A moderate TBI is characterized by a period of loss of consciousness (LOC) for 30 minutes to 6 hours and a GCS score of 9 to 12. Often but not always, focal or diffuse brain injury can be seen with a diagnostic CT or MRI scan. Post-traumatic amnesia (memory loss) may last up to 24 hours. May occur with either closed or open brain injury.	A short acute or critical care stay may be needed for close monitoring and to prevent secondary injury from brain edema, intracranial bleeding, or inadequate cerebral PERFUSION.
Severe	A severe TBI is defined by a GCS score of 3 to 8 and loss of consciousness for longer than 6 hours. Focal and diffuse damage to the brain, cerebrovascular vessels, and/or ventricles is common. Both open and closed head injuries can cause severe TBI, and injury can be focal or diffuse. CT and MRI scans can capture images of tissue damage quite early in the course of this illness.	Patients with severe TBI require management in critical care, including monitoring of hemodynamics, neurologic status, and possibly intracranial pressure (ICP). Patients with severe TBI are also at high risk for secondary brain injury from cerebral edema, hemorrhage, reduced PERFUSION, and the biomolecular cascade.

GCS, Glasgow Coma Scale.

> **CHART 45-8 Key Features**

Mild Traumatic Brain Injury

Physical Findings
- Appears dazed or stunned
- Loss of consciousness <30 minutes (unresponsive after injury)
- Headache
- Nausea
- Vomiting
- Balance or gait problems
- Dizziness
- Visual problems
- Fatigue
- Sensitivity to light
- Sensitivity to noise

Cognitive Findings
- Feeling mentally foggy
- Feeling slowed down

- Difficulty concentrating
- Difficulty remembering
- Amnesia about the events around the time of injury

Sleep Disturbances
- Drowsiness
- Sleeping less than usual
- Sleeping more than usual
- Trouble falling asleep

Emotional Changes
- Irritability
- Sadness
- Nervousness
- More "emotional"
- Depression

---

an end-tidal carbon dioxide ($EtCO_2$) monitor, or **capnography**. The early detection of changes in the patient's neurologic status enables the health care team to prevent or treat potentially life-threatening complications. Subtle changes in blood pressure, consciousness, and pupillary reaction to light can be very informative about neurologic deterioration.

Airway and Breathing Pattern Assessment. *The first priority is the assessment of the patient's ABCs—airway, breathing, and circulation.* Because TBI is occasionally associated with cervical spinal cord injuries, all patients with head trauma are treated as though they have cord injury until radiography proves otherwise. *Older adults are especially prone to cervical injuries at the first or second vertebral level, a life-threatening problem.* Assess for indicators of spinal cord injury, such as loss of MOBILITY and SENSORY PERCEPTION, tenderness along the spine, and abnormal head tilt.

> **! NURSING SAFETY PRIORITY** **QSEN**
>
> **Critical Rescue**
>
> The upper cervical spinal nerves innervate the diaphragm to control breathing. Monitor all TBI patients for respiratory problems and diaphragmatic breathing, as well as for diminished or absent reflexes in the airway (cough and gag). Hypoxia and hypercapnia are best detected through arterial oxygen levels (partial pressure of arterial oxygen [PaO_2]), oxygen saturation (SpO_2), and end-tidal volume carbon dioxide measurement ($EtCO_2$). Observe chest wall movement and listen to breath sounds. Report any sign of respiratory problems immediately to the physician!

Injuries to the brainstem may cause a major life-threatening change in the patient's breathing pattern, such as Cheyne-Stokes respirations and/or apnea. In the unconscious patient, an artificial airway provides protection from aspiration and a route for oxygenation. Mechanical ventilation may be needed to support inadequate respiratory effort.

Spine Precautions. Patients with blunt trauma to the head or neck are typically transported from the scene of the injury to the hospital with a rigid cervical collar and a long spine board. The goal is to prevent new and secondary spine injury. Spine precautions require placing the patient supine and aligning the spinal column in a neutral position so there is no rotation, flexion, or extension. The long spine board is removed as soon as possible on arrival to the emergency department (ED) or ICU. The rigid cervical collar is maintained until definitive diagnostic studies to rule out cervical spine injury are completed.

Once the spine board is removed, spinal precautions are maintained until the provider indicates that it is safe to bend or rotate the cervical, thoracic, and lumbar spine. Spinal precautions include: (1) bedrest; (2) no neck flexion with a pillow or roll; (3) no thoracic or lumbar flexion with head of bed elevation/bed controls (reverse Trendelenburg is acceptable); (4) manual control of the cervical spine anytime the rigid collar is removed; and (5) using a "log roll" procedure to reposition the patient. A hard, rigid cervical collar is used to maintain cervical spine ("C-spine") precautions and immobilization with a confirmed cervical injury. If the collar is ill-fitting or soiled, it may be changed according to hospital guidelines while a second qualified person maintains C-spine immobilization. Frequent assessment of the skin under the collar is important to monitor for skin breakdown.

Spine clearance is a clinical decision made by the health care provider, often in collaboration with the radiologist. Spine clearance includes determining the absence of acute bony, ligamentous, and neurologic abnormalities of the cervical spine based on history, physical examination, and/or negative radiologic studies.

Vital Signs Assessment. The mechanisms of autoregulation are often impaired as the result of a TBI. The more serious the injury, the more severe is the impact on *autoregulation* or the ability of cerebral vasculature to modify systemic pressure such that blood flow to the brain is sufficient. Monitor the patient's blood pressure and pulse frequently based on agency protocol and patient status. The patient may have hypotension or hypertension. **Cushing's triad,** a classic but late sign of increased ICP, is manifested by severe hypertension, a widened pulse pressure (increasing difference between systolic and diastolic values), and bradycardia. This triad of cardiovascular changes usually indicates imminent death.

Neurologic Assessment. Many hospitals use the Glasgow Coma Scale (GCS) to document neurologic status (see Chapter

41). A change of 2 points is considered clinically important; notify the primary health care provider if the change is a 2-point or more deterioration of GCS values.

The most important variable to assess with any brain injury is LOC! A decrease or change in LOC is typically the *first* sign of deterioration in neurologic status. A decrease in arousal, increased sleepiness, and increased restlessness or combativeness are all signs of declining neurologic status. *Early* indicators of a change in LOC include behavior changes (e.g., restlessness, irritability) and disorientation, which are often subtle in nature. *Report any of these signs and symptoms immediately to the primary health care provider!*

Use a bright light to assess pupillary size and reaction to light. Facial trauma may swell eyelids, making this assessment difficult. Consider whether drugs that affect pupillary dilation and constriction, such as anticholinergics or adrenergics, have been used recently.

! NURSING SAFETY PRIORITY QSEN

Critical Rescue

Check pupils of TBI patients for size and reaction to light, particularly if the patient is unable to follow directions, to assess changes in level of consciousness. *Report and document any changes in pupil size, shape, and reactivity to the primary health care provider immediately because they could indicate an increase in ICP!*

Pupillary changes or eye signs differ depending on which areas of the brain are damaged. *Pinpoint and nonresponsive pupils are indicative of brainstem dysfunction at the level of the pons.* Of particular importance is the ovoid pupil, which is regarded as the mid-stage between a normal-size and a dilated pupil. Asymmetric (uneven) pupils, loss of light reaction, or unilateral or bilateral dilated pupils are treated as herniation of the brain from increased ICP until proven differently. *Pupils that are fixed (nonreactive) and dilated are a poor prognostic sign. Patients with this problem are sometimes referred to as having "blown" pupils.*

Check gross vision if the patient's condition permits. Have the patient read any printed material (e.g., your name tag) or count the number of fingers that you hold within his or her visual field. Loss of vision is usually caused by either direct injury to the eye or injury to the occipital lobe.

Monitor for additional late signs of increased ICP. These manifestations include severe headache, nausea, vomiting (often projectile), and seizures. The provider may evaluate for papilledema (seen by ophthalmoscopic examination). Papilledema *is edema and hyperemia (increased blood flow) of the optic disc. It is always a sign of increased ICP.* Headache and seizures are a response to the injury and may or may not be associated with increased ICP. Always remember that the patient with a brain injury is at risk for potentially devastating ICP elevations during the first hours after the event and up to 3 to 4 days after injury when cerebral edema can occur.

Assess for bilateral *motor* responses. The patient's motor loss or dysfunction usually appears contralateral (opposite side) to the site of the lesion, similar to that of a stroke. For example, a left-sided hemiparesis reflects an injury to the right cerebral hemisphere. Deterioration in MOBILITY or the development of abnormal posturing (decerebrate or decorticate posturing) or flaccidity is another indicator of progressive brain injury (see

Chapter 41). These changes are the result of dysfunction within the pyramidal (motor) tracts of the spinal cord. Assess for brainstem or cerebellar injury, which may cause ataxia (loss of balance), decreased or increased muscle tone, and weakness. Remember that absence of motor function may also be an indicator of a spinal cord injury.

Carefully observe the patient's ears and nose for any signs of cerebrospinal fluid (CSF) leaks that result from a basilar skull fracture. Suspicious ear or nose fluid can be analyzed by the laboratory for glucose and electrolyte content. CSF placed on a white absorbent paper or linen can be distinguished from other fluids by the "halo" sign, a clear or yellowish ring surrounding a spot of blood. Although other body fluids can be used, a halo sign is most reliable when blood is in the center of the absorbent material because tears and saliva can also cause a clear ring in some conditions.

Palpate the patient's head gently to detect the presence of fractures or hematomas. Look for areas of ecchymosis (bruising), tender areas of the scalp, and lacerations. *Raccoon's eyes* are purplish discoloration around eyes that can follow fracture of the skull's base. When CT scans are used with head and brain injury, these fractures are often visualized before bruising appears.

Psychosocial Assessment. Patients with any level of TBI usually have varying degrees of psychosocial changes that may persist for a year or for a lifetime, depending on the severity of the injury and the individual's response. Personality changes manifested by temper outbursts, depression, risk-taking behavior, and denial of disability can occur. The patient may become talkative and develop a very outgoing personality. Memory, especially recent or short-term memory, is often affected. The patient may report difficulties in COGNITION, such as concentrating or the ability to learn new information, and may have problems with insight and planning. Aggressive behavior, agitation, and sleep disorders may interfere with the ability to return to work or school. The ability to communicate and understand the spoken and written language may be altered. Changes in MOBILITY and SENSORY PERCEPTION may necessitate rehabilitation or use of assistive devices. All these changes in health status may lead to difficulties within the family structure and with social and work-related interactions.

Laboratory Assessment. There are no established serum tests to diagnose a primary brain injury. Detection of the protein *S-100B* in serum has shown some promise as an indicator of brain injury (Defazio et al., 2013).

Imaging Assessment. The primary health care provider immediately requests CT of the brain to identify the extent and scope of injury. This diagnostic test can identify the presence of an injury that requires surgical intervention, such as an epidural or subdural hematoma. An *MRI* may be done to detect subtle changes in brain tissue and show more specific detail of the brain injury. MRI is particularly useful in the diagnosis of diffuse axonal injury, but it is not recommended for patients with ICP-monitoring devices. A functional MRI may be done to more specifically detect anoxic injury to the brain.

◆ Analysis: Interpreting

The priority collaborative problems for patients with traumatic brain injury (TBI) vary greatly, depending on the severity of the event. The most common problems include:

1. Potential for decreased cerebral tissue PERFUSION due to primary event and/or secondary brain injury

2. Potential for decreased memory, sensation, and/or mobility due to primary or secondary brain injury

◆ Planning and Implementation: Responding

Maintaining Cerebral Tissue Perfusion

Planning: Expected Outcomes. The expected outcome is that the patient will maintain adequate cerebral tissue PERFUSION with no evidence of secondary brain injury from cerebral edema and increased ICP.

Interventions. The patient with a *severe* TBI is admitted to the critical care unit or a trauma center. Patients with *moderate* TBI are admitted to either the general nursing unit or the critical care unit, where they are closely observed for at least 24 hours. Those with *mild* TBI are usually sent home from the emergency department with instructions for home-based observation and primary care provider follow-up. In some cases, the patient is hospitalized for careful observation by staff. Cerebral PERFUSION is *not* typically affected by a mild TBI.

Nonsurgical Management. *As with any critically injured patient, priority is given to maintaining a patent airway, breathing, and circulation.* Specific nursing interventions for the patient with a TBI are directed toward preventing or detecting secondary brain injury or the conditions that contribute to secondary brain injury such as increased ICP, promoting fluid and electrolyte balance, and monitoring the effects of treatments and drug therapy. Providing health teaching and emotional support for the patient and family are vital parts of the plan of care.

Preventing and Detecting Secondary Brain Injury. Take and record the patient's *vital signs* every 1 to 2 hours or more often based on patient acuity. The health care provider may prescribe IV fluids or drug therapy to prevent severe hypertension or hypotension. Dysrhythmias and nonspecific ST-segment or T-wave changes may occur, possibly in response to stimulation of the autonomic nervous system or an increase in the level of circulating catecholamines (such as epinephrine) from the stress of trauma. *Document and report the presence of cardiac dysrhythmias, hypotension, and hypertension to the primary health care provider.* Obtain the target range for blood pressure and heart rate from the health care provider and monitor parameters.

The patient with a brain injury may develop a fever as a result of systemic trauma, blood in the cranium, or a generalized inflammatory response to the injury. Fever from any cause is associated with higher morbidity and mortality rates (Madden & DeVon, 2015).

Therapeutic hypothermia may be started, regardless of the presence of fever. The purpose of therapeutic hypothermia is to rapidly cool the patient to a core temperature of 89.6° and 93.2° F (32° to 34° C) for 24 to 48 hours after the primary injury. Rewarming to a normal core temperature requires specialized knowledge and skill because rapid fluid and electrolyte shifts can cause cardiac dysrhythmias and changes to systemic and cerebral pressures. The rationale for therapeutic hypothermia is to reduce brain metabolism and prevent the cascade of molecular and biochemical events that contribute to secondary brain injury in moderate-to-severe TBI.

Arterial blood gas (ABG), oxygen saturation (SpO_2), and end-tidal carbon dioxide ($EtCO_2$) values are all used to evaluate respiratory status and guide mechanical ventilation therapy. *Hyperventilation* for the intubated patient during the first 24 hours after brain injury is usually avoided because it may produce ischemia by causing cerebral vasoconstriction. *Carbon dioxide is a very potent vasodilator that can contribute to increases in ICP.*

Prevent intermittent and sustained hypoxemia. Monitor peripheral oxygen saturation continuously in moderate-to-severe TBI. Hypoxemia damages brain tissue and contributes to cerebral vasodilation and increased ICP. Arterial oxygen levels (PaO_2) are maintained between 80 and 100 mm Hg to prevent secondary injury. If the patient is intubated, provide 100% oxygen before and after each pass of the endotracheal suction catheter. Avoid overly aggressive hyperventilation with endotracheal suctioning because of the potential for hypocarbia. Cerebral ischemia caused by even transiently decreased oxygen and either high or low carbon dioxide levels contributes to secondary brain injury. Lidocaine given IV or endotracheally may be used to suppress the cough reflex; coughing increases ICP.

⚠ NURSING SAFETY PRIORITY QSEN
Action Alert

Position the TBI patient to avoid extreme flexion or extension of the neck and to maintain the head in the midline, neutral position. Log roll him or her during turning to avoid extreme hip flexion and keep the head of the bed (HOB) elevated at least 30 degrees or as recommended by the health care provider.

Generally, HOB elevation in patients with TBI is elevated at 30 to 45 degrees to prevent aspiration. However, if increasing head elevation significantly lowers systemic blood pressure, the patient does not benefit from drainage of venous blood or CSF out of the skull from this position. If hypotension accompanies an elevated backrest position, the patient may be harmed. Avoid sudden vertical changes of the HOB in the older patient because the dura is tightly adhered to the skull and may pull away from the brain, leading to a subdural hematoma.

Patients with *severe* TBI often die. As the physiologic deterioration begins, keep in mind that the patient may be a potential organ donor. *Before* brain death is declared, contact the local organ-procurement organization. Determine if the patient consented to be an organ donor. This information is typically on a driver's license or other state-issued card or advance directive. The patient's wishes should be followed unless he or she has a medical condition that prevents organ donation. The organ donor agency representative or physician discusses the possibility of organ donation with the family. Some families may not agree with the patient's decision, which can cause an ethical dilemma. Many health care agencies have an ethics specialist of committee members who can help with these situations.

Determining Brain Death. In 2010, the American Academy of Neurology guidelines for determining brain death were updated and remain the standard in the United States today. Four prerequisites must be met to establish a brain death diagnosis (Wijdicks et al., 2010):

- Coma of known cause as established by history, clinical examination, laboratory testing, and neuroimaging
- Normal or near-normal core body temperature (higher than 96.8° F (36° C)
- Normal systolic blood pressure (higher than or equal to 100 mm Hg)
- At least one neurologic examination (some states and health care systems require two)

No consensus has been reached on who is qualified to perform head-to-toe brain-death neurologic examinations, but neurologists and critical care intensivists typically do them. Neuroimaging tests are not required to confirm brain death but are desirable. Examples of tests that may be done include cerebral angiography, bedside electroencephalography (EEG), and cerebral computed tomographic angiography (CTA).

Drug Therapy. Mannitol (Osmitrol), an osmotic diuretic, is often used to treat cerebral edema by pulling water out of the extracellular space of the edematous brain tissue. It is most effective when given in boluses rather than as a continuous infusion. Furosemide (Lasix), a loop diuretic, is often used as adjunctive therapy to reduce the incidence of rebound from mannitol. It also enhances the therapeutic action of mannitol, reduces edema and blood volume, decreases sodium uptake by the brain, and decreases the production of CSF at the choroid plexus. Although mannitol decreases intracranial pressure, research suggests that it does not improve mortality from TBI (see the Evidence-Based Practice box).

Administer *mannitol* through a filter in the IV tubing or, if given by IV push, draw it up through a filtered needle to eliminate microscopic crystals. For the patient receiving either osmotic or loop diuretics, monitor for intake and output, severe dehydration, and indications of acute renal failure, weakness, edema, and changes in urine output. Serum electrolyte and osmolarity levels are measured every 6 hours. Mannitol is used to obtain a serum osmolarity of 310 to 320 mOsm/L, depending on primary health care provider preference and the desired outcome of therapy. Insert an indwelling urinary catheter to maintain strict measurement of output every hour. Check the patient's serum and urine osmolarity daily.

Opioids such as morphine sulfate or fentanyl may be used with ventilated patients to decrease agitation and control restlessness if the agitation is caused by pain. Fentanyl has fewer effects on blood pressure and heart rate than morphine and therefore may be a safer agent to manage pain for the TBI patient. These agents may be reversed with naloxone (Narcan), but opioid reversal should be avoided if at all possible to reduce risk for withdrawal and rebound pain and agitation.

Maintaining Cognition, Sensory Perception, and Mobility

Planning: Expected Outcomes. The desired outcome is that the patient will not experience decreased memory, sensation, and/or MOBILITY. If alterations occur, the patient will receive rehabilitation to achieve optimal functioning.

Interventions. An overwhelming majority of brain injury survivors have altered COGNITION, including decreased memory and impaired judgment and reasoning ability. Cognitive impairments may interfere with the brain-injured patient's ability to function effectively in school, at work, and in his or her personal life. Cognitive rehabilitation is a way of helping brain-injured patients regain function in areas that are essential for a return to independence and a reasonable quality of life. However, these services are not widely available or accessible.

If a large lesion of the parietal lobe is present, the patient may experience a loss of SENSORY PERCEPTION for pain, temperature, touch, and proprioception (position sense), which prevents an appropriate response to environmental stimuli. A hazard-free environment is necessary to prevent injury (e.g., from burns if the patient's coffee is too hot). In collaboration with the rehabilitation therapist, integrate a sensory stimulation program into the comatose or stuporous patient's routine care activities. Sensory stimulation is done to facilitate a meaningful response to the environment. Present visual, auditory, or tactile stimuli one at a time, and explain the purpose and the type of stimulus presented. For example, show a picture of the patient's mother and say, "This is a picture of your mother." The picture is shown several times, and the same words are used to describe the picture. If auditory tapes or DVDs are used, they should be played no longer than 10 to 15 minutes. If the stimulus is presented for a longer period, it simply becomes "white" noise, or meaningless background noise.

EVIDENCE-BASED PRACTICE QSEN

Does Mannitol Reduce Mortality From Traumatic Brain Injury (TBI)?

Gottlieb, M., & Bailitz, J. (2016). Does mannitol reduce mortality from traumatic brain injury? *Annals of Emergency Medicine, 67*(1), 83–85.

Traumatic brain injury (TBI) composes more than 4.5% of all injury-related emergency department visits and 15% of annual hospitalizations. Extensive research has been conducted on prevention and treatment of TBI, including administration of mannitol. Mannitol is an osmotic diuretic that produces an initial reduction of the intracellular volume of brain tissue, resulting in transient improvement in cerebral blood flow and oxygenation. With an improvement in PERFUSION, mortality may decrease. However, there is little evidence of the effect of mannitol on mortality in patients with TBI.

In this systematic review, the researchers found four studies that met inclusion criteria to examine the effect of mannitol on mortality after severe TBI. Two of the studies compared mannitol with non-mannitol intracranial pressure (ICP)–lowering agents. Although all four trials were randomized, only three reported blinding in their

methodology. The review found that there is limited evidence that mannitol alone is sufficient to reduce mortality of severe TBI. Other agents, such as hypertonic saline, may be as effective as mannitol in decreasing ICP.

Level of Evidence: 1

The evidence in this paper was obtained in systematic review of studies about head injury in which patients sustained severe brain injury with a Glasgow Coma Scale score of less than 8.

Commentary: Implications for Practice and Research

This research questions whether traditional treatment with mannitol is sufficient for decreasing ICP while reducing mortality from severe TBI. Although staff nurses do not prescribe medications, these findings may explain a beginning shift in ICP management. More research is needed to improve survival of patients experiencing moderate-to-severe TBI.

Patients with a mild brain injury may be disoriented and have short-term memory loss. Always introduce yourself before any interaction. Keep explanations of procedures and activities short and simple, and give them immediately before and throughout patient care. To the extent possible, maintain a sleep-wake cycle with scheduled rest periods. Orient the patient to time (day, month, and year) and place, and explain the reason for the hospitalization. Reassure the patient that he or she is safe. If the client is hospitalized, ask the family to bring in familiar objects, such as pictures. Provide orientation cues within the environment, such as a large clock with numbers or a single-date calendar.

Care Coordination and Transition Management

The patient with a *mild* brain injury recovers at home after discharge from the emergency department (ED) or hospital (Chart 45-9). The patient with a *severe* brain injury requires long-term case management and ongoing rehabilitation after hospitalization. Behavioral interventions are used by cognitive and brain injury rehabilitation specialists to help both the patient and family members develop adaptive strategies. A number of specialized brain injury rehabilitation facilities are available in the United States and Canada. Communicate the patient's plan of care, including drug therapy (use best practices for drug reconciliation and transitions in care), to the receiving nurse or provider during each transition in care. Chapter 6 discusses interprofessional collaborative rehabilitative care in detail.

Home Care Management. The major overall desired outcome for rehabilitation after brain injury is to maximize the patient's ability to return to his or her highest level of functioning. Activities such as occupational therapy, physical therapy, and speech-language therapy may continue in the home after discharge

from the hospital or rehabilitation facility. Adaptation of the home environment to accommodate the patient safely may be needed. For example, smoke and fire alarms must function properly because the patient with a brain injury often loses the sense of smell. Home evaluations and referrals to outside agencies are completed before discharge. Be sure to refer the patient and family to the registered dietitian for health teaching regarding healthy nutrition to prevent weight gain from decreased activity or stress eating. About 30% of patients with TBI gain significant weight within a year of their injury, most likely because of inactivity (Duraski et al., 2014).

Self-Management Education. Collaborate with the case manager (CM) to provide the patient and family with both written and verbal instructions for discharge. The teaching plan includes a review of seizure safety at home and strategies to adapt to sensory dysfunction. Discuss issues related to personality or behavior problems that may arise and how to cope with them. Explain the purpose, dosage, schedule, and route of administration of drug therapy. Teach the family to encourage the patient to participate in activities as tolerated. Demonstrations and return demonstrations of care activities help family members become more skillful. Stress the importance of regular follow-up visits with therapists and other health care providers.

Patients with personality and behavior problems respond best to a structured and consistent environment. Instruct the family to develop a home routine that provides structure, repetition, and consistency. Remind the family about the importance of reinforcing positive behaviors rather than negative behaviors.

⚠ NURSING SAFETY PRIORITY QSEN

Action Alert

Teach the patient who has sustained a *mild* brain injury, sometimes called a *concussion*, that symptoms that disturb sleep; affect enjoyment of daily activities, work performance, mood, memory, and ability to learn new material; and cause changes in personality require follow-up care. Provide the patient and family with education materials that will alert them to symptoms and management options. A good source of written instructions is available from the CDC. Information titled "What Can I Do to Help Feel Better After a Mild Traumatic Brain Injury?" (CDC, 2017b).

Most patients with *moderate-to-severe* TBI are discharged with varied long-term physical and cognitive disabilities. Changes in personality and behavior are very common. The family must learn to cope with the patient's increased fatigue, irritability, temper outbursts, depression, loneliness, and memory problems. These patients often require constant supervision at home, and families may feel socially isolated. Provide support and encouragement for the family and patient to help them get through each day.

Teach the family about the importance of regular respite care, either in a structured day-care respite program for the patient or through relief provided by a friend or neighbor. Family members, particularly the primary caregiver, may become depressed and have feelings of loneliness. In addition, they may feel angry with the patient because of the physical, financial, and emotional responsibilities that his or her care has placed on them. To help the family cope with these problems, suggest that they join and actively participate in a local brain-injury support group.

👤 CHART 45-9 Patient and Family Education: Preparing for Self-Management

Mild Brain Injury

- Initial neurologic assessment occurs hourly until the patient returns to baseline. The frequency of ongoing assessment for mild traumatic brain injury (MTBI) is not established.
- For a headache, give acetaminophen (Tylenol) every 4 hours as needed.
- Avoid giving the person sedatives, sleeping pills, or alcoholic beverages for at least 24 hours after TBI unless the primary health care provider instructs otherwise.
- Do not allow the person to engage in strenuous activity for at least 48 hours.
- Teach the caregiver to be aware that balance disturbances cause safety concerns and that he or she should provide for monitored or assisted movement.
- If any of these symptoms occur, take the person back to the emergency department immediately:
  - Severe headache
  - Persistent or severe nausea or vomiting
  - Blurred vision
  - Drainage from the ear or nose
  - Increasing weakness
  - Slurred speech
  - Progressive sleepiness
  - Worsening headache
  - Unequal pupil size
- Keep follow-up appointments with the health care provider.

Health Care Resources. Collaborate with the CM to refer families and patients to local chapters of the Brain Injury Association of America (BIAA) (www.biausa.org) and the National Brain Injury Foundation (www.nbif.org) for information and support. The Brain Injury Association of Canada (www.braininjurycanada.ca) is available as a resource for patients in Canada. All of these organizations have a number of helpful publications on preventing and living with TBI. Other resources include religious, spiritual, and cultural leaders.

♥ VETERANS' HEALTH CONSIDERATIONS
Patient-Centered Care (QSEN)

The incidence of TBI in young veterans has increased in the past 10 years as a result of concussive blast injuries. Spouses of veterans often have the responsibility of caring for the patient at home following rehabilitation. Case management is needed to ensure transitions and continuity of care.

A qualitative study by Saban et al. (2015) found that veterans with TBI in the United States also experience depression, anxiety, and post-traumatic stress disorder (PTSD). The researchers found that family caregivers fear the anger and agitation displayed by their loved ones with TBI. In addition, the patient's children are negatively affected by the veterans' change in personality and emotional behaviors as a result of these health problems.

Suggest that the spouse or other family caregiver contact the U.S. Defense and Veterans Brain Injury Center for support groups and information. The Veterans' Health Administration has case-management services to assist with transition management and care coordination in support of both the veteran and family (Perla et al., 2013).

◆ Evaluation: Reflecting

Evaluate the care of the patient with TBI based on the identified priority problems. Expected outcomes are that the patient:

- Maintains cerebral tissue PERFUSION
- Learns to adapt to altered MOBILITY and SENSORY PERCEPTION changes, if any
- Has minimal alterations in COGNITION
- Understands how to compensate for COGNITION changes when necessary

BRAIN TUMORS

Brain tumors can arise anywhere within the brain structures and are named according to the cell or tissue where they originate; however, cerebral tumors are the most common. *Primary* tumors originate within the central nervous system (CNS) and rarely metastasize (spread) outside this area. *Secondary* brain tumors result from metastasis from other areas of the body, such as the lung, breast, kidney, and GI tract.

❖ PATHOPHYSIOLOGY
Complications of Cerebral Tumors

Regardless of location, the tumor expands and invades, infiltrates, compresses, and displaces normal brain tissue. This leads to one or more of these complications:

- Cerebral edema/brain tissue inflammation
- Increased intracranial pressure (ICP)
- Neurologic deficits (focal or diffuse)
- Hydrocephalus
- Pituitary dysfunction

Cerebral edema (vasogenic edema) results from changes in capillary endothelial tissue permeability that allows plasma to seep into the extracellular spaces. This leads to *increased ICP*

❓ CLINICAL JUDGMENT CHALLENGE 45-1
Safety; Clinical Judgment; Evidence-Based Practice (QSEN)

A 33-year-old veteran returns home from his second tour of duty from the Middle East. He is married and has two young children. His history reveals use of opioids from a previous lower back injury, two depressive episodes, and a suicide attempt during his first tour in Iraq. Since then he has become a believer in God and attends church as often as he can. He tells you that his deep faith and spirituality have helped him "turn his life around." Today he is admitted from the emergency department (ED) to the 23-hour observation unit with suspected mild traumatic brain injury as a result of a vehicular crash. A man driving under the influence of alcohol crossed the center lane of a town street and hit the car that the patient was driving. Fortunately, the patient was wearing his seat belt and was traveling at a low level of speed. His wife tells you that the car is likely totaled and they don't know where they will find the money to buy another one.

1. As this patient's nurse in the observation unit, what assessments will you perform and document, and why?
2. What diagnostic testing did this patient likely have to confirm his diagnosis?
3. After observation in the unit, the primary health care provider determines that the patient can be discharged under the care of his wife. What evidence-based discharge teaching does the patient and wife need to promote the patient's safety?
4. Using your clinical judgment, what community or support resources might you suggest that the family seek out and why?

and, depending on the location of the tumor, brain herniation syndromes. A variety of *neurologic deficits* result from edema, infiltration, distortion, and compression of surrounding brain tissue. The cerebral blood vessels may become compressed because of edema and increased ICP. This compression leads to ischemia (decreased blood flow) of the area supplied by the vessel. In addition, the tumor may enter the walls of the vessel, causing it to rupture and hemorrhage into the tumor bed or other brain tissue. Many patients who have brain tumors have headaches and seizures from interference with the brain's normal electrical activity.

Increased ICP may also result from *hydrocephalus* (increased cerebrospinal fluid [CSF]) related to obstruction of the flow of CSF or displacement of the lateral ventricles by the expanding lesion.

Pituitary dysfunction may occur as the tumor compresses the pituitary gland and causes the syndrome of inappropriate antidiuretic hormone (SIADH) or diabetes insipidus (DI). These disorders result in severe fluid and electrolyte imbalances and can be life threatening. (See Chapter 62 for a complete description of these disorders.)

Classification of Tumors

Brain tumors are usually classified as benign, malignant, or metastatic (Table 45-5). They may or may not be treated, depending on their location. Benign (noncancerous) tumors are generally associated with a favorable outcome. Malignant or metastatic tumors require more aggressive intervention, including surgery, radiation, and/or chemotherapy.

A second classification system is based on location. **Supratentorial** tumors are located within the cerebral hemispheres above the tentorium (dural fold). Located beneath the tentorium is the **infratentorial** area (i.e., the area of the brainstem structures and cerebellum).

TABLE 45-5 Classification of Brain Tumors

Benign	Malignant
• Acoustic neuroma (schwannoma)	• Astrocytoma (a *glioblastoma* is a grade 4 astrocytoma) (also called a *glioma*)
• Choroid plexus papilloma	
• Meningioma	• Oligodendroglioma
• Pituitary adenoma	• Ependymoma
• Astrocytoma	• Medulloblastoma
• Grade 1 (may undergo changes and become malignant)	• Chondrosarcoma
	• Lymphoma
• Chondroma	
• Craniopharyngioma	
• Hemangioblastoma	

⏵⏵ CHART 45-10 Key Features

Common Brain Tumors

Cerebral Tumors
- Headache (most common feature)
- Seizure
- Vomiting unrelated to food intake
- Changes in visual acuity and visual fields; diplopia (visual changes caused by papilledema)
- Hemiparesis or hemiplegia
- Hypokinesia (decreased motor ability)
- Hyperesthesia, paresthesia, decreased tactile discrimination
- Seizures
- Aphasia
- Changes in personality or behavior

Brainstem Tumors
- Hearing loss (acoustic neuroma)
- Facial pain and weakness
- Dysphagia, decreased gag reflex
- Nystagmus
- Hoarseness
- Ataxia and dysarthria (cerebellar tumors)
- Apnea
- Bradycardia
- Hypotension

Meningiomas, the most common *benign* tumors, arise from the coverings of the brain (the meninges). This tumor is capsular and well outlined and causes compression and displacement of nearby brain tissue. Although complete removal of the tumor is possible, it tends to recur.

Pituitary tumors that occur in the anterior lobe account for up to one fourth of brain tumors and may cause endocrine dysfunction. The most common type of pituitary tumor is the adenoma. These tumors are *benign* and often occur in young and middle-age adults. The presenting symptoms include visual disturbances and pituitary signs, such as loss of body hair, diabetes insipidus (DI), infertility, visual field defects, and headaches.

Acoustic neuromas arise from the sheath of Schwann cells in the peripheral part of cranial nerve VIII. They are also referred to as *cerebellar pontine angle (CPA) tumors* to describe their anatomic location. Acoustic neuromas compress brain tissue and tend to surround nearby cranial nerves (VII, V, IX, X), making surgical removal difficult without causing permanent cranial nerve dysfunction. Women are twice as likely as men to have acoustic neuromas. Common symptoms include hearing loss, **tinnitus** (ringing in the ears), and dizziness or vertigo.

Metastatic, or secondary, tumors account for many brain tumors. Cancer cells from the lung, breast, colon, pancreas, kidney, and skin can travel to the brain via the blood and the lymphatic system. Multiple metastatic lesions are fairly common.

Etiology and Genetic Risk

The exact cause of brain tumors is unknown. Several areas under investigation include genetic mutations and a variety of environmental factors. The use of cellular phones has been investigated as a cause of brain tumors, but findings are not confirmed. Brain tumors account for a small percentage of all cancer deaths. Primary brain tumors are relatively uncommon; many more patients have metastatic lesions. Malignant brain tumors are seen primarily in patients 40 to 70 years of age, and the survival rate is low compared with that of other cancers (McCance et al., 2014).

❖ INTERPROFESSIONAL COLLABORATIVE CARE

◆ Assessment: Noticing

When possible, obtain a history from both the patient and family, including current signs and symptoms. A complete neurologic assessment is needed to establish baseline data and determine the nature and extent of neurologic deficits.

The signs and symptoms of brain tumors vary with the site of the tumor (Chart 45-10). In general, assess for these symptoms of a brain tumor:

- Headaches that are usually more severe on awakening in the morning
- Nausea and vomiting
- Seizures or convulsions
- Impaired SENSORY PERCEPTION, such as facial numbness or tingling and visual changes
- Loss of balance or dizziness (ataxia)
- Weakness or paralysis in one part or one side of the body (hemiparesis or hemiplegia)
- Difficulty thinking, speaking, or articulating words
- Changes in COGNITION, mentation, or personality
- **Papilledema** (swelling of the optic disc), indicating increased ICP

Neurologic deficits result from the destruction, distortion, or compression of brain tissue. *Supratentorial (cerebral)* tumors usually result in paralysis, seizures, memory loss, cognitive impairment, language impairment, or vision problems. *Infratentorial* tumors produce ataxia, autonomic nervous system dysfunction, vomiting, drooling, hearing loss, and vision impairment. As the tumor grows, ICP increases, and the symptoms become progressively more severe.

Diagnosis is based on the history, neurologic assessment, clinical examination, and results of neurodiagnostic testing. Noninvasive diagnostic studies such as *CT* and *MRI* are conducted first. These tests identify the size, location, and extent of the tumor. The MRI may be used for initial diagnostic evaluation and is a more sensitive diagnostic study, whereas the CT is often used for follow-up during the course of illness. Skull x-rays may be done to determine any bone involvement caused by the tumor.

◆ Interventions: Responding

Interventions depend on the type, size, and location of the tumor. For example, a small benign tumor may be monitored through CT and MRI scanning to assess its growth. Malignant tumors may be managed periodically by chemotherapy, radiation, and/or surgery.

Nonsurgical Management. The desired outcomes of brain tumor management are to decrease tumor size, improve quality of life, and improve survival time. The type of treatment selected depends on the tumor size and location, patient symptoms and general condition, and whether the tumor has recurred. In addition to traditional interventions, a number of experimental treatment modalities are being investigated. These include blood-brain barrier disruption, recombinant DNA, monoclonal antibodies, new chemotherapeutic drugs, and immunotherapy. Traditional *radiation therapy* may be used alone, after surgery, or in combination with chemotherapy and surgery. Chapter 22 discusses radiation treatment for patients with cancer.

Drug Therapy. The primary health care provider may prescribe a variety of drugs to treat the tumor, manage the patient's symptoms, and prevent complications. *Chemotherapy* may be given alone, in combination with radiation and surgery, and with tumor progression. Although these drugs may control tumor growth or decrease tumor burden, the benefit does not last. Chemotherapy usually involves more than one agent that may be given orally, IV, intra-arterially, and/or intrathecally through an Ommaya reservoir placed in a cranial ventricle. When given systemically, the drug must be lipid soluble to cross the blood-brain barrier.

Commonly used oral drugs are lomustine (CCNU), temozolomide (Temodar), procarbazine (Matulane), and methotrexate (MTX). Vincristine (Oncovin) may be given IV in combination with other drugs. Monitor for side effects of these drugs, which are similar to those of any chemotherapeutic drug. Chapter 22 describes general nursing implications for care of a patient receiving chemotherapy.

Direct drug delivery to the tumor is another treatment option. Disk-shaped drug (Gliadel) wafers may be placed directly into the cavity created during surgical tumor removal (interstitial chemotherapy). The major drug in the wafer is carmustine (BCNU). This therapy is usually given for newly diagnosed high-grade malignant gliomas, but recurrent tumors may also be treated with this method. Other drugs used are molecularly targeted. Examples include erlotinib (Tarceva), gefitinib (Iressa), and bevacizumab (Avastin) (Burchum & Rosenthal, 2016).

Analgesics, such as codeine and acetaminophen (Tylenol, Ace-Tabs), are given for headache. Dexamethasone (Decadron) is given to control cerebral edema. Phenytoin (Dilantin) or other antiepileptic drugs may be given to prevent seizure activity. Proton pump inhibitors are given to decrease gastric acid secretion and prevent the development of stress ulcers.

Stereotactic Radiosurgery. Stereotactic radiosurgery (SRS) is an alternative to traditional surgery. Several techniques are used, including the modified linear accelerator (LINAC) using accelerated x-rays, a particle accelerator using beams of protons (cyclotron), and isotope seeds implanted in the tumor (brachytherapy).

The gamma knife is an SRS procedure that uses a single high dose of ionized radiation to focus multiple beams of gamma radiation produced by the radioisotope *cobalt-60* to destroy intracranial lesions selectively without damaging surrounding healthy tissue (Fig. 45-7). Combining neurodiagnostic imaging tools, including MRI, CT, magnetic resonance angiography (MRA), and angiography, with the gamma knife allows for

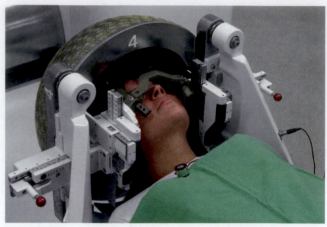

FIG. 45-7 A gamma knife treatment. The treatment beams are widely dispersed over the surface of the head to prevent damage to healthy brain tissue. The beams are intense only at the point of target. (From Flint, P. W., Haughey, B. H., Lund, V. J., Niparko, J. K., Robbins, K. T., et al. [2015]. *Cummings otolaryngology: Head & neck surgery* [6th ed.]. Philadelphia: Mosby. Courtesy Elekta, Inc.)

precise localization of deep-seated or anatomically difficult lesions. Treatment usually takes less than an hour, and patients require only overnight hospitalization. Advantages of this technique include its:

- Noninvasive nature
- Lower risk when compared with traditional craniotomy
- Surgical precision
- Decreased cost
- Decreased morbidity
- Deceased length of hospital stay
- Rapid recovery time

A disadvantage is that the device requires an uncomfortable rigid head frame. In another system, called the *CyberKnife,* no frame is needed. Both procedures are used primarily for brain tumors or arteriovenous malformations (AVMs) that are in a difficult location and therefore not removable by craniotomy. These procedures may also be used with patients who decline conventional surgery, for patients whose age and physical condition do not allow general anesthesia, as an adjunct to radiation therapy, and for recurrent or residual AVM or tumors after embolization or craniotomy.

Surgical Management. A **craniotomy** (incision into the cranium) may be performed to remove the tumor, improve symptoms related to the lesion, or decrease the tumor size (debulk). The challenge for the neurosurgeon is to remove the tumor as completely as possible without damaging normal tissue. Complete removal is possible with some benign tumors, which results in a "surgical cure." After surgery the patient is often admitted to the critical care unit or neurosurgical unit for frequent observation.

Preoperative Care. The patient having a craniotomy is typically very anxious about having his or her head opened and the brain exposed. Concerns are centered on the possibility of increased neurologic deficits after the surgery and the patient's self-image when part or all of the head is shaved. Provide reassurance that the surgeon will spare vital parts of the brain while removing or decreasing the size of the tumor. Teach the patient and family about what to expect immediately after surgery and throughout the recovery period. Some patients require short-term or long-term rehabilitation.

Check that the patient has not had alcohol, tobacco, anticoagulants, or NSAIDs for at least 5 days before surgery. Some neurosurgeons require a week or longer. Be sure that the patient has been NPO status for at least 8 hours. Other preoperative care is similar to that for any patient having surgery, as described in Chapter 14.

Operative Procedures. Surgery is performed under local or general anesthesia or sedation. Small tumors that are easily located may be removed by *minimally invasive surgery (MIS)*. For example, the trans-nasal approach using endoscopy can be performed for pituitary tumors. The patient has a short hospital stay and few complications after surgery. Stereotactic surgery using a rigid head frame can be done for tumors that are easily reached. This procedure requires only burr holes and local anesthesia because the brain has no sensory neurons for pain. Laser surgery can also be done.

For a craniotomy, the surgeon makes an incision along or behind the hairline after placing the patient's head in a skull fixation device. Several burr holes are drilled into the skull, and a saw is used to remove a piece of bone (bone flap) to expose the tumor area. The flap is stored carefully until the end of the procedure. The tumor is located using imaging technology and removed or debulked (partially removed). After the tumor removal, the bone flap is replaced and held by small screws or bolts. A drain or monitoring device may be inserted. The surgeon creates a soft dressing "cap" over the top of the head to keep the surgical area clean and prevent the patient from touching the incision site.

Postoperative Care. The focus of postoperative care is to monitor the patient to detect changes in status and prevent or minimize complications, especially increased intracranial pressure (ICP).

> **! NURSING SAFETY PRIORITY** QSEN
>
> **Action Alert**
>
> Assess neurologic and vital signs every 15 to 30 minutes for the first 4 to 6 hours after a craniotomy and then every hour. If the patient is stable for 24 hours, the frequency of these checks may be decreased to every 2 to 4 hours, depending on agency policy or the patient's condition. *Report immediately and document new neurologic deficits, particularly a decreased level of consciousness (LOC), motor weakness or paralysis, aphasia (speech and/or language problems), decreased sensation, and sluggish pupil reaction to light!* Personality changes such as agitation, aggression, or passivity can also indicate worsening neurologic status.

Managing the Patient in the Immediate Postoperative Period. Periorbital (around the eye) edema and ecchymosis of one or both eyes are not unusual and are treated with cold compresses to decrease swelling. Irrigate the affected eye with warm saline solution or artificial tears to improve patient comfort. The patient in the critical care unit has routine cardiac monitoring because dysrhythmias may occur as a result of brain–autonomic nervous system–cardiac interactions or fluid and electrolyte imbalance.

Regardless of setting, ensure recording of the patient's intake and output for the first 24 hours. Anticipate fluid restriction to 1500 mL daily if there is pituitary involvement in either the tumor or surgical site and SIADH develops. Reposition the patient, being careful not to cause pressure on the operative site. Delegate or provide repositioning and deep breathing every 2 hours. To prevent the development of venous thromboembolism (VTE), maintain intermittent sequential pneumatic devices until the patient ambulates.

For patients who have undergone *supratentorial* surgery, elevate the head of the bed 30 degrees or as tolerated to promote venous drainage from the head. *Position the patient to avoid extreme hip or neck flexion and maintain the head in a midline, neutral position to prevent increased ICP.* Turn the patient side to side or supine to prevent pressure injury and pneumonia.

Keep the patient with an *infratentorial* (brainstem) craniotomy flat or at 10 degrees, depending on the primary health care provider's prescription. Position the patient side-lying, alternating sides every 2 hours, for 24 to 48 hours or until ambulatory. This position prevents pressure on the neck-area incision site. It also prevents pressure on the internal tumor excision site from higher cerebral structures. Make sure that the patient remains NPO status until awake and alert because edema around the medulla and lower cranial nerves may also cause vomiting and aspiration.

Check the head dressing every 1 to 2 hours for signs of drainage. Mark the area of drainage once during each shift for baseline comparison, although this practice varies by health care agency. A small or moderate amount of drainage is expected. Some patients may have a Hemovac or Jackson-Pratt drain in place for 24 to 72 hours after surgery. Measure the drainage every 8 hours and record the amount and color. A typical amount of drainage is 30 to 50 mL every 8 hours. Follow the manufacturer's and neurosurgeon's instructions to maintain suction within the drain.

> **! NURSING SAFETY PRIORITY** QSEN
>
> **Critical Rescue**
>
> After craniotomy, monitor the patient's dressing for excessive amounts of drainage. Report a saturated head dressing or drainage greater than 50 mL/8 hr immediately to the surgeon! *Monitor frequently for signs of increasing ICP!*

The usual laboratory studies monitored after surgery include complete blood count (CBC), serum electrolyte levels and osmolarity, and coagulation studies. The patient's hematocrit and hemoglobin concentration may be abnormally low from blood loss during surgery, diluted from large amounts of IV fluids given during surgery, or elevated if the blood was replaced. Hyponatremia (low serum sodium) may occur as a result of fluid volume overload, syndrome of inappropriate antidiuretic hormone (SIADH), or steroid administration.

Hypokalemia (low serum potassium) may cause cardiac irritability. Weakness, a change in LOC, and confusion are symptoms of hyponatremia and hypokalemia. Hypernatremia may be caused by meningitis, dehydration, or diabetes insipidus (DI). It is manifested by muscle weakness, restlessness, extreme thirst, and dry mouth. Additional signs of dehydration such as decreased urinary output, thick lung secretions, and hypotension may be present. *Untreated hypernatremia can lead to seizure activity. DI should be considered if the patient voids large amounts of very dilute urine with an increasing serum osmolarity and electrolyte concentration.*

The patient may be mechanically ventilated for the first 24 to 48 hours after surgery to help manage the airway and maintain optimal oxygen levels. If the patient is awake or attempting to breathe at a rate other than that set on the ventilator, drugs such as dexmedetomidine (Precedex) or propofol (Diprivan) and fentanyl are given to treat pain and anxiety and promote rest and comfort. Suction the patient as needed. *Remember to hyperoxygenate the patient carefully before, during, and after suctioning!*

Drugs routinely given after surgery include antiepileptic drugs, histamine blockers or proton pump inhibitors for stress ulcer prophylaxis, and glucocorticoids such as dexamethasone (Decadron) to reduce cerebral edema. Give acetaminophen for fever or mild pain. Antibiotics are typically prescribed to prevent infection for several days after surgery.

❓ NCLEX EXAMINATION CHALLENGE 45-5
Physiological Integrity

A client returns from the postanesthesia care unit (PACU) after a surgical removal of a brainstem tumor. In what position will the nurse place the client at this time?
A. Turn the patient from side to side to prevent aspiration.
B. Keep the client flat in bed or up 10 degrees and reposition from side to side.
C. Elevate the head of the bed to at least 30 degrees at all times.
D. Keep the client in a sitting position in bed at all times.

Preventing and Managing Postoperative Complications. Postoperative complications are listed in Table 45-6. The major complications of *supratentorial* surgery are increased ICP from cerebral edema or hydrocephalus and hemorrhage.

Symptoms of *increased ICP* include severe headache, deteriorating LOC, restlessness, and irritability. Dilated or pinpoint pupils that are slow to react or nonreactive to light are late signs of increased ICP. Treatment of increased ICP is the same as that described under Interventions in the Traumatic Brain Injury section.

Hydrocephalus (increased CSF in the brain) is caused by obstruction of the normal CSF pathway from edema, an expanding lesion such as a hematoma, or blood in the subarachnoid space. Rapidly progressive hydrocephalus produces the classic symptoms of increased ICP. Slowly progressive hydrocephalus is manifested by headache, decreased LOC, irritability, blurred vision, and urinary incontinence. An intraventricular catheter (ventriculostomy) may be placed to drain CSF during surgery

or emergently after surgery for rapidly deteriorating neurologic function. If long-term treatment is required for chronic hydrocephalus, a surgical shunt is inserted to drain CSF to another area of the body. A major complication of the shunting procedure is a subdural hematoma from the tearing of bridging veins. An external lumbar drain may also be used temporarily. Additional information about shunts may be found in neuroscience nursing textbooks.

Subdural and epidural *hematomas and intracranial hemorrhage* are manifested by severe headache, a rapid decrease in LOC, progressive neurologic deficits, and herniation syndromes (brain tissue shifting, often downward). Bleeding into the posterior fossa may lead to sudden cardiovascular and respiratory arrest. Treatment of a hematoma requires surgical removal. An intracranial hemorrhage is treated with aggressive medical management (e.g., osmotic diuretics, ICP monitoring).

Respiratory complications include atelectasis, pneumonia, and neurogenic pulmonary edema. Prevent atelectasis and pneumonia by turning the patient frequently and encouraging him or her to take frequent deep breaths to expand the lungs each hour. Humidified air and incentive spirometry are also useful techniques. Other treatment modalities include endotracheal or oral tracheal suctioning and chest physiotherapy. However, these measures may cause an increase in ICP. Although not common, *neurogenic pulmonary edema* is a life-threatening complication of traumatic brain injury (TBI), brain tumors, and brain surgery. Its symptoms are the same as those of acute pulmonary edema, but there are no associated cardiac problems. In spite of aggressive treatment, most patients with neurogenic pulmonary edema do not survive.

Wound infections occur more often in older and debilitated patients and in patients with a history of diabetes, long-term steroid use, obesity, and previous infections. The patient may contribute to the problem by rubbing or scratching the wound. If infection is present, the wound appears reddened and puffy. It may begin to separate, is sensitive to touch, and feels warm. The patient may or may not be febrile. Treatment is based on the degree and extent of the infection. A localized infection may be treated by cleaning it with an antiseptic and applying a topical antibiotic. For more severe infections, systemic antibiotic administration is needed. If the underlying bone is involved, it may need to be removed.

Meningitis is an inflammation of the meninges and may occur as a result of surgery or wound infection, a cerebrospinal fluid (CSF) leak, or contamination during surgery. (See the Meningitis section in Chapter 42 for a more complete explanation of this condition.)

Syndrome of inappropriate antidiuretic hormone (SIADH) occurs when the posterior pituitary gland releases too much ADH, causing water retention. The urine output decreases dramatically with a urine output of less than 20 mL/hr. Sodium concentration in the urine is normal or elevated, whereas the serum sodium level falls. Other indications of SIADH are loss of thirst, weight gain, irritability, muscle weakness, and decreased LOC. SIADH is treated by fluid restriction, which is usually sufficient to correct the hyponatremia. Conivaptan (Vaprisol) and tolvaptan are vasopressin receptor antagonists used to increase water diuresis without serum electrolyte loss and may be useful in hypervolemic hyponatremic conditions. Slow, controlled IV infusion of hypertonic sodium may be needed for severe hyponatremia (<118 mEq/L).

TABLE 45-6 Postoperative Complications of Craniotomy

Early	Late
• Increased intracranial pressure (ICP)	• Wound infection
• Hematomas	• Meningitis
• Subdural hematoma	• Fluid and electrolyte imbalances
• Epidural hematoma	• Dehydration
• Subarachnoid hemorrhage	• Hyponatremia
• Hypovolemic shock	• Hypernatremia
• Hydrocephalus	• Seizures
• Respiratory complications	• Cerebrospinal fluid (CSF) leak
• Atelectasis	• Cerebral edema
• Hypoxia	
• Pneumonia	
• Neurogenic pulmonary edema	

Care Coordination and Transition Management

The patient with a brain tumor is managed at home if possible. Maintaining a reasonable quality of life is an important outcome for recovery and rehabilitation. Unless the patient has a significant degree of disability, no special preparation for home care is needed. Patients with hemiparesis need assistance to ensure that their home is accessible according to their method of MOBILITY (e.g., cane, walker, and wheelchair). The environment should be made safe to prevent falls. For example, teach caregivers to remove scatter rugs and to place grab bars in the bathroom.

Information about the selection of rehabilitation or chronic care facility, if needed, can be obtained from the case manager (CM) or discharge planner. The selected facility should have experience in providing care for neurologically impaired patients. A psychologist should be available to provide input in the evaluation of the cognitive disabilities that the patient may have.

It is very important that the patient and family fully understand the importance of any recommended follow-up health care appointments. Be sure that the discharge summary includes the name of the person who has been given the follow-up information.

Health teaching includes drug therapy and who to call if adverse drug events occur. Remind the patient to avoid taking any over-the-counter drugs unless approved by the primary health care provider.

Teach the patient to maintain a program of regular physical exercise within the limits of any disabilities. Referral to the dietitian may be needed to ensure adequate caloric intake for the patient receiving radiation or chemotherapy. Chapter 22 describes care of patients having radiation and chemotherapy in detail.

Seizures are a potential complication that can occur at any time for as long as 1 year or more after surgery. Provide the patient and family with information about seizure precautions and what to do if a seizure occurs. Teach the need for follow-up appointments to monitor for therapeutic levels of antiepileptic drugs (AEDs).

Be sure that the patient and family have access to resources for support. Discuss ways that they have coped with crisis in the past, such as spiritual counselors or clergy. Provide hope and help them feel empowered to make the best decisions for their care and future (Lucas, 2013). Listen to the patient's concerns and offer ideas for other community resources, depending on the patient's specific needs. Psychological support is essential because of potential changes in self-esteem, decreased ADL ability, and prognosis.

Refer the patient and the family or significant others to the American Brain Tumor Association (www.abta.org) or the National Brain Tumor Foundation (www.braintumor.org). The American Cancer Society (www.cancer.org) is also an appropriate community resource for patients with malignant tumors. In Canada, the Brain Tumor Foundation-Canada (www.braintumour.ca) can be very useful to providing information and support to patients and their families who live there. Home care agencies are available to provide both the physical and rehabilitative care that the patient may need at home. Hospice services and palliative care may be needed if he or she is terminally ill. (See Chapter 7 for additional information about end-of-life care.) Brain tumor support groups may also be a valuable asset to the patient and family.

GET READY FOR THE NCLEX® EXAMINATION!

KEY POINTS

Review these Key Points for each NCLEX Examination Client Needs Category.

Safe and Effective Care Environment
- When caring for a patient with a stroke or traumatic brain injury (TBI), assess airway, breathing, and circulation status first and implement interventions to maintain them.
- Collaborate with the interprofessional team members, including physicians, physical therapists, respiratory therapists, occupational therapists, social workers, and dietitians to ensure optimal patient function and quality of life. **QSEN: Teamwork and Collaboration**

Health Promotion and Maintenance
- Identify risk factors for new or recurrent stroke and teach patients and families about modifiable risk factors for stroke as listed in Chart 45-2. **QSEN: Evidence-Based Practice**
- Prevent secondary brain injury by protecting the airway, promoting an appropriate range of blood pressure and mean arterial pressure, maintaining fluid and electrolyte balance, promptly treating fever, avoiding sustained hypoglycemia and hyperglycemia, addressing hypoxia and hypercarbia, positioning the patient appropriately, and managing intracranial hypertension with prescribed interventions.

- Teach patients and families about community organizations, such as the National Stroke Association and the Brain Injury Association of America.

Psychosocial Integrity
- Assess the emotional reactions of families to a TBI, stroke, or brain cancer diagnosis and help them cope by providing information and including them in planning for care. **QSEN: Patient-Centered Care**

Physiological Integrity
- Perform a comprehensive, rapid, or focal neurologic assessment at regular intervals to identify changes in status. **QSEN: Evidence-Based Practice**
- Recall that decreased level of consciousness is the most sensitive indicator of adverse outcome or complication from stroke, TBI, brain tumor, or craniotomy due to decreased PERFUSION from cerebral edema or hemorrhage.
- Recall the differences between a transient ischemic attack and a brain attack (stroke) as described in Table 45-1 and Chart 45-1.
- Monitor patients with critical neurologic health problems for manifestations of increasing intracranial pressure (ICP) as described in Chart 45-6. **Clinical Judgment**

- Assess the patient's ability to swallow before providing oral intake if a stroke is suspected or diagnosed. **QSEN: Safety**
- Assess patients with strokes for SENSORY PERCEPTION changes such as unilateral neglect and impaired vision; help patients adapt to these changes, such as turning their head from side to side to see the entire meal tray. **QSEN: Patient-Centered Care**
- Provide alternate means of communication when expressive and/or receptive aphasia is present in patients who have had a stroke or brain injury in consultation with the speech-language expert. **QSEN: Teamwork and Collaboration**
- Monitor the patient on fibrinolytic therapy or anticoagulants for bleeding and abnormal coagulation studies. Best practices for fibrinolytic therapy administration are listed in Chart 45-5. **QSEN: Safety**
- Teach patients with mild TBI and their families to monitor for neurologic changes as listed in Charts 45-8 and 45-9.
- Assess for manifestations of brain tumors as listed in Chart 45-10.
- Recognize that the desired outcome for the patient with a brain tumor is to remove it if possible. Other methods may be used to decrease its size, including chemotherapy and radiation.
- Monitor patients having a craniotomy for potential complications as listed in Table 45-6.

SELECTED BIBLIOGRAPHY

Asterisk indicates a classic or definitive work on this subject.

Amarenco, P., Davis, S., Jones, E. F., et al. (2014). Clopidogrel plus aspirin versus warfarin in patients with stroke and aortic arch plaques. *Stroke; a Journal of Cerebral Circulation, 45,* 1248.

American Heart Association. (2016). Get with the guidelines® educational materials. http://www.heart.org/HEARTORG/HealthcareResearch/GetWithTheGuidelines/Get-With-The-Guidelines-Educational-Materials_UCM_310980_Article.jsp.

Beal, C. C. (2014). Women's interpretation of and cognitive and behavioral responses to the symptoms of acute ischemic stroke. *Journal of Neuroscience Nursing, 46*(5), 251–311.

Bowen, P. (2016). Early identification, rapid response, and effective treatment of acute stroke: Utilizing teleneurology to ensure optimal clinical outcomes. *Medsurg Nursing, 25*(4), 241–243.

Burchum, J. L. R., & Rosenthal, L. D. (2016). *Lehne's pharmacology for nursing care* (9th ed.). St. Louis: Elsevier.

Centers for Disease Control and Prevention (CDC). (2017). Stroke. www.cdc.gov/stroke/.

Centers for Disease Control and Prevention (CDC). (2017a). Injury prevention & control: Traumatic brain injury. www.cdc.gov/TraumaticBrainInjury.

Centers for Disease Control and Prevention (CDC). (2017b). What Can I Do to Help Feel Better After a Mild Traumatic Brain Injury? www.cdc.gov/TraumaticBrainInjury.

Chen, S., Feng, H., Sherchan, P., Klebe, D., Zhao, G., Sun, X., et al. (2014). Controversies and evolving new mechanisms in subarachnoid hemorrhage. *Progress in Neurobiology, 0,* 64–91. http://doi.org/10.1016/j.pneurobio.2013.09.002.

Defazio, M. V., Rammo, R. A., Robles, J. R., Bramlett, H. M., Dietrich, W. D., et al. (2013). The potential utility of blood-derived biochemical markers as indicators of early clinical trends following severe traumatic brain injury. *World Neurosurgery, 81*(1), 151–158.

Duraski, S. A., Lovell, L., & Roth, E. J. (2014). Nutritional intake, body-mass index, and activity in post-acute traumatic brain injury. *Rehabilitation Nursing, 39*(3), 140–146.

Focht, K. L., Gogue, A. M., & Ellis, C. (2014). Gender differences in stroke recognition among stroke survivors. *Journal of Neuroscience Nursing, 46*(1), 1–64.

Godwin, K. M., Ostwald, S. K., Cron, S. G., & Wasserman, J. (2013). Long-term health-related quality of life of stroke survivors and their spouse caregivers. *Journal of Neuroscience Nursing, 45*(2), 147–154.

Gottlieb, M., & Bailitz, J. (2016). Does mannitol reduce mortality from traumatic brain injury? *Annals of Emergency Medicine, 67*(1), 83–85.

Heart and Stroke Foundation. (2017). Statistics. www.hands.com/site.c.ikIQLcMWJtE/b.3483991/k.34A8/Statistics.htm.

*Hughes, P. (2011). Comprehensive care of adults with acute ischemic stroke. *Critical Care Nursing Clinics of North America, 23*(4), 661–675.

Lucas, M. R. (2013). What brain tumors and their families have taught me. *Journal of Neuroscience Nursing, 45*(3), 119–177.

Madden, L. K., & DeVon, H. A. (2015). A systematic review of the effects of body temperature on outcome of adult traumatic brain injury. *Journal of Neuroscience Nursing, 47*(4), 190–203.

McCance, K., Huether, S., Brashers, V., & Rote, N. (2014). *Pathophysiology: The biologic basis for disease in adults and children* (7th ed.). St. Louis: Mosby.

McKay, C., Hall, A. B., & Cortes, J. (2015). Time to blood pressure control before thrombolytic therapy in patients with acute ischemic stroke: Comparison of labetalol, nicardipine, hydralazine. *Journal of Neuroscience Nursing, 47*(6), 301–345.

*Mink, J., & Miller, J. (2011a). Opening the window of opportunity for treating acute ischemic stroke. *Nursing, 41*(1), 24–32.

*Mink, J., & Miller, J. (2011b). Stroke, Part 2: Respond aggressively to hemorrhagic stroke. *Nursing, 41*(3), 36–42.

Mosselman, M. J., Kruitwagen, C. L., Schuurmans, M. J., & Hafsteinsdottir, T. B. (2013). Malnutrition and risk of malnutrition in patients with stroke: Prevalence during hospital stay. *Journal of Neuroscience Nursing, 45*(4), 194–204.

Orion, D., Yavne, Y., Peretz, S., & Givaty, G. (2015). Diagnosing hyperperfusion syndrome: CT perfusion or transcranial Doppler? *Israel Medical Association Journal, 17*(10), 656–658.

Perla, L. Y., Jackson, P. D., Hopkins, S. L., Dagett, M. C., & Van Horn, L. J. (2013). Transitioning home: Comprehensive case management for America's heroes. *Rehabilitation Nursing, 38*(5), 231–239.

Pierce, L. L., & Steiner, V. (2013). Usage and design evaluation by family of a stroke intervention website. *Journal of Neuroscience Nursing, 45*(5), 243–317.

Ramírez-Moreno, J. M., Alonso-González, R., Peral-Pacheco, D., Millán-Núñez, M. V., & Aguirre-Sánchez, J. J. (2015). Knowledge of stroke a study from a sex perspective. *BMC Research Notes, 8,* 604. doi:10.1186/s13104-015-1582-1.

Saban, K. L., Hogan, N. S., Hogan, T. P., & Pape, T. L.-B. (2015). He looks normal but…Challenges of family caregivers of veterans diagnosed with a traumatic brain injury. *Rehabilitation Nursing, 40*(5), 277–283.

The Joint Commission. (2017). *Stroke.* http://www.jointcommission.org/specifications_manual_for_national_hospital_inpatient_quality_measures.aspx.

White, C. L., Barrientos, R., & Dunn, K. (2014). Dimensions of uncertainty of stroke: Perspectives of the stroke survivor and family caregivers. *Journal of Neuroscience Nursing, 46*(4), 197–249.

*Wijdicks, E. F., Varelas, P. N., Gronseth, G. S., Greer, D. M., & American Academy of Neurology. (2010). Evidence-based guideline update: Determining brain death in adults: Report of the Quality Standards Subcommittee of the American Academy of Neurology. *Neurology, 74*(23), 1911–1918.

CHAPTER | 46

Assessment of the Eye and Vision

Samuel A. Borchers and Andrea A. Borchers

 http://evolve.elsevier.com/Iggy/

PRIORITY AND INTERRELATED CONCEPTS

The priority concept for this chapter is SENSORY PERCEPTION.

LEARNING OUTCOMES

Safe and Effective Care Environment

1. Protect patients from injury or infection of the eye to preserve visual SENSORY PERCEPTION.

Health Promotion and Maintenance

2. Teach adults about eye health and the use of eye-protection equipment and strategies.

Psychosocial Integrity

3. Implement nursing interventions to minimize the stressors for the patient undergoing assessment testing of the eyes and vision.

Physiological Integrity

4. Apply knowledge of anatomy, physiology, pathophysiology, genetic risk, age-related changes, and psychomotor skills to perform a focused assessment of the eyes and vision.

Sensory perception is the ability to perceive and interpret sensory input into one or more meaningful responses (see Chapter 2). Many people think of vision as their most important sense because it assesses surroundings, allows independence, warns of danger, appreciates beauty, and helps them work, play, and interact with others. Visual SENSORY PERCEPTION takes place when the eye and brain work together. Vision begins when light is changed into nerve impulses in the eye and the impulses are sent on to the brain to fully perceive images (McCance et al., 2014). Many systemic conditions and eye problems change vision temporarily or permanently. Changes in the eye and vision can provide information about the patient's general health status and problems that might occur in self-care.

ANATOMY AND PHYSIOLOGY REVIEW

Structure

The eyeball, a round, ball-shaped organ, is located in the front part of the eye orbit. The orbit is the bony socket of the skull that surrounds and protects the eye along with the attached muscles, nerves, vessels, and tear-producing glands.

Layers of the Eyeball

The eye has three layers (Fig. 46-1). The external layer is the sclera (the "white" of the eye) and the transparent cornea on the front of the eye.

The middle layer, or uvea, is heavily pigmented and consists of the choroid, the ciliary body, and the iris. The choroid, a dark brown membrane between the sclera and the retina, lines most of the sclera. It has many blood vessels that supply nutrients to the retina.

The ciliary body connects the choroid with the iris and secretes aqueous humor. The iris is the colored portion of the external eye; its center opening is the pupil. The muscles of the iris contract and relax to control pupil size and the amount of light entering the eye.

The innermost layer is the retina, a thin, delicate structure made up of sensory photoreceptors that begin the transmission

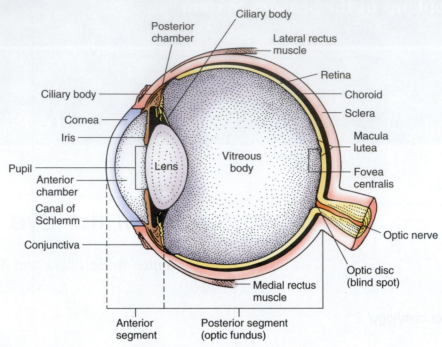

FIG. 46-1 Anatomic features of the eye.

of impulses to the optic nerve (McCance et al., 2014). The retina contains blood vessels and two types of photoreceptors called *rods* and *cones*. The rods work at low light levels and provide peripheral vision. The cones are active at bright light levels and provide color and central vision.

The **optic fundus** is the area at the inside back of the eye that can be seen with an ophthalmoscope. This area contains the **optic disc**, a pinkish-orange or white depressed area where the nerve fibers that synapse with the photoreceptors join together to form the optic nerve and exit the eyeball. The optic disc contains only nerve fibers and no photoreceptor cells. To one side of the optic disc is a small, yellowish pink area called the *macula lutea.* The center of the macula is the *fovea centralis,* where vision is most acute.

Refractive Structures and Media

Light waves pass through the cornea, aqueous humor, lens, and vitreous humor on the way to the retina. Each structure bends (*refracts*) the light waves to focus images on the retina. Together these structures are the eye's *refracting media.*

The **cornea** is the clear layer that forms the external bump on the front of the eye (see Fig. 46-1). The **aqueous humor** is a clear, watery fluid that fills the anterior and posterior chambers of the eye. This fluid is continually produced by the ciliary processes and passes from the posterior chamber, through the pupil, and into the anterior chamber. This fluid drains through the canal of Schlemm into the blood to maintain a balanced intraocular pressure (IOP), the pressure within the eye (Fig. 46-2).

The **lens** is a circular, convex structure that lies behind the iris and in front of the vitreous body. It is transparent and bends the light rays entering through the pupil to focus properly on the retina. The curve of the lens changes to focus on near or distant objects. A *cataract* (discussed in Chapter 47) is a lens that has lost its transparency.

The **vitreous body** is a clear, thick gel that fills the large vitreous chamber (the space between the lens and the retina). This gel transmits light and maintains eye shape.

The eye is a hollow organ and must be kept in the shape of a ball for vision to occur. To maintain this shape, the vitreous humor gel in the posterior segment and the aqueous humor in the anterior segment must be present in set amounts that apply pressure inside the eye to keep it inflated. This pressure is the **intraocular pressure** or **IOP**. IOP has to be precisely accurate. If the pressure is too low, the eyeball is soft and collapses, preventing light from getting to the photoreceptors on the retina in the back of the eye. If the pressure becomes too high, the extra pressure compresses capillaries in the eye and nerve fibers. Pressure on retinal blood vessels prevents blood from flowing through them; therefore the photoreceptors and nerve fibers become hypoxic. Compression of the fine nerve fibers prevents intracellular fluid flow, which also reduces nourishment to the distal portions of these thin nerve fibers. *Glaucoma* occurs with increased pressure and resulting hypoxia of photoreceptors and their synapsing nerve fibers. Continued retinal hypoxia results in necrosis and death of photoreceptors, as well as permanent nerve fiber damage. When extensive photoreceptor and nerve fiber loss occur, vision is lost, and the person is permanently blind.

External Structures

The eyelids are thin, movable skinfolds that protect the eyes and keep the cornea moist. The upper lid is larger than the lower one. The **canthus** is the place where the two eyelids meet at the corner of the eye.

The **conjunctivae** are the mucous membranes of the eye. The palpebral conjunctiva is a thick membrane with many blood vessels that lines the undersurface of each eyelid. The thin, transparent bulbar conjunctiva covers the entire front of the eye.

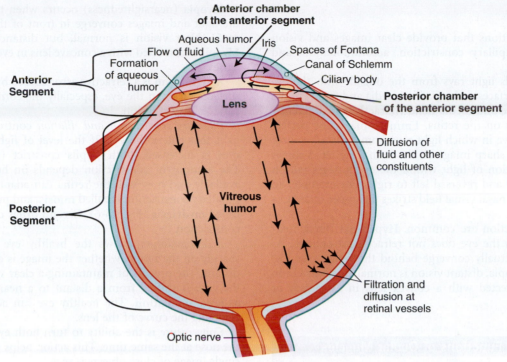

FIG. 46-2 Flow of aqueous humor.

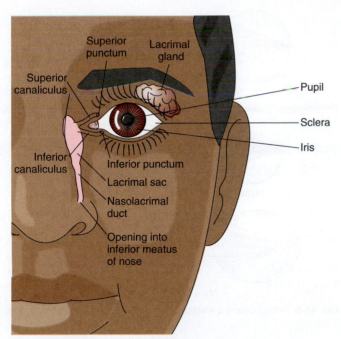

FIG. 46-3 Front view of the eye and adjacent structures.

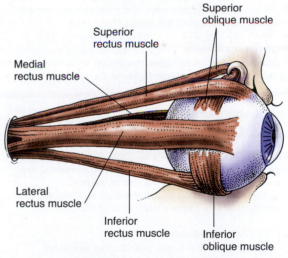

FIG. 46-4 Extraocular muscles.

A small **lacrimal gland**, which is located in the upper outer part of each orbit (Fig. 46-3), produces tears. Tears flow across the front of the eye, toward the nose, and into the inner canthus. They drain through the **punctum** (an opening at the nasal side of the lid edges) into the lacrimal duct and sac and then into the nose through the nasolacrimal duct.

Muscles, Nerves, and Blood Vessels

Six voluntary muscles rotate the eye and coordinate eye movements (Fig. 46-4 and Table 46-1). Coordinated eye movements ensure that both eyes receive an image at the same time so only a single image is seen.

The muscles around the eye are innervated by cranial nerves (CNs) III (oculomotor), IV (trochlear), and VI (abducens). The **optic nerve** (CN II) is the nerve of sight, connecting the optic disc to the brain. The trigeminal nerve (CN V) stimulates the blink reflex when the cornea is touched. The facial nerve (CN VII) innervates the lacrimal glands and muscles for lid closure.

The ophthalmic artery brings oxygenated blood to the eye and the orbit. It branches to supply blood to the retina. The ciliary arteries supply the sclera, choroid, ciliary body, and iris.

Outflow moves through several venous pathways that empty into the superior ophthalmic vein.

Function

The four eye functions that provide clear images and vision are refraction, pupillary constriction, accommodation, and convergence.

Refraction bends light rays from the outside into the eye through curved surfaces and refractive media and finally to the retina. Each surface and media bend (refract) light differently to focus an image on the retina. Emmetropia is the perfect refraction of the eye in which light rays from a distant source are focused into a sharp image on the retina. Fig. 46-5 shows the normal refraction of light within the eye. Images fall on the retina inverted and reversed left to right. For example, an object in the lower nasal visual field strikes the upper outer area of the retina.

Errors of refraction are common. Hyperopia (farsightedness) occurs when the eye does not refract light enough. As a result, images actually converge behind the retina (see Fig. 46-5). With hyperopia, distant vision is normal, but near vision is poor. It is corrected with a convex lens in eyeglasses or contact lenses.

Myopia (nearsightedness) occurs when the eye overbends the light and images converge in front of the retina (see Fig. 46-5). Near vision is normal, but distance vision is poor. Myopia is corrected with a concave lens in eyeglasses or contact lenses.

Astigmatism is a refractive error caused by unevenly curved surfaces on or in the eye, especially the cornea. These uneven surfaces distort vision.

Pupillary constriction and dilation control the amount of light that enters the eye. If the level of light to one or both eyes is increased, both pupils constrict (become smaller). The amount of constriction depends on how much light is available and how well the retina can adapt to light changes. Pupillary constriction is called miosis, and pupillary dilation is called mydriasis (Fig. 46-6). Certain drugs can alter pupillary constriction.

Accommodation allows the healthy eye to focus images sharply on the retina, whether the image is close to the eye or distant. The process of maintaining a clear visual image when the gaze is shifted from a distant to a near object is known as accommodation. The healthy eye can adjust its focus by changing the curve of the lens.

Convergence is the ability to turn both eyes inward toward the nose at the same time. This action helps ensure that only a single image of close objects is seen.

TABLE 46-1	Functions of Ocular Muscles

Superior Rectus Muscle
- Together with the lateral rectus, this muscle moves the eye diagonally upward toward the side of the head.
- Together with the medial rectus, this muscle moves the eye diagonally upward toward the middle of the head.

Lateral Rectus Muscle
- Together with the medial rectus, this muscle holds the eye straight.
- Contracting alone, this muscle turns the eye toward the side of the head.

Medial Rectus Muscle
- Contracting alone, this muscle turns the eye toward the nose.

Inferior Rectus Muscle
- Together with the lateral rectus, this muscle moves the eye diagonally downward toward the side of the head.
- Together with the medial rectus, this muscle moves the eye diagonally downward toward the middle of the head.

Superior Oblique Muscle
- Contracting alone, this muscle pulls the eye downward.

Inferior Oblique Muscle
- Contracting alone, this muscle pulls the eye upward.

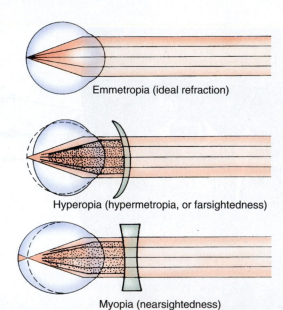

FIG. 46-5 Refraction and correction in emmetropia, hyperopia, and myopia.

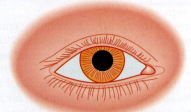

Normal pupil slightly dilated for moderate light

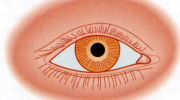

Miosis—pupil constricted when exposed to increased light or close work, such as reading

FIG. 46-6 Miosis and mydriasis.

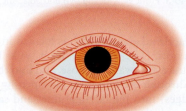

Mydriasis—pupil dilated when exposed to reduced light or when looking at a distance

Eye Changes Associated With Aging

Changes inside the eye cause visual acuity to decrease with age (Touhy & Jett, 2014). Age-related changes of the nervous system and in the eye support structures also reduce visual function (Chart 46-1).

Structural changes occur with aging, including decreased eye muscle tone that reduces the ability to keep the gaze focused on a single object. The lower eyelid may relax and fall away from the eye *(ectropion)*, leading to dry eye signs and symptoms.

Arcus senilis, an opaque, bluish-white ring within the outer edge of the cornea, is caused by fat deposits (see Fig. 24-4). This change does not affect vision.

The clarity and shape of the cornea change with age. The cornea flattens, and the curve of its surface becomes irregular. This change causes or worsens astigmatism and blurs vision.

Fatty deposits cause the sclera to develop a yellowish tinge. A bluish color may be seen as the sclera thins. With age, the iris has less ability to dilate, which leads to difficulty in adapting to dark environments. Older adults may need additional light for reading and other "close-up" work and to avoid tripping over objects.

Functional changes also occur with aging. The lens yellows with aging, reducing the ability to transmit and focus light. The lens hardens, shrinks, and loses elasticity, which reduces accommodation. The **near point of vision** (i.e., the closest distance at which the eye can see an object clearly) increases. Near objects, especially reading material, must be placed farther from the eye to be seen clearly (**presbyopia**). The **far point** (i.e., the farthest point at which an object can be distinguished) decreases. Together these changes narrow the visual field of an older adult.

General color perception decreases, especially for green, blue, and violet. More light is needed to stimulate the visual receptors. Intraocular pressure (IOP) is slightly higher in older adults.

Health Promotion and Maintenance

Vision is important for function and quality of life. Many vision and eye problems can be avoided, and others can be corrected or managed if discovered early. Teach all adults about eye-protection methods, adequate nutrition, and the importance of regular eye examinations.

The risks for cataract formation and for cancer of the eye (ocular melanoma) increase with exposure to ultraviolet (UV) light. Teach adults to protect the eyes by using sunglasses that filter UV light whenever they are outdoors or at tanning salons and when work involves UV exposure.

Vision can be affected by injury. Eye injury also increases the risk for both cataract formation and glaucoma. Urge all adults to wear eye and head protection when working with particulate matter, fluid or blood spatter, high temperatures, or sparks. Protection also should be worn during participation in sports, such as baseball, or any activity that increases the risk for the eye being hit by objects in motion. Teach adults to avoid rubbing the eyes to avoid trauma to outer eye surfaces.

Eye infections can lead to vision loss. Although the eye surface is not sterile, the sclera and cornea have no separate blood supply and thus are at risk for infection. Teach adults to wash their hands before touching the eye or eyelid. Teach patients who use eyedrops about the proper technique to use these drugs (Chart 46-2), which includes not touching the eye with the bottle tip and not sharing eyedrops with others. If an eye has a discharge, teach the patient to use a separate eyedrop

☘ CHART 46-1 Nursing Focus on the Older Adult

Changes in the Eye and Vision Related to Aging

STRUCTURE/ FUNCTION	CHANGE	IMPLICATION
Appearance	Eyes appear "sunken."	Do not use eye appearance as an indicator for hydration status.
	Arcus senilis forms.	Reassure patient that this change does not affect vision.
	Sclera yellows or appears blue.	Do not use sclera to assess for jaundice.
Cornea	Cornea flattens, which blurs vision.	Encourage older adults to have regular eye examinations and wear prescribed corrective lenses for best vision.
Ocular muscles	Muscle strength is reduced, making it more difficult to maintain an upward gaze or a focus on a single image.	Reassure patient that this is a normal happening and to re-focus gaze frequently to maintain a single image.
Lens	Elasticity is lost, increasing the near point of vision (making the near point of best vision farther away).	Encourage patient to wear corrective lenses for reading.
	Lens hardens, compacts, and forms a cataract.	Stress the importance of annual vision checks and monitoring.
Iris and pupil	Decrease in ability to dilate results in small pupil size and poor adaptation to darkness.	Teach about the need for good lighting to avoid tripping and bumping into objects.
Color vision	Discrimination among greens, blues, and violets decreases.	The patient may not be able to use color-indicator monitors of health status.
Tears	Tear production is reduced, resulting in dry eyes, discomfort, and increased risk for corneal damage or eye infections.	Teach about the use of saline eyedrops to reduce dryness. Teach patient to increase humidity in the home.

CHART 46-2   Patient and Family Education: Preparing For Self-Management

Using Eyedrops

- Check the eyedrop name, strength, expiration date, color, and clarity.
- If both eyes are to receive the same drug and one eye is infected, use two separate bottles and label each bottle with "right" or "left" for the correct eye.
- Wash your hands.
- Remove the cap from the bottle.
- Tilt your head backward, open your eyes, and look up at the ceiling.
- Using your nondominant hand, gently pull the lower lid down against your cheek, forming a small pocket.
- Hold the eyedrop bottle (with the cap off) like a pencil, with the tip pointing down, with your dominant hand.
- Rest the wrist holding the bottle against your mouth or upper lip.
- Without touching any part of the eye or lid with the tip of the bottle, gently squeeze the bottle and release the prescribed number of drops into the pocket of your lower lid.
- Release the lower lid and gently close your eye without squeezing the lids.
- Gently press and hold the corner of the eye nearest the nose to close off the punctum and prevent the drug from being absorbed systemically.
- Gently blot away any excess drug or tears with a tissue.
- Keep the eye closed for about 1 minute.
- Place the cap back on the bottle and store it as prescribed.
- Wash your hands again.

bottle for this eye and to wash the unaffected eye before washing the affected eye.

Other health problems, especially diabetes and hypertension, can seriously affect visual SENSORY PERCEPTION. Teach patients with these health problems about the importance of controlling blood glucose levels and managing blood pressure to reduce the risk for vision loss. Annual evaluation by an eye-care practitioner is needed to slow or prevent eye complications.

Teach patients who have a refractive error to have an eye examination annually. Young adults without vision problems may need an eye examination only every 3 to 5 years. Adults older than 40 years should have an eye examination annually that includes assessment of intraocular pressure and visual fields because the risk for both glaucoma and cataract formation increases with age.

! NURSING SAFETY PRIORITY (QSEN)

Action Alert

Teach adults to see a health care provider immediately when an eye injury occurs or an eye infection is suspected.

? NCLEX EXAMINATION CHALLENGE 46-1

Health Promotion and Maintenance

A 44-year-old client with diabetes asks how often a visit to the eye-care practitioner is recommended. What is the **appropriate** nursing response?

A. "Annually."
B. "Every 6 months."
C. "Only if you have vision problems."
D. "No examinations are necessary until you are 50 years old."

TABLE 46-2   Systemic Conditions and Common Drugs Affecting the Eye and Vision

Systemic Conditions and Disorders	Drugs
• Diabetes mellitus	• Antihistamines*
• Hypertension	• Decongestants*
• Lupus erythematosus	• Antibiotics
• Sarcoidosis	• Opioids
• Thyroid problems	• Anticholinergics
• Acquired immune deficiency syndrome	• Cholinergic agonists
• Cardiac disease	• Adrenergic agonists
• Multiple sclerosis	• Adrenergic antagonists (beta blockers)
• Pregnancy	• Oral contraceptives
	• Chemotherapy agents
	• Corticosteroids*

*Prescription and over-the-counter.

ASSESSMENT: NOTICING AND INTERPRETING

Patient History

Collect information to determine whether problems with the eye or vision have an impact on ADLs or other daily functions.

Age is an important factor to consider when assessing visual SENSORY PERCEPTION and eye structure. The incidence of glaucoma and cataract formation increases with aging. Presbyopia commonly begins in the 40s.

Gender may be important. Retinal detachments occur more often in men, and dry eye syndromes occur more often in women.

Occupation and leisure activities can affect visual SENSORY PERCEPTION. Ask about how the eyes are used at work. In occupations such as computer programming, constant exposure to monitors may lead to eyestrain. Machine operators are at risk for eye injury because of the high speeds at which particles can be thrown at the eye. Chronic exposure to infrared or UV light may cause photophobia and cataract formation. Teach the patient about the use of eye protection during work.

Ask whether the patient wears eye protection when participating in sports. A blow to the head near the eye, such as with a baseball, can damage external structures, the eye, the connections with the brain, or the area of the brain where vision is perceived.

Systemic health problems can affect vision. Check whether the patient has any condition listed in Table 46-2. Ask about past accidents, injuries, surgeries, or blows to the head that may have led to the present problem. Specifically ask about previous laser surgeries.

Drugs can also affect vision and the eye (see Table 46-2). Ask about the use of any prescription or over-the-counter drugs, especially decongestants and antihistamines, which tend to dry the eye and may increase intraocular pressure. Document the name, strength, dose, and scheduling for all drugs the patient uses. Ocular effects from drugs include itching, foreign body sensation, redness, tearing, photophobia (sensitivity to light), and the development of cataracts or glaucoma.

Nutrition History

Some eye problems are caused by or made worse with vitamin deficiencies. Ask the patient about food choices. For example, vitamin A deficiency can cause eye dryness, keratomalacia, and blindness. Some nutrients and antioxidants, such as lutein and beta carotene, help maintain retinal function. A diet rich in fruit and red, orange, and dark green vegetables is important to eye health. Teach adults to eat about 10 servings of these foods daily.

NCLEX EXAMINATION CHALLENGE 46-2

Health Promotion and Maintenance

Which foods will the nurse recommend to a client who wishes to enhance eye health? **Select all that apply.**
A. Kale
B. Bananas
C. Carrots
D. Ground beef
E. Shellfish
F. Spinach

Family History and Genetic Risk

Ask about a family history of eye problems because some conditions have a familial tendency and some genetic problems lead to visual impairment. When a patient tells you that other relatives, especially first-degree relatives (parents, siblings, and children), have eye problems, document the gender of the affected person, the relationship to the patient, the exact nature of the problem, and the age that the problem was first noted.

Current Health Problems

Ask the patient about the onset of visual changes. Did the change occur rapidly or slowly? Determine whether the signs and symptoms are present to the same degree in both eyes. Ask these questions if eye injury or trauma is involved:

- How long ago did the injury occur?
- What was the patient doing when it happened?
- If a foreign body was involved, what was its source?
- Was any first aid administered at the scene? If so, what actions were taken?

NURSING SAFETY PRIORITY (QSEN)

Critical Rescue

Recognize that a sudden or persistent loss of visual SENSORY PERCEPTION within the past 48 hours, eye trauma, a foreign body in the eye, or sudden ocular pain is an emergency. Respond by notifying the eye-care practitioner immediately.

Physical Assessment
Inspection

Look for head tilting, squinting, or other actions that indicate that the patient is trying to attain clear vision. For example, patients with double vision may cock the head to the side to focus the two images into one, or they may close one eye to see clearly.

Assess for symmetry in the appearance of the eyes. Check them to determine whether they are equally distant from the nose, are the same size, and have the same degree of prominence. Assess the eyes for their placement in the orbits and for symmetry of movement. **Exophthalmos** *(proptosis)* is protrusion of the eye. **Enophthalmos** is the sunken appearance of the eye.

Examine the eyebrows and eyelashes for hair distribution and determine the direction of the eyelashes. Eyelashes normally point outward and away from the eyelid. Assess the eyelids for **ptosis** (drooping), redness, lesions, or swelling. The lids normally close completely, with the lid edges touching. When the eyes are open, the upper lid covers a small portion of the iris. The edge of the lower lid lies at the iris. No sclera should be visible between the eyelid and the iris.

Scleral and corneal assessment require a penlight. Examine the sclera for color; it is usually white. A yellow color may indicate jaundice or systemic problems. In dark-skinned adults, the normal sclera may appear yellow; and small, pigmented dots may be visible (Jarvis, 2016).

The cornea is best seen by directing a light at it from the side. It should be transparent, smooth, shiny, and bright. Any cloudy areas or specks may indicate injury.

Assess the blink reflex by bringing a hand quickly toward the patient's face. Be certain to use extreme caution when performing this maneuver, especially with confused patients. Patients with vision will blink.

Pupillary assessment involves examining each pupil separately and comparing the results. The pupils are usually round and of equal size. About 5% of adults normally have a noticeable difference in the size of their pupils, which is known as **anisocoria** (Jarvis, 2016). Pupil size varies in adults exposed to the same amount of light. Pupils are smaller in older adults. Patients with myopia have larger pupils. Patients with hyperopia have smaller pupils. The normal pupil diameter is between 3 and 5 mm. Smaller pupils reduce vision in low light conditions.

Observe pupils for response to light. Increasing light causes constriction, whereas decreasing light causes dilation. Constriction of both pupils is the normal response to direct light and to accommodation. Assess pupillary reaction to light by asking the patient to look straight ahead while you quickly bring the beam of a penlight in from the side and direct it at the right pupil. Constriction of the right pupil is a direct response to shining the penlight into that eye. Constriction of the left pupil when light is shined at the right pupil is known as a **consensual response**. Assess the responses for each eye. (You may see the abbreviation "PERRLA" in a patient's electronic health record, which stands for **p**upils **e**qual, **r**ound, **r**eactive to **l**ight, and **a**ccommodation.)

Evaluate each pupil for speed of reaction. The pupil should immediately constrict when a light is directed at it (i.e., a *brisk* response). If the pupil takes more than 1 second to constrict, the response is *sluggish*. Pupils that fail to react are *nonreactive* or *fixed*. Compare the reactivity speed of right and left pupils and document any difference.

Assess for accommodation by holding your finger about 18 cm from the patient's nose and move it toward the nose. The patient's eyes normally converge during this movement, and the pupils constrict equally.

Vision Testing

Visual SENSORY PERCEPTION is measured by first testing each eye separately and then testing both eyes together. Patients who wear corrective lenses are tested both without and with their lenses.

Visual acuity tests measure both distance and near vision. The Snellen eye chart measures distance vision. This chart has letters, numbers, pictures, or a single letter presented in various positions. The chart with one letter in different positions is used for patients who cannot read, who do not speak the language used at the facility, or who cannot speak but do have adequate cognition. Have the patient stand or sit 20 feet from the chart, cover one eye, and use the other eye to read the line that appears most clear. If the patient can do this accurately, ask him or her to read the next lower line. Repeat this sequence to the last line on which the patient can correctly identify most characters. Repeat the procedure with the other eye. Record findings as a comparison between what the patient can read at 20 feet and the distance that a person with normal vision can read the same line. For example, 20/50 means that the patient sees at 20 feet from the chart what a healthy eye sees at 50 feet.

For patients who cannot see the 20/400 character, assess visual acuity by holding fingers in front of their eyes and asking them to count the number of fingers. Acuity is recorded as "counts finger vision at 5 feet," or the farthest distance at which fingers are counted correctly.

Patients who cannot count fingers are tested for hand motion (HM) acuity. Stand about 2 to 3 feet in front of the patient. Ask him or her to cover the eye not being tested. Direct a light onto your hand from behind the patient. Demonstrate the three possible directions in which the hand can move during the test (stationary, left-right, or up-down). Move your hand slowly (1 second per motion) and ask the patient, "What is my hand doing now?" Repeat this procedure five times. Visual acuity is recorded as HM at the farthest distance at which most of the HMs are identified correctly.

If the patient cannot detect HM, assess light perception (LP). Ask him or her first to cover the left eye. In a darkened room, direct the beam of a penlight at the patient's right eye from a distance of 2 to 3 feet for 1 to 2 seconds. Instruct the patient to say "on" when the beam of light is perceived and "off" when it is no longer detected. If the patient identifies the presence or absence of light three times correctly, acuity is documented as LP. If he or she is unable to identify the presence or absence of light, the test result is documented as NLP, meaning "no light perception" (Roy, 2012).

Near vision is tested for patients who have difficulty reading without using glasses or other means of vision correction. Use a small, handheld miniature eye chart called a *Rosenbaum Pocket Vision Screener* or a *Jaeger card.* Ask the patient to hold the card 14 inches away from his or her eyes and read the characters. Test each eye separately and then together. Document the lowest line on which the patient can identify more than half the characters.

Visual field testing determines the degree of peripheral vision. It can be performed with a computerized machine or with a "confrontation test" for a rapid check of peripheral vision. *Perimetry* is the computerized test. During this test, the patient is asked to look straight ahead into a viewer and then indicate, by pressing a control button, when a moving light enters the peripheral vision. This process maps the person's peripheral vision and any deficits.

During the confrontation test, sit facing the patient and ask him or her to look directly into your eyes while you look into the patient's eyes. Cover your right eye and have the patient cover his or her left eye so that you both have the same visual field. Then move a finger or an object from a nonvisible area into the patient's line of vision. The patient with normal peripheral vision notices the object at about the same time you do. Repeat this examination by covering your left eye and having the patient cover his or her right eye. Document any areas in which you can see but the patient cannot.

Extraocular muscle function is assessed using the corneal light reflex and the six cardinal positions of gaze. These tests assess smoothness of eye movements and the function of cranial nerves III, IV, and VI.

The corneal light reflex determines alignment of the eyes. After asking the patient to stare straight ahead, shine a penlight at both corneas from a distance of 12 to 15 inches. The bright dot of light reflected from the shiny surface of the cornea should be in a symmetric position (e.g., at the 1 o'clock position in the right eye and at the 11 o'clock position in the left eye). An asymmetric reflex indicates a deviating eye and possible muscle weakness.

Use the six cardinal positions of gaze to assess muscle function (Fig. 46-7). The eye will not turn to a particular position if the muscle is weak or if the controlling nerve is affected. Ask the patient to hold his or her head still and to move only the eyes to follow a small object. Move the object to the patient's right (lateral), upward and right (temporal), down and right, left (lateral), upward and left (temporal), and down and left (see Fig. 46-7). While the patient moves the eyes to these positions, note whether both eyes move in a parallel manner and any deviation of movement. **Nystagmus**, an involuntary and rapid twitching of the eyeball, is a normal finding for the far lateral gaze. It may also be caused by abnormal nerve function or problems with the inner ear or alcohol intoxication.

Color vision is usually tested using the *Ishihara chart,* which shows numbers composed of dots of one color within a circle of dots of a different color (Fig. 46-8). Test each eye separately by asking the patient what numbers he or she sees on the chart. Reading the numbers correctly indicates normal color vision.

Psychosocial Assessment

A patient with changes in visual SENSORY PERCEPTION may be anxious about possible vision loss. Patients with severe visual defects may be unable to perform ADLs. Dependency from reduced vision can affect self-esteem. Ask the patient how he or she feels about the vision changes and assess coping techniques.

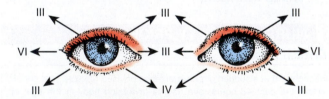

FIG. 46-7 Checking extraocular movements in the six cardinal positions indicates the functioning of cranial nerves III, IV, and VI.

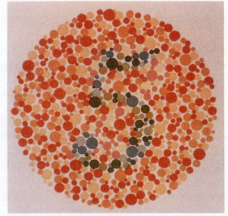

FIG. 46-8 An Ishihara chart for testing color vision.

Assess the family to determine available support. Provide information about local resources and services for patients with reduced vision.

Diagnostic Assessment

Laboratory Assessment

Cultures of corneal or conjunctival swabs and scrapings help diagnose infections. Obtain a sample of the exudate for culture before antibiotics or topical anesthetics are instilled. Take swabs from the conjunctivae and any ulcerated or inflamed areas.

Imaging Assessment

CT is useful for assessing the eyes, the bony structures around the eyes, and the extraocular muscles. It can also detect tumors in the orbital space. A contrast agent is used unless trauma is suspected. Tell the patient that this test is not painful but does require being in a confined space and keeping the head still.

MRI is often used to examine the orbits and the optic nerves and to evaluate ocular tumors. It cannot be used to evaluate injuries involving metal in the eyes. *Metal in the eye is an absolute contraindication for MRI.*

Radioisotope scanning is used to locate tumors and lesions. This test requires that the patient sign an informed consent. The patient receives a tracer dose of the radioactive isotope, either orally or by injection, and must then lie still. The scanner measures the radioactivity emitted by the radioactive atoms concentrated in the area being studied. Sedation may be used for patients who are anxious. No special follow-up care is required.

Ultrasonography is used to examine the orbit and eye with high-frequency sound waves. This noninvasive test helps diagnose trauma, intraorbital tumors, proptosis, and choroidal or retinal detachments. It is also used to determine the length of the eye and any gross outline changes in the eye and the orbit in patients with cloudy corneas or lenses that reduce direct examination of the fundus.

Inform the patient that this test is painless because it is either performed with the eyes closed or, when the eyes must remain open, anesthetic eyedrops are instilled first. He or she sits upright with the chin in the chin rest. The probe is touched against the patient's anesthetized cornea, and sound waves are bounced through the eye. The sound waves create a reflective pattern on a computer screen that can be examined for abnormalities. No special follow-up care is needed. Remind the patient not to rub or touch the eye until the anesthetic agent has worn off.

Other Diagnostic Assessment

Many tests are used to examine specific eye structures when patients have specific risks, signs and symptoms, or exposures. These tests are performed only by physicians, optometrists, or advanced practice nurses.

Slit-lamp examination magnifies the anterior eye structures (Fig. 46-9). The patient leans on a chin rest to stabilize the head. A narrow beam (slit) of light is aimed so only a segment of the eye is brightly lighted. The examiner can then locate the position of any abnormality in the cornea, lens, or anterior vitreous humor.

Corneal staining consists of placing fluorescein or other topical dye into the conjunctival sac. The dye outlines irregularities of the corneal surface that are not easily visible. This test is used for corneal trauma, problems caused by a contact lens, or the presence of foreign bodies, abrasions, ulcers, or other corneal disorders.

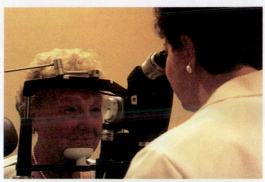

FIG. 46-9 Slit-lamp ocular examination.

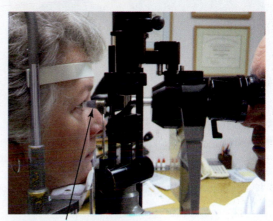

Goldmann applanation tonometer

FIG. 46-10 Use of Goldmann applanation tonometer and a slit lamp to measure intraocular pressure (IOP).

This procedure is noninvasive and is performed under aseptic conditions. The dye is applied topically to the eye, and the eye is then viewed through a blue filter. Nonintact areas of the cornea stain a bright green color.

Tonometry measures intraocular pressure (IOP) using a tonometer. This instrument applies pressure to the outside of the eye until it equals the pressure inside the eye. Normal IOP readings have always been considered to range from 10 to 21 mm Hg; however, this number is not absolute and must be considered along with corneal thickness. The thickness of the cornea affects how much pressure must be applied before indentation occurs. For example, an adult with a thicker cornea will have a higher tonometer reading that may falsely indicate increased IOP. An adult with a thinner-than-normal cornea may have a low tonometer reading even when higher IOP is present.

About 5% of patients with healthy eyes have a slightly higher pressure. Tonometer readings are indicated for all patients older than 40 years. Adults with a family history of glaucoma should have their IOP measured once or twice a year. The most common method to measure IOP by an eye-care practitioner is the Goldmann applanation tonometer used with a slit lamp (Fig. 46-10). This method involves direct eye contact. Another instrument, the Tono-Pen (Fig. 46-11), is designed for use by eye-care practitioners in extended care or long-term care facilities or for other patients unable to be positioned behind a slit lamp.

IOP varies throughout the day and typically peaks at certain times of the day. Therefore always document the type and time of IOP measurement.

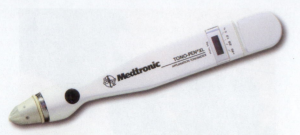

FIG. 46-11 The Tono-Pen. (Courtesy Medtronic Ophthalmics, Minneapolis, MN.)

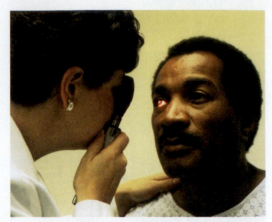

FIG. 46-12 Proper technique for direct ophthalmoscopic visualization of the retina.

TABLE 46-3 Structures Assessed by Direct Ophthalmoscopy

Red Reflex	**Fundus**
• Presence or absence	• Color
	• Tears or holes
Optic Disc	• Lesions
• Color	• Bleeding
• Margins (sharp or blurred)	
• Cup size	**Macula**
• Presence of rings or crescents	• Presence of blood vessels
	• Color
Optic Blood Vessels	• Lesions
• Size	• Bleeding
• Color	
• Kinks or tangles	
• Light reflection	
• Narrowing	
• Nicking at arteriovenous crossings	

◎ CHART 46-3 Best Practice for Patient Safety & Quality Care QSEN

Instillation of Eyedrops

- Check the name, strength, expiration date, color, and clarity of the eyedrops to be instilled.
- Check to see whether only one eye is to have the drug or if both eyes are to receive it.
- If both eyes are to receive the same drug and one eye is infected, use two separate bottles and carefully label each bottle with "right" or "left" for the correct eye.
- Wash your hands.
- Put on gloves if secretions are present in or around the eye.
- Explain the procedure to the patient.
- Have the patient sit in a chair, and you stand behind the patient.
- Ask the patient to tilt the head backward, with the back of the head resting against your body and looking up at the ceiling.
- Gently pull the lower lid down against the patient's cheek, forming a small pocket.
- Hold the eyedrop bottle (with the cap off) like a pencil, with the tip pointing down.
- Rest the wrist holding the bottle against the patient's check.
- Without touching any part of the eye or lid with the tip of the bottle, gently squeeze the bottle and release the prescribed number of drops into the pocket you have made with the patient's lower lid.
- Gently release the lower lid.
- Tell the patient to close the eye gently (without squeezing the lids tightly).
- Gently press and hold the corner of the eye nearest the nose to close off the punctum and prevent the drug from being absorbed systemically.
- Without pressing on the lid, gently blot away any excess drug or tears with a tissue.
- Remove your gloves and place the cap back on the bottle.
- Ask the patient to keep the eye closed for about 1 minute.
- Wash your hands again.

Ophthalmoscopy allows viewing of the eye's external and interior structures with an instrument called an *ophthalmoscope*. This examination can be performed by any nurse but usually is performed by an eye-care practitioner, advanced practice nurse, or physician assistant. It is easiest to examine the fundus when the room is dark because the pupil dilates. Stand on the same side as the eye being examined. Tell the patient to look straight ahead at an object on the wall behind you. Hold the ophthalmoscope firmly against your face and align it so your eye sees through the sight hole (Fig. 46-12).

When using the ophthalmoscope, move toward the patient's eye from about 12 to 15 inches away and to the side of his or her line of vision. As you direct the ophthalmoscope at the pupil, a red glare (**red reflex**) should be seen in the pupil as a reflection of the light off of the retina. An absent red reflex in an adult may indicate a lens opacity or cloudiness of the vitreous. Move toward the patient's pupil while following the red reflex. The retina should then be visible through the ophthalmoscope. Examine the optic disc, optic vessels, fundus, and macula. Table 46-3 lists the features that can be observed in each structure.

The use of an ophthalmoscope may make a confused patient or one who does not understand the language more anxious. When working with a patient who does not speak the language used at the facility, use an interpreter, when possible, to ensure the patient's understanding and cooperation with the examination.

⚠ NURSING SAFETY PRIORITY QSEN

Action Alert

Avoid using an ophthalmoscope with a confused patient to prevent accidental injury to the eye.

Fluorescein angiography, which is performed by a physician or advanced practice nurse, provides a detailed image of eye circulation. Digital pictures are taken in rapid succession after the dye is given IV. This test helps to assess problems of retinal circulation (e.g., diabetic retinopathy, retinal hemorrhage, and macular degeneration) or to diagnose intraocular tumors.

Explain the procedure to the patient, check that the patient has signed informed consent, and instill mydriatic eyedrops (cause pupil dilation) 1 hour before the test. Chart 46-3 lists the best practice for correct eyedrop instillation. Warn that the dye may cause the skin to appear yellow for several hours after the test. The stain is eliminated through the urine, which turns green.

Encourage patients to drink fluids to help eliminate the dye. Remind them that any staining of the skin will disappear in a few hours. Instruct the patient to wear dark glasses and avoid direct sunlight until pupil dilation returns to normal because the bright light will cause eye pain.

Electroretinography graphs the retina's response to light stimulation. This test is helpful in detecting and evaluating blood vessel changes from disease or drugs. The graph is obtained by placing an electrode on an anesthetized cornea. Lights at varying speeds and intensities are flashed, and the neural response is graphed. The measurement from the cornea is identical to the response that would be obtained if electrodes were placed directly on the retina.

Gonioscopy is a test performed when a high IOP is found and determines whether open-angle or closed-angle glaucoma is present. It uses a special lens that eliminates the corneal curve, is painless, and allows visualization of the angle where the iris meets the cornea.

Ultrasonic imaging of the retina and optic nerve creates a three-dimensional view of the back of the eye. It is often used for people with ocular hypertension or who are at risk for glaucoma from other problems. This computerized examination assesses the thickness and contours of the optic nerve fiber layer and retina for changes that indicate damage as a result of high IOP. It can be used serially for a patient at risk for glaucoma to detect early changes and indicate when intervention is needed.

❓ CLINICAL JUDGMENT CHALLENGE 46-1
Patient-Centered Care; Safety QSEN

You are caring for a 64-year-old patient whose last comprehensive eye examination was 8 years ago. She reports that she is having a bit of difficulty seeing out of her peripheral vision but otherwise feels healthy. She says that she has always dreaded seeing an eye-care practitioner because health care providers make her nervous.

1. What other assessment data should you collect from this patient?
2. What condition do you anticipate that this patient may be experiencing?
3. What type of test(s) do you anticipate that the eye-care practitioner may perform?
4. What recommendation about seeing an eye-care practitioner will you provide to the patient?
5. How can you address your patient's psychosocial concern about feeling nervous?

GET READY FOR THE NCLEX® EXAMINATION!

KEY POINTS

Review these Key Points for each NCLEX Examination Client Needs Category.

Safe and Effective Care Environment
- Wash your hands and don gloves before moving a patient's eyelids or instilling drugs into the eye. **QSEN: Safety**
- If a patient has discharge from one eye, examine the eye without the discharge first. **QSEN: Safety**
- Avoid using an ophthalmoscope on a confused patient. **QSEN: Safety**

Health Promotion and Maintenance
- Teach patients not to rub their eyes. **QSEN: Safety**
- Identify patients at risk for eye injury as a result of work environment or leisure activities. **QSEN: Safety**
- Teach adults to wear eye protection when they are performing yard work, working in a woodshop or metal shop, using chemicals, or in any environment in which drops or particulate matter is airborne. **QSEN: Safety**
- Teach adults to wear sunglasses outdoors in bright sunlight. **QSEN: Safety**

Psychosocial Integrity
- Provide opportunities for the patient and family to express concerns about a possible change in visual SENSORY PERCEPTION. **QSEN: Patient-Centered Care**
- Explain all diagnostic procedures, restrictions, and follow-up care to the patient scheduled for tests. **QSEN: Patient-Centered Care**

Physiological Integrity
- Ask the patient about vision problems in any other members of the family because some vision problems have a genetic component. **QSEN: Patient-Centered Care**
- Test the vision of both eyes immediately if a patient has experienced an eye injury or any sudden change in vision. **QSEN: Safety**

SELECTED BIBLIOGRAPHY

Jarvis, C. (2016). *Physical examination & health assessment* (7th ed.). St. Louis: Elsevier.

McCance, K., Huether, S., Brashers, V., & Rote, N. (2014). *Pathophysiology: The biologic basis for disease in adults and children* (7th ed.). St. Louis: Mosby.

Roy, F. H. (2012). *Ocular differential diagnosis.* Clayton, Panama: Jaypee-Highlights Medical Publishers, Inc.

Touhy, T., & Jett, K. (2014). *Ebersole and Hess' gerontological nursing and healthy aging* (4th ed.). St. Louis: Mosby.

47 CHAPTER

Care of Patients With Eye and Vision Problems

Samuel A. Borchers and Andrea A. Borchers

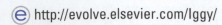 http://evolve.elsevier.com/Iggy/

PRIORITY AND INTERRELATED CONCEPTS

The priority concept for this chapter is SENSORY PERCEPTION.

✳ The SENSORY PERCEPTION concept exemplars for this chapter are:
- Cataract, below,
- Glaucoma, p. 972.

LEARNING OUTCOMES

Safe and Effective Care Environment
1. Collaborate with the interprofessional team to coordinate high-quality care for patients with eye and vision problems.
2. Protect patients with eye and vision problems from injury and infection.
3. Teach the patient with reduced visual SENSORY PERCEPTION and his or her family how to adapt the home environment for safety.

Health Promotion and Maintenance
4. Teach adults about the importance of annual eye examinations with measurement of intraocular pressure (IOP).

5. Teach patients and family members how to correctly instill ophthalmic drops and ointment.
6. Teach patients with glaucoma the relationship between increased IOP and eye problems.

Psychosocial Integrity
7. Implement nursing interventions to minimize stressors for the patient experiencing a change in visual SENSORY PERCEPTION.

Physiological Integrity
8. Prioritize care and educational needs for the patient with cataract or primary open-angle glaucoma.

Visual SENSORY PERCEPTION can be affected by many factors. Some have a gradual onset, such as cataracts or the most common form of glaucoma; others have a quick onset, such as retinal detachment. Changes in visual sensory perception, whether transient or permanent, require the patient to make adaptations in function or lifestyle. Nurses work as an integral part of the interprofessional team comprised of eye-care providers, occupational therapists, and social workers to provide high-quality care for patients with vision concerns.

✳ SENSORY PERCEPTION CONCEPT EXEMPLAR
Cataract

❖ PATHOPHYSIOLOGY

The lens is a transparent, elastic structure suspended behind the iris that focuses images onto the retina. A cataract is a lens opacity that distorts the image (Fig. 47-1). With aging, the lens gradually loses water and increases in density (Touhy & Jett,

2015). Lens density increases with drying and compression of older lens fibers and production of new fibers and lens crystals. With time, as lens density increases and transparency is lost, visual SENSORY PERCEPTION is greatly reduced. Both eyes may have cataracts, but the rate of progression in each eye is different.

Etiology and Genetic Risk
Cataracts may be present at birth or develop at any time. They may be age related or caused by trauma or exposure to toxic agents. They also occur with other diseases and eye disorders (Table 47-1).

Incidence/Prevalence
About 27.5 million adults in the United States and Canada have cataracts (Canadian National Institute for the Blind [CNIB], 2017a; National Eye Institute, 2017b). The age-related cataract is the most common type. Some degree of cataract formation is expected in all adults older than 70 years.

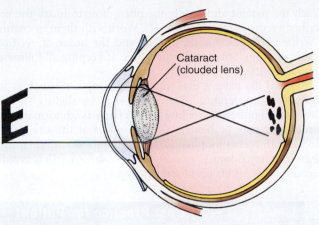

FIG. 47-1 Visual impairment produced by the presence of a cataract.

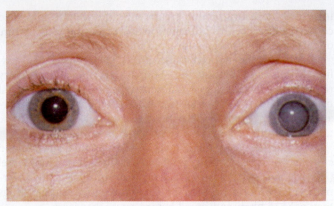

FIG. 47-2 Appearance of an eye with a mature cataract. (From Patton, K. T., & Thibodeau, G. A. [2016]. *Anatomy and physiology* [9th ed.]. St. Louis: Mosby.)

TABLE 47-1	Common Causes of Cataracts
Age-Related Cataracts	**Associated Cataracts**
• Lens water loss and fiber compaction	• Diabetes mellitus • Hypoparathyroidism • Down syndrome • Chronic sunlight exposure
Traumatic Cataracts	
• Blunt injury to eye or head • Penetrating eye injury • Intraocular foreign bodies • Radiation exposure, therapy	**Complicated Cataracts**
	• Retinitis pigmentosa • Glaucoma • Retinal detachment
Toxic Cataracts	
• Corticosteroids • Phenothiazine derivatives • Miotic agents	

Health Promotion and Maintenance

Although most cases of cataracts in North America are age related, the onset of cataract formation occurs earlier with heavy sun exposure or exposure to other sources of ultraviolet (UV) light. Teach adults to reduce the risk for cataracts by wearing sunglasses that limit exposure to UV light whenever they are outdoors in the daytime. Cataracts also may result from direct eye injury. Urge adults to wear eye and head protection during sports, such as baseball, or any activity that increases the risk for the eye being hit.

❖ INTERPROFESSIONAL COLLABORATIVE CARE

Care for the patient with cataracts is most often accomplished in the community, with the exception of the surgical procedure, which takes place in an ambulatory surgical setting.

◆ Assessment: Noticing

History. Age is important because cataracts are most prevalent in the older adult. Ask about these predisposing factors:
- Recent or past trauma to the eye
- Exposure to radioactive materials, x-rays, or UV light
- Systemic disease (e.g., diabetes mellitus, hypoparathyroidism)
- Prolonged use of corticosteroids, chlorpromazine, beta blockers, or miotic drugs
- Intraocular disease (e.g., recurrent uveitis)
- Family history of cataracts

Ask the patient to describe his or her vision. For example, you might say, "Tell me what you can see well and what you have difficulty seeing."

Physical Assessment/Clinical Signs and Symptoms. Early signs and symptoms of cataracts are slightly blurred vision and decreased color perception. At first the patient may think that his or her glasses or contact lenses are smudged. As lens cloudiness continues, blurred and double vision occurs, and the patient may have difficulty with ADLs. Without surgical intervention, visual impairment progresses to blindness. *No pain or eye redness is associated with age-related cataract formation.*

Visual SENSORY PERCEPTION is tested using an eye chart and brightness acuity testing (see Chapter 46). Examine the lens with an ophthalmoscope and describe any observed densities by size, shape, and location. As the cataract matures, the opacity makes it difficult to see the retina, and the red reflex may be absent. When this occurs, the pupil is bluish white (Fig. 47-2).

Psychosocial Assessment. Loss of vision is gradual, and the patient may not be aware of it until reading or driving is affected. The patient often has anxiety about loss of independence. Encourage the patient and family to express concerns about reduced vision.

◆ Analysis: Interpreting

The priority collaborative problems for patients with cataracts include:
1. Decreased visual acuity due to cataracts

◆ Planning and Implementation: Responding

The priority problem for the patient with cataracts is reduced visual SENSORY PERCEPTION, which is a safety risk. Patients often live with reduced vision for years before the cataract is removed.

Improving Vision

Planning: Expected Outcomes. The patient with cataracts is expected to recognize when ADLs cannot be performed safely and independently and then should have cataract surgery. This procedure is covered by Medicare for patients who are 65 years or older.

Interventions: Responding. Surgery is the only "cure" for cataracts and should be performed as soon as possible after vision is reduced to the extent that ADLs are affected.

Preoperative Care. The eye-care practitioner provides the patient with accurate information so he or she can make informed decisions about treatment and obtain informed consent. Reinforce this information and teach about the nature of cataracts, their progression, and their treatment.

Assess how the reduced vision affects ADLs, especially dressing, eating, and ambulating. Stress that care after surgery requires the instillation of different types of eyedrops several times a day for 2 to 4 weeks. Careful assessment of eye appearance is also needed. If the patient is unable to perform these tasks, help him or her make arrangements for this care.

Ask whether the patient takes any drugs that affect blood clotting, such as aspirin, warfarin (Coumadin), clopidogrel (Plavix), and dabigatran (Pradaxa). Communicate this information to the surgeon because, for some patients, these drugs may need to be discontinued before cataract surgery.

A series of ophthalmic drugs are instilled just before surgery to dilate the pupils and cause vasoconstriction. Other eyedrops are instilled to induce paralysis to prevent lens movement. When the patient is in the surgical area, a local anesthetic is injected into the muscle cone behind the eye for anesthesia and eye paralysis.

Operative Procedures. The lens is often extracted by *phacoemulsification* (Fig. 47-3), in which a probe is inserted through the capsule and high-frequency sound waves break the lens into small pieces, which are then removed by suction. The replacement intraocular lens (IOL) is placed inside the capsule to be positioned so light rays are focused in the retina. The IOL is a small, clear, plastic lens. Different types are available, and one is selected by the surgeon and patient to allow correction of a specific refractive error. Some patients have distant vision restored to 20/20 and may need glasses only for reading or close work. Some replacement lenses have multiple focal planes and may correct vision to the extent that glasses or contact lenses may not be needed.

Postoperative Care. Immediately after surgery, antibiotic and steroid ointments are instilled (see Chart 47-1 and Fig. 47-4). The patient usually is discharged within an hour after surgery. Instruct him or her to wear dark glasses outdoors or in brightly lit environments until the pupil responds to light.

Teach the patient and family members how to instill the prescribed eyedrops (see Chart 46-2). Work with them in creating a written schedule for the timing and the order of eyedrops administration. Stress the importance of keeping all follow-up appointments.

Remind the patient that mild eye itching is normal, as is a "bloodshot appearance." The eyelid may be slightly swollen. However, significant swelling or bruising is abnormal. Cool compresses may be beneficial. Discomfort at the site is controlled with acetaminophen (Tylenol, Abenol ♦) or acetaminophen with oxycodone (Percocet, Endocet ♦). Aspirin is avoided because of its effects on blood clotting.

◎ CHART 47-1 Best Practice for Patient Safety & Quality Care QSEN

Instillation of Ophthalmic Ointment

- Check the name, strength, and expiration date of the ointment to be instilled. Be sure that it is an ophthalmic (eye) preparation and not a general topical ointment.
- Check whether only one eye or both eyes are to receive the drug.
- If both eyes are to receive the same drug and one eye is infected, use two separate tubes and carefully label each tube with "right" or "left" for the correct eye.
- Wash your hands and put on gloves.
- Explain the procedure to the patient.
- Ask the patient to tilt the head backward and look up at the ceiling.
- Gently pull the lower lid down against the patient's cheek, forming a small pocket.
- Hold the tube (with the cap off) like a pencil, with the tip down.
- Rest the wrist holding the tube against the patient's cheek.
- Without touching any part of the eye or lid with the tip of the tube, gently squeeze the tube and release a small thin strip of ointment into the pocket of the lower lid. Start at the nose side of the pocket and move toward the outer edge of the pocket.
- Gently release the lower lid.
- Tell the patient to close the eye without squeezing the lid.
- While the eye is closed, gently wipe away excess ointment.
- Remind the patient that vision in that eye will be blurred and to not drive or operate heavy machinery until the ointment is removed.
- Remove your gloves and place the cap back on the tube.
- Ask the patient to keep the eye closed for about 1 minute.
- Wash your hands again.
- To remove ointment, wear gloves if drainage is present.
- Then ask the patient to close the eye; wipe the closed lids with a clean tissue from the corner of the eye nearest the nose outward. If you are wiping the same eye twice, use a different area of the tissue or use a new one.

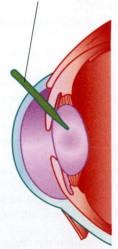

Sound wave and suctioning probe

Sound waves break up the lens, pieces are sucked out, and the capsule remains largely intact

FIG. 47-3 Cataract removal by phacoemulsification.

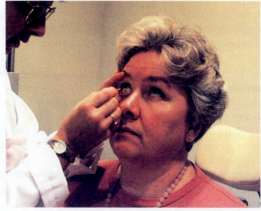

FIG. 47-4 Instillation of ophthalmic ointment

TABLE 47-2 Activities That Increase Intraocular Pressure
• Bending from the waist • Lifting objects weighing more than 10 lbs • Sneezing, coughing • Blowing the nose • Straining to have a bowel movement • Vomiting • Having sexual intercourse • Keeping the head in a dependent position • Wearing tight shirt collars

Pain early after surgery may indicate increased intraocular pressure (IOP) or hemorrhage. Instruct patients to contact the surgeon if pain occurs with nausea or vomiting.

To prevent increases in IOP, teach the patient and family about activity restrictions. Activities that can cause a sudden rise in IOP are listed in Table 47-2.

Infection is a potential and serious complication. Teach the patient and family to observe for increasing eye redness, a decrease in vision, or an increase in tears and photophobia. Creamy white, dry, crusty drainage on the eyelids and lashes is normal. However, yellow or green drainage indicates infection and must be reported. Stress the importance of proper hand-washing to reduce the potential for infection.

Patients experience a dramatic improvement in vision within a day of surgery. Remind them that final best vision will not occur until 4 to 6 weeks after surgery.

> **! NURSING SAFETY PRIORITY** QSEN
>
> **Action Alert**
>
> Instruct the patient who has had cataract surgery to immediately report any reduction of vision after surgery in the eye that had the cataract removed.

Care Coordination and Transition Management

The patient is usually discharged within an hour after cataract surgery. Nursing interventions focus on helping the patient and family plan the eyedrop schedule and daily home eye examination.

Home Care Management. If the patient has difficulty instilling eyedrops, a supportive neighbor, friend, or family member can be taught the procedure. Adaptive equipment that positions the bottle of eyedrops directly over the eye can also be purchased (Fig. 47-5).

Self-Management Education. The best outcome of cataract removal requires close adherence to the eyedrop regimen after surgery. Providing the patient or family with accurate information and demonstration of needed skills are nursing priorities. Before discharge, review these indications of complications after cataract surgery with the patient and family:

- Sharp, sudden pain in the eye
- Bleeding or increased discharge
- Green or yellow, thick drainage
- Lid swelling
- Reappearance of a bloodshot sclera after the initial appearance has cleared
- Decreased vision
- Flashes of light or floating shapes

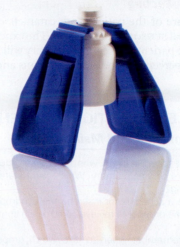

FIG. 47-5 Autosqueeze, a mechanism for self-administering eyedrops. (Courtesy Owen Mumford, Marietta, Georgia.)

> **🏠 CHART 47-2   Home Care Assessment**
> *The Patient After Cataract Surgery*
>
> Assess the eye and vision:
> • Visual acuity in both eyes using a handheld eye chart
> • Visual fields of both eyes
> • Compare operative eye with nonoperative eye for presence or absence of:
>   • Redness
>   • Tearing
>   • Drainage
> Ask the patient about:
> • Pain in or around the operative eye
> • Any change in vision (decreased or improved) in the operative eye
> • Whether any of these has been noticed in the operative eye:
>   • Dark spots
>   • Increase in the number of floaters
>   • Bright flashes of light
> Assess the home environment for:
> • Safety hazards (especially tripping and falling hazards)
> • Level of room lighting
> Assess patient adherence with and understanding of treatment and limitations, such as:
> • Manifestations to report
> • Drug regimen
> • Activity restrictions
> • Ability to perform ADLs

Remind the patient to avoid activities that might increase IOP (see Table 47-2). Some patients are prescribed to wear a light eye patch at night to prevent accidental rubbing. Instruct the patient to avoid getting water in the eye for 3 to 7 days after surgery.

Teach the patient about activity restrictions. Cooking and light housekeeping are permitted, but vacuuming should be avoided for several weeks because of the forward flexion involved and the rapid, jerky movements required. Advise him or her to refrain from driving until vision is not blurry. Chart 47-2 lists items to cover in the focused assessment of a patient at home after cataract surgery.

Health Care Resources. If the patient lives alone and has no support, arrange for a home care nurse to assess him or her and the home situation.

Evaluation: Reflecting

Evaluate the care of the patient with cataracts on the basis of improving visual SENSORY PERCEPTION. The expected outcomes include that the patient after cataract surgery will have improved visual sensory perception and recognize signs and symptoms of complications.

? NCLEX EXAMINATION CHALLENGE 47-1

Health Promotion and Maintenance

The nurse is teaching a client who must instill multiple types of eyedrops before cataract surgery. Which client statement requires **further** teaching?

A. "I will make a schedule for inserting the eyedrops."
B. "Touching the dropper to my eye could cause contamination and infection."
C. "If I can't remember when to take which drops, I'll just take them all at once."
D. "If I have trouble instilling the drops, I will have my spouse put them in for me."

✳ SENSORY PERCEPTION CONCEPT EXEMPLAR

Glaucoma

❖ PATHOPHYSIOLOGY

Glaucoma is a group of eye disorders resulting in increased intraocular pressure (IOP). As described in Chapter 46, the eye is a hollow organ. For proper eye function, the gel in the posterior segment (vitreous humor) and the fluid in the anterior segment (aqueous humor) must be present in set amounts that apply pressure inside the eye to keep it ball shaped.

In adults the volume of the vitreous humor does not change. However, the aqueous humor is continuously made from blood plasma by the ciliary bodies located behind the iris and just in front of the lens (see Fig. 46-2). The fluid flows through the pupil into the bulging area in front of the iris. At the outer edges of the iris beneath the cornea, blood vessels collect fluid and return it to the blood. Usually about 1 mL of aqueous humor is always present, but it is continuously made and reabsorbed at a rate of about 5 mL daily. *A normal IOP requires a balance between production and outflow of aqueous humor (McCance et al., 2014). If the IOP becomes too high, the extra pressure compresses retinal blood vessels and photoreceptors and their synapsing nerve fibers. This compression results in poorly oxygenated photoreceptors and nerve fibers. These sensitive nerve tissues become ischemic and die. When too many have died, vision is lost permanently.* Tissue damage starts in the periphery and moves inward toward the fovea centralis. Untreated, glaucoma can lead to complete loss of visual SENSORY PERCEPTION. Glaucoma is usually painless, and the patient may be unaware of gradual vision reduction.

There are several causes and types of glaucoma (Table 47-3), classified as primary, secondary, or associated. The most common type is primary glaucoma. **Primary open-angle glaucoma (POAG)**, the most common form of primary glaucoma, usually affects both eyes and has no signs or symptoms in the early stages. It develops slowly, with gradual loss of visual fields that may go unnoticed because central vision at first is unaffected. At times, vision is foggy, and the patient has mild eye aching or headaches. Late signs and symptoms

TABLE 47-3	Common Causes of Glaucoma
Primary Glaucoma	**Secondary Glaucoma**
• Aging	• Uveitis
• Heredity	• Iritis
	• Neovascular disorders
Associated Glaucoma	• Trauma
• Diabetes mellitus	• Ocular tumors
• Hypertension	• Degenerative disease
• Severe myopia	• Eye surgery
• Retinal detachment	• Central retinal vein occlusion

occur after irreversible damage to optic nerve function and include seeing halos around lights, losing peripheral vision, and having decreased visual SENSORY PERCEPTION that does not improve with eyeglasses. Outflow of aqueous humor through the chamber angle is reduced. Because the fluid cannot leave the eye at the same rate that it is produced, IOP gradually increases. **Primary angle-closure glaucoma** (**PACG** or *acute glaucoma*) has a sudden onset and is an emergency. The problem is a forward displacement of the iris, which presses against the cornea and closes the chamber angle, suddenly preventing outflow of aqueous humor.

Etiology and Genetic Risk

Anyone can develop glaucoma, although some adults are at higher risk, such as African Americans over 40 years old, any individual over the age of 60 (especially Mexican Americans); those who have a family history of glaucoma; and people who have high eye pressure, corneal thinness, and abnormality of the optic nerve (National Eye Institute, 2017a).

Incidence/Prevalence

Glaucoma is a common cause of blindness in North America. It is usually age related, occurring in about 3 million adults in North America (CNIB, 2017b; National Eye Institute, 2017b).

Health Promotion and Maintenance

At this time, there are no known ways to prevent glaucoma. The best prevention against damage that glaucoma can cause is for adults to have eye examinations with glaucoma checks done every 2 to 4 years before age 40, every 1 to 3 years between ages 40 and 54, every 1 to 2 years between ages 55 and 64, and every 6 to 12 months over the age of 65 (Glaucoma Research Foundation, 2016).

❖ INTERPROFESSIONAL COLLABORATIVE CARE

Care for the patient with glaucoma most often takes place in the community setting. Members of the interprofessional team who collaborate most closely to care for this patient include the eye-care practitioner and the nurse. For patients who experience psychological impact from or related to glaucoma, a psychologist or therapist will also have in important role in care.

The Concept Map addresses collaborative care issues for patients with glaucoma.

◆ Assessment: Noticing

Physical Assessment/Clinical Signs and Symptoms. Ophthalmoscopic examination shows cupping and atrophy of the optic disc. It becomes wider and deeper and turns white or gray.

CONCEPT MAP

SENSORY PERCEPTION

PRIMARY OPEN-ANGLE GLAUCOMA (POAG)

NOTICE IN THE HISTORY

80-year-old Donald Vincent has just been diagnosed with POAG. He states he has been having a gradual loss of vision, including foggy vision, with occasional eye aches. He has recently had the prescription changed on his eyeglasses but still has vision issues.

Noticing Objective Data

OBJECTIVE DATA

- PERRL with reduced accommodation
- Tonometry reading – 28 mm Hg (N = 10-21 mm Hg)
- Cupping and atrophy of the optic disk noted
- Peripheral vision decreased
- Patient instills 1 drop of travoprost (Travatan Z) 0.004% ophthalmic solution (Travatan Z) to the left eye daily

Interpreting Subjective Data

Data Synthesis

SUBJECTIVE DATA

"My vision is a little bit deteriorated. I have a little double vision sometimes. I can't read very much; that's why I like to watch the news on TV. I can't see far away. I just see a figure walking, not the facial features. I have to use a magnifying glass to read the label on the eyedrop bottle."

Data Synthesis

Interpreting Data Synthesis

PATIENT PROBLEMS

- Decreased Visual Acuity due to loss of vision
- Need for Health Teaching

Planning Expected Outcomes

EXPECTED OUTCOMES

SENSORY PERCEPTION: Prevent blindness from glaucoma by early detection, lifelong treatment, and close monitoring with follow-up care.

Remain as independent as possible while ensuring safety.

Avoid infection by instilling eyedrops correctly.

INTERVENTIONS—RESPONDING

1. Physical Assessment—Noticing

Perform an eye exam; glaucoma will show cupping and atrophy of the optic disc. *Measures visual fields to determine the extent of peripheral vision loss (SENSORY PERCEPTION).*

2. Safe Medication Administration

- Demonstrate how to instill eyedrops and evaluate the patient's ability to self-administer. If needed, suggest adaptive equipment that positions the bottle directly over the eye. *Provides psychomotor demonstration for verifying the skill is done correctly. Adaptive equipment can be used to aid patients with SENSORY PERCEPTION loss.*
- Teach the patient that most eye medications initially cause tearing and mild burning with blurred vision; the sclera may become red and itchy. *Helps the patient understand these are expected effects and not to be alarmed.*
- Emphasize instilling eyedrops on time, not skipping doses; when more than one drug is required, wait 5-10 minutes between drops. *Reinforces verbal and written instructions; prevents one drug from "washing out" or diluting the other.*

3. Nursing Safety Priority: Drug Alert!

Teach the correct technique to instill eyedrops (punctal occlusion). *Prevents drugs for glaucoma from being systemically absorbed, which can cause serious side effects.*

4. Providing Safe and Effective Care

Teach principles of infection control (e.g., hand hygiene), and teach the patient not to touch the tip of the eyedrop container to any part of the eye. *Protects the patient from transmission of infection.*

5. Blindness Prevention Strategy

Encourage the patient to keep follow-up appointments to monitor intraocular pressure (IOP). *Monitors IOP; if it becomes too high, the extra pressure can cause sensitive nerve tissues to become ischemic and die, leading to permanent blindness.*

6. Travoprost (Travatan Z) Side Effects

Teach the patient to report emergent signs of allergy—hives, difficulty breathing, angioedema. Stop using drops and call the provider for serious side effects: redness, swelling, itching, eye pain, discharge, increased light sensitivity, visual changes, or chest pain. *Educates the patient and prevents medication complications.*

7. Assessing Patterns of Psychosocial Integrity

Encourage the patient and family to express concerns about reduced vision. *Helps the patient and family to cope with fear of blindness and anxiety about loss of independence. Minimizes stressors for the patient experiencing a change in visual SENSORY PERCEPTION. Changes in vision, whether transient or permanent, require the patient to make adaptations in function or lifestyle.*

8. Health Promotion and Maintenance

Teach the patient and family how to adapt the home for patient safety. *Minimizes patient risk of injury from lack of vision.*

Concept Map by Deanne A. Blach, MSN, RN

In POAG the visual fields first show a small loss of peripheral vision that gradually progresses to a larger loss.

Symptoms of acute angle-closure glaucoma include a sudden, severe pain around the eyes that radiates over the face. Headache or brow pain, nausea, and vomiting may occur. Other symptoms include seeing colored halos around lights and sudden blurred vision with decreased light perception. The sclera may appear reddened, and the cornea foggy. Ophthalmoscopic examination reveals a shallow anterior chamber, a cloudy aqueous humor, and a moderately dilated, nonreactive pupil.

Diagnostic Assessment. An elevated intraocular pressure (IOP) is measured by tonometry. In open-angle glaucoma, the tonometry reading is often between 22 and 32 mm Hg (normal is 10 to 21 mm Hg). In angle-closure glaucoma, the tonometry reading may be 30 mm Hg or higher. Visual field testing by perimetry is performed, as is visualization by gonioscopy to determine whether the angle is open or closed. Usually the optic nerve is imaged to determine to what degree nerve damage is present. All of these diagnostic assessment techniques are described in Chapter 46.

◆ *Analysis: Interpreting*

The priority collaborative problems for patients with glaucoma include:

1. Decreased visual acuity due to glaucoma
2. Need for health teaching due to treatment regimen for glaucoma

◆ *Planning and Implementation: Responding*

Supporting Visual Acuity via Health Teaching

Planning: Expected Outcomes. With proper intervention, the patient is expected to maintain optimum visual acuity as long as possible by adhering to the treatment regimen.

Interventions

Nonsurgical Management. Teach the patient that loss of visual SENSORY PERCEPTION from glaucoma can be prevented by early detection, lifelong treatment, and close monitoring. Use of ophthalmic drugs that reduce ocular pressure can delay or prevent damage. Chart 47-3 lists ways to help the older-adult patient with reduced visual SENSORY PERCEPTION to remain as independent as possible, and Chart 47-4 provides a list of interventions to care for any patient who has reduced vision. These interventions can be very helpful when you care for hospitalized patients who have other disorders, yet also have sight problems.

Drug therapy for glaucoma works to reduce IOP in several ways. Eyedrop drugs can reduce the production of or increase the absorption of aqueous humor or constrict the pupil so the ciliary muscle is contracted, allowing better circulation of the

---

CHART 47-3 Nursing Focus on the Older Adult

Promote Independent Living in Patients With Impaired Vision

Drugs
- Having a neighbor, relative, friend, or visiting nurse visit once a week to measure the proper drugs for each day may be helpful.
  - If the patient is to take drugs more than once each day, it is helpful to use a container of a different shape (with a lid) each time. For example, if the patient is to take drugs at 9 AM, 1 PM, and 9 PM, the 9 AM drugs would be placed in a round container, the 1 PM drugs in a square container, and the 9 PM drugs in a triangular container.
  - It is helpful to place each day's drug containers in a separate box with raised letters on the side of the box spelling out the day.
- "Talking clocks" are available for the patient with low vision.
- Some drug boxes have alarms that can be set for different times.

Communication
- Telephones with large, raised block numbers may be helpful. The best models are those with black numbers on a white phone or white numbers on a black phone.
- Telephones that have a programmable automatic dialing feature ("speed dial") are very helpful. Programmed numbers should include those for the fire department, police, relatives, friends, neighbors, and 911.

Safety
- It is best to leave furniture the way the patient wants it and not move it.
- Throw rugs are best eliminated.
- Appliance cords should be short and kept out of walkways.
- Lounge-style chairs with built-in footrests are preferable to footstools.
- Nonbreakable dishes, cups, and glasses are preferable to breakable ones.
- Cleansers and other toxic agents should be labeled with large, raised letters.
- Hook-and-loop (Velcro) strips at hand level may help mark the locations of switches and electrical outlets.

Food Preparation
- Meals on Wheels is a service that many older adults find helpful. This service brings meals at mealtime, cooked and ready to eat. The cost of this service varies, depending on the patient's ability to pay.

- Many grocery stores offer a "shop by telephone" service. The patient can either complete a computer booklet indicating types, amounts, and brands of items desired; or the store will complete this booklet over the telephone by asking the patient specific information. The store then delivers groceries to the patient's door (many stores also offer a "put-away" service) and charges the patient's bank card.
- A microwave oven is a safer means of cooking than a standard stove, although many older patients are afraid of microwave ovens. If the patient has and will use a microwave oven, others can prepare meals ahead of time, label them, and freeze them for later use. Also, many microwavable complete frozen dinners that comply with a variety of dietary restrictions are available.
- Friends or relatives may be able to help with food preparation. Often relatives do not know what to give an older person for birthdays or other gift-giving occasions. One suggestion is a homemade prepackaged frozen dinner that the patient enjoys.

Personal Care
- Handgrips should be installed in bathrooms.
- The tub floor should have a nonskid surface.
- Male patients should use an electric shaver rather than a razor.
- Choosing a hairstyle that is becoming but easy to care for (avoiding parts) helps in independent living.
- Home hair-care services may be available.

Diversional Activity
- Some patients can read large-print books, newspapers, and magazines (available through local libraries and vision services).
- Books, magazines, and some newspapers are available on audiotapes or discs.
- Patients experienced in knitting or crocheting may be able to create items fashioned from straight pieces such as afghans.
- Card games, dominoes, and some board games that are available in large, high-contrast print may be helpful for patients with low vision.

CHART 47-4 Best Practice for Patient Safety & Quality Care QSEN

Care of the Patient With Reduced Vision

- Always knock or announce your entrance into the patient's room or area and introduce yourself.
- Ensure that all members of the health care team also use this courtesy of announcement and introduction.
- Ensure that the patient's reduced vision is noted in the medical record, is communicated to all staff, is marked on the call board, and is identified on the door of the patient's room.
- Determine to what degree the patient can see anything.
- Orient the patient to the environment, counting steps with him or her to the bathroom.
- Help the patient place objects on the bedside table or in the bed and around the bed and room and do not move them without the patient's permission.
- Remove all objects and clutter between the patient's bed and the bathroom.
- Ask the patient what type of assistance he or she prefers for grooming, toileting, eating, and ambulating and communicate these preferences with the staff.
- Describe food placement on a plate in terms of a clock face.
- Open milk cartons; open salt, pepper, and condiment packages; and remove lids from cups and bowls.
- Unless the patient also has a hearing problem, use a normal tone of voice when speaking.
- When walking with the patient, offer him or her your arm and walk a step ahead.

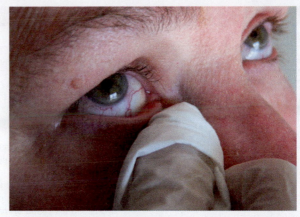

FIG. 47-6 Applying punctal occlusion to prevent systemic absorption of eyedrops. (From Workman, M. L., & LaCharity, L. [2016]. *Understanding pharmacology* [2nd ed.]. St. Louis: Saunders.)

! NURSING SAFETY PRIORITY QSEN

Drug Alert

Most eyedrops used for glaucoma therapy can be absorbed systemically and cause systemic problems. It is critical to teach punctal occlusion to patients using eyedrops for glaucoma therapy.

aqueous humor to the site of absorption. *These drugs do not improve lost vision but prevent more damage by decreasing IOP.* The prostaglandin agonist drugs reduce IOP by dilating blood vessels in the trabecular mesh, which then collects and drains aqueous humor at a faster rate. The adrenergic agonists and beta-adrenergic blockers reduce IOP by limiting the production of aqueous humor and by dilating the pupil, which improves the flow of the fluid to its absorption site. Cholinergic agonists reduce IOP by limiting the production of aqueous humor and making more room between the iris and the lens, which improves fluid outflow. Carbonic anhydrase inhibitors directly and strongly inhibit production of aqueous humor. They do not affect the flow or absorption of the fluid. Most eyedrops cause tearing, mild burning, blurred vision, and a reddened sclera for a few minutes after instilling the drug. Specific nursing implications related to drug therapy for glaucoma are listed in Chart 47-5. It is important to teach the patient about potential interactions that may exist between medications and systemic effects that may occur when using these drugs.

The priority nursing intervention for the patient with glaucoma is teaching. Teach the patient that the benefit of drug therapy occurs only when the drugs are used on the prescribed schedule, usually every 12 hours. Teach patients the importance of instilling the drops on time and not skipping doses. When more than one drug is prescribed, teach the patient to wait 5 to 10 minutes between drug instillations to prevent one drug from "washing out" or diluting another drug. Stress the need for good handwashing, keeping the eyedrop container tip clean, and avoiding touching the tip to any part of the eye. Also teach the technique of punctal occlusion (placing pressure on the corner of the eye near the nose) immediately after eyedrop instillation to prevent systemic absorption of the drug (Fig. 47-6).

Systemic osmotic drugs may be given for angle-closure glaucoma to rapidly reduce IOP. These agents include oral glycerin and IV mannitol (Osmitrol).

Surgical Management. Surgery is used when drugs for open-angle glaucoma are not effective at controlling IOP. Two common procedures are laser trabeculoplasty and trabeculectomy. A *laser trabeculoplasty* burns the trabecular meshwork, scarring it and causing the meshwork fibers to tighten. Tight fibers increase the size of the spaces between the fibers, improving outflow of aqueous humor and reducing IOP. *Trabeculectomy* is a surgical procedure that creates a new channel for fluid outflow. Both are ambulatory surgery procedures.

If glaucoma fails to respond to common approaches, an implanted shunt procedure may be used. A small tube or filament is connected to a flat plate that is positioned on the outside of the eye in the eye orbit. (The plate is not visible on the front part of the eye.) The open part of the fine tube is placed into the front chamber of the eye. The fluid then drains through or around the tube into the area around the flat plate, where it collects and is reabsorbed into the bloodstream. Potential complications of glaucoma surgery include choroidal hemorrhage and choroidal detachment.

Care Coordination and Transition Management

Home Care Management. Similar to management of cataracts, the patient with glaucoma will need to instill eyedrops as part of their home care. If the patient is unable or resistant to instilling his or her own eyedrops, teach the caregiver the proper technique or recommend adaptive equipment (see Fig. 47-5).

Self-Management Education. The patient with glaucoma is usually managed in the outpatient setting and seen every 1 to 3 months, depending on how well controlled their IOP is. Teach the importance of good handwashing and keeping the tip of the eyedrop container clean. Remind the patient to instill eyedrops on time as recommended by the eye-care provider and not to skip doses.

CHART 47-5   Common Examples of Drug Therapy (Eyedrops)

Glaucoma

DRUG CATEGORY	NURSING IMPLICATIONS

Prostaglandin Agonists
Bimatoprost (Lumigan)
Latanoprost (Xalatan)
Tafluprost (Zioptan)
Travoprost (Travatan Z)
Unoprostone (Rescula)
	Teach the patient to check the cornea for abrasions or trauma.
	   Drugs should not be used when the cornea is not intact.
	Remind the patient that, over time, the eye color darkens, and eyelashes elongate in the eye receiving the drug.
	   Knowing the side effects in advance reassures the patient that their presence is expected and normal.
	If only one eye is to be treated, teach the patient *not* to place drops in the other eye to try to make the eye colors similar.
	   Using the drug in an eye with normal IOP can cause a **lower***-than-normal IOP, which reduces vision.*
	Warn the patient that using more drops than prescribed reduces drug effectiveness.
	   Drug action is based on blocking receptors, which can increase in number when the drug is overused.

Adrenergic Agonists
Apraclonidine (Iopidine)
Brimonidine tartrate (Alphagan)
Dipivefrin hydrochloride (Propine)
	Ask whether the patient is taking any antidepressants from the MAO inhibitor class, such as phenelzine (Nardil) or tranylcypromine (Parnate).
	   These enzyme inhibitors increase blood pressure, as do the adrenergic agonists. When taken together, the patient may experience hypertensive crisis.
	Teach the patient to wear dark glasses outdoors and also indoors when lighting is bright.
	   The pupil dilates (mydriasis) and remains dilated, even when there is plenty of light, causing discomfort.
	Teach the patient not to use the eyedrops with contact lenses in place and to wait 15 minutes after using the drug to put in the lenses.
	   These drugs are absorbed by the contact lens, which can become discolored or cloudy.

Beta-Adrenergic Blockers
Betaxolol hydrochloride (Betoptic)
Carteolol (Cartrol, Ocupress)
Levobunolol (Betagan)
Timolol (Betimol, Istalol, Timoptic)
Timoptic GFS (gel-forming solution) (Timoptic-XE, Timolol-GFS)
	Ask whether the patient has moderate-to-severe asthma or COPD.
	   If these drugs are absorbed systemically, they constrict pulmonary smooth muscle and narrow airways.
	Warn patients with diabetes to check their blood glucose levels more often when taking these drugs.
	   These drugs induce hypoglycemia and also mask the hypoglycemic symptoms.
	Teach patients who also take oral beta blockers to check their pulse at least twice per day and to notify the primary health care and eye care providers if the pulse is consistently below 58 beats/min.
	   These drugs potentiate the effects of systemic beta blockers and can cause an unsafe drop in heart rate and blood pressure.

Cholinergic Agonists
Carbachol (Carboptic, Isopto Carbachol, Miostat)
Echothiophate (Phospholine Iodide)
Pilocarpine (Adsorbocarpine, Akarpine, Diocarpine ✚, Isopto Carpine, Ocu-Carpine, Ocusert, Piloptic, Pilostat)
	Teach the patient not to use more eyedrops than are prescribed and to report increased salivation or drooling to the primary health care and eye care providers.
	   These drugs are readily absorbed by conjunctival mucous membranes and can cause systemic side effects of headache, flushing, increased saliva, and sweating.
	Teach the patient to use good light when reading and to take care in darker rooms.
	   The pupil of the eye will not open more to let in more light, and it may be harder to see objects in dim light. This problem can increase the risk for falls.

Carbonic Anhydrase Inhibitors
Brinzolamide (Azopt)
Dorzolamide (Trusopt)
	Ask whether the patient has an allergy to sulfonamide antibacterial drugs.
	   Drugs are similar to the sulfonamides; and, if a patient is allergic to the sulfonamides, an allergy is likely with these drugs, even as eyedrops.
	Teach the patient to shake the drug before applying.
	   Drug separates on standing.
	Teach the patient not to use the eyedrops with contact lenses in place and to wait 15 minutes after using the drug to put in the lenses.
	   These drugs are absorbed by the contact lens, which can become discolored or cloudy.

Combination Drugs Brimonidine tartrate and timolol maleate (Combigan) Latanoprost and timolol (Xalcom)	Same as for each drug alone.

COPD, Chronic obstructive pulmonary disease; *IOP,* intraocular pressure; *MAO,* monamine oxidase.

For the patient who has had surgical management, teach the signs and symptoms of choroidal detachment and hemorrhage. These can occur after coughing, sneezing, straining at stools, or Valsalva maneuver. Serous detachment involves some degree of vision loss but is usually painless. Hemorrhagic detachment involves an immediate loss of vision with sudden, excruciating, throbbing pain. Any vision loss, particularly when accompanied by pain, should be reported immediately to the eye-care practitioner.

Health Care Resources. If needed, refer the patient and family to care services that can assist in the home situation. Support groups for individuals with vision impairment may also be helpful.

◆ Evaluation: Reflecting

Evaluate the care of the patient with glaucoma based on the identified priority patient problem. The primary expected outcomes are that the patient will have optimum visual acuity

NCLEX EXAMINATION CHALLENGE 47-2
Physiological Integrity

The nurse is caring for a client who reports slow onset of a gradual loss of vision in the center of both eyes. The client describes vision as "foggy" and reports concerns of ongoing headaches from "trying to concentrate to see." What condition does the nurse anticipate?

A. Cataract
B. Glaucoma
C. Conjunctivitis
D. Retinal detachment

as long as possible as demonstrated by adherence to the treatment regimen.

CORNEAL DISORDERS

For a sharp retinal image, the cornea must be transparent and intact. Corneal problems may be caused by irritation or infection (keratitis) with ulceration of the corneal surface, degeneration of the cornea (keratoconus), or deposits in the cornea. All corneal problems reduce visual SENSORY PERCEPTION, and some can lead to blindness.

CORNEAL ABRASION, ULCERATION, AND INFECTION
❖ PATHOPHYSIOLOGY

A corneal abrasion is a scrape or scratch injury of the cornea. This painful condition can be caused by a small foreign body, trauma, or contact lens use. Other problems contributing to corneal injury are malnutrition, dry eye syndromes, and some cancer therapies. The abrasion allows organisms to enter, leading to corneal infection. Bacterial, protozoal, and fungal infections can lead to corneal ulceration, which is a deeper injury. *This problem is an emergency because the cornea has no separate blood supply and infections that can permanently impair vision develop rapidly.*

❖ INTERPROFESSIONAL COLLABORATIVE CARE

The patient with a corneal disorder has pain, reduced vision, photophobia, and eye secretions. Cloudy or purulent fluid may be present on the eyelids or lashes. Care for patients with a corneal disorder usually takes place in the community setting. Members of the interprofessional team who collaborate most closely to care for this patient include the eye-care practitioner and the nurse.

Wear gloves when examining the eye. The cornea looks hazy or cloudy with a patchy area of ulceration. When fluorescein stain is used, the patchy areas appear green. Microbial culture and corneal scrapings are used to determine the causative organism. Anti-infective therapy is started before the organism is identified because of the high risk for vision loss. For culture, obtain swabs from the ulcer and its edges. For corneal scrapings, the cornea is anesthetized with a topical agent, and a physician or advanced practice nurse removes samples from the ulcer center and edge.

Antibiotics, antifungals, and antivirals are prescribed to eliminate the organisms. A broad-spectrum antibiotic is prescribed first and may be changed when culture results are known. Steroids may be used with antibiotics to reduce the eye inflammation. Drugs can be given topically as eyedrops or injected subconjunctivally or intravenously. Chart 46-3 lists best practices for instilling eyedrops. The nursing priorities are to begin the drug therapy, to ensure patient understanding of the drug-therapy regimen, and to prevent infection spread.

Often the anti-infective therapy involves instilling eyedrops *every hour* for the first 24 hours. Teach the patient or family member how to instill the eyedrops correctly (see Chart 46-2).

If the eye infection occurs only in one eye, teach the patient not to use the drug in the unaffected eye. Instruct him or her to wash hands after touching the affected eye and before touching or doing anything to the healthy eye. If both eyes are infected, separate bottles of drugs are needed for each eye. Teach the patient to clearly label the bottles "right eye" and "left eye" and not to switch the drugs from eye to eye. Also teach him or her to completely care for one eye, wash the hands and, using the drugs designated for the other eye, care for that eye. Remind the patient not to wear contact lenses during the entire time that these drugs are being used because the eye is more vulnerable to infection or injury and because the drugs can cloud or damage the contact lenses.

! NURSING SAFETY PRIORITY QSEN
Action Alert

Stress the importance of applying the drug as often as prescribed, even at night, and to complete the entire course of antibiotic therapy. Stopping the infection at this stage can save the vision in the infected eye. Instruct the patient to make and keep all follow-up appointments; usually the patient is seen again in 24 hours or less.

Drug therapy may continue for 3 or more weeks to ensure eradication of the infection. Warn patients to avoid using makeup around the eye until the infection has cleared. Instruct them to discard all open containers of contact lens solutions and bottles of eyedrops because these may be contaminated. Patients should not wear contact lenses for weeks to months until the infection is gone and the ulcer is healed.

! NURSING SAFETY PRIORITY QSEN
Drug Alert

Check the route of administration for ophthalmic drugs. Most are administered by the eye instillation route, not orally. Administering these drugs orally can cause systemic side effects in addition to not having a therapeutic effect on the eye.

KERATOCONUS AND CORNEAL OPACITIES
❖ PATHOPHYSIOLOGY

The cornea can permanently lose it shape, become scarred or cloudy, or become thinner, reducing useful visual SENSORY PERCEPTION. Keratoconus, the degeneration of the corneal tissue resulting in abnormal corneal shape, can occur with trauma or may be an inherited disorder (Fig. 47-7). Inadequately treated corneal infection and severe trauma can scar the cornea and lead to severe visual impairment that can be improved only by surgical interventions.

❖ INTERPROFESSIONAL COLLABORATIVE CARE

For a misshaped cornea that is still clear, surgical management involves a corneal ring implant that adjusts the shape of the cornea. During this procedure, the shape of the cornea is changed by placing a flexible ring in the outer edges of the cornea (outside of the optical zone).

The procedure is performed under local anesthesia. Improvement to best vision is immediate. Removal, replacement, or adjustment of ring tightness can enhance refraction, especially when the patient's vision changes further as a result of aging. Because the ring is placed outside of the optical zone, the risk for corneal clouding or scarring is low.

Surgery to improve clarity for a permanent corneal disorder that obscures vision is a **keratoplasty** (corneal transplant), in which the diseased corneal tissue is removed and replaced with tissue from a human-donor cornea. This process improves vision by removing corneal deformities and replacing them with healthy corneal tissue.

Preoperative care may be short, with little time for teaching because transplantation is performed when the donor cornea becomes available. Examine the eyes for signs and symptoms of infection and report any redness, drainage, or edema to the eye care practitioner. Instill prescribed antibiotic eyedrops and obtain IV access before surgery.

Operative procedures are *keratoplasties* and are usually performed with local anesthesia in an ambulatory surgical setting. The transplant may involve the entire depth of corneal tissue *(penetrating keratoplasty)* or only certain layers of the corneal tissue *(lamellar keratoplasty)*. The nerves around the eye are anesthetized so the patient cannot move the eye or see out of it. The center 7 to 8 mm of the diseased cornea is removed with an instrument that works like a cookie cutter (Fig. 47-8). The same instrument is used to cut the tissue graft from the donor cornea so the graft will be a perfect fit. The donor cornea is sutured into place on the eye. The procedure takes about an hour, and the patient is discharged to home within 1 to 2 hours.

Postoperative care involves extensive patient teaching. Local antibiotics are injected or instilled. Usually the eye is covered with a pressure patch and a protective shield until the patient returns to the surgeon.

Instruct the patient to lie on the nonoperative side to reduce intraocular pressure (IOP). If a patch is to be used for more than a day, teach the patient or family member how to apply it. Instruct the patient to wear the shield at night for the first month after surgery and whenever he or she is around small children or pets to avoid injury. Instruct him or her *not* to use an ice pack on the eye. Complications after surgery include bleeding, wound leakage, infection, and graft rejection. Teach the patient how to instill eyedrops. Teach him or her to examine the eye (or have a family member examine it) daily for the presence of infection or graft rejection. Stress that the presence of purulent discharge, a continuous leak of clear fluid from around the graft site (not tears), or excessive bleeding needs to be reported immediately to the surgeon. Other complications include decreased vision, increased reddening of the eye, pain, increased sensitivity to light, and the presence of light flashes or "floaters" in the field of vision. Teach the patient to report any of these symptoms to the surgeon if they develop after the first 48 hours and persist for more than 6 hours.

The eye should be protected from any activity that can increase the pressure on, around, or inside the eye. Teach the patient to avoid jogging, running, dancing, and any other activity that promotes rapid or jerky head motions for several weeks after surgery. Other activities that may raise IOP and should be avoided are listed in Table 47-2.

Graft rejection can occur and starts as inflammation in the cornea near the graft edge that moves toward the center. Vision is reduced, and the cornea becomes cloudy. Topical

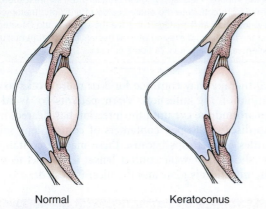

Normal   Keratoconus

FIG. 47-7 Profile of a normal cornea and one with keratoconus.

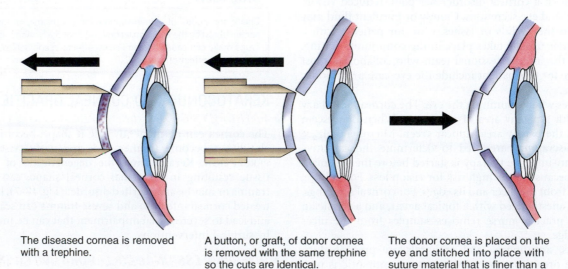

The diseased cornea is removed with a trephine.

A button, or graft, of donor cornea is removed with the same trephine so the cuts are identical.

The donor cornea is placed on the eye and stitched into place with suture material that is finer than a human hair.

FIG. 47-8 Steps involved in corneal transplantation (penetrating keratoplasty).

corticosteroids and other immunosuppressants are used to stop the rejection process. If rejection continues, the graft becomes opaque, and blood vessels branch into the opaque tissue.

Eye donation is a common procedure and needed for corneal transplantation. The Eye Banking Association of America (EBAA, 2017) has published medical standards that detail donor eligibility and contraindications. If a deceased patient is a known eye donor, follow these recommended steps:

- Raise the head of the bed 30 degrees.
- Instill prescribed antibiotic eyedrops.
- Close the eyes and apply a *small* ice pack.

RETINAL DISORDERS

MACULAR DEGENERATION

❖ PATHOPHYSIOLOGY

Macular degeneration is the deterioration of the macula (the area of central vision) and can be age related or exudative. Age-related macular degeneration (AMD) has two types. The most common type is *dry* AMD, caused by gradual blockage of retinal capillaries, allowing retinal cells in the macula to become ischemic and necrotic. Central vision declines, and patients describe mild blurring and distortion at first. Eventually the patient loses all central vision. About 2 million older adults in the United States and Canada have dry AMD (National Eye Institute, 2017b). This loss of visual SENSORY PERCEPTION affects independence, well-being, and quality of life. It is often the reason an older adult leaves his or her independent living environment and moves into an assisted-living facility (Touhy & Jett, 2015).

Dry AMD is more common and progresses at a faster rate among smokers than among nonsmokers. Other risk factors include hypertension, female gender, short stature, family history, and a long-term diet poor in carotene and vitamin E.

Another cause of AMD is the growth of new blood vessels in the macula, which have thin walls and leak blood and fluid (*wet* AMD). Exudative macular degeneration is also a type of wet macular degeneration but can occur at any age. The condition can occur in only one eye or in both eyes. The patient with dry AMD can also develop exudative macular degeneration. Patients with exudative degeneration have a sudden decrease in vision after a detachment of pigment epithelium in the macula. Newly formed blood vessels invade this injured area and cause fluid and blood to collect under the macula (like a blister), with scar formation and visual distortion.

❖ INTERPROFESSIONAL COLLABORATIVE CARE

Dry AMD has no cure. Management in the community setting is focused on slowing the progression of the vision loss and helping the patient maximize remaining vision and quality of life (Yuzawa et al., 2013). The risk for dry AMD can be reduced by increasing long-term dietary intake of antioxidants, vitamin B_{12}, and the carotenoids *lutein* and *zeaxanthin*. The same dietary therapy slows the progression of dry AMD.

Central vision loss reduces the ability to read, write, recognize safety hazards, and drive. Suggest alternatives (e.g., large-print books, public transportation) and referrals to community resources that provide adaptive equipment.

Management of patients with exudative or wet AMD is geared toward slowing the process and identifying further changes in visual perception. Fluid and blood may reabsorb in some patients. Laser therapy to seal the leaking blood vessels can limit the extent of the damage. Ocular injections with the vascular endothelial growth factor inhibitors (VEGFIs), such as bevacizumab (Avastin) or ranibizumab (Lucentis), can improve vision for the patient with wet AMD.

❓ NCLEX EXAMINATION CHALLENGE 47-3

Physiological Integrity

The nurse is caring for four clients. Which has the **highest** risk for development of age-related macular degeneration (AMD)?
A. 25-year-old, 70 inches tall, with fracture of the right femur
B. 38-year-old, 71 inches tall, who has just given birth to a healthy baby
C. 45-year-old, 67 inches tall, who is a vegetarian
D. 57-year-old, 60 inches tall, with hypertension

RETINAL HOLES, TEARS, AND DETACHMENTS

❖ PATHOPHYSIOLOGY

A retinal hole is a break in the retina. These holes can be caused by trauma or can occur with aging. A retinal tear is a jagged and irregularly shaped break in the retina. It can result from traction on the retina. A retinal detachment is the separation of the retina from the epithelium. Detachments are classified by the type and cause of their development.

One common cause of retinal holes, tears, and detachments is a *posterior vitreous detachment* (PVD). With aging, the vitreous gel often shrinks or thickens, causing it to pull away from the retina. The patient may experience small flashes of light seen as "shooting stars" or thin "lightening streaks" in one eye, most visible in a dark environment. These flashes of light may be accompanied by "floaters." In addition to aging, risk factors for PVD include extreme myopia, inflammation inside the eye, and cataract or eye laser surgery. When the PVD does not cause a retinal tear or detachment, no treatment is needed.

❖ INTERPROFESSIONAL COLLABORATIVE CARE

The onset of a retinal detachment is usually sudden and painless. Patients may suddenly see bright flashes of light (photopsia) or floating dark spots in the affected eye. During the initial phase of the detachment or if the detachment is partial, the patient may describe the sensation of a curtain being pulled over part of the visual field. The visual field loss corresponds to the area of detachment.

On ophthalmoscopic examination, detachments are seen as gray bulges or folds in the retina. Sometimes a hole or tear may be seen at the edge of the detachment.

If a retinal hole or tear is discovered before it causes a detachment, the defect may be closed or sealed. Closure prevents fluid from collecting under the retina and reduces the risk for a detachment. Treatment involves creating a scar that will bind the retina and choroid together around the break. Common methods to create the scar are with laser photocoagulation or a freezing probe (*cryopexy*).

Spontaneous reattachment of a totally detached retina is rare. Surgical repair is needed to place the retina in contact with the underlying structures. A common repair procedure is scleral buckling.

Preoperative Care

The patient is usually anxious and fearful about a possible permanent loss of vision. *Nursing priorities include providing information and reassurance to allay fears.*

Instruct the patient to restrict activity and head movement before surgery to prevent further tearing or detachment. An eye patch is placed over the affected eye to reduce eye movement. Topical drugs are given before surgery to inhibit pupil constriction and accommodation.

Operative Procedures

The surgery is performed with the patient under general anesthesia. In scleral buckling, the eye-care practitioner repairs wrinkles or folds in the retina and indents the eye surface to relieve the tugging pressure on the retina. The indentation or "buckling" is performed by placing a small piece of silicone against the outside of the sclera and holding it in place with an encircling band. This device keeps the retina in contact with the choroid for reattachment. Any fluid under the retina is drained.

A gas or silicone oil placed inside the eye can be used to promote retinal reattachment. These agents float up and against the retina to hold it in place until healing occurs.

Postoperative Care

After surgery an eye patch and shield usually are applied. Monitor the patient's vital signs, and check the eye patch and shield for any drainage.

Activity after surgery varies. If gas or oil has been placed in the eye, teach the patient to keep his or her head in the position prescribed by the surgeon to promote reattachment. Teach the patient to report any sudden increase in pain or pain occurring with nausea to the surgeon immediately. Remind him or her to avoid activities that increase intraocular pressure (IOP) (see Table 47-2).

Instruct the patient to avoid reading, writing, and close work, such as sewing, in the first week after surgery because these activities cause rapid eye movements and detachment. Teach him or her the signs and symptoms of infection and detachment (sudden reduced visual acuity, eye pain, pupil that *does not constrict* in response to light) and to notify the surgeon immediately if these symptoms occur.

❓ NCLEX EXAMINATION CHALLENGE 47-4

Health Promotion and Maintenance

A client is being discharged after surgery to correct a retinal detachment. Which symptoms will the nurse teach the client to immediately report to the eye care provider? **Select all that apply.**
A. Purulent discharge in the affected eye
B. Fever of 102° F (38.9° C)
C. Pupil that constricts in response to light
D. Improved visual acuity
E. Pain in the eye

RETINITIS PIGMENTOSA

Several types of retinal disorders can cause progressive degeneration of the retina and lead to loss of visual SENSORY PERCEPTION. Retinitis pigmentosa (RP) is a condition in which retinal nerve cells degenerate and the pigmented cells of the retina grow and move into the sensory areas of the retina, causing further degeneration.

The earliest manifestation of RP is night blindness, often occurring in childhood. Over time, decreased acuity progresses to total blindness. Examination of the retina shows heavy

---

❓ CLINICAL JUDGMENT CHALLENGE 47-1

Safety; Patient-Centered Care QSEN

You are caring for a 54-year-old male patient who drove himself to the emergency department directly from work. He reports that he is a computer programmer and that, while working this morning, he noticed bright flashes of light and "floaters" in his left eye. He says that the symptoms continued, so he covered his left eye with a patch and drove himself to the hospital. At this time, he describes his symptoms as feeling like a curtain is closing over the visual field of his left eye. He reports no other symptoms, other than feeling anxious about what is happening to him.
1. What condition involving the eye do you anticipate? Why?
2. When the patient asks if he will ever fully see out of his left eye again, what would your answer be?
3. When the patient asks if surgery will be necessary, how do you respond?
4. What nursing interventions would best address the patient's anxiety at this time?
5. The patient wants to drive himself home after the eye care provider sees him. How will you address this concern and support the patient's autonomy?

🧬 GENETIC/GENOMIC CONSIDERATIONS

Patient-Centered Care QSEN

Different forms of retinitis pigmentosa can be inherited as an autosomal-dominant (AD) trait, an autosomal-recessive (AR) trait, or an X-linked recessive trait; only one family showing possible Y-linked inheritance has been reported (Online Mendelian Inheritance in Man [OMIM], 2017). Mutations in more than 20 genes have been identified as being responsible for retinitis pigmentosa, and gene testing for more than 800 mutations of the AR and AD forms of the problem is available commercially.

---

pigmentation in a lacy pattern. Cataracts may accompany this disorder.

No current therapy is effective in preventing the degenerative process. Management strategies focus on protecting active retinal cells and slowing the progression of disease. Teach patients with RP to avoid drugs that are known to adversely affect retinal cells, such as isotretinoin (Accutane) and drugs for erectile dysfunction (e.g., sildenafil [Viagra]). Also remind them to wear eyeglasses that provide ultraviolet protection. Research has not yet definitively concluded that ingestion of supplements benefits patients with RP (Sacchetti et al., 2015). When macular edema is present, oral acetazolamide (Diamox) can reduce the edema. Cataract surgery and lens replacement are recommended when cataracts further reduce vision. Other treatments under investigation include retinal transplantation, stem cell therapy, and gene therapy (Foundation Fighting Blindness, 2017).

REFRACTIVE ERRORS

❖ PATHOPHYSIOLOGY

The ability of the eye to focus images on the retina depends on the length of the eye from front to back and the refractive power of the lens system. **Refraction** is the bending of light rays. Problems in either eye length or refraction can result in refractive errors.

Myopia is nearsightedness, in which the eye over-refracts the light and the bent images fall in front of, not on, the retina. **Hyperopia**, also called *hypermetropia,* is farsightedness, in which refraction is too weak, causing images to be focused behind the retina. Presbyopia is the age-related problem in which the lens loses its elasticity and is less able to change shape to focus the eye for close work. As a result, images fall behind the retina. This problem usually begins in adults in their 30s and 40s. Astigmatism occurs when the curve of the cornea is uneven. Because light rays are not refracted equally in all directions, the image does not focus on the retina.

❖ INTERPROFESSIONAL COLLABORATIVE CARE

Refractive errors are diagnosed through a process known as refraction. The patient is asked to view an eye chart while lenses of different strengths are systematically placed in front of the eye. With each lens strength, he or she is asked whether the lenses sharpen or worsen vision. The strength of the lens needed to focus the image on the retina is expressed in measurements called *diopters*.

Nonsurgical Management

Refractive errors are corrected with eyeglasses or contact lenses that focus light rays on the retina (see Fig. 46-5). Hyperopic vision is corrected with a convex lens that moves the image forward. Myopic vision is corrected with a concave lens that moves the image back to the retina.

Surgical Management

Surgery can correct some refractive errors and enhance vision. The most common vision-enhancing surgery is laser in-situ keratomileusis (LASIK). This procedure can correct nearsightedness, farsightedness, and astigmatism. The superficial layers of the cornea are lifted temporarily as a flap, and powerful laser pulses reshape the deeper corneal layers. After reshaping is complete, the corneal flap is placed back into its original position.

Usually both eyes are treated at the same time, which is convenient for the patient, although this practice has some risks. Many patients have improved vision within an hour after surgery, and complete healing to best vision takes up to 4 weeks. The outer corneal layer is not damaged, and pain is minimal.

Complications of LASIK include infection, corneal clouding, chronic dry eyes, and refractive errors. Some patients have developed blurred vision, halos around lights, and other refractive errors months to years after this surgery as a result of excessive laser-thinning of the cornea. The cornea then becomes unstable and does not refract appropriately.

Another procedure, corneal ring placement, can enhance vision for nearsightedness, although this procedure is usually performed for keratoconus. For more information about the procedure, see Surgical Intervention for Keratoconus.

TRAUMA

Trauma to the eye or orbital area can result from almost any activity. Care varies, depending on the area of the eye affected and whether the globe of the eye has been penetrated.

Foreign Bodies

Eyelashes, dust, dirt, and airborne particles can come in contact with the conjunctiva or cornea and irritate or abrade the surface. If nothing is seen on the cornea or conjunctiva, the eyelid is everted to examine the conjunctivae. The patient usually has a feeling of something being in the eye and may have blurred vision. Pain occurs if the corneal surface is injured. Tearing and photophobia may be present.

Visual SENSORY PERCEPTION is assessed before treatment. The eye is examined with fluorescein, followed by irrigation with normal saline (0.9%) to gently remove the particles. Best practices for ocular irrigation are listed in Chart 47-6.

If an eye patch is applied after the foreign body is removed, tell the patient how long the patch must be left in place. Follow-up as directed by the eye-care practitioner is needed to confirm that appropriate healing is taking place.

Lacerations

Lacerations are caused by sharp objects and projectiles. The injury occurs most commonly to the eyelids and cornea, although any part of the eye can be lacerated.

The patient should receive medical attention as soon as possible. Initially the eye is closed, and a small ice pack is applied to decrease bleeding. Minor lacerations of the eyelid can be sutured in an emergency department, an urgent care center, or an eye-care practitioner's office. A microscope is needed in the operating room if the patient has a laceration that involves the eyelid margin, affects the lacrimal system, involves a large area, or has jagged edges.

◎ CHART 47-6 Best Practice for Patient Safety & Quality Care QSEN

Ocular Irrigation

1. Assemble equipment:
   - Normal saline IV (1000-mL bag)
   - Macrodrip IV tubing
   - IV pole
   - Eyelid speculum
   - Topical anesthetic (proparacaine hydrochloride)
   - Gloves
   - Collection receptacle (emesis basin works well)
   - Towels
   - pH paper
2. Quickly obtain a history from the patient while flushing the tubing with normal saline:
   - Nature and time of the injury
   - Type of irritant or chemical (if known)
   - Type of first aid administered at the scene
   - Any allergies to the "caine" family of medications
3. Evaluate the patient's visual acuity *before* treatment:
   - Ask the patient to read your name tag with the affected eye while covering the good eye.
   - Ask the patient to "count fingers" with the affected eye while covering the good eye.
4. Put on gloves.
5. Place a strip of pH paper in the cul-de-sac of the patient's affected eye to test the pH of the agent splashed into the eye and to know when it has been washed out.
6. Instill proparacaine hydrochloride eyedrops as prescribed.
7. Place the patient in a supine position with the head turned slightly toward the affected eye.
8. Have the patient hold the affected eye open or position an eyelid speculum.
9. Direct the flow of normal saline across the affected eye from the nasal corner of the eye toward the outer corner of the eye.
10. Assess the patient's comfort during the procedure.
11. If both eyes are affected, irrigate them simultaneously using separate personnel and equipment.

Corneal lacerations are an emergency because eye contents may prolapse through the laceration. Symptoms include severe eye pain, photophobia, tearing, decreased vision, and inability to open the eyelid. If the laceration is the result of a penetrating injury, an object may be seen protruding from the eye.

> **! NURSING SAFETY PRIORITY** **QSEN**
>
> **Action Alert**
>
> An object protruding from the eye is removed only by an eye-care practitioner because it may be holding the eye structures in place. Improper removal can cause structures to prolapse out of the eye.

Antibiotics are given to reduce the risk for infection. Depending on the depth of the laceration, scarring may develop. If the scar alters vision, a corneal transplant may be needed later. If the eye contents have prolapsed through the laceration or if the injury is severe, enucleation (surgical eye removal) may be indicated.

Penetrating Injuries

A penetrating eye injury often leads to permanent loss of visual SENSORY PERCEPTION. Glass, high-speed metal or wood particles, BB pellets, and bullets are common causes of penetrating injuries. The particles can enter the eye and lodge in or behind the eyeball.

The patient has eye pain and reports, "I suddenly felt something hit my eye." A wound may be visible. Depending on where the object enters and rests within the eye, vision may be affected.

X-rays and CT scans of the orbit are usually performed. *MRI is contraindicated because the procedure may move any metal-containing projectile and cause more injury.*

Surgery is usually needed to remove the foreign object, and sometimes vitreal removal is needed. IV antibiotics are started before surgery, and a tetanus booster is given if necessary.

> **? NCLEX EXAMINATION CHALLENGE 47-5**
>
> **Safe and Effective Care Environment**
>
> Which action by a nurse is **most likely** to increase accurate communication with a client who has low vision?
> A. Speaking slowly and loudly
> B. Enhancing the talk using hand gestures
> C. Being very specific with descriptions and directions
> D. Marking the door of the client's room to indicate his or her vision status

---

GET READY FOR THE NCLEX® EXAMINATION

KEY POINTS

Review these Key Points for each NCLEX Examination Client Needs Category

Safe and Effective Care Environment
- Use aseptic technique when performing an eye examination or instilling drugs into the eye. **QSEN: Safety**
- Apply the principles of infection control when caring for a patient with an eye infection. **QSEN: Safety**
- Avoid performing an ophthalmoscopic examination on a confused patient. **QSEN: Safety**
- Orient the patient with reduced vision to his or her immediate surroundings, including how to call for help and where the bathroom is located. **QSEN: Safety**
- Identify the room of a patient with reduced vision. **QSEN: Safety**
- Never administer a topical ophthalmic liquid or ointment by the oral route. **QSEN: Safety**
- Teach family members who have good vision to make appropriate adaptations in the patient's home to increase his or her safety and independence (Chart 47-3). **QSEN: Safety**

Health Promotion and Maintenance
- Identify adults at risk for visual SENSORY PERCEPTION problems as a result of work environment or leisure activities and teach them specific ways to protect the eyes. **QSEN: Safety**
- Encourage all patients to wear eye protection when they are performing yard work, working in a woodshop or metal shop, using chemicals, or in any environment in which drops or particulate matter is airborne. **QSEN: Safety**
- Encourage patients over 40 years old and those with chronic disorders that affect the eye and vision to have an eye examination with measurement of intraocular pressure (IOP) every year. **QSEN: Safety**
- Encourage adults to use polarizing sunglasses whenever outdoors in the daytime. **QSEN: Safety**
- Teach all patients to wash their hands before and after touching the eyes. **QSEN: Safety**

Psychosocial Integrity
- Teach patients and family members about what to expect during procedures to correct visual SENSORY PERCEPTION and eye problems. **QSEN: Patient-Centered Care**
- Provide opportunities for the patient and family to express concerns about a change in visual SENSORY PERCEPTION. **Ethics**
- Refer the patient with reduced visual SENSORY PERCEPTION to local services, resources, and support groups for the blind and those with low vision. **QSEN: Patient-Centered Care**
- Teach the patient with reduced visual SENSORY PERCEPTION techniques to perform ADLs and self-care independently. **QSEN: Patient-Centered Care**
- Use a normal tone of voice to talk with a patient who has a vision problem and normal hearing. Knock on the door before entering the room of a patient with reduced visual SENSORY PERCEPTION and introduce yourself. **QSEN: Patient-Centered Care**

Physiological Integrity
- Ask the patient about vision problems in any other members of the family because many vision problems have a genetic component. **QSEN: Evidence-Based Practice**

- Teach patients the proper techniques for self-installation of eyedrops and eye ointment. **QSEN: Safety**
- Stress the importance of completing an antibiotic regimen for an eye infection. **QSEN: Evidence-Based Practice**
- When instilling more than one type of eyedrop into the same eye, wait 5 to 10 minutes (or as directed by the manufacturer) between instillations. **QSEN: Evidence-Based Practice**
- Teach patients who are at risk for increased IOP which activities to avoid (see Table 47-2). **QSEN: Safety**
- Teach patients with an infection of the eye or eyelid not to rub the eye (to avoid infecting the other eye). **QSEN: Safety**
- Instruct the patient who has cataract surgery to report immediately any reduction in vision after initial improvement in vision in the eye that had the surgery. **QSEN: Safety**

- Stress the importance of using antiglaucoma eyedrop agents exactly as prescribed to prevent IOP from increasing and to prevent complications of glaucoma drug therapy. **QSEN: Patient-Centered Care**
- Never attempt to remove any object protruding from the eye. **QSEN: Safety**
- Use and teach punctal occlusion technique when administering antiglaucoma eyedrops. **QSEN: Safety**
- Work with the physician, occupational therapist, social worker, and other health care professionals to increase the patient's independence and safety within the home and community. **QSEN: Teamwork and Collaboration**

SELECTED BIBLIOGRAPHY

CNIB. (2017a). *Cataracts*. http://www.cnib.ca/en/your-eyes/eye-conditions/cataracts/pages/default.aspx.

CNIB. (2017b). *Glaucoma*. http://www.cnib.ca/en/your-eyes/eye-conditions/glaucoma/Pages/default.aspx.

Eye Banking Association of America (EBAA). (2017). *Medical standards/procedures manual*. http://restoresight.org/what-we-do/publications/medical-standards-procedures-manual/.

Foundation Fighting Blindness. (2017). www.blindness.org.

Glaucoma Research Foundation. (2016). *What can I do to prevent glaucoma?* http://www.glaucoma.org/gleams/what-can-i-do-to-prevent-glaucoma.php.

McCance, K., Huether, S., Brashers, V., & Rote, N. (2014). *Pathophysiology: The biologic basis for disease in adults and children* (7th ed.). St. Louis: Mosby.

National Eye Institute of the National Institutes of Health. (2017a). *Facts about glaucoma*. https://nei.nih.gov/health/glaucoma/glaucoma_facts.

National Eye Institute of the National Institutes of Health. (2017b). *Prevalence of adult vision impairment and age-related eye diseases in America*. https://nei.nih.gov/eyedata/adultvision_usa.

Online Mendelian Inheritance in Man (OMIM). (2017). *Retinitis pigmentosa*. www.omim.org/entry/268000.

Sacchetti, M., Mantelli, F., Merlo, D., & Lambiase, A. (2015). Systematic review of randomized clinical trials on safety and efficacy of pharmacological and nonpharmacological treatments for retinitis pigmentosa. *Journal of Ophthalmology*, doi:10.1155/2015/737053. http://www.hindawi.com/journals/joph/2015/737053/abs/.

Touhy, T., & Jett, K. (2015). *Ebersole and Hess' gerontological nursing healthy aging* (9th ed.). St. Louis: Mosby.

Yuzawa, M., Fujita, K., Tanaka, E., & Wang, E. (2013). Assessing quality of life in the treatment of patients with age-related macular degeneration: Clinical research findings and recommendations for clinical practice. *Clinical Ophthalmology*, 7, 1325–1332. doi:10.2147/OPTH.S45248.

Assessment and Care of Patients With Ear and Hearing Problems

Samuel A. Borchers and Andrea A. Borchers

ⓔ http://evolve.elsevier.com/Iggy/

PRIORITY AND INTERRELATED CONCEPTS

The priority concept for this chapter is SENSORY PERCEPTION.

✳ The SENSORY PERCEPTION concept exemplars for this chapter are:
- Otitis Media, p. 991,
- Hearing Loss, p. 996.

LEARNING OUTCOMES

Safe and Effective Care Environment

1. Collaborate with the interprofessional team to protect the patient with ear and hearing problems from injury and infection.

Health Promotion and Maintenance

2. Teach adults how to protect the ear and hearing.
3. Teach patients who need them how to use hearing assistive devices.

Psychosocial Integrity

4. Implement nursing interventions to minimize stressors for the patient experiencing a potential change in auditory SENSORY PERCEPTION.

Physiological Integrity

5. Prioritize care and educational needs for the patient with SENSORY PERCEPTION problems of the ear or hearing.

Hearing is one of the five senses that is used to assess surroundings, promote independence, warn of danger, appreciate music, and communicate with others. The ear and the brain together allow auditory SENSORY PERCEPTION.

Ear and hearing problems are common in adults. Therefore assessment of the ear and hearing is an important skill for nurses practicing in any care environment. Some problems develop over long periods and may be affected by drugs or systemic health problems, whereas others occur suddenly and immediately affect auditory SENSORY PERCEPTION. These problems reduce the ability to fully communicate with the world and can lead to confusion, mistrust, and social isolation.

ANATOMY AND PHYSIOLOGY REVIEW

Structure

The external ear, the middle ear, and the inner ear make up the ear's three divisions. Each part is important to hearing.

External Ear

The external ear develops in the embryo at the same time as the kidneys and urinary tract. Thus any person with a defect of the external ear should be examined for possible problems of the kidney and urinary systems.

The *pinna* is the part of the external ear that is composed of cartilage covered by skin and attached to the head at about a 10-degree angle at the level of the eyes. The external ear extends from the pinna through the external ear canal to the *tympanic membrane* (eardrum) (Fig. 48-1). It includes the *mastoid process,* which is the bony ridge located over the temporal bone behind the pinna. The ear canal is slightly S shaped and lined with cerumen-producing glands, oil glands, and hair follicles. Cerumen (ear "wax") helps protect and lubricate the ear canal. The distance from the opening of the ear canal to the eardrum in an adult is 1 to $1\frac{1}{2}$ inches (2.5 to 3.75 cm).

Middle Ear

The eardrum separates the external ear and the middle ear. The middle ear consists of a compartment called the *epitympanum.* Located in the epitympanum are the top opening of the eustachian tube and three small bones known as the *bony ossicles,* which are the *malleus* (hammer), the *incus* (anvil), and the *stapes* (stirrup) (Fig. 48-2). The bony ossicles are joined loosely, thereby moving with vibrations created when sound waves hit the eardrum.

The eardrum is a thick sheet of tissue; is transparent, opaque, or pearly gray; and moves when air is injected into the external canal. The landmarks on the eardrum include the *annulus,* the *pars flaccida*, and the *pars tensa*. These correspond to the parts of the malleus that can be seen through the transparent eardrum. The eardrum is attached to the first bony ossicle, the malleus, at the umbo (Fig. 48-3). The umbo is seen through the eardrum membrane as a white dot and is one end of the long process of the malleus. The pars flaccida is that portion of the eardrum above the short process of the malleus. The pars tensa is that portion surrounding the long process of the malleus.

The middle ear is separated from the inner ear by the round window and the oval window. The eustachian tube begins at the floor of the middle ear and extends to the throat. The tube opening in the throat is surrounded by adenoid lymphatic tissue (Fig. 48-4). The eustachian tube allows the pressure on both sides of the eardrum to equalize. Secretions from the middle ear drain through the tube into the throat.

Inner Ear

The inner ear is on the other side of the oval window and contains the semicircular canals, the cochlea, the vestibule, and the distal end of the eighth cranial nerve (see Fig. 48-2). The *semicircular canals* arc tubes made of cartilage and contain fluid and hair cells. These canals are connected to the sensory nerve fibers of the vestibular portion of the eighth cranial nerve. The

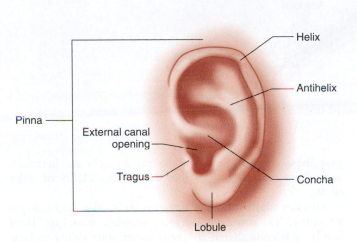

FIG. 48-1 Anatomic features of the external ear.

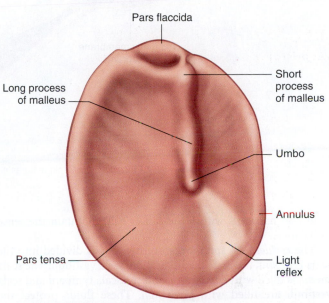

Right tympanic membrane

FIG. 48-3 Landmarks on the tympanic membrane.

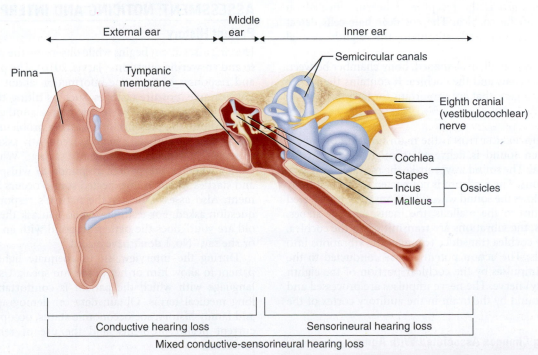

FIG. 48-2 Anatomic features of the middle and inner ear and areas involved in the three types of hearing loss.

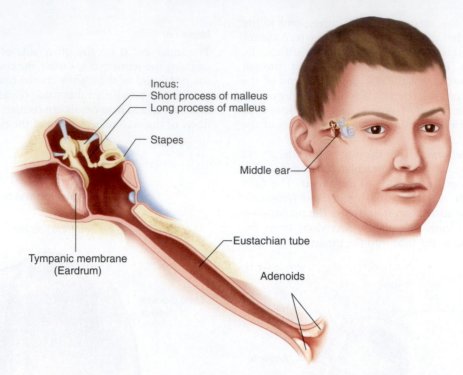

FIG. 48-4 Anatomic features and attached structures of the middle ear.

fluid and hair cells within the canals help maintain the sense of balance.

The *cochlea*, the spiral organ of hearing, is divided into the scala tympani, the scala media, and the scala vestibuli. The scala media is filled with *endolymph*, and the scala tympani and scala vestibuli are filled with *perilymph*. These fluids protect the cochlea and the semicircular canals by allowing these structures to "float" in the fluids and be cushioned against abrupt head movements.

The *organ of Corti* is the receptor of hearing located on the membrane of the cochlea. The cochlear hair cells detect vibration from sound and stimulate the eighth cranial nerve.

The *vestibule* is a small, oval-shaped, bony chamber between the semicircular canals and the cochlea. It contains the utricle and the saccule, organs that are important for balance.

Function

Auditory SENSORY PERCEPTION is the main function of the ear and occurs when sound is delivered through the air to the external ear canal. The sound waves strike the movable eardrum, creating vibrations. The eardrum is connected to the first bony ossicle, which allows the sound wave vibrations to be transferred from the eardrum to the malleus, the incus, and the stapes. From the stapes, the vibrations are transmitted to the cochlea. Receptors at the cochlea transduce (change) the vibrations into action potentials. The action potentials are conducted to the brain as nerve impulses by the cochlear portion of the eighth cranial (auditory) nerve. The nerve impulses are processed and interpreted as sound by the brain in the auditory cortex of the temporal lobe.

Ear and Hearing Changes Associated With Aging

Ear and hearing changes related to aging are listed in Chart 48-1, along with implications for care of older patients who have these changes. Some of the ear changes are harmless, and others may pose threats to the hearing ability of older adults.

All older adults should be screened for hearing acuity. Begin by asking, "Do you have a hearing problem now?" or "Have family or friends shared concerns about your ability to hear them?" In addition, family members may have noticed behaviors that suggest changes in a patient's hearing.

ASSESSMENT: NOTICING AND INTERPRETING

Patient History

Hearing assessment begins while observing the patient listening to and answering questions (Jarvis, 2016). The patient's posture and responses can provide information about hearing acuity. For example, posture changes, such as tilting the head to one side or leaning forward when listening to another person speak, may indicate the presence of a hearing problem. Other indicators of hearing difficulty include frequently asking the speaker to repeat statements or frequently saying, "What?" or "Huh?" Notice whether the patient responds to whispered questions and startles when an unexpected sound occurs in the environment. Also assess whether the patient's responses match the question asked. For example, when you ask the patient, "How old are you?" does the patient respond with an age or does he or she say, "No, I don't have a cold."

During the interview, sit in adequate light and face the patient to allow him or her to see you speak. Use short, simple language with which the patient is comfortable rather than long medical terms. Obtain data on demographics, personal and family history, socioeconomic status, occupational history, current health problems, and the use of remedies for ear problems.

The patient's gender is important. Some hearing disorders, such as otosclerosis, are more common in women. Other

CHART 48-1 Nursing Focus on the Older Adult

Age-Related Changes in the Ear and Hearing

EAR OR HEARING CHANGE	NURSING ADAPTATIONS AND ACTIONS
Pinna becomes elongated because of loss of subcutaneous tissues and decreased elasticity.	Reassure the patient that this is normal. When positioning a patient on the side, do not "fold" the ear under the head.
Hair in the canal becomes coarser and longer, especially in men.	Reassure the patient that this is normal. More frequent ear irrigation may be needed to prevent cerumen clumping.
Cerumen is drier and impacts more easily, reducing hearing function.	Teach the patient and caregiver to irrigate the ear canal weekly or whenever he or she notices a change in hearing.
Tympanic membrane loses elasticity and may appear dull and retracted.	Do not use this finding as the only indication of otitis media.
Hearing acuity decreases (in some people).	Assess hearing with the voice test or the watch test. If a deficit is present, refer the patient to a specialist to determine hearing loss and appropriate intervention. Do not assume that all older adults have a hearing loss!
The ability to hear high-frequency sounds is lost first. Older adults may have particular problems hearing the *f*, *s*, *sh*, and *pa* sounds.	Provide a quiet environment when speaking (close the door to the hallway) and face the patient. Avoid standing or sitting in front of bright lights or windows, which may interfere with the patient's ability to see your lips move. If the patient wears glasses, be sure that he or she is using them to enhance speech understanding. Speak slowly, clearly, and in a deeper voice and emphasize beginning word sounds. Some patients with a hearing loss that is not corrected may benefit from wearing a stethoscope while listening to you speak.

disorders, such as Ménière's disease, are more common in men. Age is also an important factor in hearing loss.

Personal history includes past or current signs and symptoms of ear pain, ear discharge, vertigo (spinning sensation), tinnitus (ringing), decreased hearing, and difficulty understanding people when they talk. Ask the patient about:

- Ear trauma or surgery
- Past ear infections
- Excessive cerumen
- Ear itch
- Any invasive instruments routinely used to clean the ear (e.g., Q-tip, match, bobby pin, key)
- Type and pattern of ear hygiene
- Exposure to loud noise or music during work or leisure activities
- Air travel (especially in unpressurized aircraft)
- Swimming habits and the use of ear protection when swimming
- History of health problems that can decrease the blood supply to the ear, such as heart disease, hypertension, or diabetes
- History of vitiligo (a pigment disorder that may include a loss of melanin-containing cells in the inner ear, resulting in hearing loss)
- History of smoking
- History of vitamin B_{12} and folate deficiency

If the patient uses foreign objects to clean the ear canal, explain the danger in using these objects. They can scrape the skin of the canal, push cerumen up against the eardrum, and even puncture the eardrum. If the patient says that cerumen buildup is a problem, teach him or her to use an ear irrigation syringe and proper solutions to remove it. Chart 48-2 describes techniques to teach patients how to remove cerumen safely.

If the patient uses a hearing aid, assess whether hearing is improved with its use. Obtain the date of the last hearing test, the type of test given, and the results. Ask about problems that may impair auditory SENSORY PERCEPTION such as allergies,

CHART 48-2 Patient and Family Education: Preparing for Self-Management

Self–Ear Irrigation for Cerumen Removal

- *Do not attempt to remove earwax or irrigate the ears if you have ear tubes or blood, pus, or other drainage from the ear.*
- Use an ear syringe designed for the purpose of wax removal (available at most drugstores).
- The safest type of ear syringe to use is one that has a right-angle or "elbow" in the tip.
- Irrigating your ears in the shower is an easy method.
- Always use tap water that feels just barely warm to you. Water that is warmer or colder can make you feel dizzy and nauseated.
- If your earwax is thick and sticky, you may need to place a few warm commercial eardrops that soften earwax (or baby oil or mineral oil) into the ear an hour or so before you irrigate the ear.
- Fill the syringe with the lukewarm tap water.
- If you are using a syringe with an elbow tip, place only the last part of the tip into your ear and aim it toward the roof of your ear canal.
- If you are using a straight-tipped syringe, insert the tip only about $\frac{1}{2}$ to $\frac{3}{4}$ inch into your ear canal, aiming toward the roof of the canal.
- Hold your head at a 30-degree angle to the side you are irrigating.
- Use one hand to hold the syringe and the other to push the plunger or squeeze the bulb.
- Apply gentle but firm continuous pressure, allowing the water to flow against the top of the canal.
- *Do not use blasts or bursts of sudden pressure.*
- The ear canal should fill; and water will begin to flow out, bringing earwax and debris with it.
- If a dental water-pressure irrigator is used, put it on the lowest possible setting.
- This process should not be painful! If pain occurs, decrease the pressure. If pain persists, stop the irrigation.
- Continue the irrigation until at least a cup of solution has washed into and out from your ear canal. (You may have to refill the syringe.)
- Tilting your head at a 90-degree angle to the side should allow most, if not all, of the water to drain out of your ear.
- Repeat the procedure on the other ear.
- If you feel that water is still in the canal, hold a hair dryer on a low setting near the ear.
- Irrigate your ears weekly to monthly, depending on how fast your earwax collects.

upper respiratory infections, hypothyroidism, atherosclerosis, head trauma, and recent head, facial, or dental surgery. A thorough drug history is important because many drugs are **ototoxic** (damaging to the ear), especially many antibiotics, some diuretics, NSAIDs, and many chemotherapy agents. Use a drug handbook to determine whether any of the patient's prescribed drugs are known to affect auditory SENSORY PERCEPTION.

Ask about the patient's occupation and hobbies that involve exposure to loud noise or music. Assess whether protective ear devices are used. Also ask whether any devices are consistently inserted into the ear, such as earplugs or earpiece headsets, and for how long each day they are used. Use this opportunity to teach the patient about protecting the ears from loud noises by wearing protective ear devices, such as over-the-ear headsets or foam ear inserts, when persistent loud noises are in the environment. Also suggest the use of earplugs when engaging in water sports to prevent ear infections.

Family History and Genetic Risk

Family and personal history is important in determining genetic risk for hearing loss. Although most hearing loss as a result of a genetic mutation is seen in childhood, some genetic problems can lead to progressive hearing loss in adults. For example, most people with Down syndrome develop hearing loss as adults. People with osteogenesis imperfecta have bilateral and progressive hearing loss by their 30s.

 GENETIC/GENOMIC CONSIDERATIONS

Patient-Centered Care QSEN

Mutations in several different genes are associated with hearing loss. One type of hearing loss among adults has a genetic basis with a mutation in gene GJB2 (Online Mendelian Inheritance in Man [OMIM], 2016). This mutation causes poor production of the protein connexin-26, which has a role in the function of cochlear hair cells. Other genetic variations in some of the genes for drug-metabolizing enzymes (cytochrome p450 family) slow the metabolism and excretion of drugs, including ototoxic drugs. This allows ototoxic drugs to remain in the body longer, thus increasing the risk for hearing loss.

Ask the patient:
• Who in your family has hearing problems?
• Are the hearing problems present in men and women equally, or are they present more in one gender?
• At what age was hearing loss diagnosed in your relative(s)?
• Are both ears affected?

Current Health Problems

Assess current ear-related problems by asking about any ear "trouble," ear pain, or discharge, including earwax. Ask about a change in hearing, such as **hyperacusis** (the intolerance for sound levels that do not bother other people), or tinnitus (ringing in the ears). If a change in hearing is reported, ask

whether one or both ears are involved and if the change was sudden or gradual. Also ask about problems with a feeling of fullness in the ears, dizziness, sensations of being "off-balance," or vertigo.

Physical Assessment

Begin the examination by having the patient sit or lie down. Remove any hearing aids before the examination. After the examination, inspect the hearing aid for cracks, debris, and a proper fit. An audiology specialist, physician, advanced practice nurse, or physician assistant usually performs a complete ear examination. The brief assessment of the ear and hearing usually performed by a medical-surgical nurse is described next.

External Ear and Mastoid Assessment

Inspect the entire external ear for shape, location of attachment to the head, and condition of all visible ear structures. The normal pinna has no skin tags or deformity. It should be attached to the side of the head at a posterior angle of 10 degrees or less. The normal external canal is dry, clean, free from lesions, and not reddened.

Abnormalities of the pinna include swelling, nodules, and lesions (Jarvis, 2016). In chronic gout, collections of uric acid crystals result in hard, irregular, painless nodules called *tophi* on the pinna. Other nodules on the pinna might also be from basal cell carcinoma or rheumatoid arthritis. Small, crusted, ulcerated, or indurated lesions on the pinna that fail to heal could be squamous cell carcinoma.

Inspect the mastoid process for redness and swelling. To assess for tenderness, gently tap with one finger over the mastoid process, compress the tragus with one finger, and gently move the pinna forward and backward. Any tenderness suggests an inflammation in either the external ear or the mastoid.

Assess for and record these problems:
• Furuncles
• Large amounts of cerumen
• Scaliness
• Redness
• Swelling of the ear
• Drainage amount and character

Otoscopic Assessment

The purpose of a brief otoscopic examination is to assess the patency of the external canal, identify lesions or excessive cerumen in the canal, and assess whether the tympanic membrane (eardrum) is intact or inflamed (Jarvis, 2016). An instrument called an **otoscope** is used to examine the ear. Many types are available. It consists of a light, a handle, a magnifying lens, and a pressure bulb for injecting air into the external canal to test mobility of the eardrum (Fig. 48-5). Specula of various diameters attach to the head of the otoscope. Select the largest speculum that most comfortably fits the patient's external canal.

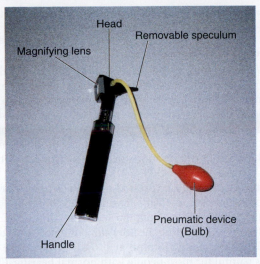

FIG. 48-5 Functional components of an otoscope.

Head

Removable speculum

Magnifying lens

Pneumatic device (Bulb)

Handle

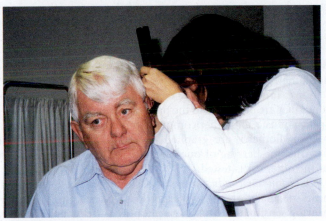

FIG. 48-6 Proper technique for an otoscopic examination.

If the patient has pain during the external ear examination, cautiously attempt an otoscopic examination. The speculum will cause extreme pain if it comes in contact with inflamed tissue in the external canal.

Tilt the patient's head slightly away and hold the otoscope upside down, like a large pen (Fig. 48-6). This position permits your hand to lie against the patient's head for support. If the patient moves, both your hand and the otoscope also move, preventing damage to the canal or eardrum. Hold the otoscope in your dominant hand and gently pull the pinna up and back with your other hand to straighten the canal. View the ear canal while you slowly insert the speculum. Use caution to avoid causing pain by touching the speculum on the walls of the canal.

> **! NURSING SAFETY PRIORITY** (QSEN)
>
> **Action Alert**
>
> Observe the ear canal through the otoscope as you insert the speculum into the external canal to avoid the risk for perforating the eardrum.

After the otoscope is comfortably in the external canal, assess for lesions and the amount, consistency, and color of cerumen and hair. The normal external canal is skin-colored, intact, and without lesions. It contains various amounts of soft cerumen and small, fine hairs.

Assess the eardrum for intactness and color. *The normal eardrum is always intact.* The eardrum is shiny, transparent or opaque, pearly gray, and without lesions. Redness is seen in otitis media. Reflection of the otoscope's light from the normal eardrum is the light reflex, and it appears as a clearly outlined triangle of light. On the right eardrum, the light reflex appears in the right lower quadrant. On the left eardrum, the light reflex appears in the left lower quadrant. The light reflex is termed diffuse when it is spotty or multiple because of a changed eardrum shape.

> **⊕ CULTURAL/SPIRITUAL CONSIDERATIONS**
>
> **Patient-Centered Care** (QSEN)
>
> Cerumen is generally moist and tan or brown in white people and black people. It is dry and light brown–to-gray in Asians and American Indians. The color of the lining of the external ear canal varies with the patient's skin tone. Variations should not be mistaken for indications of problems. Patients with more moist earwax form cerumen impactions more easily than patients with drier, flaky earwax and require more frequent ear irrigations.

General Hearing Assessment

Several rapid and simple tests for acuity of auditory SENSORY PERCEPTION can be performed at the patient's bedside. Although these tests do not determine the true extent or type of hearing loss, they can indicate a patient's functional hearing ability.

The *voice test* for hearing is conducted by asking the patient to block one external ear canal while standing 1 to 2 feet (30 to 60 cm) away. Quietly whisper a statement and ask the patient to repeat it. Test each ear separately. If the patient does not respond correctly, use a louder whisper. If you suspect that the patient is lip-reading, use your hand to block the view of your mouth or stand behind him or her while whispering. More complex hearing tests, performed by audiologists, physicians, advanced practice nurses, specialty nurses, and physician assistants, can determine the type and extent of hearing loss.

Sound is transmitted by air conduction and bone conduction. Air conduction of sound is normally more sensitive than bone conduction. If auditory SENSORY PERCEPTION is decreased, the hearing loss is categorized as:
- Conductive hearing loss, resulting from obstruction of sound wave transmission such as a foreign body in the external canal, a retracted or bulging tympanic membrane, or fused bony ossicles
- Sensorineural hearing loss, resulting from a defect in the cochlea, the eighth cranial nerve, or the brain (Exposure to loud noise or music causes this type of hearing loss by damaging the cochlear hair.)
- Mixed conductive-sensorineural hearing loss, resulting from both conductive and sensorineural hearing loss.

Audioscopy testing involves the use of a handheld device to generate tones of varying intensities to test hearing. Auditory SENSORY PERCEPTION can be measured at a 40-decibel (dB) intensity at frequencies of 500, 1000, 2000, and 4000 cycles per second (cps), or hertz (Hz).

Tuning fork tests for hearing are the Weber and Rinne tests. These tests are useful, although limited, in distinguishing between conductive and sensorineural hearing losses. The frequency range of the tuning fork used for these tests corresponds to that of normal speech.

The Weber tuning fork test is performed by placing a vibrating tuning fork on the middle of the patient's head and asking him or her to indicate in which ear the sound is louder. The normal test result is sound heard equally in both ears. The term *lateralization* is used if the sound is louder in one ear. For example, lateralization to the right means that the sound is heard louder in the right ear.

The Rinne tuning fork test compares hearing by air conduction with hearing by bone conduction. Sound is normally heard two to three times longer by air conduction than by bone conduction. Perform this test by placing the vibrating tuning fork stem on the mastoid process (bone conduction) and asking the patient to indicate when the sound is no longer heard. When the patient no longer hears the sound, bring the fork quickly in front of the pinna (air conduction) without touching the patient. He or she should then indicate when this sound is no longer heard. The patient normally continues to hear the sound two to three times longer in front of the pinna after not hearing it with the tuning fork touching the mastoid process.

Psychosocial Assessment

The patient may become frustrated and depressed by an inability to hear well. Reduced or lost hearing may lead to social isolation or mistrust of others. Be sensitive to the patient and conduct the interview at a pace appropriate for him or her.

Ask about social and work relationships to determine whether the patient is isolated because of hearing problems. Ask about any changes in feeling of enjoyment related to participation in activities with family and friends. Encourage the patient to express feelings related to hearing loss and discuss any changes in ADLs as a result of a change in hearing. Ask family members whether hearing problems have changed the patient's interactions.

💡 NCLEX EXAMINATION CHALLENGE 48-1

Safe and Effective Care Environment

For which client will the nurse avoid performing an otoscopic examination?
A. 29-year-old with abdominal pain
B. 37-year-old with vertigo
C. 45-year-old with new diagnosis of diabetes
D. 59-year-old with confusion

Diagnostic Assessment

Laboratory Assessment

Laboratory tests are helpful only when an external or internal ear infection is suspected. For an external ear infection, the typical causative organisms are known, and this infection is managed without obtaining cultures. If the usual antibiotic therapy is not successful at clearing the infection, microbial culture and antibiotic sensitivity tests may be performed.

Imaging Assessment

CT, with or without contrast enhancement, shows the structures of the ear in great detail. CT is especially helpful in diagnosing acoustic tumors.

MRI most accurately reflects soft-tissue changes. Patients with older internal metal vascular clips cannot have MRI. Newer clips are made from titanium and are not a contraindication for MRI.

Specific Auditory Assessment

Audiometry. Audiometry is the most reliable method of measuring the acuity of auditory SENSORY PERCEPTION. It is performed by audiologists, audiology technicians, or nurses with special training. **Frequency** is the highness or lowness of tones (expressed in hertz). The greater the number of vibrations per second, the higher the frequency (pitch) of the sound. The fewer the number of vibrations per second, the lower the frequency (pitch).

Intensity of sound is expressed in decibels (dB). **Threshold** is the lowest level of intensity at which pure tones and speech are heard by a patient about 50% of the time. The lowest intensity at which a young, healthy ear can detect sound about 50% of the time is 0 dB. Sound at 110 dB is so intense (loud) that it is painful for most people with normal hearing. Conversational speech is around 60 dB, and a soft whisper is around 20 dB (Table 48-1). With a hearing loss of 45 to 50 dB, speech cannot be heard without a hearing aid. A person with a hearing loss of 90 dB may not be able to hear speech even with a hearing aid.

Pure tones are generated by an audiometer to determine hearing acuity. The two types of audiometry are pure-tone audiometry and speech audiometry.

Pure-Tone Audiometry. Pure-tone audiometry generates tones that are presented to the patient at frequencies for hearing speech, music, and other common sounds. The results of pure-tone audiometry are graphed on an audiogram. For some patients, the hearing of one ear is "masked" while the hearing of the other ear is tested.

Pure-tone air-conduction testing determines whether a patient hears normally or has a hearing loss. It tests air-conduction hearing sensitivity (through earphones) at frequencies ranging from 125 to 8000 Hz. The intensities for pure tones generally range from 10 to 110 dB.

The patient sits in a sound-isolated room so background noise does not interfere with the test. Earphones are placed over his or her ears, and tones of varying frequencies and intensities

TABLE 48-1	**Decibel Intensity and Safe Exposure Time for Common Sounds**	
SOUND	**DECIBEL INTENSITY (dB)**	**SAFE EXPOSURE TIME***
Threshold of hearing	0	
Whispering	20	
Average residence or office	40	
Conversational speech	60	
Car traffic	70	>8 hr
Motorcycle	90	8 hr
Chain saw	100	2 hr
Rock concert, front row	120	3 min
Jet engine	140	Immediate danger
Rocket launching pad	180	Immediate danger

*For every 5-dB increase in intensity, the safe exposure time is cut in half.

are delivered through the earphones, testing one ear at a time. The patient presses a button or raises a hand to indicate when he or she hears a tone.

Pure-tone bone-conduction testing determines whether the hearing loss detected by air-conduction testing is caused by conductive or sensorineural factors or to a combination of the two. It is used only when air-conduction testing results are abnormal. Testing is similar to air-conduction testing except that a bone-conduction vibrator, placed firmly behind the ear on the mastoid process, is used instead of earphones.

Interpretation of audiometric evaluation determines whether hearing is within normal limits or shows a hearing impairment and, if present, whether the hearing loss is conductive, sensorineural, or mixed. The type of loss is determined by an experienced clinician who examines the shape of the audiogram after completion of pure-tone air-conduction and bone-conduction audiometry.

Speech Audiometry. In speech audiometry, the patient's ability to hear spoken words is measured. The speech reception threshold and speech discrimination are assessed.

Speech reception threshold is the minimum loudness at which a patient can repeat simple words. This test determines how intense (or loud) a simple speech stimulus must be before the patient can hear it well enough to repeat it correctly at least 50% of the time. In one common test, lists of two-syllable words called spondee are used (i.e., words in which there is equal stress on each syllable, such as *airplane, railroad,* and *cowboy*).

Speech discrimination testing determines the patient's ability to discriminate among similar sounds or among words that contain similar sounds. This test assesses the patient's *understanding* of speech. An auditory SENSORY PERCEPTION loss decreases sensitivity to sound and impairs understanding of what is being said.

A standard format contains lists of 25 to 50 *monosyllabic* (one-syllable) words, such as *carve, day, toe,* and *ran,* and phonemically balanced words, with equal word difficulty between lists. The lists are presented to the patient through earphones at a selected loudness level, generally about 30 to 40 dB above the speech reception threshold or at the patient's most comfortable listening level. The score indicates the percentage of words repeated correctly.

Tympanometry. Tympanometry assesses mobility of the eardrum and structures of the middle ear by changing air pressure in the external ear canal. The progression or resolution of serous otitis and otitis media can be accurately monitored with this procedure.

This test is helpful in distinguishing middle ear problems, such as otosclerosis, ossicular disarticulation, otitis media, and perforation of the eardrum. It is also useful for assessing patency of the eustachian tube and checking recovery of middle ear function after surgery.

Auditory Brainstem-Evoked Response. Auditory brainstem-evoked response (ABR) assesses hearing in patients who are unable to indicate their recognition of sound stimuli during standard hearing tests. It helps diagnose conductive and sensorineural hearing losses. Electrodes are placed on the scalp during the test. After the test, the patient's hair should be cleaned to remove the electrode gel.

Assessment of Balance

Electronystagmography (ENG) is a test to assess for central and peripheral disease of the vestibular system in the ear by detecting and recording nystagmus (involuntary eye movements). This response is accurate because the eyes and ears depend on one another for balance. Electrodes are taped to the skin near the eyes, and one or more procedures (caloric testing, changing gaze position, or changing head position) are performed to stimulate nystagmus. Failure of nystagmus to occur with cerebral stimulation suggests an abnormality in the vestibulocochlear apparatus, the cerebral cortex, the auditory nerve, or the brainstem.

To prepare the patient for ENG:
- Explain the procedure and its purpose. The examiners will be asking the patient to name names or do simple mathematics problems during the test to ensure that he or she stays alert.
- Instruct the patient to fast for several hours before the test and avoid caffeine-containing beverages for 24 to 48 hours before the test.
- Instruct patients with pacemakers that they should not have the test because pacemaker signals interfere with the sensitivity of ENG.
- Carefully introduce oral fluids after the test to prevent nausea and vomiting.

Caloric testing evaluates the vestibular (inner ear) portion of the auditory nerve. Water or air that is warmer or cooler than body temperature is infused into the ear. A normal response is the onset of vertigo and nystagmus within 20 to 30 seconds. Prepare the patient for caloric testing by:
- Explaining the procedure and its purpose
- Instructing the patient to fast for several hours before the test
- Explaining that he or she will be on bedrest after the procedure with careful introduction of oral fluids to prevent nausea and vomiting

✴ SENSORY PERCEPTION CONCEPT EXEMPLAR
Otitis Media

❖ PATHOPHYSIOLOGY

The common forms of otitis media are acute otitis media, chronic otitis media, and serous otitis media. Each type affects the middle ear but has different causes and pathologic changes. If otitis progresses or is untreated, permanent conductive hearing loss may occur.

Acute otitis media and chronic otitis media are similar. An infecting agent in the middle ear causes inflammation of the mucosa, leading to swelling and irritation of the ossicles within the middle ear, followed by purulent inflammatory exudate. Acute disease has a sudden onset and lasts 3 weeks or less. Chronic otitis media often follows repeated acute episodes, has a longer duration, and causes greater middle ear injury. It may be a result of the continuing presence of a biofilm in the middle ear. A *biofilm* is a community of bacteria working together to overcome host defense mechanisms to continue to survive and proliferate (see Chapter 23 for more information about biofilms). Therapy for complications associated with chronic otitis media usually involves surgical intervention.

The eustachian tube and mastoid, connected to the middle ear by a sheet of cells, are also affected by the infection. If the eardrum membrane perforates, the infection can thicken and scar the eardrum and middle ear if left untreated. Necrosis of the ossicles destroys middle ear structures and causes hearing loss.

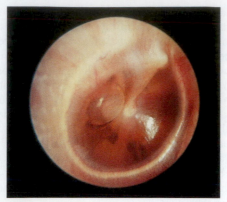

FIG. 48-7 Otoscopic view of otitis media.

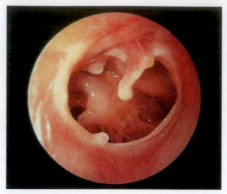

FIG. 48-8 Otoscopic view of a perforated tympanic membrane.

Health Promotion and Maintenance

Some, but not all, cases of otitis media can be prevented. Encourage adults to remain current on all immunization boosters and to receive the flu and pneumococcal vaccines as indicated. Remind adults that proper handwashing is important to minimize all types of infection.

❖ INTERPROFESSIONAL COLLABORATIVE CARE

Care of the patient with otitis media generally takes place in the outpatient (community) setting. Members of the interprofessional team who collaborate most closely to care for this patient include the primary health care provider and nurse.

◆ Assessment: Noticing

The patient with acute or chronic otitis media has ear pain. Acute otitis media causes more intense pain from increased pressure in the middle ear. Conductive hearing is reduced and distorted as sound-wave transmission is obstructed. The patient may notice tinnitus in the form of a low hum or a low-pitched sound. Headaches and systemic signs and symptoms such as malaise, fever, nausea, and vomiting can occur. As the pressure on the middle ear pushes against the inner ear, the patient may have dizziness.

Otoscopic examination findings vary, depending on the stage of the condition. The eardrum is initially retracted, which allows landmarks of the ear to be seen clearly. At this early stage, the patient has only vague ear discomfort. As the condition progresses, the eardrum's blood vessels dilate and appear red (Fig. 48-7). Later the eardrum becomes red, thickened, and bulging, with loss of landmarks. Decreased eardrum mobility is evident on inspection with a pneumatic otoscope. Pus may be seen behind the membrane.

With progression, the eardrum spontaneously perforates, and pus or blood drains from the ear (Fig. 48-8). Then the patient notices a marked decrease in pain as the pressure on middle ear structures is relieved. Eardrum perforations often heal if the underlying problem is controlled. Simple central perforation does not interfere with hearing unless the ossicles are damaged or the perforation is large. Repeated perforations with extensive scarring cause hearing loss.

◆ Analysis: Interpreting

The priority collaborative problems for patients with otitis media include:

1. Infection due to otitis media
2. Pain due to ear infection

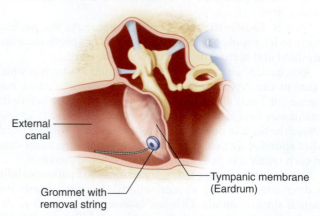

External canal

Grommet with removal string

Tympanic membrane (Eardrum)

FIG. 48-9 Grommet through the tympanic membrane. A small grommet is placed through the tympanic membrane away from the margins, which allows prolonged drainage of fluids from the middle ear.

◆ Planning and Implementation: Responding

Eliminating Infection While Reducing Pain

Nonsurgical Management. Management can be as simple as putting the patient in a quiet environment. Bedrest limits head movements that intensify the pain. Application of low heat may help reduce pain.

Systemic antibiotic therapy is prescribed. Teach the patient to complete the antibiotic therapy as prescribed and to not stop taking the drug when signs and symptoms are relieved. Analgesics such as aspirin, ibuprofen (Advil), and acetaminophen (Tylenol, Abenol ❖) relieve pain and reduce fever. For severe pain, opioid analgesics may be prescribed. Antihistamines and decongestants are prescribed to decrease fluid in the middle ear.

Surgical Management. If pain persists after antibiotic therapy and the eardrum continues to bulge, a **myringotomy** (surgical opening of the eardrum) is performed. This procedure drains middle ear fluids and immediately relieves pain.

The procedure is a small surgical incision, which is often performed in an office or clinic setting, and the incision heals rapidly. Another approach is the removal of fluid from the middle ear with a needle. For relief of pressure caused by serous otitis media and for patients who have repeated episodes of otitis media, a small **grommet** (polyethylene tube) may be surgically placed through the eardrum to allow continuous drainage of middle ear fluids (Fig. 48-9).

Priority care after surgery includes teaching the patient to keep the external ear and canal clean and dry while the incision is healing. Instruct him or her to not wash the hair or shower for several days. Other instructions after surgery are listed in Chart 48-3.

Care Coordination and Transition Management

Patients with nonsurgical otitis media are usually treated and discharged to home. Nursing interventions can focus on helping the patient and family with current treatment and reduction of risk for further infection.

Home Care Management. Remind the patient to take all antibiotics as prescribed, even if he or she begins to feel better. If the patient has been prescribed pain medication, teach about possible side effects and discourage driving and activities that require concentration.

Self-Management Education. For patients with nonsurgical otitis media, teach about signs and symptoms of eardrum perforation (see Fig. 48-8). Remind the patient that repeated perforations with scarring cause hearing loss.

Health Care Resources. If the patient lives alone and has no support, arrange for a home care nurse to assist with medication administration and adherence as needed.

◆ Evaluation: Reflecting

Evaluate the care of the patient with otitis media on the basis of elimination of infection and reduction of pain. The expected outcomes include that the patient will:

- Have absence of otitis media infection
- Recognize signs and symptoms of perforation
- Experience reduction or elimination of pain

EXTERNAL OTITIS

❖ PATHOPHYSIOLOGY

External otitis is a painful condition caused when irritating or infective agents come into contact with the skin of the external ear. The result is either an allergic response or inflammation with or without infection. Affected skin becomes red, swollen, and tender to touch or movement. Swelling of the ear canal can lead to temporary hearing loss from obstruction. Allergic external otitis is often caused by contact with cosmetics, hair sprays, earphones, earrings, or hearing aids. The most common infectious organisms are *Pseudomonas aeruginosa*, *Streptococcus*, *Staphylococcus*, and *Aspergillus*.

External otitis occurs more often in hot, humid environments, especially in the summer, and is known as **swimmer's ear** because it occurs most often in people involved in water sports. Patients who have traumatized their external ear canal with sharp or small objects (e.g., hairpins, cotton-tipped applicators) or with headphones also are more susceptible to external otitis.

Necrotizing or *malignant otitis* is the most virulent form of external otitis. Organisms spread beyond the external ear canal into the ear and skull. Death from complications such as meningitis, brain abscess, and destruction of cranial nerve VII is possible.

❖ INTERPROFESSIONAL COLLABORATIVE CARE

The care of patients with external otitis usually takes place in the outpatient setting and is managed by the primary health care provider and nurse. Signs and symptoms of external otitis range from mild itching to pain with movement of the pinna or tragus, particularly when upward pressure is applied to the external canal. Patients report feeling as if the ear is plugged and hearing is reduced. The temporary hearing loss can be severe when inflammation obstructs the canal and prevents sounds from reaching the eardrum.

Treatment focuses on reducing inflammation, edema, and pain. Nursing priorities include comfort measures, such as applying heat to the ear for 20 minutes three times a day. This can be accomplished by using towels warmed with water and then wrapped in a plastic bag or by using a heating pad placed on a low setting. Teach the patient that minimizing head movements reduces pain.

Topical antibiotic and steroid therapies are most effective in decreasing inflammation and pain. Review best practices for instilling eardrops with the patient, as shown in Chart 48-4. Observe the patient self-administer the eardrops to make sure that proper technique is used. Oral or IV antibiotics are used in severe cases, especially when infection spreads to surrounding tissue or area lymph nodes are enlarged.

Analgesics, including opioids, may be needed for pain relief during the initial days of treatment. NSAIDs, such as acetylsalicylic acid (aspirin, Entrophen ✦) and ibuprofen (Advil) or acetaminophen (Tylenol, Abenol ✦) may relieve less severe pain.

CHART 48-3 Patient and Family Education: Preparing for Self-Management

Recovery From Ear Surgery

- Avoid straining when you have a bowel movement.
- Do not drink through a straw for 2 to 3 weeks.
- Avoid air travel for 2 to 3 weeks.
- Avoid excessive coughing for 2 to 3 weeks.
- Stay away from people with respiratory infections.
- When blowing your nose, blow gently, without blocking either nostril, with your mouth open.
- Avoid getting your head wet, washing your hair, and showering for 1 week.
- Keep your ear dry for 6 weeks by placing a ball of cotton coated with petroleum jelly (e.g., Vaseline) in it. Change the cotton ball daily.
- Avoid rapidly moving the head, bouncing, and bending over for 3 weeks.
- Change your ear dressing every 24 hours or as directed.
- Report excessive drainage immediately to your health care provider.

CHART 48-4 Best Practice for Patient Safety & Quality Care QSEN

Instillation of Eardrops

- Gather the solutions to be administered.
- Check the labels to ensure correct dosage, time, and expiration date.
- Wear gloves to remove and discard any ear packing.
- Wash your hands.
- Perform a gentle otoscopic examination to determine whether the eardrum is intact.
- Irrigate the ear if the eardrum is intact (see Chart 48-4).
- Place the bottle of eardrops (with the top on tightly) in a bowl of warm water for 5 minutes.
- Tilt the patient's head in the opposite direction of the affected ear and place the drops in the ear.
- With his or her head tilted, ask the patient to gently move the head back and forth five times.
- Insert a cotton ball into the opening of the ear canal to act as packing.
- Wash your hands again.

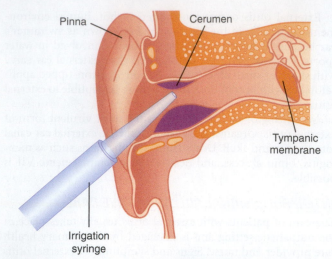

FIG. 48-10 Irrigation of the external canal. Cerumen and debris can be removed from the ear by irrigation with warm water. The stream of water is aimed above or below the impaction to allow back-pressure to push it out rather than further down the canal.

After the inflammation has subsided, a solution of 50% rubbing alcohol, 25% white vinegar, and 25% distilled water may be dropped into the ear to keep it clean and dry and prevent recurrence. Teach the patient to use preventive measures for minimizing ear-canal moisture, trauma, or exposure to materials that lead to local irritation or contact dermatitis.

CERUMEN OR FOREIGN BODIES

❖ PATHOPHYSIOLOGY

Cerumen (earwax) is the most common cause of an impacted canal. A canal can also become impacted as a result of foreign bodies that can enter or be placed in the external ear canal, such as vegetables, beads, pencil erasers, and insects. Although uncomfortable, cerumen or foreign bodies are rarely emergencies and can be removed carefully by a health care professional. Cerumen impaction in the older adult is common, and removal of the cerumen from older adults often improves hearing.

❖ INTERPROFESSIONAL COLLABORATIVE CARE

The care of patients with cerumen impaction or foreign body in the ear usually takes place in the outpatient setting and is managed by the primary health care provider and nurse. Patients may report a sensation of fullness in the ear, with or without hearing loss, and may have ear pain, itching, dizziness, or bleeding from the ear. The object may be visible with direct inspection.

When the occluding material is cerumen, management options include watchful waiting, manual removal, and the use of ceruminolytic agents followed by either manual irrigation or the use of a low-pressure electronic oral irrigation device. The canal can be irrigated with a mixture of water and hydrogen peroxide at body temperature (Fig. 48-10), following best practices for proper irrigation (Chart 48-5). Removal of a cerumen obstruction by irrigation is a slow process and may take more than one sitting. When it is the cause of hearing loss, cerumen removal may improve hearing. Between 50 and 70 mL of solution is the maximum amount that the patient usually can tolerate at one sitting.

◎ CHART 48-5   Best Practice for Patient Safety & Quality Care QSEN

Ear Irrigation

- Wash your hands.
- Use an otoscope to locate the impaction; ascertain that the eardrum is intact and that the patient does not have otitis media.
- Gather the equipment: basin, irrigation syringe, otoscope, and towel.
- Warm tap water (or other prescribed solution) to body temperature.
- Fill a syringe with the warmed irrigating solution.
- Place a towel around the patient's neck.
- Place a basin under the ear to be irrigated.
- Place the tip of the syringe at an angle so the fluid pushes to one side of and not directly on the impaction (to loosen it without moving it deeper into the canal).
- Apply gentle but firm continuous pressure, allowing the water to flow against the top of the canal.
- Do not use blasts or bursts of sudden pressure.
- If pain occurs, reduce the pressure. If pain persists, stop the irrigation.
- Watch the fluid return for cerumen plug removal.
- Continue to irrigate the ear with about 70 mL of fluid.
- If the cerumen does not drain out, wait 10 minutes and repeat the irrigation procedure.
- Monitor the patient for signs of nausea.
- If the patient becomes nauseated, stop the procedure.
- If the cerumen cannot be removed by irrigation, place mineral oil into the ear three times a day for 2 days to soften dry, impacted cerumen, after which irrigation may be repeated.
- After completion of the irrigation, have the patient turn his or her head to the side just irrigated to drain any remaining irrigation fluid.
- Wash your hands again.

❗ NURSING SAFETY PRIORITY QSEN

Action Alert

Do not irrigate an ear with an eardrum perforation or otitis media because this may spread the infection to the inner ear. Also, do not irrigate the ear when the foreign object is vegetable matter because this material expands when wet, making the impaction worse. For vegetable matter, the object needs to be physically removed by an experienced health care professional.

If the cerumen is thick and dry or cannot be removed easily, use a ceruminolytic product such as Cerumenex to soften the wax before trying to remove it. Another way to soften cerumen is to add 3 drops of glycerin or mineral oil to the ear at bedtime and 3 drops of hydrogen peroxide twice a day for several days. Then the cerumen is more easily removed by irrigation. In some cases, a small curette or cerumen spoon may be used by a health care professional to scoop out the wax. Improper use of the curette can damage the canal or the eardrum.

Discourage the use of cotton swabs and ear candles (hollow tubes coated in wax inserted into the ear and then lighted at the far end) to clean the ears or remove cerumen. Chart 48-2 describes steps to teach patients regarding ear hygiene and self-ear irrigation. Refer to Chart 48-6 for nursing care considerations of older-adult patients with cerumen impaction.

Insects are killed before removal unless they can be coaxed out by a flashlight. A topical anesthetic can be placed in the ear canal for pain relief. Mineral oil or diluted alcohol instilled into the ear can suffocate the insect, which is then removed with ear forceps.

If the patient has local irritation, an antibiotic or steroid ointment may be applied to prevent infection and reduce local irritation. Hearing acuity is tested if hearing loss is not resolved by removal of the object.

Surgical removal of the foreign object may be performed through the ear canal by a health care provider using a wire bent at a 90-degree angle. The wire is looped around the object, and the object is pulled out. Because this procedure is painful, general anesthesia is needed.

MASTOIDITIS

❖ PATHOPHYSIOLOGY

The lining of the middle ear is continuous with the lining of the mastoid air cells, which are embedded in the temporal bone. **Mastoiditis** is an infection of the mastoid air cells caused by progressive otitis media. Antibiotic therapy is used to treat the middle ear infection before it progresses to mastoiditis. If mastoiditis is not managed appropriately, it can lead to brain abscess, meningitis, and death.

❖ INTERPROFESSIONAL COLLABORATIVE CARE

The signs and symptoms of mastoiditis include swelling behind the ear and pain when moving the ear or the head. Pain is *not* relieved by myringotomy. Cellulitis develops on the skin or external scalp over the mastoid process, pushing the ear sideways and down. The eardrum is red, dull, thick, and immobile. Perforation may or may not be present. Lymph nodes behind the ear are tender and enlarged. Patients may have low-grade fever, malaise, and ear drainage. Hearing loss occurs, and CT scans show fluid in the air cells of the mastoid process.

Interventions focus on halting the infection before it spreads to other structures. IV antibiotics are used but do not easily penetrate the infected bony structure of the mastoid. Cultures of the ear drainage determine which antibiotics should be most effective. Surgical removal of the infected tissue is needed if the infection does not respond to antibiotic therapy within a few days. A simple or modified radical mastoidectomy with tympanoplasty is the most common treatment. All infected tissue must be removed so the infection does not spread to other

structures. A tympanoplasty is then performed to reconstruct the ossicles and the eardrum to restore hearing (see the later discussion in the Tympanoplasty section).

TRAUMA

Trauma and damage may occur to the eardrum and ossicles by infection, by direct damage, or through rapid changes in the middle ear pressure. Objects placed in the external canal exert pressure on the eardrum and cause perforation. If the objects continue through the canal, the ossicles may be damaged. Blunt injury to the skull and ears can also damage or fracture middle ear structures. Slapping the external ear increases the pressure in the ear canal and can tear the eardrum. Excessive nose blowing and rapid changes of pressure (*barotrauma*) can increase pressure within the middle ear, leading to damaged ossicles and a perforated eardrum.

Most eardrum perforations heal within a week or two without treatment. Repeated perforations heal more slowly, with scarring. Depending on the amount of damage to the ossicles, auditory SENSORY PERCEPTION may or may not return. Hearing aids can improve hearing in this type of hearing loss. Surgical reconstruction of the ossicles and eardrum through a tympanoplasty or a myringoplasty may also improve hearing. (See later discussion of nursing care in the Tympanoplasty section.)

Nursing care priorities focus on teaching about trauma prevention. Caution adults to avoid inserting objects into the external canal. Stress the importance of using ear protectors when blunt trauma is likely.

TINNITUS

Tinnitus (continuous ringing or noise perception in the ear) is a common ear problem that can occur in one or both ears. Diagnostic testing cannot confirm tinnitus; however, testing is performed to assess hearing and rule out other disorders. A Tinnitus and Hearing Survey (Henry et al., 2015) may be used to help patients and clinicians determine whether intervention for tinnitus is warranted.

Manifestations range from mild ringing, which can go unnoticed during the day, to a loud roaring in the ear, which can interfere with thinking and attention span. Some patients feel as if the constant ringing could drive them mad. Factors that contribute to tinnitus include age, sclerosis of the ossicles, Ménière's disease, certain drugs (aspirin, NSAIDs, high-ceiling diuretics, quinine, aminoglycoside antibiotics), exposure to loud noise, and other inner ear problems.

The problem and its management vary with the underlying cause. When no cause can be found or the disorder is untreatable, therapy focuses on ways to mask the tinnitus with background sound, noisemakers, and music during sleeping hours. Ear-mold hearing aids can amplify sounds to drown out the tinnitus during the day. A drug that is helpful to some patients is pramipexole (Mirapex), an antiparkinson drug. The American Tinnitus Association helps patients cope with tinnitus. Refer patients with tinnitus to local and online support groups to help them cope with this problem.

MÉNIÈRE'S DISEASE

Ménière's disease usually first occurs in people between the ages of 20 and 50 years. It has three features: tinnitus, one-sided sensorineural auditory SENSORY PERCEPTION loss, and *vertigo*, occurring in attacks that can last for several days. **Vertigo** is a sense of whirling or turning in space. Some patients have continuous signs and symptoms of varying intensity rather than intermittent attacks. Patients are almost totally incapacitated during an attack, and recovery takes hours to days. The pathology of Ménière's disease is an excess of endolymphatic fluid that distorts the entire inner-canal system. This distortion decreases hearing by dilating the cochlear duct, causes vertigo because of damage to the vestibular system, and stimulates tinnitus. At first, hearing loss is reversible, but repeated damage to the cochlea from increased fluid pressure leads to permanent hearing loss.

Signs and symptoms such as headache, increasing tinnitus, and fullness of the affected ear can precede the attack of vertigo. Patients often describe the tinnitus as a continuous, low-pitched roar or a humming sound, which worsens just before and during an attack. Hearing loss occurs first with the low-frequency tones but progresses to include all levels and, with repeated attacks, can become permanent. The vertigo, coupled with periods of a "whirling" sensation, may cause patients to fall. It is so intense that, even while lying down, the patient often holds the bed or ground to keep from falling. Severe vertigo usually lasts 3 to 4 hours, but the patient may feel dizzy long after the attack. Nausea and vomiting, rapid eye movement (**nystagmus**), and severe headaches often accompany vertigo.

Teach patients to move the head slowly to prevent worsening of the vertigo. Nutrition and lifestyle changes, such as reducing sodium intake, can reduce the amount of endolymphatic fluid. Encourage patients to stop smoking because of the blood vessel–constricting effects.

Drug therapy may reduce the vertigo and vomiting and restore normal balance. Mild diuretics are prescribed to decrease endolymph volume, which reduces vertigo, hearing loss, tinnitus, and aural fullness. Other drugs, such as antihistamines, antivertiginous agents, and antiemetics may be used to reduce the severity of or stop an attack and to calm the patient. Intratympanic therapy with gentamycin or corticosteroids may be attempted.

When drug therapy is not effective in controlling symptoms or attacks, other procedures may be considered. *Pressure pulse treatments,* such as the Meniett device, which use a tympanostomy tube to apply low-pressure micropulses to the inner ear several times daily, displace inner ear fluid. Surgical procedures such as a **labyrinthectomy**, which involves resection of the vestibular nerve or total removal of the labyrinth, may be done after weighing risks and benefits to the patient. This procedure results in total auditory SENSORY PERCEPTION loss on the operative side.

ACOUSTIC NEUROMA

An **acoustic neuroma** is a benign tumor of the vestibulocochlear nerve (cranial nerve VIII) that often damages other structures as it grows. Depending on the size and exact location of the tumor, damage to hearing, facial movements, and sensation can occur (McCance et al., 2014). An acoustic neuroma can cause many neurologic signs and symptoms as the tumor enlarges in the brain.

Signs and symptoms begin with tinnitus and progress to gradual sensorineural hearing loss. Later patients have constant mild-to-moderate vertigo. As the tumor enlarges, nearby cranial nerves are damaged.

The tumor is diagnosed with CT scanning and MRI. Cerebrospinal fluid assays show increased pressure and protein.

Surgical removal can be performed in a variety of ways. Usually a craniotomy is performed, and usually the remaining hearing is lost. Care is taken to preserve the function of the facial nerve (cranial nerve VII). Care after craniotomy is discussed in Chapter 45. Acoustic neuromas rarely recur after surgical removal.

✳ SENSORY PERCEPTION CONCEPT EXEMPLAR
Hearing Loss

❖ PATHOPHYSIOLOGY

Loss of auditory SENSORY PERCEPTION is common and may be conductive, sensorineural, or a combination of the two (see Fig. 48-2). Conductive hearing loss occurs when sound waves are blocked from contact with inner ear nerve fibers because of external or middle ear disorders. If the inner ear sensory nerve that leads to the brain is damaged, the hearing loss is *sensorineural*. Combined hearing loss is *mixed conductive-sensorineural*.

The differences in conductive and sensorineural hearing loss are listed in Table 48-2. Disorders that cause conductive hearing loss are often corrected with minimal or no permanent damage. Sensorineural hearing loss is often permanent.

Etiology and Genetic Risk

Conductive hearing loss can be caused by any inflammation or obstruction of the external or middle ear. Changes in the eardrum such as bulging, retraction, and perforations may damage middle ear structures and lead to conductive hearing loss. Tumors, scar tissue, and overgrowth of soft bony tissue

TABLE 48-2 Comparison of Features for Conductive and Sensorineural Hearing Loss

CONDUCTIVE HEARING LOSS	SENSORINEURAL HEARING LOSS
Causes	
Cerumen	Prolonged exposure to noise
Foreign body	Presbycusis
Perforation of the tympanic membrane	Ototoxic substance
	Ménière's disease
Edema	Acoustic neuroma
Infection of the external ear or middle ear	Diabetes mellitus
	Labyrinthitis
Tumor	Infection
Otosclerosis	Myxedema
Assessment Findings	
Evidence of obstruction with otoscope	Normal appearance of external canal and tympanic membrane
Abnormality in tympanic membrane	Tinnitus common
	Occasional dizziness
Speaking softly	Speaking loudly
Hearing best in a noisy environment	Hearing poorly in loud environment
Rinne test: air conduction greater than bone conduction	Rinne test: air conduction less than bone conduction
Weber test: lateralization to affected ear	Weber test: lateralization to unaffected ear

EVIDENCE-BASED PRACTICE QSEN

Hearing Loss Among Deployed U.S. Military in Combat (Safety)

Wells, T. S., Seeling, A. D., Ryan, M. A., Jones, J. M., Hooper, T. I., Jacobson, I. G., et al. (2015). Hearing loss associated with U.S. military combat deployment. *Noise and Health, 17*(74), 34–42.

Considering that nearly one-half million U.S. veterans currently receive over $1 billion annually from the Department of Veterans Affairs (VA) for hearing loss compensation, this study sought to explore hearing loss risk among U.S. military members relative to their deployment experiences (Wells et al., 2015). Recognizing that hearing is a critical part of a U.S. military member's preparedness, this study surveyed 48,540 participants who responded to the Millennium Cohort Study, a Department of Defense research project headquartered in San Diego, California at the Naval Health Research Center. Self-reported hearing loss was correlated with audiometry results, and new onset of hearing loss was correlated with combat deployment. Of those who reported new-onset hearing loss, correlation was made with proximity to explosives during combat and also with combat-related head injury.

Level of Evidence: 2
This research was designed as a prospective cohort study.

Commentary: Implications for Practice and Research
This study demonstrates that there was a 63% increased risk for hearing loss for military members experiencing combat situations and those with a combat-related head injury were six times more likely to experience hearing loss than those without head injury. Nurses and all members of the interdisciplinary team benefit from this information by using it to plan more effectively for predeployment prevention of hearing loss related to combat activity and to more effectively provide health care and disability planning for those already affected (Wells et al., 2015).

(otosclerosis) on the ossicles from previous middle ear surgery also lead to conductive hearing loss.

Sensorineural hearing loss occurs when the inner ear or auditory nerve (cranial nerve VIII) is damaged. Prolonged exposure to loud noise damages the hair cells of the cochlea. Many drugs are toxic to the inner ear structures, and their effects on hearing can be transient or permanent and dose related and affect one or both ears. When ototoxic drugs are given to patients with reduced kidney function, increased ototoxicity can occur because drug elimination is slower, especially among older patients.

Presbycusis is a sensorineural hearing SENSORY PERCEPTION loss that occurs with aging (McCance et al., 2014). It is caused by degeneration of cochlear nerve cells, loss of elasticity of the basilar membrane, or a decreased blood supply to the inner ear. Deficiencies of vitamin B_{12} and folic acid increase the risk for presbycusis. Other causes include atherosclerosis, hypertension, infections, fever, Ménière's disease, diabetes, and ear surgery (Touhy & Jett, 2015). Trauma to the ear, head, or brain also contributes to sensorineural hearing loss, as noted in the Evidence-Based Practice box.

Incidence/Prevalence

Because hearing loss may be gradual and affect only some aspects of hearing, many adults are unaware that their hearing is impaired. The incidence of adult hearing loss in the United States is estimated to be approximately 15% of the adult population between 20 and 69 years old; this incidence increases among people in their 70s and 80s (National Institute on Deafness and Other Communication Disorders, 2016).

Health Promotion and Maintenance

With special care to the ears, hearing can be preserved at maximum levels. Address barriers to the use of hearing protection, exposure to loud music, and other modifiable risk factors that affect hearing. Encourage everyone to have simple hearing testing performed as part of their annual health assessment.

Teach adults the danger in using objects such as bobby-pins, Q-tips, or toothpicks to clean the ear canal. These can scrape the skin of the canal, push cerumen up against the eardrum, and puncture the eardrum. If cerumen buildup is a problem, teach the person the proper technique to remove it (see Chart 48-2).

Teach adults to use protective ear devices, such as over-the-ear headsets or foam ear inserts, when exposed to persistent loud noises. Suggest using earplugs when engaging in water sports to prevent ear infections and using an over-the-counter product such as Swim-Ear to help dry the ears after swimming.

❖ INTERPROFESSIONAL COLLABORATIVE CARE

Care for the patient with hearing loss usually takes place in the community setting. Hearing loss is a common condition, especially in older adults. You will care for many patients with hearing loss who are seeking treatment for other conditions in a variety of inpatient and outpatient settings. Use the best practices strategies listed in Chart 48-7 for communicating with a hearing-impaired patient in any setting.

◆ Assessment: Noticing

History. Ask patients how long they have noticed a change in hearing and whether the changes were sudden or gradual. Age is important, because some ear and hearing changes occur with aging. Ask about exposure to loud or continuous noises,

CHART 48-7 Best Practice for Patient Safety & Quality Care QSEN

Communicating With a Hearing-Impaired Patient

- Position yourself directly in front of the patient.
- Ensure that you are not sitting or standing in front of a bright light or window, which can interfere with the patient's ability to see your lips move.
- Make sure that the room is well lighted.
- Get the patient's attention before you begin to speak.
- Move closer to the better-hearing ear.
- Speak clearly and slowly.
- Do not shout (shouting often makes understanding more difficult).
- Keep hands and other objects away from your mouth when talking to the patient.
- Have conversations in a quiet room with minimal distractions.
- Have the patient repeat your statements, not just indicate assent.
- Rephrase sentences and repeat information to aid understanding.
- Use appropriate hand motions.
- Write messages on paper if the patient is able to read.

CHART 48-8 Focused Assessment

The Patient With Suspected Hearing Loss

Assess whether the patient has any of these ear problems:
- Pain
- Feeling of fullness or congestion
- Dizziness or vertigo
- Tinnitus
- Difficulty understanding conversations, especially in a noisy room
- Difficulty hearing sounds
- The need to strain to hear
- The need to turn the head to favor one ear or the need to lean forward to hear

Assess visible ear structures, particularly the external canal and tympanic membrane:
- Position and size of the pinna
- Patency of the external canal; presence of cerumen or foreign bodies, edema, or inflammation
- Condition of the tympanic membrane: intact, edema, fluid, inflammation

Assess functional ability, including:
- Frequency of asking people to repeat statements
- Withdrawal from social interactions or large groups
- Shouting in conversation
- Failing to respond when not looking in the direction of the sound
- Answering questions incorrectly

as well as current or previous use of ototoxic drugs. Also ask about a history of ear infections and whether eardrum perforation occurred. Ask patients about any direct trauma to the ears. Because some types of hearing loss have a genetic basis, ask whether any family members are hearing impaired. When pain occurs with acute-onset hearing loss, ask about recent upper respiratory infection and allergies affecting the nose and sinuses.

The patient with hearing loss from peripheral neuropathy may have other systemic diseases, including human immune deficiency virus (HIV) disease or diabetes. Patients undergoing cancer chemotherapy or interferon therapy are at risk for neuropathic hearing loss because many of these drugs damage sensory nerves.

Physical Assessment/Signs and Symptoms. Chart 48-8 lists focused assessment techniques for patients with suspected loss of auditory SENSORY PERCEPTION. The loss may be sudden or gradual and often affects both ears. The ability to hear high-frequency consonants—especially *s, sh, f, th,* and *ch* sounds—is lost first. Patients may state that they have no problem with hearing but cannot understand specific words and that other people are mumbling. Vertigo and continuous tinnitus may be present.

Tuning fork tests help diagnose hearing loss. With the Weber test, the patient can usually hear sounds well in the ear with a conductive hearing loss because of bone conduction. With the Rinne test, the patient reports that sound transmitted by bone conduction is louder and more sustained than that transmitted by air conduction.

Otoscopic examination is used to assess the ear canal, eardrum, and middle ear structures that can be seen through the eardrum. Findings vary, depending on the cause of the hearing loss. Perform the examination as described earlier in the Otoscopic Assessment section and document the findings.

Psychosocial Assessment. For people with a loss of auditory SENSORY PERCEPTION, communication can be a struggle, and they may isolate themselves because of the difficulty in talking, listening, and interpreting what is said to them. Social isolation can lead to depression. Be sensitive to emotional changes that may be related to reduced hearing and a decline in conversational skills. Encourage the patient and family to express their feelings and concerns about an actual or potential hearing loss.

Laboratory Assessment. No laboratory test diagnoses hearing loss. However, some laboratory findings can indicate problems that affect hearing. White blood cell counts are assessed in the patient with otitis media.

Imaging Assessment. Imaging assessment can determine some problems affecting hearing ability. Skull x-rays determine bony involvement in otitis media and the location of otosclerotic lesions. CT and MRI are used to determine soft-tissue involvement and the presence and location of tumors.

Other Diagnostic Assessment. Audiometry can help determine whether hearing loss is only conductive or whether it has a sensorineural component. This is important in determining possible causes of the hearing loss and planning interventions.

◆ Analysis: Interpreting

The priority collaborative problems for the patient with any degree of hearing impairment include:
1. Decreased hearing ability due to obstruction, infection, damage to the middle ear, or damage to the auditory nerve
2. Decreased functional ability (communication) due to difficulty hearing

◆ Planning and Implementation: Responding

Increasing Hearing

Planning: Expected Outcomes. The patient with impaired auditory SENSORY PERCEPTION is expected to either have an increase in functional hearing or maintain existing hearing levels. Indicators include:
- No or minimal loss of high-pitch tones
- No or minimal loss of ability to distinguish conversation from background noise
- Turning toward sound
- Identifying discrete sounds

Interventions. Interventions are expected to identify the problem, halt the pathologic processes, and increase usable hearing. Nursing care priorities focus on teaching the patient about the use of an appropriate assistive device, providing support to the patient and family to maintain or increase communication, and helping patients find support services.

Nonsurgical Management. Interventions include early detection of impaired auditory SENSORY PERCEPTION, use of appropriate therapy, and use of assistive devices to augment the patient's usable hearing.

Early detection helps correct the problem causing the hearing loss. Assess for indications of hearing loss, as listed in Chart 48-8.

Drug therapy is focused on correcting the underlying problem or reducing the side effects of problems occurring with hearing loss. Antibiotic therapy is used to manage external otitis and other ear infections. Teach the patient the importance of taking the drug or drugs exactly as prescribed and completing the entire course. Caution him or her to not stop the drug just because signs and symptoms have improved. By treating the infection, antibiotics reduce local edema and improve hearing. When pain is also present, analgesics are used. Many ear disorders induce vertigo and dizziness with nausea and vomiting. Antiemetic, antihistamine, antivertiginous, and benzodiazepine drugs can help reduce these problems.

Assistive devices are useful for patients with permanent hearing loss. Portable amplifiers can be used while watching television to avoid increasing the volume and disturbing others. Telephone amplifiers increase telephone volume, allowing the caller to speak in a normal voice. Some telephones also have a video display of words that are being spoken by the caller. Flashing lights activated by the ringing telephone or a doorbell alert patients visually. Some patients may have a service dog to alert them to sounds (ringing telephones or doorbells, cries of other people, and potential dangers). Provide information about agencies that can assist the hearing-impaired person.

Small, portable audio amplifiers can help communicate with patients with hearing loss who do not use a hearing aid. Using amplifiers or allowing patients to use a stethoscope for listening helps you communicate with an adult who requires additional volume to hear speech.

A hearing aid is a small electronic amplifier that assists patients with conductive hearing loss but is less effective for sensorineural hearing loss. The styles vary by size, placement, and the degree to which they amplify sound. Most common hearing aids are small. Some are attached to a person's glasses and are visible to other people. Another type fits into the ear and is less noticeable. Newer devices fit completely in the canal with only a fine, clear filament visible. The cost of smaller hearing aids varies with size and quality. Some people benefit from classes that explain the best use and care of these devices.

Remind patients that hearing with a hearing aid is different from natural hearing. Teach the patient to start using the hearing aid slowly, at first wearing it only at home and only during part of the day. Listening to television and the radio and reading aloud can help the patient get used to new sounds. A difficult aspect of a hearing aid is the amplification of background noise. The patient must learn to concentrate and filter out background noises.

Teach the patient how to care for the hearing aid (Chart 48-9). Hearing aids are delicate devices that should be handled only by people who know how to care for them properly.

CHART 48-9 Patient and Family Education: Preparing for Self-Management

Hearing Aid Care

- Keep the hearing aid dry.
- Clean the ear mold with mild soap and water while avoiding excessive wetting.
- Using a toothpick, clean debris from the hole in the middle of the part that goes into your ear.
- Turn off the hearing aid when not in use.
- Check and replace the battery frequently.
- Keep extra batteries on hand.
- Keep the hearing aid in a safe place.
- Avoid dropping the hearing aid or exposing it to temperature extremes.
- Adjust the volume to the lowest setting that allows you to hear to prevent feedback squeaking.
- Avoid using hair spray, cosmetics, oils, or other hair and face products that might come into contact with the receiver.
- If the hearing aid does not work:
  - Change the battery.
  - Check the connection between the ear mold and the receiver.
  - Check the on/off switch.
  - Clean the sound hole.
  - Adjust the volume.
  - Take the hearing aid to an authorized service center for repair.

Cochlear implantation may help patients with sensorineural hearing loss. Although a superficial surgical procedure is needed to implant the device, the procedure does not enter the inner ear and thus is not considered a surgical correction for hearing impairment. A small computer converts sound waves into electronic impulses. Electrodes are placed near the internal ear, with the computer attached to the external ear. The electronic impulses then directly stimulate nerve fibers.

Surgical Management. Many surgical interventions are available for patients with specific disorders leading to hearing loss.

Tympanoplasty. Tympanoplasty reconstructs the middle ear to improve conductive hearing loss. The procedures vary from simple reconstruction of the eardrum (**myringoplasty**) to replacement of the ossicles within the middle ear (**ossiculoplasty**).

Preoperative Care. The patient requires specific instructions before surgery. Systemic antibiotics reduce the risk for infection. Teach the patient to follow other measures to decrease the risks for infection, such as avoiding people with upper respiratory infections, getting adequate rest, eating a balanced diet, and drinking adequate amounts of fluid.

Assure the patient that hearing loss immediately after surgery is normal because of canal packing and that hearing will improve when it is removed. Stress that forceful coughing increases middle ear pressure and must be avoided.

Operative Procedures. Surgery is performed only when the middle ear is free of infection. If an infection is present, the graft is more likely to become infected and not heal. Surgery of the eardrum and ossicles requires the use of a microscope and is a delicate procedure. Local anesthesia can be used, although general anesthesia is often used to prevent the patient from moving.

The surgeon can repair the eardrum with many materials, including muscle fascia, a skin graft, and venous tissue. If the ossicles are damaged, more extensive surgery is needed for

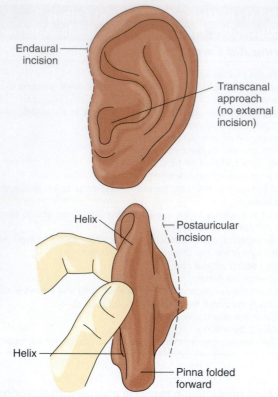

FIG. 48-11 Surgical approaches for repair of the ear and hearing structures.

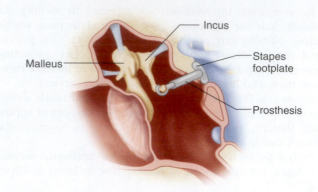

FIG. 48-12 Prosthesis used with stapedectomy. The stapes is removed, leaving the footplate. A metal or plastic prosthesis is connected to the incus and inserted through the hole to act as an artificial stapes.

repair or replacement. The ossicles can be reached in several ways—through the ear canal, with an endaural incision, or by an incision behind the ear (Fig. 48-11).

The surgeon removes diseased tissue and cleans the middle ear cavity. The patient's cartilage or bone, cadaver ossicles, stainless steel wire, or special polymers (Teflon) are used to repair or replace the ossicles.

Postoperative Care. An antiseptic-soaked gauze, such as iodoform gauze (NU GAUZE®), is packed in the ear canal. If a skin incision is used, a dressing is placed over it. Keep the dressing clean and dry, using sterile technique for changes. Keep the patient flat, with the head turned to the side and the operative ear facing up for at least 12 hours after surgery. Give prescribed antibiotics to prevent infection.

Patients often report hearing improvement after removal of the canal packing. Until that time, communicate as with a hearing-impaired patient, directing conversation to the unaffected ear. Instruct the patient in care and activity restrictions (see Chart 48-3).

Stapedectomy. A partial or complete stapedectomy with a prosthesis can correct some hearing loss, especially in patients with hearing loss related to otosclerosis. Although hearing usually improves after primary stapes surgery, some patients redevelop conductive hearing loss after surgery, and revision surgery is needed.

Preoperative Care. To prevent infection, the patient must be free from external otitis at surgery. Teach the patient to follow measures that prevent middle ear or external ear infections (Chart 48-10).

Review with the patient the expected outcomes and possible complications of the surgery. Initially hearing is worse after a

CHART 48-10 Patient and Family Education: Preparing for Self-Management

Prevention of Ear Infection or Trauma

- Do not use small objects, such as cotton-tipped applicators, matches, toothpicks, keys, or hairpins, to clean your external ear canal.
- Wash your external ear and canal daily in the shower or while washing your hair.
- Blow your nose gently.
- Do not block one nostril while blowing your nose.
- Sneeze with your mouth open.
- Wear sound protection around loud or continuous noises.
- Avoid or wear head and ear protection during activities with high risk for head or ear trauma, such as wrestling, boxing, motorcycle riding, and skateboarding.
- Keep the volume on head receivers at the lowest setting that allows you to hear.
- Frequently clean objects that come into contact with your ear (e.g., headphones, telephone receivers).
- Avoid environmental conditions with rapid changes in air pressure.

stapedectomy. The success rate of this procedure is high. However, there is always a risk for failure that might lead to total deafness on the affected side. Other possible complications include vertigo, infection, and facial nerve damage.

Operative Procedures. A stapedectomy is usually performed through the external ear canal with the patient under local anesthesia. After removal of the affected ossicles, a piston-shaped prosthesis is connected between the incus and the footplate (Fig. 48-12). Because the prosthesis vibrates with sound as the stapes did, most patients have restoration of functional hearing.

Postoperative Care. Remind the patient that improvement in hearing may not occur until 6 weeks after surgery. Drugs for pain help reduce discomfort, and antibiotics are used to prevent infection. Teach the patient about the precautions in Chart 48-3.

The surgical procedure is performed in an area where cranial nerves VII, VIII, and X can be damaged by trauma or by swelling after surgery. *Assess for facial nerve damage or muscle weakness. Indications include an asymmetric appearance or drooping of features on the affected side of the face. Ask the patient about changes in facial perception of touch and in taste.* Vertigo, nausea, and vomiting usually occur after surgery because of the nearness to inner ear structures.

Antivertiginous drugs, such as meclizine (Antivert, Bonamine ✦), and antiemetic drugs, such as droperidol (Inapsine), are given. Take care to prevent falls by assisting as needed and instructing the patient to move slowly from sitting to a standing position.

> **! NURSING SAFETY PRIORITY** **QSEN**
> **Action Alert**
>
> Prevent injury by assisting the patient with ambulation during the first 1 to 2 days after stapedectomy. Keep top bed side rails up and remind the patient to move the head slowly to avoid vertigo.

Totally Implanted Devices. Totally implanted devices, such as the Esteem®, can improve bilateral moderate-to-severe sensorineural hearing loss without any visible part (Envoy Medical, 2017). These devices have three totally implanted components: a sound processor, a sensor, and a computer. Vibrations of the eardrum and ossicles are picked up by the sensor and converted to electric signals that are processed by the sound processor. The processor is programmed to the patient's specific hearing pathology. The processor filters out some background noise and amplifies the desired sound signal. The signal is transferred to the computer, which then converts the processed signal into vibrations that are transmitted to the inner ear for auditory SENSORY PERCEPTION.

Patient criteria for totally implantable devices include:
- Bilateral stable sensorineural hearing loss
- Speech discrimination score of 40% or higher
- Healthy tympanic membrane, eustachian tube, and ossicles of the middle ear
- Large enough ear cavity to fit the device components
- At least 30 days' experience with an appropriate hearing aid
- Absence of middle ear, inner ear, or mastoid infection
- Absence of Ménière's disease or recurring vertigo
- Absence of sensitivity to device materials

The devices and the surgery may lead to possible complications, including temporary facial paralysis, changes in taste sensation, and ongoing or new-onset tinnitus. Unlike cochlear implants, the middle ear is entered, and it is considered a surgical procedure. Care before and after surgery is similar to that required with stapedectomy. The cost of the implant and procedure can exceed $40,000, which is not currently covered by Medicare or Medicaid but is covered by a few private insurers.

Maximizing Communication
Planning: Expected Outcomes. The patient with reduced auditory SENSORY PERCEPTION is expected to become proficient in hearing compensation behaviors to maintain or improve communication. Indicators include that the patient consistently demonstrates these behaviors:
- Uses hearing assistive devices
- Uses sign language, lip-reading, closed captioning, or video description (for television viewing)
- Accurately interprets messages
- Uses nonverbal language
- Exchanges messages accurately with others

Interventions. Nursing priorities focus on facilitating communication and reducing anxiety.

Use best practices that are listed in Chart 48-10 for communicating with a hearing-impaired patient. Do not shout at the patient because the sound may be projected at a higher frequency, making him or her less able to understand. Communicate by writing (if he or she is able to see, read, and write) or pictures of familiar phrases and objects. Many television programs are now closed captioned or video described (subtitled). When available, use the assistive devices described in the Nonsurgical Management section under Hearing Loss to increase communication.

Lip-reading and *sign language* can increase communication. In lip-reading, patients are taught special cues to look for when lip-reading and how to understand body language. However, the best lip-reader still misses more than half of what is being said. Because even minimal lip-reading assists hearing, urge patients to wear their eyeglasses when talking with someone to see lip movement.

> **? NCLEX EXAMINATION CHALLENGE 48-4**
> **Safe and Effective Care Environment**
>
> How should the nurse communicate with a client who is deaf?
> A. By having the client read the nurse's lips
> B. By talking more loudly to the client
> C. By using pictures and writing, if the client can see
> D. By talking exclusively with the client's caregivers

Sign languages, such as American Sign Language (ASL), combine speech with hand movements that signify letters, words, and phrases. These languages take time and effort to learn, and many people are unable to use them effectively.

Managing anxiety can increase the effectiveness of communication efforts. One source of anxiety is the possibility of permanent hearing loss. Provide accurate information about the likelihood of hearing returning. When the hearing impairment is likely to be permanent, reassure patients that communication and social interaction can be maintained.

To reduce anxiety and prevent social isolation, help patients use resources and communication to make social contact satisfying. Identify the patient's most satisfying activities and social interactions and determine the effort necessary to continue them. The patient can alter activities to improve satisfaction. Instead of large gatherings, the patient might choose smaller groups. A meal at home with friends can substitute for dining out, or consider requesting a table in a quiet area of a restaurant.

Care Coordination and Transition Management
Lengthy hospitalization is rare for ear and hearing disorders. If surgery is needed and the procedure is completed without complications, it may be performed in an ambulatory surgery center.

Home Care Management. Patients who have persistent vertigo are in danger of falling. Assess the home for potential hazards and to determine whether family or significant others are available to assist with meal preparation and other ADLs. A nurse case manager can coordinate with the home care nurse, the physical therapist, and the occupational therapist to help patients and their families determine how to maintain adequate self-care abilities, maintain a safe environment, decide about assistance needs, and provide needed care.

Self-Management Education. Provide written instructions to the patient and family about how to take drugs and when to return for follow-up care. Teach patients how to instill eardrops (see Chart 48-4) and irrigate the ears (see Chart 48-2) and obtain a return demonstration.

To prevent infection after surgery, instruct patients to follow the suggestions in Chart 48-10. Teach patients who use a hearing aid and their caregivers how to use it effectively.

Health Care Resources. If patients do not have family or friends to help before or after surgery, a referral to a home care agency is needed. Help with meal preparation, cleaning, and personal hygiene can be arranged by the case manager.

Follow-up hearing tests are scheduled when the lesions are well healed, in about 6 to 8 weeks. Audiograms done before and after treatment are compared, and evaluation for further intervention to improve hearing begins. A complication of surgery is continued disability or complete loss of hearing in the affected ear. Surgery is performed first on the ear with the greatest hearing loss. If the surgery does not improve hearing, patients must decide to either attempt surgical correction of the other ear or continue to use an amplification device. When the underlying disorder causing the hearing impairment is progressive, this decision is difficult. Support patients by listening to their concerns and giving additional information when needed.

Costs to the person with a hearing impairment can be extensive. Information and support can come from public and private agencies that specialize in counseling patients with disorders affecting auditory SENSORY PERCEPTION.

◆ *Evaluation: Reflecting*

Evaluate the care of the patient with hearing loss or hearing impairment based on the identified priority patient problems. The expected outcomes include that the patient will:

- Have at least partial improvement of hearing
- Have minimal anxiety
- Use appropriate hearing compensation behaviors
- Communicate effectively in most situations

❓ CLINICAL JUDGMENT CHALLENGE 48-1

Safety; Ethics; Teamwork and Collaboration QSEN

You are caring for an 83-year-old woman who lives on a memory-care unit at an extended-care facility. Despite the confusion associated with dementia, the patient is verbal and ambulatory. Her only other diagnoses include supraventricular tachycardia, which is well controlled with 120 mg of diltiazem (Cardizem CD) daily, and osteoarthritis. She has become progressively hard of hearing, refuses to wear hearing aids, and gets visibly frustrated when she cannot hear others talking to her.

1. How will you promote the patient's independence and autonomy?
2. Although the patient lives in a memory-care unit, which safety concerns do you identify?
3. How would you structure the patient's environment to promote effective communication?
4. Should this patient by given NSAIDs to address osteoarthritis pain? Why or why not?
5. With which other members of the interprofessional team would you consult?

GET READY FOR THE NCLEX® EXAMINATION!

KEY POINTS

Review these Key Points for each NCLEX Examination Client Needs Category.

Safe and Effective Care Environment

- Use Contact Precautions with any patient who has drainage from the ear canal. **QSEN: Safety**
- Use a separate speculum cover for each ear when conducting an otoscopic examination. **QSEN: Safety**
- Slowly and gently introduce the otoscopic speculum into the external ear canal during assessment. **QSEN: Safety**
- Do not perform an otoscopic examination on a confused patient. **QSEN: Safety**
- Use the suggestions presented in the Patient History section to enhance communication with a patient who has an impairment of auditory SENSORY PERCEPTION. **QSEN: Patient-Centered Care**
- Protect the patient with vertigo or dizziness from injury by assisting with ambulation. **QSEN: Safety**
- Follow the guidelines in Chart 48-5 when irrigating the ear canal. **QSEN: Safety**
- Use upper side rails for any patient experiencing dizziness or vertigo. **QSEN: Safety**
- Ensure that all members of the interprofessional team use a medical interpreter as indicated during communication with the patient. **QSEN: Patient-Centered Care**

- Work with members of the interprofessional team to ensure safety and optimal function for the patient with a hearing or balance problem in the community setting. **QSEN: Teamwork and Collaboration**

Health Promotion and Maintenance

- Teach adults the proper way to clean the pinna and external ear canal and how to remove cerumen from the external canal. **QSEN: Evidence-Based Practice**
- Identify adults at risk for hearing impairment as a result of work environment or leisure activities. **QSEN: Safety**
- Encourage all adults, even if they already have a hearing impairment, to use ear protection in loud environments. **QSEN: Safety**
- Inform all adults that smoking increases the risk for development of hearing problems. **QSEN: Evidence-Based Practice**
- Teach patients and caregivers how to properly care for hearing aids. **QSEN: Safety**
- Remind adults who engage in water sports and who are at risk for external otitis to wear earplugs when in the water. **QSEN: Safety**
- Teach patients and caregivers the proper techniques for self-instillation of eardrops and ear irrigation. **QSEN: Evidence-Based Practice**

Psychosocial Integrity

- Allow the patient the opportunity to express fear or anxiety about a change in hearing status. **QSEN: Patient-Centered Care**
- Assess the degree to which hearing problems interfere with the patient's ability to interact with others. **Clinical Judgment**
- Explain all diagnostic and therapeutic procedures, restrictions, and follow-up care to the patient and family. **Ethics**
- Refer patients newly diagnosed with hearing impairment or any chronic ear problem to appropriate local resources and support groups. **QSEN: Teamwork and Collaboration**
- Teach family members ways to communicate with a hearing-impaired patient with and without a hearing aid. **QSEN: Patient-Centered Care**

Physiological Integrity

- Ask the patient about hearing problems in any other members of the family because many hearing problems have a genetic component. **QSEN: Patient-Centered Care**

- Check the hearing of any patient receiving an ototoxic drug for more than 5 days. **QSEN: Evidence-Based Practice**
- Ask the patient about current and past drug use (prescribed, over-the-counter) and check with a pharmacist to evaluate for ototoxicity. **QSEN: Safety**
- Avoid ear canal irrigation if the eardrum is perforated or if the canal contains vegetative matter. **QSEN: Safety**
- Stress the importance of completing an antibiotic regimen for an ear infection. **QSEN: Evidence-Based Practice**
- Teach patients to move the head slowly after ear surgery to prevent dizziness or vertigo. **QSEN: Safety**
- Remind patients having ear surgery that hearing in the affected ear may be reduced immediately after surgery because of packing, swelling, or surgical manipulation. **QSEN: Patient-Centered Care**

SELECTED BIBLIOGRAPHY

Barton, J. (2016). *Benign paroxysmal positional vertigo.* www.uptodate.com.

Envoy Medical. (2017). *Esteem.* http://esteemhearing.com/.

Haynes, D. (2014). *Defining Ménière's disease. Hearing health,* Winter, 34–37.

Henry, J. A., Griest, S., Zaugg, T. L., Thielman, E., Kaelin, C., Galvez, G., et al. (2015). Tinnitus and hearing survey: A screening tool to differentiate bothersome tinnitus from hearing difficulties. *American Journal of Audiology, 24,* 66–77.

Jarvis, C. (2016). *Physical examination & health assessment* (7th ed.). St. Louis: Saunders.

McCance, K., Huether, S., Brashers, V., & Rote, N. (2014). *Pathophysiology: The biologic basis for disease in adults and children* (7th ed.). St. Louis: Mosby.

National Institute on Deafness and Other Communication Disorders (NIDCD). (2016). *Quick statistics about hearing.* http://www.nidcd.nih.gov/health/statistics/Pages/quick.aspx.

Online Mendelian Inheritance in Man (OMIM). (2016). *Gap junction proteins, beta-2; GJB2.* www.omim.org/entry/121011.

Touhy, T., & Jett, K. (2015). *Ebersole and Hess' gerontological nursing healthy aging* (9th ed.). St. Louis: Mosby.

49 | CHAPTER

Assessment of the Musculoskeletal System

Donna D. Ignatavicius

e http://evolve.elsevier.com/Iggy/

PRIORITY AND INTERRELATED CONCEPTS

The priority concepts for this chapter are:
- MOBILITY
- COMFORT

The interrelated concept for this chapter is SENSORY PERCEPTION.

LEARNING OUTCOMES

Safe and Effective Care Environment

1. Collaborate with the physical and occupational therapists to perform a complete musculoskeletal assessment, including functional status, as needed.

Health Promotion and Maintenance

2. Identify evidence-based health promotion activities to help prevent musculoskeletal health problems or trauma.
3. Incorporate knowledge of common physiologic aging changes associated with aging to accurately interpret musculoskeletal assessment findings and plan interventions to ensure patient safety.

Psychosocial Integrity

4. Identify potential patient reactions to musculoskeletal health problems or injuries.

Physiological Integrity

5. Apply knowledge of anatomy and physiology for a focused musculoskeletal assessment to assess patients for MOBILITY, COMFORT, and SENSORY PERCEPTION.
6. Use clinical judgment to interpret assessment findings in a patient with a musculoskeletal health problem.
7. Interpret selected laboratory tests for a patient with a musculoskeletal health problem.
8. Provide patient-centered health teaching for preparation and follow-up care for selected musculoskeletal diagnostic testing.

The musculoskeletal system is the second largest body system. It includes the bones, joints, and skeletal muscles, as well as the supporting structures needed to move them. MOBILITY is a basic human need that is essential for performing ADLs. When a patient cannot move to perform ADLs or other daily routines, self-esteem and a sense of self-worth can be diminished. Chapter 2 reviews this concept in detail.

Disease, surgery, and trauma can affect one or more parts of the musculoskeletal system, often leading to decreased mobility. When MOBILITY is impaired for a long time, other body systems can be affected. For example, prolonged immobility can lead to skin breakdown, constipation, and thrombus formation. If nerves are damaged by trauma or disease, patients may also have both impaired SENSORY PERCEPTION

TABLE 49-1   Musculoskeletal Differences in Selected Ethnic Groups

GROUP	MUSCULOSKELETAL DIFFERENCES
African Americans	Greater bone density than Europeans, Asians, and Hispanics Accounts for decreased incidence of osteoporosis
Amish	Greater incidence of dwarfism than in other populations
Chinese Americans	Bones shorter and smaller with less bone density Increased incidence of osteoporosis
Egyptian Americans	Shorter in stature than Euro-Americans and African Americans
Filipino/Vietnamese	Short in stature; adult height about 5 feet
Irish Americans	Taller and broader than other Euro-Americans Less bone density than African Americans
Navajo American Indians	Taller and thinner than other American Indians

and COMFORT (see Chapter 2 for a review of these health concepts).

ANATOMY AND PHYSIOLOGY REVIEW

Skeletal System

The skeletal system consists of 206 bones and multiple joints. The growth and development of these structures occur during childhood and adolescence and are not discussed in this text. Common physical skeletal differences among selected racial/ethnic groups are listed in Table 49-1.

Bones

Types and Structure. Bone can be classified in two ways: by shape and by structure. **Long bones,** such as the femur, are cylindric with rounded ends and often bear weight. **Short bones,** such as the phalanges, are small and bear little or no weight. **Flat bones,** such as the scapula, protect vital organs and often contain blood-forming cells. Bones that have unique shapes are known as **irregular bones**. The carpal bones in the wrist and the small bones in the inner ear are examples of **irregular bones**. The sesamoid bone is the least common type and develops within a tendon; the patella is a typical example.

The second way bone is classified is by *structure* or composition. As shown in Fig. 49-1, the outer layer of bone, or cortex, is composed of dense, compact bone tissue. The inner layer, in the medulla, contains spongy, cancellous tissue. Almost every bone has both tissue types but in varying quantities. The long bone typically has a shaft, or diaphysis, and two knoblike ends, or epiphyses.

The structural unit of the cortical compact bone is the haversian system, which is detailed in Fig. 49-1. The haversian system is a complex canal network containing microscopic blood vessels that supply nutrients and oxygen to bone and lacunae, which are small cavities that house **osteocytes** (bone cells). The canals run vertically within the hard cortical bone tissue.

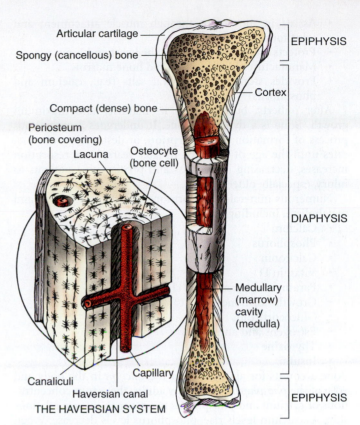

FIG. 49-1 Structure of a typical long bone. The cortex, or outer layer, is composed of dense, compact tissue. The microscopic structure of this compact cortical tissue is the haversian system.

The softer **cancellous** tissue contains large spaces, or trabeculae, which are filled with red and yellow marrow. **Hematopoiesis** (production of blood cells) occurs in the red marrow. The yellow marrow contains fat cells, which can be dislodged and enter the bloodstream to cause fat embolism syndrome (FES), a life-threatening complication. Volkmann's canals connect bone marrow vessels with the haversian system and periosteum, the outermost covering of the bone. In the deepest layer of the periosteum are osteogenic cells, which later differentiate into **osteoblasts** (bone-forming cells) and **osteoclasts** (bone-destroying cells).

Bone also contains a matrix consisting chiefly of collagen, mucopolysaccharides, and lipids. Deposits of inorganic calcium salts (carbonate and phosphate) in the matrix provide bone hardness.

Bone is a very vascular tissue. Its estimated total blood flow is between 200 and 400 mL/min. Each bone has a main nutrient artery, which enters near the middle of the shaft and branches into ascending and descending vessels. These vessels supply the cortex, the marrow, and the haversian system. Very few nerve fibers are connected to bone. Sympathetic nerve fibers control dilation of blood vessels. Sensory nerve fibers transmit pain signals experienced by patients who have primary lesions of the bone, such as bone tumors.

Function. The skeletal system:
- Provides a framework for the body and allows the body to be weight bearing, or upright
- Supports the surrounding tissues (e.g., muscle and tendons)

• Assists in movement through muscle attachment and joint formation
• Protects vital organs, such as the heart and lungs
• Manufactures blood cells in red bone marrow
• Provides storage for mineral salts (e.g., calcium and phosphorus)

After puberty, bone reaches its maturity and maximum growth. Bone is a dynamic tissue. It undergoes a continuous process of formation and resorption, or destruction, at equal rates until the age of 35 years. In later years, bone resorption increases, decreasing bone mass and predisposing patients to injury, especially older women.

Numerous minerals and hormones affect bone growth and metabolism, including:
• Calcium
• Phosphorus
• Calcitonin
• Vitamin D
• Parathyroid hormone (PTH)
• Growth hormone
• Glucocorticoids
• Estrogens and androgens
• Thyroxine
• Insulin

Bone accounts for about 99% of the *calcium* in the body and 90% of the *phosphorus*. In healthy adults, the serum concentrations of calcium and phosphorus maintain an inverse relationship. As calcium levels rise, phosphorus levels decrease. When serum levels are altered, calcitonin and PTH work to maintain equilibrium. If the calcium in the blood is decreased, the bone, which stores calcium, releases calcium into the bloodstream in response to PTH stimulation.

Calcitonin is produced by the thyroid gland and *decreases* the serum calcium concentration if it is increased above its normal level. Calcitonin inhibits bone resorption and increases renal excretion of calcium and phosphorus as needed to maintain balance in the body.

Vitamin D and its metabolites are produced in the body and transported in the blood to promote the absorption of calcium and phosphorus from the small intestine. They also seem to enhance PTH activity to release calcium from the bone. A decrease in the body's vitamin D level can result in osteomalacia (softening of bone) in the adult. Vitamin D metabolism and osteomalacia are described in Chapter 50.

When serum calcium levels are lowered, *parathyroid hormone* (PTH, or parathormone) secretion increases and stimulates bone to promote osteoclastic activity and *release* calcium to the blood. PTH reduces the renal excretion of calcium and facilitates its absorption from the intestine. If serum calcium levels increase, PTH secretion diminishes to preserve the bone calcium supply. This process is an example of the feedback loop system of the endocrine system.

Growth hormone secreted by the anterior lobe of the pituitary gland is responsible for increasing bone length and determining the amount of bone matrix formed before puberty. During childhood, an increased secretion results in gigantism, and a decreased secretion results in dwarfism. In the adult, an increase causes acromegaly, which is characterized by bone and soft-tissue deformities (see Chapter 62).

Adrenal glucocorticoids regulate protein metabolism, either increasing or decreasing catabolism to reduce or intensify the organic matrix of bone. They also aid in regulating intestinal calcium and phosphorus absorption.

Estrogens stimulate osteoblastic (bone-building) activity and inhibit PTH. When estrogen levels decline at menopause, women are susceptible to low serum calcium levels with increased bone loss (osteoporosis). *Androgens,* such as testosterone in men, promote anabolism (body tissue building) and increase bone mass.

Thyroxine is one of the principal hormones secreted by the thyroid gland. Its primary function is to increase the rate of protein synthesis in all types of tissue, including bone. *Insulin* works together with growth hormone to build and maintain healthy bone tissue.

Joints

A joint is a space in which two or more bones come together. This is also referred to as *articulation* of the joint. The major function of a joint is to provide movement and flexibility in the body.

There are three types of joints in the body:
• Synarthrodial, or completely immovable, joints (e.g., in the cranium)
• Amphiarthrodial, or slightly movable, joints (e.g., in the pelvis)
• Diarthrodial (synovial), or freely movable, joints (e.g., the elbow and knee)

Although any of these joints can be affected by disease or injury, the synovial joints are most commonly involved, as discussed in Chapter 18.

The diarthrodial, or synovial, joint is the most common type of joint in the body. Synovial joints are the only type lined with synovium, a membrane that secretes synovial fluid for lubrication and shock absorption. As shown in Fig. 49-2, the synovium lines the internal portion of the joint capsule but does not normally extend onto the surface of the cartilage at the spongy bone ends. Articular cartilage consists of a collagen fiber matrix

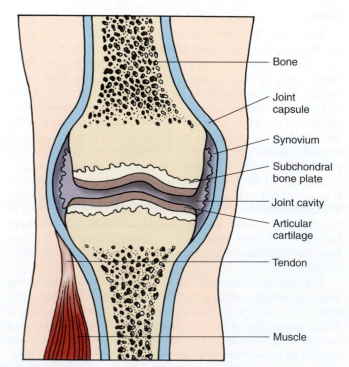

FIG. 49-2 Structure of a synovial joint. Synovium lines the joint capsule but does not extend into the articular cartilage.

Bone
Joint capsule
Synovium
Subchondral bone plate
Joint cavity
Articular cartilage
Tendon
Muscle

impregnated with a complex ground substance. Patients with inflammatory types of arthritis often have synovitis (synovial inflammation) and breakdown of the cartilage. Bursae, small sacs lined with synovial membrane, are located at joints and bony prominences to prevent friction between bone and structures adjacent to bone. These structures can also become inflamed, causing bursitis.

Synovial joints are described by their anatomic structures. *Ball-and-socket* joints (shoulder, hip) permit movement in any direction. *Hinge* joints (elbow) allow motion in one plane—flexion and extension. The knee is often classified as a hinge joint, but it rotates slightly, as well as flexes and extends. It is best described as a *condylar* type of synovial joint. The gliding movement of the wrist is characteristic of the *biaxial* joint. *Pivot* joints permit rotation only, as in the radioulnar area.

Muscular System

There are three types of muscle in the body: smooth muscle, cardiac muscle, and skeletal muscle. Smooth, or nonstriated, involuntary muscle is responsible for contractions of organs and blood vessels and is controlled by the autonomic nervous system. Cardiac or striated involuntary muscle is also controlled by the autonomic nervous system. The smooth and cardiac muscles are discussed with the body systems to which they belong in the assessment chapters.

In contrast to smooth and cardiac muscle, skeletal muscle is striated voluntary muscle controlled by the central and peripheral nervous systems. The junction of a peripheral motor nerve and the muscle cells that it supplies is sometimes referred to as a motor end plate. Muscle fibers are held in place by connective tissue in bundles, or *fasciculi*. The entire muscle is surrounded by dense fibrous tissue, or fascia, which contains the muscle's blood, lymph, and nerve supply.

The main function of skeletal muscle is *movement* of the body and its parts. When bones, joints, and supporting structures are adversely affected by injury or disease, the adjacent muscle tissue is often involved, limiting MOBILITY. During the aging process, muscle fibers decrease in size and number, even in well-conditioned adults. Atrophy results when muscles are not regularly exercised, and they deteriorate from disuse.

Supporting structures for the muscular system are very susceptible to injury. They include tendons (bands of tough, fibrous tissue that attach muscles to bones) and ligaments, which attach bones to other bones at joints.

Musculoskeletal Changes Associated With Aging

Osteopenia, or decreased bone density (bone loss), occurs as one ages. Many older adults, especially white, thin women, have severe osteopenia, a disease called *osteoporosis*. This condition causes postural and gait changes and predisposes the person to fractures. Chapter 50 discusses this health problem in detail.

Synovial joint cartilage can become less elastic and compressible as a person ages. As a result of these cartilage changes and continued use of joints, the joint cartilage becomes damaged, leading to osteoarthritis (OA). Genetic defects in cartilage may also contribute to joint disease. The most common joints affected are the weight-bearing joints of the hip, knee, and cervical and lumbar spine, but joints in the shoulder and upper extremity, feet, and hands also can be affected. Refer to Chapter 18 for a complete discussion of OA.

As one ages, muscle tissue atrophies. Increased activity and exercise can slow the progression of atrophy and restore muscle strength. Musculoskeletal changes cause decreased coordination, loss of muscle strength, gait changes, and a risk for falls with injury. (See Chapter 3 for discussion on fall prevention.) Chart 49-1 lists the major anatomic and physiologic changes and related nursing interventions to ensure patient safety.

Health Promotion and Maintenance

Many health problems of the musculoskeletal system can be prevented through health promotion strategies and avoidance of risky lifestyle behaviors. For example, women can slow the process of bone loss by taking vitamin D and calcium supplements and increasing these nutrients in their diet. Weight-bearing activities such as walking can reduce risk factors for osteoporosis and maintain muscle strength (McCance et al., 2014).

Accidents, illnesses, lifestyle, and substance abuse can contribute to the occurrence of musculoskeletal injury. Young men are at the greatest risk for trauma related to motor vehicle crashes. Older adults are at the greatest risk for falls that result in fractures and soft-tissue injury. High-impact sports, such as excessive jogging or running, can cause musculoskeletal injury

---

CHART 49-1 Nursing Focus on the Older Adult

Changes in the Musculoskeletal System Related to Aging

PHYSIOLOGIC CHANGE	NURSING INTERVENTIONS	RATIONALES
Decreased bone density	Teach safety tips to prevent falls. Reinforce need to exercise, especially weight-bearing exercise.	Porous bones are more likely to fracture. Exercise slows bone loss.
Increased bone prominence	Prevent pressure on bone prominences.	There is less soft tissue to prevent skin breakdown.
Kyphotic posture: widened gait, shift in the center of gravity	Teach proper body mechanics; instruct the patient to sit in supportive chairs with arms.	Correction of posture problems prevents further deformity; the patient should have support for bony structures.
Cartilage degeneration (arthritis)	Provide moist heat, such as a shower or warm, moist compresses.	Moist heat increases blood flow to the area.
Decreased range of motion (ROM)	Assess the patient's ability to perform ADLs and mobility.	The patient may need assistance with self-care skills.
Muscle atrophy, decreased strength	Teach isometric exercises.	Exercises increase muscle strength.
Slowed movement	Do not rush the person; be patient.	The patient may become frustrated if hurried.

to soft tissues and bone. Tobacco use slows the healing of musculoskeletal injuries. Excessive alcohol intake can decrease vitamins and nutrients that the person needs for bone and muscle tissue growth. Develop a patient-centered health promotion plan for each patient to help promote bone health and prevent musculoskeletal injury. Additional health promotion strategies can be found in other chapters of this unit related to specific health problems of the musculoskeletal system.

 NCLEX EXAMINATION CHALLENGE 49-1

Health Promotion and Maintenance

A nurse is performing a musculoskeletal assessment on an older adult living independently. What normal physiologic changes of aging does the nurse expect? **Select all that apply.**
A. Muscle atrophy
B. Slowed movement
C. Scoliosis
D. Arthritis
E. Widened gait

ASSESSMENT: NOTICING AND INTERPRETING

Patient History

In the assessment of a patient with an actual or potential musculoskeletal problem, a detailed and accurate history is helpful in identifying priority problems and nursing interventions. The history reveals information about the patient that can direct the physical assessment.

When taking a personal health history, question the patient about any traumatic injuries and sports activities, no matter when they occurred. An injury to the lumbar spine 30 years ago may have caused a patient's current low back pain. A motor vehicle crash or sports injury can cause osteoarthritis years after the event.

Previous or current illness or disease may affect musculoskeletal status. For example, a patient with diabetes who is treated for a foot ulcer is at high risk for acute or chronic osteomyelitis (bone infection). In addition, diabetes slows the healing process. Ask the patient about any previous hospitalizations and illnesses or complications. Inquire about his or her ability to perform ADLs independently or if assistive/adaptive devices are used.

Current lifestyle also contributes to musculoskeletal health. When assessing a patient with a possible musculoskeletal alteration, inquire about occupation or work life. A person's occupation can cause or contribute to an injury. For instance, fractures are not uncommon in patients whose jobs require manual labor, such as housekeepers, mechanics, and industrial workers. Certain occupations, such as computer-related jobs, may predispose a person to carpal tunnel syndrome (entrapment of the median nerve in the wrist) or neck pain.

Ask about allergies, particularly allergy to dairy products, and previous and current use of drugs (prescribed, over-the-counter, and illicit). Allergy to dairy products could cause decreased calcium intake. Some drugs, such as steroids, can negatively affect calcium metabolism and promote bone loss. Other drugs may be taken to relieve musculoskeletal pain. Inquire about herbs, vitamin and mineral supplements, or biologic compounds that may be used for arthritis and other

musculoskeletal problems, such as glucosamine and chondroitin. Complementary and integrative therapies are commonly used by patients with various types of arthritis and **arthralgias** (joint aching).

Nutrition History

A brief review of the patient's nutrition history helps determine any risks for inadequate nutrient intake. For example, most people, especially women, do not get enough calcium in their diet. Determine if the patient has had a significant weight gain or loss.

Ask the patient to recall a typical day of food intake to help identify deficiencies and excesses in the diet. Lactose intolerance is a common problem that can cause inadequate calcium intake. People who cannot afford to buy food are especially at risk for undernutrition. Some older adults and others are not financially able to buy the proper foods for adequate nutrition.

Inadequate protein or insufficient vitamin C or D in the diet slows bone and tissue healing. Obesity places excess stress and strain on bones and joints, with resulting trauma to joint cartilage. In addition, obesity inhibits MOBILITY in patients with musculoskeletal problems, which predisposes them to complications such as respiratory and circulatory problems. People with eating disorders such as anorexia nervosa and bulimia nervosa are also at risk for osteoporosis related to decreased intake of calcium and vitamin D.

Family History and Genetic Risk

Obtaining a family history helps to identify disorders that have a familial or genetic tendency. For example, osteoporosis (age-related bone loss) and gout often occur in several generations of a family. Positive family history of these types of disorders can increase risks to the patient. Chapters 18 and 50 provide a more complete description of musculoskeletal problems that have strong genetic links.

Current Health Problems

The most common reports of people with a musculoskeletal problem are impaired COMFORT and weakness, either of which can impair MOBILITY. Collect data pertinent to the patient's presenting health problem:

- Date and time of onset
- Factors that cause or exacerbate (worsen) the problem
- Course of the problem (e.g., intermittent or continuous)
- Signs and symptoms (as expressed by the patient) and the pattern of their occurrence
- Measures that improve signs and symptoms (e.g., heat, ice)

Assessment of COMFORT can present many challenges. Pain can be related to bone, muscle, or joint problems. It may be described as acute or chronic, depending on the onset and duration. Pain with movement could indicate a fracture and/or muscle or joint injury. Assess the intensity of pain by using a pain scale and asking the patient to rate the level that he or she is experiencing. Quality of pain may be described as dull, burning, aching, or stabbing. Determine the location of pain and areas to which it radiates. With any assessment, it is always best if the patient describes the pain in his or her own words and points to its location, if possible. Chapter 4 describes acute and chronic pain in detail.

Weakness may be related to individual muscles or muscle groups. Determine if weakness occurs in proximal or distal muscles or muscle groups. Proximal weakness (near trunk of body) may indicate **myopathy** (a problem in muscle tissue), whereas distal weakness (in extremities) may indicate **neuropathy** (a problem in nerve tissue). Muscle weakness in the lower extremities may increase the risk for falls and injury. Weakness in the upper extremities may interfere with MOBILITY and ADL functional ability.

Assessment of the Skeletal System

Although bones, joints, and muscles are usually assessed simultaneously in a head-to-toe approach, each subsystem is described separately for emphasis and understanding. For physical assessment of the musculoskeletal system, use inspection, palpation, and range of motion (ROM). A general assessment is described in this chapter. More specific assessment techniques are discussed in the musculoskeletal problem chapters in this unit.

General Inspection

Observe the patient's posture, gait, and general mobility for gross deformities and impairment. Note unusual findings and coordinate with the physical or occupational therapist for an in-depth physical assessment.

Posture and Gait. Posture includes the person's body build and alignment when standing and walking. Assess the curvature of the spine and the length, shape, and symmetry of extremities. Fig. 49-3 illustrates several common spinal deformities. **Lordosis** is a common finding in adults who have abdominal obesity. During screening for **scoliosis**, ask the patient to flex forward from the hips and inspect for a lateral curve in the spine.

Inspect muscle mass for size and symmetry.

Most patients with musculoskeletal problems eventually have a problem with *gait*. The nurse or therapist evaluates the patient's balance, steadiness, and ease and length of stride. Any limp or other asymmetric leg movement or deformity is noted. An abnormality in the stance phase of gait is called an **antalgic** gait. When part of one leg is painful, the patient shortens the stance phase on the affected side. An abnormality in the swing phase is called a **lurch**. This abnormal gait occurs when the muscles in the buttocks and/or legs are too weak to allow the person to change weight from one foot to the other. In this case,

the shoulders are moved either side-to-side or front-to-back for help in shifting the weight from one leg to the other. Some patients, such as those with chronic hip pain and muscle atrophy from arthritic disorders, have a combination of an antalgic gait and lurch.

If the extremities are affected by a musculoskeletal problem, assess arms or legs at the same time for side-to-side comparisons. For example, inspect and palpate both shoulders for size, swelling, deformity, poor alignment, tenderness or pain, and MOBILITY. A shoulder injury may prevent the patient from combing his or her hair with the affected arm, but severe arthritis may inhibit movement in both arms. Assess the elbows and wrists in a similar way.

Because the hand has multiple joints in a single digit, assessment of hand function is perhaps the most critical part of the examination. If the hands are affected, inspect and palpate the metacarpophalangeal (MCP), proximal interphalangeal (PIP), and distal interphalangeal (DIP) joints (Fig. 49-4). The same digits are compared on the right and left hands. Determine the range of motion (ROM) for each joint by observing active movement. If movement is not possible, evaluate passive motion. For a quick and easy assessment of ROM, ask the patient to make a fist and then appose each finger to the thumb. If he or she can perform these maneuvers, ROM of the hand is not seriously restricted.

Mobility and Functional Assessment. In collaboration with the physical or occupational therapist, assess the patient's need for ambulatory devices, such as canes and walkers, during transfer from bed to chair and while walking and climbing stairs. Observe his or her ability to perform ADLs, such as

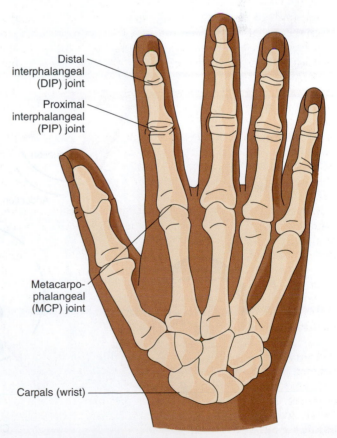

FIG. 49-4 Small joints of the hand.

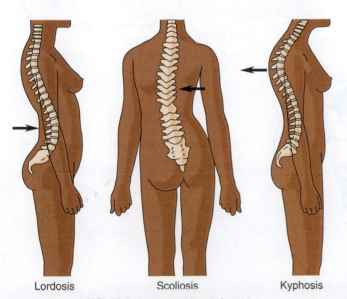

Lordosis   Scoliosis   Kyphosis

FIG. 49-3 Common spinal deformities.

dressing and bathing. Pain and deformity may limit physical MOBILITY and function. Coordinate with the physical and occupational therapists to assess the patient's functional status. A discussion of functional assessment is found in Chapter 6.

Assess major bones, joints, and muscles by inspection, palpation, and determination of ROM. Pay special attention to areas that are affected or may be affected, according to the patient's history or current problem.

A goniometer is a tool that may be used by rehabilitation therapists or nurses to provide an exact measurement of flexion and extension or joint ROM. Active range of motion (AROM) can be evaluated by asking the patient to move each joint through the ROM himself or herself. If the patient cannot actively move a joint through ROM, ask him or her to relax the muscles in the extremity. Hold the part with one hand above and one hand below the joint to be evaluated and allow passive range of motion (PROM) to evaluate joint MOBILITY. Movements shown in Fig. 49-5 may be used to evaluate active and passive ROM. Circumduction is a movement that can also be evaluated in the shoulder by having the patient move the arm in circles from the shoulder joint. As long as the patient can function to meet personal needs, a limitation in ROM may not be significant. For each anatomic location, observe the skin for color, elasticity, and lesions that may relate to musculoskeletal dysfunction. For instance, redness or warmth may indicate an inflammatory process and/or pressure injury to skin.

Evaluation of the hip joint relies primarily on determination of its degree of mobility because the joint is deep and difficult to inspect or palpate. *The patient with hip joint pain usually experiences it in the groin or has pain that radiates to the knee.* The knee is readily accessible for physical assessment, particularly when the patient is sitting and the knee is flexed. Fluid accumulation, or effusion, is easily detected in the knee joint. Limitations in movement with accompanying pain are common findings. The knees may be poorly aligned, as in genu valgum ("knock-knee") or genu varum ("bowlegged") deformities.

The ankles and feet are often neglected in the physical examination. However, they contain multiple bones and joints that can be affected by disease and injury. Observe and palpate each joint and test for ROM if feet are affected by musculoskeletal problems.

Neurovascular Assessment

While completing a physical assessment of the musculoskeletal system, perform an assessment of peripheral vascular and nerve integrity. Beginning with the injured side, always compare one extremity with the other.

> **! NURSING SAFETY PRIORITY** QSEN
>
> ***Action Alert***
>
> Perform a complete **neurovascular assessment** (also called a *circ check*), which includes palpation of pulses in the extremities below the level of injury and assessment of sensation, movement, color, temperature, and pain in the injured part. If pulses are not palpable, use a Doppler to find pulses in the extremities. See Chart 51-3 for more details about neurovascular assessment.

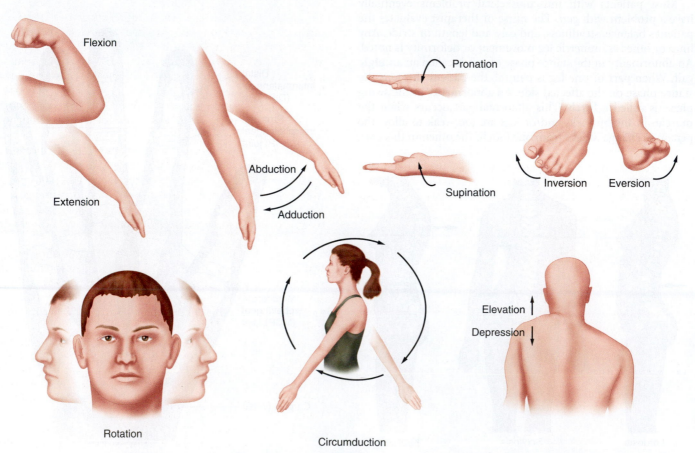

FIG. 49-5 Movements of the skeletal muscles.

Assessment of the Muscular System

During the skeletal assessment, notice the size, shape, tone, and strength of major skeletal muscles. The circumference of each muscle may be measured and compared for symmetry for an estimation of muscle mass if abnormalities are observed.

Ask the patient to demonstrate muscle strength. Apply resistance by holding the extremity and asking the patient to move against resistance. As an option, place your hands on the patient's upper arms and ask him or her to try to raise the arms. Although movement against resistance is not easily quantified, several scales used by nurses and therapists are available for grading the patient's strength. A commonly used scale is shown in Table 49-2.

Psychosocial Assessment

The data from the history and physical assessment provide clues for anticipating psychosocial problems. For instance, prolonged absence from employment or permanent disability may cause job or career loss. Further stress may be experienced if chronic pain continues and the patient cannot cope with numerous stressors. Anxiety and depression are common when patients have chronic pain. Deformities resulting from musculoskeletal disease or injury, such as an amputation, can affect a person's body image and self-concept. Help the patient identify support systems and coping mechanisms that may be useful if he or she has long-term musculoskeletal health problems. Encourage him or her to verbalize feelings related to loss and body image changes. Refer the patient and family for psychological or spiritual counseling if needed and if it is culturally appropriate.

Diagnostic Assessment

Laboratory Assessment

Chart 49-2 lists the common laboratory tests used in assessing patients with musculoskeletal disorders. There is no special patient preparation or follow-up care for any of these tests. Teach the patient about the purpose of the test and the procedure that can be expected. Additional tests performed for patients with connective tissue diseases, such as rheumatoid arthritis, are described in Chapter 18.

Disorders of bone and the parathyroid gland are often reflected in an alteration of the serum calcium or phosphorus level. Therefore these electrolytes, especially calcium, are monitored. A decrease in serum calcium could indicate bone density loss.

TABLE 49-2	Common Scale for Grading Muscle Strength
RATING	**DESCRIPTION**
5	Normal: ROM unimpaired against gravity with full resistance
4	Good: can complete ROM against gravity with some resistance
3	Fair: can complete ROM against gravity
2	Poor: can complete ROM with gravity eliminated
1	Trace: no joint motion and slight evidence of muscle contractility
0	Zero: no evidence of muscle contractility

ROM, Range of motion.

Alkaline phosphatase (ALP) is an enzyme normally present in blood. The concentration of ALP increases with bone or liver damage. In metabolic bone disease and bone cancer, the enzyme concentration rises in proportion to the osteoblastic activity, which indicates bone formation. The level of ALP is normally slightly increased in older adults (Pagana et al., 2017).

The major *muscle enzymes* affected in skeletal muscle disease or injuries are:

- Creatine kinase (CK-MM)
- Aspartate aminotransferase (AST)
- Aldolase (ALD)
- Lactic dehydrogenase (LDH)

As a result of damage, the muscle tissue releases additional amounts of these enzymes, which increases serum levels.

Imaging Assessment

The skeleton is very visible on *standard x-rays.* Anteroposterior and lateral projections are the initial screening views used most often. Other approaches, such as oblique or stress views, depend on the part of the skeleton to be evaluated and the reason for the x-ray.

Radiography. Bone density, alignment, swelling, and intactness can be seen on x-ray. The conditions of joints can be determined, including the size of the joint space, the smoothness of articular cartilage, and synovial swelling. Soft-tissue involvement may be evident but not clearly differentiated.

Inform the patient that the x-ray table is hard and cold, and instruct him or her to remain still during the filming process. Coordinate with the radiology department or clinic to keep older adults and those at risk for hypothermia as warm as possible (e.g., by using blankets).

An **arthrogram** is an x-ray study of a joint after contrast medium (air or solution) has been injected to enhance its visualization. Double-contrast arthrography, which uses both air and solution, may be performed when a traumatic injury is suspected. The physician can often determine bone chips, torn ligaments, or other loose bodies within the joint. This test is not used commonly because of newer advances in diagnostic imaging. Most joints are now studied by MRI and magnetic resonance (MR) arthrography.

CT has gained wide acceptance for detecting musculoskeletal problems, particularly those of the vertebral column and joints. The scanned images can be used to create additional images from other angles or to create three-dimensional images and view complex structures from any position. The nurse or radiology technologist should ask the patient about iodine-based contrast allergies.

Nuclear Scans. The **bone scan** is a radionuclide test in which radioactive material is injected for viewing the entire skeleton. It may be used primarily to detect tumors, arthritis, osteomyelitis, osteoporosis, vertebral compression fractures, and unexplained bone pain. Bone scans are used less commonly today as more sophisticated MRI equipment becomes more available. However, it may be very useful for detecting hairline fractures in patients with unexplained bone pain and diffuse metastatic bone disease.

The **gallium** and **thallium scans** are similar to the bone scan but are more specific and sensitive in detecting bone problems. Gallium citrate (^{67}Ga) is the radioisotope most commonly used. This substance also migrates to brain, liver, and breast tissue and therefore is used in examination of these structures when disease is suspected.

> **CHART 49-2 Laboratory Profile**
>
> *Musculoskeletal Assessment*
>
> | TEST | NORMAL RANGE FOR ADULTS | SIGNIFICANCE OF ABNORMAL FINDINGS |
> |---|---|---|
> | Serum calcium | 9.0-10.5 mg/dL (2.25-2.75 mmol/L)
 Older adults: decreased | *Hypercalcemia* (increased calcium)
 • Metastatic cancers of the bone
 • Paget's disease
 • Bone fractures in healing stage
 Hypocalcemia (decreased calcium)
 • Osteoporosis
 • Osteomalacia |
> | Serum phosphorus (phosphate) | 3.0-4.5 mg/dL (0.97-1.45 mmol/L)
 Older adults: decreased | *Hyperphosphatemia* (increased phosphorus)
 • Bone fractures in healing stage
 • Bone tumors
 • Acromegaly
 Hypophosphatemia (decreased phosphorus)
 • Osteomalacia |
> | Alkaline phosphatase (ALP) | 30-120 units/L
 Older adults: slightly increased | *Elevations* may indicate:
 • Metastatic cancers of the bone or liver
 • Paget's disease
 • Osteomalacia |
> | Serum muscle enzymes
 Creatine kinase (CK-MM) | Total CK:
 Men: 55-170 units/L
 Women: 30-135 units/L
 CK-MM: 96%-100% | *Elevations* may indicate:
 • Muscle trauma
 • Progressive muscular dystrophy
 • Effects of electromyography |
> | Lactic dehydrogenase (LDH) | Total LDH: 100-190 units/L
 LDH_1: 17%-27%
 LDH_2: 27%-37%
 LDH_3: 18%-25%
 LDH_4: 3%-8%
 LDH_5: 0%-5% | *Elevations* may indicate:
 • Skeletal muscle necrosis
 • Extensive cancer
 • Progressive muscular dystrophy |
> | Aspartate aminotransferase (AST) | 0-35 units/L
 Older adults: slightly increased | *Elevations* may indicate:
 • Skeletal muscle trauma
 • Progressive muscular dystrophy |
> | Aldolase (ALD) | 3.0-8.2 units/dL | *Elevations* may indicate:
 • Polymyositis and dermatomyositis
 • Muscular dystrophy |

For patients with osteosarcoma, thallium (^{201}Tl) is better than gallium or technetium for diagnosing the extent of the disease. Thallium has traditionally been used for the diagnosis of myocardial infarctions but can be used for additional evaluation of cancers of the bone.

Because bone takes up gallium slowly, the nuclear medicine physician or technician administers the isotope 4 to 6 hours before scanning. Other tests that require contrast media or other isotopes cannot be given during this time.

Instruct the patient that the radioactive material poses no threat because it readily deteriorates in the body. Because gallium is excreted through the intestinal tract, it tends to collect in feces after the scanning procedure.

Depending on the tissue to be examined, the patient is taken to the nuclear medicine department 4 to 6 hours after injection. The procedure takes 30 to 60 minutes, during which time the patient must lie still for accurate test results to be achieved. The scan may be repeated at 24, 48, and/or 72 hours. Mild sedation may be necessary to facilitate relaxation and cooperation during the procedure for confused older adults or those in severe pain.

No special care is required after the test. The radioisotope is excreted in stool and urine, but no precautions are taken in handling the excreta. Remind the patient to push fluids to facilitate urinary excretion.

Magnetic Resonance Imaging. MRI, with or without the use of contrast media, is commonly used to diagnose musculoskeletal disorders. It is more accurate than CT and myelography for many spinal and knee problems. MRI is most appropriate for joints, soft tissue, and bony tumors that involve soft tissue. CT is still the test of choice for injuries or pathology that involves only bone.

The image is produced through the interaction of magnetic fields, radio waves, and atomic nuclei showing hydrogen density. Simply put, the radio waves "bounce" off the body tissues being examined. Because each tissue has its own density, the computer image clearly distinguishes normal and abnormal tissues. For some tissues, the cross-sectional image is better than that produced by radiography or CT. The lack of hydrogen ions in cortical bone makes it easily distinguishable from soft tissues. The test is particularly useful in identifying problems with muscles, tendons, and ligaments.

Ensure that the patient removes all metal objects and checks for clothing zippers and metal fasteners. Although joint implants made of titanium or stainless steel are usually safe, depending on the age of the MRI equipment, pacemakers, stents, and surgical clips usually are not. Large facilities and those focused on sports medicine may have orthopedic-type MRI machines that are open design and vertically oriented (upright) to make the examination more comfortable. These machines are most useful for viewing extremity injuries but cannot be used for abdomen, brain, or spine studies because of their size and shape. Chart 49-3 lists questions that the nurse or technician should consider in preparing the patient for MRI.

MR arthrography combines arthrography and MRI. It is particularly useful for diagnosing problems of the shoulder and the type and degree of rotator cuff tears. The patient's shoulder is injected with gadolinium contrast medium under fluoroscopy. Then the patient is taken for an MRI, where the shoulder is examined.

Ultrasonography. Sound waves produce an image of the tissue in ultrasonography. An ultrasound procedure may be used to view:

- Soft-tissue disorders, such as masses and fluid accumulation
- Traumatic joint injuries
- Osteomyelitis
- Surgical hardware placement

A jellylike substance applied to the skin over the site to be examined promotes the movement of a metal probe. No special preparation or post-test care is necessary. A quantitative ultrasound (QUS) may be done for determining fractures or bone density. Bone-density testing is discussed in Chapter 50.

Other Diagnostic Assessment

Biopsies. In a **bone biopsy**, the physician extracts a specimen of the bone tissue for microscopic examination. This invasive test may confirm the presence of infection or neoplasm, but it is not commonly done today. One of two techniques may be used to retrieve the specimen: needle (closed) biopsy or incisional (open) biopsy.

Muscle biopsy is done for the diagnosis of atrophy (as in muscular dystrophy) and inflammation (as in polymyositis).

The procedure and care for patients undergoing muscle biopsy are the same as those for patients undergoing bone biopsy.

Electromyography. Although not commonly used today, electromyography (EMG) may be performed to evaluate diffuse or localized muscle weakness. EMG is usually accompanied by nerve-conduction studies for determining the electrical potential generated in an individual muscle. This test helps in the diagnosis of neuromuscular, lower motor neuron, and peripheral nerve disorders.

Inform the patient that EMG may cause temporary discomfort, especially when the patient is subjected to episodes of electrical current. For selected patients, mild sedation is prescribed. The physician may also prescribe a temporary discontinuation of skeletal muscle relaxants several days before the procedure to prevent drugs from affecting the test results.

Arthroscopy. **Arthroscopy** may be used as a diagnostic test or a surgical procedure. An arthroscope is a fiberoptic tube inserted into a joint for direct visualization of the ligaments, menisci, and articular surfaces of the joint. The knee and shoulder are most commonly evaluated. In addition, synovial biopsy and surgery to repair traumatic injury can be done through the arthroscope as an ambulatory-care or same-day surgical procedure.

Patient Preparation. Arthroscopy is performed on an ambulatory-care basis or as same-day surgery. The patient must have MOBILITY in the joint being examined. Those who cannot move the joint or who have an infected joint are not candidates for the procedure.

If the procedure is done for surgical repair, the patient may have a physical therapy consultation before arthroscopy to learn the exercises that are necessary after the test. ROM exercises are also taught but may not be allowed immediately after arthroscopic surgery. The nurse in the surgeon's office or at the surgical center can teach these exercises or reinforce the information provided by the physical therapist. The nurse also reinforces the explanation of the procedure and post-test care and ensures that the patient has signed an informed consent.

Procedure. The patient is usually given local, light general, or epidural anesthesia, depending on the purpose of the procedure. As shown in Fig. 49-6, the arthroscope is inserted through a small incision less than $\frac{1}{4}$-inch (0.6 cm) long. Multiple incisions may be required to allow inspection at a variety of angles. After the procedure, a dressing may be applied, depending on the amount of manipulation during the test or surgery.

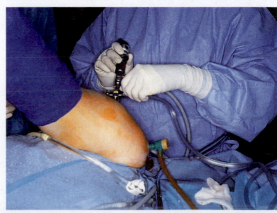

FIG. 49-6 An arthroscope is used in the diagnosis of pathologic changes in the joints. This patient is undergoing arthroscopy of the shoulder.

Follow-Up Care. The immediate care after an arthroscopy is the same for patients having the procedure for diagnostic purposes as for those having it for surgical intervention.

> ⚠️ **NURSING SAFETY PRIORITY** **QSEN**
>
> **Action Alert**
>
> The priority for postprocedure care after arthroscopy is to assess the neurovascular status of the patient's affected limb every hour or according to agency or surgeon protocol. Monitor and document distal pulses, warmth, color, capillary refill, pain, movement, and sensation of the affected extremity.

Encourage the patient to perform exercises as taught before the procedure, if appropriate. For the mild discomfort experienced after the diagnostic arthroscopy, the surgeon prescribes a mild analgesic, such as acetaminophen (Tylenol, Ace-Tabs). If postoperative, the patient may have short-term activity restrictions, depending on the musculoskeletal problem. Ice is often used for 24 hours, and the extremity should be elevated for 12 to 24 hours. When arthroscopic surgery is performed, the health care provider usually prescribes an opioid-analgesic combination, such as oxycodone and acetaminophen (Percocet, Tylox).

Although complications are not common, monitor and teach the patient to observe for:

- Swelling
- Increased joint pain attributable to mechanical injury
- Thrombophlebitis
- Infection

Severe joint or limb pain after discharge may indicate a possible complication. Teach the patient to contact the physician immediately. The surgeon usually sees the patient about 1 week after the procedure to check for complications.

> ❓ **NCLEX EXAMINATION CHALLENGE 49-2**
>
> **Safe and Effective Care Environment**
>
> A client returns to the postanesthesia care unit (PACU) after an arthroscopy to repair a knee injury. What is the nurse's priority when caring for this client?
> A. Perform passive range-of-motion exercises.
> B. Keep the affected leg immobilized.
> C. Ensure that the patient uses the patient-controlled analgesia (PCA) pump.
> D. Check the neurovascular status of the affected leg and foot.

GET READY FOR THE NCLEX® EXAMINATION!

KEY POINTS

Review these Key Points for each NCLEX Examination Client Needs Category.

Safe and Effective Care Environment

- Collaborate with the physical and/or occupational therapist to perform a complete musculoskeletal assessment, including gait, muscle strength, COMFORT, and MOBILITY, as indicated. **QSEN: Teamwork and Collaboration**

Health Promotion and Maintenance

- Be aware that older adults have physiologic changes that affect their musculoskeletal system, such as decreased bone density and joint cartilage degeneration; plan nursing interventions to ensure patient safety (see Chart 49-1). **QSEN: Patient-Centered Care; Safety**

Psychosocial Integrity

- Recall that potential patient reactions to musculoskeletal trauma or disease can include anxiety, depression, and/or altered body image and self-concept. **QSEN: Patient-Centered Care**

Physiological Integrity

- Assess the patient's COMFORT level, including pain intensity, quality, duration, and location.
- Assess and interpret the patient's MOBILITY, including gait, posture, and muscle strength status. **Clinical Judgment**
- Interpret the patient's laboratory values that are related to musculoskeletal disease (see Chart 49-2).
- Teach the patient that mild impaired COMFORT can be expected during electromyography, a test to assess the electrical potential of muscles and their innervation.
- Instruct the patient to report swelling, infection, and increased pain after an arthroscopy.
- Ask the patient questions to ensure safety before an MRI (see Chart 49-3). **QSEN: Safety**
- Ask the patient about allergy to contrast media before diagnostic testing such as CT scans.
- Evaluate the neurovascular status of the patient's affected extremity after an arthroscopic procedure as the *priority for care*. **QSEN: Safety**

SELECTED BIBLIOGRAPHY

Asterisk indicates a classic or definitive work on this subject.

Clark, S., & Santy-Tomlinson, J. (2014). *Orthopaedic and trauma nursing: An evidence-based approach to musculoskeletal care.* Hoboken, N.J.: Wiley-Blackwell.

Jarvis, C. (2014). *Physical examination & health assessment* (7th ed.). St. Louis: Elsevier Saunders.

McCance, K., Huether, S., Brashers, V., & Rote, N. (2014). *Pathophysiology: The biologic basis for disease in adults and children* (7th ed.). St. Louis: Mosby.

*Mosher, C. M. (2010). *An introduction to orthopaedic nursing* (4th ed.). Chicago: National Association of Orthopaedic Nurses.

Onubogu, U. D. (2014). Pain and depression in older adults with arthritis. *Orthopedic Nursing, 33*(2), 102–108.

Pagana, K. D., Pagana, T. J., & Pagana, T. N. (2017). *Mosby's diagnostic and laboratory test reference* (13th ed.). St. Louis: Mosby.

*Smith, M. A., & Smith, W. T. (2010). Rotator cuff tears: An overview. *Orthopaedic Nursing, 29*(5), 319–322.

CHAPTER 50

Care of Patients With Musculoskeletal Problems

Donna D. Ignatavicius

e http://evolve.elsevier.com/Iggy/

PRIORITY CONCEPTS AND EXEMPLARS

The priority concepts for this chapter are:
- CELLULAR REGULATION
- MOBILITY

✳ The CELLULAR REGULATION concept exemplar for this chapter is Osteoporosis, below.

The interrelated concepts for this chapter are:
- COMFORT
- PERFUSION

LEARNING OUTCOMES

Safe and Effective Care Environment

1. Collaborate with members of the interprofessional team to ensure safe, quality care for patients with osteoporosis.
2. Teach the patient and family about home safety when the patient has a CELLULAR REGULATION problem such as osteoporosis.

Health Promotion and Maintenance

3. Identify community resources for patients with osteoporosis.
4. Develop a patient-centered teaching plan for all adult age-groups about ways to decrease the risk for osteoporosis and possible fracture.

Psychosocial Integrity

5. Assess the patient's and family's responses to a bone cancer diagnosis and treatment options.

Physiological Integrity

6. Interpret laboratory and diagnostic findings for patients with or at risk for osteoporosis.
7. Document the presence and extent of impaired COMFORT in patients with bone tumors.
8. Educate the patient and family about common drugs used for osteoporosis, such as calcium supplements and bisphosphonates, to promote patient safety.
9. Use clinical judgment to prioritize care for patients with osteomyelitis, including neurovascular assessments to ensure adequate PERFUSION.
10. Identify patient-centered options for managing patients with primary and metastatic bone cancer.
11. Describe common disorders of the foot, including hallux valgus and plantar fasciitis, which can affect MOBILITY.

Musculoskeletal disorders include diseases of CELLULAR REGULATION (e.g., osteoporosis), bone tumors, and a variety of deformities and syndromes. Older adults are at the greatest risk for most of these problems, although *primary* bone cancer is most often found in adolescents and young adults. As technology advances and patients survive longer with primary cancers, metastatic lesions have become more prevalent among older adults. Almost all musculoskeletal health problems can cause the patient to have difficulty meeting the human need of MOBILITY. This chapter focuses on selected adult musculoskeletal health disorders not covered in Chapter 18 on arthritis or Chapter 51 on musculoskeletal trauma. Musculoskeletal problems that are seen most often in children, such as scoliosis and progressive muscular dystrophies, are not included in this chapter because they are included in pediatric or life span textbooks.

✳ CELLULAR REGULATION CONCEPT EXEMPLAR
Osteoporosis

❖ PATHOPHYSIOLOGY

Osteoporosis is a chronic disease of CELLULAR REGULATION in which bone loss causes significant decreased density and possible fracture. (See Chapter 2 for a concept review of cellular regulation.) It is often referred to as a *silent disease* or *silent thief* because the first sign of osteoporosis in most people follows

TABLE 50-1 Differential Features of Osteoporosis and Osteomalacia

CHARACTERISTIC	OSTEOPOROSIS	OSTEOMALACIA
Definition	Decreased bone mass caused by multiple factors	Bone softening caused by lack of calcification
Primary etiology	Lack of calcium and estrogen or testosterone	Lack of vitamin D
Radiographic findings	Osteopenia (bone loss), fractures	Fractures
Calcium level	Low or normal	Low or normal
Phosphate level	Normal	Low or normal
Parathyroid hormone	Normal	High or normal
Alkaline phosphatase	Normal	High

TABLE 50-2 Common Causes of Secondary Osteoporosis

Diseases/Conditions	Drugs (Chronic Use)
• Diabetes mellitus	• Corticosteroids
• Hyperthyroidism	• Antiepileptic drugs (AEDs) (e.g., phenytoin)
• Hyperparathyroidism	
• Cushing's syndrome	• Barbiturates (e.g., phenobarbital)
• Growth hormone deficiency	• Ethanol (alcohol)
• Metabolic acidosis	• Drugs that induce hypogonadism (decreased levels of sex hormones)
• Female hypogonadism	
• Rheumatoid arthritis	• High levels of thyroid hormone
• Prolonged immobilization	• Cytotoxic agents
• Bone cancer	• Immunosuppressants
• Cirrhosis	• Loop diuretics
• HIV/AIDS	• Aluminum-based antacids

AIDS, Acquired immune deficiency syndrome; *HIV,* human immune deficiency virus.

some kind of a fracture. The spine, hip, and wrist are most often at risk, although any bone can fracture.

Euro-American postmenopausal women have a 50% chance of having an osteoporotic-related (fragility) fracture in their lifetime (National Osteoporosis Foundation [NOF], 2017). A woman who experiences a hip fracture has a four times greater risk for a second fracture. Fractures as a result of osteoporosis and falling can decrease a patient's MOBILITY and quality of life. The mortality rate for older patients with hip fractures is very high, especially within the first 6 to 12 months, and the debilitating effects can be devastating (Fitton et al., 2015).

Osteoporosis is a major global health problem. In less affluent or famine countries, many individuals have both osteoporosis *and* osteomalacia as a result of dietary deficiencies. **Osteomalacia** is loss of bone related to lack of vitamin D, which causes bone softening. Vitamin D is needed for calcium absorption in the small intestines. As a result of vitamin D deficiency, normal bone building is disrupted, and calcification does not occur to harden the bone. Table 50-1 compares these two bone diseases caused by impaired cellular regulation.

Bone is a living, changing tissue that is constantly undergoing changes in a process referred to as **bone remodeling**, a type of CELLULAR REGULATION. Osteoporosis and **osteopenia** (low bone mass) occur when osteoclastic (bone resorption) activity is greater than osteoblastic (bone building) activity. The result is a decreased **bone mineral density (BMD)**. BMD determines bone strength and peaks between 25 and 30 years of age. Before and during the peak years, osteoclastic activity and osteoblastic activity work at the same rate. After the peak years, bone-resorption activity exceeds bone-building activity, and bone density decreases. BMD decreases most rapidly in postmenopausal women as serum estrogen levels diminish. Although estrogen does not build bone, it helps prevent bone loss. Trabecular, or cancellous (spongy), bone is lost first, followed by loss of cortical (compact) bone. This results in thin, fragile bone tissue that is at risk for fracture.

Standards for the diagnosis of osteoporosis are based on BMD testing that provides a T-score for the patient. A T-score represents the number of standard deviations above or below (designated with a − sign) the average BMD for young, healthy adults. The T-score in a healthy 30-year-old adult is 0. *Osteopenia is present when the T-score is at −1 and above −2.5.*

Osteoporosis is diagnosed in a person who has a T-score at or lower than −2.5 (Fitton et al., 2015; NOF, 2017). Severe or established osteoporosis is defined as a person with osteoporosis plus one or more fractures (NOF, 2017).

Osteoporosis can be classified as generalized or regional. *Generalized* osteoporosis involves many structures in the skeleton and is further divided into two categories: primary and secondary. *Primary* osteoporosis is more common and occurs in postmenopausal women and in men in their seventh or eighth decade of life. Even though men do not experience the rapid bone loss that postmenopausal women have, they do have decreasing levels of testosterone (which builds bone) and altered ability to absorb calcium. This results in a slower loss of bone mass in men, especially those older than 70 years (Fasolino & Whitright, 2015). *Secondary* osteoporosis may result from other medical conditions, such as hyperparathyroidism; long-term drug therapy, such as with corticosteroids; or prolonged immobility, such as that seen with spinal cord injury (Table 50-2). Treatment of the secondary type is directed toward the cause of the osteoporosis when possible.

Regional osteoporosis, an example of secondary disease, occurs when a limb is immobilized related to a fracture, injury, or paralysis. Immobility for longer than 8 to 12 weeks can result in this type of osteoporosis. Bone loss also occurs when people spend prolonged time in a gravity-free or weightless environment (e.g., astronauts).

Etiology and Genetic Risk

Primary osteoporosis is caused by a combination of genetic, lifestyle, and environmental factors. Chart 50-1 lists the major modifiable and nonmodifiable risk factors that contribute to the development of this disease.

The relationship of osteoporosis to nutrition is well established. For example, excessive caffeine in the diet can cause calcium loss in the urine. A diet lacking enough calcium and vitamin D stimulates the parathyroid gland to produce parathyroid hormone (PTH). PTH triggers the release of calcium from the bony matrix. Activated vitamin D is needed for calcium uptake in the body. Malabsorption of nutrients in the small intestines also contributes to low serum calcium levels. Institutionalized or homebound patients who are not exposed to sunlight may be at a higher risk because they do not receive adequate vitamin D for the metabolism of calcium.

Assessing Risk Factors for Primary Osteoporosis

Assess for these nonmodifiable risk factors:
- Older age in both genders and all races
- Parental history of osteoporosis, especially mother
- History of low-trauma fracture after age 50 years

Assess for these modifiable risk factors:
- Low body weight, thin build
- Chronic low calcium and/or vitamin D intake
- Estrogen or androgen deficiency
- Current smoking (active or passive)
- High alcohol intake (three or more drinks a day)
- Lack of physical exercise or prolonged immobility

GENETIC/GENOMIC CONSIDERATIONS

Patient-Centered Care QSEN

The genetic and immune factors that cause osteoporosis are very complex. Strong evidence demonstrates that genetics is a significant factor, with a heritability of 50% to 90% (Chang et al., 2010). Many genetic changes have been identified as possible causative factors, but there is no agreement about which ones are most important or constant in all patients. For example, changes in the vitamin D_3 receptor (*VDR*) gene and calcitonin receptor (*CTR*) gene have been found in some patients with the disease. Receptors are essential for the uptake and use of these substances by the cells (McCance et al., 2014).

The bone morphogenetic protein-2 (*BMP-2*) gene has a key role in bone formation and maintenance. Some osteoporotic patients who had fractures have changes in their *BMP-2* gene. Alterations in growth hormone-1 (GH-1) have been discovered in petite Asian-American women (i.e., those who are predisposed to developing osteoporosis.)

Hormones, tumor necrosis factor (TNF), interleukins, and other substances in the body help control osteoclasts in a very complex pathway. The identification of the importance of the cytokine receptor activator of nuclear factor kappa-B ligand (*RANKL*), its receptor *RANK*, and its decoy receptor osteoprotegerin (*OPG*) has helped researchers understand more about the activity of osteoclasts in metabolic bone disease. Disruptions in the *RANKL*, *RANK*, and *OPG* system can lead to increased osteoclast activity in which bone is rapidly broken down (McCance et al., 2014).

GENDER HEALTH CONSIDERATIONS

Patient-Centered Care QSEN

Primary osteoporosis most often occurs in women after menopause as a result of decreased estrogen levels. Obese women can store estrogen in their tissues for use as necessary to maintain a normal level of serum calcium better than thinner women.

Men also develop osteoporosis as they age because their testosterone levels decrease. Testosterone is the major sex hormone that builds bone tissue. Men are often underdiagnosed, even when they become older adults. Fasolino & Whitright (2015) conducted a pilot study to determine what other risk factors might be associated with bone loss in older men (see the Evidence-Based Practice box). These factors include smoking, alcohol consumption, and obesity.

Calcium loss occurs at a more rapid rate when phosphorus intake is high. (Chapter 11 describes the usual relationship between calcium and phosphorus in the body.) People who drink large amounts of carbonated beverages each day (over 40 ounces) are at high risk for calcium loss and subsequent osteoporosis, regardless of age or gender.

What Are the Risk Factors for Bone Loss in Men?

Fasolino, T., & Whitright, T. (2015). A pilot study to identify modifiable and nonmodifiable variables associated with osteopenia and osteoporosis in men. *Orthopaedic Nursing, 34*(5), 289–295.

The researchers conducted a pilot study to identify the variables that are associated with the development of osteopenia and osteoporosis in men. Using a self-report questionnaire, subjective data such as smoking history, alcohol use, and exercise history were collected from 101 volunteer men with a mean age of 70.7 years. Most (99%) were Caucasians. Objective data included age, height, weight (to calculate body mass index [BMI]), and bone mineral density (BMD) using dual-energy x-ray absorptiometry (DXA). Smoking history and alcohol use in men with *high* BMIs correlated with the highest risk for osteopenia and osteoporosis. These findings contradicted previous studies that found that a *low* BMI places an individual at high risk for bone loss.

Level of Evidence: 4

This research was a small, descriptive pilot study to identify risk factors for bone loss in older men.

Commentary: Implications for Practice and Research

Because osteoporosis occurs more in women than in men, most of the studies on bone loss have focused on risk factors and management of bone loss in women. This study indicates that nurses and other health care professionals need to assess for risk factors in men and teach them the importance of smoking cessation, decreasing alcohol consumption, and losing weight to help prevent osteopenia. More studies using larger and more diverse sample sizes are needed to increase generalizability of the findings.

Protein deficiency may also affect CELLULAR REGULATION. Because 50% of serum calcium is protein bound, protein is needed to use calcium. However, excessive protein intake may increase calcium loss in the urine. For example, people who are on high-protein, low-carbohydrate diets, such as the Atkins diet, may consume too much protein to replace other food not allowed.

Excessive alcohol and tobacco use are other risk factors for osteoporosis. Although the exact mechanisms are not known, these substances promote acidosis, which in turn increases bone loss. Alcohol also has a direct toxic effect on bone tissue, resulting in decreased bone formation and increased bone resorption. For people who have excessive alcohol intake, alcohol calories may decrease hunger and the need to take in adequate amounts of nutrients.

Incidence and Prevalence

Osteoporosis is a potential health problem for more than 44 million Americans. About 10 million people in the United States have the disease, and about 34 million people 50 years of age and older have osteopenia and are at risk for development of osteoporosis (NOF, 2017). As baby boomers age, these numbers are expected to increase dramatically.

Health Promotion and Maintenance

Peak bone mass is achieved by about 30 years of age in most women. *Building strong bone as a young person may be the best defense against osteoporosis in later adulthood.* Young women need to be aware of appropriate health and lifestyle practices that can prevent this potentially disabling disease. Patient-centered teaching should begin with young women because they begin to lose bone after 30 years of age. Nurses can play a vital role in patient education for women of any age to prevent and manage osteoporosis (Evenson & Sanders, 2016).

The focus of evidence-based osteoporosis prevention is to decrease modifiable risk factors to promote patient safety. For example, teach patients who do not include enough dietary calcium which foods to eat, such as dairy products and dark green leafy vegetables. Teach them to read food labels for sources of calcium content. Explain the importance of sun exposure (but not so much as to get sunburned) and adequate vitamin D in the diet. The National Osteoporosis Foundation recommends taking a vitamin D₃ supplement for all adults. Patients being treated for osteopenia or osteomalacia (vitamin D deficiency) may be prescribed high therapeutic doses up to 20,000 units a week (NOF, 2017).

Teach individuals at high risk for bone loss the importance of smoking cessation (if needed), weight loss (if needed), and excessive alcohol avoidance. Teach them the need to limit the amount of carbonated beverages consumed each day. Remind patients who have sedentary lifestyles about the importance of exercise and which types of exercise build bone tissue. Weight-bearing exercises, such as regularly scheduled walking, are preferred. Teach high-risk people to avoid activities that cause jarring, such as horseback riding and jogging, to prevent potential vertebral compression fractures.

❖ INTERPROFESSIONAL COLLABORATIVE CARE

◆ Assessment: Noticing

A complete health history with assessment of risk factors is important in the prevention, early detection, and treatment of osteoporosis. Patients who have risk factors for osteoporosis are at increased risk for fractures when falls occur. In some cases, the fracture occurs before the fall. Include a fall risk assessment in the health history, especially for older adults. Assess for fall risk factors as described in Chapter 3. **The Joint Commission's National Patient Safety Goals (NPSGs) specify the need to reduce risk for harm to patients resulting from falls. People with osteoporosis are at an increased risk for fracture if a fall occurs.**

Physical Assessment/Signs and Symptoms. When performing a musculoskeletal assessment, inspect the vertebral column. The classic "dowager's hump," or kyphosis of the dorsal spine, is often present (Fig. 50-1). The patient may state that he or she has gotten shorter, perhaps as much as 2 to 3 inches (5 to 7.5 cm), within the previous 20 years. Take or delegate height

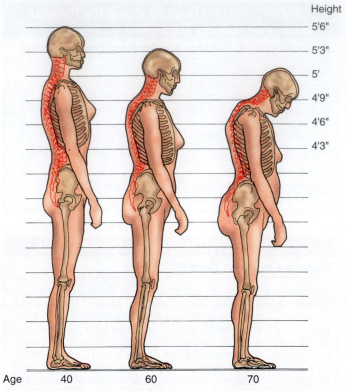

FIG. 50-1 Normal spine at age 40 years and osteoporotic changes at ages 60 and 70 years. These changes can cause a loss of as much as 6 inches in height and can result in the so-called *dowager's hump (far right)* in the upper thoracic vertebrae.

and weight measurements and compare with previous measurements if they are available.

The patient may have back pain, which often occurs after lifting, bending, or stooping. The pain may be sharp and acute in onset. Pain is worse with activity and is relieved by rest. *Back pain accompanied by tenderness and voluntary restriction of spinal movement suggests one or more compression vertebral fractures (i.e., the most common type of osteoporotic or fragility fracture).* Movement restriction and spinal deformity may result in constipation, abdominal distention, reflux esophagitis, and respiratory compromise in severe cases. The most likely area for spinal fracture is between T8 and L3, the most movable part of the vertebral column.

Fractures are also common in the distal end of the radius (wrist) and the upper third of the femur (hip). Ask the patient to locate all areas that are painful and observe for signs and symptoms of fractures, such as swelling and malalignment. Signs and symptoms of fractures are discussed in Chapter 51.

Psychosocial Assessment. Women associate osteoporosis with menopause, getting older, and becoming less independent. The disease can result in suffering, deformity, and disability that can affect the patient's well-being and life satisfaction. The quality of life may be further impacted by pain, insomnia, depression, and fear of falling (Touhy & Jett, 2014).

Assess the patient's concept of body image, especially if he or she is severely kyphotic. For example, the patient may have difficulty finding clothes that fit properly. Social interactions may be avoided because of a change in appearance or the physical limitations of being unable to sit in chairs in restaurants, movie theaters, and other places. Changes in sexuality may occur as a result of poor self-esteem or the discomfort caused by positioning during intercourse.

Because osteoporosis poses a risk for fractures, teach the patient to be extremely cautious about activities. As a result, the threat of fracture can create anxiety and fear and result in further limitation of social or physical activities. Assess for these feelings to assist in treatment decisions and health teaching. For example, the patient may not exercise as prescribed for fear that a fracture will occur.

Laboratory Assessment. Serum calcium and vitamin D$_3$ levels should be routinely monitored (at least once a year) for all women and for men older than 50 years who are at a high risk for the disease. Serum calcium should be between 9.0 and 10.5 mg/dL, or 2.25 and 2.75 mmol/L. Total 25-hydroxy D (vitamins D$_2$ +D$_3$) levels should be between 25 and 80 ng/mL, or 75 and 200 nmol/L (Pagana et al., 2017). These results help determine the need for supplements and preventive measures to slow bone loss.

No definitive laboratory tests confirm a diagnosis of primary osteoporosis, although a number of *bone turnover markers* can provide information about bone resorption and formation activity. Although not commonly tested, these markers are sensitive to bone changes and can be used to monitor effectiveness of treatment for osteoporosis or to detect bone changes early in the disease process. Examples of these markers are listed in Table 50-3.

Imaging Assessment. Conventional x-rays of the spine and long bones show decreased bone density, but only after a large amount of bone loss has occurred. Fractures can also be seen on x-ray. According to the National Osteoporosis Foundation (NOF) (2017), all postmenopausal women and men age 50 and older should be evaluated for osteoporosis risk to determine the need for BMD testing and/or vertebral imaging.

The most commonly used screening and diagnostic tool for measuring bone mineral density (BMD) is **dual x-ray absorptiometry (DXA)**. The spine and hip are most often assessed when central DXA (cDXA) scan is performed. Many health care

providers recommend that women in their 40s have a baseline screening DXA scan so later bone changes can be detected and compared. DXA is a painless scan that emits less radiation than a chest x-ray. It is the most commonly test currently used but has limitations. First, BMD alone explains only part of the bone change and provides no information on cellular activity. Second, there are variations among different DXA systems. In addition, the DXA scanner does not account for very tall or very obese patients. Finally, it is not safe for patients to have frequent scans because of radiation exposure (Fitton et al., 2015).

Tell patients that their height is taken before having a DXA scan. The patient stays dressed but is asked to remove any metallic objects such as belt buckles, coins, keys, or jewelry that might interfere with the test. The results are displayed on a computer graph, and a T-score is calculated. No special follow-up care for the test is required. However, the patient needs to discuss the results with the primary care provider for any decisions about possible preventive or management interventions.

For some patients, a *CT-based absorptiometry* (qualitative computed tomography [QCT]) may be performed. This test measures the volume of bone density and strength of the vertebral spine and hip. The peripheral QCT (pQCT) measures the same at the forearm or tibia. High-resolution pQCT (HR-pQCT) of the radius and tibia provides additional information on bone structure and architecture. These tests are predictive of spine and/or hip fractures in women; however, they require greater amounts of radiation when compared to the more traditional DXA.

Vertebral imaging can be performed using lateral spine x-rays or lateral vertebral fracture assessment (VFA), which is available as part of most DXA systems. According to the clinical guidelines outlined by NOF, vertebral imaging is indicated for these groups:

- All women age 70 and older and all men age 80 and older if BMD is less than or equal to a T-score of 1.0
- Women age 65 to 69 and men age 70 to 79 if BMD is less than or equal to 1.5
- Postmenopausal women and men age 50 and older with certain risk factors, such as significant height loss, history of low-trauma fracture, or being on long-term corticosteroids

The most promising imaging test for determining bone quality is *MRI* (see Chapter 49 for procedure). MRI does not involve radiation and can view bone in ways that other techniques cannot. To determine the presence of osteoporosis, MRI provides information about yellow bone marrow content, diffusion, and PERFUSION to the bone. Perfusion to osteoporotic bone is lower than to bone of normal bone density. Fat marrow content, sometimes referred to as *bone marrow adipose tissue (BMAT)*, is higher in patients with bone loss when compared to those with normal BMD. In addition to MRI, a more advanced imaging technique, the *magnetic resonance spectroscopy (MRS)*, is being used to create a graph for quantifying the amount of BMAT rather than merely providing an image via an MRI. Both of these tests are more reliable and offer more information about bone change than BMD measurements alone. However, they are expensive and not yet commonly used until third parties recognize their value for cost reimbursement (Fitton, et al., 2015).

Several imaging tests are available for community-based screening because these devices are more portable. However, they lack the preciseness and reliability of the previously

---

TABLE 50-3 Examples of Serum and Urinary Bone Turnover Markers

- Osteocalcin (BGP)
- Bone-specific alkaline phosphatase (BSAP)
- Procollagen Type 1 Amino Terminal Peptide (P1NP)
- Urinary total pyridinoline (Pyr)
- Urinary free deoxypyridinoline (DPyr)
- Tartrate-resistant acid phosphatase (TRAP)
- Urinary collagen type 1 cross-linked C-telopeptide (s-CTX)

discussed imaging procedures. Examples include the peripheral DXA (pDXA) and the peripheral quantitative ultrasound densitometry (pQUS). The *pDXA scan* assesses BMD of the heel, forearm, or finger. It is often used for large-scale screening purposes. The *pQUS* is an effective and low-cost screening tool that can detect osteoporosis and predict risk for hip fracture. The heel, tibia, and patella are most commonly tested. This procedure requires no special preparation, is quick, and has no radiation exposure or specific follow-up care (Pagana et al., 2017). Both tests are commonly used for screening at community health fairs, skilled nursing facilities, and women's health centers.

◆ *Analysis: Interpreting*

The priority problem for patients with osteoporosis or osteopenia is *Potential for fractures due to weak, porous bone tissue.*

◆ *Planning and Implementation: Responding*

Planning: Expected Outcomes. The expected outcome is that the patient will avoid fractures by preventing falls, managing risk factors, and adhering to preventive or treatment measures for bone loss.

Interventions. Because the patient is predisposed to fractures, nutritional therapy, exercise, lifestyle changes, and drug therapy are used to slow bone resorption and form new bone tissue. Self-management education (SME) can help prevent osteoporosis or slow the progress.

Nutrition Therapy. The nutritional considerations for the treatment of a patient with a diagnosis of osteoporosis are the same as those for preventing the disease. Teach patients about the need for adequate amounts of calcium and vitamin D for bone remodeling. Instruct them to avoid excessive alcohol and caffeine consumption. People who are lactose intolerant can choose a variety of soy and rice products that are fortified with calcium and vitamin D. In addition, calcium and vitamin D are added to many fruit juices, bread, and cereal products.

A variety of nutrients are needed to maintain bone health. *The promotion of a single nutrient will not prevent or treat osteoporosis.* Help the patient develop a nutritional plan that is most beneficial in maintaining bone health; the plan should emphasize fruits and vegetables, low-fat dairy and protein sources, increased fiber, and moderation in alcohol and caffeine (NOF, 2017).

Lifestyle Changes. Exercise is important in the prevention and management of osteoporosis. It also plays a vital role in management of impaired COMFORT, cardiovascular function, and an improved sense of well-being.

In collaboration with the primary health care provider, the physical therapist may prescribe exercises for strengthening the abdominal and back muscles for those at risk for vertebral fractures. These exercises improve posture and support for the spine. Abdominal muscle tightening, deep breathing, and pectoral stretching are stressed to increase lung capacity. Exercises for the extremity muscles include muscle-tightening, resistive, and range-of-motion (ROM) exercises to improve MOBILITY. Muscle strengthening also helps to prevent falls and promote balance. Swimming provides overall muscle exercise.

In addition to exercises for muscle strengthening, a general weight-bearing exercise program should be implemented. Teach patients that walking for 30 minutes three to five times a week is the single most effective exercise for osteoporosis prevention. Remind them to avoid any activity that would cause jarring of the body, such as jogging and horseback riding.

These activities can cause compression fractures of the vertebral column.

In addition to nutrition and exercise, other lifestyle changes may be needed. Teach the patient to avoid tobacco in any form, especially active or passive cigarette smoking (NOF, 2017). Remind women not to consume more than one alcoholic drink per day (5 ounces each); instruct men not to have more than two alcoholic drinks per day.

Hospitals and long-term care facilities have risk management programs to assess for the risk for falls. For patients at high risk, communicate this information to other members of the health care team, using colored armbands or other easy-to-recognize methods (National Patient Safety Goals). Chapter 3 discusses fall prevention in health care agencies and at home in more detail.

❓ NCLEX EXAMINATION CHALLENGE 50-2

Health Promotion and Maintenance

Which statement by the client regarding lifestyle changes to prevent osteoporosis indicates a **need for further teaching** by the nurse?

A. "I'm going to continue having my DXA scans as my doctor orders."
B. "I'll drink only a half glass of wine occasionally to help me sleep."
C. "I plan to increase calcium and vitamin D foods in my diet."
D. "I'm going to jog every day for at least 30 minutes."

Drug Therapy. The evidence shows that drug therapy should be used for postmenopausal women and men age 50 and older when the BMD T-score for the hip or lumbar spine is below or equal to −2.5 with no other risk factors, or when the T-score is below −1.5 with risk factors or previous fracture. Anyone age 50 or older who had a hip or vertebral fracture should also be treated (NOF, 2017). The health care provider may prescribe calcium and vitamin D_3 supplements, bisphosphonates, estrogen agonist/antagonists (formerly called *selective estrogen receptor modulators*), parathyroid hormone, RANKL inhibitor, or a combination of several drugs to treat or prevent osteoporosis (Chart 50-2). In addition, calcitonin may be used for some patients. Estrogen and combination hormone therapy are not used solely for osteoporosis prevention or management because they can increase other health risks such as breast cancer and myocardial infarction.

Calcium and Activated Vitamin D (D_3). Intake of *calcium* alone is not a treatment for osteoporosis, but calcium is an important part of any program to promote bone health. Most people cannot or do not have enough calcium in their diet; therefore calcium supplements are needed. NOF (2017) supports the National Academy of Medicine's research recommendation of 1000 mg daily for all postmenopausal women and men between ages 50 and 70, and 1200 mg for both women and men 71 years of age and older (NOF, 2017). Calcium carbonate, found in over-the-counter (OTC) drugs such as Os-Cal, is one of the most cost-effective supplement formulas. Teach women to start taking supplements in young adulthood to help maintain peak bone mass. Instruct patients of any age to take calcium supplements that also contain a small amount of activated vitamin D (D_3), such as Os-Cal Ultra.

Because vitamin D is needed for calcium absorption by the body, vitamin D_3 supplementation is also indicated. This drug is

CHART 50-2 Common Examples of Drug Therapy

Osteoporosis (Dietary Supplements, Bisphosphonates, Estrogen Agonist/Antagonists)

DRUG CATEGORY	NURSING IMPLICATIONS
Calcium (With Vitamin D if Needed)	
Common examples of calcium and vitamin D: • Os-Cal (with or without vitamin D) • Citracal	Take a third of the daily dose at bedtime *because no weight-bearing activity to build bone occurs while sleeping.* Encourage increased fluids, unless medically contraindicated, *to help prevent urinary calculi (stones).* Teach patient to take the drug with 6-8 ounces of water *to help dissolve it.* Assess for a history of urinary stones before giving calcium. Monitor calcium level *to determine drug effectiveness.* Observe for signs of hypercalcemia, such as calcium deposits under the skin, cardiac dysrhythmias, changes in skeletal muscle tone, and urinary stones, *which may indicate calcium excess.*
Bisphosphonates	
Common examples of bisphosphonates: • Alendronate (Fosamax or Fosamax plus D) • Ibandronate (Boniva) • Risedronate (Actonel, Actonel plus Calcium, Atelvia) • Zoledronic acid (Reclast) (IV)	Teach patients to take drug on an empty stomach first thing in the morning with a full glass of water *to help prevent esophagitis, esophageal ulcers, and gastric ulcers.* Remind patients to take drug 30 minutes before food, drink, and other drugs *to prevent interactions.* Instruct the patient to remain upright, sitting or standing, for 30 minutes after taking the drug *to help prevent esophagitis (esophageal inflammation).* Instruct the patient to have a dental examination before starting the drug *because it can cause jaw and maxillary osteonecrosis, particular if oral hygiene is poor.* Do not give the drug to patients who are sensitive to aspirin *because bronchoconstriction may occur.* For IV drug, infuse over 15-30 minutes *to prevent rare complications such as atrial fibrillation.* For IV drug, check the patient's serum creatinine before and after administering the medication *because it can cause renal insufficiency or chronic kidney disease.*
Estrogen Agonists/Antagonists	
Common example of estrogen agonist/antagonists: • Raloxifene (Evista)	Teach the patient the signs and symptoms of venous thromboembolism (VTE), especially in the first 4 months of therapy, *because these drugs can cause VTE.* Monitor liver function tests (LFTs) in collaboration with the health care provider *because the drug can increase LFT values.*

also available as an OTC medication. NOF (2017) recommends a daily dose of 800 to 1000 units for women and men age 50 or over. Up to 4000 units daily may be taken for patients who have severe bone loss or multiple nonmodifiable risk factors. Laboratory tests to measure serum calcium and vitamin D_3 are done to monitor the effectiveness of these supplements.

Bisphosphonates. Bisphosphonates (BPs) slow bone resorption by binding with crystal elements in bone, especially spongy, trabecular bone tissue. They are the most common drugs used for osteoporosis, but some are also approved for Paget's disease and hypercalcemia related to cancer. Three Food and Drug Administration (FDA)–approved BPs (alendronate [Fosamax], ibandronate [Boniva], and risedronate [Actonel, Atelvia]) are commonly used for the *prevention and treatment* of osteoporosis (Burcham & Rosenthal, 2016). These drugs are available as oral preparations, with ibandronate (Boniva) also available as an IV preparation.

The most recent additions to the bisphosphonates are IV (Reclast) and IV pamidronate (Aredia). For management of osteoporosis, zoledronic acid is needed only once a year, and pamidronate is given every 3 to 6 months. Both drugs have been linked to a complication called jaw **osteonecrosis** (also known as *avascular necrosis,* or *bone death),* in which infection and necrosis of the mandible or maxilla occur (Burcham & Rosenthal, 2016). The incidence of this serious problem is low but can be a complication of this infusion therapy.

After taking any of these drugs for 3 years, the patient has a DXA scan. If bone density has improved or is maintained, the primary care provider may discontinue the bisphosphonate until the next scan in another 2 to 3 years. At that time, the primary health care provider will determine if the drug needs to be restarted.

! NURSING SAFETY PRIORITY QSEN

Drug Alert

Do not confuse Fosamax with Flomax, a selective alpha-adrenergic blocker used for benign prostatic hyperplasia (BPH). To promote safety, teach patients to take bisphosphonates (BPs) early in the morning with 8 ounces of water and wait 30 to 60 minutes in an upright position before eating. If chest discomfort (a symptom of esophageal irritation) occurs, instruct patients to discontinue the drug and contact their health care provider. Patients with poor renal function, hypocalcemia, or gastroesophageal reflux disease (GERD) should not take BPs.

Teach patients to have an oral assessment and preventive dentistry before beginning any bisphosphonate therapy. To promote safety, instruct them to inform any dentist who is planning invasive treatment, such as a tooth extraction or implant, that they are taking a BP drug.

Estrogen Agonist/Antagonists. Formerly called the *selective estrogen receptor modulators (SERMs),* estrogen agonist/antagonists are a class of drugs designed to mimic estrogen in some parts of the body while blocking its effect elsewhere. Raloxifene (Evista) is currently the only approved drug in this class and is used for *prevention and treatment* of osteoporosis in postmenopausal women. Raloxifene increases bone mineral density (BMD), reduces bone resorption, and reduces the incidence of osteoporotic vertebral fractures. The drug should not be given to women who have a history of thromboembolism.

Other Drugs. A newer type of drug is denosumab (Prolia), a *RANKL (Receptor Activator of Nuclear Factor kappa-B Ligand) inhibitor,* which has been approved for treatment of osteoporosis when other drugs are not effective (Burcham & Rosenthal, 2016). By preventing the protein from activating its receptor, the drug decreases bone loss and increases bone mass and strength. The drug is given subcutaneously twice a year by a health care professional.

Teriparatide (Forteo) is an anabolic (bone building) drug that is given subcutaneously and can only be used up to 2 years. After the drug is stopped, the patient is usually started on a bisphosphonate (NOF, 2017).

Salmon *calcitonin* (Miacalcin or Fortical) is approved for osteoporosis in women who are at least 5 years postmenopausal when alternative drug therapy is not appropriate. Two preparations are available: an intranasal spray or subcutaneous injection. Intranasal calcitonin can cause rhinitis and epistaxis (nosebleeds). In a few patients, malignancies have been attributed to the use of calcitonin. For others, allergic responses to salmon may prevent the drug from being used or continued. Patients are usually tested for this allergy before they begin the drug. Calcitonin is less commonly used than other drugs to prevent bone loss and fractures.

CLINICAL JUDGMENT CHALLENGE 50-1

Patient-Centered Care; Evidence-Based Practice; Safety QSEN

A 61-year-old petite Euro-American woman reports that she has lost 1 inch in height over the past 8 years. She takes calcium and vitamin D_3 supplements when she remembers and works for a university as an online instructor. When reviewing her history, you note that her grandmother and older sister had osteoporosis for many years. Her sister recently died less than a year after fracturing her hip. The patient expresses her fear of having a fracture and wants to be considered for aggressive drug therapy.

1. What risk factors does this patient have for osteoporosis? What other information do you need to do a complete assessment?
2. Is this patient a good candidate for beginning drug therapy? Why or why not? Will you need more information? If so, what do you need to know?
3. What health teaching does this patient need and why?
4. How will you respond to her fear of having more fractures?

Care Coordination and Transition Management

Home Care Management. Patients with osteoporosis are usually managed at home unless they have major fragility fractures. Some patients do not know that they have osteoporosis until they experience a fall and have one or more fractures.

Part of your responsibility is to collaborate with members of the interprofessional health team to ensure that the patient's home is safe and hazard free to help prevent falling. In some cases, home modifications may be needed, such as ramps instead of stairs or handrails near toilets and bathtubs/showers. Teach patients to prevent clutter in the home for clear pathways, avoid slippery floors, wear rubber-soled shoes, and avoid scatter rugs. Chapter 3 describes fall prevention in detail.

Self-Management Education. Teach patients about lifestyle practices that can help prevent additional bone loss. For example, to help prevent vitamin D deficiency, daily sun exposure (at least 5 minutes each day) is the most important source of vitamin D. If vitamin D levels remain low, teach patients to take their vitamin D_3 and calcium supplements as described earlier. Increase calcium and vitamin D sources in the diet.

Some people are lactose intolerant or do not use dairy products because of their vegan diets. However, many products are available for people who avoid dairy products. Soy and rice milk, tofu, and soy products are substitutes, but they are expensive. Teach patients to choose products that are fortified with vitamin D. Other foods rich in the vitamin are eggs, swordfish, chicken, liver, and enriched cereals and bread products.

If the patient is on drug therapy for osteopenia or osteoporosis, teach him or her to adhere to the medication regimen and take the prescribed drug(s) as instructed. Lack of adherence to long-term therapy for osteoporosis and bone health promotion practices is a major problem that results in increased fractures, hospital stays, and health care costs. In their systematic study, Alvaro et al. (2015) found that educational interventions alone were not sufficient to promote women's adherence to their treatment plan for osteoporosis. Adherence was improved when nurses were able to follow up personally or via phone several times over a prolonged period to encourage patients and be available to answer their questions.

Health Care Resources. Refer patients to the National Osteoporosis Foundation (www.nof.org) in the United States for information regarding the disease and its treatment. The Osteoporosis Society of Canada (www.osteoporosis.ca) has similar services. Large health care systems often have osteoporosis specialty clinics and support groups for patients with osteoporosis.

OSTEOMYELITIS

❖ *PATHOPHYSIOLOGY*

Infection in bony tissue can be a severe and difficult-to-treat problem. Bone infection can result in chronic recurrence of infection, loss of function and MOBILITY, amputation, and even death.

Bacteria, viruses, or fungi can cause infection in bone, known as osteomyelitis. Invasion by one or more pathogenic microorganisms stimulates the inflammatory response in bone tissue. The inflammation produces an increased vascular leak and edema, often involving the surrounding soft tissues. Once inflammation is established, the vessels in the area become thrombosed and release exudate (pus) into bony tissue. Ischemia of bone tissue follows and results in necrotic bone. This area of necrotic bone separates from surrounding bone tissue, and sequestrum is formed. The presence of sequestrum prevents bone healing and causes superimposed infection, often in the form of bone abscess. As shown in Fig. 50-2, the cycle repeats itself as the new infection leads to further inflammation, vessel thromboses, and necrosis.

Osteomyelitis may be categorized as *exogenous,* in which infectious organisms enter from outside the body as in an open fracture, or endogenous (hematogenous), in which organisms are carried by the bloodstream from other areas of infection in the body. A third category is *contiguous,* in which bone infection results from skin infection of adjacent tissues. Osteomyelitis can be further divided into two major types: acute and chronic.

Each type of bone infection has its own causative factors. Pathogenic microbes favor bone that has a rich blood supply and a marrow cavity. Acute hematogenous infection results from bacteremia, underlying disease, or nonpenetrating trauma. Urinary tract infections, particularly in older men, tend to spread to the lower vertebrae. Long-term IV catheters can be primary sources of infection. Patients undergoing long-term

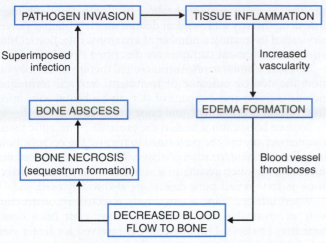

FIG. 50-2 Infection cycle of osteomyelitis.

CHART 50-3 Key Features
Acute and Chronic Osteomyelitis

CHART 50-3 **Key Features**

Acute and Chronic Osteomyelitis

Acute Osteomyelitis
- Fever; temperature usually above 101° F (38.3° C)
- Swelling around the affected area
- Possible erythema and heat in the affected area
- Tenderness of the affected area
- Bone pain that is constant, localized, and pulsating; worsens with movement

Chronic Osteomyelitis
- Foot ulcer(s) (most commonly)
- Sinus tract formation
- Localized pain
- Drainage from the affected area

hemodialysis and IV drug users are also at risk for osteomyelitis. *Salmonella* infections of the GI tract may spread to bone. Patients with sickle cell disease and other hemoglobinopathies often have multiple episodes of salmonellosis, which can cause bone infection (McCance et al., 2014).

Poor dental hygiene and periodontal (gum) infection can be causative factors in **contiguous** osteomyelitis in facial bones. Minimal nonpenetrating trauma can cause hemorrhages or small-vessel occlusions, leading to bone necrosis. Regardless of the source of infection, many infections are caused by *Staphylococcus aureus*. Treatment of infection may be complicated further by the presence of *methicillin-resistant Staphylococcus aureus* (MRSA) or other multiple drug-resistant organisms (MDROs), which are very common in hospitalized and other institutionalized patients as discussed in Chapter 23. The most common causes of MRSA in patients with musculoskeletal health problems are postoperative surgical site infections (SSIs) and infections from surgically implanted devices, such as an open-reduction, internal-fixation device (Smith, 2015). One of the major desired outcomes in health care settings today is to reduce the number of MRSA infections from any source. Preventive measures are described in Chapter 23.

CONSIDERATIONS FOR OLDER ADULTS

Patient-Centered Care **QSEN**

Malignant external otitis media involving the base of the skull is sometimes seen in older adults with diabetes. However, the most common cause of contiguous spread in older adults is found in those who have slow-healing foot ulcers. Multiple organisms tend to be responsible for the resulting osteomyelitis (McCance et al., 2014).

Penetrating trauma leads to acute osteomyelitis by direct inoculation. A soft-tissue infection may be present as well. Animal bites, puncture wounds, skin ulcerations, and bone surgery can result in osteomyelitis. The most common offending organism is *Pseudomonas aeruginosa,* but other gram-negative bacteria may be found.

If bone infection is misdiagnosed or inadequately treated, **chronic osteomyelitis** may develop, especially in older adults who have foot ulcers. Inadequate care management results when the treatment period is too short or when the treatment is delayed or inappropriate. About half of cases of chronic

osteomyelitis are caused by gram-negative bacteria. Although bacteria are the most common causes of osteomyelitis, viruses and fungal organisms also may cause infection.

❖ INTERPROFESSIONAL COLLABORATIVE CARE
◆ Assessment: Noticing
Bone pain, with or without other signs and symptoms, is a common concern of patients with osteomyelitis. The pain is described as a constant, localized, pulsating sensation that worsens with movement.

The patient with *acute* osteomyelitis has fever, usually with temperature greater than 101° F (38.3° C). *Older adults may not have an extreme temperature elevation because of a lower core body temperature and compromised immune system that occur with normal aging.* The area around the infected bone swells and is tender when palpated. Erythema (redness) and heat may also be present. When vascular compromise is severe, patients may not experience impaired COMFORT because of nerve damage from lack of adequate PERFUSION.

When vascular insufficiency is suspected, assess circulation in the distal extremities. Ulcerations may be present on the feet or hands, indicating inadequate healing ability as a result of impaired PERFUSION.

Fever, swelling, and erythema are less common in those with chronic osteomyelitis. Ulceration resulting in sinus tract formation, localized pain, and drainage is more characteristic of *chronic* infection (Chart 50-3).

The patient with osteomyelitis may have an elevated white blood cell (leukocyte) count, which may be double the normal value. The erythrocyte sedimentation rate (ESR) may be normal early in the course of the disease but rises as the condition progresses. It may remain elevated for as long as 3 months after drug therapy is discontinued.

If bacteremia (a potentially life-threatening complication that could lead to septic shock) is present, a blood culture identifies the offending organisms to determine which antibiotics should be used in treatment. Both aerobic and anaerobic blood cultures are collected before drug therapy begins.

Although bone changes cannot be detected early in the course of the disease with standard x-rays, changes in PERFUSION can be seen early by radionuclide scanning or MRI.

◆ Interventions: Responding
The specific treatment for osteomyelitis depends on the type and number of microbes present in the infected tissue. If other

measures fail to resolve the infectious process, surgical management may be needed.

Nonsurgical Management. The health care provider starts 4 to 6 weeks of antimicrobial (e.g., antibiotic) therapy as soon as possible for *acute* osteomyelitis. In the presence of copious wound drainage, use Contact Precautions to prevent the spread of the offending organism to other patients and health care personnel. Teach patients, visitors, and staff members how to use these precautions. (See Chapter 23 for a discussion of Contact Precautions.)

More than one agent may be needed to combat multiple types of organisms. The hospital or home care nurse gives the drugs at specifically prescribed times so therapeutic serum levels are achieved. Observe for the actions, side effects, and toxicity of these drugs. Teach family members or other caregivers in the home setting how to administer antimicrobials if they are continued after hospital discharge or are used only at home. Some patients may need to be admitted to a skilled nursing facility (SNF) to administer the antimicrobial. For patients with MRSA infection, IV vancomycin or linezolid (IV or oral) is used. Oral linezolid allows older patients to remain at home or assisted living rather than be admitted to an SNF.

The optimal drug regimen for patients with *chronic* osteomyelitis is not well established. Prolonged therapy for more than 3 months is typically needed to eliminate the infection. Because of the cost of lengthy hospital stays, patients are usually cared for in the home or long-term care (LTC) setting with long-term vascular access catheters, such as the peripherally inserted central catheter (PICC), for drug administration. After discontinuation of IV drugs, oral therapy may be needed. Patients and families must understand the complications of inadequate treatment or failure to follow up with their primary health care provider. Teach them that drug therapy must be continued over a long period to be effective.

! NURSING SAFETY PRIORITY **QSEN**

Drug Alert

Even when symptoms of osteomyelitis appear to be improved, teach the patient and family that the full course of IV and/or oral antimicrobials must be completed to ensure that the infection is resolved.

In addition to systemic drug therapy, the wound may be irrigated, either continuously or intermittently, with one or more antibiotic solutions. A medical technique in which beads made of bone cement are impregnated with an antibiotic and packed into the wound can provide direct contact of the antibiotic with the offending organism.

Drugs are also needed to improve patient COMFORT. Patients often experience acute and chronic pain and must receive a regimen of drug therapy for control. Chapter 4 describes pharmacologic and nonpharmacologic interventions for both acute and chronic pain.

A treatment to increase tissue PERFUSION for patients with chronic, unremitting osteomyelitis is the use of a hyperbaric chamber or portable device to administer hyperbaric oxygen (HBO) therapy. These devices are usually available in large tertiary care centers and may not be accessible to all patients who might benefit from them. With HBO therapy, the affected area is exposed to a high concentration of oxygen that diffuses

into the tissues to promote healing. In conjunction with high-dose drug therapy and surgical débridement, HBO has proven very useful in treating a number of anaerobic infections. Other wound-management therapies are described in Chapter 25.

Surgical Management. Antimicrobial therapy alone may not meet the desired outcome of treatment. Surgical techniques include incision and drainage of skin and subcutaneous infection, wound débridement, and bone excision.

Because bone cannot heal in the presence of necrotic tissue, a *sequestrectomy* may be performed to remove the necrotic bone and allow revascularization of tissue. The excision of dead and infected bone often results in a sizable cavity, or bone defect. Bone *grafts* to repair bone defects are also widely used.

When infected bone is extensively resected, reconstruction with *microvascular bone transfers* or bone graft from donor bone may be done. This procedure is reserved for larger skeletal defects. The most common donor sites are the patient's fibula and iliac crest. Nursing care of the patient after surgery is similar to that for any postoperative patient (see Chapter 16). However, the important difference is that neurovascular (NV) assessments must be done frequently because the patient experiences increased swelling after the surgical procedure. Elevate the affected extremity to increase venous return and thus control swelling. Assess and document the patient's NV status, including:

- Pain
- Movement
- Sensation
- Warmth
- Temperature
- Distal pulses
- Capillary refill (not as reliable as the above indicators)

When the previously described surgical procedures are not appropriate or successful and as a last resort, the affected limb may need to be amputated. The physical and psychological care for a patient who has undergone an amputation is discussed in Chapter 51.

BONE TUMORS

❖ *PATHOPHYSIOLOGY*

Benign Bone Tumors

Bone tumors may be classified as benign (noncancerous) or malignant (cancerous). *Benign* bone tumors are often asymptomatic and may be discovered on routine x-ray examination or as the cause of pathologic fractures. The cause of benign bone tumors is not known. Tumors may arise from several types of tissue. The major classifications include *chondrogenic* tumors (from cartilage), *osteogenic* tumors (from bone), and *fibrogenic* tumors (from fibrous tissue and found most often in children). Although many specific benign tumors have been identified, only the common ones are described here.

The most common benign bone tumor is the *osteochondroma*. Although its onset is usually in childhood, the tumor grows until skeletal maturity and may not be diagnosed until adulthood. The tumor may be a single growth or multiple growths and can occur in any bone. The femur and the tibia are most often involved.

The *chondroma,* or endochondroma, is a lesion of mature hyaline cartilage affecting primarily the hands and the feet. The ribs, sternum, spine, and long bones may also be involved. Chondromas are slow growing and often cause pathologic fractures after minor injury. They are found in people of all ages, occur in both men and women, and can affect any bone.

The origin of the *giant cell tumor* remains uncertain. This lesion is aggressive and can be extensive and may involve surrounding soft tissue. Although classified as benign, giant cell tumors can metastasize (spread) to the lung. The peak incidence occurs in patients in their 30s (McCance et al., 2014).

Malignant Bone Tumors

Malignant (cancerous) bone tumors may be primary or secondary (those that originate in other tissues and metastasize to bone). *Primary tumors* occur most often in people between 10 and 30 years of age and make up a small percentage of bone cancers. As for other forms of cancer, the exact cause of bone cancer is unknown, but genetic and environmental factors are likely causes. *Metastatic lesions* most often occur in the older age-group and account for most bone cancers in adults (McCance et al., 2014).

Osteosarcoma, or osteogenic sarcoma, is the most common type of *primary* malignant bone tumor. More than 50% of cases occur in the distal femur, followed in decreasing order of occurrence by the proximal tibia and humerus.

The tumor is relatively large, causing acute pain and swelling. The involved area is usually warm because the blood flow to the site increases. The center of the tumor is sclerotic from increased osteoblastic activity. The periphery is soft, extending through the bone cortex in the classic sunburst appearance associated with the neoplasm. An inward spread into the medullary canal is also common. Osteosarcoma typically **metastasizes** (spreads), which results in death.

Although *Ewing's sarcoma* is not as common as other tumors, it is the most malignant. Like other primary tumors, it causes pain and swelling. In addition, systemic signs and symptoms, particularly low-grade fever, leukocytosis, and anemia, characterize the lesions. The pelvis and the lower extremity are most often affected. Pelvic involvement is a poor prognostic sign. It often extends into soft tissue. Death results from metastasis to the lungs and other bones. Although the tumor can be seen in patients of any age, it usually occurs in children and young adults in their 20s. Men are affected more often than women (McCance et al., 2014). The reason for this pattern is not known.

In contrast to the patient with osteosarcoma, the patient with *chondrosarcoma* experiences dull, impaired COMFORT and swelling for a long period. The tumor typically affects the pelvis and proximal femur near the diaphysis. Arising from cartilaginous tissue, it destroys bone and often calcifies. The patient with this type of tumor has a better prognosis than one with osteogenic sarcoma. Chondrosarcoma occurs in middle-age and older people, with a slight predominance in men.

Arising from fibrous tissue, *fibrosarcomas* can be divided into subtypes, of which malignant fibrous histiocytoma (MFH) is the most malignant. Usually the clinical presentation of MFH is gradual, without specific symptoms. Local tenderness, with or without a palpable mass, occurs in the long bones of the lower extremity. As with other bone cancers, the lesion can metastasize to the lungs (McCance et al., 2014).

Primary tumors of the prostate, breast, kidney, thyroid, and lung are called *bone-seeking* cancers because they spread to the bone more often than other primary tumors. The vertebrae, pelvis, femur, and ribs are the bone sites commonly affected. Simply stated, primary tumor cells, or seeds, are carried to bone through the bloodstream. *Fragility fractures caused by metastatic bone are a major concern in patient care management.*

❖ INTERPROFESSIONAL COLLABORATIVE CARE

◆ Assessment: Noticing

Assess for pain, the most common symptom of most bone tumors. Pain can range from mild to severe. It can be caused by direct tumor invasion into soft tissue, compressing peripheral nerves, or a resulting pathologic or fragility fracture.

In addition, observe and palpate the suspected involved area. When the tumor affects the lower extremities or the small bones of the hands and feet, local swelling may be detected as the tumor enlarges. In some cases, muscle atrophy or muscle spasm may be present. Marked disability and impaired MOBILITY may occur in those with advanced metastatic bone disease.

In a patient with Ewing's sarcoma, a low-grade fever may occur because of the systemic features of the neoplasm. For this reason, it is often confused with osteomyelitis. Fatigue and pallor resulting from anemia are also common.

In performing a musculoskeletal assessment, inspect the involved area and palpate the mass, if possible, for size and tenderness. In collaboration with the physical and occupational therapists, assess the patient's ability to perform MOBILITY tasks and ADLs.

Patients with malignant bone tumors may be young adults whose productive lives are just beginning. They need strong support systems to help cope with the diagnosis and its treatment. Family, significant others, and health care professionals are major components of the needed support. Determine which systems or resources are available.

Patients often experience a loss of control over their lives when a diagnosis of cancer is made. As a result, they become anxious and fearful about the outcome of their illness. Coping with the diagnosis becomes a challenge. As patients progress through the grieving process, there may be initial denial. Identify the anxiety level and assess the stage or stages of the grieving process. Explore any maladaptive behavior, indicating ineffective coping mechanisms. Chapter 22 further describes the psychosocial assessment for patients with cancer.

Routine x-rays are used to find bone tumors and bone metastasis. CT and MRI are useful for complex anatomic areas, such as the spinal column and sacrum. These tests are particularly helpful in evaluating the extent of soft-tissue involvement. Metastatic lesions may increase or decrease bone density, depending on the amount of osteoblastic and osteoclastic activity.

In some cases a needle bone biopsy may be performed, usually under fluoroscopy to guide the surgeon. Needle biopsy is an ambulatory care procedure with rare complications. After biopsy, the cancer is staged for size and degree of spread. One popular method is the TNM system, based on tumor size and number (T), the presence of cancer cells in lymph nodes (N), and metastasis (spread) to distant sites (M) (see Chapter 21 for further discussion).

The patient with a *malignant* bone tumor typically shows elevated serum alkaline phosphatase (ALP) levels, indicating the body's attempt to form new bone by increasing osteoblastic activity. The patient with Ewing's sarcoma or metastatic bone cancer often has anemia. In addition, leukocytosis is common with Ewing's sarcoma. The progression of Ewing's sarcoma may be evaluated by elevated serum lactic dehydrogenase (LDH) levels.

In some patients with bone metastasis from the breast, kidney, or lung, the serum calcium level is elevated. Massive bone destruction stimulates release of the mineral into the bloodstream. In patients with Ewing's sarcoma and bone metastasis, the erythrocyte sedimentation rate (ESR) may be elevated because of secondary tissue inflammation (Pagana et al., 2017).

◆ *Interventions*

Because the pain is often due to direct primary tumor invasion, treatment is aimed at reducing the size of or removing the tumor. *Benign* or small primary malignant bone tumors are usually completely removed for a potential cure. The expected outcome of treating *metastatic* bone tumors is palliative rather than curative. Palliative therapies may prevent further bone destruction and improve patient function. A combination of nonsurgical and surgical management is used for bone cancer. Collaborate with members of the interprofessional health care team to plan high-quality care to achieve positive patient outcomes. The following discussion focuses on interventions for patients with malignant bone tumors or metastatic bone cancer.

Nonsurgical Management. In addition to analgesics for local pain relief, chemotherapeutic agents and radiation therapy are often administered to shrink the tumor. In patients with spinal involvement, bracing and immobilization with cervical traction may reduce back pain. Interventional radiology techniques are used to decrease vertebral pain and treat compression fractures (see Chapter 51).

Drug Therapy. The primary health care provider (PHCP) may prescribe *chemotherapy* to be given alone or in combination with radiation or surgery. Certain proliferating tumors, such as Ewing's sarcoma, are sensitive to cytotoxic drugs. Others, such as chondrosarcomas, are often totally drug resistant. Chemotherapy seems to work best for small, metastatic tumors and may be administered before or after surgery. In most cases the PHCP prescribes a combination of agents. The drugs selected are determined in part by the primary source of the cancer in metastatic disease. For example, when metastasis occurs from breast cancer, estrogen and progesterone blockers may be used. Chapter 22 describes the general nursing care of patients who receive chemotherapy. *Remember that all chemotherapeutic agents are categorized as high-alert medications* (Institute for Safe Medication Practices, 2017).

Other drugs are given for specific metastatic cancers, depending on the location of the primary site. For example, biologic agents, such as cytokines, are given to stimulate the immune system to recognize and destroy cancer cells, especially in patients with renal cancer. Zoledronic acid (Zometa) and pamidronate (Aredia) are two IV bisphosphonates that are approved for bone metastasis from the breast, lung, and prostate (Burcham & Rosenthal, 2016). These drugs help protect bones and prevent fractures. Although rare, inform patients that osteonecrosis of the jaw may also occur, especially in those who have invasive dental procedures. Monitor associated laboratory tests, such as serum creatinine and electrolytes, because these drugs can be toxic to the kidneys. Bisphosphonates are described earlier in the Osteoporosis section.

Denosumab (Prolia) is a RANKL inhibitor that is also approved for metastatic bone disease (Burcham & Rosenthal, 2016). The drug binds to a protein that is essential for the formation, function, and survival of osteoclasts and is given subcutaneously twice a year. By preventing the protein from activating its receptor, the drug decreases bone loss and increases bone mass and strength. This drug is discussed earlier in the Osteoporosis section.

Radiation Therapy. Radiation, either brachytherapy or external radiation, is used for selected types of malignant tumors. For patients with Ewing's sarcoma and early osteosarcoma, radiation may be the treatment of choice in reducing tumor size and thus pain.

For patients with metastatic disease, radiation is given primarily for palliation. The therapy is directed toward the painful sites to provide a more comfortable life. One or more treatments are given, depending on the extent of disease. With precise planning, radiation therapy can be used with minimal complications. The general nursing care for patients receiving radiation therapy is described in Chapter 22.

Interventional Radiology. Interventional radiologists can perform several noninvasive procedures to help relieve pain in the patient with metastasis to the spinal column. For example, *microwave ablation (MWA)* can be done under moderate sedation or general anesthesia to kill the targeted tissue with heat using microwaves. Most patients have pain relief or control after this ambulatory care procedure.

Surgical Management. Primary bone tumors are usually reduced or removed with surgery, and surgery may be combined with radiation or chemotherapy.

Preoperative Care. In addition to the nature, progression, and extent of the tumor, the patient's age and general health state are considered. Chemotherapy may be administered before surgery.

As for any patient preparing for cancer surgery, the patient with bone cancer needs psychological support from the nurse and other members of the health care team.

⊕ CULTURAL/SPIRITUAL CONSIDERATIONS
Patient-Centered Care [QSEN]

Assess the level of the patient's and family's understanding about the surgery and related treatments. Be present to establish a trusting relationship with the patient and be available for listening. As an advocate, encourage the patient and family to discuss concerns and questions and provide information regarding hospital routines and procedures. Provide hope but be realistic and accurate with information. Assess the patient to determine if religious and/or spiritual support is important. Contact a member of the clergy or a spiritual leader or talk with a clergy member affiliated with the hospital based on the patient's preferences.

Anticipate postoperative needs as much as possible before the patient undergoes surgery. Remind him or her what to expect after surgery and how to help ensure adequate recovery.

Operative Procedures. Wide or radical resection procedures are used for patients with bone sarcomas to salvage the affected limb. Wide excision is removal of the lesion surrounded by an intact cuff of normal tissue and leads to cure of low-grade tumors only. A radical resection includes removal of the lesion, the entire muscle, bone, and other tissues directly involved. It is the procedure used for high-grade tumors.

Large bone defects that result from tumor removal may require either:

- Total joint replacements with prosthetic implants, either whole or partial
- Custom metallic implants
- Allografts from the iliac crest, rib, or fibula

As an alternative to total replacement, an allograft may be implanted with internal fixation for patients who do not have metastases. This is a common procedure for sarcomas of the proximal femur. Allograft procedures for the knee are also performed, particularly in young adults. Preoperative chemotherapy is given to enhance the likelihood of success. **Allografts** with adjacent tendons and ligaments are harvested from cadavers and can be frozen or freeze-dried for a prolonged period. The graft is fixed with a series of bolts, screws, or plates.

Postoperative Care. The surgical incision for a limb salvage procedure is often extensive. A pressure dressing with wound suction is typically maintained for several days. The patient who has undergone a limb salvage procedure has some degree of impaired physical MOBILITY and a self-care deficit. The nature and extent of the alterations depend on the location and extent of the surgery.

> **! NURSING SAFETY PRIORITY** **QSEN**
>
> **Action Alert**
>
> For patients who have allografts, observe for signs of hemorrhage, infection, and fracture. Report these complications to the surgeon immediately.

After upper-extremity surgery, the patient can engage in active-assistive exercises by using the opposite hand to help achieve motions such as forward flexion and abduction of the shoulder. Continuous passive motion (CPM) using a CPM machine may be initiated as early as the first postoperative day for either upper-extremity or lower-extremity procedures.

After lower-extremity surgery, the emphasis is on strengthening the quadriceps muscles by using passive and active motion when possible. Maintaining muscle tone is an important prerequisite to weight bearing, which progresses from toe touch or partial weight bearing to full weight bearing by 3 months after surgery. Coordinate the patient's plan of care for ambulation and muscle strengthening with the physical therapist.

The patient who has had a bone graft may have a cast or other supportive device for several months. Weight bearing is prohibited until there is evidence that the graft is incorporated into the adjacent bone tissue.

During the recovery phase, the patient may also need assistance with ADLs, particularly if the surgery involves the upper extremity. Assist if needed but, at the same time, encourage the patient to do as much as possible unaided. Some patients need assistive/adaptive devices for a short period while they are healing. Coordinate the patient's plan of care for promoting independence in ADLs with the occupational therapist.

Surrounding tissues, including nerves and blood vessels, may be removed during surgery. Vascular grafting is common, but the lost nerve(s) is (are) usually not replaced. Assess the neurovascular status of the affected extremity and hand or foot every 1 to 2 hours immediately after surgery. Splinting or casting of the limb may also cause neurovascular (NV) compromise and needs to be checked for proper placement.

In addition to needing emotional support to cope with physical disabilities, the patient may need help coping with the surgery and its effects. Help identify available support systems as soon as possible.

As a result of most of the surgical procedures, the patient experiences an altered body image. Suggest ways to minimize cosmetic changes. For example, a lowered shoulder can be covered by a custom-made pad worn under clothing. The patient can cover lower-extremity defects with pants.

Advocate for the patient and the family to promote the physician-patient relationship. For example, the patient may not completely understand the medical or surgical treatment plan but may hesitate to question the physician. The nurse's intervention can increase communication, which is essential in successful management of the patient with cancer.

> **? NCLEX EXAMINATION CHALLENGE 50-3**
>
> **Psychosocial Integrity**
>
> A client recently diagnosed with primary bone cancer states, "My life is over. I'll never get married now!" What is the nurse's **best** action at this time?
> A. Refer the client to a clergy member or spiritual leader.
> B. Ask the client what is meant by that statement.
> C. Listen while the client expresses feelings.
> D. Provide hope that marriage will happen.

Care Coordination and Transition Management

Home Care Management. After medical treatment for a primary bone tumor, the patient is usually managed at home with follow-up care. The patient with metastatic disease may remain in the home or, when home support is not available, may be admitted to a long-term care facility for extended or hospice care. Coordinate the patient's transition and continuity of care with the case manager and other interprofessional health team members, depending on the patient's needs.

In collaboration with the occupational therapist, evaluate the patient's home environment for structural barriers that may hinder MOBILITY. The patient may be discharged with a cast, walker, crutches, or a wheelchair. Assess his or her support system for availability of assistance if needed.

Accessibility to eating and toileting facilities is essential to promote ADL independence. Because the patient with metastatic disease is susceptible to pathologic fractures, potential hazards that may contribute to falls or injury should be removed.

Self-Management Education. For the patient receiving intermittent chemotherapy or radiation on an ambulatory care basis, emphasize the importance of keeping appointments. Review the expected side and toxic effects of the drugs with the patient and family. Teach how to treat less serious side effects and when to contact the health care provider. If the drugs are administered at home via long-term IV catheter, explain and demonstrate the care involved with daily dressing changes and potential catheter complications. Chapter 13 describes the health teaching required for a patient receiving infusion therapy at home.

If the patient has undergone surgery, he or she has a wound and limited MOBILITY. Teach the patient, family, and/or significant others how to care for the wound. Help the patient learn how to perform ADLs and mobility activities independently for self-management. Coordinate with the physical and occupational therapists to assist in ADL teaching and provide or recommend assistive and adaptive devices, if necessary. The physical therapist also teaches the proper use of ambulatory aids, such as crutches, and exercises.

Pain management can be a major challenge, particularly for the patient with metastatic bone disease. Discuss the various options for pain relief, including relaxation and music therapy. Emphasize the importance of techniques that worked during hospitalization. See Chapter 4 for cancer pain assessment and management.

The patient with bone cancer may fear that the malignancy will return. Acknowledge this fear but reinforce confidence in the health care team and medical treatment chosen. Mutually establish realistic outcomes regarding returning to work and participating in recreational activities. Encourage the patient to resume a functional lifestyle but caution that it should be gradual. Certain activities, such as participating in sports, may be prohibited.

Help the patient with advanced metastatic bone disease prepare for death. The nurse and other support personnel assist the patient through the stages of death and dying. Identify resources that can help the patient write a will, visit with distant family members, or do whatever he or she thinks is needed for a peaceful death. Chapter 7 describes end-of-life care in detail.

Health Care Resources. In addition to family and significant others, cancer support groups are helpful to the patient with bone cancer. Some organizations, such as *I Can Cope,* provide information and emotional support. Others, such as *CanSurmount,* are geared more toward patient and family education. The American Cancer Society (www.cancer.org) and the Canadian Cancer Society (www.cancer.ca) can also provide education and resources for patients and families.

The hospital staff nurse, discharge planner, or case manager also ensures that follow-up care, including nursing care and physical or occupational therapy, is available in the home. The patient with terminal cancer may choose to become part of a hospice program as described in Chapter 7.

DISORDERS OF THE HAND

Specific localized health problems affecting the hand or part of the hand may affect the musculoskeletal system. Two of these problems are discussed here. Dupuytren's contracture, or deformity, is a slowly progressive thickening of the palmar fascia, resulting in flexion contracture of the fourth (ring) and fifth (little) fingers of the hand (Fig. 50-3). The third or middle finger is occasionally affected. Although Dupuytren's contracture is a common problem, the cause is unknown. It usually occurs in older Euro-American men, tends to occur in families, is most common in people with diabetes, and can be bilateral.

When function becomes impaired, surgical release is required. A partial or selective fasciectomy (cutting of fascia) is performed. After removal of the surgical dressing, a splint may be used. Nursing care is similar to that for the patient with carpal tunnel repair (see Chapter 51).

A ganglion is a round, benign cyst, often found on a wrist or foot joint or tendon. The synovium surrounding the tendon degenerates, allowing the tendon sheath tissue to become weak and distended. Ganglia are painless on palpation, but they can cause joint discomfort after prolonged joint use or minor trauma or strain. The lesion can rapidly disappear and then recur. Ganglia are most likely to develop in people between 15 and 50 years of age. With local or regional anesthesia in a physician's office or clinic, the fluid within the cyst can be aspirated through a small needle. A cortisone injection may follow. If the cyst is very large, it is removed using a small incision. Teach patients to avoid strenuous activity for 48 hours after surgery and report any signs of inflammation to their health care provider.

DISORDERS OF THE FOOT

Common Foot Deformities

The hallux valgus deformity is a common foot problem in which the great toe drifts laterally at the first metatarsophalangeal (MTP) joint (Fig. 50-4). The first metatarsal head becomes enlarged, resulting in a bunion. As the deviation worsens, the bony enlargement causes pain, particularly when shoes are worn. Women are affected more often than men. Hallux valgus often occurs as a result of poorly fitted shoes, in particular those with narrow toes and high heels. Other causes include osteoarthritis, rheumatoid arthritis, and family history.

For some patients who are of advanced age or are not surgical candidates, custom-made shoes can be made to fit the deformed feet and provide COMFORT and support. A plaster mold is made to conform to each foot from which shoes can be made. Teach the patient to consult with a podiatrist or foot clinic to be evaluated for custom shoes.

The surgical procedure, a simple bunionectomy, involves removal of the bony overgrowth and bursa and realignment.

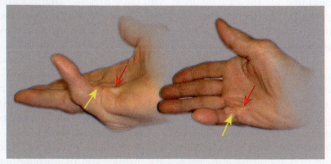

FIG. 50-3 Dupuytren's contracture. (Courtesy of School of Medicine, SUNY Stony Brook, NY. In Wolfe, S.W., Hotchkiss, R.N., Pederson, W.C., & Kozin, S.H. [2011]: *Green's operative hand surgery.* [6th ed.]. Philadelphia: Churchill Livingstone.)

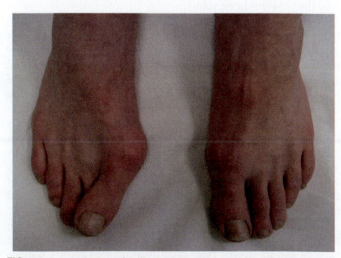

FIG. 50-4 Appearance of hallux valgus with a bunion. (From Johal, S., Sawalha, S., & Pasapula, C. [2010]. Post-traumatic acute hallux valgus: A case report. *The Foot, 29*[2], 87-89.)

When other toe deformities accompany the condition or if the bony overgrowth is large, several osteotomies, or bone resections, may be performed. Fusions may also be performed. Screws or wires are often inserted to stabilize the bones in the great toe and first metatarsal during the healing process. If both feet are affected, one foot is usually treated at a time. Surgery usually is performed as a same-day procedure. Be sure to assess neurovascular status and pain control before allowing the patient to be discharged.

Most patients are allowed partial weight bearing while wearing an orthopedic boot or shoe. Walking is difficult because the feet bear body weight. The healing time after surgery may be more than 6 to 12 weeks because the feet receive less blood flow than other parts of the body as a result of their distance from the heart.

Often patients have hammertoes and hallux valgus deformities at the same time. As shown in Fig. 50-5, a hammertoe is the dorsiflexion of any MTP joint with plantar flexion of the proximal interphalangeal (PIP) joint next to it. The second toe is most often affected. As the deformity worsens, uncomfortable corns may develop on the dorsal side of the toe, and calluses may appear on the plantar surface. Patients are uncomfortable when wearing shoes and walking.

Hammertoe may be treated by surgical correction of the deformity with osteotomies (bone resections) and the insertion of wires or screws for fixation. The postoperative course is similar to that for the patient with hallux valgus repair. The patient uses crutches or a walker until full weight bearing is allowed several weeks after surgery.

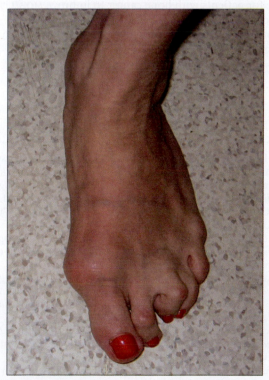

FIG. 50-5 Hammertoe of the second metatarsophalangeal joint. (From Hochberg, M., Silman, A., Smolen, J., Weinblatt, M., & Weisman, M. [2011]. *Rheumatology* [5th ed.]. Philadelphia: Mosby.)

⚡ NCLEX EXAMINATION CHALLENGE 50-4
Physiological Integrity

The nurse is caring for a client immediately after a bunionectomy. What is the nurse's **priority** action?
A. Relieve or reduce the patient's pain.
B. Assess neurovascular status in the affected foot.
C. Apply a hot compress to the surgical area.
D. Check the surgical dressing for intactness.

Plantar Fasciitis

Plantar fasciitis is an inflammation of the plantar fascia, which is located in the area of the arch of the foot. It is often seen in middle-age and older adults, as well as in athletes, especially runners. Obesity is also a contributing factor. Patients report severe pain in the arch of the foot, especially when getting out of bed. The pain is worsened with weight bearing. Although most patients have unilateral plantar fasciitis, the problem can affect both feet (McCance et al., 2014).

Most patients respond to conservative management, which includes rest, ice, stretching exercises, strapping of the foot to maintain the arch, shoes with good support, and orthotics. NSAIDs or steroids may be needed to control impaired COMFORT and inflammation. If conservative measures are unsuccessful, endoscopic surgery to remove the inflamed tissue may be required. Teach the patient about the importance of adhering to the treatment plan and coordinating care with the physical therapist for instruction in exercise.

Other Problems of the Foot

Table 50-4 lists other common foot problems and how they are managed. Although patients are usually not hospitalized for these conditions, the nurse may recognize a foot disorder and alert the physician. Even small deformities or other foot deformities can be very annoying and painful for the patient and may hinder ambulation and interfere with ADLs.

TABLE 50-4 Treatment of Common Foot Problems	
DESCRIPTION/CAUSE	**TREATMENT**
Corn	
Induration and thickening of the skin caused by friction and pressure; painful conical mass	Surgical removal by podiatrist
Callus	
Flat, poorly defined mass on the sole over a bony prominence caused by pressure	Padding and lanolin creams; overall good skin hygiene
Ingrown Nail	
Nail sliver penetration of the skin, causing inflammation	Removal of sliver by podiatrist; warm soaks; antibiotic ointment
Hypertrophic Ungual Labium	
Chronic hypertrophy of nail lip caused by improper nail trimming; results from untreated ingrown nail	Surgical removal of necrotic nail and skin; treatment of secondary infection

GET READY FOR THE NCLEX® EXAMINATION!

KEY POINTS

Review these Key Points for each NCLEX Examination Client Needs Category.

Safe and Effective Care Environment
- Collaborate with interprofessional team members when assessing patients with osteoporosis for risk for falls. **QSEN: Teamwork and Collaboration**
- Teach the patient with CELLULAR REGULATION problems (e.g., osteoporosis) and his or her family about evidence-based home safety modifications and the need to create a hazard-free environment. **QSEN: Safety; Evidence-Based Practice**
- Refer to The Joint Commission for information about National Patient Safety Goals related to fall injury prevention.

Health Promotion and Maintenance
- Develop a teaching plan for patients at risk for osteoporosis to minimize risk factors, such as stopping smoking, decreasing alcohol intake, exercising regularly, and increasing dietary calcium and vitamin D foods; for many patients, calcium and vitamin D supplementation is needed to achieve normal serum levels (see Chart 50-1). **QSEN: Informatics**
- Remind patients at risk for osteoporosis to have regular screening tests, such as the DXA scan, as needed.
- Refer patients with musculoskeletal problems to appropriate community resources, such as the National Osteoporosis Foundation (NOF).

Psychosocial Integrity
- Assess the patient's and family's responses to a diagnosis of bone cancer and treatment options. Be aware that they will progress through the grieving process due to loss.

Physiological Integrity
- Recognize that osteoporosis can be primary or secondary (see Table 50-2).

- Remind patients taking bisphosphonates (BPs) to take them early in the morning, at least 30 to 60 minutes before breakfast, with a full glass of water, and to remain sitting upright during that time to prevent esophagitis, a common complication of BP therapy (also see Chart 50-2).
- Recall that most patients are unaware that they have osteoporosis until they experience a fracture, the most common complication of the disease.
- Recognize that patients with osteopenia and osteoporosis usually have decreased calcium and vitamin D levels.
- Assess for signs and symptoms of osteomyelitis as outlined in Chart 50-3.
- Use clinical judgment to prioritize care for patients with osteomyelitis, including maintaining Contact Precautions for open wounds. For patients having surgical intervention, assess the affected extremity for neurovascular status to ensure adequate tissue PERFUSION. **Clinical Judgment**
- For patients who have surgery for bone cancer, report and document postoperative signs and symptoms of infection, dislocation, or neurovascular compromise to the surgeon promptly. **QSEN: Safety; Informatics**
- Remember that bone tumors can be benign or malignant.
- Remember that severe chronic pain is a priority for patients with metastatic bone disease.
- Be aware that even minor hand and foot problems can be very painful. Common foot problems are described in Table 50-4.
- In collaboration with the health care team (physical therapist, occupational therapist, neurologist), provide supportive care for patients with bone cancer to improve MOBILITY and function. **QSEN: Teamwork and Collaboration**
- Foot disorders can be treated with custom-made shoes or surgery to repair deformities and promote mobility.

SELECTED BIBLIOGRAPHY

Asterisk indicates a classic or definitive work on this subject.

Alvaro, R., D'Agostino, F., Cittadini, N., Zannetti, E. B., Rao, C., Feola, M., et al. (2015). Can educational interventions improve osteoporotic women's adherence to treatment? *Orthopaedic Nursing, 34*(6), 340–355.

Burcham, J. L. R., & Rosenthal, L. D. (2016). *Lehne's pharmacology for nursing care* (9th ed.). St. Louis: Elsevier.

*Chang, S. F., Yang, R. S., Chung, U. L., Chen, C. M., & Cheng, M. H. (2010). Perception of risk factors and DXA T-score among at-risk females of osteoporosis. *Journal of Clinical Nursing, 19*(13–14), 1795–1802.

*Crawford, A., & Harris, H. (2012). Balancing act: Calcium and phosphorus. *Nursing, 42*(1), 36–42.

Evenson, A. L., & Sanders, G. F. (2016). Educational intervention impact on osteoporosis knowledge, health beliefs, self-efficacy, dietary calcium, and vitamin D intakes in young adults. *Orthopaedic Nursing, 35*(1), 30–38.

Fasolino, T., & Whitright, T. (2015). A pilot study to identify modifiable and nonmodifiable variables associated with osteopenia and osteoporosis in men. *Orthopaedic Nursing, 34*(5), 289–295.

Fitton, L., Astroth, K. S., & Wilson, D. (2015). Changing measures to evaluate changing bone. *Orthopaedic Nursing, 34*(1), 12–20.

Institute for Safe Medication Practices. (2017). *ISMPs list of high-alert medications.* www.ismp.org/Tools/highalertmedications.pdf.

Jarvis, C. (2014). *Physical examination & health assessment* (7th ed.). St. Louis: Elsevier Saunders.

McCance, K., Huether, S., Brashers, V., & Rote, N. (2014). *Pathophysiology: The biologic basis for disease in adults and children* (7th ed.). St. Louis: Mosby.

National Osteoporosis Foundation (NOF) (2017). *Clinician's guide to prevention and treatment of osteoporosis.* Washington, DC: Author.

Pagana, K. D., Pagana, T. J., & Pagana, T. N. (2017). *Mosby's diagnostic and laboratory test reference* (13th ed.). St. Louis: Mosby.

Pagana, K. D., Pagana, T. J., & Pike-MacDonald, S. A. (2013). *Mosby's Canadian manual of diagnostic and laboratory tests.* Toronto, ON: Elsevier.

Saccomano, S. J., & Ferrara, L. R. (2015). Fall prevention in older adults. *Nurse Practitioner, 40*(6), 40–47.

Smith, M. A. (2015). The epidemiology of methicillin-resistant *Staphylococcus aureus* in orthopaedics. *Orthopaedic Nursing, 34*(3), 128–137.

CHAPTER 51

Care of Patients With Musculoskeletal Trauma

Roberta Goff and Donna D. Ignatavicius

PRIORITY AND INTERRELATED CONCEPTS

The priority concepts for this chapter are:
- MOBILITY
- PERFUSION

✳ The MOBILITY concept exemplar for this chapter is Fractures, p. 1032.

✳ The PERFUSION concept exemplar for this chapter is Amputations, p. 1050.

The interrelated concepts for this chapter are:
- TISSUE INTEGRITY
- COMFORT
- CLOTTING
- SENSORY PERCEPTION

LEARNING OUTCOMES

Safe and Effective Care Environment

1. Collaborate with the interprofessional health care team to ensure safe, quality care for patients with fractures and amputations.
2. Prioritize evidence-based nursing interventions for patients with fractures and amputations to promote MOBILITY, maintain PERFUSION, and increase COMFORT.
3. Prioritize nursing interventions to help prevent and monitor for complications related to fractures and/or amputations, including hemorrhage, decreased PERFUSION, increased CLOTTING, decreased SENSORY PERCEPTION, and infection due to impaired TISSUE INTEGRITY.

Health Promotion and Maintenance

4. Identify community resources for amputations for patients and their families.
5. Teach the public about ways to prevent fractures and other musculoskeletal injuries to promote safety.
6. Plan transition management and care coordination for patients with fractures and amputations.

Psychosocial Integrity

7. Assess the patient's and family's reaction to changes in body image and altered lifestyle resulting from musculoskeletal trauma.

Physiological Integrity

8. Compare and contrast nursing care for open versus closed fractures and their potential complications.
9. Use clinical judgment to provide emergency care for the patient with an extremity fracture.
10. Interpret findings from a focused neurovascular assessment for patients experiencing fractures or amputations.
11. Delineate safe, evidence-based nursing care needed to maintain casts for patients with fractures.
12. Plan nursing care needed to maintain traction and external fixation for patients with fractures.
13. Develop an evidence-based postoperative plan of care for a patient after hip fracture repair.
14. Outline emergency care for people who experience a traumatic amputation.
15. Differentiate the patient-centered care needed to manage complex regional pain syndrome and phantom limb pain.
16. Prioritize care for patients with common types of soft-tissue injuries, such as carpal tunnel syndrome and common knee injuries.

Musculoskeletal trauma accounts for about two thirds of all injuries and is one of the primary causes of disability in the United States. It ranges from simple muscle strain to multiple bone fractures with severe soft-tissue damage.

Fractures and other musculoskeletal trauma impair a patient's MOBILITY in varying degrees, depending on the severity and extent of the injury. These injuries can also result in impaired COMFORT and SENSORY PERCEPTION because of pressure on nerve endings from edema. In some cases, peripheral nerves are directly damaged as a result of musculoskeletal injury. Amputations result in impaired TISSUE INTEGRITY and are often performed because of inadequate arterial PERFUSION caused by chronic disease. These health concepts are reviewed in Chapter 2 of this text.

✳ MOBILITY CONCEPT EXEMPLAR Fractures

❖ PATHOPHYSIOLOGY

A fracture is a break or disruption in the continuity of a bone that often affects MOBILITY and causes impaired COMFORT. It can occur anywhere in the body and at any age. All fractures have the same basic pathophysiologic mechanism and require similar patient-centered, interprofessional collaborative care, regardless of fracture type or location.

Classification of Fractures

A fracture can be classified by the extent of the break:
- *Complete fracture.* The break is across the entire width of the bone in such a way that the bone is divided into two distinct sections. If bone alignment is altered or disrupted, the fracture is also referred to as a *displaced* fracture. The ends of bone sections of a displaced fracture are more likely to damage surrounding nerves, blood vessels, and other soft tissues.
- *Incomplete fracture.* The fracture does not divide the bone into two portions because the break is through only part of the bone. This type of fracture is not typically displaced.

A fracture can also be described by the extent of associated soft-tissue damage: open (or compound) or closed (or simple) (Fig. 51-1). The skin surface over the broken bone is disrupted in a *compound* fracture, which causes an external wound. These fractures are often graded to define the extent of tissue damage. A *simple* fracture does not extend through the skin and therefore has no visible wound.

In addition to being identified by type, fractures are described by their cause. A fragility fracture (also known as a pathologic or spontaneous fracture) occurs after minimal trauma to a bone that has been weakened by disease. For example, a patient with bone cancer or osteoporosis can easily have a fragility fracture (see Chapter 50 for a discussion of these disorders). A fatigue (stress) fracture results from excessive strain and stress on the bone. This problem is commonly seen in recreational and professional athletes. Compression fractures are produced by a loading force applied to the long axis of cancellous bone. They commonly occur in the vertebrae of older patients with osteoporosis and are extremely painful.

Stages of Bone Healing

When a bone is fractured, the body immediately begins the healing process to repair the injury and restore the body's

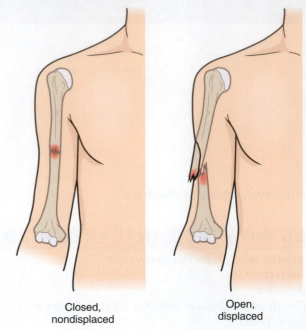

Closed, nondisplaced   Open, displaced

FIG. 51-1 Common types of fractures.

equilibrium. Fractures heal in five stages that are a continuous process and not single stages.
- In stage one, within 24 to 72 hours after the injury, a hematoma forms at the site of the fracture because bone is extremely vascular.
- Stage two occurs in 3 days to 2 weeks when granulation tissue begins to invade the hematoma. This then prompts the formation of fibrocartilage, providing the foundation for bone healing.
- Stage three of bone healing occurs as a result of vascular and cellular proliferation. The fracture site is surrounded by new vascular tissue known as a *callus* (within 3 to 6 weeks). Callus formation is the beginning of a nonbony union.
- As healing continues in stage four, the callus is gradually resorbed and transformed into bone. This stage usually takes 3 to 8 weeks.
- During the fifth and final stage of healing, consolidation and remodeling of bone continue to meet mechanical demands. This process may start as early as 4 to 6 weeks after fracture and can continue for up to 1 year, depending on the severity of the injury and the age and health of the patient. Fig. 51-2 summarizes the stages of bone healing.

In young, healthy adult bone, healing takes about 4 to 6 weeks. In the older person who has reduced bone mass, healing time is lengthened. Complete healing often takes 3 months or longer in people who are older than 70 years. Other factors also affect healing. Examples include the severity of the trauma, the type of bone injured, how the fracture is managed, infections at the fracture site, and ischemic or avascular necrosis (AVN), also called osteonecrosis.

Complications of Fractures

Regardless of the type or location of the fracture, several limb- and life-threatening acute and chronic complications can result from the injury. Signs and symptoms of beginning

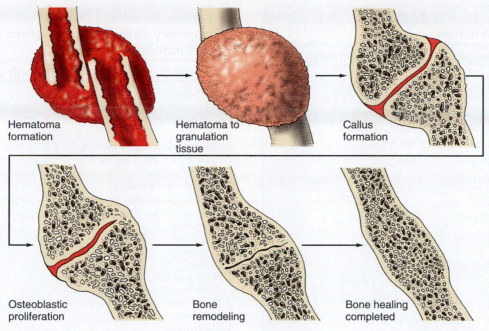

Hematoma formation

Hematoma to granulation tissue

Callus formation

Osteoblastic proliferation

Bone remodeling

Bone healing completed

FIG. 51-2 Stages of bone healing.

CONSIDERATIONS FOR OLDER ADULTS
Patient-Centered Care QSEN

Bone healing is often affected by the aging process. Bone formation and strength rely on adequate nutrition. Calcium, phosphorus, vitamin D, and protein are necessary for the production of new bone (see Chapter 50). For women, the loss of estrogen after menopause decreases the body's ability to form new bone tissue. Chronic diseases can also affect the rate at which bone heals. For instance, peripheral vascular diseases, such as arteriosclerosis, reduce arterial circulation to bone. Thus the bone receives less oxygen and fewer nutrients, both of which are needed for repair.

complications must be treated early to prevent serious consequences. In some cases, careful monitoring and assessment can prevent these complications from occurring or worsening:

- Acute compartment syndrome
- Crush syndrome
- Hemorrhage and hypovolemic shock
- Fat embolism syndrome
- Venous thromboembolism
- Infection
- Chronic complications, such as ischemic necrosis, delayed union, and complex regional pain syndrome (CRPS)

Acute Compartment Syndrome. Compartments are areas in the body in which muscles, blood vessels, and nerves are contained within fascia. Most compartments are located in the extremities. **Fascia** is an inelastic tissue that surrounds groups of muscles, blood vessels, and nerves in the body. **Acute compartment syndrome (ACS)** is a serious, limb-threatening condition in which increased pressure within one or more compartments reduces circulation to the area. The most common sites for this problem in patients with musculoskeletal trauma are the compartments in the lower leg (tibial fractures) and forearm (Hershey, 2013).

The pathophysiologic changes of increased compartment pressure are sometimes referred to as the *ischemia-edema cycle.* Capillaries within the muscle dilate, which raises capillary (arterial) and venous pressure (Hershey, 2013). Capillaries become more permeable because of the release of histamine by the ischemic muscle tissue, and venous drainage decreases. As a result, plasma proteins leak into the interstitial fluid space, and edema occurs. Edema increases pressure on nerve endings and causes severe pain. The pain experienced is greater than expected for the nature of the injury. PERFUSION to the area is reduced, and further ischemia results. SENSORY PERCEPTION deficits or paresthesia generally appears before changes in vascular or motor signs. The color of the tissue pales, and pulses begin to weaken but rarely disappear. The affected area is usually palpably tense, and pain occurs with passive motion of the extremity. If the condition is not treated, cyanosis, tingling, numbness, paresis, and necrosis can occur. Chart 51-1 summarizes the sequence of pathophysiologic events in compartment syndrome and the associated clinical assessment findings.

The pressure to the compartment can be from an external or internal source, but fracture is present in 75% of all cases of ACS (Hershey, 2013). Tight, bulky dressings and casts are examples of *external* pressure. Blood or fluid accumulation in the compartment is a common source of *internal* pressure. Crush injuries or overuse injuries are also common causes. The injury or trauma causing the problem is above the compartment involved, which decreases blood flow to the more distal area of injury. ACS is not limited to patients with musculoskeletal problems. It can also occur in those with severe burns, extensive insect bites or snakebites, or massive infiltration of IV fluids. In these situations, edema increases internal pressure in one or more compartments.

Problems resulting from compartment syndrome include infection, persistent motor weakness in the affected extremity, contracture, and myoglobinuric renal failure. In extreme cases, amputation becomes necessary (Hershey, 2013).

CHART 51-1 Key Features
Compartment Syndrome

PHYSIOLOGIC CHANGE	CLINICAL FINDINGS
Increased compartment pressure	No change
Increased capillary permeability	Edema
Release of histamine	Increased edema
Increased blood flow to area	Pulses present Pink tissue
Pressure on nerve endings	Pain
Increased tissue pressure	Referred pain to compartment
Decreased tissue perfusion	Increased edema
Decreased oxygen to tissues	Pallor
Increased production of lactic acid	Unequal pulses Flexed posture
Anaerobic metabolism	Cyanosis
Vasodilation	Increased edema
Increased blood flow	Tense muscle swelling
Increased tissue pressure	Tingling Numbness
Increased edema	Paresthesia
Muscle ischemia	Severe pain unrelieved by drugs
Tissue necrosis	Paresis/paralysis

CHART 51-2 Key Features
Pulmonary Emboli: Fat Embolism Versus Blood Clot Embolism

FAT EMBOLISM	BLOOD CLOT EMBOLISM
Definition	
Obstruction of the pulmonary vascular bed by fat globules	Obstruction of the pulmonary artery by a blood clot or clots
Origin	
95% from fractures of the long bones; occurs usually within 48 hr of injury	85% from deep vein thrombosis in the legs or pelvis; can occur anytime
Assessment Findings	
Altered mental status (earliest sign) Increased respirations, pulse, temperature Chest pain Dyspnea Crackles Decreased SaO_2 Petechiae (50%-60%) Retinal hemorrhage (not common) Mild thrombocytopenia	Same as for fat embolism, except no petechiae
Treatment	
Bedrest Gentle handling Oxygen Hydration (IV fluids) Possibly steroid therapy Fracture immobilization	Preventive measures (e.g., leg exercises, antiembolism stockings, SCDs) Bedrest Oxygen Possibly mechanical ventilation Anticoagulants Thrombolytics Possible surgery: pulmonary embolectomy, vena cava umbrella

SaO_2, Arterial oxygen saturation; *SCD*, sequential compression device.

Infection from necrosis may become severe enough that amputation of the limb is needed. *Motor weakness* from injured nerves is not reversible, and the patient may require an orthotic device for assistance in mobility. Volkmann's *contractures* of the forearm, which can begin within 12 hours of the pressure increase, result from shortening of the ischemic muscle and nerve involvement.

Hemorrhage and Hypovolemic Shock. Bone is very vascular. Therefore bleeding is a risk with bone injury. In addition, trauma can cut nearby arteries and cause hemorrhage, resulting in rapidly developing hypovolemic shock. (The pathophysiology of hypovolemic shock is described in Chapter 37.)

Fat Embolism Syndrome. **Fat embolism syndrome (FES)** is another serious complication in which fat globules are released from the yellow bone marrow into the bloodstream within 12 to 48 hours after an injury or other illness (mechanical theory). These globules clog small blood vessels that supply vital organs, most commonly the lungs, and impair organ PERFUSION. The biochemical theory for FES may be considered as a separate cause or as an additive process to the mechanical theory. The embolized fat degrades into free fatty acids and C-reactive protein, which results in capillary leakage, lipid and platelet aggregation, and clot formation (Hershey, 2013).

FES usually results from fractures or fracture repair but occasionally is seen in patients who have a total joint replacement. It may also occur, although less often, in those with pancreatitis, osteomyelitis, blunt trauma, or sickle cell disease.

The problem can occur at any age or in either gender, but young men between ages 20 and 40 years and older adults between ages 70 and 80 years are at the greatest risk. Patients with fractured hips have the highest risk, but FES is also common in those with fractures of the pelvis within 24 to 72 hours after injury or surgery (Hershey, 2013).

The earliest signs and symptoms of FES are a low arterial oxygen level (hypoxemia), dyspnea, and tachypnea (increased respirations). Headache, lethargy, agitation, confusion, decreased level of consciousness, seizures, and vision changes may follow (Hershey, 2013). Nonpalpable, red-brown **petechiae**—a macular, measles-like rash—may appear over the neck, upper arms, and/or chest. This rash is a classic manifestation but is usually the last sign to develop (Hershey, 2013).

Abnormal laboratory findings include:
- Decreased PaO_2 level (often below 60 mm Hg)
- Increased erythrocyte sedimentation rate (ESR)
- Decreased serum calcium levels
- Decreased red blood cell and platelet counts
- Increased serum level of lipids

These changes in blood values are poorly understood, but they aid in diagnosis of the condition.

The chest x-ray often shows bilateral infiltrates but may be normal. The chest CT often reveals a patchy distribution of opacities. An MRI of the brain can show evidence of neurologic deficits from hypoxemia. FES can result in respiratory failure or death, often from pulmonary edema. When the lungs are affected, the complication may be misdiagnosed as a pulmonary embolism from a blood clot (Chart 51-2).

Venous Thromboembolism. Venous thromboembolism (VTE) includes deep vein thrombosis (DVT) and its major complication, pulmonary embolism (PE). It is the most common complication of lower-extremity surgery or trauma and the most often fatal complication of musculoskeletal surgery. Factors that make patients with fractures most likely to develop VTE include:

- Cancer or chemotherapy
- Surgical procedure longer than 30 minutes
- History of smoking
- Obesity
- Heart disease
- Prolonged immobility
- Oral contraceptives or hormones
- History of VTE complications
- Older adults (especially with hip fractures)

The pathophysiology and management of VTE are described in Chapter 36.

Infection. Whenever there is trauma to tissues, the body's defense system is disrupted. Wound infections are the most common type of infection resulting from orthopedic trauma. They range from superficial skin infections to deep wound abscesses. Infection can also be caused by implanted hardware used to repair a fracture surgically, such as screws, pins, plates, or rods. Clostridia infections can result in gas gangrene or tetanus and can prevent the bone from healing properly.

Bone infection, or **osteomyelitis,** is most common with open fractures in which skin integrity is lost and after surgical repair of a fracture (see Chapter 50 for discussion of osteomyelitis). For patients experiencing this type of trauma, the risk for hospital-acquired infections is increased. These infections are common, and many are from multidrug-resistant organisms, such as methicillin-resistant *Staphylococcus aureus* (MRSA). Reducing MRSA infections is a primary desired outcome for all health care agencies.

Chronic Complications. Avascular necrosis, delayed bone healing, and chronic regional pain syndrome are later complications of musculoskeletal trauma. Blood supply to the bone is disrupted, causing decreased PERFUSION and death of bone tissue, or *avascular necrosis*. This problem is most often a complication of hip fractures or any fracture in which there is displacement of bone. Surgical repair of fractures also can cause necrosis because the hardware can interfere with circulation. Patients on long-term corticosteroid therapy, such as prednisone, are also at high risk for ischemic necrosis.

Delayed union is a fracture that has not healed within 6 months of injury. Some fractures never achieve union; that is, they never completely heal *(nonunion)*. Others heal incorrectly *(malunion)*. These problems are most common in patients with tibial fractures, fractures that involve many treatment techniques (e.g., cast, traction), and pathologic fractures. Union may also be delayed or not achieved in the older patient due to poor bone health. If bone does not heal, he or she typically has chronic pain and impaired MOBILITY from deformity.

Complex regional pain syndrome (CRPS), formerly called **reflex sympathetic dystrophy (RSD),** is a poorly understood dysfunction of the central and peripheral nervous systems that leads to severe, chronic pain. Genetic factors may play a role in the development of this devastating complication. CRPS most often results from fractures or other traumatic musculoskeletal injury and commonly occurs in the feet and hands. In some cases, specific nerve injuries are present, but in others no injury can be identified. A triad of signs and symptoms is present, including abnormalities of the autonomic nervous system (changes in color, temperature, and sensitivity of skin over the affected area, excessive sweating, edema), motor symptoms (paresis, muscle spasms, loss of function), and SENSORY PERCEPTION symptoms (intense burning pain that becomes intractable [unrelenting]).

Over time, spotty and diffuse osteoporosis can be seen on x-ray examination. Timing of diagnosis is important because the syndrome is more difficult to treat when diagnosed in the later stages.

Etiology and Genetic Risk

The primary cause of a fracture is trauma from a motor vehicle crash or fall, especially in older adults. The trauma may be a direct blow to the bone or an indirect force from muscle contractions or pulling forces on the bone. Sports, vigorous exercise, and malnutrition are contributing factors. Bone diseases, such as osteoporosis, increase the risk for a fracture in older adults (see Chapter 50). Genetic factors that increase risk for fracture are discussed with these specific health problems throughout this text.

Incidence and Prevalence

The incidence of fractures depends on the location of the injury. Rib fractures are the most common type in the adult population. Femoral shaft fractures occur most often in young and middle-age adults.

> ### CONSIDERATIONS FOR OLDER ADULTS
> **Patient-Centered Care** QSEN
>
> The incidence of proximal femur (hip) fractures is highest in older adults. Humeral fractures are also common in adults; the older the person, usually the more proximal is the fracture. Wrist (Colles') fractures are typically seen in middle and late adulthood and usually result from a fall. These fractures are sometimes referred to as *FOSH fractures* (fall outstretched hand). Middle-age and older adults, especially women, have a higher incidence of osteoporosis, which increases the risk for fragility fractures.

Health Promotion and Maintenance

Airbags and seat belts have decreased the number of severe injuries and deaths, but they have *increased* the number of leg and ankle fractures, especially in older adults. Focus health teaching on other risks for musculoskeletal injury, including:

- Osteoporosis screening and self-management education (see Chapter 50)
- Fall prevention (see Chapter 3)
- Home safety assessment and modification, if needed
- Dangers of drinking and driving
- Helmet use when riding bicycles, motorcycles, and other small motorized vehicles/devices

❖ **INTERPROFESSIONAL COLLABORATIVE CARE**

◆ **Assessment: Noticing**

History. The patient with a new fracture typically has impaired COMFORT; many patients report moderate-to-severe pain. Delay the detailed interview for a nursing history until he or she is more comfortable. Ask about the cause of the fracture. Certain types of force (e.g., incisional, crush, acceleration or deceleration), shearing, and friction lead to most musculoskeletal injuries. As a result, several body systems are often affected.

Incisional injuries, as from a knife wound, and *crush* injuries cause hemorrhage and decreased PERFUSION to major organs.

Acceleration or deceleration injuries cause direct trauma to the spleen, brain, and kidneys when these organs are moved from their fixed locations in the body. *Shearing and friction* damage TISSUE INTEGRITY and cause a high level of wound contamination.

Asking about the events leading to the injury helps identify which forces were experienced and therefore which body systems or parts of the body to assess. For example, a forward fall often results in Colles' fracture of the wrist because the person tries to catch himself or herself with an outstretched hand. Knowing the mechanism of injury also helps determine whether other types of injury, such as head and spinal cord injury, might be present.

Obtain a recent drug use history, including substance use, regardless of the patient's age. For example, a young adult may have had an excessive amount of alcohol, which contributed to a motor vehicle crash or a fall at the work site. Many older adults also consume alcohol and an assortment of prescribed and over-the-counter drugs, which can cause dizziness and loss of balance. Middle-age women, often white and affluent, may have a history of excessive opioid use.

A medical history may identify possible causes of the fracture and gives clues as to how long it will take for the bone to heal. Certain diseases such as bone cancer and osteoporosis cause fragility fractures that typically do not achieve total healing or union.

Ask about the patient's occupation and recreational activities. Some occupations are more hazardous than others. For instance, construction work is potentially more physically dangerous than office work. Certain hobbies and recreational activities are also extremely hazardous, such as skiing. Contact sports, such as football and ice hockey, often result in musculoskeletal injuries, including fractures. Other activities do not have such an obvious potential for injury but can cause fractures nonetheless. For instance, daily jogging or running can lead to fatigue fractures.

Physical Assessment/Signs and Symptoms. The patient with a fracture often has trauma to other body systems. Therefore assess all major body systems *first* for life-threatening complications, including head, chest, and abdominal trauma. Some fractures can cause internal organ damage resulting in hemorrhage. When a pelvic fracture is suspected, assess vital signs, skin color, and level of consciousness for indications of possible hypovolemic shock. Remember that if there is one pelvic fracture, there is usually another fracture in the pelvis, even if it is subtle. Check the urine for blood, which indicates possible damage to the urinary system, often the bladder. If the patient cannot void, suspect that the bladder or urethra has been damaged. Complete assessment of these areas is described elsewhere in this text.

Patients with severe or multiple fractures of the arms, legs, or pelvis have severe pain. Vertebral compression fractures are also extremely painful. Patients *with a fractured hip may have groin pain or pain referred to the back of the knee or lower back.* Pain is usually caused by muscle spasm and edema that result from the fracture.

For fractures of the shoulder and upper arm, the physical assessment is best done with the patient in a sitting or standing position, if possible, so shoulder drooping or other abnormal positioning can be seen. Support the affected arm and flex the elbow to promote COMFORT during the assessment. For more distal areas of the arm, perform the assessment with the patient

---

! NURSING SAFETY PRIORITY QSEN
Action Alert

Patients with one or more fractured ribs have severe pain when they take deep breaths. Monitor respiratory status, which may be severely compromised from pain or pneumothorax (air in the pleural cavity). Assess the patient's pain level and manage pain *before* continuing the physical assessment.

in a supine position so the extremity can be elevated to reduce swelling.

Place the patient in a supine position for assessment of the legs and pelvis. A patient with an impacted hip fracture may be able to walk for a short time after injury, although this is not recommended.

When inspecting the site of a possible fracture, look for a change in bone alignment. The bone may appear deformed, a limb may be internally or externally rotated, and/or one or more bones may also be dislocated (out of their joint capsules). Observe for extremity shortening or a change in bone shape.

If the skin is intact (closed fracture), the area over the fracture may be ecchymotic (bruised) from bleeding into the underlying soft tissues. Subcutaneous emphysema, the appearance of bubbles under the skin because of air trapping, may be present but is usually seen later.

! NURSING SAFETY PRIORITY QSEN
Action Alert

Swelling at the fracture site is rapid and can result in marked neurovascular compromise as a result of decreased arterial PERFUSION. *Gently perform a thorough neurovascular assessment and compare extremities.* Assess skin color and temperature, sensation, MOBILITY, pain, and pulses distal to the fracture site. If the fracture involves an extremity and the patient is not in severe pain, check the nails for capillary refill by applying pressure to the nail and observing for the speed of blood return (usually 3 to 5 seconds, depending on the patient's age). If nails are brittle or thick, assess the skin next to the nail. Checking for capillary refill is not as reliable as other indicators of PERFUSION. Chart 51-3 describes the procedure for a neurovascular assessment, which evaluates **c**irculation, **m**ovement, and **s**ensation (SENSORY PERCEPTION) (CMS function).

Psychosocial Assessment. The psychosocial status of a patient with a fracture depends on the extent of the injury, possible complications, coping ability, and availability of support systems. Hospitalization is not required for a single, uncomplicated fracture, and the patient returns to usual daily activities within a few days. Examples include a single fracture of a bone in the finger, wrist, foot, or toe.

In contrast, a patient suffering severe or multiple traumas may be hospitalized for weeks and may undergo many surgical procedures, treatments, and prolonged rehabilitation. These disruptions in lifestyle can create a high level of stress.

Active patients of any age or those who are older and live alone may become depressed during the healing process, especially if experiencing chronic pain that can decrease energy levels. Patients who were previously active and otherwise healthy often feel vulnerable and can become very anxious when they are not able to return to their usual level of activity. Provide hope that appropriate pain management will improve their COMFORT level and restore energy to return to their usual life

CHART 51-3 Best Practice for Patient Safety & Quality Care QSEN
Assessment of Neurovascular Status in Patients With Musculoskeletal Injury

ASSESSMENT METHOD	NORMAL FINDINGS
Skin Color Inspect the area distal to the injury.	No change in pigmentation compared with other parts of the body.
Skin Temperature Palpate the area distal to the injury (the dorsum of the hands is most sensitive to temperature).	The skin is warm.
Movement Ask the patient to move the affected area or the area distal to the injury (active motion).	The patient can move without discomfort.
Move the area distal to the injury (passive motion).	No difference in comfort compared with active movement.
Sensation Ask the patient if numbness or tingling is present (paresthesia).	No numbness or tingling.
Palpate with a paper clip (especially the web space between the first and second toes or the web space between the thumb and forefinger).	No difference in sensation in the affected and unaffected extremities. (Loss of sensation in these areas indicates peroneal nerve or median nerve damage.)
Pulses Palpate the pulses distal to the injury.	Pulses are strong and easily palpated; no difference in the affected and unaffected extremities.
Capillary Refill (Least Reliable) Press the nail beds distal to the injury until blanching occurs (or the skin near the nail if nails are thick and brittle).	Blood returns (return to usual color) within 3 sec (5 sec for older patients).
Pain Ask the patient about the location, nature, and frequency of the pain.	Pain is usually localized and is often described as stabbing or throbbing. (Pain out of proportion to the injury and unrelieved by analgesics might indicate compartment syndrome.)

CULTURAL/ SPIRITUAL CONSIDERATIONS
Patient-Centered Care QSEN

For patients experiencing long-term recovery from fractures and other trauma, stress can affect relationships between the patient and family members or friends. Assess the patient's feelings and ask how he or she coped with previously experienced stressful events. Body image and sexuality may be altered by deformity, treatment modalities for fracture repair, or long-term immobilization. Establish a trusting relationship and determine the patient's spiritual beliefs and practices. Assess the availability of love and support systems, such as family, church, or community groups, who can help patients during the acute and rehabilitation phases when multiple or severe fractures occur.

habits. Some patients may benefit from counseling or psychotherapy services to help them with symptoms of depression and/or anxiety.

Laboratory Assessment. No special laboratory tests are available for assessment of fractures. Hemoglobin and hematocrit levels may often be low because of bleeding caused by the injury. If extensive soft-tissue damage is present, the erythrocyte sedimentation rate (ESR) may be elevated, which indicates the expected inflammatory response. If this value and the white blood cell (WBC) count increase during fracture healing, the patient may have a bone infection. During the healing stages, serum calcium and phosphorus levels are often increased as the bone releases these elements into the blood.

Imaging Assessment. The primary health care provider requests standard *x-rays* to confirm a diagnosis of fracture. These reveal the bone disruption, malalignment, or deformity. If the x-ray does not show a fracture but the patient is symptomatic, the x-ray is usually repeated with additional views.

The *CT* scan is useful in detecting fractures of complex structures, such as the hip and pelvis. It also identifies compression fractures of the spine. *MRI* is useful in determining the amount of soft-tissue damage that may have occurred with the fracture.

◆ **Analysis: Interpreting**
The priority collaborative problems for patients with fractures include:
1. Acute pain due to broken bone(s), soft-tissue damage, muscle spasm, and edema
2. Decreased MOBILITY due to pain, muscle spasm, and soft-tissue damage
3. Potential for neurovascular compromise due to impaired tissue PERFUSION
4. Potential for infection due to impaired TISSUE INTEGRITY caused by an open fracture

◆ **Planning and Implementation: Responding**
Managing Acute Pain
Planning: Expected Outcomes. The patient with a fracture is expected to state that he or she has adequate pain control and improved COMFORT after fracture reduction and immobilization.

Interventions. A fracture can happen anywhere and may be accompanied by multiple injuries to vital organs or major vessels (e.g., thoracic aorta dissection or tear). Interprofessional collaborative care depends on the severity and extent of the injury and the number of fractures the patient has.

Emergency Care: Fracture. For any patient who experiences trauma in the community, first call 911 and assess for **a**irway, **b**reathing, and **c**irculation (ABCs, or primary survey). Then provide lifesaving care if needed before being concerned about the fracture (Chart 51-4). If cardiopulmonary resuscitation

Emergency Care of the Patient With an Extremity Fracture

1. Assess the patient's airway, breathing, and circulation and perform a quick head-to-toe assessment.
2. Remove the patient's clothing (cut if necessary) to inspect the affected area while supporting the area above and below the injury. Do not remove shoes because this can cause increased trauma unless the foot or ankle is injured.
3. Remove jewelry on the affected extremity in case of swelling.
4. Apply direct pressure on the area if there is bleeding and pressure over the proximal artery nearest the fracture.
5. Keep the patient warm and in a supine position.
6. Check the neurovascular status of the area distal to the fracture, including temperature, color, sensation, movement, and capillary refill. Compare affected and unaffected limbs.
7. Immobilize the extremity by splinting; include joints above and below the fracture site. Recheck circulation after splinting.
8. Cover any open areas with a dressing (preferably sterile).

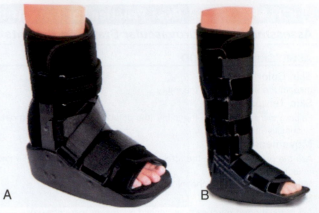

FIG. 51-3 A, Short boot. **B,** Long boot. (From Rizzone, K., & Gregory, A. [2013]. Using casts, splints, and braces in the emergency department. *Clinical Pediatric Emergency Medicine, 14*(4), 340-348. doi:10.1016/j.cpem.2013.11.003.)

(CPR) is needed, ensure circulation first, followed by airway and breathing (see Chapter 34).

If the person is clothed, cut away clothing from the fracture site and remove any jewelry from the affected extremity. Control any bleeding by direct pressure on the area and digital pressure over the artery above the fracture. To prevent shock, place the patient in a supine position and keep him or her warm.

After a head-to-toe assessment (secondary survey) and patient stabilization by the prehospital team, pain is managed with IV opioids such as fentanyl, hydromorphone (Dilaudid), or morphine sulfate. Cardiac monitoring for patients who are older than 50 years is established before drug administration. To prevent further tissue damage, reduce pain, and increase circulation, the prehospital or emergency team immobilizes the fracture by splinting. An air splint or any object or device that extends to the joints above and below the fracture to immobilize it can be used as a **splint**. Sterile gauze is placed loosely over open areas to prevent further contamination of the wound.

In the emergency department (ED), primary health care provider (PHCP) office, or urgent care center, fracture management begins with reduction and immobilization of the fracture while attending to continued pain assessment and management.

Bone reduction, or realignment of the bone ends for proper healing, is accomplished by a closed method or an open (surgical) procedure. In some cases, dislocated bones are also reduced, such as when the distal tibia and fibula are dislocated with a fractured ankle. Immobilization is achieved by the use of bandages, casts, traction, internal fixation, or external fixation.

The primary health care provider (PHCP) selects the treatment method based on the type, location, and extent of the fracture. These interventions prevent further injury and reduce pain.

Nonsurgical Management. Nonsurgical management includes closed reduction and immobilization with a bandage, splint, cast, or traction. For some small, closed incomplete or "hairline" bone fractures in the hand or foot, reduction is not required. Immobilization with an orthotic device or special orthopedic shoe or boot may be the only management during the healing process.

For each modality, the primary nursing concern is assessment and prevention of neurovascular dysfunction or compromise. Assess and document the patient's neurovascular status every hour for the first 24 hours and every 1 to 4 hours thereafter, depending on the injury and agency/PHCP protocol (see Chart 51-3). The patient usually reports impaired COMFORT that is unrelieved by analgesics if the bandage, splint, or cast is too tight. Elevate the fractured extremity higher than the heart and apply ice for the first 24 to 48 hours as needed to reduce edema.

Closed Reduction and Immobilization. Closed reduction is the most common nonsurgical method for managing a simple fracture. While applying a manual pull, or traction, on the bone, the PHCP moves the bone ends so they realign. Moderate sedation is used during this procedure to promote COMFORT. The nurse monitors the patient's oxygen saturation (and possibly end-tidal carbon dioxide [EtCO₂] level) to ensure adequate rate and depth of respirations during the procedure. *If the EtCO₂ becomes too low (30 mm Hg) and the respiratory rate falls to 10 breaths/min, rub the patient's sternum and encourage him or her to breathe.* An x-ray confirms that the bone ends are approximated (aligned) before the bone is immobilized, and a splint is usually applied to keep the bone in alignment.

Splints and Orthopedic Boots/Shoes. For certain areas of the body, such as the scapula (shoulder) and clavicle (collarbone), a commercial immobilizer may be used to keep the bone in place during healing. Because upper-extremity bones do not bear weight, splints may be sufficient to keep bone fragments in place for a closed fracture. Thermoplastic, a durable, flexible material for splinting, allows custom fitting to the patient's body part. Splints for lower extremities are also custom fitted using flexible materials and held in place with elastic bandages (e.g., ACE wrap). When possible, splints are preferred over casts to prevent the complications that can occur with casting. Splints also allow room for extremity swelling without causing decreased arterial PERFUSION.

For foot or toe fractures, orthopedic shoes may be used to support the injured area during healing. For ankles or the lower part of the leg, padded orthopedic boots supported by multiple Velcro straps to hold the boot in place may be used (Fig. 51-3). These devices are especially useful when the patient is allowed to bear weight on the affected leg.

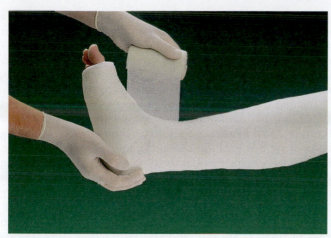

FIG. 51-4 Application of a fiberglass synthetic cast. (From Perry, A.G., Potter, P.A., & Elkin, M.K. (2012). *Nursing interventions & clinical skills* [5th ed.]. St. Louis: Mosby.)

Casts. For more complex fractures or fractures of the lower extremity, the primary health care provider or orthopedic technician may apply a cast to hold bone fragments in place after reduction. A cast is a rigid device that immobilizes the affected body part while allowing other body parts to move. It also allows early MOBILITY and reduces pain. Although its most common use is for fractures, a cast may be applied for correction of deformities (e.g., clubfoot) or for prevention of deformities (e.g., those seen in some patients with rheumatoid arthritis).

Fiberglass is the most common material used for casting and is typically the preferred method for immobilization with a cast (Fig. 51-4). Fiberglass can dry and become rigid within minutes and decreases the risk for impaired TISSUE INTEGRITY. Waterproof casting is designed to get wet in the shower or pool and is used most commonly for athletes. Plaster was the traditional material used for casts but is not as commonly used today for management of most fractures. When first applied, a plaster cast feels hot because an immediate chemical reaction occurs; it soon becomes damp and cool. This type of cast takes at least 24 hours to dry, depending on the size and location of the cast. A wet cast feels cold, smells musty, and is grayish. The cast is dry when it feels hard and firm, is odorless, and has a shiny white appearance.

If TISSUE INTEGRITY under the cast is impaired, the primary health care provider, orthopedic technician, or specially educated nurse cuts a window in the cast so the wound can be observed and cared for. The piece of cast removed to make the window must be retained and replaced after wound care to prevent localized edema in the area. This is most important when a window is cut from a cast on an extremity. Tape or elastic bandage wrap may be used to keep the "window" in place. A window is also an access for taking pulses, removing wound drains, or preventing abdominal distention when the patient is in a body or spica cast.

If the cast is too tight, it may be cut with a cast cutter to relieve pressure or allow tissue swelling. The primary health care provider may choose to bivalve the cast (i.e., cut it lengthwise into two equal pieces). Either half of the cast can be removed for inspection or for provision of care. The two halves are then held in place by an elastic bandage wrap.

When a patient has an *arm cast,* teach him or her to elevate the arm above the heart to reduce swelling. The hand should be higher than the heart. Ice may be prescribed for the first 24 to 48 hours. When the patient is walking or standing, the arm is supported with a sling placed around the neck to alleviate fatigue caused by the weight of the cast. The sling should distribute the weight over a large area of the shoulders and trunk, not just the neck. Some primary health care providers prefer that the patient not use a sling after the first few days in an arm cast, particularly a short-arm cast. This encourages normal movement of the mobile joints and enhances bone healing. For many wrist fractures, a splint is used to immobilize the area instead of a cast to accommodate for edema formation.

A *leg cast* allows MOBILITY and requires the patient to use ambulatory aids such as crutches or a walker. A cast shoe, sandal, or boot that attaches to the foot or a rubber walking pad attached to the sole of the cast assists in ambulation (if weight bearing is allowed) and helps prevent damage to the cast. Teach the patient to elevate the affected leg on several pillows to reduce swelling and to apply ice for the first 24 hours or as prescribed.

Before the cast is applied, explain its purpose and the procedure for its application. With a plaster cast, warn the patient about the heat that will be felt immediately after the wet cast is applied. Do not cover the new plaster cast. Allow for air-drying and handle the cast with the palms of the hand to prevent damage.

> **! NURSING SAFETY PRIORITY** QSEN
>
> **Action Alert**
>
> Check to ensure that any type of cast is not too tight and frequently monitor and document neurovascular status—usually every hour for the first 24 hours after application if the patient is hospitalized. You should be able to insert a finger between the cast and the skin. Teach the patient to apply ice for the first 24 to 36 hours to reduce swelling and inflammation.

Inspect the cast at least once every 8 to 12 hours for drainage, alignment, and fit. Plaster casts act like sponges and absorb drainage, whereas synthetic casts act like a wick pulling drainage away from the drainage site. Document the presence of any drainage on the cast. However, the evidence is not clear on whether drainage should be circled on the cast because it may increase anxiety and is not a reliable indicator of drainage amount. *Immediately report to the primary health care provider any sudden increases in the amount of drainage or change in the integrity of the cast.* After swelling decreases, it is not uncommon for the cast to become too loose and need replacement. If the patient is not admitted to the hospital, provide instructions regarding cast care.

During hospitalization, assess for other complications resulting from casting that can be serious and life threatening, such as infection, circulation impairment, and peripheral nerve damage. If the patient returns home after cast application, teach him or her how to monitor for these complications and when to notify the primary health care provider.

Infection most often results from impaired TISSUE INTEGRITY under the cast (pressure necrosis). If pressure necrosis occurs, the patient typically reports a very painful "hot spot" under the cast, and the cast may feel warmer in the affected area. Teach the patient or family to smell the area for mustiness or an unpleasant odor that would indicate infected material. If the infection progresses, a fever may develop. Teach the patient to never put anything down inside the cast, such as a hanger or pencil, to scratch an itch because this action can cause significant skin damage.

Circulation impairment causing decreased PERFUSION and *peripheral nerve damage* can result from tightness of the cast. Teach the patient to assess for circulation at least daily, including the ability to move the area distal to the extremity, numbness, and increased pain.

The patient with a cast may be immobilized for a prolonged period, depending on the extent of the fracture and the type of cast. In this case, assess for complications of impaired MOBILITY, such as skin breakdown, pneumonia, atelectasis, thromboembolism, and constipation. Before the cast is removed, inform the patient that the cast cutter will not injure the skin but that heat may be felt during the procedure.

Because of prolonged immobilization, a joint may become contracted, usually in a fixed state of flexion. Osteoarthritis and osteoporosis may develop from lack of weight bearing. Muscle can also atrophy from lack of exercise during prolonged immobilization of the affected body part, usually an extremity.

 NCLEX EXAMINATION CHALLENGE 51-1

Physiological Integrity

A client who has a plaster leg splint reports a painful pressure sensation under the elastic wrap that is holding the splint in place. What is the nurse's **best initial** action?
A. Remove the splint to reduce skin pressure.
B. Perform a neurovascular assessment.
C. Report the client's concern to the primary health care provider.
D. Inspect the skin under the elastic bandage.

Traction. Traction is the application of a pulling force to a part of the body to provide reduction, alignment, and rest. It is also used as a last resort to decrease muscle spasm (thus relieving pain) and prevent or correct deformity and tissue damage. A patient in traction is often hospitalized; but in some cases, home care is possible even for skeletal traction.

Traction may be classified as running traction or balanced suspension. In *running* traction, the pulling force is in one direction, and the patient's body acts as countertraction. Moving the body or bed position can alter the countertraction force. *Balanced suspension* provides the countertraction so the pulling force of the traction is not altered when the bed or patient is moved. This allows for increased movement and facilitates care (Table 51-1).

Although not used as often today, the two most common types of traction are skin and skeletal traction. *Skin traction* involves the use of a Velcro boot (Buck's traction) (Fig. 51-5), belt, or halter, which is usually secured around the affected leg. The primary purpose of skin traction is to decrease painful muscle spasms that accompany hip and proximal femur fractures. A weight is used as a pulling force, which is limited to 5 to 10 lb (2.3 to 4.5 kg) to prevent injury to the skin.

In *skeletal traction,* screws are surgically inserted directly into bone (e.g., femoral condyles for distal femur fractures). These allow the use of longer traction time and heavier weights, usually 15 to 30 lb (6.8 to 13.6 kg). Skeletal traction aids in bone realignment but impairs the patient's MOBILITY. Use pressure-reduction measures and monitor for indications of impaired TISSUE INTEGRITY. Pin site care is also an important part of nursing management to prevent infection. Keep pin sites clean and document the nature of any drainage. Follow the agency's or primary health care provider's protocol for pin care.

TABLE 51-1	Types of Traction Used for Musculoskeletal Trauma	
TYPE AND CHARACTERISTICS OF TRACTION	**USE**
Upper-Extremity Traction	
Sidearm skin or skeletal traction (the forearm is flexed and extended 90 degrees from the upper part of the body)	Fractures of the humerus with or without involvement of the shoulder and clavicle
Overhead or 90-90 traction, skin or skeletal (the elbow is flexed, and the arm is at a right angle to the body over the upper chest)	Same as above (depends on the physician's preference)
Lower-Extremity Traction	
Buck's extension traction (skin) (the affected leg is in extension)	Fractures of the hip or femur before surgery Prevention of hip flexion contractures Hip dislocation
Russell's traction (similar to Buck's traction, but a sling under the knee suspends the leg)	Fractures of the hip or distal end of the femur
Balanced skin or skeletal traction (the limb is usually elevated in a Thomas splint with Pearson's attachment, or a Böhler-Braun splint is used)	Fractures of the femur or pelvis (acetabulum)
Spinal Column and Pelvic Traction	
Cervical halter (a strap under the chin)	Cervical muscle spasms, strain/sprain, or arthritis
Cervical skeletal (e.g., halo brace)	Cervical fractures of the spine; muscle spasms
Pelvic belt (a strap around the hips at the iliac crest is attached to weights at the foot of the bed)	Pain, strain, sprain, or muscle spasms in the lower back
Pelvic sling (a wide strap around the hips is attached to an overhead bar to keep the pelvis off the bed)	Pelvic fractures; other pelvic injuries

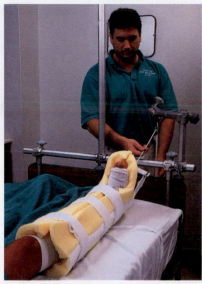

FIG. 51-5 Skin traction with a hook-and-loop fastener (Velcro) boot, commonly used for hip fractures. (Courtesy Smith & Nephew, Inc., Orthopaedics Divisions, Memphis, TN.)

The nurse may set up or assist in the setup of traction if specially educated. In larger or specialty hospitals or units, orthopedic technicians or physician assistants often set up traction.

⚠ NURSING SAFETY PRIORITY QSEN

Action Alert

When patients are in traction, weights usually are not removed without a prescription. They should not be lifted manually or allowed to rest on the floor. Weights should be freely hanging at all times. Teach this important point to unlicensed assistive personnel (UAP) on the unit, to other personnel such as those in the radiology department, and to visitors. Inspect the skin at least every 8 hours for signs of irritation or inflammation. When possible, remove the belt or boot that is used for skin traction every 8 hours to inspect under the device.

Check traction equipment frequently to ensure its proper functioning. Inspect all ropes, knots, and pulleys at least every 8 to 12 hours for loosening, fraying, and positioning. Check the weight for consistency with the primary health care provider's prescription. Sometimes one of the weights is accidentally removed by a staff member or visitor who bumps into it. Replace the weights if they are not correct and notify the primary health care provider or orthopedic technician.

If the patient reports severe pain from muscle spasm, the weights may be too heavy, or the patient may need realignment. Report the pain to the primary health care provider (PHCP) if body realignment fails to improve COMFORT. Assess neurovascular status of the affected body part per agency or health care provider protocol to detect impaired PERFUSION and TISSUE INTEGRITY. The circulation is usually monitored every hour for the first 24 hours after traction is applied and every 4 hours thereafter.

Drug Therapy. After fracture treatment, the patient often has pain for a prolonged time during the healing process. The PHCP commonly prescribes opioid and nonopioid analgesics, anti-inflammatory drugs and, possibly, muscle relaxants.

For patients with chronic, severe pain, opioid and nonopioid drugs are alternated or given together to manage pain both centrally in the brain and peripherally at the site of injury. For severe or multiple fractures, patient-controlled analgesia (PCA) with morphine, fentanyl, or hydromorphone (Dilaudid) is used. *Meperidine (Demerol) should never be used because it has toxic metabolites that can cause seizures and other complications. Most hospitals no longer use this drug.* Oxycodone and oxycodone with acetaminophen (Percocet) or hydrocodone with acetaminophen (Norco, Vicodin, Lortab) are common oral opioid drugs that are very effective for most patients with fracture pain. NSAIDs are given to decrease associated tissue inflammation; however, they can slow bone healing.

For patients who have less severe injury, the analgesic may be given on an as-needed basis. Collaborate with the patient regarding the best times for the strong analgesics to be given (e.g., before a complex dressing change, after physical therapy sessions, or at bedtime). Assess the effectiveness of the analgesic and its side effects. Constipation is a common side effect of opioid therapy, especially for older adults. Assess for frequency of bowel movements and administer stool softeners as needed. Encourage fluids and activity as tolerated.

Physical Therapy. Collaborate with the physical therapist (PT) to assist with pain control and edema reduction by using ice/heat packs, electrical muscle stimulation ("e-stim"), and special treatments such as dexamethasone iontophoresis. Iontophoresis is a method for absorbing dexamethasone, a synthetic steroid, through the skin near the painful area to decrease inflammation and edema. A small device delivers a minute amount of electricity via electrodes that are placed on the skin. The patient may describe the sensation as a pinch or slight sting. The electrical current increases the ability of the skin to absorb the drug from a topical patch into the affected soft tissue.

When acute pain is not adequately controlled, some patients experience a chronic, intense burning pain and edema that are associated with *complex regional pain syndrome (CRPS)*. This syndrome often results from fractures and other musculoskeletal trauma as described earlier in this chapter.

Management of Chronic Regional Pain Syndrome. Bone typically heals more quickly than surrounding connective tissue such as ligaments, tendons, and fascia. To facilitate soft tissue healing and prevent CRPS, the PT asks the patient to use a variety of objects with varying surfaces and apply them directly to desensitize the skin. These objects can be rough, smooth, hard, soft, sharp (but not enough to damage the skin), or dull.

The first priority for managing CRPS is pain relief. Because of the complexity of the disorder, little research has been done to demonstrate the best practices for caring for a patient with CRPS; therefore a combination of interventions is used. Nurses play an important role in interprofessional collaborative care, which includes drug therapy and a variety of nonpharmacologic modalities. Many classes of drugs may be used to manage the intense pain. These include topical and oral analgesics, antiepileptic drugs, antidepressants, corticosteroids, and bisphosphonates. Chapter 4 discusses chronic pain management in detail.

In collaboration with physical and occupational therapists, assist in maintaining adequate range of motion (ROM) and function. The skin of a patient with CRPS tends to alternate between warm, swollen, and red to cool, clammy, and bluish. Skin care needs to be gentle with minimal stimulation.

Peripheral or spinal cord neurostimulation using an external or internal implanted device delivers electrical pulses to block pain from getting to the brain where pain is perceived. The external or acupuncture method requires weekly sessions or a short-term continuous trial before the device is surgically implanted. Complications of implantable neurostimulators include spinal cord and nerve damage from hematoma, edema formation, or neurologic dysfunction.

A chemical sympathetic nerve block may be used. This procedure can be done by an IV infusion of phentolamine (Regitine), a drug that blocks sympathetic receptors, or by injecting an anesthetic agent next to the spine to block sympathetic nerves.

Minimally invasive surgical sympathectomy, or cutting of the sympathetic nerve branches via endoscopy through a small axillary incision, may be required. Topical skin adhesive is used to close the very small incision. The patient is discharged to home a few hours later with a follow-up examination the next day with the primary health care provider. Usual activities can resume a few days later.

Help the patient cope with CRPS because it often has a profound psychological effect. A referral for psychological counseling or psychotherapy may be indicated. The Reflex Sympathetic Dystrophy Syndrome Association (RSDSA) (www.rsds.org) and National Pain Association (www.nationalpainassociation.org) are available to help patients and their families organize or locate support groups and other resources. A nonprofit organization, Promoting Awareness of RSD and CRPS in Canada (PARC), is available to educate the public and health care community to increase awareness of CRPS (www.rsdcanada.org).

Surgical Management. For some types of fractures, closed reduction is not sufficient. Surgical intervention may be needed to realign the bone for the healing process.

Preoperative Care. Teach the patient and family what to expect during and after the surgery. The preoperative care for a patient undergoing orthopedic surgery is similar to that for anyone having surgery with general or epidural anesthesia. Some patients may also receive a regional nerve blockade which promotes COMFORT immediately after surgery. (See Chapter 14 for a thorough discussion of general preoperative nursing care.)

Operative Procedures. Open reduction with internal fixation (ORIF) is one of the most common methods of reducing and immobilizing a fracture. External fixation with closed reduction is used when patients have soft-tissue injury (open fracture). Although nurses do not decide which surgical technique is used, understanding the procedures enhances patient teaching and care.

Because ORIF permits early MOBILITY, it is often the preferred surgical method. Open reduction allows the surgeon to directly view the fracture site. Internal fixation uses metal pins, screws, rods, plates, or prostheses to immobilize the fracture during healing. The surgeon makes one or more incisions to gain access to the broken bone(s) and implants one or more devices into bone tissue after each fracture is reduced. A cast, boot, or splint is placed to maintain immobilization during the healing process, depending on the body part affected.

After the bone achieves union, the metal hardware may be removed, depending on the location and type of fracture. Hardware is removed most frequently in ankle fractures, depending on the severity of the injury. If the metal implants are not bothersome, they may remain in place. Examples of internal fixation devices for fractured hips are discussed later in this chapter.

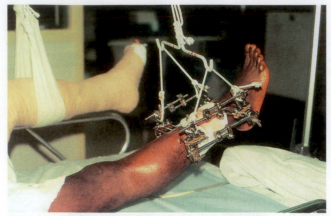

FIG. 51-6 The Hex-Fix external fixation system for tibia-fibula fractures. (From McCance, K.L., Huether, S.E., Brashers, V.L., & Rote, N.S. [2014]. *Pathophysiology: The biologic basis for disease in adults and children* [7th ed.]. St. Louis: Mosby.)

An alternative modality for the management of fractures is the external fixation apparatus, as shown in Fig. 51-6. External fixation is a system in which pins or wires are inserted through the skin and affected bone and then connected to a rigid external frame. The system may be used for upper- or lower-extremity fractures or for fractures of the pelvis, especially for open fractures when wound management is needed. After a fixator is removed, the patient may be placed in a cast, boot, or splint until healing is complete or have internal fixation.

External fixation has several advantages over other surgical techniques:

- There is minimal blood loss compared with internal fixation.
- The device allows early ambulation and exercise of the affected body part while relieving pain.
- The device maintains alignment in closed fractures that will not maintain position in a cast and stabilizes comminuted fractures that require bone grafting.

In open fractures, in which skin and tissue trauma accompany the fracture, the device permits easy access to the wound while the bone heals. This method is usually preferred over the use of a window in a cast for wound care.

A disadvantage of external fixation is an increased risk for pin-site infection. Pin-site infections can lead to osteomyelitis, which is serious and difficult to treat (see Chapter 50).

Postoperative Care. The postoperative care for a patient undergoing ORIF or external fixation is similar to that provided for any patient undergoing surgery (see Chapter 16). Because bone is a vascular, dynamic body tissue, the patient is at risk for complications specific to fractures and musculoskeletal surgery. IV ketorolac (Toradol) is often given in the postanesthesia care unit (PACU) or soon after discharge to the postsurgical area to reduce inflammation and pain. Aggressive pain management starts as soon as possible after surgery to prevent the development of chronic pain and promote early MOBILITY. Patients who had a regional nerve blockade typically have little or no pain immediately after surgery for about 18 to 24 hours. However, when the anesthetic begins to wear off, be sure that the patient is medicated to prevent severe pain. Use nonpharmacologic measures for pain management, such as imagery, distraction, music therapy, and other measures that the patient prefers and are allowed by agency policy to promote COMFORT.

Additional information about postoperative care may be found in the Selected Fractures of Specific Sites section later in this section. Depending on the fractures that are repaired, some ORIF procedures are performed as same-day surgeries. Patients stay in the hospital up to 23 hours after surgery.

For patients with an **external fixator**, pay particular attention to the pin sites for signs of inflammation or infection. In the first 48 to 72 hours, *clear* fluid drainage or weeping is expected. Although no standardized method or evidence-based protocol for pin-site care has been established, recommendations have been made based on the evidence available regarding pin-site care. Because the pins go through the skin and into bone, the risk for infection is high. Monitor the pin sites at least every 8 to 12 hours for drainage, color, odor, and severe redness, which indicate inflammation and possible infection. Follow agency policy for how to clean the pin-site areas.

The patient with an external fixator may have a disturbed body image. The frame may be large and bulky, and the affected area may have massive tissue damage with dressings. Be sensitive to this possibility in planning care. Teach about alterations to clothing that may be required while the fixator is in place.

The Ilizarov technique of circular external fixation is sometimes used to treat new fractures (closed, comminuted fractures and open fractures with bone loss) and malunion or nonunion of fractures. It may also be used to treat congenital bone deformities, especially in "little people" (e.g., dwarfs).

The circular external fixation device is used to gently pull apart the cortex of the bone and stimulate new bone growth. Unlike the traditional fixator, the Ilizarov external fixator promotes rotation, angulation, lengthening, or widening of bone to correct bony defects and allows for healing of any soft-tissue defect. The nursing care associated with this device is similar to the care of the patient with other external fixation systems with one major exception. If the device is being used for filling bone gaps, teach the patient how to manually turn the four-sided nuts (also called *clickers*) up to four times a day. Daily distraction rates vary, but 1 mm daily is common. Screening and teaching are particularly important because the patient adjusts and cares for the apparatus over a long period of up to 6 months to 1 year. Pain control is a priority outcome for patients using this device.

Procedures for Nonunion. Some management techniques are not successful because the bone does not heal. Several additional options are available to the physician to promote bone union, such as electrical bone stimulation, bone grafting, and ultrasound fracture treatment.

For selected patients, *electrical bone stimulation* may be successful. This procedure is based on research showing that bone has electrical properties that are used in healing. The exact mechanism of action is unknown. A noninvasive, external system delivers a small continuous electrical charge directed toward the nonhealed bone. There are no known risks with this system, although patients with pacemakers cannot use this device on an arm. Implanted direct-current stimulators are placed directly in the fracture site and have no external apparatus. Both systems require several months of treatment.

Another method of treating nonunion is *bone grafting*. A bone graft may also replace diseased bone or increase bone tissue for joint replacement. In most cases, chips of bone are taken from the iliac crest or other site and are packed or wired between the bone ends to facilitate union. Allografts from cadavers may also be used. These grafts are frozen or freeze-dried and stored under sterile conditions in a bone bank.

Bone banking from living donors is becoming increasingly popular. If qualified, patients undergoing total hip replacement may donate their femoral heads to the bank for later use as bone grafts for others. Careful screening ensures that the bone is healthy and that the donor has no communicable disease. The bone cannot be donated without written consent.

One of the newest modalities for fracture healing is **low-intensity pulsed ultrasound** (exogen therapy). Used for slow-healing fractures or for new fractures as an alternative to surgery, ultrasound treatment has had excellent results. The patient applies the treatment for about 20 minutes each day. It has no contraindications or adverse effects.

Increasing Mobility

Planning: Expected Outcomes. The patient with a fracture is expected to increase physical MOBILITY and be free of complications associated with immobility. The patient is also expected to move purposefully in his or her own environment independently with or without an ambulatory device unless restricted by traction or other modality.

Interventions. The interventions necessary for this diagnosis can be grouped into two types: those that help increase and promote MOBILITY and those that prevent complications of impaired MOBILITY.

Promoting Mobility. Many patients with musculoskeletal trauma, including fractures, are referred by their primary health care provider for rehabilitation therapy with a physical therapist (PT) (usually for lower-extremity injuries) and/or occupational therapist (OT) (usually for upper-extremity injuries). The timing for this referral depends on the nature, severity, and treatment modality of the fracture(s) or other musculoskeletal trauma.

For example, some patients who have an ORIF for an ankle fracture begin therapy when the incisional staples or Steri-Strips are removed and an orthopedic boot is fitted. Based on the initial evaluation, the PT performs gentle manipulative exercises to increase range of motion. The therapist may also begin to help the patient with laterality, a concept to help the brain identify the injured foot from the uninjured foot. Computer programs and mirror-box therapy can help reprogram the brain as part of *cognitive retraining*. In mirror-box therapy for an injured foot, the patient covers his or her affected foot while looking at and moving the uninjured foot in front of the mirror. The brain often perceives the foot in the mirror as the injured foot.

Stimulation by touch also helps the brain acknowledge the injured foot. The PT teaches the patient to frequently touch the injured area and use various materials and objects against the skin to desensitize it. These interventions improve MOBILITY and decrease the risk for complex regional pain syndrome, discussed earlier in this chapter.

The success of rehabilitation is affected by the patient's motivation and willingness to perform prescribed exercises and activities between PT visits. For example, rehabilitation for ankle surgery may take several months, depending on the severity of the injury and the age and general health of the patient.

When weight bearing begins for lower-extremity fractures about 6 weeks after surgery, the PT teaches the patient how to begin with toe-touch or partial weight bearing using crutches or a walker. Muscle-strengthening exercises of the affected leg help with ambulation because atrophy begins shortly after injury.

The use of crutches or a walker increases MOBILITY and assists in ambulation. The patient may progress to using a walker or cane after crutches. *Crutches* are the most commonly used ambulatory aid for many types of lower-extremity musculoskeletal trauma (e.g., fractures, sprains, amputations). In most agencies, the physical therapist or emergency department/ambulatory care nurse fits the patient for crutches and teaches him or her how to ambulate with them. Reinforce those instructions and evaluate whether the patient is using the crutches correctly.

Walking with crutches requires strong arm muscles, balance, and coordination. For this reason, crutches are not often used for older adults; walkers and canes are preferred. Crutches can cause upper-extremity bursitis or axillary nerve damage if they are not fitted or used correctly. For that reason, the top of each crutch is padded. To prevent pressure on the axillary nerve, there should be two to three finger-breadths between the axilla and the top of the crutch when the crutch tip is at least 6 inches (15 cm) diagonally in front of the foot. The crutch is adjusted so the elbow is flexed no more than 30 degrees when the palm is on the handle (Fig. 51-7). The distal tips of each crutch are rubber to prevent slipping.

There are several types of gaits for walking with crutches. The most common one for musculoskeletal injury is the three-point gait, which allows little weight bearing on the affected leg. The procedure for these gaits is discussed in fundamentals of nursing books.

A *walker* is most often used by the older patient who needs additional support for balance. The physical therapist assesses the strength of the upper extremities and the unaffected leg. Strength is improved with prescribed exercises as needed.

A *cane* is sometimes used if the patient needs only minimal support for an affected leg. The straight cane offers the least support. A hemi-cane or quad-cane provides a broader base for the cane and therefore more support. The cane is placed on the *unaffected* side and should create no more than 30 degrees of flexion of the elbow. The top of the cane should be parallel to the greater trochanter of the femur or stylus of the wrist. Chapter 6 and fundamentals textbooks describe these ambulatory devices in more detail.

Preventing Complications of Immobility. The nurse plays a vital role in preventing and assessing for complications in immobilized patients with fractures. Additional information about nursing care for preventing problems associated with immobility is found in Chapter 2 and 6.

Preventing and Monitoring for Neurovascular Compromise

Planning: Expected Outcomes. The patient with a fracture is expected to have no compromise in neurovascular status as evidenced by adequate PERFUSION (circulation), MOBILITY (movement), and SENSORY PERCEPTION (sensation) (CMS). If severe compromise occurs, the patient is expected to have early and prompt emergency treatment to prevent severe tissue damage.

Interventions. Perform neurovascular (NV) assessments (also known as *circ checks* or *CMS assessments*) frequently before and after fracture treatment. Patients who have extremity casts, splints with elastic bandage wraps, and open reduction with internal fixation (ORIF) or external fixation are especially at risk for NV compromise. If PERFUSION to the distal extremity is impaired, the patient reports impaired COMFORT, impaired MOBILITY, and decreased SENSORY PERCEPTION. If these symptoms are allowed to progress, patients are at risk for acute compartment syndrome (ACS).

Early recognition of the signs and symptoms of ACS can prevent loss of function or loss of a limb. Identify patients who may be at risk and monitor them closely. ACS can begin in 6 to 8 hours after an injury or take up to 2 days to appear.

> **! NURSING SAFETY PRIORITY** **QSEN**
>
> ### *Critical Rescue*
>
> Monitor for and document early signs of ACS. Assess for the "six Ps" (i.e., **p**ain, **p**ressure, **p**aralysis, **p**aresthesia, **p**allor, and **p**ulselessness) (rare or late stage). Pain is increased even with passive motion and may seem out of proportion to the degree of injury. Analgesics that had controlled pain become less effective or noneffective. Numbness and tingling (paresthesia) is often one of the first signs of the problem. The affected extremity then becomes pale and cool as a result of decreased arterial perfusion to the affected area. Capillary refill is an important assessment of PERFUSION but may not be reliable in an older adult because of arterial insufficiency. Losses of movement and function and decreased pulses or pulselessness are late signs of ACS! Fortunately, ACS is not common, but it creates an emergency situation when it does occur.
>
> *If ACS is suspected, notify the primary health care provider immediately and, if possible, implement interventions to relieve the pressure. For example, for the patient with tight, bulky dressings, loosen the bandage or tape. If the patient has a cast, follow agency protocol about who may cut the cast. Do not elevate or ice the extremity because that could compromise blood flow.*

In a few cases, compartment pressure may be monitored on a one-time basis with a handheld device with a digital display, or pressure can be monitored continuously. Monitoring is recommended for comatose or unresponsive high-risk patients with multiple trauma and fractures.

If ACS is verified, the surgeon may perform a **fasciotomy**, or opening in the fascia, by making an incision through the skin and subcutaneous tissues into the fascia of the affected compartment. This procedure relieves the pressure and restores

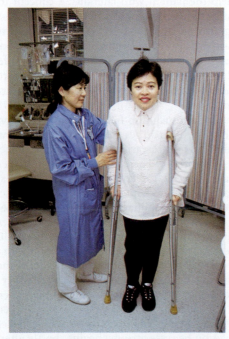

FIG. 51-7 Assisting the patient with crutch walking. Note how the therapist guards the patient and how the patient's elbows are at no more than 30 degrees of flexion.

circulation to the affected area. No consensus exists on what pressure requires fasciotomy (normal is 0 to 8 mm Hg). Compartment pressures must be considered in relation to the patient's hemodynamic status. After fasciotomy, the open wound is packed and dressed daily or more often until secondary closure occurs, usually in 4 to 5 days, depending on the patient's healing ability. Some surgeons use negative-pressure wound therapy (e.g., Wound Vac) over a fasciotomy to decrease edema and contain the blood from the site. Once the swelling has decreased in about 3 days, the surgeon may try to close the incision with sutures or may need to apply a skin graft.

Preventing Infection

Planning: Expected Outcomes. The patient with a fracture is expected to be free of wound or bone infection as evidenced by no fever, no increase in white blood cell count, and negative wound culture (if wound is present).

Interventions. When caring for a patient with an open fracture, use aseptic technique for dressing changes and wound irrigations. Check agency policy for specific protocols. *Immediately notify the primary health care provider if you observe inflammation and purulent drainage.* Other infections, such as pneumonia and urinary tract infection, may occur several days after the fracture. Monitor the patient's vital signs every 4 to 8 hours because increases in temperature and pulse often indicate systemic infection.

CONSIDERATIONS FOR OLDER ADULTS

Patient-Centered Care **QSEN**

> Older adults may not have a temperature elevation even in the presence of severe infection. An acute onset of confusion (delirium) often suggests an infection in the older-adult patient.

For most patients with an open fracture, the primary care provider prescribes one or more broad-spectrum antibiotics prophylactically and performs surgical débridement of any wounds as soon as possible after the injury. First-generation cephalosporins, clindamycin (Cleocin), and gentamycin are commonly used. In addition to systemic antibiotics, local antibiotic therapy through wound irrigation is commonly prescribed, especially during débridement.

A very effective treatment is negative-pressure wound therapy (e.g., vacuum-assisted closure [VAC] system) as a method of increasing the rate of wound healing for open fractures. This device allows quicker wound closure, which decreases the risk for infection.

When the bone is surgically repaired, hardware and/or bone grafts have typically been implanted. However, they are limited in their use. The U.S. Food and Drug Administration (FDA) approved the use of recombinant human bone morphogenetic protein-2 (rhBMP-2) for tibial and spinal fractures. This implanted genetically engineered substance increases wound healing, decreases hardware failure, and decreases the risk for infection.

Care Coordination and Transition Management

The patient with an *uncomplicated* fracture is usually discharged to home from the emergency department or urgent care center. Older adults with hip or other fractures or patients with multiple traumas are hospitalized and then transferred to home, a rehabilitation setting, or a long-term care facility

CHART 51-5 Patient and Family Education: Preparing for Self-Management

Care of the Extremity After Cast Removal

- Remove scaly, dead skin carefully by soaking; do not scrub.
- Move the extremity carefully. Expect smaller circumference, discomfort, weakness, and decreased range of motion.
- Support the extremity with pillows or your orthotic device until strength and movement return.
- Exercise slowly as instructed by your physical therapist.
- Wear support stockings or elastic bandages to prevent swelling (for lower extremity).

for rehabilitation. Collaborate with the case manager or the discharge planner in the hospital to ensure care coordination. Be sure to communicate the plan of care clearly to the health care agency receiving the patient using SBAR or other communication method.

Home Care Management. If the patient is discharged to home, the nurse, rehabilitation therapist, or case manager (CM) may assess the home environment for structural barriers to MOBILITY such as stairs. Be sure that the patient has easy access to the bathroom. Ask about small pets, scatter rugs, waxed floors, and walkway areas that could increase the risk for falls. If the patient needs to use a wheelchair or ambulatory aid, make sure that he or she can use it safely and that there is room in the house to ambulate with these devices. The physical therapist may teach the patient how to use stairs, but older adults or those using crutches may experience difficulty performing this task. Depending on the age and condition of the patient, a home health care nurse may make one or two visits to check that the home is safe and that the patient and family are able to follow the interprofessional plan of care.

Self-Management Education. The patient with a fracture may be discharged from the hospital, emergency department, office, or clinic with a bandage, splint, boot, or cast. Provide verbal and written instructions on the care of these devices. Chart 51-5 describes care of the affected extremity after removal of the cast.

The patient may also need to continue wound care at home. Instruct the patient and family about how to assess and dress the wound to promote healing and prevent infection. Teach them how to recognize complications and when and where to seek professional health care if complications occur. Additional educational needs depend on the type of fracture and fracture repair.

Encourage patients and their families to ensure adequate foods high in protein and calcium that are needed for bone and tissue healing. For patients with lower-extremity fractures, less weight bearing on long bones can cause anemia. The red bone marrow needs weight bearing to simulate red blood cell production. Encourage foods high in iron content. Teach the patient to take a daily iron-added multivitamin (take with food to prevent possible nausea) and a stool softener with a stimulant to prevent opioid-induced constipation.

Health Care Resources. Arrange for follow-up care at home. A social worker may need to help the patient apply for funds to pay medical bills. If there is severe bone and tissue damage, be realistic and help the patient and family understand the long-term nature of the recovery period. Multiple treatment techniques and surgical procedures required for complications can be mentally and emotionally draining for the patient and family. A vocational counselor may be needed to help the patient find a different type of job, depending on the extent of the fracture.

An older or incapacitated patient may need assistance with ADLs, which can be provided by home care aides if family or other caregiver is not available. In collaboration with the case manager, anticipate the patient's needs and arrange for these services.

◆ *Evaluation: Reflecting*

Evaluate the care of the patient with one or more fractures based on the identified priority patient problems. The expected outcomes include that the patient:

- States that he or she has adequate COMFORT to accomplish ADLs
- Ambulates independently with or without an assistive device (if not restricted by traction or other device)
- Is free of physiologic consequences of impaired MOBILITY
- Has adequate blood flow to maintain tissue PERFUSION and function
- Is free of infection or other complication

SELECTED FRACTURES OF SPECIFIC SITES

Upper-Extremity Fractures

In addition to the general care discussed in the previous section, management of upper-extremity fractures includes specific interventions related to the location and nature of the injury.

Fractures of the *proximal humerus*, particularly impacted or displaced fractures, are common in the older adult. A nondisplaced fracture is usually treated with a sling or other device for immobilization. A displaced fracture often requires ORIF with pins or a prosthesis. Humeral shaft fractures are generally corrected by closed reduction and a hanging-arm cast or splint. If necessary, the fracture is repaired surgically (with an intramedullary rod or metal plate and screws) or with external fixation.

The most common upper-extremity (UE) fracture is the *distal radius fracture (DRF),* which occurs in both younger and older adults. Younger adults experience this injury from high-energy (high-impact) trauma as a result of motor vehicle crashes and sports. DRFs are the most common upper-extremity fracture in adults over 65 year of age. Older adults, particularly

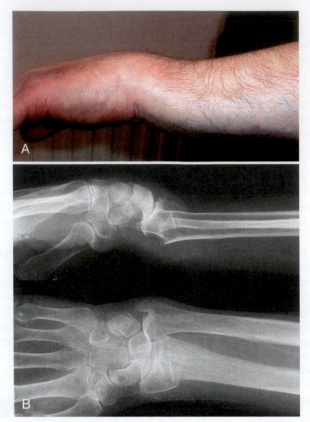

FIG. 51-8 Colles' wrist fracture showing "dinner fork" deformity. (From Douglas, G., Robertson, C., & Nicol, F. [2011]. *Macleod exploración clínica* [12th ed.]. Barcelona: Elsevier.)

active women in their eighth decade of life, typically have low-impact DRFs as a result of falls such as a "standing level fall."

Various names are used to classify DRFs, including Colles' and Smith fractures. A Colles' fracture can occur when a person attempts to break a fall by landing on the heel of the outstretched hand when the wrist is extended. The resulting deformity is often called a *dinner fork* injury (Fig. 51-8). Seen less commonly, a Smith fracture occurs from a fall on a flexed wrist.

Initial nursing interventions for a patient with a DRF include:
- Removing jewelry on the affected hand and wrist before edema worsens (Walsh, 2013)
- Performing a neurovascular assessment of the affected upper extremity
- Immobilizing the affected wrist and hand
- Elevating the affected upper extremity
- Applying ice to the affected area
- Managing pain

After initial stabilization, the most common treatment for a DRF is closed reduction. The health care provider realigns the bone ends while the patient is moderately sedated. A splint is applied and held in place with an elastic bandage. The splint may be replaced several days later with a cast after edema decreases.

For more complicated DRFs, an ORIF with pins and plates may be performed. The patient may have surgery in an ambulatory care or same-day surgical setting using general anesthesia, a peripheral/regional nerve blockade, or a combination of both. The nerve block is often given as a single injection of levobupivacaine (Chirocaine) or bupivacaine (Marcaine), which provides pain relief for 12 to 20 hours (Guarin, 2013). Teach patients having a regional nerve blockade (e.g., supraclavicular block) that temporarily they will not be able to move the affected arm. Also observe, report, and document signs and symptoms of pneumothorax, including tachypnea, decreased breath sounds, or respiratory distress (Guarin, 2013).

For all patients who experience a DRF, assess for nerve compression, especially the radial and median nerves. Be sure to perform frequent neurovascular assessment, with special attention to the presence of decreased SENSORY PERCEPTION (e.g., numbness) or decreased movement.

Fractures of the *metacarpals* and *phalanges (fingers)* are usually not displaced, which makes their treatment less difficult than that of other fractures. Metacarpal fractures are immobilized for 3 to 4 weeks. Phalangeal fractures are immobilized in finger splints for 10 to 14 days.

Lower-Extremity Fractures

Fractures of the Hip

Hip fracture is the most common injury in older adults and one of the most frequently seen injuries in any health care setting or community. It has a high mortality rate as a result of multiple complications related to surgery, depression, and prolonged immobility. Over half of older adults experiencing a hip fracture are unable to live independently, and many die within the first year (Sweitzer et al., 2013).

Hip fractures include those involving the upper third of the femur and are classified as **intracapsular** (within the joint capsule) or **extracapsular** (outside the joint capsule). These types are further divided according to fracture location (Fig. 51-9). In the area of the femoral neck, disruption of the blood supply to the head of the femur is a concern, which can result in ischemic or avascular necrosis (AVN) of the femoral head. AVN causes death and necrosis of bone tissue and results in pain and decreased MOBILITY. This problem is most likely in patients with displaced fractures.

Osteoporosis is the biggest risk factor for hip fractures (see Chapter 50). This disease weakens the upper femur (hip), which causes it to break and then causes the person to fall. This type of fall is caused from a fragility fracture. The number of people with hip fracture is expected to continue to increase as the population ages, and the associated health care costs will be tremendous.

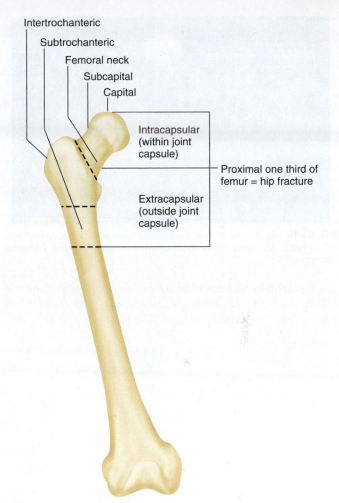

FIG. 51-9 Types of hip fractures.

The treatment of choice is surgical repair by ORIF, when possible, to reduce pain and allow the older patient to be out of bed and ambulatory. Skin (Buck's) traction may be applied before surgery to help decrease pain associated with muscle spasm. Depending on the exact location of the fracture, an ORIF may include an intramedullary rod, pins, prostheses (for femoral head or femoral neck fractures, also known as a hemiarthroplasty), or a compression screw. Figs. 51-10 and 51-11 illustrate examples of these devices. Epidural, spinal, or general anesthesia is used. Occasionally a patient will be so debilitated that surgery cannot be done. In these cases, nonsurgical options include pain management and bedrest to allow natural fracture healing.

Patients usually receive IV morphine or hydromorphone after admission to the emergency department and may receive morphine or hydromorphone PCA or epidural analgesia after surgery. In some cases, a femoral nerve block may also be performed during surgery to help relieve pain for up to 24 hours after surgery (Guarin, 2013). Meperidine (Demerol) should not be used because of its toxic metabolites that can cause seizures and other adverse drug events, especially in the older-adult population. Chapter 4 discusses the nursing care associated with pain management in detail.

After a hip repair, older adults frequently experience acute confusion, or delirium. They may pull at tubes or the surgical

CONSIDERATIONS FOR OLDER ADULTS

Patient-Centered Care QSEN

Teach older adults about the risk factors for hip fracture, including physiologic aging changes, disease processes, drug therapy, and environmental hazards. Physiologic changes include sensory changes such as diminished visual acuity and hearing; changes in gait, balance, and muscle strength; and joint stiffness. Disease processes such as osteoporosis, foot disorders, bony metastases, and changes in cardiac function increase the risk for hip fracture. Drugs, such as diuretics, antihypertensives, antidepressants, sedatives, opioids, and alcohol, are factors that increase the risks for falling in older adults. Use of three or more drugs at the same time drastically increases the risk for falls. Throw rugs, loose carpeting, floor clutter, inadequate lighting, uneven walking surfaces or steps, and pets are environmental hazards that also cause falls.

The older adult with hip fracture usually reports groin pain or pain behind the knee on the affected side. In some cases, the patient has pain in the lower back or no pain at all. However, the patient is not able to stand without pain. X-ray or other imaging assessment confirms the diagnosis.

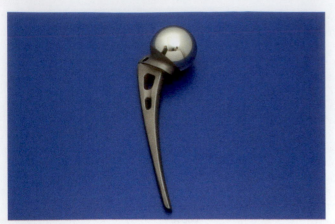

FIG. 51-10 Hip prosthesis used for femoral head or neck fractures (hemiarthroplasty). (Courtesy Smith & Nephew, Inc., Orthopaedics Divisions, Memphis, TN.)

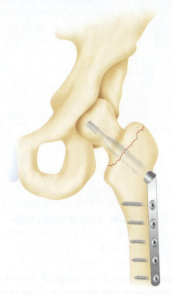

FIG. 51-11 Compression hip screw used for open reduction with internal fixation (ORIF) of the hip.

dressing or attempt to climb out of bed, possibly falling and causing self-injury. Other patients stay awake all night and sleep during the day. Keep in mind that some patients have a quiet delirium. Monitor the patient frequently to prevent falls. Use evidence-based fall prevention strategies and ask the family or other visitors to let staff know if the patient is attempting to get out of bed. Chapter 3 describes fall prevention strategies and delirium management in detail.

> **! NURSING SAFETY PRIORITY** (QSEN)
>
> **Action Alert**
>
> Patients who have a hemiarthroplasty are at risk for hip dislocation or subluxation. Be sure to prevent hip adduction and rotation to keep the operative leg in proper alignment. Regular pillows or abduction devices can be used for patients who are confused or restless. If straps are used to hold the device in place, make sure that they are not too tight and check the skin for signs of pressure. Perform neurovascular assessments to ensure that the device is not interfering with arterial circulation or peripheral nerve conduction.

The patient begins ambulating with assistance the day after surgery to prevent complications associated with immobility (e.g., pressure injuries, atelectasis, venous thromboembolism). Early MOBILITY and ambulation also decrease the chance of infection and increase surgical site healing.

Special considerations for the patient having a hip repair also include careful inspection of skin, including areas of pressure, especially the heels and sacrum. Use of skin traction to reduce muscle spasms may increase the period of bedrest before surgery. Decreased MOBILITY after surgery can increase the risk for pressure injury in this area within 24 hours.

> **! NURSING SAFETY PRIORITY** (QSEN)
>
> **Action Alert**
>
> Be sure that the patient's heels are up off the bed at all times. Inspect the heels and other high-risk bony prominence areas every 8 to 12 hours. Delegate turning and repositioning every 1 to 2 hours to unlicensed assistive personnel (UAP) and supervise this nursing activity.

Other postoperative interventions to prevent complications, such as venous thromboembolism, are similar to those for total hip replacement (see Chapter 16).

Many patients recover fully from hip fracture repair and regain their functional ability. They are typically discharged to their home, rehabilitation unit or center, or a skilled nursing facility for physical and occupational therapy. However, some patients are not able to return to their pre-fracture ADLs and MOBILITY level. Family caregivers often have unexpected responsibilities caring for patients during their recovery. Hip fracture resource centers can be very useful in providing caregiver support (see the Evidence-Based Practice box).

Other Fractures of the Lower Extremity

Other fractures of the lower extremity may or may not require hospitalization. However, if the patient has severe or multiple fractures, especially with soft-tissue damage, hospital admission is usually required. Patients who have surgery to repair their injury may also be hospitalized. Coordinate care with the physical and occupational therapists regarding MOBILITY, transfers, positioning, and ambulation. Collaborate with the case manager regarding placement after discharge. Most patients go home unless there is no support system or additional rehabilitation is needed. Health teaching and ensuring continuity of care are essential.

Fractures of the *lower two thirds of the femur* usually result from trauma, often from a motor vehicle crash. A femur fracture is seldom immobilized by casting because the powerful muscles of the thigh become spastic, which causes displacement of bone ends and significant pain. Extensive hemorrhage can occur with femur fracture.

Surgical treatment is ORIF with plates, nails, rods, or a compression screw. In a few cases in which extensive bone fragmentation or severe tissue trauma is found, external fixation may be used. Healing time for a femur fracture may be 6 months or longer. Skeletal traction, followed by a full-leg brace or cast, may be used in nonsurgical treatment.

Trauma to the lower leg most often causes fractures of both the *tibia* and the *fibula,* particularly the lower third, and is often referred to as a *tib-fib* fracture. The major treatment techniques

Are Online Resources Helpful for Caregivers of Patients After Hip Fracture?

Nahm, E-S., Resnick, B., Plummer, L., & Park, B. K. (2013). Use of discussion boards in an online hip fracture resource center for caregivers. *Orthopaedic Nursing, 32*(2), 89–96.

Family caregivers (CGs) are important for the successful recovery of patients who have hip fracture repair. In a previous study the authors found that CGs lacked knowledge in understanding how to provide care during the rehabilitation and recovery phase. The purpose of this qualitative study was to explore the experiences of CGs while they were using an online hip resource center over an 8-week period. The majority of the 27 caregivers in the study were female and white. Most had some college education, and their average age was 55.5 years. Each CG posted comments related to specific topics posted on the online discussion boards. Examples of topics included the roles of therapists, awareness of bone health, and caregiver stress. Three coders recorded and analyzed the data using well-established coding rules to ensure validity and reliability.

The analysis revealed common themes, such as need for adjustment to the fracture event, and three categories: types of care provided by the CGs, strategies used by CGs to prevent fractures, and coping mechanisms used to handle stress. The researchers concluded that discussion boards (DBs) can serve as a useful medium for CGs to share their experiences. They also noted that DBs can help health care providers identify ways to support CGs.

Level of Evidence: 4

This study was a well-designed qualitative study to gain specific information about the needs of CGs of patients with hip fractures.

Commentary: Implications for Practice and Research

Although this study was limited to a small sample size, the researchers were very careful to ensure validity and reliability of the coding process for data analysis. Additional studies with larger sample sizes that are more diverse are needed to provide generalization of results. Nurses caring for patients having surgical hip repair need to help families locate resources to provide information and support during the patients' rehabilitation and recovery period.

CLINICAL JUDGMENT CHALLENGE 51-1

Evidence-Based Practice; Safety QSEN

An 87-year-old woman living alone in a senior housing apartment complex experienced a fall resulting in a right sprained shoulder and left broken hip. Before her fall, she walked with a cane because of arthritis in her knees and hips. She has no family close by, and her best friend recently died. The patient is admitted to the emergency department and taken for surgery for an ORIF using a compression screw. Following a short stay in the ICU, she is admitted to your orthopedic unit for postoperative care. On admission she tells you that she plans to return to her apartment after her hospital stay but she is feeling very weak since her surgery. She is alert and oriented and is receiving IV fentanyl for pain control.

1. What assessment data will you need to collect from this patient on admission and why?
2. What are the priority nursing actions for her care on admission and during her stay to promote safety? Why?
3. On the second day of her hospital admission, the rehabilitation team evaluates the patient and determines that she needs intensive therapy to promote ADL functioning and mobility. When she hears this plan, she begins to cry and asks you why she can't go home to have therapy. What is your best response at this time?

---

are closed reduction with casting, internal fixation, and external fixation. If closed reduction is used, the patient may wear a cast for 6 to 10 weeks. Because of poor PERFUSION to parts of the tibia and fibula, delayed union is not unusual with this type of fracture. Internal fixation with nails or a plate and screws, followed by a long-leg cast for 4 to 6 weeks, is another option. Since the fibula is a non–weight-bearing bone, occasionally no fixation is required. When the fractures cause extensive skin and soft-tissue damage, the initial treatment may be external fixation, often for 6 to 10 weeks, usually followed by application of a cast until the fracture is completely healed. The patient is typically non–weight bearing and uses ambulatory aids such as crutches.

Ankle fractures are described by their anatomic place of injury. For example, a bimalleolar (Pott's) fracture involves the medial malleolus of the tibia and the lateral malleolus of the fibula. The small talus that makes up the rest of the ankle joint may also be broken. An ORIF is usually performed using two incisions: one on the medial (inside) aspect of the ankle and one on the lateral (outer) side. Several screws or nails are placed into the tibia, and a compression plate with multiple screws keeps the fibula in alignment. Weight bearing is restricted until the bone heals.

Treatment of fractures of the foot or phalanges (toes) is similar to that of other fractures. Phalangeal fractures may be more painful but are not as serious as most other types of fractures. Crutches are used for ambulation if weight bearing is restricted, but many patients can ambulate while wearing an orthopedic shoe or boot while the bone heals.

Fractures of the Chest and Pelvis

Chest trauma may cause fractures of the ribs or sternum. The major concern with rib and sternal fractures is the potential for puncture of the lungs, heart, or arteries by bone fragments or ends. *Assess airway, breathing, and circulation status **first** for any patient having chest trauma!* Fractures of the lower ribs may damage underlying organs, such as the liver, spleen, or kidneys. These fractures tend to heal on their own without surgical intervention. Patients are often uncomfortable during the healing process and require analgesia. They also have a high risk for pneumonia because of shallow breathing caused by pain on inspiration. Encourage them to breathe normally if possible and ensure that their pain is well managed.

Because the pelvis is very vascular and is close to major organs and blood vessels, associated internal damage is the major focus in fracture management. After head injuries, pelvic fractures are the second most common cause of death from trauma. In young adults, pelvic fractures typically result from motor vehicle crashes or falls from buildings. Falls are the most common cause in older adults. The major concern related to pelvic injury is venous oozing or arterial bleeding. Loss of blood volume leads to hypovolemic shock.

Assess for internal abdominal trauma by checking for blood in the urine and stool and by monitoring the abdomen for the development of rigidity or swelling. The trauma team may use peritoneal lavage, CT scanning, or ultrasound for assessment of hemorrhage. Ultrasound is noninvasive, rapid, reliable, and cost-effective, and it can be done at the bedside.

There are many classification systems for pelvic fractures. A system that is particularly useful divides fractures of the pelvis into two broad categories: non–weight-bearing fractures and weight-bearing fractures.

When a *non–weight-bearing* part of the pelvis is fractured, such as one of the pubic rami or the iliac crest, treatment can be as minimal as bedrest on a firm mattress or bed board. This type of fracture can be quite painful, and the patient may need stool softeners to facilitate bowel movements because of hesitancy to move. Well-stabilized fractures usually heal in 2 months.

A *weight-bearing* fracture, such as multiple fractures of the pelvic ring creating instability or a fractured acetabulum, necessitates external fixation or ORIF or both. Progression to weight bearing depends on the stability of the fracture after fixation. Some patients can fully bear weight within days of surgery, whereas others managed with traction may not be able to bear weight for as long as 12 weeks. For complex pelvic fractures with extensive soft-tissue damage, external fixation may be required.

Compression Fractures of the Spine

Most vertebral fractures are associated with osteoporosis, metastatic bone cancer, and multiple myeloma. Compression fractures result when trabecular or cancellous bone within the vertebra becomes weakened and causes the vertebral body to collapse. The patient has *severe* pain (especially when moving), deformity (kyphosis), and occasional neurologic compromise. As discussed in the Osteoporosis section of Chapter 50, the patient's quality of life is reduced by the impact of this problem.

Nonsurgical management includes bedrest, analgesics, nerve blocks, and physical therapy to maintain muscle strength. Vertebral compression fractures (VCFs) that remain painful and impair MOBILITY may be treated with vertebroplasty or kyphoplasty. These procedures are minimally invasive techniques in which bone cement is injected through the skin (percutaneously) directly into the fracture site to provide stability and immediate pain relief. In addition to vertebroplasty, radiologists and orthopedic surgeons may do a kyphoplasty (using a balloon) or the preferred vertebral augmentation (using a different cavity-creating device) to partially re-expand a compressed vertebral body.

Minimally invasive procedures can be done in an operating or interventional radiology suite by a surgeon or interventional radiologist. They can be done with moderate sedation or general anesthesia. IV ketorolac (Toradol) may be given before the procedure to reduce inflammation. Large-bore needles are placed into the fracture site using fluoroscopy or CT guidance. Then the deflated balloon is inserted through the needles and inflated in the fracture site, and the cement is injected.

Patients may have the procedures in an ambulatory care setting and return home after 2 to 4 hours or be admitted to the hospital for an overnight stay. Chart 51-6 describes the preprocedure and postprocedure care for percutaneous interventions for vertebral compression fractures.

Before discharge, teach the patient to report any signs or symptoms of infection from puncture sites. Remind him or her to not soak in a bath for 1 week, use analgesics as needed, resume activity, and contact the health care provider for questions or concerns. Surgery generally reduces preoperative pain significantly.

✳ PERFUSION CONCEPT EXEMPLAR Amputations

An amputation is the removal of a part of the body. Advances in microvascular surgical procedures, better use of antibiotic

CHART 51-6   Best Practice for Patient Safety & Quality Care QSEN

Nursing Care for Patients Having Vertebroplasty or Kyphoplasty

Provide *preprocedure care*, including:
- Check the patient's coagulation laboratory test results; platelet count should be more than 100,000/mm³.
- Make sure that all anticoagulant drugs were discontinued as requested by the physician.
- Assess and document the patient's neurologic status, especially extremity movement and sensation.
- Assess the patient's pain level.
- Assess the patient's ability to lie prone for at least 1 hour.
- Establish an IV line in a size suitable for surgery and take vital signs.

Provide *postprocedure care*, including:
- Place the patient in a flat supine position for 1 to 2 hours or as requested by the physician.
- Monitor and record vital signs and frequent neurologic assessments; report any change immediately to the physician.
- Apply an ice pack to the puncture site if needed to relieve pain.
- Assess the patient's pain level and compare it with the preoperative level; give mild analgesic as needed.
- Monitor for complications such as bleeding at the puncture site or shortness of breath; report these findings immediately if they occur.
- Assist the patient with ambulation.

Before discharge, teach the patient and family the following:
- The patient should avoid driving or operating machinery for the first 24 hours because of drugs used during the procedure.
- Monitor the puncture site for signs of infection, such as redness, pain, swelling, or drainage.
- Keep the dressing dry and remove it the next day.
- The patient should begin usual activities, including walking, the next day and should slowly increase activity level over the next few days.

therapy, and improved surgical techniques for traumatic injury and bone cancer have reduced the number of elective amputations. The psychosocial aspects of the procedure are as devastating as the physical impairments that result. The loss is complete and permanent and causes a change in body image and self-esteem. Collaborate with members of the interprofessional team, including prosthetists, rehabilitation therapists, psychologists, case managers, and physiatrists (rehabilitation physicians), when providing care to the patient who has an amputation.

❖ PATHOPHYSIOLOGY

Types of Amputation

Amputations may be elective or traumatic. Most are *elective* and are related to complications of peripheral vascular disease (PVD), arteriosclerosis, or numerous attempts to repair complex injuries. These complications result in impaired PERFUSION (ischemia) to distal areas of the lower extremity. Diabetes mellitus is often an underlying cause. Amputation is considered only after other interventions have not restored circulation to the lower extremity, sometimes referred to as *limb salvage procedures* (e.g., percutaneous transluminal angioplasty [PTA]). These procedures are discussed elsewhere in this text.

Traumatic amputations most often result from accidents or war and are the primary cause of *upper-extremity* amputation. A person may clean lawn mower blades or a snow blower without disconnecting the machine. A motor vehicle crash or industrial machine accident may also cause an amputation.

Levels of Amputation

Elective lower-extremity (LE) amputations are performed much more frequently than upper-extremity amputations. Several types of LE amputations may be performed (Fig. 51-12).

The loss of any or all of the small toes presents a minor disability. Loss of the great toe is significant because it affects balance, gait, and "push-off" ability during walking. Midfoot amputations and the Syme amputation are common procedures for peripheral vascular disease. In the Syme amputation, most of the foot is removed, but the ankle remains. The advantage of this surgery over traditional amputations below the knee is that weight bearing can occur without the use of a prosthesis and with reduced pain.

An intense effort is made to preserve knee joints with below-the-knee amputation (BKA). When the cause for the amputation extends beyond the knee, above-knee or higher amputations are performed. Hip disarticulation, or removal of the hip joint, and hemipelvectomy (removal of half of the pelvis with the leg) are more common in younger patients than in older ones who cannot easily handle the cumbersome prostheses required for ambulation. The higher the level of amputation, the more energy is required for MOBILITY. These higher-level procedures

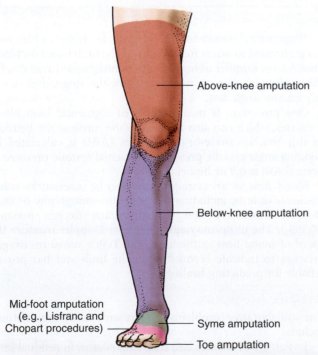

Above-knee amputation

Below-knee amputation

Mid-foot amputation (e.g., Lisfranc and Chopart procedures)

Syme amputation

Toe amputation

FIG. 51-12 Common levels of lower-extremity amputation.

are sometimes done for cancer of the bone, osteomyelitis, or trauma as a last resort.

An amputation of any part of the upper extremity is generally more incapacitating than one of the leg. The arms and hands are necessary for ADLs such as feeding, bathing, dressing, and driving a car. In the upper extremity, as much length as possible is saved to maintain function. Early replacement with a prosthetic device is vital for the patient with this type of amputation.

Complications of Amputation

The most common complications of elective or traumatic amputations are:

- Hemorrhage leading to hypovolemic shock
- Infection
- Phantom limb pain
- Neuroma
- Flexion contractures

When a person loses part or all of an extremity either by surgery or by trauma, major blood vessels are severed, which causes *hemorrhage*. If the bleeding is uncontrolled, the patient is at risk for hypovolemic shock and possibly death.

As with any surgical procedure or trauma, infection can occur in the wound or the bone (osteomyelitis). The older adult who is malnourished and confused is at the greatest risk because excreta may soil the wound or he or she may remove the dressing and pick at the incision. Preventing infection is a major emphasis in hospitals and other health care settings.

Pain is a frequent complication of amputation. Sensation is felt in the amputated part immediately after surgery and usually diminishes over time. When this SENSORY PERCEPTION persists and is unpleasant or painful, it is referred to as **phantom limb pain (PLP)**. PLP is more common in patients who had chronic limb pain before surgery and less common in those who have traumatic amputations. The patient reports pain in the removed body part shortly after surgery, usually after an above-the-knee amputation (AKA). The pain is often described as intense burning, crushing, or cramping. Some patients report that the removed part is in a distorted, uncomfortable position. They experience numbness and tingling, referred to as *phantom limb sensation,* and pain. Others state that the most distal area of the removed part feels as if it is retracted into the residual limb end. For most patients, the impaired COMFORT is triggered by touching the residual limb or by temperature or barometric pressure changes, concurrent illness, fatigue, anxiety, or stress. Routine activities such as urination can trigger the pain. If pain is long-standing, especially if it existed before the amputation, any stimulus can cause it, including touching any part of the body.

Neuroma, a sensitive tumor consisting of damaged nerve cells, forms most often in amputations of the upper extremity but can occur anywhere. The patient may or may not have pain. It is diagnosed by sonography and can be treated either surgically or nonsurgically. Surgery to remove the neuroma may be performed, but it often regrows and is more painful than before the surgery. Nonsurgical modalities include peripheral nerve blocks, steroid injections, and cognitive therapies such as hypnosis.

Flexion contractures of the hip or knee are most frequently seen in patients with amputations of the lower extremity. This complication must be avoided so the patient can ambulate with a prosthetic device. Proper positioning and active range-of-motion exercises in the early postoperative period help prevent this complication.

Health Promotion and Maintenance

The typical patient undergoing elective amputation is a middle-age or older man with diabetes and a lengthy history of smoking. He most likely has not cared for his feet properly, which has resulted in a nonhealing, infected foot ulcer and possibly gangrene. Therefore adherence to the disease management plan may help prevent the need for later amputation. Lifestyle habits such as maintaining a healthy weight, regular exercise, and avoiding smoking can help prevent chronic diseases such as diabetes and poor blood circulation.

The second largest group who has amputations consists of young men who have motorcycle or other vehicular crashes, are injured by industrial equipment, or have been in combat or accidents in war. These men may either experience a traumatic amputation or undergo a surgical amputation because of a severe crushing injury and massive soft-tissue damage. Teach young male adults the importance of taking safety precautions to prevent injury at work and to avoid speeding or driving while drinking alcohol. An increasing number of young women also tend to speed and drive while drinking, which endangers themselves and others around them.

❖ INTERPROFESSIONAL COLLABORATIVE CARE
◆ Assessment: Noticing
Physical Assessment/Signs and Symptoms. Monitor neurovascular status in the affected extremity that will be electively amputated. When the patient has peripheral vascular disease, check circulation in both legs. Assess skin color, temperature, sensation, and pulses in both affected and unaffected extremities. Capillary refill can be difficult to determine in the older adult related to thickened and opaque nails. In this situation, the skin near the nail bed can be used (see Chart 51-3). Capillary refill is not as reliable as other indicators. Observe and document any discoloration of the skin, edema, ulcerations, presence of necrosis, and hair distribution on the lower extremities.

Psychosocial Assessment. People react differently to the loss of a body part. Be aware that an amputation of only a portion of one finger, especially the thumb, can be traumatic to the patient. The thumb is needed for hand activities. Therefore the loss must not be underestimated. Patients undergoing amputation face a complete, permanent loss. Evaluate their psychological preparation for a planned amputation and expect them to go through the grieving process. Adjusting to a traumatic, unexpected amputation is often more difficult than accepting a planned one.

Attempt to determine the patient's willingness and motivation to withstand prolonged rehabilitation after the amputation. Asking questions about how he or she has dealt with previous

♥ VETERANS' HEALTH CONSIDERATIONS
Patient-Centered Care **QSEN**

The young veteran may be bitter, hostile, and depressed. In addition to loss of a body part, he or she may lose a job, the ability to participate in favorite recreational activities, or a social relationship if other people cannot accept the body change.

The patient having one or more amputations has an altered self-concept. The physical alterations that result affect body image and self-esteem. For example, a young male may think that an intimate relationship with a partner is no longer possible or desirable. An older adult may feel a loss of independence. Assess the patient's feelings about himself or herself to identify areas in which he or she needs emotional support. Consult with the certified hospital chaplain, other spiritual leader, or hospital social worker if the patient is hospitalized. Counseling resources are also available in the community and the Veterans' Administration health system in the United States.

life crises can provide clues. Adjustment to the amputation and rehabilitation is less difficult if the patient is willing to make needed changes.

🌐 CULTURAL/SPIRITUAL CONSIDERATIONS
Patient-Centered Care **QSEN**

In addition to assessing the patient's psychosocial status, assess the family's reaction to the surgery or trauma. Their response usually correlates directly with the patient's progress during recovery and rehabilitation and his or her values and beliefs. Expect the family to grieve for the loss and allow them time to adjust to the change. Establish a trusting relationship and reassure the patient and family that you are available to listen to their concerns and needs.

Assess the patient's and family's coping abilities and help them identify personal strengths and weaknesses. Assess the patient's religious, spiritual, and cultural beliefs. Some groups (e.g., Jewish) require that the amputated body part be stored for later burial with the rest of the body or buried immediately. Other cultural customs and rituals may apply, depending on the group with which the patient associates.

Diagnostic Assessment. The surgeon determines which tests are performed to assess for viability of the limb based on blood flow. A large number of noninvasive techniques are available for this evaluation. For complete accuracy, the surgeon does not rely on any single test.

One procedure is measurement of segmental limb blood pressures, which can also be used by the nurse at the bedside. In this test, an **ankle-brachial index (ABI)** is calculated by dividing ankle systolic pressure by brachial systolic pressure. A normal ABI is 0.9 or higher.

Blood flow in an extremity can also be assessed by other noninvasive tests, including Doppler ultrasonography or laser Doppler flowmetry and transcutaneous oxygen pressure ($TcPO_2$). The ultrasonography and laser Doppler measure the speed of blood flow in the limb. The $TcPO_2$ measures oxygen pressure to indicate blood flow in the limb and has proven reliable for predicting healing.

◆ Analysis: Interpreting
The collaborative problems for patients with amputations include:

1. Potential for decreased tissue PERFUSION in residual limb due to soft tissue damage, edema, and/or bleeding

2. Acute and/or chronic pain due to soft-tissue damage, muscle spasm, and edema
3. Decreased MOBILITY due to pain, muscle spasm, soft-tissue damage, and/or lack of balance due to a missing body part
4. Potential for infection due to a wound caused by surgery or trauma
5. Decreased self-esteem due to one or more ADL deficits, disturbed self-concept, and/or lack of support systems

◆ *Planning and Implementation: Responding*

Monitoring for Decreased Tissue Perfusion

Planning: Expected Outcomes. The patient with one or more amputations is expected to have adequate peripheral PERFUSION to the residual (surgical) limb(s) as evidenced by warm, usual-color skin.

Interventions. A traumatic amputation requires rapid emergency care to possibly save the severed body part for reattachment to promote PERFUSION and prevent hemorrhage.

Emergency Care: Traumatic Amputation. For a person who has a traumatic amputation in the community, first call 911. Assess the patient for airway or breathing problems. Examine the amputation site and apply direct pressure with layers of dry gauze or other cloth, using clean gloves if available. Many nurses carry gloves and first-aid kits for this type of emergency. Elevate the extremity above the patient's heart to decrease the bleeding. Do not remove the dressing to prevent dislodging the clot.

The fingers are the most likely part to be amputated and replanted. The current recommendation for prehospital care is to wrap the completely severed finger in dry sterile gauze (if available) or a clean cloth. Put the finger in a watertight, sealed plastic bag. *Place the bag in ice water, never directly on ice, at 1 part ice and 3 parts water.* Avoid contact between the finger and the water to prevent tissue damage. Do not remove any semi-detached parts of the digit. Be sure that the part goes with the patient to the hospital.

For patients with a *planned surgical amputation*, the nurse's primary focus is to monitor for signs indicating that there is sufficient tissue PERFUSION and no hemorrhage. The skin flap at the end of the residual (remaining) limb should be pink in a light-skinned person and not discolored (lighter or darker than other usual skin pigmentation) in a dark-skinned patient. The area should be warm but not hot. Assess the closest proximal pulse for presence and strength and compare it with that in the other extremity. However, if the patient has bilateral vascular disease, comparison of limbs may not be an accurate way of measuring blood flow. Use a Doppler device to determine if the affected side is being perfused. Monitor vital signs per agency protocol.

> **! NURSING SAFETY PRIORITY** QSEN
>
> **Critical Rescue**
>
> *If the patient has decreased tissue perfusion, notify the surgeon immediately to communicate your assessment findings!* If the patient's blood pressure drops and the pulse increases, suspect covert (hidden) bleeding and notify the surgeon or Rapid Response Team. *To check for the presence of overt (obvious) bleeding, be sure to lift the residual limb and feel under the pressure dressing for dampness or drainage.* If bleeding occurs, apply direct pressure and notify the Rapid Response Team or health care provider immediately. Continue to monitor the patient until help arrives.

Managing Acute and/or Chronic Pain

Planning: Expected Outcomes. The patient with an amputation is expected to state that he or she has adequate pain control and improved COMFORT after appropriate pain management.

Interventions. All patients experience pain as a result of either a traumatic or surgical (elective) amputation. Some patients also report pain in the missing body part (PLP). Be sure to determine which type the patient has, because they are managed very differently.

> **! NURSING SAFETY PRIORITY** QSEN
>
> **Action Alert**
>
> If the patient reports PLP, recognize that the pain is real and should be managed promptly and completely! It is *not* therapeutic to remind the patient that the limb cannot be hurting because it is missing. To prevent increased pain, handle the residual limb carefully when assessing the site or changing the dressing.

Opioid analgesics are not as effective for PLP as they are for residual limb pain. IV infusions of calcitonin (Miacalcin, Calcimar) during the week after amputation can reduce PLP. The primary health care provider prescribes other drugs on the basis of the type of PLP the patient experiences. For instance, beta-blocking agents such as propranolol (Inderal, Apo-Propranolol, Detensol) are used for constant, dull, burning pain. Antiepileptic drugs such as pregabalin (Lyrica) and gabapentin (Neurontin) may be used for knifelike or sharp burning (neuropathic) pain. Antispasmodics such as baclofen (Lioresal) may be prescribed for muscle spasms or cramping. Some patients improve with antidepressant drugs as adjuvant therapy.

Other pain management modalities are described in Chapter 4. Incorporate them into the plan of care if agreeable with the patient by collaborating with specialists who are trained to perform them. For example, physical therapists often use massage, heat, transcutaneous electrical nerve stimulation (TENS), and ultrasound therapy for pain control. Consult with the certified hospital chaplain or social worker to provide emotional support based on the patient's preferences and beliefs. A psychologist may be needed to provide psychotherapy.

> **? NCLEX EXAMINATION CHALLENGE 51-3**
>
> **Psychosocial Integrity**
>
> A client who had an elective below-the-knee amputation (BKA) reports pain in the foot that was amputated last week. What is the nurse's **most appropriate** response to the client's pain?
> A. "The pain will go away after the swelling decreases."
> B. "That's phantom limb pain, and every amputee has that."
> C. "Your foot has been amputated, so it's in your head."
> D. "On a scale of 0 to 10, how would you rate your pain?"

Promoting Mobility

Planning: Expected Outcomes. The patient with an amputation is expected to have adequate MOBILITY and be free of complications associated with impaired mobility. The patient is also expected to be fitted and prepared for a prosthesis, if possible, to promote MOBILITY.

Interventions. Collaborate with the physical and/or occupational therapists to begin exercises as soon as possible after surgery. If the amputation is planned, the therapist may work with the patient before surgery to start muscle-strengthening exercises and evaluate the need for ambulatory aids, such as crutches. If the patient can practice with these devices before surgery, learning how to ambulate after surgery is much easier.

Interprofessional collaborative care depends on the type and location of the amputation. For example, an above-the-knee amputation (AKA) has the potential for more postoperative complications than does a partial foot amputation. Regardless of where the amputation occurs, collaborate with the rehabilitation therapists to improve ambulation and/or enable the patient to be independent in ADLs. For many amputations, prostheses can be used to substitute for the missing body part.

Patients undergoing lower-extremity amputation today are not usually confined to a wheelchair. Advancements in the design of prosthetics have enabled them to become independent. Therefore complications from extended bedrest are not common, even for older adults.

For patients with AKAs or BKAs, teach range-of-motion (ROM) exercises for prevention of flexion contractures, particularly of the hip and knee. A trapeze and an overhead frame aid in strengthening the arms and allow the patient to move independently in bed. Teach the patient how to perform ROM exercises. Be sure to turn the patient every 2 hours or teach him or her to turn independently. Move the patient slowly to prevent muscle spasms.

A firm mattress is essential for preventing contractures with a leg amputation. Assist the patient into a prone position every 3 to 4 hours for 20- to 30-minute periods if tolerated and not contraindicated. This position may be uncomfortable initially but helps prevent hip flexion contractures. Instruct the patient to pull the residual limb close to the other leg and contract the gluteal muscles of the buttocks for muscle strengthening. After staples are removed, the physical therapist may begin resistive exercises, which should also be done at home.

For above- and below-the-knee amputations, teach the patient how to push the residual limb down toward the bed while supporting it on a soft pillow at first. Then instruct him or her to continue this activity using a firmer pillow and then progress to a harder surface. This activity helps prepare the residual limb for prosthesis and reduces the incidence of phantom limb pain and sensation.

Elevation of a lower-leg residual limb on a pillow while the patient is in a supine position is controversial. Some practitioners advocate avoiding this practice at all times because it promotes hip or knee flexion contracture. Others allow elevation for the first 24 to 48 hours to reduce swelling and subsequent impaired COMFORT. Inspect the residual limb daily to ensure that it lies completely flat on the bed.

Before an elective amputation, the patient often sees a certified prosthetist-orthotist (CPO) so planning can begin for the postoperative period. Arrangements for replacing an arm part are especially important so the patient can achieve self-management. Some patients are fitted with a temporary prosthesis at the time of surgery. Others, particularly older patients with vascular disease, are fitted after the residual limb has healed.

The patient being fitted for a leg prosthesis should bring a sturdy pair of shoes to the fitting. The prosthesis will be adjusted to that heel height.

Several devices help shape and shrink the residual limb in preparation for the prosthesis. Rigid, removable dressings are preferred because they decrease edema, protect and shape the limb, and allow easy access to the wound for inspection. The Jobst air splint, a plastic inflatable device, is sometimes used for this purpose. One of its disadvantages is air leakage and loss of compression. Wrapping with elastic bandages can also be effective in reducing edema, shrinking the limb, and holding the wound dressing in place.

For wrapping to be effective, reapply the bandages every 4 to 6 hours or more often if they become loose. *Figure-eight wrapping prevents restriction of blood flow. Decrease the tightness of the bandages while wrapping in a distal-to-proximal direction.* After wrapping, anchor the bandages to the highest joint, such as above the knee for BKAs (Fig. 51-13).

The design of and materials for prostheses have improved dramatically over the years. Computer-assisted design and manufacturing (CAD-CAM) is used for a custom fit. One of the most important developments in lower-extremity prosthetics is the ankle-foot prosthesis, such as the Flex-Foot for more active amputees.

Preventing Infection.

Planning: Expected Outcomes. The patient with an amputation is expected to be free of wound or bone infection as evidenced by no fever, no increase in white blood cell count, and negative wound culture.

Interventions. The surgeon typically prescribes a broad-spectrum prophylactic antibiotic immediately before elective surgery to prevent infection. It may be continued for patients with *traumatic* amputations or for those who have open wounds on the residual limb. The initial pressure dressing and surgical drains are usually removed by the surgeon 36 to 48 hours after surgery. Inspect the incision or wound for signs of infection. Record the appearance, amount, and odor of drainage, if present. The surgeon may want the incision open to air until staples or sutures are removed or the residual limb to have a continuous soft or rigid dressing made of fiberglass. A soft dressing is secured by an elastic bandage wrapped firmly around the residual limb.

Promoting Self-Esteem.

Planning: Expected Outcomes. The patient with an amputation is expected to adapt to the amputation to achieve a positive self-esteem and have an active and productive life.

Interventions. The patient often experiences feelings of inadequacy as a result of losing a body part, especially the older adult who was in poor health before surgery and men who are often the main providers for their families. If the patient is not able to adapt psychologically to the amputation, he or she may have difficulty adapting to a possible lifestyle change. If possible, arrange for him or her to meet with a rehabilitated, active amputee who is about the same age as the patient.

Freysteinson et al. (2016) studied a technique to help amputees get used to their body change as part of rehabilitation therapy. The authors asked the patients to view themselves in a mirror for repeated viewings. Four key themes emerged as a result of the study: mirror shock, mirror anguish, recognizing self, and acceptance as a new "normal." These themes are similar to other loss and grieving responses (see Chapter 7).

Use of the word *stump* for referring to the remaining portion of the limb (residual limb) continues to be controversial. Patients have reported feeling as if they were part of a tree when the term was used. However, some rehabilitation specialists who routinely work with amputees believe the term is appropriate because it forces the patient to realize what has happened and promotes adjustment to the amputation. *Assess the patient to determine which term is preferred.*

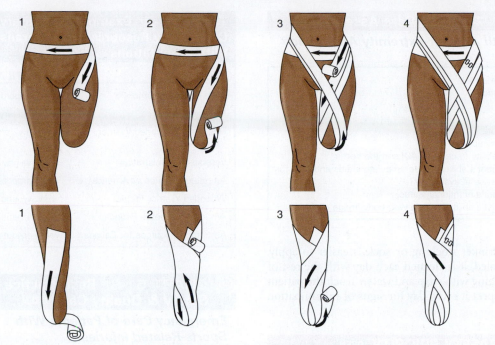

FIG. 51-13 Common method of wrapping an amputation stump. *Top,* Wrapping for above-knee amputation. *Bottom,* Wrapping for below-knee amputation.

Assess the patient's verbal and nonverbal references to the affected area. Some patients behave euphorically (extremely happy) and seem to have accepted the loss. *Do not jump to the conclusion that acceptance has occurred.* Ask the patient to describe his or her feelings about changes in body image and self-esteem. He or she may verbalize acceptance but refuse to look at the area during a dressing change. This inconsistent behavior is not unusual and should be documented and shared with other health care team members.

With advancements in prostheses and surgical techniques, most patients can return to their jobs and other activities. Professional athletes who use prostheses are often quite successful in sports. Patients with amputations ski, hike, golf, bowl, and participate in other physically demanding activities. Many amputees participate actively in organized and recreational sports.

If a job or career change is necessary, collaborate with a social worker or vocational rehabilitation specialist to evaluate the patient's skills. A supportive family or significant other is important for the adjustment to this change. The patient may also think that an intimate relationship is no longer possible because of physical changes. Discuss sexuality issues with the patient and his or her partner as needed. Professional assistance from a sex therapist, intimacy coach, or psychologist may be needed.

Help the patient and family set realistic desired outcomes and take one day at a time. Help them recognize personal strengths. If the desired outcomes are not realistic, frustration and disappointment may decrease motivation during rehabilitation. Basic principles of rehabilitation are discussed in Chapter 6.

Care Coordination and Transition Management

The patient is discharged directly to home or to a skilled facility or rehabilitation facility, depending on the extent of the amputation. When rehabilitation is not feasible, as in the debilitated

CLINICAL JUDGMENT CHALLENGE 51-2
Patient-Centered Care; Teamwork and Collaboration; Informatics **QSEN**

A 74-year-old African-American man is admitted to your surgical unit following a left below-the-knee amputation (BKA) for peripheral vascular disease and long-term diabetes mellitus. His residual limb is wrapped in a pressure dressing and slightly elevated on a towel with ice packs. The patient's wife of 50 years is at his bedside and informs you that their son and daughter-in-law are on their way to the hospital to talk with the surgeon. She also tells you that her husband is a very religious man and will likely want you to pray with him.

1. As his nurse, what is your priority action when assessing this patient? What other assessments will you perform and document in the electronic medical record (EMR)?
2. How might you respond at this time to his wife's statement about praying with the patient?
3. With what members of the interprofessional health care team will you consult and collaborate and why?

or demented older adult, he or she may be discharged to a long-term care facility. Coordinate this transfer with the case manager or discharge planner to ensure continuity of care.

Home Care Management. At home, the patient with a leg amputation needs to have enough room to use a wheelchair if the prosthesis is not yet available. He or she must be able to use toileting facilities and have access to areas necessary for self-management, such as the kitchen. Structural home modifications may be required before the patient goes home.

Self-Management Education. After the sutures or staples are removed, the patient begins residual limb care. A home care nurse may be needed to teach the patient and/or family how to care for the limb and the prosthesis if it is available (Chart 51-7). The limb should be rewrapped three times a day with an elastic bandage applied in a figure-eight manner (see Fig. 51-13). For

CHART 51-7 Home Care Assessment

The Patient With a Lower-Extremity Amputation in the Home

Assess the residual limb for:
- Adequate circulation
- Infection
- Healing
- Flexion contracture
- Dressing/elastic wrap

Assess the patient's ability to perform ADLs in the home.
- Evaluate the patient's ability to use ambulatory aids and care for the prosthetic device (if available).
- Assess the patient's nutritional status.
- Assess the patient's ability to cope with body image change.

many patients, a shrinker stocking or sock is easier to apply. After the limb is healed, it is cleaned each day with the rest of the body during bathing with soap and water. Teach the patient and/or family to inspect it every day for signs of inflammation or skin breakdown.

 NURSING SAFETY PRIORITY **QSEN**

Action Alert

Collaborate with the prosthetist to teach the patient about prosthesis care after amputation to ensure its reliability and proper function. These devices are custom made, taking into account the patient's level of amputation, lifestyle, and occupation. Proper teaching regarding correct cleansing of the socket and inserts, wearing the correct liners, and assessing shoe wear and a schedule of follow-up care are essential before discharge. This information may need to be reviewed by the home care nurse.

Health Care Resources. A patient who seems to adjust to the amputation during hospitalization may realize that it is difficult to cope with the loss after discharge from the hospital. Teach the patient and family about available resources and support from organizations such as the Amputee Coalition of America (ACA) (www.amputee-coalition.org) and the National Amputation Foundation (NAF) (www.nationalamputation.org). The NAF was originally started for veterans but has since expanded to offer services to civilians.

 VETERANS' HEALTH CONSIDERATIONS

Patient-Centered Care **QSEN**

Teach patients who are veterans about the many resources that can help them adjust to one or more amputations. In addition to specialty clinics and other services offered by the Veterans Administration in the United States, many other community and military services exist to help veterans adapt their lifestyle and remain active. Many of these services also assist families of veterans who have been injured (Table 51-2).

◆ *Evaluation: Reflecting*

Evaluate the care of the patient with one or more amputations based on the identified priority patient problems. The expected outcomes include that the patient:
- Have adequate peripheral PERFUSION to the residual limb
- State that pain is controlled to between a 2 and 3 on a 0-10 pain intensity assessment scale

TABLE 51-2 Examples of Military and Community Resources for Veterans With Amputations

RESOURCE	WEBSITE ADDRESS
Hope For The Warriors™	www.hopeforthewarriors.org
Military OneSource	www.militaryonesource.com
U.S. Army Wounded Warrior Program	www.aw2.army.mil
Veterans Administration	www.va.gov
Amputee Coalition of America	www.amputee-coalition.org
Wounded Warrior Project	www.woundedwarriorproject.org
American Amputee Foundation	www.americanamputee.org
Amputee Resources for Canada	www.amputee.ca

 CHART 51-8 Best Practice for Patient Safety & Quality Care **QSEN**

Emergency Care of Patients With Sports-Related Injuries

- Do not move the victim until spinal cord injury is ascertained (see Chapter 43 for assessment of spinal cord injury).
- Use RICE:
  - **Rest** the injured part; immobilize the joint above and below the injury by applying a splint if needed.
  - Apply **ice** intermittently for the first 24 to 48 hours (heat may be used thereafter).
  - Use **compression** for the first 24 to 48 hours (e.g., elastic wrap).
  - **Elevate** the affected limb to decrease swelling.
- Always assume that the area is fractured until x-ray studies are done.
- Assess neurovascular status in the area distal to the injury.

- Perform MOBILITY skills independently and not experience complications of decreased mobility
- Be free of surgical site infection
- Have a positive self-esteem and lifestyle adaptation to live a productive, high quality life

KNEE INJURIES

In addition to the bone and muscle problems already discussed, trauma can cause cartilage, ligament, and tendon injury. Many musculoskeletal injuries are the result of playing sports (professional and recreational) or doing other strenuous physical activities. The popularity of all-terrain vehicles (ATVs) and skateboarding has increased injuries in younger patients. Sports injuries have become so common that large metropolitan hospitals have sports medicine clinics and physicians who specialize in this field.

The principles of injury to one part of the body are similar to those of other sports injuries and accidents. For example, a tendon rupture in a knee is cared for in the same manner as a tendon rupture in the wrist. Chart 51-8 lists general emergency measures for sports-related injuries.

Because the knee is most often injured, it is discussed as a typical example of other areas of the body. Trauma to the knee results in **internal derangement**, a broad term for disturbances of an injured knee joint. When surgery is required to resolve the problem, most surgeons prefer to perform the

TABLE 51-3   Examples of Acute Soft-Tissue Musculoskeletal Injuries

ACUTE INJURY/DESCRIPTION	MANAGEMENT
Sprain: Excessive stretching of a ligament	Immobilization, RICE, possible surgery if severe
Strain: Excessive stretching of a muscle or tendon	Heat/cold, activity limitations, NSAIDs, muscle relaxants, possible tendon repair
Ligament tear (such as anterior cruciate ligament in knee): Damage to ligament most often caused by sports or vehicular crash	RICE, surgery if does not heal or is severe (usually arthroscopic)
Meniscus tear: Damage to knee cartilage caused by sports or other trauma	RICE, bracing, splinting, NSAIDs, surgery (usually arthroscopic)
Tendon rupture (such as the Achilles tendon in heel): Often caused by sports or wearing high-heeled shoes; in some cases can occur after taking fluoroquinolones such as ciprofloxacin (Cipro)	RICE, NSAIDs, orthotic devices, ultrasound, surgery if severe or does not heal
Patellofemoral pain syndrome (PFPS): Knee pain caused by overuse of the knee joint; also called *runner's knee*	Rest, splinting, bracing, NSAIDs, possibly surgery as last resort
Joint dislocation: Displacement of a bone from its usual position in a synovial joint	Manual joint relocation; possible surgery

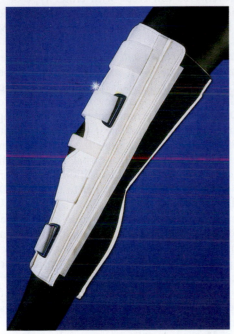

FIG. 51-14 Knee immobilizer. (Courtesy Zimmer, Inc., Warsaw, IN.)

procedure through an arthroscope when possible. A description of arthroscopy is presented in Chapter 49. Postoperative care for knee surgeries generally includes analgesics, physical therapy, and bracing or splinting, often using a knee immobilizer (Fig. 51-14). All patients require frequent neurovascular monitoring. Table 51-3 lists examples of common knee injuries and their interprofessional management.

CARPAL TUNNEL SYNDROME

❖ PATHOPHYSIOLOGY

Carpal tunnel syndrome (CTS) is a common condition in which the median nerve in the wrist becomes compressed, causing pain and numbness. The carpal tunnel is a rigid canal that lies between the carpal bones and a fibrous tissue sheet. A group of tendons surround the synovium and share space with the median nerve in the carpal tunnel. When the synovium becomes swollen or thickened, this nerve is compressed.

The median nerve supplies motor, sensory, and autonomic function for the first three fingers of the hand and the palmar aspect of the fourth (ring) finger. Because the median nerve is close to other structures, wrist flexion causes nerve impingement, and extension causes increased pressure in the lower portion of the carpal tunnel.

CTS is the most common type of **repetitive stress injury (RSI)**. RSIs are the fastest growing type of occupational injury. People whose jobs require repetitive hand activities such as pinching or grasping during wrist flexion (e.g., factory workers, computer operators, jackhammer operators) are predisposed to CTS. It can also result from overuse in sports activities such as golf, tennis, or racquetball.

CTS usually presents as a chronic problem. Acute cases are rare. Excessive hand exercise, edema or hemorrhage into the carpal tunnel, or thrombosis of the median artery can lead to acute CTS. *Patients with hand burns or a Colles' fracture of the wrist are particularly at risk for this problem.* In most cases, the cause may not result in nerve deficit for years.

CTS is also a common complication of certain metabolic and connective tissue diseases. For example, **synovitis** (inflammation of the synovium) occurs in patients with rheumatoid arthritis (RA). The hypertrophied synovium compresses the median nerve. In other chronic disorders such as diabetes mellitus, inadequate blood supply can cause median nerve neuropathy or dysfunction, resulting in CTS.

In a few cases, CTS may be a familial or congenital problem that manifests in adulthood. Space-occupying growths such as ganglia, tophi, and lipomas can also result in nerve compression.

🔴🔴 GENDER HEALTH CONSIDERATIONS
Patient-Centered Care QSEN

Women, especially those older than 50 years, are much more likely than men to experience CTS, probably due to the higher prevalence of diseases such as RA in women. The problem usually affects the dominant hand but can occur in both hands simultaneously. CTS is beginning to be found in children and adolescents as a result of the increased use of handheld mobile devices.

Health Promotion and Maintenance

Most businesses recognize the hazards of repetitive motion as a primary cause of occupational injury and disability. Both men

Health Promotion Activities to Prevent Carpal Tunnel Syndrome

- Become familiar with federal and state laws regarding workplace requirements to prevent repetitive stress injuries such as carpal tunnel syndrome (CTS).
- When using equipment or computer workstations that can contribute to developing CTS, assess that they are ergonomically appropriate, including:
  - Specially designed wrist rest devices
  - Geometrically designed computer keyboards
  - Chair height that allows good posture
- Take regular short breaks away from activities that cause repetitive stress, such as working at computers.
- Stretch fingers and wrists frequently during work hours.
- Stay as relaxed as possible when using equipment that causes repetitive stress.

and women in the labor force are experiencing increasing numbers of RSIs. Occupational health nurses have played an important role in ergonomic assessments and in the development of ergonomically designed furniture and various aids to decrease CTS and other musculoskeletal injuries.

U.S. federal and state legislation has been passed to ensure that all businesses, including health care organizations (HCOs), provide *ergonomically appropriate workstations* for their employees (Occupational Safety and Health Administration [OSHA]). The Joint Commission also requires that hospitals and other HCOs provide a safe work environment for all staff. In Canada, each province requires the work setting to have joint health and safety committees in which employees are actively involved in setting safety standards (Canadian Centre for Occupational Health and Safety). Chart 51-9 lists best practices for preventing CTS in the health care setting.

❖ INTERPROFESSIONAL COLLABORATIVE CARE

◆ Assessment: Noticing

A diagnosis is often made based on the patient's history and report of hand pain and numbness and without further assessment. Ask about the nature, intensity, and location of the pain. Patients often state that the pain is worse at night as a result of flexion or direct pressure during sleep. The pain may radiate to the arm, shoulder and neck, or chest.

In addition to reports of numbness, patients with carpal tunnel syndrome (CTS) may also have **paresthesia** (painful tingling). *Sensory* changes usually occur weeks or months before *motor* manifestations.

The primary health care provider (PHCP) performs several tests for abnormal sensory findings. Phalen's wrist test, sometimes called **Phalen's maneuver**, produces paresthesia in the median nerve distribution (palmar side of the thumb, index and middle fingers, and half of the ring finger) within 60 seconds as a result of increased internal carpal pressure. The patient is asked to relax the wrist into flexion or to place the back of the hands together and flex both wrists at the same time. The Phalen's test is positive in most patients with CTS (Jarvis, 2014).

The same sensation can be created by tapping lightly over the area of the median nerve in the wrist (**Tinel's sign**). If the test is unsuccessful, a blood pressure cuff can be placed on the

upper arm and inflated to the patient's systolic pressure (tourniquet). This often causes pain and tingling (Jarvis, 2014).

Motor changes in CTS begin with a weak pinch, clumsiness, and difficulty with fine movements. These changes progress to muscle weakness and wasting, which can impair self-management. If desired, test for pinching ability and ask the patient to perform a fine-movement task, such as threading a needle. Strenuous hand activity worsens the pain and numbness (McCance et al., 2014).

In addition to inspecting for muscle atrophy and task performance, observe the wrist for swelling. Gently palpate the area and note any unusual findings. Autonomic changes may be evidenced by skin discoloration, nail changes (e.g., brittleness), and increased or decreased hand sweating.

◆ Interventions: Responding

The PHCP uses conservative measures before surgical intervention. However, CTS can recur with either type of treatment. Management depends on the patient, but established best practices have not been determined (Skinner & McMahon, 2014).

Nonsurgical Management. Aggressive drug therapy and immobilization of the wrist are the major components of nonsurgical management. Teach the patient the importance of these modalities in the hope of preventing surgical intervention.

NSAIDs are the most commonly prescribed drugs for the relief of pain and inflammation, if present. In addition to or instead of systemic medications, the physician may inject corticosteroids directly into the carpal tunnel. If the patient responds to the injection, several additional weekly or monthly injections are given. Teach him or her to take NSAIDs with or after meals to reduce gastric irritation.

A splint or hand brace may be used to immobilize the wrist during the day, during the night, or both. Many patients experience temporary relief with these devices. The occupational therapist places the wrist in the neutral position or in slight extension.

Laser or ultrasound therapy may also be helpful. Some patients report fewer symptoms after beginning yoga or other exercise routine.

Surgical Management. Surgery can relieve the pressure on the median nerve by providing nerve decompression. Major surgical complications are rare after CTS surgery. However, in some cases, CTS recurs months to years after surgery.

The nurse in the surgeon's office or same-day surgical center reinforces the teaching provided by the surgeon regarding the nature of the surgery. Postoperative care is reviewed so the patient knows what to expect. Chapter 14 describes general preoperative care in detail.

Whatever the cause of nerve compression, the surgeon removes it either by cutting or by laser. The most common surgery is the endoscopic carpal tunnel release (ECTR). In this procedure, the surgeon makes a very small incision (less than ½ inch [1.2 cm]) through which the endoscope is inserted. He or she then uses special instruments to free the trapped median nerve. Although ECTR is less invasive and costs less than the open procedure, the patient may have a longer period of postoperative pain and numbness compared with recovery from open carpal tunnel release (OCTR). A recent systematic review showed that surgical treatment seems to be more effective than conservative measures over the long term. However, there was no evidence that one type of procedure, open or endoscopic, was more effective than the other; it is basically surgeon preference (Skinner & McMahon, 2014).

After surgery, monitor vital signs and check the dressing carefully for drainage and tightness. If ECTR has been performed, the dressing is very small. The surgeon may require that the patient's affected hand and arm be elevated above heart level for several days to reduce postoperative swelling. Check the neurovascular status of the fingers every hour during the immediate postoperative period and encourage the patient to move them frequently. Offer pain medication and assure him or her that a prescription for analgesics will be provided before discharge.

Hand movements, including lifting heavy objects, may be restricted for 4 to 6 weeks after surgery. The patient can expect weakness and discomfort for weeks or perhaps months. Teach him or her to report any changes in neurovascular status, including increased pain, to the surgeon's office immediately.

Remind the patient and family that the surgical procedure might not be a cure. For example, synovitis may recur with rheumatoid arthritis and may recompress the median nerve. Multiple surgeries and other treatments are common with CTS.

The patient may need help with self-management activities during recovery. Ensure that assistance in the home is available before discharge; this is usually provided by the family or significant others.

❓ NCLEX EXAMINATION CHALLENGE 51-4

Safe and Effective Care Environment

What is the nurse's **priority** when doing an admission for a client who returned directly from the operating suite after a carpal tunnel repair?
A. Monitor vital signs, including pulse oximetry.
B. Check the surgical dressing to ensure that it is intact.
C. Assess neurovascular assessment in the affected arm.
D. Monitor intake and output.

ROTATOR CUFF INJURIES

The musculotendinous, or rotator, cuff of the shoulder functions to stabilize the head of the humerus in the glenoid cavity during shoulder abduction. Young adults usually sustain a tear of the cuff by substantial trauma, such as may occur during a fall, while throwing a ball, or with heavy lifting. Older adults tend to have small tears related to aging, repetitive motions, or falls; and the tears are usually painless.

The patient with a torn rotator cuff has shoulder pain and cannot easily abduct the arm at the shoulder. When the arm is abducted, he or she usually drops it because abduction cannot be maintained (drop arm test). Pain is more intense at night and with overhead activities. Partial-thickness tears are more painful than full-thickness tears, but full-thickness tears result in more weakness and loss of function. Muscle atrophy is commonly seen, and MOBILITY is reduced. Diagnosis is confirmed with x-rays, MRI, ultrasonography, and/or CT scans.

The primary health care provider usually treats the patient with partial-thickness tears conservatively with NSAIDs, intermittent steroid injections, physical therapy, and activity limitations while the tear heals. Physical therapy treatments may include ultrasound, electrical stimulation, ice, and heat.

For patients who do not respond to conservative treatment in 3 to 6 months or for those who have a complete (full-thickness) tear, the surgeon repairs the cuff using mini-open or arthroscopic procedures. An interscalene nerve block may be used to extend analgesia for an open repair (Guarin, 2013). If a peripheral nerve block is used, remind the patient that the arm will feel numb and cannot be moved for up to 20 or more hours after surgery. Observe, report, and document complications of respiratory distress and neurovascular compromise.

After surgery, the affected arm is usually immobilized for several weeks. Pendulum exercises are started on the third or fourth postoperative day and progress to active exercises in about 2 weeks. Patients then begin rehabilitation in the ambulatory-care occupational therapy department. Teach them that they may not have full function for several months.

GET READY FOR THE NCLEX® EXAMINATION!

▌ KEY POINTS

Review these Key Points for each NCLEX Examination Client Needs Category.

Safe and Effective Care Environment

- Collaborate with physical and occupational therapists for care of patients with fractures to improve MOBILITY and muscle strength. **QSEN: Teamwork and Collaboration**
- Remember that the priority care for patients with fractures and amputations is to maintain PERFUSION, improve COMFORT, and prevent impaired MOBILITY.
- Monitor for potentially life-threatening complications of fractures, including hemorrhage, venous thromboembolism, fat embolism syndrome, acute compartment syndrome, and infection (see Charts 51-1 and 51-2). **Clinical Judgment**

Health Promotion and Maintenance

- Teach people to avoid musculoskeletal injury by treating or preventing osteoporosis (see Chapter 50), being cautious

when walking to prevent a fall, wearing supportive shoes, avoiding dangerous sports or activities, and decreasing time spent doing repetitive stress activities, such as using a computer keyboard.
- Several community organizations, such as the Amputee Coalition of America, are available to help patients and their families cope with the loss of a body part.
- Teach patients and their family members and significant others how to care for casts or traction at home.
- In collaboration with the interprofessional health team, reinforce teaching for ambulating with crutches, walkers, or canes; and teach exercises to patients with leg amputation to prevent hip flexion contractures. **QSEN: Teamwork and Collaboration**
- Provide special care for older adults with hip fractures, including preventing heel pressure injuries and promoting early ambulation to prevent complications of immobility. **QSEN: Patient-Centered Care**

Psychosocial Integrity

- For patients with severe trauma or amputation, assess coping skills and encourage verbalization. **QSEN: Patient-Centered Care**
- Recognize that the patient having an amputation may need to adjust to an altered lifestyle but can be active and productive. **QSEN: Patient-Centered Care**

Physiological Integrity

- Be aware that open fractures cause a higher risk for infection than do closed fractures; use strict aseptic technique when providing wound management. **QSEN: Evidence-Based Care**
- Recognize that fat embolism syndrome is different from pulmonary (blood clot) embolism as outlined in Chart 51-2.
- Provide emergency care of the patient with a fracture as described in Chart 51-4. **Clinical Judgment**
- Identify the patient at risk for acute compartment syndrome; loosen bandages or request that the patient's cast be cut if neurovascular compromise is assessed; notify the health care provider immediately. **QSEN: Evidence-Based Practice**
- As a priority, document neurovascular status frequently in patients with musculoskeletal injury, traction, or cast as described in Chart 51-3 and manage impaired comfort adequately. **QSEN: Informatics**
- Provide evidence-based appropriate cast care, depending on the type of cast (plaster or synthetic); check for pressure necrosis under the cast by feeling for heat, assessing the patient's pain level, and smelling the cast for an unpleasant odor. **QSEN: Evidence-Based Practice**
- Provide pin care for patients with skeletal traction or external fixation; assess for signs and symptoms of infection at the pin sites.
- Provide postoperative care for the patient having a fracture repair, including promoting MOBILITY and monitoring for complications of immobility.

- Provide evidence-based care for patients having a vertebroplasty or kyphoplasty as described in Chart 51-6.
- Provide emergency care for a patient having a traumatic amputation in the community. Call 911, assess the patient for ABCs, apply direct pressure on the amputation site, and elevate the extremity above the patient's heart to decrease bleeding. For finger parts, wrap the amputated part with a clean cloth and place in a sealed bag, which is lowered into ice water. **QSEN: Evidence-Based Practice**
- After surgery, assess for and promptly manage phantom limb pain in the patient who has an amputation; collaborate with specialists to incorporate complementary and integrative therapies and drug therapy into the patient's plan of care.
- Assess and document neurovascular status frequently after an endoscopic carpal tunnel release.
- Assess for and manage chronic regional pain syndrome (CRPS) in patients who have fractures or fracture repair.
- Provide emergency care for patients with a sports-related injury as outlined in Chart 51-8.
- Recall that carpal tunnel syndrome (CTS) is the most common type of repetitive stress injury (RSI) caused by certain occupations such as computer operators and factory workers.
- Many acute musculoskeletal injuries are initially treated by RICE: rest, ice, compression, and elevation. **QSEN: Evidence-Based Practice**
- The priority for managing complex regional pain syndrome (CRPS) is prompt and effective pain relief. Consult with PT, OT, and the pharmacist/pain specialist to determine the most effective pain management plan based on the patient's and family's preferences, values, and beliefs. **QSEN: Patient-Centered Care**

SELECTED BIBLIOGRAPHY

Asterisk indicates a classic or definitive work on this subject.

Freysteinson, W., Thomas, L., Sebastian-Deutsch, A., Douglas, D., Meltom, D., Celia, T., et al. (2016). A study of the amputee experience of viewing self in the mirror. *Rehabilitation Nursing*, Feb 1. doi:10.1002/mj.256. [Epub ahead of print].

Goodney, P., Holman, K., Henke, P., Travis, L., Dimick, J., Stukel, T., et al. (2013). Regional intensity of vascular care and lower-extremity amputation rates. *Journal of Vascular Surgery*, 57(6), 1471–1480.e3.

Guarin, P. L. B. (2013). How effective are nerve blocks after orthopedic surgery: A quality improvement study. *Nursing*, 43(6), 63–66.

Hershey, K. (2013). Fracture complications. *Critical Care Nursing Clinics of North America*, 25(2), 321–331.

Jarvis, C. (2014). *Physical examination & health assessment* (7th ed.). St. Louis: Elsevier Saunders.

McCance, K., Huether, S., Brashers, V., & Rote, N. (2014). *Pathophysiology: The biologic basis for disease in adults and children* (7th ed.). St. Louis: Mosby.

*Nahm, E.-S., Resnick, B., Orwig, D., Magaziner, J., & Degrezia, M. (2010). Exploration of informal caregiving following hip fractures. *Geriatric Nursing*, 31(4), 254–262.

Nahm, E.-S., Resnick, B., Plummer, L., & Park, B. K. (2013). Use of discussion boards in an online hip fracture resource center for caregivers. *Orthopaedic Nursing*, 32(2), 89–96.

Pirrung, J., & Mower-Wade, D. (2014). Early recognition and treatment of pelvic fractures. *Nursing*, 44(9), 38–46.

*Pullen, R. L. (2010). Caring for a patient after amputation. *Nursing*, 40(1), 15.

Skinner, H., & McMahon, P. (2014). *Current diagnosis & treatment: Orthopedics* (5th ed.). New York: McGraw Hill.

Sweitzer, V., Rondeau, D., Guido, V., & Rasmor, M. (2013). Interventions to improve outcomes in the elderly after hip fracture. *The Journal for Nurse Practitioners*, 9(4), 238–242.

Walsh, C. R. (2013). Wrist fractures in adults: Getting a grip. *Nursing*, 43(4), 38–44.

CHAPTER **52**

Assessment of the Gastrointestinal System

Amy Jauch

http://evolve.elsevier.com/Iggy/

PRIORITY AND INTERRELATED CONCEPTS

The priority concepts for this chapter are:
- NUTRITION
- ELIMINATION

LEARNING OUTCOMES

Safe and Effective Care Environment
1. Collaborate with the interprofessional team to assess patients for complications of esophagogastroduodenoscopy (EGD).

Health Promotion and Maintenance
2. Teach adults factors that place them at risk for GI problems.
3. Teach patients and families about pretest and posttest care for diagnostic GI testing to promote safety and comfort.

Psychosocial Integrity
4. Implement nursing interventions to minimize stressors for the patient undergoing GI diagnostic testing.

Physiological Integrity
5. Apply knowledge of anatomy, physiology, pathophysiology, genetic risk, age-related changes, and psychomotor skills to perform a focused assessment of the GI system.
6. Describe NUTRITION and ELIMINATION changes associated with aging.
7. Explain and interpret common laboratory tests for a patient with a GI health problem.
8. Describe care for patients having selected GI diagnostic tests.

The GI tract, also called the *alimentary canal,* consists of the mouth, esophagus, stomach, small and large intestines, and rectum. The salivary glands, liver, gallbladder, and pancreas secrete substances into this tract to form the GI system (Fig. 52-1). The main functions of the GI tract, with the aid of organs such as the pancreas and the liver, are the *digestion* of food to adequately meet the body's NUTRITION needs, which is required for proper body function, and the ELIMINATION of waste resulting from digestion. The GI tract is susceptible to many health problems, including structural or mechanical alterations, impaired motility, infection, inflammation or autoimmune disease, and cancer.

ANATOMY AND PHYSIOLOGY REVIEW

Structure

The lumen, or inner wall, of the GI tract consists of four layers: mucosa, submucosa, muscularis, and serosa. The *mucosa,* the innermost layer, includes a thin layer of smooth muscle and specialized exocrine gland cells. It is surrounded by the *submucosa,* which is made up of connective tissue. The *submucosa* layer is surrounded by the muscularis. The *muscularis* is composed of both circular and longitudinal smooth muscles, which work to keep contents moving through the tract. The outermost layer, the *serosa,* is composed of connective tissue. Although the

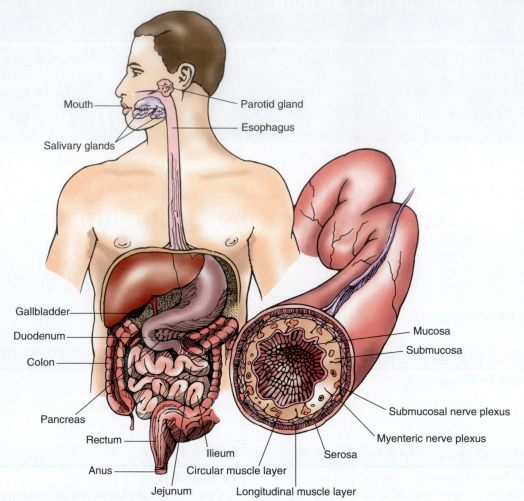

FIG. 52-1 The GI system (GI tract) can be thought of as a tube (with necessary structures) extending from the mouth to the anus for a 25-foot length. The structure of this tube *(shown enlarged)* is basically the same throughout its length.

GI tract is continuous from the mouth to the anus, it is divided into specialized regions. The mouth, pharynx, esophagus, stomach, and small and large intestines each perform a specific function. In addition, the secretions of the salivary, gastric, and intestinal glands; liver; and pancreas empty into the GI tract to aid digestion.

Function

The functions of the GI tract include secretion, digestion, absorption, motility, and ELIMINATION. Food and fluids are ingested, swallowed, and propelled along the lumen of the GI tract to the anus for elimination. The smooth muscles contract to move food from the mouth to the anus. Before food can be absorbed, it must be broken down to a liquid, called chyme. Digestion is the mechanical and chemical process in which complex foodstuffs are broken down into simpler forms that can be used by the body. During digestion, the stomach secretes hydrochloric acid, the liver secretes bile, and digestive enzymes are released from accessory organs, aiding in food breakdown. After the digestive process is complete, absorption takes place. Absorption is carried out as the nutrients produced by digestion move from the lumen of the GI tract into the body's circulatory system for uptake by individual cells (Jarvis, 2016).

Oral Cavity

The oral cavity (mouth) includes the buccal mucosa, lips, tongue, hard palate, soft palate, teeth, and salivary glands. The buccal mucosa is the mucous membrane lining the inside of the mouth. The tongue is involved in speech, taste, and mastication (chewing). Small projections called *papillae* cover the tongue and provide a roughened surface, permitting the movement of food in the mouth during chewing. The hard palate and the soft palate together form the roof of the mouth.

Adults have 32 permanent teeth: 16 each in upper and lower arches. The different types of teeth function to prepare food for digestion by cutting, tearing, crushing, or grinding the food. Swallowing begins after food is taken into the mouth and chewed. Saliva is secreted in response to the presence of food in the mouth and begins to soften the food. Saliva contains mucin and an enzyme called *salivary amylase* (also known as *ptyalin*), which begins the breakdown of carbohydrates.

Esophagus

The esophagus is a muscular canal that extends from the pharynx (throat) to the stomach and passes through the center of the diaphragm. Its primary function is to move food and fluids from

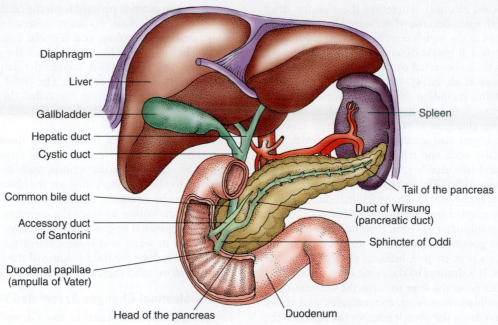

Diaphragm
Liver
Gallbladder
Hepatic duct
Cystic duct
Common bile duct
Accessory duct of Santorini
Duodenal papillae (ampulla of Vater)
Head of the pancreas

Spleen
Tail of the pancreas
Duct of Wirsung (pancreatic duct)
Sphincter of Oddi
Duodenum

FIG. 52-2 Anatomy of the pancreas, liver, and gallbladder.

the pharynx to the stomach. At the upper end of the esophagus is a sphincter referred to as the **upper esophageal sphincter (UES)**. When at rest, the UES is closed to prevent air into the esophagus during respiration. The portion of the esophagus just above the gastroesophageal (GE) junction is referred to as the **lower esophageal sphincter (LES)**. When at rest, the LES is normally closed to prevent reflux of gastric contents into the esophagus. If the LES does not work properly, gastroesophageal reflux disease (GERD) can develop (see Chapter 54).

Stomach

The stomach is located in the midline and left upper quadrant (LUQ) of the abdomen and has four anatomic regions (McCance et al., 2014). The *cardia* is the narrow portion of the stomach that is below the gastroesophageal (GE) junction. The *fundus* is the area nearest to the cardia. The main area of the stomach is referred to as the *body* or *corpus*. The *antrum* (pylorus) is the distal (lower) portion of the stomach and is separated from the duodenum by the pyloric sphincter. Both ends of the stomach are guarded by sphincters (cardiac [LES] and pyloric), which aid in the transport of food through the GI tract and prevent backflow.

Smooth muscle cells that line the stomach are responsible for gastric motility. The stomach is also richly innervated with intrinsic and extrinsic nerves. **Parietal cells** lining the wall of the stomach secrete hydrochloric acid, whereas chief cells secrete pepsinogen (a precursor to pepsin, a digestive enzyme). Parietal cells also produce **intrinsic factor**, a substance that aids in the absorption of vitamin B_{12}. Absence of the intrinsic factor causes pernicious anemia.

After ingestion of food, the stomach functions as a food reservoir where the digestive process begins, using mechanical movements and chemical secretions. The stomach mixes or churns the food, breaking apart the large food molecules and mixing them with gastric secretions to form chyme, which then

empties into the duodenum. The *intestinal phase* begins as the chyme passes from the stomach into the duodenum, causing distention. It is assisted by secretin, a hormone that inhibits further acid production and decreases gastric motility.

Pancreas

The pancreas is a fish-shaped gland that lies behind the stomach and extends horizontally from the duodenal C-loop to the spleen (Jarvis, 2016). The pancreas is divided into portions known as the *head*, the *body*, and the *tail* (Fig. 52-2).

Two major cellular bodies (exocrine and endocrine) within the pancreas have separate functions. The *exocrine* part consists of cells that secrete enzymes needed for digestion of carbohydrates, fats, and proteins (trypsin, chymotrypsin, amylase, and lipase). The *endocrine* part of the pancreas is made up of the islets of Langerhans, with alpha cells producing glucagon and beta cells producing insulin. These hormones produced are essential in the regulation of *metabolism*. Chapter 64 describes the endocrine function of the pancreas in detail.

Liver and Gallbladder

The *liver* is the largest organ in the body (other than skin) and is located mainly in the right upper quadrant (RUQ) of the abdomen. The right and left hepatic ducts transport bile from the liver. It receives its blood supply from the hepatic artery and portal vein, resulting in about 1500 mL of blood flow through the liver every minute.

The *liver* performs more than 400 functions in three major categories: storage, protection, and metabolism. It *stores* many minerals and vitamins, such as iron, magnesium, and the fat-soluble vitamins A, D, E, and K.

The *protective* function of the liver involves phagocytic **Kupffer cells**, which are part of the body's reticuloendothelial system. They engulf harmful bacteria and anemic red blood cells. The liver also detoxifies potentially harmful compounds (e.g., drugs, chemicals, alcohol). Therefore the risk for drug toxicity increases with aging because of decreased liver function.

The liver functions in the *metabolism* of proteins considered vital for human survival. It breaks down amino acids to remove ammonia, which is then converted to urea and is excreted via the kidneys (McCance et al., 2014). In addition, it synthesizes several plasma proteins, including albumin, prothrombin, and fibrinogen. The liver's role in carbohydrate metabolism involves storing and releasing glycogen as the body's energy requirements change. The organ also synthesizes, breaks down, and temporarily stores fatty acids and triglycerides.

The liver forms and continually secretes bile, which is essential for the breakdown of fat. The secretion of bile increases in response to gastrin, secretin, and cholecystokinin. Bile is secreted into small ducts that empty into the common bile duct and into the duodenum at the sphincter of Oddi. However, if the sphincter is closed, the bile goes to the gallbladder for storage.

The *gallbladder* is a pear-shaped, bulbous sac that is located underneath the liver. It is drained by the cystic duct, which joins with the hepatic duct from the liver to form the common bile duct (CBD). The gallbladder collects, concentrates, and stores the bile that has come from the liver. It releases the bile into the duodenum via the CBD when fat is present.

Small Intestine

The small intestine is the longest and most convoluted portion of the digestive tract, measuring 16 to 19 feet (5 to 6 m) in length in an adult. It is composed of three different regions: duodenum, jejunum, and ileum. The *duodenum* is the first 12 inches (30 cm) of the small intestine and is attached to the distal end of the pylorus. The common bile duct and pancreatic duct join to form the ampulla of Vater, emptying into the duodenum at the duodenal papilla. This papillary opening is surrounded by muscle known as the **sphincter of Oddi**. The 8-foot (2.5-m) portion of the small intestine that follows the sphincter of Oddi is the *jejunum*. The last 8 to 12 feet (2.5 to 4 m) of the small intestine is called the *ileum*. The ileocecal valve separates the entrance of the ileum from the cecum of the large intestine (McCance et al., 2014).

The inner surface of the small intestine has a velvety appearance because of numerous mucous membrane fingerlike projections. These projections are called *intestinal villi*. In addition to the intestinal villi, the small intestine has circular folds of mucosa and submucosa, which increase the surface area for digestion and absorption.

The small intestine has three main *functions*: movement (mixing and peristalsis), digestion, and absorption. Because the intestinal villi increase the surface area of the small intestine, it is the major organ of absorption of the digestive system. The small intestine mixes and transports the chyme to mix with many digestive enzymes. It takes an average of 3 to 10 hours for the contents to be passed by peristalsis through the small intestine. Intestinal enzymes aid the body in the digestion of proteins, carbohydrates, and lipids.

Large Intestine

The large intestine extends about 5 to 6 feet in length from the ileocecal valve to the anus and is lined with columnar epithelium that has absorptive and mucous cells. It begins with the *cecum,* a dilated, pouchlike structure that is inferior to the ileocecal opening. At the base of the cecum is the vermiform appendix, which has no known digestive function. The large

intestine then extends upward from the cecum as the colon. The colon consists of four divisions: ascending colon, transverse colon, descending colon, and sigmoid colon (McCance et al., 2014). The sigmoid colon empties into the rectum.

Following the sigmoid colon, the large intestine bends downward to form the rectum. The last 1 to 1½ inches (3 to 4 cm) of the large intestine are called the *anal canal,* which opens to the exterior of the body through the anus. Sphincter muscles surround the anal canal.

The large intestine's *functions* are movement, absorption, and ELIMINATION. Movement in the large intestine consists mainly of segmental contractions, such as those in the small intestine, to allow enough time for the absorption of water and electrolytes. In addition, peristaltic contractions are triggered by colonic distention to move the contents toward the rectum, where the material is stored until the urge to defecate occurs. Absorption of water and some electrolytes occurs in the large intestine to reduce the fluid volume of the chyme. This process creates a more solid material, the feces, for elimination.

Gastrointestinal Changes Associated With Aging

Physiologic changes occur in the GI system as people age, especially after 65 years of age. Changes in digestion and ELIMINATION that can affect NUTRITION are common (McCance et al., 2014). For example, decreased gastric hydrochloric acid (HCl) can lead to decreased absorption of essential minerals such as iron. Chart 52-1 lists common GI changes for older adults.

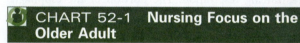

CHART 52-1 Nursing Focus on the Older Adult

Changes in the Gastrointestinal System Related to Aging

PHYSIOLOGIC CHANGE	DISORDERS RELATED TO CHANGE
Atrophy of the gastric mucosa leads to decreased hydrochloric acid levels (hypochlorhydria).	Decreased absorption of iron and vitamin B_{12} and proliferation of bacteria. Atrophic gastritis occurs as a consequence of bacterial overgrowth.
Peristalsis decreases, and nerve impulses are dulled.	Decreased sensation to defecate can result in postponement of bowel movements, which leads to constipation and impaction.
Distention and dilation of pancreatic ducts change. Calcification of pancreatic vessels occurs with a decrease in lipase production.	Decreased lipase level results in decreased fat absorption and digestion. Steatorrhea, or excess fat in the feces, occurs because of decreased fat digestion.
A decrease in the number and size of hepatic cells leads to decreased liver weight and mass. This change and an increase in fibrous tissue lead to decreased protein synthesis and changes in liver enzymes. Enzyme activity and cholesterol synthesis are diminished.	Decreased enzyme activity depresses drug metabolism, which leads to accumulation of drugs—possibly to toxic levels.

ASSESSMENT: NOTICING AND INTERPRETING

Patient History

The purpose of the health history is to determine the events related to the current health problem (Chart 52-2). Focus questions about changes in appetite, weight, and stool. Determine the patient's pain experience.

Collect data about the patient's age, gender, and culture. This information can be helpful in assessing who is likely to have particular GI system disorders. For instance, older adults are more at risk for stomach cancer than are younger adults. Younger adults are more at risk for inflammatory bowel disease (IBD). The exact reasons for these differences continue to be studied. Colon cancer is becoming more common among young people who are obese.

Question the patient about previous GI disorders or abdominal surgeries. Ask about prescription medications being taken, including how much, when the drugs are taken, and why they have been prescribed. Inquire if the patient takes over-the-counter (OTC) drugs, herbs, and/or supplements. In particular, ask whether aspirin, NSAIDs (e.g., ibuprofen), laxatives, herbal preparations, or enemas are taken routinely. Large amounts of aspirin or NSAIDs can predispose the patient to peptic ulcer disease and GI bleeding. Long term use of stimulant laxatives or enemas can cause dependence and result in constipation and electrolyte imbalance. Some herbal preparations can affect appetite, absorption, and ELIMINATION. Determine if the patient smokes, or has ever smoked, cigarettes, cigars, or pipes. Smoking is a major risk factor for most GI cancers. Chewing tobacco is a major cause of oral cancer.

Finally, investigate the patient's travel history. Ask whether he or she has traveled outside of the country recently or has been camping near lakes and streams in his or her country of residence. This information may provide clues about the cause of symptoms such as diarrhea.

Nutrition History

A NUTRITION history is important when assessing GI system function. Many conditions manifest themselves as a result of alterations in intake and absorption of nutrients. The purpose of a nutrition assessment is to gather information about how well the patient's needs are being met. Inquire about any special diet and whether there are any known food allergies. Ask the patient to describe the usual foods that are eaten daily and the times that meals are taken.

Health problems can also affect NUTRITION; therefore explore any changes that have occurred in eating habits as a result of illness. Anorexia (loss of appetite for food) can occur with GI disease. Assess changes in taste and any difficulty or pain with swallowing (dysphagia) that could be associated with esophageal disorders. Also ask if abdominal pain or discomfort occurs with eating and whether the patient has experienced any nausea, vomiting, or dyspepsia (indigestion or heartburn). Unknown food allergies may be a cause of these symptoms. Inquire about any unintentional weight loss because some cancers of the GI tract may present in this manner. Assess for alcohol and caffeine consumption because both substances are associated with many GI disorders, such as gastritis and peptic ulcer disease.

The patient's socioeconomic status may have a profound impact on his or her NUTRITION. People who have limited budgets, such as some older adults or the unemployed, may not be able to purchase foods required for a balanced diet. In addition, they may substitute less expensive and perhaps less effective OTC medications or herbs for prescription drugs.

? NCLEX EXAMINATION CHALLENGE 52-1

Health Promotion

When taking a history for a patient with GI problems, which daily client behavior requires **further** nursing assessment? **Select all that apply.**
A. Eats multiple servings of vegetables
B. Takes 800 mg of ibuprofen for arthritic pain
C. Walks 30 minutes
D. Chews tobacco
E. Takes senna to assist with bowel movements
F. Listens to music to promote relaxation

⊕ CULTURAL/SPIRITUAL CONSIDERATIONS

Patient-Centered Care QSEN

Cultural and spiritual patterns are important in obtaining a complete nutrition history. Ask if certain foods pose a problem for the patient. For example, the spices or hot pepper used in cooking in many cultures can aggravate or precipitate GI tract symptoms such as indigestion. Note religious observations such as fasting or abstinence.

Many black people and those of Asian heritage are lactose intolerant as a result either of having insufficient amounts of the enzyme lactase or producing a less active form of the enzyme. A much smaller percentage of white people also have this problem. Lactase is needed to convert lactose in milk and other dairy products to glucose and galactose. Lactose intolerance causes bloating, cramping, and diarrhea as a result of lack of the enzyme *lactase* (McCance et al., 2014).

◎ CHART 52-2 Best Practice for Patient Safety and Quality Care QSEN

Questions for Gastrointestinal Health History

- What is your typical daily food intake? Do you take any supplements? If so, what are they?
- How is your appetite? Any recent change?
- Have you lost or gained weight recently? If so, was the weight loss or gain intentional?
- Are you on a special diet?
- Do you have any difficulty chewing or swallowing?
- Do you wear dentures? How well do they fit?
- Do you ever experience indigestion or "heartburn"? How often? What seems to cause it? What helps it?
- Have you had any GI disorders or surgeries? If so, what are they?
- Is there a family history of GI health problems?
- What medications are you taking? Be sure to include prescription and over-the-counter (OTC) drugs.
- Do you smoke, or have you ever smoked? Do you chew, or have you ever chewed tobacco?
- Do you drink alcoholic beverages? If so, how many each week?
- Do you have pain, diarrhea, gas, or any other problems? Do any specific foods cause the problem?
- Have you traveled out of the country recently? If so, where?
- What is your usual bowel elimination pattern? Frequency? Character? Discomfort? Laxatives?
- Do you have any pain or bleeding associated with bowel movements?
- Have you experienced any changes in your usual bowel pattern or stool?
- Have you ever had an endoscopy or a colonoscopy?

Individuals who live in "food deserts" (i.e., places in part of the country with little access to fresh fruits and vegetables [American Nutrition Association, 2015] and other healthy foods) may also be impacted by lack of nutrition. Necessary medical care may be delayed, and patients may not seek health care until conditions are well advanced.

Family History and Genetic Risk

Ask about a family history of GI disorders. Some GI health problems have a genetic predisposition. For example, familial adenomatous polyposis (FAP) is an inherited autosomal-dominant disorder that predisposes the patient to colon cancer (McCance et al., 2014). Specific genetic risks are discussed with the GI problems in later chapters.

Current Health Problems

Because GI signs and symptoms are often vague and difficult for the patient to describe, it is important to obtain a chronologic account of the current problem, symptoms, and any treatments taken. If a patient has kept a diary of dates, symptoms, and treatments used, this can be helpful to establish patterns. Furthermore, ask about the location, quality, quantity, and timing of each symptom (onset, duration), and factors that may aggravate or alleviate it (see Chart 52-2).

For example, a change in bowel habits is a common assessment finding. Obtain this information from the patient:

- Pattern of bowel movements
- Color and consistency of the feces
- Occurrence of diarrhea or constipation
- Effective action taken to relieve diarrhea or constipation
- Presence of frank blood or tarry stools
- Presence of abdominal distention or gas

An unintentional weight gain or loss is another symptom that needs further investigation. Assess the patient's:

- Normal weight
- Weight gain or loss
- Period of time for weight change
- Changes in appetite or oral intake

Pain is a common concern of patients with GI tract disorders. Abdominal pain is often vague and difficult to evaluate. The mnemonic **PQRST** may be helpful in organizing the current problem assessment (Jarvis, 2016):

P: Precipitating or palliative. What brings it on? What makes it better? Worse? When did you first notice it? Is there a relationship of food intake to the onset or worsening of pain?

Q: Quality or quantity. How does the pain feel? Is it burning, stabbing, throbbing, shooting, dull, or achy?

R: Region or radiation. Point to where the pain is located. Does it spread anywhere? Did it start somewhere else?

S: Severity scale. How bad is it (on a scale of 0 to 10)? Is it getting better, worse, or staying the same?

T: Timing. Onset: Exactly when did it first occur? Duration: How long did it last? Frequency: How often does it occur?

Changes in the skin may result from several GI tract disorders, such as liver and biliary system obstruction. Ask about whether these clinical signs and symptoms have occurred and assess whether they are present:

- Skin discolorations or rashes
- Itching
- Jaundice (yellowing of skin caused by bilirubin pigments)
- Increased bruising
- Increased tendency to bleed

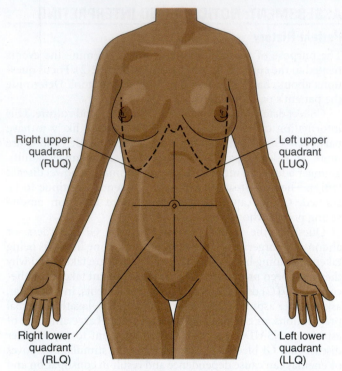

FIG. 52-3 Topographic division of the abdomen into quadrants.

Physical Assessment

Physical assessment involves a comprehensive examination of the patient's NUTRITION status, mouth, and abdomen. Nutritional assessment is discussed in detail in Chapter 60. Oral assessment is described in Chapter 53.

In preparation for examination of the *abdomen,* ask the patient to empty his or her bladder and then to lie in a supine position with knees bent, keeping the arms at the sides to prevent tensing of the abdominal muscles.

The abdominal examination usually begins at the patient's right side and proceeds in a systematic fashion (Fig. 52-3):

- Right upper quadrant (RUQ)
- Left upper quadrant (LUQ)
- Left lower quadrant (LLQ)
- Right lower quadrant (RLQ)

Table 52-1 lists the organs that lie in each of these areas.

If areas of pain or discomfort are noted from the history, they are examined last in the examination sequence. This sequence should prevent the patient from tensing abdominal muscles because of the pain, which would make the examination difficult. Examine any area of tenderness cautiously and instruct the patient to state whether it is too painful. Observe his or her face for signs of distress or pain.

The abdomen is assessed by using the four techniques of examination, but in a sequence different from that used for other body systems: inspection, auscultation, percussion, and then palpation. This sequence is preferred so palpation and percussion do not increase intestinal activity and bowel sounds. As a nurse generalist, perform inspection, auscultation, and light palpation. Health care providers, including advanced practice registered nurses (APRNs), perform percussion and deep palpation. If appendicitis or an abdominal aneurysm is suspected, palpation is not done.

TABLE 52-1 Location of Body Structures in Each Abdominal Quadrant and Midline	
Right Upper Quadrant (RUQ)	**Left Upper Quadrant (LUQ)**
• Most of the liver • Gallbladder • Duodenum • Head of the pancreas • Hepatic flexure of the colon • Part of the ascending and transverse colon	• Left lobe of the liver • Stomach • Spleen • Body and tail of the pancreas • Splenic flexure of the colon • Part of the transverse and descending colon
Midline	
• Abdominal aorta • Uterus (if enlarged) • Bladder (if distended)	
Right Lower Quadrant (RLQ)	**Left Lower Quadrant (LLQ)**
• Cecum • Appendix • Right ureter • Right ovary and fallopian tube • Right spermatic cord	• Part of the descending colon • Sigmoid colon • Left ureter • Left ovary and fallopian tube • Left spermatic cord

Inspection

Inspect the skin and note any of these findings:

- Overall asymmetry of the abdomen
- Presence of discolorations or scarring
- Abdominal distention
- Bulging flanks
- Taut, glistening skin
- Skin folds
- Subcutaneous fat noted
- Location, size, and description of any pressure injuries

Observe the shape of the abdomen by observing its contour and symmetry. The contour of the abdomen can be rounded, flat, concave, or distended. It is best determined when standing at the side of the bed or treatment table and looking down on the abdomen. View the abdomen at eye level from the side. Note whether the contour is symmetric or asymmetric. Asymmetry of the abdomen can indicate problems affecting the underlying body structures (see Table 52-1). Note the shape and position of the umbilicus for any deviations.

Finally, observe the patient's abdominal movements, including the normal rising and falling with inspiration and expiration, and note any distress during movement. Occasionally pulsations may be visible, particularly in the area of the abdominal aorta.

❗ NURSING SAFETY PRIORITY QSEN

Action Alert

If a bulging, pulsating mass is present during assessment of the abdomen, do not touch the area because the patient may have an abdominal aortic aneurysm, a life-threatening problem. Notify the primary health care provider of this finding immediately! Peristaltic movements are rarely seen unless the patient is thin and has increased peristalsis. If these movements are observed, note the quadrant of origin and the direction of peristaltic flow. Report this finding to the primary health care provider because it may indicate an intestinal obstruction.

Auscultation

Auscultation of the abdomen is performed with the diaphragm of the stethoscope, because bowel sounds are usually high pitched. Place the stethoscope lightly on the abdominal wall while listening for bowel sounds in all four quadrants.

Bowel sounds are created as air and fluid move through the GI tract. They are normally heard as relatively high-pitched, irregular gurgles every 5 to 15 seconds, with a normal frequency range of 5 to 30 per minute (Jarvis, 2016). They are characterized as normal, hypoactive, or hyperactive. They are diminished or absent after abdominal surgery or in the patient with peritonitis or paralytic ileus.

For many years, nurses have been taught to count the number of bowel sounds in each quadrant as part of routine and postoperative abdominal assessment to assess for peristalsis. However, the best, most reliable method for assessing the return of peristalsis after abdominal surgery is to ask the patient if he or she has passed flatus within the past 8 hours or a stool within the past 12 to 24 hours.

Increased bowel sounds, especially loud, gurgling sounds, result from increased motility of the bowel (**borborygmus**). These sounds are usually heard in the patient with diarrhea or gastroenteritis or above a complete intestinal obstruction.

When auscultating the abdomen, also listen for vascular sounds or **bruits** ("swooshing" sounds) over the abdominal aorta, the renal arteries, and the iliac arteries. A bruit heard over the aorta usually indicates the presence of an aneurysm. *If this sound is heard, do not percuss or palpate the abdomen. Notify the health care provider immediately of your findings!*

Percussion

Percussion may be used by APRNs and other health care providers to determine the size of solid organs; to detect the presence of masses, fluid, and air; and to estimate the size of the liver and spleen. The percussion notes normally heard in the abdomen are termed *tympanic* (the high-pitched, loud, musical sound of an air-filled intestine) or *dull* (the medium-pitched, softer, thudlike sound over a solid organ, such as the liver).

The liver and spleen can be percussed. An enlarged liver is called **hepatomegaly**. Dullness heard in the left anterior axillary line indicates enlargement of the spleen (**splenomegaly**). Mild-to-moderate splenomegaly can be detected before the spleen becomes palpable.

Palpation

The purpose of palpation is to determine the size and location of abdominal organs and to assess for the presence of masses or tenderness. Palpation of the abdomen consists of two types: light and deep. Only physicians and APRNs, such as clinical nurse specialists and nurse practitioners, should perform deep palpation. Deep palpation is used to further determine the size and shape of abdominal organs and masses.

The technique of *light palpation* is used to detect large masses and areas of tenderness. Place the first four fingers of the palpating hand close together and then place them lightly on the abdomen and proceed smoothly and systematically from quadrant to quadrant. Depress the abdomen to a depth of $\frac{1}{2}$ to 1 inch (1.25 to 2.5 cm). Proceed with a rotational movement of the palpating hand. Note any areas of tenderness or guarding because these areas will be examined last and cautiously during deep palpation. While performing light palpation, notice signs of rigidity, which, unlike voluntary guarding, is a sign of peritoneal inflammation.

 NCLEX EXAMINATION CHALLENGE 52-2

Physiological Integrity

The nurse is performing a physical assessment on a client's abdomen. The nurse inspects the abdomen and finds it asymmetrical, with a nonpulsating mass in the RUQ. What is the **priority** nursing intervention?

A. Document the findings in the electronic health record.
B. Auscultate for bowel sounds and bruits.
C. Lightly palpate the mass.
D. Notify the primary health care provider of the findings.

Psychosocial Assessment

Psychosocial assessment focuses on how the GI health problem affects the patient's life and lifestyle. Remember that patients are often reluctant to discuss ELIMINATION problems, which may be very personal and embarrassing. The interview focus is on whether usual activities have been interrupted or disturbed, including employment. Question the patient about recent stressful events. Emotional stress has been associated with the development or exacerbation (flare-up) of irritable bowel syndrome (IBS) and other GI disorders. If the patient is diagnosed with cancer, he or she is likely to experience the phases of the grieving process. Patients may be depressed, angry, or in denial. More specific psychosocial assessments are included in later GI chapters as part of each disease discussion.

Diagnostic Assessment

Laboratory Assessment

To make an accurate assessment of the many possible causes of GI system abnormalities, laboratory testing of blood, urine, and stool specimens may be performed.

A *complete blood count (CBC)* aids in the diagnosis of anemia and infection. It also detects changes in the blood's formed elements. In adults, GI bleeding is the most frequent cause of anemia. It is associated with GI cancer, peptic ulcer disease, diverticulitis, and inflammatory bowel disease.

Because the liver is the main site of all proteins involved in coagulation, *prothrombin time (PT)* is useful in evaluating the levels of these clotting factors. PT measures the rate at which prothrombin is converted to thrombin, a process that depends on vitamin K–associated clotting factors. Severe acute or chronic liver damage leads to a prolonged PT secondary to impaired synthesis of clotting proteins (Pagana et al., 2017).

Many *electrolytes* are altered in GI tract dysfunction. For example, calcium is absorbed in the GI tract and may be measured to detect malabsorption. Excessive vomiting or diarrhea causes sodium or potassium depletion, thus requiring replacement.

Assays of serum enzymes are important in the evaluation of liver damage. *Aspartate aminotransferase (AST)* and *alanine aminotransferase (ALT)* are two enzymes found in the liver and other organs. These are elevated in most liver disorders, but they are highest in conditions that cause necrosis, such as severe viral hepatitis and cirrhosis.

Elevations in serum *amylase* and *lipase* may indicate acute pancreatitis. In this disease, serum amylase levels begin to elevate within 24 hours of onset and remain elevated for up to 5 days. Serum amylase and lipase are not elevated when *extensive* pancreatic necrosis is present because there are few pancreatic cells manufacturing the enzymes (Pagana et al., 2017).

Bilirubin is the primary pigment in bile, which is normally conjugated and excreted by the liver and biliary system. It is measured as total serum bilirubin, conjugated (direct) bilirubin, and unconjugated (indirect) bilirubin. These measurements are important in the evaluation of jaundice and liver and biliary tract functioning. Elevations in direct and indirect bilirubin levels and/or gamma-glutamyl transferase (GGT) can indicate impaired secretion.

The serum level of *ammonia* may also be measured to evaluate hepatic function. Ammonia is normally used to rebuild amino acids or is converted to urea for excretion. Elevated levels are seen in conditions that cause severe hepatocellular injury, such as cirrhosis of the liver or fulminant hepatitis (Pagana et al., 2017).

Two primary *oncofetal antigens*—CA19-9 and *CEA*—are evaluated to monitor the success of cancer therapy and assess for the recurrence of cancer in the GI tract. These antigens may also be increased in benign GI conditions. Chart 52-3 lists blood tests commonly used by the health care provider in the diagnosis of GI disorders.

Additional serum tests are described in other chapters of this GI health unit.

Urine Tests. The presence of amylase can be detected in the urine. In acute pancreatitis, renal clearance of amylase is increased. Amylase levels in the urine remain high even after serum levels return to normal. This becomes an important finding in patients who are symptomatic for 3 days or longer (Pagana et al., 2017).

Urine *urobilinogen* is a form of bilirubin that is converted by the intestinal flora and excreted in the urine. Its measurement is useful in the evaluation of hepatic and biliary obstruction, because the presence of bilirubin in the urine often occurs before jaundice is seen.

Stool Tests. The American Cancer Society screening guidelines (2016) recommend a yearly guaiac fecal occult blood test (gFOBT) or fecal immunochemical test (FIT) at unspecified intervals to detect colorectal cancer early when it can be treated. These tests use a take-home, multi-sample method rather than having the test done during a digital rectal examination.

The traditionally used FOBT (e.g., Hemoccult II) requires an active component of guaiac and is therefore more likely than the FIT (e.g., HemeSelect) to yield false-positive results. In addition, patients having the guaiac-based test must avoid certain foods before the test, such as raw fruits and vegetables and red meat. Vitamin C–rich foods, juices, and tablets must also be avoided. Anticoagulants, such as warfarin (Coumadin), and NSAIDs should be discontinued for 7 days before testing begins. Patient compliance is likely to be higher with the FIT method because drugs and food do not interfere with the test results. As an alternate to the take-home test, a stool DNA test (sDNA) can be completed every 3 years (American Cancer Society [ACS], 2016).

Stool samples may also be collected to test for *ova and parasites* to aid in the diagnosis of parasitic infection. They may also be tested for *fecal fats* when steatorrhea (fatty stools) or malabsorption is suspected. Fat is normally absorbed in the small intestine in the presence of biliary and pancreatic secretions. In malabsorption, fat is abnormally excreted in the stool. Furthermore, stool samples can be tested to detect the presence of

⑤ **CHART 52-3   Laboratory Profile**

Gastrointestinal Assessment

TEST (SERUM)	NORMAL RANGE FOR ADULTS	SIGNIFICANCE OF ABNORMAL FINDINGS
Calcium (total)	9.0-10.5 mg/dL (values decrease in older adults) Canadian: Same	*Decreased* values indicate possible: Malabsorption Kidney failure Acute pancreatitis
Potassium	3.5-5.0 mEq/L or 3.5-5.0 mmol/L Canadian: Same	*Decreased* values indicate possible: Vomiting Gastric suctioning Diarrhea Drainage from intestinal fistulas
Albumin	3.5-5.0 g/dL Canadian: Same	*Decreased* values indicate possible: Hepatic disease Malnutrition
Alanine aminotransferase (ALT)	4-36 units/L (may be slightly higher in older adults) Canadian: Same	*Increased* values indicate possible: Liver disease Hepatitis Cirrhosis
Aspartate aminotransferase (AST)	0-35 units/L (may be slightly higher in older adults; women may have slightly lower levels than men) Canadian: Same	*Increased* values indicate possible: Liver disease Hepatitis Cirrhosis
Alkaline phosphatase	30-120 units/L (may be slightly higher in older adults) Canadian: Same	*Increased* values indicate possible: Cirrhosis Biliary obstruction Liver tumor
Bilirubin (total)	0.3-1.0 mg/dL Canadian: 5.1-17 mcmol/L (0.3-1.0 mg/dL)	*Increased* values indicate possible: Hemolysis Biliary obstruction Hepatic damage
Conjugated (direct) bilirubin	0.1-0.3 mg/dL Canadian: 1.7-5.1 µmol/L (0.1-0.3 mg/dL)	*Increased* values indicate possible: Biliary obstruction
Unconjugated (indirect) bilirubin	0.2-0.8 mg/dL Canadian: 3.4-12.0 µmol/L (0.2-0.8 mg/dL)	*Increased* values indicate possible: Hemolysis Hepatic damage
Ammonia	10-80 mg/dL Canadian: 6-47 µmol/L (10-80 mcg/dL)	*Increased* values indicate possible: Hepatic disease such as cirrhosis
Xylose absorption	20-57 mg/dL (60-minute plasma) 30-58 mg/dL (20-minute plasma) Canadian: >1.3 mmol/L (>20 mg/dL) (60 minute plasma) >1.6 mmol/L (>25 mg/dL) (120 minute plasma)	*Decreased* values in blood and urine indicate possible: Malabsorption in the small intestine
Serum amylase	30-220 units/L Canadian: 31-107 units/L	*Increased* values indicate possible: Acute pancreatitis
Serum lipase	0-160 units/L Canadian: Same	*Increased* values indicate possible: Acute pancreatitis
Cholesterol	<200 mg/dL Canadian: Same	*Increased* values indicate possible: Pancreatitis Biliary obstruction *Decreased* values indicate possible: Liver cell damage
Carbohydrate antigen 19-9 (CA19-9)	<37 units/mL Canadian: Same	*Increased* values indicate possible: Cancer of the pancreas, stomach, colon, gallbladder Acute pancreatitis Inflammatory bowel disease
Carcinoembryonic antigen (CEA)	<5 ng/mL Canadian: <5 mcg/L (<5 ng/mL)	*Increased* values indicate possible: Colorectal, stomach, pancreatic cancer Ulcerative colitis Crohn's disease Hepatitis Cirrhosis

infectious agents, such as *Clostridium difficile*, a common cause of diarrhea in older adults and patients on prolonged antibiotic therapy.

Imaging Assessment

Radiographic examinations and similar diagnostic procedures are useful in detecting structural and functional disorders of the GI system. Teach the patient how to prepare for the examination, provide an explanation of the procedure, and teach the required postprocedure care.

A *plain film of the abdomen* may be the first x-ray study that the health care provider requests when diagnosing a GI problem. This film can reveal abnormalities such as masses, tumors, and strictures or obstructions to normal movement. Patterns of bowel gas appear light on the abdominal film and can be useful in detecting an obstruction (ileus). No preparation is required except to wear a hospital gown and remove any jewelry or belts, which may interfere with the film.

When abdominal pain is severe or bowel perforation is suspected, an *acute abdomen series* may be requested. This procedure consists of a chest x-ray, supine abdomen film, and an upright abdomen film. The chest x-ray may reveal a hiatal hernia, and an upright abdomen film may show air in the peritoneum from a bowel perforation. Today CT and MRI scans or ultrasound scans are used more often than abdominal x-rays.

An **upper GI radiographic series** is an x-ray visualization from the mouth to the duodenojejunal junction. It may be done to detect disorders of structure or function of the esophagus (barium swallow), stomach, or duodenum. An extension of the upper GI series, the *small bowel follow-through* (SBFT), continues tracing the barium through the small intestine, up to and including the ileocecal junction, to detect disorders of the jejunum or ileum. These tests are seldom performed today because endoscopy procedures allow for direct visualization of the internal GI tract.

A **double-contrast barium enema** examination, also known as a *lower GI series,* is an x-ray of the large intestine. The 2016 American Cancer Society screening guidelines include this test every 5 years as an option to determine the presence of colorectal cancer and polyps for people older than 50 years. The other options include:

- Flexible sigmoidoscopy every 5 years, *or*
- CT colonography (virtual colonoscopy) every 5 years, *or*
- Colonoscopy every 10 years

Patient preparation is similar to that for colonoscopy. After the study is completed, the patient expels the barium. The radiology nurse or technician teaches the patient to drink plenty of fluids to assist in eliminating the barium and prevent an intestinal obstruction. A laxative is given to help remove the barium from the intestinal tract. Stools are chalky white for about 24 to 72 hours, until all barium is passed. If the patient has positive results, he or she is scheduled for a colonoscopy.

CT, also referred to as a *CT scan,* provides a noninvasive cross-sectional x-ray view that can detect tissue densities and abnormalities in the abdomen, including the liver, pancreas, spleen, and biliary tract. It may be performed with or without contrast medium. If contrast medium is to be used, ask about allergies to seafood and iodine. The patient is NPO for at least 4 hours before the test if a contrast medium is to be used. IV access will be required for injection of the contrast medium. Advise the patient that he or she may feel warm and flushed or experience a metallic taste on injection. The patient who is

somewhat claustrophobic may require a mild sedative to tolerate the study. The radiologic technician instructs the patient to lie still and to hold his or her breath when asked, as the technician takes a series of images. The test takes about 10 minutes.

Like other parts of the body, the abdomen and its organs may also be evaluated by *MRI, such as magnetic resonance cholangiopancreatography (MRCP).* Because of the use of powerful magnets, a special questionnaire and precautions are taken before the patient undergoes testing. Although this type of imaging takes longer than a CT scan, it does not expose patients to radiation.

Other Diagnostic Assessment

Endoscopy. **Endoscopy** is direct visualization of the GI tract using a flexible fiberoptic endoscope. It is commonly requested to evaluate bleeding, ulceration, inflammation, tumors, and cancer of the esophagus, stomach, biliary system, or bowel. Obtaining specimens for biopsy and cell studies (e.g., *Helicobacter pylori*) is also possible through the endoscope. There are several types of endoscopic examinations. The patient must sign an informed consent form before having these invasive studies.

Esophagogastroduodenoscopy. **Esophagogastroduodenoscopy (EGD)** is a visual examination of the esophagus, stomach, and duodenum. This procedure has largely replaced upper GI series testing. If GI bleeding is found during an EGD, the physician can use clips, thermocoagulation, injection therapy, or a topical hemostatic agent (Chen & Barkun, 2015). If the patient has an esophageal stricture, it can be dilated during an EGD. In addition, gastric lesions can be visualized using this procedure, and suspicion for celiac disease can be affirmed.

Teach the patient preparing for an upper GI endoscopic examination to remain NPO for 6 to 8 hours before the procedure. Usual drug therapy for hypertension or other diseases may be taken the morning of the test. However, patients with diabetes should consult their primary health care provider for special instructions. Usually patients are also asked to avoid anticoagulants, aspirin, or other NSAIDs for several days before the test unless it is absolutely necessary. Tell the patient that a flexible tube will be passed down the esophagus while he or she is under moderate sedation. Midazolam hydrochloride (Versed), fentanyl (Sublimaze), and/or propofol (Diprivan) are commonly used drugs for sedation. *These drugs can depress the rate and depth of the patient's respirations.* Atropine may be administered to dry secretions. In addition, a local anesthetic is sprayed to inactivate the gag reflex and facilitate passage of the tube. Explain that this anesthetic will depress the gag reflex and that swallowing will be difficult. If the patient has dentures, they are removed.

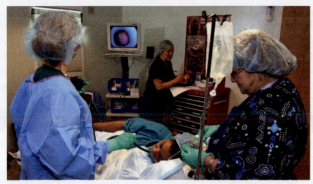

FIG. 52-4 Esophagogastroduodenoscopy allows visualization of the esophagus, the stomach, and the duodenum. If the esophagus is the focus of the examination, the procedure is called *esophagoscopy*. If the stomach is the focus, the procedure is called *gastroscopy*.

After the drugs are given, the patient is placed in a position with the head of the bed elevated. A bite block is inserted to prevent biting down on the endoscope and to protect the teeth. The physician passes the tube through the mouth and into the esophagus (Fig. 52-4). The procedure takes about 20 to 30 minutes.

During the test, the endoscopy nurse monitors the patient's respirations for rate and depth and the oxygen saturation level via pulse oximetry. Recent studies are finding benefit in using capnography as a monitoring tool to prevent hypoxemia during moderate sedation procedures (Hanlon, 2014). Shallow respirations decrease the amount of carbon dioxide that the patient exhales. *If the patient's respiratory rate is below 10 breaths/min or the exhaled carbon dioxide level falls below 20%, the nurse typically uses a stimulus such as a sternal rub to encourage deeper and faster respirations.*

After the test, the endoscopy nurse or technician checks vital signs frequently (usually every 15 to 30 minutes) until the sedation begins to wear off. The side rails of the bed are raised during this time. The patient remains NPO until the gag reflex returns (usually in 30 to 60 minutes). IV fluids that were started before the procedure are discontinued when the patient is able to tolerate oral fluids without nausea or vomiting.

! NURSING SAFETY PRIORITY QSEN

Action Alert

The priority for care to promote patient safety after esophagogastroduodenoscopy is to prevent aspiration. Do not offer fluids or food by mouth until you are sure that the gag reflex is intact! Monitor for signs of perforation, such as pain, bleeding, or fever.

Because the EGD is most often performed as an ambulatory care (outpatient) procedure requiring moderate sedation, be sure that the patient has someone to drive him or her home. Remind the patient to not drive for at least 12 to 18 hours after the procedure because of sedation. Teach him or her that a hoarse voice or sore throat may persist for several days after the test. Throat lozenges can be used to relieve throat discomfort.

Endoscopic Retrograde Cholangiopancreatography. Endoscopic retrograde cholangiopancreatography (ERCP) includes visual and radiographic examination of the liver, gallbladder, bile ducts, and pancreas to identify the cause and location of obstruction. It is commonly used today for therapeutic purposes rather than for diagnosis. After a cannula is inserted

into the common bile duct, a radiopaque dye is instilled, and several x-ray images are obtained. The physician may perform a **papillotomy** (a small incision in the sphincter around the ampulla of Vater) to remove gallstones. If a biliary duct stricture is found, plastic or metal stents may be inserted to keep the ducts open. Biopsies of tissue are also frequently taken during this test.

The patient prepares for this test in the same manner as for an EGD, including being NPO for 6 to 8 hours before the test. The patient requires IV access for moderate sedation drugs. Ask about prior exposure to x-ray contrast media and any sensitivities or allergies. If the patient has dentures, they are removed.

Ask the patient if he or she has an implantable medical device, such as a cardiac pacemaker. Modern day pacemakers generally are not affected by electrocautery; however, it is recommended that implantable defibrillators be deactivated, if possible, when electrocautery is used (Loperfido & Costamagna, 2016). Perform medication reconciliation to determine if the patient is taking anticoagulants, NSAIDs, antiplatelet drugs, or antihyperglycemic agents. The physician decides which of these drugs are safe to take and whether any will need to be stopped before the test.

The endoscopic procedure and nursing care for a patient having an ERCP are similar to those for the EGD procedure, except that the endoscope is advanced farther into the duodenum and into the biliary tract. Once the cannula is in the common duct, contrast medium is injected, and x-rays are taken to view the biliary tract. A tilt table assists in distributing the contrast medium to all areas to be assessed. The patient is placed in a left lateral position for viewing the common bile duct. Once the cannula is placed, he or she is put in a prone position. After examination of the biliary tree, the cannula is directed into the pancreatic duct for examination. The ERCP lasts from 30 minutes to 2 hours, depending on the treatment that may be done.

After the test, assess vital signs frequently, usually every 15 minutes, until the patient is stable. To prevent aspiration, check to ensure that the gag reflex has returned before offering fluids or food. Discontinue IV fluids that were started before the procedure when the patient is able to tolerate oral fluids without nausea or vomiting.

! NURSING SAFETY PRIORITY QSEN

Action Alert

Teach the patient and family to monitor for severe postprocedure complications at home, including cholangitis (gallbladder inflammation), bleeding, perforation, sepsis, and pancreatitis. The patient has severe pain if any of these complications occur. Fever is present in sepsis. These problems do not occur immediately after the procedure; they may take several hours to 2 days to develop.

Colicky abdominal pain and flatulence can result from air instilled during the procedure. Instruct the patient to report abdominal pain, fever, nausea, or vomiting that fails to resolve after returning home. Be sure that the patient has someone to drive him or her home if the test was done on an ambulatory care basis. Remind the patient to not drive for at least 12 to 18 hours after the procedure because of sedation.

Small Bowel Capsule Endoscopy. Small bowel endoscopy, or **enteroscopy**, provides a view of the small intestine. Capsule video endoscopy (M2A) is a small-bowel enteroscopy that visualizes the entire small bowel, including the distal ileum. It is used to evaluate and locate the source of GI bleeding. Before the development of the M2A capsule endoscope, viewing the small intestine was inadequate. The capsule battery lasts around 8 hours, so it is not used to view the colon.

Prepare the patient by explaining the procedure, the purpose, and what to expect during the testing. The patient must fast (water only) for 8 to 10 hours before the test and be NPO for the first 2 hours of the testing.

At the time of the procedure, the patient's abdomen is marked for the location of the sensors, and the eight-lead sensors (Sensor Array) are applied. The patient wears an abdominal belt that houses a data recorder to capture the transmitted images. After the capsule is swallowed with a glass of water, the patient may return to normal activity for the remainder of the study. He or she can resume a normal diet 4 hours after swallowing the capsule. At the end of the procedure, the patient returns to the facility with the capsule equipment for downloading to a central computer. The procedure lasts about 8 hours.

Because the M2A capsule endoscope is a single-use device that moves through the GI tract by peristalsis and is excreted naturally, explain to the patient that the capsule will be seen in the stool and is discarded after ELIMINATION. No other follow-up is necessary.

Colonoscopy. **Colonoscopy** is an endoscopic examination of the entire large bowel. The American Cancer Society recommends that, beginning at age 50 years, all healthy men and women should have a colonoscopy every 10 years or choose another equally effective recommended screening option (ACS, 2016). Evidence currently shows that younger adults with obesity are developing colon cancer, possibly due to chronic low-level inflammation that leads to cancer over a period of time (National Cancer Institute at the National Institutes of Health, 2017). Be sure to fully assess all patients who may need a colonoscopy. However, the colonoscopy is considered the gold standard test for detecting colon cancer. Those at high risk for cancer (e.g., family history) or those who had polyps removed should have the test more often. The physician may also obtain tissue biopsy specimens or remove polyps through the colonoscope. A colonoscopy can also evaluate the cause of chronic diarrhea or locate the source of GI bleeding. Topical hemostatic agents or other methods may be used to manage the bleeding.

Patient Preparation. Patients who have their first colonoscopy are often very anxious. Provide information about the procedure, level of sedation, and possibility of pain (Rollbusch et al., 2014). Reassure them that pain will be controlled with medication as needed.

To help cleanse the bowel, teach the patient to stay on a clear liquid diet the day before the scheduled colonoscopy. Instruct him or her to avoid red, orange, or purple (grape) beverages or gelatin and to drink an abundant amount of Gatorade or other sports drink to replace electrolytes that are lost during bowel preparation. The patient should be NPO (except water) 4 to 6 hours before the procedure.

Remind patients to avoid aspirin, anticoagulants, and antiplatelet drugs for several days before the procedure. Patients with diabetes should check with their primary health care provider about drug therapy requirements on the day of the test because they are NPO.

The patient may be required to drink an oral liquid preparation for cleaning the bowel (e.g., sodium phosphate [Phospho-Soda]) the evening before the examination and may repeat that procedure the morning of the study. Some physicians prescribe a gallon of GoLYTELY® to cleanse the bowel the day before. *This regimen should not be used for older adults to prevent excessive fluid and electrolyte loss.* All solutions should be chilled to improve their taste. Remind the patient to drink them quickly to prevent nausea. Watery diarrhea usually begins in about an hour after starting the bowel preparation process. In some cases, the patient may also require laxatives, suppositories (e.g., bisacodyl [Dulcolax]), or one or more small-volume cleansing enemas (e.g., Fleet's).

The failure to achieve adequate bowel preparation before a colonoscopy can lead to decreased visualization of adenoma or unsuccessful colonoscopy. Patient education and type of bowel preparation solution are critical to a successful procedure (Chen et al., 2015) (see Clinical Judgment Challenge 52-1).

Procedure. IV access is necessary for the administration of moderate sedation. The physician prescribes drugs to aid in relaxation, usually IV midazolam hydrochloride (Versed), propofol (Diprivan), and/or an opiate such as fentanyl. Alternate therapies, such as using music, can improve the individuals experience with a colposcopy, although it may not substitute the need for sedation or pain medication (Martindale et al., 2014).

Initially the patient is placed on the left side with the knees drawn up while the endoscope is placed into the rectum and moved to the cecum. Air or carbon dioxide may be instilled for better visualization. Recent literature suggests that decreased patient pain, fewer nursing interventions, and less time are needed after the procedure with the use of carbon dioxide (Lynch et al., 2015). The entire procedure lasts about 30 to 60 minutes. Atropine sulfate is kept available in case of bradycardia resulting from vasovagal response.

During the test, the endoscopy nurse monitors the patient's respirations for rate and depth and the oxygen saturation level via pulse oximetry. Shallow respirations decrease the amount of carbon dioxide that the patient exhales. *If the patient's respiratory rate is below 10 breaths/min or the exhaled carbon dioxide level falls below 20%, the nurse typically uses a stimulus such as a sternal rub to encourage deeper and faster respirations.*

Follow-Up Care. Check vital signs every 15 minutes until the patient is stable. Keep the side rails up until the patient is fully alert and maintain NPO status. Ask the patient to lie on his or her left side to promote comfort and encourage passing flatus. Observe for signs of perforation (causes severe pain) and hemorrhage, such as a rapid drop in blood pressure. Reassure the patient that a feeling of fullness, cramping, and passage of flatus is expected for several hours after the test. Fluids are permitted after the patient passes flatus to indicate that peristalsis has returned. Discontinue IV fluids that were started before the procedure when the patient is able to tolerate oral fluids without nausea or vomiting.

If a polypectomy or tissue biopsy was performed, there may be a *small* amount of blood in the first stool after the colonoscopy. Complications of colonoscopy are not common. *Report excessive bleeding or severe pain to the health care provider immediately* (Chart 52-4).

As with other endoscopic procedures, the patient will need someone to provide transportation home if the procedure was done in an ambulatory care setting. Remind the patient to avoid driving for 12 to 18 hours after the procedure because of the effects of sedation.

Virtual Colonoscopy. A noninvasive imaging procedure to obtain multi-dimensional views of the entire colon is the *CT colonography*, most popularly known as the virtual colonoscopy. The bowel preparation and dietary restrictions are similar to those for traditional colonoscopy. However, if a polyp is detected during a virtual colonoscopy or bleeding is found, the patient must have a follow-up invasive colonoscopy for treatment. Therefore the advantage of the traditional colonoscopy is that both diagnostic testing and minor surgical procedures can be done at the same time.

Sigmoidoscopy. Proctosigmoidoscopy, often referred to as a *sigmoidoscopy,* is an endoscopic examination of the rectum and sigmoid colon using a flexible scope. The purpose of this test is to screen for colon cancer, investigate the source of GI bleeding, or diagnose or monitor inflammatory bowel disease. If sigmoidoscopy is used as an alternative to colonoscopy for colorectal cancer screening, it is recommended that screening begin at 50 years of age and be done every 5 years thereafter

(ACS, 2016). Patients at high risk for cancer may require more frequent screening.

The patient should have a clear liquid diet for at least 24 hours before the test. A cleansing enema or sodium biphosphate (Fleet's) enema is usually required the morning of the procedure. A laxative may also be prescribed the evening before the test.

The patient is placed on the left side in the knee-chest position. No moderate sedation is required. The endoscope is lubricated and inserted into the anus to the required depth for viewing. Tissue biopsy may be performed during this procedure, but the patient cannot feel it. The examination usually lasts about 30 minutes.

Inform the patient that mild gas pain and flatulence may be experienced from air instilled into the rectum during the examination. If a biopsy was obtained, a small amount of bleeding may be observed. Instruct the patient that excessive bleeding should be reported immediately to the health care provider.

Ultrasonography. Ultrasonography (US) is a technique in which high-frequency, inaudible vibratory sound waves are passed through the body via a transducer. The echoes created by the sound waves are then recorded and converted into images for analysis. US is commonly used to view soft tissues, such as the liver, spleen, pancreas, and biliary system. The advantages of this test are that it is painless and noninvasive and requires no radiation.

The patient may be fasting, depending on the abdominal organs to be examined. Inform him or her that it will be necessary to lie still during the study.

The patient is usually placed in a supine position. The technician applies insulating gel to the end of the transducer and on the area of the abdomen under study. This gel allows airtight contact of the transducer with the skin. The technician moves the transducer back and forth over the skin until the desired images are obtained. The study takes about 15 to 30 minutes. No follow-up care is necessary.

Endoscopic Ultrasonography. Endoscopic ultrasonography (EUS) provides images of the GI wall and high-resolution images of the digestive organs. The ultrasonography is performed through the endoscope. This procedure is useful in diagnosing the presence of lymph node tumors; mucosal tumors; and tumors of the pancreas, stomach, and rectum. The patient preparation and follow-up care are similar to that for both endoscopy and ultrasonography.

Liver-Spleen Scan. A liver-spleen scan uses IV injection of a radioactive material that is taken up primarily by the liver and secondarily by the spleen. The scan evaluates the liver and spleen for tumors or abscesses, organ size and location, and blood flow.

Teach the patient about the need to lie still during the scanning. Assure him or her that the injection has only small amounts of radioactivity and is not dangerous. Ask female patients of childbearing age if they may be pregnant or are currently breast-feeding. The radionuclide can be found in breast milk, and radiation from x-rays or scans should be avoided in pregnancy.

The technician or the physician gives the radioactive injection through an IV line, and a wait of about 15 minutes is necessary for uptake. The patient is placed in many different positions while the scanning takes place. Tell the patient that the radionuclide is eliminated from the body through the urine in 24 hours. Careful handwashing after toileting decreases the exposure to any radiation present in the urine.

GET READY FOR THE NCLEX® EXAMINATION!

KEY POINTS

Review these Key Points for each NCLEX Examination Client Needs Category.

Safe and Effective Care Environment

- Remember that the priority for care is to check for the return of the gag reflex after an upper endoscopic procedure before offering fluids or food; aspiration may occur if the gag reflex is not intact. **QSEN: Safety**
- If an endoscopic procedure in an ambulatory care setting is scheduled, remind the patient to have someone available to drive him or her home because of the effects of moderate sedation. **QSEN: Safety**

Health Promotion and Maintenance

- Teach patients having invasive colon diagnostic procedures to follow instructions carefully for the bowel preparation before testing; the bowel must be clear to allow visualization of the colon. **QSEN: Evidence-Based Practice**
- Instruct the patient to drink plenty of fluids and take a laxative as prescribed to eliminate barium if used during diagnostic testing. **QSEN: Evidence-Based Practice**

Psychosocial Integrity

- Remember that GI health problems markedly affect lifestyle and may invoke emotions such as anger, denial, and depression. **QSEN: Patient-Centered Care**

Physiological Integrity

- Perform a focused abdominal assessment using inspection, auscultation, and light palpation. **QSEN: Evidence-Based Practice**
- Do not palpate or auscultate any abdominal pulsating mass because it could be a life-threatening aortic aneurysm. **QSEN: Safety**
- Be aware that aging causes changes in the GI system as summarized in Chart 52-1. **QSEN: Patient-Centered Care**
- Assess and report any major complications of GI testing to the health care provider. **QSEN: Safety**
- Review and interpret laboratory results and report abnormal findings to the health care provider (see Chart 52-3). **Clinical Judgment**
- Monitor vital signs carefully for the patient having any endoscopic procedure and moderate sedation. **QSEN: Safety**
- Assess patients who have endoscopies for bleeding, fever, and severe pain. **QSEN: Safety**
- For patients who have had a colonoscopy, check for passage of flatus before allowing fluids or food (see Chart 52-4). **QSEN: Safety**

SELECTED BIBLIOGRAPHY

American Cancer Society (ACS). (2016). *American Cancer Society guidelines for the early detection of cancer.* www.cancer.org/healthy/findcancerearly/cancerscreeningguidelines/american-cancer-society-guidelines-for-the-early-detection-of-cancer.

American Nutrition Association. (2015). *USDA defines food deserts.* http://americannutritionassociation.org/newsletter/usda-defines-food-deserts.

Chen, J., Athilingam, P., Saloum, Y., & Brady, P. (2015). Enhancing bowel preparation for screening colonoscopy: An evidence-based literature review. *The Journal for Nurse Practitioners, 11*(5), 519–525.

Chen, Y., & Barkun, A. N. (2015). Hemostatic powders in gastrointestinal bleeds. *Gastrointestinal Endoscopy Clinics of North America, 25*(3), 535–552.

Hanlon, P. (2014). Capnography use during endoscopy and colonoscopy. *Journal of Respiratory Care Practitioners, 27*(6), 6.

Jarvis, C. (2016). *Physical examination & health assessment* (7th ed.). St. Louis: Saunders.

Loperfido, S., & Costamagna, G. (2016). *Endoscopic retrograde cholangiopancreatography: Indications, patient preparation, and complications.* www.uptodate.com.

Lynch, I., Hayes, A., Buffum, M., & Conners, E. E. (2015). Insufflation using carbon dioxide versus room air during colonoscopy: Comparison of patient comfort, recovery time, and nursing resources. *Gastroenterology Nursing, 38*(3), 211–217.

Martindale, F., Mikocka-Walus, A., Barlomiej, P., Keage, H., & Andrews, J. M. (2014). The effect of designer music intervention on patients' anxiety, pain, and experience of colonoscopy: A short report on a pilot study. *Gastroenterology Nursing, 37*(5), 338–342.

McCance, K., Huether, S., Brashers, V., & Rote, N. (2014). *Pathophysiology: The biologic basis for disease in adults and children* (7th ed.). St. Louis: Mosby.

National Cancer Institute at the National Institutes of Health. (2017). *Obesity and cancer.* https://www.cancer.gov/about-cancer/causes-prevention/risk/obesity/obesity-fact-sheet#q4.

Pagana, K., Pagana, T. J., & Pagana, T. N. (2017). *Mosby's diagnostic and laboratory test reference* (13th ed.). St. Louis: Mosby.

Rollbusch, N., Mikocka-Walus, A. A., & Andrews, J. M. (2014). The experience of anxiety in colonoscopy outpatients: A mixed-method study. *Gastroenterology Nursing, 37*(2), 166–175.

CHAPTER 53

Care of Patients With Oral Cavity Problems

Tracy Taylor

e http://evolve.elsevier.com/Iggy/

PRIORITY AND INTERRELATED CONCEPTS

The priority concept for this chapter is TISSUE INTEGRITY.

✳ The TISSUE INTEGRITY concept exemplar for this chapter is Stomatitis, p. 1076.

The interrelated concepts for this chapter are:
- NUTRITION
- GAS EXCHANGE
- COMFORT

LEARNING OUTCOMES

Safe and Effective Care Environment

1. Collaborate with the interprofessional team to protect the patient with oral cavity problems from injury and infection.
2. Identify community resources to ensure appropriate transition management for patients with oral cavity problems.

Health Promotion and Maintenance

3. Teach adults how to maintain good oral health and prevent oral cancer.
4. Teach patients with stomatitis how to preserve TISSUE INTEGRITY, promote digestion and NUTRITION, and minimize disturbances in COMFORT.

Psychosocial Integrity

5. Implement nursing interventions to minimize stressors for the patient experiencing an oral cavity problem.

6. Refer patients with oral cancer to appropriate support groups.

Physiological Integrity

7. Apply knowledge of anatomy, physiology, pathophysiology, genetic risk, age-related changes, and psychomotor skills to perform a focused assessment of the oral cavity.
8. Describe interprofessional care and educational needs to promote NUTRITION for the patient with oral cavity problems.
9. Prioritize postoperative care for patients undergoing surgery for oral cancer to maintain GAS EXCHANGE and prevent aspiration.
10. Identify methods to help patients communicate effectively after oral surgery.

Inside the mouth, teeth tear, grind, and crush food into small particles to promote swallowing. Thus begins the process of digestion of food. Enzymes in saliva begin the breakdown of carbohydrates. The basic human need for NUTRITION may not be met by the GI tract if a person cannot take food or fluid into the mouth, cannot chew food, or cannot swallow. Adequate intake of fluids and nutrients is vital to promote function of every body organ and system.

The pharynx (throat), the portal between the mouth and GI tract where nutrients are broken down, is located just behind the mouth and has a role in both digestion and GAS EXCHANGE (oxygenation). It also is a portal for gas exchange, as inhaled air passes through the nose, into the pharynx, and down into the trachea. A blockage of the posterior oral cavity, such as a tumor, can interfere with gas exchange and digestion.

Oral cavity disorders can severely affect TISSUE INTEGRITY, NUTRITION, and GAS EXCHANGE; cause intense discomfort; and affect speech, body image, and self-esteem. These disorders commonly affect people who (World Health Organization, 2012):

- Have developmental delays or mental health disorders
- Are homeless or have less (decreased) access to care
- Reside in institutions
- Use tobacco and/or alcohol
- Consume an unhealthy diet
- Have an oral cancer
- Consume dietary excess

This chapter discusses the most common oral health problems. As a nurse, you will play an important role in maintaining and restoring oral health through nursing interventions, including

CHART 53-1 Patient and Family Education: Preparing for Self-Management

Maintaining a Healthy Oral Cavity

- Perform self-examination of your mouth every week; report any unusual finding or any noted change.
- Be sure to eat a well-balanced diet.
- Brush and floss your teeth every day. Set and maintain a consistent routine. Keeping floss where you can see it (e.g., on the countertop by the sink) will encourage you to stick to your routine.
- Manage your stress as much as possible; learn how to maintain your emotional health by using healthy coping mechanisms.
- Avoid contact with agents that may cause inflammation of the mouth, such as mouthwashes that contain alcohol.
- If possible, avoid drugs that may cause inflammation of the mouth or reduce the flow of saliva.
- Be aware of any changes in the occlusion of your teeth, mouth pain, or swelling; seek medical attention promptly if these occur.
- See your dentist regularly; have problems attended to promptly.
- If you wear dentures, make sure that they are in good repair and fit properly.

CONSIDERATIONS FOR OLDER ADULTS

Patient-Centered Care QSEN

Older adults are especially at high risk for candidiasis because aging causes a decrease in immune function. The risk increases for patients who have diabetes, are malnourished, or are under emotional stress. Many older adults take multiple medications that can contribute to oral dryness and decreased salivation as well. Those who wear dentures may use soft denture liners that provide COMFORT but can also be colonized by *C. albicans*, contributing to denture stomatitis. In addition, older adults who have poor oral hygiene are at high risk for mouth infections and aspiration pneumonia. All health care professionals in any health care setting should be educated in and aware of best practices for oral care for older adults. Improved oral care could greatly improve patient outcomes, especially for older intubated adults in critical care settings.

provision of patient and family education. Chart 53-1 lists ways to teach adults to maintain a healthy oral cavity.

❋ TISSUE INTEGRITY CONCEPT EXEMPLAR
Stomatitis

❖ PATHOPHYSIOLOGY

Stomatitis is a broad term that refers to inflammation within the oral cavity. It may present in many different ways. Painful single or multiple ulcerations (called *aphthous ulcers* or *canker sores*) that appear as inflammation and erosion of the protective lining of the mouth are one of the most common forms of stomatitis. The sores cause alterations in COMFORT, and open areas place the person at risk for bleeding and infection. Mild erythema (redness) may respond to topical treatments. Extensive stomatitis may require treatment with opioid analgesics and/or antifungal medications, depending on the source of inflammation. Stomatitis is classified according to the cause of the inflammation.

Etiology and Genetic Risk

Primary stomatitis, the most common type, includes aphthous (noninfectious) stomatitis, herpes simplex stomatitis, and traumatic ulcers. *Secondary stomatitis* generally results from infection by opportunistic viruses, fungi, or bacteria in patients who are immunocompromised. It can also result from drugs such as chemotherapy.

A common type of secondary stomatitis is caused by *Candida albicans. Candida* is sometimes present in small amounts in the mouth, especially in older adults. Long-term antibiotic therapy destroys other normal flora and allows the *Candida* to overgrow. The result can be candidiasis, also called *moniliasis,* a fungal infection that is very painful. Candidiasis is also common in those undergoing immunosuppressive therapy, such as chemotherapy, radiation, and steroids.

Stomatitis can result from infection, allergy, vitamin deficiency (complex B vitamins, folate, zinc, iron), systemic disease, and irritants such as tobacco and alcohol. Infectious agents, such as bacteria and viruses, may have a role in the development of recurrent stomatitis. Certain foods such as coffee, potatoes, cheese, nuts, citrus fruits, and gluten may trigger allergic responses that cause aphthous ulcers. In some cases, strict diets have resulted in the improvement of ulcers.

Current research regarding genetic linkage is ongoing. So far, evidence suggests that the hyperreactivity of the immune system in some patients with recurrent stomatitis is at least partially related to a genetic predisposition (Ślebioda et al., 2014).

Incidence/Prevalence

The most common type of stomatitis, recurrent aphthous ulcers (RAUs), affects more than 20% of the population of North America; incidence is higher in females than males (Mirowski, 2017).

Health Promotion and Maintenance

Proper oral hygiene can discourage the frequency and severity of stomatitis. However, it may not completely prevent all occurrences since stomatitis has been associated with numerous conditions such as bacteria or viral infections, higher stress levels, certain medications, nutrition deficiency, and oral irritants.

❖ INTERPROFESSIONAL COLLABORATIVE CARE

Care for the patient with stomatitis usually takes place in the community setting. The interprofessional team that collaborates to care for this patient generally includes the primary health care provider and nurse; a dentist and dental hygienist to provide care for the teeth, gums, and oral cavity; and an ear, nose and throat specialist if needed.

◆ Assessment: Noticing

When performing an oral assessment, ask about a history of recent infections, nutrition changes, oral hygiene habits, oral trauma, and stress. Also collect a drug history, including over-the-counter (OTC) drugs and nutrition and herbal supplements. Document the course of the current outbreak and determine if stomatitis has occurred frequently. Ask the patient if the lesions interfere with swallowing, eating, or communicating.

The symptoms of stomatitis range in severity from a dry, painful mouth to open ulcerations, placing the patient at risk for infection. These ulcerations can alter NUTRITION status because of difficulty with eating or swallowing. When they are severe, stomatitis and edema have the potential to obstruct the airway.

In oral candidiasis, white plaquelike lesions appear on the tongue, palate, pharynx (throat), and buccal mucosa (inside the cheeks) (Fig. 53-1). When these patches are wiped away, the underlying surface is red and sore. Patients may report

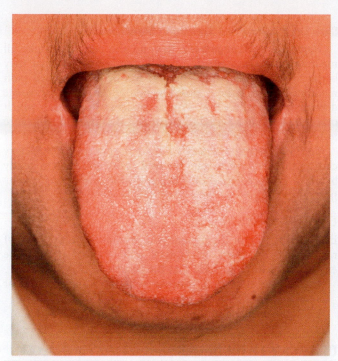

FIG. 53-1 Oral candidiasis. (From Millsop, J. W., & Fazel, N. (2016). Oral candidiasis. *Clinics in Dermatology, 34*(4), 487-494. doi:10.1016/j. clindermatol.2016.02.022.)

alterations in COMFORT, but others describe the lesions as dry or hot.

While examining the mouth, wear gloves, use a penlight to ensure adequate lighting, and use a tongue blade to aid examining the oral cavity. Assess the mouth for lesions, coating, and cracking. Document characteristics of the lesions, including their location, size, shape, odor, color, and drainage.

If lesions are seen along the pharynx and the patient reports dysphagia (difficulty on swallowing) or throat pain, the lesions might extend down the esophagus. To establish a definitive diagnosis, the primary health care provider may prescribe additional swallowing studies.

! NURSING SAFETY PRIORITY QSEN

Action Alert

When assessing the patient with stomatitis, be alert for signs and symptoms of dysphagia, such as coughing or choking when swallowing, a sensation of food "sticking" in the pharynx, or difficulty initiating the swallowing process. If dysphagia is suspected, use the PASS acronym for quick assessment: Is it **P**robable that the patient will have swallowing difficulty? **A**ccount for previous swallowing problems. **S**creen for signs and symptoms. Obtain a **S**peech-language pathologist referral (Mountain & Golles, 2017). Document all findings and report these to the primary health care provider because dysphagia can cause numerous problems, including airway obstruction, aspiration pneumonia, and malnutrition.

The physical assessment also includes palpating the cervical and submandibular lymph nodes for swelling. Advanced practice nurses and other health care providers usually perform this part of the examination.

◆ Analysis: Interpreting

The priority collaborative problems for the patient with stomatitis include:

◎ CHART 53-2 Best Practice for Patient Safety & Quality Care QSEN

Care of the Patient With Problems of the Oral Cavity

- Remove dentures if the patient has severe stomatitis or oral pain.
- Encourage the patient to perform oral hygiene or provide it after each meal and as often as needed.
- Increase mouth care to every 2 hours or more frequently if stomatitis is not controlled.
- Use a soft toothbrush or gauze for oral care.
- Encourage frequent rinsing of the mouth with warm saline, sodium bicarbonate (baking soda) solution, or a combination of these solutions.
- Teach the patient to avoid commercial mouthwashes, particularly those with high alcohol content, and lemon-glycerin swabs.
- Help the patient select soft, bland, and nonacidic foods.
- Apply topical analgesics or anesthetics as prescribed by the health care provider and monitor their effectiveness.

---

1. Compromised TISSUE INTEGRITY due to oral and/or esophageal lesions
2. Alteration in COMFORT due to oral and/or esophageal lesions

◆ Planning and Implementation: Responding

Preserving Tissue Integrity

Planning: Expected Outcomes. The patient with stomatitis is expected to regain a healthy oral cavity. Indicators include:

1. Absence of oral/esophageal lesions
2. Pink, moist, intact mucosa free from signs of inflammation or infection

Interventions. Interventions for stomatitis are targeted toward health promotion and reduced risk for infection through careful *oral hygiene* and food selection. When providing mouth care for the patient, you may delegate oral care to unlicensed assistive personnel (UAP) since this is within a UAP's scope of practice. Because you are accountable for the delegated task, remind the UAP to use a soft-bristled toothbrush or disposable foam swabs to stimulate gums and clean the oral cavity. Use toothpaste that is free of sodium lauryl sulfate (SLS), if possible, because this ingredient has been associated with stomatitis. Follow up by inspecting the patient's oral cavity after the UAP completes the task. Teach the patient to rinse the mouth every 2 to 3 hours with a sodium bicarbonate solution or warm saline solution (may be mixed with hydrogen peroxide). He or she should avoid most commercial mouthwashes because they have high alcohol content, causing a burning sensation in irritated or ulcerated areas. Health food stores sell more natural mouthwashes that are not alcohol based. Teach the patient to check the labels for alcohol content. Frequent, gentle mouth care promotes débridement of ulcerated lesions and can prevent superinfections. Chart 53-2 lists measures for best oral care.

Drug therapy used for stomatitis includes antimicrobials, immune modulators, and symptomatic topical agents. Complementary and integrative therapies may also be tried.

Antimicrobials, including antibiotics, antivirals, and antifungals, may be necessary for control of infection. Tetracycline syrup may be prescribed, especially for recurrent aphthous ulcers (RAUs). The patient rinses for 2 minutes and swallows the syrup, thus obtaining both topical and systemic therapy.

Minocycline swish/swallow and chlorhexidine mouthwashes may also be used.

A regimen of IV acyclovir (Zovirax, Xerese ✦) is prescribed for immunocompromised patients who contract herpes simplex stomatitis. Patients with healthy immune systems may be given acyclovir in oral or topical form.

For fungal infections such as yeast, nystatin (Mycostatin, Nadostine ✦, PMS-Nystatin ✦) oral suspension swish/swallow is most commonly prescribed. Ice-pop troches (lozenges) of the antifungal preparation allow the drug to slowly dissolve, and the cold provides an analgesic effect. Topical triamcinolone in benzocaine (Kenalog in Orabase) and oral dexamethasone elixir used as a swish/expectorate preparation are commonly used for stomatitis, especially RAUs.

Immune-modulating agents that may be prescribed as second-line therapy include:
- Topical amlexanox (Aphthasol)
- Topical granulocyte-macrophage colony-stimulating factor (GM-CSF)
- Thalidomide

The exact mechanism for how these drugs work is not clear. However, they may inhibit release of mediators that contribute to the inflammation seen in patients with RAUs.

Minimizing Alterations in COMFORT

Planning: Expected Outcomes. The patient with stomatitis is expected to experience restoration of oral COMFORT. Indicators include:
1. No report of oral pain or burning
2. Ability to chew and swallow without discomfort

Interventions. Dietary changes may help decrease discomfort. Cool or cold liquids can be very soothing; whereas hard, spicy, salty, and acidic foods or fluids can further irritate the ulcers. Include foods high in protein and vitamin C to promote healing, such as scrambled eggs, bananas, custards, puddings, and ice cream, unless the patient has lactose intolerance.

Over-the-counter (OTC) benzocaine anesthetics (e.g., Orabase, Anbesol) and camphor phenol (Campho-Phenique) can also control alterations in COMFORT. Viscous lidocaine may also be prescribed to use as a gargle or mouthwash. "Magic mouthwash," a mixture primarily made of lidocaine, Benadryl, Maalox, Carafate, and glucocorticoids, is also commonly prescribed for those with oral pain due to cancer treatments.

! NURSING SAFETY PRIORITY ⟨QSEN⟩

Drug Alert

Teach patients to use viscous lidocaine with extreme caution because its anesthetizing effect may cause burns from hot liquids in the mouth and/or increase the risk for choking.

? NCLEX EXAMINATION CHALLENGE 53-1

Physiological Integrity

Adequate nutrition is required for healing after treatment for recurrent aphthous ulcers (RAU). Which client response indicates that nursing teaching has been effective?
A. "I've ordered a snack of milk and pretzels."
B. "I'll try to drink orange juice twice per day."
C. "I ordered my sandwich on a crusty roll."
D. "I'd like scrambled eggs and a banana for breakfast."

Care Coordination and Transition Management

Home Care Management. Remind the patient to take all medications as prescribed, especially antibiotics, even if they begin to feel better. If the patient has been prescribed pain medication, teach about possible side effects and discourage driving and activities that require concentration. Teach which oral drugs should be used to swish and swallow and which are to be used only as a rinse.

Self-Management Education. Teach the patient about dietary choices that will not irritate the oral cavity and how to gently brush to promote good oral hygiene while preserving TISSUE INTEGRITY.

◆ Evaluation: Reflecting

Evaluate the care of the patient with stomatitis on the basis of restoration of TISSUE INTEGRITY and oral COMFORT. The expected outcomes include that the patient will:
1. Have healthy oral mucosa without inflammation or infection
2. Experience restoration of oral COMFORT

ORAL CAVITY DISORDERS

ORAL TUMORS: PREMALIGNANT LESIONS

Oral cavity tumors can be benign, precancerous, or cancerous. Whether benign or malignant, tumors of the mouth affect many daily functions, including swallowing, chewing, and speaking. Pain accompanying the tumor can also limit daily activities and self-care. Oral tumors affect body image, especially if treatment involves removal of the tongue or part of the mandible (jaw) or requires a tracheostomy.

Leukoplakia

Leukoplakia presents as slowly developing changes in the oral mucous membranes causing thickened, white, firmly attached patches that cannot easily be scraped off. These patches appear slightly raised and sharply rounded. Most of these lesions are benign. However, a small percentage of them become cancerous. Although leukoplakia can be found anywhere on the oral mucosa, lesions on the lips or tongue are more likely to progress to cancer.

Leukoplakia results from mechanical factors that cause long-term oral mucous membrane irritation, such as poorly fitting dentures, chronic cheek nibbling, or broken or poorly repaired teeth. In addition, oral hairy leukoplakia (OHL) can be found in patients with human immune deficiency virus (HIV) infection. The Joint Commission (TJC) Core Measures TOB-1 requires asking about tobacco use because tobacco products (smoked, dipped, or chewed) have been implicated in the development of leukoplakia, sometimes referred to as "smoker's patch." Oral leukoplakia can be confused with oral candidal infection. However, unlike candidal infection, leukoplakia cannot be removed by scraping.

Leukoplakia is the most common oral lesion among adults. OHL is associated with Epstein-Barr virus (EBV) and can be an early manifestation of HIV infection. When associated with HIV infection, the appearance of OHL is highly correlated with progression from HIV infection to acquired immune deficiency syndrome (AIDS). Leukoplakia not associated with HIV infection is more often seen in people older than 40 years. The incidence of leukoplakia is two times higher in men than in women; however, this ratio is changing because increasing numbers of women are smoking.

Erythroplakia

Erythroplakia appear as red, velvety mucosal lesions on the surface of the oral mucosa. There are more malignant changes in erythroplakia than in leukoplakia; therefore erythroplakia is often considered "precancerous" in presentation. As such, these lesions should be regarded with suspicion and analyzed by biopsy. Erythroplakia is most commonly found on the floor of the mouth, tongue, palate, and mandibular mucosa. It can be difficult to distinguish from inflammatory or immune reactions.

ORAL CANCER

Dentists and health care providers systematically screen patients for oral cancer. Oral assessment has become a part of the routine dental examination. People should visit a dentist at least twice a year for professional dental hygiene and oral cancer screening, which includes inspecting and palpating the mouth for lesions.

Prevention strategies for oral cancer include minimizing sun and tanning-bed exposure, tobacco cessation, and decreasing alcohol intake. Most dentists use digital technology instead of x-rays when performing the annual or biannual dental examination because excessive, prolonged radiation from x-rays has been associated with head and neck cancer (Oral Cancer Foundation [OCF], 2017). Teach adults to follow the guidelines in Chart 53-1 to maintain oral health.

❖ PATHOPHYSIOLOGY

More than 90% of oral cancers are *squamous cell carcinomas* that begin on the surface of the epithelium. Over a period of many years, premalignant (or dysplastic) changes begin. Cells begin to vary in size and shape. Alterations in the thickness of the lining of the epithelium develop, resulting in atrophy. These tumors usually grow slowly, and the lesions may be large before the onset of symptoms unless ulceration is present. *Mucosal erythroplasia is the earliest sign of oral carcinoma. Oral lesions that appear as red, raised, eroded areas are suspicious for cancer. A lesion that does not heal within 2 weeks or a lump or thickening in the cheek is a symptom that warrants further assessment* (OCF, 2017).

Squamous cell cancer can be found on the lips, tongue, buccal mucosa, and oropharynx. The major risk factors in its development are increasing age, tobacco use, and alcohol use. Most oral cancers occur in people older than 40 years. Tobacco use in any form (e.g., smoking or chewing tobacco) can increase the risk for cancer. A person who frequently consumes alcohol and uses tobacco in any form is at the highest risk

---

🧬 GENETIC/GENOMIC CONSIDERATIONS

Patient-Centered Care QSEN

Genetic variations in patients with oral cancer have been found, especially the mutation of the *TP53* gene (McCance et al., 2014). The *TP53* gene is nicknamed the "guardian of the genome" because tumor protein *p53* is essential for cell division regulation and prevention of tumor formation (National Institutes of Health, 2017). Because mutations in this gene are linked to various cancers, always ask about a personal and family history of **any** type of cancer when assessing the patient with oral cavity problems.

An increased rate of squamous cell cancer is found in people with occupations such as textile workers, plumbers, and coal and metal workers, mainly as a result of prolonged exposure to polycyclic aromatic hydrocarbons (PAHs). People with periodontal (gum) disease in which mandibular (jaw) bone loss has occurred are especially at risk for cancer of the mouth. Additional factors, such as sun exposure, poor NUTRITION habits, poor oral hygiene, and infection with the human papilloma virus (HPV16) may also contribute to oral cancer (OCF, 2017).

Research indicates a correlation between specific strains of the human papilloma virus (HPV) and oral cancer. Oral cancer associated with HPV appears in the tonsillar area or along the base of the tongue in younger people. Because HPV-positive oral cancers account for a large number of oral cancer diagnoses, routine oral assessment is essential. Oral cavity inspection combined with neck palpation is recommended yearly to aid in early detection (OCF, 2017).

Basal cell carcinoma of the mouth occurs primarily on the lips. The lesion is asymptomatic and resembles a raised scab. With time, it evolves into a characteristic ulcer with a raised, pearly border. Basal cell carcinomas do not metastasize (spread) but can aggressively involve the skin of the face. The major risk factor for this type of cancer is excessive sunlight exposure.

Basal cell carcinoma occurs as a result of the failure of basal cells to mature into keratinocytes. It is the second most common type of oral cancer, but it is much less common than squamous cell carcinoma.

Kaposi's sarcoma is a malignant lesion in blood vessels, appearing as a raised, purple nodule or plaque, which is usually painless. In the mouth, the hard palate is the most common site of Kaposi's sarcoma, but it can be found also on the gums, tongue, or tonsils. It is most often associated with AIDS. (See Chapter 19 for a complete discussion of Kaposi's sarcoma.)

As a group, oral cancers account for about 3% of all cancers in men and 2% of all cancers in women in the United States. Over 45,000 new cases are diagnosed each year, and over 8000 deaths occur (OCF, 2017). Most cancers occur in middle-age and older people, although in recent years, younger adults have been affected, probably as a result of sun exposure and HPV.

💡 NCLEX EXAMINATION CHALLENGE 53-2

Health Promotion and Maintenance

The nurse is caring for four clients. Which is at the **highest** risk for development of oral cancer?
A. 32-year-old client with ankle fracture
B. 41-year-old with human papilloma virus (HPV) infection
C. 60-year-old who quit smoking 20 years ago
D. 83-year-old who lives in a warm climate during the winter

❖ INTERPROFESSIONAL COLLABORATIVE CARE

Care of the patient with oral cancer takes place in a variety of settings ranging from the hospital to the community, depending on the degree of treatment needed. The interprofessional team that treats and cares for a patient with oral cancer may include the health care provider, dentist, surgeon, oncologist, nurse, speech therapist, dietician, social worker, and spiritual leader of the patient's choosing.

◆ Assessment: Noticing

Begin by assessing the patient's routine oral hygiene regimen and use of dentures or oral appliances, which might add to discomfort or mechanically irritate the mucosa. Ask about oral bleeding, which might indicate an ulcerative lesion or periodontal (gum) disease. Determine the patient's past and current appetite and NUTRITION state, including difficulty chewing or swallowing. A continuing trend of weight loss may be related to metastasis, heavy alcohol intake, difficulty eating or chewing, or an underlying health problem (Chart 53-3).

An examination of the oral cavity requires adequate lighting. Thoroughly inspect the oral cavity for any lesions, evidence of alterations in COMFORT, or restriction of movement. Gently using a tongue blade and penlight, examine all areas of the mouth. Carefully note any change in speech caused by tongue movement. Notice any change in voice or swallowing and assess for thick or absent saliva. After inspection, the advanced practice nurse, specialty nurse, or other health care provider uses bimanual palpation of any visible nodules to determine size and fixation. The cervical lymph nodes are also palpated (Fig. 53-2).

The functioning and appearance of the mouth are strongly linked with body image and quality of life. Therefore it is important to assess the impact of oral lesions on the patient's self-concept. Assess for any educational, cultural, and/or spiritual needs that might affect health teaching or treatment. Evaluate the patient's support system and past coping mechanisms.

OralCDx is a diagnostic procedure usually performed by a dentist during a routine dental examination. The procedure involves brushing of a lesion and is helpful in determining whether the lesion is precancerous (OralCDx, 2017). However, biopsy is the definitive method for diagnosis of oral cancer. The health care provider obtains a needle-biopsy specimen of the abnormal tissue to assess for malignant or premalignant changes. Incisional biopsies may also be performed. An intraoral biopsy can be done under local anesthesia. In very small lesions, an excisional biopsy can permit complete tumor removal. MRI is useful in detecting perineural involvement and evaluating thickness in cancers of the tongue. Both CT and MRI can be used to determine spread to the liver or lungs if further staging of the disease is warranted.

◆ **Interventions**

Both the presence of tumors of the oral cavity and the effects of their treatment threaten the integrity of the oral mucosa and the patient's airway. Oral cavity lesions can be treated by surgical excision, nonsurgical treatments such as radiation or chemotherapy, or a combination of treatments (referred to as *multimodal therapy*). Chemotherapy is currently not used independently in the treatment of oral cancers but is used in addition to other modes of treatment to sensitize malignant cells to radiation, shrink a malignancy before surgery, or decrease the potential for malignancy (OCF, 2017). Multimodal

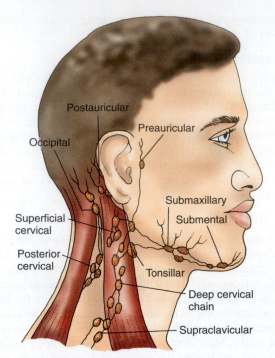

FIG. 53-2 The lymph nodes of the cervical region.

therapy is the most costly treatment option, yet it is more frequently used (OCF, 2017). *If the patient has extensive tumor involvement and copious, tenacious (thick and "stringy") secretions, maintaining an open airway is your priority for care to promote GAS EXCHANGE.* Other nursing interventions focus on restoring and maintaining oral health.

Nonsurgical Management. Implement interventions to *manage the patient's airway* by increasing air exchange, removing secretions, and preventing aspiration as needed. Assess for dyspnea resulting from the tumor obstruction or from excessive secretions. Assess the quality, rate, and depth of respirations. Auscultate the lungs for adventitious sounds, such as wheezes caused by aspiration. Listen for stridor caused by partial airway obstruction. Promote deep breathing to help produce an effective cough to mobilize the patient's secretions.

To promote GAS EXCHANGE, place the patient in a semi-Fowler's or high-Fowler's position. If the patient is able to swallow and gag reflexes are intact, it is beneficial to encourage fluids to liquefy secretions for easier removal. Chest physiotherapy also increases air exchange and promotes effective coughing. If available, collaborate with the respiratory therapist about performing this procedure. If needed, use oral suction equipment with a dental tip or a tonsil tip (Yankauer catheter) to remove secretions that obstruct the airway. Teach the patient and family to use the catheters as needed.

If edema occurs with oral cavity lesions, the patient may receive steroids to reduce inflammation. Antibiotics may be prescribed if infection is present because it can increase inflammation and edema. A cool mist supplied by a face tent may help with oxygen transport and control of edema.

It is important to work with the patient to *establish an oral hygiene routine.* Perform oral hygiene every 2 hours for ulcerated lesions or infection or in the immediate postoperative period. Modifications might be needed because of oral discomfort, bleeding, or edema. Oral care with a soft-bristled toothbrush is preferred. If the platelet count falls below 40,000/mm³, switch the

Aspiration Precautions prevent or reduce the risk factors for aspiration. Assess the patient's level of consciousness (LOC), gag reflex, and ability to swallow. To prevent aspiration, place the patient sitting upright at 90 degrees (high-Fowler's position). As a precaution, keep suction equipment nearby. For patients at high risk, assess the gag reflex before giving any fluids. Remind UAP to feed patients at risk for aspiration in small amounts. Teach visitors to speak with you before offering any type of food or drink to the patient. Provide thickened liquids as an aid to prevent aspiration. Referral to the speech/language pathologist can be beneficial for patients who are experiencing aspiration with swallowing. A swallow study may be needed to fully assess the risk for aspiration.

patient to an ultrasoft "chemobrush." The use of "Toothettes" or a disposable foam brush is discouraged because these products may not adequately control bacteremia-promoting plaque and may further dry the oral mucosa. Lubricant can be applied to moisten the lips and oral mucosa as needed.

Teach patients and their families that the patient should avoid using commercial mouthwashes and lemon-glycerin swabs. Commercial mouthwashes contain alcohol, and lemon-glycerin swabs are acidic. These substances can cause a burning sensation and contribute to dry oral mucous membranes. Encourage frequent rinsing of the mouth with sodium bicarbonate solution or warm saline (see also Chart 53-2). Follow hospital or health care provider protocol if available.

Radiation therapy for oral cancers can be given by external beam or interstitial implantation to reduce the size of the tumor before surgery. *External-beam* radiation passes through the skin or mucous membrane to the tumor site. Typically, treatments are given as five daily treatments per week, with a 2-day break each week, over a 6- to 9-week period. Each treatment lasts only about 10 to 15 minutes, with more time being dedicated to undertaking special precautions to minimize the dose of radiation to the brain or spinal cord (OCF, 2017).

Another option is the implantation of radioactive substances (*interstitial radiation therapy* or *brachytherapy*) to either boost the dosage or deliver a radiation dose close to the tumor bed. This form of implant therapy can be curative in early-stage lesions in the floor of the mouth or anterior tongue. It may also add a boost of radiation to a tumor that received external-beam radiation.

With the exception of radioactive seeds, which have a low level of emission, patients receiving interstitial radiation are usually hospitalized for the duration of treatment. *Place patients on radiation transmission precautions while the materials are active or in place.* Patients need to be placed in a private room with lead-lined walls or movable panels. When permitted, visitors may stay only 30 minutes or less each day and must sit or stand away from the patient in designated areas. Pregnant women and children younger than 18 years should not be permitted to visit. A tracheostomy may be required with interstitial implants because of edema and increased oral secretions. (See Chapter 22 for general nursing care of patients undergoing radiation therapy.)

Teach the patient undergoing *chemotherapy* and family members about the side effects of these agents, which vary with each drug. Give antiemetics as prescribed and provide other comfort measures as needed. (See Chapter 22 for general care of patients receiving chemotherapy.)

Patients who are undergoing radiation and/or chemotherapy treatment may experience a decreased ability to tolerate prescribed and over-the-counter medications as a result of being immunocompromised. Teach patients about expected side effects and remind them to not take any medication (including over-the-counter medications, herbs, or vitamin supplements) without first discussing them with their health care provider.

One of the most recent advances in the use of drugs for oral cancer is targeted therapy. Hormone-like substances known as *growth factors (GFs)* occur in the body's cells. Oral tumor cells, along with other types of cancers, grow quickly because they have more GF receptors than does normal healthy tissue. One of these GFs is called *epidermal growth factor (EGF)*, which has been associated with oral cancers. Newer drugs that can target and block EGF receptors (EGF-R) are being tested, and more than a dozen have been approved, including cetuximab (Erbitux), erlotinib (Tarceva), and panitumumab (Vectibix). (Chapter 22 describes targeted molecular therapy.)

? NCLEX EXAMINATION CHALLENGE 53-3
Health Promotion and Maintenance

The nurse is caring for a client who is concerned about developing oral tumors. Which client statement requires **immediate** nursing intervention?
A. "I used to chew tobacco but quit 5 years ago."
B. "I use sunscreen to cover my face and body when I'm at the beach."
C. "I don't have dental insurance, so I can't get dental check-ups."
D. "I only drink alcohol on special occasions like my birthday and anniversary."

Surgical Management. The health care provider can often remove small, noninvasive lesions of the oral cavity in an ambulatory surgical center with local anesthesia. The surgical opening is usually small enough to be closed by sutures. These smaller lesions may also be responsive to carbon dioxide laser therapy or **cryotherapy** (extreme cold application), as well as photodynamic therapy. These procedures can be performed as an ambulatory care procedure in a surgical center but may require general anesthesia.

Small oral cancers are equally responsive to radiation or photodynamic therapy and to surgery. More invasive lesions (stages III and IV) require more extensive surgical excision and result in a greater loss of function and disfigurement. Not all lesions can be excised by the peroral approach (through the mouth). The goal of surgical resection is removal of the tumor with a surgical margin that is free of cancer cells.

Preoperative Care. Before excision of a lesion in the oral cavity, assess and document the patient's level of understanding of the disease process, the rationale for the surgery, and the planned intervention. Problems associated with cancer therapy can be reduced or optimally managed by collaborating with the patient and family regarding preparation and instruction. Reinforce information as needed. Include family members or other caregivers in the health teaching unless culturally or spiritually inappropriate.

EVIDENCE-BASED PRACTICE QSEN

Preoperative Oral Care Contributes to Better Postsurgical Outcomes (Safety)

Shigeishi H., et al. (2016). Preoperative oral health care reduces postoperative inflammation and complications in oral cancer patients. *Experimental and Therapeutic Medicine, 12,* 1922-1928.

This study reviewed the records of 70 patients with oral cancer who were treated at one institution between 2008 and 2014, focusing on body temperature, white blood cell count, and C-reactive protein (CRP) levels between those who received preoperative oral care versus those who did not. Those who received professional teeth cleaning and were instructed in self-care had lower incidences of inflammation and postoperative complications.

Level of Evidence: 2

This research was designed as a retrospective review.

Commentary: Implications for Practice and Research

Patients who received oral care in the form of professional teeth cleaning or scaling at least 3 days before surgery and who received oral care at least once daily following surgery experienced a significantly lower CRP on days 3 to 5 after surgery. Although body temperature and white blood cell counts were not statistically different between those who received oral care before surgery versus those who did not, the data suggest that preoperative oral care contributes to lesser postoperative inflammation in patients who have invasive surgery for oral cancer. Nurses must teach patients to seek professional oral care before surgery, to perform ongoing oral care after surgery while hospitalized, and about home oral care before discharge, all of which contribute to better patient outcomes.

For small, local excisions, postoperative restrictions include a liquid diet for a day and then advancing as tolerated. There are no activity limitations, and postoperative analgesics are prescribed. Research shows that preoperative oral health reduces postoperative inflammation and complications, so teach patients how to perform proper oral care before procedures take place (see the Evidence-Based Practice box).

Instructions for the patient undergoing large surgical resections may include but are not limited to these expectations after surgery:

- Placement of a temporary tracheostomy, oxygen therapy, and suctioning
- Temporary loss of speech because of the tracheostomy
- Frequent monitoring of postoperative vital signs
- NPO status until intraoral suture lines are healed
- Need to have IV lines in place for drug delivery and hydration
- Postoperative drug therapy and activity (out of bed on the day or surgery or first postoperative day)
- Possibility of surgical drains

Because communication is interrupted, assess the patient's ability to read, write, and draw pictures to communicate. In coordination with the patient, select the method of communication to use after surgery with staff and family members (e.g., Magic Slate, handheld mobile device, computer, picture board, or pad and pencil). Preprinted flashcards may be used to communicate the patient's needs, such as "I'm tired," "I'm in pain," or "I'm hungry." Urge the patient to practice the chosen method before surgery to reduce frustration after surgery.

Operative Procedures. Three factors influence the extent of surgery performed for oral cancers: the size and location of the

CHART 53-4 Focused Assessment

The Postoperative Older Adult With Oral Cancer

- Assess the mouth and surrounding tissues for candidiasis, mucositis, and pain; assess for loss of appetite and taste.
- Monitor the patient's weight.
- Monitor nutrition and fluid intake.
- Assess for difficulty in eating or speech.
- Assess pain status and measures used to control pain.
- Monitor the patient's response to medications.
- Identify psychosocial problems, such as depression, anxiety, and fear.
- Assess the patient's overall physiologic condition and how this may affect pharmacologic therapy.

tumor, tumor invasion into the bone, and whether there has been metastasis (cancer spread) to neck lymph nodes. Small, noninvasive tumors can be removed perorally (through the mouth). Otherwise an external approach may be used. The most extensive oral operations are composite resections, which combine partial or total **glossectomy** (tongue removal) and partial **mandibulectomy** (jaw removal). In the **commando** (co-mandible) **procedure** (**COM**bined neck dissection, **MAN**Dibulectomy, and **O**ropharyngeal resection), the surgeon removes a segment of the mandible with the oral lesion and performs a radical neck dissection (see Chapter 29).

Metastasis to cervical lymph nodes usually indicates a poor prognosis for patients with cancer of the oral cavity. In those with cervical node metastasis, a neck dissection may also be performed. A radical neck dissection usually involves the removal of all cervical lymph nodes on the affected side, along with cranial nerve XI (the accessory nerve), the internal jugular vein, and the sternocleidomastoid (front neck) muscle. Modified and selective neck dissections may be performed in patients with minimal lymph node involvement.

Postoperative Care. The patient may have a temporary or permanent tracheostomy, requiring intensive nursing care to promote airway clearance. In addition, care must be taken to protect the surgical incision site from mechanical damage and infection (see Chapter 29). Nursing interventions to relieve discomfort and promote NUTRITION are also important. Older adults are a special risk for surgery and need to be monitored very carefully (Chart 53-4).

! NURSING SAFETY PRIORITY QSEN

Action Alert

After extensive excision or resection for oral cancer, the most important nursing intervention is maintaining the patient's airway to promote GAS EXCHANGE! On awakening from anesthesia, the patient may not recall, or realize, that a tracheostomy tube is in place and may initially panic because of the inability to speak. Remind the patient why he or she cannot speak and provide reassurance that the vocal cords are intact (unless a total laryngectomy has been performed, in which case the loss of voice is permanent).

Ensure that the predetermined method of communication is available for the patient, family members, and staff. When the patient has an adequate airway and can effectively clear secretions by coughing, the tracheostomy tube may be removed. When the tube is removed, an airtight dressing is placed over the site, and the tracheostomy incision heals without the need for sutures.

Patients who have undergone extensive resection may have slurred speech or difficulty in speaking as a result of nerve damage or tongue removal. Collaborate with the speech-language pathologist if speech is altered.

Protect the incision site to avoid infection. Provide gentle mouth care for cleaning away thick secretions and stimulating the flow of saliva. The delivery of oral care depends on the nature and extent of the surgical procedure. Give oral care at least every 4 hours in the early postoperative phase. The presence of unusual odors from the mouth can indicate infection; therefore continual assessment of the oral cavity is very important. In the early postoperative phase, take care to avoid disruption of the suture line during oral hygiene.

Elevate the head of the bed to assist in decreasing edema by gravity. If skin grafting was done, inspect the donor site (generally on the anterior thigh) every 8 hours for bleeding or signs of infection. (See Chapter 29 for specific nursing care of the patient with a radical neck dissection.)

To provide optimal pain relief in the postoperative period, rely on subjective and objective data to assess the need for analgesics and their effectiveness. The desired outcome of drug therapy during this period is to promote COMFORT while allowing the patient to function at an optimal level. Those who have undergone surgery for oral cancer describe their pain as throbbing or pounding. IV morphine is usually the initial pain medication given with acetaminophen or ibuprofen to decrease inflammation. Percocet (oxycodone plus acetaminophen) may be used for systemic relief of moderate pain after the IV morphine is discontinued.

Patients who have undergone extensive resections of the oral cavity remain on NPO status for several days. This time allows healing in the oral cavity before food comes in contact with the incision. Nasogastric feeding or total parenteral NUTRITION may be needed until oral nutrition can begin (see Chapter 60).

> **! NURSING SAFETY PRIORITY** **QSEN**
>
> **Action Alert**
>
> When oral fluid intake is started, assess for and document signs of difficulty swallowing, aspiration, or leakage of saliva or fluids from the suture line. Monitor daily weights and hydration. NUTRITION supplementation may improve the patient's quality of life. Patients who have weight loss or who are having difficulty maintaining hydration may be candidates for the placement of a gastrostomy tube. Coordinate NUTRITION care with the dietitian.

Encourage the patient to perform swallowing exercises. Collaborate with the speech-language pathologist to assist with swallowing techniques. Thickened fluids may be needed to prevent aspiration. A swallowing impairment may be temporary or permanent.

Care Coordination and Transition Management

Continuing care for the patient with an oral tumor depends on the severity of the tumor, its collaborative care, and available support systems. Most patients are maintained at home during follow-up care. Ongoing NUTRITION management remains a vital part of the treatment plan. In addition, the patient and family may benefit from a community-based support group for cancer patients.

Home Care Management. If radiation therapy is part of the patient's treatment plan, home care considerations include health teaching and management strategies. Complications from radiation to the head or neck can be acute or delayed. Acute effects include treatment-related mucositis, stomatitis, and alterations in taste. Long-term effects such as xerostomia (excessive mouth dryness) and dental decay require ongoing oral care, the use of saliva substitutes, and follow-up dental visits. Although ongoing dental care is important, the possible adverse effects that radiation has on bone make elective oral surgical procedures, such as tooth extraction, impossible in the area of the radiation. Fatigue is a common side effect of radiation and chemotherapy.

The patient whose tracheostomy tube has been removed is often placed on a soft diet by mouth before discharge. However, occasionally patients are discharged from the hospital while still requiring tracheostomy suction, oral suction, and nasogastric feedings. Suction equipment, NUTRITION supplies, and nursing care can be provided by home care companies. (See Chapter 60 for home care preparation for the patient receiving home parenteral nutrition and Chapter 28 for home care preparation for the patient with a tracheostomy.)

Self-Management Education. Before hospital discharge, teach the patient and family about drug therapy, NUTRITION therapies, any treatments (e.g., tracheostomy care, suture line care, dressing changes), and early symptoms of infection (Chart 53-5). Alterations in taste and dysphagia make maintaining adequate nutrition a challenge for the oral cancer patient. Alterations in taste occur when the taste buds are included in the radiation treatment field. Taste sensation may begin to return several weeks after the completion of treatment. Some types of chemotherapy can also affect the patient's taste. Sometimes the loss of taste is permanent.

Changes in taste include dislike of meat, such as beef or pork, and metallic tastes in the mouth. Teach patients to add seasonings to foods, to use gravies or sauces to make foods more palatable, and to use high-protein foods such as cheeses, milk, eggs, puddings, and legumes in place of meat. Instruct patients with dysphagia in swallowing exercises. Recommend thickened liquids because thin liquids, such as water, are difficult to control during swallowing. Collaborate with the dietitian to teach the family how to assess the NUTRITION intake of the patient who is just beginning to eat. Liquid dietary supplements are usually recommended at this time. If bleeding or stomatitis is present, recommend soft foods to prevent further injury to the mucous membranes.

> **CHART 53-5 Patient and Family Education: Preparing for Self-Management**
>
> *Care of the Patient With Oral Cancer at Home*
>
> - Follow the treatment plan for cancer therapies.
> - Remember that taste sensation may be decreased; add nonspicy seasonings to food to better enjoy it.
> - Use a thickening agent for liquids if dysphagia is present.
> - Eat soft foods if stomatitis occurs.
> - Inspect the mouth every day for changes, such as redness or lesions.
> - Continue meticulous oral hygiene at home using a chemobrush and frequent rinsing; clean brush after every use.
> - Use saliva substitute as prescribed.
> - Avoid sun or tanning-bed exposure if radiation is part of therapy.
> - Clean with a gentle, nondeodorant soap, such as Ivory.

Teach the patient or family members to inspect the oral cavity daily for areas of redness, which can indicate the onset of stomatitis. Meticulous oral hygiene should be continued at home, especially with adjuvant chemotherapy or radiation. Reinforce the oral hygiene routine, emphasizing the need for frequent mouth rinsing to reduce the number of microorganisms and to maintain adequate hydration. The patient should use a chemobrush (an extra-soft type of toothbrush), rinse the chemobrush with hydrogen peroxide and water or with a diluted bleach solution after each use, and change chemobrushes weekly. The brush may also be cleaned in a dishwasher.

Saliva production is greatly reduced as a consequence of radiation. The resulting xerostomia (dry mouth) causes the inability to eat dry foods and may be permanent. Teach the patient regarding the use of saliva substitutes.

Skin reactions are also a common side effect of radiation. Instruct the patient to avoid sun exposure, to avoid perfumed lotions and powders, and to cleanse the face and neck area with a gentle nondeodorant soap. Teach individuals to use an electric razor for shaving and to avoid alcohol-based aftershave lotions to prevent further skin irritation.

> ### ❓ NCLEX EXAMINATION CHALLENGE 53-4
> #### *Physiological Integrity*
>
> A client completing radiation treatment has developed dysphagia and stomatitis. What teaching will the nurse provide? **Select all that apply.**
> A. Brush teeth twice daily with chemobrush.
> B. Thin liquids will make it easier to swallow.
> C. Limit alcohol consumption to three drinks per day.
> D. Rinse mouth with mild saline and water mix before and after eating.
> E. Refrain from using liquid dietary supplements because these will irritate mucous membranes.
> F. Plan to eat soft foods such as cheese, well-cooked legumes, peanut butter, and pudding.

Health Care Resources. Patients who have undergone composite resection often require community services because they have both physical and psychosocial needs. Depression related to a change in body image is common. Excision of part of the jaw can leave a facial defect that may be difficult to hide. Assess for depression and other behavioral responses such as anxiety, fear, anger, shame, and/or loneliness. A social worker or other health care professional may be needed for patient and family counseling. Those who have undergone a total glossectomy may be able to speak with special training and the use of an intraoral prosthesis created by a maxillofacial prosthodontist. The prosthesis is similar to dentures.

Collaborate with the case manager to provide assistance in obtaining special equipment or NUTRITION resources needed by the patient at home. The case manager assesses the patient's financial needs and makes referrals to government, community, and religious organizations as needed. Refer the patient to the American Cancer Society (ACS) (www.cancer.org), the Oral Cancer Foundation (www.oralcancerfoundation.org), and/or the Canadian Cancer Society (www.cancer.ca/en/region-selector-page/) for local support groups and resources, including additional information. The ACS often provides dressing supplies and transportation to and from follow-up visits or medical treatments.

> ### ❓ CLINICAL JUDGMENT CHALLENGE 53-1
> #### *Safety; Patient-Centered Care* **QSEN**
>
> A 55-year-old patient is beginning outpatient radiation therapy for a small mass near the submaxillary lymph node. She has transportation and sees a local dentist yearly. You are preparing to teach the patient methods of self-care management.
> 1. What are your teaching priorities for her before the radiation treatment?
> 2. For what complications is this patient most at risk?
> 3. What would you teach the patient that would be most helpful to minimize radiation side effects?
> 4. Considering that this is a female patient, what psychosocial or sociocultural concerns would you anticipate that she may experience after beginning radiation therapy?
> 5. What follow-up care will you recommend for this patient?

DISORDERS OF THE SALIVARY GLANDS

ACUTE SIALADENITIS

❖ PATHOPHYSIOLOGY

Acute sialadenitis, the inflammation of a salivary gland, can be caused by infectious agents, irradiation, or immunologic disorders. Salivary gland inflammation can have a bacterial or viral cause, such as infection with cytomegalovirus (CMV). The most common bacterial organisms are *Staphylococcus aureus, Staphylococcus pyogenes, Streptococcus pneumoniae,* and *Escherichia coli.* This disorder most commonly affects the parotid or submandibular gland in adults.

A decrease in the production of saliva (as in dehydrated or debilitated patients or in those who are on NPO status after surgery for an extended time) can lead to acute sialadenitis. The bacteria or viruses enter the gland through the ductal opening in the mouth. Systemic drugs, such as phenothiazines and the tetracyclines, can also trigger an episode of acute sialadenitis. Untreated infections of the salivary glands can evolve into abscesses, which can rupture and spread infection into the tissues of the neck and the mediastinum.

Patients who receive radiation for the treatment of cancers of the head and neck or thyroid may develop decreased salivary flow, predisposing them to acute or persistent sialadenitis. The effect of radiation on the salivary glands is rapid and dose related. Immunologic disorders such as HIV infection can cause enlargement of the parotid gland that results from secondary infection. Sjögren's syndrome, an autoimmune disorder, is characterized by chronic salivary gland enlargement and inflammation that cause a very dry mouth (see Chapter 20).

❖ INTERPROFESSIONAL COLLABORATIVE CARE

The primary individuals who will care for the patient with acute sialadenitis include the health care provider, nurse, and radiological specialist. During the initial interview, assess for any predisposing factors for sialadenitis, such as ionizing radiation to the head or neck area. Collect a thorough drug history and ask about systemic illnesses, such as HIV infection.

Dehydration can be assessed by examining the oral membrane for dryness and the skin for turgor. Other assessment findings include pain and swelling of the face over the affected gland. Assess facial function because the branches of cranial nerve VII (the facial nerve) lie close to the salivary glands. Fever and general malaise also occur, and purulent drainage can often be massaged from the affected duct in the oral cavity.

Collaborative care includes the administration of IV fluids and measures such as these to treat the underlying cause and increase the flow of saliva:

- Hydration
- Application of warm compresses
- Massage of the gland
- Use of a saliva substitute
- Use of sialagogues (substances that stimulate the flow of saliva)

Sialagogues include lemon slices and citrus- and other fruit-flavored candy. Massage is accomplished by milking the edematous gland with the fingertips toward the ductal opening. Elevation of the head of the bed promotes gravity drainage of the edematous gland.

Acute sialadenitis is best prevented by adherence to routine oral hygiene. This practice prevents infection from ascending to the salivary glands from the mouth.

POST-IRRADIATION SIALADENITIS

The salivary glands are sensitive to ionizing radiation, such as from radiation therapy or radioactive iodine treatment of thyroid cancers. Exposure of the glands to radiation produces a type of sialadenitis known as xerostomia (very dry mouth caused by a severe reduction in the flow of saliva) within 24 hours. Radiation to the salivary glands can also cause alterations in COMFORT and edema, which generally abate after several days.

Xerostomia may be temporary or permanent, depending on the dose of radiation and the percentage of total salivary gland tissue irradiated. Little can be done to relieve the patient's dry mouth during the course of radiation therapy. Frequent sips of water and frequent mouth care, especially before meals, are the most effective interventions. After the course of radiation therapy has been completed, saliva substitutes may provide moisture for 2 to 4 hours at a time. Over-the-counter solutions are available; or methylcellulose (Cologel), glycerin, and saline may be mixed to form a solution.

SALIVARY GLAND TUMORS

Of all oral tumors, those of the salivary glands are relatively rare. Initially malignant tumors present as slow-growing, painless masses. Involvement of the facial nerve results in facial weakness or paralysis (partial or total) on the affected side.

Collect information about any prior radiation exposure, because radiation to the head and neck areas is associated with the occurrence of salivary gland tumors. Salivary gland tumors present as localized, firm masses. Submandibular and minor salivary gland tumors may be tender or painful. Tumor invasion of the hypoglossal nerve causes impaired movement of the tongue, and a loss of sensation can follow. *Pay particular attention to assessment of the facial nerve because of its proximity to the salivary glands.* Assess the patient's ability to:

- Wrinkle the brow
- Raise the eyebrows
- Squeeze and hold the eyes shut while you gently pull upward on the eyebrows and cheeks beneath the orbit to check for symmetry
- Wrinkle the nose
- Pucker the lips
- Puff out the cheeks
- Grimace or smile

Be aware of any asymmetry when the patient performs these motions. The treatment of choice for both benign and malignant tumors of the salivary glands is surgical excision. However, radiation therapy is often used for salivary gland cancers that are large, have recurred, show evidence of residual disease after excision, or are highly malignant.

> ### ❓ NCLEX EXAMINATION CHALLENGE 53-5
> *Physiological Integrity*
>
> Which facial assessment finding in a client with a salivary gland tumor prompts the nurse to notify the health care provider?
> A. Loss of sensation in tongue
> B. Alternates smiling and grimacing
> C. Wrinkles brows on command
> D. Holds eyes shut as the nurse pulls gently on the eyebrows

Patients who have undergone parotidectomy (surgical removal of the parotid glands) or submandibular gland surgery are at risk for weakness or loss of function of the facial nerve because the nerve courses directly through the gland. Facial nerve repair with grafting can be done at the time of surgery. A combination of surgery followed by radiation is common for advanced disease. Care for patients after parotidectomy is similar to that required for those having oral cancer surgery, which is described in the Surgical Management discussion in the Oral Cavity Disorders section.

GET READY FOR THE NCLEX® EXAMINATION!

▌ KEY POINTS

Review these key points for each NCLEX Examination Client Needs Category.

Safe and Effective Care Environment

- Be aware that airway management is the priority of care for patients having surgery for oral cancer. **QSEN: Safety**
- Place patients having oral cancer surgery in a high-Fowler's position to facilitate breathing and prevent aspiration. **QSEN: Safety**
- Assess for swallowing ability to prevent aspiration by checking the gag reflex before offering liquids or food to the patient who has had oral cancer surgery. **QSEN: Safety**
- Plan transition management to meet the patients' needs when they are transferred from the hospital to community-based agencies. **QSEN: Teamwork and Collaboration**

Health Promotion and Maintenance

- Remind adults to visit their dentist regularly for dental hygiene and oral examinations and to seek medical or dental attention for oral lesions that do not heal.

- Follow the best practice recommendations for maintaining oral health as listed in Chart 53-1.
- Instruct patients to avoid harsh commercial mouthwashes if they have oral lesions.
- In keeping with The Joint Commission (TJC) Core Measures TOB-2, teach adults to avoid tobacco or offer a cessation plan, alcohol, and sun exposure to decrease their chance of having oral cancer. **QSEN: Evidence-Based Practice**
- Instruct patients with acute sialadenitis to use sialagogues to stimulate saliva, such as citrus foods or candies.

Psychosocial Integrity

- Assess the patient's and family's response to an oral cancer diagnosis, which may include feelings of anger, depression, anxiety, and/or fear. **QSEN: Patient-Centered Care**
- Help the patient and family identify and use strengths and coping mechanisms to deal with changes in body image and altered self-esteem. **QSEN: Patient-Centered Care**
- Refer patients with oral cancer to support groups, such as those available through the American Cancer Society.

Physiological Integrity

- Remember that stomatitis usually begins as painful single or multiple ulcerations within the mouth.

- Recognize that stomatitis can be caused by a variety of organisms; *Candida* infections are common in patients who receive antibiotic therapy and in those who are immunocompromised.
- Provide gentle oral care for patients with oral lesions by using chemobrushes and warm saline or sodium bicarbonate solution. **QSEN: Safety**
- Be aware that patients with stomatitis receive antimicrobials, anti-inflammatory agents, immune modulators, and topical agents for relief of symptoms. **QSEN: Evidence-Based Practice**
- Differentiate leukoplakia and erythroplakia: leukoplakia presents as thin, white patches; and erythroplakia presents as red, velvety lesions. **Clinical Judgment**
- Be aware that patients with oral cancer may undergo chemotherapy, radiation, surgery, or a combination of these treatment methods.
- Recognize that sialadenitis can occur as a result of radiation therapy.
- Assess for facial nerve involvement for patients with salivary gland tumors. **QSEN: Safety**
- Remember that a parotidectomy involves the removal of the salivary glands; postoperative care is similar to that for patients who have oral cancer surgery.

SELECTED BIBLIOGRAPHY

Kiyoshi-Teo, H., & Blegen, M. (2015). Influence of institutional guidelines on oral hygiene practices in intensive care units. Results of a section of a larger survey study. *American Journal of Critical Care Nurses*, 24(4), 309–317.

McCance, K., Huether, S., Brashers, V., & Rote, N. (2014). *Pathophysiology: The biologic basis for disease in adults and children* (7th ed.). St. Louis: Mosby.

Mirowski, G. (2017). *Aphthous stomatitis*. http://emedicine.medscape.com/article/1075570-overview#a6.

Mountain, C., & Golles, K. (2017). Detecting dysphagia. *American Nurse Today*, (12)5. https://www.americannursetoday.com/detecting-dysphagia/.

National Institutes of Health (2017). *Genetics home reference: TP53.* www.ghr.nlm.nih.gov/gene/TP53.

Oral Cancer Foundation (OCF) (2017). *Oral cancer facts.* www.oralcancerfoundation.org.

OralCDx (2017). *The OralCDx brush test.* www.cdxdiagnostics.com/OralCDx.html.

Ślebioda, Z., Szponar, E., & Kowalska, A. (2014). Etiopathogenesis of recurrent aphthous stomatitis and the role of immunologic aspects: Literature review. *Archivum Immunologiae et Therapiae Experimentalis*, 62(3), 205–215. http://doi.org/10.1007/s00005-013-0261-y.

World Health Organization (2012). *Oral health.* www.who.int/mediacentre/factsheets/fs318/en/.

CHAPTER 54

Care of Patients With Esophageal Problems

Tracy Taylor

PRIORITY AND INTERRELATED CONCEPTS

The priority concept for this chapter is NUTRITION.

✳ The NUTRITION concept exemplars for this chapter are:
- Gastroesophageal Reflux Disease (GERD), below
- Esophageal Tumors, p. 1095

The interrelated concept for this chapter is COMFORT.

LEARNING OUTCOMES

Safe and Effective Care Environment
1. Collaborate with the interprofessional team to protect the patient with esophageal problems from injury and infection.
2. Identify appropriate community resources to ensure appropriate transition management for patients with esophageal problems.

Health Promotion and Maintenance
3. Teach patients about lifestyle changes that decrease gastroesophageal reflux disease (GERD) and alterations in COMFORT associated with hiatal hernias.

Psychosocial Integrity
4. Implement nursing interventions to minimize stressors for the patient and family who have received a diagnosis of esophageal cancer.

Physiological Integrity
5. Apply knowledge of anatomy, physiology, pathophysiology, genetic risk, age-related changes, and psychomotor skills to perform a focused assessment for patients with esophageal health problems.
6. Evaluate the impact of esophageal problems on the patient's NUTRITION status.
7. Prioritize care for patients with esophageal problems.
8. Develop an evidence-based postoperative teaching plan for the patient who has had esophageal surgery.

The esophagus moves partially digested food from the mouth to the stomach. Without this process, adults cannot meet their basic human need for NUTRITION. Food nutrients are necessary for normal body cell function. Common esophageal problems that can interfere with digestion and NUTRITION are caused by inflammation, structural defects or obstruction, and cancer. Interprofessional collaborative care involves dietary and lifestyle changes and may include medical and surgical therapies.

✳ NUTRITION CONCEPT EXEMPLAR
Gastroesophageal Reflux Disease (GERD)

❖ PATHOPHYSIOLOGY

Gastroesophageal reflux disease (GERD), the most common upper GI disorder in the United States, occurs most often in middle-age and older adults but can affect people of any age.

Gastroesophageal reflux (GER) occurs as a result of backward flow of stomach contents into the esophagus. GERD is the chronic and more serious condition that arises from persistent GER.

Reflux produces symptoms by exposing the esophageal mucosa to the irritating effects of gastric or duodenal contents, resulting in inflammation. A patient with acute symptoms of inflammation is often described as having mild or severe **reflux esophagitis** (McCance et al., 2014).

The reflux of gastric contents into the esophagus is normally prevented by the presence of two high-pressure areas that remain contracted at rest. A 1.2-inch (3-cm) segment at the proximal end of the esophagus is called the *upper esophageal sphincter (UES)*, whereas another small portion at the gastroesophageal junction (near the cardiac sphincter) is called the **lower esophageal sphincter (LES)**. The function of the LES is supported by its anatomic placement in the abdomen, where the surrounding pressure is significantly higher than in the low-pressure thorax. Sphincter function is also supported by the acute angle (angle of His) that is formed as the esophagus enters the stomach.

The most common cause of GERD is excessive relaxation of the LES, which allows the reflux of gastric contents into the esophagus and exposure of the esophageal mucosa to acidic gastric contents. Patients who are overweight or obese are at highest risk for development of GERD because increased weight increases intra-abdominal pressure, which contributes to reflux of stomach contents into the esophagus. Nighttime reflux tends to cause prolonged exposure of the esophagus to acid because lying supine decreases peristalsis and the benefit of gravity. Hiatal hernias also increase the risk for development of GERD due to the creation of increased intra-abdominal pressure. *Helicobacter pylori* may contribute to reflux (McCance et al., 2014) by causing gastritis and thus poor gastric emptying. This increases frequency of GER events and acid exposure to the esophagus.

A person having reflux may be asymptomatic. However, the esophagus has limited resistance to the damaging effects of the acidic GI contents. The pH of acid secreted by the stomach ranges from 1.5 to 2.0, whereas the pH of the distal esophagus is normally neutral (6.0 to 7.0).

Refluxed material is returned to the stomach by a combination of gravity, saliva, and peristalsis. The inflamed esophagus cannot eliminate the refluxed material as quickly as a healthy one; therefore the length of exposure increases with each reflux episode. Hyperemia (increased blood flow) and erosion (ulceration) occur in the esophagus in response to the chronic inflammation. Gastric acid and pepsin injure tissue. Minor capillary bleeding often occurs with erosion, but hemorrhage is rare.

During the process of healing, the body may substitute Barrett's epithelium (columnar epithelium) for the normal squamous cell epithelium of the lower esophagus. Although this new tissue is more resistant to acid and therefore supports esophageal healing, it is considered premalignant and is associated with an increased risk for cancer in patients with prolonged GERD. The fibrosis and scarring that accompany the healing process can produce esophageal stricture (narrowing of the esophageal opening). The stricture leads to progressive difficulty swallowing. Uncontrolled esophageal reflux also increases the risk for other complications such as asthma, laryngitis, dental decay, cardiac disease, as well as serious concerns for hemorrhage and aspiration pneumonia.

Gastric distention caused by eating very large meals or delayed gastric emptying predisposes the patient to reflux. Certain foods and drugs, smoking, and alcohol influence the tone function of the LES (Table 54-1).

Patients who have a nasogastric tube also have decreased esophageal sphincter function. The tube keeps the cardiac sphincter open and allows acidic contents from the stomach to enter the esophagus. Other factors that increase intra-abdominal and intragastric pressure (e.g., pregnancy, wearing tight belts or girdles, bending over, ascites) overcome the gastroesophageal pressure gradient maintained by the LES and allow reflux to occur. Many patients with obstructive sleep apnea report frequent episodes of GERD. Patients with hiatal hernias often have reflux because the upper portion of the stomach protrudes through the diaphragm into the thorax, which allows acid to reach the esophagus (see later discussion of hiatal hernia).

Health Promotion and Maintenance

Adults who have gastroesophageal reflux (GER) may initially be asymptomatic. Teach patients to engage in healthy eating habits that include consuming small, frequent meals and limiting intake of fried, fatty, and spicy foods, and caffeine. Sitting upright for at least 1 hour after eating can promote proper digestion and reduce the risk for reflux.

? NCLEX EXAMINATION CHALLENGE 54-1

Health Promotion and Maintenance

On assessment of a client with GERD, which statement requires nursing intervention?
A. "I quit smoking several years ago."
B. "Sometimes I wake up gasping for air in the middle of the night."
C. "My family likes to eat small meals every 3 to 4 hours throughout the day."
D. "When I buy meat, I ask for the leanest cut that is available."

❖ INTERPROFESSIONAL COLLABORATIVE CARE

Care for the patient with GERD usually takes place in the community setting. Only infrequently is surgery needed to correct the problem. The interprofessional team that usually collaborates to care for this patient includes the primary health care provider, nurse, and dietician.

◆ Assessment: Noticing

Ask the patient about a history of heartburn or atypical chest pain associated with the reflux of GI contents. Ask whether he or she has been newly diagnosed with asthma or has experienced morning hoarseness or pneumonia. These symptoms may indicate severe reflux reaching the pharynx or mouth or pulmonary aspiration.

Physical Assessment/Signs and Symptoms. Dyspepsia, also known as *indigestion,* and regurgitation are the main symptoms of GERD, although symptoms may vary in severity (Chart 54-1). Symptoms associated with "indigestion" may include abdominal discomfort, feeling uncomfortably full, nausea, and burping.

TABLE 54-1   Factors Contributing to Decreased Lower Esophageal Sphincter Pressure

- Caffeinated beverages, such as coffee, tea, and cola
- Chocolate
- Citrus fruits
- Tomatoes and tomato products
- Smoking and use of other tobacco products
- Calcium channel blockers
- Nitrates
- Peppermint, spearmint
- Alcohol
- Anticholinergic drugs
- High levels of estrogen and progesterone
- Nasogastric tube placement

▶▶ CHART 54-1   Key Features

Gastroesophageal Reflux Disease

- Dyspepsia (indigestion)
- Regurgitation (may lead to aspiration or bronchitis)
- Coughing, hoarseness, or wheezing at night
- Water brash (hypersalivation)
- Dysphagia
- Odynophagia (painful swallowing)
- Epigastric pain
- Generalized abdominal pain
- Belching
- Flatulence
- Nausea
- Pyrosis (heartburn)
- Globus (feeling of something in back of throat)
- Pharyngitis
- Dental caries (severe cases)

Because indigestion might not be viewed as a serious concern, patients may delay seeking treatment. The symptoms typically worsen when the patient bends over, strains, or lies down. If the indigestion is severe, the pain may radiate to the neck or jaw or may be referred to the back, mimicking cardiac pain. Patients may come to the emergency department (ED) fearing that they are having a myocardial infarction ("heart attack").

With severe GERD, pain generally occurs after each meal and lasts for 20 minutes to 2 hours. Discomfort may worsen when the patient lies down. Drinking fluids, taking antacids, or maintaining an upright posture usually provides prompt relief.

Regurgitation (backward flow into the throat) of food particles or fluids is common. Risk for aspiration is increased if regurgitation occurs when the patient is lying down. Even if the patient is in an upright position, he or she may experience warm fluid traveling up the throat without nausea. If the fluid reaches the level of the pharynx, he or she notes a sour or bitter taste in the mouth. A reflex salivary hypersecretion known as water brash occurs in response to reflux. Water brash is different from regurgitation. The patient reports a sensation of fluid in the throat, but unlike with regurgitation, there is no bitter or sour taste.

Ask the patient if he or she experiences eructation (belching), flatulence (gas), and bloating after eating; these are other common symptoms. Nausea and vomiting rarely occur; unplanned weight loss is not common.

Assess for crackles in the lung, which can be an indication of associated aspiration. Patients who have had long-term regurgitation may experience coughing, hoarseness, or wheezing at night, which may be associated with bronchitis.

Chronic GERD can cause dysphagia (difficulty swallowing), a narrowing of the esophagus because of stricture or inflammation, which can interfere with NUTRITION. Assess the patient for degree of dysphagia, whether ingesting solids and/or liquids induces dysphagia, and whether dysphagia occurs intermittently or with each swallowing effort. See Chapter 53 for more information on assessing for dysphagia.

Odynophagia (painful swallowing) can also occur with chronic GERD, but it is rare in patients with uncomplicated reflux disease. Severe and long-lasting chest pain may be present if esophageal spasms cause the muscle to contract with excess force. The resulting pain can be agonizing and may last for hours.

Other symptoms include atypical chest pain, symptoms of asthma, and chronic cough that occurs mostly at night or when the patient is lying down. Cough and symptoms of asthma occur when refluxed acid is spilled over into the tracheobronchial tree. *Atypical chest pain* is thought to be caused by stimulation of pain receptors in the esophageal wall and by esophageal spasm. This type of chest pain can mimic angina and needs to be carefully distinguished from cardiac pain.

CONSIDERATIONS FOR OLDER ADULTS

Patient-Centered Care QSEN

Older adults are at risk for developing severe complications associated with GERD caused by age-related physiologic changes, medication side effects, and an increased prevalence of hiatal hernias (Solomon & Reynolds, 2012). Instead of heartburn associated with GERD, this population experiences more severe complications of the disease such as atypical chest pain; ear, nose, and throat infections; and pulmonary problems, such as aspiration pneumonia, sleep apnea, and asthma. Barrett's esophagus and esophageal erosions are also more common in older adults.

Diagnostic Assessment. A definitive diagnostic test for GERD does not exist; however, health care providers may use one or more options to attempt to establish a diagnosis when GERD is suspected (The Ohio State University Wexner Medical Center [OSUWMC], 2017).

Patients may drink a solution and then have x-rays performed as part of a *barium swallow,* which shows hiatal hernias, strictures, and other structural or anatomic esophageal problems. Although this test, when conducted by itself, does not confirm GERD, it can be helpful when used in combination with other diagnostic procedures.

Upper endoscopy (also called esophagogastroduodenoscopy [EGD]) involves insertion of an endoscope (a flexible plastic tube equipped with a light and lens) down the throat, which allows the health care provider to see the esophagus and look for abnormalities. A biopsy can be taken while the patient undergoes endoscopy (see Chapter 52) (OSUWMC, 2017). This test requires the use of moderate sedation during the procedure, and patients must have someone accompany them home after recovery.

A pH monitoring examination is the most accurate method of diagnosing GERD. This involves either (1) placing a small catheter through the nose into the distal esophagus or (2) temporarily attaching a small capsule to the wall of the esophagus during an upper endoscopy (the 48-hour Bravo esophageal pH test). The patient is asked to keep a diary of activities and symptoms over 24 to 48 hours (depending on diagnostic method), and the pH is continuously monitored and recorded. Ambulatory pH monitoring is especially useful in diagnosing patients with atypical symptoms. A wireless monitoring device may be used to promote patient COMFORT (OSUWMC, 2017).

Although not as common, *esophageal manometry,* or motility testing, may be performed when the diagnosis is uncertain. Water-filled catheters are inserted in the patient's nose or mouth and slowly withdrawn while measurements of LES pressure and peristalsis are recorded. When used alone, manometry is not sensitive or specific enough to establish a diagnosis of GERD (National Institutes of Health, 2015). A Gastric Emptying Study can also be done while a patient is in the radiology/nuclear medicine department. He or she is given a meal mixed with radiolucent dye, and imaging is performed to determine how well the stomach empties over the next few hours. If food stays too long in the stomach, it can reflux back into the esophagus, causing symptoms. Imaging of the lungs can also be conducted 24 hours later to visualize whether the patient has aspirated stomach contents.

◆ Analysis: Interpreting

The priority collaborative problems for the patient with gastroesophageal reflux disease (GERD) include:
1. Potential for compromised NUTRITION status due to dietary selection
2. Acute pain due to reflux of gastric contents

◆ Planning and Implementation: Responding

Balancing Nutrition

Planning: Expected Outcomes. The patient with imbalanced NUTRITION is expected to have improvement in nutrition status, which allows esophagitis to heal and prevents complications such as strictures or Barrett's esophagus. Indicators include:
- Selection of food items that minimize symptoms of GERD
- No report of reflux after eating

Interventions. Interventions are designed to optimize NUTRITION status, decrease symptoms experienced with GERD, and prevent complications. Nursing care priorities focus on teaching the patient about proper dietary selections that provide optimum nutrients and that do not contribute to reflux.

Nonsurgical Management. For most patients, GERD can be controlled by NUTRITION therapy, lifestyle changes, and drug therapy. *The most important role of the nurse is patient and family education. Teach the patient that GERD is a chronic disorder that requires ongoing management. The disease should be treated more aggressively in older adults.*

NUTRITION therapy is used to relieve symptoms in patients with relatively mild GERD. Ask about the patient's basic meal patterns and food preferences. Coordinate with the dietitian, patient, and family about how to adapt to changes in eating that may decrease reflux symptoms.

Teach the patient to limit or eliminate foods that decrease LES pressure and irritate inflamed tissue, causing heartburn, such as peppermint, chocolate, alcohol, fatty foods (especially fried), caffeine, and carbonated beverages. The patient should also restrict spicy and acidic foods (e.g., orange juice, tomatoes) until esophageal healing can occur. Patients who are smart phone users may find different types of applications ("apps") that can help them follow a healthier diet, such as MyFitnessPal (www.myfitnesspal.com). In keeping with The Joint Commission Core Measures, teach patients that smoking and alcohol use should also be avoided, because these can also decrease LES pressure. Explore the possibility and methods for smoking cessation and make appropriate referrals. Ask the patient about his or her use of alcoholic beverages and, if appropriate, help the patient find alcohol-cessation programs.

Large meals increase the volume of and pressure in the stomach and delay gastric emptying. Remind the patient to eat four to six small meals each day rather than three large ones. Encourage patients to avoid eating at least 3 hours before going to bed because reflux episodes are most damaging at night. Advise the patient to eat slowly and chew thoroughly to facilitate digestion and prevent eructation (belching).

CONSIDERATIONS FOR OLDER ADULTS

Patient-Centered Care QSEN

Research has also found that long-term use of proton pump inhibitors (PPIs) may increase the risk for hip fracture, especially in older adults. PPIs can interfere with calcium absorption and protein digestion and therefore reduce available calcium to bone tissue. Decreased calcium makes bones more brittle and likely to fracture, especially as adults age.

NCLEX EXAMINATION CHALLENGE 54-2

Health Promotion and Maintenance

A client reports ongoing episodes of heartburn. The nurse educates the client on prevention and control of reflux by recommending dietary elimination of which food item?
A. Lean steak
B. Carrot sticks
C. Chocolate candy
D. Air-popped popcorn

Improving Comfort
Planning: Expected Outcomes. The patient with alterations in COMFORT is expected to have relief of signs and symptoms of pain. Indicators include:
- Decrease in level of reported pain

Interventions. Interventions are designed to optimize the patient's perceived level of COMFORT. Nursing care priorities focus on teaching the patient about lifestyle modifications that will alleviate pain.

Nonsurgical Management. In addition to appropriate dietary selections that promote NUTRITION and allow esophageal tissues to heal, patients should be empowered to adhere to other methods of controlling symptoms associated with GERD to minimize COMFORT alterations.

Lifestyle Changes. The control of GERD involves *lifestyle changes* to promote health and control reflux (Chart 54-2). Teach the patient to elevate the head of the bed by 6 to 12 inches for sleep to prevent nighttime reflux. This can be done by placing blocks under the head of the bed or by using a large, wedge-style pillow instead of a standard pillow. Teach the patient to sleep in the right side-lying position to promote gas exchange and to swallow frequently to clear the esophagus. Help the patient examine approaches to weight reduction. Decreasing intra-abdominal pressure often reduces reflux symptoms. Teach the patient to avoid wearing constrictive clothing, lifting heavy objects or straining, and working in a bent-over or stooped position. Emphasize that these general adaptations are an essential and effective part of disease management and can produce prompt results in uncomplicated cases.

Patients with obesity often have both obstructive sleep apnea and GERD. Those who receive continuous positive airway pressure (CPAP) treatment report improved sleeping and decreased episodes of reflux at night. See Chapter 29 for a discussion of CPAP.

Drug Therapy. Some drugs lower LES pressure and *cause* reflux, such as oral contraceptives, anticholinergic agents, sedatives, NSAIDs (e.g., ibuprofen), nitrates, and calcium channel blockers. The possibility of eliminating the drugs causing reflux should be explored with the primary health care provider. Drug

---

 CHART 54-2 **Patient and Family Education: Preparing for Self-Management**

Health Promotion and Lifestyle Changes to Control Reflux

- Eat four to six small meals a day.
- Limit or eliminate fatty foods, coffee, tea, cola, and chocolate.
- Reduce or eliminate from your diet any food or spice that increases gastric acid and causes pain.
- Limit or eliminate alcohol and tobacco and reduce exposure to secondhand smoke.
- Do not snack in the evening and do not eat for 2 to 3 hours before you go to bed.
- Eat slowly and chew your food thoroughly to reduce belching.
- Remain upright for 1 to 2 hours after meals, if possible.
- Elevate the head of your bed 6 to 12 inches using wooden blocks or elevate your head using a foam wedge. Never sleep flat in bed.
- If you are overweight, lose weight.
- Do not wear constrictive clothing.
- Avoid heavy lifting, straining, and working in a bent-over position.
- Chew "chewable" antacids thoroughly and follow with a glass of water.

therapy for GERD management includes three major types: antacids, histamine blockers, and proton pump inhibitors. These drugs, which are also used for peptic ulcer disease, have one or more of these functions (see Chart 55-3).

- Inhibit gastric acid secretion
- Accelerate gastric emptying
- Protect the gastric mucosa

In response to these actions, the pain or discomfort that a patient experiences should decrease. In uncomplicated cases of GERD, *antacids* may be effective for *occasional* episodes of heartburn discomfort. Antacids act by elevating the pH level of the gastric contents, thereby deactivating pepsin. They are not helpful in controlling frequent symptoms because their length of action is too short and their nighttime effectiveness is minimal. They also *increase* LES pressure and therefore are not given for long-term use.

Antacids containing aluminum hydroxide or magnesium hydroxide may be used. Maalox and Mylanta consist of a combination of these two agents. Patients often tolerate them better because they produce fewer side effects, such as constipation and diarrhea. Liquid forms of these medications are preferred, since they coat the esophagus to provide pain relief and buffer acid. Teach the patient to take the antacid 1 hour before and 2 to 3 hours after each meal.

Gaviscon, a combination of alginic acid and sodium bicarbonate, is often a very effective drug for GERD. It forms thick foam that floats on top of the gastric contents and theoretically decreases the incidence of reflux. If reflux occurs, the foam enters the esophagus first and buffers the acid in the refluxed material, causing less pain and decreasing the risk for further mucosal irritation. Remind the patient to take this drug when food is in the stomach.

Histamine receptor antagonists, commonly called *histamine blockers,* such as famotidine (Pepcid), cimetidine (Tagamet), and ranitidine (Zantac), decrease acid, are long acting, have fewer side effects, and allow less-frequent dosing. Although these drugs do not affect the occurrence of reflux directly, they do reduce gastric acid secretion, improve symptoms, and promote healing of inflamed esophageal tissue so COMFORT is improved. With these drugs available over-the-counter (OTC) and widely advertised for heartburn, many patients self-medicate before seeking professional assistance from their primary health care provider. Encourage patients to speak with their primary health care provider to determine whether long-term use of these medications is appropriate.

Proton pump inhibitors (PPIs), such as omeprazole (Prilosec), rabeprazole (AcipHex), pantoprazole (Protonix), lansoprazole (Prevacid), and esomeprazole (Nexium), are the *main* treatment for more severe GERD. Some PPIs are available as OTC drugs. These agents provide effective, long-acting inhibition of gastric acid secretion by affecting the proton pump of the gastric parietal cells. PPIs reduce gastric acid secretion and can be given in a single daily dose. If once-a-day dosing fails to control symptoms, twice-daily dosing may be used (National Guideline Clearinghouse [NGC], 2013). An omeprazole/sodium bicarbonate combination, Zegerid, is the first immediate-release PPI and is designed for short-term use. Dexlansoprazole (Kapidex) is a dual-release (delayed-release) drug that is available in several dosages but has more side and adverse effects than other PPIs.

Some PPIs, such as Nexium and Protonix, may be administered in IV form for short-term use to treat or prevent stress ulcers that can result from surgery. PPIs promote rapid tissue healing, but recurrence is common when the drug is stopped. Long-term use may mask reflux symptoms, and stopping the drug determines if reflux has been resolved. Long-term use may also cause community-acquired pneumonia and GI infections such as those caused by *Clostridium difficile.*

Endoscopic Therapies. The Stretta procedure, a nonsurgical method, can replace surgery for GERD when other measures are not effective. Patients who are very obese or have severe symptoms may not be candidates for this procedure. In the Stretta procedure, the physician applies radiofrequency (RF) energy through the endoscope using needles placed near the gastroesophageal junction. The RF energy decreases vagus nerve activity, thus reducing discomfort for the patient. Postoperative instructions for patients who have undergone the Stretta procedure can be found in Chart 54-3.

Surgical Management. A very small percentage of patients with GERD require anti-reflux surgery. It is usually indicated for otherwise healthy patients who have failed to respond to medical treatment or have developed complications related to GERD. Various surgical procedures may be used through conventional open techniques or laparoscope.

Laparoscopic Nissen fundoplication (LNF) is a minimally invasive surgery (MIS) and is the standard surgical approach for treatment of severe GERD (Buckley, 2016). Information about this procedure can be found in the next section (Hiatal Hernia) in the Surgical Management discussion. Patients who have surgery are encouraged to continue following the basic anti-reflux regimen of antacids and NUTRITION therapy because the rate of recurrence is high.

Care Coordination and Transition Management

Patients with nonsurgical GERD are usually managed in the community setting. Nursing interventions focus on helping the patient and family with current treatment and reducing risk for continuing symptoms and complications.

Home Care Management. Remind the patient to make appropriate dietary selections that enhance NUTRITION and decrease symptoms associated with GERD.

Self-Management Education. For patients with nonsurgical GERD, teach about signs and symptoms of more serious complications such as esophageal stricture and Barrett's esophagus.

CHART 54-3 Patient and Family Education: Preparing for Self-Management

Postoperative Instructions for Patients Having Stretta Procedure

- Remain on clear liquids for 24 hours after the procedure.
- After the first day, consume a soft diet, such as custard, pureed vegetables, mashed potatoes, and applesauce.
- Avoid NSAIDs and aspirin for 10 days.
- Continue drug therapy as prescribed, usually proton pump inhibitors.
- Use liquid medications whenever possible.
- Do not allow nasogastric tubes for at least 1 month because the esophagus could be perforated.
- Contact the health care provider immediately if these problems occur:
  - Chest or abdominal pain
  - Bleeding
  - Dysphagia
  - Shortness of breath
  - Nausea or vomiting

Health Care Resources. Patients may find it helpful to work with a dietitian or a support group for meal-planning purposes. Refer the patient to a dietitian as necessary. Inform him or her of local support groups for patients with GERD and also of credible online communities that provide a forum for ongoing management of this condition.

◆ Evaluation: Reflecting

Evaluate the care of the patient with GERD on the basis of adherence to plan of care, reduction of symptoms, and prevention of complications. The expected outcomes include that the patient will:

- Exhibit adherence to choosing appropriate dietary selections, taking drugs as prescribed, and making appropriate lifestyle modifications
- Report decrease of reflux signs and symptoms associated with GERD
- Avoid complications resulting from GERD

HIATAL HERNIAS

Hiatal hernias, also called *diaphragmatic hernias,* involve the protrusion of the stomach through the esophageal hiatus of the diaphragm into the chest. The esophageal hiatus is the opening in the diaphragm through which the esophagus passes from the thorax to the abdomen. Most patients with hiatal hernias are asymptomatic, but some may have daily symptoms similar to those with GERD (McCance et al., 2014).

❖ PATHOPHYSIOLOGY

The two major types of hiatal hernias are sliding hernias (which are most common) and paraesophageal (rolling) hernias. The esophagogastric junction and a portion of the fundus of the stomach slide upward through the esophageal hiatus into the chest, usually as a result of weakening of the diaphragm (Fig. 54-1). The hernia generally moves freely and slides into and out of the chest during changes in position or intra-abdominal pressure. Although **volvulus** (twisting of a GI structure) and

obstruction do occur rarely, the major concern for a sliding hernia is the development of esophageal reflux and associated complications (see the Gastroesophageal Reflux Disease section earlier in this chapter). The development of reflux is related to chronic exposure of the lower esophageal sphincter (LES) to the low pressure of the thorax, which significantly reduces the effectiveness of the LES. Symptoms associated with decreased LES pressure are worsened by positions that favor reflux, such as bending or lying supine. Coughing, obesity, and ascites also increase reflux symptoms.

With *rolling hernias,* also known as *paraesophageal hernias,* the gastroesophageal junction remains in its normal intra-abdominal location; but the fundus (and possibly portions of the stomach's greater curvature) rolls through the esophageal hiatus and into the chest beside the esophagus (see Fig. 54-1). The herniated portion of the stomach may be small or quite large. In rare cases, the stomach completely inverts into the chest. Reflux is not usually present because the LES remains anchored below the diaphragm. However, the risks for volvulus (twisting of a GI structure), obstruction (blockage), and strangulation (stricture) are high. The development of iron deficiency anemia is common because slow bleeding from venous obstruction causes the gastric mucosa to become engorged and ooze. Significant bleeding or hemorrhage is rare.

Rolling hernias are thought to develop from an anatomic defect occurring when the stomach is not properly anchored below the diaphragm rather than from muscle weakness. They can also be caused by previous esophageal surgeries, including sliding hernia repair.

❖ INTERPROFESSIONAL COLLABORATIVE CARE

Care for the patient with a hiatal hernia usually takes place in the community setting, unless surgery is needed to correct the problem. The interprofessional team that collaborates to care for this patient includes the health care provider, nurse, surgeon, dietitian, and spiritual leader of the patient's choice if surgery is needed.

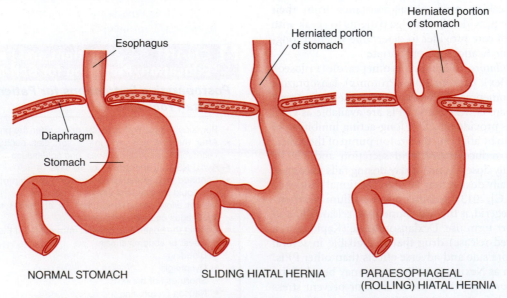

FIG. 54-1 Comparison of the normal stomach and sliding and paraesophageal (rolling) hiatal hernias.

◆ Assessment: Noticing

Ask the patient if he or she has heartburn, regurgitation (backward flow of food into the throat), pain, dysphagia (difficulty swallowing), and eructation (belching). Assess general physical appearance and NUTRITION status. Note the location, onset, duration, and quality of pain and factors that relieve it or make it worse. The primary symptoms of sliding hiatal hernias are associated with reflux. Auscultate the lungs because pulmonary symptoms similar to those of asthma may be triggered by episodes of aspiration, particularly at night. A detailed history is crucial in attempting to differentiate angina from noncardiac chest pain caused by reflux. Symptoms resulting from hiatal hernia typically worsen after a meal or when the patient is in a supine position (Chart 54-4).

In those with rolling hernias, assess for symptoms related to stretching or displacement of thoracic contents by the hernia. Patients may report a feeling of fullness after eating or have breathlessness or a feeling of suffocation if the hernia interferes with breathing. Some may experience chest pain associated with reflux that mimics angina.

The *barium swallow study with fluoroscopy* is the most specific diagnostic test for identifying hiatal hernia. Rolling hernias are usually clearly visible, and sliding hernias can often be observed when the patient moves through a series of positions that increase intra-abdominal pressure. To visualize sliding hernias, an esophagogastroduodenoscopy (EGD) may be performed to view both the esophagus and gastric lining (see Chapter 52).

◆ Interventions: Responding

Patients with hiatal hernias may be managed either medically or surgically. Collaborative care is based on the severity of symptoms and the risk for serious complications. Sliding hiatal hernias are most commonly treated medically. Large rolling hernias can become strangulated or obstructed; therefore early surgical repair is preferred.

Nonsurgical Management. The collaborative interventions for patients with hiatal hernia are similar to those for GERD and include drug therapy, NUTRITION therapy, and lifestyle changes. The primary health care provider typically recommends antacids and a proton-pump inhibitor such as lansoprazole (Prevacid), omeprazole (Prilosec), or esomeprazole (Nexium) in an attempt to control reflux and its symptoms. NUTRITION therapy is also important and follows the guidelines discussed earlier for GERD.

Surgical Management. Surgery may be required when the risk for complications is high or when damage from chronic reflux becomes severe.

! **NURSING SAFETY PRIORITY** QSEN

Action Alert

The most important role of the nurse in caring for a patient with a hiatal hernia is health teaching. Encourage the patient to avoid eating in the late evening and avoid foods associated with reflux. Teach the patient and family that the patient should follow a restricted diet and exercise regularly. Reducing body weight is beneficial because obesity increases intra-abdominal pressure and worsens both the hernia and the symptoms of reflux. Teach about positioning, including:

*   Sleep at night with the head of the bed elevated 6 inches
*   Remain upright for several hours after eating
*   Avoid straining or excessive vigorous exercise
*   Refrain from wearing clothing that is tight or constrictive around the abdomen

---

Preoperative Care. If the surgery is not urgent, the surgeon instructs patients who are overweight to lose weight before surgery. They are also advised to quit or significantly reduce smoking. As part of preoperative teaching, reinforce the surgeon's instructions and prepare the patient for what to expect after surgery.

Operative Procedures. Several types of hiatal hernia repair procedures are used, each of which involves reinforcement of the lower esophageal sphincter (LES) by fundoplication. The surgeon wraps a portion of the stomach fundus around the distal esophagus to anchor it and reinforce the LES (Fig. 54-2).

Laparoscopic Nissen fundoplication (LNF) is a minimally invasive surgery commonly used for hiatal hernia repair (Buckley, 2016). Complications after LNF occur less frequently compared with those seen in patients having the more traditional open surgical approach. A small percentage of patients are not candidates for LNF and therefore require a conventional open fundoplication.

For the trans-thoracic surgical approach, teach the patient about chest tubes. Inform him or her that a nasogastric tube will be inserted during surgery and will remain in place for several days. Oral intake is started gradually with clear liquids after peristalsis is re-established or to stimulate peristalsis. Instruct the patient how to deep breathe and use the incentive spirometer. These measures are essential to prevent postoperative respiratory complications. The high incision makes deep

---

» **CHART 54-4** **Key Features**

Hiatal Hernias

Sliding Hiatal Hernias	Paraesophageal Hernias
• Heartburn	• Feeling of fullness after eating
• Regurgitation	• Breathlessness after eating
• Chest pain	• Feeling of suffocation
• Dysphagia	• Chest pain that mimics angina
• Belching	• Worsening of manifestations in a recumbent position

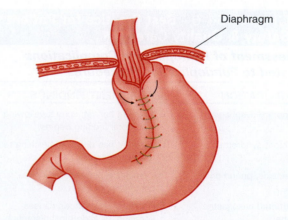

FIG. 54-2 Open surgical approach for Nissen fundoplication for gastroesophageal reflux disease or hiatal hernia repair.

breathing extremely painful. Teach the patient about postoperative pain and assure him or her that adequate postoperative analgesic will be given promptly. Pain levels must be monitored continuously.

In paraesophageal repair (a laparoscopic surgery), several $\frac{1}{2}$-inch incisions are made in the abdomen, through which the hernia is closed and typically reinforced using mesh. Less commonly, a conventional open procedure is used in which the surgeon uses a high trans-thoracic approach that requires a large chest incision for access to the surgical area.

Postoperative Care. Patients having the *LNF procedure* or paraesophageal repair via laparoscope are at risk for bleeding and infection, although these problems are not common. *The nursing care priority is to observe for these complications and provide health teaching as described in* Chart 54-5.

Postoperative care after *conventional open repair* closely follows that required after any esophageal surgery. Complications after open surgery are more common and potentially serious. Carefully assess for complications of open fundoplication surgery, described next, and report any complications to the health care provider (Chart 54-6).

CHART 54-5 Patient and Family Education: Preparing for Self-Management

Postoperative Instructions for Patients Having Laparoscopic Nissen Fundoplication (LNF) or Paraesophageal Repair via Laparoscope

- Stay on a soft diet for about a week, including mashed potatoes, puddings, custard, and milkshakes; avoid carbonated beverages, tough foods, and raw vegetables that are difficult to swallow.
- Remain on anti-reflux medications as prescribed for at least a month.
- Do not drive for a week after surgery; do not drive if taking opioid pain medication.
- Walk every day but do not do any heavy lifting.
- Remove small dressings 2 days after surgery and shower; do not remove Steri-Strips until 10 days after surgery.
- Wash incisions with soap and water, rinse well, and pat dry; report any redness or drainage from the incisions to your surgeon.
- Report fever above 101°F (38.3°C), nausea, vomiting, or uncontrollable bloating or pain. For patients older than 65 years, report elevations above 100°F (37.8°C).
- Schedule an appointment for follow-up with your surgeon in 3 to 4 weeks.

CHART 54-6 Best Practice for Patient Safety & Quality Care QSEN

Assessment of Postoperative Complications Related to Fundoplication Procedures

COMPLICATION	ASSESSMENT FINDINGS
Temporary dysphagia	The patient has difficulty swallowing when oral feeding begins.
Gas bloat syndrome	The patient has difficulty belching to relieve distention.
Atelectasis, pneumonia	The patient experiences dyspnea, chest pain, or fever.
Obstructed nasogastric tube	The patient experiences nausea, vomiting, or abdominal distention. The nasogastric tube does not drain.

! NURSING SAFETY PRIORITY QSEN

Action Alert

The primary focus of care after conventional surgery for a hiatal hernia repair is the prevention of respiratory complications. Elevate the head of the patient's bed at least 30 degrees to lower the diaphragm and promote lung expansion. Assist the patient out of bed and begin ambulation as soon as possible. Be sure to support the incision during coughing to reduce pain and prevent excessive strain on the suture line, especially with obese patients.

Incentive spirometry and deep breathing are routinely used after surgery to maintain patency of the airways and lung expansion. Adequate pain control with analgesics is essential for postoperative deep breathing and coughing. Patients with a smoking history or chronic airway limitation (e.g., chronic obstructive pulmonary disease, asthma) require more aggressive management by the respiratory therapist to prevent atelectasis and pneumonia. Patients with large hiatal hernias are at the highest risk for developing respiratory complications.

For patients who have extensive head-neck cancer or who have had trauma to this area, a gastric feeding tube may have been placed through the abdominal wall to provide a temporary or permanent means for NUTRITION intake. This can be preferable to a nasogastric (NG) tube since it can provide longer-term access for nutrition intake. It can be placed percutaneously by an interventional radiologist, through an open incision, or endoscopically by a surgeon, into the stomach, stomach and jejunum, or jejunum only. Patients with this type of catheter can receive feedings through this tube by a family member or home health nurse with minimal care needed.

Alternately, the patient having the conventional surgery usually has a large-bore (diameter) nasogastric (NG) tube to prevent the fundoplication wrap from becoming too tight around the esophagus. Initially the NG drainage should be dark brown with old blood. The drainage should become normal yellowish green within the first 8 hours after surgery. Check the NG tube every 4 to 8 hours for proper placement in the stomach. It should be properly anchored so it is not displaced, because reinsertion could perforate the fundoplication. Follow the surgeon's directions for care of the patient with an NG tube.

Monitor patency of the NG tube to keep the stomach decompressed. This prevents retching or vomiting, which can strain or rupture the stomach sutures. The NG tube is irritating. Therefore provide frequent oral hygiene to increase COMFORT. Assess the patient's hydration status regularly, including accurate measures of intake and output. Adequate fluid replacement helps thin respiratory secretions.

After open fundoplication, the patient may begin clear fluids when peristalsis is re-established or in an effort to stimulate peristalsis. Some surgeons create a temporary gastrostomy for feeding to allow for undisturbed healing of the repair. The patient gradually progresses to a near-normal diet during the first 4 to 6 weeks. Some foods, especially caffeinated or carbonated beverages and alcohol, are either restricted or eliminated. The food storage area of the stomach is reduced by the surgery, and meals need to be both smaller and more frequent.

Carefully supervise the first oral feedings because temporary dysphagia is common. Continuous dysphagia usually indicates that the fundoplication is too tight, and dilation may be required.

Another common complication of this surgery is *gas bloat syndrome,* in which patients are unable to voluntarily eructate (belch). The syndrome is usually temporary but may persist, even in those who have the laparoscopic approach. Teach the patient to avoid drinking carbonated beverages and eating gas-producing foods (especially high-fat foods), chewing gum, and drinking with a straw.

Other patients have *aerophagia* (air swallowing) from attempting to reverse or clear acid reflux. Teach them to relax consciously before and after meals, to eat and drink slowly, and to chew all food thoroughly. Air in the stomach that cannot be removed by belching can be extremely uncomfortable. Frequent position changes and ambulation are often effective interventions for eliminating air from the GI tract. If gas pain is still present, patients are taught to take simethicone, which dissolves in the mouth.

Care Coordination and Transition Management

Patients undergoing one of the open surgical repairs require activity restrictions during the 3- to 6-week postoperative recovery period. For laparoscopic surgery, activity is typically restricted for a shorter time, and the patient can return to his or her usual lifestyle more quickly, usually in a few days to a week.

For long-term management, teach the patient and family about appropriate NUTRITION modifications. The use of stool softeners or bulk laxatives is recommended for the first postoperative weeks until healing is complete. Instruct the patient to avoid straining and prevent constipation. Teach him or her to inspect the healing incision daily and notify the health care provider if swelling, redness, tenderness, discharge, or fever occurs. Advise the patient to avoid contact with individuals with a respiratory infection and to contact the health care provider if symptoms of a cold or influenza develop. Continuous coughing can cause the incision or the fundoplication to dehisce ("break open").

If needed, collaborate with the dietitian to educate the patient and family about dietary changes. Encourage the patient to eat smaller and more frequent meals. Few ongoing diet restrictions are needed, but overeating or eating the wrong types of foods can produce discomfort if the patient cannot belch. Instruct the patient to report reflux symptoms to the primary health care provider.

Although severe surgical complications are rare, conditions such as gas bloat syndrome and dysphagia may continue. Prepare the patient for these problems and for the potential that reflux may not be completely controlled or may occur again. Although surgery controls the condition, a cure is rare, and lifestyle modifications need to be ongoing.

✳ NUTRITION CONCEPT EXEMPLAR
Esophageal Tumors

❖ PATHOPHYSIOLOGY

Although esophageal tumors can be benign, most are malignant (cancerous), and the majority arise from the epithelium. Squamous cell carcinomas of the esophagus are located in the upper two thirds of the esophagus. Adenocarcinomas are more commonly found in the distal third and at the gastroesophageal junction and are now the most common type of esophageal cancer (McCance et al., 2014). Esophageal tumors grow rapidly because there is no serosal layer to limit their extension. Because the esophageal mucosa is richly supplied with lymph tissue,

there is early spread of tumors to lymph nodes. Esophageal tumors can protrude into the esophageal lumen and can cause thickening or invade deeply into surrounding tissue. In rare cases, the lesion may be confined to the epithelial layer (in situ). In most cases, the tumor is large and well established on diagnosis. More than half of esophageal cancers metastasize (spread throughout the body).

Primary risk factors associated with the development of esophageal cancer are smoking and obesity. The compounds in tobacco smoke may be responsible for the genetic mutations seen in many squamous cell carcinomas of the esophagus. Increased abdominal pressure associated with obesity is linked to reflux and Barrett's esophagus (a premalignant condition). Both conditions can contribute to changes in cellular structure in the esophagus, increasing the potential for adenocarcinoma of the esophagus (ACS, 2016c). In addition to these primary risk factors, malnutrition, untreated gastroesophageal reflux disease (GERD), and excessive alcohol intake are also associated with esophageal cancer. Barrett's esophagus results from exposure to acid and pepsin, which leads to the replacement of normal distal squamous mucosa with columnar epithelium as a response to tissue injury. This tissue undergoes dysplasia (cell appearance changes) and ultimately becomes cancerous. In parts of the world where esophageal cancer is more common, the incidence of squamous cell carcinoma appears to be linked to high levels of nitrosamines (which are found in pickled and fermented foods) and foods high in nitrate. Diets that are chronically deficient in fresh fruits and vegetables have also been implicated in the development of squamous cell carcinoma.

🧬 GENETIC/GENOMIC CONSIDERATIONS
Patient-Centered Care (QSEN)

Certain genetic factors may have a role in the development of esophageal cancers. It is thought that these cancers result from mutations in tumor suppressor genes. Tumor suppressor genes are normal genes that control cell growth and division. When this type of gene is mutated and does not work properly, cells are unable to stop growing and dividing, and tumors can result. (See Chapter 21 for discussion of suppressor gene activity.)

Overexpression and mutations of the *Tp53*, *Tp16* and tumor suppressor genes have been found in patients with esophageal cancer (National Center for Biotechnology Information, 2017). In addition, the presence of the mutated *Tp53* gene may be an indication of advanced disease, especially in those with adenocarcinomas.

Overexpression of *cyclin D1*, a protein that promotes cell growth and division, has also been found in patients with esophageal squamous cell cancers. Cyclins are products of oncogenes, which are normal genes involved in cell division and are controlled by suppressor genes. Prolonged exposure to carcinogens, such as tobacco, can cause oncogenes to escape the control of suppressor genes, leading to overexpression of cyclins and uncontrolled cell growth (cancer).

❓ NCLEX EXAMINATION CHALLENGE 54-3
Health Promotion and Maintenance

The community clinic nurse is discussing risk factors for esophageal cancer with a group of clients. Which client behavior requires **further** teaching?
A. Smokes one pack of cigarettes daily
B. Walks at the shopping mall three times weekly
C. Elevates pillows at night
D. Eats a small snack each night before bedtime

❖ INTERPROFESSIONAL COLLABORATIVE CARE

Care for the patient with esophageal tumors usually takes place in the hospital, followed by the community setting. The interprofessional team that collaborates to care for this patient generally includes the health care provider, nurse, surgeon, dietitian, respiratory therapist, social worker, and spiritual leader of the patient's choice.

◆ Assessment: Noticing

History. Assess for risk factors related to the development or symptoms of esophageal cancer, such as gender, history of alcohol consumption, tobacco use, dietary habits, and other esophageal problems (e.g., dysphagia, reflux). In the United States, adenocarcinoma of the esophagus is more common than squamous cell carcinoma (National Cancer Institute at the National Institutes of Health, 2014). Men, regardless of race or ethnicity, have higher incidence and mortality rates associated with esophageal cancer (National Cancer Institute, 2014). Ask the patient about consumption of smoked and/or pickled foods, changes in appetite, changes in taste, or weight loss.

Physical Assessment/Signs and Symptoms. Cancer of the esophagus is a silent tumor in its early stages, with few observable signs. By the time the tumor causes symptoms, it usually has spread extensively.

Dysphagia *(difficulty swallowing) is the most common symptom of esophageal cancer, but it may not be present until the esophageal opening has gotten much smaller.* Dysphagia is persistent and progressive when stricture (narrowing) occurs. It is initially associated with swallowing solids, particularly meat, and then progresses rapidly over a period of weeks or months to difficulty swallowing soft foods and liquids. Late in the disease, even saliva can cause choking. Patients usually report a sensation of food sticking in the throat or in the substernal area. Careful assessment of dysphagia is important because dysphagia associated with other esophageal disorders is not usually continuous. Weight loss often accompanies dysphagia and can exceed 20 lb over several months.

Odynophagia (painful swallowing) is reported by many patients as a steady, dull, substernal pain that may radiate. It occurs most often when the patient drinks cold liquids. The presence of severe or persistent pain often indicates tumor invasion of the mediastinal structures. Assess for regurgitation, vomiting, halitosis (foul breath), and chronic hiccups, which often accompany advanced disease. In most patients, pulmonary problems develop. Assess for chronic cough, increased secretions, and a history of recent infections. Tumors in the upper esophagus may involve the larynx and thus cause hoarseness. Chart 54-7 summarizes the common clinical symptoms of esophageal tumors.

Psychosocial Assessment. The diagnosis of esophageal cancer causes high patient anxiety. The disease is accompanied by distressing symptoms and is often terminal. The fear of choking can place unusual stress, especially at mealtimes. The loss of pleasure and social aspects of eating may affect relationships with family and friends. Assess the patient's response to the diagnosis and prognosis. Ask about his or her usual coping strengths and resources. Assess the impact of the disease on the patient's usual daily activity routine. Determine the availability of support systems and the potential financial impact of the disease and its treatment. Refer the patient and

---

> ⟫ **CHART 54-7**   **Key Features**
> ### *Esophageal Tumors*
>
> - Persistent and progressive dysphagia (most common feature)
> - Feeling of food sticking in the throat
> - Odynophagia (painful swallowing)
> - Severe, persistent chest or abdominal pain or discomfort
> - Regurgitation
> - Chronic cough with increasing secretions
> - Hoarseness
> - Anorexia
> - Nausea and vomiting
> - Weight loss (often more than 20 lb)
> - Changes in bowel habits (diarrhea, constipation, bleeding)

> ❓ **NCLEX EXAMINATION CHALLENGE 54-4**
> ### *Psychosocial Integrity*
>
> The nurse is caring for a client who has been diagnosed with esophageal cancer. The client appears anxious and asks the nurse, "Does this mean I'm going to die?" Which nursing responses are appropriate? **Select all that apply.**
> A. "No, surgery can cure you."
> B. "It sounds like death frightens you."
> C. "Let me call the hospital chaplain to talk with you."
> D. "You can beat this disease if you just put your mind to it."
> E. "Let me sit with you for a while and we can discuss how you're feeling about this."

---

family members to psychological counseling, pastoral care, and/or the social worker or case manager as needed. Chapter 7 describes end-of-life care for patients in the terminal stage of the disease.

Diagnostic Assessment. A *barium swallow* study with fluoroscopy may be the first diagnostic test requested to evaluate dysphagia. In a barium swallow, the margins of a tumor may be seen. The definitive diagnosis of esophageal cancer is made by *esophageal ultrasound (EUS)* with fine-needle aspiration to examine the tumor tissue. An *esophagogastroduodenoscopy (EGD)* may also be performed to inspect the esophagus and obtain tissue specimens for cell studies and disease staging. A complete cancer staging workup is performed to determine the extent of the disease and plan appropriate therapy.

Positron emission tomography (PET) may identify metastatic disease with more accuracy than a CT scan. PET can also help evaluate response to chemotherapy to treat the cancer.

◆ Analysis: Interpreting

The most specific common problem for patients with esophageal cancer is *Potential for compromised nutrition due to impaired swallowing and possible metastasis.* Many patients with cancer also have pain and are fearful because of the diagnosis of cancer. Chapter 22 describes problems that are typically seen with any patient with cancer.

◆ Planning and Implementation: Responding

Promoting Nutrition

Planning: Expected Outcomes. The major concern for a patient with esophageal cancer is weight loss secondary to dysphagia. Therefore he or she is expected to maintain adequate nutrient intake and weight either orally or via an alternative method.

Interventions. Interventions to maintain or improve NUTRI-TION status focus on treatments that remove or shrink the obstructive tumor. Methods to reduce the effects of treatment that can impact NUTRITION are also a priority. Surgery is the most definitive intervention for esophageal cancer.

Nonsurgical Management. The treatment of esophageal cancer often involves a combination of therapies. Patients with cancer of the esophagus experience many physical problems, and symptom management becomes essential.

Nonsurgical treatment options for cancer of the esophagus that can assist in both disease and NUTRITION management include:

- Nutrition therapy
- Swallowing therapy
- Chemotherapy
- Radiation therapy
- Chemoradiation
- Targeted therapies
- Photodynamic therapy
- Esophageal dilation
- Endoscopic therapies

Nutrition and Swallowing Therapy. The purpose of NUTRITION *therapy is to administer food and fluids to support the patient who is malnourished or at high risk for becoming malnourished.* Conduct a screening assessment to provide information about the patient's NUTRITION status. The dietitian determines the caloric needs of the patient to meet daily requirements. Be sure that the patient is weighed daily before breakfast on the same scale each day. To keep the esophagus patent, careful positioning is essential for a patient who is experiencing frequent reflux or who has tubes. Teach him or her to remain upright for several hours after meals and avoid lying completely flat. Remind unlicensed assistive personnel (UAP) and other health care team members to keep the head of the bed elevated to a 30-degree angle or more to prevent reflux.

Semisoft foods and thickened liquids are preferred because they are easier to swallow. Record the amount of food and fluid intake every day to monitor progress in meeting desired NUTRI-TION outcomes. Liquid NUTRITION supplements (e.g., Boost, Ensure) are used between feedings to increase caloric intake. Ongoing efforts are made to preserve the ability to swallow, but enteral feedings (tube feedings) may be needed temporarily when dysphagia is severe. In patients with complete esophageal obstruction or life-threatening fistulas, the surgeon may create a gastrostomy or jejunostomy for feeding. Encourage the patient and family to meet with the dietitian for diet teaching and planning. Chapter 60 describes care for patients receiving enteral feeding.

Collaborate with the speech-language pathologist (SLP) to assist the patient with oral exercises to improve swallowing *(swallowing therapy)* and with the occupational therapist (OT) for feeding therapy. Ask the patient to suck on a lollipop to enhance tongue strength. Teach him or her to reach for food particles on the lips or chin using the tongue. In preparation for swallowing, remind the patient to position the head in forward flexion (chin tuck). Then tell him or her to place food at the back of the mouth. Monitor the patient for sealing of the lips and tongue movements while eating. Check for pocketing of food in the cheeks after swallowing.

Chemotherapy and Radiation. The use of *chemotherapy* in the treatment of esophageal cancer has been only moderately effective. It can be given as a primary treatment if the patient

is not a candidate for surgery or given for palliation (control of symptoms). However, in most cases, chemotherapy is given in combination with radiation therapy to provide the patient the best chance of cure. The rationale for this approach is to shrink the primary tumor and eliminate any other tumor that may be in the local lymph nodes, improving the odds for a complete surgical resection. The most commonly used paired chemotherapeutic agents for esophageal cancer are carboplatin and paclitaxel (Taxol) or cisplatin and 5-fluorouracil (5-FU). These drugs are often combined with radiation because they make the tumor cells more sensitive to radiation effects (American Cancer Society [ACS], 2016a). Because chemotherapeutic drugs affect both healthy cells and cancer cells, they have many side effects that cause discomfort to the patient. Chapter 22 describes chemotherapy in detail and discusses the role of the nurse in caring for patients receiving these drugs.

Radiation therapy to manage esophageal cancer is only moderately effective and can be used alone or in combination with other treatments. Radiation alone can provide palliation of symptoms by shrinking the tumor. It is contraindicated for patients with tracheoesophageal fistula, mediastinitis, mediastinal hemorrhage, or infiltration of the cancer to the trachea or bronchus. Normal esophageal tissue is very sensitive to the effects of radiation. Although high doses of radiation demonstrate the best results for tumor shrinkage, esophageal stricture or stenosis can result in many patients, which then requires esophageal dilation. Chapter 22 describes radiation methods and the general nursing care for the patient having radiation therapy.

Chemoradiation is a treatment for esophageal cancer that involves the use of chemotherapy at the same time as radiation therapy. One cycle of chemotherapy is given during the first week of radiation, and another is delivered during the fifth week of radiation. Additional drug cycles are given after radiation therapy is complete.

Other Therapies. Targeted therapies may be used in combination with radiation and chemotherapy. Unlike chemotherapy, these therapies interfere with cancer cell growth in a variety of ways with less impact on healthy cells. Many of these drugs focus on proteins that are involved in signaling cells when to grow and divide. A key to success with targeted therapy is that the cancer cells must overexpress the targeted protein. Thus each patient's cancer cells are first examined for the overexpression to determine if targeted therapy is appropriate and which drug to use. Trastuzumab (Herceptin) is a commonly used drug that is used for patients whose esophageal cancer tests positive for an excess of the *HER2* protein on the cell surface. It is given by IV injection once every 3 weeks, in addition to chemotherapy (ACS, 2016b). Chapter 22 describes targeted therapies in detail, including nursing implications for patient safety and quality care.

Photodynamic therapy (PDT) is used as a palliative treatment for patients with advanced esophageal cancer who are not candidates for surgery. It may be used also as a cure for patients who have very small, localized tumors. The patient is injected with porfimer sodium (Photofrin), a light-sensitive drug that collects in cancer cells. Two days after the injection, a fiberoptic probe with a light at the tip is threaded into the esophagus through an endoscope. The light activates the Photofrin, destroying only cancer cells. PDT is far less invasive than surgery and is performed on an ambulatory care basis under moderate sedation. Endoscopy nurses observe the patient's rate and depth of respirations and monitor his or her oxygen saturation and end-tidal (exhaled) carbon dioxide to ensure adequate gas exchange.

The side effects of Photofrin are rare but include nausea, fever, and constipation. Before the procedure, the patient is given written guidelines concerning photosensitivity measures. Remind him or her to avoid exposure to sunlight for 1 to 3 months. Sunglasses and protective clothing that covers all exposed body areas are essential. The patient may experience chest pain secondary to tissue damage and will require pain relief with opioid analgesics for a short time. Teach the patient to follow a clear liquid diet for 3 to 5 days after the procedure and advance to full liquids as tolerated. Warn the patient that tissue particles may release from the tumor site and be present in the sputum. Chapter 22 describes in detail the health teaching needed to promote patient safety associated with PDT.

Esophageal dilation may be performed as necessary throughout the course of the disease to achieve temporary but immediate relief of dysphagia. It is usually performed on an ambulatory care basis. Dilators are used to tear soft tissue, thereby widening the esophageal lumen (opening). In most cases, malignant tumors can be dilated safely, but perforation remains a significant risk. Large metal stents may be used to keep the esophagus open for longer periods. A stent covered with graft material can be used to seal a perforation. Bacteremia can also occur. To reduce the risk for endocarditis, antibiotics are given. The treatment is repeated as often as needed to preserve the patient's ability to swallow. Prolonged stent embedment into benign esophageal tissue can cause ulceration, bleeding, fistula, dysphagia, and formation of a new stricture if the stent is not removed (Patel & Siddiqui, 2013).

When patients are not candidates for surgery or the tumor is too large to remove surgically, laser therapy or electrocoagulation using endoscopy may be performed as a palliative measure. Both of these methods destroy some cancer cells and reduce tumor size to improve swallowing. The procedures are done in ambulatory care settings or same-day surgery centers using moderate sedation.

Surgical Management. The purposes of surgical resection vary from palliation to cure. **Esophagectomy** is the removal of all or part of the esophagus. An **esophagogastrostomy** involves the removal of part of the esophagus and proximal stomach. The remaining stomach may be "pulled up" to take the place of the esophagus, or a section of the jejunum or colon may be placed as a conduit. Conventional open surgical techniques are lengthy and associated with many complications or death. Fistula formation between the trachea and esophagus, abscess, and respiratory complications are common.

For patients with early-stage cancer, a laparoscopic-assisted **minimally invasive esophagectomy (MIE)** may be performed.

However, most patients require the conventional open surgery because of tumor size and metastasis by the time they are diagnosed with the disease.

Preoperative Care. Preoperative preparation for patients undergoing esophagectomy or esophagogastrostomy can be quite extensive, especially before conventional techniques. Advise the patient to stop smoking 2 to 4 weeks before surgery to enhance pulmonary function. Patient preparation may include 5 days to 2 to 3 weeks of NUTRITION support to decrease the risk for postoperative complications. Ideally this supplementation is given orally, but many patients require tube feeding or parenteral NUTRITION. Teach the patient and family to monitor the patient's weight and intake and output. A preoperative evaluation may be required to treat dental disease. Teach the patient to practice meticulous oral care four times daily to decrease the risk for postoperative infection.

Preoperative nursing care focuses on teaching and psychological support regarding the surgical procedure and preoperative and postoperative instructions. Teach the patient about:

- The number and sites of all incisions and drains
- The placement of a jejunostomy tube for initial enteral feedings
- The need for chest tubes if the pleural space is entered
- The purpose of the nasogastric tube
- The need for IV infusion

Teach the patient about regularly turning, coughing, deep breathing, and having chest physiotherapy. Emphasize the crucial nature of postoperative respiratory care. If colon interposition (resecting a piece of colon and creating an esophagus) is planned, the patient also has a complete bowel preparation before surgery.

The patient facing a serious illness and extensive surgery can be expected to experience grief and anxiety. Encourage him or her to talk about personal feelings and fears and involve the family or significant others in all preoperative teaching and discussions. A social worker, certified hospital chaplain, or case manager can be extremely helpful in providing continuity of care and support to the entire family.

Operative Procedures. In the MIE procedure, the surgeon makes four or five small incisions in the chest and abdomen using a video-assisted thoracoscope and laparoscope. The lower esophagus and gastric fundus are removed. The remaining portion of the esophagus is then anastomosed (reconnected) to the stomach.

For most patients, the surgeon performs an open subtotal or total esophagectomy because tumors are often large and involve distant lymph nodes. For a subtotal (partial) removal, the diseased portion of the esophagus is removed, and the cervical portion is anastomosed (connected) to the stomach (Fig. 54-3). A **pyloromyotomy** is done by cutting and suturing the pylorus. Finally, a jejunostomy tube may be placed for postoperative enteral feeding.

For patients with early-stage tumors of the lower third of the esophagus, a transhiatal esophagectomy is the preferred surgical approach. The surgery is performed through an upper midline cervical incision. With this approach, the pleural space is not entered, reducing respiratory complications. For patients with tumors in the upper esophagus, a radical neck dissection and laryngectomy may also be needed if the disease has spread to the larynx. Chapter 29 discusses the care of patients having these procedures.

The surgeon may perform a **colon interposition** when the tumor involves the stomach or the stomach is otherwise

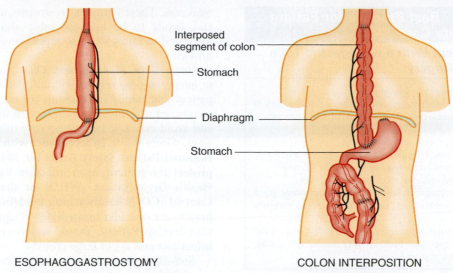

ESOPHAGOGASTROSTOMY   COLON INTERPOSITION

FIG. 54-3 Open surgical approaches to the treatment of esophageal cancer.

unsuitable for anastomosis. A section of right or left colon is removed and brought up into the thorax to substitute for the esophagus (see Fig. 54-3).

Postoperative Care. The patient requires intensive postoperative care and is at risk for multiple serious complications. The patient having an MIE has the same risk for postoperative complications as one having the open procedure. The advantages of MIE include:

- Less blood loss during surgery; fewer blood transfusions
- Decreased healing and recovery time
- Decreased trauma to the body
- No large incisions
- Less postoperative pain
- Shorter hospital stay (5 to 7 days rather than 7 to 10 days)

> **! NURSING SAFETY PRIORITY** **QSEN**
>
> **Action Alert**
>
> Respiratory care is the highest postoperative priority for patients having an esophagectomy. For those who had traditional surgery, intubation with mechanical ventilation is needed for at least the first 16 to 24 hours. Pulmonary complications include atelectasis and pneumonia. The risk for postoperative pulmonary complications is increased in the patient who has received preoperative radiation. Once the patient is extubated, begin deep breathing, turning, and coughing every 1 to 2 hours. Assess the patient for decreased breath sounds and shortness of breath every 1 to 2 hours. Provide incisional support and adequate analgesia for effective coughing.

Remind all staff to keep the patient in a semi-Fowler's or high-Fowler's position to support ventilation and prevent reflux. The health care provider prescribes prophylactic antibiotics and supplemental oxygen. *Ensure the patency of the chest tube drainage system and monitor for changes in the volume or color of the drainage.*

Cardiovascular complications, particularly hypotension during surgery, can occur as a result of pressure placed on the posterior heart and usually respond well to IV fluid administration.

> **! NURSING SAFETY PRIORITY** **QSEN**
>
> **Action Alert**
>
> Monitor for symptoms of fluid volume overload, particularly in older patients and those who have undergone lymph node dissection. Assess for edema, crackles in the lungs, and increased jugular venous pressure. In the immediate postoperative phase, the patient is often admitted to the intensive care unit. Critical care nurses assess hemodynamic parameters such as cardiac output, cardiac index, and systemic vascular resistance every 2 hours to monitor for myocardial ischemia. Observe for atrial fibrillation that results from irritation of the vagus nerve during surgery and manage according to agency protocol.

The patient with poor NUTRITION or prior radiation or chemotherapy is at risk for infection. For those who undergo more radical surgical procedures, there is a serious risk for leakage at the anastomosis (surgical connection) sites. This situation is especially true with colon interpositions because several sites are stressed by the effects of tension, poor blood supply, and delayed healing. *Mediastinitis* (inflammation of the mediastinum) resulting from an anastomotic leak can lead to fatal sepsis.

Wound management is another major postoperative concern for conventional surgery because the patient typically has multiple incisions and drains. *Provide direct support to the incision during turning and coughing to prevent dehiscence.* Wound infection can occur 4 to 5 days after surgery. Leakage from the site of anastomosis is a dreaded complication that can appear 2 to 10 days after surgery. If an anastomotic leak occurs, all oral intake is discontinued and is not resumed until the site of the leak has healed.

> **! NURSING SAFETY PRIORITY** **QSEN**
>
> **Critical Rescue**
>
> After esophageal surgery, recognize if the patient has signs of fever, fluid accumulation, signs of inflammation, and symptoms of early shock (e.g., tachycardia, tachypnea). Respond immediately by reporting any of these findings to the surgeon **and** Rapid Response Team!

Managing the Patient With a Nasogastric Tube After Esophageal Surgery

- Check for tube placement every 4 to 8 hours.
- Ensure that the tube is patent (open) and draining; drainage should turn from bloody to yellowish green by the end of the first postoperative day.
- Secure the tube well to prevent dislodgment.
- Do not irrigate or reposition the tube without a physician's request.
- Provide meticulous oral and nasal hygiene every 2 to 4 hours.
- Keep the head of the bed elevated to at least 30 degrees.
- When the patient is permitted to have a small amount of water, place him or her in an upright position and observe for dysphagia (difficulty swallowing).
- Observe for leakage from the anastomosis site, as indicated by fever, fluid accumulation, and manifestations of early shock (tachycardia, tachypnea, altered mental status).

A nasogastric (NG) tube is placed intraoperatively to decompress the stomach to prevent tension on the suture line. Monitor the NG tube for patency and carefully secure the tube to prevent dislodgment, which can disrupt the sutures at the anastomosis. *Do not irrigate or reposition the NG tube in patients who have undergone esophageal surgery unless requested by the surgeon!* The initial nasogastric drainage is bloody but should change to a greenish-yellow color by the end of the first postoperative day. The continued presence of blood may indicate internal bleeding at the suture line. Commonly an antacid will be prescribed to support the patient's healing. Provide oral hygiene for the patient every 2 to 4 hours while the tube is in place or delegate and appropriately supervise this activity (Chart 54-8).

NUTRITION management of the patient who has undergone esophageal surgery is an early postoperative concern. After conventional surgery, on the second postoperative day, initial feedings usually begin through the jejunostomy tube (J tube). Do not aspirate for residual because this increases the risk for mucosal tearing. Feedings are slowly increased over the next several days. Feeding by this method can be discontinued once the patient is taking adequate oral NUTRITION.

Before beginning oral feedings, a cine-esophagram study is performed to detect any anastomotic leaks, strictures, or signs of aspiration. If no leaks are seen, a liquid diet is started. If liquids are well tolerated, the patient's diet is advanced to include semi-solid foods and then solid foods.

Place the patient in an upright position and supervise all initial swallowing efforts. The food storage area of the stomach has been radically decreased, and gravity is the only defense against reflux. *Teach the patient and/or family the importance of the patient eating six to eight small meals per day. Fluids should be taken between, rather than with, meals to prevent diarrhea.* Diarrhea can occur 20 minutes to 2 hours after eating and can be managed with loperamide (Imodium) before meals. The diarrhea is thought to be the result of *vagotomy syndrome*, which develops as a result of interrupted vagal fibers to the abdominal organs during surgery.

Care Coordination and Transition Management

Patients with esophageal cancer have many challenges to face once they are discharged home. The combination treatment regimens cause long-lasting side effects, such as fatigue and weakness. These complex treatments also require the patient and family to be knowledgeable about symptom management and to know when to report concerns to the health care provider.

Home Care Management. *Once the patient is discharged to home, ongoing respiratory care remains a priority.* Give the patient and family instructions for ambulation and incentive spirometer use. Encourage the patient to be as active as possible and avoid excessive bedrest because this can lead to complications of immobility. In accordance with The Joint Commission National Patient Safety Goals for 2017, teach the family to protect the patient from infection by following the World Health Organization (WHO) or the Centers for Disease Control (CDC) handwashing guidelines and to contact the health care provider immediately if signs of respiratory infection develop. Patients should stay away from individuals with infections and avoid large crowds.

Self-Management Education. Remind the patient and family to wash their hands frequently and teach them to inspect the incisions daily for redness, tenderness, swelling, odor, and discharge because proper wound healing is still a concern at the time of discharge. Instruct them to report a temperature greater than 101° F (38.3° C), or 100° F (37.8° C) for older adults, which may be a sign of infection. Prepare written instructions about the signs of anastomosis leakage. *Teach the patient or family to immediately report to the health care provider the presence of fever and a swollen, painful neck incision.*

NUTRITION support is important. Encourage the patient to continue increasing oral feedings as tolerated. Remind him or her to eat small, frequent meals containing high-calorie, high-protein foods that are soft and easily swallowed. Teach the value of using supplemental milkshakes between meals and instruct the patient to eat slowly. Patients who have undergone esophageal resection can lose up to 10% of their body weight. Teach the patient to monitor his or her weight at home and to report a weight loss of 5 lb or more in 1 month. If sufficient oral intake is not possible, the patient and family may need instruction about tube feedings or parenteral NUTRITION at home.

Emphasize the importance of remaining upright after meals. Dysphagia or odynophagia may recur because of stricture, reflux, or cancer recurrence. These symptoms should be reported to the health care provider promptly. Despite radical surgery, the patient with cancer of the esophagus often still has a terminal illness and a relatively short life expectancy. Emphasis is placed on maximizing quality of life. Realistic planning is important as the patient's condition eventually worsens and the patient and family are assisted to plan for the future together. Help family members explore formal and informal sources of support. Help the family or significant others arrange for hospice care when it is needed. Chapter 7 describes end-of-life care, including hospice.

Health Care Resources. Referrals to community or home care organizations help the family provide care in the home. The patient may need transportation to the radiation treatment center five times per week for up to 6 weeks. Oncology nursing care may be needed to monitor and evaluate the patient who is receiving chemotherapy at home through venous access devices or portable infusion pumps. Inform the patient and family about the services available through the American Cancer Society (www.cancer.org), including support groups and transportation. Familiarize the family with area hospice services for future planning. Coordinate resource referrals with the case manager or home care agency.

◆ **Evaluation: Reflecting**

Evaluate the care of the patient with esophageal cancer based on the identified priority patient problems. The major expected outcome is that the patient will be able to consume adequate NUTRITION and maintain a stable weight.

⊘ CLINICAL JUDGMENT CHALLENGE 54-1

Teamwork and Collaboration; Safety; Evidence-Based Practice **QSEN**

A 58-year-old patient has undergone a Laparoscopic Nissen Fundoplication (LNF) for a hiatal hernia. Before discharge, you are preparing to teach the patient and family about self-management.
1. For what postoperative complications will you monitor, and why could they occur after this surgery?
2. What type of diet will the patient need to eat, and for how long will the diet be recommended?
3. What types of activities will you recommend for the patient? Are there any restrictions in activity that you should teach the patient?
4. The patient will have a postoperative incision. What will you teach the patient about wound care?
5. What type of follow-up instructions will you provide?

ESOPHAGEAL DIVERTICULA

Diverticula are sacs resulting from the herniation of esophageal mucosa and submucosa into surrounding tissue. They may develop anywhere along the length of the esophagus. No environmental risk factors are known to be involved in their development. The incomplete or late opening of swallowing muscles can cause high pressure in the hypopharynx and lead to *Zenker's diverticula*, the most common form. This type occurs most often in older adults. Patients report dysphagia (difficulty swallowing), regurgitation (reflux), nocturnal cough, and halitosis (bad breath). They can also be at risk for perforation because the mucosa is without the protection of the normal esophageal muscle layer.

Esophageal diverticula are diagnosed most often by *esophagogastroduodenoscopy (EGD)*. This procedure must be performed with strict care because of the risk for perforation. NUTRITION therapy and positioning are the major interventions for controlling symptoms related to diverticula. Collaborate with the dietitian to help the patient explore variations in the size and frequency of meals and food texture and consistency. Semisoft foods and smaller meals are often best tolerated and may reduce or relieve the symptoms of pressure and reflux. Nocturnal reflux associated with diverticula is managed by teaching the patient to sleep with the head of the bed elevated and to avoid the supine position for at least 2 hours after eating. Advise the patient to avoid vigorous exercise after meals. Teach him or her to avoid restrictive clothing and frequent stooping or bending.

Surgical management is aimed at removing the diverticula. After surgery, the patient is NPO status for several days to promote healing. During that period, he or she receives IV fluids for hydration and tube feedings; after that, he or she is given oral fluid and food. Provide pain relief measures and monitor for complications such as bleeding or perforation. *A nasogastric (NG) tube is placed during surgery for decompression*

and is not irrigated or repositioned unless specifically requested by the surgeon.

Care coordination and transition management include teaching the patient and family about:
• Nutrition therapy
• Positioning guidelines to prevent reflux
• Warning signs of complications, such as bleeding or infection

ESOPHAGEAL TRAUMA

Trauma to the esophagus can result from blunt injuries, chemical burns, surgery or endoscopy (rare), or the stress of continuous severe vomiting (Table 54-2). Trauma may affect the esophagus directly, impairing swallowing and NUTRITION, or it may create problems in related structures such as the lungs or mediastinum. The incidence of most forms of esophageal trauma is low in adults. When excessive force is exerted on the esophageal mucosa, it may perforate or rupture, allowing the caustic acid secretions to enter the mediastinal cavity. These tears are associated with a high mortality rate related to shock, respiratory impairment, or sepsis.

Chemical injury is usually a result of the accidental or intentional ingestion of caustic substances. The damage to the mouth and esophagus is rapid and severe. Acid burns tend to affect the superficial mucosal lining, whereas alkaline substances cause deeper penetrating injuries. Strong alkalis can cause full perforation of the esophagus within 1 minute. Additional problems may include aspiration pneumonia and hemorrhage. Esophageal strictures may develop as scar tissue forms.

Patients with esophageal trauma are initially evaluated and treated in the emergency department. Assessment focuses on the nature of the injury and the circumstances surrounding it. *Assess for airway patency, breathing, chest pain, dysphagia, vomiting, and bleeding as the priorities for patient care.* If the risk for extending the damage is not excessive, an endoscopic study may be requested to evaluate tears or perforation. A CT scan of the chest can be done to assess for the presence of mediastinal air.

After the injury, keep the patient NPO to prevent further leakage of esophageal secretions. Esophageal and gastric suction can be used for drainage and to rest the esophagus. Esophageal rest is maintained for more than a week after injury to allow for initial healing of the mucosa. Total parenteral NUTRITION (TPN) is prescribed to provide calories and protein for wound healing while the patient is not eating.

To prevent sepsis, the health care provider prescribes broad-spectrum antibiotics. High-dose corticosteroids may be administered to suppress inflammation and prevent strictures (esophageal narrowing). In addition, opioid and nonopioid analgesics are prescribed for pain management. When caustic burns involve the mouth, topical agents such as lidocaine (Xylocaine Viscous) may be used for analgesia and local anti-inflammatory action.

TABLE 54-2 Common Causes of Esophageal Perforation

• Straining	• Instrument or tubes
• Seizures	• Chemical injury
• Trauma	• Complications of esophageal surgery
• Foreign objects	• Ulcers

If nonsurgical management is not effective in healing traumatized esophageal tissue, the patient may need surgery to remove the damaged tissue. Those with severe injuries may require resection of part of the esophagus with a gastric pull-through and repositioning or replacement by a bowel segment; also, gastrostomy tube (G-tube) placement may be needed to meet NUTRITION needs while healing.

GET READY FOR THE NCLEX® EXAMINATION!

KEY POINTS

Review these Key Points for each NCLEX Examination Client Needs Category.

Safe and Effective Care Environment

- Consult with the dietitian, patient, and family regarding NUTRITION modifications for patients with GERD. **QSEN: Teamwork and Collaboration**
- Collaborate with the interprofessional team to care for the patient with impaired swallowing and/or limited NUTRITION. **QSEN: Teamwork and Collaboration**
- Teach the patient and family to recognize the symptoms of dysphagia. **QSEN: Safety**
- Remain with the patient with dysphagia during meals to prevent choking episodes or intervene quickly. **QSEN: Safety**

Health Promotion and Maintenance

- Teach the patient oral exercises to improving swallowing.
- Stress the importance of controlling reflux through NUTRITION and drug therapy to avoid further esophageal damage that could lead to Barrett's esophagus. **QSEN: Safety**
- Teach the patient to elevate the head of the bed by 6 inches for sleep and to lie in the right side-lying position to minimize or prevent nighttime reflux. **QSEN: Evidence-Based Practice**
- Teach the patient with esophageal cancer to monitor body weight and to notify the health care provider of weight loss.
- Teach the patient to avoid alcoholic beverages, smoking, and other substances listed in Chart 54-2 because they lead to increased gastroesophageal reflux. **QSEN: Evidence-Based Practice**
- Teach the patient to prevent gas bloat syndrome by avoiding carbonated beverages and gas-producing foods, chewing gum, and drinking with a straw.

- Review postprocedure instructions for patients having the Stretta procedure for GERD as outlined in Chart 54-3. **QSEN: Safety**

Psychosocial Integrity

- Allow the patient the opportunity to express fear or anxiety regarding the diagnosis of esophageal cancer. **QSEN: Patient-Centered Care**
- Explain all procedures, restrictions, drug therapy, and follow-up care to the patient and family. **Ethics**
- Refer the patient or family members to psychological counseling, hospice, spiritual care, and the case manager as needed. **QSEN: Teamwork and Collaboration**

Physiological Integrity

- For patients with GERD, teach the importance of strict adherence to anti-reflux agents in preventing esophageal damage (see Chart 55-3). **QSEN: Evidence-Based Practice**
- Assess for complications and provide postoperative care for patients having the common surgical procedures for esophageal problems, as described in Chart 54-6. **QSEN: Safety**
- Be sure to frequently monitor the NUTRITION status of the patient with esophageal cancer. **Clinical Judgment**
- Teach the patient having open conventional esophageal surgery about incisions, drains, and jejunostomy tube placement before he or she undergoes surgery for esophageal cancer.
- For the patient with a nasogastric (NG) tube, check the NG tube every 4 to 8 hours for proper placement and anchorage; follow guidelines outlined in Chart 54-8.
- Assess patients for key features of esophageal tumors listed in Chart 54-7. **Clinical Judgment**

SELECTED BIBLIOGRAPHY

American Cancer Society (ACS) (2015). *Cancer facts and figures 2015.* http://www.cancer.org/research/cancerfactsstatistics/cancerfacts figures2015/index.

American Cancer Society (ACS). (2016a). *Chemotherapy for cancer of the esophagus.* www.cancer.org/cancer/esophaguscancer/detailedguide/esophagus-cancer-treating-chemotherapy.

American Cancer Society (ACS). (2016b). *Targeted therapy for cancer of the esophagus.* www.cancer.org/cancer/esophaguscancer/detailedguide/esophagus-cancer-treating-targeted-therapy.

American Cancer Society (ACS). (2016c). *What are the risk factors for cancer of the esophagus?* https://www.cancer.org/cancer/esophagus-cancer/causes-risks-prevention/risk-factors.html.

Buckley, F. (2016). *Laparoscopic Nissen fundoplication.* http://emedicine.medscape.com/article/1892517-overview.

McCance, K., Huether, S., Brashers, V., & Rote, N. (2014). *Pathophysiology: The biologic basis for disease in adults and children* (7th ed.). St. Louis: Mosby.

National Cancer Institute at the National Institutes of Health (2014). *A snapshot of esophageal cancer.* www.cancer.gov/researchandfunding/snapshots/esophageal.

National Center for Biotechnology Information. (2017). *TP tumor protein p53.* http://www.ncbi.nlm.nih.gov/gene/7157.

National Guideline Clearinghouse (NGC) (2013). *Guideline synthesis: Diagnosis and management of gastroesophageal reflux disease (GERD).* http://www.guideline.gov/content.aspx?id=43847&search=gerd.

National Institutes of Health (2015). *Esophageal manometry.* www.nlm.nih.gov/medlineplus/ency/article/003884.htm.

Patel, D., & Siddiqui, R. (2013). *Fully covered esophageal stents: Role in benign disease. Practical Gastroenterology,* 39-46, www.practicalgastro.com/pdf/May13/D-Patel.pdf.

Solomon, M., & Reynolds, J. (2012). Esophageal reflux disease and its complications. In *Geriatric gastroenterology.* New York: Springer.

The Joint Commission (2017). *The 2017 National Patient Safety Goals.* https://www.jointcommission.org/assets/1/6/NPSG_Chapter_OME_Jan2017.pdf.

The Ohio State University Wexner Medical Center (OSUWMC). (2017). *Esophageal disorders.* https://internalmedicine.osu.edu/digestivediseases/about-the-division/esodisease/.

CHAPTER 55

Care of Patients With Stomach Disorders

Lara Carver

PRIORITY AND INTERRELATED CONCEPTS

The priority concept for this chapter is IMMUNITY.

✻ The IMMUNITY concept exemplar for this chapter is Peptic Ulcer Disease (PUD), p. 1107.

The interrelated concepts for this chapter are:
- NUTRITION
- COMFORT

LEARNING OUTCOMES

Safe and Effective Care Environment

1. Collaborate with the interprofessional team to protect the patient with a stomach disorder from injury and infection.
2. Identify community resources to ensure appropriate transition management for patients with stomach disorders.

Health Promotion and Maintenance

3. Teach adults how to promote GI health and prevent gastritis.
4. Teach patients with a stomach disorder how to enhance NUTRITION, promote digestion, and minimize disturbances in COMFORT.

Psychosocial Integrity

5. Implement nursing interventions to minimize stressors for the patient with a stomach disorder.

6. Identify end-of-life care needs for patients with advanced gastric cancer.

Physiological Integrity

7. Apply knowledge of anatomy, physiology, pathophysiology, genetic risk, age-related changes, and psychomotor skills to perform a focused assessment of the GI system.
8. Describe interprofessional care and educational needs to promote NUTRITION for the patient with a stomach disorder.
9. Prioritize care and educational needs for the patient with a stomach disorder to prevent complications associated with altered IMMUNITY.
10. Develop an evidence-based plan of care for the patient undergoing gastric surgery.

The stomach is part of the upper GI system that is responsible for a large part of the digestive process. It is only affected by a few diseases, including gastritis, peptic ulcer disease (PUD), and cancer, yet these conditions can be very serious and sometimes life threatening. Each of these health problems can result in impaired or altered *digestion* and NUTRITION. Inflammation and infection can create disturbances in COMFORT. Interprofessional collaborative care for stomach disorders often includes therapies to meet the patient's need for adequate nutrition.

GASTRITIS

Gastritis is the inflammation of gastric mucosa (stomach lining) (see discussion of Inflammation in Chapter 17). Inflammation, an alteration in IMMUNITY, can be scattered or localized; thus gastritis can be classified according to cause, cellular changes, or distribution of the lesions. It can be erosive (causing ulcers) or nonerosive. Although the mucosal changes that result from *acute* gastritis typically heal after several months, this is not true for *chronic* gastritis.

❖ PATHOPHYSIOLOGY

Prostaglandins provide a protective mucosal barrier that prevents the stomach from digesting itself by a process called acid autodigestion. If there is a break in the protective barrier, mucosal injury occurs. The resulting injury is worsened by histamine release and vagus nerve stimulation. Hydrochloric acid can then diffuse back into the mucosa and injure small vessels. This back-diffusion causes edema, hemorrhage, and erosion of the stomach's lining, which alters IMMUNITY. The pathologic changes of gastritis include vascular congestion, edema, acute inflammatory cell infiltration, and degenerative changes in the superficial epithelium of the stomach lining.

Types of Gastritis

Inflammation of the gastric mucosa or submucosa after exposure to local irritants or other causes can result in acute gastritis. The early pathologic manifestation of gastritis is a thickened, reddened mucous membrane with prominent rugae, or folds. Various degrees of mucosal necrosis and inflammatory reaction occur in acute disease. The diagnosis cannot be based solely on clinical symptoms. Complete regeneration and healing usually occur within a few days. If the stomach muscle is not involved, complete recovery usually occurs with no residual evidence of gastric inflammatory reaction. If the muscle is affected, hemorrhage may occur during an episode of acute gastritis.

Chronic gastritis appears as a patchy, diffuse (spread out) inflammation of the mucosal lining of the stomach. As the disease progresses, the walls and lining of the stomach thin and atrophy. With progressive gastric atrophy from chronic mucosal injury, the function of the parietal (acid-secreting) cells decreases, and the source of intrinsic factor is lost. Intrinsic factor is critical for absorption of vitamin B_{12}. When body stores of vitamin B_{12} are eventually depleted, pernicious anemia results. The amount and concentration of acid in stomach secretions gradually decrease until the secretions consist of only mucus and water.

Chronic gastritis is associated with an increased risk for gastric cancer. The persistent inflammation extends deep into the mucosa, causing alteration in IMMUNITY by destruction of the gastric glands and cellular changes. Chronic gastritis may be categorized as type A, type B, or atrophic (McCance et al., 2014).

Type A (nonerosive) chronic gastritis refers to an inflammation of the glands and the fundus and body of the stomach. Type B chronic gastritis usually affects the glands of the antrum but may involve the entire stomach. In atrophic chronic gastritis, diffuse inflammation and destruction of deeply located glands accompany the condition. Chronic atrophic gastritis affects all layers of the stomach, thus decreasing the number of cells. The muscle thickens, and inflammation is present. Chronic atrophic gastritis is characterized by total loss of fundal glands, minimal inflammation, thinning of the gastric mucosa, and intestinal metaplasia (abnormal tissue development). These cellular changes can lead to peptic ulcer disease (PUD) and gastric cancer (McCance et al., 2014).

Etiology and Genetic Risk

The onset of infection with *Helicobacter pylori* can result in acute gastritis. *H. pylori* is a gram-negative bacterium that penetrates the mucosal gel layer of the gastric epithelium. Although less common, other forms of bacterial gastritis from organisms such as staphylococci, streptococci, *Escherichia coli,* or salmonella can cause life-threatening problems such as sepsis and extensive tissue necrosis (death), greatly altering a patient's IMMUNITY.

Long-term NSAID use creates a high risk for acute gastritis. NSAIDs inhibit prostaglandin production in the mucosal barrier. Other risk factors include use of alcohol, coffee, caffeine, and corticosteroids. Acute gastritis is also caused by local irritation from radiation therapy and accidental or intentional ingestion of corrosive substances, including acids or alkalis (e.g., lye and drain cleaners).

Type A gastritis has been associated with the presence of antibodies to parietal cells and intrinsic factor. Therefore an autoimmune cause for this type of gastritis is likely. Parietal cell antibodies have been found in most patients with pernicious anemia and in more than one half of those with type A gastritis. A genetic link to this disease, with an autosomal-dominant pattern of inheritance, has been found in the relatives of patients with pernicious anemia (McCance et al., 2014).

The most common form of chronic gastritis is type B gastritis, caused by *H. pylori* infection. A direct correlation exists between the number of organisms and the degree of cellular abnormality present. The host response to the *H. pylori* infection is activation of lymphocytes and neutrophils. Release of inflammatory cytokines, such as interleukin (IL)-1, IL-8, and tumor necrosis factor (TNF)–alpha, damages the gastric mucosa (McCance et al., 2014).

Chronic local irritation and toxic effects caused by alcohol ingestion, radiation therapy, and smoking have been linked to chronic gastritis. Surgical procedures that involve the pyloric sphincter, such as a pyloroplasty, can lead to gastritis by causing reflux of alkaline secretions into the stomach. Other systemic disorders such as Crohn's disease, graft-versus-host disease, and uremia can also precipitate the development of chronic gastritis.

Atrophic gastritis is a type of chronic gastritis that is seen most often in older adults. It can occur after exposure to toxic substances in the workplace (e.g., benzene, lead, nickel) or *H. pylori* infection, or it can be related to autoimmune factors. Atrophic gastritis can lead to two types of cancer: gastric cancer and gastric mucosa-associated lymphoid tissue (MALT) lymphoma. See Gastric Cancer later in this chapter for a more detailed explanation.

Health Promotion and Maintenance

Gastritis is a very common health problem in the United States. A balanced diet, regular exercise, and stress-reduction techniques can help prevent it (Chart 55-1). A balanced diet includes following the recommendations of the U.S. Department of Agriculture (USDA) and limiting intake of foods and spices that can cause gastric distress, such as caffeine, chocolate, mustard, pepper, and other strong or hot spices. Alcohol and tobacco should also be avoided. Regular exercise maintains peristalsis, which helps prevent gastric contents from irritating the gastric mucosa. Stress-reduction techniques can include aerobic exercise, meditation, reading, and/or yoga, depending on individual preferences.

CHART 55-1   Patient and Family Education: Preparing for Self-Management

Gastritis Prevention

- Eat a well-balanced diet.
- Avoid drinking excessive amounts of alcoholic beverages.
- Use caution in taking large doses of aspirin, other NSAIDs (e.g., ibuprofen), and corticosteroids.
- Avoid excessive intake of coffee (even decaffeinated).
- Be sure that foods and water are safe to avoid contamination.
- Manage stress levels using complementary and integrative therapies such as relaxation and meditation techniques.
- Stop smoking.
- Protect yourself against exposure to toxic substances in the workplace such as lead and nickel.
- Seek medical treatment if you are experiencing symptoms of esophageal reflux (see Chapter 54).

⏩ **CHART 55-2** **Key Features**

Gastritis

Acute Gastritis	Chronic Gastritis
• Rapid onset of epigastric pain or discomfort	• Vague report of epigastric pain that is relieved by food
• Nausea and vomiting	• Anorexia
• Hematemesis (vomiting blood)	• Nausea or vomiting
• Gastric hemorrhage	• Intolerance of fatty and spicy foods
• Dyspepsia (heartburn)	• Pernicious anemia
• Anorexia	

Excessive use of aspirin and other NSAIDs should also be avoided. If a family member has *H. pylori* infection or has had it in the past, patient testing should be considered. This test can identify the bacteria before they cause gastritis.

❖ **INTERPROFESSIONAL COLLABORATIVE CARE**

Care of the patient with gastritis usually takes place in the community setting. However, if symptoms are severe, the patient may be hospitalized. The interprofessional team that collaborates to care for this patient generally includes the primary health care provider and nurse.

◆ **Assessment: Noticing**

Symptoms of *acute* gastritis range from mild to severe. The patient may report epigastric alterations in COMFORT or pain, anorexia, cramping, nausea, and vomiting (Chart 55-2). Assess for abdominal tenderness and bloating, **hematemesis** (vomiting blood), or **melena** (dark, sticky feces, as evidence of blood in the stool). Symptoms last only a few hours or days and vary with the cause. Aspirin/NSAID–related gastritis may result in **dyspepsia** (heartburn). Gastritis or food poisoning caused by endotoxins, such as staphylococcal endotoxin, has an abrupt onset. Severe nausea and vomiting often occur within 5 hours of ingestion of the contaminated food. *In some cases gastric hemorrhage is the presenting symptom, which is a life-threatening emergency.*

Chronic gastritis causes few symptoms unless ulceration occurs. Patients may report nausea, vomiting, or upper abdominal discomfort. Periodic epigastric pain may occur after a meal. Some patients have anorexia (see Chart 55-2).

Esophagogastroduodenoscopy (EGD) via an endoscope with biopsy is the gold standard for diagnosing gastritis. (See Chapter 52 for discussion of nursing care associated with this diagnostic procedure.) The physician performs a biopsy to establish a definitive diagnosis of the type of gastritis. If lesions are patchy and diffuse, biopsy of several suspicious areas may be necessary to avoid misdiagnosis. A *cytologic examination* of the biopsy specimen is performed to confirm or rule out gastric cancer. Tissue samples can also be taken to detect *H. pylori* infection using *rapid urease testing.* The results of these tests are more reliable if the patient has discontinued taking antacids for at least a week (Pagana et al., 2017).

◆ **Interventions: Responding**

Patients with gastritis are not often seen in the acute care setting unless they have an exacerbation ("flare-up") of acute or chronic gastritis that results in fluid and electrolyte imbalance, bleeding, or increased pain. Collaborative care is directed toward supportive care for relieving the symptoms and removing or reducing the cause of discomfort.

Acute gastritis is treated symptomatically and supportively because the healing process is spontaneous, usually occurring within a few days. When the cause is removed, pain and discomfort usually subside. If bleeding is severe, a blood transfusion may be necessary. Fluid replacement is prescribed for patients with severe fluid loss. Surgery, such as partial gastrectomy, pyloroplasty, and/or vagotomy, may be needed for patients with major bleeding or ulceration. Treatment of *chronic* gastritis varies with the cause. The approach to management includes the elimination of causative agents, treatment of any underlying disease (e.g., uremia, Crohn's disease), avoidance of toxic substances (e.g., alcohol, tobacco), and health teaching.

Eliminating the causative factors, such as *H. pylori* infection if present, is the primary treatment approach. Drugs and nutritional therapy are also used. In the *acute* phase the primary health care provider prescribes drugs that block and buffer gastric acid secretions to relieve pain.

H₂-receptor antagonists, such as famotidine (Pepcid) and nizatidine (Axid), are typically used to block gastric secretions. Sucralfate (Carafate, Sulcrate), a *mucosal barrier fortifier,* may also be prescribed. *Antacids* used as buffering agents include aluminum hydroxide combined with magnesium hydroxide (Maalox) and aluminum hydroxide combined with simethicone and magnesium hydroxide (Mylanta). Antisecretory agents (**proton pump inhibitors [PPIs]**) such as omeprazole (Prilosec) or pantoprazole (Protonix) may be prescribed to suppress gastric acid secretion (Chart 55-3).

❗ **NURSING SAFETY PRIORITY** ᴏꜱᴇɴ

Drug Alert

Teach the patient to monitor for symptom relief and side effects of drugs to treat gastritis and to notify the primary health care provider of any adverse effects or worsening of gastric distress. The dose, frequency, or type of drug may need to be changed if symptoms of gastric irritation appear or persist. *Remind patients not to take additional over-the-counter (OTC) drugs such as Pepcid AC or Axid AR if they are taking similar prescribed drugs.*

Patients with *chronic* gastritis may require vitamin B₁₂ for prevention or treatment of pernicious anemia. If *H. pylori* is found, the primary health care provider treats the infection. Current practice for infection treatment is described in the Drug Therapy discussion in the Peptic Ulcer Disease section.

The nurse, primary health care provider, or pharmacist teaches patients to avoid drugs and other irritants that are associated with gastritis episodes, if possible. These drugs include corticosteroids, erythromycin (E-Mycin, Erythro-ES 🍁), ASA (aspirin), and NSAIDs such as naproxen (Naprosyn, Maxidol 🍁) and ibuprofen (Motrin, Advil). NSAIDs are also available as OTC drugs and should not be used. Teach patients to read all OTC drug labels because many preparations contain aspirin or other NSAID.

Teach the patient to limit intake of any foods and spices that cause distress, such as those that contain caffeine or high acid content (e.g., tomato products, citrus juices) or those that are heavily seasoned with strong or hot spices. Bell peppers and onions are also commonly irritating foods. Most patients seem to progress better with a bland, nonspicy diet and smaller, more frequent meals. Alcohol and tobacco should also be avoided.

CHART 55-3   Common Examples of Drug Therapy

Peptic Ulcer Disease

CLASS AND COMMON EXAMPLES	SELECTED NURSING IMPLICATIONS
Antacids—Increase pH of gastric contents by deactivating pepsin	
Magnesium hydroxide with aluminum hydroxide	Give 2 hours after meals and at bedtime. *Hydrogen ion load is high after ingestion of foods.* Use liquid rather than tablets. *Suspensions are more effective than chewable tablets.* Do not give other drugs within 1-2 hours of antacids. *Antacids interfere with absorption of other drugs.* Assess patients for a history of renal disease. *Hypermagnesemia may result, especially in patients with poorly functioning kidneys, thus causing toxicity.* Assess the patient for a history of heart failure. *Inadequate renal perfusion from heart failure decreases the ability of the kidneys to excrete magnesium, thus causing toxicity.* Observe the patient for the side effect of diarrhea. *Magnesium often causes diarrhea.*
Aluminum hydroxide (Gaviscon, Alugel ✦)	Give 1 hour after meals and at bedtime. *Hydrogen ion load is high after ingestion of food.* Use liquid rather than tablets if palatable. *Suspensions are more effective than chewable tablets.* Do not give other drugs within 1-2 hours of antacids. *Antacids interfere with absorption of other drugs.* Observe patients for the side effect of constipation. If constipation occurs, consider alternating with magnesium antacid. *Aluminum causes constipation, and magnesium has a laxative effect.* Use for patients with renal failure. *Aluminum binds with phosphates in the GI tract. This antacid does not contain magnesium.*
H₂ Antagonists (Blockers)—Decrease gastric acid secretions by blocking histamine receptors in parietal cells	
Ranitidine (Zantac) Famotidine (Pepcid) Nizatidine (Axid) **NOTE:** IV famotidine or IV ranitidine may also be given to prevent surgical stress ulcers.	Give single dose at bedtime for treatment of GI ulcers, heartburn, and PUD. *Bedtime administration suppresses nocturnal acid production.*
Mucosal Barrier Fortifiers—Protect stomach mucosa	
Sucralfate (Carafate, Sulcrate ✦)	Give 1 hr before and 2 hr after meals and at bedtime. *Food may interfere with drug's adherence to mucosa.* Do not give within 30 min of giving antacids or other drugs. *Antacids may interfere with effect.*
Bismuth subsalicylate (Pepto-Bismol)	Remind patient to refrain from taking aspirin while on this drug. *Aspirin is a salicylic acid and can lead to overdose.*
Proton Pump Inhibitors—Suppress HK–ATPase enzyme system of gastric acid secretion	
Omeprazole (Prilosec, Losec ✦, Olex ✦)	Have patients take capsule whole; do not crush. *Delayed-release capsules allow absorption after granules leave the stomach.* Give 30 minutes before the main meal of the day. *The proton pump is activated by the presence of food. Therefore the drug needs a chance to work before the patient eats.*
Lansoprazole (Prevacid)	Give 30 min before the main meal of the day. *The proton pump is activated by the presence of food. Therefore the drug needs a chance to work before the patient eats.*
Rabeprazole (Aciphex, Pariet ✦)	Take after the morning meal. *This drug promotes healing and symptom relief of duodenal ulcers.* Do not crush capsule. *This drug is a sustained-release capsule.*
Pantoprazole (Protonix, Pantoloc ✦, Panto IV ✦, Tecta ✦)	Do not crush. *This drug is enteric coated.* IV form must be given on a pump with a filter and in a separate line. *Given IV, this drug precipitates easily.* Do not give Protonix IV with other IV drugs. Monitor for adverse drug interactions if patient is on other medications. *The IV form is not compatible with most other drugs. This drug will alter how other drugs are metabolized, either increasing or decreasing their effectiveness.*
Esomeprazole (Nexium)	Assess for hepatic impairment. *Patients with severe hepatic problems need a low dose.* Do not give Nexium IV with other IV drugs. *The IV form is not compatible with most other drugs.* Monitor for adverse drug interactions if patient is on other medications. *This drug will alter how other drugs are metabolized, either increasing or decreasing the effectiveness.*
Prostaglandin Analogs—Stimulate mucosal protection and decrease gastric acid secretions	
Misoprostol (Cytotec)	Avoid magnesium-containing antacids. *Misoprostol and magnesium-containing antacids can cause diarrhea.* Do not administer to pregnant women. *This drug can cause abortion, premature birth, or birth defects.*

CHART 55-3 Common Examples of Drug Therapy—cont'd

Peptic Ulcer Disease

CLASS AND COMMON EXAMPLES	SELECTED NURSING IMPLICATIONS
Antimicrobials—Treat *H. pylori* infection	
Clarithromycin (Biaxin)	Give with caution to patients with renal impairment; monitor renal function laboratory values. *This drug can increase the patient's BUN level and should be monitored.*
Amoxicillin (Amoxil, Novamoxin)	Teach patients to take the drug with food or immediately after a meal. *This drug can cause GI disturbances, including nausea, vomiting, and diarrhea.*
Tetracycline	Teach patients to take the drug at least 1 hour before meals or 2 hours after meals. *Dairy products and other foods may interfere with drug absorption.* Teach patients to avoid direct sunlight and wear sunscreen when outdoors. *This drug can cause the skin to burn as a result of photosensitivity.*
Metronidazole (Flagyl, Nidagel ❖, Novo-Nidazol ❖)	Teach patients to take the drug with food. *This drug can cause GI disturbances, especially nausea.* Teach patients to avoid alcohol during drug therapy and for at least 3 days after therapy is completed. *The patient can experience a drug-alcohol reaction, including severe nausea, vomiting, and headache.*

BUN, Blood urea nitrogen.

TABLE 55-1 Commonly Used Complementary and Integrative Therapies for Gastritis and Peptic Ulcer Disease (PUD)

Herbs and Vitamins	Homeopathy
• Cranberry	• Carbo vegetabilis
• Deglycyrrhizinated licorice (DGL)	• Ipecacuanha
• Ginger	• Nux vomica
• Probiotics	• Pulsatilla
• Slippery elm	
• Vitamin C	

❓ NCLEX EXAMINATION CHALLENGE 55-1

Safe and Effective Care Environment

The nurse is performing medication reconciliation for a newly admitted client. The nurse recognizes which drugs contribute to signs and symptoms of gastritis? **Select all that apply.**
A. Aspirin, taken once daily to prevent cardiac concerns
B. Naproxen, taken once daily for joint pain associated with arthritis
C. Amoxicillin, taken over a 10-day period for an acute sinus infection
D. Bacitracin ointment (over the counter), applied to minor scrapes on arms and legs
E. Prednisone, tapered over a 14-day period to decrease inflammation associated with an acute sinus infection

Teach the patient about various techniques that reduce stress and discomfort, such as progressive relaxation, cutaneous stimulation, guided imagery, and distraction. Table 55-1 lists commonly used complementary and integrative therapies for gastritis and peptic ulcer disease.

✳ IMMUNITY CONCEPT EXEMPLAR
Peptic Ulcer Disease (PUD)

A **peptic ulcer** is a mucosal lesion of the stomach or duodenum. **Peptic ulcer disease (PUD)** results when mucosal defenses become impaired and no longer protect the epithelium from the effects of acid and pepsin.

❖ PATHOPHYSIOLOGY

Types of Ulcers

Three types of ulcers may occur: gastric ulcers, duodenal ulcers, and stress ulcers (less common). Many ulcers are caused by *H. pylori* infection (National Institute of Diabetes and Digestive and Kidney Diseases, 2017). Although it is not certain how *H. pylori* is transmitted, it is believed to be spread through contaminated food or water. Studies have also suggested that interpersonal transmission appears to be the main route of transmission (Eusebi et al., 2014).

As a response to the bacteria, cytokines, neutrophils, and other substances are activated and cause epithelial cell necrosis. These bacteria produce substances that damage the mucosa. Urease produced by *H. pylori* breaks down urea into ammonia, which neutralizes the acidity of the stomach. Urease can be detected through laboratory testing to confirm the *H. pylori* infection. In addition, the helical shape of *H. pylori* allows the bacterium to burrow into the mucus layer of the stomach and become undetectable by the body's immune cells. Although this bacterium does not cause illness in most individuals, it is a major risk factor for peptic and duodenal ulcers and gastric cancer (McCance et al., 2014).

Gastric ulcers usually develop in the antrum of the stomach near acid-secreting mucosa. When a break in the mucosal barrier occurs (such as that caused by *H. pylori* infection), hydrochloric acid injures the epithelium. Gastric ulcers may then result from back-diffusion of acid or dysfunction of the pyloric sphincter (Fig. 55-1). Without normal functioning of the pyloric sphincter, bile refluxes (backs up) into the stomach. This reflux of bile acids may break the integrity of the mucosal barrier, which leads to mucosal inflammation and compromise in IMMUNITY. Toxic agents and bile then destroy the membrane of the gastric mucosa.

Gastric emptying is often delayed in patients with gastric ulceration. This causes regurgitation of duodenal contents, which worsens the gastric mucosal injury. Decreased blood flow to the gastric mucosa may also alter the defense barrier and thereby allow ulceration to occur. Gastric ulcers are deep and penetrating, and they usually occur on the lesser curvature of the stomach, near the pyloric sphincter (Fig. 55-2).

Most *duodenal ulcers* occur in the upper portion of the duodenum. They are deep, sharply demarcated lesions that

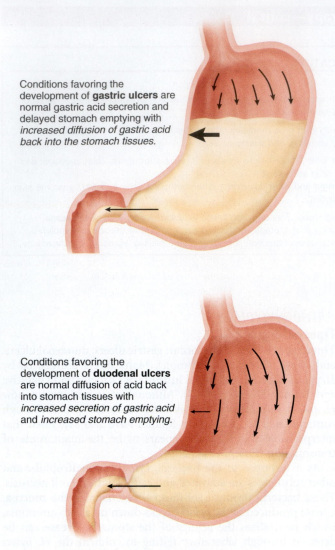

Conditions favoring the development of **gastric ulcers** are normal gastric acid secretion and delayed stomach emptying with *increased diffusion of gastric acid back into the stomach tissues.*

Conditions favoring the development of **duodenal ulcers** are normal diffusion of acid back into stomach tissues with *increased secretion of gastric acid* and *increased stomach emptying.*

FIG. 55-1 Pathophysiology of peptic ulcer.

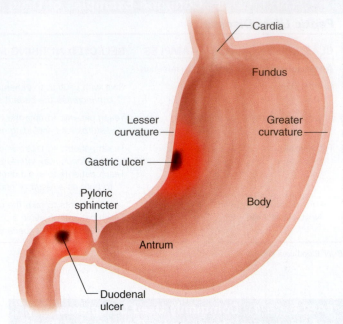

FIG. 55-2 Most common sites for peptic ulcers.

penetrate through the mucosa and submucosa into the muscularis propria (muscle layer). The floor of the ulcer consists of a necrotic area residing on granulation tissue and surrounded by areas of fibrosis (McCance et al., 2014).

The main feature of a duodenal ulcer is high gastric acid secretion, although a wide range of secretory levels are found. In patients with duodenal ulcers, pH levels are low (excess acid) in the duodenum for long periods. Protein-rich meals, calcium, and vagus nerve excitation stimulate acid secretion. Combined with hypersecretion, a rapid emptying of food from the stomach reduces the buffering effect of food and delivers a large acid bolus to the duodenum. Inhibitory secretory mechanisms and pancreatic secretion may be insufficient to control the acid load.

Stress ulcers are acute gastric mucosal lesions occurring after an acute medical crisis or trauma, such as sepsis or a head injury. In the patient who is NPO for major surgery, gastritis may lead to **stress ulcers**, which are multiple shallow erosions of the stomach and occasionally the proximal duodenum. Patients who are critically ill, especially those with extensive burns (**Curling's ulcer**), sepsis (ischemic ulcer), or increased

intracranial pressure (**Cushing's ulcer**), are also susceptible to these ulcers.

Bleeding caused by gastric erosion is the main manifestation of acute stress ulcers. Multifocal lesions associated with stress ulcers occur in the stomach and proximal duodenum. These lesions begin as areas of ischemia and evolve into erosions and ulcerations that may progress to massive hemorrhage. Little is known of the exact etiology of stress ulcers. Stress ulcers are associated with lengthened hospital stay and increased mortality rates. Therefore most patients who have major trauma or surgery receive IV drug therapy (e.g., PPI) to prevent stress ulcer development.

Complications of Ulcers

The most common complications of PUD are hemorrhage, perforation, pyloric obstruction, and intractable disease. *Hemorrhage is the most serious complication.* It tends to occur more often in patients with *gastric* ulcers and in older adults. Many patients have a second episode of bleeding if underlying infection with *H. pylori* remains untreated or if therapy does not include an H_2 antagonist. With massive bleeding the patient vomits bright red or coffee-ground blood (**hematemesis**). Hematemesis usually indicates bleeding at or above the duodenojejunal junction (upper GI bleeding) (Chart 55-4).

Minimal bleeding from ulcers is manifested by occult blood in a dark, "tarry" stool (**melena**). The digestion of blood within the duodenum and small intestine may result in this black stool. Melena may occur in patients with gastric ulcers but is more common in those with duodenal ulcers. Gastric acid digestion of blood typically results in a granular dark vomitus (*coffee-ground appearance*).

Gastric and duodenal ulcers can perforate and bleed (Fig. 55-3). *Perforation* occurs when the ulcer becomes so deep that the entire thickness of the stomach or duodenum is worn away. The stomach or duodenal contents can then leak into the peritoneal cavity. Sudden, sharp pain begins in the

CHART 55-4 Key Features

Upper GI Bleeding

- Bright red or coffee-ground vomitus (hematemesis)
- Melena (tarry or dark, sticky) stools
- Decreased blood pressure
- Increased heart rate
- Weak peripheral pulses
- Acute confusion (in older adults)
- Vertigo
- Dizziness or light-headedness
- Syncope (loss of consciousness)
- Decreased hemoglobin and hematocrit

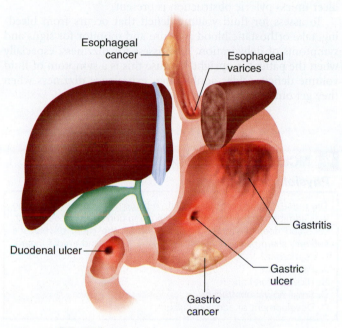

FIG. 55-3 Common causes of upper GI bleeding.

mid-epigastric region and spreads over the entire abdomen. The amount of pain correlates with the amount and type of GI contents spilled. The classic pain causes the patient to be apprehensive. The abdomen is tender, rigid, and boardlike (**peritonitis**). The patient often assumes a "fetal" position to decrease the tension on the abdominal muscles. He or she can become severely ill within hours. Bacterial septicemia and hypovolemic shock follow. Peristalsis diminishes, and paralytic ileus develops. *Peptic ulcer perforation is a surgical emergency and can be life threatening!*

NCLEX EXAMINATION CHALLENGE 55-2

Safe and Effective Care Environment

When caring for a patient who has just had an upper GI endoscopy, the nurse assesses that the client has developed a temperature of 101.8° F (38.8° C). What is the **appropriate** nursing intervention?
A. Promptly assess the client for potential perforation.
B. Ask the nursing assistant to bathe the client with tepid water.
C. Administer acetaminophen (Tylenol) to lower the temperature.
D. Delegate to an unlicensed assistive personnel (UAP) to retake the temperature.

Pyloric (gastric outlet) obstruction (blockage) occurs in a small percentage of patients and is manifested by vomiting caused by stasis and gastric dilation. Obstruction occurs at the pylorus (the gastric outlet) and is caused by scarring, edema, inflammation, or a combination of these factors.

Symptoms of obstruction include abdominal bloating, nausea, and vomiting. When vomiting persists, the patient may have hypochloremic (metabolic) alkalosis from loss of large quantities of acid gastric juice (hydrogen and chloride ions) in the vomitus. Hypokalemia may also result from the vomiting or metabolic alkalosis.

Many patients with ulcers have a single episode with no recurrence. However, *intractability* may develop from complications of ulcers, excessive stressors in the patient's life, or an inability to adhere to long-term therapy. He or she no longer responds to conservative management, or recurrences of symptoms interfere with ADLs. In general, the patient continues to have recurrent pain and alteration in COMFORT, despite treatment. Those who fail to respond to traditional treatments or who have a relapse after discontinuation of therapy are referred to a gastroenterologist.

Etiology and Genetic Risk

Peptic ulcer disease is caused most often by bacterial infection with *H. pylori* and NSAIDs. NSAIDs (e.g., ibuprofen) break down the mucosal barrier and disrupt the mucosal protection mediated systemically by cyclooxygenase (COX) inhibition. COX-2 inhibitors (celecoxib [Celebrex]) are less likely to cause mucosal damage but place patients at high risk for cardiovascular events, such as myocardial infarction. In addition, NSAIDs cause decreased endogenous prostaglandins, resulting in local gastric mucosal injury (Lilley et al., 2017). GI complications from NSAID use can occur at any time, even after long-term uncomplicated use. NSAID-related ulcers are difficult to treat, even with long-term therapy, because they have a high rate of recurrence.

Certain substances may contribute to gastroduodenal ulceration by altering gastric secretion, which produces localized damage to mucosa and interferes with the healing process. For example, corticosteroids (e.g., prednisone), theophylline (Theo-Dur), and caffeine stimulate hydrochloric acid production. Patients receiving radiation therapy may also develop GI ulcers. Other risk factors for PUD are the same as for gastritis (see Chart 55-1).

Incidence and Prevalence

PUD affects millions of adults across the world. However, health care provider visits, hospitalizations, and the mortality rate for PUD have decreased in the past few decades due in part to the use of proton pump inhibitors and earlier treatment for *H. pylori*.

❖ INTERPROFESSIONAL COLLABORATIVE CARE

Care of the patient with PUD generally takes place in the community setting, unless the patient develops a more serious condition such as upper GI bleeding, which requires hospitalization for management. The interprofessional team that collaborates to care for this patient generally includes the primary or specialty health care provider and nurse and may include the surgeon, case manager, and dietitian if the patient requires surgery.

◆ Assessment: Noticing

History. Collect data related to the causes and risk factors for peptic ulcer disease (PUD). Question the patient about factors that can influence the development of PUD, including alcohol intake and tobacco use. Note if certain foods such as tomatoes or caffeinated beverages precipitate or worsen symptoms. Information regarding actual or perceived daily stressors should also be obtained.

A history of current or past medical conditions focuses on GI problems, particularly any history of diagnosis or treatment for *H. pylori* infection. Review all prescription and OTC drugs the patient is taking. Specifically inquire whether the patient is taking corticosteroids, chemotherapy, or NSAIDs. Also ask whether he or she has ever undergone radiation treatments. Assess whether the patient has had any GI surgeries, especially a partial gastrectomy, which can cause chronic gastritis.

A history of GI upset, pain and its relationship to eating and sleep patterns, and actions taken to relieve pain are also important. Inquire about any changes in the character of the pain because this may signal the development of complications. For example, if pain that was once intermittent and relieved by food and antacids becomes constant and radiates to the back or upper quadrant, the patient may have ulcer perforation. However, many adults with active duodenal or gastric ulcers report having no ulcer symptoms.

Physical Assessment/Signs and Symptoms. Physical assessment findings may reveal epigastric tenderness, usually located at the midline between the umbilicus and the xiphoid process. *If perforation into the peritoneal cavity is present, the patient typically has a rigid, boardlike abdomen accompanied by rebound tenderness and pain.* Initially, auscultation of the abdomen may reveal hyperactive bowel sounds, but these may diminish with progression of the disorder.

Dyspepsia *(indigestion) is the most commonly reported symptom associated with PUD.* It is typically described as sharp, burning, or gnawing pain. Some patients may perceive discomfort as a sensation of abdominal pressure or of fullness or hunger. Specific differences between gastric and duodenal ulcers are listed in Table 55-2.

Gastric ulcer pain often occurs in the upper epigastrium with localization to the left of the midline and is aggravated by food. *Duodenal* ulcer pain is usually located to the right of or below the epigastrium. The pain associated with a duodenal ulcer occurs 90 minutes to 3 hours *after* eating and often awakens the patient at night (McCance et al., 2014). Pain may also be exacerbated (made worse) by certain foods (e.g., tomatoes, hot spices, fried foods, onions, alcohol, caffeine drinks) and certain drugs (e.g., NSAIDs, corticosteroids). Perform a comprehensive pain assessment.

Nausea and vomiting may be symptoms accompanying ulcer disease, most commonly with pyloric sphincter dysfunction. It may result from gastric stasis associated with pyloric obstruction. Appetite is generally maintained in patients with a peptic ulcer unless pyloric obstruction is present.

To assess for fluid volume deficit that occurs from bleeding, take orthostatic blood pressure and monitor for signs and symptoms of dehydration. Also assess for dizziness, especially when the patient is upright, because this is a symptom of fluid volume deficit. Older adults often experience dizziness when they get out of bed and are at risk for falls.

? NCLEX EXAMINATION CHALLENGE 55-3

Physiological Integrity

The nurse is caring for a client with a bleeding duodenal ulcer who was admitted to the hospital after vomiting bright, red blood. Which condition does the nurse anticipate when the client develops a sudden, sharp pain in the mid-epigastric region and a rigid, board-like abdomen?

A. Pancreatitis
B. Ulcer perforation
C. Small bowel obstruction
D. Development of additional ulcers

TABLE 55-2   Differential Features of Gastric and Duodenal Ulcers

FEATURE	GASTRIC ULCER	DUODENAL ULCER
Age	Usually 50 yr or older	Usually 50 yr or older
Gender	Male/female ratio of 1.1 : 1	Male/female ratio of 1 : 1
Blood group	No differentiation	Most often type O
General nourishment	May be malnourished	Usually well nourished
Stomach acid production	Normal secretion or hyposecretion	Hypersecretion
Occurrence	Mucosa exposed to acid-pepsin secretion	Mucosa exposed to acid-pepsin secretion
Clinical course	Healing and recurrence	Healing and recurrence
Pain	Occurs 30-60 min after a meal; at night: rarely Worsened by ingestion of food	Occurs 1½-3 hr after a meal; at night: often awakens patient between 1 and 2 AM Relieved by ingestion of food
Response to treatment	Healing with appropriate therapy	Healing with appropriate therapy
Hemorrhage	Hematemesis more common than melena	Melena more common than hematemesis
Malignant change	Perhaps in less than 10%	Rare
Recurrence	Tends to heal and recurs often in the same location	60% recur within 1 yr; 90% recur within 2 yr
Surrounding mucosa	Atrophic gastritis	No gastritis

Psychosocial Assessment. Assess the impact of ulcer disease on the patient's lifestyle, occupation, family, and social and leisure activities. Evaluate the impact that lifestyle changes will have on the patient and family. This assessment may reveal information about the patient's ability to adhere to the prescribed treatment regimen and obtain the needed social support to alter his or her lifestyle.

Laboratory Assessment. There are three simple, noninvasive tests to detect *H. pylori* in the patient's blood, breath, or stool. Although the breath and stool tests are considered more accurate, *serologic testing* for *H. pylori* antibodies is the most common method to confirm *H. pylori* infection. The *urea breath test* involves swallowing a capsule, liquid, or pudding that contains urea with a special carbon atom. After a few minutes the patient exhales; and, if the special carbon atom is found, the bacterium is present. The *stool antigen test* is performed on a stool sample provided by the patient and is tested for *H. pylori* antigens. Patients who have venous bleeding from a peptic ulcer may have *decreased hemoglobin and hematocrit* values. The stool may also be positive for occult (not seen) blood if bleeding is present (Pagana et al., 2017).

Imaging Assessment. If perforation is suspected, the health care provider may request a *chest and abdomen x-ray series,* but other diagnostic tests are more helpful in diagnosis.

Other Diagnostic Assessment. The major diagnostic test for PUD is esophagogastroduodenoscopy (EGD), which is the most accurate means of establishing a diagnosis. Direct visualization of the ulcer crater by EGD allows the health care provider to take specimens for *H. pylori* testing and biopsy and cytologic studies for ruling out gastric cancer. The rapid urease test can confirm a quick diagnosis because urease is produced by the bacteria in the gastric mucosa. EGD may be repeated at 4- to 6-week intervals while the health care provider evaluates the progress of healing in response to therapy. Chapter 52 describes this test in more detail.

GI bleeding may be tested using a *nuclear medicine scan.* No special preparation is required for this scan. The patient is injected with a contrast medium (usually ^{99m}Tc), and the GI system is scanned for the presence of bleeding after a waiting period. A second scan may be done 1 to 2 days after the bleeding is treated to determine if the interventions were effective.

◆ **Analysis: Interpreting**

The priority collaborative problems for patients with peptic ulcer disease (PUD) include:
1. Acute pain or chronic noncancer pain due to gastric and/or duodenal ulceration
2. Potential for upper GI bleeding due to gastric and/or duodenal ulceration

◆ **Planning and Implementation: Responding**

Managing Acute Pain or Chronic Noncancer Pain

Planning: Expected Outcomes. The patient with PUD is expected to report pain control as evidenced by no more than a 3 on a 0-to-10 pain intensity scale.

Interventions. PUD causes significant discomfort that impacts many aspects of daily living. Interventions to manage pain focus on drug therapy and dietary changes.

Drug Therapy. The primary purposes of drug therapy in the treatment of PUD are to (1) provide pain relief, (2) eliminate *H. pylori* infection, (3) heal ulcerations, and (4) prevent recurrence. Several different regimens can be used. In selecting a therapeutic drug regimen, the health care provider considers the efficacy of the treatment, the anticipated side effects, the ability of the patient to adhere to the regimen, and the cost of the treatment.

Although numerous drugs have been evaluated for the treatment of *H. pylori* infection, no single agent has been used successfully against the organism. A common drug regimen for *H. pylori* infection is PPI–triple therapy, which includes a proton pump inhibitor (PPI) such as lansoprazole (Prevacid) plus two antibiotics such as metronidazole (Flagyl, Novonidazol) and tetracycline (Ala-Tet, Panmycin, Nu-Tetra) or clarithromycin (Biaxin, Biaxin XL) and amoxicillin (Amoxil, Amoxi) for 10 to 14 days. Some health care providers may prefer to use quadruple therapy, which contains combination of a proton pump inhibitor (PPI), any two commonly used antibiotics as described previously, with the addition of bismuth (Pepto-Bismol). Bismuth therapy is often used in patients who are allergic to penicillin-based medications.

⬡ CONSIDERATIONS FOR OLDER ADULTS

Patient-Centered Care QSEN

Many older adults have *H. pylori* infection that is undiagnosed because of vague symptoms associated with physiologic changes of aging and comorbidities that mask dyspepsia. Because the average age of gastric cancer diagnosis is 70 years, it is important to teach older adults about the symptoms of PUD and to consider *H. pylori* screening. Early detection and aggressive treatment can prevent PUD and gastric cancer.

Hyposecretory drugs reduce gastric acid secretions and are therefore used for both peptic ulcer disease (PUD) and gastritis management. The primary prescribed drugs include proton pump inhibitors and H_2-receptor antagonists (see Chart 55-3).

Proton pump inhibitor (PPI) is the drug class of choice for treating patients with acid-related disorders. Examples include omeprazole (Prilosec), lansoprazole (Prevacid), rabeprazole (Aciphex), pantoprazole (Protonix), and esomeprazole (Nexium). These drugs suppress the HK–ATPase enzyme system of gastric acid production, and several of them are available as over-the-counter (OTC) drugs (Lilley et al., 2017).

Omeprazole, lansoprazole, and esomeprazole are each available as delayed-release capsules designed to release their contents after they pass through the stomach. Omeprazole and lansoprazole may be dissolved in a sodium bicarbonate solution and given through any feeding tube. Bicarbonate protects the dissolved omeprazole and lansoprazole granules in gastric acid. Therefore the drugs are still absorbed correctly. These capsules can also be opened. The enteric-coated capsules can be put in apple juice or orange juice and given through a large-bore feeding tube. Rabeprazole (Aciphex) and pantoprazole (Protonix) are enteric-coated tablets that quickly dissolve after the tablet has moved through the stomach and should not be crushed before giving them. Several of the PPIs are also available in an IV form, which may be helpful for patients who are NPO.

Some patients use PPIs for years and perhaps a lifetime; these patient should be assessed periodically to determine the necessity of PPI use. Some studies have suggested there may be an increased risk of osteoporotic fractures related to long-term PPI use, yet current research is ongoing to determine if there is a definitive link between the two (Mulcahy, 2015). Omeprazole (Prilosec and Prilosec OTC) reduces the effect of clopidogrel (Plavix), an antiplatelet drug. Teach patients to tell their health care provider if they are taking clopidogrel. PPIs should not be discontinued abruptly to prevent rebound activation of the proton pump. Therefore a step-down approach over several days is recommended (Haastrup et al., 2014).

H₂-receptor antagonists are drugs that block histamine-stimulated gastric secretions. These drugs may also be used for indigestion and gastritis. Lower-dose forms are available in over-the-counter (OTC) products. H₂-receptor antagonists block the action of the H₂ receptors of the parietal cells, thus inhibiting gastric acid secretion. Two of the most common drugs are famotidine (Pepcid) and nizatidine (Axid) and are available as Pepcid OTC and Axid AR in OTC form. These drugs are typically administered in a single dose at bedtime and are used for 4 to 6 weeks in combination with other therapy.

Antacids buffer gastric acid and prevent the formation of pepsin. They may help small duodenal ulcers heal but are usually not used alone as drug therapy. Liquid suspensions are the most therapeutic form, but tablets may be more convenient and enhance adherence. The most widely used preparations are mixtures of aluminum hydroxide and magnesium hydroxide. This combination overcomes the unpleasant GI side effects of either of these preparations when used alone. Mylanta and Maalox are examples of this type of combination antacid formulation. The aluminum and magnesium hydroxide combination products neutralize well at small doses. These products must be administered cautiously to patients with renal impairment because elimination is reduced and excessive amounts are retained in the body.

> ## ! NURSING SAFETY PRIORITY **QSEN**
>
> ### Drug Alert
>
> Teach the patient that, to achieve a therapeutic effect, sufficient antacid must be ingested to neutralize the hourly production of acid. For optimal effect, take antacids about 2 hours after meals to reduce the hydrogen ion load in the duodenum. Antacids may be effective from 30 minutes to 3 hours after ingestion. If taken on an empty stomach, they are quickly evacuated. Thus the neutralizing effect is reduced (Lilley et al., 2017).

Calcium carbonate (Tums) is a potent antacid, but it triggers gastrin release, causing a rebound acid secretion. Therefore its use in acid inhibition is not recommended.

Antacids can interact with certain drugs such as phenytoin (Dilantin), tetracycline (Ala-Tet, Nu-Tetra), and ketoconazole (Nizoral) and interfere with their effectiveness. Ask what other drugs the patient is using before a specific antacid is prescribed. Other drugs are given 1 to 2 hours before or after the antacid. Inform the patient that flavored antacids, especially wintergreen, should be avoided. The flavoring increases the emptying time of the stomach. Thus the desired effect of the antacid is negated.

Teach the patient with past or present heart failure to avoid antacids with high sodium content, such as aluminum hydroxide, magnesium hydroxide, sodium bicarbonate, and simethicone combination products (Gelusil and Mylanta). Magaldrate (Riopan) has the lowest sodium concentration.

Sucralfate (Carafate) is a *mucosal barrier fortifier* (protector) that forms complexes with proteins at the base of a peptic ulcer. This protective coat prevents further digestive action of both acid and pepsin. Sucralfate does not inhibit acid secretion. Rather, it binds bile acids and pepsins, reducing injury from these substances. The drug may be used in conjunction with H₂-receptor antagonists and antacids but should not be administered within 1 hour of the antacid. Sucralfate is given on an empty stomach 1 hour before each meal and at bedtime. The main side effect of this drug is constipation.

Bismuth subsalicylate (Pepto-Bismol) inhibits *H. pylori* from binding to the mucosal lining and stimulates mucosal protection and prostaglandin production. Teach patients that they cannot take aspirin while on this drug because aspirin is a salicylic acid and could cause an overdose of salicylates. Patients should also be taught that this medication may cause the stools to be discolored black. This discoloration is temporary and harmless.

Nutrition Therapy. The role of diet in the management of ulcer disease is controversial. There is no evidence that dietary restriction reduces gastric acid secretion or promotes tissue healing, although a bland diet may assist in relieving symptoms. Food itself acts as an antacid by neutralizing gastric acid for 30 to 60 minutes. An increased rate of gastric acid secretion, called *rebound,* may follow.

> ## ! NURSING SAFETY PRIORITY **QSEN**
>
> ### Action Alert
>
> Teach the patient with peptic ulcer disease to avoid substances that increase gastric acid secretion. This includes caffeine-containing beverages (coffee, tea, cola). Both caffeinated and decaffeinated coffees should be avoided because coffee contains peptides that stimulate gastrin release (McCance et al., 2014).

Teach the patient to exclude any foods that cause discomfort. A bland, nonirritating diet is recommended during the acute symptomatic phase. Bedtime snacks are avoided because they may stimulate gastric acid secretion. Eating six smaller meals daily may help, but this regimen is no longer a regular part of therapy. No evidence supports the theory that eating six meals daily promotes healing of the ulcer. This practice may actually stimulate gastric acid secretion. Patients should avoid alcohol and tobacco because of their stimulatory effects on gastric acid secretion.

Complementary and Integrative Health. Teach patients about complementary and integrative therapies that can reduce stress, including hypnosis and imagery. For example, the use of yoga and meditation techniques has demonstrated a beneficial effect on anxiety disorders. Many have suggested that GI disorders result from the dysfunction of both the GI tract itself and the brain. This means that emotional stress is thought to worsen GI disorders such as peptic ulcer disease. Yoga may alter the activities of the central and autonomic nervous systems.

Many herbs, such as powders of slippery elm and marshmallow root, quercetin, and licorice, are used commonly by patients with gastritis and PUD. These herbs may help heal inflamed tissue and increase blood flow to the gastric mucosa. Other substances include zinc, vitamin C, essential fatty acids, acidophilus, vitamin A, and glutamine. Table 55-1 provides a list of therapies that have been used by many patients with gastric disorders. Many of them have been scientifically supported in animal studies but have not been thoroughly studied in humans.

> ### ! NURSING SAFETY PRIORITY QSEN
> #### *Action Alert*
>
> Teach the patient who has peptic ulcer disease to seek immediate medical attention if experiencing any of these symptoms:
> - Sharp, sudden, persistent, and severe epigastric or abdominal pain
> - Bloody or black stools
> - Bloody vomit or vomit that looks like coffee grounds

Managing Upper GI Bleeding

Planning: Expected Outcomes. The patient with upper GI bleeding (often called *upper GI hemorrhage* or *UGH*) is expected to have bleeding promptly and effectively controlled and vital signs within normal limits.

Interventions. Blood loss from PUD results in high morbidity and mortality. Fluid volume loss secondary to vomiting can lead to dehydration and electrolyte imbalances. Interventions aimed at managing complications associated with PUD include prevention and/or management of bleeding, perforation, and gastric outlet obstruction. In some cases surgical treatment of complications becomes necessary.

Nonsurgical Management. Because prevention or early detection of complications is needed to obtain a positive clinical outcome, monitor the patient carefully and immediately report changes to the health care provider. The type of intervention selected will depend on the type and severity of the complication.

Emergency: Upper GI Bleeding. The patient who is actively bleeding has a life-threatening emergency. He or she needs supportive therapy to prevent hypovolemic shock and possible death.

> ### ! NURSING SAFETY PRIORITY QSEN
> #### *Critical Rescue*
>
> *Recognize that your priority for care of the patient with upper GI bleeding is to maintain **a**irway, **b**reathing, and **c**irculation (ABCs).* Respond to these needs by providing oxygen and other ventilatory support as needed, starting two large-bore IV lines for replacing fluids and blood, and monitoring vital signs, hematocrit, and oxygen saturation.

The purpose of managing hypovolemia is to expand intravascular fluid in a patient who is volume depleted. Carefully monitor the patient's fluid status, including intake and output. *Fluid replacement in older adults should be closely monitored to prevent fluid overload.* Serum electrolytes are also assessed because depletions from vomiting or nasogastric suctioning must be replaced. Volume replacement with isotonic solutions (e.g., 0.9% normal saline solution, lactated Ringer's solution) should be started immediately. The health care provider may prescribe blood products such as packed red blood cells to expand volume and correct a low hemoglobin and hematocrit. For patients with active bleeding, fresh frozen plasma may be given if the prothrombin time is 1.5 times higher than the midrange control value.

Continue to monitor the patient's hematocrit, hemoglobin, and coagulation studies for changes from the baseline measurements. With mild bleeding (less than 500 mL), slight feelings of weakness and mild perspiration may be present. When blood loss exceeds 1 L/24 hr, manifestations of shock may occur, such as hypotension, chills, palpitations, diaphoresis, and a weak, thready pulse.

A combination of several different treatments, including nasogastric tube (NGT) placement and lavage, endoscopic therapy, interventional radiologic procedures, and acid suppression, can be used to control acute bleeding and prevent rebleeding. If the patient is actively bleeding at home, he or she is usually admitted to the emergency department for GI lavage. If the patient is already a patient in the hospital, lavage can be done at the bedside. After the bleeding has stopped, H_2-receptor antagonists, proton pump inhibitors, and antacids are the primary drugs used.

Nasogastric Tube Placement and Lavage. Upper GI bleeding often requires the primary care provider or nurse to insert a large-bore NGT to:
- Determine the presence or absence of blood in the stomach
- Assess the rate of bleeding
- Prevent gastric dilation
- Administer lavage

Although not performed as commonly today, **gastric lavage** requires the insertion of a large-bore NGT with instillation of a room-temperature solution in volumes of 200 to 300 mL. There is no evidence that sterile saline or sterile water is better than tap water for this procedure. Follow agency protocol for the solution that is required. The solution and blood are repeatedly withdrawn manually until returns are clear or light pink and without clots. Instruct the patient to lie on the left side during this procedure. The NGT may remain in place for a few days or be removed after lavage.

Endoscopic Therapy. Endoscopic therapy via an esophagogastroduodenoscopy (EGD) can assist in achieving homeostasis during an acute hemorrhage by isolating the bleeding artery to embolize (clot) it. A physician can insert instruments through the endoscope during the procedure to stop bleeding in three different ways: (1) inject chemicals into the bleeding site; (2) treat the bleeding area with heat, electric current, or laser; or (3) close the affected blood vessels with a band or clip. During the EGD, a specialized endoscopy nurse and technician assist the physician with the procedure.

Pre-EGD nursing care involves inserting one or two large-bore IV catheters if they are not in place. A large catheter allows the patient to receive IV moderate sedation (e.g., midazolam [Versed] and an opioid) and possibly a blood transfusion. Keep the patient NPO for 4 to 6 hours before the procedure. This prevents the risk for aspiration and allows the endoscopist to view and treat the ulcer. A patient must sign a consent form before the EGD *after* the physician informs him or her about the procedure.

Endoscopic therapy is beneficial for most patients with active bleeding. However, ulcers that continue to bleed or continue to rebleed despite endoscopic therapy may require an interventional radiologic procedure or surgical repair.

Interventional Radiologic Procedures. For patients with persistent, massive upper GI bleeding or those who are not surgical candidates, catheter-directed embolization may be performed. This endovascular procedure is usually done if endoscopic procedures are not successful or available. A femoral approach is most often used, but brachial access may be used. An arteriogram is performed to identify the arterial anatomy and find the exact location of the bleeding. The physician injects medication or other material into the blood vessels to stop the bleeding. Care of the patient following an arteriogram is similar to care following a percutaneous vascular intervention, which is described in Chapters 36 and 38. Post-arteriogram nursing care should be provided after the procedure.

Acid Suppression. Aggressive acid suppression is used to prevent rebleeding. When acute bleeding is stopped and clot formation has taken place within the ulcer crater, the clot remains in contact with gastric contents. Acid-suppressive agents are used to stabilize the clot by raising the pH level of gastric contents. Several types of drugs are used. H_2-receptor antagonists prevent acid from being produced by parietal cells. Proton pump inhibitors prevent the transport of acid across the parietal cell membrane, whereas antacids buffer acid produced in the stomach.

Perforation is managed by immediately replacing fluid, blood, and electrolytes, administering antibiotics, and keeping the patient NPO. Maintain nasogastric suction to drain gastric secretions and thus prevent further peritoneal spillage. Carefully monitor intake and output and check vital signs at least hourly. Monitor the patient for signs and symptoms of septic shock, such as fever, alterations in COMFORT, tachycardia, lethargy, or anxiety.

Pyloric obstruction is caused by edema, spasm, or scar tissue. Symptoms of obstruction related to difficulty in emptying the stomach include feelings of fullness, distention, or nausea after eating, as well as vomiting copious amounts of undigested food.

Treatment of obstruction is directed toward restoring fluid and electrolyte balance and decompressing the dilated stomach. Obstruction related to edema and spasm generally responds to medical therapy. First, the stomach must be decompressed with nasogastric suction. Next, interventions are directed at correcting metabolic alkalosis and dehydration. The NGT is clamped after about 72 hours. Check the patient for retention of gastric contents. If the amount retained is not more than 50 mL in 30 minutes, the health care provider may allow oral fluids. In some cases, surgical intervention may be required to treat PUD.

Surgical Management. Evidence-based guidelines for the treatment of PUD that include *H. pylori* treatment and the development of nonsurgical means of controlling bleeding have led to a decline in the need for surgical intervention. In PUD, surgical intervention may be used to:

- Treat patients who do not respond to medical therapy or other nonsurgical procedures
- Treat a surgical emergency that develops as a complication of PUD, such as perforation

Two general surgical approaches are available for PUD: minimally invasive surgery and conventional open surgery.

Minimally invasive surgery (MIS) via laparoscopy (a type of endoscope) may be used to remove a chronic gastric ulcer or treat hemorrhage from perforation. Several small incisions allow access to the stomach and duodenum. The patient may have partial stomach removal (subtotal gastrectomy), pyloroplasty (to open the pylorus), and/or a vagotomy (vagus nerve cutting) to control acid secretion. Acid-reduction surgery may not be necessary because of the increased use of PPIs and endoscopic procedures in the treatment of PUD. The advantages of MIS over traditional open surgical procedures include a shorter hospital stay, fewer complications, less pain, and better, quicker recovery.

Care Coordination and Transition Management

Patients may be discharged from the hospital if there is no evidence of ongoing bleeding, orthostatic changes, or cardiopulmonary distress or compromise. Those discharged after treatment for peptic ulcer disease (PUD) and/or complications secondary to the disease must face several challenges to manage the disease successfully. Long-term adherence to drug therapy may require the patient to take several drugs each day. Permanent lifestyle alterations in NUTRITION habits must also be made.

Home Care Management. Most patients are discharged to home to continue their recovery. Those who have had major surgery or complications, such as hemorrhage, may require one or two visits from a home care nurse to assess clinical progress, especially if the patient is an older adult (Chart 55-5).

Self-Management Education. The primary focus of home care preparation is patient and family teaching regarding risk factors for the recurrence of PUD. Teach them how to recognize new complications and what to do if they occur, especially abdominal pain; nausea and vomiting; black, tarry stools; and weakness or dizziness.

CHART 55-5 Home Care Assessment

The Patient With Ulcer Disease

Assess gastrointestinal and cardiovascular status, including:
- Vital signs, including orthostatic vital signs
- Skin color
- Presence of abdominal pain (location, severity, character, duration, precipitating factors, and relief measures)
- Character, color, and consistency of stools
- Changes in bowel elimination pattern
- Hemoglobin and hematocrit
- Bowel sounds; palpate for areas of tenderness

Assess nutritional status, including:
- Dietary patterns and habits
- Intake of coffee and alcohol
- Relationship of food ingestion to symptoms

Assess medication history:
- Use of steroids
- Use of NSAIDs
- Use of over-the-counter medications

Assess patient's coping style:
- Recent stressors
- Past coping style

Assess patient's understanding of illness and ability to adhere to the therapeutic regimen:
- Symptoms to report to health care provider
- Expected and side effects of medications
- Food and drug interactions
- Need for smoking cessation

Help the patient plan ways to make needed lifestyle changes. For postsurgical patients, especially those who have undergone partial stomach removal, smaller meals may be required. Other postoperative nutrition changes are described in the Self-Management Education discussion in the Gastric Cancer section.

NURSING SAFETY PRIORITY (QSEN)

Action Alert

Teach the patient who has had surgery for PUD to avoid any OTC product containing aspirin or other NSAID. Emphasize the importance of following the treatment regimen for *H. pylori* infection and healing the ulcer and of keeping all follow-up appointments. Help the patient identify situations that cause stress, describe feelings during stressful situations, and develop a plan for coping with stressors.

Health Care Resources. If needed, refer the patient and family to the National Digestive Diseases Information Clearinghouse (www.digestive.niddk.nih.gov/). This group provides information and support to patients who have digestive disorders.

◆ Evaluation: Reflecting

Evaluate the care of the patient with peptic ulcer disease (PUD) based on the identified priority patient problems. The expected outcomes are that the patient:
- Does not have active PUD or associated complications
- Verbalizes relief or control of pain and alterations in COMFORT
- Adheres to the drug regimen and lifestyle changes to prevent recurrence and heal the ulcer
- Does not experience an upper GI bleed; if bleeding occurs, it will be promptly and effectively managed

GASTRIC CANCER

Most cancers of the stomach are adenocarcinomas. This type of cancer develops in the mucosal cells that form the innermost lining of any portion or all of the stomach. *Often there are no symptoms in the early stages, and the disease is advanced when detected.*

❖ PATHOPHYSIOLOGY

Gastric cancer usually begins in the glands of the stomach mucosa. Atrophic gastritis and intestinal metaplasia (abnormal tissue development) are precancerous conditions. Inadequate acid secretion in patients with atrophic gastritis creates an alkaline environment that allows bacteria (especially *H. pylori*) to multiply. This infection causes mucosa-associated lymphoid tissue (MALT) lymphoma, which starts in the stomach (McCance et al., 2014).

Gastric cancers spread by direct extension through the gastric wall and into regional lymphatics, which carry tumor deposits to lymph nodes. Direct invasion of and adherence to adjacent organs (e.g., the liver, pancreas, and transverse colon) may also result. Hematogenous spread via the portal vein to the liver and via the systemic circulation to the lungs and bones is the most common mode of metastasis. Peritoneal seeding of cancer cells from the tumor areas to the omentum, peritoneum, ovary, and pelvic cul-de-sac can also occur.

In adults with *advanced* gastric cancer, there is invasion of the muscularis (stomach muscle) or beyond. These lesions are not cured by surgical resection. The overall 5-year survival rate of adults with stomach cancer in the United States is poor because most patients have no symptoms until the disease advances.

Etiology and Genetic Risk

Infection with *H. pylori* is the largest risk factor for gastric cancer because it carries the cytotoxin-associated gene A (*CagA*) gene. Patients with pernicious anemia, gastric polyps, chronic atrophic gastritis, and achlorhydria (absence of secretion of hydrochloric acid) are two to three times more likely to develop gastric cancer.

The disease also seems to be positively correlated with eating pickled foods, nitrates from processed foods, and salt added to food. The ingestion of these foods over a long period can lead to atrophic gastritis, a precancerous condition. A low intake of fruits and vegetables is also a risk factor for cancer (McCance et al., 2014).

Gastric surgery seems to increase the risk for gastric cancer because of the eventual development of atrophic gastritis, which results in changes to the mucosa. Patients with Barrett's esophagus from prolonged or severe gastroesophageal reflux disease (GERD) have an increased risk for cancer in the cardia (at the point where the stomach connects to the esophagus).

Incidence and Prevalence

Generally, stomach cancer is more common in males than in females, and there is a sharp increase in adults over 50, with most diagnosed between ages 60 and 80. Across the world, the highest incidence rates are in Japan, China, Southern and Eastern Europe, and South and Central America. In the United States, according to ethnicity, Hispanic Americans, African Americans, and Asian/Pacific Islanders have more incidence of stomach cancer than non-Hispanic whites. The average age for an adult diagnosed with gastric cancer is 69 years old (American Cancer Society, 2017).

Nurses are uniquely positioned to improve gastric cancer survival rates by ensuring that patients with high risk and suspicious symptoms are assessed and diagnosed early. Maintaining functional status and quality of life during gastric cancer care is a priority for nursing care.

Health Promotion and Maintenance

Teach patients with gastritis and/or *H. pylori* infection to follow the treatment regimen to ensure that gastritis heals and *H. pylori* infection is eliminated. *Stress the need for eating a well-balanced diet and limiting pickled, salted, and processed foods to help prevent gastric cancer.*

❖ INTERPROFESSIONAL COLLABORATIVE CARE

Care of the patient with gastric cancer takes place in all settings, ranging from the home and community environment to the inpatient setting, depending on the stage of disease and the immediate course of treatment. The interprofessional team that collaborates to care for this patient generally includes the surgeon, nurse, case manager, dietitian, social worker, and spiritual leader of the patient's choice.

◆ Assessment: Noticing

Question the patient about known risk factors for the development of gastric cancer. Ask about preferred foods, especially pickled, salted, or smoked foods. Inquire whether the patient has ever been diagnosed with or treated for *H. pylori* infection, gastritis, or pernicious anemia. Note whether he or she has a history of gastric surgery or polyps. Also ask whether any of the patient's immediate relatives have gastric cancer.

Although patients with *early* gastric cancer may be asymptomatic, indigestion (heartburn) and abdominal discomfort are the *most* common symptoms (Chart 55-6). However, these symptoms are often ignored, or a change in diet or use of antacids relieves them. As the tumor grows, these symptoms become more severe and do not respond to nutrition changes or antacids. Epigastric or back pain is also an early symptom that may go unrecognized.

In *advanced* gastric cancer, progressive weight loss, nausea, and vomiting can occur. Vomiting represents pronounced dilation, thickening of the stomach wall, or pyloric obstruction. Obstructive symptoms appear earlier with tumors located near the pylorus than with those in the fundus. Patients with advanced disease may have weakness, fatigue, and anemia. Physical assessment findings in advanced disease may be

absent, or a palpable epigastric mass may suggest hepatomegaly (liver enlargement) from metastatic disease. Hard, enlarged lymph nodes in the left supraclavicular chain, left axilla, or umbilicus result from metastasis from gastric cancer. Masses on the right suggest metastasis in the perigastric lymph nodes or liver.

In patients with advanced disease, anemia is evidenced by *low hematocrit* and hemoglobin values. Patients may have macrocytic or microcytic anemia associated with decreased iron or vitamin B_{12} absorption. *The stool may be positive for occult blood. Hypoalbuminemia* and *abnormal results of liver tests* (e.g., bilirubin and alkaline phosphatase) occur with advanced disease and hepatic metastasis. The level of carcinoembryonic antigen (CEA) is elevated in advanced cancer of the stomach (Pagana et al., 2017).

The health care provider uses esophagogastroduodenoscopy (EGD) with biopsy for definitive diagnosis of gastric cancer. (See Chapter 52 for a discussion of nursing care associated with this diagnostic test.) The lesion can be viewed directly, and biopsies of all visible lesions can be obtained to determine the presence of cancer cells. During the endoscopy, an endoscopic (endoluminal) ultrasound (EUS) of the gastric mucosa can also be performed. This technology allows the health care provider to evaluate the depth of the tumor and the presence of lymph node involvement, which permits more accurate staging of the disease. CT, positron emission tomography (PET), and MRI scans of the chest, abdomen, and pelvis are used in determining the extent of the disease and planning therapy.

◆ Interventions: Responding

Management of gastric cancer includes drug therapy, radiation, and/or surgery. Drug therapy and radiation may be used instead of surgery or as an adjunct before and/or after surgery.

Nonsurgical Management. The treatment of gastric cancer depends highly on the stage of the disease. Radiation and chemotherapy commonly prolong survival of patients with advanced gastric disease.

Combination *chemotherapy* with multiple cycles of drugs such as cisplatin (Platinol) and epirubicin (Ellence) before and after surgery may be given. Bone marrow suppression, nausea, and vomiting are common adverse drug effects. Chapter 22 discusses the general nursing care of patients receiving chemotherapy.

Although gastric cancers are somewhat sensitive to the effects of radiation, the use of this treatment is limited because the disease is often widely spread to other abdominal organs on diagnosis. Organs such as the liver, kidneys, and spinal cord can endure only a limited amount of radiation. Intraoperative radiotherapy (IORT) is available in large tertiary care health care systems. Radiation may be used for palliative management when surgery is not an option.

The most common side effects of radiation include impaired skin integrity, fatigue, and anorexia. Nausea, vomiting, and diarrhea may occur about 1 week after treatment is initiated and diminish a month or more after treatment ends. (See Chapter 22 for more information on radiation therapy.)

Surgical Management. Surgical resection by removing the tumor is the preferred method for treating gastric cancer. The primary surgical procedures for the treatment of gastric cancer are total and subtotal (partial) gastrectomy. In early stages, laparoscopic surgery (minimally invasive surgery [MIS]) plus

---

▶ CHART 55-6   Key Features

Early versus Advanced Gastric Cancer

Early Gastric Cancer*	Advanced Gastric Cancer
• Indigestion	• Nausea and vomiting
• Abdominal discomfort initially relieved with antacids	• Obstructive symptoms
• Feeling of fullness	• Iron deficiency anemia
• Epigastric, back, or retrosternal pain	• Palpable epigastric mass
	• Enlarged lymph nodes
	• Weakness and fatigue
	• Progressive weight loss

*NOTE: Many patients with early gastric cancer have no signs or symptoms.

adjuvant chemotherapy or radiation may be curative. Patients having MIS have less pain, shorter hospital stays, rare postoperative complications, and quicker recovery. However, MIS is seldom performed because very few patients are diagnosed in the early stage of the disease.

Most patients with advanced disease are candidates for palliative surgical treatment. Metastasis in the supraclavicular lymph nodes, inguinal lymph nodes, liver, umbilicus, or perirectal wall indicates that the opportunity for cure by resection has been lost. Palliative resection may significantly improve the quality of life for a patient suffering from obstruction, hemorrhage, or pain.

Preoperative Care. Before conventional open-approach surgery, a nasogastric tube (NGT) is often inserted and connected to suction to remove secretions and empty the stomach. This allows surgery to take place without contamination of the peritoneal cavity by gastric secretions. The NGT remains in place for a few days *after surgery* to prevent the accumulation of secretions, which may lead to vomiting or GI distention and pressure on the incision. Patients having laparoscopic surgery (minimally invasive surgery [MIS]) do not require an NGT.

Because weight loss is problematic for patients with gastric cancer, NUTRITION therapy is a vital aspect of preoperative and postoperative management. Before surgery, compression by the tumor can prevent adequate nutritional intake. To correct malnutrition before surgery, the health care provider may prescribe enteral supplements to the diet and/or total parenteral nutrition (TPN). Vitamin, mineral, iron, and protein supplements are essential to correct nutritional deficits.

Other preoperative nursing measures for the patient undergoing open gastric surgery are the same as those for any patient undergoing abdominal surgery and general anesthesia (see Chapter 14).

Operative Procedures. The surgeon usually removes part or all of the stomach to take out the tumor. When the tumor is located in the mid-portion or distal (lower) portion of the stomach, a subtotal (partial) gastrectomy is typically performed. The omentum, spleen, and relevant nodes are also removed. The surgery may be performed as an MIS procedure or as an open conventional surgical technique, with or without robotic assistance.

For the patient with a removable growth in the proximal (upper) third of the stomach, a total gastrectomy is performed (Fig. 55-4). In this procedure the surgeon removes the entire stomach along with the lymph nodes and omentum. The surgeon sutures the esophagus to the duodenum or jejunum to reestablish continuity of the GI tract. More radical surgery involving removal of the spleen and distal pancreas is controversial, although the Whipple procedure may be used to prolong life. However, the complications of this drastic surgery are very serious and common. For patients with advanced disease, total gastrectomy is performed only when gastric bleeding or obstruction is present.

Patients with tumors at the gastric outlet who are not candidates for subtotal or total gastrectomy may undergo gastroenterostomy for palliation. The surgeon creates a passage between the body of the stomach and the small bowel, often the duodenum.

Postoperative Care. Provide the usual postoperative care for patients who have had general anesthesia to prevent atelectasis,

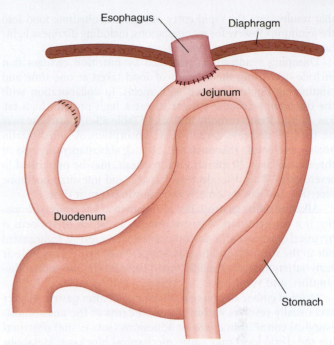

FIG. 55-4 Total gastrectomy with anastomosis of the esophagus to the jejunum (esophagojejunostomy) is the principal surgical intervention for extensive gastric cancer.

paralytic ileus, wound infection, and peritonitis (see Chapter 16). Document and report any signs and symptoms of these complications immediately to the surgeon. Patients who have laparoscopic surgery usually have less postoperative pain, fewer complications, and a shorter stay in the hospital.

Auscultate the lungs for adventitious sounds (crackles or reduced breath sounds) and monitor for the return of bowel sounds. Take vital signs as appropriate to detect signs of infection or bleeding. Aggressive pulmonary exercises and early ambulation can help prevent respiratory complications and deep vein thrombosis. Also inspect the operative site every 8 to 12 hours for the presence of redness, swelling, or drainage, which indicate wound infection. Keep the head of the bed elevated to prevent aspiration from reflux.

Decreased patency caused by a clogged NGT can result in *acute gastric dilation* after surgery. This problem is characterized by epigastric pain and a feeling of fullness, hiccups, tachycardia, and hypotension. Notify the surgeon to obtain an order for irrigation or replacement of the NGT to relieve these symptoms.

Dumping syndrome is a term that refers to a group of vasomotor symptoms that occur after eating. This syndrome is believed to occur as a result of the rapid emptying of food contents into the small intestine, which shifts fluid into the gut, causing abdominal distention. Observe for *early* manifestations of this syndrome, which typically occur within 30 minutes of eating. Symptoms include vertigo, tachycardia, syncope, sweating, pallor, palpitations, and the desire to lie down. Report these manifestations to the surgeon, and encourage the patient to lie down. Monitor the patient for late symptoms.

Late dumping syndrome, which occurs 90 minutes to 3 hours after eating, is caused by a release of an excessive amount of insulin. The insulin release follows a rapid rise in the blood glucose level that results from the rapid entry of high-carbohydrate food into the jejunum. Observe for manifestations, including dizziness, light-headedness, palpitations, diaphoresis, and confusion.

Dumping syndrome is managed by nutrition changes that include decreasing the amount of food taken at one time and eliminating liquids ingested with meals. In collaboration with the dietitian, teach the patient to eat a high-protein, high-fat, low- to moderate-carbohydrate diet (Table 55-3). Acarbose may be used to decrease carbohydrate absorption. A somatostatin analog, octreotide (Sandostatin), 50 mcg subcutaneously two or three times daily 30 minutes before meals, may be prescribed in severe cases. This drug decreases gastric and intestinal hormone secretion and slows stomach and intestinal transit time.

Alkaline reflux gastropathy, also known as *bile reflux gastropathy*, is a complication of gastric surgery in which the pylorus is bypassed or removed. Endoscopic examination reveals regurgitated bile in the stomach and mucosal hyperemia. Symptoms include early satiety (satisfied quickly with little food), abdominal discomfort, and vomiting.

Delayed gastric emptying is often present after gastric surgery and usually resolves within 1 week. Edema at the anastomosis (surgical connection areas) or adhesions (scar tissue) obstructing the distal loop may cause mechanical blockage. Metabolic causes (e.g., hypokalemia, hypoproteinemia, or hyponatremia) should be considered. The edema is resolved with nasogastric suction, maintenance of fluid and electrolyte balance, and proper nutrition.

Several problems related to NUTRITION develop as a result of partial removal of the stomach, including deficiencies of vitamin B_{12}, folic acid, and iron; impaired calcium metabolism; and reduced absorption of calcium and vitamin D. These problems are caused by a reduction of intrinsic factor. The decrease results from the resection and from inadequate absorption because of rapid entry of food into the bowel. In the absence of intrinsic factor, signs and symptoms of pernicious anemia may occur. Assess for the development of atrophic glossitis secondary to vitamin B_{12} deficiency. In atrophic glossitis, the tongue takes on a shiny, smooth, and "beefy" appearance. The patient may also have signs of anemia secondary to folic acid and iron deficiency. Monitor the complete blood count (CBC) for signs of megaloblastic anemia (low red blood cell [RBC] level) and leukopenia (low white blood cell [WBC] level). These manifestations are corrected by the administration of vitamin B_{12}. The health care provider may also prescribe folic acid or iron preparations.

Care Coordination and Transition Management

Patients who have undergone total gastrectomy and those who are debilitated with advanced gastric cancer are discharged to home with maximal assistance and support or to a transitional

TABLE 55-3	**Diet for Dumping Syndrome**		
FOOD GROUP	**FOODS ALLOWED OR ENCOURAGED**	**FOODS TO USE WITH CAUTION**	**FOODS THAT MUST BE EXCLUDED**
Soups		Fluids 1 hr before and after meals	Spicy soups
Meat and meat substitutes	8 oz or more per day: fish, poultry, beef, pork, veal, lamb, eggs, cheese, and peanut butter		Spicy meats or meat substitutes
Potatoes	Potato, rice, pasta, starchy vegetables (small amount)		Highly spiced potatoes or potato substitutes
Bread and cereal	White bread, rolls, muffins, crackers, and cereals (small amount)	Whole-grain bread, rolls, crackers, and cereals	Breads with frosting or jelly, sweet rolls, and coffee cake
Vegetables	Two or more cooked vegetables	Gas-producing vegetables, such as cabbage, onions, broccoli, or raw vegetables	
Fruits	Limit three per day: unsweetened cooked or canned fruits	Unsweetened juice or fruit drinks 30-45 min after meals; fresh fruit	Sweetened fruit or juice
Beverages	Dietetic drinks	Limit to 1 hr after meals; caffeine-containing beverages, such as coffee, tea, and cola; if tolerated, diet carbonated beverages	Milk shakes, malts, and other sweet drinks; regular carbonated beverages and alcohol
Fats	Margarine, oils, shortening, butter, bacon, and salad dressings	Mayonnaise	Any fats with milk products
Desserts	Fruit (see Fruits)	Sugar-free gelatin, pudding, and custard	All sweets, cakes, pies, cookies, candy, ice cream, and sherbet
Seasonings and miscellaneous	Diet jelly, diet syrups, sugar substitutes	Excessive amounts of salt	Excessive amounts of spices, sugar, jelly, honey, syrup, or molasses

General Principles for Patients to Follow
- Several small meals daily
- Relatively high fat and protein content
- Low roughage
- Relatively low carbohydrate content
- No milk, sweets, or sugars
- Liquid between meals *only*

NCLEX EXAMINATION CHALLENGE 55-4

Psychosocial Integrity

Which client statement regarding treatment for gastric cancer requires the nurse to intervene **immediately**?

A. "I understand my treatment regimen."

B. "My prognosis is frightening to me and my partner."

C. "Life just doesn't seem to be worth living anymore."

D. "There is a list of community resources stored in my computer for when I need them."

care unit or skilled nursing facility. Patients who have undergone subtotal gastrectomy and are not debilitated may be discharged to home with partial assistance for ADLs. Recurrence of cancer is common, and patients need regular follow-up examinations and imaging assessments. Collaborate with the case manager (CM) to ensure continuity of care and thorough follow-up with diagnostic testing.

Home Care Management. Gastric cancer is a life-threatening illness. Therefore the patient and family members require physical and emotional care. Assess their ability to cope with the disease and the possible need for end-of-life care. The adverse effects of gastric cancer treatment can be debilitating, and patients need to learn symptom-management strategies. Hospice programs can help both the patient and the family cope with these physical and emotional needs.

Patients may fear returning home because of their inability for self-management. Enlisting family and health care resources for the patient may ease some of this anxiety. Provide the family with adequate information about community support systems to make the transition to home care easier. If the prognosis is poor, they need continued professional support from case managers, social workers, and/or nurses to cope with death and dying. (See Chapter 7 for a discussion of end-of-life care.)

Self-Management Education. Educate the patient and family about any continuing needs, drug therapy, and nutrition therapy. If patients are discharged to home with surgical dressings, teach the patient and family how to change them. Review the manifestations of incisional infection (e.g., fever, redness, and drainage) that they should report to their surgeon.

Patients who will be receiving radiation therapy or chemotherapy require instructions related to the side effects of these treatments. Nausea and vomiting are common side effects of chemotherapy, and instruction in the use of prescribed antiemetics may be needed. (See Chapter 22 for health teaching for patients receiving chemotherapy or radiation therapy.)

In collaboration with the dietitian, teach the patient and family about the type and quantity of foods that will provide optimal nutritional value. Interventions to minimize dumping syndrome and decrease gastric stimulants are also emphasized (see Table 55-3). Remind the patient to:

- Eat small, frequent meals
- Avoid drinking liquids with meals
- Avoid foods that cause discomfort
- Eliminate caffeine and alcohol consumption
- Begin a smoking-cessation program, if needed
- Receive B_{12} injections, as prescribed
- Lie flat after eating for a short time

Health Care Resources. A home care referral provides continued assessment, assistance, and encouragement to the patient and family. A home care nurse can help with care procedures and provide valuable psychological support. Additional referrals to a dietitian, professional counselor, or clergy/spiritual leader may be necessary. Referral to a hospice agency can be of great assistance for the patient with advanced disease. Hospice care may be delivered in the home or in an institutional setting. Appropriate support groups (e.g., I Can Cope, provided by the American Cancer Society [http://www.cancer.org/treatment/index]) can be a major resource.

GET READY FOR THE NCLEX® EXAMINATION!

KEY POINTS

Review these Key Points for each NCLEX Examination Client Needs Category.

Safe and Effective Care Environment

- When caring for patients with gastric health problems, collaborate with the members of the interprofessional team, including the pharmacist, dietitian, health care provider, and/or case manager. **QSEN: Teamwork and Collaboration**

Health Promotion and Maintenance

- Refer the patient with gastric cancer to the American Cancer Society.
- Identify patients at risk for gastritis and PUD, especially those with *H. pylori* and older adults who take large amounts of NSAIDs. **QSEN: Safety**
- Teach adults to prevent PUD by avoiding excess consumption of caffeine, alcohol, coffee, aspirin, NSAIDs, and contaminated food and water and by avoiding smoking (see Chart 55-1). **QSEN: Evidence-Based Practice**

- Teach patients the importance of adhering to *H. pylori* treatment to prevent development of gastric cancer. **QSEN: Evidence-Based Practice**

Psychosocial Integrity

- Allow patients with gastric cancer to express feelings of grief, fear, and anxiety. **QSEN: Patient-Centered Care**
- For patients with advanced gastric cancer, identify end-of-life care needs, including referral to hospice care. **Ethics**

Physiological Integrity

- Recall that *acute* gastritis causes a rapid onset of epigastric pain and dyspepsia; *chronic* gastritis causes vague epigastric pain (usually relieved with food) and intolerance to fatty and spicy foods (see Chart 55-2).
- Remember that patients with gastric ulcers may be malnourished and have pain that is worsened by ingestion of food; patients with duodenal ulcers are usually well nourished,

have pain that is relieved by ingestion of food, and awaken with pain during the night (see Table 55-2).

- For patients who have undergone a gastrectomy, collaborate with the dietitian and instruct the patient regarding diet changes to avoid abdominal distention and dumping syndrome. **QSEN: Teamwork and Collaboration**
- Teach patients with abnormal abdominal symptoms to consult with their health care provider immediately. **QSEN: Safety**
- Teach that hematemesis is a medical emergency and refer to the emergency department for prompt treatment. **QSEN: Safety**
- Teach the proper administration of antacids (one or two after meals), reminding patients that antacids can interfere with the effectiveness of certain drugs, such as phenytoin (Dilantin). **QSEN: Evidence-Based Practice**
- Teach the proper administration of H_2 antagonists and explain that they should be taken at bedtime (see Chart 55-3). **QSEN: Evidence-Based Practice**

- Teach the proper administration of antisecretory agents, noting that most cannot be crushed because they are sustained-release or enteric-coated tablets. **QSEN: Evidence-Based Practice**
- Monitor patients with ulcers for signs and symptoms of upper GI bleeding that are listed in Chart 55-4. Report any of these symptoms to the health care provider immediately. **QSEN: Safety**
- After an EGD, monitor vital signs, heart rhythm, and oxygen saturation frequently until they return to baseline. To prevent aspiration, assess the gag reflex and ensure that it is intact before giving the patient food or fluids. **QSEN: Safety**
- Observe for signs and symptoms of dumping syndrome after gastric surgery; teach characteristics and management of this syndrome. **QSEN: Evidence-Based Practice**

SELECTED BIBLIOGRAPHY

American Cancer Society. (2017). *Stomach Cancer*. http://www.cancer.org/cancer/stomachcancer/detailedguide/stomach-cancer-key-statistics.

Eusebi, L., Zagari, R., & Bazzoli, F. (2014). Epidemiology of helicobacter pylori infection. *Helicobacter, 19*(Suppl.), 1–5. doi:10.1111/hel.12165.

Haastrup, P., Paulsen, M. S., Begtrup, L. M., Hansen, J. M., & Jarbol, D. E. (2014). Strategies for discontinuation of proton pump inhibitors: A systematic review. *Family Practice, 31*(6), 625–630.

Lilley, L., Rainforth Collins, S., & Snyder, J. (2017). *Pharmacology and the nursing process* (8th ed.). St. Louis: Elsevier.

McCance, K., Huether, S., Brashers, V., & Rote, N. (2014). *Pathophysiology: the biologic basis for disease in adults and children* (7th ed.). St. Louis: Mosby.

Mulcahy, E. A. (2015). Nursing perspectives: The state of the science of proton pump inhibitors causing osteoporotic changes in postmenopausal women. *Society of Gastroenterology Nurses and Associates, 38*(2), 129–133.

National Institute of Diabetes and Digestive and Kidney Diseases. (2017). *Definitions and facts for peptic ulcers (stomach ulcers)*. https://www.niddk.nih.gov/health-information/health-topics/digestive-diseases/peptic-ulcer/pages/definition-facts.aspx.

Pagana, K., Pagana, T. J., & Pagana, T. N. (2017). *Mosby's diagnostic and laboratory test reference* (13th ed.). St. Louis: Mosby.

CHAPTER 56

Care of Patients With Noninflammatory Intestinal Disorders

Keelin Cromar

PRIORITY AND INTERRELATED CONCEPTS

The priority concepts for this chapter are:
- ELIMINATION
- CELLULAR REGULATION

✳ The ELIMINATION concept exemplar for this chapter is Intestinal Obstruction, below.

✳ The CELLULAR REGULATION concept exemplar for this chapter is Colorectal Cancer, p. 1126.

The interrelated concepts for this chapter are:
- NUTRITION
- COMFORT
- FLUID AND ELECTROLYTE BALANCE

LEARNING OUTCOMES

Safe and Effective Care Environment

1. Collaborate with the interprofessional team to protect the patient with a noninflammatory intestinal disorder from injury and infection.
2. Identify community resources to ensure appropriate transition management for patients with a noninflammatory intestinal disorder.

Health Promotion and Maintenance

3. Teach adults health promotion practices to prevent noninflammatory intestinal disorders.
4. Teach patients with a colostomy about self-management.

Psychosocial Integrity

5. Implement nursing interventions to minimize stressors for the patient with a noninflammatory intestinal disorder.

Physiological Integrity

6. Apply knowledge of anatomy, physiology, pathophysiology, genetic risk, age-related changes, and psychomotor skills to perform a focused assessment of the gastrointestinal system.
7. Prioritize care for patients with colorectal cancer (CRC).
8. Describe interprofessional care and educational needs to promote NUTRITION and COMFORT for the patient with a noninflammatory intestinal disorder.
9. Differentiate between assessment findings associated with small-bowel and large-bowel obstructions.
10. Develop an evidence-based plan of care for the patient undergoing an intestinal surgical procedure.

If not diagnosed and managed early, certain intestinal problems can lead to inadequate absorption of vital nutrients and affect the need for NUTRITION and ELIMINATION. If these disorders become severe or progress, COMFORT and/or CELLULAR REGULATION alterations and problems with FLUID AND ELECTROLYTE BALANCE may occur. Intestinal health problems are classified as inflammatory or noninflammatory; this chapter focuses on disorders that are noninflammatory in origin.

✳ ELIMINATION CONCEPT EXEMPLAR
Intestinal Obstruction

❖ PATHOPHYSIOLOGY

Intestinal obstructions can be partial or complete and are classified as mechanical or nonmechanical. With either condition, ELIMINATION is compromised by this common and serious disorder.

Types of Intestinal Obstructions

In **mechanical obstruction**, the bowel is physically blocked by problems outside the intestine (e.g., adhesions), in the bowel wall (e.g., Crohn's disease), or in the intestinal lumen (e.g., tumors). **Nonmechanical obstruction** (also known as **paralytic ileus** or *adynamic ileus)* does not involve a physical obstruction in or outside the intestine. Instead, peristalsis is decreased or absent as a result of neuromuscular disturbance, resulting in a slowing of the movement or a backup of intestinal contents (McCance et al., 2014).

Intestinal contents are composed of ingested fluid, food, and saliva; gastric, pancreatic, and biliary secretions; and swallowed air. In both mechanical and nonmechanical obstructions, the intestinal contents accumulate at and above the area of obstruction. Distention results from the intestine's inability to absorb the contents and move them down the intestinal tract. To compensate for the lag, peristalsis increases in an effort to move the intestinal contents forward. This increase stimulates more secretions, which then leads to additional distention. The bowel then becomes edematous, and increased capillary permeability results. Plasma leaking into the peritoneal cavity and fluid trapped in the intestinal lumen decrease the absorption of fluid and electrolytes into the vascular space. Reduced circulatory blood volume (hypovolemia) and electrolyte imbalances typically occur. Hypovolemia ranges from mild to extreme (hypovolemic shock).

Complications of Intestinal Obstruction

Specific problems related to FLUID AND ELECTROLYTE BALANCE and acid-base balance result, depending on the part of the intestine that is blocked. An obstruction high in the small intestine causes a loss of gastric hydrochloride, which can lead to *metabolic alkalosis.* Obstruction below the duodenum but above the large bowel results in a loss of both acids and bases so that acid-base balance is usually not compromised. Obstruction at the end of the small intestine and lower in the intestinal tract causes loss of alkaline fluids, which can lead to *metabolic acidosis* (McCance et al., 2014).

If hypovolemia is severe, acute kidney injury or even death can occur. Bacterial peritonitis with or without actual perforation can also result. Bacteria in the intestinal contents lie stagnant in the obstructed intestine. This is not a problem unless the blood flow to the intestine is compromised. However, with *closed-loop obstruction* (blockage in two different areas) or a **strangulated obstruction** (obstruction with compromised blood flow), the risk for peritonitis is greatly increased. Bacteria without blood supply can form and release an endotoxin into the peritoneal or systemic circulation and cause septic shock. With a strangulated obstruction, major blood loss into the intestine and the peritoneum can occur. Sepsis and bleeding can result in an increased intra-abdominal pressure (IAP) or acute compartment syndrome.

Etiology

Intestinal obstruction is caused by a variety of conditions and associated with significant morbidity. It can occur anywhere in the intestinal tract, although the ileum in the small intestine (the narrowest part of the intestinal tract) is the most common site.

Mechanical obstruction can result from:
- Adhesions (scar tissue from surgeries or pathology)
- Benign or malignant tumor

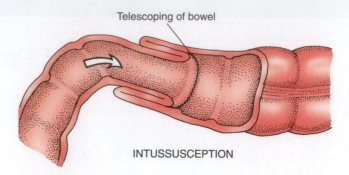

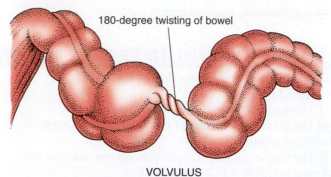

FIG. 56-1 Two major types of mechanical obstruction.

- Complications of appendicitis
- Hernias
- Fecal impactions (especially in older adults)
- Strictures due to Crohn's disease (an inflammatory condition) or previous radiation therapy
- **Intussusception** (telescoping of a segment of the intestine within itself) (Fig. 56-1)
- **Volvulus** (twisting of the intestine) (see Fig. 56-1)
- Fibrosis due to disorders such as endometriosis
- Vascular disorders (e.g., emboli and arteriosclerotic narrowing of mesenteric vessels)

In people ages 65 years or older, diverticulitis, tumors, and fecal impaction are the most common causes of obstruction (McCance et al., 2014).

Postoperative ileus (POI) (paralytic ileus), or *nonmechanical* obstruction, is most commonly caused by handling of the intestines during abdominal surgery. In patients with POI, intestinal function is lost for a few hours to several days. Electrolyte disturbances, especially hypokalemia, predispose the patient to this problem. The ileus can also be a consequence of **peritonitis** because leakage of colonic contents causes severe irritation and triggers an inflammatory response and infection (see discussion of the Concept Exemplar of peritonitis in Chapter 57). Vascular insufficiency to the bowel, also referred to as *intestinal ischemia,* is another potential cause of an ileus. It results when arterial or venous thrombosis or an embolus decreases blood flow to the mesenteric blood vessels surrounding the intestines, as in heart failure or severe shock. Severe insufficiency of blood supply can result in infarction of surrounding organs (e.g., bowel infarction).

❖ *INTERPROFESSIONAL COLLABORATIVE CARE*

Care for the patient with an intestinal obstruction takes place in the hospital setting. The interprofessional team that collaborates to care for this patient generally includes the surgeon, nurse, and dietitian.

◆ **Assessment: Noticing**

History. Collect information about a history of GI disorders, surgeries, and treatments. Question the patient about recent nausea and vomiting and the color of emesis, noting if vomitus is described as green, bilious, or hematemesis. Perform a thorough pain assessment with particular attention to the onset, aggravating factors, alleviating factors, and patterns or rhythms of the pain. Severe pain that then stops and changes to tenderness on palpation may indicate perforation and should be reported promptly to the physician. Ask about the passage of flatus and the time, character, and consistency of the last bowel movement. Singultus (hiccups) is common with all types of intestinal obstruction. When an obstruction is suspected, keep the patient NPO and contact the physician promptly for further direction.

Assess for a family history of colorectal cancer (CRC) and ask about blood in the stool or a change in bowel pattern. Body temperature with uncomplicated obstruction is rarely higher than 100° F (37.8° C). A temperature higher than this, with or without guarding and tenderness, and a sustained elevation in pulse could indicate a strangulated obstruction or peritonitis. A fever, tachycardia, hypotension, increasing abdominal pain, abdominal rigidity, or change in color of skin overlying the abdomen should be reported to the health care provider immediately.

Physical Assessment/Signs and Symptoms. The patient with *mechanical* obstruction in the *small intestine* often has mid-abdominal pain or cramping. The pain can be sporadic, and the patient may feel comfortable between episodes. If strangulation is present, the pain becomes more localized and steady. Vomiting often accompanies obstruction and is more profuse with obstructions in the proximal small intestine. The vomitus may contain bile and mucus or be orange-brown and foul smelling as a result of bacterial overgrowth with low ileal obstruction. Prolonged vomiting can result in a disruption in FLUID AND ELECTROLYTE BALANCE. **Obstipation** (no passage of stool) and failure to pass flatus are signs of ELIMINATION concerns associated with complete obstruction; diarrhea may be present in partial obstruction.

Mechanical colonic obstruction causes a milder, more intermittent colicky abdominal pain than is seen with small-bowel obstruction. Lower abdominal distention and obstipation may be present, or the patient may have ribbonlike stools if obstruction is partial. ELIMINATION alterations in bowel patterns and blood in the stools may accompany the obstruction if colorectal cancer or diverticulitis is the cause.

On examination of the abdomen, observe for abdominal distention, which is common in all forms of intestinal obstruction. Peristaltic waves may also be visible. Auscultate for proximal high-pitched bowel sounds **(borborygmi)**, which are associated with cramping early in the obstructive process as the intestine tries to push the mechanical obstruction forward. In later stages of mechanical obstruction, bowel sounds are absent, especially distal to the obstruction. Abdominal tenderness and rigidity are usually minimal. The presence of a tense, fluid-filled bowel loop mimicking a palpable abdominal mass may signal a closed-loop, strangulating small-bowel obstruction.

In most types of *nonmechanical* obstruction, the pain is described as a constant, diffuse discomfort. Colicky cramping is not characteristic of this type of obstruction. Pain associated with obstruction caused by vascular insufficiency or infarction

 CHART 56-1 Key Features

Small-Bowel and Large-Bowel Obstructions

SMALL-BOWEL OBSTRUCTIONS	LARGE-BOWEL OBSTRUCTIONS
Abdominal discomfort or pain possibly accompanied by visible peristaltic waves in upper and middle abdomen	Intermittent lower abdominal cramping
Upper or epigastric abdominal distention	Lower abdominal distention
Nausea and early, profuse vomiting (may contain fecal material)	Minimal or no vomiting
Obstipation	Obstipation or ribbonlike stools
Severe fluid and electrolyte imbalances	No major fluid and electrolyte imbalances
Metabolic alkalosis	Metabolic acidosis (not always present)

is usually severe and constant. On inspection, abdominal distention is typically present. On auscultation of the abdomen, note and document decreased bowel sounds in early obstruction and absent bowel sounds in later stages. Vomiting of gastric contents and bile is frequent, but the vomitus rarely has a foul odor and is rarely profuse. Obstipation may or may not be present. Chart 56-1 compares small- and large-bowel obstructions.

Diagnostic Assessment. There is no definitive laboratory test to confirm a diagnosis of mechanical or nonmechanical obstruction. *White blood cell (WBC) counts* are normal unless there is a strangulated obstruction, in which case there may be leukocytosis (increased WBCs). *Hemoglobin, hematocrit, creatinine, and blood urea nitrogen (BUN)* values are often elevated, indicating dehydration. Serum sodium, chloride, and potassium are decreased. Elevations in serum amylase levels may be found with strangulating obstructions, which can damage the pancreas.

The health care provider obtains imaging information in the form of an *abdominal CT scan* or MRI as soon as an obstruction is suspected. Distention with fluid and gas in the small intestine with the absence of gas in the colon indicates an obstruction in the small intestine.

The diagnostic examination chosen depends on the suspected location of the obstruction. As an initial assessment, the health care provider may order an *abdominal ultrasound* to evaluate the potential cause of the obstruction. The health care provider may perform endoscopy (sigmoidoscopy or colonoscopy) to determine the cause of the obstruction, except when perforation or complete obstruction is suspected.

◆ **Analysis: Interpreting**

The priority collaborative problems for patients with intestinal obstruction include:

1. Potential for injury (e.g., peritonitis, acute kidney injury) due to obstruction
2. Acute pain due to obstruction

◆ **Planning and Implementation: Responding**

Interventions are aimed at uncovering the cause and relieving the obstruction. Relieving the obstruction simultaneously

CHART 56-2　Best Practice for Patient Safety & Quality Care QSEN

Nursing Care of Patients Who Have an Intestinal Obstruction

- Monitor vital signs, especially blood pressure, for indications of fluid balance.
- Assess the patient's abdomen at least twice a day for bowel sounds, distention, and passage of flatus.
- Monitor fluid and electrolyte status, including laboratory values.
- Manage the patient who has a nasogastric tube (NGT):
  - Monitor drainage.
  - Ensure tube patency.
  - Check tube placement.
  - Irrigate tube as prescribed.
  - Maintain the patient on NPO status.
  - Provide frequent mouth and nares care.
  - Maintain the patient in a semi-Fowler's position.
- Give analgesics for pain as prescribed.
- Give alvimopan (Entereg) as prescribed for patients with a postoperative ileus.
- Maintain parenteral NUTRITION if prescribed.

decreases the potential for injury and reduces pain. Intestinal obstructions can be relieved by nonsurgical or surgical means. If the obstruction is partial and there is no evidence of strangulation, nonsurgical management may be the treatment of choice (Chart 56-2). Once the obstruction has been addressed effectively, expected ELIMINATION patterns should resume.

Reducing Potential for Injury and Reducing Pain

Nonsurgical Management. Paralytic ileus responds well to nonsurgical methods of relieving obstruction. Nonsurgical approaches are also preferred in the treatment of patients with terminal disease associated with bowel obstruction. In addition to being NPO, patients typically have a nasogastric tube (NGT) inserted to decompress the bowel by draining fluid and air. The tube is attached to suction.

Nasogastric Tubes. Most patients with an obstruction have an NGT unless the obstruction is mild. A **Salem sump tube** is inserted through the nose and placed into the stomach. It is attached to low continuous suction. This tube has a vent ("pigtail") that prevents the stomach mucosa from being pulled away during suctioning. Levin tubes do not have a vent and therefore should only be connected to low intermittent suction. They are used much less often than the Salem sump tubes.

❗ NURSING SAFETY PRIORITY QSEN

Action Alert

At least every 4 hours, assess the patient with an NGT for proper placement of the tube, tube patency, and output (quality and quantity). Monitor the nasal skin around the tube for irritation. Use a device that secures the tube to the nose to prevent accidental removal. Assess for peristalsis by auscultating for bowel sounds with the suction disconnected (suction masks peristaltic sounds).

Ask the patient about the passage of flatus and record flatus and the character of bowel movements daily. Flatus or stool means that peristalsis has returned. Assess for nausea and ask the patient to report this symptom if he or she begins to experience it.

Monitor any NGT for proper functioning. Occasionally NGTs move out of optimal drainage position or become plugged. In this case, note a decrease in gastric output or stasis of the tube's contents. Assess the patient for nausea, vomiting, increased abdominal distention, and placement of the tube. If the NGT is repositioned or replaced, confirmation of proper placement may be obtained by x-ray before use. After appropriate placement is established, aspirate the contents and irrigate the tube with 30 mL of normal saline every 4 hours or as requested by the health care provider.

Other Nonsurgical Interventions. Most types of nonmechanical obstruction respond to nasogastric decompression with medical treatment of the primary disorder. Incomplete mechanical obstruction can sometimes be treated successfully without surgery. Obstruction caused by lower fecal impaction usually resolves after disimpaction and enema administration. Intussusception may respond to hydrostatic pressure changes during a barium enema.

For patients with a postoperative ileus (POI), alvimopan (Entereg) may be given for short-term use. This drug is an oral, peripherally acting mu opioid receptor antagonist that increases GI motility (Bragg et al., 2015).

IV fluid replacement and maintenance are indicated for all patients with intestinal obstruction because the patient is NPO and FLUID AND ELECTROLYTE BALANCE is lost (particularly potassium) through vomiting and nasogastric suction. On the basis of serum electrolytes and blood urea nitrogen (BUN) levels, the health care provider prescribes aggressive fluid replacement with 2 to 4 L of an isotonic solution (normal saline or lactated Ringer's solution) with potassium added. Use care with patients who are susceptible to fluid overload (e.g., older adults with a history of heart or kidney failure). Monitor lung sounds, weight, and intake and output daily. Weight is the most reliable indicator of fluid balance. Blood replacement may be indicated in strangulated obstruction because of blood loss into the bowel or peritoneal cavity.

Monitor vital signs and other measures of fluid status (e.g., urine output, skin turgor, mucous membranes) every 2 to 4 hours, depending on the severity of the patient's symptoms. In collaboration with the dietitian, the health care provider may prescribe parenteral NUTRITION (PN), especially if the patient has had chronic nutritional problems and has been NPO for an extended period. Chapter 60 discusses the nursing care of patients receiving PN.

The patient with intestinal obstruction is usually thirsty, although some older adults have a decreased thirst response. Delegate frequent mouth care to unlicensed assistive personnel (UAP) to help maintain moist mucous membranes. Be sure to supervise this activity. A few ice chips may be allowed if the patient is not having surgery. Follow agency protocol or the health care provider's request regarding ice chips.

Abdominal distention can cause a great deal of pain, especially when it is severe. The colicky, crampy pain that comes and goes with mechanical obstruction, as well as the nausea, vomiting, dry mucous membranes, and thirst contribute to the patient's alteration in COMFORT. Continually assess the character and location of the pain and immediately report any pain that significantly increases or changes from colicky and intermittent to a constant discomfort. These changes can indicate perforation of the intestine or peritonitis.

Opioid analgesics may be temporarily withheld in the diagnostic workup period so signs and symptoms of perforation or peritonitis are not masked. Explain to the patient and family the rationale for not giving analgesics. In addition, if analgesics such as morphine are given, they may slow intestinal motility and can cause vomiting. Be alert to this side effect because nausea and vomiting are also signs of NGT obstruction or worsening bowel obstruction. Consider the importance of nonpharmacologic pain control measures when withdrawing this type of medication.

Help the patient obtain a position of COMFORT with frequent position changes to promote increased peristalsis. A semi-Fowler's position helps alleviate the pressure of abdominal distention on the chest and promotes thoracic excursion to facilitate breathing.

Discomfort is generally lesser with nonmechanical obstruction than with mechanical obstruction. With both types of obstruction, COMFORT alterations are aggravated by taking in food or fluids.

If strangulation is thought to be likely, the health care provider prescribes IV broad-spectrum antibiotics. In addition, in cases of partial obstruction or paralytic ileus, drugs that enhance gastric motility such as octreotide acetate (Sandostatin) may be used.

Surgical Management. In patients with complete mechanical obstruction and in some cases of incomplete mechanical obstruction, surgical intervention is necessary to relieve the obstruction. A strangulated obstruction is complete, and surgical intervention is always required. An **exploratory laparotomy** (a surgical opening of the abdominal cavity to investigate the cause of the obstruction) is initially performed for many patients with obstruction. More specific surgical procedures depend on the cause of the obstruction.

Preoperative Care. Provide general preoperative teaching for both the patient and family as discussed in Chapter 14. In cases of complete obstruction, the patient may feel too ill to absorb and understand the information. In this case, reinforce the information with the family or other caregiver. Depending on the cause and severity of the obstruction and the expertise of the surgeon, patients have either minimally invasive surgery (MIS) via laparoscopy or a conventional open approach.

Operative Procedures. In the *conventional open surgical approach*, the surgeon makes a large incision, enters the abdominal cavity, and explores for obstruction and its cause, if possible (exploratory laparotomy). If adhesions are found, they are lysed (cut and released). Obstruction caused by a tumor or diverticulitis requires a colon resection with primary anastomosis or a temporary or permanent colostomy. If obstruction is caused by intestinal infarction, an embolectomy, thrombectomy, or resection of the gangrenous small or large bowel may be necessary. In severe cases a colectomy (removal of the entire colon) may be needed.

For the *MIS* approach, the specially trained surgeon makes several small incisions in the abdomen and places a video camera to view the abdominal contents to determine the extent of the obstruction. A laparoscope (type of endoscope) with a lighted end is inserted along with various surgical instruments to address and remove the problem. This procedure takes longer than the open approach, but blood loss is less, and healing is faster. Robotic assistance may be used, depending on the experience of the surgeon and available equipment.

Postoperative Care. General postoperative care for the patient undergoing an *exploratory laparotomy* with lysis of adhesions, colon resection, thrombectomy, or embolectomy is similar to that described in Chapter 16. In addition, patients who had an open surgical approach have an NGT in place until peristalsis resumes. A clear liquid diet may be prescribed to encourage peristalsis return. As liquids are started, the NGT can be disconnected from suction and capped for 1 to 2 hours after the patient has taken clear liquids to determine if he or she is able to tolerate them. If the patient vomits after liquids, the suction is resumed. When the patient has return of peristalsis, the NGT suction is discontinued, and the tube is clamped for a scheduled amount of time. If the patient does not experience nausea while the NGT is clamped, the tube is removed.

Most patients today have laparoscopic surgery (MIS) for mechanical intestinal obstructions. They usually do *not* have an NGT and can recover more quickly than those with the open surgical approach. The hospital stay for a patient having MIS to remove tumors, adhesions, and other obstructions may be as short as 1 to 2 days compared with 3 days or longer for the conventional surgical patients. Recovery is much quicker because there is less pain and there are fewer postoperative complications among those who had laparoscopic surgery.

❓ CLINICAL JUDGMENT CHALLENGE 56-1

Patient-Centered Care; Teamwork and Collaboration; Informatics QSEN

You receive a 40-year-old woman on your medical-surgical unit after being admitted from the emergency department for a bowel obstruction. When the patient arrives, she has a Salem sump nasogastric tube (NGT) in place that is currently clamped. She also has IV normal saline running at 125 mL/hr. The patient's vital signs are stable, except for her blood pressure, which remains low at 90/45. She reports a pain score of 8/10 in her lower abdomen. The patient currently does not have orders related to her NGT.

1. After the patient arrives, what are your primary assessments?
2. What nursing intervention is appropriate related to the patient's incomplete NGT orders?
3. Using SBAR, how will you communicate the information about this patient to the health care provider?
4. What immediate evidence-based collaborative interventions are appropriate for this patient?
5. What information will you document in the electronic health record?

Care Coordination and Transition Management

All patients with intestinal obstruction are hospitalized for monitoring and treatment. The length of stay varies according to the type of obstruction, the treatment, and the presence of complications. Patients who have complicated obstruction, such as strangulation or incarceration, are at greater risk for peritonitis, sepsis, and shock.

Patients with nonmechanical (adynamic) intestinal obstruction are less likely to require a lengthy hospitalization because of the obstruction alone. Nonmechanical obstruction generally responds to nasogastric suction and possible drug therapy within a few days. However, if the ileus occurs as a complication of an abdominal surgery, the hospital stay could be lengthy.

Home Care Management. Preparation for home care depends on the cause of the obstruction and the treatment required. Those who have resolution of obstruction without surgical intervention are assessed for their knowledge of strategies to avoid recurrent obstruction. For example, if fecal impaction was the cause of the obstruction, assess the patient's ability to carry out a bowel regimen independently (Chart 56-3). For those who have had surgery, evaluate their ability to function at home with the added tasks of incision care and possibly colostomy care.

Preventing Fecal Impaction

- Teach the patient to eat high-fiber foods, including plenty of raw fruits and vegetables and whole-grain products.
- Encourage the patient to drink adequate amounts of fluids, especially water.
- Do not routinely administer a laxative; teach the patient that laxative abuse decreases abdominal muscle tone and contributes to an atonic colon.
- Encourage the patient to exercise regularly, if possible. Walking every day is an excellent exercise for promoting intestinal motility.
- Use natural foods to stimulate peristalsis, such as warm beverages and prune juice.
- Take bulk-forming products, such as Metamucil, to provide fiber.
- Check the patient's stool for amount and frequency; oozing of soft or diarrheal stool often indicates a fecal impaction.
- Have the patient sit on a toilet or bedside commode rather than on a bedpan for ELIMINATION.

Self-Management Education. Instruct the patient to report any abdominal pain or distention, nausea, or vomiting, with or without constipation, because these symptoms might indicate recurrent obstruction. However, the patient should be reassured that recurrent paralytic ileus is not common.

Teach the patient who has had surgery about incision care, drug therapy, and activity limitations. Drug therapy consists of an oral opioid analgesic, such as oxycodone hydrochloride with acetaminophen (Percocet), to be taken as needed for incisional discomfort. As with any opioid therapy, an over-the-counter laxative with a softener (e.g., docusate with senna) or polyethylene glycol (MiraLax) may be added to prevent constipation and possible recurrent obstruction.

The patient who had curative treatment of the underlying cause most likely requires less support than one who had treatment of obstruction related to a serious disease that will require further management. Encourage the patient to express fears and concerns about the future. Assess the patient's understanding and needs with regard to treatment plans.

Health Care Resources. The need for follow-up appointments depends on the cause of the obstruction and the treatment required. In collaboration with the case manager, make arrangements for a home care nurse if the patient needs help with incision or colostomy care.

◆ **Evaluation: Reflecting**

Evaluate the care of the patient with intestinal obstruction based on the identified priority patient problems. The expected outcomes are that the patient will have relief of the obstruction and no evidence of injury (e.g., development of peritonitis or acute kidney injury) and report that pain is controlled.

POLYPS

❖ PATHOPHYSIOLOGY

Polyps in the intestinal tract are small growths covered with mucosa and attached to the surface of the intestine. Although most are benign, they are significant because some have the potential to become malignant.

Polyps can be classified as an adenomatous, malignant, or hyperplastic. Hyperplastic polyps have little chance of becoming cancerous; whereas adenomas have the potential to become malignant. A very small number of adenomas progress to cancer; almost all colorectal cancers develop from an adenoma. Adenomas are further classified as villous or tubular. Of these, villous adenomas pose a greater cancer risk. Malignant polyps are those that contain cancerous cells when they are discovered.

Familial adenomatous polyposis (FAP) and hereditary nonpolyposis colorectal cancer (HNPCC) are inherited syndromes characterized by progressive development of colorectal adenomas. Unless these syndromes are treated, colorectal cancer (CRC) inevitably occurs by the fourth to fifth decade of life. These conditions are discussed in the Genetic/Genomic Considerations feature in the Colorectal Cancer section.

❖ INTERPROFESSIONAL COLLABORATIVE CARE

Polyps are usually asymptomatic and are discovered during routine colonoscopy screening. However, they can cause gross rectal bleeding, intestinal obstruction, or intussusception (telescoping of the bowel). Biopsy specimens of polyps can be obtained, and the entire polyp can be removed (polypectomy) during this procedure with the use of a snare that fits through the sigmoidoscope or colonoscope. This often eliminates the need for abdominal surgery to remove a suspicious or definitely malignant polyp. The patient with FAP often requires a total colectomy (colon removal) to prevent the development of cancer (see the Genetic/Genomic Considerations box).

Psychosocial Integrity

A client with rectal bleeding who is preparing to undergo a colonoscopy tells the nurse, "I'm very afraid of having polyps and cancer." What is the appropriate nursing response?
A. "Let's worry about that after the procedure."
B. "Polyps are never cancerous, so you don't need to worry."
C. "Unfortunately all polyps are malignant, so you may already have cancer."
D. "It's understandable that you are fearful. Tell me what frightens you most."

Nursing care focuses on patient education. Instruct the patient about:

- The nature of the polyp
- Signs and symptoms to report to the health care provider
- The need for regular, routine monitoring or screening

If the patient has had a polypectomy, follow-up sigmoidoscopic or colonoscopic examinations are needed because of an increased risk for developing multiple polyps.

Nursing care of the patient after a polypectomy of the colorectal area includes monitoring for abdominal distention and pain, rectal bleeding, mucopurulent drainage from the rectum, and fever. A small amount of blood might appear in the stool after a polypectomy, but this should be temporary.

✳ CELLULAR REGULATION CONCEPT EXEMPLAR
Colorectal Cancer

❖ PATHOPHYSIOLOGY

Colorectal refers to the colon and rectum, which together make up the large intestine, also known as the *large bowel*. Colorectal

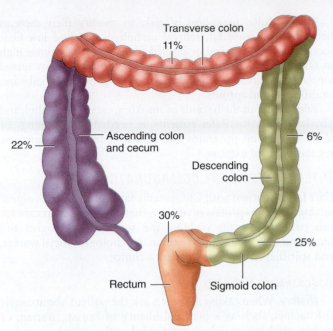

FIG. 56-2 Incidence of cancer in relation to colorectal anatomy.

cancer (CRC) is cancer of the colon or rectum. This CELLULAR REGULATION concern (see Chapter 2) is a major health problem worldwide. In the United States, it is one of the most common malignancies. Patients often consider a diagnosis of cancer as a "death sentence," but colon cancer is highly curable for many patients, especially if caught early.

Tumors occur in different areas of the colon, with about two thirds occurring within the rectosigmoid region as shown in Fig. 56-2. Most CRCs are **adenocarcinomas,** which are tumors that arise from the glandular epithelial tissue of the colon. Abnormal CELLULAR REGULATION develops as a multi-step process affecting immunity, resulting in a number of molecular changes. These changes include loss of key tumor suppressor genes and activation of certain oncogenes that alter colonic mucosa cell division. The increased proliferation of the colonic mucosa forms polyps that can transform into malignant tumors. Most CRCs are believed to arise from adenomatous polyps that present as visible protrusions from the mucosal surface of the bowel (McCance et al., 2014).

CRC can metastasize by direct extension or by spreading through the blood or lymph. The tumor may spread locally into the four layers of the bowel wall and into neighboring organs. It may enlarge into the lumen of the bowel or spread through the lymphatics or the circulatory system. CRC enters the circulatory system directly from the primary tumor through blood vessels in the bowel or via the lymphatic system. The liver is the most common site of metastasis from circulatory spread. Metastasis to the lungs, brain, bones, and adrenal glands may also occur. Colon tumors can also spread by peritoneal seeding during surgical resection of the tumor. Seeding may occur when a tumor is excised and cancer cells break off from the tumor into the peritoneal cavity. For this reason, special techniques are used during surgery to decrease this possibility.

Complications related to the abnormal CELLULAR REGULATION in the increasing growth of the tumor locally or through metastatic spread include bowel obstruction or perforation with resultant peritonitis, abscess formation, and fistula formation

to the urinary bladder or the vagina. The tumor may invade neighboring blood vessels and cause frank bleeding. Gradual obstruction of the intestine can occur when tumors grow; these tumors can eventually block it completely. Tumors extending beyond the bowel wall may place pressure on neighboring organs (uterus, urinary bladder, and ureters) and cause symptoms that mask those of the cancer. Chapter 21 discusses cancer pathophysiology in more detail.

Etiology and Genetic Risk

The major risk factors for the development of colorectal cancer (CRC) include being older than 50 years, genetic predisposition, personal or family history of cancer, and/or diseases that predispose the patient to cancer such as familial adenomatous polyposis (FAP), Crohn's disease, and ulcerative colitis (McCance et al., 2014). Only a small percentage of colorectal cancers are familial and transmitted genetically.

❓ NCLEX EXAMINATION CHALLENGE 56-2

Health Promotion and Maintenance

The community nurse is talking with a group of individuals about colorectal cancer (CRC) risk factors. Which community participant is at the **highest risk** for development of CRC?
A. 23-year-old vegetarian
B. 30-year-old with Crohn's disease
C. 39-year-old with no family history of cancer
D. 46-year-old with genetic predisposition to cancer

🧬 GENETIC/GENOMIC CONSIDERATIONS

Patient-Centered Care **QSEN**

People with a first-degree relative (parent, sibling, or child) diagnosed with colorectal cancer (CRC) have three to four times the risk for developing the disease. An autosomal-dominant inherited genetic disorder known as *familial adenomatous polyposis (FAP)* accounts for 1% of CRCs. FAP is the result of one or more mutations in the adenomatous polyposis coli (APC) gene. In very young patients, thousands of adenomatous polyps develop over the course of 10 to 15 years and have nearly a 100% chance of becoming malignant. By 20 years of age, most patients require surgical intervention, usually a colectomy with ileostomy or ileoanal pull-through, to prevent cancer. Chemotherapy may also be used for cancer prevention (Roncucci & Mariani, 2015).

Lynch Syndrome, also known as hereditary nonpolyposis colorectal cancer (HNPCC), is another autosomal-dominant disorder and accounts for approximately 3% of all CRCs. Lynch Syndrome is also caused by gene mutations, including *MLH1* and *MLH2*. People with these mutations have an 80% chance of developing CRC at an average of 45 years of age. They also tend to have a higher incidence of endometrial, ovarian, stomach, small bowel, brain, and ureteral cancers (Lynch et al., 2009). Genetic testing is available for both of these familial CRC syndromes. Refer patients for genetic counseling and testing if the patient prefers.

The role of infectious agents in the development of colorectal and anal cancer continues to be investigated. Some lower GI cancers are related to *Helicobacter pylori, Streptococcus bovis,* John Cunningham (JC) virus, and human papilloma virus (HPV) infections.

There is also strong evidence that long-term smoking, obesity, physical inactivity, and heavy alcohol consumption are risk factors for CRC (American Cancer Society [ACS], 2016a).

A high-fat diet, particularly animal fat from red meats, increases bile acid secretion and anaerobic bacteria, which are thought to be carcinogenic for the bowel. Diets with large amounts of refined carbohydrates that lack fiber decrease bowel transit time.

Incidence and Prevalence

Colorectal cancer (CRC) is the third most common cause of cancer death in the United States (ACS, 2016). The overall incidence of CRC has decreased over the past 20 years, probably as a result of increased cancer screenings (Wilkes, 2013). The disease is most common in African Americans, and their survival rate is lower than that of Euro-Americans (Caucasians). The possible reasons for this difference include less use of diagnostic testing (especially colonoscopy), increased biological susceptibilities, decreased access to health care, lack of health insurance, cultural or spiritual beliefs, and lack of education about the need for early cancer detection (Haddad & You, 2016; Tammana & Laiyemo, 2014).

Health Promotion and Maintenance

People at risk can take action to decrease their chance of getting CRC and/or increase their chance of surviving it. For example, those whose family members have had hereditary CRC should be genetically tested for FAP and Lynch Syndrome. If gene mutations are present, the individual at risk can collaborate with the health care team to decide which prevention or treatment plan to implement.

Teach adults about the need for diagnostic screening. When an adult turns 40 years of age, he or she should discuss with the primary health care provider the need for colon cancer screening. The interval depends on level of risk. Adults of average risk who are 50 years of age and older and without a family history should undergo regular CRC screening. The screening includes fecal occult blood testing (FOBT) every year, colonoscopy every 10 years, or double-contrast barium enema every 5 years. Adults who have a personal or family history of the disease should begin screening earlier and more frequently. Teach all patients to follow the American Cancer Society (ACS, 2016b) recommendations for CRC screening listed in Chart 56-4.

> ### ⊚ CHART 56-4 Best Practice for Patient Safety & Quality Care QSEN
>
> **Screening Recommendations for Men and Women Ages 50 Years and Older at Average Risk for Colorectal Cancer**
>
> | PROCEDURE | FREQUENCY | NOTES |
> |---|---|---|
> | Fecal occult blood test (FOBT) | Yearly | FOBT procedure: two or three samples from three consecutive bowel movements obtained at home; tested by physician or nurse |
> | **and** (chose one of the following) | | |
> | Sigmoidoscopy | Every 5 years | |
> | Double-contrast barium enema | Every 5 years | |
> | Colonoscopy | Every 10 years | |

Teach adults, regardless of risk, to modify their diets as needed to decrease fat, refined carbohydrates, and low-fiber foods. Encourage baked or broiled foods, especially those high in fiber and low in animal fat. Remind adults to eat increased amounts of brassica vegetables, including broccoli, cabbage, cauliflower, and sprouts.

Educate about the hazards of smoking, excessive alcohol, and physical inactivity. Refer patients as needed for smoking- or alcohol-cessation programs and recommend ways to increase regular physical exercise.

❖ INTERPROFESSIONAL COLLABORATIVE CARE

Care for the patient with CRC usually takes place in the hospital setting. The interprofessional team that collaborates to care for this patient generally includes the surgeon, oncologist, and nurse and may include the dietitian, psychologist, social worker, and spiritual leader of the patient's choice.

◆ Assessment: Noticing

History. When taking a history, ask the patient about major risk factors, such as a personal history of breast, ovarian, or endometrial cancer (which can spread to the colon); ulcerative colitis; Crohn's disease; familial polyposis or adenomas; polyps; or a family history of CRC. In addition, assess the patient's participation in age-specific cancer screening guidelines. Ask about whether the patient uses tobacco and/or alcohol. Assess his or her usual physical activity level. Explore cultural preferences because food choices may contribute to development of colon cancer.

Ask whether vomiting and changes in bowel ELIMINATION habits, such as constipation or change in shape of stool with or without blood, have been noted. The patient may also report fatigue (related to anemias), abdominal fullness, vague abdominal pain, or unintentional weight loss. These symptoms suggest advanced disease.

Physical Assessment/Signs and Symptoms. The signs and symptoms of CRC depend on the location of the tumor. *However, the most common signs are rectal bleeding, anemia, and a change in stool consistency or shape.* Stools may contain microscopic amounts of blood that are occult (hidden), or the patient may have mahogany (dark)-colored or bright red stools (Fig. 56-3). Gross blood is not usually detected with tumors of the right side of the colon, but it is common (but not massive) with tumors of the left side of the colon and the rectum.

Tumors in the transverse and descending colon result in symptoms of obstruction as growth of the tumor blocks the passage of stool. The patient may report "gas pains," cramping, or incomplete evacuation. Tumors in the rectosigmoid colon are associated with **hematochezia** (the passage of red blood via the rectum), straining to pass stools, and narrowing of stools. Patients may report dull pain. Right-sided tumors can grow quite large without disrupting bowel patterns or appearance because the stool consistency is more liquid in this part of the colon. These tumors ulcerate and bleed intermittently; thus stools can contain mahogany (dark)-colored blood. A mass may be palpated in the lower right quadrant, and the patient often has anemia secondary to blood loss.

Examination of the abdomen begins with assessment for obvious distention or masses. Visible peristaltic waves accompanied by high-pitched or "tinkling" bowel sounds may indicate a partial bowel obstruction from the tumor. With auscultation, total absence of bowel sounds indicates a complete bowel

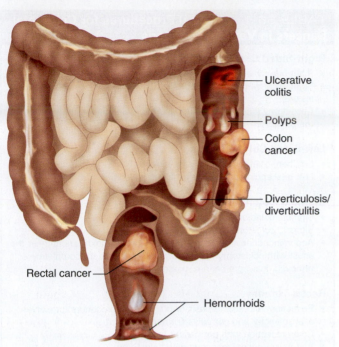

FIG. 56-3 Common causes of lower gastrointestinal bleeding.

Labels: Ulcerative colitis · Polyps · Colon cancer · Diverticulosis/diverticulitis · Rectal cancer · Hemorrhoids

obstruction. Palpation and percussion are performed by the advanced practice nurse or other health care provider to determine whether the spleen or liver is enlarged or whether masses are present along the colon. The examiner may also perform a digital rectal examination to palpate the rectum and lower sigmoid colon for masses. Fecal occult blood testing (FOBT) should not be done with a specimen from a rectal examination because it is not reliable. A positive result could occur as a consequence of tissue trauma during the examination.

Psychosocial Assessment. The psychological consequences associated with a diagnosis of colorectal cancer (CRC) are numerous. Patients must cope with a diagnosis that instills fear and anxiety about treatment, feelings that life has been disrupted, a need to search for ways to deal with the diagnosis, and concern about family. They also have questions about why colon cancer affected them, as well as concerns about pain, possible body changes, and possible death. In addition, if the cancer is believed to have a genetic origin, there is anxiety concerning implications for immediate family members.

Laboratory Assessment. Hemoglobin and hematocrit values are often decreased as a result of the intermittent bleeding associated with the tumor. For some patients, that may be the first indication that a tumor is present. CRC that has metastasized to the liver causes liver enzymes to be elevated.

A positive test result for occult blood in the stool (**fecal occult blood test [FOBT]**) indicates bleeding in the GI tract. These tests can yield false-positive results if certain vitamins or drugs are taken before the test. Depending on the age of the test being used, the patient may need to avoid aspirin, vitamin C, iron, and red meat for 48 hours before giving a stool specimen. Also assess whether the patient is taking anti-inflammatory drugs (e.g., ibuprofen, corticosteroids, or salicylates). These drugs should be discontinued for a designated period before the test. Two or three separate stool samples should be tested on 3 consecutive days. Negative results do not completely rule out

the possibility of CRC; for this reason additional testing may be suggested (see Chart 56-4).

Carcinoembryonic antigen (CEA), an oncofetal antigen, is elevated in many people with CRC. The normal value is less than 5 ng/mL (Pagana et al., 2017). This protein is not specifically associated with the CRC, and it may be elevated in the presence of other benign or malignant diseases and in smokers. CEA is often used to monitor the effectiveness of treatment and to identify disease recurrence.

Imaging Assessment. A *double-contrast barium enema* (air and barium are instilled into the colon) or colonoscopy provides better visualization of polyps and small lesions than does a barium enema alone. These tests may show an occlusion in the bowel where the tumor is decreasing the size of the lumen.

CT or *MRI* of the chest, abdomen, pelvis, lungs, or liver helps confirm the existence of a mass, the extent of disease, and the location of distant metastases. CT-guided virtual colonoscopy is growing in popularity and may be more thorough than traditional colonoscopy. However, treatments, biopsies, or surgeries cannot be performed when a virtual colonoscopy is used.

Other Diagnostic Assessment. A *sigmoidoscopy* provides visualization of the lower colon using a fiberoptic scope. Polyps can be visualized, and tissue samples can be taken for biopsy. Polyps are usually removed during the procedure. A *colonoscopy* provides views of the entire large bowel from the rectum to the ileocecal valve. As with sigmoidoscopy, polyps can be seen and removed, and tissue samples can be taken for biopsy. Colonoscopy is the definitive test for the diagnosis of colorectal cancer. These procedures and associated nursing care are discussed in Chapter 52.

◆ Analysis: Interpreting

The priority collaborative problems for patients with colorectal cancer (CRC) include:
1. Potential for metastasis due to colorectal cancer
2. Potential for grieving due to cancer diagnosis

◆ Planning and Implementation: Responding

The primary approach to treating CRC is to remove the entire tumor or as much of the tumor as possible to prevent or slow metastatic spread of the disease. A patient-centered collaborative care approach is essential to meet the desired outcomes.

Preventing or Controlling Metastasis

Planning: Expected Outcomes. The patient with colorectal cancer (CRC) is expected to not have the cancer spread to vital organs. Thus the patient's life expectancy will be increased, and the quality of life will be improved. However, if metastasis is present, the desired outcome is to limit further metastasis and to ensure that the patient is as comfortable as possible and pain is well managed.

Interventions. Although surgical resection is the primary method used to control the disease, several adjuvant (additional) therapies are used. Adjuvant therapies are administered before or after surgery to achieve a cure and prevent recurrence, if possible.

Nonsurgical Management. The type of therapy used is based on the pathologic staging of the disease. The staging system used most often in colorectal cancer is the TNM (tumor, nodes, metastasis) classification; more information on the use of this system can be found in Chapter 21.

The administration of preoperative *radiation therapy* has not improved overall survival rates for colon cancer, but it has been effective in providing local or regional control of the disease. Postoperative radiation has not demonstrated any consistent improvement in survival or recurrence. However, as a palliative measure, radiation therapy may be used to control pain, hemorrhage, bowel obstruction, or metastasis to the lung in advanced disease. For rectal cancer, unlike colon cancer, radiation therapy is almost always a part of the treatment plan. Reinforce information about the radiation therapy procedure to the patient and family and monitor for possible side effects (e.g., diarrhea, fatigue). Chapter 22 describes the general nursing care of patients undergoing radiation therapy.

Adjuvant *chemotherapy* after primary surgery is recommended for patients with stage II or stage III disease to interrupt the DNA production of cells and destroy them. The drugs of choice are IV 5-fluorouracil (5-FU) with leucovorin (LV) (folinic acid) (5-FU/LV), capecitabine (Xeloda), or a combination of drugs referred to as *FOLFOX4*. The most frequently used FOLFOX4 combination for metastatic CRC is fluorouracil (5-FU), leucovorin (LV), and oxaliplatin (Eloxatin), a platinum analog. These drugs cannot discriminate between cancer and healthy cells. Therefore common side effects are diarrhea, mucositis, leukopenia, mouth ulcers, and peripheral neuropathy (Cutsem et al., 2014).

Bevacizumab (Avastin) and panitumumab (Vectibix) are antiangiogenesis drugs, also known as *vascular endothelial growth factor (VEGF) inhibitors,* approved for advanced CRC. These drugs reduce blood flow to the growing tumor cells, thereby depriving them of necessary nutrients needed to grow (Cutsem et al., 2014). A VEGF inhibitor is usually given in combination with other chemotherapeutic agents.

Cetuximab (Erbitux), a monoclonal antibody known as an *epidermal growth factor receptor (EGFR) inhibitor (EGFRI),* may also be given in combination with other drugs for advanced disease (Cutsem et al., 2014). This drug works by blocking factors that promote cancer cell growth.

Intrahepatic arterial chemotherapy, often with 5-FU, may be administered to patients with liver metastasis. Patients with CRC also receive drugs for relief of symptoms, such as opioid analgesics and antiemetics. Chapter 22 describes care of patients receiving chemotherapy in detail.

Surgical Management. Surgical removal of the tumor with margins free of disease is the best method of ensuring removal of CRC. The size of the tumor, its location, the extent of metastasis, the integrity of the bowel, and the condition of the patient determine which surgical procedure is performed for colorectal cancer (Table 56-1). Many regional lymph nodes are removed and examined for presence of cancer. The number of lymph nodes that contain cancer is a strong predictor of prognosis. The most common surgeries performed are **colon resection** (removal of the tumor and regional lymph nodes) with reanastomosis, **colectomy** (colon removal) with *colostomy (temporary or permanent)* or *ileostomy/ileoanal pull-through,* and **abdominoperineal (AP) resection**. A **colostomy** is the surgical creation of an opening of the colon onto the surface of the abdomen. An AP resection is performed when rectal tumors are present. The surgeon removes the sigmoid colon, rectum, and anus through combined abdominal and perineal incisions.

For patients having a colon resection, minimally invasive surgery (MIS) via laparoscopy is commonly performed today. This procedure results in shorter hospital stays, less pain, fewer complications, and quicker recovery compared with the conventional open surgical approach (Kapritsou et al., 2013).

TABLE 56-1 **Surgical Procedures for Colorectal Cancers in Various Locations**

Right-Sided Colon Tumors
- Right hemicolectomy for smaller lesions
- Right ascending colostomy or ileostomy for large, widespread lesions
- Cecostomy (opening into the cecum with intubation to decompress the bowel)

Left-Sided Colon Tumors
- Left hemicolectomy for smaller lesions
- Left descending colostomy for larger lesions

Sigmoid Colon Tumors
- Sigmoid colectomy for smaller lesions
- Sigmoid colostomy for larger lesions
- Abdominoperineal resection for large, low sigmoid tumors (near the anus) with colostomy (the rectum and the anus are completely removed, leaving a perineal wound)

Rectal Tumors
- Resection with anastomosis or pull-through procedure (preserves anal sphincter and normal ELIMINATION pattern)
- Colon resection with permanent colostomy
- Abdominoperineal resection with colostomy

Preoperative Care. Reinforce the physician's explanation of the planned surgical procedure. The patient is told as accurately as possible what anatomic and physiologic changes will occur with surgery. The location and number of incision sites and drains are also discussed.

Before evaluating the tumor and colon during surgery, the surgeon may not be able to determine whether a colostomy (or less commonly, an ileostomy) will be necessary. The patient is told that a colostomy is a possibility. If a colostomy is planned, the surgeon consults a certified wound, ostomy, continence nurse (CWOCN) to recommend optimal placement of the ostomy. The CWOCN teaches the patient about the rationale and general principles of ostomy care. In many settings, the CWOCN marks the patient's abdomen to indicate a potential ostomy site that will decrease the risk for complications such as interference of the undergarments or a prosthesis with the ostomy appliance. Table 56-2 describes the role of the CWOCN.

The patient who requires low rectal surgery (e.g., AP resection) is faced with the risk for postoperative sexual dysfunction and urinary incontinence after surgery as a result of nerve damage during surgery. The surgeon discusses the risk for these problems with the patient before surgery and allows him or her to verbalize concerns and questions related to this risk before he or she gives informed consent. Reinforce teaching about abdominal surgery performed for the patient under general anesthesia and review the routines for turning and deep breathing (see Chapter 14). Teach the patient about the method of pain management to be used after surgery such as IV patient-controlled analgesia (PCA), epidural analgesia, or other method.

If the bowel is not obstructed or perforated, elective surgery is planned. The patient may be instructed to thoroughly clean the bowel, or "bowel prep," to minimize bacterial growth and prevent complications. Mechanical cleaning is accomplished with laxatives and enemas or with "whole-gut lavage." The use of bowel preps is controversial, and some surgeons do not recommend it because alterations in COMFORT may arise. Older adults may become dehydrated from this process.

To reduce the risk for infection, the surgeon may prescribe one dose of oral or IV antibiotics to be given before the surgical incision is made. Teach patients that a nasogastric tube (NGT) may be placed for decompression of the stomach after surgery.

A peripheral IV or central venous catheter is also placed for fluid and electrolyte replacement while the patient is NPO after surgery. Patients having minimally invasive surgeries do not need an NGT.

The patient with colorectal cancer faces a serious illness with long-term consequences of the disease and treatment. A case manager or social worker can be very helpful in identifying patient and family needs and ensuring continuity of care and support.

Operative Procedures. For the conventional open surgical approach, the surgeon makes a large incision in the abdomen and explores the abdominal cavity to determine whether the tumor can be removed. For a colon resection, the portion of the colon with the tumor is excised, and the two open ends of the bowel are irrigated before **anastomosis** (reattachment) of the colon. If an anastomosis is not feasible because of the location of the tumor or inflammation of the bowel, a colostomy is created.

A temporary or permanent colostomy may be created in the ascending, transverse, descending, or sigmoid colon (Fig. 56-4). One of several techniques is used to construct a colostomy. A loop **stoma** (surgical opening) is made by bringing a loop of colon to the skin surface, severing and everting the anterior wall, and suturing it to the abdominal wall. Loop colostomies are usually performed in the transverse colon and are usually temporary. An external rod may be used to support the loop until the intestinal tissue adheres to the abdominal wall. Care must be taken to avoid displacing the rod, especially during appliance changes.

TABLE 56-2 **Preoperative Assessment by the CWOCN Before Ostomy Surgery**
Key Points of Psychosocial Assessment
• Patient's and family's level of knowledge of disease and ostomy care
• Patient's educational level
• Patient's physical limitations (particularly sensory)
• Support available to patient
• Patient's type of employment
• Patient's involvement in activities such as hobbies
• Financial concerns regarding purchase of ostomy supplies
Key Points of Physical Assessment
• Before marking the placement for the ostomy, the nurse specialist considers:
• Contour of the abdomen in lying, sitting, and standing positions
• Presence of skinfolds, creases, bony prominences, and scars
• Location of belt line
• Location that is easily visible to the patient
• Possible location in the rectus muscle

CWOCN, Certified wound, ostomy, continence nurse.

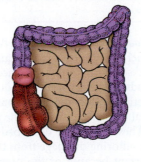

The **ascending colostomy** is done for right-sided tumors.

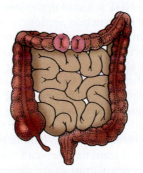

The **transverse (double-barrel) colostomy** is often used in such emergencies as intestinal obstruction or perforation because it can be created quickly. There are two stomas. The proximal one, closest to the small intestine, drains feces. The distal stoma drains mucus.

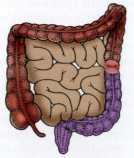

The **descending colostomy** is done for left-sided tumors.

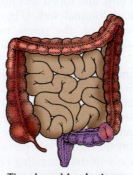

The **sigmoid colostomy** is done for rectal tumors.

FIG. 56-4 Different locations of colostomies in the colon.

An end stoma is often constructed, usually in the descending or sigmoid colon, when a colostomy is intended to be permanent. It may also be done when the surgeon oversews the distal stump of the colon and places it in the abdominal cavity, preserving it for future reattachment. An end stoma is constructed by severing the end of the proximal portion of the bowel and bringing it out through the abdominal wall.

The least common colostomy is the **double-barrel stoma**, which is created by dividing the bowel and bringing both the proximal and distal portions to the abdominal surface to create two stomas. The proximal stoma (closest to the patient's head) is the functioning stoma and eliminates stool. The distal stoma (farthest from the head) is considered nonfunctioning, although it may secrete some mucus. The distal stoma is sometimes referred to as a *mucous fistula.*

Laparoscopic (MIS) colon resection or total colectomy allows complete tumor removal with an adequate surgical margin and removal of associated lymph nodes. Several small incisions are made, and a miniature video camera is placed within the abdomen to help see the area that is involved. This technique takes longer than the conventional procedure and requires specialized training. However, blood loss is reduced.

Postoperative Care. Patients who have an *open colon resection* without a colostomy receive care similar to that of those having any abdominal surgery (see Chapter 16). Other patients have surgeries that also require colostomy management. They typically have a nasogastric tube (NGT) after open surgery and receive IV PCA for the first 24 to 36 hours. After NGT removal, the diet is slowly progressed from liquids to solid foods as tolerated. The care of patients with an NGT is found in the Interventions discussion in the Intestinal Obstruction section.

By contrast, patients who have *laparoscopic (MIS) surgery* can eat solid foods very soon after the procedure. Because they usually have less pain, they are able to ambulate earlier than those who have the conventional approach. The hospital stay is usually shorter for the patient with MIS—typically 1 to 2 days, depending on the patient's age and general condition.

Colostomy Management. The patient who has a colostomy may return from surgery with a clear ostomy pouch system in place. A clear pouch allows the health care team to observe the stoma. If no pouch system is in place, a petrolatum gauze dressing is usually placed over the stoma to keep it moist. This is covered with a dry, sterile dressing. In collaboration with the CWOCN, place a pouch system as soon as possible. The colostomy pouch system, also called an *appliance,* allows more convenient and suitable collection of stool than a dressing does.

Assess the color and integrity of the stoma frequently. A healthy stoma should be reddish pink and moist and protrude about ¾ inch (2 cm) from the abdominal wall (Fig. 56-5). During the initial postoperative period, the stoma may be slightly edematous. A small amount of bleeding at the stoma is common.

The colostomy should start functioning in 2 to 3 days after surgery. When it begins to function, the pouch may need to be emptied frequently because of excess gas collection. It should be emptied when it is one-third to one-half full of stool. Stool is liquid immediately after surgery but becomes more solid, depending on where in the colon the stoma was placed. For example, the stool from a colostomy in the ascending colon is liquid, the stool from a colostomy in the transverse colon is pasty, and the stool from a colostomy in the descending colon is more solid (similar to stool expelled from the rectum).

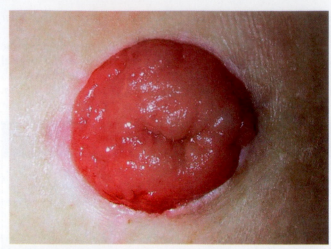

FIG. 56-5 Mature colostomy. (From Evans, S. [2009]. *Surgical pitfalls.* Philadelphia: Saunders.)

Wound Management. For an AP resection, the perineal wound is generally surgically closed, and two bulb suction drains such as Jackson-Pratt drains are placed in the wound or through stab wounds near the wound. The drains help prevent drainage from collecting within the wound and are usually left in place for several days, depending on the character and amount of drainage. These drains are described in more detail in Chapter 16.

Monitoring drainage from the perineal wound and cavity is important because of the possibility of infection and abscess formation. Serosanguineous drainage from the perineal wound may be observed for 1 to 2 months after surgery. Complete healing of the perineal wound may take 6 to 8 months. This wound can be a greater source of COMFORT alteration than the abdominal incision and ostomy, and more care may be required. The patient may experience phantom rectal sensations because sympathetic innervation for rectal control has not been interrupted. Rectal pain and itching may occasionally occur after healing. Interventions may include use of antipruritic drugs, such as benzocaine, and warm compresses. Continually assess for signs of infection, abscess, or other complications and implement methods for promoting wound drainage and comfort (Chart 56-5).

Assisting With the Grieving Process

Planning: Expected Outcomes. The expected outcomes are that the patient will verbalize feelings about the diagnosis and treatment and progress through the normal stages of grief.

Interventions. The patient and family are faced with a possible loss of or alteration in body functions. Medical and surgical interventions for the treatment of colorectal cancer may result in cure, disease control, or palliation. Nursing interventions are

NCLEX EXAMINATION CHALLENGE 56-3

Physiological Integrity

A client had an open partial colectomy and ascending colostomy 3 days ago. Which assessment findings does the nurse expect? **Select all that apply.**
A. Black, moist stoma
B. Gas inside the pouch
C. Pain controlled with analgesics
D. Small amount of formed stool from the colostomy
E. Serosanguineous fluid draining from two Jackson-Pratt drains

designed to help the patient and family plan effective strategies for expressing feelings of grief and developing coping skills.

Observe and identify:
- The patient's and family's current methods of coping
- Effective sources of support used in past crises
- The patient's and family's present perceptions of the health problem
- Signs of anticipatory grief, such as denial, crying, anger, and withdrawal from usual relationships

Encourage the patient and family to verbalize feelings about the diagnosis, treatment, and anticipated alteration in body functions if a colostomy is planned. (See the Operative Procedures discussion in the Surgical Management section.) Denial, sadness, anger, feelings of loss, and depression are common responses to this change in body function. The patient will need to learn new methods for toileting and how to cope with these changes.

If a colostomy is planned, instruct the patient on what to expect about the appearance and care of the colostomy. After surgery, encourage him or her to look at and touch the stoma. When the patient is physically able, ask him or her to participate in colostomy care. Participation helps restore the patient's sense of control over his or her lifestyle and thus facilitates improved self-esteem. If culturally appropriate, encourage participation of family or other caregivers in colostomy care.

Help the patient identify the nature of and reaction to the loss. Encourage the patient and family to verbalize feelings and identify fears to help move them through the appropriate phases of the grief process. Establish a trusting, ongoing relationship with the patient and family and provide support through the personal grieving stages.

In collaboration with the social worker or chaplain, help the patient identify personal coping strategies. Encourage him or her to implement cultural, spiritual, and social customs associated with the loss and identify sources of community support. Modifications in lifestyle are needed for patients with CRC. Help the patient and family identify these changes and how best to make them. The spiritual leader of the patient's choice, social worker, or case manager assists in discussions and decisions with them concerning treatment, the prognosis, and end-of-life decisions as appropriate.

GENETICS/GENOMICS CONSIDERATIONS

Patient-Centered Care QSEN

Refer patients who are at risk for or have familial CRC for genetic counseling. Specially trained nurses can discuss the purposes and goals of genetic testing. Ensure privacy and confidentiality. A review of the family history may provide important information concerning the pattern of CRC inheritance. To make an informed decision, the patient and family need information about the advantages, risks, and costs of appropriate genetic tests. Monitor the patient's response regarding genetic risk factors.

Care Coordination and Transition Management

Patients undergoing a colon resection by open approach are typically hospitalized for 2 to 3 days or longer, depending on the age of the patient and any complications or concurrent health problems. Collaborate with the case manager to help patients and their families cope with the immediate postoperative phase of recovery. After hospitalization for surgery, the patient is usually managed at home. Radiation therapy or chemotherapy is typically administered on an ambulatory care basis. For the patient with advanced cancer, hospice care may be an option (see Chapter 7).

Home Care Management. Assess all patients for their ability for self-management within limitations. For those requiring assistance with care, home care visits by nurses or assistive nursing personnel can be provided.

For the patient who has undergone a colostomy, review the home situation to help the patient arrange for care. Ostomy products should be kept in an area (preferably the bathroom) where the temperature is neither hot nor cold (skin barriers may become stiff or melt in extreme temperatures) to ensure proper functioning.

No changes are needed in sleeping accommodations. A moisture-proof covering may initially be placed over the bed mattress if patients feel insecure about the pouch system. They may consume their usual diet on discharge.

Self-Management Education. Before discharge, teach the patient to avoid lifting heavy objects or straining on defecation to prevent tension on the anastomosis site. If he or she had the open surgical approach, the patient should avoid driving and vigorous physical activity for 4 to 6 weeks while the incision heals. Patients who have had laparoscopy can usually return to all usual activities in 1 to 2 weeks.

Colostomy Care. Rehabilitation after surgery requires that patients and family members learn how to perform colostomy care. Provide adequate opportunity before discharge for patients to learn the psychomotor skills involved in this care. Plan sufficient practice time for learning how to handle, assemble, and apply all ostomy equipment. Teach patients and families or other caregivers about:

- Appearance of a normal stoma
- Signs and symptoms of complications
- Measurement of the stoma
- Choice, use, care, and application of the appropriate appliance to cover the stoma
- Measures to protect the skin adjacent to the stoma
- NUTRITION changes to control gas and odor
- What to expect in terms of stool consistency
- Resumption of normal activities, including work, travel, and sexual intercourse

The appropriate pouch system must be selected and fitted to the stoma. Patients with flat, firm abdomens may use either flexible (bordered with paper tape) or nonflexible (full skin barrier wafer) pouch systems. A firm abdomen with lateral creases or folds requires a flexible system. Patients with deep creases, flabby abdomens, a retracted stoma, or a stoma that is flush or concave to the abdominal surface can benefit from a convex appliance with a stoma belt. This type of system presses into the skin around the stoma, causing the stoma to protrude. This protrusion helps tighten the skin and prevents leaks around the stoma opening onto the peristomal skin.

Measurement of the stoma is necessary to determine the correct size of the stomal opening on the appliance. The opening should be large enough not only to cover the peristomal skin but also to avoid stomal trauma. The stoma will shrink within 6 to 8 weeks after surgery. Therefore it needs to be measured at least once weekly during this time to gauge appliance fit and COMFORT. Measurements are also necessary if the patient gains or loses weight. Teach the patient and family caregiver to trace the pattern of the stomal area on the wafer portion of the appliance and to cut an opening about $\frac{1}{8}$- to $\frac{1}{16}$-inch larger than the stomal pattern to ensure that stomal tissue will not be constricted.

Skin preparation may include clipping peristomal hair or shaving the area (moving from the stoma outward) to achieve a smooth surface, prevent unnecessary discomfort when the wafer is removed, and minimize the risk for infected hair follicles. Advise the patient to clean around the stoma with mild soap and water before putting on an appliance. He or she should avoid using moisturizing soaps to clean the area because the lubricants can interfere with adhesion of the appliance.

Control of gas and odor from the colostomy is often an important outcome for patients with new ostomies. Although a leaking or inadequately closed pouch is the usual cause of odor, flatus can also contribute to it. Remind the patient with an ostomy that, although generally no foods are forbidden, certain foods (such as vegetables) can cause flatus or contribute to odor when the pouch is open. Charcoal filters, pouch deodorizers, or placement of a breath mint in the pouch helps eliminate odors. The patient should be cautioned to not put aspirin tablets in the pouch because they may cause ulceration of the stoma. Vents that allow release of gas from the ostomy bag through a deodorizing filter are available and may decrease the patient's level of self-consciousness about odor.

The patient with a sigmoid colostomy may benefit from colostomy irrigation to regulate ELIMINATION. However, most patients with a sigmoid colostomy can become regulated through diet. An irrigation is similar to an enema but is administered through the stoma rather than the rectum.

In addition to teaching the patient about the signs and symptoms of obstruction and perforation, ask him or her to report any fever or sudden onset of pain or swelling around the stoma. Other home care assessment is listed in Chart 56-6.

Psychosocial Concerns. The diagnosis of cancer can be emotionally immobilizing for the patient and family or significant others, but treatment may be welcomed because it may provide hope for control of the disease. Explore reactions to the illness and perceptions of planned interventions.

The patient's reaction to ostomy surgery may include:

- Fear of not being accepted by others
- Feelings of grief related to disturbance in body image
- Concerns about sexuality

Encourage the patient and family to verbalize their feelings. Education about how to physically manage the ostomy will empower both the family and patient to begin restoration of self-esteem and improvement of body image. Inclusion of family and significant others in the rehabilitation process may help preserve relationships and raise self-esteem. Anticipatory instruction includes information on leakage accidents, odor control measures, and adjustments to resuming sexual relationships.

Health Care Resources. Several resources are available to maintain continuity of care in the home environment and provide for patient needs that the nurse is not able to meet. Make referrals to community-based case managers or social workers who can provide further emotional counseling, aid in managing financial concerns, or arrange for services in the home or long-term care facility as needed.

Provide information about the United Ostomy Associations of America, Inc. (www.uoaa.org), a self-help group of people with ostomies. This group has literature such as the organization's publication (*Ostomy Quarterly*) and information about local chapters. The organization conducts a visitor program that sends specially trained visitors (who have an ostomy [ostomate]) to talk with patients. After obtaining consent, make a referral to the visitor program so the volunteer ostomate can see the patient both before and after surgery. A health care provider's consent for visitation may be necessary.

The local division or unit of the American Cancer Society (ACS) (www.cancer.org) can help provide necessary medical equipment and supplies, home care services, travel accommodations, and other resources for the patient who is having cancer treatment or surgery. Inform the patient and family of the programs available through the local division or unit. Other excellent Internet resources include Cancer Care (www.cancercare.org), Colon Cancer Alliance (www.ccalliance.org), and the National Cancer Institute (www.nci.gov).

Because of short hospital stays, patients with new ostomies receive much health teaching from nurses working for home health care agencies. This resource also helps provide physical care needs, medication management, and emotional support. If the patient has advanced colorectal cancer, a referral for hospice services in the home, nursing home, or other long-term care setting may be appropriate. The home health care nurse informs the patient and family about which ostomy supplies are needed and where they can be purchased. Price and location are considered before recommendations are made.

◆ **Evaluation: Reflecting**

Evaluate the care of the patient with colorectal cancer based on the identified priority patient problems. The expected outcomes are that the patient:
- Adjusts to actual or impending loss
- Is free of complications or metastasis associated with CRC
- States that he or she has well-controlled pain and is as comfortable as possible (if metastasis is present)

IRRITABLE BOWEL SYNDROME

❖ PATHOPHYSIOLOGY

Irritable bowel syndrome (IBS) is a functional GI disorder that causes chronic or recurrent diarrhea, constipation, and/or abdominal pain and bloating. It is sometimes referred to as *spastic colon, mucous colon,* or *nervous colon* (Fig. 56-6). *IBS is the most common digestive disorder seen in clinical practice and*

may affect as many as one in five people in the United States (McCance et al., 2014).

In patients with IBS, bowel motility changes, and increased or decreased bowel transit times result in changes in the normal *bowel* ELIMINATION pattern to one of these classifications: diarrhea (IBS-D), constipation (IBS-C), alternating diarrhea and constipation (IBS-A), or a mix of diarrhea and constipation (IBS-M). Symptoms of the disease typically begin to appear in young adulthood and continue throughout the patient's life.

The etiology of IBS remains unclear. Research suggests that a combination of environmental, immunologic, genetic, hormonal, and stress factors play a role in the development and course of the disorder. Examples of environmental factors

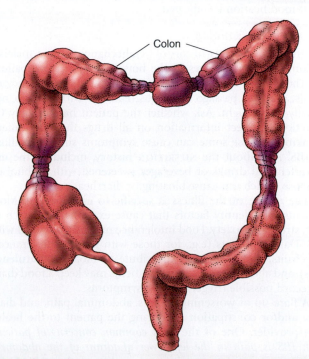

FIG. 56-6 Spastic contractions of the colon as they occur with irritable bowel syndrome.

include foods and fluids such as caffeinated or carbonated beverages and dairy products. Infectious agents have also been identified. Several studies have found that patients with IBS often have small-bowel bacterial overgrowth, which causes bloating and abdominal distention. Multiple normal flora and pathogenic agents have been identified, including *Pseudomonas aeruginosa* (Kerckhoffs et al., 2011). Other researchers believe that these agents are less causative and serve as measurable biomarkers for the disease (Berry & Reinisch, 2013).

Immunologic and genetic factors have also been associated with IBS, especially cytokine genes, including pro-inflammatory interleukins (IL), such as IL-6, IL-8, and tumor necrosis factor (TNF)–alpha. These findings may provide the basis of targeted drug therapy for the disease.

In the United States, women are two times more likely to have IBS than are men. This difference may be the result of hormonal differences. However, in other areas of the world, this distribution pattern may not occur.

Considerable evidence relates the role of stress and mental or behavioral illness, especially anxiety and depression, to IBS. Many patients diagnosed with IBS meet the criteria for at least one primary mental health disorder. However, the pain and other chronic symptoms of the disease may lead to secondary mental health disorders. For example, when diarrhea is predominant, patients fear that there will be no bathroom facilities available and can become very anxious. As a result, they may not want to leave their homes or travel on trips where bathrooms are not available at all times. The long-term nature of dealing with a chronic disease for which there is no cure can lead to secondary depression in some patients.

❖ INTERPROFESSIONAL COLLABORATIVE CARE

Care for the patient with IBS usually takes place in the outpatient setting, although patients with severe cases of IBS may be hospitalized for a period of time. The interprofessional team that collaborates to care for this patient generally includes the health care provider, nurse, and possibly the dietitian if NUTRITION modification is indicated.

◆ Assessment: Noticing

Ask the patient about a history of weight change, fatigue, malaise, abdominal pain, changes in the bowel pattern (constipation, diarrhea, or an alternating pattern of both) or consistency of stools, and the passage of mucus. Patients with IBS do not usually lose weight. Ask whether the patient has had any GI infections. Collect information on all drugs that the patient is taking because some can cause symptoms similar to those of IBS. Ask about the NUTRITION history, including the use of caffeinated drinks or beverages sweetened with sorbitol or fructose, which can cause bloating or diarrhea.

The course of the illness is specific to each patient. Most patients can identify factors that cause exacerbations, such as diet, stress, or anxiety. Food intolerance may be associated with IBS. Dairy products (e.g., for those with lactose intolerance), raw fruits, and grains can contribute to bloating, flatulence (gas), and abdominal distention. Patients may keep a food diary to record possible triggers for IBS symptoms.

A flare-up of worsening cramps, abdominal pain, and diarrhea and/or constipation may bring the patient to the health care provider. One of the *most common concerns of patients with IBS is pain in the left lower quadrant of the abdomen.* Assess the location, intensity, and quality of the pain. Some

patients have internal visceral (organ) hypersensitivity that can cause or contribute to it. Nausea may be associated with mealtime and defecation. The constipated stools are small and hard and are generally followed by several softer stools. The diarrheal stools are soft and watery, and mucus is often present. Patients with IBS often report belching, gas, anorexia, and bloating.

The patient generally appears well, with a stable weight, and nutritional and fluid status is within normal ranges. Inspect and auscultate the abdomen. Bowel sounds vary but are generally within normal range. With constipation, bowel sounds may be hypoactive; with severe diarrhea, they may be hyperactive.

Routine laboratory values (including a complete blood count [CBC], serum albumin, erythrocyte sedimentation rate [ESR], and stools for occult blood) remain normal in IBS. Some health care providers request a *hydrogen breath test* (Rana & Malik, 2014) or small-bowel bacterial overgrowth breath test. When small-intestinal bacterial overgrowth or malabsorption of nutrients is present, an excess of hydrogen is produced. Some of this hydrogen is absorbed into the bloodstream and travels to the lungs where it is exhaled. Patients with IBS often exhale an increased amount of hydrogen.

Teach the patient that he or she will need to be NPO (may have water) for at least 12 hours before the hydrogen breath test. At the beginning of the test, the patient blows into a hydrogen analyzer. Then, small amounts of test sugar are ingested, depending on the purpose of the test, and additional breath samples are taken every 15 minutes for 1 to 5 hours (Pagana et al., 2017).

◆ Interventions: Responding

The patient with IBS is usually managed on an ambulatory care basis and learns self-management strategies. Interventions include health teaching, drug therapy, and stress reduction. Some patients also use complementary and integrative therapies. A holistic approach to patient care is essential for positive outcomes (Chey et al., 2015).

Dietary fiber and bulk help produce bulky, soft stools and establish regular bowel ELIMINATION habits. The patient should ingest about 30 to 40 g of fiber each day. Eating regular meals, drinking 8 to 10 glasses of water each day, and chewing food slowly help promote normal bowel function.

Drug therapy depends on the main symptom of IBS. The health care provider may prescribe bulk-forming or antidiarrheal agents and/or newer drugs to control symptoms.

For the treatment of *constipation-predominant IBS (IBS-C)*, bulk-forming laxatives, such as *psyllium* hydrophilic mucilloid (Metamucil), are generally taken at mealtimes with a glass of water. The hydrophilic properties of these drugs help prevent dry, hard, or liquid stools. *Lubiprostone* (Amitiza) is an oral laxative approved for women with IBS-C, which increases fluid in the intestines to promote bowel ELIMINATION. Teach the patient to take the drug with food and water. Linaclotide (Linzess) is the newest drug for IBS-C, which works by simulating receptors in the intestines to increase fluid and promote bowel transit time. The drug also helps relieve pain and cramping that are associated with IBS. Teach patients to take this drug once a day about 30 minutes before breakfast.

Diarrhea-predominant IBS (IBS-D) may be treated with antidiarrheal agents, such as loperamide (Imodium), and psyllium (a bulk-forming agent). *Alosetron* (Lotronex), a selective serotonin (5-HT3) receptor antagonist, may be used with caution in women with IBS-D as a last resort when they have not responded to conventional therapy (Nee et al., 2015). Patients taking this drug must agree to report symptoms of colitis or constipation early because it is associated with potentially life-threatening bowel complications, including ischemic colitis (lack of blood flow to the colon).

> **! NURSING SAFETY PRIORITY** (QSEN)
> ### Drug Alert
>
> Before the patient begins alosetron (Lotronex), take a thorough drug history (including alternative treatments), both prescribed and over the counter, because it interacts with many drugs in a variety of classes. Remind patients that they should not take psychoactive drugs and antihistamines while taking alosetron. Teach patients to report severe constipation, fever, increasing abdominal pain, increasing fatigue, darkened urine, bloody diarrhea, or rectal bleeding as soon as it occurs and to stop the drug immediately (Lilley et al., 2017).

Many patients with IBS who have bloating and abdominal distention without constipation have success with *rifaximin* (Xifaxan), an antibiotic that works locally with little systemic absorption. The U.S. Food and Drug Administration (FDA) originally approved this drug for "traveler's diarrhea," and only recently has it been approved for use in IBS-D (Nee et al., 2015).

A newer group of drugs called *muscarinic-receptor antagonists* also inhibit intestinal motility. Some of these agents have been approved for people with overactive bladder but have not yet received FDA approval for IBS. Examples in this group currently undergoing clinical trials for IBS are darifenacin (Enablex) and fesoterodine (Toviaz).

For IBS in which pain is the predominant symptom, tricyclic antidepressants such as amitriptyline (Elavil) have also been used successfully. It is unclear whether their effectiveness is the result of the antidepressant or anticholinergic effects of the drugs. If patients have postprandial (after eating) alterations in COMFORT, they should take these drugs 30 to 45 minutes before mealtime.

Complementary and Integrative Health. For patients with increased intestinal bacterial overgrowth, recommend daily probiotic supplements. *Probiotics* have been shown to be effective for reducing bacteria and successfully alleviating GI symptoms of IBS (Quigley, 2015). There is also evidence that peppermint oil capsules may be effective in reducing symptoms for patients with IBS (Grundmann & Yoon, 2014).

Stress management is also an important part of holistic care. Suggest relaxation techniques, meditation, and/or yoga to help the patient decrease GI symptoms. If the patient has a stressful work or family situation, personal counseling may be helpful. Based on patient preference, make appropriate referrals or assist in making appointments if needed. The opportunity to discuss problems and attempt creative problem solving is often helpful. Teach the patient that regular exercise is important for managing stress and promoting regular bowel ELIMINATION.

HERNIATION

❖ PATHOPHYSIOLOGY

A **hernia** is a weakness in the abdominal muscle wall through which a segment of the bowel or other abdominal structure protrudes. Hernias can also penetrate through any other defect in the abdominal wall, through the diaphragm, or through other structures in the abdominal cavity.

The most important elements in the development of a hernia are congenital or acquired muscle weakness and increased intra-abdominal pressure. The most significant factors contributing to increased intra-abdominal pressure are obesity, pregnancy, and lifting heavy objects.

The most common types of abdominal hernias (Fig. 56-7) are indirect, direct, femoral, umbilical, and incisional (McCance et al., 2014).

- An **indirect inguinal hernia** is a sac formed from the peritoneum that contains a portion of the intestine or omentum. The hernia pushes downward at an angle into the inguinal canal. In males, indirect inguinal hernias can become large and often descend into the scrotum.
- **Direct inguinal hernias**, in contrast, pass through a weak point in the abdominal wall.
- **Femoral hernias** protrude through the femoral ring. A plug of fat in the femoral canal enlarges and eventually pulls the peritoneum and often the urinary bladder into the sac.
- **Umbilical hernias** are congenital or acquired. Congenital umbilical hernias appear in infancy. Acquired umbilical hernias directly result from increased intra-abdominal pressure. They are most commonly seen in people who are obese.

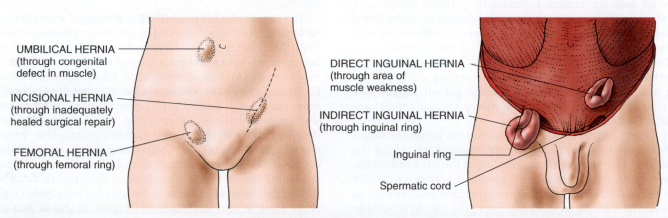

FIG. 56-7 Types of abdominal hernias.

- **Incisional**, or **ventral**, **hernias** occur at the site of a previous surgical incision. These hernias result from inadequate healing of the incision, which is usually caused by postoperative wound infections, inadequate NUTRITION, and obesity.

Hernias may also be classified as reducible, irreducible (incarcerated), or strangulated. A hernia is **reducible** when the contents of the hernial sac can be placed back into the abdominal cavity by application of gentle pressure. An **irreducible** (incarcerated) hernia cannot be reduced or placed back into the abdominal cavity. *Any hernia that is not reducible requires immediate surgical evaluation.*

A hernia is **strangulated** when the blood supply to the herniated segment of the bowel is cut off by pressure from the hernial ring (the band of muscle around the hernia). If a hernia is strangulated, there is ischemia and obstruction of the bowel loop. *This can lead to necrosis of the bowel, sepsis, and possibly bowel perforation. Signs of strangulation are abdominal distention, nausea, vomiting, pain, fever, and tachycardia.*

Indirect inguinal hernias, the most common type, occur mostly in men because they follow the tract that develops when the testes descend into the scrotum before birth. Direct hernias occur more often in older adults. Femoral and adult umbilical hernias are most common in pregnant women or those with obesity. Incisional hernias can occur in people who have undergone abdominal surgery.

❖ INTERPROFESSIONAL COLLABORATIVE CARE

Care for the patient with a hernia usually takes place in the outpatient setting while the hernia is monitored. Patients with inguinal hernias often need surgery and will be hospitalized following this procedure. The interprofessional team that collaborates to care for this patient generally includes the health care provider (or surgeon, if the hernia requires surgical repair) and nurse.

◆ Assessment: Noticing

The patient with a hernia typically comes to the health care provider's office, clinic, or the emergency department with a report of a "lump" or protrusion felt at the involved site. The development of the hernia may be associated with straining or lifting.

Perform an abdominal assessment inspecting the abdomen when the patient is lying and again when he or she is standing. If the hernia is reducible, it may disappear when the patient is lying flat. The advanced practice nurse or other health care provider asks the patient to strain or perform the Valsalva maneuver and observes for bulging. Auscultate for active bowel sounds. *Absent bowel sounds may indicate obstruction and strangulation, which are considered medical emergencies.*

To palpate an inguinal hernia, the health care provider gently examines the ring and its contents by inserting a finger in the ring and noting any changes when the patient coughs. *The hernia is never forcibly reduced; this maneuver could cause strangulated intestine to rupture.*

If a male patient suspects a hernia in his groin, the health care provider has him stand for the examination. Using the right hand for the patient's right side and the left hand for the patient's left side, the examiner pushes in the loose scrotal skin with the index finger, following the spermatic cord upward to the external inguinal cord. At this point, the patient is asked to cough, and any palpable herniation is noted.

◆ Interventions: Responding

The type of treatment selected depends on patient factors such as age and the type and severity of the hernia.

Nonsurgical Management. If the patient is not a surgical candidate (often an older man with multiple health problems), the health care provider may prescribe a truss for an inguinal hernia, usually for men. A **truss** is a pad made with firm material. It is held in place over the hernia with a belt to help keep the abdominal contents from protruding into the hernial sac. If a truss is used, it is applied only after the physician has reduced the hernia if it is not incarcerated. The patient usually applies the truss on awakening. Teach him to assess the skin under the truss daily and to protect it with a light layer of powder.

Surgical Management. Most hernias are inguinal, and surgical repair is the treatment of choice. Surgery is usually performed on an ambulatory care basis for patients who have no pre-existing health conditions that would complicate the operative course. In same-day surgery centers, anesthesia may be regional or general, and the procedure is typically laparoscopic. If bowel strangulation and tissue death occur, more extensive surgery, such as a bowel resection or temporary colostomy, may be necessary. Patients undergoing this extensive surgery are hospitalized for a longer period.

Surgical repair of a hernia is called **herniorrhaphy**. A **minimally invasive inguinal hernia repair (MIIHR)** through a laparoscope is the surgery of choice. A conventional open herniorrhaphy may be performed when laparoscopy is not appropriate. Patients having minimally invasive surgery (MIS) recover more quickly, have less pain, and develop fewer postoperative complications compared with those having a conventional open surgery.

In addition to patient education about the procedure, the most important preoperative preparation is to teach the patient to remain NPO for the number of hours before surgery that the surgeon specifies. If same-day surgery is planned, remind the patient to arrange for someone to take him or her home and for that adult to be available for the rest of the day at home. For patients having a conventional open approach, provide general preoperative care as described in Chapter 14.

During an MIIHR, the surgeon makes several small incisions, identifies the defect, and places the intestinal contents back into the abdomen. During a conventional open herniorrhaphy, the surgeon makes an abdominal incision to perform this procedure. When a **hernioplasty** is also performed, the surgeon reinforces the weakened outside abdominal muscle wall with a mesh patch.

The patient who has had MIIHR is discharged from the surgical center in 3 to 5 hours, depending on recovery from anesthesia. Teach him or her to avoid strenuous activity for several days before returning to work and a normal routine. A stool softener may be needed to prevent constipation. Caution patients who are taking oral opioids for pain management to not drive or operate heavy machinery. Teach them to observe incisions for redness, swelling, heat, drainage, and increased pain and promptly report their occurrence to the surgeon. Remind patients that soreness and alterations in COMFORT (rather than severe, acute pain) are common after MIIHR. Be sure to make a follow-up telephone call on the day after surgery to check on the patient's status.

General postoperative care of patients having a hernia repair is the same as that described in Chapter 16 *except that they should avoid coughing.* To promote lung expansion, encourage deep breathing and ambulation. With repair of an indirect inguinal hernia, the physician may suggest a scrotal support and ice bags applied to the scrotum to prevent swelling, which often contributes to pain. Elevation of the scrotum with a soft pillow helps prevent and control swelling.

In the immediate postoperative period, male patients who have had an inguinal hernia repair may experience difficulty voiding. Encourage them to stand to allow a more natural position for gravity to facilitate voiding and bladder emptying. Urine output of less than 30 mL per hour should be reported to the surgeon. Techniques to stimulate voiding such as allowing water to run may also be used. A fluid intake of at least 1500 to 2500 mL daily prevents dehydration, maintains urinary function, and minimizes constipation. A "straight" or intermittent ("in and out") catheterization is required if the patient cannot void. Chart 56-7 summarizes best nursing practices for postoperative care after an MIIHR.

Most patients have uneventful recoveries after a hernia repair. Surgeons generally allow them to return to their usual activities after surgery, with avoidance of straining and lifting for several weeks while subcutaneous tissues heal and strengthen.

On discharge, provide oral instructions and a written list of symptoms to be reported, including fever, chills, wound drainage, redness or separation of the incision, and increasing incisional pain. Teach the patient to keep the wound dry and clean with antibacterial soap and water. Showering is usually permitted in a few days (see Chart 56-7).

HEMORRHOIDS

❖ PATHOPHYSIOLOGY

Hemorrhoids are unnaturally swollen or distended veins in the anorectal region. The veins involved in the development of hemorrhoids are part of the normal structure in the anal region. With limited distention, the veins function as a valve overlying the anal sphincter that assists in continence. Increased intra-abdominal pressure causes elevated systemic and portal venous pressure, which is transmitted to the anorectal veins. Arterioles in the anorectal region shunt blood directly to the distended anorectal veins, which increases the pressure. With repeated elevations in pressure from increased intra-abdominal pressure and engorgement from arteriolar shunting of blood, the distended veins eventually separate from the smooth muscle surrounding them. The result is prolapse of the hemorrhoidal vessels.

Hemorrhoids can be internal or external (Fig. 56-8). Internal hemorrhoids, which cannot be seen on inspection of the perineal area, lie above the anal sphincter. External hemorrhoids lie below the anal sphincter and can be seen on inspection of the anal region. Prolapsed hemorrhoids can become thrombosed or inflamed, or they can bleed (McCance et al., 2014).

Hemorrhoids are common and not significant unless they cause pain or bleeding. Because of the increase in abdominal pressure, the condition worsens during pregnancy, or with

---

? NCLEX EXAMINATION CHALLENGE 56-4

Physiological Integrity

The emergency department nurse is assessing a client with a known inguinal hernia. Which assessment findings indicate that the hernia may have strangulated? **Select all that apply.**
A. Fever
B. Tachycardia
C. Abdominal distention
D. Mild abdominal pain
E. Nausea and vomiting

◎ CHART 56-7 Best Practice for Patient Safety & Quality Care QSEN

Nursing Care of the Postoperative Patient Having a Minimally Invasive Inguinal Hernia Repair (MIIHR)

- Monitor vital signs, especially blood pressure, for indications of internal bleeding.
- Assess and manage incisional pain with oral analgesics; report and document severe pain that does not respond to drug therapy immediately.
- Encourage deep breathing after surgery; avoid excessive coughing.
- Encourage ambulation with assistance as soon as possible after surgery (within the first few hours).
- Apply ice packs as prescribed to the surgical area.
- Assist the patient to void by standing the first time after surgery.
- Teach patients at discharge to:
  - Rest for several days after surgery.
  - Observe the incision sites for redness or drainage and report these findings to the surgeon.
  - Shower after 24 to 36 hours after removing any bandage (do not remove Steri-Strips); be aware that the Steri-Strips will fall off in about a week.
  - Monitor temperature for the first few days and report the occurrence of a fever.
  - Do not lift more than 10 lb until allowed by the surgeon.
  - Avoid constipation by eating high-fiber foods and drinking extra fluids.
  - Return to work when allowed by the surgeon, usually in 1 to 2 weeks, depending on the patient's work responsibilities.

PROCEDURE: CHOICE OF ONE OF THE FOLLOWING	INTERVAL AFTER SCREENING INITIATED AT AGE 50 YEARS	COMMENTS
FOBT and sigmoidoscopy	Every 5 years	FOBT procedure: two or three samples from three consecutive bowel movements obtained at home; tested by physician or nurse
or Double-contrast barium enema	Every 5 years	
or Colonoscopy	Every 10 years	

FOBT, Fecal occult blood testing.

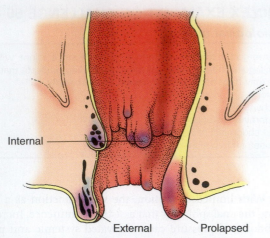

FIG. 56-8 Internal, external, and prolapsed hemorrhoids. *Internal hemorrhoids* lie above the anal sphincter and cannot be seen on inspection of the anal area. *External hemorrhoids* lie below the anal sphincter and can be seen on inspection of the anal region. Hemorrhoids that enlarge, fall down, and protrude through the anus are called *prolapsed hemorrhoids.*

constipation with straining, obesity, heart failure, prolonged sitting or standing, and strenuous exercise and weight lifting. Decreased fluid intake can also cause hemorrhoids because of the development of hard stool and subsequent constipation. Straining while evacuating stool causes hemorrhoids to enlarge.

Health Promotion and Maintenance

Prevention of constipation is the most essential measure to address hemorrhoids. It can be prevented by increasing fiber in the diet, such as eating more whole grains and raw vegetables and fruits. Encourage patients to drink plenty of water unless otherwise contraindicated (e.g., kidney disease, heart disease). Remind the patient to avoid straining at stool. Remind him or her to exercise regularly with a gradual buildup in intensity. Maintaining a healthy weight also helps prevent hemorrhoids.

❖ INTERPROFESSIONAL COLLABORATIVE CARE

Care of the patient with hemorrhoids usually takes place in the outpatient setting and is delivered by the health care provider and nurse. If surgery is required, the patient will be admitted to an inpatient facility, and care is provided by the surgeon and nurse. The dietitian may be consulted to recommend nutrition sources that normalize bowel patterns and minimize constipation.

◆ Assessment: Noticing

The most common symptoms of hemorrhoids are bleeding, swelling, and prolapse (bulging). Blood is characteristically bright red and is present on toilet tissue or streaked in the stool. Pain is a common symptom and is often associated with thrombosis, especially if thrombosis occurs suddenly. Other symptoms include itching and a mucous discharge. Diagnosis is usually made by inspection and digital examination.

◆ Interventions: Responding

Interventions are typically conservative and are aimed at reducing symptoms with minimal discomfort, cost, and time lost from usual activities. Local treatment and NUTRITION therapy are used when symptoms begin. Cold packs applied to the anorectal region for a few minutes at a time beginning with the onset of pain and tepid sitz baths three or four times per day are often enough to relieve discomfort, even if the hemorrhoids are thrombosed.

Topical anesthetics, such as lidocaine (Xylocaine), are useful for severe pain. Dibucaine (Nupercainal) ointment and similar products are available over the counter and may be applied for mild-to-moderate pain and itching. However, this ointment should be used only temporarily, because it can mask worsening symptoms and delay diagnosis of a severe disorder. If itching or inflammation is present, the primary health care provider prescribes a steroid preparation, such as hydrocortisone. Cleansing the anal area with moistened cleansing tissues rather than standard toilet tissue helps avoid irritation. The anal area should be cleansed gently by dabbing rather than wiping.

Diets high in fiber and fluids are recommended to promote regular bowel movements without straining. Stool softeners, such as docusate sodium (Colace) or polyethylene glycol (Miralax), can be used temporarily. Irritating laxatives are avoided, as are foods and beverages that can make hemorrhoids worse. Spicy foods, nuts, coffee, and alcohol can be irritating. Remind patients to avoid sitting for long periods. The primary health care provider may prescribe mild oral analgesics for pain if the hemorrhoids are thrombosed.

Conservative treatment should alleviate symptoms in 3 to 5 days. If symptoms continue or recur frequently, the patient may require surgical intervention.

The surgeon can perform several procedures in an ambulatory care setting to remove symptomatic hemorrhoids (**hemorrhoidectomy**). The type of surgery (e.g., ultrasound or laser removal) depends on the degree of prolapse, whether there is thrombosis, and the overall condition of the patient. Complications of these procedures include pain, thrombosis of other hemorrhoids, infection, bleeding, and abscess formation. If the hemorrhoid is prolapsed, a circular stapling device may be used to excise a band of mucosa above the prolapse and restore the hemorrhoidal tissue back into the anal canal.

Teach patients with hemorrhoids about the need to eat high-fiber, high-fluid diets to promote regular bowel patterns before and after surgery. Advise them to avoid stimulant laxatives, which can be habit forming.

For patients who undergo any type of surgical intervention, monitor for bleeding and pain after surgery and teach them to report these problems to their health care provider. Using moist heat (e.g., sitz baths or warm compresses) three or four times per day can help promote COMFORT.

> **! NURSING SAFETY PRIORITY** QSEN
>
> **Action Alert**
>
> *Tell the patient who has had surgical intervention for hemorrhoids that the first postoperative bowel movement may be very painful.* Be sure that someone is with or near the patient when this happens. Some patients become light-headed and diaphoretic and may have syncope related to a vasovagal response (Moss & Bordeianou, 2013).

The health care provider usually prescribes stool softeners such as docusate sodium (Colace) to begin before surgery and continue after surgery. Analgesics and anti-inflammatory drugs are prescribed. A mild laxative should be administered if the patient has not had a bowel movement by the third postoperative day.

MALABSORPTION SYNDROME

❖ PATHOPHYSIOLOGY

Malabsorption is a syndrome associated with a variety of disorders and intestinal surgical procedures. This syndrome can be caused by inflammation, intrinsic disease, or injury to the lining of the intestine. With various disorders, physiologic mechanisms limit absorption of nutrients because of one or more of these abnormalities:

- Bile salt deficiencies
- Enzyme deficiencies
- Presence of bacteria
- Disruption of the mucosal lining of the small intestine
- Altered lymphatic and vascular circulation
- Decrease in the gastric or intestinal surface area

The nutrient involved in malabsorption depends on the type and location of the abnormality in the intestinal tract.

Deficiencies of bile salts can lead to malabsorption of fats and fat-soluble vitamins. Bile salt deficiencies can result from decreased synthesis of bile in the liver, bile obstruction, or alteration of bile salt absorption in the small intestine.

Enzymes normally found in the intestine split disaccharides (complex sugars) to monosaccharides (simple sugars). Examples of these enzymes are lactase, sucrase, maltase, and isomaltase. Lactase deficiency is the most common disaccharide enzyme deficiency. Without sufficient amounts of this enzyme, the body is not able to break down lactose. Lactase deficiency can be the result of genetic inheritance, injury to intestinal mucosa from viral hepatitis, or excessive bacteria in the intestine. Deficiencies of the other disaccharide enzymes are rare.

Pancreatic enzymes are also necessary for absorption of vitamin B_{12}. With destruction or obstruction of the pancreas or insufficient pancreatic stimulation, this nutrient is not well absorbed. Chronic pancreatitis, pancreatic carcinoma, resection of the pancreas, and cystic fibrosis can cause these malabsorption problems.

Loops of bowel can accumulate intestinal contents, resulting in bacterial overgrowth, when peristalsis is decreased. Bacteria at these sites break down bile salts, and fewer salts are available for fat absorption. These bacteria can also ingest vitamin B_{12}, which contributes to vitamin B_{12} deficiency. This process can occur after a gastrectomy.

Obstruction to lymphatic flow in the intestine can lead to loss of plasma proteins along with loss of minerals (e.g., iron, copper, calcium), vitamin B_{12}, folic acid, and lipids. Lymphatic obstruction can be caused by many conditions. Certain cancers such as lymphoma, inflammatory states, radiation enteritis, Crohn's disease, heart failure, and constrictive pericarditis are causes of lymphatic obstruction.

Interference with blood flow to the intestinal mucosa results in malabsorption. With intestinal surgery, there is loss of the surface area needed to facilitate absorption. Resection of the ileum results in vitamin B_{12}, bile salt, and other nutrient deficiencies. Gastric surgery is one of the most common causes of malabsorption and maldigestion. Other conditions associated with poor digestion and malabsorption include small-bowel ischemia and radiation enteritis.

❖ INTERPROFESSIONAL COLLABORATIVE CARE

Care of the patient with malabsorption syndrome may take place in the inpatient or outpatient setting depending on severity, and it is usually delivered by the health care provider and nurse.

◆ Assessment: Noticing

Chronic diarrhea is a classic symptom of malabsorption. It occurs as a result of unabsorbed nutrients, which add to the bulk of the stool, and unabsorbed fat. **Steatorrhea** (greater than normal amounts of fat in the feces) is a common sign. It is a result of bile salt deconjugation, nonabsorbed fats, or bacteria in the intestine. Not all patients with malabsorption have diarrhea. Instead some have an increased stool mass. Other symptoms include:

- Unintentional weight loss
- Bloating and flatus (carbohydrate malabsorption)
- Decreased libido
- Easy bruising (purpura)
- Anemia (with iron and folic acid or vitamin B_{12} deficiencies)
- Bone pain (with calcium and vitamin D deficiencies)
- Edema (caused by hypoproteinemia)

Serum laboratory studies reveal a decrease in mean corpuscular volume (MCV), mean corpuscular hemoglobin (MCH), and mean corpuscular hemoglobin concentration (MCHC). These decreases indicate hypochromic microcytic anemia resulting from iron deficiency. Increased MCV and variable MCH and MCHC values indicate macrocytic anemia (pernicious anemia) resulting from vitamin B_{12} and folic acid deficiencies. Serum iron levels are low in protein malabsorption because of insufficient gastric acid for use of iron. Serum cholesterol levels may be low from decreased absorption and digestion of fat. Low serum calcium levels may indicate malabsorption of vitamin D and amino acids. Low levels of serum vitamin A (retinol) and carotene, its precursor, indicate a bile salt deficiency and malabsorption of fat. Serum albumin and total protein levels are low if protein is lost.

A quantitative *fecal fat analysis* is often elevated in either malabsorption or maldigestive disorders (Pagana et al., 2017).

A *lactose tolerance test* is a type of disaccharidase analysis that may show an inability to digest foods and beverages that contain lactose. A hydrogen breath test can also be performed to detect this problem. The D-xylose absorption test can reveal low urine and serum D-xylose levels if malabsorption in the small intestine is present (Pagana et al., 2017).

The *Schilling test* measures urinary excretion of vitamin B_{12} for diagnosis of pernicious anemia and a variety of other malabsorption syndromes. The *bile acid breath test* assesses the absorption of bile salt. If the patient has bacterial overgrowth, the bile salts will become deconjugated, and the carbon dioxide level in the breath will peak earlier than expected.

Ultrasonography is used to diagnose pancreatic tumors and tumors in the small intestine that are causing malabsorption. X-rays of the GI tract reveal pancreatic calcifications, tumors, or other abnormalities that cause malabsorption. A CT scan may also be done.

◆ Interventions: Responding

Interventions for most malabsorption syndromes focus on (1) avoidance of substances that aggravate malabsorption, and (2) supplementation of nutrients. Surgical management of the primary disease may be indicated. Drug therapy may also improve or resolve malabsorption.

NUTRITION management includes a low-fat diet for patients who have gallbladder disease, severe steatorrhea, or cystic fibrosis. A low-fat diet may or may not be indicated for pancreatic insufficiency because this disorder improves with enzyme replacement. Some clinicians believe that limitation of fat intake is not necessary with enzyme replacement. Dietary intake of fat is actually beneficial to the patient because it has a high number of calories. After a total gastrectomy, a high-protein, high-calorie diet and small, frequent meals are recommended. Lactose-free or lactose-restricted diets are available for patients with lactase deficiency, and gluten-free diets are available for those with celiac disease, discussed in Chapter 57.

The health care provider prescribes NUTRITION supplements according to the specific deficiency. Common supplements include:

- Water-soluble vitamins, such as folic acid and vitamin B complex
- Fat-soluble vitamins, such as vitamins A, D, and K
- Minerals, such as calcium, iron, and magnesium
- Pancreatic enzymes, such as pancrelipase (Pancrease, Viokase)

Antibiotics are used to treat disorders involving bacterial overgrowth. Bacterial overgrowth can be caused by a variety of disorders but is often treated with tetracycline and metronidazole (Flagyl, Novonidazol).

Drug therapy is used to control the signs and symptoms of malabsorption. Antidiarrheal agents, such as diphenoxylate hydrochloride and atropine sulfate (Lomotil, N-Lomotil), are often used to control diarrhea and steatorrhea. Anticholinergics, such as dicyclomine hydrochloride (Bentyl, Bentylol), may be

 CHART 56-8 **Best Practice for Patient Safety & Quality Care** QSEN

Special Skin Care for Patients With Chronic Diarrhea

- Use medicated wipes or premoistened disposable wipes rather than toilet tissue to clean the perineal area.
- Clean the perineal area well with mild soap and warm water after each stool; rinse soap from the area well.
- If the physician allows, provide a sitz bath several times per day.
- Apply a thin coat of A+D ointment or other medicated protective barrier, such as aloe products, after each stool.
- Keep the patient off the affected buttock area.
- Cover open areas with thin DuoDerm or Tegaderm occlusive dressing to promote rapid healing.
- Observe for fungal or yeast infections, which appear as dark red rashes with "satellite" lesions. Obtain prescription for medication if this problem occurs.

given before meals to inhibit gastric motility. IV fluids may be necessary to replenish fluid losses associated with diarrhea.

Provide special measures to protect the skin when chronic diarrhea occurs (Chart 56-8). Conduct an ongoing assessment for signs and symptoms of malabsorption and relate these to activities and dietary intake. For example, patients with steatorrhea are monitored for FLUID AND ELECTROLYTE BALANCE and are encouraged to drink electrolyte-rich liquids liberally. Teach them the rationale for dietary, drug, and surgical management of nutritional deficiencies and evaluate interventions on the basis of changes in or resolution of signs and symptoms.

GET READY FOR THE NCLEX® EXAMINATION!

KEY POINTS

Review these Key Points for each NCLEX Examination Client Needs Category.

Safe and Effective Care Environment
- Collaborate with the certified wound, ostomy, continence nurse (CWOCN) or enterostomal therapist (ET) when a patient is scheduled for or has a new colostomy. **QSEN: Teamwork and Collaboration**
- Collaborate with the case manager/discharge planner, health care provider, and CWOCN to plan care for the patient with colorectal cancer (CRC). **QSEN: Teamwork and Collaboration**

Health Promotion and Maintenance
- Refer patients with familial CRC syndromes for genetic counseling and testing. **QSEN: Evidence-Based Practice**
- Refer ostomy patients to the United Ostomy Associations of America, Inc. and the American Cancer Society for additional information and support groups. **QSEN: Patient-Centered Care**
- Teach patients with irritable bowel syndrome (IBS) to avoid GI stimulants, such as caffeine, alcohol, and milk and milk products, and to manage stress. **QSEN: Evidence-Based Practice**
- Instruct patients on dietary modifications to decrease the occurrence of CRC, such as eating a diet high in fiber and avoiding red meat. **QSEN: Evidence-Based Practice**

- Teach adults 50 years and older to have routine screening for CRC as listed in Chart 56-4; people with genetic predispositions should have earlier and more frequent screening. **QSEN: Evidence-Based Practice**
- Teach people to prevent or manage constipation to help avoid hemorrhoids; teach patients the importance of maintaining a healthy weight to decrease the risk for hemorrhoids. **QSEN: Evidence-Based Practice**
- Teach patients and caregivers how to provide colostomy care, including dietary measures, skin care, and ostomy products. **QSEN: Patient-Centered Care**

Psychosocial Integrity
- Assist the patient with CRC with the grieving process. **QSEN: Patient-Centered Care**
- Be aware that having a colostomy is a life-altering event that can severely impact one's body image; issues related to sexuality and fear of acceptance should be discussed. **QSEN: Patient-Centered Care**

Physiological Integrity
- Be aware that minimally invasive inguinal hernia repair is an ambulatory care procedure done via laparoscopy; postoperative management requires health teaching regarding rest for a few days and inspection of incisions for signs of infection (see Chart 56-7). **QSEN: Evidence-Based Practice**

- Be aware that a strangulated hernia can cause ischemia and bowel obstruction, requiring immediate intervention. **QSEN: Safety**
- Monitor patients who have conventional open herniorrhaphy for ability to void. **QSEN: Safety**
- Recall that changes in bowel habits or stool characteristics and/or rectal bleeding are often associated with a diagnosis of CRC. **QSEN: Safety**
- Keep the peristomal skin clean and dry; observe for leakage around the pouch seal. **QSEN: Evidence-Based Practice**
- Provide meticulous perineal wound care for patients having an abdominoperineal (AP) resection, as described in Chart 56-5. **QSEN: Safety**
- Recognize characteristics of the colostomy stoma, which should be reddish pink and moist; report abnormalities such as ischemia and necrosis (purplish or black) or unusual bleeding to the surgeon. **Clinical Judgment**
- Recall that bowel sounds are altered in patients with obstruction; absent bowel sounds imply total obstruction. **QSEN: Safety**

- Assess the patient's nasogastric tube for proper placement, patency, and output at least every 4 hours. **QSEN: Safety**
- Monitor patients with bowel obstruction for signs and symptoms of fluid, electrolyte, and acid-base imbalances; patients with small bowel obstruction are at greater risk for problems with FLUID AND ELECTROLYTE BALANCE. **QSEN: Safety**
- Teach patients having hemorrhoid surgery to take stool softeners before and after surgery to decrease discomfort during ELIMINATION. **QSEN: Evidence-Based Practice**
- Provide COMFORT measures for the patient who has chronic diarrhea associated with malabsorption as described in Chart 56-8. **QSEN: Patient-Centered Care**
- Reinforce teaching regarding supplements or dietary restrictions needed for malabsorption management. **QSEN: Evidence-Based Practice**

SELECTED BIBLIOGRAPHY

Asterisk indicates a classic or definitive work on this subject.

American Cancer Society (ACS) (2016a). *Colorectal cancer risk factors.* Atlanta: ACS.

American Cancer Society (ACS) (2016b). *Recommendations for colorectal cancer early detection.* Atlanta: ACS.

Bragg, D., El-Sharkawy, A. M., Psaltis, E., Maxwell-Armstrong, C. A., & Lobo, D. N. (2015). Postoperative ileus: Recent developments in pathophysiology and management. *Clinical Nutrition : Official Journal of the European Society of Parenteral and Enteral Nutrition, 34,* 367–376.

Berry, D., & Reinisch, W. (2013). Intestinal microbiota: A source of novel biomarkers in inflammatory bowel disease? *Best Practice & Research. Clinical Gastroenterology, 27*(1), 47–58.

Chey, W. D., Kurlander, J., & Eswaran, S. (2015). Irritable bowel syndrome: A clinical review. *Journal of the American Medical Association, 313*(9), 949–958.

Cutsem, E. V., Cervantes, A., Nordlinger, B., & Arnold, D. (2014). Metastatic colorectal cancer: ESMO clinical practice guidelines for diagnosis, treatment and follow-up. *Annals of Oncology, 25*(Suppl. 3), iii1–iii9.

Grundmann, O., & Yoon, S. L. (2014). Complementary and alternative medicines in irritable bowel syndrome: An integrative view. *World Journal of Gastroenterology, 20*(2), 346–362.

Haddad, J. D., & You, D. M. (2016). Colorectal cancer screening and race an equal access medical system. *Journal of Community Health, 41,* 78–81.

Kapritsou, M., Korkolis, D. P., & Knostantinou, E. A. (2013). Open or laparoscopic surgery for colorectal cancer: A retrospective comparative study. *Gastroenterology Nursing, 36*(1), 37–41.

*Kerckhoffs, A. P., Ben-Amor, K., Samsom, M., van der Rest, M. E., de Vogel, J., Knol, J., et al. (2011). Molecular analysis of faecal and duodenal samples reveals significantly higher prevalence and numbers of *Pseudomonas aeruginosa* in irritable bowel syndrome. *Journal of Medical Microbiology, 60,* 236–245.

Lilley, L. L., Rainforth-Collins, S., & Snyder, J. S. (2017). *Pharmacology and the nursing process.* St. Louis: Elsevier.

*Lynch, H. T., Lynch, P. M., Lanspa, S. J., Snyder, C. L., Lynch, J. F., & Boland, C. R. (2009). Review of the Lynch syndrome: History, molecular genetics, screening, differential diagnosis, and medico-legal ramifications. *Clinical Genetics, 76,* 1–18.

McCance, K., Huether, S., Brashers, V., & Rote, N. (2014). *Pathophysiology: The biologic basis for disease in adults and children* (7th ed.). St. Louis: Mosby.

Moss, A. K., & Bordeianou, L. (2013). Outpatient management of hemorrhoids. *Seminars in Colon and Rectal Surgery, 24*(2), 76–80.

Nee, J., Zakari, M., & Lembo, A. J. (2015). Novel therapies in IBS-D treatment. *Current Treatment Options in Gastroenterology, 13,* 432–440.

Quigley, E. M. (2015). Probiotics in irritable bowel syndrome: The science and the evidence. *Journal of Clinical Gastroenterology, 49*(1), S60–S64.

Pagana, K., Pagana, T. J., & Pagana, T. N. (2017). *Mosby's diagnostic and laboratory test reference* (13th ed.). St. Louis: Mosby.

Rana, S. V., & Malik, A. (2014). Breath tests and irritable bowel syndrome. *World Journal of Gastroenterology, 20*(24), 7587–7601. http://doi.org/10.3748/wjg.v20.i24.7587.

Roncucci, L., & Mariani, F. (2015). Prevention of colorectal cancer: How many tools do we have in our basket? *European Journal of Internal Medicine, 26,* 752–756.

Tammana, V. S., & Laiyemo, A. O. (2014). Colorectal cancer disparities: Issues, controversies and solutions. *World Journal of Gastroenterology, 20*(4), 869–876.

Wilkes, G. (2013). *What's new in colon cancer: Update for the practicing nurse.* www.nursingconsult.com.

Wilkes, G., & Hartshorn, K. (2012). Clinical update: Colon, rectal, and anal cancers. *Seminars in Oncology Nursing, 28*(4), 1–22.

Care of Patients With Inflammatory Intestinal Disorders

Keelin Cromar

PRIORITY AND INTERRELATED CONCEPTS

The priority concepts for this chapter are:
- IMMUNITY
- ELIMINATION

✳ The IMMUNITY concept exemplar for this chapter is Peritonitis, below.

✳ The ELIMINATION concept exemplar for this chapter is Ulcerative Colitis, p. 1150.

The interrelated concepts for this chapter are:
- NUTRITION
- COMFORT
- FLUID AND ELECTROLYTE BALANCE

LEARNING OUTCOMES

Safe and Effective Care Environment

1. Collaborate with the interprofessional team to protect and provide care for the patient with an inflammatory bowel disorder (IBD).
2. Identify community resources to ensure appropriate transition management for patients with an inflammatory bowel disorder (IBD).

Health Promotion and Maintenance

3. Teach patients how to self-care for an ileostomy or other surgical diversion.
4. Discuss ways to prevent gastroenteritis.

Psychosocial Integrity

5. Implement nursing interventions to minimize stressors for the patient with an inflammatory bowel disorder (IBD) who has ileostomy or other surgical diversion.

Physiological Integrity

6. Differentiate pathophysiology and presentation of common types of acute inflammatory bowel disorders (IBDs).
7. Prioritize care for patients with inflammatory bowel disorders (IBDs).
8. Discuss the purpose of, and nursing implications related to, drug therapy for patients with an inflammatory bowel disorder (IBD).
9. Create an evidence-based plan of care for the patient undergoing surgery for an inflammatory bowel disorder (IBD).
10. Explain the role of NUTRITION therapy in caring for a patient with diverticular disease.
11. Describe nursing interventions that promote IMMUNITY, COMFORT, and ELIMINATION and maintain FLUID AND ELECTROLYTE BALANCE for patients with an inflammatory bowel disorder (IBD).

The *intestinal tract* is made up of the small intestine and large intestine (colon). Continued digestion of food and absorption of nutrients occurs primarily in the small intestine to meet the body's needs for energy. Water is reabsorbed in the large intestine to help maintain a fluid balance and promote the passage of waste products. When the intestinal tract and its nearby structures become inflamed, NUTRITION may be inadequate to meet a patient's needs. Bowel ELIMINATION changes, COMFORT is altered, and IMMUNITY concerns and/or problems with FLUID AND ELECTROLYTE BALANCE can arise.

ACUTE INFLAMMATORY BOWEL DISORDERS

Appendicitis, gastroenteritis, and peritonitis are the most common acute inflammatory bowel problems. These disorders are potentially life threatening and can have major systemic complications if not treated promptly.

✳ IMMUNITY CONCEPT EXEMPLAR Peritonitis

Peritonitis is a life-threatening, acute inflammation and infection of the visceral/parietal peritoneum and endothelial lining of the abdominal cavity. This type of acute inflammation and infection alters the body's process of IMMUNITY (see Chapter 2). Primary peritonitis is rare (and thus not discussed here) and indicates that the peritoneum is infected via the bloodstream.

❖ PATHOPHYSIOLOGY

Normally the peritoneal cavity contains about 50 mL of sterile fluid (transudate), which prevents friction in the abdominal cavity during peristalsis. When the peritoneal cavity is contaminated by bacteria, the body first begins an inflammatory reaction, walling off a localized area to fight the infection. The body's IMMUNITY is immediately affected by this local reaction, which involves vascular dilation and increased capillary permeability, allowing transport of leukocytes and subsequent phagocytosis of the offending organisms. If the process of walling-off fails, the inflammation spreads, and contamination becomes massive, resulting in diffuse (widespread) peritonitis.

Peritonitis is most often caused by contamination of the peritoneal cavity by bacteria or chemicals. Bacteria gain entry into the peritoneum by perforation (from appendicitis, diverticulitis, peptic ulcer disease) or from an external penetrating wound, a gangrenous gallbladder, bowel obstruction, or ascending infection through the genital tract. Less common causes include perforating tumors, leakage or contamination during surgery, and infection by skin pathogens in patients undergoing continuous ambulatory peritoneal dialysis (CAPD).

When diagnosis and treatment of peritonitis are delayed, blood vessel dilation continues. The body responds to the continuing infectious process by shunting extra blood to the area of inflammation (hyperemia). Fluid is shifted from the extracellular fluid compartment into the peritoneal cavity, connective tissues, and GI tract (*"third spacing"*). This shift of fluid can result in a significant decrease in circulatory volume and *hypovolemic shock*. Severely decreased circulatory volume can result in insufficient perfusion of the kidneys, leading to acute kidney injury with impaired FLUID AND ELECTROLYTE BALANCE (McCance et al., 2014). Assess for signs and symptoms of these life-threatening problems.

Peristalsis slows or *stops* in response to severe peritoneal inflammation, and the lumen of the bowel becomes distended with gas and fluid. Fluid that normally flows to the small bowel and the colon for reabsorption accumulates in the intestine in volumes of 7 to 8 L daily. The toxins or bacteria responsible for the peritonitis can also enter the bloodstream from the peritoneal area and lead to bacteremia or **septicemia** (bacterial invasion of the blood), a life-threatening condition when the body's IMMUNITY is compromised.

Respiratory problems can occur as a result of increased abdominal pressure against the diaphragm from intestinal distention and fluid shifts to the peritoneal cavity. Pain can interfere with respirations at a time when the patient has an increased oxygen demand because of the infectious process.

Etiology

Common bacteria responsible for peritonitis include *Escherichia coli, Streptococcus, Staphylococcus, Pneumococcus,* and *Gonococcus.* Chemical peritonitis results from leakage of bile, pancreatic enzymes, and gastric acid (McCance et al., 2014), all of which can greatly alter the patient's IMMUNITY.

Incidence and Prevalence

Peritonitis is the dominant cause of death from surgical infections, with a mortality rate of up to 20% (Doklestić et al., 2014).

❖ INTERPROFESSIONAL COLLABORATIVE CARE

Patients with peritonitis are hospitalized because of the severe nature of the illness. If complications are extensive, the patients are often admitted to a critical care unit. The interprofessional team that collaborates to care for this patient generally includes

CHART 57-1 Key Features

Peritonitis

- Rigid, boardlike abdomen (classic)
- Abdominal pain (localized, poorly localized, or referred to the shoulder or chest)
- Distended abdomen
- Nausea, anorexia, vomiting
- Diminishing bowel sounds
- Inability to pass flatus or feces
- Rebound tenderness in the abdomen
- High fever
- Tachycardia
- Dehydration from high fever (poor skin turgor)
- Decreased urine output
- Hiccups
- Possible compromise in respiratory status

the health care provider (and/or surgeon), nurse, respiratory therapist, and social worker to facilitate transition.

◆ Assessment: Noticing

History. Ask the patient about abdominal pain and determine the character of the pain (e.g., cramping, sharp, aching), location of the pain, and whether the pain is localized or generalized. Ask about a history of a low-grade fever or recent spikes in temperature.

Physical Assessment/Signs and Symptoms. Physical findings of peritonitis (Chart 57-1) depend on several factors: the stage of the disease, the ability of the body to localize the process by walling off the infection, and whether the inflammation has progressed to generalized peritonitis. The patient most often appears acutely ill, lying still, possibly with the knees flexed. Movement is guarded, and he or she may report and show signs of pain (e.g., facial grimacing) with coughing or movement of any type. During inspection, observe for progressive abdominal distention, often seen when the inflammation markedly reduces intestinal motility. Auscultate for bowel sounds, which usually disappear with progression of the inflammation.

The cardinal signs of peritonitis are abdominal pain, tenderness, and distention. In the patient with *localized* peritonitis, the abdomen is tender on palpation in a well-defined area with rebound tenderness in this area. With *generalized* peritonitis, tenderness is widespread.

Psychosocial Assessment. The patient with peritonitis may be very fearful and anxious about the implications of a diagnosis of peritonitis and may be distressed regarding the physical pain that he or she feels. Provide a calm, nonanxious presence and reassure the patient that you will stay with him or her during this time. Allow the patient to express feelings of fear and anxiety, and provide nonjudgmental listening and presence.

❗ NURSING SAFETY PRIORITY QSEN

Action Alert

For patients with peritonitis, assess for abdominal wall rigidity, which is a classic finding that is sometimes referred to as a "boardlike" abdomen. Monitor the patient for a high fever because of the infectious process. Assess for tachycardia occurring in response to the fever and decreased circulating blood volume. Observe whether he or she has dry mucous membranes and a low urine output seen with third spacing. Nausea and vomiting may also be present. Hiccups may occur as a result of diaphragmatic irritation. Be sure to document all assessment findings.

Laboratory Assessment. White blood cell (WBC) counts are often elevated to 20,000/mm³ with a high neutrophil count. *Blood culture* studies may be done to determine whether septicemia has occurred and to identify the causative organism to enable appropriate antibiotic therapy. The health care provider may request laboratory tests to assess FLUID AND ELECTROLYTE BALANCE and renal status, including blood urea nitrogen (BUN), creatinine, hemoglobin, and hematocrit. Oxygen saturation and end–carbon dioxide monitoring may be obtained to assess respiratory function and acid-base balance.

Imaging Assessment. Abdominal x-rays can assess for free air or fluid in the abdominal cavity, indicating perforation. The x-rays may also show dilation, edema, and inflammation of the small and large intestines. An *abdominal ultrasound* may also be performed.

◆ Analysis: Interpreting

The priority collaborative problems for patients with peritonitis include:

1. Potential for infection due to peritonitis
2. Potential for fluid volume shift due to fluid moving into interstitial or peritoneal space
3. Acute pain due to peritonitis

◆ Planning and Implementation: Responding

Decreasing Potential for Infection

Planning: Expected Outcomes. The patient will be free from infection.

Interventions

Nonsurgical Management. Assess vital signs frequently, noting any change that may indicate septic shock, such as unresolved or progressive hypotension, decreased pulse pressure, tachycardia, fever, skin changes, and/or tachypnea. Monitor mental changes for any sign of confusion or altered level of consciousness. Practice proper handwashing and maintain strict asepsis when caring for wounds, drains, and dressings to decrease chance of infection. If the patient has or requires a urinary catheter, maintain strict sterile technique and provide appropriate catheter care. Observe and document wound drainage; report any changes immediately to the health care provider. Administer broad-spectrum antibiotics as prescribed to treat known or potential pathogens. Apply oxygen as ordered and according to the patient's respiratory status and oxygen saturation via pulse oximetry (e.g., SpO₂ less than 93%).

Surgical Management. Abdominal surgery may be needed to identify and repair the cause of the peritonitis to decrease further chance for infection. If the patient is critically ill and surgery would be life threatening, it may be delayed. Surgery focuses on controlling the contamination, removing foreign material from the peritoneal cavity, and draining collected fluid.

Exploratory laparotomy (surgical opening into the abdomen) or laparoscopy is used to remove or repair the inflamed or perforated organ (e.g., appendectomy for an inflamed appendix; a colon resection, with or without a colostomy, for a perforated diverticulum). Before the incision(s) is closed, the surgeon irrigates the peritoneum with antibiotic solutions. Several catheters may be inserted to drain the cavity and provide a route for irrigation after surgery.

If an open surgical procedure is needed, the infection may slow healing of an incision, or the incision may be partially open to heal by second or third intention. These wounds require special care involving manual irrigation or packing as prescribed

by the surgeon. If the surgeon requests peritoneal irrigation through a drain, *maintain sterile technique during manual irrigation* to prevent further risk for infection. The preoperative care is similar to that described in Chapter 14 for patients having general anesthesia. Chapter 16 describes general postoperative care.

> **⚠ NURSING SAFETY PRIORITY** QSEN
>
> **Action Alert**
>
> Monitor the patient's level of consciousness, vital signs, respiratory status (respiratory rate and breath sounds), and intake and output at least hourly immediately after abdominal surgery. Maintain the patient in a semi-Fowler's position to promote drainage of peritoneal contents into the lower region of the abdominal cavity. This position also helps increase lung expansion.

Restoring Fluid Volume Balance

Planning: Expected Outcomes. The patient will experience restoration of fluid volume balance.

Interventions. The health care provider prescribes hypertonic IV fluids and broad-spectrum antibiotics immediately after establishing the diagnosis of peritonitis. IV fluids are used to replace fluids collected in the peritoneum and bowel. Monitor daily weight and intake and output carefully. A nasogastric tube (NGT) decompresses the stomach and the intestine, and the patient is NPO.

Multi-system complications can occur with peritonitis. Loss of fluids and electrolytes from the extracellular space to the peritoneal cavity, NGT suctioning, and NPO status require that the patient receives IV fluid replacement. Be sure that unlicensed assistive personnel (UAP) carefully measure intake and output. Fluid rates may be changed frequently based on laboratory values, assessment findings, and patient condition.

Assess whether the patient retains fluid used for irrigation by comparing and recording the amount of fluid returned with the amount of fluid instilled. Fluid retention could cause abdominal distention or pain.

Managing Acute Pain

Planning: Expected Outcomes. The patient with peritonitis is expected to report pain control as evidenced by no more than a 3 on a 0-to-10 pain intensity scale.

Interventions. Peritonitis causes significant alteration in COMFORT. Interventions to manage pain focus on drug therapy. Administer analgesics and monitor for pain control. Document all pain assessments and interventions implemented to promote comfort thoroughly.

Care Coordination and Transition Management

Home Care Management. The length of hospitalization for a patient with peritonitis depends on the extent and severity of the infectious process. Patients who have a localized abscess drained and who respond to antibiotics and IV fluids without multi-system complications are discharged in several days. Others may require mechanical ventilation or hemodialysis with longer hospital stays. Some patients may be transferred to a transitional care unit to complete their antibiotic therapy and recovery. Convalescence is often longer than for other surgeries because of multi-system involvement.

Self-Management Education. When discharged home, assess the patient's ability for self-management at home with the added task of incision care and a reduced activity tolerance.

Provide the patient and family with written and oral instructions to report the following problems to the health care provider immediately:

- Unusual or foul-smelling drainage
- Swelling, redness, or warmth or bleeding from the incision site
- A temperature higher than 101°F (38.3°C)
- Abdominal pain
- Signs of wound dehiscence or ileus

Patients with large incisions heal by second or third intention and may require dressings, solution, and catheter-tipped syringes to irrigate the wound. A home care nurse may be needed to assess, irrigate, or pack the wound and change the dressing as needed until the patient and family feel comfortable with the procedure. If the patient needs assistance with ADLs, a home care aide or temporary placement in a skilled care facility may be indicated.

Review information about antibiotics and analgesics. For patients taking oral opioid analgesics such as oxycodone with acetaminophen (Percocet, Endocet) for any length of time, a stool softener such as docusate sodium (Colace) may be prescribed with a laxative such as Senna. Older adults are especially at risk for constipation from codeine-based drugs. Remind patients to avoid taking additional acetaminophen (Tylenol) to prevent liver toxicity.

Teach patients to refrain from any lifting for *at least* 6 weeks after an open surgical procedure. Other activity limitations are made on an individual basis with the health care provider's recommendation. Patients who have laparoscopic surgery can resume activities within a week or two and may not have any major restrictions.

Health Care Resources. Patients with peritonitis may benefit from a social services consultation. Social workers can help patients locate the most appropriate and affordable supplies that will be needed for ongoing care. Collaborate with the case manager (CM) to determine the appropriate setting for seamless continuing care in the community.

💡 NCLEX EXAMINATION CHALLENGE 57-1

Safe and Effective Care Environment

A client who recently had laparoscopic surgery to treat a ruptured appendix has developed subsequent peritonitis. The client currently has two Jackson Pratt drains placed in the abdomen. Which finding(s) would the nurse report **immediately** to the surgeon? **Select all that apply.**
A. Serosanguineous drainage
B. Fever
C. Cloudy drainage
D. Painful abdominal distention
E. Pain level 3 on a scale of 1 to 10

◆ **Evaluation: Reflecting**

Evaluate the care of the patient with peritonitis based on the identified priority patient problems. The expected outcomes are that the patient:

- Does not develop further infection
- Experiences restoration of fluid balance
- Verbalizes relief or control of pain and alterations in COMFORT

APPENDICITIS

❖ PATHOPHYSIOLOGY

Appendicitis is an acute inflammation of the vermiform appendix that occurs most often among young adults. It is the most common cause of right lower quadrant (RLQ) pain. The appendix usually extends off the proximal cecum of the colon just below the ileocecal valve. Inflammation occurs when the lumen (opening) of the appendix is obstructed (blocked), leading to infection as bacteria invade the wall of the appendix. The initial obstruction is usually a result of fecaliths (very hard pieces of feces) composed of calcium phosphate–rich mucus and inorganic salts. Less common causes are malignant tumors, helminthes (worms), or other infections (McCance et al., 2014).

When the lumen is blocked, the mucosa secretes fluid, increasing the internal pressure and restricting blood flow, which results in pain. If the process occurs slowly, an abscess may develop, but a rapid process may result in peritonitis (inflammation and infection of the peritoneum). *All complications of peritonitis are serious. Gangrene and sepsis can occur within 24 to 36 hours, are life threatening, and are some of the most common indications for emergency surgery. Perforation may develop within 24 hours, but the risk rises rapidly after 48 hours.* Perforation of the appendix also results in peritonitis with a temperature of greater than 101°F (38.3°C) and a rise in pulse rate.

🔲 CONSIDERATIONS FOR OLDER ADULTS

Patient-Centered Care QSEN

Appendicitis is relatively rare at extremes in age. However, perforation is more common in older adults, causing a higher mortality rate. The diagnosis of appendicitis is difficult to establish in older adults because symptoms of pain and tenderness may not be as pronounced in this age-group. This difference results in treatment delay and an increased risk for perforation, peritonitis, and death.

❖ INTERPROFESSIONAL COLLABORATIVE CARE

Patients with appendicitis are hospitalized because of the severe nature of the illness. The interprofessional team that collaborates most closely to care for this patient generally includes the health care provider, surgeon, and nurse.

◆ **Assessment: Noticing**

History taking and tracking the sequence of symptoms are important because nausea or vomiting before abdominal pain can indicate gastroenteritis. Abdominal pain followed by nausea and vomiting can indicate appendicitis. Ask about risk factors such as age, familial tendency, and intra-abdominal tumors. Classically, patients with appendicitis have cramping pain in the epigastric or periumbilical area. Anorexia is a frequent symptom, with nausea and vomiting occurring in many cases.

Perform a complete pain assessment. Initially pain can present anywhere in the abdomen or flank area. As the inflammation and infection progress, the pain becomes more severe and steady and shifts to the RLQ between the anterior iliac crest and the umbilicus. This area is referred to as *McBurney's point* (Fig. 57-1). *Abdominal pain that increases with cough or movement and is relieved by bending the right hip or the knees suggests perforation and peritonitis.* An advanced practice nurse or other health care provider will assess for muscle rigidity and guarding

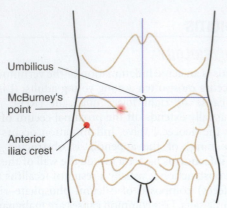

Umbilicus

McBurney's point

Anterior iliac crest

FIG. 57-1 McBurney's point is located midway between the anterior iliac crest and the umbilicus in the right lower quadrant. This is the classic area for localized tenderness during the later stages of appendicitis.

on palpation of the abdomen. The patient may report pain after release of pressure. This is referred to as *rebound* tenderness.

Laboratory findings do not establish the diagnosis, but often there is a moderate elevation of the *white blood cell (WBC) count* (leukocytosis) to 10,000 to 18,000/mm³ with a "shift to the left" (an increased number of immature WBCs). A WBC elevation to greater than 20,000/mm³ may indicate a perforated appendix. An *ultrasound* study may show the presence of an enlarged appendix. If symptoms are recurrent or prolonged, a CT scan can be used for diagnosis and may reveal the presence of a fecaloma (a small "stone" of feces).

◆ Interventions: Responding

All patients with suspected or confirmed appendicitis are hospitalized, and most have surgery to remove the inflamed appendix.

Nonsurgical Management. Keep the patient with suspected or known appendicitis NPO to prepare for the possibility of surgery and to avoid making the inflammation worse. Before surgical intervention be sure that the patient's pain is adequately managed.

❗ NURSING SAFETY PRIORITY **QSEN**

Action Alert

For the patient with suspected appendicitis, administer IV fluids as prescribed to maintain FLUID AND ELECTROLYTE BALANCE and replace fluid volume. If tolerated, advise the patient to maintain a semi-Fowler's position so abdominal drainage can be contained in the lower abdomen. Once the diagnosis of appendicitis is confirmed and surgery is scheduled, administer opioid analgesics and antibiotics as prescribed. *The patient with suspected or confirmed appendicitis should not receive laxatives or enemas, which can cause perforation of the appendix. Do not apply heat to the abdomen because this may increase circulation to the appendix and result in increased inflammation and perforation!*

Surgical Management. Surgery is required as soon as possible. An **appendectomy** is the removal of the inflamed appendix by one of several surgical approaches. Uncomplicated appendectomy procedures are done via laparoscopy. A **laparoscopy** is a minimally invasive surgery (MIS) with one or more small incisions near the umbilicus through which a small endoscope is placed. Patients having this type of surgery for appendix removal have few postoperative complications (see Chapter 15). A procedure known as natural orifice transluminal endoscopic surgery (NOTES) (e.g., transvaginal endoscopic appendectomy)

TABLE 57-1	Common Types of Gastroenteritis and Their Characteristics
TYPE	**CHARACTERISTICS**
Viral Gastroenteritis	
Epidemic viral	Caused by many parvovirus-type organisms
	Transmitted by the fecal-oral route in food and water
	Incubation period 10-51 hr
	Communicable during acute illness
Norovirus (Norwalk viruses)	Transmitted by the fecal-oral route and possibly the respiratory route (vomitus)
	Incubation in 48 hr
	Affects adults of all ages
	Older adults can become hypovolemic and experience electrolyte imbalances
Bacterial Gastroenteritis	
Campylobacter enteritis	Transmitted by the fecal-oral route or by contact with infected animals or infants
	Incubation period 1-10 days
	Communicable for 2-7 weeks
Escherichia coli diarrhea	Transmitted by fecal contamination of food, water, or fomites
Shigellosis	Transmitted by direct and indirect fecal-oral routes
	Incubation period 1-7 days
	Communicable during the acute illness to 4 weeks after the illness
	Humans possibly carriers for months

does not require an external skin incision. In this procedure the surgeon places the endoscope into the vagina or other orifice and makes a small incision to enter the peritoneal space. Patients having any type of laparoscopic procedure are typically discharged the same day of surgery with less pain and few complications after discharge. Most patients can return to usual activities in 1 to 2 weeks.

If the diagnosis is not definitive but the patient is at high risk for complications from suspected appendicitis, the surgeon may perform an exploratory laparotomy to rule out appendicitis. A **laparotomy** is an open surgical approach with a large abdominal incision for complicated or atypical appendicitis or peritonitis.

Preoperative teaching is often limited because the patient is in pain or may be admitted quickly for emergency surgery. The patient is prepared for general anesthesia and surgery as described in Chapter 14. After surgery, care of the patient who has undergone an appendectomy is the same as that required for anyone who has received general anesthesia (see Chapter 16).

If complications such as peritonitis or abscesses are found during *open* traditional surgery, wound drains are inserted, and a nasogastric tube may be placed to decompress the stomach and prevent abdominal distention. Administer IV antibiotics and opioid analgesics as prescribed. Help the patient out of bed on the evening of surgery to help prevent respiratory complications, such as atelectasis. He or she may be hospitalized for as long as 3 to 5 days and return to normal activity in 4 to 6 weeks.

GASTROENTERITIS

❖ PATHOPHYSIOLOGY

Gastroenteritis is a very common health problem worldwide that causes diarrhea and/or vomiting as a result of inflammation of the mucous membranes of the stomach and intestinal tract. It affects mainly the small bowel and can be caused by either viral (more common) or bacterial infection. Table 57-1 lists common types of gastroenteritis and their primary characteristics.

Norovirus (also known as a *Norwalk-like virus*) is the leading foodborne disease that causes gastroenteritis. It occurs most often between November and April because it is resistant to low temperatures and has a long viral shedding before and after the illness. Norovirus is transmitted (spread) through the fecal-oral route from person to person and from contaminated food and water. Infected individuals can also contaminate surfaces and objects in the environment. Vomiting may cause the virus to become airborne. The incubation time is 1 to 2 days.

In most cases of gastroenteritis, the illness is self-limiting and lasts about 3 days. However, in those who are immunosuppressed or in older adults, dehydration and hypovolemia can occur as complications requiring medical attention and possibly hospitalization.

Health Promotion and Maintenance

Outbreaks of norovirus have occurred in prisons, on cruise ships, and in nursing homes, college dormitories, and other places where large groups of people are in close proximity. Handwashing and sanitizing surfaces and other environmental items help prevent the spread of the illness. Hand sanitizers are often placed in public areas so hands can be cleaned when washing with soap and water is inconvenient. Proper food and beverage preparation is also important to prevent contamination.

❖ INTERPROFESSIONAL COLLABORATIVE CARE

Patients with gastroenteritis are generally cared for in the community setting and self-manage at home. Those who develop the more severe types of this condition, or become extremely dehydrated during it course, may be hospitalized. The interprofessional team that collaborates to care for this patient generally includes the health care provider and nurse.

◆ Assessment: Noticing

The patient history can provide information related to the potential cause of the illness. Ask about recent travel, especially to tropical regions of Asia, Africa, Mexico, or Central or South America, because these areas historically have been a source of gastroenteritis. Inquire if the patient has eaten at any restaurant in the past 24 to 36 hours. Some have acquired gastroenteritis from eating in "fast-food" restaurants or from food items purchased at a farmer's market or grocery store. Bacterial infections have caused large outbreaks that resulted from contaminated spinach and lettuce in the United States.

The patient who has gastroenteritis usually looks ill. Nausea and vomiting typically occur first, followed by abdominal cramping and diarrhea.

For patients who are older or for those who have inadequate immune systems, weakness and cardiac dysrhythmias may occur from loss of potassium (hypokalemia) from diarrhea. Monitor for and document manifestations of hypokalemia and hypovolemia (dehydration).

◆ Interventions: Responding

For any type of gastroenteritis, encourage fluid replacement. The amount and route of fluid administration are determined by the patient's hydration status and overall health condition. Teach patients to drink extra fluids to replace fluid lost through vomiting and diarrhea. Oral rehydration therapy (ORT) may be

> **! NURSING SAFETY PRIORITY** QSEN
>
> **Action Alert**
>
> For patients with gastroenteritis, note any abdominal distention and listen for hyperactive bowel sounds. Depending on the amount of fluids and electrolytes lost through diarrhea and vomiting, patients may have varying degrees of dehydration manifested by:
> - Poor skin turgor
> - Fever (not common in older adults)
> - Dry mucous membranes
> - Orthostatic blood pressure changes (which can cause a fall, especially for older adults)
> - Hypotension
> - Oliguria (decreased or absent urinary output)
>
> In some cases, dehydration may be severe. It occurs rapidly in older adults. Monitor mental status changes, such as acute confusion, that result from hypoxia in the older adult. These changes may be the only signs and symptoms of dehydration in older adults.

needed for some patients to replace fluids and electrolytes. Examples of ORT solutions include Gatorade, Pedialyte, and Powerade. Depending on the patient's age and severity of dehydration, he or she may be treated in the hospital with IV fluids to restore hydration.

Drugs that suppress intestinal motility may not be given for bacterial or viral gastroenteritis. *Use of these drugs can prevent the infecting organisms from being eliminated from the body.* If the health care provider determines that antiperistaltic agents are necessary, loperamide (Imodium) may be recommended.

> **! NURSING SAFETY PRIORITY** QSEN
>
> **Drug Alert**
>
> Diphenoxylate hydrochloride with atropine sulfate (Lomotil, Lomanate) reduces GI motility but is used sparingly because of its habit-forming ability. *The drug should not be used for older adults because it also causes drowsiness and could contribute to falls.*

Treatment with antibiotics may be needed if the gastroenteritis is caused by bacterial infection with fever and severe diarrhea. Depending on the type and severity of the illness, examples of drugs that may be prescribed include ciprofloxacin (Cipro) or azithromycin (Zithromax). If the gastroenteritis is caused by shigellosis, anti-infective agents such as trimethoprim/sulfamethoxazole (Septra DS, Bactrim DS) or ciprofloxacin (Cipro) are prescribed (Fhogartaigh & Dance, 2013).

Frequent stools that are rich in electrolytes and enzymes and frequent wiping and washing of the anal region can irritate the skin. Teach the patient to avoid toilet paper and harsh soaps. Ideally, he or she can gently clean the area with warm water or an absorbent material, followed by thorough but gentle drying. Cream, oil, or gel can be applied to a damp, warm washcloth to remove stool that sticks to open skin. Special prepared skin wipes can also be used. Protective barrier cream can be applied to the skin between stools. Sitz baths for 10 minutes two or three times daily can also relieve discomfort.

If leakage of stool is a problem, the patient can use an absorbent cotton or panty liner and keep it in place with snug underwear. For patients who are incontinent, the use of incontinent pads at night instead of briefs allows air to circulate to the skin and prevents irritation. Remind unlicensed assistive personnel (UAP) to keep the perineal and buttock areas clean and dry and that frequent changes will be necessary.

During the acute phase of the illness, teach the patient and family about the importance of fluid replacement. Patient and family education regarding risk for transmission of gastroenteritis is also important (Chart 57-2).

CHRONIC INFLAMMATORY BOWEL DISEASE

Ulcerative colitis and Crohn's disease are the two most common inflammatory bowel diseases (IBDs) that affect adults. Comparisons and differences are listed in Table 57-2. Many other infectious mechanisms can cause symptoms similar to those of IBD, and other problems must be ruled out before a definitive diagnosis is made. The approach to each patient is individualized. Encourage patients to self-manage their disease by learning about the illness, treatment, drugs, and complications.

✳ ELIMINATION CONCEPT EXEMPLAR
Ulcerative Colitis

❖ PATHOPHYSIOLOGY

Ulcerative colitis (UC) creates widespread inflammation of mainly the rectum and rectosigmoid colon but can extend to the entire colon when the disease is extensive. Distribution of the disease can remain constant for years. UC is a disease that is associated with periodic remissions and exacerbations (flare-ups). Many factors can cause exacerbations, including intestinal infections. Most patients who are affected have mild-to-moderate disease, but 10% to 15% of patients present with severe symptoms (Macken & Blaker, 2015). Older adults with UC are at high risk for impaired FLUID AND ELECTROLYTE BALANCE as a result of diarrhea, including dehydration and hypokalemia.

The intestinal mucosa becomes hyperemic (has increased blood flow), edematous, and reddened. In more severe inflammation, the lining can bleed, and small erosions, or ulcers, occur. Abscesses can form in these ulcerative areas and result in tissue necrosis (cell death). Continued edema and mucosal thickening can lead to a narrowed colon and possibly a partial bowel obstruction. Table 57-3 lists the categories of the severity of UC.

The patient's stool typically contains blood and mucus. Patients report tenesmus (an unpleasant and urgent sensation to defecate) and lower abdominal colicky pain relieved with defecation. Malaise, anorexia, anemia, dehydration, fever, and weight loss are common. Extraintestinal manifestations such as migratory polyarthritis, ankylosing spondylitis, and erythema nodosum are present in a large number of patients. The common and extraintestinal complications of UC are listed in Table 57-4.

Etiology and Genetic Risk

The exact cause of UC is unknown; but a combination of genetic, immunologic, and environmental factors likely contributes to disease development. A genetic basis of the disease has been supported because it is often found in families and twins. Immunologic causes, including autoimmune dysfunction, are likely the etiology of extraintestinal manifestations of the disease. Epithelial antibodies in the immunoglobulin G

👤 CHART 57-2 Patient and Family Education: Preparing for Self-Management

Preventing Transmission of Gastroenteritis

Advise the patient to:
- Wash hands well for at least 30 seconds with an antibacterial soap, especially after a bowel movement, and maintain good personal hygiene.
- Restrict the use of glasses, dishes, eating utensils, and tubes of toothpaste for his or her own use. In severe cases, disposable utensils may be wise.
- Maintain clean bathroom facilities to avoid exposure to stool.
- Inform the health care provider if symptoms persist beyond 3 days.
- Do not prepare or handle food that will be consumed by others. If you (the patient) are employed as a food handler, the public health department should be consulted for recommendations about the return to work.

TABLE 57-2 Differential Features of Ulcerative Colitis and Crohn's Disease

FEATURE	ULCERATIVE COLITIS	CROHN'S DISEASE
Location	Begins in the rectum and proceeds in a continuous manner toward the cecum	Most often in the terminal ileum, with patchy involvement through all layers of the bowel
Etiology	Unknown	Unknown
Peak incidence at age	15-25 yr and 55-65 yr	15-40 yr
Number of stools	10-20 liquid, bloody stools per day	5-6 soft, loose stools per day, nonbloody
Complications	Hemorrhage Nutritional deficiencies	Fistulas (common) Nutritional deficiencies
Need for surgery	Infrequent	Frequent

TABLE 57-3 American College of Gastroenterologists Classification of UC Severity

SEVERITY	STOOL FREQUENCY	SIGNS/SYMPTOMS
Mild	<4 stools/day with/without blood	Asymptomatic Laboratory values usually normal
Moderate	>4 stools/day with/without blood	Minimal symptoms Mild abdominal pain Mild intermittent nausea Possible increased C-reactive protein* or ESR†
Severe	>6 bloody stools/day	Fever Tachycardia Anemia Abdominal pain Elevated C-reactive protein* and/or ESR†
Fulminant	>10 bloody stools/day	Increasing symptoms Anemia may require transfusion Colonic distention on x-ray

UC, Ulcerative colitis.
*C-reactive protein is a sensitive acute-phase serum marker that is evident in the first 6 hours of an inflammatory process.
†*ESR*, erythrocyte sedimentation rate; may be helpful but is less sensitive than C-reactive protein.

TABLE 57-4 Complications of Ulcerative Colitis and Crohn's Disease

COMPLICATION	DESCRIPTION
Hemorrhage/ perforation	Lower GI bleeding results from erosion of the bowel wall.
Abscess formation	Localized pockets of infection develop in the ulcerated bowel lining.
Toxic megacolon	Paralysis of the colon causes dilation and subsequent colonic ileus, possibly perforation.
Malabsorption	Essential nutrients cannot be absorbed through the diseased intestinal wall, causing anemia and malnutrition (most common in Crohn's disease).
Nonmechanical bowel obstruction	Obstruction results from toxic megacolon or cancer.
Fistulas	In Crohn's disease in which the inflammation is transmural, fistulas can occur anywhere but usually track between the bowel and bladder, resulting in pyuria and fecaluria.
Colorectal cancer	Patients with ulcerative colitis with a history longer than 10 years have a high risk for colorectal cancer. This complication accounts for about one third of all deaths related to ulcerative colitis.
Extraintestinal complications	Complications include arthritis, hepatic and biliary disease (especially cholelithiasis), oral and skin lesions, and ocular disorders, such as iritis. The cause is unknown.
Osteoporosis	Osteoporosis occurs especially in patients with Crohn's disease.

(IgG) class have been identified in the blood of some patients with UC (McCance et al., 2014).

With long-term disease, cellular changes can occur that increase the risk for colon cancer. Damage from pro-inflammatory cytokines, such as specific interleukins (ILs) (e.g., IL-1, IL-6, IL-8) and tumor necrosis factor (TNF)–alpha, have cytotoxic effects on the colonic mucosa (McCance et al., 2014).

Incidence and Prevalence

Chronic inflammatory bowel disease (IBD) affects about 1.4 million individuals in the United States and is split about equally between ulcerative colitis (UC) and Crohn's disease (discussed later). Although diagnosis can occur at any age, most people are diagnosed between 15 and 35 years of age (Crohn's and Colitis Foundation, 2017). Women are more often affected than men in their younger years, but men have the disease more often as middle-age and older adults (McCance et al., 2014).

⊕ CULTURAL/SPIRITUAL CONSIDERATIONS

Patient-Centered Care QSEN

Ulcerative colitis is more common among Askenazki Jewish individuals than among those who are not Jewish and among whites more than nonwhites (McCance et al., 2014). The reasons for these cultural differences are not known.

❖ INTERPROFESSIONAL COLLABORATIVE CARE

Patients with UC may be self-managed at home, cared for in the community setting, or hospitalized, depending on their immediate condition related to this chronic bowel disease. The interprofessional team that collaborates to care for this patient generally includes the health care provider (and/or surgeon), nurse, psychologist, social worker, and spiritual leader of the patient's choice.

◆ Assessment: Noticing

History. Collect data on family history of IBD, previous and current therapy for the illness, and dates and types of surgery. Obtain a NUTRITION history, including intolerance of milk and milk products and fried, spicy, or hot foods. Ask about usual bowel ELIMINATION pattern (color, number, consistency, and character of stools), abdominal pain, tenesmus, anorexia, and fatigue. Note any relationship between diarrhea, timing of meals, emotional distress, and activity. Inquire about recent (past 2 to 3 month) exposure to antibiotics to rule out a *Clostridium difficile* infection. Has the patient traveled to or emigrated from tropical areas? Ask about recent use of NSAIDs because these can cause a flare-up of the disease. Inquire about any extraintestinal symptoms such as arthritis, mouth sores, vision problems, and skin disorders.

Physical Assessment/Signs and Symptoms. Symptoms vary with an acuteness of onset. Vital signs are usually within normal limits in mild disease. In more severe cases, the patient may have a low-grade fever (99° to 100° F [37.2° to 37.8° C]). The physical assessment findings are usually nonspecific, and in milder cases the physical examination may be normal. Viral and bacterial infections can cause symptoms similar to those of UC.

Note any abdominal distention along the colon. Fever associated with tachycardia may indicate dehydration, peritonitis, and bowel perforation. Assess for signs and symptoms associated with extraintestinal complications, such as inflamed joints and lesions inside the mouth.

Psychosocial Assessment. Many patients are very concerned about the frequency of stools and the presence of blood. *The inability to control the disease symptoms, particularly diarrhea, can be disruptive and anxiety producing.* Severe illness may limit the patient's activities outside the home with fear of fecal incontinence resulting in feeling "tied to the toilet." Severe anxiety and depression may result. Eating may be associated with pain and cramping and an increased frequency of stools. This can make mealtimes an unpleasant experience. Frequent visits to health care providers and close monitoring of the colon mucosa for abnormal cell changes can be anxiety provoking.

Assess the patient's understanding of the illness and its impact on his or her lifestyle. Encourage and support the patient while exploring:

- The relationship of life events to disease exacerbations
- Stress factors that produce symptoms
- Family and social support systems
- Concerns regarding the possible genetic basis and associated cancer risks of the disease
- Internet access for reliable education information

Laboratory Assessment. As a result of chronic blood loss, hematocrit and hemoglobin levels may be low, which indicates anemia and a chronic disease state. *An increased WBC count, C-reactive protein, or erythrocyte sedimentation rate (ESR) is consistent with inflammatory disease.* Blood levels of sodium, potassium, and chloride may be *low* as a result of frequent diarrheal stools and malabsorption through the diseased bowel (Pagana et al., 2017). Hypoalbuminemia (decreased serum albumin) is found in patients with extensive disease from losing protein in the stool.

Other Diagnostic Assessment. Magnetic resonance enterography (MRE) is the main examination used to study the bowel in patients who have IBD. An MRE allows the primary provider to visualize the bowel lumen and wall, mesentery, and surrounding abdominal organs. Teach the patient that he or she will need to fast for 4 to 6 hours before the test. As part of the test the patient drinks a large amount of contrast medium; this can cause abdominal discomfort and diarrhea. Be sure that the patient has the opportunity to go to the restroom before positioning on the MRI table. The patient then lies prone while the first of two doses of glucagon are given subcutaneously. This substance helps to slow the bowel's activity and motility (Sinha, 2015).

An upper endoscopy and/or *colonoscopy* may be done to aid in diagnosis, but the bowel prep can be especially uncomfortable for patients with inflammatory bowel disease (IBD). Frequent colonoscopies are recommended when patients have longer than a 10-year history of UC involving the entire colon because they are at high risk for colorectal cancer. In some cases, a *CT scan* may be done to confirm the disease or its complications. *Barium enemas* with air contrast can show differences between UC and Crohn's disease and identify complications, mucosal patterns, and the distribution and depth of disease involvement. In early disease, the barium enema may show incomplete filling as a result of inflammation and fine ulcerations along the bowel contour, which appear deeper in more advanced disease.

◆ *Analysis: Interpreting*

The priority collaborative problems for patients with UC include:

1. Diarrhea due to inflammation of the bowel mucosa
2. Acute pain or chronic noncancer pain due to inflammation and ulceration of the bowel mucosa and skin irritation
3. Potential for lower GI bleeding and resulting anemia due to UC

◆ *Planning and Implementation: Responding*

Decreasing Diarrhea

Planning: Expected Outcomes. The major concern for a patient with ulcerative colitis is the occurrence of frequent, bloody diarrhea and fecal incontinence from tenesmus. Therefore the goal of treatment is for the patient to have decreased diarrhea, formed stools, and control of bowel movements, which allow for mucosal healing.

Interventions. Many measures are used to relieve symptoms and reduce intestinal motility, decrease inflammation, and promote intestinal healing. Nonsurgical and/or surgical management may be needed.

Nonsurgical Management. Nonsurgical management includes drug and NUTRITION therapy. The use of physical and emotional rest is also an important consideration. Teach the patient to record color, volume, frequency, and consistency of stools, either on paper or via an electronic app, to determine severity of the problem.

Monitor the skin in the perianal area for irritation and ulceration resulting from loose, frequent stools. Stool cultures

may be sent for analysis if diarrhea continues. Have the patient weigh himself or herself one or two times per week. If the patient is hospitalized, remind unlicensed assistive personnel to weigh him or her on admission and daily in the morning before breakfast and document all weights.

? NCLEX EXAMINATION CHALLENGE 57-2

Physiological Integrity

The nurse is caring for an older adult client who experiences an exacerbation of ulcerative colitis with severe diarrhea that have lasted a week. For which complications will the nurse assess? **Select all that apply.**

A. Dehydration
B. Hypokalemia
C. Skin breakdown
D. Deep vein thrombus
E. Hyperkalemia

Drug Therapy. Common drug therapy for UC includes aminosalicylates, glucocorticoids, antidiarrheal drugs, and immunomodulators. Teach patients about side effects and adverse drug events (ADEs) and when to call their health care provider.

The *aminosalicylates* are drugs commonly used to treat mild-to-moderate UC and/or maintain remission. Several aminosalicylic acid compounds are available. These drugs, also called *5-ASAs*, are thought to have an anti-inflammatory effect on the lining of the intestine by inhibiting prostaglandins and are usually effective in 2 to 4 weeks.

Sulfasalazine (Azulfidine, Azulfidine EN-tabs), the first aminosalicylate approved for UC, is metabolized by the intestinal bacteria into 5-ASA, which delivers the beneficial effects of the drug, and sulfapyridine, which is responsible for unwanted side effects. Teach patients to take a folic acid supplement, because sulfa decreases its absorption.

! NURSING SAFETY PRIORITY **QSEN**

Drug Alert

Teach patients taking sulfasalazine to report nausea, vomiting, anorexia, rash, and headache to the health care provider. With higher doses, hemolytic anemia, hepatitis, male infertility, or agranulocytosis can occur. This drug is in the same family as sulfonamide antibiotics. Therefore assess the patient for an allergy to sulfonamide or other drugs that contain sulfa *before* the patient takes the drug. The use of a thiazide diuretic may be a contraindication for sulfasalazine (Pfizer, 2016).

Mesalamine (Apriso, Asacol HD, Asacol 800 ♦, Canasa, Lialda, Pentasa, Rowasa) is better tolerated than sulfasalazine because none of its preparations contain sulfapyridine. Asacol is a delayed-release drug and is released in the terminal ileum and beyond within the colon. Pentasa is an extended-release drug that works throughout the colon and rectum. Rowasa can be given as an enema, and Canasa can be given as a suppository. These preparations have minimal systemic absorption and therefore have fewer side effects. Table 57-5 lists these commonly used 5-ASA drugs.

Glucocorticoids, such as prednisone and prednisolone, are corticosteroid therapies prescribed during exacerbations of the disease. Prednisone is typically prescribed, and the dose may be increased as acute flare-ups occur. Once clinical improvement occurs, the corticosteroids are tapered because of the adverse effects that commonly occur with long-term steroid therapy (e.g., hyperglycemia, osteoporosis, peptic ulcer disease, increased potential for infection, adrenal insufficiency). For patients with rectal inflammation, topical steroids in the form of small

TABLE 57-5   5-ASA Medications Used to Treat Mild to Moderate Ulcerative Colitis

GENERIC NAME	TRADE NAME
Sulfasalazine	Azulfidine
	Azulfidine EN-tabs
Mesalamine	Apriso
	Asacol HD
	Asacol 800 🍁
	Lialda
	Pentasa
	Rowasa

5-ASA, 5-aminosalicylic acid.

retention enemas or suppositories may be prescribed. Medications such as budesonide (Uceris or Entocort EC), steroids that are thought to work mostly in the bowel, produce less systemic side effects.

To provide symptomatic management of diarrhea, *antidiarrheal drugs* may be prescribed. However, these drugs are given very cautiously because they can cause colon dilation and toxic megacolon. Common antidiarrheal drugs include diphenoxylate hydrochloride and atropine sulfate (Lomotil) and loperamide (Imodium).

Immunomodulators are drugs that alter an individual's immune response. Alone, they are often not effective in the treatment of ulcerative colitis. However, in combination with steroids, they may offer a synergistic effect to a quicker response, thereby decreasing the amount of steroids needed. Biologic response modifiers (BRMs) used for UC (and Crohn's disease, discussed later in this chapter) include infliximab (Inflectra 🍁, Remicade, Remsima 🍁) and adalimumab (Humira). Although not approved as a first-line therapy for UC, infliximab may be used for refractory disease or for severe complications, such as **toxic megacolon** (massive dilation of the colon that can lead to gangrene and peritonitis) and extraintestinal manifestations. Remicade (Inflectra 🍁, Remsima 🍁) is an immunoglobulin G (IgG) monoclonal antibody that reduces the activity of tumor necrosis factor (TNF) to decrease inflammation. Adalimumab (Humira) is another monoclonal antibody approved for refractory (not responsive to other therapies) cases. BRMs are used more commonly in management of Crohn's disease. These drugs cause immunosuppression and should be used with caution. Teach the patient to report any signs of a beginning infection, including a cold, and to avoid large crowds or others who are sick.

Several newer monoclonal antibodies have recently been approved by the U.S. Food and Drug Administration (FDA) for use in patients with IBD. One of these drugs, vedolizumab (Entyvio), is an intestinal-specific leukocyte traffic inhibitor in that it prevents white blood cells from migrating to inflamed bowel tissue (Randall et al., 2015).

Nutrition Therapy and Rest. Patients with severe symptoms who are hospitalized are kept NPO to ensure bowel rest. The physician may prescribe total parenteral NUTRITION (TPN) for severely ill and malnourished patients during severe exacerbations. Chapter 60 describes this therapy in detail. Patients with less severe symptoms may drink elemental formulas such as Vivonex Plus or Vivonex T.E.N., which have components that are absorbed in the small bowel and reduce bowel stimulation.

Diet is not a major factor in the inflammatory process, but some patients with ulcerative colitis (UC) find that caffeine and alcohol increase diarrhea and cramping. For some patients, raw vegetables and other high-fiber foods can cause GI symptoms. Lactose-containing foods may be poorly tolerated and should be reduced or eliminated. Teach patients that carbonated beverages, pepper, nuts and corn, dried fruits, and smoking are common GI stimulants that could cause discomfort. Each patient differs in his or her food and fluid tolerances.

During an exacerbation of the disease, patient activity is generally restricted because rest can reduce intestinal activity, provide COMFORT, and promote healing. Ensure that the patient has easy access to a bedpan, bedside commode, or bathroom in case of urgency or tenesmus.

Complementary and Integrative Health. In addition to dietary changes, complementary and integrative therapies may be used to supplement traditional management of UC. Examples include herbs (e.g., flaxseed), selenium, and vitamin C. Biofeedback, hypnosis, yoga, acupuncture, and ayurveda (a combination of diet, yoga, herbs, and breathing exercises) may also be helpful. These therapies need further study to validate their effectiveness, but some patients find them helpful.

Surgical Management. Some patients with UC require surgery to help manage their disease when medical therapies alone are not effective. In some cases, surgery is performed for complications of UC such as toxic megacolon, hemorrhage, bowel perforation, dysplastic biopsy results, and colon cancer.

Preoperative Care. General preoperative teaching related to abdominal surgery is described in Chapter 14. If a temporary or permanent ileostomy is planned, provide an in-depth explanation to the patient and family. An **ileostomy** is a procedure in which a loop of the ileum is placed through an opening in the abdominal wall (**stoma**) for drainage of fecal material into a pouching system worn on the abdomen. The external pouching system consists of a solid skin barrier (wafer) to protect the skin and a fecal collection device (pouch), similar to the system used for patients with colostomies (discussed in Chapter 56).

If an ileostomy is planned, the surgeon consults with a certified wound, ostomy, continence nurse (CWOCN) before surgery for recommendations on the best location of the stoma. A visit before surgery from an **ostomate** (a patient with an ostomy) may be helpful. **Parenteral antibiotics are given within 1 hour of surgical opening based on current best evidence and per The Joint Commission's National Patient Safety Goals.**

Operative Procedures. Any one of several surgical approaches may be used for the patient with UC. Minimally invasive procedures, such as laparoscopic, laparoscopic-assisted, hand-assisted, and robotic-assisted surgery, are common for patients with UC in large tertiary care centers (Seifarth et al., 2015). Laparoscopic surgery usually involves one or several small incisions but often takes longer to perform than the open surgical approach. The natural orifice transluminal endoscopic surgery (NOTES) procedure can be performed via the anus or vagina for certain patients. The availability of this type of procedure depends greatly on the training of the surgeon. Patients may have moderate sedation or general anesthesia for minimally invasive surgical procedures and because of this are not typically admitted to critical care units for continuing postoperative care.

Patients who are obese, have had previous abdominal surgeries, or have dense scar tissue (adhesions) may not be candidates for laparoscopic procedures. The conventional open surgical

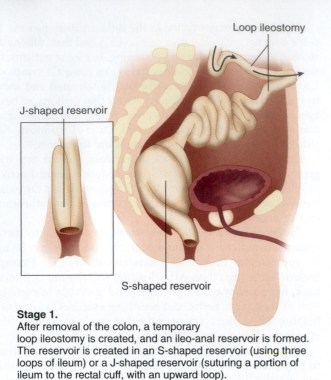

Loop ileostomy

J-shaped reservoir

S-shaped reservoir

Stage 1.
After removal of the colon, a temporary
loop ileostomy is created, and an ileo-anal reservoir is formed.
The reservoir is created in an S-shaped reservoir (using three
loops of ileum) or a J-shaped reservoir (suturing a portion of
ileum to the rectal cuff, with an upward loop).

Loop ileostomy
reversed

Stage 2.
After the reservoir has had
time to heal—usually several months—the temporary
loop ileostomy is reversed, and stool is allowed to drain
into the reservoir.

FIG. 57-2 Creation of an ileo-anal reservoir.

approach involves an abdominal incision and is completed under
general anesthesia. Patients with open procedures are typically
admitted to critical care units for short-term stabilization.

*Restorative Proctocolectomy With Ileo Pouch–Anal Anastomosis
(RPC-IPAA).* This procedure has become the gold standard for
patients with UC. In some centers, the surgery is performed via
laparoscopy (laparoscopic RPC-IPAA). It is usually a two-stage
procedure that includes the removal of the colon and most of
the rectum (Fig. 57-2). The anus and anal sphincter remain
intact. The surgeon then surgically creates an internal pouch
(reservoir) using the last $1\frac{1}{2}$ feet of the small intestine. The
pouch, sometimes called a *J-pouch, S-pouch,* or *pelvic pouch,* is
then connected to the anus. A temporary ileostomy through the
abdominal skin is created to allow healing of the internal pouch
and all anastomosis sites. It also allows for an increase in the
capacity of the internal pouch. In the *second* surgical stage, the
loop ileostomy is closed. The time interval between the first and
second stages varies, but many patients have the second surgical
stage to close the ileostomy within 1 to 2 months of the first
surgery.

Usually bowel continence is excellent after this procedure,
but some patients report leakage of stool during sleep. They
may take antidiarrheal drugs to help control this problem. Reassure the patient that it is not unusual to have frequent stools
and urgency after this procedure.

Total Proctocolectomy With a Permanent Ileostomy. Total proctocolectomy with a permanent ileostomy is done for patients
who are not candidates for or do not want the ileo-anal pouch.
The procedure involves the removal of the colon, rectum, and
anus with surgical closure of the anus (Fig. 57-3A). The surgeon
brings the end of the ileum out through the abdominal wall and
forms a stoma, or ostomy.

Initially after surgery the output from an ileostomy is a loose,
dark green liquid that may contain some blood. Over time, a

NURSING SAFETY PRIORITY (QSEN)

Critical Rescue

The ileostomy stoma (Fig. 57-3B) is usually placed in the right lower
quadrant of the abdomen below the belt line. It should not be prolapsed
or retract into the abdominal wall. *Assess the stoma frequently after
stoma placement. Recognize that it should be pinkish to cherry red to
ensure an adequate blood supply. If the stoma looks pale, bluish, or
dark, respond by reporting these findings to the health care provider
immediately!*

process called *ileostomy adaptation* occurs. The small intestine
begins to perform some of the functions that had previously
been done by the colon, including the absorption of increased
amounts of sodium and water. Stool volume decreases, becomes
thicker (pastelike), and turns yellow-green or yellow-brown.
The effluent (fluid material) usually has little odor or a sweet
odor. Any foul or unpleasant odor may be a symptom of a
problem such as blockage or infection.

The ostomy drains frequently, and the stool is irritating. *The
patient with an ostomy must wear a pouch system at all times.*
The stool from the small intestine contains many enzymes and
bile salts, which can quickly irritate and excoriate the skin. *Skin
care around the stoma is a priority!* A pouch system with a skin
barrier (gelatin or pectin) provides sufficient protection for
most patients. Other products are also available.

Postoperative Care. Provide general postoperative care after
surgery, as described in Chapter 16. The few patients requiring
open-approach surgery for UC will have a large abdominal
incision. At first they are NPO, and a nasogastric tube (NGT)
is used for suction. The tube is removed in 1 to 2 days as the
drainage decreases, and fluids and food are slowly introduced.

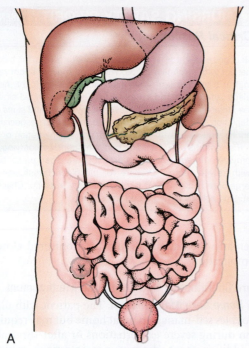

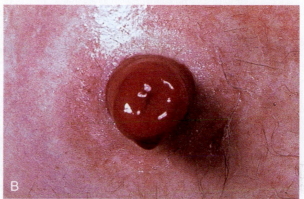

FIG. 57-3 A, Total proctocolectomy with a permanent ileostomy. This involved removal of the colon, the rectum, and the anus with closure of the anus. Note the missing colon, rectum, and anus with the resultant stoma **(B)** in the right lower quadrant. **(B** from Perry, A.G., & Potter, P.A. (2006). *Clinical nursing skills & techniques* [6th ed.]. St. Louis: Mosby. Courtesy ConvaTec, a Bristol-Myers Squibb Company, Princeton, NJ.)

The patient having minimally invasive surgery (MIS) usually does not have an NGT.

In collaboration with the CWOCN, help the patient adjust and learn the required care. The ileostomy usually begins to drain stool within 24 hours after surgery at more than 1 liter per day. Be sure that fluids are replaced by adding an additional 500 mL or more each day to prevent dehydration. After about a week of high-volume output, the stool drainage slows and becomes thicker. During this period, some patients need antidiarrheal drugs.

The hospital stay is usually from 1 to 4 days, depending on whether the patient has laparoscopic or conventional open surgery. Patients having MIS have less pain from surgery and faster restoration of bowel function when compared with other surgical patients (Hata et al., 2015).

For those who have the RPC-IPAA procedure, remind them that the internal pouch can become inflamed. This problem is usually effectively treated with metronidazole (Flagyl) for 7 to 10 days. VSL#3, a probiotic, has also been shown in some studies to reduce incidence of pouchitis (Singh et al., 2015). Teach patients that, after the second stage of surgery, they might have burning during bowel ELIMINATION because gastric acid cannot be absorbed well by the ileum. Also instruct them to omit foods that can cause odors or gas, such as cabbage, asparagus, Brussels sprouts, and beans. Teach patients to eliminate foods that cannot be digested well, such as nuts and corn. Each patient differs in which foods he or she can tolerate.

Surgery for UC may result in altered body image. However, it may be viewed as positive because the patient will have fewer symptoms and feel more comfortable than before the procedure. Patients have to adjust to having an ostomy before they can resume their presurgery activities.

Minimizing Pain

Planning: Expected Outcomes. The desired outcome for the patient is that he or she will verbalize decreased pain and an improvement in COMFORT as a result of collaborative, evidence-based pain management interventions. Take into consideration the effects of opioid-based pain medications on intestinal function.

Interventions. Pain control requires pharmacologic and nonpharmacologic measures. Physical discomfort can contribute to emotional distress. A variety of symptom-reducing interventions and supportive measures are used. Surgery also reduces pain for many patients.

The purpose of pain management is alleviation of pain or a reduction in pain to a level of comfort that is acceptable to the patient. Increases in pain may indicate the development of complications such as peritonitis (see earlier discussion in this chapter). Assist the patient in reducing or eliminating factors that can cause or increase the pain experience. For example, he or she may benefit from NUTRITION changes to decrease abdominal discomfort such as cramping and bloating.

CHART 57-3   Best Practice for Patient Safety & Quality Care QSEN

Pain Control and Skin Care for Patients With Inflammatory Bowel Disease

PATIENT PROBLEM	INTERVENTIONS
Abdominal pain (particularly with exacerbations of the disease)	Administer analgesics. Assist with frequent positioning. Identify foods that increase pain. Perform a comprehensive pain assessment. Observe for signs and symptoms of peritonitis. Evaluate effectiveness of pain management. Teach music therapy, guided imagery.
Skin excoriation and/or irritation from frequent bowel movements	Encourage good skin care with a mild soap and water after each bowel movement. Gently pat the area dry. Identify foods that increase diarrhea. Sitz baths may be of benefit. Apply a thin coat of A+D Ointment or aloe cream. Use medicated wipes instead of tissue. Ensure appropriate ostomy supplies that fit well. Antidiarrheal medications may help, but use with caution. Observe for symptoms related to megacolon (fever, leukocytosis, tachycardia, distended abdomen with three-view abdominal x-ray noting an enlarged colon).

! NURSING SAFETY PRIORITY QSEN
Critical Rescue

Recognize that it is important to monitor stools for blood loss for the patient with ulcerative colitis. The blood may be bright red (frank bleeding) or black and tarry (melena). Monitor hematocrit, hemoglobin, and electrolyte values and assess vital signs. Prolonged slow bleeding can lead to anemia. Observe for fever, tachycardia, and signs of fluid volume depletion. Changes in mental status may occur, especially among older adults, and may be the first indication of dehydration or anemia.

If symptoms of GI bleeding begin, respond by notifying the health care provider immediately. Blood products are often prescribed for patients with severe anemia. Prepare for the blood transfusion by inserting a large-bore IV catheter if it is not already in place. Chapter 40 outlines nursing actions during blood transfusion.

Antidiarrheal drugs may be needed to control diarrhea, thus reducing the discomfort. However, they must be used with caution and for a short time because toxic megacolon can develop.

Perineal skin can be irritated by contact with loose stools and frequent cleaning. Explain special measures for skin care. Use of medicated wipes is soothing if the rectal area is tender or sensitive from the use of toilet tissue (Chart 57-3). A number of ostomy manufacturers (e.g., Hollister, ConvaTec) produce a system for skin care that may help prevent and heal perineal skin irritation. These systems usually include a skin-cleaning solution, a moisturizing and healing cream, and a petroleum jelly–like barrier that prevents contact of moisture and stool with the skin.

Monitoring for Lower GI Bleeding

Planning: Expected Outcomes. The patient with UC is expected to have a reduction in or cessation of bleeding with prompt collaborative care. If possible, patients are expected to remain free of complications that can cause bleeding, such as perforation or anemia.

Interventions. The nursing priority is to monitor the patient closely for signs and symptoms of GI bleeding resulting from the disease or its complications.

If the patient has lower GI bleeding of more than 0.5 mL per minute, a *GI bleeding scan* may be useful to localize the site of the bleeding (Pagana et al., 2017). However, this test cannot indicate the cause of the bleeding and may take several hours to administer. Patients in the critical care unit are not candidates for the test because they must leave the unit for it. Keep in mind that a GI bleeding is considered a medical emergency;

therefore the patient should be monitored closely to prevent complications.

Care Coordination and Transition Management

Home Care Management. The patient with ulcerative colitis provides self-management at home but may require hospitalization during severe exacerbations or after surgical intervention. In addition, those who have extraintestinal problems often need ongoing collaborative care for joint and/or skin problems.

Home care management focuses on controlling signs and symptoms and monitoring for complications. For patients returning home or transferring to nursing home or transitional care after surgery, ongoing respiratory care, incision care (if applicable), ostomy care, and pain management should be continued.

Self-Management Education. Teach the patient about the nature of ulcerative colitis, including its acute episodes, remissions, and symptom management. Also stress that, even though the cause is unknown, relapses can be prevented with proper health care. Teach patients taking immunosuppressive drugs, such as corticosteroids and biologic response modifiers—more commonly known as *biologics* (monoclonal antibodies), to report signs of possible infection, such as sore throat, to the health care provider. Remind them to avoid crowds and anyone who has an infection. Review the purpose of drug therapy, when drugs should be taken, side effects, and adverse drug events.

Instruct the patient about measures to reduce or control abdominal pain, cramping, and diarrhea. Also teach the patient and family about symptoms associated with disease exacerbation that should be reported to the health care provider, such as fever higher than 101°F (38.3°C), tachycardia, palpitations, and an increase in diarrhea, abdominal pain, or nausea/vomiting. Provide written information and contact numbers for the health care provider.

There is no special diet for a patient with an ileostomy. However, teach the patient to avoid any foods that cause gas. Examples include high-fiber foods such as nuts, raw cabbage, corn, celery, apples with peels, and popcorn. The patient needs to learn which foods he or she tolerates best and adjust the diet accordingly.

If the patient has undergone a temporary or permanent surgical diversion, collaborate with the CWOCN to explain and demonstrate required care so he or she can self-manage or the family/caregiver can assist. Also teach the importance of including adequate amounts of salt and water in the diet because the ileostomy increases the loss of these substances. Urge the patient to be cautious in situations that lead to heavy sweating or fluid loss, such as strenuous physical activity, high environmental heat, and episodes of diarrhea and vomiting.

Finding the best ostomy pouching system is a major issue for many patients. An effective system is one that:

- Protects the skin
- Contains the effluent (drainage) and reduces odor, if any
- Remains securely attached to the skin for a dependable period of time

Most patients desire an adhesive barrier that will last for 3 to 7 days. The barrier must create a solid seal to prevent the enzymes in the drainage from irritating the skin. Solid barriers are classified as "regular wear" or "extended wear." An adult with a high output may want an extended-wear barrier. A special cream can be used to help fill any uneven skin surfaces and provide a consistent seal. Pouches can also be individualized by the patient. Large pouches can hold more but are heavy when full. Patients also have to consider the costs of the various systems and if or how much their insurance will pay for them. Chart 57-4 describes the main aspects of ileostomy care, including skin care.

A patient with an ileostomy may have many concerns about management at home and about sexual and social adjustments. Considering possible sexual issues helps the patient identify and discuss these concerns with the sex partner. For example, a change in positioning during intercourse may alleviate apprehension. Social situations may cause anxiety related to decreased self-esteem and a disturbance in body image. Encourage the patient to discuss possible concerns in addressing and resolving these potentially stressful events. Clinical depression is common among patients with ulcerative colitis. Refer patients to appropriate mental health resources if depression is suspected.

Some hospitals provide community support groups for their patients with inflammatory bowel disease (IBD). These groups help patients and their families cope with the psychological impact of IBD and educate them about NUTRITION and complementary and integrative therapies.

Health Care Resources. If the patient needs assistance with self-management at home, collaborate with the case manager or social worker to arrange the services of a home care aide or nurse. A home care nurse can provide assessment and guidance in integrating ostomy care into the patient's lifestyle. The nurse may also teach about wound care, including monitoring wound healing, if needed (Chart 57-5). The patient and family need to know where to purchase ostomy supplies, along with the name, size, and manufacturer's order number.

For patients with a permanent ileostomy, locate a community ostomy support group by contacting the United Ostomy Associations of America (www.uoaa.org). The United Ostomy Association of Canada serves the needs of Canadian patients (www.ostomycanada.ca). A local support group or the Crohn's and Colitis Foundation of America (www.ccfa.org) may be helpful in obtaining supplies and providing education for ostomates. Inform the patient and family members of available ostomy ambulatory care clinics and ostomy specialists. If the patient agrees, a visit from an ostomate can be continued after discharge to home.

◆ **Evaluation: Reflecting**

Evaluate the care of the patient with ulcerative colitis based on the identified priority patient problems. Expected outcomes may include that the patient will:

👤 CHART 57-4 Patient and Family Education: Preparing for Self-Management

Ileostomy Care

Skin Protection
- Use a skin barrier to protect your skin from contact with contents from the ostomy.
- Use skin-care products, such as skin sealants and ostomy skin creams. If your skin continues to come into contact with ostomy contents, select a product to fill in problem areas and provide an even skin surface.
- Watch your skin for any irritation or redness.

Pouch Care
- Empty your pouch when it is one-third to one-half full.
- Change the pouch during inactive times, such as before meals, before retiring at night, on waking in the morning, and 2 to 4 hours after eating.
- Change the entire pouch system every 3 to 7 days.

Nutrition
- Chew food thoroughly.
- Be cautious of high-fiber and high-cellulose foods. You may need to eliminate these from the diet if they cause severe problems (diarrhea, constipation, or blockage). Examples include corn, peanuts, coconut, Chinese vegetables, string beans, tough-fiber meats, shrimp and lobster, rice, bran, and vegetables with skins (tomatoes, corn, and peas).

Drug Therapy
- Avoid taking enteric-coated and capsule medications.
- Inform any health care provider who is prescribing medications for you that you have an ostomy. Before having prescriptions filled, inform your pharmacist that you have an ostomy.
- Do not take any laxative or enemas. You should usually have loose stool and should contact a physician if no stool has passed in 6 to 12 hours.

Symptoms to Watch
- Report any drastic increase or decrease in drainage to your health care provider.
- If stomal swelling, abdominal cramping, or distention occurs or if ileostomy contents stop draining:
  - Remove the pouch with faceplate.
  - Lie down, assuming a knee-chest position.
  - Begin abdominal massage.
  - Apply moist towels to the abdomen.
  - Drink hot tea.
  - If none of these maneuvers is effective in resuming ileostomy flow or if abdominal pain is severe, call your health care provider right away.

- Experience no diarrhea or a decrease in diarrheal episodes
- Verbalize decreased pain
- Gain control over bowel ELIMINATION
- Have absence of lower GI bleeding
- Self-manage the ileostomy (temporary or permanent)
- Maintain peristomal skin integrity
- Demonstrate behaviors that integrate ostomy care into his or her lifestyle if a permanent ileostomy is performed

CROHN'S DISEASE

❖ **PATHOPHYSIOLOGY**

Crohn's disease (CD) is a chronic inflammatory disease of the small intestine (most often), the colon, or both. It can affect the

GI tract from the mouth to the anus but most commonly affects the terminal ileum. CD is a slowly progressive and unpredictable disease with involvement of multiple regions of the intestine with normal sections in between (called *skip lesions* on x-rays). Like ulcerative colitis (UC), this disease is recurrent, with remissions and exacerbations.

CD presents as inflammation that causes a thickened bowel wall. Strictures and deep ulcerations (cobblestone appearance) also occur, which put the patient at risk for developing bowel fistulas (abnormal openings between two organs or structures). The result is severe diarrhea and malabsorption of vital nutrients. Anemia is common, usually from iron deficiency or malabsorption issues (McCance et al., 2014).

The complications associated with CD are similar to those of UC (see Table 57-4). Hemorrhage is more common in UC, but it can occur in CD as well. Severe malabsorption by the small intestine is more common in patients with CD versus UC that may not involve the small bowel to any significant extent. Therefore patients with CD can become very malnourished and debilitated.

CHART 57-5 Home Care Assessment
The Patient With Inflammatory Bowel Disease

Assess gastrointestinal function and nutritional status, including:
- Abdominal cramping or pain
- Bowel elimination pattern, specifically frequency, characteristics, and amount of stools and presence or absence of blood in stools
- Food and fluid intake (include relationship of specific foods to cramping and stools)
- Weight gain or loss
- Signs and symptoms of dehydration
- Presence or absence of fever, rectal tenesmus, or urgency
- Bowel sounds
- Condition of perianal skin, including presence or absence of perianal fistula or abscess

Assess patient's and family's coping skills, including:
- Current and ongoing stress level and coping style
- Availability of support system

Assess home environment, including:
- Adequacy and availability of bathroom facilities
- Opportunity for rest and relaxation

Assess ability to self-manage therapeutic regimen, including:
- Drug therapy
- Signs and symptoms to report
- Nutrition therapy
- Availability of community resources
- Importance of follow-up care

Rarely, cancer of the small bowel and colon develop but can occur after the disease has been present for 15 to 20 years. Fistula formation is a common complication of CD but is rare in UC. Fistulas can occur between segments of the intestine or manifest as cutaneous fistulas (opening to the skin) or perirectal abscesses. They can also extend from the bowel to other organs and body cavities, such as the bladder or vagina (Fig. 57-4). Some patients develop intestinal obstruction, which at first is secondary to inflammation and edema. Over time, fibrosis and scar tissue develop, and obstruction results from a narrowing of the bowel. Most patients with CD require surgery at some point.

GENETIC/GENOMIC CONSIDERATIONS
Patient-Centered Care **QSEN**

The exact cause of CD is unknown. A combination of genetic, immune, and environmental factors may contribute to its development. About 20% of patients have a positive family history for the disease (Cleynen et al., 2016). The discovery of a mutation in the *NOD2/CARD15* gene on chromosome 16 seems to be associated with some patients who have CD. This gene is found in monocytes that normally recognize and destroy bacteria.

Pro-inflammatory cytokines, such as tumor necrosis factor–alpha (TNF-alpha) and interleukins (ILs) (e.g., IL-6 and IL-8), are immunologic factors that contribute to the etiology of CD (McCance et al., 2014). Many of the drugs used for the disease inhibit or block one or more of these factors.

Other risk factors include tobacco use, Jewish ethnicity, and living in urban areas (McCance et al., 2014). CD is more common in individuals of Ashkenazi Jewish background than in any other group. Current research has found genetic markers in this population that contribute to higher rates of CD (Zhang et al., 2013). It was once thought that stress and nutrition play a role in the development of CD, but these factors have not been proven. However, inadequate NUTRITION can exacerbate the patient's symptoms.

Almost a million individuals in the United States have Crohn's disease, and Canada has one of the highest incidences of Crohn's and colitis worldwide (Crohn's and Colitis Canada, 2016). Most have symptoms and are diagnosed as adolescents or young adults between 15 and 35 years of age (Crohn's and Colitis Foundation, 2017).

❖ INTERPROFESSIONAL COLLABORATIVE CARE

Similar to patients with ulcerative colitis, patients with Crohn's disease may be self-managed at home, cared for in the community setting, or hospitalized depending on their immediate condition related to this chronic bowel disease. The interprofessional team that collaborates to care for this patient generally

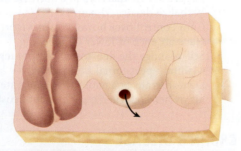

External enterocutaneous
(between skin and intestine)

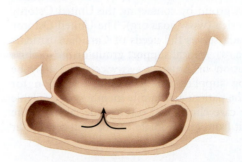

Enteroenteric
(between intestine and intestine)

FIG. 57-4 Types of fistulas that are complications of Crohn's disease.

includes the health care provider (and/or surgeon), nurse, psychologist, social worker, dietitian, and spiritual leader of the patient's choice.

◆ Assessment: Noticing

Crohn's disease can be exacerbated by bacterial infection. A detailed history is needed to identify manifestations specific to the disease. Ask about recent unintentional weight loss, the frequency and consistency of stools, the presence of blood in the stool, fever, and abdominal pain.

Perform a thorough abdominal assessment. Assess for manifestations of the disease, and evaluate the patient's NUTRITION and hydration status.

When inspecting the abdomen, assess for distention, masses, or visible peristalsis. Inspection of the perianal area may reveal ulcerations, fissures, or fistulas. During auscultation, bowel sounds may be decreased or absent with severe inflammation or obstruction. An increase in high-pitched or rushing sounds may be present over areas of narrowed bowel loops. Muscle guarding, masses, rigidity, or tenderness may be noted on palpation by the advanced practice nurse or health care provider.

The signs and symptoms associated with Crohn's disease vary greatly from person to person. Most patients report diarrhea, abdominal pain, and low-grade fever. Fever is common with fistulas, abscesses, and severe inflammation. If the disease occurs in only the ileum, diarrhea occurs five or six times per day, often with a soft, loose stool. Steatorrhea (fatty diarrheal stools) is common. Stools may contain bright red blood.

Abdominal pain from the inflammatory process is usually constant and often located in the right lower quadrant. The patient also may have pain around the umbilicus before and after bowel movements. If the lower colon is diseased, pain is common in both lower abdominal quadrants.

Most patients with Crohn's disease have *weight loss.* Nutritional problems are the result of increased catabolism from chronic inflammation, anorexia, malabsorption, or self-imposed dietary restrictions. These problems result in impaired FLUID AND ELECTROLYTE BALANCE and vital nutrient deficiencies.

The inflammatory bowel changes decrease the small bowel's ability to absorb nutrients, which may be made worse by surgery and fistulas.

! NURSING SAFETY PRIORITY QSEN

Action Alert

For the patient with Crohn's disease, be especially alert for signs and symptoms of peritonitis (discussed earlier in this chapter), small-bowel obstruction, and nutritional and fluid imbalances. Early detection of a change in the patient's status helps reduce these life-threatening complications.

The patient who has Crohn's disease (CD) needs a complete psychosocial assessment. The chronic nature of the problem and the associated complications can greatly affect patients and their families. Lifestyle changes are necessary to cope with such a disruptive and painful chronic illness. Assess the patient's coping skill and help identify support systems. Similar to problems associated with other chronic diseases, clinical depression and severe anxiety disorders are common among patients with CD.

The health care provider requests many laboratory studies for patients with CD. The results of laboratory tests often indicate the extent and severity of inflammation or complications that occur with the disease.

Anemia is common as a result of slow bleeding and poor nutrition. Serum levels of folic acid and vitamin B$_{12}$ are generally low because of malabsorption, further contributing to anemia. Amino acid malabsorption and protein-losing enteropathy may result in *decreased albumin* levels. C-reactive protein and ESR may be elevated to indicate inflammation. White blood cells (WBCs) in the urine may show infection (pyuria), which is caused by ureteral obstruction or an enterovesical (bowel to bladder) fistula. If severe diarrhea or fistula is present, the patient may have fluid and electrolyte losses, particularly potassium and magnesium. Assess the patient for signs and symptoms that can occur as a result of electrolyte losses (see Chapter 11).

X-rays show the narrowing, ulcerations, strictures, and fistulas common with Crohn's disease. *Magnetic resonance enterography (MRE)* is performed to determine bowel activity and motility as discussed under Other Diagnostic Assessment in the Ulcerative Colitis concept exemplar. An *abdominal ultrasound or CT* scan may also be performed. In acute illness, these tests may be deferred until the risk for perforation lessens. If the patient has lower GI bleeding of more than 0.5 mL per minute, a *GI bleeding scan* may be useful to localize the site of the bleeding (Pagana et al., 2017).

◆ Interventions: Responding

Collaborative care for patients with Crohn's disease is similar to that described in the Nonsurgical Management discussion in the Ulcerative Colitis section. Specific interventions vary with the severity of disease and the complications that are present.

Nonsurgical Management

Drug Therapy. Drugs used to manage Crohn's disease (CD) are similar to those used in the treatment of ulcerative colitis (UC). For mild-to-moderate disease, 5-ASA drugs may be effective, although research shows that their usage for CD has produced mixed results (see the Drug Therapy discussion in the Ulcerative Colitis section).

Most patients have moderate-to-severe disease and need stronger drug therapy to control their symptoms. Two agents that may be prescribed for CD are azathioprine (Azasan, Imuran) and mercaptopurine (Purinethol). These drugs suppress the immune system and can lead to serious infections. Methotrexate may also be given to suppress immune activity of the disease.

A group of biologic response modifiers (BRMs), also known as *monoclonal antibody drugs,* have been approved for use in CD when other drugs have been ineffective. These drugs inhibit tumor necrosis factor (TNF)–alpha, which decreases the inflammatory response. Examples of commonly used drugs for patients with CD include infliximab (Inflectra ✤, Remicade, Remsima ✤), adalimumab (Humira), natalizumab (Tysabri), certolizumab pegol, (Cimzia), and vedolizumab (Entyvio) (Randall et al., 2015). These agents are not given to patients with a history of cancer, heart disease, or multiple sclerosis.

Although glucocorticoids can be effective for patients with CD, sepsis can result from abscesses or fistulas that may be present. These drugs mask the symptoms of infection. Therefore they must be used with caution and only on a short-term basis. Monitor the patient closely for signs of infection. Teach the patient not to stop the steroids abruptly because of the potential for adrenal insufficiency. Ciprofloxacin (Cipro) and metronidazole (Flagyl, Novo-Nidazol ✤) have been helpful in patients with fistulas and infections related to CD.

Nutrition Therapy. Long-standing nutritional deficits can have severe consequences for the patient with Crohn's disease.

Drug Alert

Both infliximab and certolizumab pegol must be given in a health care setting, such as a physician's office, via parenteral routes. Adalimumab (Humira) is self-administered by subcutaneous injection every other week. Teach patients how to give themselves a subcutaneous injection. Teach them to report injection site reactions, including redness and swelling. Remind them that headache, abdominal pain, and nausea and vomiting are common side effects. Teach them to avoid crowds and people with infection. Reinforce the need to report any infection, including a cold or sore throat, to the health care provider immediately.

Natalizumab is given IV under medical supervision every 4 weeks for moderate-to-severe CD and when other drugs are not effective. Natalizumab can cause **progressive multifocal leukoencephalopathy** (PML), a deadly infection that affects the brain. Before giving the drug, be sure that the patient is free of all infections. Teach patients the importance of reporting any cognitive, motor, or sensory changes immediately to the health care provider.

Vedolizumab (Entyvio) is used for treatment of moderate-to-severe CD. This drug is administered IV at weeks 0, 2, 6, and then 8 weeks afterward. Clinical trials verify that it does not increase risk for PML; but, because of its mechanism action, the FDA strongly encourages education regarding this possible complication (Randall et al., 2015).

Poor NUTRITION can lead to inadequate fistula and wound healing, loss of lean muscle mass, decreased immune responses, and increased morbidity and mortality. During severe exacerbations of the disease, the patient may be hospitalized to provide bowel rest and nutritional support with total parenteral nutrition (TPN). Nutritional supplements such as Ensure or Sustacal can be given to provide nutrients and more calories. Teach the patient to avoid GI stimulants, such as caffeinated beverages and alcohol.

Fistula Management. Fistulas (abnormal tracts between two or more body areas) are common with acute exacerbations of Crohn's disease. They can be between the bowel and bladder (enterovesical), between two segments of bowel (enteroenteric), between the skin and bowel (enterocutaneous), or between the bowel and vagina (enterovaginal) (see Fig. 57-4). The patient with one or more fistulas often has complications such as systemic infections, skin problems, malnutrition, and impaired FLUID AND ELECTROLYTE BALANCE. Treatment of the patient with a fistula is complicated and includes nutrition and electrolyte therapy, skin care, and prevention of infection.

Action Alert

Adequate NUTRITION and FLUID AND ELECTROLYTE BALANCE are priorities in the care of the patient with a fistula. GI secretions are high in volume and rich in electrolytes and enzymes. The patient is at high risk for malnutrition, dehydration, and hypokalemia (decreased serum potassium). Assess for these complications and collaborate with the health care team to manage them. Monitor urinary output and daily weights. A decrease indicates possible dehydration, which should be treated immediately by providing additional fluids.

The patient requires at least 3000 calories daily to promote healing of the fistula. If he or she cannot take adequate oral fluids and nutrients, total enteral nutrition (TEN) or TPN may be prescribed. For patients who do not require TEN or TPN, collaborate with the dietitian to:

- Carefully monitor the patient's tolerance of the prescribed diet
- Help the patient select high-calorie, high-protein, high-vitamin, low-fiber meals
- Offer enteral supplements, such as Ensure and Vivonex PLUS
- Record food intake for accurate calorie counts

Providing enteral supplements, recording intake and output, and taking daily weights may be delegated to unlicensed assistive personnel (UAP) under the supervision of the registered nurse (RN). Collaborate with the certified wound, ostomy, and continence nurse (CWOCN) to select the most appropriate wound management for each patient.

Action Alert

For patients with fistulas, preserving and protecting the skin are the nursing priorities. Be sure that wound drainage is not in direct contact with skin because intestinal fluid enzymes are caustic! Clean the skin promptly to prevent skin breakdown or fungal infection, which can cause major discomfort for the patient.

Enzymes and bile in the stool contribute to the problem of skin irritation and excoriation. Skin irritation needs to be prevented. This may be accomplished through the use of skin barriers, pouching systems, and insertion of drains (Fig. 57-5). Skin barriers or dressings are used when the fistula drainage is less than 100 mL in 24 hours. A pouch is used for heavily draining fistulas to reduce the risk for skin breakdown and measure the **effluent** (drainage). However, they are very challenging because of location and drainage amount. Treatment with an antifungal powder applied to the skin around the fistula is often very helpful to prevent or treat *Candida* infection.

For some fistulas, pouching may not be possible because of their location. Drainage may need to be managed using regulated wall suction or a negative-pressure wound therapy device. Continuous low wall suction is attached to a suction catheter in the wound bed of the fistula, not into the fistula tract. These systems are not meant for long-term management.

Negative-pressure wound therapy (e.g., vacuum-assisted closure, or wound VAC therapy) promotes wound healing by secondary intention as it prepares the wound bed for closure, reduces edema, promotes granulation and perfusion, and removes exudate and infectious material. It should not be used for patients who are at risk for bleeding or only for the purpose of drainage containment.

Patients with fistulas are also at high risk for intra-abdominal abscesses and sepsis. Antibiotic therapy is commonly prescribed. Observe for signs of sepsis (systemic infection), such as fever, abdominal pain, or a change in mental status. Monitor for increased WBC levels that could indicate a systemic infection.

Other helpful interventions for the patient with CD are those that relax the patient and soothe the GI tract. Such therapies may include naturopathy, herbs (e.g., ginger), acupuncture, hypnotherapy, and ayurveda (a combination of diet, herbs, yoga, and breathing exercises). The evidence supporting the use of these substances for CD is lacking, but many patients find them helpful for overall physical and emotional health. Teach patients about the availability of these therapies and recommend that they include them in their collaborative plan of care.

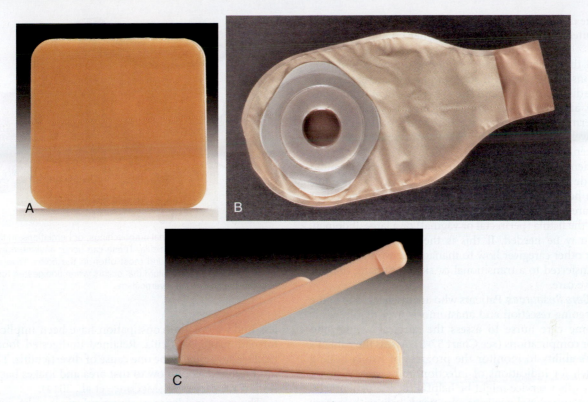

FIG. 57-5 Skin barriers, such as wafers **(A)** are cut to fit ⅛ inch around the fistula. A drainable pouch **(B)** is applied over the wafer and clamped **(C)** until the pouch is to be emptied. Effluent should drain into the bag and not contact the skin. (Courtesy ConvaTec, a Bristol-Myers Squibb Company, Princeton, NJ.)

❓ CLINICAL JUDGMENT CHALLENGE 57-1

Patient-Centered Care; Evidence-Based Practice; Teamwork and Collaboration QSEN

A 19-year-old man has a new diagnosis of Crohn's disease. This patient reports that he recently started college and that his stress levels have been higher than ever. He has been prescribed and is taking prednisone to control his flare-up but currently has not made any other modifications. The patient is concerned because he has very little knowledge about his new diagnosis and how it might impact his current lifestyle.

1. What is your therapeutic response to the patient at this time?
2. Based on the patient data provided, what priority problems do you identify?
3. What lifestyle modifications might be helpful for this patient?
4. What complementary and/or integrative therapies would be available?
5. Using best current evidence, how will you plan care with other members of the health care team? What members of the health care team will be involved in this patient's care?

Surgical Management. Surgery for Crohn's disease may be performed for patients who have not improved with medical management or for those who have complications from the disease. Surgery to manage Crohn's disease is not as successful as that for ulcerative colitis because of the extent of the disease. The patient with a fistula may undergo resection of the diseased area. Other indications for surgical treatment include perforation, massive hemorrhage, intestinal obstruction or strictures, abscesses, or cancer.

In some cases, a resection (removal of part of the small bowel) can be performed as minimally invasive surgery (MIS) via laparoscopy. This surgery involves one or more small incisions, less pain, and a quicker surgical recovery when compared with traditional open surgery. Both small-bowel resection (usually the ileum) and ileocecal resection can be done using this procedure. For other patients, an open surgical approach is used to allow for better visual access to the bowel.

Strictureplasty may be performed for bowel strictures related to Crohn's disease. This procedure increases the bowel diameter. Care before and after each of these surgical procedures is similar to care for patients undergoing other types of abdominal surgery (see Chapters 14 and 16).

Care Coordination and Transition Management

Home Care Management. The discharge care plan for the patient with Crohn's disease is similar to that for the patient with ulcerative colitis (see the Care Coordination and Transition Management discussion in the Ulcerative Colitis section). Collaborate with the case manager and CWOCN or wound nurse to help the patient plan self-management.

Self-Management Education. Reinforce measures to control the disease and related symptoms and manage NUTRITION. Teach the patient and family to make arrangements for the patient to have easy access to the bathroom and privacy to perform fistula care, if needed.

The health teaching plan for Crohn's disease is similar to that for the patient with ulcerative colitis. Teach the patient about the usual course of the disease, symptoms of complications, and when to notify the health care provider. Provide health teaching for drug therapy, including purpose, dose, and side effects. In addition to other drugs, vitamin supplements, including monthly vitamin B_{12} injections, may be needed because of the inability of the ileum to absorb these nutrients. In collaboration with the dietitian, instruct the patient to follow a low-residue, high-calorie diet and to avoid foods that cause discomfort, such as milk, gluten (wheat products), and other GI stimulants like caffeine.

Remind the patient to take rest periods, especially during exacerbations of the disease. If stress appears to increase symptoms of the disease, recommend stress-management techniques, counseling, and/or physical activity to improve quality of life. For long-term follow-up, teach the patient about the increased risk for bowel cancer and the importance of frequent colorectal cancer screening (see Chapter 56).

If a patient has a fistula, explain and demonstrate wound care. Provide the opportunity for the patient to practice this care in the hospital. Ideally, he or she should be independent in fistula care before leaving the hospital. However, because of location of the fistula (perirectal or vaginal) or a large abdomen, assistance may be needed. If this is the case, teach a family member or other caregiver how to manage the wound. Patients may be transferred to a transitional or skilled nursing unit for collaborative care.

Health Care Resources. Patients who are discharged to home after undergoing resection and anastomosis may require visits from a home care nurse to assess the surgical wound and monitor for complications (see Chart 57-5). Assess the patient's and family's ability to monitor the progress of fistula healing and to watch for indications of infection and sepsis. A home care aide or other service might be helpful for the patient who cannot meet nutritional needs or who needs help with grocery shopping and meal preparation.

In collaboration with the case manager, assist with obtaining the equipment and supplies for fistula care, such as skin barriers and wound drainage bags. A support group sponsored by the United Ostomy Associations of America (www.uoaa.org) or a local hospital in the community may also be available to help with meeting physical and psychosocial needs.

DIVERTICULAR DISEASE

Diverticula are pouchlike herniations of the mucosa through the muscular wall of any part of the gut but most commonly the colon. **Diverticulosis** is the presence of many abnormal pouchlike herniations (diverticula) in the wall of the intestine. Acute **diverticulitis** is the inflammation or infection of diverticula.

❖ PATHOPHYSIOLOGY

Diverticula can occur in any part of the small or large intestine, but usually occur in the sigmoid colon (Fig. 57-6). The muscle of the colon hypertrophies, thickens, and becomes rigid, and herniation of the mucosa and submucosa through the colon wall is seen. Diverticula seem to occur at points of weakness in the intestinal wall, often at areas where blood vessels interrupt the muscle layer. Muscle weakness develops as part of the aging process or as a result of a lack of fiber in the diet.

Diverticula without inflammation cause few problems. However, if undigested food or bacteria become trapped in a diverticulum, blood supply to that area is reduced. Bacteria invade the diverticulum, resulting in diverticulitis, which then can perforate and develop a local abscess. A perforated diverticulum can progress to an intra-abdominal perforation with peritonitis (inflammation of the peritoneum). Lower GI bleeding may also occur.

High intraluminal pressure forces the formation of a pouch in the weakened area of the mucosa. Diets low in fiber that cause

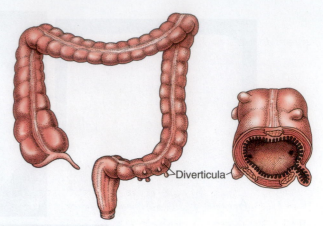

FIG. 57-6 Several abnormal outpouchings, or herniations, in the wall of the intestine, which are diverticula. These can occur anywhere in the small or large intestine but are found most often in the colon. Diverticulitis is the inflammation of a diverticulum that occurs when undigested food or bacteria become trapped in the diverticulum.

less bulky stool and constipation have been implicated in the formation of diverticula. Retained undigested food in diverticula is suggested to be one cause of diverticulitis. The retained food reduces blood flow to that area and makes bacterial invasion of the sac easier (McCance et al., 2014).

The exact incidence of diverticulosis is unknown, but millions are affected by the problem. It is found in two thirds of adults older than 80 years, with more men than women affected.

❖ INTERPROFESSIONAL COLLABORATIVE CARE

Patients with diverticular disease are self-managed at home, cared for in the community setting, or hospitalized if surgery is needed to correct the concern. The interprofessional team that collaborates to care for this patient generally includes the health care provider (and/or surgeon) and nurse.

◆ Assessment: Noticing

The patient with *diverticulosis* usually has no symptoms. Unless pain or bleeding develops, the condition may go undiagnosed. Diverticula are most often diagnosed during routine colonoscopy. Occasionally diverticulosis will cause symptoms. For the patient with uncomplicated diverticulosis, ask about intermittent pain in the left lower quadrant and a history of constipation. If diverticulitis is suspected, ask about a history of low-grade fever, nausea, and abdominal pain. Inquire about recent bowel ELIMINATION patterns because constipation may develop as a result of intestinal inflammation. Also ask about any bleeding from the rectum.

The patient with *diverticulitis* may have abdominal pain, most often localized to the left lower quadrant. It is intermittent at first but becomes progressively steady. Occasionally pain may be just above the pubic bone or may occur on one side. Abdominal pain is generalized if peritonitis has occurred. Nausea and vomiting are common. The patient's temperature is elevated, ranging from a low-grade fever to 101°F (38.3°C). Chills may be present. Often an increased heart rate (tachycardia) occurs with fever (Almerie & Simpson, 2015).

On examination of the abdomen, observe for distention. The patient may report tenderness over the involved area. Localized muscle spasm, guarded movement, and rebound tenderness may be present with peritoneal irritation. If generalized

The first sign of peritonitis in older adults may be a sudden change in mental status (e.g., acute confusion). For those who have dementia, the confusion worsens. Fever and chills may not be present because of normal physiologic changes associated with aging.

🔵 **CHART 57-6** **Nursing Focus on the Older Adult**

Diverticulitis

- Provide antibiotics, analgesics, and anticholinergics as prescribed. Observe older patients carefully for side effects of these drugs, especially confusion (or increased confusion), urinary retention or failure, and orthostatic hypotension.
- Do not give laxatives or enemas. Teach the patient and family about the importance of avoiding these measures.
- Encourage the patient to rest and to avoid activities that may increase intra-abdominal pressure, such as straining and bending.
- While diverticulitis is active, provide a *low*-fiber diet. When the inflammation resolves, provide a *high*-fiber diet. Teach the patient and family about these diets and when they are appropriate.
- Because older patients do not always experience the typical pain or fever expected, observe carefully for other signs of active disease, such as a sudden change in mental status.
- Perform frequent abdominal assessments to determine distention and tenderness on palpation.
- Check stools for occult or frank bleeding.

peritonitis is present, profound guarding occurs; rebound tenderness is more widespread; and sepsis, hypotension, or hypovolemic shock can occur. If the perforated diverticulum is close to the rectum, the health care provider may palpate a tender mass during the rectal examination. Blood pressure checks may show orthostatic changes. *If bleeding is massive, the patient may have hypovolemia and hypotension that result in shock.*

For the patient with uncomplicated diverticulosis, laboratory studies are not indicated. However, the patient with diverticulitis has an *elevated white blood cell (WBC) count. Decreased hematocrit and hemoglobin* values are common if chronic or severe bleeding occurs. Stool tests for occult blood, if requested, are sometimes positive. Abdominal x-rays may be done to evaluate for free air and fluid indicating perforation. A CT scan may be performed to diagnose an abscess or thickening of the bowel related to diverticulitis.

Abdominal ultrasonography, a noninvasive test, may also reveal bowel thickening or an abscess. The health care provider may recommend a colonoscopy 4 to 8 weeks *after the acute phase* of the illness to rule out a tumor in the large intestine, particularly if the patient has rectal bleeding.

◆ *Interventions: Responding*

Patients are managed on an ambulatory care basis if the symptoms are mild. Monitor the patient for any prolonged or increased fever, abdominal pain, or blood in the stool. The patient with moderate-to-severe diverticulitis may be hospitalized, especially if he or she is older or has complications. Manifestations suggesting the need for admission are a temperature higher than 101°F (38.3°C), persistent and severe abdominal pain for more than 3 days, and/or lower GI bleeding.

Nonsurgical Management. A combination of drug and NUTRITION therapy with rest is used to decrease the inflammation associated with diverticular disease. Broad-spectrum antimicrobial drugs, such as metronidazole (Flagyl) in conjunction with trimethoprim/sulfamethoxazole (TMZ) (Bactrim or Bactrim DS, Septra) or ciprofloxacin (Cipro), are often prescribed. A mild analgesic may be given for pain. Chart 57-6 lists nursing interventions needed for care of older adults with diverticulitis.

The patient with more severe pain may be admitted to the hospital for IV fluids to correct dehydration and IV drug therapy. For patients with moderate-to-severe diverticulitis, an opioid analgesic may alleviate pain.

Laxatives and enemas are avoided because they increase intestinal motility. Assess the patient on an ongoing basis for manifestations of impaired FLUID AND ELECTROLYTE BALANCE.

Teach the patient to rest during the acute phase of illness. Remind him or her to refrain from lifting, straining, coughing, or bending to avoid an increase in intra-abdominal pressure, which can result in perforation of the diverticulum. NUTRITION

therapy should be restricted to low fiber or clear liquids based on symptoms. The patient with more severe symptoms is NPO. A nasogastric tube (NGT) is inserted if nausea, vomiting, or abdominal distention is severe. Infuse IV fluids as prescribed for hydration. In collaboration with a dietitian, the patient increases dietary intake slowly as symptoms subside. When inflammation has resolved and bowel function returns to normal, a fiber-containing diet is introduced gradually.

Surgical Management. Diverticulitis can result in rupture of the diverticulum with peritonitis, pelvic abscess, bowel obstruction, fistula, persistent fever or pain, or uncontrolled bleeding. The surgeon performs emergency surgery if peritonitis, bowel obstruction, or pelvic abscess is present. Colon resection, with or without a colostomy, is the most common surgical procedure for patients with diverticular disease. Chapter 56 discusses the nursing care for patients with this procedure.

Care Coordination and Transition Management

Discharge plans vary according to the treatment. The patient who has surgical intervention has the added responsibilities of incision care and possibly colostomy care with temporary limitations placed on activities.

Patients with diverticular disease need education regarding a high-fiber diet. Encourage the patient with *diverticulosis* to eat a diet high in cellulose and hemicellulose types of fiber. These substances can be found in wheat bran, whole-grain breads, and cereals. Teach the patient to eat at least 25 to 35 grams of fiber per day. Fresh fruits and vegetables with high fiber content are added to provide bulk to stools.

If not accustomed to eating high-fiber foods, teach the patient to add them to the diet gradually to avoid flatulence and abdominal cramping. If he or she cannot tolerate the recommended fiber requirement, a bulk-forming laxative, such as psyllium hydrophilic mucilloid (Metamucil), can be taken to increase fecal size and consistency. Teach the patient to drink plenty of fluids to help prevent bloating that may occur with a high-fiber diet. Alcohol should be avoided because it irritates the bowel. Foods containing seeds or indigestible material that may block a diverticulum, such as nuts, corn, popcorn, cucumbers, tomatoes, figs, and strawberries, may need to be eliminated.

Teach the patient that dietary fat intake should not exceed 30% of the total daily caloric intake.

The patient should be instructed to avoid all fiber when symptoms of *diverticulitis* are present, because high-fiber foods can be irritating. As inflammation resolves, fiber can gradually be added until progression to a high-fiber diet is established. The patient who has undergone surgery is usually taking solid food by the time of discharge from the hospital.

Provide oral and written instructions on incision care and the signs and symptoms to report to the health care provider for the patient who had abdominal surgery. If a colostomy was created, reinforce ostomy care as needed. Encourage the patient to express concerns about body image. Allow time and address sexual concerns regarding the changed body image.

Instruct the patient with any type of diverticular disease about the manifestations of acute diverticulitis, including fever, abdominal pain, and bloody, mahogany, or tarry stools. Advise patients to avoid the use of laxatives (other than bulk-forming types) and enemas. Reassure them that this disorder should not cause problems if a proper diet is followed.

In collaboration with the case manager, arrange for a home care nurse, if needed, to assess wound healing and proper functioning of the ostomy and the appliance. If the patient is interested, arrange for a visit from an ostomy volunteer (ostomate) or an ostomy nurse. For information about other community resources, remind the patient to contact the United Ostomy Associations of America (www.uoaa.org).

 NCLEX EXAMINATION CHALLENGE 57-4

Physiological Integrity

The nurse is teaching a client about nutrition and diverticulosis. Which food will the nurse teach the client to avoid?
A. Popcorn
B. Oatmeal
C. Bran
D. Lettuce

CELIAC DISEASE

Celiac disease (CD) was once thought to be a rare disease but, as a result of improved diagnostic testing, many cases have been diagnosed in the past 10 to 15 years. CD is a multi-system autoimmune disease with an estimated incidence as high as 1 in 250 of the world's population (Mavrinac et al., 2014). Patients who have other autoimmune diseases, such as rheumatoid arthritis and diabetes mellitus type 1, are at the highest risk for the disease.

CD is a chronic inflammation of the small intestinal mucosa that can cause bowel wall atrophy, malabsorption, and diarrhea. Like many inflammatory disorders, it is thought to be caused by a combination of genetic, immunologic, and environmental factors. The primary complication of CD is cancer, specifically non-Hodgkin's lymphoma or GI cancers and NUTRITION deficiencies.

Patients with CD have varying signs and symptoms with cycles of remission and exacerbation (flare-up), usually related to how well they monitor their diet. Classic symptoms include anorexia, diarrhea and/or constipation, steatorrhea (fatty stools), abdominal pain, abdominal bloating and distention, and weight loss. Some patients have no symptoms. Still others have atypical symptoms that affect every body system (Chart

 CHART 57-7   **Key Features**
Celiac Disease

Classic Symptoms	Atypical Symptoms
• Weight loss	• Osteoporosis
• Anorexia	• Joint pain and inflammation
• Diarrhea and/or constipation	• Lactose intolerance
• Steatorrhea	• Iron deficiency anemia
• Abdominal pain and distention	• Depression
• Vomiting	• Migraines
	• Epilepsy
	• Autoimmune disorders
	• Stomatitis
	• Early menopause
	• Protein-calorie malnutrition
	• Infertility

57-7). Diagnosis is usually made by obtaining a screening blood test and endoscopy.

NCLEX EXAMINATION CHALLENGE 57-5

Physiological Integrity

The nurse is caring for a client who has celiac disease. Which food will the nurse remove from the client's dietary tray? **Select all that apply.**
A. Rice
B. Graham crackers
C. Croissant
D. Fresh peaches
E. Chicken breast

Dietary management is the only available treatment for achieving disease remission. In most cases, a gluten-free diet (GFD) results in healing the intestinal mucosa after about 2 years (Mavrinac et al., 2014). Gluten is the primary substance in wheat and wheat-based products. Teach patients to carefully check for hidden sources of gluten that are in foods, food additives, drugs, and cosmetics. Patients often take vitamin and mineral supplements to replace those lost in avoiding gluten foods. A registered dietitian should be included in the patient's long-term planning and overall treatment.

ANAL DISORDERS

ANORECTAL ABSCESS

Anorectal abscess is a localized area of induration and pus caused by inflammation of the soft tissue near the rectum or anus. It is most often the result of obstruction of the ducts of glands in the anorectal region. Feces, foreign bodies, or trauma can be the cause of the obstruction and stasis, leading to infection that spreads into nearby tissue.

Rectal pain is often the first symptom. There may be no other signs or symptoms at first, but local swelling, redness, and tenderness are present within a few days after the onset of pain. If the abscess becomes chronic, discharge, bleeding, and pruritus (itching) may exist. Fever occurs if larger abscesses are present.

Anorectal abscesses are managed by surgical incision and drainage (I&D). The physician can often excise (surgically remove) simple perianal and ischiorectal abscesses using a local anesthetic. For patients with a more extensive abscess, a regional or general anesthetic may be needed. Systemic antibiotics are given only for patients who are immunocompromised, have diabetes, have valvular disease or a prosthetic valve, or are obese.

> ### ! NURSING SAFETY PRIORITY (QSEN)
> **Action Alert**
>
> For patients with an anorectal abscess, nursing interventions are focused on COMFORT and helping the patient maintain optimal perineal hygiene. Encourage the use of warm sitz baths, analgesics, bulk-producing agents, and stool softeners after the surgery to promote healing. *Stress the importance of good perineal hygiene after all bowel movements and the maintenance of a regular bowel pattern with a high-fiber diet.*

Patients are often embarrassed about having anal problems. Provide privacy and maintain the patient's dignity during the examination and treatment.

ANAL FISSURE

An anal fissure is a tear in the anal lining, which can be very painful. Smaller fissures occur with straining to have a stool, such as with diarrhea or constipation. Larger, deeper fissures may occur as a result of another disorder (e.g., Crohn's disease, tuberculosis, leukemia, neoplasm) or from trauma (e.g., from a foreign body, anal intercourse, perirectal surgery).

An *acute* anal fissure is superficial and usually resolves on its own or heals with conservative treatment. It can take up to 6 weeks for a fissure to heal. *Chronic* fissures recur, and surgical treatment may be needed. Pain during and after defecation and bright red blood in the stool are the most common symptoms. Other manifestations include pruritus, urinary frequency or retention, dysuria, and dyspareunia (painful intercourse).

The diagnosis is made by stretching and inspecting the perianal skin. If the patient is having pain at the time of the examination, diagnostic testing is usually limited to inspection. If he or she is not in severe pain, a digital examination and possibly a sigmoidoscopy are performed. When painless or multiple fissures are present, a colonoscopy may be performed to rule out any inflammatory bowel disorder.

Management of an acute fissure is usually aimed at local pain relief and softening of stools to reduce trauma to the area. Teach the patient to use warm sitz baths, analgesics, and bulk-producing agents (e.g., psyllium hydrophilic mucilloid [Metamucil]) to help minimize the pain from defecation. Topical anti-inflammatory agents (hydrocortisone creams and suppositories) may be helpful for some patients.

Explain pain control measures to the patient. Remind him or her to notify the health care provider if pain is not relieved within a few days. If fissures do not respond to management within several days to weeks, surgical repair under a local anesthetic may be needed. Teach the patient to report any drainage or bleeding from the rectum to the health care provider.

ANAL FISTULA

An anal fistula, or *fistula in ano*, is an abnormal tract leading from the anal canal to the perianal skin. Most anal fistulas result from anorectal abscesses, which are caused by obstruction of anal glands (see the Anorectal Abscess section). Fistulas can also occur with tuberculosis, Crohn's disease, or cancer. Intermittent discharge is usually noted over the perianal area.

The patient with an anal fistula has pruritus (itching), purulent discharge, and tenderness or pain that worsens with bowel movements. A proctoscope may be used to identify the source of symptoms and to locate the fistula. Because fistulas do not heal spontaneously, surgery is necessary. To perform a fistulotomy, the surgeon opens the tissue over the tract and scrapes the base. The incision site then heals by secondary intention. For a fistula higher in the anus, a special surgical technique is used to preserve important sphincters. After surgery, instruct the patient about sitz baths, analgesics, and the use of bulk-producing agents or stool softeners to reduce pain.

PARASITIC INFECTION

❖ PATHOPHYSIOLOGY

Parasites can enter and invade the GI tract and cause infection. They commonly enter through the mouth (oral-fecal transmission) from contaminated food or water, oral-anal sexual practices, or contact with feces from a contaminated person. Common parasites that cause infection in humans are *Giardia lamblia*, which causes giardiasis; *Entamoeba histolytica*, which causes amebiasis (amoebic dysentery); and *Cryptosporidium*. *Handwashing is the best way to prevent the spread of parasitic infections.*

Giardia lamblia is a protozoal parasite that causes superficial invasion, destruction, and inflammation of the mucosa in the small intestine. This organism occurs in cysts and trophozoites (sporozoan parasites). Trophozoites die rapidly after they leave the body in stool; but cysts can remain alive in the right type of environment for weeks or months. Humans who eliminate cysts are infectious. Flies can spread the cysts, and the problem is more common in areas that use human excrement for fertilizer. Humans are hosts to this organism, but beavers and dogs may be reservoirs for infection.

Giardiasis is a well-recognized problem in international travelers, campers, and immunosuppressed patients. In the United States, it is prevalent and is the most common parasitic infection. This disorder affects only the intestinal system, causing acute diarrhea, chronic diarrhea, or malabsorption syndrome. The acute phase usually is self-limiting, lasting days or weeks. The chronic phase can last for years. Diarrhea is usually mild in both forms, but it can be severe. As stools increase in frequency, they become more watery, greasy, frothy, and malodorous with mucus. Weight loss and weakness are also common. Malabsorption can occur with diarrhea that continues for longer than 3 weeks. Manifestations result from malabsorption of fat, protein, and vitamin B_{12} and lactase deficiency.

Humans are the only known hosts for *E. histolytica* (also known as *amebiasis*). This organism also occurs in cysts and trophozoites. Amebiasis occurs worldwide, but it is most common in tropical areas. Prevalence rates are high in areas with poor sanitation, crowding, and poor NUTRITION. Amebiasis causes tens of thousands of deaths annually worldwide. The disease causes less severe symptoms and often goes undiagnosed in temperate climates. *E. histolytica* either feeds on bacteria in the intestine or invades and ulcerates the mucosa of the large intestine. The parasite can be limited to the GI tract (intestinal amebiasis), or it can extend outside the intestines (extraintestinal amebiasis). Individuals can have intestinal amebiasis without having any symptoms, or symptoms can range from mild to severe.

Cryptosporidium is manifested by diarrhea. This infection occurs most commonly in immunosuppressed patients, particularly those with human immune deficiency virus (HIV). It can also occur in children and older adults from contaminated swimming pools. (See Chapter 19 for a discussion of HIV infection.)

Chagas disease is caused by the *Trypanosoma cruzi* parasite, which is most commonly transmitted in impoverished areas of Latin America by the triatomine (kissing) bug. Patients first develop an acute infection, followed by an intermediate asymptomatic period and a chronic infection. Patients with chronic Chagas disease often develop cardiac dysrhythmias or heart failure and colon or esophagus dilation, causing impaired digestion and bowel ELIMINATION. An estimated 300,000 individuals in the United States have the disease (most in the southern areas of the United States), which can be transmitted through blood transfusions and organ transplantations. The Centers for Disease Control and Prevention (CDC) has targeted Chagas disease as one of five neglected parasitic infections that require public health action as the number of cases is expected to increase (CDC, 2016).

❖ **INTERPROFESSIONAL COLLABORATIVE CARE**

◆ **Assessment: Noticing**

A thorough history can help determine potential sources of exposure to parasitic infection. A history of travel to parts of the world where such infections are prevalent increases suspicion for infection with parasites. GI symptoms related to travel may be delayed as long as 1 to 2 weeks after the return home. Immigrants (newcomers) may have the infection on entering a new country. A NUTRITION history is especially helpful if several people in a group become ill. Common water supplies or bodies of water may be infected with *Giardia* or *Cryptosporidium*. Trichinosis should be considered if the patient has eaten pork products.

Mild-to-moderate *E. histolytica* infestation causes the daily passage of several strongly foul-smelling stools, possibly with mucus but without blood, accompanied by abdominal cramping, flatulence (gas), fatigue, and weight loss.

The infected patient usually experiences remissions and recurrences. Severe amoebic dysentery is manifested by frequent, more liquid, and foul-smelling stools with mucus *and* blood. Fever up to 104°F (40°C), tenesmus (feeling the urge to defecate), generalized abdominal tenderness, and vomiting can also occur. The ulcerations of invading amebiasis that occur in the colon can cause pain, bleeding, and obstruction. Ulcerations can also occur in the rectum, resulting in formed stool with blood. Complications are rare but include appendicitis and bowel perforation.

Extraintestinal amebiasis can occur without symptoms of intestinal infection. The most common form is amoebic liver abscess, which causes symptoms of fever, pain, and an enlarged liver. The abscess can rupture, and death can result if the infection and complications are not treated.

The diagnosis of *amebiasis* is made by examining the stool for parasites. Because *E. histolytica* is difficult to detect, serial stool examinations are needed if the disease is suspected. The use of sigmoidoscopy may detect ulcerations in the rectum or colon. Exudate obtained during sigmoidoscopic examination is studied for the parasite. The white blood cell (WBC) count can be very high when severe dysentery is present.

The diagnosis of *giardiasis* is also confirmed by the presence of parasites in the stool. Because organisms may not be detected for at least 1 week after symptoms appear, multiple stool samples should be examined.

◆ **Interventions: Responding**

Treatment for all types of *amebiasis* involves the use of amebicide drugs. Metronidazole (Flagyl, Novo-Nidazol ✦), followed by a luminal agent such as paromomycin, is commonly prescribed (Leder & Weller, 2016). The patient with severe amoebic dysentery requires IV fluid replacement and possibly an opiate-like drug, such as diphenoxylate hydrochloride and atropine sulfate (Lomotil), to control bowel motility. The patient with extraintestinal amebiasis or severe dehydration, especially the older adult, is hospitalized. The patient with asymptomatic, mild, or moderate disease is treated with drug therapy on an ambulatory care basis. Therapy effectiveness is based on the examination of at least three stools at 2- to 3-day intervals, starting 2 to 4 weeks after drug therapy has been completed. *Teach patients the importance of keeping their follow-up appointments and taking all drugs as prescribed.*

Treatment for *giardiasis* is drug therapy. Metronidazole (Flagyl, Novo-Nidazol ✦) is the drug of choice. Tinidazole can be used as an alternative. Stools are examined 2 weeks after treatment to assess for drug effectiveness.

! **NURSING SAFETY PRIORITY** QSEN

Action Alert

Explain modes of transmission of parasitic infections and means to avoid the spread of infection and recurrent contact with parasitic organisms. *Inform the patient that the infection can be transmitted to others until amebicides effectively kill the parasites. Teach the patient to:*
- Avoid contact with stool
- Keep toilet areas clean
- Wash hands meticulously with an antimicrobial soap after bowel movements
- Maintain good personal hygiene by bathing or showering daily
- Avoid stool from dogs and beavers

Advise the patient to avoid sexual practices that allow rectal contact until drug therapy is completed. *All household and sexual partners should have stool examinations for parasites.* If the water supply is suspected as the source, a sample is obtained and sent for analysis. Multiple infections are common in households, often as a result of contaminated water supplies. Well water and water from areas with inadequate or no filtration equipment can be sources of contamination.

Infection with *Cryptosporidium* is usually self-limiting in adults who have normal immune function. Drug therapy for patients who are immunosuppressed may include paromomycin, an aminoglycoside antibiotic. Teach patients that this drug can cause dizziness.

GET READY FOR THE NCLEX® EXAMINATION!

KEY POINTS

Review these Key Points for each NCLEX Examination Client Needs Category.

Safe and Effective Care Environment

- Collaborate with a CWOCN, health care provider, and case manager to plan care for patients with IBD. **QSEN: Teamwork and Collaboration**
- When transitioning care, remind patients and families about community resources for IBD, including the United Ostomy Associations of America and the Crohn's and Colitis Foundation of America. **QSEN: Teamwork and Collaboration**

Health Promotion and Maintenance

- Teach patients to use infection control measures to prevent transmission of gastroenteritis as stated in Chart 57-2. **QSEN: Safety**
- Teach patients how to self-manage an ileostomy or other surgical diversion, including skin care, pouch management, and stoma assessment (see Chart 57-4).

Psychosocial Integrity

- Be aware that all IBDs (acute and chronic) are very disruptive to one's daily routine; living with IBD requires a lifetime of modifications. **QSEN: Patient-Centered Care**
- Recognize that having a chronic bowel disease or an ileostomy impacts the patient's body image and self-esteem; assess for coping strategies that the patient has previously used, and identify personal support systems, such as family members, to assist in coping. **Clinical Judgment**

Physiological Integrity

- Assess for the classic signs and symptoms of appendicitis, which include abdominal pain, nausea and vomiting, and abdominal tenderness on palpation (McBurney's point); some patients also have leukocytosis. **QSEN: Safety**
- Recognize that perforation (rupture) of the appendix requires prompt intervention and can result in peritonitis. **QSEN: Safety**
- Assess for the key features of peritonitis as listed in Chart 57-1.
- Assess for signs and symptoms of dehydration in patients who have acute and chronic inflammatory bowel disorders.
- Administer antidiarrheal medications as prescribed to decrease stools and therefore prevent dehydration in patients with acute and chronic inflammatory bowel disorders. **QSEN: Evidence-Based Practice**

- Differentiate between two major types of chronic inflammatory bowel disease (IBD): ulcerative colitis (UC) and Crohn's disease (see Table 57-2). **Clinical Judgment**
- Be alert for GI bleeding in the patient with chronic IBD. **QSEN: Safety**
- Be aware that patients with Crohn's disease are at high risk for malnutrition as a result of an inability to absorb nutrients via the small intestine. **Clinical Judgment**
- Priority problems for patients with UC include diarrhea, pain, and potential for lower GI bleeding.
- Monitor for complications of UC as listed in Table 57-4.
- Provide nursing interventions for patients with IBD as listed in Chart 57-3.
- Teach patients with IBD to avoid GI stimulants, such as alcohol and caffeine. **QSEN: Evidence-Based Practice**
- Administer 5-aminosalicylic acid (5-ASA) drugs as prescribed to decrease inflammation in patients with UC.
- Administer infliximab (Inflectra ♣, Remicade, Remsima ♣) or other monoclonal antibody agent as prescribed for patients with Crohn's disease; these drugs may also be useful for those with UC in selected cases.
- Observe for signs and symptoms of lower GI bleeding in patients with chronic inflammatory and diverticular disease. **QSEN: Safety**
- Teach patients with diverticulosis to eat a high-fiber diet; diverticulitis requires a low-fiber diet. **QSEN: Evidence-Based Practice**
- Teach older patients how to self-manage diverticulitis as outlined in Chart 57-6.
- Instruct patients with diverticulosis about NUTRITION modifications, such as avoiding nuts, foods with seeds, and GI stimulants. **QSEN: Evidence-Based Practice**
- Be aware that patients with celiac disease (CD) have various signs and symptoms; some have no symptoms, some have classic symptoms, and some have atypical symptoms (see Chart 57-7).
  Teach patients with CD about the need to consume a strict gluten-free diet, which avoids wheat and wheat-based products. **QSEN: Evidence-Based Practice**
- Be aware that GI problems, including diarrhea, may be caused by parasites and food poisoning.
- Instruct patients with anorectal disorders to use sitz baths, bulk-forming agents (e.g., Metamucil), and stool softeners to decrease pain.

SELECTED BIBLIOGRAPHY

Almerie, M. Q., & Simpson, J. (2015). Diagnosing and treating diverticular disease. *The Practitioner, 259*(1785), 29.

Centers for Disease Control and Prevention (CDC). (2016). *Parasites—American trypanosomiasis.* http://www.cdc.gov/parasites/chagas.

Cleynen, I., Boucher, G., Jostins, L., Schumm, L. P., Zeissig, S., Ahmad, T., et al. (2016). Inherited determinants of Crohn's disease and ulcerative colitis phenotypes: A genetic association study. *Lancet, 387,* 156–167.

Crohn's and Colitis Canada. (2016). *What are Crohn's and colitis?* http://www.crohnsandcolitis.ca/About-Crohn-s-Colitis/What-are-Crohns-and-Colitis.

Crohn's and Colitis Foundation. (2017). *Crohn's disease and ulcerative colitis: Who gets IBD?* http://www.crohnscolitisfoundation.org/resources/guide-for-parents.html?referrer=https://www.google.com/.

Doklestić, S., Bajec, D., Djukić, R., Bumbaširević, V., Detanac, A. D., Detanac, S. D., et al. (2014). Secondary peritonitis—evaluation of 204 cases and literature review. *Journal of Medicine and Life*, 7(2), 132–138.

Fhogartaigh, C. N., & Dance, D. A. (2013). Bacterial gastroenteritis. *Medicine*, 41(12), 693–699.

Hata, K., Kazama, S., Nozawa, H., Kawai, K., Kiyomatsu, T., Tanaka, J., et al. (2015). Laparoscopic surgery for ulcerative colitis: A review of the literature. *Surgery Today*, 45, 933–938.

Leder, K., & Weller, P. (2016). Intestinal *Entamoeba histolytica* amebiasis. Retrieved from www.uptodate.com.

Macken, L., & Blaker, P. A. (2015). Management of acute severe ulcerative colitis (NICE CG 166). *Clinical Medicine*, 15(5), 473–476. doi:10.7861/clinmedicine.15-5-473.

Mavrinac, M. A., Ohannessian, A., Dowling, E., & Dowling, P. (2014). Why is celiac disease so easy to miss? *The Journal of Family Practice*, 63(9), 508–513.

McCance, K., Huether, S., Brashers, V., & Rote, N. (2014). *Pathophysiology: The biologic basis for disease in adults and children* (7th ed.). St. Louis: Mosby.

Pagana, K., Pagana, T. J., & Pagana, T. N. (2017). *Mosby's diagnostic and laboratory test reference* (13th ed.). St. Louis: Mosby.

Pfizer. (2016). *Azulfidine*. Retrieved from http://labeling.pfizer.com/ShowLabeling.aspx?id=524.

Randall, C. W., Vizuete, J. A., Martinez, N., Alvarez, J. J., Garapati, K. V., Malakouti, M., et al. (2015). From historical perspective to modern therapy: A review of current and future biological treatment for Crohn's disease. *Therapeutic Advances in Gastroenterology*, 8(3), 143–159.

Seifarth, C., Ritz, J. P., Kroesen, A., & Groene, J. (2015). Effects of minimizing access trauma in laparoscopic colectomy in patients with IBD. *Surgical Endoscopy*, 29, 1413–1418.

Singh, S., Stroud, A., Holubar, S., Sandborn, W., & Pardi, D. (2015). *Therapy for treatment and prevention of pouchitis*. http://www.cochrane.org/CD001176/IBD_therapy-treatment-and-prevention-pouchitis.

Sinha, R. (2015). Magnetic resonance enterography. In R. Kozarek & J. A. Leighton (Eds.), *Endoscopy in small bowel disorders* (pp. 65–90). New York: Springer.

Zhang, W., Hui, K. Y., Gusev, A., Warner, N., Ng, S. M., Ferguson, J., et al. (2013). Extended haplotype association study in Crohn's disease identifies a novel, Ashkenazi Jewish-specific missense mutation in the NF-kB pathway gene, HEATR3. *Genes and Immunity*, 14, 310–316.

CHAPTER 58

Care of Patients With Liver Problems

Lara Carver and Jennifer Powers

 http://evolve.elsevier.com/Iggy/

PRIORITY AND INTERRELATED CONCEPTS

The priority concepts for this chapter are:
- CELLULAR REGULATION
- IMMUNITY

✳ The CELLULAR REGULATION concept exemplar for this chapter is Cirrhosis, below.

✳ The IMMUNITY concept exemplar for this chapter is Hepatitis, p. 1180.

The interrelated concepts for this chapter are:
- COMFORT
- FLUID AND ELECTROLYTE BALANCE
- NUTRITION

LEARNING OUTCOMES

Safe and Effective Care Environment
1. Collaborate with the interprofessional team to provide care for the patient with liver inflammation and necrosis.
2. Identify community resources to ensure appropriate transition management for patient with chronic liver disease.

Health Promotion and Maintenance
3. Teach adults how to prevent hepatitis and its spread to others.
4. Teach patients how to prevent or slow the progress of alcohol-induced cirrhosis.

Psychosocial Integrity
5. Implement nursing interventions to minimize stressors for the patient with liver problems.

Physiological Integrity
6. Differentiate among assessment findings associated with cirrhosis, hepatitis, and other liver problems.
7. Prioritize care for patients with liver problems.
8. Create an evidence-based plan of care for the patient with late-stage cirrhosis.
9. Describe nursing interventions to address life-threatening complications associated with liver problems.
10. Explain the role of the nurse in assisting with paracentesis.
11. Describe nursing interventions that promote IMMUNITY, CELLULAR REGULATION, COMFORT, and FLUID AND ELECTROLYTE BALANCE for patients with liver problems.

As the largest and one of the most vital internal organs, the liver performs more than 400 functions and affects every bodily system. When the liver is diseased or damaged, IMMUNITY, CELLULAR REGULATION, *digestion*, NUTRITION, *and metabolism* can be severely affected. Liver diseases range in severity from mild hepatic inflammation to chronic end-stage cirrhosis.

✳ CELLULAR REGULATION CONCEPT EXEMPLAR
Cirrhosis

Cirrhosis is extensive, irreversible scarring of the liver, usually caused by a chronic reaction to hepatic inflammation and necrosis. This scarring process directly impairs CELLULAR REGULATION. The disease typically develops slowly and has a progressive, prolonged, destructive course resulting in end-stage liver disease. The most common causes for cirrhosis in the United States are chronic alcoholism, chronic viral hepatitis, nonalcoholic steatohepatitis (NASH), bile duct disease, and genetic diseases (Table 58-1).

❖ PATHOPHYSIOLOGY

Cirrhosis is characterized by widespread fibrotic (scarred) bands of connective tissue that change the liver's normal makeup and its associated CELLULAR REGULATION. Inflammation caused by either toxins or disease results in extensive degeneration and destruction of **hepatocytes** (liver cells). As

TABLE 58-1	Common Causes of Cirrhosis
• Alcoholic liver disease	• Drugs and chemical toxins
• Viral hepatitis	• Gallbladder disease
• Autoimmune hepatitis	• Metabolic/genetic causes
• Steatohepatitis (from fatty liver)	• Cardiovascular disease

cirrhosis develops, the tissue becomes nodular. These nodules can block bile ducts and normal blood flow throughout the liver. Impairments in blood and lymph flow result from compression caused by excessive fibrous tissue. In early disease, the liver is usually enlarged, firm, and hard. As the pathologic process continues, the liver shrinks in size, resulting in decreased liver function, which can occur in weeks to years. Some patients with cirrhosis have no symptoms until serious complications occur. The impaired liver function results in elevated serum liver enzymes (Pagana et al., 2017).

Cirrhosis of the liver can be divided into several common types, depending on the cause of the disease (McCance et al., 2014):

- Postnecrotic cirrhosis (caused by viral hepatitis [especially hepatitis C] and certain drugs or other toxins)
- Laennec's or alcoholic cirrhosis (caused by chronic alcoholism)
- Biliary cirrhosis (also called *cholestatic;* caused by chronic biliary obstruction or autoimmune disease)

Complications of Cirrhosis

Common problems and complications associated with hepatic cirrhosis depend on the amount of damage sustained by the liver. In **compensated cirrhosis**, the liver is scarred and CELLULAR REGULATION is impaired, but the organ can still perform essential functions without causing major symptoms. In **decompensated cirrhosis**, liver function is impaired with obvious signs and symptoms of liver failure.

The loss of hepatic function contributes to the development of metabolic abnormalities. Hepatic cell damage may lead to these common complications:

- Portal hypertension
- Ascites and esophageal varices
- Coagulation defects
- Jaundice
- Portal-systemic encephalopathy (PSE) with hepatic coma
- Hepatorenal syndrome
- Spontaneous bacterial peritonitis

Portal Hypertension. **Portal hypertension**, a persistent increase in pressure within the portal vein greater than 5 mm Hg, is a major complication of cirrhosis. It results from increased resistance to or obstruction (blockage) of the flow of blood through the portal vein and its branches. The blood meets resistance to flow and seeks collateral (alternative) venous channels around the high-pressure area.

Blood flow backs into the spleen, causing **splenomegaly** (spleen enlargement). Veins in the esophagus, stomach, intestines, abdomen, and rectum become dilated. Portal hypertension can result in ascites (excessive abdominal [peritoneal] fluid), esophageal varices (distended veins), prominent abdominal veins (caput medusae), and hemorrhoids.

Ascites and Gastroesophageal Varices. **Ascites** is the collection of free fluid within the peritoneal cavity caused by increased hydrostatic pressure from portal hypertension (McCance et al.,

2014). The collection of plasma protein in the peritoneal fluid reduces the amount of circulating plasma protein in the blood. When this decrease is combined with the inability of the liver to produce albumin because of impaired liver cell functioning, the serum colloid osmotic pressure is decreased in the circulatory system. The result is a fluid shift from the vascular system into the abdomen, a form of "third spacing." As a result, the patient may have hypovolemia and edema at the same time.

Massive ascites may cause renal vasoconstriction, triggering the renin-angiotensin system. This results in sodium and water retention, which increases hydrostatic pressure and the vascular volume and leads to more ascites.

As a result of portal hypertension, the blood backs up from the liver and enters the esophageal and gastric veins. **Esophageal varices** occur when fragile, thin-walled esophageal veins become distended and tortuous from increased pressure. The potential for varices to bleed depends on their size; size is determined by direct endoscopic observation. Varices occur most often in the distal esophagus but can be present also in the stomach and rectum.

Bleeding esophageal varices are a life-threatening medical emergency. Severe blood loss may occur, resulting in shock from hypovolemia. The bleeding may be either **hematemesis** (vomiting blood) or **melena** (black, tarry stools). Loss of consciousness may occur before any observed bleeding. Variceal bleeding can occur spontaneously with no precipitating factors. However, any activity that increases abdominal pressure may increase the likelihood of a variceal bleed, including heavy lifting or vigorous physical exercise. In addition, chest trauma or dry, hard food in the esophagus can cause bleeding.

Patients with portal hypertension may also have **portal hypertensive gastropathy**. This complication can occur with or without esophageal varices. Slow gastric mucosal bleeding occurs, which may result in chronic slow blood loss, occult-positive stools, and anemia.

Splenomegaly (enlarged spleen) results from the backup of blood into the spleen. The enlarged spleen destroys platelets, causing thrombocytopenia (low serum platelet count) and increased risk for bleeding. Thrombocytopenia is often the first clinical sign that a patient has liver dysfunction.

Biliary Obstruction. In patients with cirrhosis, the production of bile in the liver is decreased. This prevents the absorption of fat-soluble vitamins (e.g., vitamin K). Without vitamin K, clotting factors II, VII, IX, and X are not produced in sufficient quantities, and the patient is susceptible to bleeding and easy bruising. These abnormalities are confirmed by coagulation studies. Some patients have a genetic predisposition to obstruction of the bile duct that leads to biliary cirrhosis—usually from gallbladder disease or an autoimmune form of the disease called *primary biliary cirrhosis (PBC)*.

Jaundice (yellowish coloration of the skin) in patients with cirrhosis is caused by one of two mechanisms: hepatocellular disease or intrahepatic obstruction (Fig. 58-1). *Hepatocellular* jaundice develops because the liver cells cannot effectively excrete bilirubin. This decreased excretion results in excessive circulating bilirubin levels. *Intrahepatic obstructive* jaundice results from edema, fibrosis, or scarring of the hepatic bile channels and bile ducts, which interferes with normal bile and bilirubin excretion. Patients with jaundice often report pruritus (itching).

Hepatic Encephalopathy. **Hepatic encephalopathy** (also called **portal-systemic encephalopathy [PSE]**) is a complex

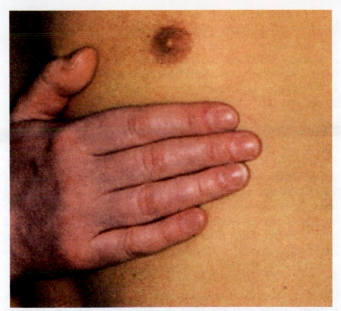

FIG. 58-1 Jaundice as a result of liver dysfunction such as cirrhosis and hepatitis. (From Leonard, P. [2011]. *Quick & easy medical terminology* (6th ed.). St. Louis: Saunders.)

TABLE 58-2	Stages of Hepatic Encephalopathy

Stage I
- Subtle manifestations that may not be recognized immediately
- Personality changes
- Behavior changes (agitation, belligerence)
- Emotional lability (euphoria, depression)
- Impaired thinking
- Inability to concentrate
- Fatigue, drowsiness
- Slurred or slowed speech
- Sleep pattern disturbances

Stage II
- Continuing mental changes
- Mental confusion
- Disorientation to time, place, or person
- Asterixis (hand flapping)

Stage III
- Progressive deterioration
- Marked mental confusion
- Stuporous, drowsy but arousable
- Abnormal electroencephalogram tracing
- Muscle twitching
- Hyperreflexia
- Asterixis (hand flapping)

Stage IV
- Unresponsiveness, leading to death in most patients progressing to this stage
- Unarousable, obtunded
- Usually no response to painful stimulus
- No asterixis
- Positive Babinski's sign
- Muscle rigidity
- Fetor hepaticus (characteristic liver breath—musty, sweet odor)
- Seizures

cognitive syndrome that results from liver failure and cirrhosis. Patients report sleep disturbance, mood disturbance, mental status changes, and speech problems early as this complication begins. Hepatic encephalopathy may be reversible with early intervention. Later neurologic symptoms include an altered level of consciousness, impaired thinking processes, and neuromuscular problems.

Hepatic encephalopathy may develop slowly in patients with chronic liver disease and go undetected until the late stages. Symptoms develop rapidly in acute liver dysfunction. Four stages of development have been identified (Table 58-2). The patient's symptoms may gradually progress to coma or fluctuate among the four stages.

The exact mechanisms causing hepatic encephalopathy are not clearly understood but probably are the result of the shunting of portal venous blood into the central circulation so the liver is bypassed. As a result, substances absorbed by the intestine are not broken down or detoxified and may lead to metabolic abnormalities, such as elevated serum ammonia and gamma-aminobutyric acid (GABA). Elevated serum ammonia results from the inability of the liver to detoxify protein by-products and is common in patients with hepatic encephalopathy. However, it is not a clear indicator of the presence of encephalopathy. Some patients may have major impairment without high elevations of serum ammonia, and elevations of ammonia can occur without evidence of encephalopathy.

Factors that may lead to hepatic encephalopathy in patients with cirrhosis include:
- High-protein diet
- Infection
- Hypovolemia (decreased fluid volume)
- Hypokalemia (decreased serum potassium)
- Constipation
- GI bleeding (causes a large protein load in the intestines)
- Drugs (e.g., hypnotics, opioids, sedatives, analgesics, diuretics, illicit drugs)

The prognosis depends on the severity of the underlying cause, the precipitating factors, and the degree of liver dysfunction.

Other Complications. The development of **hepatorenal syndrome (HRS)** indicates a poor prognosis for the patient with liver failure. It is often the cause of death in these patients. This syndrome is manifested by:
- A sudden decrease in urinary flow (<500 mL/24 hr) (oliguria)
- Elevated blood urea nitrogen (BUN) and creatinine levels with abnormally decreased urine sodium excretion
- Increased urine osmolarity

HRS often occurs after clinical deterioration from GI bleeding or the onset of hepatic encephalopathy. It may also complicate other liver diseases, including acute hepatitis and fulminant liver failure.

Patients with cirrhosis and ascites may develop acute *spontaneous bacterial peritonitis* (SBP). Those who are particularly susceptible are patients with very advanced liver disease. This may be the result of low concentrations of proteins; proteins normally provide some protection against bacteria.

The bacteria responsible for SBP are typically from the bowel and reach the ascitic fluid after migrating through the bowel wall and transversing the lymphatics. Symptoms vary but may include fever, chills, alterations in COMFORT (especially in the abdomen), and tenderness. However, indications can also be minimal with only mild symptoms in the absence of fever. Worsening encephalopathy and increased jaundice may also be present without abdominal symptoms.

The diagnosis of SBP is made when a sample of ascitic fluid is obtained by paracentesis for cell counts and culture. An ascitic fluid leukocyte count of more than 250 polymorphonuclear (PMN) leukocytes may indicate the need for treatment.

Etiology and Genetic Risk

Hepatitis C is a leading cause of cirrhosis and liver failure in the United States (Centers for Disease Control and Prevention, 2017). It is an infectious bloodborne illness that usually causes chronic disease and compromises the body's IMMUNITY. Inflammation caused by infection over time leads to progressive scarring of the liver, which impedes CELLULAR REGULATION. It usually takes decades for cirrhosis to develop, although alcohol use in combination with hepatitis C may speed the process.

Hepatitis B and hepatitis D are the most common causes of cirrhosis worldwide. Hepatitis B also causes inflammation and low-grade damage over decades that can ultimately lead to cirrhosis. Hepatitis D virus can infect the liver but only in people who already have hepatitis B (see discussion in Immunity Concept Exemplar: Hepatitis).

Cirrhosis may also occur as a result of nonalcoholic fatty liver disease (NAFLD), a rapidly growing health care concern. NAFLD is associated with obesity, diabetes mellitus type 2, and metabolic syndrome. It is the most common cause of liver disease in the world (World Gastroenterology Organisation, 2012). This disease can progress to liver cancer, cirrhosis, or failure, causing premature death. Up to 30% of Americans may have NAFLD (American Liver Foundation, 2017a). The Patatin-like phospholipase domain-containing 3 gene (*PNPLA3*) has been identified as a risk gene for the disease. Hispanics have this gene more often than other ethnic groups and therefore are at the highest risk for NAFLD (Houghton-Rahrig et al., 2014).

Another common cause of cirrhosis is excessive and prolonged alcohol use. Alcohol has a direct toxic effect on the hepatocytes and causes liver inflammation (alcoholic hepatitis). The liver becomes enlarged, with cellular degeneration and infiltration by fat, leukocytes, and lymphocytes. Over time, the inflammatory process decreases, and the destructive phase increases, as the ability to maintain appropriate CELLULAR REGULATION decreases. Early scar formation is caused by fibroblast infiltration and collagen formation. Damage to the liver tissue progresses as malnutrition and repeated exposure to the alcohol continue. If alcohol is withheld, the fatty infiltration and inflammation are reversible. If alcohol use continues, widespread scar tissue formation and fibrosis infiltrate the liver as a result of cellular necrosis. The long-term use of illicit drugs, such as cocaine, has similar effects on the liver.

GENDER HEALTH CONSIDERATIONS

Patient-Centered Care (QSEN)

The amount of alcohol necessary to cause cirrhosis varies widely from individual to individual, and there are gender differences. In women, it may take as few as two or three drinks per day over a minimum of 10 years. In men, perhaps six drinks per day over the same time period may be needed to cause disease. However, a smaller amount of alcohol over a long period of time can increase memory loss from alcohol toxicity of the cerebral cortex. Binge drinking can increase risk for hepatitis and fatty liver.

Incidence and Prevalence

Approximately 3.2 million Americans have hepatitis C (American Liver Foundation, 2017b), and 1 in 7 Americans have hepatitis B, which can particularly affect Asian American and Pacific Islander-born individuals (Immunization Action Coalition, 2016).

Combined, the incidence of chronic liver disease and cirrhosis are a major common cause of death in the United States. The national prevalence of hepatitis B in Canada is 270,000 individuals (Canadian Digestive Health Association, 2017). It is more challenging to quantify the exact number of Canadians with liver disease, since these statistics are grouped with other digestive disorders; however, it is known that approximately 7000 Canadians die annually after being affected with a liver disorder (Canadian Digestive Health Association, 2017.)

❖ INTERPROFESSIONAL COLLABORATIVE CARE

Care for the patient with cirrhosis can take place in various settings. These patients may, at different times, self-manage at home, be hospitalized for immediate concerns, need rehabilitative care, or be cared for in the community setting. Members of the interprofessional team that collaborate most closely to care for the patient with cirrhosis include the primary and specialty health care providers, nurse, dietitian, social worker, pharmacist, and spiritual leader of the patient's choice.

◆ Assessment: Noticing

History. Obtain data from patients with suspected cirrhosis, including age, gender, and employment history, especially history of exposure to alcohol, drugs (prescribed and illicit), use of herbal preparations, and chemical toxins. Keep in mind that all exposures are important, regardless of how long ago they occurred. Determine whether there has ever been a needlestick injury. Sexual history and orientation may be important in determining an infectious cause for liver disease, because men having sex with men (MSM) are at high risk for hepatitis A, hepatitis B, and hepatitis C. People with hepatitis can develop cirrhosis.

Inquire about whether there is a family history of alcoholism and/or liver disease. Ask the patient to describe his or her alcohol intake, including the amount consumed during a given period. Is there a history of illicit drug use, including oral, IV, and intranasal forms? Is there a history of obtaining tattoos? If so, when and where were they done? Has the patient been in the military or in prison? Is the patient a health care worker, firefighter, or police officer? For patients previously or currently in an alcohol or drug recovery program, how long have they been sober? This information is sensitive and often difficult for the patient to answer. Be sure to establish why you are asking these questions and accept answers in a nonjudgmental manner. Provide privacy during the interview. For many people, the behaviors causing the liver disease occurred years before the onset of their current illness, and they are regretful and often embarrassed.

Ask the patient about previous medical conditions, such as an episode of jaundice or acute viral hepatitis, biliary tract disorders (such as cholecystitis), viral infections, surgery, blood transfusions, autoimmune disorders, obesity, altered lipid profile, heart failure, respiratory disorders, or liver injury.

Physical Assessment/Signs and Symptoms. Because cirrhosis has a slow onset, many of the *early* signs and symptoms are vague and nonspecific. Assess for:

- Fatigue
- Significant change in weight
- GI symptoms, such as anorexia and vomiting
- Comfort alterations in the abdominal area and liver tenderness (both of which may be ignored by the patient)

Liver function problems are often found during a routine physical examination or when laboratory tests are completed for an unrelated illness or problem. The patient with *compensated cirrhosis* may be completely unaware that there is a liver problem. The first sign may present before the onset of symptoms when routine laboratory tests, presurgical evaluations, or life and health insurance assessments show abnormalities. These tests could indicate abnormal liver function or thrombocytopenia, requiring a more thorough diagnostic workup.

The development of late signs of *advanced cirrhosis* (also called *end-stage liver failure*) usually causes the patient to seek medical treatment. GI bleeding, jaundice, ascites, and spontaneous bruising indicate poor liver function and complications of cirrhosis.

Thoroughly assess the patient with liver dysfunction or failure because it affects every body system. The clinical picture and course vary from patient to patient, depending on the severity of the disease. Assess for:

- Obvious yellowing of the skin (jaundice) and sclerae (icterus)
- Dry skin
- Rashes
- Purpuric lesions, such as **petechiae** (round, pinpoint, red-purple lesions) or **ecchymoses** (large purple, blue, or yellow bruises)
- Warm and bright red palms of the hands (palmar erythema)
- Vascular lesions with a red center and radiating branches, known as **spider angiomas** (telangiectases, spider nevi, or vascular spiders), on the nose, cheeks, upper thorax, and shoulders
- Ascites (abdominal fluid)
- Peripheral dependent edema of the extremities and sacrum
- Vitamin deficiency (especially fat-soluble vitamins A, D, E, and K)

Abdominal Assessment. *Massive* ascites can be detected as a distended abdomen with bulging flanks (Fig. 58-2). The umbilicus may protrude, and dilated abdominal veins (caput medusae) may radiate from the umbilicus. Ascites can cause physical problems. For example, orthopnea and dyspnea from increased abdominal distention can interfere with lung expansion. The patient may have difficulty maintaining an erect body posture, and problems with balance may affect walking. Inspect and palpate for the presence of inguinal or umbilical hernias, which are likely to develop because of increased intra-abdominal pressure. *Minimal* ascites is often more difficult to detect, especially in the obese patient.

When performing an assessment of the abdomen, keep in mind that **hepatomegaly** (liver enlargement) occurs in many cases of early cirrhosis. Splenomegaly is common in nonalcoholic causes of cirrhosis. As the liver deteriorates, it may become hard and small.

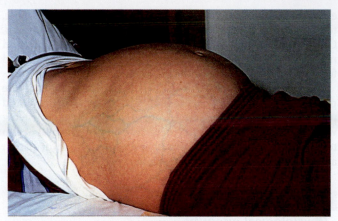

FIG. 58-2 Patient with abdominal ascites in late-stage cirrhosis. (From Talley, N., & O'Connor, S. [2010]. *Clinical examination: A systematic guide to physical diagnosis* (6th ed.). Sydney: Churchill Livingstone Australia.)

Measure the patient's abdominal girth to evaluate the progression of ascites (see Fig. 58-2). To measure abdominal girth, the patient lies flat while the nurse or other examiner pulls a tape measure around the largest diameter (usually over the umbilicus) of the abdomen. The girth is measured at the end of exhalation. Mark the abdominal skin and flanks to ensure the same tape measure placement on subsequent readings. *However, taking daily weights is the most reliable indicator of fluid retention.*

Other Physical Assessment. Observe vomitus and stool for blood. This may be indicated by frank blood in the excrement or by a positive fecal occult blood test (FOBT) (Hema-Check, Hematest). Gastritis, stomach ulceration, or oozing esophageal varices may be responsible for the blood in the stool. Note the presence of **fetor hepaticus,** which is the distinctive breath odor of chronic liver disease and hepatic encephalopathy and is characterized by a fruity or musty odor.

Amenorrhea (no menstrual period) may occur in women; and men may exhibit testicular atrophy, **gynecomastia** (enlarged breasts), and impotence as a result of inactive hormones. Patients with problems of the hematologic system caused by hepatic failure may have bruising and petechiae (small, purplish hemorrhagic spots on the skin).

Continually assess the patient's neurologic function; it may also be helpful to include family members in conversations about the patient's baseline mental status if the patient is unable to effectively communicate. Subtle changes in mental status and personality often progress to coma—a late complication of encephalopathy. Monitor for **asterixis**—a coarse tremor characterized by rapid, nonrhythmic extensions and flexions in the wrists and fingers (hand-flapping).

Psychosocial Assessment. The patient with hepatic cirrhosis may undergo subtle or obvious personality, cognitive, and behavior changes, such as agitation. He or she may experience sleep pattern disturbances or exhibit signs of emotional lability (fluctuations in emotions), euphoria (a very elevated mood), or depression. A psychosocial assessment identifies needs and helps guide care.

Repeated hospitalizations are common for patients with cirrhosis. It is a life-altering chronic disease, impacting not only the patient but also the immediate and extended family members and significant others. There are significant emotional, physical, and financial changes. Substance use may continue even as health worsens. It is important, whenever possible, to use resources available to these patients and their families. Collaborate with social workers, substance use counselors, and mental health/behavioral health care professionals as needed for patient assessment and management.

Part of the psychosocial assessment is determining if the patient is alcohol dependent. If this is the case, observe and prepare for alcohol withdrawal. Care of the patient experiencing withdrawal can be a medical emergency. Consult mental health textbooks or references for this chapter for more information about caring for the alcohol-dependent patient.

❓ NCLEX EXAMINATION CHALLENGE 58-1

Physiological Integrity

The nurse is caring for a client who is jaundiced and reports pruritus. Which intervention will the nurse include in the plan of care?
A. Monitor the client's vital signs and intake and output
B. Instruct the client to scratch with knuckles instead of nails
C. Assist the client with a hot bath and apply moisturizer
D. Encourage the client to eat a high-protein, high-cholesterol diet

---

Laboratory Assessment. Laboratory study abnormalities are common in patients with liver disease (Table 58-3). Serum levels of *aspartate aminotransferase* (AST), *alanine aminotransferase* (ALT), and *lactate dehydrogenase* (LDH) typically are elevated because these enzymes are released into the blood during hepatic inflammation. However, as the liver deteriorates, the hepatocytes may be unable to create an inflammatory response, and the AST and ALT may be normal. ALT levels are more specific to the liver, whereas AST can be found in muscle, kidney, brain, and heart. An AST/ALT ratio greater than 1.0 is usually found in alcoholic liver disease (Pagana et al., 2017).

Increased *alkaline phosphatase* and gamma-glutamyl transpeptidase (GGT) levels are caused by biliary obstruction and therefore may increase in patients with cirrhosis. Alkaline phosphatase is a nonspecific bone, intestinal, and liver enzyme. However, alkaline phosphatase also increases when bone disease, such as osteoporosis, is present. Total serum *bilirubin* levels also rise. Indirect bilirubin levels increase in patients with cirrhosis because of the inability of the failing liver to excrete bilirubin. Therefore bilirubin is present in the urine (urobilinogen) in increased amounts. Fecal urobilinogen concentration is decreased in patients with biliary tract obstruction. These patients have light- or clay-colored stools.

Total serum *albumin* levels are decreased in patients with severe or chronic liver disease as a result of decreased synthesis by the liver (Pagana et al., 2017). Loss of osmotic "pull" proteins such as albumin promotes the movement of intravascular fluid into the interstitial tissues (e.g., ascites). Prothrombin time/*international normalized ratio* (PT/INR) is prolonged because the liver decreases the production of prothrombin. The platelet count is low, resulting in a characteristic thrombocytopenia of cirrhosis. Anemia may be reflected by decreased red blood cell (RBC), hemoglobin, and hematocrit values. The white blood cell (WBC) count may also be decreased. *Ammonia* levels are usually elevated in patients with advanced liver disease. Serum creatinine may be elevated in patients with deteriorating kidney function. Dilutional hyponatremia (low serum sodium) may occur in patients with ascites.

TABLE 58-3 Assessment of Abnormal Laboratory Findings in Liver Disease

ABNORMAL FINDING	SIGNIFICANCE
Serum Enzymes	
Elevated serum aspartate aminotransferase (AST)	Hepatic cell destruction, hepatitis
Elevated serum alanine aminotransferase (ALT)	Hepatic cell destruction, hepatitis (most specific indicator)
Elevated lactate dehydrogenase (LDH)	Hepatic cell destruction
Elevated serum alkaline phosphatase	Obstructive jaundice, hepatic metastasis
Elevated gamma-glutamyl transpeptidase (GGT)	Biliary obstruction, cirrhosis
Bilirubin	
Elevated serum total bilirubin	Hepatic cell disease
Elevated serum direct conjugated bilirubin	Hepatitis, liver metastasis
Elevated serum indirect unconjugated bilirubin	Cirrhosis
Elevated urine bilirubin	Hepatocellular obstruction, viral or toxic liver disease
Elevated urine urobilinogen	Hepatic dysfunction
Decreased fecal urobilinogen	Obstructive liver disease
Serum Proteins	
Increased serum total protein	Acute liver disease
Decreased serum total protein	Chronic liver disease
Decreased serum albumin	Severe liver disease
Elevated serum globulin	Immune response to liver disease
Other Tests	
Elevated serum ammonia	Advanced liver disease or portal-systemic encephalopathy (PSE)
Prolonged prothrombin time (PT) or international normalized ratio (INR)	Hepatic cell damage and decreased synthesis of prothrombin

---

Imaging Assessment. Plain x-rays of the abdomen may show hepatomegaly, splenomegaly, or massive ascites. A CT scan may be requested.

MRI is another test used to diagnose the patient with liver disease. It can reveal mass lesions, giving additional specific information. This information is helpful in determining whether the condition is malignant or benign. *MR elastography* is a type of MRI that provides a way to assess liver elasticity, which helps the health care provider determine the amount of liver disease present.

Other Diagnostic Assessment. Ultrasound (US) of the liver is often the first assessment for an adult with suspected liver disease to detect ascites, hepatomegaly, and splenomegaly. It can also determine the presence of biliary stones or biliary duct obstruction. Liver US with Doppler is useful in detecting portal vein thrombosis and evaluating whether the direction of portal blood flow is normal.

Some patients being assessed for liver disease require biopsies to determine the exact pathology and the extent of disease progression. This procedure can be problematic because a large number of patients are at risk for bleeding. Even a **percutaneous** (through the skin) biopsy can pose a significant risk to the patient. To minimize this risk, an interventional radiologist can perform a liver biopsy using a long sheath through a jugular vein that then is threaded into the hepatic vein and liver. A tissue sample is obtained for microscopic evaluation. If a biopsy procedure is not possible, a radioisotope liver scan may be used to identify cirrhosis or other diffuse disease.

The health care provider may request *arteriography* if US is not conclusive in finding portal vein thrombosis. To evaluate the portal vein and its branches, a portal venogram may be performed instead, by passing a catheter into the liver and into the portal vein. This procedure is described in the Transjugular Intrahepatic Portal-Systemic Shunt (TIPS) section.

The health care provider may perform an **esophagogastroduodenoscopy (EGD)** to directly visualize the upper GI tract to detect complications of liver failure. These complications may include bleeding or oozing esophageal varices, stomach irritation and ulceration, or duodenal ulceration and bleeding. EGD is performed by introducing a flexible fiberoptic endoscope into the mouth, esophagus, and stomach while the patient is under moderate sedation. A camera attached to the scope permits direct visualization of the mucosal lining of the upper GI tract. An **endoscopic retrograde cholangiopancreatography (ERCP)** uses the endoscope to inject contrast material via the sphincter of Oddi to view the biliary tract and allow for stone removals, sphincterotomies, biopsies, and stent placements if required. These procedures are described in more detail in Chapter 52.

◆ Analysis: Interpreting

The priority collaborative problems for patients with cirrhosis include:

1. Fluid overload due to third spacing of abdominal and peripheral fluid
2. Potential for hemorrhage due to portal hypertension
3. Potential for hepatic encephalopathy due to shunting of portal venous blood and/or increased serum ammonia levels

◆ Planning and Implementation: Responding

Managing Fluid Volume

Planning: Expected Outcomes. The patient with cirrhosis is expected to have less excess fluid volume as evidenced by decreased ascites and peripheral edema and adequate circulatory volume. If ascites continues, the patient will not have respiratory distress and will manage ascites by adhering to the collaborative plan of care (see the Concept Map for liver failure caused by cirrhosis).

Interventions. Fluid accumulations are minimal during the early stages of ascites. Therefore interventions are aimed at preventing the accumulation of additional fluid and moving the existing fluid collection. Nonsurgical treatment measures are used to treat ascites in most cases.

Supportive measures to control abdominal ascites include NUTRITION therapy, drug therapy, paracentesis, and respiratory support. The patient's FLUID AND ELECTROLYTE BALANCE is also carefully monitored. If the patient is jaundiced, he or she will likely scratch the skin because the excess bilirubin products cause irritation and pruritus (itching).

Nutrition Therapy. The health care provider usually places the patient with abdominal ascites on a low-sodium diet as an

---

> **! NURSING SAFETY PRIORITY** QSEN
>
> **Action Alert**
>
> For skin irritation and pruritus associated with jaundice, teach the patient to use cool rather than warm water on the skin and to use a small amount of soap. Teach unlicensed assistive personnel to use lotion to soothe the skin. Assess for open skin areas from scratching, which could become infected.

initial means of controlling fluid accumulation in the abdominal cavity. The amount of daily sodium (Na$^+$) intake restriction varies, but a 1- to 2-g (2000 mg) Na$^+$ restriction may be tried first. In collaboration with the dietitian, explain the purpose of the restriction and advise the patient and family to read the sodium content labels on all food and beverages. Table salt should be completely excluded. Low-sodium diets may be distasteful, so suggest alternative flavoring additives such as lemon, vinegar, parsley, oregano, and pepper. Remind the patient that seasoned and salty food is an acquired taste; in time, he or she will become used to the decrease in dietary sodium.

In general, patients with late-stage cirrhosis are malnourished and have multiple dietary deficiencies. Vitamin supplements such as thiamine, folate, and multivitamin preparations are typically added to the IV fluids because the liver cannot store vitamins. For patients with biliary cirrhosis, bile may not be available for fat-soluble vitamin transport and absorption. Oral vitamins are prescribed when IV fluid administration is discontinued.

Drug Therapy. The health care provider usually prescribes a *diuretic* to reduce fluid accumulation and prevent cardiac and respiratory problems. Monitor the effect of diuretic therapy by weighing the patient daily, measuring daily intake and output, measuring abdominal girth, documenting peripheral edema, and assessing electrolyte levels. Serious fluid and electrolyte imbalances, such as dehydration, hypokalemia (decreased potassium), and hyponatremia (decreased sodium), may occur with loop diuretic therapy. Depending on the diuretic selected, the provider may prescribe an oral or IV potassium supplement. Some clinicians prescribe furosemide (Lasix) and spironolactone (Aldactone) as a combination diuretic therapy for the treatment of ascites. Because these drugs work differently, they are used for maintenance of sodium and potassium balance. For example, furosemide causes potassium loss, whereas spironolactone conserves it in the body.

All patients with ascites have the potential to develop **spontaneous bacterial peritonitis (SBP)** from bacteria in the collected ascitic fluid. In some patients, mild symptoms such as low-grade fever and loss of appetite occur. In others, there may be abdominal pain, fever, and change in mental status. When performing an abdominal assessment, listen for bowel sounds and assess for abdominal wall rigidity. Treatment involves IV cefotaxime or other third-generation cephalosporins or fluoroquinolones (Runyon, 2016).

Paracentesis. For some patients, abdominal **paracentesis** may be needed. Nursing implications associated with this procedure are described in Chart 58-1. The procedure is performed at the bedside, in an interventional radiology department, or in an ambulatory care setting. The health care provider inserts a trocar catheter or drain into the abdomen to remove the ascitic fluid from the peritoneal cavity. This procedure is done using ultrasound for added safety. In some situations, a short-term

CONCEPT MAP

IMMUNITY

NUTRITION

FLUID & ELECTROLYTE BALANCE

CELLULAR REGULATION

COMFORT

CIRRHOSIS

NOTICE IN THE HISTORY

Ray Jones, a 62-year-old farmer, has a 30-year history of heavy alcoholic intake. He arrives in the ED with hematemesis and melena.

Noticing Objective Data

- Patient states he feels light-headed and dizzy when he stands.
- Vital signs on admission: BP – 100/60; HR – 116, T – 100.8° F; RR – 24
- Pulse ox – 92%; HGB – 11 g/dL; HCT – 33%
- Platelets 100,000
- Ascites with peripheral edema, jaundice and icterus, petechiae on arms, & spider angiomas on nose and cheeks.

Interpreting Data Synthesis

- Widespread scarring disrupts normal liver function.
- Inflammation destroys liver cells, & nodular tissue blocks bile ducts & normal blood flow.
- IMMUNITY, NUTRITION, and CELLULAR REGULATION severely affected.
- Eventually end-stage liver failure occurs.

Pathophysiology of Cirrhosis

PATIENT PROBLEMS

- Fluid overload due to third spacing of abdominal and peripheral fluid
- Potential for hemorrhage due to portal hypertension
- Potential for hepatic encephalopathy due to shunting of portal venous blood and/or increased serum ammonia levels

Interpreting Data Synthesis

EXPECTED OUTCOMES

- Decrease fluid volume as evidenced by decreased ascites and peripheral edema and adequate circulatory volume
- If ascites continues, respiratory distress will not develop
- Manage ascites by adhering to the collaborative plan of care
- Remain free of bleeding episodes or managed immediately if bleeding occurs
- Lab values within normal limits
- No development of encephalopathy or decrease in LOC; immediate management if it occurs possible
- Achieve highest quality of life possible
- Abstain from alcohol or drugs

Planning and Responding for

INTERVENTIONS—RESPONDING

1 **Physical Assessment: Noticing**
Assess for jaundice and icterus; dry skin; rashes; petechiae; ecchymosis; palmar erythema; spider angiomas on the nose, cheeks, upper thorax, and shoulders; ascites; peripheral dependent edema of the extremities and sacrum. Listen to bowel sounds; assess for abdominal wall rigidity. *Evaluates the effects of chronic inflammation and necrosis resulting from cirrhosis.*

2 **Nursing Safety Priority—Action Alert!**
Monitor for and manage potentially life-threatening complications of cirrhosis with ascites, esophageal varices, coagulation defects, jaundice, encephalopathy, hepatic coma, hepatorenal syndrome, spontaneous bacterial peritonitis. *Prevents hemorrhage and death.*

3 **Preventing Infection**
Monitor for signs of acute spontaneous bacterial peritonitis (SBP) (low-grade fever, loss of appetite, abdominal pain, change in mental state) that can result from low concentrations of proteins. *Proteins provide some protection against bacteria.*

4 **Recognizing and Responding to Critical Lab Values**
Monitor blood urea nitrogen (BUN), serum protein, hemoglobin, hematocrit, platelets, and electrolytes. *Helps determine fluid and electrolyte status. Elevated BUN, decreased serum proteins, and increased hematocrit may indicate hypovolemia. Indicates destroyed platelets caused by splenomegaly (which causes thrombocytopenia and increased risk for bleeding).*

5 **Drug Therapy**
Administer antibiotics, propranolol (Inderal), and vasoconstrictive drugs as prescribed. *Prevents or controls infection and bleeding in patients with esophageal varices.*

6 **Fluid and Electrolyte Balance**
Monitor the effect of diuretic therapy by taking daily weights, measuring daily intake and output, measuring abdominal girth, documenting peripheral edema, and assessing electrolyte levels. *Identifies serious problems with FLUID AND ELECTROLYTE BALANCE such as dehydration, hypokalemia, and hypernatremia.*

7 **Sodium Restriction**
Teach the patient about decreasing sodium in the diet (1 to 2 g). Review how to read nutritional labels. Avoid table salt; use lemon, vinegar, parsley, oregano, and pepper instead. *Helps to manage electrolyte imbalance of hypernatremia with low-sodium diet controlling fluid accumulation in the abdominal cavity.*

8 **Promoting COMFORT—Regulating Activity**
Decrease activity that increases abdominal pressure, such as heavy lifting or vigorous physical exercise, chest trauma, or dry, hard food in the esophagus. *Such increased activity can cause bleeding and increases the likelihood of a variceal bleed.*

9 **Nursing Safety Priority—Action Alert!**
Use cool rather than warm water on the skin and only a small amount of soap. Teach UAP to use lotion to soothe the skin. Assess for open skin areas from scratching. *Maintains skin integrity and prevents infection.*

10 **Nursing Safety Priority—Action Alert!**
For patient with hepatopulmonary syndrome, monitor O_2 sat with pulse ox. Apply O_2 therapy as needed. Elevate head of the bed 30 degrees or higher, elevate feet and weigh daily. *Relieves dyspnea, decreases dependent ankle edema, and monitors FLUID BALANCE.*

Concept Map by Deanne A. Blach, MSN, RN

CHART 58-1 Best Practice for Patient Safety & Quality Care QSEN

The Patient With Paracentesis

- Explain the procedure and answer patient questions.
- Obtain vital signs, including weight.
- *Ask the patient to void before the procedure to prevent injury to the bladder!*
- Position the patient in bed with the head of the bed elevated.
- Monitor vital signs per protocol or physician's request.
- Measure the drainage and record accurately.
- Describe the collected fluid.
- Label and send the fluid for laboratory analysis; document in the patient record that specimens were sent.
- After the physician removes the catheter, apply a dressing to the site; assess for leakage.
- Maintain bedrest per protocol.
- Weigh the patient after the paracentesis; document in the patient record weight both before and after paracentesis.

ascites drain catheter may be placed while the patient is awaiting surgical intervention, or tunneled ascites drains (e.g., PleurX drains) can allow a patient or family caregiver to drain ascitic fluid at home.

If SBP is suspected, a sample of fluid is withdrawn and sent for cell count and culture. If the patient has symptoms of infection, the health care provider may prescribe antibiotics while awaiting the culture results.

Respiratory Support. Excessive ascitic fluid volume may cause the patient to have respiratory problems. He or she may develop *hepatopulmonary syndrome.* Dyspnea develops as a result of increased intra-abdominal pressure, which limits thoracic expansion and diaphragmatic excursion. Auscultate lungs every 4 to 8 hours for crackles that could indicate pulmonary complications, depending on the patient's overall condition.

! NURSING SAFETY PRIORITY QSEN

Action Alert

For the patient with hepatopulmonary syndrome, monitor his or her oxygen saturation with pulse oximetry. If needed, apply oxygen therapy to ease breathing. Elevate the head of the bed to at least 30 degrees or as high as the patient wants to improve breathing. This position, with his or her feet elevated to decrease dependent ankle edema, often relieves dyspnea. Weigh the patient daily or delegate and supervise this activity.

FLUID AND ELECTROLYTE BALANCE problems are common as a result of the disease or treatment. Laboratory tests, such as blood urea nitrogen (BUN), serum protein, hematocrit, and electrolytes, help determine fluid and electrolyte status. An elevated BUN, decreased serum proteins, and increased hematocrit may indicate hypovolemia.

If medical management fails to control ascites, the health care provider may choose to divert ascites into the venous system by creating a shunt. Patients with ascites are poor surgical risks. The transjugular intrahepatic portal-systemic shunt (TIPS) is a nonsurgical procedure that is used to control long-term ascites and reduce variceal bleeding. This procedure is described in the discussion of Interventions in the Preventing or Managing Hemorrhage section that follows.

? NCLEX EXAMINATION CHALLENGE 58-2

Physiological Integrity

The nurse is caring for a client who has had paracentesis performed. Which nursing intervention is appropriate? **Select all that apply.**
A. Keep head of bed flat
B. Measure, describe, and record drainage
C. Ambulate 30 minutes postprocedure
D. Weigh client
E. Label fluid container and send for laboratory analysis

Preventing or Managing Hemorrhage

Planning: Expected Outcomes. The patient is expected to be free of bleeding episodes. However, if he or she has a hemorrhage, it is expected to be controlled by prompt, evidence-based interdisciplinary interventions. Esophageal variceal bleeds are the most common type of upper GI bleeding.

Interventions. All patients with cirrhosis should be screened for esophageal varices by endoscopy to detect them early *before they bleed.* If patients have varices, they are placed on preventive therapy. If acute bleeding occurs, early interventions are used to manage it. *Because massive esophageal bleeding can cause rapid blood loss, emergency interventions are needed.*

Drug Therapy. The role of early drug therapy is to *prevent* bleeding and infection in patients who have varices. A nonselective *beta-blocking agent* such as propranolol (Inderal) is usually prescribed to prevent bleeding. By decreasing heart rate and the hepatic venous pressure gradient, the chance of bleeding may be reduced (World Gastroenterology Organisation, 2012).

Up to 20% of cirrhotic patients who are admitted to the hospital as a result of upper GI bleeding have bacterial infections, and even more patients develop health care–associated infections, usually urinary tract infections or pneumonia (McCance et al., 2014). Infection is one of the most common indicators that patients will have an acute variceal bleed (AVB). Therefore cirrhotic patients with GI bleeding should receive *antibiotics* when admitted to the hospital.

If bleeding occurs, the health care team intervenes quickly to control it by combining vasoactive drugs with endoscopic therapies. *Vasoactive* drugs, such as vasopressin and octreotide acetate (Sandostatin), reduce blood flow through vasoconstriction to decrease portal pressure. Octreotide also suppresses secretion of gastrin, serotonin, and intestinal peptides, which decreases GI blood flow to help with pressure reduction within the varices (World Gastroenterology Organisation, 2012).

Endoscopic Therapies. Endoscopic therapies include ligation of the bleeding veins or sclerotherapy. Both procedures have been very effective in controlling bleeding and improving patient survival rates. Esophageal varices may be managed with endoscopic variceal ligation (EVL) (banding). This procedure involves the application of small "O" bands around the base of the varices to decrease the blood supply to the varices. The patient is unaware of the bands, and they cause no discomfort.

Endoscopic sclerotherapy (EST), also called injection sclerotherapy, may be done to stop bleeding. The varices are injected with a sclerosing agent via a catheter. This procedure is associated with complications such as mucosal ulceration, which could result in further bleeding.

Rescue Therapies. If rebleeding occurs, rescue therapies are used. These procedures include a second endoscopic procedure, balloon tamponade and esophageal stents, and shunting procedures. Short-term esophagogastric balloon tamponade with esophageal stents is a very effective way to control bleeding. However, the procedure can cause potentially life-threatening complications, such as aspiration, asphyxia, and esophageal perforation (World Gastroenterology Organisation, 2012). Similar to a nasogastric tube, the tube is placed through the nose and into the stomach. An attached balloon is inflated to apply pressure to the bleeding variceal area. Before this tamponade, the patient is usually intubated and placed on a mechanical ventilator to protect the airway. This therapy is used if the patient is not able to have a second endoscopy or TIPS procedure.

Transjugular Intrahepatic Portal-Systemic Shunt. The transjugular intrahepatic portal-systemic shunt (TIPS) is a nonsurgical procedure performed in interventional radiology departments. This procedure is used for patients who have not responded to other modalities for hemorrhage or long-term ascites. If time permits, patients have a Doppler ultrasound to assess jugular vein anatomy and patency. The patient receives heavy IV sedation or general anesthesia for this procedure. The radiologist places a large sheath through the jugular vein. A needle is guided through the sheath and pushed through the liver into the portal vein. A balloon enlarges this tract, and a stent keeps it open. Most patients also have a Doppler ultrasound study of the liver after the TIPS procedure to record the blood flow through the shunt. Treating patients with TIPS who have esophageal/gastric varix hemorrhage problems may also require esophageal/gastric vein embolization as a part of the procedure. Patients with a highly cirrhotic liver usually have little flow through the liver parenchyma. These patients develop large portal-esophageal (or portal-gastric) veins diverting blood away from the diseased liver. Even after a successful TIPS, the diverting veins may persist and must be embolized (intentionally blocked) so they will not rebleed.

Serious complications of TIPS are not common. Patients are usually discharged in 1 or 2 days and are followed up with ultrasounds for the first year after the shunt is placed to ensure continued patency. Patients must also be monitored for hepatic encephalopathy, which can be cause by a TIPS. After creation of the TIPS, blood now bypasses most of the liver's filtration processes, allowing toxins to circulate throughout the body. For some patients, this can cause disturbances in consciousness and behavior. Lactulose or other medications may be given to counteract this affect, and dietary modification may also be helpful. In some cases, a TIPS shunt may have to have the flow reduced or closed completely to reverse the encephalopathy. This is done by deploying a smaller stent or occluding device inside the original TIPS shunt. This is a delicate decision for the health care provider to make, because reduction of flow through the shunt will likely cause the initial esophageal hemorrhaging to recur.

Patients receiving TIPS can also have significant elevation of their pulmonary artery pressure. This is a result of the sudden increase of blood flow to the right heart. Diuretics may help to treat this problem. For this reason, patients must be carefully evaluated for right heart failure before TIPS placement.

Other Interventions. Depending on the procedure done to control esophageal bleeding, patients usually have a nasogastric tube (NGT) inserted to detect any new bleeding episodes. They often receive packed red blood cells, fresh frozen plasma, dextran, albumin, and platelets through large-bore IV catheters.

Monitor vital signs every hour and check coagulation studies, including prothrombin time (PT), partial thromboplastin time (PTT), platelet count, and international normalized ratio (INR). Additional interventions for upper GI bleeding are discussed in Chapter 55.

Preventing or Managing Hepatic Encephalopathy

Planning: Expected Outcomes. The patient is expected to be free of encephalopathy. However, if it occurs, it is expected that the interdisciplinary team will intervene early to prevent further health problems or death.

Interventions. The poorly functioning liver cannot convert ammonia and other by-products of protein metabolism to a less toxic form. They are carried by the circulatory system to the brain, where they affect cerebral function. Interventions are planned around the management of slowing or stopping the accumulation of ammonia in the body.

Because ammonia is formed in the GI tract by the action of bacteria on protein, nonsurgical treatment measures to decrease ammonia production include dietary limitations and drug therapy to reduce bacterial breakdown.

Nutrition Therapy. Patients with cirrhosis have increased nutritional requirements—high-carbohydrate, moderate-fat, and high-protein foods. However, the diet may be changed for those who have elevated serum ammonia levels with signs of encephalopathy. Patients should have a moderate amount of protein and fat foods and simple carbohydrates. Strict protein restrictions are not required because patients need protein for healing. In collaboration with the dietitian, be sure to include family members or significant others in NUTRITION counseling. The patient is often weak and unable to remember complicated guidelines. Brief, simple directions regarding dietary dos and don'ts are recommended. Keep in mind any financial, cultural, or personal implications and the patient's food allergies when discussing food choices.

Drug Therapy. Drugs are used sparingly because they are difficult for the failing liver to metabolize. In particular, opioid analgesics, sedatives, and barbiturates should be restricted, especially for the patient with a history of encephalopathy.

However, several types of drugs may eliminate or reduce ammonia levels in the body. These include lactulose (e.g., Evalose, Heptalac) or lactitol and nonabsorbable antibiotics (AASLD practice guideline, 2014). The health care provider may prescribe *lactulose* (or lactitol) to promote the excretion of ammonia in the stool. This drug is a viscous, sticky, sweet-tasting liquid that is given either orally or by NG tube. The purpose is to obtain a laxative effect. Cleansing the bowels may rid the intestinal tract of the toxins that contribute to encephalopathy. It works by increasing osmotic pressure to draw fluid into the colon and prevents absorption of ammonia in the colon. The drug may be prescribed to the patient who has manifested signs of encephalopathy, regardless of the stage. The desired effect of the drug is production of two or three soft stools per day and a decrease in patient confusion caused by this complication.

Observe for response to lactulose. The patient may report intestinal bloating and cramping. Serum ammonia levels may be monitored but do not always correlate with symptoms. Hypokalemia and dehydration may result from excessive stools. Remind unlicensed nursing personnel to help the patient with skin care if needed to prevent breakdown caused by excessive stools.

Several *nonabsorbable antibiotics* may be given if lactulose does not help the patient meet the desired outcome or if he or she cannot tolerate the drug. These drugs should not be given together. Older adults can become weak and dehydrated from having multiple stools. Neomycin sulfate or rifaximin (Xifaxan), both broad-spectrum antibiotics, may be given to act as an intestinal antiseptic. These drugs destroy the normal flora in the bowel, diminishing protein breakdown and decreasing the rate of ammonia production. Maintenance doses of neomycin are given orally but may also be administered as a retention enema. Long-term use has the potential for kidney toxicity and therefore is not commonly used. It cannot be used for patients with existing kidney disease.

Metronidazole (Flagyl, Nidagel ✚, Novo-Nidazol ✚) is another broad-spectrum antibiotic with similar action to neomycin, but it can cause peripheral neuropathy. Vancomycin (Vancocin) may also be given, but its long-term use can lead to resistance (AASLD practice guideline, 2014).

Frequently assess for changes in level of consciousness and orientation. Check for asterixis (liver flap) and fetor hepaticus (liver breath). These signs suggest worsening encephalopathy. Thiamine supplements and benzodiazepines may be needed if the patient is at risk for alcohol withdrawal.

❓ CLINICAL JUDGMENT CHALLENGE 58-1

Safety; Evidence-Based Practice QSEN

You are caring for a 45-year-old man who arrived at the emergency department. He reports having abdominal pain for 3 weeks and states that he drinks three to five mixed alcoholic drinks daily. He has no known history of liver disease. He denies fever, chills, nausea and vomiting, or discolored stools. His last drink was last night. Assessment reveals yellowed skin, blood pressure of 100/58 mm Hg, and pulse rate of 102 beats/min. His abdomen is distended, and he is having some difficulty breathing; his respirations are 34 breaths/min, and room air pulse oximetry is 87%. The emergency department health care provider orders an ECG, chest x-ray, CT scan of abdomen/pelvis, oxygen at 2L/NC, and IV access.

1. For which complications is this patient at risk, and why?
2. Into what position will you place the patient, and why? What evidence supports your answer?
3. You anticipate that the patient has acute liver failure. What assessment findings support this suspicion?
4. What laboratory findings do you anticipate that would support the diagnosis of liver failure?

Care Coordination and Transition Management

If the patient with late-stage cirrhosis survives life-threatening complications, he or she is usually discharged to home or to a long-term care facility after treatment measures have managed the acute medical problems. A home care referral may be needed if the patient is discharged to home. These chronically ill patients are often readmitted multiple times; and community-based care is aimed at optimizing COMFORT, promoting independence, supporting caregivers, and preventing rehospitalization. Patients with end-stage disease may benefit from hospice care. Collaborate with the case manager (CM) or other discharge planner to coordinate interdisciplinary continuing care.

Home Care Management. In collaboration with the patient, family, and case manager, assess physical adaptations needed to prepare the patient's home for recovery. Referrals for physical therapy, nutrition therapy, and transportation for health care provider and laboratory follow-up may be needed. The patient's rest area needs to be close to a bathroom because diuretic and/or lactulose therapy increases the frequency of urination and stools. If the patient has difficulty reaching the toilet, additional equipment (e.g., bedside commode) is necessary. Special adult-size incontinence pads or briefs may be helpful if the patient has an altered mental status and incontinence. If the patient has shortness of breath from massive ascites, elevating the head of the bed and maintaining him or her in a semi-Fowler's to high-Fowler's position may help alleviate respiratory distress. Alternatively, a reclining chair with an elevated foot rest may be used.

Self-Management Education. The patient is discharged to the home setting with an individualized teaching plan (Chart 58-2) that includes NUTRITION therapy, drug therapy, and alcohol abstinence, if needed. The patient who has a tunneled ascites drain (e.g., PleurX drain) will need to be taught how to access the drain and remove excess fluid. *Review the home care instructions that are provided with the drainage system with both the patient and family/caregiver. Remind them not to remove more than 2000 mL from the abdomen at one time to prevent hypovolemic shock.*

The patient with encephalopathy often finds that small, frequent meals are best tolerated. If his or her nutritional intake or albumin/prealbumin is decreased after discharge, multivitamin supplements and supplemental liquid feedings (e.g., Ensure, Boost) are usually needed. Teach patients to avoid excessive vitamins and minerals that can be toxic to the liver, such as fat-soluble vitamins, excessive iron supplements, and niacin. Remind patients to check with their health care provider before taking any vitamin supplement.

The patient is often discharged while receiving diuretics. Provide instructions regarding the health care provider's prescription for the diuretic. Teach about side effects of therapy, such as hypokalemia. The patient may need to take a potassium supplement if he or she is taking a diuretic that is not potassium sparing.

If the patient has had problems with bleeding from gastric ulcers, the health care provider may prescribe an H_2-receptor

---

👤 CHART 58-2 Patient and Family Education: Preparing for Self-Management

Cirrhosis

Nutrition Therapy
- Consume a diet that adheres to the guidelines set by your physician, nurse, or dietitian.
- If you have excessive fluid in your abdomen, follow the low-sodium diet prescribed for you.
- Eat small, frequent meals that are nutritionally well balanced.
- Include in your diet daily supplemental liquids (e.g., Ensure or Ensure Plus) and a multivitamin.

Drug Therapy
- Take the diuretic or preventive beta blocker prescribed for you. If you experience muscle weakness, irregular heartbeat, or light-headedness, contact your health care provider right away.
- Take the medication prescribed for you that helps prevent GI bleeding.
- Take the lactulose syrup as prescribed to maintain two or three bowel movements every day.
- Do *not* take any other medication (prescribed or over the counter) unless specifically prescribed by your health care provider.

Alcohol Abstinence
- Do not consume any alcohol.
- Seek support services for help if needed.

antagonist agent or proton pump inhibitor to reduce acid reflux (see Chapter 55). Patients who have had episodes of spontaneous bacterial peritonitis (SBP) may be on a daily maintenance antibiotic.

Teach family members how to recognize signs of encephalopathy and to contact the health care provider if these signs develop. Reinforce that constipation, bleeding, and infections can increase the risk for encephalopathy.

Advise the patient to avoid all over-the-counter drugs, especially NSAIDs and hepatic toxic herbs, vitamins, and minerals. Reinforce the need to keep appointments for follow-up medical care. Remind the patient and family to notify the health care provider immediately if any GI bleeding (overt bleeding or melena) is noted so re-evaluation can begin quickly.

> **! NURSING SAFETY PRIORITY** QSEN
>
> **Action Alert**
>
> One of the most important aspects of ongoing care for the patient with cirrhosis is to stress the need to avoid acetaminophen (Tylenol), alcohol, smoking, and illicit drugs. By avoiding these substances, the patient may:
> - Prevent further fibrosis of the liver from scarring
> - Allow the liver to heal and regenerate
> - Prevent gastric and esophageal irritation
> - Reduce the incidence of bleeding
> - Prevent other life-threatening complications

Health Care Resources. The patient with chronic cirrhosis may require a home care nurse for several visits after hospital discharge. The home care nurse can monitor the effectiveness of treatment in controlling ascites. The encephalopathic patient may need to be monitored for adherence to drug therapy and alcohol abstinence, if appropriate. Individual and group therapy sessions may be arranged to help patients deal with alcohol abstinence if they are too ill to attend a formal treatment program. Because some patients may have alienated relatives over the years because of substance use, it may be necessary to help them identify a friend, neighbor, or adult in their recovery group for support. If needed, refer the patient and family to self-help groups, such as Alcoholics Anonymous and Al-Anon.

The patient with cirrhosis may also desire spiritual or other psychosocial support. Finances are frequently a problem for the chronically ill patient and family; social support and community services need to be identified. The American Liver Foundation (www.liverfoundation.org) and American Gastroenterological Association (www.gastro.org) are excellent sources for more information about liver disease.

For patients who are not candidates for liver transplantation, address end-of-life issues. Discuss options such as hospice care with patients and their families (see Chapter 7). Be aware that they will go through a grieving process and will perhaps be in denial or very angry.

◆ Evaluation: Reflecting

Evaluate the care of the patient with cirrhosis based on the identified priority patient problems. The expected outcomes include that the patient will:
- Have a decrease in or have no ascites
- Have electrolytes within normal limits (WNL)

- Not have hemorrhage or will be managed immediately if bleeding occurs
- Not develop encephalopathy or will be managed immediately if it occurs
- Successfully abstain from alcohol or drugs (if disease is caused by these substances)

✳ IMMUNITY CONCEPT EXEMPLAR Hepatitis

❖ PATHOPHYSIOLOGY

Hepatitis is the widespread inflammation of liver cells. *Viral* hepatitis, which can be acute or chronic, is the most common type. Less common types of hepatitis are caused by chemicals, drugs, and some herbs. This section discusses hepatitis caused by a virus. Viral hepatitis results from an infection caused by one of five major categories of viruses:
- Hepatitis A virus (HAV)
- Hepatitis B virus (HBV)
- Hepatitis C virus (HCV)
- Hepatitis D virus (HDV)
- Hepatitis E virus (HEV)

Some cases of viral hepatitis are not caused by any of these viruses. These patients have non–A-E hepatitis.

Liver injury with inflammation can develop after exposure to a number of drugs and chemicals by inhalation, ingestion, or parenteral (IV) administration. Toxic and drug-induced hepatitis can result from exposure to hepatotoxins (e.g., industrial toxins, alcohol, and drugs). Hepatitis may also occur as a secondary infection during the course of infections with other viruses, such as Epstein-Barr, herpes simplex, varicella-zoster, and cytomegalovirus. Occurrence of any type of hepatitis affects the body's IMMUNITY and ability to protect itself.

After the liver has been exposed to any causative agent (e.g., a virus), it becomes enlarged and congested with inflammatory cells, lymphocytes, and fluid, resulting in right upper quadrant pain and discomfort. As the disease progresses, the liver's normal lobular pattern becomes distorted as CELLULAR REGULATION is compromised as a result of widespread inflammation, necrosis, and hepatocellular regeneration. This distortion increases pressure within the portal circulation, interfering with the blood flow into the hepatic lobules. Edema of the liver's bile channels results in obstructive jaundice (yellowing of the skin).

Classification of Hepatitis and Etiologies

The five major types of acute viral hepatitis vary by mode of transmission, manner of onset, and incubation periods. Hepatitis cases must be reported to the local public health department, which then notifies the Centers for Disease Control and Prevention (CDC).

Hepatitis A. The causative agent of hepatitis A, hepatitis A virus (HAV), is a ribonucleic acid (RNA) virus of the enterovirus family. *It is a hardy virus and survives on human hands.* The virus is resistant to detergents and acids but is destroyed by chlorine (bleach) and extremely high temperatures.

Hepatitis A usually has a mild course similar to that of a typical flu-like infection and often goes unrecognized. It is spread most often by the fecal-oral route by fecal contamination either from person-to-person contact (e.g., oral-anal sexual activity) or by consuming contaminated food or water. Common sources of infection include shellfish caught in contaminated water and food contaminated by food handlers infected with HAV. The incubation period of hepatitis A is usually 15 to 50 days, with a peak of 25 to 30 days. The disease is usually not life threatening, but its course may be more severe in adults older than 40 years and those with pre-existing liver disease such as hepatitis C (McCance et al., 2014).

In a small percentage of hepatitis A cases, severe illness with extrahepatic signs and symptoms can occur. Advanced age and conditions such as chronic liver disease may cause widespread damage that requires a liver transplant. In some cases when the patient's IMMUNITY is irreparably affected, death may occur. The incidence of hepatitis A is particularly high in nonaffluent countries in which sanitation is poor; however, cases are diagnosed internationally across the globe (World Health Organization, 2016). Some adults have hepatitis A and do not know it. The course is similar to that of a GI illness, and the disease and recovery are usually uneventful.

Hepatitis B. The **hepatitis B** virus (HBV) is not transmitted like HAV. It is a double-shelled particle containing DNA composed of a core antigen (HBcAg), a surface antigen (HBsAg), and another antigen found within the core (HBeAg) that circulates in the blood. HBV may be spread through these common modes of transmission (CDC, 2016):

- Unprotected sexual intercourse with an infected partner
- Sharing needles, syringes, or other drug-injection equipment
- Sharing razors or toothbrushes with an infected individual
- Accidental needlesticks or injuries from sharp instruments primarily in health care workers (low incidence)
- Blood transfusions (that have not been screened for the virus, before 1992)
- Hemodialysis
- Direct contact with the blood or open sores of an infected individual
- Birth (spread from an infected mother to baby during birth)

In addition, patients whose IMMUNITY is compromised either by disease or drug therapy are more likely to develop hepatitis B.

❓ NCLEX EXAMINATION CHALLENGE 58-3

Physiological Integrity

The nurse is caring for four clients. Which client is at the **highest** risk for hepatitis B infection?

A. 24-year-old with abdominal pain who just returned from Central America

B. 40-year-old who is 2 days postpartum and is breastfeeding

C. 65-year-old who reports using street drugs 10 years ago when homeless

D. 81-year-old who donated own blood before a surgical procedure

---

The clinical course of hepatitis B may be varied. Symptoms usually occur within 25 to 180 days of exposure and include (McCance et al., 2014):

- Anorexia, nausea, and vomiting
- Fever
- Fatigue
- Right upper quadrant pain
- Dark urine with light stool
- Joint pain
- Jaundice

Blood tests confirm the disease, although many individuals with hepatitis B have no symptoms.

Most adults who get hepatitis B recover, clear the virus from their body, and develop IMMUNITY. However, a small percentage of people do not develop immunity and become carriers. **Hepatitis carriers** can infect others even though they are not sick and have no obvious signs of hepatitis B. Chronic carriers are at high risk for cirrhosis and liver cancer. Because of the high number of newcomers from endemic areas, the incidence of hepatitis B has increased in the United States.

Hepatitis C. The causative virus of **hepatitis C** (HCV) is an enveloped, single-stranded RNA virus. Transmission is blood to blood. The rate of sexual transmission is very low in a single-couple relationship but increases with multiple sex partners. HCV is spread most commonly by:

- Illicit IV drug needle sharing (highest incidence)
- Blood, blood products, or organ transplants received before 1992
- Needlestick injury with HCV-contaminated blood (health care workers at high risk)
- Unsanitary tattoo equipment
- Sharing of intranasal cocaine paraphernalia

The disease is **not** transmitted by casual contact or intimate household contact. However, those infected are advised not to share razors, toothbrushes, or pierced earrings because microscopic blood may be on these items.

The average incubation period is 7 weeks. Acute infection and illness are not common. Most people are completely unaware that they have been infected. They are asymptomatic and not diagnosed until many months or years after the initial exposure when an abnormality is detected during a routine laboratory evaluation or when liver problems occur. Unlike with hepatitis B, most people infected with hepatitis C do not clear the virus, and a chronic infection develops.

HCV usually does its damage to the body's IMMUNITY over decades by causing a chronic inflammation in the liver that eventually causes the liver cells to scar. This scarring may progress to cirrhosis (McCance et al., 2014).

Hepatitis D. **Hepatitis D** (delta hepatitis) is caused by a defective RNA virus that needs the helper function of HBV. It occurs only with HBV to cause viral replication. This usually develops into chronic disease. The incubation period is about 14 to 56 days. As with hepatitis B, the disease is transmitted primarily by parenteral routes, especially in patients who are IV drug users. Having sexual contact with someone with HDV is also a high risk factor (McCance et al., 2014).

Hepatitis E. The **hepatitis E** virus (HEV) causes a waterborne infection associated with epidemics in the Indian subcontinent, Asia, Africa, the Middle East, Mexico, and Central and South America. Many large outbreaks have occurred after heavy rains and flooding. Like hepatitis A, hepatitis E is caused by fecal contamination of food and water.

In the United States, hepatitis E has been found only in international travelers. It is transmitted via the fecal-oral route, and the clinical course resembles that of hepatitis A. Hepatitis E has an incubation period of 15 to 64 days. There is no evidence at this time of a chronic form of the disease. The disease tends to be self-limiting and resolves on its own (McCance et al., 2014).

Complications of Hepatitis

Failure of the liver cells to regenerate, with progression of the necrotic process, results in a severe acute and often fatal form of hepatitis known as **fulminant hepatitis**. Hepatitis is considered to be chronic when liver inflammation lasts longer than 6 months. **Chronic hepatitis** usually occurs as a result of hepatitis B or hepatitis C. Superimposed infection with hepatitis D virus (HDV) in patients with chronic hepatitis B may also result in chronic hepatitis. Chronic hepatitis can lead to cirrhosis and liver cancer. Many patients have multiple infections, especially a combination of HBV with HCV, HDV, or HIV infections (McCance et al., 2014).

Incidence and Prevalence

The incidence of hepatitis A and hepatitis B is declining as a result of CDC recommendations for vaccination. However, hepatitis B and hepatitis C are a concern because of their association with cirrhosis and liver cancer. Although exact numbers are not known, it is estimated that about 71 million people worldwide have the hepatitis C virus (HCV) (World Health Organization, 2017). Currently there is no vaccine for HCV; however, patients may be treated with antiviral drug therapies. The goal of treatment of HCV-infected patients is to reduce mortality and liver-related health adverse consequences, including end-stage liver disease and liver cancer (AASLD, HCV Guidance, 2016). It is expected that the cases of HCV may rise over the next several decades as a result of increasing illicit drug use. Any increase will require a major increase in transplantations and lead to many more deaths.

Health Promotion and Maintenance

Hepatitis vaccines for infants, children, and adolescents have helped to protect the population's IMMUNITY by decreasing the incidence of hepatitis A and hepatitis B. Some adults also are advised to receive these immunizations.

Measures for preventing hepatitis A in adults include:
- Proper handwashing, especially after handling shellfish
- Avoiding contaminated food or water (including tap water in countries with high incidence)
- Receiving immunoglobulin within 14 days if exposed to the virus
- Receiving the HAV vaccine before traveling to areas where the disease is common (e.g., Mexico, Caribbean)
- Receiving the vaccine if living or working in enclosed areas with others, such as college dormitories, correctional institutions, day-care centers, and long-term care facilities

Several HAV vaccines are available (e.g., Havrix and Vaqta). Both of these vaccines are made of inactivated hepatitis A virus and are given in the deltoid muscle.

Several vaccines can also provide protection against hepatitis B (HBV) infection (e.g., Engerix-B and Recombivax-HB). Twinrix is a combination HAV and HBV vaccine that is also available for adults. Examples of groups for whom immunization against HBV should be used include:
- People who have sexual intercourse with more than one partner
- People with sexually transmitted infection (STI) or a history of STI
- Men having sex with men (MSM)

- People with any chronic liver disease (such as hepatitis C or cirrhosis)
- Patients with human immune deficiency virus (HIV) infection
- People who are exposed to blood or body fluids in the workplace, including health care workers, firefighters, and police
- People in correctional facilities
- Patients needing immunosuppressant drugs
- Family members, household members, and sexual contacts of people with HBV infection

Additional measures to prevent viral hepatitis for health care workers and others in contact with infected patients are listed in Charts 58-3 and 58-4.

❖ INTERPROFESSIONAL COLLABORATIVE CARE

Care for the patient with hepatitis can take place in various settings. These patients may, at different times, self-manage at home, be hospitalized for immediate concerns, or be cared for in the community setting. Members of the interprofessional team that collaborates most closely to care for the patient with hepatitis include the health care provider, nurse, and dietitian.

◎ CHART 58-3   Best Practice for Patient Safety & Quality Care QSEN

Prevention of Viral Hepatitis in Health Care Workers

- Use Standard Precautions to prevent the transmission of disease between patients or between patients and health care staff (see Chapter 23).
- Eliminate needles and other sharp instruments by substituting needleless systems. (Needlesticks are the major source of hepatitis B transmission in health care workers.)
- Take the hepatitis B vaccine (e.g., Recombivax HB), which is given in a series of three injections. This vaccine also prevents hepatitis D by preventing hepatitis B.
- For postexposure prevention of hepatitis A, seek medical attention immediately for immunoglobulin (Ig) administration.
- Report all cases of hepatitis to the local health department.

▊ CHART 58-4   Patient and Family Education: Preparing for Self-Management

Health Practices to Prevent Viral Hepatitis

- Maintain adequate sanitation and personal hygiene. Wash your hands before eating and after using the toilet.
- Drink water treated by a water purification system.
- If traveling in underdeveloped or nonindustrialized countries, drink only bottled water. Avoid food washed or prepared with tap water, such as raw vegetables, fruits, and soups. Avoid ice.
- Use adequate sanitation practices to prevent the spread of the disease among family members.
- Do not share bed linens, towels, eating utensils, or drinking glasses.
- Do not share needles for injection, body piercing, or tattooing.
- Do not share razors, nail clippers, toothbrushes, or Waterpiks®
- Use a condom during sexual intercourse or abstain from this activity.
- Cover cuts or sores with bandages.
- If ever infected with hepatitis, never donate blood, body organs, or other body tissue.

◆ **Assessment: Noticing**

History. Begin by asking the patient whether or not he or she has had known exposure to a person with hepatitis. For the patient who presents with few or no symptoms of liver disease but has abnormal laboratory tests (e.g., elevated alanine aminotransferase [ALT] or aspartate aminotransferase [AST] level), the history may need to include additional questions regarding risk factors such as:

- Exposure to either inhaled or ingested chemical
- Use of herbal supplements
- Use of any new prescribed drug or over-the-counter (OTC) medication
- Recent ingestion of shellfish
- Exposure to a possibly contaminated water source
- Travel to another country
- Sexual activities with men, women, or both and whether it was protected or unprotected
- Illicit drug use, IV or intranasal
- For health care workers, recent needlestick exposure
- Body piercing or tattooing
- Close living accommodations (e.g., military barracks, correctional institutions, overcrowded dormitories, long-term care facilities, day-care centers) or employment in any such setting
- Blood or blood products or organ transplants received before 1992
- Military service
- Place of birth (United States or other country) and parents' place of birth
- Family history of liver disease
- History of alcohol use (how many drinks each day or week)
- Human immune deficiency virus (HIV)

Physical Assessment/Signs and Symptoms. Assess whether the patient has:

- Abdominal pain
- Changes in skin or sclera (icterus)
- Arthralgia (joint pain) or myalgia (muscle pain)
- Diarrhea/constipation
- Changes in color of urine or stool
- Fever
- Lethargy
- Malaise
- Nausea/vomiting
- Pruritus (itching)

Lightly palpate the right upper abdominal quadrant to assess for liver tenderness. The patient may report right upper quadrant pain with jarring movements. Inspect the skin, sclerae, and mucous membranes for jaundice. He or she may present for medical treatment only after jaundice appears, believing that other vague symptoms are related to a flu-like syndrome.

Jaundice in hepatitis results from intrahepatic obstruction and is caused by edema of the liver's bile channels. Dark urine and clay-colored stools are often reported by the patient. If possible, obtain a urine and stool specimen for visual inspection and laboratory analysis. The patient may also have skin abrasions from scratching because of pruritus (itching).

Psychosocial Assessment. Viral hepatitis has various presentations, but for most infected people the initial course is mild with few or no symptoms. The long-term complications

EVIDENCE-BASED PRACTICE   QSEN

Caring for Military Veterans With Hepatitis C

Phillips, F., & Barnes, D. (2016). Social support and adherence for military veterans with hepatitis C. *Clinical Nurse Specialist, 30*(1), 38–44.

This qualitative study's aim was to describe military veterans' experience of support after diagnosis of hepatitis C and how support impacted their adherence to treatment.

A convenience sample of 21 veterans was used for this phenomenological study. Inclusion criteria were comprised of veterans who were over 18 years of age; were receiving standard care for hepatitis C; and could read, write, and communicate in English. In keeping with a phenomenological design, researchers collected data during a one-time, in-depth interview with each participant. Follow-up phone calls were used to verify that the themes identified were congruent with the lived experience of subjects.

Results indicated that veterans selectively tell only certain individuals about their diagnosis due to fear of stigma. In turn, this limits the amount of people in their circle of support. Veterans found some level of support, yet some level of burden, when disclosing their status to family members, friends, and health care providers.

Level of Evidence: 3

This qualitative research was designed as a phenomenological study.

Commentary: Implications for Practice and Research

Nurses must use empathy and concern while assessing availability of support systems for patients. In absence of a personal support network, or in addition to an existing support system, nurses should recommend support groups or counseling to help the patient adhere to treatment and management of hepatitis C.

of fibrosis and cirrhosis cause the more serious problem. This is especially true for patients who have chronic HBV and HCV infection.

Emotional problems for affected patients may center on their feeling sick and fatigued. General malaise, inactivity, and vague symptoms contribute to depression. Some patients often feel guilty and are remorseful about decisions made that caused the disease. These feelings are most likely to occur when the source of infection is from drug use.

Infectious diseases such as hepatitis continue to have a social stigma. (See the Evidence-Based Practice box on caring for military veterans with hepatitis C.) The patient may feel embarrassed by the precautions that are imposed in the hospital and continue to be necessary at home. This embarrassment may cause the patient to limit social interactions. Patients may be afraid that they will spread the virus to family and friends.

Family members are sometimes afraid of getting the disease and may distance themselves from the patient. Allow them to verbalize these feelings and explore the reasons for these fears. Educate the patient and family members about modes of transmission, and clarify information as needed.

Patients may be unable to return to work for several weeks during the acute phases of illness. The loss of wages and the cost of hospitalization for a patient without insurance coverage may produce great anxiety and financial burden. This situation may last for months or years if hepatitis becomes chronic.

Laboratory Assessment. Hepatitis A, hepatitis B, and hepatitis C are usually confirmed by acute elevations in levels of liver enzymes, indicating liver cellular damage, and by specific serologic markers.

Levels of ALT and AST may possibly rise into the thousands in acute or fulminant cases of hepatitis. Alkaline phosphatase levels may be normal or elevated. Serum total bilirubin levels are elevated and are consistent with the clinical appearance of jaundice.

The presence of *hepatitis A* is established when hepatitis A virus (HAV) antibodies (anti-HAV) are found in the blood. Ongoing inflammation of the liver by HAV is indicated by the presence of immunoglobulin M (IgM) antibodies, which persist in the blood for 4 to 6 weeks. Previous infection is identified by the presence of immunoglobulin G (IgG) antibodies. These antibodies persist in the serum and provide permanent IMMUNITY to HAV.

The presence of the *hepatitis B* virus (HBV) is established when serologic testing confirms the presence of hepatitis B antigen-antibody systems in the blood and a detectable viral count (HBV polymerase chain reaction [PCR] DNA). Antigens located on the surface (shell) of the virus (HBsAg) and IgM antibodies to hepatitis B core antigen (anti-HBcAg IgM) are the most significant serologic markers. The presence of these markers establishes the diagnosis of hepatitis B. *The patient is infectious as long as hepatitis B surface antigen (HBsAg) is present in the blood.* Persistence of this serologic marker after 6 months or longer indicates a carrier state or chronic hepatitis. HBsAg levels normally decline and disappear after the acute hepatitis B episode. The presence of antibodies to HBsAg in the blood indicates recovery and immunity to hepatitis B. *People who have been vaccinated against HBV have a positive HBsAg because they also have immunity to the disease.*

To detect HCV infection, blood is tested for anti-HCV antibodies to HCV recombinant core antigen, *NS3 gene*, NS4 antigen, and NS5 antibody (Pagana et al., 2017). The antibodies can be detected within 4 weeks of the infection (Pagana et al., 2017). To identify the actual circulating virus, the HCV RNA test is used. This confirms active virus and can measure the viral load. A diagnostic tool called the *OraQuick HCV Rapid Antibody Test* has the advantage of providing a quick diagnosis of the disease as a point-of-care test.

The presence of *hepatitis D* virus (HDV) can be confirmed by the identification of intrahepatic delta antigen or, more often, by a rise in the hepatitis D virus antibodies (anti-HDV) titer. This increase can be seen within a few days of infection (Pagana et al., 2017).

Hepatitis E virus (HEV) testing is usually reserved for travelers in whom hepatitis is present but the virus cannot be detected. Hepatitis E antibodies (anti-HEV) are found in people infected with the virus.

Other Diagnostic Assessment. *Liver biopsy* may be used to confirm the diagnosis of hepatitis and establish the stage and grade of liver damage. Characteristic changes help the pathologist distinguish among a virus, drug, toxin, fatty liver, iron, and other disease. It is usually performed in an ambulatory care setting as a percutaneous procedure (through the skin) after a local anesthetic is given. However, if coagulation is abnormal, it may be done using either a CT-guided or transjugular route to reduce the risk for pneumothorax or hemothorax. *Ultrasound* also may be used.

◆ Analysis: Interpreting

The priority collaborative problems for patients with hepatitis include:

1. Weight loss due to complications associated with inflammation of the liver
2. Fatigue due to decreased metabolic energy production
3. Potential for infection due to state of immunocompromise

◆ Planning and Implementation: Responding

The patient with viral hepatitis can be mildly or acutely ill, depending on the severity of the inflammation. Most patients are not hospitalized, although older adults and those with dehydration may be admitted for a short-term stay. The plan of care for all patients with viral hepatitis is based on measures to rest the liver, promote CELLULAR REGULATION and regeneration, strengthen IMMUNITY, and prevent complications, if possible.

Promoting Nutrition

Planning: Expected Outcomes. The patient will maintain appropriate weight and NUTRITION status as evidenced by laboratory reports free of signs of malnutrition.

Interventions. The patient with hepatitis may decline food because of general malaise, anorexia, abdominal discomfort, or nausea. The patient's diet should be high in carbohydrates and calories with moderate amounts of fat and protein added after nausea and anorexia subside. Small, frequent meals are often preferable to three standard meals daily. Ask the patient about appealing food preferences because favorite foods are tolerated better than randomly selected foods. High-calorie snacks may be needed. Supplemental vitamins are often prescribed.

Addressing Fatigue

Planning: Expected Outcomes. The patient will progressively exhibit increasing energy as evidenced by participation in ADLs and self-reported decrease in level of fatigue.

Interventions

Rest. During the acute stage of viral hepatitis, interventions are aimed at resting the inflamed liver to promote hepatic cell regeneration. *Rest* is an essential intervention to reduce the liver's metabolic demands and increase its blood supply. Collaborative care is generally supportive. The patient is usually tired and expresses feelings of general malaise. Complete bedrest is usually not required, but rest periods alternating with periods of activity are indicated and are often enough to promote hepatic healing. Individualize the patient's plan of care and change it as needed to reflect the severity of symptoms, fatigue, and the results of liver function tests and enzyme determinations. Activities such as self-care and ambulating are gradually added to the activity schedule as tolerated.

Drug Therapy. Drugs of any kind are used sparingly for patients with hepatitis to allow the liver to rest. An antiemetic to relieve nausea may be prescribed. However, because of the life-threatening nature of chronic hepatitis B and hepatitis C, a number of drugs are given, including antiviral and immunomodulating drugs (Table 58-4). Similar to patients with other chronic diseases, patients with hepatitis often use complementary and integrative therapies to promote general well-being and improve quality of life. Be sure to ask patients about their use of these therapies and incorporate them into the collaborative plan of care.

Reducing the Potential for Infection

Planning: Expected Outcomes. The patient will be free from infection as evidenced by remaining fever free with laboratory values that are free from indications of infection.

TABLE 58-4 Drug Therapy for Chronic Hepatitis B and Hepatitis C

DRUG	NURSING INTERVENTIONS	RATIONALES
Chronic Hepatitis B		
Tenofovir (Viread)	Monitor kidney function.	Drug is excreted through kidneys; monitoring for renal impairment is important.
	Teach risk for falls to prevent fractures.	Can cause bone de-mineralization.
Adefovir (Hepsera)	Monitor kidney function.	Drug is excreted through kidneys; monitoring for renal impairment is important.
Lamivudine (Epivir-HBV, 3TC , Heptovir)	Monitor kidney function.	Drug is excreted through kidneys; monitoring for renal impairment is important.
	Remind patient to not discontinue drug without consulting with health care provider.	Discontinuation of drug can cause flareup of HBV.
Entecavir (Baraclude)	Monitor kidney function.	Drug is excreted through kidneys; monitoring for renal impairment is important.
Chronic Hepatitis C		
Telaprevir (Incivek)	Monitor complete blood count (CBC).	Anemia can be a side effect of this drug.
Boceprevir (Victrelis) in combination with HIV medications if co-infection present	Monitor chemistry panel.	Kidney and liver function may become impaired, and electrolyte imbalances may occur when taking this drug.
PEG-IFN/RBV (interferon/ribavirin)	Instruct patients that they cannot miss a dose.	Efficacy of treatment diminishes when doses are missed.

HBV, Hepatitis B virus; *HIV,* human immune deficiency virus.

Interventions. Teach the patient and caregivers about proper handwashing and any implemented isolation precautions. Restrict visitors who have active infections or have recently been exposed to such. Monitor for development of fever; report increasing temperature and any changes in white blood cell laboratory values to the health care provider.

Care Coordination and Transition Management

Home Care Management. Home care management varies according to the type of hepatitis and whether the disease is acute or chronic. A primary focus in any case is preventing the spread of the infection. For hepatitis transmitted by the fecal-oral route, careful handwashing and sanitary disposal of feces are important. Therefore education is very important.

> **! NURSING SAFETY PRIORITY** **QSEN**
>
> **Action Alert**
>
> Teach the patient with viral hepatitis and the family to use measures to prevent infection transmission (see Chart 58-4). In addition, instruct the patient to avoid alcohol and to check with the health care provider before taking any medication or vitamin, supplement, or herbal preparation.

Self-Management Education. Encourage the patient to increase activity gradually to prevent fatigue. Suggest that the patient eats small, frequent meals of high-carbohydrate foods (Chart 58-5).

Health Care Resources. Collaborate with the certified infection control practitioner and infectious disease specialist if needed in caring for these patients. These experts can suggest appropriate resources for the patient and family.

◆ *Evaluation: Reflecting*

Evaluate the care of the patient with hepatitis based on the identified priority patient problems. The expected outcomes include that the patient will:

> **CHART 58-5** **Patient and Family Education: Preparing for Self-Management**
>
> ***Viral Hepatitis***
>
> - Avoid all medications, including over-the-counter drugs such as acetaminophen (Tylenol), unless prescribed by your physician.
> - Avoid all alcohol.
> - Rest frequently throughout the day, and get adequate sleep at night.
> - Eat small, frequent meals with a high-carbohydrate, moderate-fat, and moderate-protein content.
> - Avoid sexual intercourse until antibody testing results are negative.
> - Follow the guidelines for preventing transmission of the disease (see Chart 58-4).

- Maintain nutritional status adequate for body requirements
- Report increasing energy levels as the liver rests
- Remain infection-free

FATTY LIVER (STEATOSIS)

Fatty liver is caused by the accumulation of fats in and around the hepatic cells. It may be caused by alcohol use or other factors. Nonalcoholic fatty liver disease (NAFLD) and nonalcoholic steatohepatitis (NASH) are types of fatty liver disease. Causes include:

- Diabetes mellitus
- Obesity
- Elevated lipid profile
- Genetic contribution via the Patatin-like phospholipase domain-containing 3 gene (PNPLA3) (Houghton-Rahrig et al., 2014).

Fatty infiltration of the liver may result from faulty fat metabolism in the liver and the movement of fatty acids from adipose tissue (fat). Many patients are asymptomatic. The most

---

❓ CLINICAL JUDGMENT CHALLENGE 58-2

Patient-Centered Care; Safety **QSEN**

You are caring for a 39-year-old woman who returned to the United States 3 weeks ago from a month-long humanitarian mission trip to South America. Since that time, she reports that she has been experiencing periodic fevers, abdominal pain, nausea, and fatigue. At first, she states that thought she had the flu, but she now thinks that something else "must be terribly wrong" because of how long her symptoms have persisted. She confirms that she is a nonsmoker and only drinks one to two alcoholic drinks monthly when out to dinner with friends. When asked about her dietary habits in South America, the patient reports that she and several of her friends often enjoyed fresh shrimp prepared by a street vendor.

1. Based on the patient's dietary intake in South America and current symptoms, what condition do you anticipate?
2. Other than fever, abdominal pain, nausea, and fatigue, what signs and symptoms do you anticipate you will find on physical assessment?
3. Which laboratory findings do you anticipate will be abnormal for this patient?
4. How do you respond to the patient's concern about something being "terribly wrong?"

▶ CHART 58-6   Key Features

Liver Trauma

- Right upper quadrant pain with abdominal tenderness
- Abdominal distention and rigidity
- Guarding of the abdomen
- Increased abdominal pain exaggerated by deep breathing and referred to the right shoulder (Kehr's sign)
- Indicators of hemorrhage and hypovolemic shock:
  - Hypotension
  - Tachycardia
  - Tachypnea
  - Pallor
  - Diaphoresis
  - Cool, clammy skin
  - Confusion or other change in mental state

---

common and typical finding is an elevated ALT and AST or normal ALT and elevated AST (part of a group of liver function tests [LFTs]).

MRI, ultrasound, and nuclear medicine examinations can be used to suggest excessive fat in the liver. A percutaneous biopsy can confirm the diagnosis. Interventions are aimed at removing the underlying cause of the infiltration. Weight loss, glucose control, and aggressive treatment using lipid-lowering agents are recommended. Monitoring liver function tests is essential in disease management.

LIVER TRAUMA

The liver is one of the most common organs to be injured in patients with abdominal trauma. Damage or injury should be suspected whenever any upper abdominal or lower chest trauma is sustained. The liver is often injured by steering wheels in vehicular crashes. Common injuries include simple lacerations, multiple lacerations, avulsions (tears), and crush injuries.

The liver is a highly vascular organ and receives almost a third of the body's cardiac output. When hepatic trauma occurs, blood loss can be massive. *Observe for early signs of hypovolemic shock* (Chart 58-6).

An ultrasound or CT scan of the abdomen is often done to determine the presence of a hematoma (blood clot). A decreased hematocrit may confirm suspected blood loss. Clinical signs and symptoms include right upper quadrant pain with abdominal tenderness, distention, guarding, and rigidity. COMFORT alterations exaggerated by deep breathing and referred to the right shoulder may indicate diaphragmatic irritation.

Liver trauma is managed in a conservative manner through new diagnostic and therapeutic modalities such as enhanced critical care monitoring and damage control surgery. The condition of the patient, grade of liver injury, and presence of other injuries will determine the management strategy (i.e., whether to operate or not). Patients with hepatic trauma may require multiple blood products such as packed red blood cells

and fresh frozen plasma, as well as massive volume infusion to maintain adequate hydration. After surgery, the patient is admitted to a critical care unit. Monitor the patient for persistent or new bleeding. Closely monitor complete blood count and coagulation studies for trends in changes.

CANCER OF THE LIVER

❖ PATHOPHYSIOLOGY

Cancers may be *primary* tumors (hepatocellular carcinoma) starting in the liver, or they may be *metastatic* cancers that spread from another organ to the liver. Liver cancer is one of the most fatal types of cancer, and according to the American Cancer Society (2017), its incidence has more than tripled since 1980, likely because there continues to be an increase in cases of hepatitis C.

Chronic infection with HBV and HCV frequently lead to cirrhosis, which is a risk factor for developing liver cancer. It is important to remember that cirrhosis from any cause, including alcoholic liver disease, increases the risk for cancer.

❖ INTERPROFESSIONAL COLLABORATIVE CARE

Care for the patient with cancer of the liver can take place in various settings. At different times, these patients may self-manage at home, be hospitalized for immediate concerns, need rehabilitative care, be cared for in the community setting, or be under the care of hospice. Members of the interprofessional team who collaborate most closely to care for the patient with liver cancer include the health care provider, surgeon, nurse, dietitian, psychologist, social worker, and spiritual leader of the patient's choice.

◆ Assessment: Noticing

In the early stage of cancer, most patients are without symptoms. Later in the disease, they report weight loss, anorexia, and weakness. Ask the patient if he or she has or has had recent alterations in abdominal COMFORT, the most common concern. It is most often felt in the right upper quadrant before jaundice, bleeding, ascites, and edema develop. Palpation may reveal an enlarged, nodular liver.

Elevated serum *alpha-fetoprotein* (AFP) (a tumor marker for cancers of the liver, testis, and ovary) and increased *alkaline phosphatase* are also common (Pagana et al., 2017). Ultrasound (US) and contrast-enhanced CT are both useful in detecting metastasis. If the primary tumor site is not known, a CT- or US-guided liver biopsy can confirm the diagnosis, although this procedure is risky because of possible bleeding and spread of the cancer cells.

◆ Interventions: Responding

Surgical resection and liver transplantation offer the only treatments for long-term survival from liver cancer. Unfortunately, most patients are not candidates for surgical removal because their tumors are unresectable. Tunneled abdominal drains, such as the PleurX drainage system, may be used at home by the patient and family to remove excess ascitic fluid. *Teach them how to empty the drain and maintain the system. Remind them not to remove more than 2000 mL of fluid at one time to prevent hypovolemic shock.*

The primary treatment for nonresectable liver cancer is a TACE (transarterial chemoembolization). In this procedure, an interventional radiologist injects microscopic-size embolic beads that have absorbed a chemotherapy drug directly. An angiographic catheter is advanced from the femoral artery and maneuvered into the liver and then directly into the blood vessel feeding the tumor. From there, the beads are injected. These beads clog up the tumor arteries, arresting blood flow as they release the chemotherapy. It is now becoming accepted practice to immediately follow the TACE with a microwave ablation (MWA) of the same tumor. This burns (ablates) the tumor to further slow any regrowth.

Selective internal radiation therapy (SIRT) is reserved for patients with nonresectable liver cancer and an occluded portal vein. Occluding some of the hepatic artery (TACE procedure) with an absence of portal flow reduces overall blood flow to the liver to an unacceptable level. SIRT therapy is quite expensive, and insurance companies limit its use to specific tumor types.

Other palliative approaches include hepatic artery embolization, ablation techniques, and drug therapy. *Hepatic artery embolization* causes cell death by blocking blood supply to the tumor in the liver. It is performed under moderate sedation by an interventional radiologist who threads a catheter through the femoral artery to inject small beads into the hepatic artery to block blood flow. The patient usually stays overnight in the hospital for observation in case of bleeding. This procedure may be followed by infusing a chemotherapy agent directly into the hepatic artery (chemoembolization).

Common *ablation* procedures include radiofrequency ablation (RFA) and cryotherapy. RFA uses energy waves to heat cancer cells and kill them. It is most often performed as an ambulatory care procedure using a percutaneous laparoscopic approach. Cryotherapy uses liquid nitrogen to freeze and destroy liver tumors. The general nursing care for patients having cryotherapy is described in Chapter 22.

Chemotherapy may be administered orally or IV. However, it is not effective in many cases. Examples of drugs used are doxorubicin (Adriamycin), 5-fluorouracil (5-FU), and cisplatin. Sorafenib (Nexavar) is a kinase inhibitor that is approved for inoperable liver cancer. Other drugs are targeted therapies that are being investigated and used with some success.

Another drug route is a catheter-directed method directly into the hepatic artery, a procedure called *hepatic arterial infusion (HAI)*. The interventional radiologist places a catheter into the artery that supplies the tumor and injects a mixture of chemotherapy and contrast agent into the tumor. This procedure has the unique effect of depositing chemotherapeutic drugs directly into the tumor without causing major systemic effects. Chapter 22 describes the general nursing care for patients receiving chemotherapy.

Patients with advanced liver cancer usually need end-of-life care and hospice services. Collaborate with the case manager to help patients and their families find the best community resources that meet their needs. Chapter 7 describes end-of-life care and hospice services in detail.

LIVER TRANSPLANTATION

❖ PATHOPHYSIOLOGY

Liver transplantation has become a common procedure worldwide. The patient with end-stage liver disease or acute liver failure who has not responded to conventional medical or surgical intervention is a potential candidate for liver transplantation. Many diseases can cause liver failure. Cirrhosis (scarring of the liver) is the most common reason for liver transplants. Other common reasons are chronic hepatitis B and hepatitis C, bile duct diseases, autoimmune liver disease, primary liver cancer, alcoholic liver disease, and fatty liver disease.

Transplantation Considerations

The patient for potential transplantation has extensive physiologic and psychological assessment and evaluation by health care providers and transplant coordinators. Alternative treatment should be extensively explored before committing a patient for a liver transplant. Patients who are *not* considered candidates for transplantation are those with:

- Severe cardiovascular instability with advanced cardiac disease
- Severe respiratory disease
- Metastatic tumors
- Inability to follow instructions regarding drug therapy and self-management

Liver transplantation has become the most effective treatment for an increasing number of patients with acute and chronic liver diseases. Inclusion and exclusion criteria vary among transplantation centers and are continually revised as treatment options change and surgical techniques improve.

Donor livers are obtained primarily from trauma victims who have not had liver damage. They are distributed through a nationwide program, the United Network of Organ Sharing (UNOS). This system distributes donor livers based on regional considerations and patient acuity. Candidates with the highest level of acuity receive highest priority.

The donor liver is transported to the surgery center in a solution that preserves the organ for up to 8 hours. The diseased liver is removed through an incision made in the upper abdomen. The new liver is carefully put in its place and attached to the patient's blood vessels and bile ducts. The procedure can take many hours to complete and requires a highly specialized team and large volumes of fluid and blood replacement.

Living donors have also been used and are usually close family members or spouse. This is done on a voluntary basis after careful psychological and physiologic preparation and testing. The donor's liver is resected (usually removal of one lobe) and implanted into the recipient after removal of the diseased liver. In both the donor and the recipient, the liver regenerates and grows in size to meet the demands of the body.

Transplantation Complications

Although liver transplantations are commonly performed, complications can occur. Some problems can be managed medically, whereas others require removal of the transplant. The most common complications are acute graft rejection, infection, and bleeding (Lynn, 2016).

The success rate for transplantations has greatly improved since the introduction many years ago of cyclosporine (cyclosporin A), an immunosuppressant drug. Today many other anti-rejection drugs are used. (See Chapter 17 for a complete discussion of rejection and preventive drug therapy.)

! NURSING SAFETY PRIORITY QSEN

Action Alert

For the patient who has undergone liver transplantation, monitor for clinical signs and symptoms of rejection, which may include tachycardia, fever, COMFORT alterations in the right upper quadrant or flank, decreased bile pigment and volume, and increasing jaundice. Laboratory findings include elevated serum bilirubin, rising ALT and AST levels, elevated alkaline phosphatase levels, and increased prothrombin time/international normalized ratio (PT/INR).

Transplant rejection is treated aggressively with immunosuppressive drugs. As with all rejection treatments, the patient is at a greater risk for infection. If therapy is not effective, liver function rapidly deteriorates. Multi-system organ failure, including respiratory and renal involvement, develops along with diffuse coagulopathies and portal-systemic encephalopathy (PSE). The only alternative for treatment is emergency retransplantation.

Infection is another potential threat to the transplanted graft and the patient's survival. Vaccinations and prophylactic antibiotics are helpful in prevention. Immunosuppressant therapy, which must be used to prevent and treat organ rejection, significantly increases the patient's risk for infection. Other risk factors include the presence of multiple tubes and intravascular lines, immobility, and prolonged anesthesia.

In the early post-transplantation period, common infections include pneumonia, wound infections, and urinary tract infections. Opportunistic infections usually develop after the first postoperative month and include cytomegalovirus, mycobacterial infections, and parasitic infections. Latent infections such as tuberculosis and herpes simplex may be reactivated.

The health care provider prescribes broad-spectrum antibiotics for prophylaxis during and after surgery. Obtain culture specimens from all lines and tubes and collect specimens for culture at predetermined time intervals as dictated by the agency's policy. If an infection is detected, the health care provider prescribes organism-specific anti-infective agents. The patient should be taught to contact the health care provider at any time that signs of infection are present.

The biliary anastomosis is susceptible to breakdown, obstruction, and infection. If leakage occurs or if the site becomes necrotic or obstructed, an abscess can form; or peritonitis, bacteremia, and cirrhosis may develop. Observe for potential complications, which are listed in Table 58-5.

TABLE 58-5 Assessment and Prevention of Common Postoperative Complications Associated With Liver Transplantation

ASSESSMENT	PREVENTION
Acute Graft Rejection	
Occurs from the 4th to 10th postoperative day	Prophylaxis with immunosuppressant agents, such as cyclosporine
Manifested by tachycardia, fever, right upper quadrant (RUQ) or flank pain, diminished bile drainage or change in bile color, or increased jaundice	Early diagnosis to treat with more potent anti-rejection drugs
Laboratory changes: (1) increased levels of serum bilirubin, transaminases, and alkaline phosphatase; (2) prolonged prothrombin time	
Infection	
Can occur at any time during recovery	Antibiotic prophylaxis; vaccinations
Manifested by fever or excessive, foul-smelling drainage (urine, wound, or bile); other indicators depend on location and type of infection	Frequent cultures of tubes, lines, and drainage
	Early removal of invasive lines
	Good handwashing
	Early diagnosis and treatment with organism-specific anti-infective agents
Hepatic Complications (Bile Leakage, Abscess Formation, Hepatic Thrombosis)	
Manifested by decreased bile drainage, increased RUQ abdominal pain with distention and guarding, nausea or vomiting, increased jaundice, and clay-colored stools	If present, keep T-tube in dependent position and secure to patient; empty frequently, recording quality and quantity of drainage
Laboratory changes: increased levels of serum bilirubin and transaminases	Report manifestations to physician immediately
	May necessitate surgical intervention
Acute Renal Failure	
Caused by hypotension, antibiotics, cyclosporine, acute liver failure, or hypothermia	Monitor all drug levels with nephrotoxic side effects
Indicators of hypothermia: shivering, hyperventilation, increased cardiac output, vasoconstriction, and alkalemia	Prevent hypotension
Early indicators of renal failure: changes in urine output, increased blood urea nitrogen (BUN) and creatinine levels, and electrolyte imbalance	Observe for early signs of renal failure and report them immediately to the physician

---

❖ INTERPROFESSIONAL COLLABORATIVE CARE

Care of the patient undergoing liver transplantation requires an interprofessional team approach. Receiving a transplant has a major psychosocial impact. Transplant complications cause patients to be very anxious. In collaboration with the members of the health care team, assure them and their families that these problems are common and usually treated successfully.

After the patient is identified as a candidate and a donor organ is procured, the actual liver transplantation surgical procedure usually takes many hours. The length of the procedure can vary greatly.

In the immediate postoperative period, the patient is managed in the critical care unit and requires aggressive monitoring and care. Assess for signs and symptoms of complications of surgery and immediately report them to the surgeon (see Table 58-5).

Post–liver transplant patients are living longer today than ever. Teach patients to be aware of side effects of immunosuppressive drugs, such as hypertension, nephrotoxicity, and gastrointestinal disturbances. Remind them that long-term management of care includes surveillance for malignancy, metabolic syndrome, and diabetes. Teaching the patient self-examination for skin, breast, and testicular malignancies and reminders for annual Papanicolaou (Pap) smears and other cancer screening tests are

! NURSING SAFETY PRIORITY (QSEN)

Action Alert

For the patient who has had a liver transplantation, monitor the temperature frequently per hospital protocol and report elevations, increased abdominal pain, distention, and rigidity, which are indicators of peritonitis. Nursing assessment also includes monitoring for a change in neurologic status that could indicate encephalopathy from a nonfunctioning liver. Report signs of clotting problems (e.g., bloody oozing from a catheter, petechiae, ecchymosis) to the surgeon immediately because they may indicate impaired function of the transplanted liver.

important. Post-transplant patients need to maintain lifestyle changes to increase their longevity after surgery.

GET READY FOR THE NCLEX® EXAMINATION!

KEY POINTS

Review these Key Points for each NCLEX Examination Client Needs Category.

Safe and Effective Care Environment

- When caring for patients with cirrhosis, collaborate with the health care provider, dietitian, pharmacist, social worker, and spiritual leader of the patient's choice to provide comprehensive interprofessional care. **QSEN: Teamwork and Collaboration**
- Refer patients with liver disorders to the American Liver Foundation; refer dying patients to hospice and other community resources as needed. **QSEN: Patient-Centered Care**

Health Promotion and Maintenance

- Follow the guidelines listed in Chart 58-3 to prevent viral hepatitis in the workplace. **QSEN: Evidence-Based Practice**
- Teach patients to take precautions to prevent viral hepatitis in the community as described in Chart 58-4. QSEN: **Evidence-Based Practice**
- For patients with viral hepatitis, instruct them to follow the guidelines listed in Chart 58-5. **QSEN: Safety**
- Teach patients to avoid alcohol and illicit drugs to prevent or slow the progression of alcohol-induced cirrhosis; remind them not to take any medication (including over-the-counter drugs) without checking with their health care provider. **QSEN: Safety**

Psychosocial Integrity

- Recognize that patients with cirrhosis have mental and emotional changes due to hepatic encephalopathy. **QSEN: Patient-Centered Care**
- Be aware that patients with cirrhosis and/or chronic hepatitis may feel guilty about their disease because of past habits such as drug and alcohol use. Allow patients to express feelings openly. **Ethics**
- Be aware that family members and friends may fear getting hepatitis from the patient.
- Be aware that patients having liver transplantation have major concerns about the possibility of complications, such as organ rejection. **QSEN: Patient-Centered Care**

Physiological Integrity

- Be aware that cirrhosis has many causes other than alcohol use (see Table 58-1).
- Observe for clinical signs and symptoms of hepatic encephalopathy (PSE) as listed in Table 58-2. **QSEN: Safety**
- Monitor laboratory values of patients suspected of or diagnosed with cirrhosis of the liver as listed in Table 58-3. **Clinical Judgment**
- Monitor the patient with cirrhosis for bleeding and neurologic changes. **QSEN: Safety**
- Provide care for the patient having a paracentesis as described in Chart 58-1. **QSEN: Safety**
- Administer drug therapy to decrease ammonia levels (that cause PSE) in patients with cirrhosis, such as lactulose and nonabsorbable antibiotics. **QSEN: Safety**
- Differentiate the five major types of hepatitis: A, B, C, D, and E. Hepatitis D occurs only with hepatitis B and is transmitted most commonly by blood and body fluid exposure. Hepatitis A is transmitted via the fecal-oral route. Hepatitis C is the most common type and is also transmitted via blood and body fluids. **QSEN: Evidence-Based Practice**
- Be aware that patients with chronic viral hepatitis often develop cirrhosis and cancer of the liver. **QSEN: Evidence-Based Practice**
- Recognize that potent immunomodulators and antivirals are given to treat hepatitis B and hepatitis C; teach patients on immunomodulators to avoid large crowds and people who have infections. **QSEN: Safety**
- Monitor for bleeding in the patient with liver trauma; assume that any abdominal trauma has damaged the liver. **QSEN: Safety**
- Monitor the patient having a liver transplantation for complications, such as those described in Table 58-5. **QSEN: Safety**
- Report and document elevated temperature, increased abdominal pain and rigidity, bleeding, and/or neurologic status changes as possible indicators of liver transplantation complications. **QSEN: Safety**

SELECTED BIBLIOGRAPHY

American Association for the Study of Liver Diseases (AASLD). (2014). *Practice guidelines.* https://www.aasld.org/sites/default/files/guideline_documents/hepaticencephenhanced.pdf.

American Association for the Study of Liver Diseases (AASLD). (2016). *Recommendations for testing, managing and treating hepatitis C.* http://hcvguidelines.org/sites/default/files/HCV-Guidance_February_2016_a1.pdf.

American Cancer Society. (2017). *Key statistics about liver cancer.* http://www.cancer.org/cancer/livercancer/detailedguide/liver-cancer-what-is-key-statistics.

American Liver Foundation. (2017a). *Non-alcoholic fatty liver disease.* http://www.liverfoundation.org/abouttheliver/info/nafld/.

American Liver Foundation. (2017b). *Hepatitis C.* http://hepc.liverfoundation.org/.

American Liver Foundation. (2017c). *Liver transplant.* http://www.liverfoundation.org/abouttheliver/info/transplant/.

Canadian Digestive Health Association. (2017). *Statistics.* http://www.cdhf.ca/en/statistics#19.

Centers for Disease Control and Prevention (CDC). (2016). *Hepatitis B FAQs for the public.* http://www.cdc.gov/hepatitis/hbv/bfaq.htm#bFAQ10.

Centers for Disease Control and Prevention (CDC). (2017). *Liver cancer.* https://www.cdc.gov/cancer/liver/index.htm.

Houghton-Rahrig, L., Schutte, D., Fenton, J. I., & Awad, J. (2014). Nonalcoholic fatty liver disease and the *PNPLA3* gene. *Medsurg Nursing, 23*(2), 101–106.

Immunization Action Coalition. (2016). *Hepatitis B information for Asian Americans and Pacific Islanders.* http://www.immunize.org/catg.d/p4190.pdf.

Lynn, S. (2016). How to help patients with liver failure. *American Nurse Today, 11*(9), 26–29.

McCance, K., Huether, S., Brashers, V., & Rote, N. (2014). *Pathophysiology: The biologic basis for disease in adults and children* (7th ed.). St. Louis: Mosby.

Pagana, K., Pagana, T. J., & Pagana, T. N. (2017). *Mosby's diagnostic and laboratory test reference* (13th ed.). St. Louis: Mosby.

Runyon, B. (2016). *Spontaneous bacterial peritonitis in adults: Treatment and prophylaxis.* http//www.uptodate.com.

World Gastroenterology Organisation (WGO). (2012). *World Gastroenterology Organisation global guidelines: Nonalcoholic fatty liver disease and nonalcoholic steatohepatitis.* http://www.worldgastroenterology.org/guidelines/global-guidelines/nafld-nash.

World Health Organization. (2016). *Hepatitis A.* http://www.who.int/mediacentre/factsheets/fs328/en/.

World Health Organization. (2017). *Global hepatitis report 2017.* http://apps.who.int/iris/bitstream/10665/255016/1/9789241565455-eng.pdf?ua=1.

CHAPTER 59

Care of Patients With Problems of the Biliary System and Pancreas

Lara Carver and Jennifer Powers

PRIORITY AND INTERRELATED CONCEPTS

The priority concepts for this chapter are:

- NUTRITION
- IMMUNITY

✳ The NUTRITION concept exemplar for this chapter is Cholecystitis, below.

✳ The IMMUNITY concept exemplar for this chapter is Acute Pancreatitis, p. 1197.

The interrelated concept for this chapter is COMFORT.

LEARNING OUTCOMES

Safe and Effective Care Environment

1. Collaborate with the interprofessional team members to provide care for the patient with a gallbladder or pancreatic disorder.
2. Identify community resources to ensure appropriate transition management for the patient with a gallbladder or pancreatic disorder.

Health Promotion and Maintenance

3. Teach adults evidence-based health promotion practices to prevent gallbladder disease and pancreatitis.

Psychosocial Integrity

4. Implement nursing interventions to minimize stressors for the patient with a gallbladder or pancreatic disorder.

Physiological Integrity

5. Differentiate between assessment findings associated with various gallbladder and pancreatic disorders.
6. Prioritize care for patients with a gallbladder or pancreatic disorder.
7. Create an evidence-based plan of care for the patient with a gallbladder or pancreatic disorder.
8. Describe nursing interventions to address postoperative care of patients undergoing a cholecystectomy or Whipple procedure.
9. Describe nursing interventions that promote NUTRITION, IMMUNITY, and COMFORT for patients with a gallbladder or pancreatic disorder.

The liver, gallbladder, and pancreas make up the biliary system. This chapter focuses on problems of the gallbladder and pancreas. Liver disorders are described in Chapter 58. The biliary system secretes enzymes and other substances that promote food digestion in the stomach and small intestine. When these organs do not work properly, IMMUNITY is impaired; and individuals experience impaired *digestion,* which may result in inadequate NUTRITION.

Disorders of the gallbladder and pancreas may extend to other organs because of the close anatomic location of these organs, if the primary health problem is not treated early. Inflammation, which impairs IMMUNITY, is caused by obstruction (blockage) in the biliary system from gallstones, edema, stricture, or tumors. For example, gallstones in the cystic duct

cause cholecystitis. Gallstones lodged in the ampulla of Vater block the flow of bile and pancreatic secretions, which can result in pancreatitis. These problems frequently cause the patient to have moderate-to-severe alterations in abdominal COMFORT.

✳ NUTRITION CONCEPT EXEMPLAR Cholecystitis

❖ PATHOPHYSIOLOGY

Cholecystitis is an inflammation of the gallbladder that affects many adults, very commonly in affluent countries. It may be either acute or chronic, although most patients have the acute type.

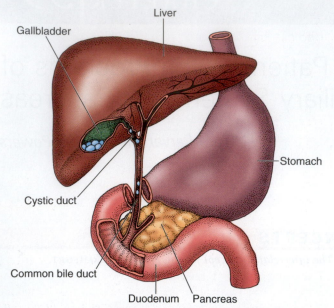

FIG. 59-1 Gallstones within the gallbladder and obstructing the common bile and cystic ducts.

Acute Cholecystitis

Two types of acute cholecystitis can occur: calculous and acalculous cholecystitis. The most common type is **calculous cholecystitis,** in which chemical irritation and inflammation result from gallstones (**cholelithiasis**) that obstruct the cystic duct (most often), gallbladder neck, or common bile duct (choledocholithiasis) (Fig. 59-1). When the gallbladder is inflamed, trapped bile is reabsorbed and acts as a chemical irritant to the gallbladder wall. Reabsorbed bile, in combination with impaired circulation, edema, and distention of the gallbladder, causes ischemia and infection. The result is tissue sloughing with necrosis and gangrene within the gallbladder itself. The gallbladder wall may eventually perforate (rupture). If the perforation is small and localized, an abscess may form. **Peritonitis,** infection of the peritoneum, may result if the perforation is large.

The exact mechanism of gallstone formation is not clearly understood, but abnormal metabolism of cholesterol and bile salts plays an important role. The gallbladder provides an excellent environment for the production of stones because it only occasionally mixes its normally abundant mucus with its highly viscous, concentrated bile. Impaired gallbladder motility can lead to stone formation by delaying bile emptying and causing biliary stasis.

Gallstones are composed of substances normally found in bile, such as cholesterol, bilirubin, bile salts, calcium, and various proteins. They are classified as either cholesterol stones or pigment stones. Cholesterol calculi form as a result of metabolic imbalances of cholesterol and bile salts. They are the most common type found in adults in the United States (McCance et al., 2014).

Bacteria can collect around the stones in the biliary system. Severe bacterial invasion can lead to life-threatening *suppurative* cholangitis when symptoms are not recognized quickly and pus accumulates in the ductal system.

Acalculous cholecystitis (inflammation occurring without gallstones) is typically associated with biliary stasis caused by any condition that affects the regular filling or emptying of the gallbladder. For example, a decrease in blood flow to the gallbladder or anatomic problems such as twisting or kinking

of the gallbladder neck or cystic duct can result in pancreatic enzyme reflux into the gallbladder, causing inflammation. Sphincter of Oddi dysfunction (SOD) can also occur to cause reflux and inflammation. Most cases of this type of cholecystitis occur in patients with:

- Sepsis
- Severe trauma or burns
- Long-term total parenteral NUTRITION
- Multiple organ dysfunction syndrome (MODS)
- Major surgery
- Hypovolemia

Chronic Cholecystitis

Chronic cholecystitis results when repeated episodes of cystic duct obstruction cause chronic inflammation. Calculi are almost always present. In chronic cholecystitis, the gallbladder becomes fibrotic and contracted, which results in decreased motility and deficient absorption.

Pancreatitis and cholangitis (bile duct inflammation) can occur as chronic complications of cholecystitis. These problems result from the backup of bile throughout the biliary tract. Bile obstruction leads to jaundice.

Jaundice (yellow discoloration of the skin and mucous membranes) and **icterus** (yellow discoloration of the sclera) can occur in patients with acute cholecystitis but are most commonly seen in those with the *chronic* form of the disease. Obstructed bile flow caused by edema of the ducts or gallstones contributes to *extrahepatic* **obstructive jaundice.** Jaundice in cholecystitis may also be caused by direct liver involvement. Inflammation of the liver's bile channels or bile ducts may cause *intrahepatic* obstructive jaundice, resulting in an increase in circulating levels of bilirubin, the major pigment of bile.

In an adult with obstructive jaundice, the normal flow of bile into the duodenum is blocked, and excessive bile salts accumulate in the skin. This accumulation of bile salts leads to **pruritus** (itching) or a burning sensation. The bile flow blockage also prevents bilirubin from reaching the large intestine, where it is converted to urobilinogen. Because urobilinogen accounts for the normal brown color of feces, clay-colored stools result. Water-soluble bilirubin is normally excreted by the kidneys in the urine. When an excess of circulating bilirubin occurs, the urine becomes dark and foamy because of the kidneys' effort to clear the bilirubin.

Etiology and Genetic Risk

A familial or genetic tendency appears to contribute to the development of cholelithiasis, but this may be partially related to familial nutrition habits (excessive dietary cholesterol intake) and sedentary lifestyles. Gene-environment interactions may contribute to gallstone production. For example, some gene variations program some individuals to make and secrete more cholesterol into bile, leading to the increase in cholesterol-containing gallstones. The main risk factors for developing gallstones are obesity, type 2 diabetes, dyslipidemia, and insulin resistance. Independent risk factors for developing gallstones are increase in age, female gender, and family history (Agostino et al., 2013). Also, individuals who experience rapid weight loss and intestinal diseases affecting the normal absorption of nutrients, such as Crohn's disease, are at risk for gallstones. The highest frequency of gallstone production lies among the American-Indian and Mexican-American populations (McCance et al., 2014). Risk factors for cholecystitis are listed in Table 59-1.

TABLE 59-1	Risk Factors for Cholecystitis
• Women	• Cholesterol-lowering drugs
• Aging	• Family history of gallstones
• American Indian, Mexican American, or Caucasian	• Prolonged total parenteral nutrition
• Obesity	• Crohn's disease
• Rapid weight loss or prolonged fasting	• Gastric bypass surgery
• Increased serum cholesterol	• Sickle cell disease
• Women on hormone replacement therapy (HRT)	• Glucose intolerance/diabetes mellitus
	• Pregnancy
	• Genetic factors

 NCLEX EXAMINATION CHALLENGE 59-1

Health Promotion and Maintenance

The community nurse is talking with four clients who have reported digestive concerns. Which client does the nurse recognize as **most** likely to experience gallstone production? **Select all that apply.**

A. 23-year-old Caucasian vegetarian who is a dancer
B. 35-year-old American Indian who works in construction
C. 48-year-old Canadian who manages a fast-food restaurant
D. 59-year-old Asian American who is an investment banker
E. 64-year-old Mexican American who resides with grandchildren

---

GENDER HEALTH CONSIDERATIONS

Patient-Centered Care QSEN

Women between 20 and 60 years of age are twice as likely to develop gallstones as men. Obesity is a major risk factor for gallstone formation, especially in women. Pregnancy and drugs such as hormone replacements and birth control pills alter hormone levels and delay muscular contraction of the gallbladder, decreasing the rate of bile emptying. The incidence is higher in women who have had multiple pregnancies. Combinations of causative factors increase the incidence of stone formation, especially in women. Therefore some clinicians refer to the patient most at risk for acute cholecystitis and gallstones by the four **F**s:
• **F**emale
• **F**orty
• **F**at
• **F**ertile

Incidence and Prevalence

The incidence of chronic cholecystitis is increased in young, thin women, especially those who are athletic (e.g., ballerinas and gymnasts). These women have chronic pain that is often misdiagnosed as gastritis.

❖ INTERPROFESSIONAL COLLABORATIVE CARE

Care for the patient with cholecystitis primarily takes place by self-management at home, in the community, or within the hospital setting if surgery is required. Members of the interprofessional team who collaborate most closely to care for the patient with cholecystitis include the health care provider, surgeon if surgery is required, nurse, and dietitian.

◆ Assessment: Noticing

Physical Assessment/Signs and Symptoms. Obtain the patient's height, weight, and vital signs; or delegate these activities to unlicensed assistive personnel (UAP) with appropriate supervision. Ask about food preferences and determine whether excessive fat and cholesterol are part of the diet, since

---

▶▶ CHART 59-1   Key Features

Cholecystitis

- Episodic or vague upper abdominal pain or discomfort that can radiate to the right shoulder
- Pain triggered by a high-fat or high-volume meal
- Anorexia
- Nausea and/or vomiting
- Dyspepsia (indigestion)
- Eructation (belching)
- Flatulence (gas)
- Feeling of abdominal fullness
- Rebound tenderness (Blumberg's sign)
- Fever
- Jaundice, clay-colored stools, dark urine, steatorrhea (most common with chronic cholecystitis)

NUTRITION intake often contributes to cholecystitis and may affect care that is provided for this disorder. Typically, diets high in fat, high in calories, low in fiber, and high in refined white carbohydrates place patients at higher risk for developing gallstones. Inquire if intake of certain foods causes pain. Question whether any GI symptoms occur when fatty food is eaten: flatulence (gas), dyspepsia (indigestion), eructation (belching), anorexia, nausea, vomiting, and abdominal alterations in COMFORT.

Patients with cholecystitis have abdominal pain, although symptoms vary in intensity and frequency (Chart 59-1). Ask the patient to describe the pain, including its intensity and duration, precipitating factors, and any measures that relieve it. Pain may be described as indigestion of varying intensity, ranging from a mild, persistent ache to a steady, constant pain in the right upper abdominal quadrant. It may radiate to the right shoulder or scapula. In some cases the abdominal pain of chronic cholecystitis may be vague and nonspecific. The usual pattern is episodic. Patients often refer to acute pain episodes as "gallbladder attacks."

👵 CONSIDERATIONS FOR OLDER ADULTS

Patient-Centered Care QSEN

Older adults and patients with diabetes mellitus may have atypical symptoms of cholecystitis, including the absence of pain and fever. Localized tenderness may be the only presenting sign. The older patient may become acutely confused (delirium) as the first symptom of gallbladder disease.

The severe pain of biliary colic is produced by obstruction of the cystic duct of the gallbladder or movement of one or more stones. When a stone is moving through or is lodged within the duct, tissue spasm occurs in an effort to get the stone through the small duct.

❗ NURSING SAFETY PRIORITY QSEN

Critical Rescue

Biliary colic may be so severe that it occurs with tachycardia, pallor, diaphoresis, and prostration (extreme exhaustion). Assess the patient for possible shock caused by biliary colic. **Notify the health care provider or Rapid Response Team if these symptoms occur.** Stay with the patient and keep the head of the bed flat.

Ask patients to describe their daily activity or exercise routines to determine whether they are sedentary. Sedentary lifestyle, rapid weight loss, prolonged fasting, and pregnancy are risk factors for developing gallstones. Question whether there is a family history of gallbladder disease. Ask the patient about taking current or previous hormone replacement therapy (HRT). If the patient is female, ask if she is taking or has recently been on oral contraceptives (birth control pills).

Assessment for rebound tenderness (Blumberg's sign) and deep palpation are performed only by physicians and advanced practice nurses. To elicit rebound tenderness, the health care provider pushes his or her fingers deeply and steadily into the patient's abdomen and then quickly releases the pressure. Pain that results from the rebound of the palpated tissue may indicate peritoneal inflammation. Deep palpation below the liver border in the right upper quadrant may reveal a sausage-shaped mass, representing the distended, inflamed gallbladder. Percussion over the posterior rib cage worsens localized abdominal pain.

In *chronic* cholecystitis, patients may have slowly developing symptoms and may not seek medical treatment until late symptoms such as jaundice (yellowing of the skin), clay-colored stools, and dark urine occur from biliary obstruction. Yellowing of the sclera (icterus) and oral mucous membranes may also be present. Steatorrhea (fatty stools) occurs because fat absorption is decreased as a result of the lack of bile. Bile is needed for the absorption of fats and fat-soluble vitamins in the intestine. As with any inflammatory process, the patient may have an elevated temperature of 99° to 102° F (37.2° to 38.9° C), tachycardia, and dehydration from fever and vomiting. He or she often will decline NUTRITION intake because of pain or symptoms that arise when food is eaten.

CONSIDERATIONS FOR OLDER ADULTS
Patient-Centered Care QSEN

Older adults become dehydrated much quicker than other age-groups, and they may not present with a fever. Monitor for a new onset of disorientation or acute confusion due to decreased blood volume available to oxygenate the cells of the brain (hypoxia)

Diagnostic Assessment. A differential diagnosis rules out other diseases that may cause similar symptoms, such as peptic ulcer disease, hepatitis, and pancreatitis. An increased *white blood cell (WBC)* count indicates inflammation. Serum levels of *alkaline phosphatase, aspartate aminotransferase (AST),* and *lactate dehydrogenase (LDH)* may be elevated, indicating abnormalities in liver function in patients with severe biliary obstruction. The direct (conjugated) and indirect (unconjugated) *serum bilirubin levels* are also elevated. If the pancreas is involved, serum amylase and lipase levels are elevated.

Calcified gallstones are easily viewed on abdominal x-ray. Stones that are not calcified cannot be seen. *Ultrasonography (US) of the right upper quadrant is the best initial diagnostic test for cholecystitis.* It is safe, accurate, and painless. Acute cholecystitis is seen as edema of the gallbladder wall and pericholecystic fluid.

A hepatobiliary scan (sometimes called an *HIDA scan*) can be performed to visualize the gallbladder and determine patency of the biliary system. In this nuclear medicine test, a radioactive tracer or chemical is injected IV. About 20 minutes after the injection, a gamma camera tracks the flow of the tracer from the gallbladder to determine the ejection rate of bile into the biliary duct. A decreased bile flow indicates gallbladder disease with obstruction. Teach patients having this test to have nothing by mouth before the procedure. Remind the patient that the camera is large and close to the body for most of the procedure.

When the cause of cholecystitis or cholelithiasis is not known or the patient has symptoms of biliary obstruction (e.g., jaundice), an *endoscopic retrograde cholangiopancreatography (ERCP)* may be performed. Some patients have the less invasive and safer *magnetic resonance cholangiopancreatography (MRCP),* which can be performed by an interventional radiologist. For this procedure, the patient is given oral or IV contrast material (gadolinium) before having an MRI scan.

Before the test, ask the patient about any history of urticaria (hives) or other allergy. MRI is also contraindicated in patients with pacemaker or other incompatible devices. Gadolinium does not contain iodine, which decreases the risk for an allergic response. Chapter 52 discusses these tests in more detail.

◆ Analysis: Interpreting

The priority collaborative problems for patients with cholecystitis include:

1. Weight loss due to decreased intake because of pain, nausea, and inflammation
2. Acute pain due to cholecystitis

◆ Planning and Implementation: Responding

Acute cholecystitis is diagnosed on the basis of clinical findings, laboratory tests, and abdominal imaging. If acute gallbladder infection is diagnosed, an emergency cholecystectomy is usually performed the same or the following day. Laparoscopic cholecystectomy is the treatment of choice for patients with acute and long-term chronic cholecystitis. This minimally invasive procedure achieves the desired outcomes of shorter recovery time, decreased expense, less postoperative pain, and minimal scarring after surgery. NUTRITION status, pain levels, and risk for infection must be addressed before and after surgery.

Promoting Nutrition

Planning: Expected Outcomes. The patient will maintain appropriate weight and NUTRITION status as evidenced by laboratory reports free of signs of malnutrition and stabilized weight.

Interventions. The patient with cholecystitis may decline food because of abdominal discomfort, nausea, and anorexia. Collaborate with the dietitian to structure a plan for enhancement of NUTRITION. The patient's diet should be high in fiber and low in fat. Gas-producing foods should be avoided. Small, frequent meals are often preferable to three standard meals daily. Ask the patient about appealing food preferences because favorite foods are tolerated more readily than randomly selected foods. Weigh the patient regularly to assess for stabilization of weight or concerns associated with weight loss. Monitor laboratory results such as blood urea nitrogen (BUN), prealbumin, albumin, and total protein and transferrin levels to assess ongoing NUTRITION status; report abnormal findings to the health care provider right away. See information later in this chapter that addresses postoperative NUTRITION interventions.

Managing Acute Pain

Planning: Expected Outcomes. The patient with acute pancreatitis is expected to report a decrease in, or absence of, alterations in abdominal COMFORT, as evidenced by a pain intensity scale measurement.

Interventions. The priorities for patient care to address pain include providing supportive care by relieving symptoms, increasing COMFORT, and decreasing inflammation. Pain assessment to measure the effectiveness of these interventions is an essential part of nursing care.

Nonsurgical Management. Many patients with gallstones have no symptoms. Acute pain is present when gallstones partially or totally obstruct the cystic or common bile duct. Most patients find that they need to avoid fatty foods to prevent further episodes of biliary colic, which causes variations in COMFORT. Withhold food and fluids if nausea and vomiting occur. IV therapy is used for hydration.

Drug Therapy. Acute biliary pain requires opioid analgesia, such as morphine or hydromorphone (Dilaudid). All opioids may cause some degree of sphincter of Oddi spasm.

Ketorolac (Toradol), an NSAID, may be used for mild-to-moderate alterations in COMFORT. Be sure to monitor the patient for signs and symptoms of GI distress and pain because the drug can cause GI bleeding. The health care provider prescribes antiemetics to control nausea and vomiting. IV antibiotic therapy may also be given, depending on the cause of cholecystitis or as a one-time dose for surgery.

An option for a small number of patients with cholelithiasis (gallstones) is the use of oral bile acid dissolution or gallstone-stabilizing agents. Drugs such as ursodiol (Actigall) and chenodiol (Chenodal) may be given as long-term therapy to dissolve or stabilize gallstones. A gallbladder ultrasound is required every 6 months for the first year of therapy to determine the effectiveness of the drug. Teach patients on this type of drug therapy to report diarrhea, vomiting, or severe abdominal pain, especially if it radiates to the shoulders, to their health care provider immediately. Remind them to take the medication with food and milk.

Other Nonsurgical Interventions. For some patients with small stones or for those who are not good surgical candidates, a treatment that is commonly used for kidney stones can be used to break up gallstones—*extracorporeal shock wave lithotripsy (ESWL)*. This procedure can be used only for patients who have a normal weight, cholesterol-based stones, and good gallbladder function. The patient lies on a water-filled pad, and shock waves break up the large stones into smaller ones that can be passed through the digestive system. During the procedure, the patient might have alterations in COMFORT experienced from the movement of the stones or duct or gallbladder spasms. A therapeutic bile acid, such as ursodeoxycholic acid (UDCA), may be used after the procedure to help dissolve the remaining stone fragments.

Another treatment option for patients who cannot have surgery is the insertion of a percutaneous transhepatic biliary catheter (drain) using CT or ultrasound guidance to open the blocked duct(s) so bile can flow (cholecystostomy). Catheters can be placed several ways, depending on the condition of the biliary ducts, in an internal, external, or internal/external drain. Biliary catheters usually divert bile from the liver into the duodenum to bypass a stricture. When all of the bile enters the duodenum, it is called an *internal* drain. However, in some cases a patient has an *internal/external* drain in which part of the bile empties into a drainage bag. Patients who need this drain for an extended period may have the external drain capped. If jaundice or leakage around the catheter site occurs, teach the patient to reconnect the catheter to a drainage bag and have a follow-up cholangiogram injection done by an interventional radiologist. An *external*-only catheter is connected either temporarily or permanently to a drainage bag. A reduction in bile drainage indicates that the drain is no longer working.

Surgical Management. **Cholecystectomy** is the surgical removal of the gallbladder. One of two procedures is performed: the laparoscopic cholecystectomy and, far less often, the traditional open-approach cholecystectomy.

Laparoscopic Cholecystectomy. Laparoscopic cholecystectomy, a minimally invasive surgery (MIS), is the "gold standard" and is performed far more often than the traditional open approach. The advantages of MIS when compared with the open approach include:

- Complications are not common.
- The death rate is very low.
- Bile duct injuries are rare.
- Patient recovery is quicker.
- Postoperative pain is less severe.

The laparoscopic procedure (often called a *lap chole*) is commonly done on an ambulatory-care basis in a same-day surgery suite. The surgeon explains the procedure, and the nurse answers questions and reinforces the instructions. Reinforce what to expect after surgery and review pain management, deep-breathing exercises, incisional care, and leg exercises to prevent deep vein thrombosis. There is no special preoperative preparation other than the routine preparation for surgery under general anesthesia described in Chapter 14. Evidence regarding the use of prophylactic antibiotics before a laparoscopic cholecystectomy is mixed (Soper & Malladi, 2017); check facility policy when caring for a patient who will undergo this procedure.

During the surgery the surgeon makes a very small midline puncture at the umbilicus. Additional small incisions may be needed, although single-incision laparoscopic cholecystectomy (SILC) using a flexible endoscope is often done. The abdominal cavity is insufflated with 3 to 4 liters of carbon dioxide. Gasless laparoscopic cholecystectomy using abdominal wall–lifting devices are used in some centers. This technique results in improved pulmonary and cardiac function. A trocar catheter is inserted, through which a laparoscope is introduced. The laparoscope is attached to a video camera, and the abdominal organs are viewed on a monitor. The gallbladder is dissected from the liver bed, and the cystic artery and duct are closed. The surgeon aspirates the bile and crushes any large stones, if present, and then extracts the gallbladder through the umbilical port.

Removing the gallbladder with the laparoscopic technique reduces the risk for wound complications. Some patients have mild-to-severe discomfort from carbon dioxide retention in the abdomen, which may be felt throughout the thorax and shoulders.

> ⚠ **NURSING SAFETY PRIORITY** QSEN
>
> **Action Alert**
>
> After a laparoscopic cholecystectomy, assess the patient's oxygen saturation level frequently until the effects of the anesthesia have passed. Remind the patient to perform deep-breathing exercises every hour.

Other postoperative care for the patient after a laparoscopic procedure is similar to that for any patient having minimally invasive endoscopic surgery (see Chapter 16). Offer the patient food and water when fully awake, and monitor for the nausea and/or vomiting that often results from anesthesia. If needed, administer an antiemetic drug, such as ondansetron hydrochloride (Zofran), either IV push or as a disintegrating tablet. Several drug doses may be needed. Maintain an IV line to administer fluids until nausea and/or vomiting subside. Be sure to have the head of the bed elevated in the same-day surgery unit to prevent aspiration from vomiting. After nausea subsides, assist the patient to the bathroom to void. Early ambulation also promotes absorption of the carbon dioxide, which can decrease postoperative discomfort.

Administer an oral or IV push opioid as needed immediately after surgery. Continuous IV pain control is usually not required because there is only one or a few small incisions, which are covered with Steri-Strips and small adhesive bandages (e.g., Band-Aids) or are surgically glued. The glue or Steri-Strips lose their adhesiveness in about a week to 10 days and can be removed or fall off as the incision heals.

The patient is usually discharged from the hospital or surgery center the same day, although older and obese patients may stay overnight. Provide postoperative teaching regarding pain management, incision care, and follow-up appointments. Teach the patient to use ice and oral opioids for incisional pain, if needed, for a few days. For abdominal or thoracic discomfort from carbon dioxide retention, many patients report that heat application is helpful. The patient is typically allowed to bathe or shower the day after surgery.

After laparoscopic surgery, the patient can return to usual activities much sooner than those having an open cholecystectomy. Instruct the patient to rest for the first 24 hours and then begin to resume usual activities Most patients are able to resume usual activities within a week.

Some patients are able to return to their usual diet after surgery, whereas others must carefully monitor their diet to avoid high-fat foods. A large intake of fatty foods may result in abdominal pain and diarrhea, which could result in a mild post-cholecystectomy syndrome (PCS) (see later discussion of PCS in the Traditional Cholecystectomy section). Teach patients to introduce foods high in fat one at a time to determine which foods are best tolerated.

A new minimally invasive surgical procedure is *natural orifice transluminal endoscopic surgery (NOTES)* for removal or repair of organs. Surgery can be performed on many body organs through the mouth, vagina, and rectum. For removal of the gallbladder, the vagina is used most often in women because it can be easily decontaminated with Betadine or other antiseptic and allows easy access into the peritoneal cavity. The surgeon makes a small internal incision through the cul-de-sac of Douglas between the rectum and uterine wall to access the gallbladder. The main advantages of this procedure are the lack of visible incisions and minimal, if any, postoperative complications (Roberts & Kate, 2016).

Traditional Cholecystectomy. Use of the open surgical approach (abdominal laparotomy) has greatly declined during the past several decades. Patients who have this type of surgery usually have severe biliary obstruction, and the ducts are explored to ensure patency.

The surgical nurse provides the usual preoperative care and teaching in the operating suite on the day of surgery (see Chapter 14). The surgeon removes the gallbladder through an incision and explores the biliary ducts for the presence of stones or other cause of obstruction. The surgeon usually inserts a drainage tube such as a Jackson-Pratt (JP) drain. This tube is placed in the gallbladder bed to prevent fluid accumulation. The

drainage is usually serosanguineous (serous fluid mixed with blood) and is stained with bile in the first 24 hours after surgery. Antibiotic therapy is given to prevent infection.

Patient care for a patient who has had a traditional open cholecystectomy is similar to the care for any patient who has had abdominal surgery under general anesthesia as described in Chapter 16. Postoperative incisional pain after a traditional cholecystectomy is controlled with opioids using a patient-controlled analgesia (PCA) pump. Encourage the patient to use coughing and deep-breathing exercises when pain is controlled and the incision is splinted.

Antiemetics may be necessary for episodes of postoperative nausea and vomiting. Administer the antiemetic early, as prescribed, to prevent retching associated with vomiting and thus to decrease pain related to muscle straining.

Provide care for the incision and the surgical drain. The surgeon typically removes the surgical dressing and drain within 24 hours after surgery.

The patient is NPO until fully awake after surgery. Document his or her level of consciousness, vital signs, and pain level. Assess the surgical incision for signs of infection, such as excessive redness or purulent drainage. Report changes to the surgeon immediately. Begin ambulation as soon as possible to prevent deep vein thrombosis and promote peristalsis.

Advance the diet from clear liquids to solid foods as peristalsis returns to promote enhanced NUTRITION status. The patient usually resumes solid foods and is discharged to home 1 to 2 days after surgery, depending on any complications and the patient's general condition. In the early postoperative period, if bile flow is reduced, a low-fat diet may reduce discomfort and prevent nausea. For most patients, a special diet is not required. Advise them to eat nutritious meals and avoid excessive intake of fatty foods, especially fried food, butter, and "fast food." If the patient is obese, recommend a weight-reduction program.

Teach the patient to keep the incision clean and report any changes that may indicate infection. Remind him or her to report repeated abdominal or epigastric pain with vomiting and/or diarrhea that may occur several weeks to months after surgery. These symptoms indicate possible **post-cholecystectomy syndrome (PCS)**. There are multiple causes of PCS, some of which are related to the biliary system, and others are not. Common causes of PCS are listed in Table 59-2. Not all patients experience PCS. Often the pain returns because of one of the underlying conditions listed in Table 59-2, not as a result of the cholecystectomy itself.

Management depends on the exact cause but usually involves the use of endoscopic retrograde cholangiopancreatography

TABLE 59-2 **Common Causes of Postcholecystectomy Syndrome**	
BILIARY	**NONBILIARY**
• Pseudocyst	• Coronary artery disease
• Common bile duct (CBD) leak	• Intercostal neuritis
• CBD or pancreatic duct stricture or obstruction	• Unexplained pain syndrome
• Sphincter of Oddi dysfunction	• Psychiatric or neurologic disorder
• Retained or new CBD gallstone	
• Pancreatic or liver mass	
• Primary sclerosing cholangitis	
• Diverticular compression	

(ERCP) to find the cause of the problem and repair it. This procedure and related nursing care are described in Chapter 52. Collaborative care includes pain management, antibiotics, NUTRITION and hydration therapy (possibly short-term parenteral nutrition), and control of nausea and vomiting.

❓ NCLEX EXAMINATION CHALLENGE 59-2

Physiological Integrity

The nurse will include what postoperative teaching when caring for the client who is preparing to undergo endoscopic cholecystectomy? **Select all that apply.**
A. "You'll have a small, midline abdominal incision."
B. "You can't eat or drink for a few days after the procedure."
C. "You won't be able to return to regular activity for several weeks."
D. "Generally the pain associated with this procedure is minimal."
E. "This procedure has a low incidence of infection."
F. "The hospital stay after this procedure is typically 3 to 4 days."

Care Coordination and Transition Management

Some patients may have uncomfortable experiences with cholecystitis that can be managed by nutrition intervention; others may require surgery and subsequent hospitalization. Home care preparation is individual, based on each patient's circumstances. Collaborate with the case manager to plan the best recovery for the patient and anticipate resources that may be needed.

Education needs to be started as soon as a patient has an initial experience with cholecystitis and has been provided appropriate pain relief. Assess the patient's and family's knowledge of the disease and provide teaching as needed. The desired outcomes for discharge planning and education are to avoid further episodes of cholecystitis. Key teaching points include reminding the patient to avoid fatty, fried, and "fast" food and to report any signs of postoperative complications to the health care provider immediately (see Chapter 16).

◆ Evaluation: Reflecting

Evaluate the care of the patient with cholecystitis based on the identified priority patient problems. The expected outcomes include that the patient will:

- Have adequate NUTRITION available to meet metabolic needs
- Report control of abdominal pain, as indicated by self-report and pain scale measurement

✳ IMMUNITY CONCEPT EXEMPLAR
Acute Pancreatitis

❖ PATHOPHYSIOLOGY

Acute pancreatitis is a serious and, at times, life-threatening inflammation of the pancreas. This process, which affects the body's IMMUNITY, is caused by a premature activation of excessive pancreatic enzymes that destroy ductal tissue and pancreatic cells, resulting in autodigestion and fibrosis of the pancreas. The pathologic changes occur in different degrees. The severity of pancreatitis depends on the extent of inflammation and tissue damage. Pancreatitis can range from mild involvement evidenced by edema and inflammation to **necrotizing hemorrhagic pancreatitis (NHP)**. NHP is diffusely bleeding pancreatic tissue with fibrosis and tissue death.

The pancreas is unusual in that it functions as both an exocrine gland and an endocrine gland. The primary *endocrine* disorder is diabetes mellitus and is discussed in Chapter 64. The *exocrine* function of the pancreas is responsible for secreting enzymes that assist in the breakdown of starches, proteins, and fats. These enzymes are normally secreted in the inactive form and become activated once they enter the small intestine. Early activation (i.e., activation within the pancreas rather than the intestinal lumen) results in the inflammatory process of pancreatitis. Direct toxic injury to the pancreatic cells and the production and release of pancreatic enzymes (e.g., trypsin, lipase, elastase) result from the obstructive damage. After pancreatic duct obstruction, increased pressure may contribute to ductal rupture, allowing spillage of trypsin and other enzymes into the pancreatic parenchymal tissue. Autodigestion of the pancreas occurs as a result (Fig. 59-2). In *acute* pancreatitis, four major pathophysiologic processes occur: lipolysis, proteolysis, necrosis of blood vessels, and inflammation, all of which impact the body's IMMUNITY.

The hallmark of pancreatic necrosis is enzymatic fat necrosis of the endocrine and exocrine cells of the pancreas caused by the enzyme *lipase*. Fatty acids are released during this *lipolytic process* and combine with ionized calcium to form a soaplike product. The initial rapid lowering of serum calcium levels is not readily compensated for by the parathyroid gland. Because the body needs ionized calcium and cannot use bound calcium, hypocalcemia occurs (McCance et al., 2014).

Proteolysis involves the splitting of proteins by hydrolysis of the peptide bonds, resulting in the formation of smaller polypeptides. Proteolytic activity may lead to thrombosis and gangrene of the pancreas. Pancreatic destruction may be localized and confined to one area or may involve the entire organ.

Elastase is activated by trypsin and causes elastic fibers of the blood vessels and ducts to dissolve. The *necrosis of blood vessels* results in bleeding, ranging from minor bleeding to massive hemorrhage of pancreatic tissue. Another pancreatic enzyme, kallikrein, causes the release of vasoactive peptides, bradykinin, and a plasma kinin known as *kallidin*. These substances contribute to vasodilation and increased vascular permeability, further compounding the hemorrhagic process. This massive destruction of blood vessels by necrosis may lead to generalized hemorrhage, with blood escaping into the retroperitoneal tissues. *The ultimate impact to a patient's IMMUNITY occurs in the presence of hemorrhagic pancreatitis. The patient with this disorder is critically ill, and extensive pancreatic destruction and shock may lead to death. The majority of deaths in patients with acute pancreatitis result from irreversible shock.*

The *inflammatory stage* occurs when leukocytes cluster around the hemorrhagic and necrotic areas of the pancreas. A secondary bacterial process may lead to suppuration (pus formation) of the pancreatic parenchyma or the formation of an abscess. (See the following discussion of Pancreatic Abscess.) Mild infected lesions may be absorbed. When infected lesions are severe, calcification and fibrosis occur. If the infected fluid becomes walled off by fibrous tissue, a pancreatic pseudocyst is formed. (See the following discussion of Pancreatic Pseudocyst.)

Complications of Acute Pancreatitis

Acute pancreatitis may result in severe, life-threatening complications (Table 59-3) that affect the body's ability to protect itself via its IMMUNITY. Jaundice occurs from swelling of the head

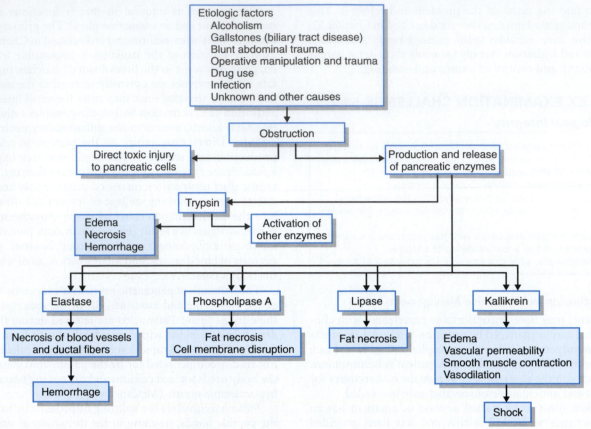

FIG. 59-2 The process of autodigestion in acute pancreatitis.

TABLE 59-3 Potential Complications of Acute Pancreatitis

- Pancreatic infection (causes septic shock)
- Hemorrhage (necrotizing hemorrhagic pancreatitis [NHP])
- Acute kidney failure
- Paralytic ileus
- Hypovolemic shock
- Pleural effusion
- Acute respiratory distress syndrome (ARDS)
- Atelectasis
- Pneumonia
- Multi-organ system failure
- Disseminated intravascular coagulation (DIC)
- Type 2 diabetes mellitus

---

of the pancreas, which slows bile flow through the common bile duct. The bile duct may also be compressed by calculi (stones) or a pancreatic pseudocyst. The resulting total bile flow obstruction causes severe jaundice. Intermittent hyperglycemia occurs from the release of glucagon, as well as the decreased release of insulin due to damage to the pancreatic islet cells. Total destruction of the pancreas may occur, leading to type 1 diabetes mellitus (McCance et al., 2014).

Left lung pleural effusions frequently develop in the patient with acute pancreatitis. *Atelectasis and pneumonia may occur also, especially in older patients.*

Multi-system organ failure is caused by necrotizing hemorrhagic pancreatitis (NHP). The patient is at risk for acute respiratory distress syndrome (ARDS). This severe form of

pulmonary edema is caused by disruption of the alveolar-capillary membrane and is a serious complication of acute pancreatitis. (See Chapter 32 for a discussion of ARDS.) In acute pancreatitis, pulmonary failure accounts for more than half of all deaths that occur in the first week of the disease.

Coagulation defects are another major potential complication and may result in death. Complex physiologic changes in the pancreas cause the release of necrotic tissue and enzymes into the bloodstream, resulting in altered coagulation. Disseminated intravascular coagulation (DIC) involves hypercoagulation of the blood, with consumption of clotting factors and the development of microthrombi.

Shock in acute pancreatitis results from peripheral vasodilation from the released vasoactive substances and the retroperitoneal loss of protein-rich fluid from proteolytic digestion. Hypovolemia may result in decreased renal perfusion and acute renal failure. Paralytic (adynamic) ileus results from peritoneal irritation and seepage of pancreatic enzymes into the abdominal cavity.

❓ NCLEX EXAMINATION CHALLENGE 59-3

Physiological Integrity

The nurse closely monitors the client with acute pancreatitis for which life-threatening complication?

A. Jaundice
B. Type I diabetes mellitus
C. Abdominal pain
D. Disseminated intravascular coagulation (DIC)

Etiology and Genetic Risk

In many cases the cause of pancreatitis is not known, but many factors can injure the pancreas. The most common cause is biliary tract disease, with gallstones accounting for almost half of the cases of obstructive pancreatitis (McCance et al., 2014). Acute pancreatitis may occur as a result of trauma from surgical manipulation after biliary tract, pancreatic, gastric, and duodenal procedures, such as cholecystectomy, the Whipple procedure, and partial gastrectomy. The trauma may also occur as a complication of the diagnostic procedure *endoscopic retrograde cholangiopancreatography (ERCP)*, although this rarely occurs.

Other causative factors include:

- Trauma: external (blunt trauma, stab wounds, gunshot wounds [GSWs])
- Pancreatic obstruction: tumors, cysts, or abscesses; abnormal organ structure
- Metabolic disturbances: hyperlipidemia, hyperparathyroidism, or hypercalcemia
- Renal disturbances: failure or transplantation
- Familial, inherited pancreatitis
- Penetrating gastric or duodenal ulcers, resulting in peritonitis
- Viral infections such as coxsackievirus B and human immune deficiency virus [HIV] infection
- Alcoholism
- Toxicities of drugs, including opiates, sulfonamides, thiazides, steroids, and oral contraceptives (less common)
- Cigarette smoking
- Cystic fibrosis
- Gallstones
- Abdominal surgery

Incidence and Prevalence

Pancreatic "attacks" are especially common during holidays and vacations when alcohol consumption may be high, especially in men. Women are affected most often after cholelithiasis and biliary tract problems. They are also most at risk for pancreatitis within several months after childbirth.

Death occurs in a small percentage of patients with acute pancreatitis, but with early diagnosis and treatment, mortality can be reduced. It occurs at a higher rate in *older adults* and in patients with postoperative pancreatitis. The prognosis for recovery is usually good for pancreatitis associated with biliary tract disease and poor if pancreatitis accompanies alcoholism.

❖ INTERPROFESSIONAL COLLABORATIVE CARE

Care for the patient with acute pancreatitis usually takes place in the hospital setting for pain control and possible surgical intervention. Members of the interprofessional team who collaborate most closely to care for the patient with acute pancreatitis include the health care provider, surgeon if surgery is required, nurse, and dietitian.

◆ Assessment: Noticing

History. Most often the patient reports severe and constant abdominal pain. Conduct the interview *after pain is controlled*. Ask whether the abdominal pain occurs when drinking alcohol or eating a high-fat meal. Obtain information about alcohol usage, including the amount of alcohol consumed during what period of time (i.e., years of consumption, how much usually consumed over a particular period). Question the patient about a family or personal history of alcoholism, pancreatitis, trauma, or biliary tract disease. Ask whether any abdominal surgical interventions such as cholecystectomy, or diagnostic procedures such as ERCP, have been performed recently.

Ask about other medical problems known to cause pancreatitis, including peptic ulcer disease, renal failure, vascular disorders, hyperparathyroidism, and hyperlipidemia. Inquire about recent viral infections. Ask the patient or family member to list all prescription and over-the-counter (OTC) drugs taken recently, including nutritional and herbal supplements.

Physical Assessment/Signs and Symptoms. The diagnosis of pancreatitis is made based on the clinical presentation combined with the results of diagnostic studies, both laboratory and imaging assessments. Symptoms of acute pancreatitis vary widely and depend on the severity of the inflammation. Typically, a patient is diagnosed after presenting with severe abdominal pain in the mid-epigastric area or left upper quadrant. Assess the intensity and quality of pain. The patient often states that the pain had a sudden onset and radiates to the back, left flank, or left shoulder. The pain is described as intense, **boring** (feeling that it is going through the body), and continuous and is worsened by lying in the supine position. Often the patient finds relief by assuming the fetal position (with the knees drawn up to the chest and the spine flexed) or by sitting upright and bending forward. He or she may report weight loss resulting from nausea and vomiting. Obtain the patient's weight.

When performing an abdominal assessment, inspect for:

- Generalized jaundice
- Gray-blue discoloration of the abdomen and periumbilical area
- Gray-blue discoloration of the flanks, caused by pancreatic enzyme leakage to cutaneous tissue from the peritoneal cavity

Listen for bowel sounds; absent or decreased bowel sounds usually indicate paralytic (adynamic) ileus. On light palpation, note abdominal tenderness, rigidity, and guarding as a result of peritonitis. A palpable mass may be found if a pancreatic pseudocyst is present. Pancreatic ascites creates a dull sound on percussion.

Monitor and record vital signs frequently to assess for elevated temperature, tachycardia, and decreased blood pressure or delegate and closely supervise this activity. Respiratory problems, such as left lung pleural effusions, atelectasis, and pneumonia, are common in patients with acute pancreatitis. Auscultate the lung fields for adventitious sounds or diminished breath sounds and observe for dyspnea or orthopnea.

> ### ❗ NURSING SAFETY PRIORITY QSEN
> #### *Critical Rescue*
>
> For the patient with acute pancreatitis, monitor for significant changes in vital signs that may indicate the life-threatening complication of shock. Hypotension and tachycardia may result from pancreatic hemorrhage, excessive fluid volume shifting, or the toxic effects of abdominal sepsis from enzyme damage. Observe for changes in behavior and level of consciousness (LOC) that may be related to alcohol withdrawal, hypoxia, or impending sepsis with shock.

Psychosocial Assessment. If excessive alcohol is a causative factor, tactfully explore the patient's alcohol intake history. Provide patient privacy and establish a trusting relationship. Discuss the intake of alcohol and the reasons for overindulging. Using the CAGE questionnaire to assist with determining alcohol use may be beneficial. Ask the patient when increased drinking episodes occur and, in particular, whether binges occur during holidays, vacations, or weekends or revolve around particular activities, such as television viewing. Question him or her about any recent traumatic or stressful event that may have contributed to increased alcohol consumption, such as the death of a family member or a job loss.

Laboratory Assessment. Diagnostic laboratory abnormalities are typical in patients with acute pancreatitis (Table 59-4). A variety of pancreatic and nonpancreatic disorders can cause increased serum amylase levels. In patients with pancreatitis, *amylase* levels usually increase within 12 to 24 hours and remain elevated for 2 to 3 days. Persistent elevations may be an indicator of duct obstruction or pancreatic duct leak (Pagana et al., 2017).

Lipase also helps determine the presence of acute pancreatitis. Serum levels may rise later than amylase and remain elevated for up to 2 weeks. Because these levels stay elevated for such a long time, the health care provider may find this test useful in diagnosing patients who are not examined until several days after the initial onset of symptoms. An increase in lipase and amylase in the urine is also expected (Pagana et al., 2017).

If pancreatitis is accompanied by biliary dysfunction (biliary pancreatitis), serum *bilirubin* and *alkaline phosphatase* levels are usually elevated. A sensitive indicator of biliary obstruction in acute pancreatitis is serum *alanine aminotransferase (ALT)*. A threefold or greater rise in concentration indicates that the diagnosis of acute biliary pancreatitis is valid. Elevated *white blood cell (WBC) count and differential, erythrocyte sedimentation rate (ESR),* and serum *glucose* levels are also common in acute pancreatitis. The levels often correlate with disease severity.

TABLE 59-4 Causes of Diagnostic Laboratory Abnormalities in Acute Pancreatitis

ABNORMAL FINDING	CAUSE
Cardinal Diagnostic Tests	
Increased *serum* amylase	Pancreatic cell injury
Elevated *serum* lipase	Pancreatic cell injury
Elevated *serum* trypsin	Pancreatic cell injury
Elevated *serum* elastase	Pancreatic cell injury
Other Diagnostic Tests	
Elevated serum glucose	Pancreatic cell injury, resulting in impaired carbohydrate metabolism; decreased insulin release
Decreased serum calcium and magnesium	Fatty acids combined with calcium; seen in fat necrosis
Elevated bilirubin	Hepatobiliary obstructive process
Elevated alanine aminotransferase (ALT)	Hepatobiliary involvement
Elevated aspartate aminotransferase (AST)	Hepatobiliary involvement
Elevated leukocyte count	Inflammatory response

Decreased serum *calcium* and *magnesium* levels are seen with fat necrosis. Calcium levels may fall and remain decreased for 7 to 10 days. Those that consistently remain below 8 mg/dL are associated with a poor prognosis. Other tests include the basic metabolic panel (BMP), complete blood count (CBC), triglycerides, serum total protein, and albumin. The blood urea nitrogen (BUN), serum glucose, and triglycerides are usually elevated. Hemoconcentration is common as a result of third-space fluid loss. Leukocytosis (elevated WBCs) and thrombocytopenia (decreased platelets) are common. Albumin levels are decreased because cytokines (e.g., tumor necrosis factor [TNF]) released as part of the inflammatory response allow it to move from the bloodstream into the extravascular space. The presence of C-reactive protein suggests possible pancreatic inflammation and necrosis.

Imaging Assessment. Abdominal ultrasound is the most sensitive test to diagnose causes of pancreatitis, such as gallstones, and can be performed at the bedside. However, it is not helpful in viewing the pancreas because of overlying bowel gas. Therefore *contrast-enhanced CT* provides a more reliable image and diagnosis of acute pancreatitis. This noninvasive technique may also be used to rule out pancreatic pseudocyst or ductal calculi.

An abdominal x-ray may also reveal gallstones. A chest x-ray may show elevation of the left side of the diaphragm or pleural effusion. Pancreatic stones are best diagnosed through ERCP.

◆ Analysis: Interpreting

The priority collaborative problems for patients with acute pancreatitis include:

1. Acute pain due to pancreatic inflammation and enzyme leakage
2. Weight loss due to inability to ingest food and absorb nutrients

◆ Planning and Implementation: Responding

Managing Acute Pain

Planning: Expected Outcomes. The patient with acute pancreatitis is expected to state that he or she has a decrease in or absence of abdominal pain, as evidenced by a pain intensity scale measurement.

Interventions. The priorities for patient care are to provide supportive care by relieving symptoms, to decrease inflammation, and to anticipate or treat complications. *As for any patient, continually assess for and support the ABCs (**a**irway, **b**reathing, and **c**irculation).* In collaboration with the respiratory therapist, if available, provide oxygen and other respiratory support as needed. The collaborative plan of care depends on the severity of the illness.

Abdominal pain is the most common symptom of pancreatitis. The main focus of nursing care is aimed at controlling pain by interventions that decrease GI tract activity, thus decreasing pancreatic stimulation. Pain assessment to measure the effectiveness of these interventions is an essential part of nursing care.

Nonsurgical Management. *Mild* pancreatitis requires hydration with IV fluids, pain control, and drug therapy. The health care team initially attempts to relieve pain with nonsurgical interventions, which include fasting and rest, drug therapy, and COMFORT measures. If the patient has a life-threatening complication or requires frequent assessment, he or she is admitted to a critical care unit for invasive hemodynamic monitoring.

To rest the pancreas and reduce pancreatic enzyme secretion, withhold food and fluids (NPO) during the acute period. The health care provider prescribes IV isotonic fluid administration to maintain hydration. IV replacement of calcium and magnesium may also be needed. Measure and document intake and output. Some patients have an indwelling urinary catheter to obtain accurate measurements.

Nasogastric drainage and suction are reserved for more *severely ill* patients who have continuous vomiting or biliary obstruction. Gastric decompression using a nasogastric tube (NGT) prevents gastric juices from flowing into the duodenum.

> **! NURSING SAFETY PRIORITY** **QSEN**
>
> **Action Alert**
>
> Because paralytic (adynamic) ileus is a common complication of acute pancreatitis, prolonged nasogastric intubation may be necessary. Assess frequently for the return of peristalsis by asking the patient if he or she has passed flatus or had a stool. The return of bowel sounds is not reliable as an indicator of peristalsis return; passage of flatus or a bowel movement is the most reliable indicator. See the discussion of intestinal obstructions in Chapter 56.

To decrease pain, the primary drug class used is opioid. Other drugs may also be prescribed. Pain management for acute pancreatitis typically begins with the administration of opioids by patient-controlled analgesia (PCA). Drugs such as morphine or hydromorphone (Dilaudid) are typically used because meperidine (Demerol) can cause seizures, especially in older adults. Other options that have been used successfully to manage acute pain include IV or transdermal fentanyl and epidural analgesia.

In *mild* pancreatitis, the pain usually subsides in 2 to 3 days. However, with *severe* acute pancreatitis, the abdominal pain and tenderness may persist for up to 2 weeks. Drug dosages and intervals are individualized according to the severity of the disease and the symptoms.

Histamine receptor antagonists (e.g., ranitidine [Zantac]) and proton pump inhibitors (e.g., omeprazole [Prilosec]) help decrease gastric acid secretion. Antibiotics may be used, but they are indicated primarily for patients with acute necrotizing pancreatitis. The health care provider will prescribe appropriate antibiotics, if needed.

Helping the patient assume a side-lying position (with the legs drawn up to the chest) may decrease the abdominal pain of pancreatitis ("fetal position"). Sitting with the knees flexed toward the chest is also helpful.

If the patient is NPO or has an NGT, remind assistive nursing personnel to implement frequent oral and nares hygiene measures to keep mucous membranes moist and free of inflammation or crusting. Because of the drying effect of drugs and the absence of oral fluids, the mouth and oral cavity may be extremely dry, resulting in considerable discomfort and possibly parotitis (inflammation of the parotid [salivary] glands).

Observe for signs and symptoms of hypocalcemia by assessing for Chvostek's and Trousseau's signs. These tests cause muscle spasms after stimulating the associated nerves. Chapter 11 discusses assessment and care of patients with hypocalcemia in more detail.

Lowering the patient's anxiety level may also substantially reduce pain. Explain all procedures and other aspects of patient

> **! NURSING SAFETY PRIORITY** **QSEN**
>
> **Action Alert**
>
> For the patient with acute pancreatitis, monitor his or her respiratory status every 4 to 8 hours or more often as needed and provide oxygen to promote comfort in breathing. Respiratory complications such as pleural effusions increase patient discomfort. Fluid overload can be detected by assessing for weight gain, listening for crackles, and observing for dyspnea. Carefully monitor for signs of respiratory failure.

care thoroughly. Provide reassurance, offer diversional activities such as music and reading material, and encourage visitors to direct attention away from the pain.

If pancreatitis was caused by gallstones, an ERCP with a **sphincterotomy** (opening of the sphincter of Oddi) may be performed on an urgent or emergent basis. If this procedure is not successful, surgery is required. ERCP is described in detail in Chapter 52.

Surgical Management. Surgical intervention for acute pancreatitis is usually not indicated. However, if an ERCP is not successful in removing gallstones, a laparoscopic cholecystectomy may be performed as described in the Surgical Management discussion in the Cholecystitis section.

Complications of pancreatitis, such as pancreatic pseudocyst and abscess, may also require surgical intervention. Laparoscopy (minimally invasive surgery [MIS]) may be done to drain an abscess or pseudocyst. For patients who are high surgical risks, pseudocysts or abscesses can be treated by percutaneous drainage under CT guidance.

Promoting Nutrition

Planning: Expected Outcomes. The patient with acute pancreatitis is expected to have adequate NUTRITION to meet his or her metabolic needs.

Interventions. The patient is maintained on NPO status in the early stages of pancreatitis. Antiemetics for nausea and vomiting are prescribed as needed. Patients who have severe pancreatitis and are unable to eat for 24 to 48 hours after illness onset may begin jejunal tube feeding unless paralytic ileus is present. *Early* NUTRITION intervention enhances immune system functioning and may prevent complications and worsening inflammation. Enteral feeding is preferred over total parenteral nutrition (TPN) because it causes fewer episodes of glucose elevation and other complications associated with TPN. Be sure that the patient is weighed every day. Collaborate with the health care provider, dietitian, and pharmacist to plan and implement the most appropriate nutritional intervention. Chapter 60 describes collaborative care of patients receiving enteral feeding and TPN.

When food is tolerated during the healing phase, the health care provider prescribes small, frequent, moderate- to high-carbohydrate, high-protein, low-fat meals. Food should be bland with little spice. GI stimulants such as caffeine-containing food (tea, coffee, cola, and chocolate), as well as alcohol, should be avoided. Monitor the patient beginning to resume oral food intake for nausea, vomiting, and diarrhea. *If any of these symptoms occur, notify the health care provider immediately.*

To boost caloric intake, commercial liquid nutritional preparations supplement the diet. The health care provider may also prescribe fat-soluble and other vitamin and mineral replacement supplements. Glutamine, omega-3 fatty acids, fiber, antioxidants, and/or nucleotides may be added to the patient's nutrition plan.

Care Coordination and Transition Management

Home Care Management. Home care preparation is individualized for each patient's circumstances. Some patients may be severely weakened from their acute illness and need to confine activity to one floor, limiting stair climbing and other strenuous activities until they regain their strength. Collaborate with the case manager to plan the best place for the patient to recover and resources that may be needed.

Self-Management Education. Education needs to be started early in the hospitalization period—as soon as the acute episodes of pain have subsided. Assess the patient's and family's knowledge of the disease.

The desired outcomes for discharge planning and education are to avoid further episodes of pancreatitis and prevent progression to a chronic disease. If the patient uses alcohol, instruct him or her to abstain from drinking to prevent further pain attacks and extension of inflammation and pancreatic insufficiency. Tell the patient that, if alcohol is consumed, acute pain will return, and further autodigestion of the pancreas may lead to chronic pancreatitis.

Teach the patient to notify the health care provider after discharge to home if acute abdominal pain or biliary tract disease (as evidenced by jaundice, clay-colored stools, or darkened urine) occurs. These signs and symptoms are possible indicators of complications or disease progression.

Health Care Resources. Patients with acute pancreatitis may require several visits by a home care nurse if the hospital course was complicated. In these cases, home care may be needed for wound care and assistance with ADLs. The patient requires medical follow-up with the primary care provider to monitor the disease process. For those with alcoholism, provide information about groups such as Alcoholics Anonymous (AA). Family members may attend support groups such as Al-Anon and Alateen.

◆ Evaluation: Reflecting

Evaluate the care of the patient with acute pancreatitis based on the identified priority patient problems. The expected outcomes include that the patient will:

- Have control of abdominal pain, as indicated by self-report and pain scale measurement
- Have adequate NUTRITION available to meet metabolic needs

CHRONIC PANCREATITIS

❖ PATHOPHYSIOLOGY

Chronic pancreatitis is a progressive, destructive disease of the pancreas that has remissions and exacerbations ("flare-ups"). Inflammation and fibrosis of the tissue contribute to pancreatic insufficiency and diminished function of the organ.

Chronic pancreatitis can be classified into several categories. *Alcoholism* is the primary risk factor for chronic calcifying pancreatitis (CCP), the most common type. In the early stages of the disease, pancreatic secretions precipitate as insoluble proteins that plug the pancreatic ducts and flow of pancreatic juices. As the protein plugs become more widespread, the cellular lining of the ducts changes and ulcerates. This inflammatory process causes fibrosis of the pancreatic tissue. Intraductal calcification and marked pancreatic tissue destruction (necrosis) develop in the late stages. The organ becomes hard and firm as a result of cell atrophy and pancreatic insufficiency.

Chronic calcifying pancreatitis is found predominantly in men, but the incidence in women is increasing. In women, chronic pancreatitis occurs more commonly among those with biliary tract disease (cholecystitis and cholelithiasis).

Chronic obstructive pancreatitis develops from inflammation, spasm, and obstruction of the sphincter of Oddi, often from cholelithiasis (gallstones). Inflammatory and sclerotic lesions occur in the head of the pancreas and around the ducts, causing an obstruction and backflow of pancreatic secretions. (See the Complications of Acute Pancreatitis section.)

Autoimmune pancreatitis is a chronic inflammatory process in which immunoglobulins invade the pancreas. Other organs may also be infiltrated, including the lungs and liver. There is evidence to show that autoimmune pancreatitis puts the patient at risk for pancreatic cancer (Kawa et al., 2013).

Idiopathic and hereditary chronic pancreatitis may be associated with *SPINK1* and *CFTR* gene mutations and with mutations in the *BRCA2* gene. Individuals with hereditary pancreatitis have been shown to have a 53-fold increased risk of pancreatic cancer (Klein, 2012).

The protein encoded by the *SPINK1* gene is a trypsin inhibitor. The *CFTR* gene is associated with cystic fibrosis. Research on these gene mutations can help develop targeted drug therapy for treatment of these diseases.

Pancreatic insufficiency in any type of chronic pancreatitis causes loss of *exocrine* function. Most patients with chronic pancreatitis have decreased pancreatic secretions and bicarbonate. Pancreatic enzyme secretion must be greatly reduced to produce steatorrhea resulting from severe malabsorption of fats. These characteristic stools are pale, bulky, and frothy and have an offensive odor. The action of colonic bacteria on unabsorbed lipids and proteins is responsible for the extremely foul odor. On inspection of the stools, the fat content is visible. In severe chronic pancreatitis, stool fat output may be more than 40 g/day.

Fat malabsorption also contributes to weight loss and muscle wasting (a decrease in muscle mass) and leads to general debilitation. Protein malabsorption results in a "starvation" edema of the feet, legs, and hands caused by decreased levels of circulating albumin.

The loss of pancreatic *endocrine* function is responsible for the development of diabetes mellitus in patients with chronic pancreatic insufficiency. (See Chapter 64 for a complete discussion of diabetes mellitus.)

The patient with chronic pancreatitis may have pulmonary complications, such as pleuritic pain, pleural effusions, and pulmonary infiltrates. Pancreatic ascites may decrease diaphragmatic excursion and lung expansion, resulting in impaired ventilation. In the ill patient with chronic pancreatitis, acute respiratory distress syndrome (ARDS) may develop.

❖ INTERPROFESSIONAL COLLABORATIVE CARE

Care for the patient with chronic pancreatitis takes place in the home or community setting but moves to the hospital setting for pain control and possible surgical intervention. Members of the interprofessional team who collaborate most closely to care for the patient with chronic pancreatitis include the health care provider, surgeon if surgery is required, nurse, and dietitian.

◆ Assessment: Noticing

Many symptoms of chronic pancreatitis differ from those of an acute inflammation. Abdominal pain is the major symptom

> **CHART 59-2   Key Features**
>
> **Chronic Pancreatitis**
>
> - Intense abdominal pain, a major symptom, that is continuous and burning or gnawing
> - Abdominal tenderness
> - Ascites
> - Possible left upper quadrant mass (if pseudocyst or abscess is present)
> - Respiratory compromise manifested by adventitious or diminished breath sounds, dyspnea, or orthopnea
> - Steatorrhea; clay-colored stools
> - Weight loss
> - Jaundice
> - Dark urine
> - Polyuria, polydipsia, polyphagia (diabetes mellitus)

> **CHART 59-3   Patient and Family Education: Preparing for Self-Management**
>
> **Enzyme Replacement for the Patient With Chronic Pancreatitis**
>
> - Take pancreatic enzymes with meals and snacks and follow with a glass of water.
> - Administer enzymes after antacid or H₂ blockers. (Decreased pH inactivates drug.)
> - Swallow the tablets or capsules without chewing to minimize oral irritation and allow the drug to be released slowly.
> - If you cannot swallow the capsule, pierce the gelatin casing and place contents in applesauce.
> - Do not mix enzyme preparations in protein-containing foods.
> - Wipe your lips after taking enzymes to avoid skin irritation.
> - Do not crush enteric-coated preparations.
> - Follow up on all scheduled laboratory testing. (Pancrelipase can cause an increase in uric acid levels.)

for most types of pancreatitis (Chart 59-2). For those with chronic pancreatitis, pain is typically described as a continuous burning or gnawing dullness with periods of acute exacerbation (flare-ups). The pain is very intense and relentless. The frequency of acute exacerbations may increase as the pancreatic fibrosis develops.

Perform an abdominal assessment. Abdominal tenderness is less intense in patients with chronic pancreatitis than in those with acute pancreatitis. A mass may be palpated in the left upper quadrant, which may suggest a pancreatic pseudocyst or abscess. Massive pancreatic ascites may be present, producing dullness on abdominal percussion. Because respiratory complications can occur, auscultate the lung fields for adventitious sounds or decreased aeration and observe for dyspnea or orthopnea.

Ask the patient to collect a random stool specimen if able or ask him or her to describe the stools. The specimen may show steatorrhea (foul-smelling fatty stools that may increase in volume as pancreatic insufficiency progresses and lipase production decreases). Assess for unintentional weight loss; muscle wasting; jaundice; dark urine; and the symptoms of diabetes mellitus, such as polyuria (increased urinary output), polydipsia (excessive thirst), and polyphagia (increased appetite).

Diagnosis is based on the patient's symptoms and laboratory and imaging assessment. *Endoscopic retrograde cholangiopancreatography* (ERCP) is done to visualize the pancreatic and common bile ducts. *Imaging studies* such as CT scanning, contrast-enhanced MRI, abdominal ultrasound (US), and endoscopic ultrasound (EUS) are also useful in making the diagnosis. In chronic pancreatitis, laboratory findings include normal or moderately elevated serum *amylase* and *lipase* levels. Obstruction of the intrahepatic bile duct can cause elevated serum *bilirubin* and *alkaline phosphatase* levels. Intermittent elevations in serum *glucose* levels are common and can be detected by blood glucose monitoring, both fasting and nonfasting.

◆ Interventions: Responding

The focuses of caring for the patient with chronic pancreatitis are to manage pain, assist in maintaining sufficient NUTRITION, and prevent recurrence.

Nonsurgical Management. Nonsurgical interventions include drug and NUTRITION therapy. The major intervention for the pain of chronic pancreatitis is drug therapy. Medicate the patient as prescribed according to the assessment of the intensity of pain. Evaluate the effectiveness of the drug intervention.

Initially opioid analgesia is used most frequently, but dependency may occur. Nonopioid analgesics may be tried to relieve pain. (See Chapter 4 for other interventions for chronic pain.)

Pancreatic-enzyme replacement therapy (PERT) is the standard of care to prevent malnutrition, malabsorption, and excessive weight loss (Chart 59-3). Pancrelipase is usually prescribed in capsule or tablet form and contains varying amounts of amylase, lipase, and protease. Teach patients not to chew or crush pancrelipase delayed-release capsules (Creon) or enteric tablets and teach them to take the medications with all meals and snacks.

The dosage of pancreatic enzymes depends on the severity of the malabsorption. Record the number and consistency of stools per day to monitor the effectiveness of enzyme therapy. If pancreatic enzyme treatment is effective, the stools should become less frequent and less fatty.

> **! NURSING SAFETY PRIORITY** QSEN
>
> **Action Alert**
>
> If the patient has diabetes, insulin or oral antidiabetic agents for glucose control are prescribed. Patients maintained on total parenteral nutrition (TPN) are particularly susceptible to elevated glucose levels and require regular insulin additives to the solution. Monitor blood glucose to control hyperglycemia. Check fingerstick blood glucose (FSBG) or sugar (FSBS) levels every 2 to 4 hours. Chapter 60 describes in detail the care associated with TPN.

The health care provider may also prescribe drug therapy to decrease gastric acid. Gastric acid destroys the lipase needed to break down fats. Controlling the acidity of the stomach with H₂ blockers or proton pump inhibitors or neutralizing stomach acid with oral sodium bicarbonate may enhance the effectiveness of PERT.

Protein and fat malabsorption result in significant weight loss and decreased muscle mass in the patient with chronic pancreatitis. Therefore the nutritional interventions for acute pancreatitis are also used for chronic pancreatitis. The patient often limits food intake to avoid increased pain. For this reason, nutrition maintenance is often difficult to achieve. Patients receive either total parenteral nutrition (TPN) or total enteral nutrition (TEN), including vitamin and mineral replacement.

Collaborate with the dietitian to teach the patient about long-term dietary management. He or she needs an increased number of calories, up to 4000 to 6000 calories/day, to maintain weight. Food high in carbohydrates and protein also assists in the healing process. Food high in fat is avoided because it causes or increases diarrhea. Teach all patients to avoid alcohol. Alcohol-cessation programs may be recommended.

Surgical Management. Surgery is not a primary intervention for the treatment of chronic pancreatitis. However, it may be indicated for ongoing abdominal pain, incapacitating relapses of pain, or complications such as abscesses and pseudocysts.

The underlying pathologic changes determine the procedure indicated. Using laparoscopy, the surgeon incises and drains an abscess or pseudocyst. Laparoscopic cholecystectomy or choledochotomy (incision of the common bile duct) may be indicated if biliary tract disease is an underlying cause of pancreatitis. If the pancreatic duct sphincter is fibrotic, the surgeon performs a sphincterotomy (incision of the sphincter) to enlarge it. Endoscopic sphincterotomy may be used for patients who are poor surgical candidates.

In some cases laparoscopic distal pancreatectomy may be appropriate for resection of the distal pancreas or pancreas head. Endoscopic pancreatic necrosectomy and natural orifice transluminal endoscopic surgery (NOTES) are becoming more common for removing necrosed pancreatic tissue. Both procedures are performed through the GI wall without a visible skin incision. The NOTES procedure is discussed in Surgical Management in the Cholecystitis section.

In a few cases, pancreas transplantation may be done. However, this procedure is performed most often for patients with severe, uncontrolled diabetes. Chapter 64 discusses pancreas transplantation.

Care Coordination and Transition Management

Home Care Management. Collaborate with the hospital-based case manager (CM) or discharge planner about home care or follow-up in another setting. A community-based CM may continue to follow the patient after hospital discharge. If the patient is discharged to home, the living area should be limited to one floor until he or she regains strength and can increase activity. Teach patients and families that toilet facilities must be easily accessible because of chronic steatorrhea and frequent defecation. If they are not easily accessible, a bedside commode is obtained for the home.

Self-Management Education. Because there is no known cure for chronic pancreatitis, patient and family education is aimed at preventing acute episodes of the disease, providing long-term care, and promoting health maintenance (Chart 59-4). Teach the patient to avoid known irritating substances, such as caffeinated beverages (stimulates the GI system) and alcohol. Collaborate with the dietitian in diet teaching, which focuses on eating bland, low-fat, frequent meals and avoiding rich, fatty foods. Stress the importance of adhering to the nutritional recommendations. Written instructions are essential, with consideration of personal and cultural food preferences.

Remind the patient and family members or significant others of the importance of adhering to pancreatic enzyme replacement. The patient must take the prescribed enzymes with meals and snacks to aid in the digestion of food and promote the absorption of fats and proteins. Teach the patient to take the enzymes before or at the beginning of the meal. Instruct him or her to report any increase in abdominal distention, cramping,

---

CHART 59-4 Patient and Family Education: Preparing for Self-Management

Prevention of Exacerbations of Chronic Pancreatitis

- Avoid things that make your symptoms worse, such as drinking caffeinated beverages.
- Avoid alcohol ingestion; refer to self-help group for assistance.
- Avoid nicotine.
- Eat bland, low-fat, high-protein, and moderate-carbohydrate meals; avoid gastric stimulants such as spices.
- Eat small meals and snacks high in calories.
- Take the pancreatic enzymes that have been prescribed for you with meals.
- Rest frequently; restrict your activity to one floor until you regain your strength.

---

and foul-smelling, frothy, fatty stools to the health care provider so these supplements may be increased as needed. Remind the patient to report any skin breakdown so therapeutic interventions to promote skin integrity can be started. Abdominal fistulas are common and present a difficult challenge because pancreatic secretions irritate the skin.

The frequency of defecation (whether continent or incontinent) poses challenging skin care problems. Instruct the patient to keep the skin dry and free of the abrasive fatty stools, which damage the skin. The skin should be cleaned thoroughly after each stool, and a moisture barrier applied to prevent breakdown and maintain skin integrity. Many products on the market actively repel stool from the skin.

If the patient develops diabetes mellitus as a result of chronic pancreatitis, management of elevated glucose levels after discharge from the hospital may require oral antidiabetic agents or insulin injections. If this is the case, collaborate with the certified diabetic educator (CDE) to provide in-depth teaching concerning diabetes, its signs and symptoms, medical management, drug therapy, nutrition therapy, blood glucose monitoring, and general care.

Chronic illnesses are devastating for families. The high costs of medical insurance, medical treatment, and drug therapy cause serious financial problems. Often the patient with chronic pancreatitis is unable to work. Collaborate with the CM about ways to assist the patient with resources for financial help.

Health Care Resources. The patient may require several home visits by nurses, depending on the severity of the chronic health problems and home maintenance and support needs. The nurse assesses the patient for pain, enzyme therapy, and psychosocial adaptation to a chronic illness. Refer him or her and the family to a counselor or a self-help group, such as Alcoholics Anonymous (www.aa.org) and Al-Anon (www.al-anon.org), if appropriate.

NCLEX EXAMINATION CHALLENGE 59-4

Physiological Integrity

Which teaching will the nurse provide when discharging a client with chronic pancreatitis?

A. Weight reduction and daily exercise regimen
B. Constipation precautions, including daily laxative use
C. Dietary adjustments to include avoiding high-fat food, caffeine, and alcohol
D. Relaxation techniques and stress management

PANCREATIC ABSCESS

Pancreatic abscesses are the most serious complication of acute necrotizing pancreatitis. If untreated, they are always fatal. After surgery, the recurrence rate is high. The abscesses form from collections of purulent liquefaction of the necrotic pancreas.

Patients with pancreatic abscesses often appear more seriously ill than those with pseudocysts. Signs and symptoms are similar. However, the temperature in patients with abscesses may spike to as high as 104° F (40° C). Drainage via the percutaneous method or laparoscopy should be performed as soon as possible to prevent sepsis. Antibiotic treatment alone does not resolve the abscess. Death rates remain high even after surgical drainage. Many patients require multiple drainage procedures for repeated abscesses.

PANCREATIC PSEUDOCYST

❖ PATHOPHYSIOLOGY

Pancreatic pseudocysts, or false cysts, are so named because, unlike true cysts, they do not have an epithelial lining. They are encapsulated, saclike structures that form on or surround the pancreas. The pseudocyst wall is inflamed, vascular, and fibrotic. It may contain up to several liters of straw-colored or dark brown viscous fluid, the enzymatic exudate of the pancreas (McCance et al., 2014). Risk factors for pseudocysts are acute pancreatitis, abdominal trauma, and chronic pancreatitis.

❖ INTERPROFESSIONAL COLLABORATIVE CARE

Care for the patient with pancreatic pseudocyst takes place in the hospital setting when surgical intervention is required. Members of the interprofessional team who collaborate most closely to care for the patient with pancreatic pseudocyst include the health care provider, surgeon, and nurse.

◆ Assessment: Noticing

A pseudocyst can be palpated as an epigastric mass in about half of all cases. The primary presenting symptom is epigastric pain radiating to the back. Other common symptoms include abdominal fullness, nausea, vomiting, and jaundice. Pseudocysts are diagnosed, and their growth and resolution monitored by serial pancreatic diagnostic testing. Complications of pseudocyst formation include:

- Hemorrhage
- Infection
- Obstruction of the bowel, biliary tract, or splenic vein
- Abscess
- Fistula formation
- Pancreatic ascites

◆ Interventions: Responding

Pseudocysts may resolve spontaneously, or they may rupture and produce hemorrhage. Surgical intervention is necessary if the pseudocyst does not resolve within 6 to 8 weeks or if complications develop. To provide external drainage, the surgeon inserts a sump drainage tube to remove pancreatic secretions and exudate. Pancreatic fistulas are common after surgery, and skin breakdown from corrosive pancreatic enzymes in patients who have external drainage presents a major nursing care challenge.

PANCREATIC CANCER

❖ PATHOPHYSIOLOGY

Cancer of the pancreas is a leading cause of cancer deaths each year in the United States. It is difficult to diagnose early because the pancreas is hidden and surrounded by other organs. Treatment has limited results, and 5-year survival rates are low (American Cancer Society, 2017).

Pancreatic tumors usually originate from epithelial cells of the pancreatic ductal system. If the tumor is discovered in the early stages, the tumor cells may be localized within the glandular organ. However, this is highly unlikely. Most often, the tumor is discovered in the late stages of development and may be a well-defined mass or diffusely spread throughout the pancreas.

The tumor may be a primary cancer, or it may result from metastasis from cancers of the lung, breast, thyroid, kidney, or skin. Primary tumors are generally adenocarcinomas and grow in well-differentiated glandular patterns. They grow rapidly and spread to surrounding organs (stomach, duodenum, gallbladder, and intestine) by direct extension and invasion of lymphatic and vascular systems. This highly metastatic lesion may eventually invade the lung, peritoneum, liver, spleen, and lymph nodes.

Signs and symptoms depend on the site of origin or metastasis. The head of the pancreas is the most common site. The tumors are usually small lesions with poorly defined margins. Jaundice results from tumor compression and obstruction of the common bile duct and from gallbladder dilation, causing the organ to enlarge.

Cancers of the body and tail of the pancreas are usually large and invade the entire tail and body. These tumors may be palpable abdominal masses, especially in the thin patient. Through metastatic spread via the splenic vein, metastasis to the liver may cause hepatomegaly (enlargement of the liver up to two to three times its normal size). Cancers of the body and tail spread more extensively than do pancreatic head carcinomas, with invasion of the retroperitoneum, vertebral column, spleen, adrenal glands, colon, or stomach. Regardless of where it originates, it spreads rapidly through the lymphatic and venous systems to other organs.

Venous thromboembolism is a common complication of pancreatic cancer. Necrotic products of the pancreatic tumor are believed to have thromboplastic properties resulting in the blood's hypercoagulable state. In addition, the patient is at high risk because of decreased mobility and extensive surgical manipulation.

The exact cause of pancreatic cancer is unknown. High-risk populations are those in their sixth to eighth decades of life and those with a personal history of smoking.

⚕ GENETIC/GENOMIC CONSIDERATIONS
Patient-Centered Care QSEN

A small number of those with pancreatic cancer have an inherited risk. Mutations in certain oncogenes have been identified. Mutations have also been revealed in tumor suppressor genes, such as *p16* and *BRCA2*—the same mutation that makes some women susceptible to breast and ovarian cancer. Genes responsible for hereditary nonpolyposis colorectal cancer can also increase an individual's risk for pancreatic cancer (Ducreux et al., 2015).

Other risk factors associated with the disease include:

- Diabetes mellitus
- Chronic pancreatitis
- Cirrhosis
- High intake of red meat, especially processed meat such as steak
- Long-term exposure to chemicals such as gasoline and pesticides
- Obesity
- Older age
- Male gender
- Cigarette smoking
- Family history
- Genetic syndromes

❖ INTERPROFESSIONAL COLLABORATIVE CARE

Care for the patient with pancreatic cancer usually takes place in the hospital setting, and eventually with hospice. Members of the interprofessional team who collaborate most closely to care for the patient with pancreatic cancer include the health care provider, surgeon if surgery is required, nurse, dietitian, social worker, and spiritual leader of the patient's choice.

◆ Assessment: Noticing

Pancreatic cancer often presents in a slow and vague manner. The presenting symptoms depend somewhat on the location of the tumor. The first sign may be jaundice, which suggests late, advanced disease (Chart 59-5). Jaundice occurs because the gallbladder and liver are commonly involved. As the tumor spreads, the yellow skin color associated with obstructive jaundice progressively worsens. Ask the patient whether the color of the stool and urine has changed. As a result of the obstructive process, the stool is clay colored, and the urine is dark and frothy. Inspect the skin for dryness and scratch marks, indicating pruritus from jaundice caused by bile salt collection. Assess the sclera for icterus (yellowing) and the mucous membranes for signs of jaundice.

The enlarged gallbladder and liver may be palpable. In advanced cases of pancreatic carcinoma, the tumor may be felt as a firm, fixed mass in the left upper abdominal quadrant or epigastric region.

The most common concern is fatigue, which is described as a diminished energy level and an increased need for rest relative

---

CHART 59-5   Key Features

Pancreatic Cancer

- Jaundice
- Clay-colored (light) stools
- Dark urine
- Abdominal pain: usually vague, dull, or nonspecific that radiates into the back
- Weight loss
- Anorexia
- Nausea or vomiting
- Glucose intolerance
- Splenomegaly (enlarged spleen)
- Flatulence
- Gastrointestinal bleeding
- Ascites (abdominal fluid)
- Leg or calf pain (from thrombophlebitis)
- Weakness and fatigue

---

to the level of activity. The patient notices an inability to perform usual physical or intellectual activities.

Question the patient about abdominal pain, which is usually described as a vague, constant dullness in the upper abdomen and nonspecific in nature. Pain also indicates advanced stages of the disease and may be related to eating or activity. Ask whether the patient has pain in other areas of the body. Referred back pain may be caused by pressure on the nerve plexus. Some patients have leg or calf pain with swelling and redness as a result of deep vein thrombosis or thrombophlebitis.

Weigh the patient to determine the extent of weight loss and whether it has occurred rapidly. Ask about food intake and intolerances. Anorexia accompanied by early satiety, nausea, flatulence (gas), and vomiting is common. GI bleeding may develop from esophageal or gastric varices caused by the tumor pressing on the portal vein. A new diagnosis of diabetes is found in some patients.

In addition to the focused history, perform a general abdominal assessment. In particular, observe for distention and swelling, which may be ascites (abdominal fluid). Percussion over the ascitic abdomen elicits dullness, seen in the advanced stages of the disease process.

No specific blood tests diagnose pancreatic cancer. Serum *amylase* and *lipase* levels and *alkaline phosphatase* and *bilirubin* levels are increased. The degree of elevation depends on the acuteness or chronicity of the pancreatic and biliary damage. Elevated *carcinoembryonic antigen* (CEA) levels occur in most patients with pancreatic cancer. This test may provide early information about the presence of tumor cells. The tumor marker CA 19-9 has been found to be a useful serologic test for monitoring a proven diagnosis and continuing surveillance for potential spread or recurrence (Pagana et al., 2017).

Abdominal *ultrasound* and *contrast-enhanced CT* are the most commonly used imaging techniques for confirming a tumor and can differentiate the tumor from a cyst. Endoscopic ultrasonography can also be performed to sample tissue for diagnosis and provide information on tumor type and size (Ducreux et al., 2015). Contrast harmonic echo-endoscopic ultrasound increases the accuracy of diagnosing solid pancreatic masses (Ducreux et al., 2015).

Endoscopic retrograde cholangiopancreatography (ERCP) also provides visual diagnostic data. An alternative to ERCP is a percutaneous transhepatic biliary cholangiogram with placement of a percutaneous transhepatic biliary drain (PTBD). This drain decompresses the blocked biliary system by draining bile, internally, externally, or both. Aspiration of pancreatic ascitic fluid by abdominal paracentesis may reveal cancer cells and elevated amylase levels.

◆ Interventions: Responding

Management of the patient with pancreatic cancer is geared toward preventing tumor spread and decreasing pain. These measures are not curative, only palliative. The cancers are often metastatic and recur despite treatment.

Nonsurgical Management. As in other types of cancer, chemotherapy or radiation is used to relieve pain by shrinking the tumor. It may be used before, after, or instead of surgery. *Chemotherapy* has had limited success in increasing survival time. In most cases, combining agents has been more successful than single-agent chemotherapy. 5-Fluorouracil (5-FU), a commonly used drug, may be given alone or with gemcitabine (Gemzar) for locally advanced, or unresectable, pancreatic cancers. Observe for adverse drug effects, such as fatigue, rash, anorexia, and diarrhea. Chapter 22 discusses nursing implications of chemotherapy in more detail.

Other targeted therapies being investigated include growth factor inhibitors, anti-angiogenesis factors, and kinase inhibitors (also known as *tyrosine kinase inhibitors*). Kinase inhibitors are a newer group of drugs that focus on cancer cells with little or no effect on healthy cells. Chapter 22 describes general nursing interventions associated with chemotherapy.

To control pain, the patient takes high doses of opioid analgesics (usually morphine) as prescribed and uses other COMFORT measures before the pain escalates and peaks. Because of the poor prognosis, drug dependency is not a consideration. Chapter 4 describes in detail the care of the patient with chronic cancer pain.

Intensive external beam *radiation* therapy to the pancreas may offer pain relief by shrinking tumor cells, alleviating obstruction, and improving food absorption. It does not improve survival rates. The patient may experience discomfort during and after the radiation treatments. Chapter 22 describes radiation therapy in more detail.

For patients experiencing biliary obstruction who are high surgical risks, **biliary stents** placed percutaneously (through the skin) can ensure patency to relieve pain. These stents are devices made of plastic materials that keep the ducts of the biliary system open. Using another approach, self-expandable stents may be inserted endoscopically to relieve obstruction.

Surgical Management. Complete surgical resection of the pancreatic tumor offers the patient with pancreatic cancer the only effective treatment, but it is done only in patients with small tumors. *Partial pancreatectomy* is the preferred surgery for tumors smaller than 3 cm in diameter, depending on location and length of time since diagnosis. Recent technologic advances have expanded the role of **minimally invasive surgery (MIS)** via laparoscopy in the staging, palliation, and removal of pancreatic cancers. The procedure selected depends on the purpose of the surgery and stage of the disease. For example, if the patient has a biliary obstruction, a laparoscopic procedure to relieve it is performed. This procedure diverts bile drainage into the jejunum.

For larger tumors, the surgeon may perform either a *radical pancreatectomy* or the *Whipple procedure (pancreaticoduodenectomy)*. These procedures have traditionally been done using an open surgical approach. Because of new advances in laparoscopic technology using a hand-assist device, this method is beginning to replace the conventional method. Some surgeons are not yet trained in how to perform this technique. Therefore the traditional open surgical approach remains the most common method of performing these surgeries.

Preoperative Care. The patient with pancreatic cancer may be a poor surgical risk because of malnutrition and debilitation. Specific care depends on the type of surgical approach being used.

Often, in the late stages of pancreatic cancer or before the Whipple procedure, the physician inserts a small catheter into the jejunum (**jejunostomy**) so enteral feedings may be given. This feeding method is preferred to prevent reflux and facilitate absorption. Feedings are started in low concentrations and volumes and gradually increased as tolerated. Provide feedings using a pump to maintain a constant volume and assess for diarrhea frequency to determine tolerance. Chapter 60 provides additional information about enteral feeding.

For optimal NUTRITION, TPN may be necessary in addition to tube feedings or as a single measure to provide NUTRITION. When central venous access is required, a peripherally inserted central catheter (PICC) or other type of IV catheter may be necessary. Meticulous IV line care is an important nursing measure to prevent catheter sepsis. Sterile dressing changes and site observation are extremely important. Additional nursing care measures for the patient receiving TPN are given in Chapter 60. Monitor nutrition indicators such as serum prealbumin and albumin.

For the laparoscopic procedure, no bowel preparation is needed. However, either approach requires that the patient have nothing by mouth (NPO) for at least 6 to 8 hours before surgery. Surgeon preference and agency policy determine the preferred protocol for preoperative preparation.

Operative Procedures. The **Whipple procedure (radical pancreaticoduodenectomy)** involves extensive surgical manipulation and is used most often to treat cancer of the head of the pancreas. The procedure entails removal of the proximal head of the pancreas, the duodenum, a portion of the jejunum, the stomach (partial or total **gastrectomy**), and the gallbladder, with anastomosis of the pancreatic duct (**pancreaticojejunostomy**), the common bile duct (**choledochojejunostomy**), and the stomach (**gastrojejunostomy**) to the jejunum (Fig. 59-3). In addition, the surgeon may remove the spleen (**splenectomy**).

Postoperative Care. In addition to routine postoperative care measures, the patient who has undergone an open radical pancreaticoduodenectomy requires intensive nursing care and is usually admitted to a surgical critical care unit. Observe for multiple potential complications of the open Whipple procedure as listed in Table 59-5.

The primary benefits of MIS for the patient are a shorter postoperative recovery and less pain than with traditional open procedures. The patient having the laparoscopic Whipple surgery or radical pancreatectomy is also less at risk for severe

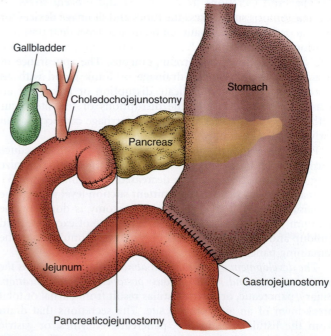

FIG. 59-3 The three anastomoses that constitute the Whipple procedure: choledochojejunostomy, pancreaticojejunostomy, and gastrojejunostomy.

TABLE 59-5	Potential Complications of the Whipple Procedure

Cardiovascular Complications
- Hemorrhage at anastomosis sites with hypovolemia
- Myocardial infarction
- Heart failure
- Thrombophlebitis

Pulmonary Complications
- Atelectasis
- Pneumonia
- Pulmonary embolism
- Acute respiratory distress syndrome
- Pulmonary edema

Metabolic Complications
- Unstable diabetes mellitus
- Renal failure

GI Complications
- Adynamic (paralytic) ileus
- Gastric retention
- Gastric ulceration
- Bowel obstruction from peritonitis
- Acute pancreatitis
- Hepatic failure
- Thrombosis to mesentery

Wound Complications
- Infection
- Dehiscence
- Fistulas: pancreatic, gastric, and biliary

complications. For patients having one of these procedures, observe for and implement preventive measures for these surgical complications:

- Diabetes (Check blood glucose often.)
- Hemorrhage (Monitor pulse, blood pressure, skin color, and mental status [e.g., LOC].)
- Wound infection (Monitor temperature and assess wounds for redness and induration [hardness].)
- Bowel obstruction (Check bowel sounds and stools.)
- Intra-abdominal abscess (Monitor temperature and patient's report of severe pain.)

Immediately after surgery the patient is NPO and usually has a nasogastric tube (NGT) to decompress the stomach. Monitor GI drainage and tube patency. In open surgical approaches, biliary drainage tubes are placed during surgery to remove drainage and secretions from the area and prevent stress on the anastomosis sites. Assess the tubes and drainage devices for tension or kinking and maintain them in a dependent position.

Monitor the drainage for color, consistency, and amount. The drainage should be serosanguineous. The appearance of clear, colorless, bile-tinged drainage or frank blood with an increase in output may indicate disruption or leakage of an anastomosis site. Most of the disruptions of the site occur within 7 to 10 days after surgery. Hemorrhage can occur as an early or late complication.

Place the patient in the semi-Fowler's position to reduce tension on the suture line and anastomosis site and to optimize lung expansion. Stress can be decreased by maintaining NGT drainage at a low or high intermittent suction level to keep the remaining stomach (if a partial gastrectomy is done) or the jejunum (if a total gastrectomy is done) free of excessive fluid buildup and pressure. The NGT also reduces stimulation of the remaining pancreatic tissue.

The development of a fistula (an abnormal passageway) is the most common and most serious postoperative complication. Biliary, pancreatic, or gastric fistulas result from partial or total breakdown of an anastomosis site. The secretions that drain from the fistula contain bile, pancreatic enzymes, or gastric secretions, depending on which site is ruptured. *These secretions, particularly pancreatic fluid, are corrosive and irritating to*

the skin; and internal leakage causes chemical peritonitis. **Peritonitis** (inflammation and infection of the peritoneum causing boardlike abdominal rigidity) requires treatment with multiple antibiotics. *If you suspect any postoperative complications resulting from MIS or open surgical approaches, call the surgeon immediately and provide assessment findings that support your concerns.*

Because the *open* Whipple procedure is extensive and can take many hours to complete, maintaining fluid and electrolyte balance can be difficult. Patients often have significant intraoperative blood loss and postoperative bleeding. The intestine is exposed to air for long periods, and fluid evaporates. Significant losses of fluid and electrolytes occur from the NGT and other drainage tubes. In addition, these patients may be malnourished and have low serum levels of protein and albumin, which maintain colloid osmotic pressure within the circulating system. Reduction in the serum osmotic pressure makes the patient likely to develop third spacing of body fluids, with fluid moving from the vascular to the interstitial space, resulting in shock. These problems are less likely to occur when MIS is used. Therefore, when possible, the trained surgeon prefers to perform laparoscopic Whipple procedures to shorten operating time and prevent the many complications that can occur.

> ⚠️ **NURSING SAFETY PRIORITY** QSEN
>
> **Action Alert**
>
> To detect early signs of hypovolemia and prevent shock, closely monitor vital signs for decreased blood pressure and increased heart rate, decreased vascular pressures with a pulmonary artery catheter (Swan-Ganz catheter) (in ICU setting), and decreased urine output. Be alert for pitting edema of the extremities, dependent edema in the sacrum and back, and an intake that far exceeds output. Maintain sequential compression devices to prevent deep vein thrombosis.

Maintenance of prescribed IV isotonic fluid replacement with colloid replacements is important. Monitor hemoglobin and hematocrit values to assess for blood loss and the need for blood transfusions. Review electrolyte values for decreased serum levels of sodium, potassium, chloride, and calcium. IV fluid concentrations must be altered to correct these electrolyte imbalances. The physician prescribes replacement of electrolytes as needed.

Immediately after the Whipple procedure, the patient may have hyperglycemia or hypoglycemia as a result of stress and surgical manipulation of the pancreas. Most of the endocrine cells (responsible for insulin and glucagon secretion) are located in the body and tail of the pancreas. In some patients, up to half of the gland remains, and diabetes does not develop. However, a large number of patients have diabetes before surgery. For patients having a radical pancreatectomy, administer insulin as prescribed because the entire pancreas is removed. Monitor glucose levels frequently during the early postoperative period and administer insulin injections as prescribed.

Care Coordination and Transition Management

The patient with pancreatic cancer is usually followed by a case manager (CM), both in the hospital and in the home or other community-based setting. Collaborate with the CM to ensure that the patient receives cost-effective treatment and that his or her needs are met.

CLINICAL JUDGMENT CHALLENGE 59-1

Patient-Centered Care; Evidence-Based Practice; Teamwork and Collaboration; Informatics QSEN

You are the nurse on a critical care unit, caring for a 79-year-old woman who has had a Whipple procedure after being diagnosed with pancreatic cancer. She is sleeping soundly, and vital signs are stable. While you continue your assessment, the patient's 82-year-old husband states, "I'm so glad she had this surgery, but I'm exhausted from taking care of her and don't know how I'll manage when she is allowed to go home."

1. What specific assessment findings will you document in the electronic health record?
2. For which conditions will you monitor the patient, recognizing the surgical procedure she has just had?
3. What laboratory values will you closely follow, and why?
4. What is your response to the patient's husband?

NCLEX EXAMINATION CHALLENGE 59-5

Psychosocial Integrity

The hospice nurse is caring for a client with pancreatic cancer who has been given 2 to 3 months to live. What is the appropriate nursing response when the client's wife states, "I know he's going to get better."?

A. Use therapeutic silence and say nothing.
B. "Your spouse will die in 2 to 3 months."
C. "Let's talk about how you're feeling about your spouse's prognosis."
D. "If your spouse adheres to the entire treatment plan, recovery is possible."

Home Care Management. The stage of progression of pancreatic cancer and available home care resources determine whether the patient can be discharged to home or whether additional care is needed in a skilled nursing facility or with a hospice provider. Home care preparations depend on the patient's physical and activity limitations and should be tailored to his or her needs. Coordinate care with the patient, family, or whoever will be providing care after discharge from the hospital (i.e., home care provider, hospice care provider, or extended-care provider).

The patient and family need compassionate emotional support to deal with issues related to this illness. The diagnosis of pancreatic cancer can frighten and overwhelm the patient and family. Help family members look realistically and objectively at the amount of physical care required. Tell family members that their own physical and emotional health is at risk during this stressful period and that supportive counseling may be needed. If the family does not have a religious affiliation or a spiritual leader (e.g., a minister or a rabbi) to provide support, suggest alternative counseling options. Refer patients and families to the certified hospital chaplain if desired. It is appropriate for the nurse to make the initial contact or appointment according to the patient's or family's wishes.

Self-Management Education. When the patient is discharged to home, many interventions are palliative and aimed at managing symptoms such as pain. In many cases the diagnosis of pancreatic cancer is made a few months before death occurs. The patient needs time to adjust to the diagnosis, which is usually made too late for cure or prolonged survival. Help the patient identify what needs to be done to prepare for death, including end-of-life care. For example, he or she may want to write a will or see family members and friends whom he or she has not seen recently. The patient needs to make known to family members or others his or her specific requests for the funeral or memorial service. These actions help prepare for death in a dignified manner. Chapter 7 discusses in detail anticipatory grieving and preparation for death, as well as symptom management during the end of life.

Health Care Resources. Regular home care nursing and assistive nursing personnel visits may be scheduled to assist the patient and family by providing physical, psychological, and supportive care. Supply information about local palliative and hospice care (see Chapter 7) and cancer support groups.

GET READY FOR THE NCLEX® EXAMINATION!

KEY POINTS

Review these Key Points for each NCLEX Examination Client Needs Category.

Safe and Effective Care Environment

- Collaborate with the dietitian, pharmacist, health care provider, and case manager when planning care for patients with pancreatic cancer. **QSEN: Teamwork and Collaboration**
- Refer patients with end-stage pancreatic cancer for palliative and hospice care. **Ethics**
- Refer patients with pancreatitis who use alcohol to community resources such as Alcoholics Anonymous. **QSEN: Patient-Centered Care**

Health Promotion and Maintenance

- Recognize that obese, middle-age women are most likely to have gallbladder disease. **QSEN: Patient-Centered Care**

- Teach patients to avoid losing weight too quickly and to keep weight under control to help prevent gallbladder disease. **QSEN: Evidence-Based Practice**
- Teach patients to avoid alcohol consumption to help prevent alcohol-induced acute pancreatitis. **QSEN: Evidence-Based Practice**
- Instruct patients about ways to prevent exacerbations of chronic pancreatitis as outlined in Chart 59-4.

Psychosocial Integrity

- Refer patients with pancreatic cancer to support services such as spiritual leaders and counselors for coping strategies and facilitation of the grieving process. **Ethics**
- Help prepare the pancreatic cancer patient and family for the death and dying process. **Ethics**

Physiological Integrity

- Be aware that autodigestion of the pancreas causes severe pain in patients with acute pancreatitis (see Fig. 59-2).
- Monitor serum laboratory values, especially amylase and lipase (both elevated), in patients with pancreatitis (see Table 59-4). **QSEN: Evidence-Based Practice**
- Assess for common symptoms of cholecystitis as listed in Chart 59-1.
- Provide pain management, including opioid analgesia, for patients with acute pancreatitis. **QSEN: Patient-Centered Care**
- Recognize that acute pain relief is the first priority of care for patients with acute pancreatitis. **QSEN: Evidence-Based Practice**

- Be aware that patients with biliary and pancreatic disorders are at high risk for biliary obstruction, a serious and painful complication. **QSEN: Safety**
- Assess for common symptoms of chronic pancreatitis as listed in Chart 59-2.
- Document health teaching about enzyme replacement therapy as described in Chart 59-3. **QSEN: Informatics**
- Assess patients with symptoms of pancreatic cancer as described in Chart 59-5.
- Observe for and implement interventions to prevent life-threatening complications of the Whipple procedure as outlined in Table 59-5. **QSEN: Safety**

SELECTED BIBLIOGRAPHY

Agostino, D. I., Wang, D. Q., Bonfrate, L., & Portincasa, P. (2013). Current views on genetics and epigenetics of cholesterol gallstone disease. *Cholesterol,* doi:10.1155/2013/298421.

American Cancer Society (ACS) (2017). *Cancer facts and figures—2017.* Atlanta: Author.

Ducreux, M., Cuhna, A. S., Caramella, C., Hollebecque, A., Burtin, P., Goéré, D., et al. (2015). Cancer of the pancreas: ESMO Clinical Practice Guidelines for diagnosis, treatment and follow-up. *Annals of Oncology, 26*(5), v56–v68.

Girometti, R., Brondani, G., Cereser, L., Como, G., Del Pin, M., Bazzocchi, M., et al. (2010). Post-cholecystectomy syndrome: Spectrum of biliary findings at magnetic resonance cholangiopancreatography. *The British Journal of Radiology, 83,* 351–361.

Kawa, S., Maruyama, M., & Watanabe, T. (2013). Prognosis and long-term outcomes of autoimmune pancreatitis. *Pancreapedia: American Pancreatic Association,* version 1.0, doi:10.3998/panc.2013.21.

Klein, A. P. (2012). Genetic susceptibility to pancreatic cancer. *Molecular Carcinogenesis, 51*(1), 14–24.

McCance, K., Huether, S., Brashers, V., & Rote, N. (2014). *Pathophysiology: The biologic basis for disease in adults and children* (7th ed.). St. Louis: Mosby.

Pagana, K., Pagana, T. J., & Pagana, T. N. (2017). *Mosby's diagnostic and laboratory test reference* (13th ed.). St. Louis: Mosby.

Papp, K., Angst, E., Seidel, S., Flury-Frei, R., & Hetzer, F. H. (2015). The diagnostic challenges of autoimmune pancreatitis. *Case Reports in Gastroenterology, 9,* 56–61.

Roberts, K. E., & Kate, V. (2016). *Transvaginal cholecystectomy.* http://emedicine.medscape.com/article/1900692-overview#a5.

Soper, N., & Malladi, P. (2017). *Laparoscopic cholecystectomy.* www.uptodate.com.

CHAPTER 60

Care of Patients With Malnutrition: Undernutrition and Obesity

Laura M. Willis and Cherie Rebar

PRIORITY AND INTERRELATED CONCEPTS

The priority concept for this chapter is NUTRITION.

✳ The NUTRITION concept exemplars for this chapter are:
- Malnutrition, p. 1215
- Obesity, p. 1225

The interrelated concept for this chapter is FLUID AND ELECTROLYTE BALANCE.

LEARNING OUTCOMES

Safe and Effective Care Environment

1. Collaborate with the interprofessional team members to protect and provide care for the patient with undernutrition or obesity.
2. Identify community resources to ensure appropriate transition management for the patient with undernutrition or obesity.

Health Promotion and Maintenance

3. Teach adults the importance of lifestyle habits that promote NUTRITION health.
4. Perform and interpret a nutrition screening for adults.

Psychosocial Integrity

5. Implement nursing interventions to minimize stressors for the patient with undernutrition or obesity.

Physiological Integrity

6. Interpret assessment findings associated with undernutrition or obesity.
7. Prioritize care for the patient with undernutrition or obesity.
8. Create an evidence-based plan of care for the patient with undernutrition or obesity.
9. Describe nursing interventions to prevent complications of total parenteral nutrition (TPN) and maintain FLUID AND ELECTROLYTE BALANCE.
10. Describe nursing interventions to address postoperative care of the patient having bariatric surgery.
11. Identify the role of supplements and drug therapy in restoring or maintaining NUTRITION status.

In healthy adults, most energy supplied by carbohydrates, protein, and fat undergo digestion and are absorbed from the GI tract. Proper NUTRITION plays a major role in promoting and maintaining health; and this helps the body to maintain temperature, respiration, cardiac output, muscle function, protein synthesis, and the storage and metabolism of food sources. The relationship between energy used and energy stored is referred to as *energy balance*. Weight is gained when food intake is more than energy used, and weight loss occurs when energy used is more than intake. The body attempts to meet its calorie requirements even if it is at the expense of protein needs; when calorie intake is insufficient, body proteins are used for energy.

NUTRITION STANDARDS FOR HEALTH PROMOTION AND MAINTENANCE

Current focuses on NUTRITION are targeted toward health promotion and the prevention of disease by healthy eating and exercise. The entity formerly known as the Institute of Medicine, now known as the Health Medicine Division of the National Academies of Sciences, Engineering, and Medicine (HMDN-ASEM) developed the **Dietary Reference Intakes (DRIs)** to serve as a nutrition guide that provides a scientific basis for food guidelines in the United States and Canada. Age, gender, and life stage influence the nutrient reference values of more than 40 nutrient substances (United States Department of Agriculture [USDA], 2017). In the United States, the **Dietary Guidelines for Americans** are revised by the U.S. Department of Agriculture (USDA) and the U.S. Department of Health and Human Services (DHHS) every 5 years. The 2015-2020 guidelines emphasize the need to focus on "shifts," which involves making active choices to consumer nutrient-dense foods and beverages instead of less healthy ones. Examples of other guidelines are listed in Table 60-1.

To remind adults about healthy eating habits, the USDA designed "MyPlate," a picture to demonstrate that half of each

TABLE 60-1   Examples of *2015-2020 Dietary Guidelines for Americans*

- Follow a healthy eating pattern across the lifespan.
- Focus on variety, nutrient density, and amount.
- Limit calories from added sugars and saturated fats and reduce sodium intake.
- Shift to healthier food and beverage choices.
- Support healthy eating patterns for all.

Source: *Dietary Guidelines for Americans 2015-2020* (8th ed.). (2015). http://health.gov/dietaryguidelines/2015/resources/2015-2020_Dietary_Guidelines.pdf.

meal should consist of fruits and vegetables (Fig. 60-1). When grains are consumed, half of them should be whole grains rather than refined grain products.

Some adults follow vegetarian diet patterns for health, environmental, or moral reasons. In general, vegetarians are leaner than those who consume meat. The lacto-vegetarian eats milk, cheese, and dairy foods but avoids meat, fish, poultry, and eggs. The lacto-ovo-vegetarian includes eggs in his or her diet. The vegan eats only foods of plant origin. Some adults among these groups eat fish as well. Vegans can develop anemia as a result of vitamin B_{12} deficiency. Therefore they should include a daily source of vitamin B_{12} in their diets, such as a fortified breakfast cereal, fortified soy beverage, or meat substitute. All vegetarians should ensure that they get adequate amounts of calcium, iron, zinc, and vitamins D and B_{12}. Well-planned vegetarian diets can provide adequate NUTRITION. The Academy of Nutrition and Dietetics (2016) publishes a number of credible resources regarding vegetarian health at www.eatright.org.

Health Canada publishes the Canada Food Guide, which was originally created in 2011. Compared with previous documents, it includes more culturally diverse foods, information on *trans* fats, customized individual recommendations, and exercise guidelines. Several booklets can be purchased to help adults select the best foods and nutrients from the new guide, such as *Eating Well with Canada's Food Guide* (Minister of Health Canada, 2016). In addition, Canada has published a separate booklet in 2007 to address the special needs of some of its Aboriginal population, which places emphasis on cultural, spiritual, and physical importance of food (Health Canada, 2016).

NUTRITION ASSESSMENT

Nutrition status reflects the balance between nutrient requirements and intake. Common factors that affect these requirements

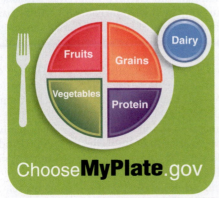

FIG. 60-1 The U.S. Department of Agriculture MyPlate. (From U.S. Department of Agriculture, 2011, www.ChooseMyPlate.gov.)

⊕ CULTURAL/SPIRITUAL CONSIDERATIONS
Patient-Centered Care QSEN

Many adults have specific food preferences based on their ethnicity or race. For example, for adults of Hispanic descent, tortillas, beans, and rice *may* be desired over pasta, risotto, and potatoes. *Never assume that an adult's racial or ethnic background means that he or she eats only foods associated with his or her primary ethnicity.* Health teaching about nutrition should incorporate any cultural preferences.

Some adults have food allergies or intolerances. For instance, lactose intolerance (lactose is found in milk and milk products) is a common problem that occurs in a number of ethnic groups. It is found more often in Mexican Americans and black adults and in some American Indian groups, Asian Americans, and Ashkenazi Jews. A small percentage of white adults, particularly those of Mediterranean descent (e.g., Greek, Italian), are also lactose intolerant. The cause of lactose intolerance is an inadequate amount of the lactase enzyme, which converts lactose into absorbable glucose. Patients may benefit from learning more about the management of lactose intolerance from resources provided by organizations such as the American Dietetic Association or the Dietitians of Canada.

♻ CONSIDERATIONS FOR OLDER ADULTS
Patient-Centered Care QSEN

The USDA recommends that older adults drink eight glasses of water a day and eat plenty of fiber to prevent or manage constipation. It also suggests daily calcium and vitamins D and B_{12} supplements and a reduction in sodium and cholesterol-containing foods.

include age, gender, disease, infection, and psychological stress. Eating behavior, economic implications, emotional stability, disease, drug therapy, and cultural factors influence nutrient intake. Malnutrition (also called *undernutrition)* and obesity, discussed later in this chapter, are common nutrition health problems that may lead to many comorbidities and complications, including death.

Evaluation of nutrition status is an important part of total patient assessment and includes:

- Review of the nutrition history
- Food and fluid intake record
- Laboratory data
- Food-drug interactions
- Health history and physical assessment
- Anthropometric measurements
- Psychosocial assessment

Monitor the NUTRITION status of a patient during hospitalization as an important part of your initial assessment. Collaborate with the interdisciplinary health care team to identify patients at risk for nutrition problems.

Initial Nutrition Screening

An initial screening provides an inexpensive, quick way of determining which patients need more extensive nutrition assessment by the health care team. The Joint Commission Patient Care Standards require that a nutrition screening occur within 24 hours of the patient's hospital admission. If indicated, an in-depth nutrition assessment should be performed. When patients are in the hospital for more than a week, nutrition assessment should be part of the daily plan of care.

The initial nutrition screening includes inspection, measured height and weight, weight history, usual eating habits, ability to chew and swallow, and any recent changes in appetite

⊙ **CHART 60-1** **Best Practice for Patient Safety & Quality Care** QSEN

Nutrition Screening Assessment

General
- Does the patient have any conditions that cause nutrient loss, such as malabsorption syndromes, draining abscesses, wounds, fistulas, or prolonged diarrhea?
- Does the patient have any conditions that increase the need for nutrients, such as fever, burns, injury, sepsis, or antineoplastic therapies?
- Has the patient been NPO for 3 days or more?
- Is the patient receiving a modified diet or a diet restricted in one or more nutrients?
- Is the patient being enterally or parenterally fed?
- Does the patient describe food allergies, lactose intolerance, or limited food preferences?
- Has the patient experienced a recent unexplained weight loss?
- Is the patient on drug therapy—either prescription, over-the-counter, or herbal/natural products?

Gastrointestinal
- Does the patient report nausea, indigestion, vomiting, diarrhea, or constipation?
- Does the patient exhibit glossitis (tongue inflammation), stomatitis (oral inflammation), or esophagitis?
- Does the patient have difficulty chewing or swallowing?
- Does the patient have a partial or total GI obstruction?
- What is the patient's state of dentition?

Cardiovascular
- Does the patient have ascites or edema?
- Is the patient able to perform ADLs?
- Does the patient have heart failure?

Genitourinary
- Is fluid intake about equal to fluid output?
- Does the patient have an ostomy?
- Is the patient hemodialyzed or peritoneally dialyzed?

Respiratory
- Is the patient receiving mechanical ventilatory support?
- Is the patient receiving oxygen via nasal prongs?
- Does the patient have chronic obstructive pulmonary disease (COPD) or asthma?

Integumentary
- Does the patient have abnormal nail or hair changes?
- Does the patient have rashes or dermatitis?
- Does the patient have dry or pale mucous membranes or decreased skin turgor?
- Does the patient have pressure areas on the sacrum, hips, heels, or ankles?

Extremities
- Does the patient have pedal edema?
- Does the patient have cachexia?

Modified Courtesy Ross Products Division, Abbott Laboratories, Columbus, OH.

or food intake. Examples of questions that help identify patients at risk for nutrition problems are part of the history and physical assessment (Chart 60-1).

The Mini Nutritional Assessment (MNA), a two-part tool that has been tested worldwide, provides a reliable, rapid assessment for patients in the community and in any health care setting. The *first* part (A-F) is a screening section that takes 3 minutes to complete and asks about food intake, mobility, and body mass index (BMI) (described in Anthropometric Measurements). It also screens for weight loss, acute illness, and psychological health problems. If the patient scores 11 points or less, the *second* part (G-R) of the MNA is completed, for an additional 12 questions. The entire assessment takes only minutes to complete (Fig. 60-2). The MNA Short Form can be used as a stand-alone tool to evaluate whether the older patient is well nourished, at risk for malnutrition, or malnourished. The alternative is to take the patient's calf circumference, which can be a reliable alternative if BMI is unavailable.

Anthropometric Measurements

Anthropometric measurements are noninvasive methods of evaluating NUTRITION status. These measurements include height and weight and assessment of BMI.

Obtain a current *height and weight* to provide a baseline. Be sure to obtain accurate measurements because patients tend to overestimate height and underestimate weight. Measurements taken days or weeks later may indicate an early change in nutrition status. You may delegate this activity to unlicensed assistive personnel (UAP) under your supervision.

Patients should be measured and weighed while wearing minimal clothing and no shoes. Determine the height in inches or centimeters using the measuring stick of a weight scale if the patient can stand. He or she should stand erect and look straight ahead, with the heels together and the arms at the sides. For patients who cannot stand or those who cannot stand erect (e.g., some older adults), use a sliding-blade **knee height caliper**, if available. This device uses the distance between the patient's patella and heel to estimate height. It is especially useful for patients who have knee or hip contractures.

Remind UAP to weigh ambulatory patients with an upright balance-beam or digital scale. Nonambulatory patients can be weighed with a digital wheelchair or bed scale. If a bed scale is used, document in the electronic health record the number of sheets, pillows, and blankets that were on the bed during baseline measurement. The patient should be wearing the same clothing and have the same bedding on the bed from day to day thereafter to ensure accurate measurement. Lines, devices, and equipment should be lifted off the bed when the measurement is taking place.

! **NURSING SAFETY PRIORITY** QSEN
Action Alert

For daily or sequential weights, obtain the weight at the same time each day, if possible, preferably before breakfast. Conditions such as congestive heart failure and renal disease cause weight gain; dehydration and conditions such as cancer cause weight loss. *Weight is the most reliable indicator of fluid gain or loss, so accurate weights are essential!*

Mini Nutritional Assessment
MNA®

Nestlé
Nutrition Institute

Last name:		First name:		
Sex:	Age:	Weight, kg:	Height, cm:	Date:

Complete the screen by filling in the boxes with the appropriate numbers.
Add the numbers for the screen. If score is 11 or less, continue with the assessment to gain a Malnutrition Indicator Score.

Screening

A Has food intake declined over the past 3 months due to loss of appetite, digestive problems, chewing or swallowing difficulties?
0 = severe decrease in food intake
1 = moderate decrease in food intake
2 = no decrease in food intake ☐

B Weight loss during the last 3 months
0 = weight loss greater than 3kg (6.6lbs)
1 = does not know
2 = weight loss between 1 and 3kg (2.2 and 6.6 lbs)
3 = no weight loss ☐

C Mobility
0 = bed or chair bound
1 = able to get out of bed / chair but does not go out
2 = goes out ☐

D Has suffered psychological stress or acute disease in the past 3 months?
0 = yes   2 = no ☐

E Neuropsychological problems
0 = severe dementia or depression
1 = mild dementia
2 = no psychological problems ☐

F Body Mass Index (BMI) = weight in kg / (height in m)^2
0 = BMI less than 19
1 = BMI 19 to less than 21
2 = BMI 21 to less than 23
3 = BMI 23 or greater ☐

Screening score (subtotal max. 14 points) ☐☐

12-14 points: Normal nutritional status
8-11 points: At risk of malnutrition
0-7 points: Malnourished

For a more in-depth assessment, continue with questions G-R

Assessment

G Lives independently (not in nursing home or hospital)
1 = yes   0 = no ☐

H Takes more than 3 prescription drugs per day
0 = yes   1 = no ☐

I Pressure sores or skin ulcers
0 = yes   1 = no ☐

J How many full meals does the patient eat daily?
0 = 1 meal
1 = 2 meals
2 = 3 meals ☐

K Selected consumption markers for protein intake
• At least one serving of dairy products
  (milk, cheese, yoghurt) per day   yes ☐ no ☐
• Two or more servings of legumes
  or eggs per week   yes ☐ no ☐
• Meat, fish or poultry every day   yes ☐ no ☐
0.0 = if 0 or 1 yes
0.5 = if 2 yes
1.0 = if 3 yes ☐.☐

L Consumes two or more servings of fruit or vegetables per day?
0 = no   1 = yes ☐

M How much fluid (water, juice, coffee, tea, milk...) is consumed per day?
0.0 = less than 3 cups
0.5 = 3 to 5 cups
1.0 = more than 5 cups ☐.☐

N Mode of feeding
0 = unable to eat without assistance
1 = self-fed with some difficulty
2 = self-fed without any problem ☐

O Self view of nutritional status
0 = views self as being malnourished
1 = is uncertain of nutritional state
2 = views self as having no nutritional problem ☐

P In comparison with other people of the same age, how does the patient consider his / her health status?
0.0 = not as good
0.5 = does not know
1.0 = as good
2.0 = better ☐.☐

Q Mid-arm circumference (MAC) in cm
0.0 = MAC less than 21
0.5 = MAC 21 to 22
1.0 = MAC greater than 22 ☐.☐

R Calf circumference (CC) in cm
0 = CC less than 31
1 = CC 31 or greater ☐

Assessment (max. 16 points) ☐☐.☐
Screening score ☐☐
Total Assessment (max. 30 points) ☐☐.☐

Malnutrition Indicator Score
24 to 30 points   ☐   Normal nutritional status
17 to 23.5 points   ☐   At risk of malnutrition
Less than 17 points   ☐   Malnourished

References
1. Vellas B, Villars H, Abellan G, et al. Overview of the MNA® - Its History and Challenges. J Nutr Health Aging. 2006; **10:456**-465.
2. Rubenstein LZ, Harker JO, Salva A, Guigoz Y, Vellas B. Screening for Undernutrition in Geriatric Practice: Developing the Short-Form Mini Nutritional Assessment (MNA-SF). J. Geront. 2001; **56A**: M366-377
3. Guigoz Y. The Mini-Nutritional Assessment (MNA®) Review of the Literature - What does it tell us? J Nutr Health Aging. 2006; **10:**466-487.

For more information: www.mna-elderly.com

FIG. 60-2 The Mini Nutritional Assessment (MNA). (®Société des Produits Nestlé S.A., Vevey, Switzerland, Trademark Owners.)

Normal weights for adult men and women are available from several reference standards, such as the Metropolitan Life tables. Some health care professionals prefer these tables because they consider body-build differences by gender and body frame size.

Changes in body weight can be expressed by three different formulas:

Weight as a percentage of ideal body weight (IBW):

$$\% \, IBW = \frac{Current \; weight}{Ideal \; body \; weight} \times 100$$

Current weight as a percentage of usual body weight (UBW):

$$\% \, UBW = \frac{Current \; weight}{Usual \; body \; weight} \times 100$$

Change in weight:

$$Weight \; change = \frac{Usual \; weight - Current \; weight}{Usual \; weight} \times 100$$

An unintentional weight loss of 10% over a 6-month period at any time significantly affects nutrition status and should be evaluated. Depending on the patient's needs, weights may need to be taken daily, several times a week, or weekly for monitoring status and the effectiveness of nutrition support.

In the health care setting, *assessment of body fat* is usually calculated by the dietitian. For adults who participate in a structured exercise program in the community, this assessment is typically performed by a fitness trainer or physical therapist.

The **body mass index (BMI)** is a measure of nutrition status that does not depend on frame size (Centers for Disease Control and Prevention [CDC], 2015). It indirectly estimates total fat stores within the body by the relationship of weight to height. *Therefore an accurate height is as important as an accurate weight.*

A simple calculation for estimating BMI can be programmed into handheld computers or calculators using one of these two formulas:

$$BMI = \frac{Weight \; (lb)}{Height \; (in \; inches)^2} \times 703$$

$$BMI = \frac{Weight \; (kg)}{Height \; (in \; meters)^2}$$

BMI can also be determined using a table that is linked with height and weight. The least risk for malnutrition is associated with scores between 18.5 and 25. BMIs above and below these values are associated with increased health risks (CDC, 2015).

CONSIDERATIONS FOR OLDER ADULTS

Patient-Centered Care QSEN

Body weight and BMI usually increase throughout adulthood until about 60 years of age. As adults get older, they often become less hungry and eat less, even if they are healthy. Ideally, older adults should have a BMI between 23 and 27.

The average daily energy intake expended by this group tends to be more than the average energy intake. This physiologic change has been called the "anorexia of aging" (Martone et al., 2013). Many older adults are underweight, leading to undernutrition and increased risk for illness.

❓ NCLEX EXAMINATION CHALLENGE 60-1

Health Promotion and Maintenance

An older adult is admitted to the hospital. The client's height is 5 feet, 10 inches (1.78 meters), and weight is 286 lb (129.7 kg). The nurse calculates the client's current body mass index (BMI) as _____. **Fill in the blank. Round your answer to the nearest whole number.**

Skinfold measurements estimate body fat and can be measured by either the nurse or the dietitian. The *triceps and subscapular* skinfolds are most commonly measured with a special caliper. Both are compared with standard measurements and recorded as percentiles.

The *midarm circumference (MAC) and calf circumference (CC)* can be obtained to measure muscle mass and subcutaneous fat. These measurements are needed if the Mini Nutritional Assessment tool is used. To measure MAC, place a flexible tape around the upper arm at the midpoint, taking care to hold the tape firmly but gently to avoid compressing the tissue. This measurement is usually recorded in centimeters. The midarm muscle mass (MAMM) measures the amount of muscle in the body and is a sensitive indicator of protein reserves. It can be computed from the MAC and the triceps skinfold measure. The CC is obtained using a similar procedure on the calf.

✳ NUTRITION CONCEPT EXEMPLAR Malnutrition

❖ PATHOPHYSIOLOGY

Protein-energy malnutrition (PEM), also known as **protein-calorie malnutrition (PCM),** may present in three forms:

Marasmus: a calorie malnutrition in which body fat and protein are wasted. Serum proteins are often preserved.

Kwashiorkor: a lack of protein quantity and quality in the presence of adequate calories. Body weight is more normal, and serum proteins are low.

Marasmic-kwashiorkor: a combined protein and energy malnutrition. This problem often presents clinically when metabolic stress is imposed on a chronically starved patient.

The outcome of unrecognized or untreated PEM is often dysfunction or disability and increased morbidity and mortality.

Malnutrition (also called *undernutrition*) is a multinutrient problem because foods that are good sources of calories and protein are also good sources of other nutrients. In the malnourished patient many problems may be identified such as:

- Protein catabolism that exceeds protein intake and synthesis
- Negative nitrogen balance
- Weight loss
- Decreased muscle mass
- Weakness
- Decrease in serum proteins (**hypoproteinemia**) as protein synthesis in the liver decreases
- Vital capacity reduced as a result of respiratory muscle atrophy
- Diminished cardiac output
- Malabsorption because of atrophy of GI mucosa and the loss of intestinal villi

Common complications of *severe* malnutrition in adults include:

- Leanness and cachexia (muscle wasting with prolonged malnutrition)
- Decreased activity tolerance
- Lethargy
- Intolerance to cold
- Edema
- Dry, flaking skin and various types of dermatitis
- Poor wound healing
- Infection, particularly postoperative infection and sepsis
- Possible death

Malnutrition results from inadequate nutrient intake, increased nutrient losses, and increased nutrient requirements. Inadequate nutrient intake can be linked to:

- Poverty
- Lack of education
- Substance abuse
- Decreased appetite
- Vomiting
- Decline in functional ability to eat independently
- Infectious diseases, such as tuberculosis and human immune deficiency virus (HIV) infection
- Diseases that produce diarrhea and infections leading to anorexia. (Anorexia then leads to poor food intake.)
- Medical treatments such as chemotherapy
- Catabolic processes, such as prolonged immobility, that increase nutrient requirements and metabolic losses

Inadequate nutrient intake can also result when an adult is admitted to the hospital or long-term care facility. For example, decreased staffing may not allow time for patients who need to be fed, especially older adults, who may eat slowly. Many diagnostic tests, surgery, trauma, and unexpected medical complications require a period of NPO or cause anorexia (loss of appetite).

🌐 CULTURAL/SPIRITUAL CONSIDERATIONS
Patient-Centered Care QSEN

In some cases, malnutrition results when the provided meals are different from what the patient usually eats. Be sure to identify specific food preferences that the patient can eat and enjoy that are in keeping with his or her cultural practices.

CONSIDERATIONS FOR OLDER ADULTS
Patient-Centered Care QSEN

Older adults in the community or in any health care setting are most at risk for poor nutrition, especially PEM. Risk factors include physiologic changes of aging, environmental factors, and health problems. Chart 60-2 lists some of these major factors. Chapter 3 discusses NUTRITION for older adults in more detail.

Acute PEM may develop in patients who were adequately nourished before hospitalization but experience starvation while in a catabolic state from infection, stress, or injury. *Chronic* PEM can occur in those who have cancer, end-stage kidney or liver disease, or chronic neurologic disease.

Eating disorders such as anorexia nervosa and bulimia nervosa, which are seen most often in teens and young adults, also lead to malnutrition. Anorexia nervosa is a self-induced starvation resulting from a fear of fatness, even though the

---

CHART 60-2 Nursing Focus on the Older Adult
Risk Assessment for Malnutrition

Assess for:
- Decreased appetite
- Weight loss
- Poor-fitting or no dentures/poor dental health
- Poor eyesight
- Dry mouth
- Limited income
- Lack of transportation
- Inability to prepare meals because of functional decline or fatigue
- Loneliness and/or depression
- Chronic constipation (e.g., in patients with Alzheimer's disease)
- Decreased meal enjoyment
- Chronic physical illness
- "Failure to thrive" (a combination of three of five symptoms, including weakness, slow walking speed, low physical activity, unintentional weight loss, exhaustion)
- Prescription and over-the-counter (OTC) drugs (including herbs, vitamins, and minerals)
- Acute or chronic pain

---

patient is underweight. Bulimia nervosa is characterized by episodes of binge eating in which the patient ingests a large amount of food in a short time. The binge eating is followed by some form of purging behavior, such as self-induced vomiting or excessive use of laxatives and diuretics. If not treated, death can result from starvation, infection, or suicide. Information about eating disorders can be found in textbooks on mental/behavioral health nursing.

Health Promotion and Maintenance

One in three patients in health care settings is malnourished. This may be caused by inadequate intake before being hospitalized or lack of nutrition while hospitalized because of the illness or injury. Those diagnosed with malnutrition have a length of stay that may be three times higher than those who do not have altered nutrition. The annual burden of disease-associated malnutrition across eight diseases in the United States is over $156 billion (American Society for Parenteral and Enteral Nutrition [ASPEN], 2016). Nurses can have a significant impact on patient length of stay when adequately advocating for their client's nutrition status.

Incidence and Prevalence

At the World Food Summit in 1996, a target was set to reduce the number of undernourished people in the world by 50% by 2015 (Bhutta, 2013). At that time, an estimated 824 million people were undernourished (Bhutta, 2013). In 2010, it was estimated that 925 million people worldwide were undernourished (Bhutta, 2013).

❖ INTERPROFESSIONAL COLLABORATIVE CARE

Care for the patient with malnutrition takes place in a variety of settings (i.e., the home, the community, and the hospital setting) if more comprehensive management is needed. Members of the interprofessional team who collaborate most closely to care for the patient with malnutrition include the health care provider, nurse, and dietitian. For patients who experience psychological impact from or related to malnutrition, a psychologist or therapist will also have in important role in care.

Assessment: Noticing

History. Review the medical history to determine the possibility of increased metabolic needs or NUTRITION losses, chronic disease, trauma, recent surgery of the GI tract, drug and alcohol use, and recent significant weight loss. Each of these conditions can contribute to malnutrition. For older adults, explore mental status changes; note poor eyesight, diseases affecting major organs, constipation or incontinence, and slowed reactions. Review prescription and over-the-counter (OTC) drugs, including vitamin, mineral, herbal, and other nutrition supplements.

For patients who live independently in the community, the nurse may assess their performance of *instrumental activities of daily living* (IADLs). Functional status can best be evaluated for institutionalized patients by assessing their ADL performance. Poor NUTRITION is a major contributing factor to decreased functional ability.

In collaboration with the dietitian, obtain information about the patient's:

- Usual daily food intake
- Eating behaviors
- Change in appetite
- Recent weight changes.

Ask the patient or family if patient cannot communicate, about:

- Usual foods eaten
- Cultural food preferences
- Times of meals and snacks

The dietitian can more thoroughly analyze the diet, if necessary, based on your initial nutrition screening.

Ask about changes in eating habits as a result of illness and document any change in appetite, taste, and weight loss. A weight loss of 5% or more in 30 days, a weight loss of 10% in 6 months, or a weight that is below ideal may indicate malnutrition.

> **⚠ NURSING SAFETY PRIORITY** QSEN
>
> **Action Alert**
>
> When assessing for malnutrition, assess for difficulty or pain chewing or swallowing. Unrecognized dysphagia is a common problem among nursing home residents and can cause malnutrition, dehydration, and aspiration pneumonia. Ask the patient whether any foods are avoided and why. Ask UAP to report any choking while the patient eats. Record the occurrence of nausea, vomiting, heartburn, or any other symptoms of discomfort with eating.

Ask the patient about dental health problems, including the presence of dentures. Dentures or partial plates that do not fit well interfere with food intake. Dental caries (decay) or missing teeth may also cause discomfort while eating.

Physical Assessment/Signs and Symptoms. Assess for signs and symptoms of various nutrient deficiencies (Table 60-2). Inspect the patient's hair, eyes, oral cavity, nails, and musculoskeletal and neurologic systems. Examine the condition of the skin, including any reddened or open areas. Anthropometric measurements may also be obtained as described in the section of the same name. The nurse or UAP monitors all food and fluid intake and notes any mouth pain or difficulty chewing or swallowing. A 3-day caloric intake may be collected and then calculated by the dietitian.

Psychosocial Assessment. The psychosocial history provides information about the patient's economic status, occupation, educational level, gender orientation, ethnicity/race, living and cooking arrangements, and mental status. Determine whether financial resources are adequate for providing the necessary food. If resources are inadequate, the social worker or case manager may refer the patient and family to available community services. Chapter 3 discusses NUTRITION in older adults in more detail.

Laboratory Assessment. Laboratory tests supply objective data that can support subjective data and identify deficiencies. Interpret laboratory data carefully with regard to the total patient; focusing on an isolated value may yield an inaccurate conclusion.

A low *hemoglobin* level may indicate anemia, recent hemorrhage, or hemodilution caused by fluid retention. Hemoglobin may also be decreased secondary to conditions such as low serum albumin, infection, catabolism, or chronic disease. High levels may indicate hemoconcentration or dehydration or may be found secondary to liver disease.

Low *hematocrit* levels may reflect anemia, hemorrhage, excessive fluid, renal disease, or cirrhosis. High hematocrit levels may indicate dehydration or hemoconcentration.

Serum albumin, thyroxine-binding prealbumin, and transferrin are measures of **visceral proteins**. Serum *albumin* is a plasma protein that reflects the nutrition status of the patient a few weeks before testing; therefore it is not considered to be a sensitive test. Patients who are dehydrated often have high levels of albumin, and those with fluid excess have a lowered value. The normal serum albumin level for men and women is 3.5 to 5.0 g/dL or 35 to 50 g/L (SI units) (Pagana et al., 2017).

Thyroxine-binding **prealbumin (PAB)** is a plasma protein that provides a more sensitive indicator of nutrition deficiency because of its short half-life of 2 days. Depending on the laboratory test used, the normal PAB range is 15 to 36 mg/dL or 150 to 360 mg/L (SI units) (Pagana et al., 2017). Although not used as commonly, serum **transferrin**, an iron-transport protein, can be measured directly or calculated as an indirect measurement of total iron-binding capacity (TIBC). It has a short half-life of 8 to 10 days and therefore is also a more sensitive indicator of protein status than albumin.

Cholesterol levels normally range between 160 and 200 mg/dL in adult men and women. Values are typically low with malabsorption, liver disease, pernicious anemia, end-stage cancer, or sepsis. A cholesterol level below 160 mg/dL has been identified as a possible indicator of malnutrition. Cholesterol levels are discussed in more detail in Chapter 36.

Total lymphocyte count (TLC) can be used to assess immune function. Malnutrition suppresses the immune system and leaves the patient more likely to get an infection. When a patient is malnourished, the TLC is usually decreased to below 1500/mm^3.

Analysis: Interpreting

The priority collaborative problem for the patient with malnutrition is:

1. Weight loss due to inability to ingest or digest food or absorb nutrients

Planning and Implementation: Responding

Improving Nutrition

Planning: Expected Outcomes. The patient with malnutrition is expected to have nutrients available to meet his or her

TABLE 60-2   Manifestations of Nutrient Deficiencies

SIGN/SYMPTOM	POTENTIAL NUTRIENT DEFICIENCY	SIGN/SYMPTOM	POTENTIAL NUTRIENT DEFICIENCY
Hair		**Extremities**	
Alopecia	Zinc	Subcutaneous fat loss	Calories
Easy to remove	Protein	Muscle wastage	Calories, protein
Lackluster hair	Protein	Edema	Protein
"Corkscrew" hair	Vitamin C	Osteomalacia, bone pain, rickets	Vitamin D
Decreased pigmentation	Protein	**Hematologic**	
Eyes		Anemia	Vitamin B_{12}, iron, folic acid, copper, vitamin E
Xerosis of conjunctiva	Vitamin A	Leukopenia, neutropenia	Copper
Corneal vascularization	Riboflavin	Low prothrombin time, prolonged clotting time	Vitamin K, manganese
Keratomalacia	Vitamin A	**Neurologic**	
Bitot's spots	Vitamin A	Disorientation	Niacin, thiamine
GI Tract		Confabulation	Thiamine
Nausea, vomiting	Pyridoxine	Neuropathy	Thiamine, pyridoxine, chromium
Diarrhea	Zinc, niacin	Paresthesia	Thiamine, pyridoxine, vitamin B_{12}
Stomatitis	Pyridoxine, riboflavin, iron	**Cardiovascular**	
Cheilosis	Pyridoxine, iron	Congestive heart failure, cardiomegaly, tachycardia	Thiamine
Glossitis	Pyridoxine, zinc, niacin, folic acid, vitamin B_{12}	Cardiomyopathy	Selenium
Magenta tongue	Vitamin A, riboflavin	Cardiac dysrhythmias	Magnesium
Swollen, bleeding gums	Vitamin C		
Fissured tongue	Niacin		
Hepatomegaly	Protein		
Skin			
Dry and scaling	Vitamin A		
Petechiae/ecchymoses	Vitamin C		
Follicular hyperkeratosis	Vitamin A		
Nasolabial seborrhea	Niacin		
Bilateral dermatitis	Niacin		

Courtesy Ross Products Division, Abbott Laboratories, Columbus, OH.

metabolic needs as evidenced by normal serum proteins and adequate hydration.

Interventions. The preferred route for food intake is through the GI tract because it enhances the immune system and is safer, easier, less expensive, and more enjoyable.

Meal Management. The dietitian calculates the nutrients required daily and plans the patient's diet. In collaboration with the health care provider and dietitian, provide high-calorie, nutrient-rich foods (e.g., milkshakes, cheese, supplement drinks such as Boost or Ensure). Assess the patient's food likes and dislikes. A feeding schedule of six small meals may be tolerated better than three large ones. A pureed or dental soft diet may be easier for those who have problems chewing or are edentulous (toothless).

Nutrition Supplements. If the patient cannot take in enough nutrients in food, fortified medical nutrition supplements (MNSs) (e.g., Ensure, Sustacal, Carnation Instant Breakfast [also available as lactose-free supplement]) may be given, especially to older adults. Many commercial enteral products

! NURSING SAFETY PRIORITY QSEN
Action Alert

Malnourished ill patients often need to be encouraged to eat. Instruct UAP who are feeding patients to keep food at the appropriate temperature and to provide mouth care before feeding. Assess for other needs, such as pain management, and provide interventions to make the patient comfortable. Pain can prevent patients from enjoying their meals. Remove bedpans, urinals, and emesis basins from sight. Provide a quiet environment, which is conducive to eating. Soft music may calm those with advanced dementia or delirium. Appropriate time should be taken so the patient does not feel rushed through a meal.

are available. For patients with medical diagnoses such as liver and renal disease or diabetes, special products that meet these needs are available (e.g., Glucerna for patients with diabetes). Nutrition supplements used in acute care, long-term care, and home care can be costly. In addition, patients may refuse them, and the supplements are then wasted. In a classic study, Bender

CONSIDERATIONS FOR OLDER ADULTS
Patient-Centered Care (QSEN)

Some patients, especially older adults, may take a long time to eat even small quantities of food because they tend to be less hungry than younger adults. If available, suggest that family members bring in favorite or ethnic foods that the patient might be more likely to eat. Teach them about ways to encourage the patient to increase food intake. Chart 60-3 describes additional interventions to promote food intake in older adults.

Restorative feeding programs help nursing home residents who need special assistance. These residents often eat in a separate dining area so time and attention can be given to them. Some nursing homes have designated food and nutrition nursing assistants and/or trained volunteers who are primarily responsible for promoting and maintaining nutrition and hydration. Delegate and supervise appropriate feeding tasks to UAPs during resident mealtime.

et al. (2000) found that a more successful alternative to having the MNS given by nursing assistant staff in the nursing home was to have the supplements delivered by nurses during their usual medication passes. In this study, the nurses gave 60 mL or more of the MNS at least four times a day with the residents'

CHART 60-3 Nursing Focus on the Older Adult
Promoting Nutrition Intake

- Be sure that patient is toileted and receives mouth care before mealtime.
- Be sure that patient has glasses and hearing aids in place, if appropriate, during meals.
- Be sure that bedpans, urinals, and emesis basins are removed from sight.
- Give analgesics to control pain and/or antiemetics for nausea at least 1 hour before mealtime.
- Remind unlicensed assistive personnel (UAP) to have patient sit in chair, if possible, at mealtime.
- If needed, open cartons and packages and cut up food at the patient's and/or family's request.
- Observe the patient during meals for food intake.
- Ask the patient about food likes and dislikes and ethnic food preferences.
- Encourage self-feeding or feed the patient slowly; *delegate* this activity to UAP if desired and provide appropriate supervision.
- If feeding patient, sit at eye level if culturally appropriate.
- Create an environment that is conducive to eating and socialization and relaxation, if possible.
- Decrease distractions, such as environmental noise from television, music, or other people.
- Provide adequate, nonglaring lighting.
- Keep patient away from offensive or medicinal odors.
- Keep eye contact with the patient during the meal if culturally appropriate.
- Serve snacks with activities, especially in long-term care settings; *delegate* this activity to UAP if desired.
- Document the percentage of food eaten at each meal and snack; *delegate* this activity to UAP if appropriate.
- Ensure that meals are visually appealing, appetizing, appropriately warm or cold, and properly prepared.
- Do not interrupt patients during mealtime for nonurgent procedures or rounds.
- Assess for need for supplements between meals and at bedtime.
- Review the patient's drug profile and discuss with the health care provider the use of drugs that might be suppressing appetite.
- If the patient is depressed, be sure that the depression is treated by the health care provider.

medications. As a result, the patients gained weight and had fewer pressure injuries, thus making the program very cost-effective and providing positive clinical outcomes.

NUTRITION supplements are supplied as liquid formulas, powders, soups, coffee, and puddings in a variety of flavors. They come in different degrees of sweetness and are also available as modular supplements that provide single nutrients. Examples of modular supplements are Polycose glucose polymers for carbohydrates and Resource Beneprotein for protein, both available in liquid and powder form. Carbohydrate modulars are useful only if additional calories are needed. Protein modulars are indicated when metabolic stress causes a need for higher protein intake.

The dietitian may ask the nursing staff to keep a food and fluid intake record for at least 3 consecutive days to help assess the patient's nutrition status. Delegate this activity to UAP under your ongoing supervision. UAPs also weigh the patient daily, every 3 days, or once a week, depending on the health care setting and severity of malnutrition; review this information, and supervise and intervene accordingly.

Drug Therapy. Multivitamins, zinc, and an iron preparation are often prescribed to treat or prevent anemia. Monitor the patient's hemoglobin and hematocrit levels. Drug therapy can affect nutrition and elimination. For example, iron can cause constipation, and zinc can cause nausea and vomiting.

If the patient still does not receive enough nutrition by mouth using the interventions just mentioned, request nutrition therapy in the form of **specialized nutrition support (SNS)**. SNS consists of either total enteral nutrition (TEN) or total parenteral nutrition (TPN).

Total Enteral Nutrition. Patients often cannot meet the desired outcomes of adequate nutrition via their usual oral intake because of increased metabolic demands or a decreased ability to eat. Therefore TEN using enteral tube feeding may be necessary to supplement oral intake or to provide total nutrition.

Patients likely to receive TEN can be divided into three groups:

- Those who can eat but cannot maintain adequate NUTRITION by oral intake of food alone
- Those who have permanent neuromuscular impairment and cannot swallow
- Those who do not have permanent neuromuscular impairment but cannot eat because of their condition

Patients in the first group are often older adults or patients receiving cancer treatment who cannot meet their calorie and protein needs. In some cases, this artificial nutrition and hydration may not be desired. For example, some patients have advance directives stating that they do not want to be kept alive by artificial nutrition and hydration if certain conditions exist. *However, legal and ethical questions arise when patients are not able to make their wishes known!*

For many years it was believed that withholding food and fluids would cause discomfort. Terminally or chronically ill patients who do not eat and drink may not suffer. In fact, they may be more comfortable if food and fluids are withheld. *The decision to feed is complex, and there is no clear right or wrong answer. To compound this legal and ethical dilemma, medical complications (e.g., aspiration, pressure injuries) are common in older adults who are tube-fed.*

Decisions about these dilemmas are aided by the advice of interdisciplinary ethics committees in health care facilities. When clinicians are making decisions about the desirability of tube feedings in these cases, the focus should be on achieving consensus by:

- Reviewing what is known about tube feedings, especially their risks and benefits
- Reviewing the medical facts about the patient
- Investigating any available evidence that would help understand the patient's wishes
- Obtaining the opinions of all stakeholders in the situation
- Delaying any action until consensus is achieved

Those in the second group of patients likely to receive TEN usually have permanent swallowing problems and require some type of feeding tube for delivery of the enteral product on a long-term basis. Examples of conditions that can cause permanent swallowing problems are strokes, severe head trauma, and advanced multiple sclerosis. Patients in the third group receive enteral NUTRITION for as long as their illness lasts. The feeding is discontinued when the patient's condition improves and he or she can eat again. Many commercially prepared enteral products are available. A therapeutic combination of carbohydrates, fat, vitamins, minerals, and trace elements is available in liquid form. Differences among products allow the dietitian to select the right formula for each patient. A prescription from the health care provider is required for enteral nutrition, but the dietitian usually makes the recommendation and computes the amount and type of product needed for each patient.

Methods of Administering Total Enteral Nutrition. TEN is administered as "tube feedings" through one of the available GI tubes, either through a nasoenteric or enterostomal tube. It can be used in the patient's home or any health care setting.

A **nasoenteric tube (NET)** is any feeding tube inserted nasally and then advanced into the GI tract, such as a Keofeed, Entriflex, or Dobbhoff tube. Commonly used NETs include the

nasogastric (NG) tube and the smaller (small-bore) **nasoduodenal tube (NDT)** (Fig. 60-3A).

A nasojejunal tube (NJT) is also available but is used less often than the other NETs.

The NDTs are used for delivering *short-term* enteral feedings (usually less than 4 weeks) because they are easy to use and safer for the patient at risk for aspiration *if the tip of the tube is placed below the pyloric sphincter of the stomach and into the duodenum.* Small-bore polyurethane or silicone tubes from 8 to 12 Fr external diameter are preferred. The smaller tubes are more comfortable and are less likely to cause complications such as nasal irritation, sinusitis, tissue erosion, and pulmonary compromise.

Enterostomal feeding tubes are used for patients who need *long-term* enteral feeding. The most common types are

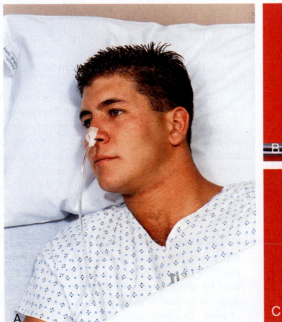
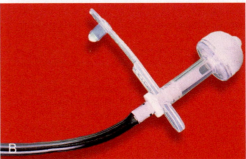
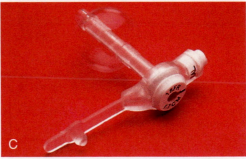

FIG. 60-3 Feeding tubes used for total enteral nutrition. **A,** Nasoduodenal tube. **B** and **C,** Gastrostomy tubes. (**A** from Lilley, L., Rainforth Collins, S., Harrington, S., & Snyder, J. [2011]. *Pharmacology and the nursing process* [6th ed.]. St. Louis: Mosby; **B** from Harkreader, H. [2007]). *Fundamentals of nursing* [3rd ed.]. St. Louis: Saunders; courtesy C.R. Bard, Inc., Billerica, MA; **C** from Harkreader, H. [2007]. *Fundamentals of nursing* [3rd ed.]. St. Louis: Saunders; courtesy Ballard Medical Products, Draper, UT.)

gastrostomies and jejunostomies. The surgeon directly accesses the GI tract using various surgical, endoscopic, and laparoscopic techniques.

A **gastrostomy** is a stoma created from the abdominal wall into the stomach, through which a short feeding tube is inserted by the surgeon. It may require a small abdominal incision or be placed endoscopically. This tube is called a **percutaneous endoscopic gastrostomy (PEG)** or dual-access gastrostomy-jejunostomy (PEG/J) tube. The PEG requires monitored conscious sedation for placement and is secure and durable. An alternative to either device is the **low-profile gastrostomy device (LPGD)** (Fig. 60-3B-C). The LPGD is available with a firm or balloon-style internal bumper or retention disk. An anti-reflux valve keeps GI contents from leaking onto the skin. This device is less irritating to the skin, longer lasting, and more cosmetically pleasing. It also allows greater patient independence. However, skin-level devices do not allow easy access for checking **residuals** (the amount of feeding that remains in the stomach).

Jejunostomies are used less often than gastrostomies. A **jejunostomy** is used for long-term feedings when it is desirable to bypass the stomach, such as with gastric disease, upper GI obstruction, and abnormal gastric or duodenal emptying.

Tube feedings are administered by bolus feeding, continuous feeding, and cyclic feeding. **Bolus feeding** is an intermittent feeding of a specified amount of enteral product at set intervals during a 24-hour period, typically every 4 hours. This method can be accomplished manually or by infusion through a mechanical pump or controller device. Another method of tube feeding is continuous enteral feeding. **Continuous feeding** is similar to IV therapy in that small amounts are continuously infused (by gravity drip or by a pump or controller device) over a specified time. The most commonly seen method, **cyclic feeding**, is the same as continuous feeding except that the infusion is stopped for a specified time in each 24-hour period, usually 6 hours or longer ("down time"). Down time typically occurs in the morning to allow bathing, treatments, and other activities.

Infusion rates for cyclic feedings (and to some extent for intermittent bolus feeding) vary with the total amount of solution to be infused, the specific composition of the product, and the response of the patient to the feeding. The health care provider and dietitian usually decide the type, rate, and method of tube feeding, as well as the amount of additional water ("free water") needed. If the patient can swallow small amounts of food, he or she may also eat orally while the tube is in place.

The nurse is responsible for the care and maintenance of the feeding tube and the enteral feeding. Chart 60-4 lists best practices for the patient receiving TEN.

Complications of Total Enteral Nutrition. The nursing priority for care is patient safety, including preventing, assessing, and managing complications associated with tube feeding. Some complications of therapy result from the type of tube used to administer the feeding, and others result from the enteral product itself. The most common problem is the development of an obstructed ("clogged") tube. Use the tips in Chart 60-5 to maintain tube patency.

Patients receiving TEN are at risk for several other complications, including refeeding syndrome; tube misplacement and dislodgment; abdominal distention and nausea/vomiting; and FLUID AND ELECTROLYTE imbalance, often associated with

---

◎ CHART 60-4 Best Practice for Patient Safety & Quality Care QSEN

Tube-Feeding Care and Maintenance

- If nasogastric or nasoduodenal feeding is prescribed, use a soft, flexible, small-bore feeding tube (smaller than 12 Fr). *The initial placement of the tube should be confirmed by x-ray study.* Secure the tube with tape or a commercial attachment device after applying a skin protectant; change the tape regularly.
- Check tube placement by x-ray study when the correct position of the tube is in question; *an x-ray study is the most reliable method.*
- **Per The Joint Commission's National Patient Safety Goals, if a gastrostomy or jejunostomy tube is used, assess the insertion site for signs of infection or excoriation (e.g., excessive redness, drainage). Rotate the tube 360 degrees each day and check for in-and-out play of about ¼ inch (0.6 cm). If the tube cannot be moved, notify the health care provider immediately because the retention disk may be embedded in the tissue. Cover the site with a dry, sterile dressing and change the dressing at least once a day.**
- Check and record the residual volume every 4 to 6 hours or per facility policy by aspirating stomach contents into a syringe. If residual feeding is obtained, check with the health care provider for the appropriate intervention (usually to slow or stop the feeding for a time) or use the American Society of Parenteral and Enteral Nutrition (ASPEN) best practice recommendations.
- Check the feeding pump to ensure proper mechanical operation.
- Ensure that the enteral product is infused at the prescribed rate (mL/hr).
- Change the feeding bag and tubing every 24 to 48 hours; label the bag with the date and time of the change with your initials. Use an irrigation set for no more than 24 hours.
- For continuous or cyclic feeding, add only 4 hours of product to the bag at a time to prevent bacterial growth. *A closed system is preferred, and each set should be used no longer than 24 hours.*
- Wear clean gloves when changing or opening the feeding system or adding product; wipe the lid of the formula can with clean gauze; wear sterile gloves for critically ill or immunocompromised patients.
- Label open cans with date and time opened; cover and keep refrigerated. Discard any unused open cans after 24 hours.
- *Do not use blue (or any color) food dye in formula because it does not assess aspiration and can cause serious complications.*
- To prevent aspiration, keep the head of the bed elevated at least 30 degrees during the feeding and for at least 1 hour after the feeding for bolus feeding; continuously maintain semi-Fowler's position for patients receiving cyclic or continuous feeding.
- Monitor laboratory values, especially blood urea nitrogen (BUN), serum electrolytes, hematocrit, prealbumin, and glucose.
- Monitor for complications of tube feeding, especially diarrhea.
- Monitor and carefully record the patient's weight and intake and output as requested by the physician or dietitian.

---

diarrhea. These problems can be prevented if the patient is monitored carefully and complications are detected early.

Refeeding Syndrome. **Refeeding syndrome** is a potentially life-threatening metabolic complication that can occur when nutrition is restarted for a patient who is in a *starvation* state. When a patient is starved for nutrition, the body breaks down fat and protein, rather than carbohydrates, for energy. Protein catabolism leads to muscle and cell loss, often in major organs such as the heart, liver, and lungs. The body's cells lose valuable electrolytes, including potassium and phosphate, into the plasma. Insulin secretion decreases in response to these changes. When *refeeding* begins, insulin production resumes; and the cells take up glucose and electrolytes from the bloodstream, thus depleting serum levels.

CHART 60-5 Best Practice for Patient Safety & Quality Care QSEN

Maintaining a Patent Feeding Tube

- Flush the tube with 20 to 30 mL of water (or the amount prescribed by the health care provider or dietitian):
  - At least every 4 hours during a continuous tube feeding
  - Before and after each intermittent tube feeding
  - Before and after drug administration (use warm water)
  - After checking residual volume
- If the tube becomes clogged, use 30 mL of water for flushing, applying gentle pressure with a 50-mL piston syringe.
- Avoid the use of a carbonated beverage, except for existing clogs *when water is not effective.* Do not use cranberry juice.
- Whenever possible, use liquid medications instead of crushed tablets unless liquid forms cause diarrhea; make sure that the drug is compatible with the feeding solution.
- Do not mix drugs with the feeding product before giving. Crush tablets as finely as possible and dissolve in warm water. *(Check to see which tablets are safe to crush. For example, do not crush slow-acting [SA] or slow-release [SR] drugs.)*
- Consider use of automatic-flush feeding pump such as Flexiflo or Kangaroo.

! NURSING SAFETY PRIORITY QSEN

Critical Rescue

Recognize that the electrolyte shift of refeeding syndrome can cause cardiovascular, respiratory, and neurologic problems, primarily as a result of hypophosphatemia, according to a classic study by Mehanna et al. (2008). Observe for signs and symptoms to recognize this electrolyte imbalance, including shallow respirations, weakness, acute confusion, seizures, and increased bleeding tendency. Respond by reporting to the health care provider and documenting your findings immediately. More information on FLUID AND ELECTROLYTE imbalance can be found in Chapter 11.

Refeeding syndrome can be prevented if patients are carefully assessed and managed for nutrition needs. Interventions to supplement or replace NUTRITION should be implemented early before the patient is in a starvation state. Patients receiving parenteral nutrition (described later in this chapter) also may experience refeeding syndrome.

Tube Misplacement and Dislodgment. A serious complication is misplacement or dislodgment of the tube, *which can cause aspiration and possible death. Immediately remove any tube that you suspect is dislodged!* **The Joint Commission's National Patient Safety Goals and the Centers for Medicare and Medicaid Services require all health care facilities to establish and implement procedures and systems to prevent patient harm from medical complications.**

Several techniques should be used to confirm proper placement to prevent harm and to keep the patient safe. *An x-ray is the most accurate confirmation method and should always be done on initial tube insertion.* After the initial placement is confirmed, check the placement before each intermittent feeding or at least every 4 to 8 hours during feeding. Also check placement before each drug administration.

The traditional auscultatory method for checking tube placement may not be reliable, especially for patients with small-bore tubes. In this method, the nurse instills 20 to 30 mL of air into the tube ("insufflation") while listening over the epigastric area

(stomach) with a stethoscope. *The resulting "whooshing" sound does not guarantee correct tube placement!*

Several safer procedures have been recommended for checking tube placement *after the initial placement has been confirmed by x-ray.* These methods include:

- Testing aspirated contents for pH, bilirubin, trypsin, or pepsin
- Assessing for carbon dioxide using capnometry

Some hospitals and nursing homes support testing the *pH of GI contents* at the bedside. To perform this procedure, aspirate a sample of the GI content, observe its color, and test its pH. When aspirating fluid, wait at least 1 hour after drug administration and then flush the tube with 20 mL of air to clear it. Collect the aspirate and test it with pH paper. The pH of gastric fluid ranges from 0 to 4.0. If the tube has moved down into the intestines, the pH will be between 7.0 and 8.0. If the tube is in the lungs, the pH will be greater than 6.0. The pH may also be as high as 6.0 if the patient takes certain drugs, such as H_2 blockers (e.g., ranitidine [Zantac] and famotidine [Pepcid]). Because these drugs affect pH, bilirubin testing or capnometry may be a more reliable and valid method for predicting tube location.

Capnometry can determine if carbon dioxide is emitted from the tube (Kodali & Urman, 2014). A device to measure the presence of the gas is attached to the end of the tube after placement. The test is positive for carbon dioxide if the tube is placed into the lungs rather than the stomach. *The tube should be removed immediately if the gas is detected.*

! NURSING SAFETY PRIORITY QSEN

Action Alert

If enteral tubes are misplaced or become dislodged, the patient is likely to aspirate. Aspiration pneumonia is a life-threatening complication associated with TEN, especially for older adults. Observe for increasing temperature and pulse and for other signs of dehydration such as dry mucous membranes and decreased urinary output. Auscultate lungs every 4 to 8 hours to check for diminishing breath sounds, especially in lower lobes. Patients may become short of breath and report chest discomfort. A chest x-ray confirms this diagnosis, and treatment with antibiotics is started.

Abdominal Distention and Nausea/Vomiting. Abdominal distention, nausea, and vomiting during tube feeding are often caused by overfeeding. To *prevent* overfeeding, check gastric residual volumes every 4 to 6 hours, depending on facility policy and the needs of the patient. The American Society of Parenteral and Enteral Nutrition (ASPEN) (2011) recommends holding a feeding if the gastric residual volumes are more than 200 mL on two consecutive assessments. In some facilities, feedings are temporarily held if the gastric residual is 100 mL or more, depending on the patient. After a period of rest, the feeding can be restarted at a lower flow rate.

Fluid and Electrolyte Imbalances. Patients receiving enteral nutrition therapy are at an increased risk for fluid imbalances. They are often older or debilitated and may also have cardiac or renal problems. Fluid imbalances associated with enteral nutrition are usually related to the body's response to increased serum osmolarity, but *fluid overload* from too much tube feeding can also occur.

Osmolarity is the amount or concentration of particles dissolved in solution. This concentration exerts a specific osmotic pressure within the solution. Normal osmolarity of extracellular fluid (ECF) ranges between 270 and 300 mOsm. Enteral feeding products range in osmolarity from isotonic (about 300 mOsm) to extremely hypertonic (600 mOsm). Electrolytes (including sodium) contribute to this hypertonicity, but more of the osmolarity is determined by the concentration of proteins and sugar molecules in the enteral product. Even when the product is isotonic, the ECF can become hyperosmolar unless some hypotonic fluids are also administered to the patient. This situation is most likely to develop in patients who are unconscious, unable to respond to the thirst reflex, on fluid restrictions, or receiving hyperosmotic enteral preparations.

Because increased plasma osmolarity is largely a result of extra glucose and proteins (which tend to remain in the plasma rather than move to interstitial spaces), the plasma osmotic pressure (water-pulling pressure) is increased. In this situation, intracellular and interstitial water move into and expand the plasma volume. This volume expansion results in an increased renal excretion of water (in patients with normal renal function) and leads to osmotic *dehydration*.

CONSIDERATIONS FOR OLDER ADULTS
Patient-Centered Care QSEN

If patients do *not* have normal renal and cardiac function, expansion of the plasma volume can lead to circulatory overload and pulmonary edema, especially in older adults. Therefore early identification of patients at risk for impairment of renal and/or cardiac function is important. Assess for signs and symptoms of circulatory overload, such as peripheral edema, sudden weight gain, crackles, dyspnea, increased blood pressure, and bounding pulse. Collaborate with the dietitian and health care provider to plan the correct amount of fluid to be provided.

Excessive *diarrhea* may develop when hyperosmolar enteral preparations are delivered quickly. This situation can also lead to *dehydration* through excessive water loss. Collaborate with the health care provider and dietitian for recommendations to prevent diarrhea. The dietitian usually changes the feeding to a more iso-osmolar formula. Most of these formulas can be started full strength but slowly at 15 to 20 mL/hr. The rate is gradually increased as the patient tolerates and as the expected nutrition outcome is achieved.

If diarrhea continues, especially if it has a very foul odor, evaluate the patient for *Clostridium difficile* or other infectious organisms. Contamination can occur because of repeated and often faulty handling of the feeding solution and system. **Per The Joint Commission's National Patient Safety Goals, wear clean gloves when changing systems and adding product. Sterile gloves may help prevent infection in critically ill or immunocompromised patients.** *A closed feeding system is preferred over an open one because the chance of contamination is lessened* (see Chart 60-4). Tubes with ports also minimize contamination by eliminating the need to open the feeding system to administer drugs.

In some cases, diarrhea may be the result of multiple liquid medications, such as elixirs and suspensions that have a very high osmolarity. Examples include acetaminophen (Tylenol), furosemide (Lasix), and phenytoin (Dilantin). Patients receiving multiple liquid drugs should be evaluated by the health care provider to determine whether their drug regimen can be

changed to prevent diarrhea. Diluting these liquids may also be an option.

Depending on the patient's state of health, some electrolyte imbalances can be avoided. This is achieved by the use of enteral preparations containing lower concentrations of the electrolytes that the patient cannot handle well. For example, renal patients with high potassium levels receive a special formula that is used for this imbalance.

The two most common electrolyte imbalances associated with enteral nutrition therapy are hyperkalemia and hyponatremia. Both of these conditions may be related to hyperglycemia-induced hyperosmolarity of the plasma and the resultant osmotic diuresis. Risks for disturbances in FLUID AND ELECTROLYTE BALANCE are discussed in detail in Chapter 11.

Parenteral Nutrition. When a patient cannot effectively use the GI tract for NUTRITION, either partial or total parenteral nutrition therapy may be needed. This form of IV therapy differs from standard IV therapy in that any or all nutrients (carbohydrates, proteins, fats, vitamins, minerals, and trace elements) can be given. One liter of IV fluid containing 5% dextrose, which is often used as standard therapy, provides only 170 kcal. A hospitalized patient typically receives 3 to 4 L a day, for a total number of calories ranging between 500 and 700 a day. This calorie intake is not sufficient when the patient requires IV therapy for a prolonged period and cannot eat an adequate diet or has increased calorie needs for tissue repair and building.

Partial Parenteral Nutrition. Partial, or peripheral, parenteral nutrition (PPN) is usually given through a cannula or catheter in a large distal vein of the arm or through a peripherally inserted central catheter (PICC line). (See Chapter 13 for care of patients with PICC lines.) The alternative is used for some patients who can eat but are not able to take in enough nutrients to meet their needs. The patient must have adequate peripheral vein access and be able to tolerate large volumes of fluid to have PPN. Two types of solutions are commonly used in various combinations for PPN: IV fat (lipid) emulsions (IVFEs) and amino acid–dextrose solutions. IVFEs are usually given using a piggyback method.

! NURSING SAFETY PRIORITY QSEN
Critical Rescue

Recognize that you must monitor patients receiving fat emulsions for fever, increased triglycerides, clotting problems, and multi-system organ failure to recognize indications of fat overload syndrome, especially in those who are critically ill. If any of these signs and symptoms is present, respond by discontinuing the IVFE infusion and reporting the changes to the health care provider immediately.

Most IVFEs (20% fat emulsion) are isotonic, but the tonicity of commercially prepared amino acid–dextrose solutions ranges from 300 mOsm to nearly 900 mOsm for PPN. Amino acid–dextrose solutions are considered more stable than IVFEs; therefore additives (e.g., vitamins, minerals, electrolytes, trace elements) tend to be mixed with them. These solutions must be delivered through an in-line filter and are administered by an infusion pump for an accurate and constant delivery rate.

Some PPN products are a *mixture* of lipids (10% or 20% fat emulsion) and an amino acid–dextrose (usually 10%) solution.

This mixture of three types of nutrients is referred to as a *3:1, total nutrient admixture (TNA)*, or *triple-mix solution*.

Total Parenteral Nutrition. When the patient requires intensive NUTRITION support for an extended time, the health care provider prescribes centrally administered **total parenteral nutrition (TPN)**. TPN is delivered through access to central veins, usually through a PICC line or the subclavian or internal jugular veins. Central venous catheters and associated nursing care are described in detail in Chapter 13.

Total parenteral nutrition solutions contain higher concentrations of dextrose and proteins, usually in the form of synthetic amino acids or protein hydrolysates (3% to 5%). These solutions are hyperosmotic (three to six times the osmolarity of normal blood). The base solutions are available as commercially prepared solutions. The hospital or community pharmacist adds components (specific electrolytes, minerals, trace elements, and insulin) according to the patient's nutrition needs. This therapy provides needed calories and spares body proteins from catabolism for energy requirements.

The TPN solutions are administered with an infusion pump. The osmolarity of the fluid and the concentrations of the specific components make controlled delivery essential.

Patients receiving parenteral nutrition fluids are at risk for a wide variety of serious and potentially life-threatening complications. Complications may result from the solutions or from the peripheral or central venous catheter. The following discussion is limited to the complications that involve FLUID AND ELECTROLYTE BALANCE. Complications of IV cannulas and central venous catheters are discussed in Chapter 13, including infection and sepsis.

Patients receiving parenteral nutrition therapy are at high risk for fluid imbalance. If the patient also has cardiac or renal dysfunction, he or she may develop fluid overload, congestive heart failure, and pulmonary edema. Monitor the infusion rate of the parenteral fluid, and give insulin as prescribed. Monitor for these complications by taking daily weights and documenting accurate intake and output while the patient is receiving parenteral nutrition. Serum glucose and electrolyte values are also monitored (Chart 60-6). Report any major changes or abnormalities to the health care provider and document all assessments and interventions.

Patients receiving TPN are at an increased risk for many different disturbances of FLUID AND ELECTROLYTE BALANCE, depending on the composition of the solution and whether a fluid imbalance occurs. The health care provider usually requests frequent determinations of serum electrolyte levels to detect these imbalances. The risk for metabolic and electrolyte complications is reduced when the rate of administration is carefully controlled and patients are closely monitored for response to treatment. Potassium and sodium imbalances are common, especially when insulin is also administered as part of the therapy. Calcium imbalances, particularly hypercalcemia, are associated with TPN.

Care Coordination and Transition Management

Malnourished patients can be cared for in a variety of settings, including the acute care hospital, transitional care unit, nursing home, or their own home. Malnutrition is often diagnosed when the patient is admitted to the acute care hospital or shortly after hospitalization if complications such as poor wound healing or sepsis occur. If the patient is severely compromised, he or she may require admission to a traditional nursing home for either transitional or long-term care. If adequate home support is

---

◎ CHART 60-6 Best Practice for Patient Safety & Quality Care QSEN

Care and Maintenance of Total Parenteral Nutrition

- Check each bag of total parenteral nutrition (TPN) solution for accuracy by comparing it with the physician's or pharmacist's prescription.
- Monitor the IV pump for accuracy in delivering the prescribed hourly rate.
- If the TPN solution is temporarily unavailable, give 10% dextrose/water ($D_{10}W$) or 20% dextrose/water ($D_{20}W$) until the TPN solution can be obtained.
- If the TPN administration is not on time ("behind"), do not attempt to "catch up" by increasing the rate.
- Monitor the patient's weight daily or according to facility protocol.
- Monitor serum electrolytes and glucose daily or per facility protocol. (Many facilities require fingerstick blood sugars [FSBSs] every 4 hours, especially if the patient is receiving insulin. Urine testing for ketones may also be requested.)
- Monitor for, report, and document complications, including fluid and electrolyte imbalances.
- Monitor and carefully record the patient's intake and output.
- Assess the patient's IV site for signs of infection or infiltration (see Chapter 13).
- Change the IV tubing every 24 hours or per facility protocol.
- Change the dressing around the IV site every 48 to 72 hours or per facility protocol.
- Before administering TPN, have a second nurse check the prescription and solution to prevent patient harm.

---

available, he or she may be discharged to home in the care of a family member or other caregiver. Home care nurses may be needed to monitor and direct the care.

Home Care Management. The malnourished patient needs a variety of resources at home to continue aggressive NUTRITION support. If he or she can consume food by the oral route, the case manager or other discharge planner determines whether financial resources are available for the necessary nutrition supplements. If the hospital provides ambulatory nutrition counseling services, the patient is scheduled for follow-up after discharge for assessment of weight gain.

Self-Management Education. The dietitian teaches the malnourished patient and family about high-calorie, high-protein diet and NUTRITION supplements. It is important to educate the patient and family about the following:

- Reinforce the importance of adhering to the prescribed diet.
- Review any drugs the patient may be taking.
- If using an iron preparation, teach the importance of taking the drug immediately before or during meals.
- Caution the patient that iron tends to cause constipation.
- For the patient already susceptible to constipation, emphasize the importance of measures for prevention, including adequate fiber intake, adequate fluids, and exercise. Teach the family or other caregiver how to continue these therapies.
- Remind caregivers to consider the psychosocial aspects of these alternative methods for nutrition.
- Moving the feeding equipment out of view of the patient when it is not in use is also helpful.

Health Care Resources. The malnourished patient discharged to home on enteral or parenteral nutrition support needs the specialized services of a home nutrition therapy team. This team generally consists of the physician, nurse, dietitian, pharmacist, and case manager or social worker. Several commercial companies supply these services to patients at home in addition to the feeding supplies and formulas and health teaching.

◆ Evaluation: Reflecting

Evaluate the care of the malnourished patient based on the identified priority patient problem. The primary expected outcome is that the patient consumes available nutrients to meet the metabolic demands for maintaining weight and total protein and has adequate hydration.

✳ NUTRITION CONCEPT EXEMPLAR Obesity

❖ PATHOPHYSIOLOGY

Obesity is not just one disease; it includes many conditions with varying causes. The terms *obesity* and *overweight* are often used interchangeably, but they refer to different health problems. For both problems, the patient often does not consume enough healthy nutrients and may not receive adequate NUTRITION. Overweight is an increase in body weight for height compared with a reference standard, or up to 10% greater than ideal body weight (IBW) and a body mass index (BMI) of 25 to 29. This weight may not reflect excess body fat. For example, well-developed athletes may appear overweight because of increased muscle (lean) mass, in which the proportion of muscle to fat is greater than average.

Obesity refers to an excess amount of body fat when compared with lean body mass. The normal amount of body fat in *men* is between 15% and 20% of body weight. For *women,* the normal amount is 18% to 32%. An obese adult weighs at least 20% above the upper limit of the normal range for ideal body weight and has a BMI of 30 or more. Morbid obesity refers to a weight that has a severely negative effect on health—usually more than 100% above IBW and a BMI over 40.

More than one third of Americans have obesity (CDC, 2016). About 10% or more of adults are morbidly obese. *This problem is the second leading cause of preventable deaths in the United States, second only to smoking, and has become a national crisis.* Obesity across the life span is considered an epidemic in the United States and Canada. Worldwide, it is recognized as a major global health problem, costing billions of dollars for health care and lost productivity.

The pathophysiology of obesity is very complex. A number of chemicals in the body, including hormones known as *adipokines,* work together to affect appetite and fat metabolism:

- **Leptin**: a hormone released by fat cells and possibly by gastric cells; it also acts on the hypothalamus to control appetite
- **Adiponectin**: an anti-inflammatory and insulin-sensitizing hormone
- **Resistin**: a hormone produced by fat cells that creates resistance to insulin activity
- **Inflammatory cytokines**: such as inflammatory interleukins and tumor necrosis factor–alpha
- **Apolipoprotein E**: one of several regulators of lipoprotein metabolism
- **Cholecystokinin**: a hormone that stimulates digestive juices and may work with leptin to increase or decrease appetite
- **Ghrelin**: the "hunger hormone" that is secreted in the stomach; increases in a fasting state and decreases after a meal

Some adipokines are neuropeptides, including orexins and anorexins, which play a role in body weight. Orexins are appetite stimulants; examples are ghrelin secreted by the stomach and peptide YY from the intestines. Anorexins decrease appetite and include leptin and insulin (McCance et al., 2014). Increased circulating plasma levels of orexins are associated with the development of obesity. However, in some, adults high levels of leptin may not be effective in suppressing appetite—a condition known as *leptin resistance.* In this case, overeating and excessive weight gain can result. Hyperleptinemia also stimulates the autonomic nervous system and contributes to blood vessel inflammation and ventricular hypertrophy. Obesity is also associated with insulin resistance, which predisposes patients with obesity to type 2 diabetes mellitus (see Chapter 64).

The distribution of excess body fat rather than the degree of obesity has been used to predict increased health risks. For example, the waist circumference (WC) is a stronger predictor of coronary artery disease (CAD) than is the BMI. A WC greater than 35 inches (89 cm) in women and greater than 40 inches (102 cm) in men indicates central obesity (National Institute of Diabetes and Digestive and Kidney Diseases, 2017). Central obesity is a major risk factor for CAD, stroke, type 2 diabetes, some cancers (e.g., colon, breast), sleep apnea, and early death.

The waist-to-hip ratio (WHR) is also a predictor of CAD. This measure differentiates peripheral lower body obesity from central obesity. A WHR of 0.95 or greater in men (0.8 or greater in women) indicates android obesity with excess fat at the waist and abdomen.

Complications of Obesity

The major complications of obesity affect primarily the cardiovascular and respiratory systems. However, excess weight can also cause degeneration of the musculoskeletal system, especially the weight-bearing joints such as hips and knees (osteoarthritis). Obese adults are also more susceptible to infections and infectious diseases than are thinner adults and tend to heal more slowly. Table 60-3 lists some of the most common complications of obesity.

Etiology and Genetic Risk

The causes of obesity involve complex interrelationships of many environmental, genetic, and behavioral factors. One

---

TABLE 60-3 Common Complications of Obesity

- Type 2 diabetes mellitus
- Hypertension
- **Hyperlipidemia** (increased serum lipids)
- Coronary artery disease (CAD)
- Stroke
- Peripheral artery disease (PAD)
- Metabolic syndrome
- Obstructive sleep apnea
- Obesity hypoventilation syndrome
- Depression and other mental health/behavioral health problems
- Urinary incontinence
- **Cholelithiasis** (gallstones)
- Gout
- Chronic back pain
- Early osteoarthritis
- Decreased wound healing

of the most common causes of being overweight or obese is eating *high-fat and high-cholesterol diets*. Obesity is associated with diet when it contains a significant amount of *saturated* fat, which increases low-density lipoproteins (LDL, or LDL-C for low-density lipoproteins cholesterol). *Trans* fatty acids (TFAs), saturated fats, and cholesterol are linked to a higher risk for heart disease (American Heart Association, 2017). By contrast, monounsaturated and polyunsaturated fats are healthy fats.

Physical inactivity has been identified as another cause of overweight and obesity. The major barriers to increasing physical activity include:

- Lack of time
- Learned behaviors regarding a sedentary lifestyle
- Decreased mobility associated with prolonged illness.

Regular exercise is associated with:

- Lower death rates for adults of any age
- Increased lean muscle
- Decreased body fat
- Weight control
- Enhanced psychological well-being.

Some adults think that regular exercise has to include joining a fitness program or exercising for long periods; simple forms of exercise such as walking 20 minutes provide the same type of benefit. Older adults can engage in this type of exercise. It does not cost money (like joining a program) and provides health benefits such as strengthening joints and improving cardiovascular health.

Another cause of obesity is *drug therapy*. Some prescribed drugs contribute to weight gain when they are taken on a long-term basis. Examples include:

- Corticosteroids
- Estrogens and certain progestins
- NSAIDs
- Antihypertensives
- Antidepressants and other psychoactive drugs
- Antiepileptic drugs
- Certain oral antidiabetic agents

🧬 GENETIC/GENOMIC CONSIDERATIONS

Patient-Centered Care (QSEN)

Familial and genetic factors play an important role in obesity. When both parents are overweight, about 80% of their children will be overweight. If neither parent is overweight, fewer than 10% of the children will be overweight. In studies of nonidentical twins, when one twin is obese, the second twin also is obese about 30% of the time. In studies of identical twins, when one twin is obese, the second twin also is obese about 80% of the time. These results indicate a strong genetic component to obesity along with lifestyle (environmental) influences. Genome-wide association studies indicate that mutations in many genes are associated with the development of obesity (Online Mendelian Inheritance in Man [OMIM], 2016).

Genetic composition may predispose some adults but not others to obesity. Leptin, the hormone encoded by the *ob* gene, appears to send a message to the brain that the body has stored enough fat. This message serves as a signal to stop eating. An abnormality of this gene has been found in some adults with obesity. In some obese adults, other gene mutations have been identified that appear to contribute to obesity (e.g., activation of the melanocortin-4 receptor, which normally inhibits appetite). In some families with a history of obesity, an abnormality in the gene coding for this receptor causes appetite to be less inhibited.

TABLE 60-4 Meeting *Healthy People 2020* Sample Objectives and Targets: Nutrition and Weight Status

- Reduce the proportion of adults who are obese (by 10%).
- Increase the proportion of adults who are at a healthy weight (by 10%).
- Increase the proportion of physician visits made by adult patients that include counseling about nutrition or diet (by 15.2%).
- Increase the proportion of primary care physicians who regularly assess body mass index (BMI) in their adult patients (by 10%).
- Increase the contribution of total vegetables to the diets of the population age 2 years and older (to 1.1 cups per 1000 calories).
- Increase the contribution of fruits to the diets of the population age 2 years and older (to 0.9 cups per 1000 calories).
- Reduce consumption of saturated fat in the population age 2 years and older (by 9.5%).

Health Promotion and Maintenance

Obesity is a major public health problem and is associated with many complications, including death. As a result of this increasing problem, the *Healthy People 2020* agenda addresses the need to reduce the proportion of children, adolescents, and adults who are obese. *Healthy People 2020 Objectives for Nutrition and Weight Status* include specific population targets related to obesity and healthy nutrition habits (Table 60-4). In collaboration with the dietitian, teach the importance of weight management and exercise to improve health. Even a 5% weight loss can drastically decrease the risk for coronary artery disease (CAD) and diabetes mellitus. Nurses who practice healthful behaviors and value a healthy lifestyle are more likely to be seen by patients as credible teachers of this information (Marchiondo, 2014).

Incidence and Prevalence

Between 2011 and 2014, 36.5% of U.S. adults were identified as obese, with the prevalence of obesity being greater in women than in men and greater in adults 40 to 59 years of age than in younger adults (National Center for Health Statistics, 2015). Worldwide, approximately 2.8 million people die annually from complications associated with overweight or obesity (World Health Organization, 2017).

❓ NCLEX EXAMINATION CHALLENGE 60-3

Psychosocial Integrity

A client with obesity tells the nurse, "I wouldn't be overweight if it weren't for my genes." What is the appropriate nursing response? **Select all that apply.**
A. "Genes are responsible for obesity."
B. "Tell me about your family history."
C. "Let's talk about your nutrition intake."
D. "How do you feel about exercise?"
E. "You should get bariatric surgery."

❖ *INTERPROFESSIONAL COLLABORATIVE CARE*

Care for the patient with obesity takes place in a variety of settings, from the home, to the community, and in the hospital setting if more comprehensive management or surgery is needed. Members of the interprofessional team who collaborate most closely to care for the patient with malnutrition include the health care provider, surgeon if surgery is required, nurse, social worker, and dietitian. For patients who experience psychological impact from or related to obesity, a psychologist or therapist will also have in important role in care.

◆ **Assessment: Noticing**

History. Patients with obesity may be embarrassed or reluctant to talk about their weight or fear judgment because of the stigma that can be attached to this condition. Approach patients with obesity by using the acronym RESPECT, created by The Ohio State University (Budd & Peterson, 2015). Create a **r**apport with them in an **e**nvironment that is **s**afe. Ensure their safety and **p**rivacy, **e**ncourage them to set realistic goals (in the planning phase), provide **c**ompassion, and use **t**act in conversation. In addition to taking a complete history regarding present and past health problems, collect this information about the patient in collaboration with the dietitian:

- Economic status
- Usual food intake
- Eating behavior
- Cultural background
- Attitude toward food
- Appetite
- Chronic diseases
- Drugs (prescribed and over-the-counter [OTC], including herbal preparations)
- Physical activity/functional ability
- Family history of obesity
- Developmental level

A nutrition history usually includes a 24-hour recall of food intake and the frequency with which foods are consumed. The adequacy of the diet can be evaluated by comparing the amount and types of foods consumed daily with the established standards. The dietitian then provides a more detailed analysis of nutrition intake. You should be aware that patients who live in food deserts (i.e., urban areas where fresh, healthy food is in low supply or unaffordable) may have difficulty obtaining food that is densely nutritious.

Physical Assessment/Signs and Symptoms. Obtain an accurate height and weight. The dietitian calculates the percentage of ideal body weight (% IBW) and the body mass index (BMI). He or she may also:

- Measure the waist circumference
- Calculate the waist-to-hip ratio
- Determine arm and calf circumferences

Examine the skin of the patient with obesity for reddened or open areas. Lift skinfold areas, such as pendulous breasts and abdominal aprons (**panniculus**), to observe for *Candida* (yeast) (a condition called *intertrigo)* or other infections or lesions. Infection of the panniculus is referred to as **panniculitis**.

Psychosocial Assessment. Obtain a psychosocial history to determine the patient's circumstances and emotional factors that might prevent successful therapy or that might be worsened by therapy. Interview the patient to determine his or her perception of current weight and weight reduction. Some patients do not view weight as a problem, which affects planning, treatment, and outcome. Ask the patient questions about his or her health beliefs related to being overweight, such as:

- What does food mean to you?
- Do you want to lose weight?
- What prevents you from losing weight?
- What do you think will motivate you to lose weight?
- How do you think you might benefit from losing weight?

Many patients report that they have tried multiple diets to lose weight but either the diets have not worked or they regained the weight they had initially lost. Adults who attempt restrictive diets become easy targets for the billion-dollar weight-loss industry, yet most dieters regain lost weight. This problem can be even more concerning for the older adult who loses weight and then regains it.

The results of dieting and other efforts can lead to a sense of failure and lowered self-esteem, which often stimulates more overeating. Many overweight and obese adults eat in response to environmental and emotional stressors rather than because they are hungry. Ask patients to identify their perceived stressors and what triggers their need for food.

Lifestyle changes are difficult without adequate family and community support. Assess useful coping strategies and support systems that the patient can use during treatment for obesity. Explore the patient's history to assess:

- Attempts at weight-reduction diets and outcomes
- Effects of obesity on lifestyle
- Effects of obesity on social interactions
- Mental health/behavioral health problems, such as depression
- Effects of obesity on intimate relationships, especially sexuality

Obese men often experience erectile dysfunction (ED), which can cause or worsen depression. Women often experience changes in their menstrual cycles and may have problems getting pregnant.

◆ **Analysis: Interpreting**

The priority collaborative problem for the patient with obesity is:

1. Weight gain due to excessive intake of calories

◆ **Planning and Implementation: Responding**

Improving Nutrition. Weight is lost when energy used is greater than intake. Weight loss may be accomplished by nutrition modification with or without the aid of drugs and in combination with a regular exercise program. Patients who may be candidates for surgical treatment include those who have:

- Repeated failure of nonsurgical interventions
- A BMI equal to or greater than 40
- Weight more than 100% above IBW (i.e., morbidly obese)

Nonsurgical Management. Various nutrition approaches and drug therapy have been attempted to help patients with obesity achieve permanent weight loss.

Diet Programs. Diets for helping adults lose weight include fasting, very-low-calorie diets, balanced and unbalanced low-energy diets, and novelty diets.

Short-term fasting programs have not been successful in treating morbidly obese patients, and prolonged fasting does not produce permanent benefits. Most patients regain the weight that was lost by this method. In addition, the risks associated with fasting (e.g., severe ketosis) require close medical supervision.

Very-low-calorie diets generally provide 200 to 800 calories/day. Two types of these diets are the *protein-sparing modified fast* and the *liquid formula diet*. The protein-sparing modified fast provides protein of high biologic value (1.5 g/kg of desirable body weight daily) within a limited number of calories. This diet produces rapid weight loss while preserving lean body mass. The liquid formula diet provides between 33 and 70 g of protein daily.

Both diets require an initial cardiac evaluation, supervision by an interdisciplinary health care team with monitoring by a physician, nutrition counseling by a dietitian, and supplementation with vitamins and minerals. Patients who are on these diets should receive nutrition education, psychological counseling, exercise, and behavior therapy. Comparable weight losses have been achieved with both diets; but, again, most patients regain the weight they lost.

Nutritionally balanced diets generally provide about 1200 calories/day with a conventional distribution of carbohydrate, protein, and fat. Vitamin and mineral supplements may be necessary if energy intakes fall below 1200 calories for women and 1800 calories for men. These diets provide conventional food that is economical and easy to obtain. Thus the outcome of weight loss is facilitated, and it is hoped that loss is maintained. For example, Weight Watchers is an organization that provides education about nutritionally balanced diets based on a point system. They offer on-site weekly group support meetings or the option of an online community.

Unbalanced low-energy diets, such as the low-carbohydrate diet (e.g., Atkins or South Beach diet), restrict one or more nutrients. Protein and vegetables are encouraged, but certain carbohydrates and high-fat foods are not. Although they remain controversial in the medical community, these diets are extremely popular. Scientific outcome data have been conflicting.

Novelty diets, such as the grapefruit diet, the Cookie diet, and the Hollywood diet, are often nutritionally *inadequate.* This type of diet implies that a certain food or liquid increases metabolic rate or accelerates the oxidation of body fat. Weight loss is achieved because energy is restricted by food choice, but patients do not sustain weight loss after stopping the diet.

Nutrition Therapy. Nutrition recommendations for each patient are developed through close interaction among the patient, family, physician, nurse, and dietitian. The diet must meet the patient's needs, habits, and lifestyle and should be realistic.

The dietitian develops a diet plan and instructs the patient. At a minimum, the diet should:

* Have a scientific rationale
* Be nutritionally adequate for all nutrients
* Have a low risk-benefit ratio
* Be practical and conducive to long-term success

Calorie estimates are easily calculated. Resting metabolic rate is determined using a gender-specific formula that incorporates the appropriate activity factor. This figure reflects the total calories needed daily for maintaining current weight. To encourage a weight loss of 1 lb (0.45 kg) a week, the dietitian subtracts 500 calories each day. To encourage a weight loss of 2 lb (0.9 kg) a week, 1000 calories each day are subtracted. The amount of weight lost varies with the patient's food intake, level of physical activity, and water losses. A reasonable expected outcome of 5% to 10% loss of body weight has been shown to improve glycemic control and reduce cholesterol and blood pressure. These benefits continue if the weight loss is sustained.

Exercise Program. Along with change in eating habits, a major intervention to manage obesity is to increase the type and amount of daily exercise to burn calories. For most adults, adding exercise to a nutrition intervention produces more weight loss than just dieting alone. More of the weight lost is fat, which preserves lean body mass. An increase in exercise can reduce the waist circumference and the waist-to-hip ratio.

A minimum-level workout should be developed so consistency can be achieved. The expected outcome is to maintain a lifetime of increased physical activity. The patient is likely to be less fatigued and discouraged with a low-intensity, short-duration program. Encourage sedentary (physically inactive) patients to increase their activity by walking 30 to 40 minutes at least 5 days each week. The activity may be performed all at once or divided over the course of the day. Structured national programs with support staff may be helpful for some patients. The staff typically offers diet counseling and cardiovascular and muscle-toning activities.

Drug Therapy. A BMI of 30 or a BMI of 27 with comorbidities is one indicator for the use of drug therapy. **Anorectic drugs** suppress appetite, which reduces food intake and, over time, may result in weight loss. Over the years, the U.S. Food and Drug Administration (FDA) has removed several drugs from the market and not approved other drugs because of concerns about cardiovascular complications associated with long-term use. Prescription drugs still available for longer-term treatment of obesity include orlistat (Xenical), lorcaserin (Belviq), phentermine-topiramate (Qsymia), naltrexone SR/bupropion SR (Contrave), and liraglutide (Saxenda, Victoza ✦).

Orlistat (Xenical) inhibits lipase and leads to partial hydrolysis of triglycerides. Because fats are only partially digested and absorbed, calorie uptake is decreased. Most patients taking this drug have GI symptoms that include loose stools, abdominal cramps, and nausea unless they reduce their fat intake to less than 30% of their food intake each day. Therefore the drug should be used with caution and limited to adults between 18 and 75 years of age. Treatment is usually not extended beyond 12 months. A lower-dose 60-mg orlistat tablet (Alli) is the only *over-the-counter* weight-loss aid product that has received FDA approval for long-term use.

Lorcaserin (Belviq) works by activating the serotonin 2C receptor in the brain to help decrease appetite and create a sense of feeling full after eating small amounts of food. Side effects may include headaches, dizziness, dry mouth, and constipation. Teach patients to report the signs of the rare but serious side effect of serotonin syndrome, including suicidal thoughts, psychiatric concerns, and problems with memory or comprehension.

Phentermine-topiramate (Qsymia) combines a short-term weight-loss drug (phentermine) with a drug that is used to control seizures (topiramate). Side effects may include an increased heart rate, hand and feet tingling, insomnia, dizziness, dry mouth, and constipation. Teach patients that a rare but serious side effect associated with this drug is suicidal thoughts, which should immediately be reported to the prescribing health care provider.

Naltrexone HCl/bupropion HCl (Contrave) combines the opioid antagonist naltrexone with the antidepressant bupropion. Patients with uncontrolled hypertension or seizure disorders should not take this drug. Teach patients about the possibility of an onset or increase in suicidal ideation and behaviors, as well as neuropsychiatric reactions.

Liraglutide (Saxenda, Victoza ✦) injection activates appetite regulation in the brain, which decreases caloric intake. Patients taking insulin should not take this medication. Serious side effects can include a risk for medullary thyroid carcinoma, hypoglycemia, renal impairment, suicidal behaviors, and acute pancreatitis.

Other sympathomimetic drugs suppress appetite for *short-term* use along with a structured weight-management and exercise program. These drugs act on the central nervous system, including suppressing the appetite center in the hypothalamus.

! NURSING SAFETY PRIORITY QSEN

Drug Alert

Patients with hypertension, heart disease, and hyperthyroidism should not take anorectic drugs because they may worsen their symptoms. These drugs are not prescribed for any patient taking psychoactive agents because they cause similar side effects. Teach patients who are candidates for sympathomimetic drugs about side effects, which include:

- Palpitations
- Diarrhea or constipation
- Restlessness
- Insomnia
- Dry mouth
- Blurred vision (especially with Bontril PDM)
- Change in sex drive or activity
- Anxiety

Examples include phentermine hydrochloride (Adipex-P), diethylpropion hydrochloride (Tenuate, Tenuate Dospan), and phendimetrazine tartrate (Bontril PDM).

Behavioral Management. Behavioral management of obesity helps the patient change daily eating habits to lose weight. Self-monitoring techniques include keeping a record of foods eaten (food diary), exercise patterns, and emotional and situational factors. Stimulus control involves controlling the external cues that promote overeating. Reinforcement techniques are used to self-reward the behavior change. Cognitive restructuring involves modifying negative beliefs by learning positive coping self-statements. Counseling by health care professionals must continue before, during, and after treatment. The 12-step program offered by Overeaters Anonymous (www.oa.org) has helped many adults lose weight, especially those who are compulsive eaters.

Complementary and Integrative Health. Many complementary and integrative therapies have been tested and used for obesity. These modalities aim to suppress appetite and therefore limit food intake to lose weight:

- Acupuncture
- Acupressure
- Ayurveda (a combination of holistic approaches)
- Hypnosis

Surgical Management. At any weight, some patients seek to improve their appearance by having a variety of cosmetic procedures to reduce the amount of adipose tissue in selected areas of the body. A typical example of this type of surgery is **liposuction**, which can be done in a physician's office or ambulatory surgery center. Although the patient's appearance improves, if weight gain continues, the fatty tissue will return. This procedure is not a solution for adults who are morbidly obese.

Morbidly obese adults who do not respond to traditional interventions may be considered for a major surgical procedure aimed at producing permanent weight loss. Patients with a body mass index (BMI) of 40 or greater or a BMI of 35 or greater along with additional risk factors are considered for surgery. Surgery has been perceived as a last resort to address weight issues, but it *is the only method that has a long-term impact on morbid obesity.*

Bariatrics. **Bariatrics** is a branch of medicine that manages patients with obesity and its related diseases. Surgical procedures include these three types: gastric restrictive, malabsorption, or both. *Restrictive* surgeries decrease the volume capacity of the stomach to limit the amount of food that can be eaten at one time. As the name implies, *malabsorption* procedures interfere with the absorption of food and nutrients from the GI tract.

In 2014, more than 179,000 adults in the United States had bariatric surgical procedures (American Society for Metabolic and Bariatric Surgery, 2014), and that number continues to increase. The surgeon may use a conventional open approach or minimally invasive surgery (MIS). Most patients have MIS by having either the laparoscopic adjustable gastric band (LAGB) procedure or the laparoscopic sleeve gastrectomy (LSG). Both procedures are classified as restrictive surgeries. The decision of whether the patient is a candidate for the MIS is based on weight, body build, history of abdominal surgery, and co-existing medical complications. With any surgical approach, patients must agree to modify their lifestyle and follow stringent protocols to lose weight and keep the weight off. After bariatric surgery, many patients no longer have complications of obesity, such as diabetes mellitus, hypertension, depression, or sleep apnea.

Preoperative Care. Preoperative care is similar to that for any patient undergoing abdominal surgery or laparoscopy (see Chapter 14). However, patient with obesity are at increased surgical risks of pulmonary and thromboembolitic complications, as well as death. Some surgeons require limited weight loss before bariatric surgery to decrease these complications. Patients also have a thorough psychological assessment and testing to detect depression, substance abuse, or other mental health/behavioral health problems that could interfere with their success after surgery. Cognitive ability, coping skills, development, motivation, expectations, and support systems are also assessed. Patients who are not alert and oriented or do not have sufficient strength and mobility are not considered for bariatric surgery. *The primary role of the nurse is to reinforce health teaching in preparation for surgery.* Most bariatric surgical centers provide education sessions for groups of patients who plan to have the procedure.

Operative Procedures. *Gastric restriction* surgeries allow for normal digestion without the risk for nutrition deficiencies. In the LAGB procedure, the surgeon places an adjustable band to create a small proximal stomach pouch through a laparoscope (Fig. 60-4A). The band may or may not be inflatable. For example, the REALIZE® band requires that saline be injected into a balloon to control the tightness of the band. This type of procedure is considered to be restrictive; malabsorption complications usually do not occur. For the LSG, the surgeon removes the portion of the stomach where ghrelin, the "hunger hormone," is secreted. Restrictive surgeries are the easiest to perform. However, weight lost is often regained after a period of time. By contrast, patients having the malabsorption procedures maintain 60% to 70% of their weight loss even after 20 years.

The most common *malabsorption surgery* performed in the United States is the *Roux-en-Y gastric bypass (RNYGB)*, which is often done as a robotic-assistive surgical procedure. This procedure results in quick weight loss, but it is more invasive with a higher risk for postoperative complications. In RNYGB, most commonly just called a **gastric bypass**, gastric resection is combined with malabsorption surgery. The patient's stomach, duodenum, and part of the jejunum are bypassed so fewer calories can be absorbed (Fig. 60-4B).

Postoperative Care. Postoperative care depends on the type of surgery (i.e., the conventional open approach or the minimally invasive technique). Although many patients have MIS, they are considered as having major abdominal surgery along with all its risks and are cared for accordingly. These patients may require less than 24 hours in the hospital; some may need 1 to

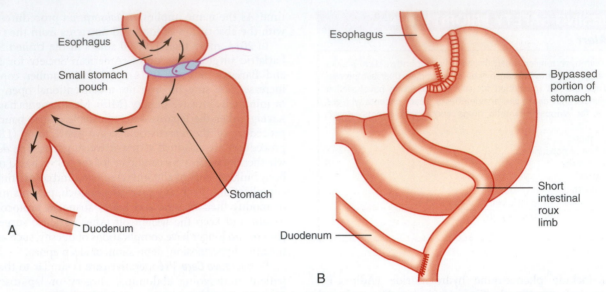

FIG. 60-4 Bariatric surgical procedures. **A,** Adjustable banded gastroplasty. **B,** Roux-en-Y gastric bypass (RNYGB).

2 days. Patients with open procedures may need several days to recover.

Patients having one of the MIS procedures have less pain, scarring, and blood loss. They typically have a faster recovery time and a faster return to daily activities.

The priority for immediate care of postoperative bariatric surgery patients is airway management. Patients with short and thick necks often have compromised airways and need aggressive respiratory support—possibly mechanical ventilation in the critical care unit.

All patients experience some degree of pain, but it is usually less severe when MIS is done. Patients may use patient-controlled analgesia (PCA) with morphine for up to the first 24 hours. All patients receive oral opioid analgesic agents as prescribed after the PCA is discontinued. Liquid forms of drug therapy are preferred. Acute pain management is discussed in detail in Chapter 4.

Care of the bariatric surgical patient is similar to that of any patient having abdominal or laparoscopic surgery. *A major focus is patient and staff safety.* Special bariatric equipment and accommodations, including an extra-wide bed and additional personnel for moving the patient, are needed for both the surgical suite and postoperative care units. Weight-rated beds must be wide enough to allow the patient to turn. Bed rails should not be touching the body because they can cause pressure areas. Pressure between skinfolds and tubes and catheters can also cause skin breakdown. Monitor the skin in these areas and keep it clean and dry.

> ### ! NURSING SAFETY PRIORITY QSEN
> #### Action Alert
> Some patients who have bariatric surgery have a nasogastric (NG) tube put in place, especially after open surgical procedures. In gastroplasty procedures, the NG tube drains both the proximal pouch and the distal stomach. Closely monitor the tube for patency. *Never reposition the tube because its movement can disrupt the suture line!* The NG tube is removed on the second day if the patient is passing flatus.

Clear liquids are introduced slowly if the patient can tolerate water, and 1-ounce cups are used for each serving. Pureed foods; juice; and soups thinned with broth, water, or milk are added to the diet 24 to 48 hours after clear liquids are tolerated. Typically, the patient can increase the volume to 1 ounce over 5 minutes or until satisfied, but the diet is limited to liquids or pureed food for 6 weeks. The patient then progresses to regular food, with an emphasis on nutrient-dense foods. Nausea, vomiting, or discomfort occurs if too much liquid is ingested.

> ### ! NURSING SAFETY PRIORITY QSEN
> #### Critical Rescue
> Anastomotic leaks are the most common serious complication and cause of death after gastric bypass surgery. Recognize that you must monitor for symptoms of this life-threatening problem, which includes increasing back, shoulder, or abdominal pain; restlessness; and unexplained tachycardia and oliguria (scant urine). If any of these findings is present, report it to the surgeon immediately!

In addition to the postoperative complications typically associated with abdominal and laparoscopic surgeries, bariatric patients have special needs and risks, such as the risk for anastomotic leaks (a leak of digestive juices and partially digested food through an anastomosis).

Implement these measures to prevent complications:
- Apply an abdominal binder to prevent wound dehiscence for open surgical procedures.
- Place the patient in semi-Fowler's position or use bi-level or continuous positive airway pressure (BiPAP or CPAP) ventilation at night to improve breathing and decrease risk for sleep apnea or other pulmonary complications, such as pneumonia and atelectasis.
- Monitor oxygen saturation; provide oxygen at 2 L/min as prescribed.
- Apply sequential compression stockings and administer prophylactic anticoagulant (usually heparin) therapy as

prescribed to help prevent thromboembolitic complications, including pulmonary embolism (PE). These are The Joint Commission Core Measure interventions to prevent venous thromboembolism (VTE).

- Observe skin areas and folds for redness, excoriation, or breakdown to treat these problems early.
- Use absorbent padding between folds to prevent pressure areas and skin breakdown; make sure that tubes and catheters are not causing pressure as well.
- **Remove urinary catheter within 24 hours after surgery to prevent urinary tract infection per the National Patient Safety Goals.**
- Assist the patient out of bed on the day of surgery; encourage and assist with turning every 2 hours using an appropriate weight-bearing overhead trapeze. Collaborate with the physical or occupational therapist if needed for transfers or ambulation assistive devices, such as walkers.
- Ambulate patient as soon as possible to prevent postoperative complications, such as deep vein thrombosis and pulmonary embolus.
- Measure and record abdominal girth daily, as requested.
- In collaboration with the dietitian, provide six small feedings and plenty of fluids to prevent dehydration.
- Observe for signs and symptoms of dumping syndrome (caused by food entering the small intestine instead of the stomach) after *gastric bypass,* such as tachycardia, nausea, diarrhea, and abdominal cramping.

CLINICAL JUDGMENT CHALLENGE 60-1

Patient-Centered Care; Evidence-Based Practice; Teamwork and Collaboration; Informatics QSEN

A 53-year-old woman with morbid obesity had a Roux-en-Y gastric bypass (RNYGB) a month ago. At a follow-up examination, the patient reports frequent problems with nausea, diarrhea, and a feeling like her heart is "racing."
1. What patient problem do you anticipate that the patient is having? What data support your answer?
2. What priority assessment will you perform at this time, and why?
3. What patient teaching will you provide?
4. With whom will you collaborate to care for this patient?
5. What information will you document in the electronic health record?

Care Coordination and Transition Management

Obesity is a chronic, lifelong problem. Diets, drug therapy, exercise, and behavior modification can produce short-term weight losses with reasonable safety. However, many patients who do lose weight often regain it. Treatment of obesity should focus on the long-term reduction of health risks and medical problems associated with obesity, improving quality of life, and promoting a health-oriented lifestyle.

Home Care Management. The most important features of health teaching for any patient with obesity and family focus on health-related behavior patterns. In collaboration with the dietitian, counsel the patient on a healthful eating pattern. The physical therapist or exercise physiologist recommends an appropriate exercise program. A psychologist may recommend cognitive restructuring approaches that help alter dysfunctional eating patterns.

CHART 60-7 Patient and Family Education: Preparing for Self-Management

Discharge Teaching for the Patient After Bariatric Surgery

Nutrition: Diet progression, nutrient (including vitamin and mineral) supplements, hydration guidelines
Drug therapy: Analgesics and antiemetic drugs, if needed; drugs for other health problems
Wound care: Clean procedure for open or laparoscopic wounds; cover during shower or bath
Activity level: Restrictions, such as avoiding lifting; activity progression; return to driving and work
Signs and symptoms to report: Fever; excessive nausea or vomiting; epigastric, back, or shoulder pain; red, hot, and/or draining wound(s); pain, redness, or swelling in legs; chest pain; difficulty breathing
Follow-up care: Health care provider office or clinic visits, support groups and other community resources, counseling for patient and family
Continuing education: Nutrition and exercise classes; follow-up visits with dietitian

For patients who have surgery, additional discharge teaching is needed. Chart 60-7 lists the important areas that should be reviewed. Bariatric surgery results in a major lifestyle change and a variety of emotions. During weight loss, the patient may become depressed or anxious. Some experience a "hibernation phase" for about a month after surgery because of physical and emotional adjustments. Patients are usually followed closely by the surgeon and dietitian for several years. Encourage them to keep all appointments and to adhere to the community-based treatment plan to ensure success. Plastic surgery, such as panniculectomy (removal of the abdominal apron, or panniculus), may be performed after weight is stabilized, usually in about 18 to 24 months.

Self-Care Management. Remind patients to coordinate with their health care provider to create a manageable and appropriate physical activity plan. Focus should be placed on monitoring diet for a decrease in overall fat intake and reliance on appetite-reducing drugs. Ask patients to consider keeping a food journal that also documents mood and events that take place with eating. This can be helpful for the patient to identify eating patterns and then strive to establish a normal eating pattern in response to physiologic hunger.

Teach patients that bowel changes are common after surgery, including constipation. Vitamin and mineral supplements are often needed after surgery, especially vitamin D, B-complex vitamins, iron, and calcium.

Health Care Resources. Provide the patient with a list of available community resources, such as Overeaters Anonymous (www.oa.org) and the American Obesity Association (www.obesity.org). For surgical patients, the American Society for Metabolic and Bariatric Surgery (www.asmbs.org) may be helpful.

◆ Evaluation: Reflecting

Evaluate the care of the patient with obesity based on the identified priority patient problem. The primary expected outcome is that the patient consumes appropriate, nutrient-dense foods to meet metabolic demands without overeating. For surgical patients, an additional expected outcome is that the patient remains free of infection following bariatric surgery.

GET READY FOR THE NCLEX® EXAMINATION!

KEY POINTS

Review these Key Points for each NCLEX Examination Client Needs Category.

Safe and Effective Care Environment
- Collaborate with the interdisciplinary health care team, especially the dietitian, health care provider, and case manager, when caring for patients with malnutrition or obesity. **QSEN: Teamwork and Collaboration**
- Be sure that bariatric furniture and equipment are available for the patient with obesity in the hospital or other health care setting; avoid pressure on skinfold areas. **QSEN: Safety**

Health Promotion and Maintenance
- Perform nutrition screening for all patients to determine if they are at risk (see Charts 60-1 and 60-2). **QSEN: Evidence-Based Practice**
- Recognize that older patients are at increased risk for malnutrition (see Chart 60-2).
- Implement interventions to promote nutrition intake in older adults as specified in Chart 60-3. **QSEN: Patient-Centered Care**

Psychosocial Integrity
- Be aware that some patients with malnutrition or obesity may not view their weight as a problem and may be reluctant to be part of a NUTRITION plan.
- Recognize that malnutrition and obesity can contribute to depression or anxiety, low self-esteem, and a disturbed body image. **QSEN: Patient-Centered Care**
- Be aware of legal and ethical issues related to tube-feeding older adults with chronic or terminal illness. **Ethics**

Physiological Integrity
- Review serum prealbumin, hemoglobin, and hematocrit levels to identify patients at NUTRITION risk. **Clinical Judgment**
- Assess patients with severe malnutrition for complications such as edema, lethargy, and dry, flaking skin.
- Provide evidence-based nursing interventions for managing total enteral nutrition as listed in Chart 60-4. **QSEN: Evidence-Based Practice**
- Maintain feeding tube patency for patients receiving total enteral nutrition as described in Chart 60-5. **QSEN: Safety**
- Ensure that feeding tube placement is verified by x-ray; check placement every 4 to 8 hours by aspirating gastric contents and assessing pH for nasogastric tubes. **QSEN: Safety**

- Place patients receiving tube feeding in a semi-Fowler's position at all times to prevent aspiration; check residual contents every 4 hours or as designated per facility policy. **QSEN: Safety**
- Use gloves when changing feeding system tubing or adding product; use sterile gloves when working with critically ill or immunocompromised patients. **QSEN: Evidence-Based Practice**
- Use a feeding pump when the patient receives continuous or cyclic tube feeding.
- Teach family members or other caregivers of patients receiving enteral or parenteral nutrition at home how to provide NUTRITION while avoiding complications. **QSEN: Safety**
- Teach patients who are undernourished to eat high-protein, high-calorie food and nutrition supplements. **QSEN: Evidence-Based Practice**
- Provide care for patients receiving total parenteral nutrition as specified in Chart 60-6. **QSEN: Evidence-Based Practice**
- Recall that normal body mass index (BMI) for adults should be between 18.5 and 25; older adults should have a BMI between 23 and 27. A BMI of 27 to 30 indicates overweight, over 30 indicates obesity, and 40 and greater indicates morbid obesity.
- Recall that obesity contributes to early onset of many chronic illnesses, such as osteoarthritis, diabetes mellitus, hypertension, coronary artery disease, pulmonary problems, delayed wound healing, and infection.
- Instruct patients with obesity about the importance of a health care provider–approved exercise plan for weight reduction.
- Recognize that many adults are following low-carbohydrate rather than low-fat diets to lose weight.
- Remember that bariatric surgery includes gastric restriction procedures or gastric bypass; a panniculectomy may be performed to remove skinfolds once weight is stabilized.
- Be alert for signs and symptoms of anastomotic leak after bariatric surgery, including severe pain, restlessness, anxiety, and unexplained tachycardia. **QSEN: Safety**
- Provide postoperative care for patients having bariatric surgery to prevent complications such as wound dehiscence, respiratory distress, skin breakdown, and thromboembolitic complications, such as pulmonary embolism. Establishing and maintaining an airway is the priority for patients having bariatric surgery! **QSEN: Safety**
- Observe for complications, such as dumping syndrome in patients who have a gastric bypass. Tachycardia, nausea, diarrhea, and abdominal cramping are common symptoms of dumping syndrome.
- Provide discharge teaching for patients having bariatric surgery as described in Chart 60-7.

SELECTED BIBLIOGRAPHY

Asterisk indicates a classic or definitive work on this subject.

Academy of Nutrition and Dietetics. (2016). *Vegetarianism: The basic facts.* http://www.eatright.org/resource/food/nutrition/vegetarian-and-special-diets/vegetarianism-the-basic-facts.

American Heart Association. (2017). *The skinny on fats.* www.heart.org/HEARTORG/Conditions/Cholesterol/PreventionTreatmentofHighCholesterol/Know-Your-Fats_UCM_305628_Article.jsp.

American Society for Metabolic and Bariatric Surgery (2014). *New procedure estimates for bariatric surgery.* http://connect.asmbs.org/may-2014-bariatric-surgery-growth.html.

American Society of Parenteral and Enteral Nutrition (ASPEN). (2016). *Overview: Did you know?* https://www.nutritioncare.org/Malnutrition/.

*Bender, S., Pusateri, M., Cook, A., Ferguson, M., & Hall, J. C. (2000). Malnutrition: Role of the TwoCal® HN Med Pass Program. *Medsurg Nursing, 9*(6), 284–296.

Bhutta, Z. (2013). Nutrition epidemiology. *Annals of Nutrition & Metabolism, 61*(Suppl. 1), 1–5. https://www.nestlenutrition-institute.org/resources/library/Free/annales/annales_70_3/Documents/Editorial.pdf.

Budd, G., & Peterson, J. (2015). The obesity epidemic, part 2: Nursing assessment and intervention. *American Journal of Nursing, 115*(1), 38–46.

Centers for Disease Control and Prevention (CDC). (2015). *About Adult BMI.* www.cdc.gov/healthyweight/assessing/bmi/adult_bmi/.

Centers for Disease Control and Prevention (CDC). (2016). *Adult obesity facts.* http://www.cdc.gov/obesity/data/adult.html.

Health Canada. (2016). *Eating well with Canada's food guide.* www.hc-sc.gc.ca/fn-an/food-guide-aliment/index_e.html.

Kodali, B. S., & Urman, R. D. (2014). Capnography during cardiopulmonary resuscitation: Current evidence and future directions. *Journal of Emergencies, Trauma, and Shock, 7*(4), 332–340. http://doi.org/10.4103/0974-2700.142778.

Marchiondo, K. (2014). Stemming the obesity epidemic: Are nurses credible coaches? *Medsurg Nursing, 23*(3), 155–158.

Martone, A. M., Onder, G., Vetrano, D. L., Ortolani, E., Tosato, M., Marzetti, E., et al. (2013). Anorexia of aging: A modifiable risk factor for frailty. *Nutrients, 5*(10), 4126–4133. http://doi.org/10.3390/nu5104126.

McCance, K., Huether, S., Brashers, V., & Rote, N. (2014). *Pathophysiology: The biologic basis for disease in adults and children* (7th ed.). St. Louis: Mosby.

*Mehanna, H. M., Moledina, J., & Travis, J. (2008). Refeeding syndrome: What it is, and how to prevent and treat it. *BMJ (Clinical Research Ed.), 336*, 1495–1498.

Minister of Health Canada. (2016). *Eating well with Canada's food guide.* http://healthycanadians.gc.ca/eating-nutrition/healthy-eating-saine-alimentation/food-guide-aliment/index-eng.php.

National Academies of Science, Engineering, Medicine. (2016). *Dietary references intakes and application tables.* http://www.nationalacademies.org/hmd/Activities/Nutrition/SummaryDRIs/DRI-Tables.aspx.

National Center for Health Statistics. (2015). *Prevalence of obesity among adults and youth: United States, 2011-2014.* https://www.cdc.gov/nchs/data/databriefs/db219.pdf.

National Institute of Diabetes and Digestive and Kidney Diseases. (2017). *Diabetes, heart disease and stroke.* http://www.niddk.nih.gov/health-information/health-topics/Diabetes/diabetes-heart-disease-stroke/Pages/index.aspx.

Nestle Nutrition Institute. (n.d.). *Mini nutritional assessment (MNA).* http://www.mna-elderly.org/forms/MNA_english.pdf.

Online Mendelian Inheritance in Man (OMIM). (2016). *Obesity,* https://www.omim.org/entry/601665.

Pagana, K., Pagana, T. J., & Pagana, T. N. (2017). *Mosby's diagnostic and laboratory test reference* (13th ed.). St. Louis: Mosby.

U.S. Department of Agriculture (USDA). (2015). *2015-2020 Dietary guidelines for Americans.* http://www.cnpp.usda.gov/2015-2020-dietary-guidelines-americans.

U.S. Department of Agriculture (USDA). (2017). *Dietary References Intakes.* https://fnic.nal.usda.gov/dietary-guidance/dietary-reference-intakes.

World Health Organization. (2017). *Global Health Observatory (GHO) data: Obesity.* http://www.who.int/gho/ncd/risk_factors/obesity_text/en/.

61 | CHAPTER

Assessment of the Endocrine System

M. Linda Workman

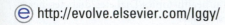 http://evolve.elsevier.com/Iggy/

PRIORITY AND INTERRELATED CONCEPTS

The priority concepts for this chapter are:
- NUTRITION
- ELIMINATION

The interrelated concept for this chapter is FLUID AND ELECTROLYTE BALANCE.

LEARNING OUTCOMES

Safe and Effective Care Environment

1. Collaborate with the interprofessional team to perform a complete endocrine assessment, including issues with NUTRITION, ELIMINATION, and FLUID AND ELECTROLYTE BALANCE.

Health Promotion and Maintenance

2. Teach adults about factors that increase the risk for endocrine problems.
3. Teach patients and families about pretest and post-test care for assessment of endocrine function.

Psychosocial Integrity

4. Implement patient-centered nursing interventions to help patients and families cope with the psychosocial impact caused by changes in endocrine function.

Physiological Integrity

5. Apply the principles of anatomy, physiology, and the aging process to perform an evidence-based assessment for the patient with a problem of the endocrine system.
6. Explain and interpret assessment findings for the patient with an endocrine problem.
7. Coordinate appropriate care for patients and proper handling of specimens before, during, and after testing of the endocrine system.
8. Monitor for complications of diagnostic procedures used to assess endocrine function.

The endocrine system is composed of tissues and organs (glands) that are located in many body areas (Fig. 61-1) and affect all other body systems. The purpose of endocrine glands and tissues is to secret **hormones**, which are natural chemicals that exert their effects on specific tissues known as **target tissues**. Target tissues are usually located some distance from the endocrine gland, with no connecting duct between the endocrine gland and its target tissue. For this reason, endocrine glands are called *ductless* glands and use the blood to transport secreted hormones to the target tissues (McCance et al., 2014). The major endocrine glands are:

- Hypothalamus (a neuroendocrine gland)
- Pituitary gland
- Adrenal glands
- Thyroid gland
- Islet cells of the pancreas
- Parathyroid glands
- Gonads

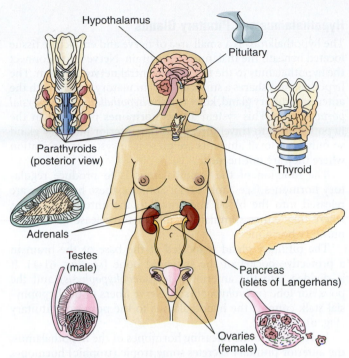

FIG. 61-1 Locations of various glands within the endocrine system.

TABLE 61-1 Principal Hormones of the Endocrine Glands

GLAND	HORMONES
Hypothalamus	Corticotropin-releasing hormone (CRH)
	Thyrotropin-releasing hormone (TRH)
	Gonadotropin-releasing hormone (GnRH)
	Growth hormone–releasing hormone (GHRH)
	Growth hormone–inhibiting hormone (somatostatin GHIH)
	Prolactin-inhibiting hormone (PIH)
	Melanocyte-inhibiting hormone (MIH)
Anterior pituitary	Thyroid-stimulating hormone (TSH), also known as *thyrotropin*
	Adrenocorticotropic hormone (ACTH, corticotropin)
	Luteinizing hormone (LH), also known as *Leydig cell–stimulating hormone (LCSH)*
	Follicle-stimulating hormone (FSH)
	Prolactin (PRL)
	Growth hormone (GH)
	Melanocyte-stimulating hormone (MSH)
Posterior pituitary	Vasopressin (antidiuretic hormone [ADH])
	Oxytocin
Thyroid	Triiodothyronine (T_3)
	Thyroxine (T_4)
	Calcitonin
Parathyroid	Parathyroid hormone (PTH)
Adrenal cortex	Glucocorticoids (cortisol)
	Mineralocorticoids (aldosterone)
Ovary	Estrogen
	Progesterone
Testes	Testosterone
Pancreas	Insulin
	Glucagon
	Somatostatin

The endocrine system works with the nervous system to control overall body function and regulation, including metabolism, NUTRITION, ELIMINATION, temperature, FLUID AND ELECTROLYTE BALANCE, growth, and reproduction. Many interactions must occur between the endocrine system and all other body systems to ensure that each system maintains a constant normal balance (**homeostasis**) in response to environmental changes. For example, this regulation keeps the internal body temperature at or near 98.6° F (37° C), even when environmental temperatures vary. Other actions keep the serum sodium level between 136 and 145 mEq/L (mmol/L), regardless of whether a healthy adult eats 2 g or 12 g of sodium per day.

Table 61-1 lists hormones secreted by various endocrine glands. Hormones travel through the blood to all body areas but exert their actions only on target tissues. They recognize their target tissues and exert their actions by binding to receptors on or within the target tissue cells. In general, each receptor site type is specific for only one hormone. Hormone-receptor actions work in a "lock and key" manner in that only the correct hormone (key) can bind to and activate the receptor site (lock) (Fig. 61-2). Binding a hormone to its receptor causes the target tissue to change its activity, producing specific responses (Lazar & Birnbaum, 2016).

Disorders of the endocrine system usually are related to:
- An excess of a specific hormone
- A deficiency of a specific hormone
- Poor hormone-receptor interactions resulting in decreased responsiveness of the target tissue

ANATOMY AND PHYSIOLOGY REVIEW

The control of cellular function by any hormone depends on a series of reactions working through *negative-feedback control mechanisms*. Hormone secretion usually depends on the body's need for the final action of that hormone. When a body

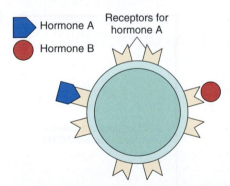

FIG. 61-2 "Lock and Key" hormone-receptor binding. *Hormone A* fits and binds to its receptors, causing a change in cell action. *Hormone B* does not fit or bind to receptors; no change in cell action results.

condition starts to move away from the normal range and a specific response is needed to correct this change, secretion of the hormone capable of starting the correcting action or response is stimulated until the need (demand) is met and the body condition returns to the normal range. As the correction occurs, hormone secretion decreases (and may halt). This control of hormone synthesis is **negative feedback** because the hormone causes the *opposite* action of the initial condition change.

An example of a simple negative-feedback hormone response is the control of insulin secretion. When blood glucose levels start to rise above normal, the hormone *insulin* is secreted. Insulin increases glucose uptake by the cells, causing a *decrease* in blood glucose levels. Thus the action of insulin (decreasing blood glucose levels) is the opposite of or negative to the condition that stimulated insulin secretion (elevated blood glucose levels).

Some hormones have more complex interactions for negative feedback. These interactions involve a series of reactions in which more than one endocrine gland, as well as the final target tissues, are stimulated. In this situation, the first hormone in the series may have another endocrine gland or glands as its target tissue. The final result of complex negative feedback for endocrine function is still opposite of the initiating condition.

An example of complex control is the interaction of the hypothalamus and the anterior pituitary with the adrenal cortex (Fig. 61-3). Low blood levels of cortisol from the adrenal cortex stimulate the secretion of corticotropin-releasing hormone (CRH) in the hypothalamus. CRH stimulates the anterior pituitary gland to secrete adrenocorticotropic hormone (ACTH). ACTH then triggers the release of cortisol from the adrenal cortex, the final endocrine gland in this series. The rising blood levels of cortisol inhibit CRH release from the hypothalamus. Without CRH, the anterior pituitary gland stops secretion of ACTH. In response, normal blood cortisol levels are maintained.

The normal blood level range of each hormone is well defined. Excesses or deficiencies of hormone secretion can lead to pathologic conditions affecting many body systems.

Hypothalamus and Pituitary Glands

The hypothalamus is a small area of nerve and endocrine tissue located beneath the thalamus in the brain. Nerve fibers connect the hypothalamus to the rest of the central nervous system. The hypothalamus shares a small, closed circulatory system with the anterior pituitary gland, known as the *hypothalamic-hypophysial portal system*. This system allows hormones produced in the hypothalamus to travel directly to the anterior pituitary gland so only very small amounts are present in systemic circulation where they are not needed.

The function of the hypothalamus is to produce regulatory hormones (see Table 61-1). Some of these hormones are released into the blood and travel to the anterior pituitary, where they either stimulate or inhibit the release of anterior pituitary hormones.

The pituitary gland is located at the base of the brain in a protective pocket of the sphenoid bone (see Fig. 61-1). It is divided into the anterior lobe *(adenohypophysis)* and the posterior lobe *(neurohypophysis)*. Nerve fibers in the hypophysial stalk connect the hypothalamus to the posterior pituitary (Fig. 61-4).

In response to the releasing hormones of the hypothalamus, the anterior pituitary secretes some tropic (trophic) hormones that stimulate other endocrine glands. Other pituitary hormones, such as prolactin, produce their effect directly on final target tissues (Table 61-2).

The hormones of the posterior pituitary—vasopressin (antidiuretic hormone [ADH]) and oxytocin—are produced in the hypothalamus and delivered to the posterior pituitary where

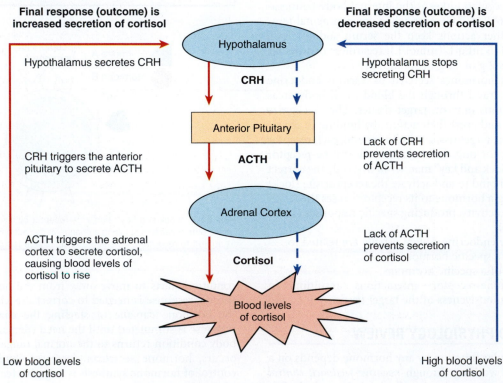

FIG. 61-3 Examples of positive and negative feedback control of hormone secretion. *ACTH,* Adrenocorticotropic hormone; *CRH,* corticotropin-releasing hormone.

TABLE 61-2   Pituitary Hormones: Target Tissues and Subsequent Actions

HORMONE	TARGET TISSUE	ACTIONS
Anterior Pituitary		
Thyroid-stimulating hormone or thyrotropin (TSH)	Thyroid	Stimulates synthesis and release of thyroid hormone
Adrenocorticotropic hormone, corticotropin (ACTH)	Adrenal cortex	Stimulates synthesis and release of corticosteroids and adrenocortical growth
Luteinizing hormone (LH) (known as *Leydig cell–stimulating hormone* in males)	Ovary Testis	Stimulates ovulation and progesterone secretion Stimulates testosterone secretion
Follicle-stimulating hormone (FSH) (known as *interstitial cell–* or *Sertoli cell–stimulating hormone* in males)	Ovary Testis	Stimulates estrogen secretion and follicle maturation Stimulates spermatogenesis
Prolactin (PRL)	Mammary glands	Stimulates breast milk production
Growth hormone (GH)	Bone and soft tissue	Promotes growth through lipolysis, protein anabolism, and insulin antagonism
Melanocyte-stimulating hormone (MSH)	Melanocytes	Promotes pigmentation
Posterior Pituitary*		
Vasopressin (antidiuretic hormone [ADH])	Kidney	Promotes water reabsorption
Oxytocin	Uterus and mammary glands	Stimulates uterine contractions and ejection of breast milk

*These hormones are synthesized in the hypothalamus and are stored in the posterior pituitary gland. They are transported from the hypothalamus down the hypothalamic stalk to the posterior pituitary while bound to proteins known as *neurophysins.*

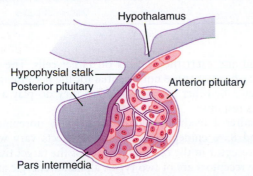

FIG. 61-4 Hypothalamus, hypophysial stalk, anterior pituitary gland, and posterior pituitary gland. (From Guyton, A., & Hall, J. (2006). *Textbook of medical physiology* (11th ed.). Philadelphia: Saunders.)

they are stored. These hormones are released from the posterior pituitary into the blood when needed.

Other factors affect hormone release from the pituitary gland. Drugs, diet, lifestyle, and pathologic conditions can change pituitary hormone secretion (McCance et al., 2014).

Gonads

The **gonads** are the male and female reproductive endocrine glands. Male gonads are the testes, and female gonads are the ovaries. Function of the gonads is dormant until puberty when, under the influence of gonadotropic hormones secreted by the anterior pituitary, the glands and external genitalia mature. The testes are stimulated to produce testosterone, and the ovaries are stimulated to produce estrogen. These changes are responsible for the development of secondary sexual characteristics. The function of the gonads is detailed in Chapter 69.

Adrenal Glands

The adrenal glands are vascular, tent-shaped organs on the top of each kidney. They have an outer cortex and an inner medulla (see Fig. 61-1). Adrenal hormones affect the entire body.

Adrenal Cortex

The adrenal cortex makes up about 90% of the adrenal gland and has cells divided into three layers. The main hormone types secreted by the cortex are the mineralocorticoids and the glucocorticoids. In addition, the cortex also secretes small amounts of sex hormones.

Mineralocorticoids are produced and secreted by the adrenal cortex to help control FLUID AND ELECTROLYTE BALANCE. **Aldosterone** is the mineralocorticoid that maintains extracellular fluid volume. It promotes sodium and water reabsorption and potassium excretion in the kidney. Aldosterone secretion is regulated by the renin-angiotensin system, serum potassium ion level, and adrenocorticotropic hormone (ACTH).

Renin is produced by specialized cells of the kidney arterioles. Its release is triggered by a decrease in extracellular fluid volume from blood loss, sodium loss, or posture changes. Renin converts renin substrate (angiotensinogen), a plasma protein, to angiotensin I. Angiotensin I is converted by an enzyme to form angiotensin II, the active form. In turn, angiotensin II stimulates the secretion of aldosterone. Chapter 11 (see Fig. 11-6) further explains the renin-angiotensin-aldosterone system (RAAS). Aldosterone causes the kidney to reabsorb sodium and water to bring the plasma volume and osmolarity back to normal.

Serum potassium level also controls aldosterone secretion. It is secreted whenever the serum potassium level increases above normal by as little as 0.1 mEq/L (mmol/L). Aldosterone then enhances kidney excretion of potassium to reduce the blood potassium level back to normal.

Glucocorticoids are produced by the adrenal cortex and are essential for life. The main glucocorticoid produced by the adrenal cortex is **cortisol**. Cortisol affects:

- The body's response to stress
- Carbohydrate, protein, and fat metabolism
- Emotional stability
- Immune function
- Sodium and water balance

TABLE 61-3 **Functions of Glucocorticoid Hormones**
• Prevent hypoglycemia by increasing liver glucose production (gluconeogenesis) and inhibiting peripheral glucose use
• Maintain excitability and responsiveness of cardiac muscle
• Increase lipolysis, releasing glycerol and free fatty acids
• Increase protein catabolism
• Degrade collagen and connective tissue
• Increase the number of mature neutrophils released from bone marrow
• Exert anti-inflammatory effects that decrease the migration of inflammatory cells to sites of injury
• Maintain behavior and cognitive functions

TABLE 61-4 **Catecholamine Receptors and Effects of Adrenal Medullary Hormone Stimulation on Selected Organs and Tissues**		
ORGAN OR TISSUE	**RECEPTORS**	**EFFECTS**
Heart	Beta$_1$	Increased heart rate Increased contractility
Blood vessels	Alpha Beta$_2$	Vasoconstriction Vasodilation
GI tract	Alpha Beta	Increased sphincter tone Decreased motility
Kidneys	Beta$_2$	Increased renin release
Bronchioles	Beta$_2$	Relaxation; dilation
Bladder	Alpha Beta$_2$	Sphincter contractions Relaxation of detrusor muscle
Skin	Alpha	Increased sweating
Fat cells	Beta	Increased lipolysis
Liver	Alpha	Increased gluconeogenesis and glycogenolysis
Pancreas	Alpha Beta	Decreased glucagon and insulin release Increased glucagon and insulin release
Eyes	Alpha	Dilation of pupils

Cortisol also influences other important body processes. For example, it must be present for epinephrine and norepinephrine action and maintaining the normal excitability of the heart muscle cells (McCance et al., 2014). Glucocorticoid functions are listed in Table 61-3.

Glucocorticoid release is regulated directly by the anterior pituitary hormone *ACTH* and indirectly by the hypothalamic corticotropin-releasing hormone *(CRH)*. The release of CRH and ACTH is affected by the serum level of free cortisol, the normal sleep-wake cycle, and stress.

As described earlier and shown in Fig. 61-3, when blood cortisol levels are low, the hypothalamus secretes CRH, which triggers the pituitary to release ACTH. Then ACTH triggers the adrenal cortex to secrete cortisol. Adequate or elevated blood levels of cortisol *inhibit* the release of CRH and ACTH. This inhibitory effect is an example of a negative-feedback system.

Glucocorticoid release peaks in the morning and reaches its lowest level 12 hours after the peak. Emotional, chemical, or physical stress increases the release of glucocorticoids.

Sex hormones (androgens and estrogens) are secreted in low levels by the adrenal cortex in both genders. Adrenal secretion of these hormones is usually not significant because the gonads (ovaries and testes) secrete much larger amounts of estrogens and androgens. However, in women the adrenal gland is the major source of androgens.

❓ NCLEX EXAMINATION CHALLENGE 61-1

Physiological Integrity

Which hormone changes does the nurse expect when a client receives a continuous cortisol infusion for 24 hours when his or her endocrine feedback mechanisms are functioning normally?
A. Lower than normal adrenocorticotropic hormone (ACTH) levels; lower than normal corticotropin-releasing hormone (CRH) levels
B. Lower than normal adrenocorticotropic hormone (ACTH) levels; higher than normal corticotropin-releasing hormone (CRH) levels
C. Higher than normal adrenocorticotropic hormone (ACTH) levels; lower than normal corticotropin-releasing hormone (CRH) levels
D. Higher than normal adrenocorticotropic hormone (ACTH) levels; higher than normal corticotropin-releasing hormone (CRH) levels

Adrenal Medulla

The adrenal medulla is a sympathetic nerve ganglion that has secretory cells. Stimulation of the sympathetic nervous system causes the release of adrenal medullary hormones, the catecholamines (which include epinephrine and norepinephrine). These hormones travel to all areas of the body through the blood and exert their effects on target cells. The adrenal medullary hormones are not essential for life because they also are secreted by other body tissues, but they do play a role in the stress response.

The adrenal medulla secretes about 15% norepinephrine (NE) and 85% epinephrine. Hormone effects vary with the specific receptor in the cell membranes of the target tissue.

These receptors are of two types: alpha adrenergic and beta adrenergic, which are further classified as alpha$_1$ and alpha$_2$ receptors and beta$_1$, beta$_2$, and beta$_3$ receptors. NE acts mainly on alpha-adrenergic receptors, and epinephrine acts mainly on beta-adrenergic receptors.

Catecholamines exert their actions on many target organs (Table 61-4). Activation of the sympathetic nervous system, which then releases adrenal medullary catecholamines, is an important part of the stress response. Catecholamines are secreted in small amounts at all times to maintain homeostasis. Stress triggers increased secretion of these hormones, resulting in the "fight-or-flight" response, a state of heightened physical and emotional awareness.

Thyroid Gland

The thyroid gland is in the anterior neck, directly below the cricoid cartilage (Fig. 61-5). It has two lobes joined by a thin strip of tissue *(isthmus)* in front of the trachea.

The thyroid gland is composed of follicular and parafollicular cells. Follicular cells produce the thyroid hormones thyroxine (T$_4$) and triiodothyronine (T$_3$). Parafollicular cells produce thyrocalcitonin (TCT or calcitonin), which helps regulate serum calcium levels.

Control of metabolism occurs through T$_3$ and T$_4$. Both hormones increase metabolism, which causes an increase in oxygen use and heat production in all tissues. Most circulating T$_4$ and

T_3 are bound to plasma proteins. The free hormone moves into the cell, where it binds to its receptor in the cell nucleus. Once in the cell, T_4 is converted to T_3, the most active thyroid hormone. Conversion of T_4 to T_3 is impaired by stress, starvation, dyes, and some drugs. Cold temperatures increase the conversion. Table 61-5 lists thyroid hormone functions.

Secretion of T_3 and T_4 is controlled by the hypothalamic-pituitary-thyroid gland axis negative-feedback mechanism. The hypothalamus secretes thyrotropin-releasing hormone (TRH). TRH triggers the anterior pituitary gland to secrete thyroid-stimulating hormone (TSH), which then stimulates the thyroid gland to make and release thyroid hormones. If thyroid hormone levels are high, release of TRH and TSH is inhibited. If thyroid hormone levels are low, TRH and TSH release is increased. Cold and stress are two factors that cause the hypothalamus to secrete TRH, which then stimulates the anterior pituitary to secrete TSH.

TABLE 61-5	Functions of Thyroid Hormones in Adults

- Control metabolic rate of all cells
- Promote sufficient pituitary secretion of growth hormone and gonadotropins
- Regulate protein, carbohydrate, and fat metabolism
- Exert effects on heart rate and contractility
- Increase red blood cell production
- Affect respiratory rate and drive
- Increase bone formation and decrease bone resorption of calcium
- Act as insulin antagonists

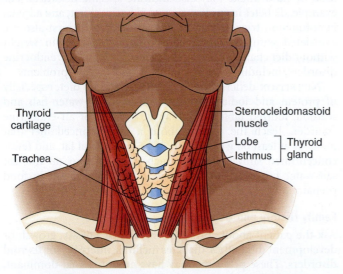

Thyroid cartilage
Trachea
Sternocleidomastoid muscle
Lobe
Isthmus
Thyroid gland

FIG. 61-5 Anatomic location of the thyroid gland.

Dietary intake of protein and iodine is needed to produce thyroid hormones. Iodine is absorbed from the intestinal tract as iodide. The thyroid gland draws iodide from the blood and concentrates it. After iodide is in the thyroid, it combines with the amino acid *tyrosine* to form T_4 and T_3. These hormones bind to thyroglobulin and are stored in thyroid follicular cells. When stimulated, T_4 and T_3 are released into the blood. They enter all cells, where they bind to DNA receptors and turn on genes important in metabolism to regulate basal metabolic rate (BMR).

Calcium and phosphorus balance occurs partly through the actions of calcitonin (thyrocalcitonin [TCT]), which also is produced in the thyroid gland. Calcitonin lowers serum calcium and serum phosphorus levels by reducing bone resorption (release) of these minerals. Its actions are opposite of parathyroid hormone.

The serum calcium level determines calcitonin secretion. Low serum calcium levels suppress the release of calcitonin. Elevated serum calcium levels increase its secretion.

Parathyroid Glands

The parathyroid glands consist of four small glands located close to or within the back surface of the thyroid gland (see Fig. 61-1). These cells secrete parathyroid hormone (PTH).

Parathyroid hormone regulates calcium and phosphorus metabolism by acting on bones, the kidneys, and the GI tract (Fig. 61-6). Bone is the main storage site of calcium. PTH increases **bone resorption** (bone release of calcium into the blood from bone storage sites), thus increasing serum calcium. In the kidneys, PTH activates vitamin D, which then increases the absorption of calcium and phosphorus from the intestines. In the kidney tubules, PTH allows calcium to be reabsorbed and put back into the blood.

Serum calcium levels determine PTH secretion. Secretion decreases when serum calcium levels are high, and it increases when serum calcium levels are low. PTH and calcitonin work together to maintain normal calcium levels in the blood and extracellular fluid.

Pancreas

The pancreas has exocrine and endocrine functions. The exocrine function of the pancreas involves the secretion of digestive enzymes through ducts that empty into the duodenum. The cells in the islets of Langerhans perform the pancreatic endocrine functions (Fig. 61-7). About one million islet cells are found throughout the pancreas.

The islets have three distinct cell types: alpha cells, which secrete glucagon; beta cells, which secrete insulin; and delta cells, which secrete somatostatin. Glucagon and insulin affect carbohydrate, protein, and fat metabolism.

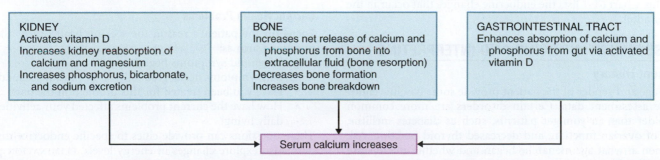

KIDNEY	BONE	GASTROINTESTINAL TRACT
Activates vitamin D Increases kidney reabsorption of calcium and magnesium Increases phosphorus, bicarbonate, and sodium excretion	Increases net release of calcium and phosphorus from bone into extracellular fluid (bone resorption) Decreases bone formation Increases bone breakdown	Enhances absorption of calcium and phosphorus from gut via activated vitamin D

Serum calcium increases

FIG. 61-6 Effects of parathyroid hormone on target tissues to maintain calcium balance.

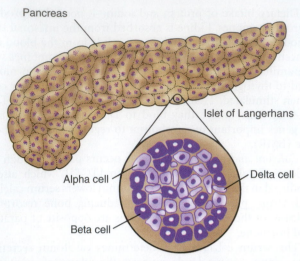

Pancreas

Islet of Langerhans

Alpha cell

Delta cell

Beta cell

FIG. 61-7 Cells of the islets of Langerhans of the pancreas.

Glucagon is a hormone that increases blood glucose levels. It is triggered by decreased blood glucose levels and increased blood amino acid levels. This hormone helps prevent hypoglycemia. Chapter 64 discusses glucagon function in more detail.

Insulin promotes the movement and storage of carbohydrate, protein, and fat. It lowers blood glucose levels by enhancing glucose movement across cell membranes and into the cells of many tissues. Insulin secretion rises in response to an increase in blood glucose levels. More information on insulin is presented in Chapter 64.

Somatostatin, which is secreted not only in the pancreas but also in the intestinal tract and the brain, inhibits the release of glucagon and insulin from the pancreas. It also inhibits the release of gastrin, secretin, and other GI peptides.

Endocrine Changes Associated With Aging

The effects of aging on the endocrine system vary but usually result in reduced glandular function and decreased hormone secretion. The three endocrine tissues that usually have reduced function with aging are the gonads, the thyroid gland, and the endocrine pancreas (Lamberts & van den Beld, 2016; Touhy & Jett, 2016). It is difficult to distinguish normal from abnormal endocrine activity in older adults because of chronic illness, changes in diet and activity, sleep disturbances, decreased metabolism, and the use of drugs that may affect hormone function. Consider these factors when assessing the older adult with endocrine dysfunction.

Encourage the older adult to participate in regular screening examinations, including fasting and random blood glucose checks, calcium level determinations, and thyroid function testing. Chart 61-1 lists the endocrine changes that occur in the older adult.

ASSESSMENT: NOTICING AND INTERPRETING

Patient History

The age and gender of the patient provide some baseline endocrine assessment data. Certain disorders are more common in older than in younger patients, such as diabetes mellitus, loss of ovarian function, and decreased thyroid function. Ask women at what age menarche began and whether menopause has occurred.

? NCLEX EXAMINATION CHALLENGE 61-2

Physiological Integrity

Which problems does the nurse expect in an older adult as a result of age-related changes in endocrine function? **Select all that apply.**
A. Increased basal metabolic rate (BMR)
B. Decreased core body temperature
C. Dehydration
D. Diarrhea
E. Hyperglycemia
F. Polyuria

Symptoms of endocrine disorders can be gender related, such as the sexual effects of hyperpituitarism and hypopituitarism (see Chapter 62). Thyroid problems are more common in women (McCance et al., 2014). Assess for a history of endocrine problems, symptoms that could indicate a disorder, and hospitalizations. Ask about past and current drugs, such as cortisone, levothyroxine, oral contraceptives, and antihypertensive agents. The use of exogenous hormone drugs, when not needed for hormone replacement, can cause serious dysfunction in many endocrine glands. Use the opportunity to warn patients about the dangers of misusing hormone-based drugs such as androgens and thyroid hormones (Burchum & Rosenthal, 2016).

Nutrition History

NUTRITION changes or GI tract disturbances may reflect many different endocrine problems. Ask about a history of nausea, vomiting, and abdominal pain. An increase or decrease in food or fluid intake may also indicate specific disorders. For example, diabetes insipidus triggers excessive thirst, and adrenal hypofunction triggers salt craving. Hunger and thirst also are associated with diabetes mellitus. Rapid changes in weight without diet changes are often associated with many endocrine disorders, including diabetes mellitus and thyroid problems.

NUTRITION deficiencies from an inadequate diet, especially of protein and iodide-containing foods (salt-water fish and seafood, iodized table salt), may be a cause of an endocrine disorder. Teach the patient about a well-balanced diet that includes at least 60 g of protein daily, less animal fat, and fewer concentrated simple sugars. Teach patients who do not eat salt-water fish on a regular basis to use iodized salt in food preparation.

Family History and Genetic Risk

Ask the patient about any family history of obesity, growth or development difficulties, diabetes mellitus, infertility, or thyroid disorders. These problems may have an autosomal-dominant, recessive, or cluster pattern of inheritance.

Current Health Problems

Focus on the patient's reason for seeking health care, asking questions such as:
- When did symptoms begin?
- Did symptoms occur gradually, or was the onset sudden?
- Have you been treated for this problem in the past?
- How have the current problems affected your activities of daily living?

These questions can provide clues to specific endocrine disorders. Also explore changes in energy levels, ELIMINATION patterns, sexual and reproductive functions, and physical features.

CHART 61-1 Nursing Focus on the Older Adult

Changes in the Endocrine System Related to Aging

CHANGES	CLINICAL FINDINGS	NURSING ACTIONS/ADAPTATIONS
Decreased antidiuretic hormone (ADH) production	Urine is more dilute and may not concentrate when fluid intake is low.	The patient is at greater risk for dehydration. Assess the older patient more frequently for dehydration. If fluids are not restricted because of another health problem, teach unlicensed assistive personnel (UAP) to offer fluids at least every 2 hours while awake.
Decreased ovarian production of estrogen	Bone density decreases.	Teach the patient to engage in regular exercise and weight-bearing activity to maintain bone density. Handle the patient carefully to avoid injury from pathologic fractures.
	Skin is thinner, drier, and at greater risk for injury.	Avoid pulling or dragging the patient. Use minimal tape on the skin. Help patients confined to bed or chairs change positions at least every 2 hours. Teach patients to use skin moisturizers.
	Perineal and vaginal tissues become drier, and the risk for cystitis increases.	Perform or assist the patient to perform perineal care at least twice daily. Unless another health problem requires fluid restriction, encourage all women to drink at least 2 liters of fluids daily. Teach sexually active older women to urinate immediately after sexual intercourse. Teach sexually active women that using vaginal lubricants with sexual activity can reduce discomfort and the risk for tissue damage.
Decreased glucose tolerance	Weight becomes greater than ideal along with: • Elevated fasting blood glucose level • Elevated random blood glucose level • Slow wound healing • Frequent yeast infections • Polydipsia • Polyuria	Obtain a family history of obesity and type 2 diabetes. Encourage the patient to engage in regular exercise and to keep body weight within 10 lb (4.5 kg) of ideal. Teach patients the signs and symptoms of diabetes and instruct them to report any of these to the primary health care provider. Suggest diabetes testing for any patient with: • Persistent vaginal candidiasis • Failure of a foot or leg skin wound to heal in 2 weeks or less • Increased hunger and thirst • Noticeable decrease in energy level
Decreased general metabolism	There is less tolerance for cold. Appetite is decreased. Heart rate and blood pressure (BP) are decreased.	Can be difficult to distinguish from hypothyroidism. Check for additional signs and symptoms of: • Lethargy • Constipation (as a change from usual bowel habits) • Decreased cognition • Slowed speech • Body temperature consistently below 97°F (36°C) • Heart rate below 60 beats/min Teach patients to dress warmly in cool or cold weather.

Energy level changes occur with many endocrine problems, especially thyroid problems (see Chapter 63) and adrenal problems (see Chapter 62). Ask the patient about any change in ability to perform ADLs and assess his or her current energy level. For instance, has he or she been sleeping longer or are fatigue and generalized weakness present?

ELIMINATION is affected by the endocrine system. Identify the patient's past pattern of elimination to determine deviations from the normal routine. Ask about the amount and frequency of urination. Does he or she urinate frequently in large amounts? Does the patient wake during the night to urinate (**nocturia**)? Information about the frequency of bowel movements and their consistency and color may provide clues to problems in FLUID AND ELECTROLYTE BALANCE or metabolic rate (i.e., thyroid function).

Sexual and reproductive functions are greatly affected by endocrine disturbances. Ask about any changes in the menstrual cycle, such as increased flow, duration, and frequency of menses or a change in the regularity of menses. Ask men whether they have experienced impotence. Ask men and women about a change in libido (sexual desire) or fertility issues.

Physical appearance changes can reflect an endocrine problem. Discuss any changes that the patient perceives in physical features. Ask about changes in:

- Hair texture and distribution
- Facial contours and eye protrusion
- Voice quality
- Body proportions
- Secondary sexual characteristics

For example, ask a man whether he is shaving less often or a woman if she has noticed an increase in facial hair. These changes may be associated with pituitary, thyroid, parathyroid, or adrenal dysfunction.

Physical Assessment

Inspection

An endocrine problem can change physical features because of its effect on growth and development, sex hormone levels, FLUID AND ELECTROLYTE BALANCE, and metabolism. Different findings can occur with many endocrine disorders or with nonendocrine problems.

Observe the patient's general appearance, and assess height, weight, fat distribution, and muscle mass in relation to age. Heredity and age rather than health problems may be responsible for some physical features (e.g., short stature). Assess scalp and body hair growth patterns.

When examining the head, focus on abnormalities of facial structure, features, and expression, such as:

- Prominent forehead or jaw
- Round or puffy face
- Dull or flat expression
- Exophthalmos (protruding eyeballs and retracted upper lids)

Check the lower neck for a visible enlargement of the thyroid gland. Normally the thyroid tissue cannot be observed. The isthmus may be noticeable when the patient swallows. Jugular vein distention may be seen on inspection of the neck and can indicate fluid overload.

Observe skin color and look for areas of pigment loss (hypopigmentation) or excess (hyperpigmentation). Fungal skin infections, slow wound healing, bruising, and petechiae are often seen in patients with adrenal hyperfunction. Skin infections, foot ulcers, and slow wound healing often occur with diabetes mellitus. With some types of adrenal gland dysfunction, the skin over the joints, as well as any scar tissue, may show increased pigmentation due to increased levels of adrenocorticotropic hormone (ACTH) and melanocyte-stimulating hormone.

Vitiligo (patchy areas of pigment loss) is seen with primary hypofunction of the adrenal glands and is caused by autoimmune destruction of melanocytes in the skin. It is seen most often on the face, neck, arms, hands, legs, and fold areas (Jarvis, 2016). Mucous membranes may have large areas of uneven pigmentation. Document the location, color, distribution, and size of skin color changes.

Inspect the fingernails for malformation, thickness, or brittleness, all of which may suggest thyroid gland problems. Examine the extremities and the base of the spine for edema, which suggests impaired FLUID AND ELECTROLYTE BALANCE.

Check the trunk for any abnormalities in chest size and symmetry. Truncal obesity and the presence of a "buffalo hump" between the shoulders on the back may indicate adrenocortical excess. Hormonal imbalance may also change secondary sexual characteristics. Inspect the breasts of both men and women for size, symmetry, pigmentation, and discharge. Striae (reddish-purple "stretch marks") on the breasts or abdomen are often seen with adrenocortical excess.

Assess the patient's hair distribution for signs of endocrine gland dysfunction. Changes can include hirsutism (excessive body hair growth, especially on the face, chest, and the center abdominal line of women), excessive scalp hair loss, or changes in hair texture (Jarvis, 2016).

Examination of the genitalia may reveal a dysfunction in hormone secretion. Observe the size of the scrotum and penis or of the labia and clitoris in relation to standards for the patient's age. The distribution and quantity of pubic hair are often affected in hypogonadism.

Palpation

The thyroid gland and the testes can be examined by palpation. Chapters 69 and 72 discuss examination of the testes. The thyroid gland is palpated for size, symmetry, general shape, and the presence of nodules or other irregularities.

Palpate the thyroid gland by standing either behind or in front of the patient. The posterior approach may be easier (Jarvis, 2016). Having the patient swallow sips of water during the examination helps you palpate the thyroid gland, which is not easily felt when normal.

Ask the patient to sit and to lower the chin. Using the posterior approach, place both your thumbs on the back of the patient's neck, with the fingers curved around to the front of the neck on either side of the trachea. Ask the patient to swallow, and locate the thyroid as you feel it rising. To examine the right lobe, turn the patient's head to the right and gently displace the trachea to the right with your left fingers. Palpate the right lobe with your right hand. Reverse this procedure to examine the left lobe (Jarvis, 2016).

⚠ NURSING SAFETY PRIORITY QSEN

Action Alert

Always palpate the thyroid gently in an adult who has or is suspected to have hyperthyroidism because vigorous palpation can stimulate a sudden release of thyroid hormones and cause a thyroid storm.

Auscultation

Auscultate the chest to assess cardiac rate and rhythm to use later as a means of assessing treatment effectiveness. Some endocrine problems induce dysrhythmias. Many endocrine problems can cause dehydration and volume depletion. Document any difference in the patient's blood pressure and pulse in the lying, standing, or sitting positions (orthostatic vital signs).

If an enlarged thyroid gland is palpated, auscultate the area of enlargement for bruits. Hypertrophy of the thyroid gland causes an increase in vascular flow, which may result in bruits.

Psychosocial Assessment

Many endocrine problems can change a patient's behaviors, personality, and psychological responses. Assess the patient's coping skills, support systems, and health-related beliefs. Ask whether the patient has noticed a change in how stress is handled, frequency of crying, or degree of patience and anger expression. Patients may not recognize these changes in themselves. Ask the family about changes in the patient's behaviors or personality.

A number of endocrine disorders affect the patient's perception of self. For example, body features can change greatly in disorders of the pituitary, adrenal, and thyroid glands. Infertility, impotence, and other changes in sexual function may result from endocrine problems. Encourage the patient to express his or her feelings and concerns about a change in appearance or in sexual function. Ask about any difficulty in coping with these changes.

Patients with endocrine problems may require lifelong drugs and follow-up care. Assess their readiness to learn and ability to carry out specific self-management skills. Patients may also face financial difficulties resulting from a prolonged medical regimen or loss of employment. A referral to social service agencies may be needed.

Diagnostic Assessment
Laboratory Tests

Laboratory tests are an essential part of the diagnostic process for possible endocrine problems. Fluids commonly used for these tests include blood, urine, and saliva. Salivary levels of the steroid hormones (cortisol, testosterone, progesterone, and estradiol) accurately reflect blood levels of these hormones (Sluss & Hayes, 2016). Protein hormones, such as those from the pituitary gland and thyroid gland, cannot be accurately assessed using saliva. Always check with the agency's laboratory for proper collection and handling of the specimen. The specialized testing for specific disorders is described in Chapters 62 to 64. Best practices for the collection of specimens for general endocrine testing are listed in Chart 61-2.

Assays. An assay measures the level of a specific hormone in blood or other body fluid. The most common assays for endocrine testing are antibody-based immunologic assays and chromatographic assays, which include mass spectrometry. These assays are very sensitive and can detect even minute quantities of a given hormone. Many different hormone concentrations can be analyzed at the same time by the mass spectrometry method.

Provocative/Suppression Tests. Measurement of specific hormone blood levels does not always distinguish between the normal and the abnormal. The wide normal range for some hormones makes it necessary to trigger responses by provocative ("stimulation") or suppression tests.

For the patient who might have an underactive endocrine gland, a stimulus may be used to determine whether the gland is capable of normal hormone production. This method is called *provocative testing.* Measured amounts of selected hormones are given to stimulate the target gland to maximum production. Hormone levels are then measured and compared with expected normal values. Failure of the hormone level to rise with provocation indicates hypofunction.

Suppression tests are used when hormone levels are high or in the upper range of normal. Drugs or other substances known to normally suppress hormone production are administered. Failure of suppression of hormone production during testing indicates hyperfunction.

Urine Tests. Hormone levels and their metabolites in the urine can be measured to determine endocrine function. Because many of the endocrine hormones are secreted in a pulsatile fashion, measurement of a specific hormone in a 24-hour urine collection, rather than as a single blood or urine sample, better reflects specific gland function, such as the adrenal gland. Teach the patient how to collect a 24-hour urine sample (see also Chart 61-2).

Certain hormones require additives in the container at the beginning of the collection. Instruct the patient not to discard the preservative from the container and to use caution when handling it because some are caustic. Remind him or her that this collection is timed for *exactly* 24 hours. Instruct the patient to avoid taking any unnecessary drugs during endocrine testing because some drugs can interfere with the assay.

Genetic Testing. When some hormone levels are too low to be measured, genetic testing may be performed. DNA analysis or RNA assessment can determine whether a genetic mutation is responsible for the lack of hormone production or the absence of hormone receptors (Sluss & Hayes, 2016).

Tests for Glucose. Tests for functions of the islet cells of the pancreas measure the *result* of pancreatic islet cell function. Blood glucose values and the oral glucose tolerance test help diagnose diabetes mellitus. The glycosylated hemoglobin (A1C) value indicates the *average* blood glucose level over a period of 2 to 3 months. (See Chapter 64 for diabetes mellitus testing.)

Imaging Assessment

Anterior, posterior, and lateral skull x-rays may be used to view the sella turcica, the bony pocket in the skull where the pituitary gland rests. Erosion of the sella turcica indicates invasion of the wall from an abnormal growth.

MRI with contrast is the most sensitive method of imaging the pituitary gland, although CT scans can also be used to evaluate it. The thyroid, parathyroid glands, ovaries, and testes are evaluated by ultrasound. CT scans are used to evaluate the adrenal glands, ovaries, and pancreas.

Other Diagnostic Assessment

Needle biopsy is a safe and quick ambulatory surgery procedure used to indicate the composition of thyroid nodules. It is used to determine whether surgical intervention is needed.

CHART 61-2 Best Practice for Patient Safety & Quality Care QSEN

Endocrine Testing

For Blood Tests:

- Check your laboratory's method of handling hormone test samples for tube type, timing, drugs to be administered as part of the test, etc. For example, blood samples drawn for catecholamines must be placed on ice and taken to the laboratory immediately.
- Explain the procedure and any restrictions to the patient.
- If you are drawing blood samples from an IV line, clear the line thoroughly. Do not use a double- or triple-lumen line to obtain samples; contamination or dilution from another port is possible.
- Emphasize the importance of taking a drug prescribed for the test on *time.* Tell the patient to set an alarm if the drug is to be taken during the night.

For Urine Tests:

- Instruct the patient to begin the urine collection (whether for 2, 4, 8, 12, or 24 hours) by first emptying his or her bladder.
- Remind the patient to *not* save the urine specimen that begins the collection. The timing for the urine collection begins *after* this specimen.
- Tell the patient to note the time of the discarded specimen and to plan to collect all urine from this time until the end of the urine collection period.
- To end the collection, instruct the patient to empty his or her bladder at the end of the timed period and *add* that urine to the collection.
- Check with the laboratory to determine any special handling of the urine specimen (e.g., Is a preservative needed? Does the container need to be kept cold?).
- If needed, make sure that the preservative has been added to the collection container at the *beginning* of the collection.
- Tell the patient about any preservative and the need to avoid splashing urine from the container because some preservatives make the urine caustic.
- If the specimen must be kept cool or cold, instruct the patient to place the container in an inexpensive cooler with ice. The specimen container should not be kept with food or drinks.

GET READY FOR THE NCLEX® EXAMINATION!

KEY POINTS

Review these Key Points for each NCLEX Examination Client Needs Category.

Safe and Effective Care Environment
- Be aware that assessment of endocrine problems requires a systematic approach because of the variety and combination of signs and symptoms. **QSEN: Evidence-Based Practice**
- Physical, psychosocial, and laboratory findings are needed for a complete and accurate endocrine assessment to avoid overlooking any problems. **QSEN: Safety**

Health Promotion and Maintenance
- Teach all patients that abusing or misusing hormones or steroids can have an adverse effect on endocrine function. **QSEN: Patient-Centered Care**
- Explain all diagnostic procedures, restrictions, and follow-up care to the patient scheduled for endocrine tests. **QSEN: Patient-Centered Care**

Psychosocial Integrity
- Encourage the patient to express concerns about a change in appearance, sexual function, or fertility as a result of a possible endocrine problem. **QSEN: Patient-Centered Care**

- Ask family members about changes in the patient's personality or behavior. **QSEN: Patient-Centered Care**

Physiological Integrity
- Be aware that the onset of endocrine problems can be slow and insidious or abrupt and life threatening.
- The presence of excess hormone production in an older adult is more likely to be caused by an actual endocrine problem than by age-related changes.
- Ask the patient about other family members with endocrine disorders, because some problems have a genetic component. **QSEN: Evidence-Based Practice**
- Ask the patient what prescribed and over-the-counter drugs are taken on a regular basis because some drugs can alter endocrine function. **QSEN: Patient-Centered Care**
- Follow the laboratory's procedures for collecting and handling specimens for endocrine function studies. **QSEN: Evidence-Based Practice**
- Differentiate normal from abnormal laboratory test findings and signs and symptoms for patients with possible endocrine problems. **QSEN: Patient-Centered Care**

SELECTED BIBLIOGRAPHY

Burchum, J., & Rosenthal, L. (2016). *Lehne's pharmacology for nursing care* (9th ed.). St. Louis: Elsevier.

Jarvis, C. (2016). *Physical examination & health assessment* (7th ed.). St. Louis: Saunders.

Lamberts, S., & van den Beld, A. (2016). Endocrinology and aging. In S. Melmed, K. Polonsky, P. R. Larsen, & H. Kronenberg (Eds.), *Williams' textbook of endocrinology* (13th ed.). Philadelphia: Elsevier.

Lazar, M., & Birnbaum, M. (2016). Principles of hormone actions. In S. Melmed, K. Polonsky, P. R. Larsen, & H. Kronenberg (Eds.), *Williams' textbook of endocrinology* (13th ed.). Philadelphia: Elsevier.

McCance, K., Huether, S., Brashers, V., & Rote, N. (2014). *Pathophysiology: The biologic basis for disease in adults and children* (7th ed.). St. Louis: Mosby.

Melmed, S., Polonsky, K., Larsen, P. R., & Kronenberg, H. (Eds.), (2016). *Williams' textbook of endocrinology* (13th ed.). Philadelphia: Elsevier.

Pagana, K., Pagana, T., & Pike-MacDonald, S. (2013). *Mosby's Canadian manual of diagnostic and laboratory tests*. St. Louis: Mosby.

Pagana, K., Pagana, T. J., & Pagana, T. N. (2017). *Mosby's diagnostic and laboratory test reference* (13th ed.). St. Louis: Mosby.

Sluss, P., & Hayes, F. (2016). Laboratory techniques for recognition of endocrine disorders. In S. Melmed, K. Polonsky, P. R. Larsen, & H. Kronenberg (Eds.), *Williams' textbook of endocrinology* (13th ed.). Philadelphia: Elsevier.

Touhy, T., & Jett, K. (2016). *Ebersole and Hess' toward healthy aging: Human needs and nursing response* (9th ed.). St. Louis: Mosby.

CHAPTER 62

Care of Patients With Pituitary and Adrenal Gland Problems

M. Linda Workman

PRIORITY AND INTERRELATED CONCEPTS

The priority concept for this chapter is FLUID AND ELECTROLYTE BALANCE.

✷ The FLUID AND ELECTROLYTE BALANCE concept exemplar for this chapter is Hypercortisolism (Cushing's Disease), p. 1255.

The interrelated concepts for this chapter are:
• CELLULAR REGULATION
• IMMUNITY

LEARNING OUTCOMES

Safe and Effective Care Environment

1. Collaborate with the interprofessional team to coordinate high-quality care and promote FLUID AND ELECTROLYTE BALANCE, CELLULAR REGULATION, and IMMUNITY in patients who have pituitary or adrenal disorders.
2. Teach the patient and caregiver(s) about how impaired FLUID AND ELECTROLYTE BALANCE, CELLULAR REGULATION, and IMMUNITY resulting from pituitary or adrenal problems affect home safety.

Health Promotion and Maintenance

3. Identify community resources for patients requiring assistance with any disorder of the pituitary or adrenal gland.

Psychosocial Integrity

4. Implement nursing interventions to help the patient and family cope with the psychosocial impact caused by acute or chronic problems of the pituitary or adrenal gland.

Physiological Integrity

5. Apply knowledge of anatomy, physiology, and pathophysiology to assess patients with impaired pituitary or adrenal gland function affecting FLUID AND ELECTROLYTE BALANCE, CELLULAR REGULATION, or IMMUNITY.
6. Interpret clinical changes and laboratory data to determine the effectiveness of therapy for diabetes insipidus (DI) and syndrome of inappropriate antidiuretic hormone (SIADH).
7. Prioritize evidence-based nursing care for the patient with acute adrenal insufficiency.
8. Teach the patient and caregiver(s) about common drugs and other management strategies used for pituitary or adrenal gland problems.
9. Prioritize evidence-based care for the patient with hyperaldosteronism or pheochromocytoma.

The pituitary and adrenal glands secrete hormones that affect the CELLULAR REGULATION of the entire body, including FLUID AND ELECTROLYTE BALANCE. When too much or too little of one or more hormones is secreted, physical and psychological changes are induced. The anterior pituitary hormones regulate growth, metabolism, and sexual development. The posterior pituitary hormone, vasopressin (antidiuretic hormone [ADH]), helps maintain FLUID AND ELECTROLYTE BALANCE. Adrenal gland hormones are life sustaining.

A complete assessment is performed to detect specific clinical findings. The patient also often undergoes many diagnostic tests and relies on the nurse for explanations. Surgical intervention may be indicated. Nursing care for the patient with pituitary or adrenal disorders includes assessment,

patient education, evaluating patient response to therapy, and providing support. The patient often needs lifelong hormone replacement therapy, and physical and emotional support is critical.

DISORDERS OF THE ANTERIOR PITUITARY GLAND

HYPOPITUITARISM

❖ *PATHOPHYSIOLOGY*

As discussed in Chapter 61, the anterior pituitary gland (adeno-hypophysis) secretes these hormones to maintain homeostasis:

- Growth hormone (GH; somatotropin)
- Thyrotropin (thyroid-stimulating hormone [TSH])
- Corticotropin (adrenocorticotropic hormone [ACTH])
- Follicle-stimulating hormone (FSH)
- Luteinizing hormone (LH)
- Melanocyte-stimulating hormone (MSH)
- Prolactin (PRL)

An adult with hypopituitarism usually has a deficiency of one pituitary hormone, a condition known as *selective hypopituitarism.* Decreased production of *all* of the anterior pituitary hormones *(panhypopituitarism)* is rare.

Deficiencies of *adrenocorticotropic hormone (ACTH)* or *thyroid-stimulating hormone (TSH)* are the *most* life threatening because they cause a decrease in the secretion of vital hormones from the adrenal and thyroid glands. Adrenal gland hypofunction is discussed later in this chapter; hypothyroidism is discussed in Chapter 63.

Deficiency of the **gonadotropins** (luteinizing hormone [LH] and follicle-stimulating hormone [FSH]—hormones that stimulate the gonads to produce sex hormones) changes sexual function in both men and women. In men, gonadotropin deficiency results in testicular failure with decreased testosterone production that may cause sterility. In women, gonadotropin deficiency results in ovarian failure, amenorrhea, and infertility.

Growth hormone (GH) deficiency changes tissue growth patterns by reducing liver production of *somatomedins.* These substances, especially somatomedin C, trigger growth and maintain bone, cartilage, and other tissues throughout life.

GH deficiency results from decreased GH production, failure of the liver to produce somatomedins, or a failure of tissues to respond to the somatomedins. In adults GH deficiency alters CELLULAR REGULATION by increasing the rate of bone destructive activity, leading to thinner bones (**osteoporosis**) and an increased risk for fractures.

The cause of hypopituitarism varies. Benign or malignant pituitary tumors can compress and destroy pituitary tissue. Pituitary function can be impaired by malnutrition or rapid loss of body fat. Shock or severe hypotension reduces blood flow to the pituitary gland, leading to hypoxia, infarction, and reduced hormone secretion. Other causes of hypopituitarism include head trauma, brain tumors or infection, radiation or surgery of the head and brain, and AIDS. *Idiopathic hypopituitarism* has an unknown cause.

Postpartum hemorrhage is the most common cause of pituitary infarction, which results in decreased hormone secretion. This clinical problem is known as *Sheehan's syndrome.* The pituitary gland normally enlarges during pregnancy; and, when hypotension during delivery results from hemorrhage, ischemia and necrosis of the gland occur.

❖ INTERPROFESSIONAL COLLABORATIVE CARE

Patients with hypopituitarism often require lifelong hormone replacement therapy (HRT). Such patients can be found in the community and in any care setting. It is important that HRT continues when they are admitted to an acute care setting for any reason.

◆ Assessment: Noticing

Changes in physical appearance and target organ function occur with deficiencies of specific pituitary hormones (Chart 62-1). Gonadotropin (LH and FSH) deficiency results in the loss of

 CHART 62-1   **Key Features**

Pituitary Hypofunction

DEFICIENT HORMONE	SIGNS AND SYMPTOMS
Anterior Pituitary Hormones	
Growth hormone (GH)	Decreased bone density Pathologic fractures Decreased muscle strength Increased serum cholesterol levels
Gonadotropins (luteinizing hormone [LH], follicle-stimulating hormone [FSH])	Women: • Amenorrhea • Anovulation • Low estrogen levels • Breast atrophy • Loss of bone density • Decreased axillary and pubic hair • Decreased libido Men: • Decreased facial hair • Decreased ejaculate volume • Reduced muscle mass • Loss of bone density • Decreased body hair • Decreased libido • Impotence
Thyroid-stimulating hormone (thyrotropin) (TSH)	Decreased thyroid hormone levels Weight gain Intolerance to cold Scalp alopecia Hirsutism Menstrual abnormalities Decreased libido Slowed cognition Lethargy
Adrenocorticotropic hormone (ACTH)	Decreased serum cortisol levels Pale, sallow complexion Malaise and lethargy Anorexia Postural hypotension Headache Hypoglycemia Hyponatremia Decreased axillary and pubic hair (women)
Posterior Pituitary Hormones	
Vasopressin (antidiuretic hormone [ADH])	Diabetes insipidus: • Greatly increased urine output • Low urine specific gravity (<1.005) • Hypotension • Dehydration • Increased plasma osmolarity • Increased thirst • Output does not decrease when fluid intake decreases

or change in secondary sex characteristics in men and women. In male patients, look for facial and body hair loss. Ask about impotence and decreased *libido* (sex drive). Women may report **amenorrhea** (absence of menstrual periods), **dyspareunia** (painful intercourse), infertility, and decreased libido. In female patients, check for dry skin, breast atrophy, and a decrease or absence of axillary and pubic hair.

Neurologic symptoms of hypopituitarism as a result of tumor growth often first occur as changes in vision. Assess the patient's visual acuity, especially peripheral vision, for changes or loss. Headaches, diplopia (double vision), and limited eye movement are common.

Laboratory findings vary widely. Some pituitary hormone levels may be measured directly. As described in Chapter 61, laboratory assessment of some pituitary hormones involves measuring the *effects* of the hormones rather than the actual hormone levels. For example, blood levels of triiodothyronine (T_3) and thyroxine (T_4) from the thyroid, testosterone and estradiol from the gonads, and prolactin levels are measured easily. If levels of any of these hormones are low, further pituitary evaluation is necessary.

Pituitary problems may cause changes in the *sella turcica* (the bony nest where the pituitary gland rests) that can be seen with skull x-rays (McCance et al., 2014). Changes may include enlargement, erosion, and calcifications as a result of pituitary tumors. CT and MRI can more distinctly define bone or soft-tissue lesions. An angiogram may be used to rule out the presence of an aneurysm or other vascular problems in the area before surgery.

◆ *Interventions: Responding*

Management of the adult with hypopituitarism focuses on replacement of deficient hormones to ensure appropriate CEL-LULAR REGULATION. Men who have gonadotropin deficiency receive sex steroid replacement therapy with androgens (testosterone). The most effective routes of androgen replacement are parenteral and transdermal. Therapy begins with high-dose testosterone and is continued until virilization (presence of male secondary sex characteristics) is achieved, with responses that include increases in penis size, libido, muscle mass, bone size, and bone strength. Chest, facial, pubic, and axillary hair growth also increase. Patients usually report improved body image after therapy is initiated. The dose may then be decreased, but therapy continues throughout life. Therapy to increase fertility requires gonadotropin-releasing hormone (GnRH) injections, rather than testosterone therapy (Kaiser & Ho, 2016).

Androgen therapy is avoided in men with prostate cancer to prevent enhancing tumor cell growth. Side effects of therapy include gynecomastia (male breast tissue development), acne, baldness, and prostate enlargement.

Women who have gonadotropin deficiency receive HRT with a combination of estrogen and progesterone. The risk for hypertension or *thrombosis* (formation of blood clots in deep veins) is increased with estrogen therapy, especially among smokers. Emphasize measures to reduce risk and the need for regular health visits. For inducing pregnancy, specific hormones may be given to trigger ovulation.

Adult patients with GH deficiency may be treated with subcutaneous injections of human GH (hGH). Injections are given at night to mimic normal GH release (Kaiser & Ho, 2016).

HYPERPITUITARISM

❖ *PATHOPHYSIOLOGY*

Hyperpituitarism is hormone oversecretion that occurs with anterior pituitary tumors or tissue hyperplasia (tissue overgrowth). Tumors occur most often in the anterior pituitary cells that produce growth hormone (GH), prolactin (PRL), and adrenocorticotropic hormone (ACTH). Overproduction of PRL also may occur in response to tumors that overproduce

GH and ACTH. Excess ACTH may occur with increased secretion of melanocyte-stimulating hormone (MSH).

🧬 GENETIC/GENOMIC CONSIDERATIONS
Patient-Centered Care QSEN

> One cause of hyperpituitarism is multiple endocrine neoplasia, type 1 (MEN1), in which there is inactivation of the suppressor gene *MEN1* (Online Mendelian Inheritance in Man [OMIM], 2016b). MEN1 has an autosomal-dominant inheritance pattern and may result in a benign tumor of the pituitary, parathyroid glands, or pancreas. In the pituitary, this problem causes excessive production of growth hormone and acromegaly. Ask a patient with acromegaly whether either parent also has this problem or has had a tumor of the pancreas or parathyroid glands.

The most common cause of hyperpituitarism is a pituitary adenoma—a benign tumor of one or more tissues within the anterior pituitary (Melmed et al., 2016). Adenomas are classified by the hormone secreted. As an adenoma gets larger and compresses brain tissue, neurologic changes, as well as endocrine problems, may occur. Symptoms may include visual disturbances, headache, and increased intracranial pressure.

Prolactin (PRL)-secreting tumors are the most common type of pituitary adenoma. Excessive PRL inhibits the secretion of gonadotropins and sex hormones in men and women, resulting in *galactorrhea* (breast milk production), amenorrhea, and infertility.

Overproduction of GH in adults results in *acromegaly* (Fig. 62-1). The onset may be gradual with slow progression, and changes may remain unnoticed for years before diagnosis of the disorder. Early detection and treatment are essential to prevent irreversible enlargement of the face, hands, and feet. Other changes include increased skeletal thickness, hypertrophy of the skin, and enlargement of many organs such as the liver and heart. Some changes may be reversible after treatment, but skeletal changes are permanent.

Bone thinning and bone cell overgrowth occur slowly. Breakdown of joint cartilage and hypertrophy of ligaments, vocal cords, and eustachian tubes are common. Nerve entrapment and hyperglycemia (elevated blood glucose levels) are common.

Excess ACTH overstimulates the adrenal cortex. The result is excessive production of glucocorticoids, mineralocorticoids, and androgens, which leads to the development of Cushing's disease (see Hypercortisolism [Cushing's Disease]).

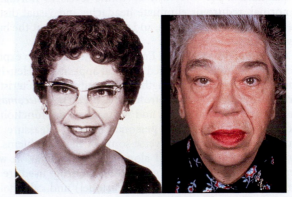

FIG. 62-1 Progression of acromegaly. (Courtesy of the Group for Research in Pathology Educations [GRIPE], Oklahoma City, OK.)

Usually hyperpituitarism is caused by benign tumors (*adenomas*) from one pituitary cell type (Melmed & Kleinberg, 2016). It can also be caused by a hypothalamic problem of excessive production of releasing hormones, which then overstimulate a normal pituitary gland.

❖ INTERPROFESSIONAL COLLABORATIVE CARE

Most care of a patient with hyperpituitarism occurs on an outpatient basis. When surgical intervention is required, hospitalization is necessary.

◆ Assessment: Noticing

Symptoms of hyperpituitarism vary with the hormone produced in excess. Obtain the patient's age, gender, and family history. Ask about any change in hat, glove, ring, or shoe size and the presence of fatigue. The patient with high GH levels may have backache and joint pain from bone changes. Ask specifically about headaches and changes in vision.

The patient with hypersecretion of PRL often reports sexual function difficulty. Ask women about menstrual changes, decreased libido, painful intercourse, and any difficulty in becoming pregnant. Men may report decreased libido and impotence.

Changes in appearance and target organ function occur with excesses of specific anterior pituitary hormones (Chart 62-2). Symptoms of GH excess are increases in lip and nose sizes, a prominent brow ridge, and increases in head, hand, and foot sizes. The patient often seeks health care because of these dramatic changes in appearance.

In a patient with hyperpituitarism, usually only one hormone is produced in excess because the cell types within the pituitary gland are so individually organized. The most common hormones produced in excess with hyperpituitarism are PRL, ACTH, and GH.

MRI is the best imaging assessment for diagnosis of hyperpituitarism (Melmed & Kleinberg, 2016). Skull x-rays may be used to identify abnormalities of the sella turcica.

Suppression testing can help diagnose hyperpituitarism. High blood glucose levels usually suppress the release of GH. Giving 100 g of oral glucose or 0.5 g/kg of body weight is followed by serial GH level measurements. GH levels that do not fall below 5 ng/mL (mcg/L) indicate a positive (abnormal) result.

◆ Interventions: Responding

The expected outcomes of management for the patient who has hyperpituitarism are to return hormone levels to normal or near normal, reduce or eliminate headache and visual disturbances, prevent complications, and reverse as many of the body changes as possible.

Nonsurgical Management. Encourage the patient to express concerns about his or her altered physical appearance. Help him or her identify personal strengths and positive characteristics. *Galactorrhea* (fluid leakage from the breast), *gynecomastia* (breast enlargement in men), and reduced sexual functioning can disturb self-image and personal identity. Reassure the patient that treatment may reverse some of these problems.

Drug therapy may be used alone or in combination with surgery and/or radiation. The most common drugs used are the dopamine agonists bromocriptine (Parlodel) and cabergoline (Dostinex). These drugs stimulate dopamine receptors in the brain and inhibit the release of GH and PRL. In most cases,

---

> **» CHART 62-2 Key Features**
> **Anterior Pituitary Hyperfunction**
>
> **Prolactin (PRL)**
> - Hypogonadism (loss of secondary sexual characteristics)
> - Decreased gonadotropin levels
> - Galactorrhea
> - Increased body fat
> - Increased serum prolactin levels
>
> **Growth Hormone (GH)**
> *Acromegaly*
> - Thickened lips
> - Coarse facial features
> - Increasing head size
> - Lower jaw protrusion
> - Enlarged hands and feet
> - Joint pain
> - Barrel-shaped chest
> - Hyperglycemia
> - Sleep apnea
> - Enlarged heart, lungs, and liver
>
> **Adrenocorticotropic Hormone (ACTH)**
> *Cushing's Disease (Pituitary)*
> - Elevated plasma cortisol levels
> - Weight gain
> - Truncal obesity
> - "Moon face"
> - Extremity muscle wasting
> - Loss of bone density
> - Hypertension
> - Hyperglycemia
> - Striae and acne
>
> **Thyrotropin (Thyroid-Stimulating Hormone [TSH])**
> - Elevated plasma TSH and thyroid hormone levels
> - Weight loss
> - Tachycardia and dysrhythmias
> - Heat intolerance
> - Increased GI motility
> - Fine tremors
>
> **Gonadotropins (Luteinizing Hormone [LH], Follicle-Stimulating Hormone [FSH])**
> *Men:*
> - Elevated LH and FSH levels
> - Hypogonadism or hypergonadism
>
> *Women:*
> - Normal LH and FSH levels

small tumors decrease until the pituitary gland is of normal size. Large pituitary tumors usually decrease to some extent.

Side effects of bromocriptine include orthostatic (postural) hypotension, headaches, nausea, abdominal cramps, and constipation. Give bromocriptine with a meal or a snack to reduce GI side effects. Treatment starts with a low dose and is gradually increased until the desired level is reached. *If pregnancy occurs, the drug is stopped immediately.*

> **! NURSING SAFETY PRIORITY** **QSEN**
> **Drug Alert**
>
> Teach patients taking bromocriptine to seek medical care immediately if chest pain, dizziness, or watery nasal discharge occurs because of the possibility of serious side effects, including cardiac dysrhythmias, coronary artery spasms, and cerebrospinal fluid leakage.

Other agents used for acromegaly are the somatostatin analogs, especially octreotide (Sandostatin) and lanreotide (Somatuline), and a growth hormone receptor blocker, pegvisomant (Somavert). Octreotide inhibits GH release through negative feedback. Pegvisomant blocks growth hormone (GH) receptor activity and blocks production of insulin-like growth factor (IGF). Combination therapy with monthly injections of a somatostatin analog and weekly injections of pegvisomant has provided good control of the disease.

Radiation therapy does not have immediate effects in reducing pituitary hormone excesses, and months to years may pass before a therapeutic effect can be seen. It is not recommended to manage acromegaly (Melmed & Kleinberg, 2016). The use of the gamma knife or stereotactic confocal radiotherapy method of delivering radiation to pituitary tumors has reduced the long-term side effects of this therapy.

Surgical Management. Surgical removal of the pituitary gland and tumor (**hypophysectomy**) is the most common treatment for hyperpituitarism. Successful surgery decreases hormone levels, relieves headaches, and may reverse changes in sexual functioning.

Preoperative Care. Explain that, because nasal packing is present for 2 to 3 days after surgery, it will be necessary to breathe through the mouth, and a "mustache" dressing ("drip" pad) will be placed under the nose. Instruct the patient not to brush teeth, cough, sneeze, blow the nose, or bend forward after surgery. These activities can increase intracranial pressure (ICP) and delay healing.

Operative Procedures. Depending on tumor size and location, a transsphenoidal approach or a minimally invasive endoscopic transnasal approach with smaller instruments is used instead of a more invasive procedure. General anesthesia is used. Nasal packing is inserted after the transsphenoidal incision is closed, and a mustache dressing is applied. These are not needed for the minimally invasive transnasal procedure. If the tumor cannot be reached by either the endoscopic transnasal or the transsphenoidal approach, a craniotomy may be indicated (Melmed & Kleinberg, 2016) (see Chapter 45).

Postoperative Care. Monitor the patient's neurologic response and document any changes in vision or mental status, altered level of consciousness, or decreased strength of the extremities. Observe the patient for complications such as transient diabetes insipidus (discussed later in this chapter), cerebrospinal fluid (CSF) leakage, infection, and increased ICP.

Teach the patient to report any postnasal drip or increased swallowing, which may indicate leakage of CSF. Keep the head of the bed elevated after surgery. Assess nasal drainage for quantity, quality, and the presence of glucose (which indicates that the fluid is CSF). A light yellow color at the edge of the clear drainage on the dressing is called the *halo sign* and indicates CSF. If the patient has persistent, severe headaches, CSF fluid may have leaked into the sinus area. Most CSF leaks resolve with bedrest, and surgical intervention is rarely needed.

Teach the patient to avoid coughing early after surgery because it increases pressure in the incision area and may lead to a CSF leak. Remind him or her to perform deep-breathing exercises hourly while awake to prevent pulmonary problems. Patients may have mouth dryness from mouth breathing. Instruct the patient to rinse the mouth frequently and to apply a lubricating jelly to dry lips.

Assess for indications of infection, especially meningitis, such as headache, fever, and nuchal (neck) rigidity. The surgeon may prescribe antibiotics, analgesics, and antipyretics.

If the entire pituitary gland has been removed, replacement of thyroid hormones and glucocorticoids is lifelong. Best practices for care after surgery are listed in Chart 62-3.

After surgery the patient needs daily self-management regimens and frequent checkups. Chart 62-4 lists areas for a focused

---

 CHART 62-3 **Best Practice for Patient Safety & Quality Care** QSEN

The Patient After Hypophysectomy

- Monitor the patient's neurologic status hourly for the first 24 hours and then every 4 hours.
- Monitor fluid balance, especially for output greater than intake.
- Encourage the patient to perform deep-breathing exercises.
- Instruct the patient not to cough, blow the nose, or sneeze.
- Instruct the patient to use dental floss and oral mouth rinses rather than toothbrushing until the surgeon gives permission.
- Instruct the patient to avoid bending at the waist to prevent increasing intracranial pressure.
- Monitor the nasal drip pad for the type and amount of drainage.
- Teach the patient methods to avoid constipation and subsequent "straining."
- Teach the patient self-administration of the prescribed hormones.

CHART 62-4 **Focused Assessment**

The Patient Who Has Undergone Nasal Hypophysectomy for Hyperpituitarism

Assess cardiovascular status:
- Vital signs, including apical pulse, pulse pressure, presence or absence of orthostatic hypotension, and the quality/rhythm of peripheral pulses

Assess cognition and mental status

Assess condition of operative site:
- Observe nasal area for drainage:
  - If present, note color, clarity, and odor
  - Test clear drainage for the presence of glucose

Assess neuromuscular status:
- Reactivity of patellar and biceps reflexes
- Oral temperature
- Handgrip strength
- Steadiness of gait
- Distant and near visual acuity
- Pupillary responses to light

Assess kidney function:
- Observe urine specimen for color, odor, cloudiness, and amount
- Ask about:
  - Headaches or visual disturbances
  - Ease of bowel movements
  - 24-hour fluid intake and output
  - Over-the-counter and prescribed drugs taken

Assess patient's understanding of illness and adherence with treatment:
- Symptoms to report to health care provider
- Drug plan (correct timing and dose)

---

assessment for the patient at home after a hypophysectomy. Review drug regimens and symptoms of infection and cerebral edema with the family.

After a hypophysectomy, advise the patient to avoid activities that might interfere with healing or increase intracranial pressure (ICP). Teach him or her to avoid bending over from the waist to pick up objects or tie shoes because this position increases ICP. Teach the patient to bend the knees and then lower the body to pick up fallen objects. ICP also increases when the patient strains to have a bowel movement. Suggest techniques to prevent constipation, such as eating high-fiber foods, drinking plenty of fluids, and using stool softeners or laxatives.

Teach the patient to avoid toothbrushing for about 2 weeks after transsphenoidal surgery. Frequent mouth care with mouthwash and daily flossing provide adequate oral hygiene. A decreased sense of smell is expected after surgery and usually lasts 3 to 4 months.

Hormone replacement with vasopressin may be needed to maintain fluid balance (see discussion of Interventions in the Diabetes Insipidus section). If the anterior portion of the pituitary gland is removed, instruct the patient in cortisol, thyroid, and gonadal hormone replacement. Teach the patient to report the return of any symptoms of hyperpituitarism immediately to the primary health care provider.

DISORDERS OF THE POSTERIOR PITUITARY GLAND

DIABETES INSIPIDUS

❖ PATHOPHYSIOLOGY

Diabetes insipidus (DI) is a disorder of the posterior pituitary gland in which water loss is caused by either an antidiuretic hormone (ADH) deficiency or an inability of the kidneys to respond to ADH. The result of DI is the excretion of large volumes of dilute urine because the distal kidney tubules and collecting ducts do not reabsorb water; this leads to polyuria (excessive water loss through urination), dehydration, and disturbed FLUID AND ELECTROLYTE BALANCE.

Dehydration from massive water loss increases plasma osmolarity and serum sodium levels, which stimulate the sensation of thirst. Thirst promotes increased fluid intake and aids in maintaining hydration. *If the thirst mechanism is poor or absent or if the adult is unable to obtain water independently, dehydration becomes more severe and can lead to death* (Robinson & Verbalis, 2016).

! NURSING SAFETY PRIORITY **QSEN**

Action Alert

Ensure that no patient suspected of having DI is deprived of fluids for more than 4 hours because he or she cannot reduce urine output and severe dehydration can result.

ADH deficiency is classified as neurogenic (primary or secondary), nephrogenic, or drug-related, depending on whether the problem is caused by insufficient production of ADH or an inability of the kidney to respond to the presence of ADH.

Primary neurogenic diabetes insipidus is caused by a defect in the hypothalamus or pituitary gland, resulting in a lack of ADH production or release. *Secondary neurogenic diabetes insipidus* is not caused by a direct problem with the posterior pituitary but is a result of tumors in or near the hypothalamus or pituitary gland, head trauma, infectious processes, brain surgery, or metastatic tumors.

Nephrogenic diabetes insipidus is a problem with the kidney's response to ADH rather than a problem with ADH production or release. Any severe kidney injury can reduce the ability of the kidney tubules to respond to ADH. In this situation, as long as the kidney is able to continue to produce urine, DI results. In some cases, a mutation in the gene responsible for producing the ADH receptor interferes with kidney response to ADH.

Drug-related diabetes insipidus is usually caused by lithium carbonate (Eskalith, Lithobid, Carbolith ♣) and demeclocycline (Declomycin) (Robinson & Verbalis, 2016). These drugs can interfere with the response of the kidneys to ADH.

GENETIC/GENOMIC CONSIDERATIONS
Patient-Centered Care **QSEN**

Nephrogenic diabetes insipidus can be a genetic disorder in which the ADH receptor (vasopressin receptor) has a defect that prevents kidney tubules from interacting with ADH. The result is poor water reabsorption by the kidney, although the actual amount of hormone produced is not deficient. This problem is most commonly inherited as an X-linked recessive disorder in which the *AVPR2* gene coding for the ADH receptor is mutated and only males are affected (Online Mendelian Inheritance in Man [OMIM], 2016a). There is also an autosomal form of the disorder in which the *AQP2* gene is mutated and both males and females are affected. When assessing a patient with DI, always ask whether anyone else in the family has ever had this disorder.

❖ INTERPROFESSIONAL COLLABORATIVE CARE

Management of patients with chronic DI occurs in the community unless acute problems develop. Also, whenever patients are in an acute care setting for other health problems, care must include continuing DI management.

◆ Assessment: Noticing

Most symptoms of DI are related to dehydration (Chart 62-5). Key symptoms are an increase in urination and excessive thirst. Ask about a history of recent surgery, head trauma, or drug use (e.g., lithium). Although increased fluid intake prevents serious volume depletion, the patient who is deprived of fluids or who cannot increase oral fluid intake may develop shock from fluid loss. Symptoms of dehydration (e.g., poor skin turgor, dry or cracked mucous membranes) may be present. (See Chapter 11 for discussion of dehydration.)

Water loss changes blood and urine tests. The 24-hour fluid intake and output is measured without restricting food or fluid intake. DI is considered if urine output is more than 4 L during this period and is greater than the volume ingested. The amount of urine excreted in 24 hours by patients with DI may vary from 4 to 30 L/day. Urine is dilute with a low specific gravity (less than 1.005) and low osmolarity (50 to 200 mOsm/kg) or osmolality (50 to 200 mOsm/L).

CHART 62-5 Key Features
Diabetes Insipidus

Cardiovascular Symptoms
- Hypotension
- Tachycardia
- Weak peripheral pulses
- Hemoconcentration

Kidney/Urinary Symptoms
- Increased urine output
- Dilute, low specific gravity

Skin Symptoms
- Poor turgor
- Dry mucous membranes

Neurologic Symptoms
- Decreased cognition*
- Ataxia*
- Increased thirst
- Irritability*

*Occurs when access to water is limited and rapid dehydration results.

CLINICAL JUDGMENT CHALLENGE 62-1

Safety; Patient-Centered Care QSEN

A 36-year-old man is admitted to your unit 4 hours after a surgical reduction of a compound fracture of the femur. His other health problems include hypercholesterolemia, for which he takes atorvastatin (Lipitor) 80 mg once daily, and bipolar disorder for which he takes lithium (Eskalith) 600 mg once daily. He has an IV of dextrose 5% in 0.45% saline infusing at a rate of 150 mL/hr. His blood pressure is now 96/70, down from the last reading of 128/80 obtained in the postanesthesia recovery area. His pulse is 84 and regular, and his pulse oximetry is 99%. In assessing him for possible shock, you note that the catheter drainage bag contains 800 mL of pale urine. His last output, measured 1 hour ago, was 1100 mL. According to the operative record, his output during the 3-hour surgery was 1800 mL. His total IV intake for the surgical and postoperative period was 1500 mL. He is to have his IV and Foley catheter removed when stable.

1. Is his output cause for concern? Provide a rationale for your response.
2. Will you discontinue the IV and/or the Foley? Why or why not?
3. What symptoms of shock are present?
4. What are the possible causes of his urine output volume?
5. What is your best course of action?

Interventions: Responding

Management focuses on controlling symptoms with drug therapy. The most preferred drug is desmopressin acetate (DDAVP), a synthetic form of vasopressin given orally, as a sublingual "melt," or intranasally in a metered spray (Robinson & Verbalis, 2016). The frequency of dosing varies with patient responses. Teach patients that each metered spray delivers 10 mcg and those with mild DI may need only one or two doses in 24 hours. For more severe DI, one or two metered doses two or three times daily may be needed. During severe dehydration, ADH may be given IV or IM. Ulceration of the mucous membranes, allergy, a sensation of chest tightness, and lung inhalation of the spray may occur with use of the intranasal preparations. If side effects occur or if the patient has an upper respiratory infection, oral or subcutaneous vasopressin is used.

! NURSING SAFETY PRIORITY QSEN

Drug Alert

The parenteral form of desmopressin is 10 times stronger than the oral form, and the dosage must be reduced.

For the hospitalized patient with DI, nursing management focuses on early detection of dehydration and maintaining adequate hydration. Interventions include accurately measuring fluid intake and output, checking urine specific gravity, and recording the patient's weight daily.

Urge the patient to drink fluids in an amount equal to urine output. If fluids are given IV, ensure the patency of the access catheter and accurately monitor the amount infused hourly.

The patient with permanent DI requires lifelong drug therapy. Check his or her ability to assess symptoms and adjust dosages as prescribed for changes in conditions. Teach that polyuria and polydipsia are signals of the need for another dose.

Drugs for DI induce water retention and can cause fluid overload (see Chapter 11). *Teach all patients taking these drugs*

to weigh themselves daily to identify weight gain. Stress the importance of using the same scale and weighing at the same time of day while wearing a similar amount of clothing. If weight gain of more than 2.2 lb (1 kg) along with other signs of water toxicity occur (e.g., persistent headache, acute confusion, nausea, vomiting), instruct the patient or family that the patient must go to the emergency department or call 911. Instruct him or her to wear a medical alert bracelet identifying the disorder and drugs.

NCLEX EXAMINATION CHALLENGE 62-1

Health Promotion and Maintenance

Which statements made by a client who has diabetes insipidus indicates to the nurse that more teaching is needed? **Select all that apply.**

A. If I gain more than 2 lb (1 kg) in a day, I'll limit my fluid intake.
B. If I become thirstier, I'll take another dose of the drug.
C. I'll avoid aspirin and aspirin-containing substances.
D. I'll stop taking the drug for 24 hours before I have any dental work performed.
E. I'll limit my intake of salt and sodium to no more than 2 g daily.
F. I'll wear my medical alert bracelet at all times.

SYNDROME OF INAPPROPRIATE ANTIDIURETIC HORMONE

❖ PATHOPHYSIOLOGY

The **syndrome of inappropriate antidiuretic hormone (SIADH)** or *Schwartz-Bartter syndrome* is a problem in which vasopressin (antidiuretic hormone [ADH]) is secreted even when plasma osmolarity is low or normal. A decrease in plasma osmolarity normally inhibits ADH production and secretion. SIADH occurs with many conditions (e.g., cancer therapy, pulmonary infection or impairment) and with specific drugs, including selective serotonin reuptake inhibitors (Robinson & Verbalis, 2016). Table 62-1 lists common causes of SIADH.

In SIADH, ADH continues to be released even when plasma is hypo-osmolar, leading to disturbances of FLUID AND ELECTROLYTE BALANCE. Water is *retained*, which results in dilutional **hyponatremia** (a decreased serum sodium level) and fluid overload. The increase in blood volume increases the kidney filtration and inhibits the release of renin and aldosterone, which increase urine sodium loss and lead to greater hyponatremia.

❖ INTERPROFESSIONAL COLLABORATIVE CARE

Severe or sudden onset SIADH usually requires management in an acute care setting. Mild SIADH is managed in the community.

◆ Assessment: Noticing

Ask the patient about his or her medical history, which may reveal conditions that can cause SIADH. Information about these conditions should be obtained:

- Recent head trauma
- Cerebrovascular disease
- Tuberculosis or other pulmonary disease
- Cancer
- All past and current drug use

TABLE 62-1 **Conditions Causing the Syndrome of Inappropriate Antidiuretic Hormone**	
Malignancies	**CNS Disorders**
• Small cell lung cancer	• Trauma
• Pancreatic, duodenal, and GU carcinomas	• Infection
• Thymoma	• Tumors (primary or metastatic)
• Hodgkin's lymphoma	• Strokes
• Non-Hodgkin's lymphoma	• Porphyria
	• Systemic lupus erythematosus
Pulmonary Disorders	**Drugs**
• Viral and bacterial pneumonia	• Exogenous ADH
• Lung abscesses	• Chlorpropamide
• Active tuberculosis	• Vincristine
• Pneumothorax	• Cyclophosphamide
• Chronic lung diseases	• Carbamazepine
• Mycoses	• Opioids
• Positive-pressure ventilation	• Tricyclic antidepressants
	• General anesthetics
	• Fluoroquinolone antibiotics

ADH, Antidiuretic hormone; *CNS,* central nervous system; *GU,* genitourinary.

Early symptoms of SIADH are related to the water-retention dilution of serum sodium levels (hyponatremia). GI disturbances, such as loss of appetite, nausea, and vomiting, may occur first, as discussed in Chapter 11. Weigh the patient and document any recent weight gain. Use this information to monitor responses to therapy. In SIADH, free water (not salt) is retained; and dependent edema is not usually present, even though water is retained.

Water retention, hyponatremia, and fluid shifts affect central nervous system function, especially when the serum sodium level is below 115 mEq/L (mmol/L). The patient may have lethargy, headaches, hostility, disorientation, and a change in level of consciousness. Lethargy and headaches can progress to decreased responsiveness, seizures, and coma. Assess deep tendon reflexes, which are usually decreased.

Vital sign changes include full and bounding pulse (caused by the increased fluid volume) and hypothermia (caused by central nervous system disturbance). Chapter 11 presents other findings that occur with hyponatremia.

Water retention causes urine volume to decrease and urine osmolarity to increase. At the same time, plasma volume increases, and plasma osmolarity decreases. Elevated urine sodium levels and specific gravity reflect increased urine concentration. Serum sodium levels are decreased, often as low as 110 mEq/L (mmol/L), because of fluid retention and sodium loss.

◆ *Interventions: Responding*

Medical interventions for SIADH focus on restricting fluid intake, promoting the excretion of water, replacing lost sodium, and interfering with the action of ADH. Nursing interventions focus on monitoring response to therapy, preventing complications, teaching the patient and family about fluid restrictions and drug therapy, and preventing injury.

Fluid restriction is essential because fluid intake further dilutes plasma sodium levels. In some cases, fluid intake may be kept as low as 500 to 1000 mL/24 hr (Robinson & Verbalis, 2016). Dilute tube feedings with saline rather than water and use saline to irrigate GI tubes. Mix drugs to be given by GI tube with saline.

Measure intake, output, and daily weights to assess the degree of fluid restriction needed. A weight gain of 2.2 lb (1 kg) or more per day or a gradual increase over several days is cause for concern. A 2.2-lb (1-kg) weight increase is equal to a 1000-mL fluid retention (1 kg = 1 L). Keep the mouth moist by offering frequent oral rinsing (warn patients not to swallow the rinses).

Drug therapy with vasopressin receptor antagonists (vaptans), such as tolvaptan (Samsca) or conivaptan (Vaprisol), is used to treat SIADH when hyponatremia is present in hospitalized patients. These drugs promote water excretion without causing sodium loss. Tolvaptan is an oral drug, and conivaptan is given IV. Tolvaptan has a black box warning that rapid increases in serum sodium levels (those greater than a 12-mEq/L [mmol/L] increase in 24 hours) have been associated with central nervous system demyelination that can lead to serious complications and death. In addition, when this drug is used at higher dosages or for longer than 30 days, there is a significant risk for liver failure and death (Robinson & Verbalis, 2016).

> **! NURSING SAFETY PRIORITY** **QSEN**
>
> **Drug Alert**
>
> Administer tolvaptan or conivaptan only in the hospital setting so serum sodium levels can be monitored closely for the development of hypernatremia.

Diuretics may be used on a limited basis to manage SIADH when sodium levels are near normal and heart failure is present. With diuretics sodium loss can be potentiated, further contributing to the problems caused by SIADH. For milder SIADH, demeclocycline (Declomycin), an oral antibiotic, may help reach FLUID AND ELECTROLYTE BALANCE, although the drug is not approved for this problem.

Hypertonic saline (i.e., 3% sodium chloride [3% NaCl]) is used to treat SIADH when the serum sodium level is very low (Robinson & Verbalis, 2016). Give IV saline cautiously because it may add to existing fluid overload and promote heart failure. If the patient needs routine IV fluids, a saline solution rather than a water solution is prescribed to prevent further sodium dilution.

Monitor the patient's response to therapy to prevent the fluid overload from becoming worse, leading to pulmonary edema and heart failure. Any patient with SIADH, regardless of age, is at risk for these complications. The older adult or one who also has cardiac, kidney, pulmonary, or liver problems is at greater risk.

Monitor for increased fluid overload (bounding pulse, increasing neck vein distention, crackles in lungs, dyspnea, increasing peripheral edema, reduced urine output) at least every 2 hours. *Pulmonary edema can occur very quickly and can lead to death.* Notify the primary health care provider of any change that indicates the fluid overload is not responding to therapy or is worse.

Providing a safe environment is needed when the serum sodium level falls below 120 mEq/L (mmol/L). The risk for neurologic changes and seizures increases as a result of osmotic fluid shifts into brain tissue. Observe for and document changes in the patient's neurologic status. Assess for subtle changes, such as muscle twitching, increasing irritability, or restlessness before they progress to seizures or coma. Check orientation to time, place, and person every 2 hours because disorientation or confusion may be present. Reduce environmental noise and lighting to prevent overstimulation.

Flow sheets recording neurologic assessments and laboratory data are helpful in detecting neurologic trends. The frequency of neurologic checks depends on the patient's status. For the patient being treated for SIADH who is hyponatremic but alert, awake, and oriented, checks every 2 to 4 hours may be sufficient. For the patient who has had a change in level of consciousness, perform neurologic checks at least every hour or as prescribed. Inspect the environment every shift, making sure that basic safety measures, such as side rails being securely in place, are observed.

 NCLEX EXAMINATION CHALLENGE 62-2

Safe and Effective Care Environment

When reviewing the laboratory values of a client who has chronic obstructive pulmonary disease and pneumonia, the nurse observes these findings. Which one does the nurse report to the provider immediately?

A. International normalized ratio (INR) 2.1
B. Serum chloride 96 mEq/L (mmol/L)
C. Serum sodium 117 mEq/L (mmol/L)
D. pH 7.28

DISORDERS OF THE ADRENAL GLAND

ADRENAL GLAND HYPOFUNCTION

❖ PATHOPHYSIOLOGY

Adrenocortical steroid production may decrease as a result of inadequate secretion of adrenocorticotropic hormone (ACTH), dysfunction of the hypothalamic-pituitary control mechanism, or direct dysfunction of adrenal gland tissue. Symptoms may develop gradually or occur quickly with stress. In acute adrenocortical insufficiency (adrenal crisis), life-threatening symptoms may appear without warning.

Insufficiency of adrenocortical steroids causes problems through the loss of aldosterone and cortisol action. Decreased cortisol levels result in hypoglycemia. Gastric acid production and glomerular filtration decrease. Decreased glomerular filtration leads to excessive blood urea nitrogen levels, which cause anorexia and weight loss.

Reduced aldosterone secretion causes disturbances of FLUID AND ELECTROLYTE BALANCE. Potassium excretion is decreased, causing hyperkalemia. Sodium and water excretion are increased, causing hyponatremia and hypovolemia. Potassium retention also promotes reabsorption of hydrogen ions, which can lead to acidosis.

Low adrenal androgen levels decrease the body, axillary, and pubic hair, especially in women, because the adrenals produce most of the androgens in females. The severity of symptoms is related to the degree of hormone deficiency.

Acute adrenal insufficiency (Addisonian crisis) is a life-threatening event in which the need for cortisol and aldosterone is greater than the body's supply (McCance et al., 2014). It often occurs in response to a stressful event (e.g., surgery, trauma,

severe infection), especially when the adrenal hormone output is already reduced. Problems are the same as those of chronic insufficiency but are more severe. *However, unless intervention is initiated promptly, sodium levels fall, and potassium levels rise rapidly (Pereira, 2016). Severe hypotension results from the blood volume depletion that occurs with the loss of aldosterone.* Best practices for emergency care of patients with acute adrenal insufficiency are listed in Chart 62-6.

Adrenal insufficiency (Addison's disease) is classified as primary or secondary. Causes of primary and secondary adrenal insufficiency are listed in Table 62-2. A common cause of secondary adrenal insufficiency is the sudden cessation of long-term glucocorticoid therapy. This therapy suppresses production of glucocorticoids through negative feedback by causing atrophy

---

⊙ CHART 62-6 Best Practice for Patient Safety & Quality Care QSEN

Emergency Care of the Patient With Acute Adrenal Insufficiency

Hormone Replacement
- Start rapid infusion of normal saline or dextrose 5% in normal saline.
- Initial dose of hydrocortisone sodium (Solu-Cortef) is 100 to 300 mg or dexamethasone 4 to 12 mg as an IV bolus.
- Administer additional 100 mg of hydrocortisone sodium by continuous IV infusion over the next 8 hours.
- Give hydrocortisone 50 mg IM concomitantly with hydration every 12 hours.
- Initiate an H_2 histamine blocker (e.g., ranitidine) IV for ulcer prevention.

Hyperkalemia Management
- Administer insulin (20 to 50 units) with dextrose (20 to 50 mg) in normal saline to shift potassium into cells.
- Administer potassium binding and excreting resin (e.g., Kayexalate).
- Give loop or thiazide diuretics.
- Avoid potassium-sparing diuretics, as prescribed.
- Initiate potassium restriction.
- Monitor intake and output.
- Monitor heart rate, rhythm, and ECG for signs and symptoms of hyperkalemia (slow heart rate; heart block; tall, peaked T waves; fibrillation; asystole).

Hypoglycemia Management
- Administer IV glucose as prescribed.
- Administer glucagon as needed and prescribed.
- Maintain IV access.
- Monitor blood glucose level hourly.

TABLE 62-2 Causes of Primary and Secondary Adrenal Insufficiency

Primary Causes	Secondary Causes
• Autoimmune disease*	• Pituitary tumors
• Tuberculosis	• Postpartum pituitary necrosis
• Metastatic cancer	• Hypophysectomy
• AIDS	• High-dose pituitary or whole-brain radiation
• Hemorrhage	• Cessation of long-term corticosteroid drug therapy*
• Gram-negative sepsis	
• Adrenalectomy	
• Abdominal radiation therapy	
• Drugs (mitotane) and toxins	

AIDS, Acquired immune deficiency syndrome.
*Most common cause.

> **CHART 62-7**   **Key Features**
>
> ### Adrenal Insufficiency
>
> **Neuromuscular Symptoms**
> - Muscle weakness
> - Fatigue
> - Joint/muscle pain
>
> **Gastrointestinal Symptoms**
> - Anorexia
> - Nausea, vomiting
> - Abdominal pain
> - Constipation or diarrhea
> - Weight loss
> - Salt craving
>
> **Skin Symptoms**
> - Vitiligo
> - Hyperpigmentation
>
> **Cardiovascular Symptoms**
> - Anemia
> - Hypotension
> - Hyponatremia
> - Hyperkalemia
> - Hypercalcemia

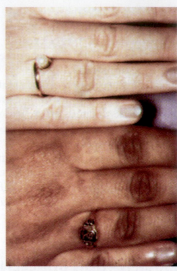

FIG. 62-2 Increased pigmentation seen in primary adrenocortical insufficiency. (From Wilson, J.D., Foster, D., Kronenberg, H., & Larsen, P.R. [1998]. *Williams' textbook of endocrinology* [9th ed.]. Philadelphia: Saunders. Courtesy Dr. H. Patrick Higgins.)

of the adrenal cortex. Glucocorticoid drugs must be withdrawn gradually to allow for pituitary production of ACTH and activation of adrenal cells to produce cortisol.

❖ INTERPROFESSIONAL COLLABORATIVE CARE

Acute adrenal insufficiency is an emergency and managed in an acute care setting. When detected early at a less severe stage, it is managed in the community.

◆ Assessment: Noticing

History. Ask about symptoms and factors that cause adrenal hypofunction. Ask about any change in activity level because lethargy, fatigue, and muscle weakness are often present. Include questions about salt intake, because salt craving often occurs with hypofunction.

GI problems, such as anorexia, nausea, vomiting, diarrhea, and abdominal pain, often occur. Ask about weight loss during the past months. Women may have menstrual changes related to weight loss, and men may report impotence.

Ask whether the patient has had radiation to the abdomen or head. Abdominal radiation could directly damage the adrenal glands, whereas cranial radiation could interfere with hypothalamic or pituitary influences on adrenal function. Document medical problems (e.g., tuberculosis or previous intracranial surgery) and all past and current drugs, especially steroids, anticoagulants, opioids, and cancer drugs.

Physical Assessment/Signs and Symptoms. Symptoms of adrenal insufficiency vary, and the severity is related to the degree of hormone deficiency (Chart 62-7). In patients with primary insufficiency (problem with adrenal gland function), plasma ACTH and melanocyte-stimulating hormone (MSH) levels are elevated in response to the adrenal-hypothalamic-pituitary feedback system. (Both ACTH and MSH are made from the same prehormone molecule. Anything that stimulates increased production of ACTH also leads to increased production of MSH.) Elevated MSH levels result in areas of increased pigmentation (Fig. 62-2). In primary autoimmune disease, patchy areas of decreased pigmentation may occur because of destruction of skin melanocytes. Body hair may also be decreased. In secondary adrenal insufficiency (problem in the hypothalamus or pituitary gland leading to decreased ACTH and MSH levels), skin pigmentation is not changed.

Assess for hypoglycemia (e.g., sweating, headaches, tachycardia, and tremors) and fluid depletion (postural hypotension and dehydration). **Hyperkalemia** (elevated blood potassium levels) can cause dysrhythmias with an irregular heart rate and result in cardiac arrest. **Hyponatremia** (low blood sodium levels) leading to hypotension and decreased cognition is often one of the first indicators of adrenal insufficiency (Pereira, 2016).

Psychosocial Assessment. Depending on the degree of imbalance, patients may appear lethargic, depressed, confused, and even psychotic. Assess the patient's orientation to person, place, and time. Families may report that the patient has wide mood swings and is forgetful.

Diagnostic Assessment. Laboratory findings include low serum and low salivary cortisol levels, low fasting blood glucose, low sodium, elevated potassium, and increased blood urea nitrogen (BUN) levels (Chart 62-8). In primary disease, the eosinophil count and ACTH level are elevated. Plasma cortisol levels do not rise during provocation tests (see Chapter 61).

Urinary 17-hydroxycorticosteroids are the glucocorticoid metabolites, and 17-ketosteroid levels reflect the adrenal androgen metabolites. Both levels are in the low or low-normal range in adrenal hypofunction.

An ACTH stimulation (provocation) test is the most definitive test for adrenal insufficiency. ACTH 0.25 to 1 mg is given IV, and plasma cortisol levels are obtained at 30-minute and 1-hour intervals. In primary insufficiency, the cortisol response is absent or very decreased. In secondary insufficiency, it is increased. When acute adrenal insufficiency is suspected, treatment is started without stimulation testing (Stewart & Newell-Price, 2016).

Imaging Assessment. CT, MRI, and arteriography may help determine the cause of pituitary problems leading to adrenal insufficiency. CT scans may show adrenal gland atrophy.

◆ Interventions: Responding

Nursing interventions focus on promoting fluid balance, monitoring for fluid deficit, and preventing hypoglycemia. *Because hyperkalemia can cause dysrhythmias with an irregular heart rate*

CHART 62-8 Laboratory Profile

Adrenal Gland Assessment

TEST	NORMAL RANGE FOR ADULTS	SIGNIFICANCE OF ABNORMAL FINDINGS	
		HYPOFUNCTION OF THE ADRENAL GLAND	HYPERFUNCTION OF THE ADRENAL GLAND
Sodium	136-145 mEq/L (mmol/L)	Decreased	Increased
Potassium	3.5-5.0 mEq/L (mmol/L)	Increased	Decreased
Glucose	Fasting: 70-110 mg/dL (4-6 mmol/L) *Older adults:* slightly increased	Normal to decreased	Normal to increased
Calcium	Total: 9-10.5 mg/dL (2.25-2.75 mmol/L) Ionized: 4.5-5.6 mg/dL (1.05-1.30 mmol/L) *Older adults:* slightly decreased	Increased	Decreased
Bicarbonate	23-30 mEq/L (mmol/L)	Increased	Decreased
BUN	10-20 mg/dL (3.6-7.1 mmol/L) *Older adults:* may be slightly higher	Increased	Normal
Cortisol (serum)	6 AM to 8 AM: 5-23 mcg/dL (138-635 nmol/L) 4 PM to 6 PM: 3-13 mcg/dL (83-359 nmol/L)	Decreased	Increased
Cortisol (salivary)	7 AM to 9 AM: 180-750 ng/dL 3 PM to 5 PM: <401 ng/dL 11 PM to midnight: <100 ng/dL	Decreased	Increased

Data from Pagana, K., Pagana, T., & Pike-MacDonald, S. (2013). *Mosby's Canadian manual of diagnostic and laboratory tests.* St. Louis: Mosby; and Pagana, K., Pagana, T.J., & Pagana, T.N. (2017). *Mosby's diagnostic and laboratory test reference* (13th ed.). St. Louis: Mosby.
BUN, Blood urea nitrogen.

and result in cardiac arrest, assessing cardiac function is a nursing priority. Assess vital signs every 1 to 4 hours, depending on the patient's condition and the presence of dysrhythmias or postural hypotension. Weigh the patient daily and record intake and output. Monitor laboratory values to identify hemoconcentration (e.g., increased hematocrit or BUN). Chapter 11 discusses dehydration in detail.

Cortisol and aldosterone deficiencies are corrected by hormone replacement therapy. Hydrocortisone corrects glucocorticoid deficiency (Chart 62-9). Oral cortisol replacement regimens and dosages vary. The most common drug used for this purpose is prednisone. Generally, divided doses are given, with two thirds given on arising in the morning and one third at 6:00 PM to mimic the normal release of this hormone.

! NURSING SAFETY PRIORITY QSEN

Drug Alert

Prednisone and prednisolone are sound-alike drugs, and care is needed not to confuse them. Although they are both corticosteroids, they are not interchangeable because prednisolone is several times more potent than prednisone and dosages are not the same.

An additional mineralocorticoid hormone, such as fludrocortisone (Florinef), may be needed to maintain or restore FLUID AND ELECTROLYTE BALANCE (especially sodium and potassium). Dosage adjustment may be needed, especially in hot weather when more sodium is lost because of excessive perspiration. *Salt restriction or diuretic therapy should not be started without considering whether it might lead to an adrenal crisis.*

CHART 62-9 Common Examples of Drug Therapy

Hypofunction of the Adrenal Gland

DRUGS	NURSING IMPLICATIONS
Cortisone	Instruct the patient to take the drug with meals or a snack *to avoid gastric irritation.*
Hydrocortisone (Cortef, Hycort)	Instruct the patient to report the following signs or symptoms of excessive drug therapy, *which indicate Cushing's syndrome and a possible need for a dosage adjustment:* • Rapid weight gain • Round face • Fluid retention
Prednisone (Winpred)	Instruct the patient to report illness *because the usual daily dosage may not be adequate during periods of illness or severe stress.*
Fludrocortisone (Florinef)	Monitor the patient's blood pressure *to assess for the potential side effect of hypertension.* Instruct the patient to report weight gain or edema *because sodium intake may need to be restricted.*

✳ FLUID AND ELECTROLYTE BALANCE CONCEPT EXEMPLAR Hypercortisolism (Cushing's Disease)

❖ PATHOPHYSIOLOGY

Cushing's disease is the excess secretion of cortisol from the adrenal cortex, causing many problems. It is caused by a problem in the adrenal cortex itself, a problem in the anterior pituitary gland, or a problem in the hypothalamus. In addition, glucocorticoid therapy can cause hypercortisolism.

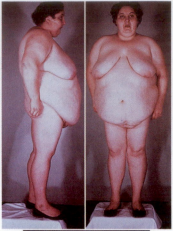

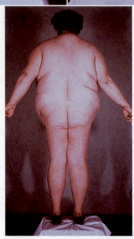

FIG. 62-3 Typical appearance of a patient with Cushing's disease or syndrome. Note truncal obesity, moon face, buffalo hump, thinner arms and legs, and abdominal striae. (From Wenig, B.M., Heffess, C.S., & Adair, C.F. [1997]. *Atlas of endocrine pathology.* Philadelphia: Saunders.)

The presence of excess glucocorticoids, regardless of the cause, affects metabolism and all body systems. An increase in total body fat results from slow turnover of plasma fatty acids. This fat is redistributed, producing truncal obesity, "buffalo hump," and "moon face" (Fig. 62-3). Increases in the breakdown of tissue protein result in decreased muscle mass and muscle strength, thin skin, and fragile capillaries. The effects on minerals lead to bone density loss.

High levels of corticosteroids reduce lymphocyte production and shrink organs containing lymphocytes, such as the spleen and the lymph nodes. White blood cell cytokine production is decreased. These changes reduce IMMUNITY and increase the risk for infection.

In most cases, increased androgen production also occurs and causes acne, **hirsutism** (increased body hair growth), and occasionally clitoral hypertrophy. Increased androgens disrupt the normal ovarian hormone feedback mechanism, decreasing the ovary's production of estrogens and progesterone. **Oligomenorrhea** (scant or infrequent menses) occurs as a result.

Etiology

Cushing's disease or syndrome is a group of clinical problems caused by an excess of cortisol. Table 62-3 lists causes of cortisol excess. When the anterior pituitary gland oversecretes

TABLE 62-3 Conditions Causing Increased Cortisol Secretion

Endogenous Secretion (Cushing's Disease)
- Bilateral adrenal hyperplasia*
- Pituitary adenoma increasing the production of ACTH (pituitary Cushing's disease)
- Malignancies: carcinomas of the lung, GI tract, pancreas
- Adrenal adenomas or carcinomas

Exogenous Administration (Cushing's Syndrome)
- Therapeutic use of ACTH or glucocorticoids—most commonly for treatment of:
  - Asthma
  - Autoimmune disorders
  - Organ transplantation
  - Cancer chemotherapy
  - Allergic responses
  - Chronic fibrosis

ACTH, Adrenocorticotropic hormone.
*Most common cause.

adrenocorticotropic hormone (ACTH), this hormone causes hyperplasia of the adrenal cortex in both adrenal glands and an excess of glucocorticoid production (see Fig. 61-3). This problem is **pituitary Cushing's disease** because the tissue causing the problem is the pituitary, not in the adrenal gland. When excess glucocorticoids are caused by an actual problem in the actual adrenal cortex, usually a benign tumor (adrenal adenoma), the problem is called **adrenal Cushing's disease** (or primary Cushing's disease) and usually occurs in only one adrenal gland. When glucocorticoid excess results from drug therapy for another health problem, it is known as **Cushing's syndrome** (also called *secondary Cushing's syndrome*).

Incidence and Prevalence

The most common cause of Cushing's disease is a pituitary adenoma. Women are more likely than men to develop Cushing's disease. Cushing's syndrome from chronic use of exogenous corticosteroids is more common because these drugs are often used to control serious chronic inflammatory conditions.

❖ INTERPROFESSIONAL COLLABORATIVE CARE

Cushing's syndrome is usually managed in the community. Cushing's disease is initially managed in an acute care setting.

◆ Assessment: Noticing

History. Ask about the patient's other health problems and drug therapies because glucocorticoid therapy is common. Regardless of cause, the patient has many changes because of the widespread effect of excessive cortisol. He or she may report weight gain and an increased appetite. Ask about changes in activity or sleep patterns, fatigue, and muscle weakness. Ask about bone pain or a history of fractures, because osteoporosis is common in hypercortisolism. Ask about a history of frequent infections and easy bruising. Women often stop menstruating. GI problems include ulcer formation from increased hydrochloric acid secretion and decreased production of protective gastric mucus.

Physical Assessment/Signs and Symptoms. The patient with hypercortisolism has specific physical changes, although all body systems are affected (see Fig. 62-3; Chart 62-10). Changes

CHART 62-10 Key Features

Hypercortisolism (Cushing's Disease/Syndrome)

General Appearance
- Moon face
- Buffalo hump
- Truncal obesity
- Weight gain

Cardiovascular Symptoms
- Hypertension
- Frequent dependent edema
- Bruising
- Petechiae

Musculoskeletal Symptoms
- Muscle atrophy (most apparent in extremities)
- Osteoporosis (bone density loss)
  - Pathologic fractures
  - Decreased height with vertebral collapse
  - Aseptic necrosis of the femur head
  - Slow or poor healing of bone fractures

Skin Symptoms
- Thinning skin
- Striae and increased pigmentation

Immune System Symptoms
- Increased risk for infection
- Reduced IMMUNITY
- Decreased inflammatory responses
- Signs and symptoms of infection/inflammation possibly masked

in fat distribution may result in fat pads on the neck, back, and shoulders ("buffalo hump"); an enlarged trunk with thin arms and legs; and a round face ("moon face"). Other changes include muscle wasting and weakness. Assess for and document changes and use these findings to prioritize patient problems.

Skin changes result from blood vessel fragility and include bruises, thin or translucent skin, and wounds that have not healed. Reddish-purple striae ("stretch marks") occur on the abdomen, thighs, and upper arms because of the destructive effect of cortisol on collagen.

Acne and a fine coating of hair may occur over the face and body. In women, look for the presence of hirsutism, clitoral hypertrophy, and male pattern balding related to androgen excess.

Cardiac changes occur as a result of disturbed FLUID AND ELECTROLYTE BALANCE. Both sodium and water are reabsorbed and retained, leading to hypervolemia and edema formation. Blood pressure is elevated, and pulses are full and bounding.

Musculoskeletal changes occur as a result of nitrogen depletion and mineral loss. Muscle mass decreases, especially in arms and legs (see Fig. 62-3). Muscle weakness increases the risk for falls. Bone is thinner, and osteoporosis is common, increasing the risk for fractures.

Glucose metabolism is affected by hypercortisolism. Fasting blood glucose levels are high because the liver releases glucose and the insulin receptors are less sensitive; therefore blood glucose does not move as easily into the tissues.

Immune changes caused by excess cortisol result in reduced IMMUNITY. Excess cortisol reduces the number of circulating lymphocytes, inhibits macrophage activity, reduces antibody synthesis, and inhibits production of cytokines and inflammatory chemicals (e.g., histamine). Infection risk is increased; and the patient may not have fever, purulent exudate, or redness in the affected area when an infection is present.

Psychosocial Assessment. Hypercortisolism can result in emotional instability, and patients often say that they do not feel like themselves. Ask about mood swings, irritability, confusion, or depression. Ask the patient whether he or she has been crying or laughing inappropriately or has had difficulty concentrating. Family members often report changes in the patient's mental or emotional status. The excess hormones stimulate the central nervous system, heightening the awareness of and responses to sensory stimulation. The patient often reports sleep difficulties and fatigue.

Laboratory Assessment. Laboratory tests include blood, salivary, and urine cortisol levels. These are high in patients with any type of hypercortisolism. Plasma ACTH levels vary, depending on the cause of the problem. In pituitary Cushing's disease, ACTH levels are elevated. In adrenal Cushing's disease or when Cushing's syndrome results from chronic steroid use, ACTH levels are low.

Salivary cortisol levels may be used to detect hypercortisolism because these levels accurately reflect blood levels, especially late-night specimens (Elias et al., 2014; Raff, 2015). A normal salivary cortisol level is lower than 2.0 ng/mL. Higher levels indicate hypercortisolism.

Urine is tested to measure levels of free cortisol and the metabolites of cortisol and androgens (17-hydroxycorticosteroids and 17-ketosteroids). In Cushing's disease, levels of urine cortisol and androgens are all elevated in a 24-hour specimen. Cortisol-to-creatinine ratios in the first specimen of the day can replace the 24-hour test for screening. A ratio greater than 25 nmol/mmol is a positive test (Stewart & Newell-Price, 2016)

Dexamethasone suppression testing can screen for hypercortisolism and may take place overnight or over a 3-day period. Set doses of dexamethasone are given. A 24-hour urine collection follows drug administration. When urinary 17-hydroxycorticosteroid excretion and cortisol levels are suppressed by dexamethasone, Cushing's disease is not present.

Additional laboratory findings that accompany hypercortisolism include:
- Increased blood glucose level
- Decreased lymphocyte count
- Increased sodium level
- Decreased serum calcium level

Imaging Assessment. Imaging for hypercortisolism includes CT scans, MRI, and arteriography. These images can identify lesions of the adrenal or pituitary glands, lung, GI tract, or pancreas.

◆ Analysis: Interpreting

The priority collaborative problems for patients with Cushing's disease or Cushing's syndrome are:
1. Fluid overload due to hormone-induced water and sodium retention
2. Potential for injury due to skin thinning, poor wound healing, and bone density loss
3. Potential for infection due to hormone-induced reduced IMMUNITY
4. Potential for acute adrenal insufficiency

◆ Planning and Implementation: Responding

Expected outcomes of hypercortisolism management are the reduction of plasma cortisol levels, removal of tumors, and restoration of normal or acceptable body appearance. When the disorder is caused by pituitary or adrenal problems, cure is possible.

When caused by drug therapy for another health problem, the focus is to prevent complications from hypercortisolism.

Restoring Fluid Volume Balance

Planning: Expected Outcomes. The patient with hypercortisolism is expected to achieve and maintain a normal or near-normal FLUID AND ELECTROLYTE BALANCE. Indicators include that these parameters are within or close to the normal range:

- Blood pressure
- Stable body weight
- Serum electrolytes, especially sodium and potassium

Interventions. Interventions for patients with fluid volume excess focus on ensuring patient safety, restoring FLUID AND ELECTROLYTE BALANCE, and providing supportive care. Depending on the cause, surgical management may be used to reduce cortisol production.

Nonsurgical Management. Patient safety, drug therapy, nutrition therapy, and monitoring are the basis of nonsurgical interventions for hypercortisolism and fluid overload.

Patient safety includes preventing fluid overload from becoming worse, leading to pulmonary edema and heart failure. Any patient with fluid overload, regardless of age, is at risk for these complications. The older adult or one who has coexisting cardiac problems, kidney problems, pulmonary problems, or liver problems is at greater risk.

Monitor for indicators of fluid overload (bounding pulse, increasing neck vein distention, lung crackles, increasing peripheral edema, reduced urine output) at least every 2 hours. *Pulmonary edema can occur very quickly and lead to death.* Notify the primary health care provider of any change that indicates the fluid overload either is not responding to therapy or is worse.

The patient with fluid volume excess and dependent edema is at risk for skin breakdown. Use a pressure-reducing or pressure-relieving overlay on the mattress. Assess skin pressure areas, especially the coccyx, elbows, hips, and heels, daily for redness or open areas. For patients receiving oxygen by mask or nasal cannula, check the skin around the mask, nares, and ears and under the elastic band. Help the patient change positions every 2 hours or ensure that others delegated to perform the intervention are diligent in this action.

Drug therapy involves the use of drugs that interfere with adrenocorticotropic hormone (ACTH) production or adrenal hormone synthesis for temporary relief. Metyrapone (Metopirone), aminoglutethimide (Elipten, Cytadren), and ketoconazole use different pathways to decrease cortisol production (Stewart & Newell-Price, 2016). For patients with hypercortisolism resulting from increased ACTH production, cyproheptadine (Periactin) may be used because it interferes with ACTH production. Mitotane (Lysodren) is an adrenal cytotoxic agent used for inoperable tumors causing hypercortisolism. For adults with increased ACTH production who have type 2 diabetes and who do not respond to other drug therapies, another drug is mifepristone (Korlym), which is a synthetic steroid that blocks glucocorticoid receptors.

⚠ NURSING SAFETY PRIORITY QSEN

Drug Alert

Mifepristone (Korlym) cannot be used during pregnancy because it also blocks progesterone receptors and would cause termination of the pregnancy.

A drug to manage hypercortisolism resulting from a pituitary adenoma is pasireotide (Signifor). This subcutaneous drug binds to somatostatin receptors on the adenoma and inhibits tumor production of corticotropin. Lower levels of corticotropin lead to lower levels of cortisol production in the adrenal glands (McKeage, 2013). The drug is ineffective for patients whose tumors do not have somatostatin receptors.

Monitor the patient for response to drug therapy, especially weight loss and increased urine output. Observe for symptoms of problems with FLUID AND ELECTROLYTE BALANCE, especially changes in electrocardiogram (ECG) patterns. Assess laboratory findings, especially sodium and potassium values, whenever they are drawn.

Nutrition therapy for the patient with hypercortisolism may involve restrictions of both fluid and sodium intake to control fluid volume. Review the patient's serum sodium levels whenever fluid overload is present. Often sodium restriction involves only "no added salt" to ordinary table foods when fluid overload is mild. For more pronounced fluid overload, the patient may be restricted to anywhere from 2 g/day to 4 g/day of sodium. When sodium restriction is ongoing, teach the patient and family how to check food labels for sodium content and how to keep a daily record of sodium ingested. Explain to the patient and family the reason for any fluid restriction and the importance of adhering to the prescribed restriction.

Monitor intake and output and weight to assess therapy effectiveness. Ensure that unlicensed assistive personnel (UAP) understand that these measurements need to be accurate, not just estimated, because treatment decisions are based on the findings. Schedule fluid offerings throughout the 24 hours. Teach UAP to check urine for color and character and to report these findings. Check the urine specific gravity (a specific gravity below 1.005 may indicate fluid overload). If IV therapy is used, infuse only the amount prescribed.

Fluid retention may not be visible. Rapid weight gain is the best indicator of fluid retention and overload. Each 1 lb (about 500 g) of weight gained (after the first half pound) equates to 500 mL of retained water. Weigh the patient at the same time daily (before breakfast), using the same scale. Have the patient wear the same type of clothing for each weigh-in.

Surgical Management. The surgical treatment of adrenocortical hypersecretion depends on the cause of the problem. When adrenal hyperfunction is due to increased pituitary secretion of ACTH, removal of a pituitary adenoma using minimally invasive techniques may be attempted. Sometimes a total *hypophysectomy* (surgical removal of the pituitary gland) is needed. (See earlier discussion of Hypophysectomy in the Hyperpituitarism section.) If hypercortisolism is caused by an adrenal tumor, an *adrenalectomy* (removal of the adrenal gland) may be needed.

Preoperative Care. Disturbances of FLUID AND ELECTROLYTE BALANCE are corrected before surgery. Continue to monitor blood potassium, sodium, and chloride levels. Dysrhythmias from potassium imbalance may occur, and cardiac monitoring is needed. Hyperglycemia is controlled before surgery.

The patient with hypercortisolism is at risk for complications of infections and fractures. Prevent infection with handwashing and aseptic technique. Decrease the risk for falls by raising top side rails and encouraging the patient to ask for assistance when getting out of bed. A high-calorie, high-protein diet is prescribed before surgery.

Glucocorticoid preparations are given before surgery. The patient continues to receive glucocorticoids during surgery to prevent adrenal crisis because the removal of the tumor results in a sudden drop in cortisol levels. Before surgery, discuss the need for long-term drug therapy.

Operative Procedures. A unilateral adrenalectomy is performed when one gland is involved. A bilateral adrenalectomy is needed when ACTH-producing tumors cannot be treated by other means or when both adrenal glands are diseased. Surgery is most often performed by laparoscopic adrenalectomy, a minimally invasive surgical approach. If necessary, an open surgery through the abdomen or the lateral flank can be performed.

Postoperative Care. After an adrenalectomy, the patient is monitored in an ICU. Immediately after surgery, assess the patient every 15 minutes for shock (e.g., hypotension; a rapid, weak pulse; and a decreasing urine output) resulting from insufficient glucocorticoid replacement. Monitor vital signs, central venous pressure, pulmonary wedge pressure, intake and output, daily weights, and serum electrolyte levels.

After a bilateral adrenalectomy, patients require lifelong glucocorticoid and mineralocorticoid replacement, starting immediately after surgery. In unilateral adrenalectomy, hormone replacement continues until the remaining adrenal gland increases hormone production. This therapy may be needed for up to 2 years after surgery.

🔎 NCLEX EXAMINATION CHALLENGE 62-3

Physiological Integrity

In the preoperative holding area, the client who is scheduled to have an adrenalectomy for hypercortisolism is prescribed to receive cortisol by IV infusion. What is the nurse's **best** action?

A. Request a "time-out" to determine whether this is a valid prescription.

B. Ask the client whether he or she usually takes prednisone.

C. Hold the dose because the client has a high cortisol level.

D. Administer the drug as prescribed.

Preventing Injury. The patient is at risk for injury from skin breakdown, bone fractures, and GI bleeding. Prevention of these injuries is a major nursing care focus.

Planning: Expected Outcomes. The patient with hypercortisolism is expected to avoid injury. Indicators include:

- Skin is intact.
- Minimal or no bruising is present.
- Bones are intact.
- Stools, vomitus, and other GI secretions contain no gross or occult blood.

Interventions. Priority nursing interventions for prevention of injury focus on skin assessment and protection, coordinating care to ensure gentle handling, and patient teaching regarding drug therapy for prevention of GI ulcers.

Skin injury is a continuing risk even after surgery has corrected the cortisol excess because the changes induced in the skin and blood vessels remain for weeks to months. Assess the skin for reddened areas, excoriation, breakdown, and edema. If mobility is decreased, turn the patient every 2 hours and pad bony prominences.

Instruct the patient to avoid activities that can result in skin trauma. Teach him or her to use a soft toothbrush and an electric shaver. Instruct patients to keep the skin clean and dry it thoroughly after washing. Excessive dryness can be prevented by using a moisturizing lotion.

Adhesive tape often causes skin breakdown. Use tape sparingly and remove it carefully. After venipuncture, the patient may have increased bleeding because of blood vessel fragility. Exert pressure over the site until bleeding has stopped.

Pathologic fractures from bone density loss and osteoporosis are possible for months to years after cortisol levels return to normal. Teach the patient about safety issues and dietary needs. When helping the patient move in bed, use a lift sheet instead of grasping him or her. Remind the patient to call for help when walking. Review the use of walkers or canes, if needed. Teach UAP to use a gait belt when walking with a patient who has bone density loss.

Coordinate with a dietitian to teach the patient about nutrition therapy. A high-calorie diet that includes increased amounts of calcium and vitamin D is needed. Milk, cheese, yogurt, and green leafy and root vegetables add calcium to promote bone density. Advise the patient to avoid caffeine and alcohol, which increase the risk for GI ulcers and reduce bone density.

GI bleeding is common with hypercortisolism. Cortisol (1) inhibits production of the thick, gel-like mucus that protects the stomach lining, (2) decreases blood flow to the area, and (3) triggers the release of excess hydrochloric acid. Although surgery reduces cortisol levels, the normal mucus and increased blood flow may take weeks to return. Interventions focus on drug therapy to reduce irritation, protect the GI mucosa, and decrease secretion of hydrochloric acid.

Antacids buffer stomach acids and protect the GI mucosa. Teach the patient that these drugs should be taken on a regular schedule rather than on an as-needed basis.

Some agents block the H_2 receptors in the gastric mucosa. When histamine binds to these receptors, a series of actions release hydrochloric acid. Drugs that block the H_2-receptor site include cimetidine (Tagamet, Peptol ♣, Novo-Cimetine ♣), ranitidine (Zantac, Apo-Ranitidine ♣), famotidine (Pepcid), and nizatidine (Axid). Omeprazole (Losec ♣, Prilosec) and esomeprazole (Nexium) inhibit the gastric proton pump and prevent the formation of hydrochloric acid.

Instruct the patient to reduce alcohol or caffeine consumption, smoking, and fasting because these actions cause gastric irritation. NSAIDs and drugs that contain aspirin or other salicylates can cause gastritis and intensify GI bleeding. These should be avoided or limited.

Preventing Infection. Glucocorticoids reduce both the inflammation and the immune responses of IMMUNITY, increasing the risk for infection. For the patient who is taking glucocorticoid replacement therapy, the risk is ongoing. For the patient who is recovering from surgery to prevent hypercortisolism, the infection risk continues for weeks after surgery.

Planning: Expected Outcomes. The patient with hypercortisolism is expected to remain free from infection and avoid situations that increase the risk for infection. Indicators include these symptoms and behaviors:

- Does not have fever and foul-smelling or purulent drainage
- Does not have cough, chest pain, and dyspnea
- Does not have urinary frequency, urgency, or pain and burning
- Avoids crowds and large gatherings
- Obtains appropriate vaccinations
- Washes hands frequently

Interventions. Protect the patient with reduced IMMUNITY from infection. All personnel must use extreme care during all nursing procedures. Thorough handwashing is important. Anyone with an upper respiratory tract infection who enters the patient's room must wear a mask. Observe strict aseptic technique when performing dressing changes or any invasive procedure.

Continually assess the patient for possible infection. Symptoms may not be obvious because excess cortisol suppresses infection indicators. Fever and pus formation depend on the presence of white blood cells (WBCs). The patient who has reduced IMMUNITY may have a severe infection without pus and with only a low-grade fever.

Monitor the patient's daily complete blood count (CBC) with differential WBC count, especially neutrophils. Inspect the mouth during every shift for lesions and mucosa breakdown. Assess the lungs every 8 hours for crackles, wheezes, or reduced breath sounds. Assess all urine for odor and cloudiness. Ask about any urgency, burning, or pain on urination.

Take vital signs at least every 4 hours to assess for fever. A temperature elevation of even 1° F (or 0.5° C) above baseline is significant for a patient who has reduced IMMUNITY and indicates infection until it has been proven otherwise.

Skin care is important for preventing infection because the skin may be the patient's only intact defense. Teach him or her about hygiene and urge daily bathing. If the patient is immobile, turn him or her every hour and apply skin lubricants.

Perform pulmonary hygiene every 2 to 4 hours. Listen to the lungs for crackles, wheezes, or reduced breath sounds. Urge the patient to deep breathe or use an incentive spirometer every hour while awake.

Preventing Acute Adrenal Insufficiency. The patient most at risk for acute adrenal insufficiency is the one who has Cushing's syndrome as a result of glucocorticoid drug therapy. The exogenous drug inhibits the feedback control pathway (see Figure 61-3), preventing the hypothalamus from secreting corticotropin-releasing hormone (CRH). The lack of CRH inhibits secretion of ACTH from the anterior pituitary gland. Without normal levels of ACTH, the adrenal glands atrophy and completely stop production of the corticosteroids. As a result, the patient completely depends on the exogenous drug. If the drug is stopped, even for a day or two, the atrophied adrenal glands cannot produce the glucocorticoids; and the patient develops acute adrenal insufficiency, a life-threatening condition. Management of this problem is described in the Adrenal Gland Hypofunction section.

> **! NURSING SAFETY PRIORITY** QSEN
>
> **Drug Alert**
>
> Teach patients who are taking a corticosteroid for more than a week not to stop the drug suddenly. The drug should be tapered gradually under the care of the primary health care provider.

Care Coordination and Transition Management

Home Care Management. The patient with hypercortisolism usually has muscle weakness and fatigue for some weeks after surgery and remains at risk for falls and other injury. These problems may necessitate one-floor living for a short time; and a home health aide may be needed to assist with hygiene, meal preparation, and maintenance.

Self-Management Education. The patient taking exogenous glucocorticoids who is discharged to home remains at

> **CHART 62-11   Patient and Family Education: Preparing for Self-Management**
>
> ***Cortisol Replacement Therapy***
>
> - Take your medication in divided doses, as prescribed (e.g., the first dose in the morning and the second dose between 4 PM and 6 PM).
> - Take your medication with meals or snacks.
> - Weigh yourself daily and keep a record to show your primary health care provider.
> - Increase your dosage as directed by your primary health care provider for increased physical stress or severe emotional stress.
> - Never skip a dose of medication. If you have persistent vomiting or severe diarrhea and cannot take your medication by mouth for 24 to 36 hours, call your physician. If you cannot reach your primary health care provider, go to the nearest emergency department. You may need an injection to take the place of your usual oral medication.
> - Always wear your medical alert bracelet or necklace.
> - Make regular visits for health care follow-up.
> - Learn how to give yourself an intramuscular injection of hydrocortisone.

continuing risk for impaired FLUID AND ELECTROLYTE BALANCE, especially fluid volume excess. Teach him or her and the family to monitor the patient's weight. Suggest that a record of these daily weights be kept to show the primary health care provider at any checkups. Also instruct the patient to call the health care provider if more than 3 lb are gained in a week or more than 1 to 2 lb are gained in a 24-hour period.

Lifelong hormone replacement is needed after bilateral adrenalectomy. Teach the patient and family about adherence to the drug regimen and its side effects (Chart 62-11).

Protecting the patient with reduced IMMUNITY from infection at home is important. Urge him or her to use proper hygiene and to avoid crowds or others with infections. Encourage the patient and all people living in the same home with him or her to have yearly influenza vaccinations. Stress that the patient should immediately notify the primary health care provider if he or she has a fever or any other sign of infection. Chart 40-10 lists guidelines for patients for infection prevention.

Health Care Resources. Immediately after returning home, the patient may need a support person to stay and provide more attention than could be given by a visiting nurse or home care aide. Contact with the health care team is needed for follow-up and identification of potential problems. The patient taking corticosteroid therapy may have symptoms of adrenal insufficiency if the dosage is inadequate. Suggest that the patient obtain and wear a medical alert bracelet listing the condition and the drug replacement therapy.

◆ Evaluation: Reflecting

Evaluate the care of the patient with hypercortisolism based on the identified priority patient problems. The expected outcomes are that the patient will:

- Maintain fluid and electrolyte balance
- Remain free from injury
- Remain free from infection
- Not experience acute adrenal insufficiency

HYPERALDOSTERONISM

❖ PATHOPHYSIOLOGY

Hyperaldosteronism is an increased secretion of aldosterone with mineralocorticoid excess. Primary hyperaldosteronism

(*Conn's syndrome*) diagnosed in adults results from excessive secretion of aldosterone from one or both adrenal glands, usually caused by an adrenal adenoma. In secondary hyperaldosteronism, excessive secretion of aldosterone is caused by the high levels of angiotensin II that are stimulated by high plasma renin levels. Some causes include kidney hypoxia, diabetic nephropathy, and excessive use of some diuretics.

Increased aldosterone levels cause disturbances of FLUID AND ELECTROLYTE BALANCE, which then trigger the kidney tubules to retain sodium and excrete potassium and hydrogen ions. Hypernatremia, hypokalemia, and metabolic alkalosis result. Sodium retention increases blood volume, which raises blood pressure, increasing the risk for strokes, heart attacks, and kidney damage. (See Chapter 11 for discussion of specific electrolyte imbalances.)

❖ INTERPROFESSIONAL COLLABORATIVE CARE

Patients are hospitalized for surgery. After surgery, they self-manage hormone replacement therapy in the community.

◆ Assessment: Noticing

Hypokalemia and elevated blood pressure are the most common problems that patients with hyperaldosteronism develop. He or she may have headache, fatigue, muscle weakness, dehydration, and loss of stamina. Polydipsia (excessive fluid intake) and polyuria (excessive urine output) occur less frequently. Paresthesias (sensations of numbness and tingling) may occur if potassium depletion is severe.

Hyperaldosteronism is diagnosed on the basis of laboratory studies and imaging with CT or MRI. Serum potassium levels are decreased, and sodium levels are elevated. Plasma renin levels are low, and aldosterone levels are high. Hydrogen ion loss leads to metabolic alkalemia (elevated blood pH). Urine has a low specific gravity and high aldosterone levels.

◆ Interventions: Responding

Surgery is a common treatment for hyperaldosteronism. One or both adrenal glands may be removed. The patient's potassium level must be corrected before surgery. Drugs used to increase potassium levels include spironolactone (Aldactone, Spirono, Sincomen ✦), a potassium-sparing diuretic and aldosterone antagonist. Potassium supplements may be prescribed to increase potassium levels before surgery. The patient may also benefit from a low-sodium diet before surgery.

The patient who has undergone a unilateral adrenalectomy may need temporary glucocorticoid replacement. Replacement is lifelong if both adrenal glands are removed. Glucocorticoids are given before surgery to prevent adrenal crisis. The patient receiving long-term replacement therapy should wear a medical alert bracelet. (See the discussion of adrenalectomy in the Hypercortisolism [Cushing's disease] section for more information about care after surgery and patient education.)

When surgery cannot be performed, spironolactone therapy is continued to control hypokalemia and hypertension. *Because spironolactone is a potassium-sparing diuretic, hyperkalemia can occur in patients who have impaired kidney function or excessive potassium intake.* Advise the patient to avoid potassium supplements and food rich in potassium (see Chapter 11). Hyponatremia can occur with spironolactone therapy, and the patient may need increased dietary sodium. Instruct patients to report symptoms of hyponatremia, such as mouth dryness, thirst, lethargy, or drowsiness. Teach them to report any additional side effects of spironolactone therapy, including gynecomastia, diarrhea, drowsiness, headache, rash, urticaria (hives), confusion, erectile dysfunction, hirsutism, and amenorrhea. Additional drug therapy to control hypertension is often needed.

PHEOCHROMOCYTOMA

❖ PATHOPHYSIOLOGY

Pheochromocytoma is a catecholamine-producing tumor of the adrenal medulla. These tumors usually occur in one adrenal gland, although they can be bilateral or in the abdomen. Pheochromocytomas are usually benign, but about 10% are malignant (Young, 2016).

The tumors produce, store, and release epinephrine and norepinephrine (NE). Excessive epinephrine and NE stimulate adrenergic receptors and can have wide-ranging adverse effects mimicking the action of the sympathetic nervous system.

The cause is unknown, but some pheochromocytomas occur with inherited disorders such as neurofibromatosis (type 1), multiple endocrine neoplasia (MEN-2), von Hippel-Lindau disease, and pheochromocytoma-paraganglioma syndrome (OMIM, 2016c). These tumors are rare and appear most commonly in patients between 30 and 50 years of age (Young, 2016).

❖ INTERPROFESSIONAL COLLABORATIVE CARE

Although most pheochromocytomas are benign, they must be surgically removed to prevent life-threatening complications. Because intensive monitoring is required immediately after surgery, this treatment takes place in an ICU.

◆ Assessment: Noticing

The patient often has intermittent episodes of hypertension or attacks that range from a few minutes to several hours. During these episodes, the patient has severe headaches, palpitations, profuse diaphoresis, flushing, apprehension, or a sense of impending doom. Pain in the chest or abdomen, with nausea and vomiting, can also occur. Increased abdominal pressure, defecation, and vigorous abdominal palpation can provoke a hypertensive crisis. Drugs such as tricyclic antidepressants, droperidol, glucagon, metoclopramide, phenothiazines, and naloxone can induce a hypertensive crisis in the patient with pheochromocytoma. Foods or beverages high in tyramine (e.g., aged cheese, red wine) also induce hypertension. The patient may also report heat intolerance, weight loss, and tremors.

The most common diagnostic test is blood and 24-hour urine collection for fractionated metanephrine and catecholamine levels, all of which are elevated in the presence of a pheochromocytoma. Another test that may be conducted when catecholamine levels are not consistent is the clonidine suppression test (Young, 2016). MRI or CT scans can precisely locate tumors in the adrenal gland, as well as in the chest or abdomen.

◆ Interventions: Responding

Surgery is the main treatment for a pheochromocytoma. One or both adrenal glands are removed (depending on whether the tumor is bilateral). After surgery, nursing interventions focus on promoting adequate tissue perfusion, nutritional needs, and comfort measures.

Hypertension is the main sign of the disease and the most common complication after surgery. Monitor the blood pressure regularly and place the cuff consistently on the same arm, with the patient in lying and standing positions. Teach the patient not to smoke, drink caffeine-containing beverages, or change position suddenly, which can stimulate blood pressure changes. Provide a diet rich in calories, vitamins, and minerals.

> ⚠️ **NURSING SAFETY PRIORITY** QSEN
>
> **Action Alert**
>
> Do not palpate the abdomen of a patient with a pheochromocytoma, because this action could stimulate a sudden release of catecholamines and trigger severe hypertension.

The patient is hydrated before surgery because decreased blood volume increases the risk for hypotension during and after surgery. Assess the patient's hydration status and report symptoms of dehydration or fluid overload.

The patient's blood pressure is stabilized with adrenergic blocking agents such as phenoxybenzamine (Dibenzyline) starting 7 to 10 days before surgery because of the increased risk for severe hypertension during surgery. Drug dosages are adjusted until blood pressure is controlled and hypertensive attacks do not occur. The blood volume expands, and blood pressure in the supine position returns to normal.

Anesthetic agents and touching the tumor during surgery can cause a catecholamine release. Short-acting alpha-adrenergic blockers are given by IV bolus or continuous infusion for a hypertensive crisis.

Nursing care after surgery is similar to that for the patient who has undergone an adrenalectomy (see the Hypercortisolism [Cushing's Disease] section). Monitor the patient for hypertension and hypotension (from the sudden decrease in catecholamine levels) and for hypovolemia. Hemorrhage and shock are possible, and plasma expanders or fluids may be needed. Monitor vital signs, as well as fluid intake and output. If opioids are given, check for their effect on blood pressure.

When tumors are inoperable, management is medical, with alpha-adrenergic and beta-adrenergic blocking agents. For these patients, self-measurement of blood pressure with home-monitoring equipment is essential. (See Chapter 36 for teaching priorities and community-based care of the patient with chronic hypertension.)

GET READY FOR THE NCLEX® EXAMINATION!

KEY POINTS

Review these Key Points for each NCLEX Examination Client Needs Category.

Safe and Effective Care Environment
- Handle all patients with bone density loss carefully, using lift sheets whenever possible. **QSEN: Safety**
- Use good handwashing techniques before providing any care to a patient who has reduced IMMUNITY. **QSEN: Safety**
- Ensure that hormone replacement drugs are given as close to the prescribed times as possible. **QSEN: Safety**
- Teach the patient with diabetes insipidus the indicators of dehydration.

Health Promotion and Maintenance
- Instruct the patient with adrenal insufficiency to wear a medical alert bracelet and to carry simple carbohydrates with him or her at all times. **QSEN: Patient-Centered Care**
- Teach the patient and family about the symptoms of infection and when to seek medical advice. **QSEN: Patient-Centered Care**
- Teach patients who have permanent endocrine hypofunction the proper techniques and timing of hormone replacement therapy. **QSEN: Patient-Centered Care**
- Teach patients taking bromocriptine to seek medical care immediately if chest pain, dizziness, or watery nasal discharge occurs. **QSEN: Safety**

Psychosocial Integrity
- Encourage the patient and family to express concerns about a change in health status. **QSEN: Patient-Centered Care**
- Explain all treatment procedures, restrictions, and follow-up care to the patient. **QSEN: Patient-Centered Care**
- Allow patients who experience a change in physical appearance to mourn this change. **QSEN: Patient-Centered Care**

Physiological Integrity
- During the immediate period after a hypophysectomy, teach the patient to avoid activities that increase intracranial pressure (e.g., bending at the waist, straining to have a bowel movement, coughing). **QSEN: Patient-Centered Care**
- Measure intake and output accurately on patients who have either diabetes insipidus or syndrome of inappropriate antidiuretic hormone (SIADH). **QSEN: Evidence-Based Practice**
- Teach patients who are taking a corticosteroid for more than a week not to stop the drug suddenly. **QSEN: Safety**
- Ensure that no patient suspected of having DI is deprived of fluids for more than 4 hours. **QSEN: Evidence-Based Practice**
- Do not confuse prednisone with prednisolone. **QSEN: Safety**
- Do not palpate the abdomen of a patient who has a pheochromocytoma. **QSEN: Safety**
- Teach patients with diabetes insipidus the proper way to self-administer desmopressin orally or by nasal spray. **QSEN: Patient-Centered Care**

SELECTED BIBLIOGRAPHY

Burchum, J., & Rosenthal, L. (2016). *Lehne's pharmacology for nursing care* (9th ed.). St. Louis: Elsevier.

Capatina, C., & Wass, J. (2015). Hypopituitarism: Growth hormone and corticotrophin deficiency. *Endocrinology and Metabolism Clinics of North America, 44*(1), 127–141.

Elias, P., Martinez, E., Barone, B., Mermejo, L., Castro, M., & Moreira, A. (2014). Late-night salivary cortisol has a better performance than urinary free cortisol in the diagnosis of Cushing's syndrome. *Journal of Clinical Endocrinology & Metabolism, 99*(6), 2045–2051.

Galati, S. (2015). Primary aldosteronism. *Endocrinology and Metabolism Clinics of North America, 44*(2), 355–369.

Hahner, S., Spinnler, C., Fassnacht, M., Burger-Stritt, S., Lang, K., Milovanovic, D., et al. (2015). High incidence of adrenal crisis in educated patients with chronic adrenal insufficiency: A prospective study. *Journal of Clinical Endocrinology & Metabolism, 100*(2), 407–416.

Jarvis, C. (2016). *Physical examination & health assessment* (7th ed.). St. Louis: Elsevier.

Kaiser, U., & Ho, K. (2016). Pituitary physiology and diagnostic evaluation. In S. Melmed, K. Polonsky, P. R. Larsen, & H. Kronenberg (Eds.), *Williams' textbook of endocrinology* (13th ed.). Philadelphia: Saunders.

McCance, K., Huether, S., Brashers, V., & Rote, N. (2014). *Pathophysiology: The biologic basis for disease in adults and children* (7th ed.). St. Louis: Mosby.

McKeage, K. (2013). Pasireotide: A review of its use in Cushing's disease. *Drugs, 73*(6), 563–574.

Melmed, S., & Kleinberg, D. (2016). Pituitary masses and tumor. In S. Melmed, K. Polonsky, P. R. Larsen, & H. Kronenberg (Eds.), *Williams' textbook of endocrinology* (13th ed.). Philadelphia: Saunders.

Melmed, S., Polonsky, K., Larsen, P. R., & Kronenberg, H. (Eds.), (2016). *Williams' textbook of endocrinology* (13th ed.). Philadelphia: Saunders.

Michels, A., & Michels, N. (2014). Addison disease: Early detection and treatment principles. *American Family Physician, 89*(7), 563–568.

Online Mendelian Inheritance in Man (OMIM). (2016a). *Diabetes insipidus, nephrogenic, X-linked.* www.omim.org/entry/304800.

Online Mendelian Inheritance in Man (OMIM). (2016b). *Multiple endocrine neoplasia type 1.* www.omim.org/entry/131100.

Online Mendelian Inheritance in Man (OMIM). (2016c). *Pheochromocytoma, susceptibility to.* www.omim.org/entry/171300.

Pagana, K., Pagana, T. J., & Pagana, T. N. (2017). *Mosby's diagnostic and laboratory test reference* (13th ed.). St. Louis: Mosby.

Pagana, K., Pagana, T., & Pike-MacDonald, S. (2013). *Mosby's Canadian manual of diagnostic and laboratory tests.* St. Louis: Mosby.

Pereira, K. (2016). Hyponatremia signals acute adrenal insufficiency. *American Nurse Today, 11*(7), 30.

Raff, H. (2015). Cushing syndrome: Update on testing. *Endocrinology and Metabolism Clinics of North America, 44*(1), 43–50.

Robinson, A., & Verbalis, J. (2016). Posterior pituitary. In S. Melmed, K. Polonsky, P. R. Larsen, & H. Kronenberg (Eds.), *Williams' textbook of endocrinology* (13th ed.). Philadelphia: Saunders.

Stewart, P., & Newell-Price, J. (2016). The adrenal cortex. In S. Melmed, K. Polonsky, P. R. Larsen, & H. Kronenberg (Eds.), *Williams' textbook of endocrinology* (13th ed.). Philadelphia: Saunders.

Tucci, V., & Sokari, T. (2014). The clinical manifestations, diagnosis, and treatment of adrenal emergencies. *Emergency Medicine Clinics of North America, 32*(2), 465–484.

Young, W. (2016). Endocrine hypertension. In S. Melmed, K. Polonsky, P. R. Larsen, & H. Kronenberg (Eds.), *Williams' textbook of endocrinology* (13th ed.). Philadelphia: Saunders.

Care of Patients With Problems of the Thyroid and Parathyroid Glands

M. Linda Workman

e http://evolve.elsevier.com/Iggy/

PRIORITY AND INTERRELATED CONCEPTS

The priority concept for this chapter is Cellular Regulation.

✳ The Cellular Regulation concept exemplar for this chapter is Hypothyroidism, p. 1270.

The interrelated concepts for this chapter are:
- Nutrition
- Gas Exchange

LEARNING OUTCOMES

Safe and Effective Care Environment

1. Collaborate with the interprofessional team to coordinate high-quality care and promote cellular regulation and optimal nutrition in patients who have thyroid or parathyroid disorders.
2. Teach the patient and caregiver(s) about home safety issues affected by inadequate nutrition or cellular regulation resulting from thyroid or parathyroid problems.

Health Promotion and Maintenance

3. Identify community resources for patients requiring assistance with any disorder of the thyroid or parathyroid glands.

Psychosocial Integrity

4. Implement nursing interventions to help the patient and family cope with the psychosocial impact caused by acute or chronic problems of the thyroid gland or parathyroid glands.

Physiological Integrity

5. Apply knowledge of anatomy, physiology, and pathophysiology to assess patients with impaired thyroid or adrenal parathyroid function affecting nutrition or cellular regulation.
6. Interpret clinical changes and laboratory data to determine the effectiveness of therapy for hyperthyroidism and hypothyroidism.
7. Prioritize evidence-based nursing care for the patient with thyroid storm.
8. Teach the patient and caregiver(s) about common drugs and other management strategies used for thyroid gland or parathyroid gland problems.
9. Prioritize evidence-based care for the patient with myxedema coma.

The hormones secreted by the thyroid gland and parathyroid glands affect whole-body metabolism, cellular regulation, nutrition, gas exchange, electrolyte balance, and excitable membrane activity. Because of the widespread effects of these hormones, problems of either gland can lead to symptoms in many body systems and can range from mild to life-threatening.

THYROID DISORDERS

HYPERTHYROIDISM

❖ *PATHOPHYSIOLOGY*

Hyperthyroidism is excessive thyroid hormone secretion from the thyroid gland. The symptoms of hyperthyroidism are called **thyrotoxicosis**, regardless of the origin of the thyroid hormones. This term is correct even when an adult takes a large amount of synthetic thyroid hormones and has symptoms of thyrotoxicosis although his or her thyroid gland is normal. Thyroid hormones increase metabolism in all body organs, producing many different symptoms. Hyperthyroidism can be temporary or permanent, depending on the cause.

The excessive thyroid hormones stimulate most body systems, causing hypermetabolism and increased sympathetic nervous system activity. Symptoms are listed in Chart 63-1.

Thyroid hormones stimulate the heart, increasing rate and stroke volume. These responses increase cardiac output, blood pressure, and blood flow (McCance et al., 2014).

Elevated thyroid hormone levels affect protein, fat, and glucose metabolism. Protein buildup and breakdown are increased; but breakdown exceeds buildup, causing a net loss

CHART 63-1 Key Features

Hyperthyroidism

Skin Symptoms
- Diaphoresis (excessive sweating)
- Fine, soft, silky body hair
- Smooth, warm, moist skin
- Thinning of scalp hair

Cardiopulmonary Symptoms
- Palpitations
- Chest pain
- Increased systolic blood pressure
- Tachycardia
- Dysrhythmias
- Rapid, shallow respirations

Gastrointestinal Symptoms
- Weight loss
- Increased appetite
- Increased stools

Neurologic Symptoms
- Blurred or double vision
- Eye fatigue
- Increased tears
- Injected (red) conjunctiva
- Photophobia
- Exophthalmos*
- Eyelid retraction, eyelid lag
- Globe lag
- Hyperactive deep tendon reflexes
- Tremors
- Insomnia

Metabolic Symptoms
- Increased basal metabolic rate
- Heat intolerance
- Low-grade fever
- Fatigue

Psychological/Emotional Symptoms
- Decreased attention span
- Restlessness and irritability
- Emotional instability
- Manic behavior

Reproductive Symptoms
- Amenorrhea
- Increased libido

Other Symptoms
- Goiter
- Wide-eyed or startled appearance (exophthalmos)*
- Enlarged spleen
- Muscle weakness and wasting

*Present in Graves' disease only.

of body protein known as a **negative nitrogen balance**. Glucose tolerance is decreased, and the patient has **hyperglycemia** (elevated blood glucose levels). Fat metabolism is increased, and body fat decreases. Although the patient has an increased appetite, the increased metabolism causes weight loss and NUTRITION deficits.

Thyroid hormones are produced in response to the stimulation hormones secreted by the hypothalamus and anterior pituitary glands. Thus oversecretion of thyroid hormones changes the secretion of hormones from the hypothalamus and the anterior pituitary gland through negative feedback (see Chapter 61). Thyroid hormones also have some influence over sex hormone production. Women have menstrual problems and decreased fertility. Both men and women with hyperthyroidism have an increased **libido** (sexual interest).

Etiology and Genetic Risk

Hyperthyroidism has many causes. The most common form of the disease is Graves' disease, also called *toxic diffuse goiter*. **Graves' disease** is an autoimmune disorder resulting from Hashimoto's thyroiditis (HT) (Davies et al., 2016). HT results in the production of autoantibodies to different substances and structures within the thyroid gland. In Graves' disease, these antibodies (thyroid-stimulating immunoglobulins [TSIs]) attach to the thyroid-stimulating hormone (TSH) receptors on

the thyroid gland. This increases the number of glandular cells, which enlarges the gland, forming a **goiter**, and overproduces thyroid hormones (**thyrotoxicosis**). When HT causes production of antibodies to other structures within the thyroid gland, hypothyroidism results (see the discussion of Etiology in the Hypothyroidism section).

In Graves' disease, all the general symptoms of hyperthyroidism are present. In addition, other changes specific to Graves' disease may occur, including **exophthalmos** (abnormal protrusion of the eyes) and **pretibial myxedema** (dry, waxy swelling of the front surfaces of the lower legs that resembles benign tumors or keloids).

Hyperthyroidism caused by multiple thyroid nodules is termed **toxic multinodular goiter**. The nodules may be enlarged thyroid tissues or benign tumors (adenomas). These patients usually have had a goiter for years. The symptoms are milder than those seen in Graves' disease, and the patient does not have exophthalmos or pretibial myxedema.

Hyperthyroidism also can be caused by excessive use of thyroid replacement hormones. This type of problem is called **exogenous hyperthyroidism**.

GENETIC/GENOMIC CONSIDERATIONS
Patient-Centered Care QSEN

Susceptibility to Graves' disease is associated with several gene mutations (*GRD1, GRD2, GRDX1, GRDX2*). The pattern of inheritance is autosomal-recessive with sex limitation to females. Graves' disease is associated with other autoimmune disorders, such as diabetes mellitus, vitiligo, and rheumatoid arthritis and often occurs in both members of identical twins (Online Mendelian Inheritance in Man [OMIM], 2016). Ask the patient with Graves' disease whether any other family members also have the problem.

Incidence and Prevalence

Hyperthyroidism is a common endocrine disorder. Graves' disease can occur at any age but is diagnosed most often in women between 20 and 40 years of age (Davies et al., 2016). Toxic multinodular goiter usually occurs after the age of 50 years and affects women four times more often than men (McCance et al., 2014).

❖ INTERPROFESSIONAL COLLABORATIVE CARE

Depending on the severity of the hyperthyroid symptoms at the time of diagnosis, initial therapy may start in an acute care environment or in the community. When thyroid storm is present, an intensive care environment may be required. Once the disorder is controlled, the patient manages his or her disorder in the community.

◆ Assessment: Noticing

History. Many changes and problems occur because hyperthyroidism affects all body systems, although changes may occur over such a long period that patients may be unaware of them. Record age, gender, and usual weight. The increased metabolic rate affects NUTRITION. The patient may report a recent unplanned weight loss, an increased appetite, and an increase in the number of bowel movements per day.

A hallmark of hyperthyroidism is heat intolerance. The patient may have increased sweating even when environmental temperatures are comfortable for others. He or she often wears lighter clothing in cold weather. The patient may also report

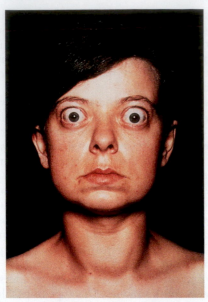

FIG. 63-1 Exophthalmos.

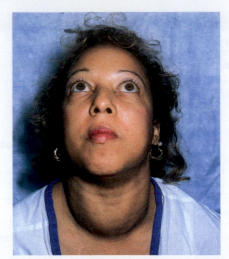

FIG. 63-2 Goiter.

TABLE 63-1	Goiter Classification
GOITER GRADE	**DESCRIPTION**
0	There is no palpable or visible goiter.
1	Mass is not visible with neck in the normal position. Goiter can be palpated and moves up when the patient swallows.
2	Mass is visible as swelling when the neck is in the normal position. Goiter is easily palpated and is usually asymmetric.

palpitations or chest pain as a result of the cardiovascular effects. Ask about changes in breathing patterns because dyspnea (with or without exertion) is common.

Visual changes may be the earliest problem the patient or family notices, especially exophthalmos with Graves' disease (Fig. 63-1). Ask about changes in vision, such as blurring or double vision and tiring of the eyes.

Ask about changes in energy level or in the ability to perform ADLs. Fatigue and insomnia are common. Families may report that the patient has become irritable or depressed.

Ask women about changes in menses, because amenorrhea or a decreased menstrual flow is common. Initially both men and women may have an increase in libido, but this changes as the patient becomes more fatigued.

Ask about previous thyroid surgery or radiation therapy to the neck, because some adults remain hyperthyroid after surgery or are resistant to radiation therapy. Ask about past and current drugs, especially the use of thyroid hormone replacement or antithyroid drugs.

Physical Assessment/Signs and Symptoms. Exophthalmos is common in patients with Graves' disease. The wide-eyed or "startled" look is due to edema in the extraocular muscles and increased fatty tissue behind the eye, which pushes the eyeball forward and may cause problems with focusing. Pressure on the optic nerve may impair vision. If the eyelids fail to close completely and the eyes are unprotected, they may become dry, and corneal ulcers may develop. Observe the eyes for excessive tearing and a bloodshot appearance. Ask about sensitivity to light (**photophobia**).

Two other eye problems are common in all types of hyperthyroidism: eyelid retraction (eyelid lag) and globe (eyeball) lag. In eyelid lag, the upper eyelid fails to descend when the patient gazes slowly downward. In globe lag, the upper eyelid pulls back faster than the eyeball when the patient gazes upward. During assessment, ask the patient to look down and then up and document the response.

Observe the size and symmetry of the thyroid gland. Palpate the thyroid gland to assess its consistency. In goiter, a generalized thyroid enlargement, the thyroid gland may increase to four times its normal size (Fig. 63-2). Goiters are common in Graves' disease and are classified by size (Table 63-1). *Not*

all patients with a goiter have hyperthyroidism. Bruits (turbulence from increased blood flow) may be heard in the neck with a stethoscope. (See Chapter 61 for thyroid palpation and auscultation.)

The cardiovascular problems of hyperthyroidism include increased systolic blood pressure, tachycardia, and dysrhythmias. Usually the diastolic pressure is decreased, causing a widened pulse pressure.

Inspect the hair and skin. Fine, soft, silky hair and smooth, warm, moist skin are common. Many patients notice thinning of scalp hair. Muscle weakness and hyperactive deep tendon reflexes are common. Observe motor movements of the hands for tremors. The patient may appear restless, irritable, and fatigued.

Psychosocial Assessment. The patient often has wide mood swings, irritability, decreased attention span, and manic behavior. Hyperactivity often leads to fatigue because of the inability to sleep well. Some patients describe their activity as having two modes (i.e., either "full speed ahead" or "completely stopped"). Ask whether he or she cries or laughs without cause or has difficulty concentrating. Family members often report a change in the patient's mental or emotional status.

Laboratory Assessment. Testing for hyperthyroidism involves measurement of blood levels for triiodothyronine (T_3), thyroxine (T_4), and thyroid-stimulating hormone (TSH). Antibodies to the TSH receptor (thyrotropin receptor [TRAbs]) are measured to diagnose Graves' disease. The most common changes in laboratory tests for hyperthyroidism are listed in Chart 63-2.

Other Diagnostic Assessment. Thyroid scan evaluates the position, size, and functioning of the thyroid gland. Radioactive

CHART 63-2 Laboratory Profile

Thyroid Function for Adults

TEST	NORMAL RANGE FOR ADULTS	SIGNIFICANCE OF ABNORMAL FINDINGS	
		HYPERTHYROIDISM	HYPOTHYROIDISM
Serum T_3	70-205 ng/dL (1.7-5.2 pmol/L)	Increased	Decreased
Serum T_4 (total)	4-12 mcg/dL (51-154 nmol/L)	Increased	Decreased
Free T_4 index	0.8-2.8 ng/dL, (10-36 pmol/L)	Increased	Decreased
TSH stimulation test (thyroid stimulation test)	>10% in RAIU or >1.5 mcg/dL	N/A (test differentiates primary from secondary hypothyroidism)	No response in primary hypothyroidism Normal response in secondary hypothyroidism
Thyroid-stimulating immunoglobulins (TSI)	<130% of basal activity	Elevated in Graves' disease Normal in other types of hyperthyroidism	No change
Thyrotropin receptor antibodies (TRAb)	Titer: 0%	80%-95% indicates Graves' disease	No response
TSH	0.3-5 µU/mL (0.3-5 mU/L)	Low in Graves' disease High in secondary or tertiary hyperthyroidism	High in primary disease Low in secondary or tertiary disease

Data from Pagana, K., Pagana, T., & Pike-MacDonald, S. (2013). *Mosby's Canadian manual of diagnostic and laboratory tests.* St. Louis: Mosby, and Pagana, K., Pagana, T.J., & Pagana, T.N. (2017). *Mosby's diagnostic and laboratory test reference* (13th ed.). St. Louis: Mosby.
T_3, Triiodothyronine; *T_4*, thyroxine; *TSH*, thyroid-stimulating hormone.

iodine (RAI [^{123}I]) is given by mouth, and the uptake of iodine by the thyroid gland (radioactive iodine uptake [RAIU]) is measured. The half-life of ^{123}I is short, and radiation precautions are not needed. Pregnancy should be ruled out before the scan is performed. The normal thyroid gland has an uptake of 5% to 35% of the given dose at 24 hours. RAIU is increased in hyperthyroidism and can be used to identify active thyroid nodules. It is no longer the most common test for thyroid function (Davies et al., 2016).

Ultrasonography of the thyroid gland can determine its size and the general composition of any masses or nodules. This outpatient procedure takes about 30 minutes to perform and is painless. No special instructions are required.

ECG usually shows supraventricular tachycardia. Other ECG changes include atrial fibrillation, dysrhythmias, and premature ventricular contractions.

◆ Interventions: Responding

Because Graves' disease is the most common form of hyperthyroidism, the interventions discussed in the following sections include those specific for the problems that occur with Graves' disease. In North America, the most common interventions are drug therapy and radioablation. Surgery is reserved for severe disease that is not responsive to other forms of management. Medical management is used to decrease the effect of thyroid hormone on cardiac function and to reduce thyroid hormone secretion. The priorities for nursing care focus on monitoring for complications, reducing stimulation, promoting comfort, and teaching the patient and family about therapeutic drugs and procedures.

Nonsurgical Management. Monitoring includes measuring the patient's apical pulse, blood pressure, and temperature at least every 4 hours. Instruct the patient to report immediately any palpitations, dyspnea, vertigo, or chest pain. Increases in temperature may indicate a rapid worsening of the patient's condition and the onset of *thyroid storm*, a life-threatening event that occurs with uncontrolled hyperthyroidism and is

characterized by high fever and severe hypertension (discussed later in the Hyperthyroidism section). *Immediately report a temperature increase of even 1 degree Fahrenheit.* If this task is delegated to unlicensed assistive personnel (UAP), instruct them to report the patient's temperature to you as soon as it has been obtained. If temperature is elevated, immediately assess the patient's cardiac status. If the patient has a cardiac monitor, check for dysrhythmias.

Reducing stimulation helps prevent increasing the symptoms of hyperthyroidism and the risk for cardiac complications. Encourage the patient to rest. Keep the environment as quiet as possible by closing the door to the room, limiting visitors, and eliminating or postponing nonessential care or treatments.

Promoting comfort includes reducing the room temperature to decrease discomfort caused by heat intolerance. Instruct UAP to ensure that the patient always has a fresh pitcher of ice water and to change the bed linen whenever it becomes damp from diaphoresis. Suggest that the patient take a cool shower or sponge bath several times each day. For patients with exophthalmos, prevent eye dryness by encouraging the use of artificial tears.

Drug therapy with antithyroid drugs is the initial treatment for hyperthyroidism and causes some patients to go into remission for as long as 10 years (Davies et al., 2016). Chart 63-3 lists teaching priorities for the patient receiving drug therapy for hyperthyroidism. The preferred drugs are the thionamides, especially methimazole (Tapazole). Propylthiouracil (PTU) is used less often because of its liver toxic effects (Davies et al., 2016). These drugs block thyroid hormone production by preventing iodide binding in the thyroid gland. The response to these drugs is delayed because the patient may have large amounts of stored thyroid hormones that continue to be released.

Iodine preparations may be used for short-term therapy before surgery. They decrease blood flow through the thyroid gland, reducing the production and release of thyroid hormone. Improvement usually occurs within 2 weeks, but it may be

CHART 63-3   Common Examples of Drug Therapy

Hyperthyroidism

DRUGS	NURSING IMPLICATIONS
Propylthiouracil (PTU, Propyl-Thyracil) Methimazole (Northyx, Tapazole)	Teach patient to avoid crowds and people who are ill *because the drug reduces the immune response, increasing the risk for infection.* Teach patients to check for weight gain, slow heart rate, and cold intolerance, *which are indications of hypothyroidism and the need for a lower drug dose.* Teach patients taking propylthiouracil to report darkening of the urine or a yellow appearance to the skin or whites of the eyes, *which indicate possible liver toxicity or failure, a serious side effect of propylthiouracil.* Remind women taking methimazole to notify their primary health care providers if they become pregnant *because the drug causes birth defects and should not be used during pregnancy.*
Lugol's solution Saturated solution of potassium iodide (SSKI)	Administer these drugs orally 1 hour *after* a thionamide has been given *because initially the iodine agents can cause an increase in the production of thyroid hormones. Giving a thionamide first prevents this initial increase in thyroid hormone production.* Check patient for a fever or rash and ask about a metallic taste, mouth sores, sore throat, or GI distress *as these are indications of iodism, a toxic effect of the drugs, and may require that the drug be discontinued.*

! NURSING SAFETY PRIORITY QSEN

Drug Alert

Although similar in action, methimazole and propylthiouracil are not interchangeable. The dosages for propylthiouracil are much higher than those for methimazole.

! NURSING SAFETY PRIORITY QSEN

Drug Alert

Methimazole can cause birth defects and should not be used during pregnancy, especially during the first trimester. Instruct women to notify their primary health care provider if pregnancy occurs.

weeks before metabolism returns to normal. This treatment can result in hypothyroidism, and the patient is monitored closely for the need to adjust the drug regimen.

Beta-adrenergic blocking drugs, such as propranolol (Inderal, Detensol ✦) may be used as supportive therapy. These drugs relieve diaphoresis, anxiety, tachycardia, and palpitations but do not inhibit thyroid hormone production. See Chapters 34 and 36 for a discussion of the actions and nursing implications of these agents.

Radioactive iodine (RAI) therapy is not used in pregnant women because ^{131}I crosses the placenta and can damage the fetal thyroid gland. The patient with hyperthyroidism may receive RAI in the form of oral [131]I. The dosage depends on the thyroid gland's size and sensitivity to radiation. The thyroid gland picks up the RAI, and some of the cells that produce thyroid hormone are destroyed by the local radiation. Because the thyroid gland stores thyroid hormones to some degree, the patient may not have complete symptom relief until 6 to 8 weeks after RAI therapy. Additional drug therapy for hyperthyroidism is still needed during the first few weeks after RAI treatment.

RAI therapy is performed on an outpatient basis. One dose may be sufficient, although some patients need a second or third dose. The radiation dose is low and is usually completely eliminated within a month; however, the source is unsealed, and some radioactivity is present in the patient's body fluids and

stool for a few weeks after therapy. Radiation precautions are needed to prevent exposure to family members and other people. Chart 63-4 lists precautions to teach the patient during the first few weeks after receiving [131]I.

The degree of thyroid destruction varies. Some patients become hypothyroid as a result of treatment. The patient then needs lifelong thyroid hormone replacement. All patients who have undergone RAI therapy should be monitored regularly for changes in thyroid function.

? NCLEX EXAMINATION CHALLENGE 63-1

Health Promotion and Maintenance

Which statement by a client undergoing radioactive iodine (RAI) therapy demonstrates to the nurse **correct understanding** of postprocedure precautions?
A. "I'll wear a wig until my hair grows back in."
B. "I'll be sure to use only one toilet and not let others use it for 2 weeks."
C. "I'll avoid crowds and people who are ill to reduce the risk for an infection."
D. "I'll avoid having a manicure or pedicure during the first month after treatment."

CULTURAL/SPIRITUAL CONSIDERATIONS

Patient-Centered Care QSEN

A potentially life-threatening complication of thyrotoxicosis is periodic paralysis (thyrotoxic periodic paralysis, TPP), which results from low blood potassium levels caused by increased skeletal muscle uptake of potassium. The potassium movement is thought to result from direct thyroid hormone action or the increased adrenergic response of hyperthyroidism. The change in both intracellular and extracellular potassium levels reduces skeletal muscle membrane excitability and leads to temporary paralysis, including paralysis of the respiratory muscles. TPP is most common in men of Chinese and Japanese descent (Patel et al., 2013).

Emergency management involves treating the thyrotoxicosis and the hypokalemia. In addition to antithyroid drug therapy, potassium is replaced IV. This condition is increasing in frequency in North America and is not always recognized. Be alert to any adult male of Asian descent who has lower limb paralysis or weakness along with signs and symptoms of hyperthyroidism.

CHART 63-4 Patient and Family Education: Preparing for Self-Management

Safety Precautions for the Patient Receiving an Unsealed Radioactive Isotope

- Use a toilet that is not used by others for at least 2 weeks after receiving the radioactive iodine.
- Sit to urinate (males and females) to avoid splashing the seat, walls, and floor.
- Flush the toilet three times after each use.
- If urine is spilled on the toilet seat or floor, use paper tissues or towels to clean it up, bag them in sealable plastic bags, and take them to the hospital's radiation therapy department.
- Men with urinary incontinence should use condom catheters and a drainage bag rather than absorbent gel-filled briefs or pads.
- Women with urinary incontinence should use facial tissue layers in their clothing to catch the urine rather than absorbent gel-filled briefs or pads. These tissues should then be flushed down the toilet exclusively used by the patient.
- Using a laxative on the second and third days after receiving the radioactive drug helps you excrete the contaminated stool faster (this also decreases the exposure of your abdominal organs to radiation).
- Wear only machine-washable clothing and wash these items separately from others in your household.
- After washing your clothing, run the washing machine for a full cycle on empty before it is used to wash the clothing of others.
- Avoid close contact with pregnant women, infants, and young children for the first week after therapy. Remain at least 3 feet (about 1 meter) away from these people and limit your exposure to them to no more than 1 hour daily.
- Some radioactivity will be in your saliva during the first week after therapy. Precautions to avoid exposing others to this contamination (both household members and trash collectors) include:
  - Not sharing toothbrushes or toothpaste tubes
  - Using disposable tissues rather than cloth handkerchiefs and either flushing used ones down the toilet or keeping them in a plastic bag and turning them in to the radiation department of the hospital for disposal
  - Using disposable utensils, plates, and cups
  - Selecting foods that can be eaten completely and that do not result in a saliva-coated remnant (Foods to avoid are fruit with a core that can be contaminated, meat with a bone [e.g., chicken wings or legs, ribs]. Consider preparing these foods by cutting out the core and removing the bone before eating.)

Data from Al-Shakhrah, I. (2008). Radioprotection using iodine-131 for thyroid cancer and hyperthyroidism: A review. *Clinical Journal of Oncology Nursing, 12*(6), 905-912.

Surgical Management. Surgery to remove all or part of the thyroid gland is used for Graves' disease that does not respond to other therapies. It is also used when a large goiter causes tracheal or esophageal compression. Removal of all (**total thyroidectomy**) or part (**subtotal thyroidectomy**) of the thyroid tissue decreases the production of thyroid hormones. After a total thyroidectomy, patients must take lifelong thyroid hormone replacement.

Preoperative Care. The patient is treated with thionamide drug therapy first to have near-normal thyroid function (**euthyroid**) before thyroid surgery. Iodine preparations also are used to decrease thyroid size and vascularity, thereby reducing the risk for hemorrhage and the potential for thyroid storm during surgery. (Thyroid storm is discussed in the Hyperthyroid section.)

Hypertension, dysrhythmias, and tachycardia must be controlled before surgery. The patient with hyperthyroidism may need to follow a high-protein, high-carbohydrate diet for days or weeks before surgery.

Teach the patient to perform deep-breathing exercises. Stress the importance of supporting the neck when coughing or moving by placing both hands behind the neck to reduce strain on the incision. Explain that hoarseness may be present for a few days as a result of endotracheal tube placement during surgery.

Explain the surgery and the care after surgery to the patient. Remind him or her that a drain and a dressing may be in place after surgery. Answer any questions the patient and family have.

Operative Procedures. Many thyroidectomies are now performed as minimally invasive surgeries or mini-incision surgeries. With these surgeries, as with the traditional open approach, the parathyroid glands and recurrent laryngeal nerves are avoided to reduce the risk for complications and injury.

With a subtotal thyroidectomy, the remaining thyroid tissues are sutured to the trachea. With a total thyroidectomy, the entire thyroid gland is removed, but the parathyroid glands are left with an intact blood supply to prevent causing hypoparathyroidism.

Postoperative Care. *Monitoring the patient for complications is the most important nursing action after thyroid surgery.* Monitor vital signs every 15 minutes until the patient is stable and then every 30 minutes. Increase or decrease the monitoring of vital signs based on changes in the patient's condition.

Assess the patient's level of discomfort. Use pillows to support the head and neck. Place the patient, while he or she is awake, in a semi-Fowler's position. Avoid positions that cause neck extension. Give prescribed drugs for pain control as needed.

Help the patient deep-breathe every 30 minutes to 1 hour. Suction oral and tracheal secretions when necessary.

Thyroid surgery can cause hemorrhage, respiratory distress with reduced GAS EXCHANGE, parathyroid gland injury (resulting in **hypocalcemia** [low serum calcium levels] and **tetany** [hyperexcitability of nerves and muscles]), damage to the laryngeal nerves, and thyroid storm. Remain alert to the potential for complications and identify symptoms early.

Hemorrhage is most likely to occur during the first 24 hours after surgery. Inspect the neck dressing and behind the patient's neck for blood. A drain may be present, and a moderate amount of serosanguineous drainage is normal. Hemorrhage may be seen as bleeding at the incision site or as respiratory distress caused by tracheal compression.

Respiratory distress and reduced GAS EXCHANGE can result from swelling, tetany, or damage to the laryngeal nerve, resulting in spasms. Laryngeal **stridor** (harsh, high-pitched respiratory sounds) is heard in acute respiratory obstruction. Keep emergency tracheostomy equipment in the patient's room. Check that oxygen and suctioning equipment are nearby and in working order.

! NURSING SAFETY PRIORITY QSEN

Critical Rescue

Monitor the patient to identify symptoms of obstruction and poor GAS EXCHANGE (stridor, dyspnea, falling oxygen saturation, inability to swallow, drooling) after thyroid surgery. If any indications of obstruction are present, respond by immediately notifying the Rapid Response Team.

Hypocalcemia and tetany may occur if the parathyroid glands are removed or damaged or their blood supply is impaired during thyroid surgery, resulting in decreased parathyroid hormone (PTH) levels. Ask the patient hourly about tingling around the mouth or of the toes and fingers. Assess for muscle twitching as a sign of calcium deficiency. Calcium gluconate or calcium chloride for IV use should be available in an emergency situation. (For information on the later signs of hypocalcemia, see the discussion of postoperative care in the Hyperparathyroidism section and the Assessment discussion in the Hypoparathyroidism section. Hypocalcemia is also discussed in Chapter 11.)

Laryngeal nerve damage may occur during surgery. This problem results in hoarseness and a weak voice. Assess the patient's voice at 2-hour intervals and document any changes. Reassure the patient that hoarseness is usually temporary.

🔮 NCLEX EXAMINATION CHALLENGE 63-2

Safe and Effective Care Environment

Which assessment finding of a client 10 hours after a subtotal thyroidectomy indicates to the nurse possible airway obstruction?
A. The client is drooling.
B. The oxygen saturation is 97%.
C. The dressing has a moderate amount of serosanguinous drainage.
D. The client responds to questions correctly but does not open the eyes while talking.

Thyroid storm or **thyroid crisis** is a life-threatening event that occurs in patients with uncontrolled hyperthyroidism, most often with Graves' disease. Symptoms develop quickly, and the problem is fatal if left untreated (Devereaux & Tewelde, 2014). It is often triggered by stressors such as trauma, infection, diabetic ketoacidosis, and pregnancy. Other conditions that can lead to thyroid storm include vigorous palpation of the goiter, exposure to iodine, and radioactive iodine (RAI) therapy. Although thyroid storm after surgery is less common because of drug therapy before thyroid surgery, it can still occur.

Symptoms of thyroid storm are caused by excessive thyroid hormone release, which dramatically increases metabolic rate. *Key symptoms include fever, tachycardia, and systolic hypertension.* The patient may have abdominal pain, nausea, vomiting, and diarrhea. Often he or she is very anxious and has tremors. As the crisis progresses, the patient may become restless, confused, or psychotic and may have seizures, leading to coma. *Even with treatment, thyroid storm may lead to death.*

❗ NURSING SAFETY PRIORITY QSEN

Critical Rescue

When caring for a patient with hyperthyroidism, even after a thyroidectomy, assess temperature often because an increase of even 1°F may indicate an impending thyroid crisis. If an increase occurs, respond by reporting it immediately to the primary health care provider.

Emergency measures to prevent death vary with the intensity and type of changes. Interventions focus on maintaining airway patency, promoting adequate ventilation and GAS EXCHANGE, reducing fever, and stabilizing the hemodynamic status. Chart 63-5 outlines the best practices for emergency management of thyroid storm.

Eye and vision problems of Graves' disease are not corrected by treatment for hyperthyroidism, and management

⊙ CHART 63-5 Best Practice for Patient Safety & Quality Care QSEN

Emergency Care of the Patient During Thyroid Storm

- Maintain a patent airway and adequate ventilation.
- Give oral antithyroid drugs as prescribed: methimazole (Tapazole), up to 60 mg daily; propylthiouracil (PTU, Propyl-Thyracil), 300 to 900 mg daily.
- Administer sodium iodide solution, 2 g IV daily as prescribed.
- Give propranolol (Inderal, Detensol), 1 to 3 mg IV as prescribed. Give slowly over 3 minutes. The patient should be connected to a cardiac monitor, and a central venous pressure catheter should be in place.
- Give glucocorticoids as prescribed: hydrocortisone, 100 to 500 mg IV daily; prednisone, 4 to 60 mg orally daily; or dexamethasone, 2 mg IM every 6 hours.
- Monitor continually for cardiac dysrhythmias.
- Monitor vital signs every 30 minutes.
- Provide comfort measures, including a cooling blanket.
- Give nonsalicylate antipyretics as prescribed.
- Correct dehydration with normal saline infusions.
- Apply cooling blanket or ice packs to reduce fever.

is symptomatic. Teach the patient with mild problems to elevate the head of the bed at night and use artificial tears. If **photophobia** (sensitivity to light) is present, dark glasses may be helpful. For those who cannot close the eyelids completely, recommend gently taping the lids closed at bedtime. These actions prevent irritation and injury. If pressure behind the eye continues and forces the eye forward, blood supply to the eye can be compromised, leading to ischemia and blindness.

In severe cases, short-term glucocorticoid therapy is prescribed to reduce swelling and halt the infiltrative process. Prednisone (Deltasone, Winpred ♦) is given in high doses (often 120 mg daily) at first and then is tapered down according to the patient's response. Explain the need to reduce the prednisone gradually and review its side effects with the patient.

Other management strategies include external radiation combined with lower-dose glucocorticoid therapy. Surgical intervention (orbital decompression) may be needed if loss of sight or damage to the eyeball is possible. Rituximab injections have been successful on a limited basis for this problem (Davies et al., 2016).

Health teaching includes reviewing with the patient and family the symptoms of hyperthyroidism and instructing the patient to report any increase or recurrence of these. Also teach about the symptoms of hypothyroidism (discussed in the next section) and the need for thyroid hormone replacement. Reinforce the need for regular follow-up because hypothyroidism can occur several years after radioactive iodine therapy.

The discharged patient may continue to have mood changes. Explain the reason for mood swings to the patient and family and reassure them that these will decrease with continued treatment.

✴ CELLULAR REGULATION CONCEPT EXEMPLAR
Hypothyroidism

❖ *PATHOPHYSIOLOGY*

Symptoms of hypothyroidism (Chart 63-6) are the result of decreased metabolism from low levels of thyroid hormones.

CHART 63-6 Key Features

Hypothyroidism

Skin Symptoms
- Cool, pale or yellowish, dry, coarse, scaly skin
- Thick, brittle nails
- Dry, coarse, brittle hair
- Decreased hair growth, with loss of eyebrow hair
- Poor wound healing

Pulmonary Symptoms
- Hypoventilation
- Pleural effusion
- Dyspnea

Cardiovascular Symptoms
- Bradycardia
- Dysrhythmias
- Enlarged heart
- Decreased activity tolerance
- Hypotension

Metabolic Symptoms
- Decreased basal metabolic rate
- Decreased body temperature
- Cold intolerance

Psychological/Emotional Symptoms
- Apathy
- Depression
- Paranoia

Gastrointestinal Symptoms
- Anorexia
- Weight gain
- Constipation
- Abdominal distention

Neuromuscular Symptoms
- Slowing of intellectual functions:
  - Slowness or slurring of speech
  - Impaired memory
  - Inattentiveness
- Lethargy or somnolence
- Confusion
- Hearing loss
- Paresthesia (numbness and tingling) of the extremities
- Decreased tendon reflexes
- Muscle aches and pain

Reproductive Symptoms

Women
- Changes in menses (amenorrhea or prolonged menstrual periods)
- Anovulation
- Decreased libido

Men
- Decreased libido
- Impotence

Other Symptoms
- Periorbital edema
- Facial puffiness
- Nonpitting edema of the hands and feet
- Hoarseness
- Goiter (enlarged thyroid gland)
- Thick tongue
- Increased sensitivity to opioids and tranquilizers
- Weakness, fatigue
- Decreased urine output
- Easy bruising
- Iron deficiency anemia
- Vitamin deficiencies

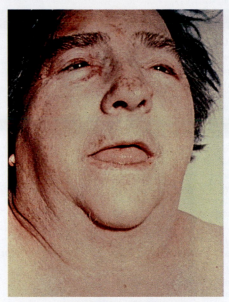

FIG. 63-3 Myxedema.

GAG buildup increases the mucus and water, forms cellular edema, and changes organ texture. The edema is mucinous and called **myxedema**, rather than edema caused by water alone. This edema changes the patient's appearance (Fig. 63-3). Nonpitting edema forms everywhere, especially around the eyes, in the hands and feet, and between the shoulder blades. The tongue thickens; and edema forms in the larynx, making the voice husky. General physiologic function is decreased.

Myxedema coma, sometimes called *hypothyroid crisis,* is a rare, serious complication of untreated or poorly treated hypothyroidism and has a mortality rate of 60% (Dubbs & Spangler, 2014). The decreased metabolism causes the heart muscle to become flabby and the chamber size to increase. The result is decreased cardiac output with decreased perfusion and GAS EXCHANGE in the brain and other vital organs, which makes the already slowed cellular metabolism worse, resulting in tissue and organ failure. *The mortality rate for myxedema coma is extremely high, and this condition is a life-threatening emergency.* Myxedema coma can be caused by a variety of events, drugs, or conditions.

Etiology

Most cases of hypothyroidism in the United States occur as a result of thyroid surgery and radioactive iodine (RAI) treatment of hyperthyroidism. Worldwide, hypothyroidism is common in areas where the soil and water have little natural iodide, causing endemic goiter. Hypothyroidism is also caused by a variety of other conditions (Table 63-2).

Incidence and Prevalence

Hypothyroidism occurs most often in women between 30 and 60 years of age. Women are affected 7 to 10 times more often than men (McCance et al., 2014).

❖ INTERPROFESSIONAL COLLABORATIVE CARE

Depending on the severity of the symptoms at the time of diagnosis, initial therapy for hypothyroidism may start in an acute care environment or in the community. When symptoms are severe or if myxedema coma is present, an

Thyroid cells may fail to produce sufficient levels of thyroid hormones (THs) for several reasons. Sometimes the cells themselves are damaged and no longer function normally. At other times the thyroid cells are functional, but the adult does not ingest enough of the substances needed to make thyroid hormones, especially iodide and tyrosine. When the production of thyroid hormones is too low or absent, the blood levels of TH are very low, and the patient has a decreased metabolic rate. This lowered metabolism causes the hypothalamus and anterior pituitary gland to make stimulatory hormones, especially thyroid-stimulating hormone (TSH), in an attempt to trigger hormone release from the poorly responsive thyroid gland. The TSH binds to thyroid cells and causes the thyroid gland to enlarge, forming a goiter, although thyroid hormone production does not increase.

Most tissues and organs are affected by the low metabolic rate caused by hypothyroidism. Cellular energy is decreased, and metabolites that are compounds of proteins and sugars called *glycosaminoglycans (GAGs)* build up inside cells. This

TABLE 63-2 Causes of Hypothyroidism

Primary Causes
Decreased Thyroid Tissue
- Surgical or radiation-induced thyroid destruction
- Autoimmune thyroid destruction
- Congenital poor thyroid development
- Cancer (thyroidal or metastatic)

Decreased Synthesis of Thyroid Hormone
- Endemic iodine deficiency
- Drugs:
  - Lithium
  - Propylthiouracil
  - Sodium or potassium perchlorate
  - Aminoglutethimide

Secondary Causes
Inadequate Production of Thyroid-Stimulating Hormone
- Pituitary tumors, trauma, infections, or infarcts
- Congenital pituitary defects
- Hypothalamic tumors, trauma, infections, or infarcts

intensive care environment may be required. Drug therapy is lifelong, and patients learn to manage their disorders in the community.

◆ **Assessment: Noticing**

History. A decrease in thyroid hormones produces many symptoms related to decreased metabolism. However, changes may have occurred slowly, and the patient may not have noticed them. Ask him or her to compare activity now with that of a year ago. The patient often reports an increase in time spent sleeping, sometimes up to 14 to 16 hours daily. Generalized weakness, anorexia, muscle aches, and paresthesias may also be present. Constipation and cold intolerance are common. Ask whether more blankets at night or extra clothing, even in warm weather, has been needed. Some changes may be subtle and are often missed, especially in older adults.

Both men and women may report a decreased libido. Women may have had difficulty becoming pregnant or have changes in menses (heavy, prolonged bleeding or amenorrhea). Men may have problems with impotence and infertility.

Ask about current or previous use of drugs, such as lithium, thiocyanates, aminoglutethimide, sodium or potassium perchlorate, or cobalt. All of these drugs can impair thyroid hormone production. In particular, the cardiac drug amiodarone (Cordarone) often has damaging effects on the thyroid gland (Brent & Weetman, 2016; Devereaux & Tewelde, 2014). Also ask whether the patient has ever been treated for hyperthyroidism and what specific treatment was used.

Physical Assessment/Signs and Symptoms. Observe the patient's overall appearance. Fig. 63-3 shows the typical appearance of an adult with hypothyroidism. Common changes include coarse features, edema around the eyes and face, a blank expression, and a thick tongue. The patient's overall muscle movement is slow. He or she may not speak clearly and may take a longer time to respond to questions.

Cardiac and respiratory functions are decreased, leading to reduced GAS EXCHANGE. Heart rate may be below 60 beats/min, and respiratory rate may be slow. Body temperature is often lower than 97°F (36.1°C).

Weight gain is very common, even when the adult is not overeating. Weigh the patient and ask whether the result is the same or different from his or her weight a year ago.

Depending on the cause of hypothyroidism, the patient may have a goiter. However, some types of hypothyroidism do not induce a goiter, and some types of hyperthyroidism do. The presence of a goiter *suggests* a thyroid problem but does not indicate whether the problem is excessive hormone secretion or too little hormone secretion.

Psychosocial Assessment. Hypothyroidism causes many problems in psychosocial functioning. Depression is the most common reason for seeking medical attention. Family members often bring the patient for the initial evaluation. The patient may be too lethargic, apathetic, or drowsy to recognize changes in his or her condition. Families may report that the patient is withdrawn and has reduced cognition. Assess his or her attention span and memory, both of which can be impaired by hypothyroidism. The mental slowness can contribute to social isolation.

Laboratory Assessment. Laboratory findings for hypothyroidism are the opposite of those for hyperthyroidism. Triiodothyronine (T_3) and thyroxine (T_4) serum levels are decreased. TSH levels are high in primary hypothyroidism but can be decreased or near normal in patients with secondary hypothyroidism (see Chart 63-2). Patients older than 80 years may have lower-than-normal levels of thyroid hormones without symptoms of hypothyroidism, and hormone replacement is not used until other symptoms are present (Touhy & Jett, 2016).

❓ NCLEX EXAMINATION CHALLENGE 63-3
Physiological Integrity

Which symptoms are **most** often seen in hypothyroidism? **Select all that apply.**
A. Increased appetite
B. Cold intolerance
C. Constipation
D. Hypotension
E. Exophthalmia
F. Palpitations
G. Tremors
H. Weight gain

◆ **Analysis: Interpreting**

The priority collaborative problems for patients who have hypothyroidism are:
1. Decreased GAS EXCHANGE and oxygenation due to decreased energy, obesity, muscle weakness, and fatigue
2. Hypotension and reduced perfusion due to decreased heart rate from decreased myocardial metabolism
3. Reduced cognition due to reduced brain metabolism and formation of edema
4. Potential for the complication of myxedema coma

◆ **Planning and Implementation: Responding**

Respiratory and cardiac problems are serious, and their management is a priority. *The most common cause of death among patients with myxedema coma is respiratory failure.*

Improving Gas Exchange

Planning: Expected Outcomes. With appropriate management, the patient with hypothyroidism is expected to have improved GAS EXCHANGE. Indicators include:

- Maintenance of Spo₂ of at least 90%
- Absence of cyanosis
- Maintenance of cognitive orientation

Interventions. Observe and record the rate and depth of respirations and adequacy of GAS EXCHANGE. Measure oxygen saturation by pulse oximetry and apply oxygen if the patient has hypoxemia. Auscultate the lungs for a decrease in breath sounds or presence of crackles. If hypothyroidism is severe, the patient may require ventilatory support. Severe respiratory distress occurs with myxedema coma.

Sedating a patient with hypothyroidism can make GAS EXCHANGE worse and is avoided if possible. When sedation is needed, the dosage is reduced because hypothyroidism increases sensitivity to these drugs. For the patient receiving sedation, assess for adequate gas exchange.

Preventing Hypotension

Planning: Expected Outcomes. The patient is expected to have adequate cardiovascular function and tissue perfusion with GAS EXCHANGE. Indicators include that the patient:

- Maintains heart rate above 60 beats/min
- Maintains blood pressure within normal limits for his or her age and general health
- Has no dysrhythmias, peripheral edema, or neck vein distention

Interventions. The patient may have decreased blood pressure, bradycardia, and dysrhythmias. Nursing priorities are monitoring for condition changes and preventing complications. Monitor blood pressure and heart rate and rhythm and observe for indications of shock (e.g., hypotension, decreased urine output, changes in mental status).

If hypothyroidism is chronic, the patient may have cardiovascular disease. *Instruct the patient to report episodes of chest pain or chest discomfort immediately.*

The patient requires lifelong thyroid hormone replacement. Synthetic hormone preparations are usually prescribed. The most common is levothyroxine sodium (Synthroid, T₄, Eltroxin ✦). Therapy is started with low doses and gradually increased over a period of weeks. *The patient with more severe symptoms of hypothyroidism is started on the lowest dose of thyroid hormone replacement.* This precaution is especially important when the patient has known cardiac problems. Starting at too high a dose or increasing the dose too rapidly can cause severe hypertension, heart failure, and myocardial infarction. With myxedema coma, the drug may need to be given IV because of the severely reduced motility and absorption of the GI tract (Hampton, 2013).

> ### ! NURSING SAFETY PRIORITY (QSEN)
> #### Drug Alert
>
> Teach patients and families who are beginning thyroid replacement therapy to take the drug exactly as prescribed and not to change the dose or schedule without consulting the primary health care provider. Instruct them not to switch brands because the response to different drug brands can vary.

Assess the patient for chest pain and dyspnea during initiation of therapy. The final dosage is determined by blood levels of TSH and the patient's physical responses. The dosage and time required for symptom relief vary with each patient. Monitor for and teach the patient and family about the symptoms

of hyperthyroidism (see Chart 63-1), which can occur with replacement therapy.

Supporting Cognition

Planning: Expected Outcomes. The patient is expected to return to the same level of cognitive function as before the thyroid problem started. Indicators include that the patient:

- Demonstrates immediate memory
- Communicates clearly and appropriately for age and ability
- Is attentive during conversations

Interventions. Observe for and record the presence and severity of lethargy, drowsiness, memory deficit, poor attention span, and difficulty communicating. These problems should decrease with thyroid hormone treatment, and mental awareness usually returns to the patient's normal level within 2 weeks. Orient the patient to person, place, and time and explain all procedures slowly and carefully. Provide a safe environment.

Family members may have difficulty coping with the patient's behavior. Encourage them to accept the mood changes and mental slowness as symptoms of the disease. Remind the family that these problems should improve with therapy.

Preventing Myxedema Coma.
Any patient with hypothyroidism who has any other health problem or who is newly diagnosed is at risk for myxedema coma. Factors leading to myxedema coma include acute illness, surgery, chemotherapy, discontinuing thyroid replacement therapy, and the use of sedatives or opioids. Problems that often occur with this condition include:

- Coma
- Respiratory failure
- Hypotension
- Hyponatremia
- Hypothermia
- Hypoglycemia

> ### ! NURSING SAFETY PRIORITY (QSEN)
> #### Action Alert
>
> Myxedema coma can lead to shock, organ damage, and death. Assess the patient with hypothyroidism at least every 8 hours for changes that indicate increasing severity, especially changes in mental status, and report these promptly to the primary health care provider.

Treatment is instituted quickly according to the patient's symptoms and without waiting for laboratory confirmation. Best practices for emergency care of the patient with myxedema coma are listed in Chart 63-7.

Care Coordination and Transition Management

Hypothyroidism is usually chronic. Patients usually live in the community and are managed on an outpatient basis. Patients in acute care settings, subacute care settings, and rehabilitation centers may have long-standing hypothyroidism in addition to other health problems. Ensure that whoever is responsible for overseeing the patient's daily care is aware of the condition and understands its management.

Home Care Management.
The patient with hypothyroidism does not usually require changes in the home unless cognition has decreased to the point that he or she poses a danger to himself or herself. Activity intolerance and fatigue may necessitate one-floor living for a short time. If symptoms

CHART 63-7 Best Practice for Patient Safety & Quality Care QSEN

Emergency Care of the Patient During Myxedema Coma

- Maintain a patent airway.
- Replace fluids with IV normal or hypertonic saline as prescribed.
- Give levothyroxine sodium IV as prescribed.
- Give glucose IV as prescribed.
- Give corticosteroids as prescribed.
- Check the patient's temperature hourly.
- Monitor blood pressure hourly.
- Cover the patient with warm blankets.
- Monitor for changes in mental status.
- Turn every 2 hours.
- Institute Aspiration Precautions.

CHART 63-8 Nursing Focus on the Older Adult

Thyroid Problems

Teach the patient these facts about changes in the thyroid gland related to aging:

- Thyroid hormone secretion decreases with age, but the hormone level remains stable because storage site clearance of the hormone also decreases with age.
- The basal metabolic rate decreases with age, which changes body composition from predominantly muscular to predominantly fatty.
- Older patients require lower doses of replacement thyroid hormone. Too large a dose may adversely affect the heart muscle.

have not improved before discharge, discuss the need for extra heat or clothing because of cold intolerance. The patient may need help with the drug regimen. Discuss this issue with the family and patient and develop a plan for drug therapy. One person should be clearly designated as responsible for drug preparation and delivery so doses are neither missed nor duplicated.

Self-Management Education. The most important educational need for the patient with hypothyroidism is about hormone replacement therapy and its side effects. Emphasize the need for lifelong drugs and review the symptoms of both hyperthyroidism and hypothyroidism. Teach the patient to wear a medical alert bracelet. Teach the patient and family when to seek medical interventions for dosage adjustment and the need for periodic blood tests of hormone levels. Instruct the patient not to take any over-the-counter (OTC) drugs without consulting his or her primary health care provider because thyroid hormone preparations interact with many other drugs. Older patients may need additional information about the effects of aging on the thyroid gland (Chart 63-8).

Advise the patient to maintain NUTRITION by eating a well-balanced diet with adequate fiber and fluid intake to prevent constipation. Caution him or her that use of fiber supplements may interfere with the absorption of thyroid hormone. Thyroid hormones should be taken on an empty stomach, at least 4 hours before or after a meal. Remind the patient about the importance of adequate rest.

Help the family understand that the time required for resolution of hypothyroidism varies. During this time the patient may

continue to have mental slowness. Teach the family to orient the patient often and to explain everything clearly, simply, and as often as needed.

Teach the patient to monitor himself or herself for therapy effectiveness. The two easiest parameters to check are need for sleep and bowel elimination. When the patient requires more sleep and is constipated, the dose of replacement hormone may need to be increased. When the patient has difficulty getting to sleep and has more bowel movements than normal for him or her, the dose may need to be decreased.

Health Care Resources. Immediately after returning home, the patient may need a support person to stay and provide day and night attention. Contact with the health care team is needed for follow-up and identification of potential problems. The patient taking thyroid drugs may have symptoms of hypothyroidism if the dosage is inadequate or symptoms of hyperthyroidism if the dose is too high. A home care nurse performs a focused assessment at every home visit for the patient with thyroid dysfunction (Chart 63-9).

◆ Evaluation: Reflecting

Evaluate the care of the patient with hypothyroidism based on the identified priority patient problems. The expected outcomes are that with proper management the patient should:

- Maintain normal cardiovascular function
- Maintain adequate respiratory function and GAS EXCHANGE
- Experience improvement in thought processes

CHART 63-9 Focused Assessment

The Patient With Thyroid Dysfunction

Assess cardiovascular status:
- Vital signs, including apical pulse, pulse pressure, presence or absence of orthostatic hypotension, and the quality and rhythm of peripheral pulses
- Presence or absence of peripheral edema
- Weight gain or loss

Assess cognition and mental status:
- Level of consciousness
- Orientation to time, place, and person
- Ability to accurately read a seven-word sentence containing no words greater than three syllables
- Ability to count backward from 100 by 3s

Assess condition of skin and mucous membranes:
- Moistness of skin, most reliable on chest and back
- Skin temperature and color

Assess neuromuscular status:
- Reactivity of patellar and biceps reflexes
- Oral temperature
- Handgrip strength
- Steadiness of gait
- Presence or absence of fine tremors in the hand

Ask about:
- Sleep in the past 24 hours
- Patient warm enough or too warm indoors
- 24-hour diet recall
- 24-hour activity recall
- Over-the-counter and prescribed drugs taken
- Last bowel movement

Assess patient's understanding of illness and adherence with therapy:
- Symptoms to report to primary health care provider
- Drug therapy plan (correct timing and dose)

THYROIDITIS

❖ PATHOPHYSIOLOGY

Thyroiditis is an inflammation of the thyroid gland. There are three types: acute, subacute, and chronic. Chronic thyroiditis (Hashimoto's disease) is the most common type.

Acute thyroiditis is caused by bacterial invasion of the thyroid gland. Symptoms include pain, neck tenderness, malaise, fever, and dysphagia (difficulty swallowing). It usually resolves with antibiotic therapy.

Subacute or granulomatous thyroiditis results from a viral infection of the thyroid gland after a cold or other upper respiratory infection. Symptoms include fever, chills, dysphagia, and muscle and joint pain. Pain can radiate to the ears and the jaw. The thyroid gland feels hard and enlarged on palpation. Thyroid function can remain normal, although hyperthyroidism or hypothyroidism may develop.

Chronic thyroiditis (Hashimoto's disease) is a common type of hypothyroidism that affects women more often than men. Hashimoto's disease is an autoimmune disorder that is usually triggered by a bacterial or viral infection. The thyroid is invaded by antithyroid antibodies and lymphocytes, causing selective thyroid tissue destruction. When large amounts of the gland are destroyed, serum thyroid hormone levels are low, and secretion of thyroid-stimulating hormone (TSH) is increased.

❖ INTERPROFESSIONAL COLLABORATIVE CARE

Symptoms of Hashimoto's disease include dysphagia and painless enlargement of the gland. Diagnosis is based on circulating antithyroid antibodies and needle biopsy of the thyroid gland. Serum thyroid hormone levels and TSH levels vary with disease stage.

The patient is given thyroid hormone to prevent hypothyroidism and to suppress TSH secretion, which decreases the size of the thyroid gland. Surgery (subtotal thyroidectomy) is needed if the goiter does not respond to thyroid hormone, is disfiguring, or compresses other structures. Nursing interventions focus on promoting comfort and teaching the patient about hypothyroidism, drugs, and surgery.

THYROID CANCER

❖ PATHOPHYSIOLOGY

The four distinct types of thyroid cancer are papillary, follicular, medullary, and anaplastic (American Cancer Society, 2017;

Canadian Cancer Society, 2016). The initial sign of thyroid cancer is a single, painless lump or nodule in the thyroid gland. Additional signs and symptoms depend on the presence and location of metastasis (spread of cancer cells).

Papillary carcinoma, the most common type of thyroid cancer, occurs most often in younger women. It is a slow-growing tumor that can be present for years before spreading to nearby lymph nodes. When the tumor is confined to the thyroid gland, the chance for cure is good with a partial or total thyroidectomy.

Follicular carcinoma occurs most often in older adults. It invades blood vessels and spreads to bone and lung tissue. When it adheres to the trachea, neck muscles, great vessels, and skin, dyspnea (difficulty breathing) and dysphagia (difficulty swallowing) result. When the tumor involves the recurrent laryngeal nerves, the patient may have a hoarse voice.

Medullary carcinoma is most common in patients older than 50 years. It often occurs with multiple endocrine neoplasia (MEN) type 2, a familial endocrine disorder (OMIM, 2014). The tumor usually secretes a variety of hormones.

Anaplastic carcinoma is a rapidly growing, aggressive tumor that invades nearby tissues. Symptoms include stridor (harsh, high-pitched respiratory sounds), hoarseness, and dysphagia.

A hallmark of thyroid cancer is an elevated serum thyroglobulin (Tg) level. The normal Tg level is 0.5 to 53.0 ng/mL (mcg/L) for men and 0.5 to 43.0 ng/mL (mcg/L) for women.

❖ INTERPROFESSIONAL COLLABORATIVE CARE

Radiation therapy is used most often for anaplastic carcinoma because this cancer has usually metastasized at diagnosis. The patient is treated with ablative (enough to destroy the tissue) amounts of RAI. (See Chart 63-4 for precautions to teach the patient receiving unsealed RAI therapy.) If spread has occurred to the neck or mediastinum, external radiation is also used. If thyroid cancer does not respond to RAI, chemotherapy is initiated.

Surgery is the treatment of choice for other types of thyroid cancer. A total thyroidectomy is usually performed with dissection of lymph nodes in the neck if regional lymph nodes are involved. (See the postoperative care discussion in the Surgical Management section for Hyperthyroidism.) Suppressive doses of thyroid hormone are usually taken for 3 months after surgery. Thyroglobulin levels are monitored after surgery. A rising level indicates probable presence of cancer cells.

The patient is hypothyroid after treatment for thyroid cancer. Nursing interventions then focus on teaching him or her about the management of hypothyroidism. (See the discussion of patient-centered collaborative care in the Hypothyroidism section.)

PARATHYROID DISORDERS

HYPERPARATHYROIDISM

❖ PATHOPHYSIOLOGY

The parathyroid glands maintain calcium and phosphate balance (see Fig. 61-6). Serum calcium level is normally maintained within a narrow range. Increased levels of parathyroid hormone (PTH) act directly on the kidney, causing increased kidney reabsorption of calcium and increased phosphorus excretion. In hyperparathyroidism, these processes cause *hypercalcemia* (excessive calcium) and *hypophosphatemia* (inadequate phosphorus).

In bone, excessive PTH levels increase bone *resorption* (bone loss of calcium) by decreasing *osteoblastic* (bone production) activity and increasing *osteoclastic* (bone destruction) activity. This process releases calcium and phosphorus into the blood and reduces bone density. With chronic calcium excess and hypercalcemia, calcium is deposited in soft tissues.

Although the exact trigger is unknown, primary hyperparathyroidism results when one or more parathyroid glands do not respond to the normal feedback of serum calcium levels. The most common cause is a benign tumor in one parathyroid gland. Table 63-3 lists other causes.

❖ INTERPROFESSIONAL COLLABORATIVE CARE

◆ Assessment: Noticing

Symptoms of hyperparathyroidism may be related to the effects of either excessive PTH or the accompanying hypercalcemia.

Ask about any bone fractures, recent weight loss, arthritis, or psychological stress. Ask whether the patient has received radiation treatment to the head or neck. The patient with chronic disease may have a waxy pallor of the skin and bone deformities in the extremities and back.

High levels of PTH cause kidney stones and deposits of calcium in the soft tissue of the kidney. Bone lesions are caused by an increased rate of bone destruction and may result in fractures, bone cysts, and osteoporosis.

GI problems (e.g., anorexia, nausea, vomiting, epigastric pain, constipation, weight loss) are common when serum calcium levels are high. Elevated serum gastrin levels are caused by hypercalcemia and lead to peptic ulcer disease. Fatigue and lethargy may be present and worsen as the serum calcium levels increase. When serum calcium levels are greater than 12 mg/dL (3.0 mmol/L), the patient may have psychosis with confusion, followed by coma and death if left untreated. (See Chapter 11 for more information about hypercalcemia.)

Serum PTH, calcium, and phosphorus levels and urine cyclic adenosine monophosphate (cAMP) levels are the laboratory tests used to detect hyperparathyroidism (Chart 63-10). X-rays may show kidney stones, calcium deposits, and bone lesions. Loss of bone density occurs in the patient with chronic hyperparathyroidism. Other diagnostic tests include arteriography, (CT scans, venous sampling of the thyroid for blood PTH levels, and ultrasonography). Explain the procedures and care for the patient undergoing diagnostic tests.

◆ Interventions: Responding

Surgical management is the treatment of choice for patients with hyperparathyroidism. For those who are not candidates for surgery, drug therapy can help control the problems. Priority nursing interventions focus on monitoring and preventing injury.

Nonsurgical Management. Diuretic and hydration therapies help reduce serum calcium levels in patients who have milder disease. Usually furosemide (Lasix, Uritol ✦), a diuretic that increases kidney excretion of calcium, is used along with IV saline in large volumes to promote calcium excretion.

Drug therapy for patients who have more severe symptoms of hyperparathyroidism or who have hypercalcemia related to parathyroid cancer involves the use of cinacalcet (Sensipar), a calcimimetic. When taken orally, the drug binds to calcium-sensitive receptors on parathyroid tissue, reducing PTH production and release. The result is decreased serum calcium levels, stabilization of other minerals, and decreased progression of PTH-induced bone complications. The patient's serum calcium

TABLE 63-3	**Causes of Parathyroid Dysfunction**
Causes of Hyperparathyroidism	**Causes of Hypoparathyroidism**
• Parathyroid tumor or cancer • Congenital hyperplasia • Neck trauma or radiation • Vitamin D deficiency • Chronic kidney disease with hypocalcemia • Parathyroid hormone–secreting carcinomas of the lung, kidney, or GI tract	• Surgical or radiation-induced thyroid ablation • Parathyroidectomy • Congenital dysgenesis • Idiopathic (autoimmune) hypoparathyroidism • Hypomagnesemia

⚡ CHART 63-10 **Laboratory Profile**

Parathyroid Function

TEST	NORMAL RANGE FOR ADULTS	SIGNIFICANCE OF ABNORMAL FINDINGS	
		HYPERPARATHYROIDISM	HYPOPARATHYROIDISM
Serum calcium	Total: 9.0-10.5 mg/dL (2.25-2.75 mmol/L) units Ionized (active): 4.5-5.6 mg/dL (1.05-1.30 mmol/L)	Increased in primary hyperparathyroidism	Decreased
Serum phosphorus	3.0-4.5 mg/dL (0.97-1.45 mmol/L) *Older adults:* May be slightly lower	Decreased	Increased
Serum magnesium	1.8-2.6 mEq/L (0.74-1.07 mmol/L)	Increased	Decreased
Serum parathyroid hormone	C-terminal: 50-330 pg/mL (ng/L) N-terminal: 8-25 pg/mL (ng/L) Whole: 10-65 pg/mL (ng/L)	Increased	Decreased
Vitamin D (calciferol)	25-80 ng/mL (75-200 nmol/L)	Variable	Decreased
Urine cAMP	18.3-45.4 nmol/L in a 24-hour urine collection specimen	Increased	Decreased

Pagana, K., Pagana, T., & Pike-MacDonald, S. (2013). *Mosby's Canadian manual of diagnostic and laboratory tests.* St. Louis: Mosby; and Pagana, K., Pagana, T.J., & Pagana, T.N. (2017). *Mosby's diagnostic and laboratory test reference* (13th ed.). St. Louis: Mosby.
cAMP, Cyclic adenosine monophosphate.

must be monitored for hypocalcemia on a regular basis for the duration of therapy.

For patients who do not respond to cinacalcet, oral phosphates are used to inhibit bone resorption and interfere with calcium absorption. IV phosphates are used only when serum calcium levels must be lowered rapidly. Calcitonin decreases the release of skeletal calcium and increases kidney excretion of calcium. It is not effective when used alone because of its short duration of action. Therapeutic effects are enhanced if calcitonin is given with glucocorticoids.

Monitor cardiac function and intake and output every 2 hours during hydration therapy. Continuous cardiac monitoring may be necessary. Compare recent ECG tracings with the patient's baseline tracings. Especially look for changes in the T waves and the QT interval, as well as changes in the rate and rhythm. Monitor serum calcium levels and immediately report any sudden drop to the primary health care provider. Sudden drops in calcium levels may cause tingling and numbness in the muscles.

Preventing injury is important because the patient with chronic hyperparathyroidism often has significant bone density loss and is at risk for fractures. Teach unlicensed assistive personnel (UAP) to handle the patient carefully and to use a lift sheet to reposition the patient rather than pulling him or her.

Surgical Management. Surgical management of hyperparathyroidism is a parathyroidectomy. Before surgery the patient is stabilized, and calcium levels are decreased to near normal.

The operative procedure can be performed as minimally invasive surgery or mini-incision surgery or with a traditional transverse incision in the lower neck. All four parathyroid glands are examined for enlargement. If a tumor is present on one side but the other side is normal, the surgeon removes the glands containing tumor and leaves the remaining glands on the opposite side intact. If all four glands are diseased, they are all removed.

Nursing care before and after surgical removal of the parathyroid glands is the same as that for thyroidectomy. See the Preoperative Care and Postoperative Care sections of hyperthyroidism for specific nursing interventions.

The remaining glands, which may have atrophied as a result of PTH overproduction, require several days to several weeks to return to normal function. A hypocalcemic crisis can occur during this critical period, and the serum calcium level is assessed frequently after surgery. Check serum calcium levels whenever they are drawn until calcium levels stabilize. Monitor for indications of hypocalcemia, such as tingling and twitching in the extremities and face. Check for Trousseau's and Chvostek's signs, either of which indicates potential tetany (see Figs. 11-13 and 11-14).

The recurrent laryngeal nerve can be damaged during surgery. Assess the patient for changes in voice patterns and hoarseness.

When hyperparathyroidism is caused by *hyperplasia* (tissue overgrowth), three glands plus half of the fourth gland are usually removed. If all four glands are removed, a small portion of a gland may be implanted in the forearm, where it produces PTH and maintains calcium homeostasis. If all these maneuvers fail, the patient will need lifelong treatment with calcium and vitamin D because the resulting hypoparathyroidism is permanent (see next section).

HYPOPARATHYROIDISM

❖ PATHOPHYSIOLOGY

Hypoparathyroidism is a rare disorder in which parathyroid function is decreased. Problems are directly related to a lack of

parathyroid hormone (PTH) secretion or to decreased effectiveness of PTH on target tissue. Whether the problem is a lack of PTH secretion or an ineffectiveness of PTH on tissues, the result is the same: *hypocalcemia.*

Iatrogenic hypoparathyroidism, the most common form, is caused by the removal of all parathyroid tissue during total thyroidectomy or surgical removal of the parathyroid glands.

Idiopathic hypoparathyroidism can occur spontaneously. The exact cause is unknown, but an autoimmune basis is suspected, and it may occur with other autoimmune disorders.

Hypomagnesemia (decreased serum magnesium levels) may cause hypoparathyroidism. Low magnesium levels are seen in patients with malabsorption syndromes, chronic kidney disease, and malnutrition. Low magnesium levels suppress PTH secretion and may interfere with the effects of PTH on the bones, kidneys, and calcium regulation.

❖ INTERPROFESSIONAL COLLABORATIVE CARE

◆ Assessment: Noticing

Ask about any head or neck surgery or radiation therapy because these treatments may injure the parathyroid glands and cause hypoparathyroidism. Also ask whether the neck has ever sustained a serious injury in a car crash or by strangulation. Assess whether the patient has any symptoms of hypoparathyroidism, which may range from mild tingling and numbness to muscle tetany. Tingling and numbness around the mouth or in the hands and feet reflect mild-to-moderate hypocalcemia. Severe muscle cramps, spasms of the hands and feet, and seizures (with no loss of consciousness or incontinence) reflect a more severe hypocalcemia. The patient or family may notice mental changes ranging from irritability to psychosis.

The physical assessment may show excessive or inappropriate muscle contractions that cause finger, hand, and elbow flexion. This can signal an impending attack of tetany. Check for Chvostek's sign and Trousseau's sign; positive responses indicate potential tetany (see Figs. 11-13 and 11-14). Bands or pits may encircle the teeth, which indicates a loss of tooth calcium and enamel.

Diagnostic tests for hypoparathyroidism include electroencephalography (EEG), blood tests, and CT scans. EEG changes revert to normal with correction of hypocalcemia. Serum calcium, phosphorus, magnesium, vitamin D, and urine cyclic adenosine monophosphate (cAMP) levels may be used in the diagnostic workup for hypoparathyroidism (see Chart 63-10). The CT scan can show brain calcifications, which indicate chronic hypocalcemia.

◆ Interventions: Responding

Nonsurgical management of hypoparathyroidism focuses on correcting hypocalcemia, vitamin D deficiency, and hypomagnesemia. For patients with acute and severe hypocalcemia, IV calcium is given as a 10% solution of calcium chloride or calcium gluconate over 10 to 15 minutes. Acute vitamin D deficiency is treated with oral calcitriol (Rocaltrol), 0.5 to 2 mg daily. Acute hypomagnesemia is corrected with 50% magnesium sulfate in 2-mL doses (up to 4 g daily) IV. Long-term oral therapy for hypocalcemia involves the intake of calcium, 0.5 to 2 g daily, in divided doses.

Long-term therapy for vitamin D deficiency is 50,000 to 400,000 units of oral ergocalciferol daily. The dosage is adjusted to keep the patient's calcium level in the low-normal range (slightly hypocalcemic), enough to prevent symptoms of hypocalcemia. It must also be low enough to prevent increased urine calcium levels, which can lead to stone formation.

Nursing management includes teaching about the drug regimen and interventions to reduce anxiety. Teach the patient to eat food high in calcium but low in phosphorus. Milk, yogurt, and processed cheeses are avoided because of their high phosphorus content. *Stress that therapy for hypocalcemia is lifelong.* Advise the patient to wear a medical alert bracelet. With adherence to the prescribed drug and diet regimen, the calcium level usually remains high enough to prevent a hypocalcemic crisis.

 NCLEX EXAMINATION CHALLENGE 63-4

Safe and Effective Care Environment

The nurse reviewing the laboratory work of a client with hypoparathyroidism finds all the following blood values. For which value does the nurse immediately assess the client's reflexes?
A. Sodium 131 mEq/L (mmol/L)
B. Potassium 5.1 mEq/L (mmol/L)
C. Calcium 7.8 mg/dL (1.76 mmol/L)
D. pH 7.33

GET READY FOR THE NCLEX® EXAMINATION

KEY POINTS

Review these Key Points for each NCLEX Examination Client Needs Category.

Safe and Effective Care Environment
- Keep the environment of a patient at risk for thyroid storm cool, dark, and quiet. **QSEN: Safety**
- Keep emergency suctioning and tracheotomy equipment in the room of a patient who has had thyroid or parathyroid surgery. **QSEN: Safety**
- Use a lift sheet to move or reposition a patient with hypocalcemia. **QSEN: Safety**

Health Promotion and Maintenance
- Teach all patients to take antithyroid drugs or thyroid hormone replacement therapy as prescribed. **QSEN: Patient-Centered Care**
- Teach patients to use signs and symptoms (e.g., the number of bowel movements per day, the ability to sleep) as indicators of therapy effectiveness and when the dose of thyroid hormone replacement may need to be adjusted. **QSEN: Patient-Centered Care**
- Include the person who prepares the patient's meals when teaching about dietary electrolyte restrictions. **QSEN: Patient-Centered Care**
- Collaborate with the registered dietitian to teach patients about diets that are restricted in calcium or phosphorus. **QSEN: Teamwork and Collaboration**

Psychosocial Integrity
- Be accepting of patient behavior. **QSEN: Patient-Centered Care**
- Remind patients and family members that changes in cognition and behavior related to thyroid problems are usually temporary. **QSEN: Patient-Centered Care**

- Encourage the patient who has a permanent change in appearance (e.g., exophthalmia) to mourn the change. **QSEN: Patient-Centered Care**

Physiological Integrity
- Be aware that:
  - The presence of a goiter indicates a problem with the thyroid gland but can accompany either hyperthyroidism or hypothyroidism.
  - Although similar in action, methimazole and propylthiouracil are not interchangeable.
  - Methimazole can cause birth defects and should not be used during pregnancy, especially during the first trimester. Instruct women to notify their primary health care provider if pregnancy occurs.
- When stridor, dyspnea, or other symptoms of obstruction appear after thyroid surgery, notify the Rapid Response Team. **QSEN: Safety**
- When caring for a patient with hyperthyroidism, even after a thyroidectomy, immediately report a temperature increase of even 1°F because it may indicate an impending thyroid crisis. **QSEN: Evidence-Based Practice**
- Assess the cardiopulmonary status of any patient with hypothyroidism for decreased perfusion or decreased GAS EXCHANGE at least every 8 hours. **QSEN: Patient-Centered Care**
- Use sedating drugs or opioids sparingly with patients who have hypothyroidism. **QSEN: Patient-Centered Care**
- Monitor the hydration status of patients who have hypercalcemia. **QSEN: Patient-Centered Care**
- Assess the patient with hypoparathyroidism for manifestations of hypocalcemia, especially numbness or tingling around the mouth and a positive Chvostek's sign or Trousseau's sign (see Figs. 11-13 and 11-14). **QSEN: Patient-Centered Care**

SELECTED BIBLIOGRAPHY

American Cancer Society. (2017). *Cancer facts and figures 2017.* Report No. 00-300M–No. 500817. Atlanta: Author.

Brent, G., & Weetman, A. (2016). Hypothyroidism and thyroiditis. In S. Melmed, K. Polonsky, P. R. Larsen, & H. Kronenberg (Eds.), *Williams' textbook of endocrinology* (13th ed.). Philadelphia: Saunders.

Bringhurst, F. R., Demay, M., & Kronenberg, H. (2016). Hormones and disorders of mineral metabolism. In S. Melmed, K. Polonsky, P. R. Larsen, & H. Kronenberg (Eds.), *Williams' textbook of endocrinology* (13th ed.). Philadelphia: Saunders.

Burchum, J., & Rosenthal, L. (2016). *Lehne's pharmacology for nursing care* (9th ed.). St. Louis: Elsevier.

Canadian Cancer Society, Statistics Canada. (2016). *Canadian Cancer Statistics, 2016*. Toronto: Canadian Cancer Society.

Davies, T., Laurberg, P., & Bahn, R. (2016). Thyrotoxicosis. In S. Melmed, K. Polonsky, P. R. Larsen, & H. Kronenberg (Eds.), *Williams' textbook of endocrinology* (13th ed.). Philadelphia: Saunders.

Devereaux, D., & Tewelde, S. (2014). Hyperthyroidism and thyrotoxicosis. *Emergency Medicine Clinics of North America, 32*(2), 277–292.

Dubbs, S., & Spangler, R. (2014). Hypothyroidism: Causes, killers, and life-saving treatments. *Emergency Medicine Clinics of North America, 32*(2), 303–317.

Hampton, J. (2013). Thyroid gland emergencies: Thyroid storm and myxedema coma. *AACN Advanced Critical Care, 24*(3), 325–332.

McCance, K., Huether, S., Brashers, V., & Rote, N. (2014). *Pathophysiology: The biologic basis for disease in adults and children* (7th ed.). St. Louis: Mosby.

Melmed, S., Polonsky, K., Larsen, P. R., & Kronenberg, H. (Eds.), (2016). *Williams' textbook of endocrinology* (13th ed.). Philadelphia: Saunders.

Online Mendelian Inheritance in Man (OMIM). (2014). *Multiple endocrine neoplasia, Type II A; MEN2A*. www.omim.org/entry/171400.

Online Mendelian Inheritance in Man (OMIM). (2016). *Graves disease, susceptibility to, 1*. www.omim.org/entry/275000.

Pagana, K., Pagana, T., & Pike-MacDonald, S. (2013). *Mosby's Canadian manual of diagnostic and laboratory tests*. St. Louis: Mosby.

Pagana, K., Pagana, T. J., & Pagana, T. N. (2017). *Mosby's diagnostic and laboratory test reference* (13th ed.). St. Louis: Mosby.

Patel, H., Wilches, V., & Guerro, J. (2013). Thyrotoxic periodic paralysis: Diversity in America. *The Journal of Emergency Medicine, 46*(6), 760–762.

Salvatore, D., Davies, T., Schlumberger, M., Hay, I., & Larsen, P. R. (2016). Thyroid physiology and diagnostic evaluation of patients with thyroid disorders. In S. Melmed, K. Polonsky, P. R. Larsen, & H. Kronenberg (Eds.), *Williams' textbook of endocrinology* (13th ed.). Philadelphia: Saunders.

Touhy, T., & Jett, K. (2016). *Ebersole and Hess' Toward nursing healthy aging* (9th ed.). St. Louis: Mosby.

Care of Patients With Diabetes Mellitus

Saundra Hendricks

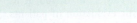
http://evolve.elsevier.com/Iggy/

PRIORITY AND INTERRELATED CONCEPTS

The priority concept for this chapter is GLUCOSE REGULATION.

❋ The GLUCOSE REGULATION concept exemplar for this chapter is Diabetes Mellitus, below.

The interrelated concepts for this chapter are:

- NUTRITION
- TISSUE INTEGRITY
- SENSORY PERCEPTION
- PERFUSION
- IMMUNITY
- FLUID AND ELECTROLYTE BALANCE
- ACID-BASE BALANCE

LEARNING OUTCOMES

Safe and Effective Care Environment

1. Collaborate with the interprofessional team to coordinate high-quality care and promote GLUCOSE REGULATION in patients who have diabetes mellitus (DM).
2. Teach the patient and caregiver(s) about how impaired GLUCOSE REGULATION from DM and its complications affect home safety.
3. Prioritize evidence-based care for patients with common complications of DM affecting GLUCOSE REGULATION.

Health Promotion and Maintenance

4. Identify community resources for patients with DM.
5. Teach adults how to decrease the risk for complications of DM.
6. Teach adults at risk for impaired GLUCOSE REGULATION how to prevent or delay development of type 2 DM.

Psychosocial Integrity

7. Implement nursing interventions to help the patient and family cope with the psychosocial impact caused by DM and its complications.

Physiological Integrity

8. Apply knowledge of pathophysiology to assess patients for problems associated with impaired GLUCOSE REGULATION and DM.
9. Implement evidence-based nursing interventions to improve GLUCOSE REGULATION and prevent complications of DM.
10. Teach the patient and caregiver(s) about common drugs and other therapies used to manage DM and its complications.
11. Implement evidence-based interprofessional collaborative care to manage patients experiencing hypoglycemia, ketoacidosis, or hyperglycemic-hyperosmolar state (HHS).

❋ GLUCOSE REGULATION CONCEPT EXEMPLAR
Diabetes Mellitus

GLUCOSE REGULATION is the process of maintaining optimal blood glucose levels (Fig. 64-1) (Giddens, 2017). Diabetes mellitus (DM), once known as *sugar* diabetes, is a very common chronic endocrine disorder of impaired glucose regulation that affects the function of all cells and tissues. Complications of DM, especially hypertension and hyperlipidemia (high blood lipid levels), are responsible for many associated life-shortening health problems in the United States, Canada, and other affluent countries. Many adults have undiagnosed diabetes and,

among those who are diagnosed, many continue to have high blood glucose levels. The complications of DM can be greatly reduced with glycemic (blood glucose) control along with management of hypertension and hyperlipidemia. Nursing priorities focus on helping the patient with DM achieve and maintain permanent lifestyle changes that keep blood glucose levels and cholesterol levels as close to normal as possible to slow or prevent long-term complications.

An interprofessional collaborative management approach helps the patient achieve desired outcomes successfully. In addition to primary health care providers, other professionals commonly involved in planning and providing continuing care

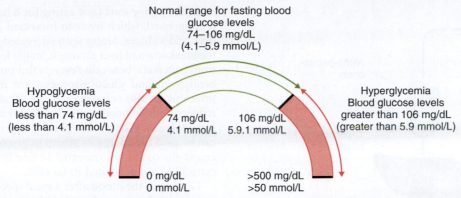

Normal range for fasting blood
glucose levels
74–106 mg/dL
(4.1–5.9 mmol/L)

Hypoglycemia
Blood glucose levels
less than 74 mg/dL
(less than 4.1 mmol/L)

Hyperglycemia
Blood glucose levels
greater than 106 mg/dL
(greater than 5.9 mmol/L)

74 mg/dL
4.1 mmol/L

106 mg/dL
5.9.1 mmol/L

0 mg/dL
0 mmol/L

>500 mg/dL
>50 mmol/L

FIG. 64-1 Fasting blood glucose levels. When GLUCOSE REGULATION is adequate, fasting levels remain in the normal range. With insufficient insulin usage, hyperglycemia results. Excess insulin or insufficient glucose results in hypoglycemia.

TABLE 64-1 Classification of Diabetes Mellitus

Type 1 Diabetes (T1DM)
- Beta-cell destruction leading to absolute insulin deficiency
- Autoimmune
- Idiopathic

Type 2 Diabetes (T2DM)
- Ranges from insulin resistance with relative insulin deficiency to secretory deficit with insulin resistance

Other Conditions Resulting in Hyperglycemia
- Genetic defects of beta-cell function
- Genetic defects in insulin action
- Pancreatic diseases (pancreatitis, trauma, cancer, cystic fibrosis, hemochromatosis)
- Endocrine problems (acromegaly, Cushing's disease, hyperthyroidism, aldosteronism)
- Drug- or chemical-induced hyperglycemia
- Infections: congenital rubella, cytomegalovirus, human immune deficiency virus
- Genetic syndromes associated with diabetes: Down syndrome, Klinefelter syndrome, Turner syndrome, Huntington disease, and others

Gestational Diabetes Mellitus (GDM)
- Glucose intolerance with onset or first recognition during pregnancy. (All pregnant women should be screened.)

for patients with diabetes include endocrinologists, diabetes educators, ophthalmologists, other medical practitioners, pharmacists, registered dietitians, podiatrists, physical therapists, wound care specialists, and home health nurses. As part of the team, you will help plan, organize, and coordinate care with other team members to promote the patient's health and well-being. These activities may take place in almost any setting.

❖ PATHOPHYSIOLOGY
Classification of Diabetes
For all types of diabetes mellitus (DM), the main feature is chronic hyperglycemia (high blood glucose level) resulting from problems with GLUCOSE REGULATION that include reduced insulin secretion or reduced insulin action or both. The disease is classified by the underlying problem causing a lack of insulin or its action and the severity of the insulin deficiency. Table 64-1 outlines the types of DM.

The Endocrine Pancreas
The pancreas has both endocrine and exocrine functions. The exocrine functions are related to digestion, and endocrine functions ensure blood GLUCOSE REGULATION. The endocrine portion of the pancreas has about 1 million small glands, the islets of Langerhans, scattered through the organ. The islet cells are only a small portion of the gland, and most of the pancreatic tissue is devoted to the production and delivery of digestive acids. Inside the islet cells are two types of cells important to glucose regulation. These are the *alpha* cells, which secrete glucagon, and the *beta* cells, which produce insulin and amylin. Glucagon is a "counterregulatory" hormone that has actions opposite those of insulin. It prevents *hypoglycemia* (low blood glucose levels) by triggering the release of glucose from storage sites in the liver and skeletal muscle. Insulin prevents *hyperglycemia* by allowing body cells to take up, use, and store carbohydrate, fat, and protein.

Active insulin is a protein made up of 51 amino acids. It is initially produced as inactive *proinsulin*, a prohormone that contains an additional amino acid chain (the C-peptide chain). Proinsulin is converted in the liver to active insulin by removal of the C-peptide (Fig. 64-2).

Insulin is secreted daily directly into liver circulation in a two-step manner. It is secreted at low levels during fasting (basal insulin secretion) and in a two-phase release after eating (**prandial**). An early burst of insulin secretion occurs within 10 minutes of eating, followed by an increasing release that lasts until the blood glucose level has returned to normal.

Glucose Regulation and Homeostasis
As stated earlier, GLUCOSE REGULATION is the process of maintaining optimal blood glucose levels. Although glucose is a critical nutrient, chronically high blood glucose levels cause many serious problems, and low blood glucose levels can rapidly lead to death. Thus maintaining blood glucose levels within a relatively normal range is important for health (see Fig. 64-2). Several organs and hormones play a role in maintaining glucose regulation. During fasting, when the stomach is empty, blood glucose is maintained between 60 and 150 mg/dL (3.3 and 8.3 mmol/L) by a balance between glucose uptake by cells and glucose production by the liver. Insulin plays a pivotal role in this process.

Glucose is the main fuel for central nervous system (CNS) cells. Because the brain cannot produce or store much glucose,

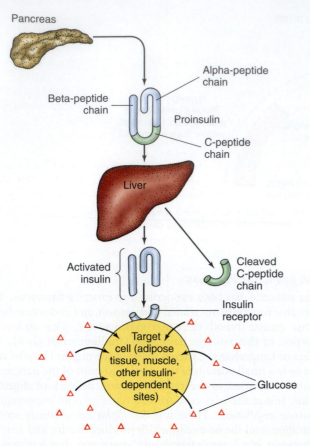

FIG. 64-2 Proinsulin, secreted by and stored in the beta cells of the islets of Langerhans in the pancreas, is transformed by the liver into active insulin. Insulin attaches to receptors on target cells, where it promotes glucose transport into the cells through the cell membranes.

it needs a continuous supply from the blood to prevent neuron dysfunction and cell death. Other organs can use both glucose and fatty acids to generate energy. Glucose is stored as glycogen in the liver and skeletal muscles, and free fatty acids are stored as triglyceride in fat cells. During a prolonged fast or after illness, proteins are broken down, and some of the amino acids are converted into glucose.

Movement of glucose into most cells requires the presence of specific membrane receptors along with insulin. Insulin is like a "key" that opens "locked" membranes to glucose, allowing blood glucose to move into cells to generate energy. Insulin starts this action by binding to membrane insulin receptors, which changes membrane permeability to glucose.

Insulin exerts many effects on metabolism and cellular processes in all tissues and organs. The main metabolic effects of insulin are to stimulate glucose uptake in skeletal muscle and heart muscle and to suppress liver production of glucose and very-low-density lipoprotein (VLDL). In the liver, insulin promotes the production and storage of glycogen (**glycogenesis**) at the same time that it inhibits glycogen breakdown into glucose (**glycogenolysis**). It increases protein and lipid (fat) synthesis and inhibits **ketogenesis** (conversion of fats to acids) and **gluconeogenesis** (conversion of proteins to glucose). In muscle, insulin promotes protein and glycogen synthesis. In fat cells, it promotes triglyceride storage. Overall, insulin keeps blood glucose levels from becoming too high and helps keep blood lipid levels in the normal range.

In the *fasting state* (not eating for 8 hours), insulin secretion is suppressed, which leads to increased gluconeogenesis in the liver and kidneys, along with increased glucose generation by the breakdown of liver glycogen. In the fed state, insulin released from pancreatic beta cells reverses this process. Instead, glycogen breakdown and gluconeogenesis are inhibited. At the same time, insulin also enhances glucose uptake and use by cells and reduces both fat breakdown (**lipolysis**) and protein breakdown (**proteolysis**). When more glucose is present in liver cells than can be used for energy or stored as glycogen, insulin causes the excess glucose to be converted to free fatty acids (FFAs). These extra FFAs are deposited in fat cells.

Glucose in the blood after a meal is controlled by the emptying rate of the stomach and delivery of nutrients to the small intestine, where they are absorbed into circulation. Incretin hormones (e.g., GLP-1), secreted in response to food in the stomach, have several actions. They increase insulin secretion, inhibit glucagon secretion, and slow the rate of gastric emptying, thereby preventing hyperglycemia after meals.

Counterregulatory hormones increase blood glucose by actions opposite those of insulin when more energy is needed. Glucagon is the main counterregulatory hormone. Other hormones that increase blood glucose levels are epinephrine, norepinephrine, growth hormone, and cortisol. The combined actions of insulin and counterregulatory hormones (discussed in the next section) participate in GLUCOSE REGULATION and keep blood glucose levels in the range of 60 to 100 mg/dL (3.3 to 5.6 mmol/L) to support brain function. When blood glucose levels fall, insulin secretion stops and glucagon is released. Glucagon causes glucose release from the liver. Liver glucose is made through breakdown of glycogen to glucose (glycogenolysis) and conversion of amino acids into glucose. When liver glucose is unavailable, the breakdown of fat (lipolysis) and the breakdown of proteins (proteolysis) provide fuel for energy.

> ### ❓ NCLEX EXAMINATION CHALLENGE 64-1
> #### *Physiological Integrity*
>
> Which physiologic actions result from normal insulin secretion?
> **Select all that apply.**
> A. Increased liver storage of glucose as glycogen
> B. Increased gluconeogenesis
> C. Increased cellular uptake of blood glucose
> D. Increased breakdown of lipids (fats) for fuel
> E. Increased production and release of epinephrine
> F. Decreased storage of free fatty acids in fat cells
> G. Decreased blood glucose levels
> H. Decreased blood cholesterol levels

Absence of Insulin

Insulin for GLUCOSE REGULATION is needed to move glucose into many body tissues. The lack of insulin in diabetes, from either a lack of production or a problem with insulin use at its cell receptor, prevents some cells from using glucose for energy. The body then breaks down fat and protein in an attempt to provide energy and increases levels of counterregulatory hormones to make glucose from other sources. Table 64-2 outlines responses to insufficient insulin.

Without insulin, glucose builds up in the blood, causing **hyperglycemia** (high blood glucose levels). Hyperglycemia disturbs FLUID AND ELECTROLYTE BALANCE, leading to

TABLE 64-2   **Physiologic Response to Insufficient Insulin**
• Decreased glycogenesis (conversion of glucose to glycogen)
• Increased glycogenolysis (conversion of glycogen to glucose)
• Increased gluconeogenesis (formation of glucose from noncarbohydrate sources such as amino acids and lactate)
• Increased lipolysis (breakdown of triglycerides to glycerol and free fatty acids)
• Increased ketogenesis (formation of ketones from free fatty acids)
• Proteolysis (breakdown of protein with amino acid release in muscles)

the classic symptoms of diabetes: polyuria, polydipsia, and polyphagia.

Polyuria is frequent and excessive urination and results from an osmotic diuresis caused by excess glucose in the urine. With diuresis, electrolytes are excreted in the urine, and water loss is severe. Dehydration results, and polydipsia (excessive thirst) occurs. Because the cells receive no glucose, cell starvation triggers polyphagia (excessive eating). Despite eating, the adult with diabetes remains in metabolic starvation until insulin is available to move glucose into the cells.

With insulin deficiency, the body turns to stored fat for energy, releasing free fatty acids. When this stored fat is used for energy, *ketone bodies* (small acids) provide a backup energy source. Ketone bodies ("ketones") are abnormal breakdown products that collect in the blood when insulin is not available, leading to the ACID-BASE BALANCE problem of metabolic acidosis.

Dehydration with DM leads to *hemoconcentration* (increased blood concentration); *hypovolemia* (decreased blood volume); poor tissue PERFUSION; and *hypoxia* (poor tissue oxygenation), especially to the brain. Hypoxic cells do not metabolize glucose efficiently, the Krebs' cycle is blocked, and lactic acid production increases, causing more acidosis.

The excess acids caused by absence of insulin increase hydrogen ion (H^+) and carbon dioxide (CO_2) levels in the blood, causing anion-gap metabolic acidosis. These products trigger the brain to increase the rate and depth of respiration in an attempt to "blow off" carbon dioxide and acid. This type of breathing is known as Kussmaul respiration. Acetone is exhaled, giving the breath a "rotting citrus fruit" odor. When the lungs can no longer offset acidosis, the blood pH drops. Arterial blood gas studies show a metabolic acidosis (decreased pH with decreased arterial bicarbonate [HCO_3^-] levels) and compensatory respiratory alkalosis (decreased partial pressure of arterial carbon dioxide [$Paco_2$]).

Insulin lack initially causes potassium depletion. With the increased fluid loss from hyperglycemia, excessive potassium is excreted in the urine, leading to low serum potassium levels. High serum potassium levels may occur in acidosis because of the shift of potassium from inside the cells to the blood. Serum potassium levels in DM, then, may be low (hypokalemia), high (hyperkalemia), or normal, depending on hydration, the severity of acidosis, and the patient's response to treatment. Chapter 12 discusses ACID-BASE BALANCE and acidosis in more detail.

Acute Complications of Diabetes

Three glucose-related emergencies can occur in patients with diabetes (DM):

- Diabetic ketoacidosis (DKA) caused by absence of insulin and generation of ketoacids
- Hyperglycemic-hyperosmolar state (HHS) caused by insulin deficiency and profound dehydration
- Hypoglycemia from too much insulin or too little glucose

All three problems require emergency treatment and can be fatal if treatment is delayed or incorrect. These problems and their interventions are described later in this chapter.

Chronic Complications of Diabetes

Diabetes mellitus (DM) can lead to organ complications and early death because of changes in large blood vessels (*macrovascular*) and small blood vessels (*microvascular*) in tissues and organs. These blood vessel changes lead to complications from poor tissue PERFUSION and cell ischemia. Macrovascular complications include coronary heart disease, cerebrovascular disease, and peripheral vascular disease, all of which lead to early morbidity and mortality. Microvascular complications of blood vessel structure and function lead to nephropathy (kidney dysfunction), neuropathy (nerve dysfunction), and retinopathy (vision problems). Such problems are responsible for increased morbidity and reduced quality of life. Causes of these diabetic vascular complications include:

- Chronic hyperglycemia thickens basement membranes, which causes organ damage.
- Glucose toxicity directly or indirectly affects functional cell integrity.
- Chronic ischemia in small blood vessels causes connective tissue hypoxia and micro-ischemia.

Chronic high blood glucose levels are the main cause of microvascular complications and allow premature development of macrovascular complications. Additional risk factors contributing to poor health outcomes for adults with DM include smoking, physical inactivity, obesity, hypertension, and high blood fat and cholesterol levels (Frank & Gerhardt, 2015). Many of these factors can be modified to reduce complications related to DM.

Hyperglycemia from poor GLUCOSE REGULATION leads to long-term complications of DM. Intensive therapy to maintain blood glucose levels as close to normal as possible delays the onset and progression of retinopathy, nephropathy, neuropathy, and macrovascular disease for patients with DM. For every percentage point decrease in A1C (glycosylated hemoglobin A1C), a 35% reduction of kidney and eye complications has been shown (ADA, 2014a).

Macrovascular Complications

Cardiovascular Disease. Patients with diabetes, prediabetes, or metabolic syndrome are at increased risk for cardiovascular disease (CVD) (McCance et al., 2014). This risk affects women to a greater degree than men and is influenced by the patient's ethnic group. DM is a "coronary heart disease risk equivalent" and a target for aggressive reduction of risk factors.

Patients with DM often have the traditional CVD risk factors of obesity, high blood lipid levels, hypertension, and sedentary lifestyle. Cigarette smoking and a positive family history also increase risk for CVD. Kidney disease, indicated by albuminuria (presence of albumin in the urine), and retinopathy are markers of increased risk for coronary heart disease and mortality from coronary artery disease. Patients with DM often have higher levels of C-reactive protein (CRP), an inflammatory marker associated with increased risk for cardiovascular inflammation and death.

Cardiovascular complication rates can be reduced through aggressive management of hyperglycemia, hypertension, and hyperlipidemia. The American Diabetes Association (ADA) recommends that blood pressure (BP) be measured at every routine visit and confirmed on a separate day if elevated. The ADA also recommends that BP be maintained below 140/90 mm Hg, with a target of 130/80 in younger adults if that level can be achieved without excessive burden. Lipid profile screening is recommended at first diagnosis, at the initial medical evaluation, and/or at the age of 40 years and every 1 to 2 years thereafter. Patients with DM who do not have overt CVD are recommended to maintain low-density lipoprotein (LDL) cholesterol below 100 mg/dL (2.60 mmol/L), and patients with indications of CVD are recommended to maintain LDLs at less than 70 mg/dL (1.8 mmol/L) (ADA, 2017a). Lifestyle modifications that focus on reducing saturated fat, *trans* fat, and cholesterol intake; increasing intake of omega-3 fatty acids, fiber, and plant sterols; weight loss (if indicated); and increasing physical activity are recommended to improve the lipid profile for patients with DM (ADA, 2017a).

Priority nursing actions focus on interventions to reduce modifiable risk factors associated with CVD, such as smoking cessation, diet, exercise, blood pressure control, maintaining prescribed aspirin use, and maintaining prescribed lipid-lowering drug therapy. Teach patients to report subtle indications of ischemia, such as dyspnea with or without cough, extreme fatigue, and sudden onset of nausea and vomiting, to their primary health care provider for evaluation.

Cerebrovascular Disease. The risk for stroke is two to four times higher in adults with DM compared with those who do not have the disease (McCance et al., 2014). Diabetes also increases the likelihood of severe carotid atherosclerosis. Hypertension, hyperlipidemia, nephropathy, peripheral vascular disease, and alcohol and tobacco abuse further increase the risk for stroke in adults with DM.

DM also affects stroke outcomes. Patients with DM are likely to suffer brain injury with carotid emboli that produce only transient ischemic attacks in adults without DM. Elevated blood glucose levels at the time of the stroke may lead to greater brain injury and higher mortality from the event.

Reduced Immunity. The combination of vascular changes and hyperglycemia reduce IMMUNITY by reducing white blood cell activity, inhibiting gas exchange in tissues, and promoting the growth of microorganisms. As a result, any adult who has DM is at an increased risk for developing an infection on exposure to bacteria and other organisms. In addition, infections become serious more quickly and can lead to major complications and sepsis (McCance et al., 2014).

Microvascular Complications

Eye and Vision Complications. Legal blindness (a corrected visual acuity of 20/200 or less) is 25 times more common in patients with DM (National Institute of Diabetes and Digestive and Kidney Diseases [NIDDKD], 2014). Diabetic retinopathy (DR) is strongly related to the duration of diabetes. After 20 years of DM, nearly all patients with the disease have some degree of retinopathy (ADA, 2014a). Unfortunately, DR has few symptoms until vision loss occurs.

The cause and progression of DR are related to problems that block retinal blood vessels and cause them to leak, leading to retinal hypoxia. Nonproliferative diabetic retinopathy causes structural problems in retinal vessels, including areas of poor retinal circulation, edema, hard fatty deposits in the eye, and retinal hemorrhages. Fluid and blood leak from the retinal vessels and cause retinal edema and hard exudates. Nonproliferative DR develops slowly and rarely reduces vision to the point of blindness.

Proliferative diabetic retinopathy is the growth of new retinal blood vessels, also known as *neovascularization*. When retinal blood flow is poor and hypoxia develops, retinal cells secrete vascular endothelial growth factors that stimulate formation of new blood vessels in the eye. These new vessels are thin, fragile, and bleed easily, leading to vision loss.

Other retinal problems are optic nerve atrophy from hypoxia and *venous beading,* which is the abnormal appearance of retinal veins with areas of swelling and constriction that resemble links of sausage. Venous beading occurs in areas of retinal ischemia.

Visual SENSORY PERCEPTION loss from DR has several mechanisms. Central vision may be impaired by macular edema, characterized by increased blood vessel permeability and deposits of hard exudates at the center of the retina. This problem is the main cause of vision loss in the adult with DM. Injections of ranbizumab (Lucentis) or aflibercept (Eylea) into the vitreous monthly can improve vision for some adults with macular edema. Vision loss also occurs from macular degeneration, corneal scarring, and changes in lens shape or clarity.

Hyperglycemia may cause blurred vision, even with eyeglasses. Because hypoglycemia can cause temporary vision changes, it is important to wait until blood glucose levels are normal before assessing for refractory changes. Cataracts occur at a younger age and progress faster among patients with DM. Open-angle glaucoma also is more common in patients with DM. The management of cataracts and glaucoma is discussed in Chapter 47.

Control of blood glucose, blood pressure, and blood lipid level is important in preventing DR. Thus patients with DM should have routine ophthalmic evaluations to detect vision problems early before vision loss occurs. The ADA recommends eye-care examinations with an ophthalmologist every year after an adult has been diagnosed with type 2 diabetes and yearly for an adult who has had type 1 diabetes for more than 5 years. The silent nature of many eye problems causes some adults with DM to not recognize the importance of annual screenings.

CONSIDERATIONS FOR OLDER ADULTS
Patient-Centered Care QSEN

The older patient with diabetic retinopathy also has general age-related vision changes, and the ability to perform self-care may be seriously affected. He or she may have blurred vision, distorted central vision, fluctuating vision, loss of color perception, and mobility problems resulting from loss of depth perception. When a patient has visual changes, it is especially important to assess his or her ability to measure and inject insulin and to monitor blood glucose levels to determine if adaptive devices are needed to assist in self-management (Touhy & Jett, 2016).

Diabetic Peripheral Neuropathy. Diabetic peripheral neuropathy (DPN) is a progressive deterioration of nerve function that results in loss of SENSORY PERCEPTION. It is a common complication of DM and often involves all parts of the body. Damage to sensory nerve fibers results in pain followed by loss of sensation. Damage to motor nerve fibers results in muscle weakness. Damage to nerve fibers in the autonomic nervous system can cause dysfunction in every part of the body. The combination of factors leading to the nerve damage in diabetic neuropathy are:

- Hyperglycemia, long duration of DM, hyperlipidemia
- Damaged blood vessels leading to reduced neuronal oxygen and other nutrients
- Autoimmune neuronal inflammation
- Increased genetic susceptibility to nerve damage
- Smoking and alcohol use

Hyperglycemia leads to DPN through blood vessel changes and reduced tissue PERFUSION that cause nerve hypoxia. Both the axon and its myelin sheath are damaged by reduced blood flow, resulting in blocked nerve impulse transmission. Excessive glucose is converted to sorbitol, which collects in nerves and impairs motor nerve conduction (McCance et al., 2014). Common diabetic neuropathies are listed in Table 64-3.

Diabetic neuropathy can be focal or diffuse. *Diffuse neuropathies* are the most common neuropathies in DM and involve widespread nerve function loss and SENSORY PERCEPTION loss. The onset is slow, affects both sides of the body, involves motor and sensory nerves, progresses slowly, and is permanent. Late complications include foot ulcers and deformities.

Focal neuropathies in DM affect a single nerve or nerve group and usually are caused by an acute ischemic event that leads to nerve damage or nerve death. Ischemic neuropathies occur when the blood supply to a nerve or nerve group is disrupted. Symptoms begin suddenly, affect only one side of the body area, and are self-limiting. The most common neuropathies affect the nerves that control the eye muscles. Symptoms begin with pain on one side of the face near the affected eye. The eye muscles become paralyzed, resulting in double vision. The problem usually resolves in 2 to 3 months.

Diabetic Autonomic Neuropathy. Cardiovascular autonomic neuropathy (CAN) affects sympathetic and parasympathetic nerves of the heart and blood vessels. This problem contributes to left ventricular dysfunction, painless myocardial infarction, and exercise intolerance. Most often, CAN leads to orthostatic (postural) hypotension and syncope (brief loss of consciousness on standing). These problems are from failure of the heart and arteries to respond to position changes by increasing heart rate and vascular tone. As a result, blood flow to the brain is interrupted briefly. Orthostatic hypotension and syncope increase the risk for falls, especially among older adults.

Autonomic neuropathy can affect the entire GI system. Common GI problems from diabetic neuropathy include gastroesophageal reflex, delayed gastric emptying and gastric retention, early satiety, heartburn, nausea, vomiting, and anorexia. Sluggish movement of the small intestine can lead to bacterial overgrowth, which causes bloating, gas, and diarrhea. Diarrhea caused by DM is chronic, may be severe, and often occurs at night. Constipation, the most common GI problem with DM, is intermittent and may alternate with bouts of diarrhea. Gastroparesis (delay in gastric emptying) is a cause of hypoglycemia related to the mismatch of nutrient absorption and insulin action.

Urinary problems from neuropathy result in incomplete emptying and urine retention, which leads to urinary infection and kidney problems. Early symptoms include frequency and urgency. Later symptoms include an inability to sense bladder fullness and incontinence.

❓ NCLEX EXAMINATION CHALLENGE 64-2

Health Promotion and Maintenance

Which precaution is **most important** for the nurse to teach a client who has cardiovascular autonomic neuropathy (CAN) from diabetes?
A. "Avoid drinking ice-cold beverages."
B. "Be sure to check your blood pressure twice daily."
C. "Change positions slowly when moving from sitting to standing."
D. "Check your hands and feet weekly for areas of numbness or sensation change."

TABLE 64-3 Features of Diabetic Neuropathy

	COMPLICATION	SYMPTOM
Diffuse Neuropathies		
Distal symmetric polyneuropathy	Sensory alterations	Paresthesias: burning/tingling sensations, starting in toes and moving up legs
		Dysesthesias: burning, stinging, or stabbing pain
		Anesthesia: loss of sensation
	Motor alterations in intrinsic muscles of foot	Foot deformities: high arch, claw toes, hammertoes; shift of weight bearing to metatarsal heads and tips of toes
Autonomic neuropathy	Anhidrosis	Drying, cracking of skin
	Gastrointestinal	Delayed gastric emptying, gastric retention, early satiety, bloating, nausea, vomiting, anorexia, constipation, diarrhea, diffuse sweating while eating
		Nocturnal diarrhea
	Neurogenic bladder	Atonic bladder, urinary retention
	Impotence	Erectile dysfunction
	Cardiovascular autonomic neuropathy	Early fatigue, weakness with exercise, orthostatic hypotension
	Defective counterregulation	Loss of warning signs of hypoglycemia
Focal Neuropathies		
Focal ischemia	Thoracolumbar radiculopathy with sensory and reflex loss	Pain radiating across back, side, and front of chest or abdomen
	Cranial nerve palsies, third and sixth nerves	Sudden diplopia or ptosis; eye pain
	Amyotrophy	Pain; asymmetric weakness; wasting of iliopsoas, quadriceps, and adductor muscles

Diabetic Nephropathy. Nephropathy is a pathologic change in the kidney that reduces kidney function and leads to kidney failure. Diabetes is the leading cause of end-stage kidney disease (ESKD) and kidney failure in the United States (NIDDKD, 2014). Risk factors include a 10- to 15-year history of DM, poor blood glucose control, uncontrolled hypertension, and genetic predisposition. The onset of diabetic kidney disease may be prevented, and the progression to ESKD can be delayed by maintaining optimum blood GLUCOSE REGULATION, keeping blood pressure within the normal ranges, and using drug therapy to protect the kidneys (ADA, 2017b). Drugs used to protect the kidneys in patients who meet specific criteria are the angiotensin-converting enzyme inhibitors (ACEIs) and the angiotensin receptor blockers (ARBs).

Kidney disease causes progressive albumin excretion and declining glomerular filtration rate (GFR). Annual testing for urine albumin is recommended for patients who have had type 1 DM for at least 5 years and in everyone with type 2 DM (ADA, 2017b).

Chronic high blood glucose levels cause hypertension in kidney blood vessels and excess kidney tissue PERFUSION. The increased pressure damages the kidney in many ways. The blood vessels become leakier, especially in the glomerulus. This leakiness allows filtration of albumin and other proteins, which then form deposits in the kidney tissues and blood vessels. Blood vessels narrow, decreasing kidney oxygenation and leading to kidney cell hypoxia and cell death. These processes worsen over time, with scarring of glomerular blood vessels and loss of urine filtration ability, leading to chronic kidney disease (see Chapter 68 for a detailed presentation of chronic kidney disease and end-stage kidney disease).

Kidney damage is also related to hypertension for patients with DM and cardiovascular disease. Both systolic and diastolic hypertension speed the progression of diabetic nephropathy.

Sexual Dysfunction. Both men and women with diabetes can develop sexual dysfunction as a result of damage to both nerve tissue and vascular tissue. This is made worse by poorly controlled blood glucose levels. Other factors include obesity, hypertension, tobacco use, and some prescribed drugs.

In men sexual dysfunction is manifested by both erectile dysfunction (ED) and retrograde ejaculation. Women may experience deceased vaginal lubrication, uncomfortable or painful sexual intercourse, and decreases in libido and sexual response.

Cognitive Dysfunction. Adults age 65 or older with DM are at a significantly higher risk for developing all types of dementia compared with adults who do not have the disease (ADA, 2017h). Chronic hyperglycemia with microvascular disease contributes to neuron damage, brain atrophy, and cognitive impairment. These problems are more frequent and more severe in patients with longer-duration DM and increase the complications of neuropathy and retinopathy. Depression is highly prevalent in adults with diabetes and is associated with worse outcomes.

Etiology and Genetic Risk

Type 1 Diabetes. Type 1 diabetes mellitus (DM) is an autoimmune disorder in which beta cells are destroyed in a genetically susceptible person (Table 64-4). The immune system fails to recognize normal body cells as "self," and immune system cells and antibodies take destructive actions against the insulin-secreting cells in the islets. People with certain tissue types are

TABLE 64-4 Differentiation of Type 1 and Type 2 Diabetes

Features	Type 1	Type 2
Former names	Juvenile-onset diabetes Ketosis-prone diabetes Insulin-dependent diabetes mellitus (IDDM)	Adult-onset diabetes Ketosis-resistant diabetes Non–insulin-dependent diabetes mellitus (NIDDM)
Age at onset	Usually younger than 30 yr	May occur at any age in adults
Symptoms	Abrupt onset, thirst, hunger, increased urine output, weight loss	Frequently none; thirst, fatigue, blurred vision, vascular or neural complications
Etiology	Viral infection, autoimmunity	Not known
Pathology	Pancreatic beta-cell destruction	Insulin resistance Dysfunctional pancreatic beta cell
Antigen patterns	*HLA-DR, HLA-DQ*	None
Antibodies	Present at diagnosis	None
Endogenous insulin and C-peptide	None	Low, normal, or high
Inheritance	Complex	Autosomal-dominant, multifactorial
Nutritional status	Usually nonobese	60% to 80% obese
Insulin	All dependent on insulin	Required for 20% to 30%
Medical therapy	Mandatory	Mandatory

more likely to develop autoimmune diseases, including type 1 DM. Viral infections, such as mumps and coxsackie virus infection, may trigger autoimmune destructive actions (McCance et al., 2014).

🧬 GENETIC/GENOMIC CONSIDERATIONS

Evidence-Based Practice QSEN

Risk for type 1 DM is determined by inheritance of genes coding for the HLA-DR and HLA-DQA and DQB tissues types (McCance et al., 2014). However, inheritance of these genes only increases the risk, and most people with these genes do not develop type 1 DM. Development of DM is an interactive effect of genetic predisposition and exposure to certain environmental factors. When assessing adults, always ask whether any family members have been diagnosed with either type 1 or type 2 diabetes.

Type 2 Diabetes and Metabolic Syndrome. Type 2 DM is a progressive disorder in which the person initially has insulin resistance that progresses to decreased beta cell secretion of insulin. *Insulin resistance* (a reduced cell response to insulin) develops from obesity and physical inactivity in a genetically susceptible adult. It occurs before the onset of type 2 DM and often is accompanied by the cardiovascular risk factors of hyperlipidemia, hypertension, and increased clot formation.

Many but not all patients with type 2 DM are obese. The specific causes of type 2 DM are not known, although insulin resistance and beta-cell failure have many genetic and nongenetic causes. Heredity plays a major role in the development of type 2 DM, although not all gene variations that increase the risk for type 2 DM are known.

Metabolic syndrome is the simultaneous presence of metabolic factors known to increase risk for developing type 2 DM and cardiovascular disease (Frazer, 2015). Features of the syndrome include:

- Abdominal obesity: waist circumference of 40 inches (100 cm) or more for men and 35 inches (88 cm) or more for women
- Hyperglycemia: fasting blood glucose level of 100 mg/dL or more or on drug treatment for elevated blood glucose levels
- Hypertension: systolic BP of 130 mm Hg or more or diastolic blood pressure of 85 mg Hg or more or on drug treatment for hypertension
- Hyperlipidemia: triglyceride level of 150 mg/dL or more or on drug treatment for elevated triglycerides; high-density lipoprotein (HDL) cholesterol less than 40 mg/dL for men or less than 50 mg/dL for women

Any one of these health problems increases the rate of atherosclerosis and the risk for stroke, coronary heart disease, and early death. Teach patients about the lifestyle changes that can improve health. (See the Health Promotion and Maintenance section.)

♥ VETERANS' HEALTH CONSIDERATIONS
Patient-Centered Care QSEN

A suggestive risk factor for type 2 DM independent of other risk factors is exposure to the main component of agent orange, dioxin, which was used during the military conflicts in Korea and Vietnam. The risk for type 2 diabetes appears higher among U.S. military personnel deployed in those geographic areas. The risk increases with higher exposures (United States Department of Veterans Affairs, 2016). Development of DM among veterans who served in areas where agent orange was used occurs at earlier ages and with less obesity.

Assess veterans who were exposed to agent orange at every health care encounter for subtle indications of diabetes so the disease can be identified early and interventions implemented to prevent or delay complications. Also encourage them to use DM prevention strategies of maintaining a healthy weight and engaging in regular physical activity.

Incidence and Prevalence

In the United States, more than 29 million people are living with DM, and 27.8% (8.1 million) are undiagnosed. Another 86 million have prediabetes (CDC, 2016). (**Prediabetes** is defined as impaired fasting glucose (IGF) or impaired glucose tolerance [IGT]. Over a 3- to 5-year period, adults with prediabetes have a 5-fold to 15-fold higher risk for developing type 2 DM than do those with normal blood glucose levels.). In Canada, nearly 2 million adults have diabetes, which represents about 6% of the population (Statistics Canada, 2015).

About 90% to 95% of adults with diabetes have type 2 DM (CDC, 2016). It can be diagnosed even in preadolescents but is most often diagnosed among middle-age and older adults, affecting about 12.3% of adults over the age of 20 years and 25.9% of adults 65 years or older (Touhy & Jett, 2016). It is more common among men than women (CDC, 2015). With the prevalence of obesity rising in North America, diabetes will become even more common.

🌐 CULTURAL/SPIRITUAL CONSIDERATIONS
Patient-Centered Care QSEN

Racial and ethnic minorities have a higher prevalence and greater burden of DM compared with non-Hispanic whites, and some minority groups also have higher rates of complications. The rate of DM is 13% among African Americans and 12.8% in the Hispanic population compared with non-Hispanic white Americans. At nearly 16.1%, American Indians and Alaska Indians have the highest age-adjusted prevalence of DM among U.S. racial and ethnic groups (CDC, 2015). *The increase in obesity and sedentary lifestyles in the North American population intensifies this growing problem. The ADA has identified patients who should be tested for diabetes in Table 64-5.*

The outcomes for minority patients with diabetes is worse than for non-Hispanic whites with DM. Factors for these outcome differences include lack of access to health care, lifestyle issues, mistrust of the health care system, reduced financial resources, and lack of knowledge about GLUCOSE REGULATION and complications. Be alert to the risk for DM whenever you are interviewing or assessing adults who belong to these higher-risk groups.

Health Promotion and Maintenance

Diabetes mellitus (DM) causes many preventable but devastating complications and is a major health problem. Control of DM and its complications is a major focus for health promotion activities. No interventions prevent type 1 DM, but health promotion activities that focus on controlling hyperglycemia can reduce its long-term complications.

TABLE 64-5 Indications for Testing People for Type 2 Diabetes

- Testing for diabetes is considered at any age in adults with a BMI greater than 25 kg/m² (or greater than 23 kg/m² in Asian Americans) with one or more of these additional risk factors:
  - Have a first-degree relative with diabetes
  - Are physically inactive
  - Are members of a high-risk ethnic population (e.g., African American, Hispanic American, American Indian, or Pacific Islander)
  - Have a baby weighing more than 9 lb or have been diagnosed with GDM
  - Are hypertensive (>140/90 mm Hg)
  - Have a high-density lipoprotein (HDL) cholesterol level less than 35 mg/dL
  - (0.90 mmol/L) and/or a triglyceride level greater than 250 mg/dL (2.82 mmol/L)
  - Have polycystic ovary syndrome
  - Have A1C greater than 5.7%, or IFG or IGT on previous testing
  - Have a history of vascular disease
- If the tested adult has normal glucose values at this time but other conditions and risk factors remain the same, testing should be repeated at 3-year intervals.

BMI, Body mass index; *GDM,* gestational diabetes mellitus; *IFG,* impaired fasting glucose, *IGT,* impaired glucose tolerance.
Data from American Diabetes Association (ADA). (2017). Classification and diagnosis of diabetes. *Diabetes Care, 40*(Suppl. 1), S11-S24; and American Diabetes Association (ADA). (2017). Standards of medical care in diabetes—2017: Prevention or delay of type 2 diabetes. *Diabetes Care, 40*(Suppl. 1), S44-S47.

Adopting a healthy lifestyle that includes a low-calorie diet and increasing physical activity with weight loss improves metabolic and cardiac risk factors (Watts & Howard, 2016). These improvements include reducing hypertension, increasing heart rate variability between resting rate and exercise rate, lowering triglyceride levels, increasing high-density lipoprotein cholesterol ("good" cholesterol) levels, and reducing low-density lipoprotein cholesterol ("bad" cholesterol) levels.

Teach all patients with DM that tight control of blood glucose levels can prevent many complications. Urge them to regularly follow up with their primary health care provider or endocrinologist, to have their eyes and vision tested yearly by an ophthalmologist, and to have urine albumin levels assessed yearly. Early detection of changes in the eye or kidney permits adjustments in treatment regimens that can slow or halt progression of retinopathy and nephropathy. Encourage all adults to maintain weight within an appropriate range for height and body build and to engage in physical activity at least 150 minutes per week (American Association of Diabetes Educators [AADE], 2015.

❖ INTERPROFESSIONAL COLLABORATIVE CARE

Although adults who have DM are often hospitalized for complications of the disease, diagnosis and management generally occur in a clinic or health care provider's office. Much of the essential teaching about management is performed in the community as is the overall management of the disorder. Because DM is a chronic disorder, you can expect to interact with and care for these patients in any health care setting.

◆ Assessment: Noticing

History. Ask about risk factors and symptoms related to DM. Age is important because, although type 2 DM is more common in older patients, it is now being diagnosed increasingly in younger adults. Ask women how large their children were at birth, because many women who develop type 2 DM had gestational diabetes mellitus (GDM) or glucose intolerance during pregnancy (ADA, 2017b). Women with a history of GDM and found to have prediabetes should receive education on lifestyle interventions to prevent DM (ADA, 2017b).

Assessing weight and weight change is important, because excess weight and obesity are risk factors for type 2 DM. The patient with type 1 DM often has weight loss with increased appetite during the weeks before diagnosis. For both types of DM, patients usually have fatigue, polyuria, and polydipsia. Ask about recent major or minor infections and assess overall IMMUNITY. In particular, ask women about frequent vaginal yeast infections. Ask all patients whether they have noticed that small skin injuries become infected more easily or take longer to heal. Also ask whether they have noticed any changes in vision or in the sense of touch. Determine whether the patient is up-to-date on his or her immunizations.

Laboratory Assessment

Diagnosis of Diabetes. Diabetes can be diagnosed by assessing blood glucose levels. The ADA defines normal blood glucose values in Chart 64-1. A test result indicating DM should be repeated to rule out laboratory error unless symptoms of hyperglycemia or hyperglycemic crisis are also present. Table 64-6 lists criteria for the diagnosis of DM.

TABLE 64-6   Criteria for the Diagnosis of Diabetes

A1C >6.5%. The test should be performed in a laboratory using a method that is NGSP certified and standardized to the DCCT assay.

Or

Fasting blood glucose greater than or equal to 126 mg/dL (7.0 mmol/L). *Fasting* is defined as no caloric intake for at least 8 hours.

Or

Two-hour blood glucose equal to or greater than 200 mg/dL (11.1 mmol/L) during oral glucose tolerance test. The test should be performed using a glucose load containing the equivalent of 75 g anhydrous glucose dissolved in water.

Or

In a patient with classic manifestations of hyperglycemia or hyperglycemic crisis, a random blood glucose concentration greater than 200 mg/dL (11.1 mmol/L). *Casual* is defined as any time of the day without regard to time since last meal. The classic symptoms of diabetes include polyuria, polydipsia, and unexplained weight loss. **NOTE:** In the absence of unequivocal hyperglycemia, the first three criteria should be confirmed by repeat testing.

Data from American Diabetes Association (ADA). (2017). Classification and diagnosis of diabetes. *Diabetes Care, 40*(Suppl. 1), S11-S24.
DCCT, Diabetes Control and Complications Trial; *NGSP,* National Glycohemoglobin Standardization Program.

🔬 CHART 64-1   Laboratory Profile

Blood Glucose Values

TEST	NORMAL RANGE FOR ADULTS	SIGNIFICANCE OF ABNORMAL RESULTS
Fasting blood glucose test	<100 mg/dL (5.6 mmol/L) Older adults: Levels rise 1 mg/dL per decade of age	Levels >100 mg/dL (5.6 mmol/L) but <126 mg/dL (7.0 mmol/L) indicate impaired fasting glucose (IFG). Levels >126 mg/dL (7.0 mmol/L) obtained on at least two occasions are diagnostic of diabetes, even in older adults.
Glucose tolerance test (2-hr post-load result)	<140 mg/dL (7.8 mmol/L)	Levels >140 mg/dL (7.8 mmol/L) and <200 mg/dL (11.1 mmol/L) indicate impaired glucose tolerance (IGT). Levels >200 mg/dL (11.1 mmol/L) indicate provisional diagnosis of diabetes.
Glycosylated hemoglobin (A1C) test	4%-6%	Levels of 5.7% to 6.4% indicate increased risk for development of diabetes. Levels >6.5% indicate diabetes. Levels >8% indicate poor diabetes control and need for adherence to regimen or changes in therapy.

Data from Pagana, K., Pagana, T.J., & Pagana, T.N. (2017). *Mosby's diagnostic and laboratory test reference* (13th ed.). St. Louis: Mosby; and Pagana, K., Pagana, T., & Pike-MacDonald, S. (2013). *Mosby's Canadian manual of diagnostic and laboratory tests.* St. Louis: Mosby.

The diagnosis of DM includes elevated glycosylated hemoglobin levels. **Glycosylated hemoglobin (A1C)** is a standardized test that measures how much glucose permanently attaches to the hemoglobin molecule. Because glucose binds to many proteins, including hemoglobin, through a process called *glycosylation,* the higher the blood glucose level is over time, the more glycosylated hemoglobin becomes. The ADA defines A1C levels greater than or equal to 6.5% as diagnostic of DM (ADA, 2017b).

Fasting plasma glucose (FPG) (fasting blood glucose [FBG]) can be used to diagnose DM in nonpregnant adults. The patient should have no caloric intake for at least 8 hours (water is permitted). A diagnosis of DM is made with two separate test results greater than 126 mg/dL (7 mmol/L) (ADA, 2017b). *Random* or *casual plasma* glucose greater than 200 mg/dL (7.0 mmol/L) is used to diagnose DM in patients with classic hyperglycemia symptoms or hyperglycemic crisis.

Oral glucose tolerance testing (OGTT) is a sensitive test for the diagnosis of DM. It is often used to diagnose gestational diabetes mellitus (GMD) during pregnancy and is not routinely used for general diagnosis.

Other blood tests for diabetes can help determine whether a patient has type 1 or type 2 DM. Type 1 DM results from autoimmune destruction of the beta cells of the pancreas. Markers of this destruction include islet cell autoantibodies (ICAs), autoantibodies to insulin, and autoantibodies to glutamic acid decarboxylase (GAD65). ICAs are present in 85% to 90% of patients with new-onset type 1 DM (McCance et al., 2014).

Measurement of C-peptide levels indicates beta secretory function of the pancreas. Low-to-absent C-peptide levels diagnose type 1 DM as well as late-stage type 2 DM when the ability of the pancreas to secrete insulin is severely impaired.

Screening for Diabetes. Testing to detect prediabetes and type 2 DM should be considered in patients older than 45 years and those defined as overweight (BMI greater than 25 kg/m²) (Touhy & Jett, 2016). Testing is considered for patients who are younger than 45 years and are overweight if they have additional risk factors for DM or other health problems associated with it. Screening for DM usually is done with either hemoglobin A1C levels or fasting plasma glucose levels (ADA, 2017b). The use of portable glucose meters for the diagnosis of DM is *not* recommended for screening because of imprecise results and variance in results among the different glucose monitors.

Ongoing Assessment. *Glycosylated hemoglobin assays* are useful as a good indicator of the average blood glucose levels. Measurement of A1C shows the average blood glucose level during the previous 120 days—the life span of red blood cells. A1C testing can help assess long-term glycemic control and predict the risk for complications. *Unlike the fasting blood glucose test, A1C test results are not altered by eating habits the day before the test.* This testing is performed at diagnosis and at specific intervals to evaluate the treatment plan. A1C testing is recommended at least twice yearly in patients who are meeting expected treatment outcomes and have stable blood glucose control. Quarterly assessment is recommended for patients whose therapy has changed or who are not meeting prescribed glycemic levels (ADA, 2017d). Table 64-7 shows the correlation between A1C and mean blood glucose levels.

Fructosamine assays are useful for short-term follow-up of treatment changes or in patients with hemoglobin abnormalities

TABLE 64-7 Correlation Between A1C Level and Mean Blood Glucose Levels

A1C (%)	MEAN BLOOD GLUCOSE	
	mg/dL	mmol/L
6	126	7.0
7	154	8.6
8	183	10.2
9	212	11.8
10	240	13.4
11	269	14.9
12	298	16.5

in which A1C does not accurately reflect glucose levels. When glucose binds to amino groups on serum proteins, especially albumin, the glycosylated protein product is called *fructosamine.* This product increases with elevated blood glucose levels like hemoglobin does but can indicate blood glucose control over a shorter period.

💡 NCLEX EXAMINATION CHALLENGE 64-3
Physiological Integrity

The laboratory values of a client who has diabetes mellitus include a fasting blood glucose level of 82 mg/dL (mmol/L) and hemoglobin A1C of 5.9%. What is the nurse's interpretation of these findings?
A. The client's glucose control for the past 24 hours has been good, but the overall control is poor.
B. The client's glucose control for the past 24 hours has been poor, but the overall control is good.
C. The values indicate that the client has poorly managed his or her disease.
D. The values indicate that the client has managed his or her disease well.

◆ *Analysis: Interpreting*

The priority collaborative problems for patients with diabetes DM include:
1. Potential for injury due to hyperglycemia
2. Potential for impaired wound healing due to endocrine and vascular effects of diabetes
3. Potential for injury due to diabetic neuropathy
4. Pain due to diabetic neuropathy
5. Potential for injury due to diabetic retinopathy–induced reduced vision
6. Potential for kidney disease due to impaired kidney circulation
7. Potential for hypoglycemia
8. Potential for diabetic ketoacidosis
9. Potential for hyperglycemic-hyperosmolar state and coma

◆ *Planning and Implementation: Responding*

The management of diabetes mellitus (DM) is complex and involves extensive patient education. The Concept Map highlights care issues for the patient with type 2 DM.

CONCEPT MAP

ACID-BASE BALANCE

IMMUNITY

GLUCOSE REGULATION

PERFUSION

FLUID AND ELECTROLYTE BALANCE

TISSUE INTEGRITY

SENSORY PERCEPTION

NUTRITION

DIABETES MELLITUS TYPE 2

EXPECTED OUTCOMES

- Manage DM and prevent progression by maintaining BG levels in expected range
- Seek care if BG levels fluctuate outside normal parameters
- Meet recommended activity level
- Use drugs as prescribed
- Maintain optimum weight
- Problem solve about barriers to self-management

Planning Expected Outcomes

PATIENT PROBLEMS

- Potential for injury due to hyperglycemia; diabetic retinopathy
- Potential for impaired wound healing due to endocrine and vascular effects
- Pain due to diabetic neuropathy
- Potential for kidney disease due to impaired kidney circulation, hypoglycemia, diabetic ketoacidosis, hyperglycemic-hyperosmolar state, and coma

Interpreting Data Synthesis

LAB VALUES

- Hyperglycemia
  – BG 330 mg/dL
- Central obesity
  – waist 39 inches
- Drug treatment for ↑ BG
- Hypertension: 160/90 mm Hg
- Triglycerides ↑ level 250 mg/dL
- HDL cholesterol 40 mg/dL

Interpreting Data Synthesis

Noticing Objective Data

NOTICE IN THE HISTORY

Emma Gomez is an Hispanic woman with a 20-year history of diabetes type 2. She has peripheral vascular disease and vision changes. She is admitted for gastroenteritis and a blood glucose (BG) level of 330 mg/dL.

Noticing Subjective Data

SUBJECTIVE DATA

"My vision is blurred, and I have trouble with my central vision. Sometimes my vision gets a little better. I'm scared I'm going to fall when I come down the stairs because I can't tell how deep the steps are."

INTERVENTIONS—RESPONDING

1 **Nursing Safety Priority: Critical Rescue!**
Assess vital signs, provide fluids for hydration, intervene to manage BP of 160/90 mm Hg, and treat high BG level. *Treats gastroenteritis and reduces the risk of a CVA and continued vascular damage. Drug therapy may be required to achieve desired outcomes.*

2 **Early Detection**
Teach about tight control of BG, regular eye checkups, and urine assessment for microalbumin and ketones. *Checks for early detection of SENSORY PERCEPTION (retinopathy) and PERFUSION issues (hypertensive kidney disease, nephropathy), which permits adjustments in treatment.*

3 **Interpreting Laboratory Values**
- Monitor K+ levels closely (it can be decreased, increased, or normal). *Potassium levels vary depending on hydration, the severity of any acidosis, and the patient's response to treatment.*
- Teach the patient to keep BG in the range of 60-100 mg/dL and maintain A1C levels below 7%. *Monitors history of glucose regulation. Maintaining near-normal levels delays problems with visual SENSORY PERCEPTION, PERFUSION, and TISSUE INTEGRITY (retinopathy, nephropathy, neuropathy, macrovascular disease).*

4 **GLUCOSE REGULATION**
Review with the patient the treatment regimen including nutrition, monitoring BG, when to seek medical care, recommended activity levels, using drug therapy correctly, optimum weight, and problem solving about barriers to self-management. *Prevents injury from hyperglycemia.*

5 **Nursing Safety Priority: Drug Alert!**
Teach the patient who is taking an antidiabetic drug to consult with the health care provider or pharmacist before using any over-the-counter drugs. *Prevents adverse drug interactions.*

6 **Maintaining Nutrition**
Evaluate an individualized nutritional plan in collaboration with dietitian: food intake during illness; activity level; amount of carbohydrates, fat, and fiber; consumption of alcohol; weight, and financial constraints. *Determines whether present habits are effective, need reinforcement, or require change.*

7 **Preventing Complications**
Teach the patient to recognize symptoms of poor GLUCOSE REGULATION, hypoglycemia or hyperglycemia (and treatments), and when to call the health care provider. *Prevents development of diabetic ketoacidosis (ACID-BASE IMBALANCE), prevents frequent episodes of hypoglycemia. Establishes what dietary changes are needed during illness.*

8 **Health Promotion Activities – Risk Factors**
Teach the patient to report decreased TISSUE PERFUSION: dyspnea, cough, extreme fatigue, and sudden onset of nausea and vomiting. *Improves CVD risk factors if the patient addresses smoking cessation, nutrition, exercise, blood pressure control, aspirin use, and adhering to prescribed lipid-lowering drug therapy.*

9 **Racial and Ethnic Considerations**
Explore issues related to lack of access to health care, lifestyle, mistrust of the health care system, limited financial resources, and lack of knowledge. *Racial and ethnic differences affect clinical outcomes for patients with diabetes.*

10 **Decreased IMMUNITY**
Teach the client about the increased risk for infection and to monitor closely for evidence of infection. *Vascular changes and hyperglycemia reduce IMMUNITY; infections become serious quickly and can lead to major complications including sepsis and greater mortality.*

Concept Map by Deanne A. Blach, MSN, RN

Preventing Injury From Hyperglycemia

Planning: Expected Outcomes. The patient is expected to manage DM and prevent disease progression by maintaining blood glucose levels in his or her target range. Indicators are that the patient consistently demonstrates these behaviors:

- Performs treatment regimen as prescribed
- Follows recommended diet
- Monitors blood glucose using correct testing procedures
- Seeks health care if blood glucose levels fluctuate outside of recommended parameters
- Meets recommended activity levels
- Follows prescribed drug regimen
- Reaches and maintains optimum body weight
- Problem solves about barriers to self-management

Interventions

Nonsurgical Management. Management of DM involves NUTRITION interventions, blood glucose monitoring, a planned exercise program, and often drugs to lower blood glucose levels. The nurse and other interprofessional team members (e.g., primary health care provider, dietitian, pharmacist, case manager), along with the patient, plan, coordinate, and deliver care.

The American Diabetes Association (ADA) has proposed these treatment outcomes for glycosylated hemoglobin (A1C) and blood glucose levels (ADA, 2017d):

- A1C levels are maintained at 7.0% or below. A lower goal may be recommended for patients who can achieve a lower goal without adverse effects. A less stringent goal may be needed for patients who have hypoglycemic unawareness, advanced microvascular or macrovascular disease, or a limited life expectancy.
- The majority of premeal blood glucose levels are 70 to 130 mg/dL (3.9 to 7.2 mmol/L).
- Peak after-meal blood glucose levels are less than 180 mg/dL (< 10.0 mmol/L).

Drug Therapy. Drug therapy is indicated when a patient with type 2 DM does not achieve blood glucose control with diet changes, regular exercise, and stress management. Several categories of drugs are available to lower blood glucose levels. Patients with type 1 DM require insulin therapy for blood glucose control.

Drugs are started at the lowest effective dose and increased every 1 to 2 weeks until the patient reaches desired blood glucose control or the maximum dosage. If the maximum dosage of one agent does not control blood glucose levels, a second agent with a different mechanism of action may be added. Insulin therapy is indicated for the patient with type 2 DM when blood glucose goals cannot be met with the use of two or three different antidiabetic agents.

Antidiabetic drugs are not a substitute for dietary modification and exercise. Teach the patient about the need for continuing dietary changes and regular exercise while taking antidiabetic drugs.

Drug Selection. The choice of antidiabetic drug is based on cost, the patient's ability to manage multiple drug dosages, age, and response to the drugs. Shorter-acting agents (e.g., glitinides) are preferable in older patients, those with irregular eating schedules, or those with liver, kidney, or cardiac dysfunction. Longer-acting agents (e.g., glyburide, glimepiride) with once-a-day dosing are better for adherence. Beta-cell function in type 2 DM often declines over time, reducing the effectiveness of some drugs. The treatment regimen for patients with type 2 DM may eventually require insulin therapy either alone or with other antidiabetic drugs.

Antidiabetic Drugs. Some antidiabetic drugs are oral agents, and others require subcutaneous injection. Chart 64-2 lists common antidiabetic drugs in each category.

Insulin Stimulators. Insulin stimulators (also known as insulin secretagogues) stimulate insulin release from pancreatic beta cells and are used for patients who are still able to produce insulin. Drugs in this class include the sulfonylureas and the meglitinide analogs.

> *Sulfonylurea agents* lower fasting blood glucose levels by triggering the release of insulin from beta cells. Many drugs interact with sulfonylureas. Be sure to consult a drug reference book or pharmacologist when instructing patients who are prescribed a drug from this class.
>
> *Meglitinide analogs* are insulin secretagogues and have actions and adverse effects similar to those of sulfonylureas. They tend to increase meal-related insulin secretion.

Biguanides. Metformin (Glucophage) does not increase insulin secretion. It decreases liver glucose production and decreases intestinal absorption of glucose. It also improves insulin sensitivity by increasing peripheral glucose uptake and utilization.

! NURSING SAFETY PRIORITY QSEN

Drug Alert

Metformin can cause lactic acidosis in patients with kidney impairment and should not be used by anyone with kidney disease. To prevent lactic acidosis and acute kidney injury, the drug is withheld before and after using contrast medium or any surgical procedure requiring anesthesia until adequate kidney function is established.

Insulin Sensitizers. Thiazolidinediones (TZDs, or "glitazones") increase cellular utilization of glucose, which lowers blood glucose levels. Both of the TZDs, rosiglitazone (Avandia) and pioglitazone (Actos), are associated with an increased risk for heart-related deaths, bone fracture, and macular edema. The Food and Drug Administration (FDA) has issued a black box warning indicating that these drugs are not to be used by patients who have symptomatic heart failure or other specific types of cardiovascular disease. (A black box warning is a government designation indicating that a drug has at least one serious side effect and must be used with caution.)

! NURSING SAFETY PRIORITY QSEN

Drug Alert

To avoid drug interactions, teach the patient who is taking an antidiabetic drug to consult with his or her primary health care provider or pharmacist before using *any* over-the-counter drugs.

! NURSING SAFETY PRIORITY QSEN

Drug Alert

Do not confuse Actos with Actonel. Actos is an oral antidiabetic drug from the thiazolidinedione class, and Actonel is a drug that prevents calcium loss from bones.

CHART 64-2 **Common Examples of Drug Therapy**

Diabetes Mellitus

DRUG CATEGORY	NURSING IMPLICATIONS
Insulin Stimulators (Secretagogues)—These drugs lower blood glucose levels by triggering the release of preformed insulin from beta cells.	
Second-Generation Sulfonylurea Agents (Oral) • Glipizide (Glucotrol) • Glyburide (Diabeta, Micronase) • Glimepiride (Amaryl) *Meglitinide Analogs (Oral)* • Repaglinide (Prandin) • Nateglinide (Starlix)	Teach patients the signs and symptoms of hypoglycemia (hunger, headache, tremors, sweating, confusion) *because these drugs lower blood glucose levels even when hyperglycemia is not present.* Instruct patients to take these drugs with or just before meals *to prevent hypoglycemia.* Instruct patients taking a sulfonylurea to check with his or her primary health care provider or a pharmacist before taking any over-the-counter drug or supplement *because these drugs interact with many other drugs.* Warn patients that nausea, headache, and weight gain are common side effects of these drugs *because knowing the expected side effects decreases anxiety when they appear.*
Biguanides—These drugs lower blood glucose levels by inhibiting liver glucose production, decreasing intestinal absorption of glucose, and increasing insulin sensitivity.	
• Metformin (Glucophage)	Instruct patients not to drink alcoholic beverages while taking this drug *to reduce the risk for lactic acidosis.* Remind patients that this drug must be discontinued before certain imaging tests using contrast agents and not started again for 48 hours after testing *because of the increased risk for kidney damage and lactic acidosis.* Warn patients that diarrhea, nausea, flatulence, indigestion, and abdominal pain are common side effects of this drug class *because knowing the expected side effects decreases anxiety when they appear.*
Insulin Sensitizers—These drugs lower blood glucose levels by decreasing liver glucose production and improving the sensitivity of insulin receptors.	
Thiazolidinediones (TZDs) (Oral) • Pioglitazone (Actos) • Rosiglitazone (Avandia)	Teach patients with any cardiovascular disease to weigh themselves daily and report a weight gain of more than 2 lb (1 kg) in one day or 4 lb (2 kg) in a week to the primary health care provider *because this class of drugs increases the risk for heart failure. These drugs carry a black box warning from the FDA and are not to be given to anyone with symptomatic heart failure.* Instruct patients to report vision changes immediately *because these drugs increase the risk for macular edema.* Warn women about an increased risk for bone fractures because *these drugs decrease bone density in women.* Warn patients that weight gain and peripheral edema are common side effects of this drug class *because knowing the expected side effects decreases anxiety when they appear.*
Alpha-Glucosidase Inhibitors—These oral drugs prevent after-meal hyperglycemia by inhibiting enzymes in the intestinal tract from breaking down starches into glucose. This action delays the digestion of starches and the absorption of glucose from the small intestine.	
• Acarbose (Precose) • Miglitol (Glyset)	Teach patients to take these drugs only with a meal because the action is in the intestinal tract. If a meal is skipped, so is the drug. Warn patients that abdominal discomfort and bloating, flatulence, nausea, diarrhea, and indigestion are common side effects of this drug class *because knowing the expected side effects decreases anxiety when they appear.*
Incretin Mimetics (GLP-1 Agonists)—These drugs act like natural "gut" hormones that work with insulin to lower blood glucose levels by reducing pancreatic glucagon secretion; reducing liver glucose production; and delaying gastric emptying, which slows the rate of nutrient absorption into the blood.	
• Albiglutide (Tanzeum) • Dulaglutide (Trulicity) • Exenatide (Byetta) • Exenatide extended-release (Bydureon) • Liraglutide (Victoza) • Lixisenatide (Adlyxin)	Teach patients the signs and symptoms of hypoglycemia (hunger, headache, tremors, sweating, confusion) *because these drugs lower blood glucose levels even when they are not elevated.* Instruct patients how to inject themselves *because these drugs are only available as subcutaneous formulations.* Teach patients to inspect injection sites for redness, warmth, or hard nodules because *injection site reactions are common.* Instruct patients to read exenatide, albiglutide, and dulaglutide pens carefully *because the extended-release form is only injected weekly (compared with others given at least daily). Injecting the extended-release form daily may cause serious harm.* Teach patients to report persistent abdominal pain and nausea to the health care provider *because these drugs increase the risk for pancreatitis.*

CHART 64-2 Common Examples of Drug Therapy—cont'd

Diabetes Mellitus

DRUG CATEGORY	NURSING IMPLICATIONS
DPP-4 Inhibitors—DPP-4 is an enzyme that breaks down the natural gut hormones (GLP-1 and GIP). DPP-4 inhibitors are oral agents that prevent the enzyme DPP-4 from breaking down the natural gut hormones (GLP-1 and GIP), which then allows these natural substances to work with insulin to lower glucagon secretion from the pancreas, leading to reduced liver glucose production. These oral drugs also reduce blood glucose levels by delaying gastric emptying, slowing the rate of nutrient absorption into the blood, and reducing food intake.	
• Alogliptin (Nesina) • Linagliptin (Tradjenta) • Saxagliptin (Onglyza) • Sitagliptin (Januvia)	Teach patients the signs and symptoms of hypoglycemia (hunger, headache, tremors, sweating, confusion) *because these drugs lower blood glucose levels even when hyperglycemia is not present.* Instruct patients to be alert and observe for rash or other sign of allergic reaction *because this class of drugs is associated with a moderate incidence of drug allergy.* Teach patients to report persistent abdominal pain and nausea to the primary health care provider *because these drugs increase the risk for pancreatitis.*
Amylin Analogs—These drugs are similar to amylin, a naturally occurring hormone from beta cells in the pancreas that is co-secreted with insulin and lowers blood glucose levels by decreasing endogenous glucagon, delaying gastric emptying and triggering satiety.	
• Pramlintide (Symlin)	Teach patients the signs and symptoms of hypoglycemia (hunger, headache, tremors, sweating, confusion) *because these drugs lower blood glucose levels even when hyperglycemia is not present.* Instruct patients how to inject themselves *because these drugs are only available as subcutaneous formulations.* Teach patients to inspect injection sites for redness, warmth, or hard nodules *because injection site reactions are common.* Warn patients that nausea and vomiting are common side effects of this drug class *because knowing the expected side effects decreases anxiety when they appear*
Sodium-Glucose Cotransport Inhibitors—These oral drugs lower blood glucose levels by preventing kidney reabsorption of glucose and sodium that was filtered from the blood into the urine. This filtered glucose is excreted in the urine rather than moved back into the blood.	
• Canagliflozin (Invokana) • Dapagliflozin (Farxiga) • Empagliflozin (Jardiance)	Teach patients the signs and symptoms of hypoglycemia (hunger, headache, tremors, sweating, confusion) *because these drugs lower blood glucose levels even when they are not elevated.* Teach patients the signs and symptoms of dehydration (increased thirst, light-headedness, dry mouth and mucous membranes, orthostatic hypotension) *because these drugs increase urine output and increase dehydration risk.* Teach patients the signs and symptoms of hyponatremia (muscle weakness, decreased ability to concentrate, abdominal cramping, rapid heart rate, orthostatic hypotension) *because these drugs increase sodium excretion.* Teach patients the signs and symptoms of urinary tract infection (frequency, pain and burning on urination, foul urine odor) *because the increased glucose in the urinary tract predisposes to infection.* Instruct women to be alert for genital itching and vaginal discharge *because these drugs increase the risk for genital yeast infection.*
Combination Products—Many fixed combinations of oral drugs are available. Each ingredient has the same mechanism of action and nursing implications as the parent drug class. When a drug that has the side effect of hypoglycemia is combined with a drug that does not alone produce hypoglycemia, the development of hypoglycemia is still very much a risk for the combination agent.	

FDA, Food and Drug Administration.

Alpha-Glucosidase Inhibitors. Alpha-glucosidase inhibitors prevent after-meal hyperglycemia by delaying absorption of carbohydrate from the small intestine. These drugs inhibit enzymes in the intestinal tract, reducing the rate of starch digestion and glucose absorption. These actions prevent a sudden blood glucose surge after meals. These drugs do not cause hypoglycemia unless given with sulfonylureas or insulin.

Incretin Mimetics. Incretin mimetics work like the natural "gut" hormones, glucagon-like peptide-1 (GLP-1) and glucose-dependent insulinotropic polypeptide (GIP), that are released by the intestine in response to food intake and act with insulin for GLUCOSE REGULATION. Drugs in this class include the GLP-1 agonists *albiglutide* (Tanzeum), *dulaglutide* (Trulicity), *exenatide* (Byetta), *exenatide extended-release* (Bydureon), *liraglutide* (Victoza), and *lixisenatide* (Adlyxin). These drugs are used in addition to diet and exercise to improve glycemic control in adults with type 2 DM.

DPP-4 Inhibitors. The incretins GLP and GIP produced by the body are rapidly metabolized and inactivated by the enzyme

! NURSING SAFETY PRIORITY QSEN

Drug Alert

Albiglutide (Tanzeum), extended-release exenatide (Bydureon), and dulaglutide (Trulicity) are administered subcutaneously once *weekly.*

DPP-4. Drugs that inhibit the DPP-4 enzyme work by reducing the inactivation of the incretin hormones so they remain available for blood GLUCOSE REGULATION. The four DPP-4 inhibitors used to control type 2 DM are sitagliptin (Januvia), saxagliptin (Onglyza), linagliptin (Tradjenta), and alogliptin (Nesina).

Amylin Analogs. Amylin analogs are drugs similar to amylin, a naturally occurring hormone produced by pancreatic beta cells that works with and is co-secreted with insulin in response to blood glucose elevation. Amylin levels are deficient in patients with type 1 DM who are also deficient in insulin. Pramlintide (Symlin), an analog of amylin, is approved for patients with DM

! **NURSING SAFETY PRIORITY** QSEN

Drug Alert

DPP-4 inhibitors and the incretin mimetics may be associated with an increased risk for pancreatitis. Warn patients taking these drugs to immediately report signs of jaundice; sudden onset of intense abdominal pain that radiates to the back, left flank, or left shoulder; or gray-blue discoloration of the abdomen or periumbilical area to the primary health care provider.

who are treated with insulin. It works by three mechanisms: delaying gastric emptying; reducing after-meal blood glucose levels; and triggering satiety (in the brain). (Satiety leads to decreased caloric intake and eventual weight loss.)

! **NURSING SAFETY PRIORITY** QSEN

Drug Alert

Do not mix pramlintide and insulin in the same syringe because the pH of the two drugs is not compatible.

Sodium-Glucose Cotransport Inhibitors. Sodium-glucose co-transport inhibitors lower blood glucose levels by preventing kidney reabsorption of glucose that was filtered from the blood into the urine. The filtered glucose is excreted in the urine rather than moved back into the blood. These oral drugs include *canagliflozin* (Invokana), *dapagliflozin* (Farxiga), and *empagliflozin* (Jardiance).

! **NURSING SAFETY PRIORITY** QSEN

Drug Alert

The Food and Drug Administration (FDA) has issued a warning that the use of empagliflozin increases the risk for acute kidney injury and impaired renal function (Aschenbrenner, 2017).

Combination Agents. Combination agents combine drugs with different mechanisms of action. For example, Glucovance combines glyburide with metformin. Combining drugs with different mechanisms of action may be highly effective in maintaining desired blood glucose control. Some patients may need a combination of antidiabetic agents and insulin to control blood glucose levels.

Insulin Therapy. Insulin therapy is required for type 1 DM and may be used for type 2 DM. The safety of insulin therapy in older patients may be affected by reduced vision, mobility and coordination problems, and decreased memory. Many types of insulin and regimens are available to achieve normal blood glucose levels. Because insulin is a small protein that is quickly digested and inactivated in the GI tract, it is usually administered as an injection.

Types of Insulin. Insulin is manufactured using DNA technology to produce pure human insulin. Insulin analogs are synthetic human insulins in which the structure of the insulin molecule is altered to change the rate of absorption and duration of action within the body. An example is Lispro insulin, a rapid-acting insulin analog that is created by switching the positions of lysine and proline in one area of the insulin molecule.

Rapid-, short-, intermediate-, and long-acting forms of insulin can be injected separately; and some can be mixed in the same syringe. Insulin is available in concentrations of 100 units/mL (U-100), 200 units/mL (U-200), 300 units/mL (U-300), and 500 units/mL (U-500). Insulin concentrations above 100 units/mL are usually reserved for patients who require large doses of insulin.

Teach the patient that the insulin types, the injection technique, and the site of injection can all affect the absorption, onset, degree, and duration of insulin activity. Reinforce that changing insulins may affect blood glucose control and should be done only under supervision of the primary health care provider. Table 64-8 outlines the timed activity of human insulin.

Insulin Regimens. Insulin regimens try to replicate the normal insulin release pattern from the pancreas. The pancreas produces a constant *(basal)* amount of insulin that balances liver glucose production with glucose use and maintains normal blood glucose levels between meals. The pancreas also produces additional mealtime *(prandial)* insulin to prevent blood glucose elevation after meals. The insulin dose required for blood glucose control varies among patients. A usual starting dose is between 0.5 and 1 unit/kg of body weight per day. For multiple-dose regimens or continuous subcutaneous insulin infusion (CSII), basal insulin makes up about 40% to 50% of the total daily dosage, with the remainder divided into premeal doses of rapid-acting insulin analogs or regular insulin. Basal insulin coverage is provided by intermediate-acting insulin or long-acting insulin analogs such as insulin glargine (Lantus), insulin detemir (Levemir), or insulin degludec (Tresiba). Dosages are adjusted based on the results of blood glucose monitoring.

Single daily injection protocols require insulin injection only once daily. This protocol may include one injection of intermediate- or long-acting insulin or an injection of combination short- and intermediate-acting insulin. Many patients with type 2 diabetes combine once-daily insulin injection with oral agent therapy to stimulate mealtime insulin secretion.

Multiple-component insulin therapy combines short- and intermediate-acting insulin injected twice daily. Two thirds of the daily dose is given before breakfast, and one third before the evening meal. Ratios of intermediate-acting and regular insulin are based on results of blood glucose monitoring.

Intensified regimens include a basal dose of intermediate- or long-acting insulin and a mealtime bolus dose of short- or rapid-acting insulin designed to bring the *next* blood glucose value into the target range. Blood glucose elevations above the target range are treated with "correction" doses of short- or rapid-acting insulin. The patient's blood glucose patterns determine insulin dosage. Frequency of blood glucose monitoring is based on the timed action of insulin and may occur as often as eight times daily. Blood glucose testing 1 to 2 hours after meals and within 10 minutes before the next meal helps determine the adequacy of the previous bolus dose. The patient determines the effects of basal insulin by monitoring blood glucose levels before breakfast (fasting) and before the evening meal.

Patients on intensified insulin regimens need extensive education to achieve target blood glucose values. They need to know how to adjust insulin doses and understand NUTRITION therapy for dietary flexibility and meeting target blood glucose values. Patients must also be able to accurately monitor blood glucose levels so therapy decisions are based on accurate data.

Regardless of the specific insulin regimen, adherence to insulin injection schedules is critical in achieving glycemic control and maintaining A1C levels below the 7% needed to reduce long-term complications. At times, skipping an

TABLE 64-8   Timed Activity of Pharmaceutical Insulin

PREPARATION	BRAND	ONSET (hr)	PEAK (hr)	DURATION (hr)
Rapid-Acting Insulin Analogs				
Insulin aspart injection	NovoLog	0.25	1-3	3-5
Insulin glulisine injection	Apidra	0.3	0.5-1.5	3-4
Human lispro injection	Humalog	0.25	0.5-1.5	5
Human lispro injection U-200	Humalog U-200	0.25	0.5-1.5	5
Insulin human inhalation powder	Afrezza	0.25	1-1.25	2.5
Short-Acting Insulin				
Regular human insulin injection	Humulin R	0.5	2-4	5-7
	Novolin R	0.5	2.5-5	8
	ReliOn R	0.5	2.5-5	8-12
Humulin R (Concentrated U-500)	Humulin R (U-500)	1.5	4-12	24
Intermediate-Acting Insulin				
Isophane insulin NPH injection	Humulin N	1.5	4-12	16-24+
	Novolin N	1-4	4-14	10-24+
	ReliOn N	1-4	4-14	10-24+
70% human insulin isophane suspension/30% human insulin injection	Humulin 70/30 Novolin 70/30 ReliOn 70/30	0.5	2-12	24
70% insulin aspart protamine suspension/30% insulin aspart injection	NovoLog Mix 70/30	0.25	1-4	24
75% insulin lispro protamine suspension/25% insulin lispro injection	Humalog Mix 75/25	0.25	1-2	24
Long-Acting Insulin Analogs				
Insulin glargine injection	Lantus	2-4	None	24
Insulin glargine injection U-300	Toujeo	2-4	12	24
Insulin detemir injection	Levemir	1	6-8	5.7-24
Insulin degludec injection U-100, U-200	Tresiba U-100 Tresiba U-200	1 1	9 9	42 42

occasional insulin dose may be related to an unusual meal pattern for a day or a change in exercise.

Factors Influencing Insulin Absorption. Many factors affect insulin absorption and availability, including injection site; timing, type, or dose of insulin used; and physical activity.

Injection site area affects the speed of insulin absorption. Fig. 64-3 shows common insulin injection areas. Absorption is fastest in the abdomen and, except for a 2-inch radius around the navel, is the preferred injection site. Rotating injection sites allows each injection site to heal completely before the site is used again. Rotation *within* one anatomic site is preferred to rotation from one area to another to prevent day-to-day variability in absorption.

Absorption rate is determined by insulin properties. The longer the duration of action, the more unpredictable is absorption. Larger doses of insulin also prolong the absorption. Factors that increase blood flow from the injection site, such as local application of heat, massage of the area, and exercise of the injected area, increase insulin absorption. Scarred sites often become favorite injection sites because they are less sensitive to pain, but these areas usually slow the rate of insulin absorption.

Injection depth changes insulin absorption. Usually injections are made into the subcutaneous tissue. IM injection has a

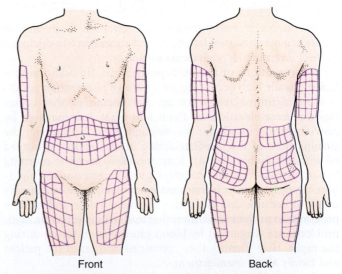

Front   Back

FIG. 64-3 Common insulin injection areas and sites.

faster absorption and is not used for routine insulin use. Most patients lightly grasp a fold of skin and inject at a 90-degree angle; however, a 45-degree angle is advised for frail older adults and those who are cachexic. Aspiration for blood is not needed. Patients with high body mass index (BMI) levels can use 4-mm or 5-mm needles to inject insulin at a 90-degree angle without pinching a skinfold before injection. Assess the older patient's ability to inject insulin and arrange for assistance when self-care is no longer possible.

Timing of injection affects blood glucose levels. The interval between premeal injections and eating, known as *"lag time,"* affects blood glucose levels after meals. Insulin lispro, insulin aspart, and insulin glulisine have rapid onsets of action and are to be given within 10 minutes before mealtime when blood glucose is in the target range. If hyperglycemia or hypoglycemia is not present, these insulins can be given at any time from 10 minutes before mealtime to just before eating or even immediately after eating. Regular insulin is given at least 20 to 30 minutes before eating when glucose levels are within the target range. When blood glucose levels are above the target range, the lag time is increased to permit insulin to begin to have a glucose-lowering effect before food enters the stomach. When blood glucose levels are below the target range, injection of regular insulin should be delayed until immediately before eating, and injection of rapid-acting insulin should be delayed until sometime *after* eating the meal.

Mixing insulins can change the time of peak action. Mixtures of short- and intermediate-acting insulins produce a more normal blood glucose response in some patients than does a single dose. The patient's response to mixed insulin may differ from the response to the same insulins given separately.

> ### ⚠ NURSING SAFETY PRIORITY (QSEN)
> #### Drug Alert
>
> Do not mix any other insulin type with insulin glargine, insulin detemir, or any of the premixed insulin formulations such as Humalog Mix 75/25.

Complications of Insulin Therapy. Hypoglycemia from insulin excess has many causes. Its effects and treatment are discussed in the Preventing Hypoglycemia section.

Two conditions of fasting hyperglycemia (in addition to a lack of insulin) can occur (Fig. 64-4). *Dawn phenomenon* results from a nighttime release of adrenal hormones that causes blood glucose elevations at about 5 to 6 AM. It is managed by providing more insulin for the overnight period (e.g., giving the evening dose of intermediate-acting insulin at 10 PM instead of with the evening meal). *Somogyi phenomenon* is morning hyperglycemia from the counterregulatory response to nighttime hypoglycemia. It is managed by ensuring adequate dietary intake at bedtime and evaluating the insulin dose and exercise programs to prevent conditions that lead to hypoglycemia. Both problems are diagnosed by blood glucose monitoring during the night. Help identify these problems and teach the patient and family about management.

Alternative Methods of Insulin Administration. Many methods of insulin delivery are available in addition to traditional subcutaneous injections.

Continuous subcutaneous infusion of a basal dose of insulin (CSII) with additional insulin at mealtimes is more effective in controlling blood glucose levels than other schedules. It allows

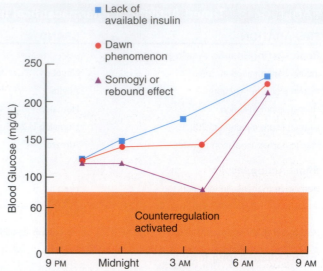

FIG. 64-4 Three blood glucose phenomena in patients with diabetes.

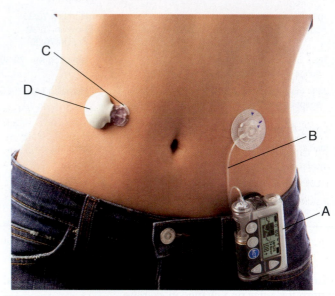

FIG. 64-5 MiniMed Paradigm REAL-Time Insulin Pump and Continuous Glucose Monitoring System. **A,** Pump. **B,** Injection cannula. **C,** Glucose sensor. **D,** Data transmitter. (Courtesy Medtronic Diabetes, Northridge, CA.)

flexibility in meal timing because, if a meal is skipped, the additional mealtime dose of insulin is not given. CSII is given by an externally worn pump containing a reservoir of rapid-acting insulin and is connected to the patient by an infusion set. Teach him or her to adjust the amount of insulin based on data from blood glucose monitoring. Rapid-acting insulin analogs are used with insulin infusion pumps (Fig. 64-5).

Problems with CSII include skin infections that can occur when the infusion site is not cleaned or the infusion set is not changed every 2 to 3 days. Ketoacidosis may occur more often because of inexperience in pump use, infection, accidental cessation or obstruction of the infusion, or mechanical pump problems. Stress the importance of testing for ketones when blood glucose levels are greater than 300 mg/dL (16.7 mmol/L).

Patients using CSII need intensive and extensive education (Lampe, 2015). They must be able to operate the pump, adjust the settings, and respond appropriately to alarms. Removing the pump for any length of time can result in hyperglycemia.

Provide supplemental insulin schedules for times when the pump is not operational.

Injection devices include a needleless system and an insulin pen in addition to traditional insulin syringes. With a needleless device, the needle is replaced by an ultrathin liquid stream of insulin forced through the skin under high pressure. Insulin given by jet injection is absorbed at a faster rate and has a shorter duration of action. Most types of insulin are available in pen devices, which are more convenient for multiple daily injection regimens.

Patient Education: Drugs. Provide specific instructions about insulin therapy, new drug therapies, and self-monitoring of blood glucose levels.

Insulin storage varies by use. Teach patients to refrigerate insulin that is not in use to maintain potency, prevent exposure to sunlight, and inhibit bacterial growth. Insulin in use may be kept at room temperature for up to 28 days to reduce injection site irritation from cold insulin.

To prevent loss of drug potency, teach the patient to avoid exposing insulin to temperatures below 36°F (2.2°C) or above 86 F° (30°C), to avoid excessive shaking, and to protect insulin from direct heat and light. Insulin should not be allowed to freeze. Insulin glargine (Lantus) should be stored in a refrigerator (36° to 46°F [2.2° to 7.8°C]) even when in use. Teach patients to discard any unused insulin after 28 days.

Teach patients to always have a spare supply of each type of insulin used. A slight loss in potency may occur for bottles in use for more than 30 days, even when the expiration date has not passed. Prefilled syringes are stable up to 30 days when refrigerated. Store prefilled syringes in the upright position, with the needle pointing upward or flat, so insulin particles do not clog it. Teach patients to roll prefilled syringes between the hands before using.

Proper dose preparation is critical for insulin effectiveness and patient safety. Teach patients that the person giving the insulin needs to inspect the vial before each use for changes (e.g., clumping, frosting, precipitation, or change in clarity or color) that may indicate loss in potency. Preparations containing NPH insulin are uniformly cloudy after gently rolling the vial between the hands. Other insulins should be clear when inspected in good lighting. If potency is questionable, another vial or pen of the same insulin type should be used.

Syringes may be used to administer insulin. The standard insulin syringes are marked in insulin units. They are available in 1-mL (100-U), ½-mL (50-U), and ³⁄₁₀-mL (30-U) sizes. The unit scale on the barrel of the syringe differs with the syringe size and manufacturer. Insulin syringe needles are measured in 28-, 29-, 30-, and 31-gauge and in lengths of 6 mm, 8 mm, and 12.7 mm. To ensure accurate insulin measurement, instruct the patient to always buy the same type of syringe. Chart 64-3 reviews instructions for drawing up a single insulin injection.

Disposable needles are used only once. Teach the patient to discard the syringe and needle after one use. Information on needle disposal can be obtained at www.safeneedledisposal.org.

Pen-type injectors hold small, lightweight, prefilled insulin cartridges. The injectors are easy to carry and make intensive therapy with multiple injections easier. These devices allow greater accuracy than traditional insulin syringes, especially when measuring small doses. Discuss proper storage for prefilled insulin pens or cartridges. Ensure that the product is appropriate for the patient's unique needs. *Pen-type injectors are not designed for independent use by visually impaired patients or by those with cognitive impairment.* Ensure that the patient has

---

CHART 64-3 Patient and Family Education: Preparing for Self-Management

Subcutaneous Insulin Administration

With Vial and Syringe
- Wash your hands.
- Inspect the bottle for the type of insulin and the expiration date.
- Gently roll the bottle of intermediate-acting insulin in the palms of your hands to mix the insulin.
- Clean the rubber stopper with an alcohol swab.
- Remove the needle cover and pull back the plunger to draw air into the syringe. The amount of air should be equal to the insulin dose. Push the needle through the rubber stopper and inject the air into the insulin bottle.
- Turn the bottle upside down and draw the insulin dose into the syringe.
- Remove air bubbles in the syringe by tapping on the syringe or injecting air back into the bottle. Redraw the correct amount.
- Make certain the tip of the plunger is on the line for your dose of insulin. Magnifiers are available to assist in measuring accurate doses of insulin.
- Remove the needle from the bottle. Recap the needle if the insulin is not to be given immediately.
- Select a site within your injection area that has not been used in the past month.
- Clean your skin with an alcohol swab. Lightly grasp an area of skin and insert the needle at a 90-degree angle.
- Push the plunger all the way down. This will push the insulin into your body. Release the pinched skin.
- Pull the needle straight out quickly. Do not rub the place where you gave the shot.
- Dispose of the syringe and needle without recapping in a puncture-proof container.

With a Pen Device
- Wash your hands.
- Check the drug label to be sure it is what was prescribed.
- Remove the cap.
- Look at the insulin to be sure it is evenly mixed if it contains NPH and that there is no clumping of particles.
- Wipe the tip of the pen where the needle will attach with an alcohol swab.
- Remove the protective pull tab from the needle and screw it onto the pen until snug.
- Remove both the plastic outer cap and inner needle cap.
- Look at the dose window and turn the dosage knob to the appropriate dose.
- Holding the pen with the needle pointing upward, press the button until at least a drop of insulin appears. This is the "cold shot," "air shot," or "safety shot." Repeat this step if needed until a drop appears.
- Dial the number of units needed.
- Hold the pen perpendicular to and against the intended injection site with the thumb on the dosing knob.
- Press the dosing knob slowly all the way to dispense the dose.
- Hold the pen in place for 6-10 seconds; then withdraw from the skin.
- Replace the outer needle cap; unscrew until the needle is removed and dispose of the needle in a hard plastic or metal container.
- Replace the cap on the insulin pen.

---

received education on its use. Each syringe or cartridge has specific requirements. **The Institute for Safe Medication Practices (ISMP) and The Joint Commission's National Patient Safety Goals identify insulin as a *High-Alert* drug. (High-Alert drugs are those that have an increased risk for causing patient harm if given in error.) The ISMP cautions that digital displays on some of the newer insulin pens can be misread. If the pen is held upside down, as a left-handed person might do, a**

dose of 52 units actually appears to be a dose of 25 units, and a dose of 12 units looks like a dose of 21 units.

Patient Education: Blood Glucose Monitoring. Self-monitoring of blood glucose (SMBG) levels provides information to assess effectiveness of the management plan and assists the patient in self-care decisions. Results of SMBG are useful in preventing hypoglycemia and hyperglycemia by adjusting drug therapy, diet therapy, and physical activity (Greenwood, 2015). Assessment of blood glucose levels is very important for these situations:

- Symptoms of hypoglycemia/hyperglycemia
- Hypoglycemic unawareness
- Periods of illness
- Before and after exercise
- Gastroparesis
- Adjustment of antidiabetes drugs
- Evaluation of other drug therapies (e.g., steroids)
- Preconception planning
- Pregnancy

Techniques for SMBG follow principles that are the same for most self-monitoring systems. Meter systems now require a very small blood sample, which allows for alternate testing sites (e.g., arm, thigh, hand). The finger or alternate site is pricked, a drop of blood flows over or is drawn into a testing strip or disc impregnated with chemicals, and the glucose value is displayed in mg/dL or mmol/L on a screen. For vision-impaired patients, "talking-meters" are available to allow independence in blood glucose monitoring.

Data obtained from SMBG are evaluated along with other measures of blood glucose (e.g., glycosylated hemoglobin [A1C] values) or periodic laboratory blood glucose tests. Even when SMBG is performed correctly, the results are affected by hematocrit values (anemia falsely elevates glucose values; polycythemia falsely depresses them) and may be unreliable in the hypoglycemic or severe hyperglycemic ranges.

Accuracy of the blood glucose monitor is ensured when the manufacturer's directions are followed. The most common source of error is related to the skill of the user and not to errors of the instrument. Common errors involve failure to obtain a sufficient blood drop, poor storage of test strips, using expired strips, and not changing the code number on the meter to match the strip bottle code. Help the patient select a meter based on cost of the meter and strips, ease of use, and availability of repair and servicing. Provide training, explain and demonstrate procedures, assess visual acuity, and check the patient's ability to perform the procedure using "teach-back" strategies. Glucose meters are designed to reduce user error as much as possible. Newer meters have fewer steps, include error signals for inadequate sample size, and can store hundreds of SMBG results. (See the Consumer Guide published yearly in the January edition of Diabetes Forecast [forecast.diabetes.org] for information to help patients determine which blood glucose meter best meets their needs.)

Accuracy and precision vary widely among capillary blood glucose monitoring devices. If the meter requires calibration, teach patients to properly calibrate the machine. Instruct them to recheck the calibration and retest if they obtain a test result that is unusual for them and whenever they are in doubt about test accuracy. Continued retraining of patients performing SMBG helps ensure accurate results because performance accuracy deteriorates over time. Laboratory glucose determinations are more accurate than SMBG.

Frequency of testing varies with the drug schedules, the patient's prescribed therapy, and his or her target outcomes. The ADA recommends that patients taking multiple insulin injections or using insulin pump therapy monitor glucose levels three or more times daily. For patients taking less-frequent injections of insulin, noninsulin therapy, or diet therapy alone, SMBG is useful for evaluation of therapy.

Blood glucose therapy target goals are set individually for each patient based on duration of disease, age and life expectancy, comorbid conditions, severity of cardiovascular disease, and presence of hypoglycemia unawareness. The health care team works with him or her to reach target blood glucose levels. The ADA recommends that patients with type 1 DM aim for A1C values less than 7%, premeal glucose levels of 70 to 130 mg/dL (3.9 to 7.2 mmol/L), and postmeal glucose levels less than 180 mg/dL (10.0 mmol/L) (ADA, 2017d).

Infection control measures are needed for SMBG. The chance of becoming infected from blood glucose monitoring processes is reduced by handwashing before monitoring and by not reusing lancets. *Instruct patients to not share their blood glucose monitoring equipment.* The hepatitis B virus can survive in a dried state for at least 1 week. Infection can be spread by the lancet holder even when the lancet itself has been changed. Small particles of blood can stick to the device and infect multiple users. Regular cleaning of the meter is critical for infection control. Remind health care staff who perform blood glucose testing and family members who help with testing to wear gloves.

Many meters allow data to be downloaded to a computer that has diabetes management software. Some meters allow entry of additional data such as insulin dose, amounts of carbohydrate eaten, or exercise. A radio link to an insulin pump allows automatic transfer of glucose readings to a calculator that helps the patient decide on an appropriate insulin dose. Some patients use smart phone applications to record and trend or graph serial blood glucose levels, insulin dosages, food intake, and other data. This information can be sent to the primary health care provider electronically or downloaded and printed.

Once the patient learns the technical aspects of meter use, help him or her use the results of SMBG to achieve glycemic control. Postmeal glucose monitoring provides information about the effects of the size and content of their meals. SMBG allows the patient to assess effects of exercise on glucose control and provides critical information to help patients who take insulin to exercise safely. Teach patients how to use SMBG results to adjust the treatment plan. Patients should make agreed-on adjustments in the treatment plan when results are consistently out of range for a 3-day period when no change in meal plan, drugs, or activity has occurred.

Alternate site testing uses blood obtained from sites other than the fingertip and is available on many meters. However, use caution when interpreting results obtained from alternate sites. Studies have shown wide variation between fingertip and alternate sites, and variation is most evident during times when glucose levels change rapidly. Teach patients about the lag time for blood glucose levels between the fingertip and other sites when blood glucose levels are changing rapidly and that the fingertip reading is the only safe choice at those times.

Continuous blood glucose monitoring (CGM) systems monitor glucose levels in interstitial fluid to provide real-time glucose information to the user. The system consists of three parts: a

Action Alert

Teach patients with a history of hypoglycemic unawareness **not** to test at alternative sites.

disposable sensor that measures glucose levels, a transmitter that is attached to the sensor, and a receiver that displays and stores glucose information. After an initiation or warm-up period, the sensor gives glucose values every 1 to 5 minutes. Sensors may be used for 3 to 7 days, depending on the manufacturer. CGM provides information about the current blood glucose level, short-term feedback about results of treatment, and warnings when glucose readings become dangerously high or low. Most available sensors require at least two capillary glucose readings per day for calibration of the sensor. Sensor accuracy depends on these calibrations. There may be a lag time between the capillary glucose measurement and the glucose sensor value. If the blood glucose value is changing rapidly, the time between capillary and interstitial glucose values may be as long as 30 minutes. For this reason, capillary glucose readings need to be checked on all extreme values or if symptoms of hypoglycemia are present before any corrective treatment is given. *Continuous glucose monitoring is meant to supplement, not replace, fingerstick tests. Give insulin only after confirming the results of any continuous glucose monitoring system.*

? NCLEX EXAMINATION CHALLENGE 64-4

Health Promotion and Maintenance

Which client does the nurse caution to **avoid** self-monitoring of blood glucose (SMBG) at alternate sites?
A. 75-year-old client whose blood glucose levels show little variation
B. 55-year-old client who has hypoglycemic unawareness
C. 80-year-old client with type 2 diabetes mellitus
D. 45-year-old client with type 1 diabetes mellitus

Nutrition Therapy. Effective self-management of DM requires that NUTRITION, including the meal plan, education, and counseling programs, be individualized for each patient. A registered dietitian (RD) is a member of the interprofessional team. The nurse, RD, patient, and family work together on all aspects of the meal plan, which must be realistic and as flexible as possible. Plans that consider the patient's cultural background, financial status, and lifestyle are more likely to be successful. The desired outcomes of NUTRITION and diet therapy are listed in Table 64-9.

Principles of Medical Nutrition Therapy in Diabetes. Medical Nutrition Management (MNT) is recommended for all adults with DM. For overweight or obese adults with Type 2 DM, even modest weight loss through reduced caloric intake is beneficial. Blood pressure, blood glucose levels, and lipid profiles are improved by weight loss (ADA, 2017c).

The dietitian develops a meal plan based on the patient's usual food intake, weight-management expectations, and lipid and blood glucose patterns. Consistency in the daily timing and amount of food eaten helps control blood glucose. Patients using insulin therapy need to eat at times that are coordinated with the timed action of insulin. Teach patients using intense

TABLE 64-9 Desired Outcomes of Nutrition Therapy for the Patient With Diabetes

- Achieving and maintaining blood glucose levels in the normal range or as close to normal as is safely possible
- Achieving and maintaining a blood lipid profile that reduces the risk for vascular disease
- Achieving blood pressure levels in the normal range or as close to normal as is safely possible
- Preventing or slowing the rate of development of the chronic complications of diabetes by modifying nutrient intake and lifestyle
- Addressing patient NUTRITION needs, taking into account personal and cultural preferences and willingness to change
- Maintaining the pleasure of eating by limiting food choices only when indicated by scientific evidence
- Meeting the NUTRITION needs of unique times of the life cycle, particularly for pregnant and lactating women and for older adults with diabetes
- Providing self-management training for patients treated with insulin or insulin stimulators (secretagogues) for exercising safely, including the prevention and treatment of hypoglycemia and managing diabetes during acute illness

insulin therapy to adjust premeal insulin to allow for timing and quantity changes in their meal plan.

Current evidence indicates that no specific percentage of calories from carbohydrates, protein, or fat is ideal for all adults with DM. Recommendations for the distribution of these macronutrients is individualized based on food preferences, eating patterns, and metabolic goals (ADA, 2017c; Nwankwo & Funnell, 2016; Watts & Howard, 2016).

Carbohydrate intake avoids nutrient deficient sources ("empty calories") and focuses on sources from vegetables, fruits, whole grains, legumes, and dairy products. Adults with diabetes are recommended to consume at least 25 g of fiber daily. Teach those who are at risk for or who have DM to avoid sugar-sweetened beverages (including high fructose corn syrup) and sucrose to prevent weight gain and adverse effects on metabolism (ADA, 2017c; ADA, 2017j).

Dietary fat and cholesterol intake for adults with DM focuses on the quality of fat rather than on the quantity of fat. A Mediterranean-style diet rich in monounsaturated fatty acids (MUFAs) often is beneficial to lower cardiometabolic risk factors. MUFA diets include avocados, nuts and seeds, olives, and dark chocolate. Omega-3 fatty acids, including EPA (eicosapentaenoic acid) and DHA (docosahexaenoic acid) from fish or fish oil supplements are recommended as part of a healthy diet to prevent heart disease, as is ALA (alpha linolenic acid) derived from plant sources. Current recommendations from the ADA to limit trans fats, saturated fats, and cholesterol are the same as for the general population (ADA, 2017a; ADA 2017c).

Alcohol consumption affects blood glucose levels. Levels are not affected by *moderate* use of alcohol when DM is well controlled. Teach patients that two alcoholic beverages for men and one for women can be ingested with, and in addition to, the usual meal plan. (One alcoholic beverage equals 12 ounces of beer, 5 ounces of wine, or 1½ ounces of distilled spirits.) When alcohol is consumed by adults taking insulin or an insulin secretagogue, the risk for delayed hypoglycemia is increased.

Patient Education: Prescribed Nutrition Plan. No one meal plan is right for all patients with DM. Each patient's NUTRITION recommendations are based on blood glucose monitoring results, total blood lipid levels, and A1C levels. These tests help

NURSING SAFETY PRIORITY QSEN

Action Alert

Because of the potential for alcohol-induced delayed hypoglycemia, instruct the patient with DM to ingest alcohol only with or shortly after meals.

determine whether current meal and exercise patterns need adjustment or whether present habits need reinforcement. A specific nutritional prescription is developed for each patient.

Reinforce NUTRITION information provided by the dietitian. The patient with DM must understand how to adjust food intake during illness, planned exercise, and social occasions and when the usual time of eating is delayed. He or she may be unable to follow the prescribed plan because of an inability to read or understand printed materials. Share dietary information with the person who prepares the meals. The dietitian sees each patient yearly to identify changes in lifestyle and make appropriate diet therapy changes. Some patients, such as those with weight-control problems or low incomes, may need more frequent dietary evaluation and counseling.

Meal Planning Strategies. Many meal planning approaches for good NUTRITION are available. Each approach emphasizes different aspects of nutrition.

Carbohydrate (CHO) counting is a simple approach to NUTRITION and meal planning that uses label information of the nutritional content of packaged food items. Because fat and protein have little effect on after-meal blood glucose levels, CHO counting focuses on the nutrient that has the greatest impact on these levels. It uses total grams of CHO, regardless of the food source. This method is effective in achieving blood glucose control when daily CHO intake is consistent.

Patients using intensive insulin or pump therapies can use CHO counting to determine insulin coverage. After the amount of insulin needed to cover the usual meal is determined, insulin may be added or subtracted for changes in CHO intake. An initial formula of 1 unit of rapid-acting insulin for each 15 g of CHO provides flexibility to meal plans. The patient determines the grams of CHO in a specific meal or snack by reading labels or weighing and measuring each item. The total grams of CHO are used to calculate the bolus dose of insulin based on the prescribed insulin-to-carbohydrate ratio.

Special considerations for type 1 diabetes include developing insulin regimens that conform to the patient's preferred meal routines, food preferences, and exercise patterns. Patients using rapid-acting insulin by injection or an insulin pump should adjust insulin doses based on the CHO content of the meals and snacks. Insulin-to-carbohydrate ratios are developed and are used to provide mealtime insulin doses. Blood glucose monitoring before and 2 hours after meals determines whether the insulin-to-carbohydrate ratio is correct. For patients who are on fixed insulin regimens and do not adjust premeal insulin dosages, consistency of timing of meals and the amount of CHO eaten at each meal is important to prevent hypoglycemia.

Exercise can cause hypoglycemia if insulin is not decreased before activity. For planned exercise, reduction in insulin dosage is used for hypoglycemia prevention. For unplanned exercise, intake of additional CHO is usually needed. Moderate exercise increases glucose utilization by 2 to 3 mg/kg/min. A 70-kg adult would need about 10 to 15 g additional CHO per hour of moderate-intensity activity. More CHO is needed for intense activity.

It is important for patients using insulin to avoid weight gain. **Hyperinsulinemia** (chronic high blood insulin levels) can occur with intensive management schedules and may result in weight gain. These patients may need to manage hyperglycemia by restricting calories rather than increasing insulin. Weight gain can be minimized by following the prescribed meal plan, getting regular exercise, and avoiding overtreatment of hypoglycemia.

Special considerations for type 2 DM focus on lifestyle changes. Many patients with type 2 DM are overweight and insulin resistant. NUTRITION therapy stresses lifestyle changes that reduce calories eaten and increase calories expended through physical activity. Many patients also have abnormal blood fat levels and hypertension (metabolic syndrome), making reductions of saturated fat, cholesterol, and sodium desirable. A moderate caloric restriction (250 to 500 calories less daily) and an increase in physical activity improve GLUCOSE REGULATION and weight control. Decreases of more than 10% of body weight can significantly improve A1C.

When patients with type 2 DM need insulin, consistency in timing and CHO content of meals is important. Division of the total daily calories into three meals or into smaller meals and snacks is based on patient preference.

CONSIDERATIONS FOR OLDER ADULTS

Patient-Centered Care QSEN

Older patients are at increased risk for poor NUTRITION, reduced awareness of either hypoglycemia and hyperglycemia, and dehydration, a factor in the development of hyperglycemic-hyperosmolar state (HHS) (Touhy & Jett, 2016). Nutrition needs of the older adult change as his or her taste, smell, and appetite diminish and the ability to obtain and prepare food decreases. Older patients who prepare their own food or have dental issues may not eat enough food. Neuropathy with gastric retention or diarrhea compounds poor food intake. Impaired cognition may disrupt self-care. Older patients may have a marginal food supply because of low income, may have poor understanding of meal-planning needs, or may live alone and not care to prepare or eat proper meals. They may eat in restaurants or live in situations in which they have little control over meal preparation. Visits by home health nurses can help older patients follow a diabetic meal plan.

A realistic approach to NUTRITION therapy is essential for the older patient with DM. Changing the eating habits of 60 to 70 years is very difficult. The nurse, dietitian, and patient assess the patient's usual eating patterns. Teach the older patient taking antidiabetic drugs the importance of eating meals and snacks at the same time every day, eating the same amount of food from day to day, and eating all food allowed on the diet.

Exercise Therapy. Regular exercise is an essential part of DM management. It has beneficial effects on carbohydrate metabolism and insulin sensitivity. Programs of increased physical activity and weight loss reduce the risk for type 2 DM in patients with impaired glucose tolerance (AADE, 2015).

Plasma glucose levels remain stable in physically active patients without diabetes because of the balance between glucose use by exercising muscles and glucose production by the liver. The patient with type 1 DM cannot make the hormonal changes needed to maintain stable blood glucose levels during exercise. Without an adequate insulin supply, cells cannot use glucose. Low insulin levels trigger release of glucagon and epinephrine (counterregulatory hormones) to increase liver glucose production, further raising blood glucose levels. In the absence of insulin, free fatty acids become the source of energy. Exercise in the patient with uncontrolled DM results in further hyperglycemia and the formation of ketone bodies. He or she may have prolonged elevated blood glucose levels after vigorous exercise.

Exercise in the adult with DM can cause hypoglycemia because of increased muscle glucose uptake and inhibited glucose release from the liver. It can occur during exercise and for up to 24 hours after exercise. Replacement of muscle and liver glycogen stores, along with increased insulin sensitivity after exercise, causes insulin requirements to drop.

Benefits of Exercise. Appropriate exercise results in better blood GLUCOSE REGULATION and reduced insulin requirements for patients with type 1 DM. Exercise also increases insulin sensitivity, which enhances cell uptake of glucose and promotes weight loss.

Regular exercise decreases risk for cardiovascular disease. It decreases most blood lipid levels and increases high-density lipoproteins (HDLs, the "good" cholesterol). Exercise decreases blood pressure and improves cardiovascular function. Regular vigorous physical activity prevents or delays type 2 DM by reducing body weight, insulin resistance, and glucose intolerance.

Adjustments for Diabetes Complications. Exercise in the presence of long-term DM complications may require adjustment. Vigorous aerobic or resistance exercise should be avoided in the presence of proliferative diabetic retinopathy or severe nonproliferative diabetic retinopathy. Teach the patient with retinopathy to avoid the *Valsalva maneuver* (breath holding while bearing down) and activities that increase blood pressure. Heavy lifting, rapid head motion, or jarring activities can cause vitreous hemorrhage or retinal detachment. Decreased pain sensation in the extremities increases the risk for skin breakdown and joint damage. Teach patients with peripheral neuropathy to wear proper footwear and examine their feet daily for lesions or injury. Teach anyone with a foot injury or open sore to engage in non–weight-bearing activities such as swimming, bicycling, or arm exercises. Those with autonomic neuropathy are at increased risk for exercise-induced injury from impaired temperature control, postural hypotension, and impaired thirst with risk for dehydration. Physical activity also can increase urine protein excretion. Encourage high-risk patients to start with short periods of low-intensity exercise and increase the intensity and duration slowly.

Safety Assessment. Although current ADA guidelines do not recommend routine screening for patients with DM who have no indications of cardiovascular disease, conditions that might predispose to injury or that contraindicate certain types of exercise include:

- Uncontrolled hypertension
- Severe autonomic neuropathy
- Severe peripheral neuropathy or foot lesions
- Unstable proliferative retinopathy

Advise adults with DM to perform at least 150 min/week of moderate-intensive (50% to 70% maximum heart rate) aerobic physical activity divided into 3 days, or 75 min/week of vigorous aerobic physical activity, or an equivalent combination of the two. Teach patients to avoid going more than 2 consecutive days without aerobic physical activity. In the absence of contraindications, patients with type 2 DM are urged to perform resistance exercise at least twice weekly, targeting all major muscle groups.

A 5- to 10-minute warm-up period with stretching and low-intensity exercise before exercise prepares the muscles, heart, and lungs for a progressive increase in exercise intensity. After

---

CHART 64-4 Patient and Family Education: Preparing for Self-Management

Exercise

- Teach the patient about the relationship between regularly scheduled exercise and blood glucose levels, blood lipid levels, and complications of diabetes.
- Reinforce the level of exercise recommended for the patient based on his or her physical health.
- Instruct the patient to wear appropriate footwear designed for exercise.
- Remind the patient to examine his or her feet daily and after exercising.
- Remind the patient to stay hydrated and not to exercise in extreme heat or cold.
- Warn the patient not to exercise within 1 hour of insulin injection or near the time of peak insulin action.
- Teach patients how to prevent hypoglycemia during exercise:
  - Do not exercise unless blood glucose level is at least 80 and less than 250 mg/dL.
  - Have a carbohydrate snack before exercising if 1 hour has passed since the last meal or if the planned exercise is high intensity.
  - Carry a simple sugar to eat during exercise if symptoms of hypoglycemia occur.
  - Ensure that identification information about diabetes is carried during exercise.
- Remind the patient to check blood glucose levels more frequently on days in which exercise is performed and that extra carbohydrate and less insulin may be needed during the 24-hour period after extensive exercise.

---

exercising, a cool-down of at least 5 to 10 minutes is performed to gradually bring the heart rate down to pre-exercise level.

Guidelines for exercise are based on blood glucose levels and urine ketone levels. Recommend that the patient test blood glucose before exercise, at intervals during exercise, and after exercise to determine if it is safe to exercise and to evaluate the effects of exercise. The absence of urine ketones indicates that enough insulin is available for glucose transport. *When urine ketones are present, the patient should not exercise.* Ketones indicate that current insulin levels are not adequate and that exercise would elevate blood glucose levels. Carbohydrate foods should be ingested to raise blood glucose levels above 100 mg/dL (5.6 mmol/L) before engaging in exercise. Chart 64-4 lists tips to teach the patient and family about exercise.

! NURSING SAFETY PRIORITY QSEN

Action Alert

Teach patients with type 1 DM to perform vigorous exercise only when blood glucose levels are 100 to 250 mg/dL (5.6 to 13.8 mmol/L) and no ketones are present in the urine.

Blood Glucose Control in Hospitalized Patients. Hyperglycemia in hospitalized patients occurs for many reasons and is associated with poor outcomes. It may result from decline in basic level of GLUCOSE REGULATION and control caused by illness, decreased physical activity, withholding of antidiabetic drugs, use of drugs that cause hyperglycemia such as corticosteroids, and initiation of tube feedings or parenteral NUTRITION.

Hyperglycemia among medical-surgical patients is linked to reduced IMMUNITY, higher infection rates, longer hospital stays, increased need for intensive care, and greater mortality. Admission glucose levels greater than 198 mg/dL (10.9 mmol/L)

CONSIDERATIONS FOR OLDER ADULTS

Evidence-Based Practice QSEN

With age, the ability of the heart and lungs to deliver oxygen to tissues and organs declines. Muscle strength and power decline gradually. Connective tissue becomes less elastic, affecting range of motion and flexibility. Limited range of motion can alter gait, increasing risk for falls. Older adults who remain active can limit losses in muscle mass and function.

Emphasize that the focus for any activity program is on changing sedentary behavior to active behavior at any level. Encourage sedentary older adults to begin with low-intensity physical activity. Start low-intensity activities in short sessions (less than 10 minutes); include warm-up and cool-down components with active stretching. Changes in activity levels should be gradual. Formal evaluation by a physical therapist or occupational therapist may be needed. Examples of specific exercise can be found at www.geri.com.

CLINICAL JUDGMENT CHALLENGE 64-1

Patient-Centered Care; Teamwork and Collaboration; Evidence-Based Practice QSEN

A 33-year-old woman has just returned from a 5-year mission trip to a less affluent country and is having a complete check-up. She is 25 lb (11.3 kg) overweight and had an 11 lb (5 kg) baby 2 years ago while on the mission trip. Her fasting blood glucose level is 119 mg/dL (6.5 mmol/L), and her A1C is 5.8. She reports that her mother, sister, and maternal grandmother all have type 2 DM. She asks what she can do about this possible health problem.

1. Does she have diabetes? Provide a rationale for your response.
2. What risk factors does she have for type 2 DM?
3. What additional assessment information should you obtain?
4. In addition to yourself and the primary health care provider, what other interprofessional health team members would be appropriate to consult at this time?
5. What lifestyle recommendations are appropriate for this patient?

are associated with greater risk for mortality and complications. Hypoglycemia, defined as blood glucose values lower than 40 mg/dL (2.2 mmol/L), is an independent risk factor for mortality.

Current American Association of Clinical Endocrinologists (AACE) and ADA guidelines recommend treatment protocols that maintain blood glucose levels between 140 and 180 mg/dL (7.8 and 10.0 mmol/L) for critically ill patients. For the majority of non–critically ill patients, premeal glucose targets should be lower than 140 mg/dL (7.8 mmol/L), with random blood glucose values less than 180 mg/dL (10.0 mmol/L). To prevent hypoglycemia, insulin regimens should be reviewed if blood glucose levels fall below 100 mg/dL (5.6 mmol/L) and should be modified when blood glucose levels are less than 70 mg/dL (3.9 mmol/L) (ADA, 2017d).

Continuous IV insulin solutions are the most effective method for achieving glycemic targets in the intensive care setting. Scheduled subcutaneous injection with basal, meal, and correction elements is the preferred method for achieving and maintaining glucose control in non–critically ill patients. Using correction dose or "supplemental insulin" to correct premeal hyperglycemia in addition to scheduled prandial and basal insulin is recommended. The correction dose is determined by the patient's insulin sensitivity and current blood glucose level.

Prevention of hypoglycemia is also part of managing blood glucose levels. Causes of inpatient hypoglycemia include an inappropriate insulin type, mismatch between insulin type and/or timing of food intake, and altered eating plan without insulin dosage adjustment. Many facilities have protocols for hypoglycemia treatment that direct staff to provide carbohydrate replacement if the patient is alert and able to swallow or to administer 50% dextrose IV or glucagon by subcutaneous injection if the patient cannot swallow.

There is confusion about whether to give or to hold insulin from a patient who is NPO. Administration of rapid-acting or short-acting insulin, as well as amylin and incretin mimetics, will cause hypoglycemia if a patient is not eating. Basal insulin should be administered when the patient is NPO because it controls baseline glucose levels. Insulin mixtures are not administered because they contain some short-acting or rapid-acting insulin and will cause hypoglycemia.

Surgical Management. Surgical interventions for DM include a pancreas transplantation or islet cell transplantation. When successful, these procedures eliminate the need for insulin injections, blood glucose monitoring, and many dietary restrictions. They can eliminate the acute complications related to blood GLUCOSE REGULATION but are only partially successful in reversing long-term complications. Pancreatic transplant is successful when the patient no longer needs insulin therapy and all blood measures of glucose are normal.

Transplantation requires lifelong drug therapy to prevent graft rejection. These drug regimens have toxic side effects that restrict their use to patients who have serious progressive complications from DM. Some antirejection drugs increase blood glucose levels. A pancreas-alone transplant is most often considered for patients with severe metabolic complications and for those with consistent failure of insulin-based therapy to prevent acute complications.

Pancreas transplantation is considered in patients with DM and end-stage kidney disease (ESKD) who have had or plan to have a kidney transplant. Normal blood glucose levels after pancreas transplantation improve kidney graft survival. Pancreas graft survival is better when performed at the time of the kidney transplant.

Whole-Pancreas Transplantation. The 1-year survival rate for patients in North America is above 95%, with more than 83% of patients remaining free of insulin injection and diet restrictions after 1 year (Kidney Foundation of Canada, 2015; U.S. Department of Health and Human Services [USDHHS], 2015). The degree of HLA tissue-type matching affects the results.

Pancreatic transplantation is performed in one of three ways: pancreas transplant alone (PTA), pancreas after kidney transplant (PAK), and simultaneous pancreas and kidney transplant (SPK). SPK is the ideal procedure for patients with DM and uremia.

Operative Procedure. Most pancreatic transplants are from cadaver donors using a total pancreas still attached to the exit of the pancreatic duct. The recipient's pancreas is left in place, and the donated pancreas is placed in the pelvis. The insulin released by the pancreas graft is secreted into the bloodstream. The new pancreas also produces about 800 to 1000 mL of fluid daily, which is diverted to either the bladder or the bowel.

Excretion of pancreatic fluids can impair FLUID AND ELECTROLYTE BALANCE, and drainage of these fluids into the urinary bladder causes irritation. When the pancreas is attached to the bladder, the loss of fluid rich in bicarbonate may cause acidosis.

Rejection Management. A combination of drugs is used to reverse rejection. (See Chapter 17 for a listing of agents used to prevent or manage transplant rejection.) Patients undergoing antirejection therapy first receive drugs to prevent viral, bacterial, and fungal infection because of the risk for opportunistic infections from overall reduced IMMUNITY. Most patients receiving high-dose steroids, as well as those on chronic long-term steroid therapy, will require dosage adjustments in insulin to achieve desired levels of glucose control.

In most episodes of rejections, kidney problems occur before pancreatic problems. An increase in serum creatinine indicates rejection of both the transplanted kidney and the pancreas. In patients with bladder drainage of pancreatic hormones, a decrease in the urine amylase level by 25% is an indication to treat rejection. High blood glucose levels are a later marker of rejection and usually indicate irreversible graft failure.

Long-Term Effects. Long-term antirejection therapy reduces IMMUNITY even further and increases the risk for infection, cancer, and atherosclerosis. When insulin drains into systemic rather than portal (liver) circulation, blood insulin levels rise (hyperinsulinemia) and increase the risk for hypertension and macrovascular disease.

Complications. Complications are common in patients taking long-term antirejection therapy. Monitor laboratory values, FLUID AND ELECTROLYTE BALANCE, physical changes, and changes in vital signs to identify possible complications. Early removal of IV and intra-arterial lines, use of sterile technique with dressing changes and catheter irrigations, strict handwashing by all personnel, and good pulmonary hygiene help prevent infection.

Immediate complications include thrombosis, pancreatitis, anastomosis leak with infection, and rejection of the transplanted pancreas. Pancreatic blood vessel thrombosis occurs in about 30% of patients after transplantation. Observe for and report any sudden drop in urine amylase levels, rapid increases in blood glucose, gross **hematuria** (bloody urine), and tenderness or pain in the graft area. Pancreatitis in the transplanted organ occurs to some degree in all patients after surgery. Report elevations in serum amylase that persist after 48 to 96 hours.

The most serious complication of enteric-drained pancreas transplantation is leaking and intra-abdominal abscess. Observe for and report temperature elevation, abdominal discomfort, and elevation in white blood cell (WBC) count. Drainage of bicarbonate-rich fluid with pancreatic enzymes into the urinary bladder can cause urinary tract infections, cystitis, urethritis, and balanitis rather than intra-abdominal abscess. Metabolic acidosis occurs from the loss of large amounts of alkaline pancreatic secretions.

Assess for and document indications of rejection. In acute rejection, decreased kidney function is indicated by increased serum creatinine, decreased urine output, hypertension, weight gain, graft tenderness, and fever. Proteinuria is the first indicator of chronic graft rejection. Check for increased blood amylase, lipase, or glucose; decreased urine amylase; graft tenderness; hyperglycemia; and fever. *It is especially important to assess for infection and start appropriate therapy. Fever can indicate both infection and rejection.*

Monitor for side effects of the antirejection drugs. Cyclosporine (Neoral) is toxic to the kidney. Signs of toxicity are elevated creatinine and decreased urine output. Monitor WBC counts daily because azathioprine (Imuran) can suppress bone marrow function. Common side effects of tacrolimus (Prograf) are hypertension, kidney toxicity, neurotoxicity, GI toxicity, and

glucose intolerance. Prednisone has many side effects, including elevated blood glucose levels.

Islet Cell Transplantation. Islet cell transplantation has had limited success. Wider use of this procedure is hindered by the limited supply of beta cells available for transplantation and by issues related to rejection. Islet cells from tissue-typed (HLA-matched) cadaver pancreas glands are injected into the portal vein. The new cells lodge in the liver and begin to function, secreting insulin and maintaining near-perfect blood GLUCOSE REGULATION.

Currently most patients undergoing this procedure eventually have a progressive loss of islet cell function over time. Very few islet cell transplant recipients have remained insulin free for more than 4 years. The reasons for this gradual loss of function are not known and make this procedure a long-term but temporary intervention.

Enhancing Surgical Recovery

Planning: Expected Outcomes. The patient with DM undergoing a surgical procedure is expected to recover completely without complications. Indicators include:

- Wound healing
- Absence of infection
- Maintenance of blood glucose levels within expected range

Interventions. Surgery is a physical and emotional stressor, and the patient with DM is at higher risk for complications. Anesthesia and surgery cause a stress response with release of counterregulatory hormones that elevate blood glucose. Stress hormones suppress insulin action, increasing the risk for ketoacidosis acidosis. Hyperglycemic-hyperosmolar state (HHS) is a serious complication after surgery and is associated with increased mortality. Diuresis from hyperglycemia can cause dehydration and increases the risk for acute kidney injury.

Complications of DM increase the risk for surgical problems. Patients with DM are at higher risk for hypertension, ischemic heart disease, cerebrovascular disease, myocardial infarction (MI), and cardiomyopathy. Heart failure is a serious risk factor and must be optimized before surgery. Autonomic neuropathy may result in sudden tachycardia, bradycardia, or postural hypotension. The patient with DM is at risk for acute kidney injury and urinary retention after surgery, especially if he or she has albumin in the urine (indicator of kidney damage). Nerves to the intestinal wall and sphincters can be impaired, leading to delayed gastric emptying and reflux of gastric acid, which increases the risk for aspiration with anesthesia. Autonomic neuropathy may cause paralytic ileus after surgery.

Preoperative Care. Before surgery, blood glucose levels are optimized to reduce the risk for complications. Sulfonylureas are discontinued 1 day before surgery. Metformin is stopped at least 24 hours before surgery and restarted only after kidney function is documented as normal. All other oral drugs are stopped the day of surgery. Patients taking long-acting insulin may need to be switched to intermediate-acting insulin forms 1 to 2 days before surgery.

Preoperative blood glucose levels should be less than 200 mg/dL (11.1 mmol/L). Higher levels are associated with increased infection rates and impaired wound healing.

Plan ahead for pain control after surgery. Pain, a stressor, triggers the release of counterregulatory hormones, increasing blood glucose levels and insulin needs. Opioid analgesics slow GI motility and alter blood glucose levels. The older patient who receives opioids is more at risk for confusion, paralytic ileus, hypoventilation, hypotension, and urinary retention. Patient-controlled analgesia (PCA) systems reduce respiratory complications and confusion. (See Chapter 3 for pain interventions and Chapter 14 for general preoperative care.)

Intraoperative Care. IV infusion of insulin, glucose, and potassium is standard therapy for perioperative management of DM. The object is to keep the glucose level between 140 and 180 mg/dL (7.8 and 10.0 mmol/L) during surgery to prevent hypoglycemia and reduce risks from hyperglycemia. Insulin/glucose infusion rates are based on hourly capillary glucose tests. Higher insulin doses may be needed because stress releases glucagon and epinephrine. Patients with DM usually receive about 5 g of glucose per hour during surgery to prevent hypoglycemia, ketosis, and protein breakdown.

Monitor the patient's temperature—it may be lowered deliberately in some surgical procedures and inadvertently in others. Low operating room temperatures and large incisions also lower body temperature. Hypothermia decreases metabolic needs, depresses heart rate and contractility, causes vasoconstriction, and impairs insulin release, resulting in high blood glucose levels. Monitor arterial blood gas values for acidosis.

Postoperative Care. Hyperglycemia leads to increased mortality after surgical procedures. AACE and ADA guidelines recommend insulin dosing to maintain blood glucose between 140 and 180 mg/dL (7.8 and 10.0 mmol/L) for critically ill patients (ADA, 2017d).

Protocols and computer-based programs can be used to determine the insulin infusion rate required to maintain blood glucose levels within a defined target range. Many insulin infusion algorithms are implemented by nursing staff. Continue glucose and insulin infusions as prescribed until the patient is stable and can tolerate oral feedings. Short-term insulin therapy may be needed after surgery for the patient who usually uses oral agents. For those receiving insulin therapy, dosage adjustments may be required until the stress of surgery subsides.

Monitoring. Patients with autonomic neuropathy or vascular disease need close monitoring to avoid hypotension or respiratory arrest. Those who take beta blockers for hypertension need close monitoring for hypoglycemia because these drugs mask symptoms of hypoglycemia. Patients with increased blood protein or nitrogens in the blood may have problems with fluid management. Check central venous pressure or pulmonary artery pressure as needed.

Glucose levels are a sensitive marker of counterregulatory hormones, which are often activated before patients become febrile. *Hyperglycemia often occurs before a fever.*

> **! NURSING SAFETY PRIORITY** QSEN
>
> ***Action Alert***
>
> When a patient who has had reasonably controlled blood glucose levels in the hospital develops an unexpected rise in blood glucose values, check for wound infection.

Hyperkalemia (high blood potassium level) is common in patients with mild to moderate kidney failure and can lead to cardiac dysrhythmia. In other patients, hypokalemia (low blood potassium level) may occur and be made worse by insulin and glucose given during surgery. Monitor the cardiac rhythm and serum potassium values.

Cardiovascular monitoring by continuous ECG is recommended for older patients with DM, those with long-standing type 1 DM, and those with heart disease. Patients with DM are at higher risk for MI after surgery with a higher mortality rate. Changes in ECG or potassium level may indicate a silent MI.

Kidney monitoring, especially observing fluid balance, helps detect acute kidney injury. Diagnosis of kidney impairment may require the use of x-ray studies using contrast medium, which may be nephrotoxic. Management of infections may require the use of nephrotoxic antibiotics. Ensure adequate hydration when these drugs are used. Check for impending kidney failure by assessing FLUID AND ELECTROLYTE BALANCE.

Nutrition. Patients requiring clear or full liquid diets should receive about 200 g of carbohydrate daily in equally divided amounts at meals and snack times. Initial liquids should ***not*** be sugar free. Most patients require 25 to 35 calories per kilogram of body weight every 24 hours. After surgery, food intake is initiated as quickly as possible, with progression from clear liquids to solid foods occurring as rapidly as tolerated. Returning to a normal meal plan as soon as possible after surgery promotes healing and metabolic balance. When oral foods are tolerated, make sure the patient eats at least 150 to 200 g of carbohydrate daily to prevent hypoglycemia.

If total parenteral NUTRITION (TPN) is used after surgery, severe hyperglycemia may occur. Monitor blood glucose often to determine the need for supplemental insulin.

Preventing Injury From Peripheral Neuropathy

Planning: Expected Outcomes. The patient with DM is expected to identify factors that increase the risk for injury, practice proper foot care, and maintain intact skin on the feet. Indicators include that the patient consistently demonstrates these behaviors:

- Cleanses and inspects the feet daily
- Wears properly fitting shoes
- Avoids walking in bare feet
- Trims toenails properly
- Reports nonhealing breaks in the skin of the feet to the primary health care provider

Interventions. Patients with DM need intensive teaching about foot care because foot injury is a common complication. Once a failure of TISSUE INTEGRITY has occurred and an ulcer has developed, there is an increased risk for wound progression that may eventually lead to amputation. Most lower-extremity amputations in adults with DM are preceded by foot ulcers, and the 5-year mortality rate after leg or foot amputation is high (Centers for Disease Control and Prevention [CDC], 2015). Neuropathy is the main factor for development of a diabetic ulcer, and an inadequate vascular supply is the main cause of poor healing.

Motor neuropathy damages the nerves of foot muscles, resulting in foot deformities. These deformities create pressure points that gradually reduce TISSUE INTEGRITY with skin breakdown and ulceration. Thinning or shifting of the fat pad under the metatarsal heads decreases cushioning and increases areas of pressure. In claw toe deformity, toes are hyperextended and increase pressure on the metatarsal heads ("ball" of the foot). These changes predispose the patient to callus formation, ulceration, and infection. The Charcot foot is a type of diabetic foot deformity with many abnormalities, often including a *hallux valgus* (turning inward of the great toe) (Fig. 64-6). The foot is warm, swollen, and painful. Walking collapses the arch, shortens the foot, and gives the foot a "rocker bottom" shape.

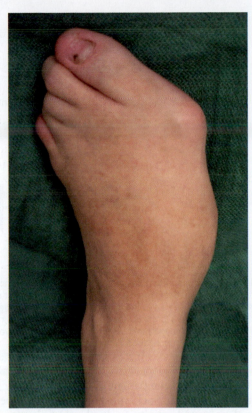

FIG. 64-6 "Charcot foot" type of diabetic foot deformity. (From Frykberg, R.G., Zgonis, T., Armstrong, D.G., Driver, V.R., Giurini, J.M., Kravitz, S.R., et al. (2006). Diabetic foot disorders: A clinical practice guideline—2006 revision. *The Journal of Foot and Ankle Surgery, 45*(5), S1-S66.)

TABLE 64-10	Foot Risk Categories
RISK CATEGORIES	**MANAGEMENT CATEGORIES**
Risk Category 0 • Has protective sensation • No evidence of peripheral vascular disease • No evidence of foot deformity or loss of TISSUE INTEGRITY	**Management Category 0** • Comprehensive foot examination once a year • Patient education to include advice on appropriate footwear
Risk Category 1 • Does not have protective sensation • May have evidence of foot deformity	**Management Category 1** • Evaluation every 3-6 months • Consider referral to a specialist to assess need for specialized treatment and follow-up • Patient education
Risk Category 2 • Does not have protective sensation • Evidence of peripheral vascular disease	**Management Categories 2 & 3** • Evaluation every 1-3 months • Referral to a specialist • Prescription footwear • Consider vascular consultation for combined follow-up • Patient education
Risk Category 3 • History of ulcer or amputation	

Data from American Diabetes Association (ADA). (2017). Classification and diagnosis of diabetes. *Diabetes Care, 40*(Suppl 1), S11-S24.

Autonomic neuropathy causes loss of normal sweating and skin temperature regulation, resulting in dry, thinning skin. Skin cracks and fissures increase the infection risk. Sensory neuropathy may cause tingling or burning, but more often it produces numbness and reduced SENSORY PERCEPTION. Without sensation, the patient does not notice injury and loss of TISSUE INTEGRITY in the foot. Peripheral arterial disease reduces blood flow to the foot, increasing the risk for ulcer formation and slowing ulcer healing (McCance et al., 2014).

Foot injuries are caused by walking barefoot, wearing ill-fitting shoes, sustaining thermal injuries from heat (e.g., hot water bottles, heating pads, baths), or chemical burns from over-the-counter corn treatments. These injuries lead to loss of TISSUE INTEGRITY and to amputation.

Ulcers result from continued pressure. Plantar ulcers (on the sole, usually the ball) are from standing or walking. Those on the top or sides of the foot usually are from shoes. The increased pressure causes calluses. Ulcers usually form over or around the great toe, under the metatarsal heads, and on the tops of claw toes.

Loss of TISSUE INTEGRITY with broken skin increases the risk for infection. Skin tends to break in areas of pressure. Infection is common in diabetic foot ulcers and, once present, is difficult to treat. Infection also impairs GLUCOSE REGULATION, leading to higher blood glucose levels and reduced IMMUNITY, which further increases the risk for infection.

Prevention of High-Risk Conditions. Neuropathy of the feet and legs can be delayed by keeping blood glucose levels near normal. Poor glucose control increases the risk for neuropathy

and amputation. Urge smoking cessation to reduce the risk for vascular complications.

The risk for ulcers or amputation increases with duration of diabetes. Other risk factors are male gender; poor glucose control; and cardiovascular, retinal, or kidney complications. Foot-related risks include poor gait and stepping mechanics, peripheral neuropathy, increased pressure (callus, erythema, hemorrhage under a callus, limited joint mobility, foot deformities, or severe nail pathology), peripheral vascular disease, and a history of ulcers or amputation.

Peripheral Neuropathy Management. The feet should be evaluated closely at least annually. Chart 22-9 lists self-management activities for prevention of injury from peripheral neuropathy, and Table 64-10 lists foot risk categories.

Complete a full foot assessment as outlined in Chart 64-5. Sensory examination with Semmes-Weinstein monofilaments is a practical measure of the risk for foot ulcers. The nylon monofilament is mounted on a holder standardized to exert a 10-g force. An adult who cannot feel the 10-g pressure at any point is at increased risk for ulcers. To perform the examination:

- Ask the patient to close his or her eyes during the test.
- Test the monofilament on the patient's cheek so he or she knows what to expect.
- Test the sites noted in Fig. 64-7.
- Apply the monofilament at a right angle to the skin surface.
- Apply enough force to bend the filament using a smooth, not jabbing, motion (Fig. 64-8).
- The approach, contact, and removal of the filament at each site should take 1 to 2 seconds.
- Apply the filament along the perimeter and **not** on an ulcer site, callus, scar, or necrotic tissue. Do not slide the

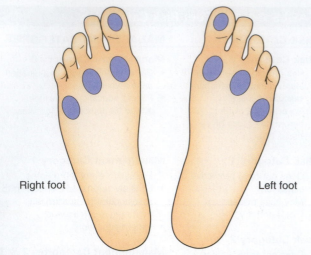

FIG. 64-7 Placement sites of monofilaments for testing of protective sensation.

Right foot   Left foot

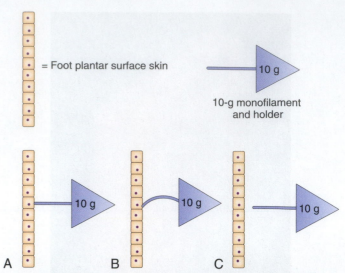

= Foot plantar surface skin

10-g monofilament and holder

A   B   C

FIG. 64-8 Correct technique for sensation testing with 10-g monofilament. **A,** Apply monofilament to designated areas of the foot sole (intact skin only; see Fig. 64-7). **B,** Apply pressure to the filament either until the patient states that he or she can feel the pressure or until the filament bends (see the Peripheral Neuropathy Management section). **C,** Quickly remove the filament without sliding it or touching other areas of the foot.

CHART 64-5   Focused Assessment

The Diabetic Foot

Assess the patient's risk for diabetic foot problems:
- History of previous ulcer
- History of previous amputation

Assess the foot for abnormal skin and nail conditions:
- Dry, cracked, fissured skin
- Ulcers
- Toenails: thickened, long nails; ingrown nails
- Tinea pedis; onychomycosis (mycotic nails)
- Assess the foot for status of circulation:
- Symptoms of claudication
- Presence or absence of dorsalis pedis or posterior tibial pulse
- Prolonged capillary filling time (greater than 25 seconds)
- Presence or absence of hair growth on the top of the foot

Assess the foot for evidence of deformity:
- Calluses, corns
- Prominent metatarsal heads (metatarsal head is easily felt under the skin)
- Toe contractures: clawed toes, hammertoes
- Hallux valgus or bunions
- Charcot foot ("rocker bottom")

Assess the foot for loss of strength:
- Limited ankle joint range of motion
- Limited motion of great toe

Assess the foot for loss of protective sensation:
- Numbness, burning, tingling
- Semmes-Weinstein monofilament testing at 10 points on each foot

Data from American Diabetes Association (ADA). (2017). Standards of medical care in diabetes—2017: Microvascular complications and foot care. *Diabetes Care, 40*(Suppl. 1), S88-S98.

---

filament across the skin or make repeated contact at the test site.

- Randomize the sequence of applying the filament throughout the examination. Have the patient identify where the filament touched rather than asking, "Do you feel this?"

Footwear. Patients with any degree of peripheral neuropathy are at risk for loss of TISSUE INTEGRITY and need to wear protective shoes fitted by an experienced shoe fitter, such as a certified podiatrist. The shoe should be ½ to ⅝ inch longer than the longest toe. Heels should be less than 2 inches high. Tight shoes

damage tissue. Instruct the patient to change shoes by midday and again in the evening. Socks must fit properly and be appropriate for the planned activity. Socks should feel soft and have no thick seams, creases, or holes. They should pad the foot and absorb excess moisture. Teach patients to avoid tight stockings or those that have constricting bands. Patients with toe deformities need custom shoes with high, wide toe boxes and extra depth. Those with severely deformed feet need specially molded shoes. New shoes need a long break-in period with frequent foot inspection for irritation or blistering.

Foot Care. Teach patients about preventive foot care and the need for examination of the feet and legs at each visit to a primary health care provider. A mirror placed on the floor can help the patient visually examine the plantar surface (sole) of the foot. Identify patients with high-risk foot conditions. Explain problems caused by loss of protective sensation, the importance of monitoring the feet daily, proper care of the feet (including nail and skin care), and how to select appropriate footwear.

Assess the patient's ability to inspect all areas of the foot and to perform foot care. Teach family members how to inspect and care for the patient's feet if the patient cannot. Chart 64-6 lists foot care instructions for self-management.

Wound Care. The standards of care for diabetic ulcers are a moist wound environment, débridement of necrotic tissue, and elimination of pressure (offloading). Proper wound care and débridement are discussed in Chapter 25.

Eliminating pressure on an infected area is essential for wound healing. Teach patients with foot ulcers to not wear a shoe on the affected foot while the ulcer is healing. Those with poor SENSORY PERCEPTION may keep walking on an ulcer because it does not hurt. This results in pressure necrosis that delays healing and increases ulcer size. Pressure is reduced by specialized orthotic devices, custom-molded shoe inserts, or shoe adjustments that redistribute weight.

Offloading redistributes force away from ulcer sites and pressure points to wider areas of the foot. Available products

CHART 64-6 Patient and Family Education: Preparing for Self-Management

Foot Care Instructions

- Inspect your feet daily, especially the area between the toes.
- Wash your feet daily with lukewarm water and soap. Dry thoroughly.
- Apply moisturizing cream to your feet after bathing. Do not apply to the area between your toes.
- Change into clean cotton socks every day.
- Do not wear the same pair of shoes 2 days in a row and wear only shoes made of breathable materials, such as leather or cloth.
- Check your shoes for foreign objects (nails, pebbles) before putting them on. Check inside the shoes for cracks or tears in the lining.
- Purchase shoes that have plenty of room for your toes. Buy shoes later in the day, when feet are normally larger. Break in new shoes gradually.
- Wear socks to keep your feet warm.
- Trim your nails straight across with a nail clipper. Smooth the nails with an emery board.
- See your physician or nurse immediately if you have blisters, sores, or infections. Protect the area with a dry, sterile dressing. Do not use adhesive tape to secure dressing to the skin.
- Do not treat blisters, sores, or infections with home remedies.
- Do not smoke.
- Do not step into the bathtub without checking the temperature of the water with your wrist or thermometer. Optimal temperature is 95° F (35° C). Maximum temperature is 110° F (43° C).
- Do not use very hot or cold water. Never use hot-water bottles, heating pads, or portable heaters to warm your feet.
- Do not treat corns, blisters, bunions, calluses, or ingrown toenails yourself.
- Do not go barefooted.
- Do not wear sandals with open toes or straps between the toes.
- Do not cross your legs or wear garters or tight stockings that constrict blood flow.
- Do not soak your feet.

Data from American Diabetes Association (ADA). (2017). Standards of medical care in diabetes—2017: Microvascular complications and foot care. *Diabetes Care, 40*(Suppl. 1), S88-S98.

include total-contact casting, half shoes, removable cast walkers, wheelchairs, and crutches. Total-contact casts redistribute pressure over the bottom of the foot. Casting material is molded to the foot and leg to spread pressure along the entire surface of contact, reducing vertical force. The almost complete elimination of motion of the total-contact cast reduces plantar shear forces. The cast is removed 24 to 48 hours after application to inspect the foot and cast fit. It is replaced and then reapplied weekly until the ulcer is healed. *Teach the patient that foot ulcers will recur unless weight is permanently redistributed.*

Managing Pain

Planning: Expected Outcomes. The patient with neuropathic pain is expected to experience relief of pain. Indicators include these consistent behaviors:

- Uses preventive measures
- Uses available resources to increase comfort
- Reports pain controlled

Interventions. Neuropathic pain results from damage anywhere along the nerve. Many patients with DM suffer from the painful neuropathy. Symptoms of diabetic neuropathy include:

- Burning, tingling, numbness, and loss of proprioception in lower extremities
- Muscle cramps
- Piercing, stabbing, or darting pain
- Metatarsalgia (feeling as if you are walking on marbles)

- Hyperalgesia (exaggerated pain response)
- Allodynia (pain in response to normally nonpainful stimuli)

Maintaining normal blood glucose levels and avoiding extreme fluctuations prevent chronic neuropathy and relieve symptoms. Rapid improvement in blood glucose control may actually trigger acute peripheral neuropathy.

Several pharmacologic agents are used to manage neuropathic pain, such as the anticonvulsants gabapentin (Neurontin) and pregabalin (Lyrica) and the serotonin-norepinephrine reuptake inhibitor (SNRI) duloxetine (Cymbalta). Tricyclic antidepressants such as amitriptyline hydrochloride (Elavil, Levate ♣) and nortriptyline (Pamelor) have been used for neuropathic pain but are not approved for this purpose and have significant side effects. Their use is contraindicated for older adults and those with cardiovascular disease.

The burning of neuropathy may respond to capsaicin cream 0.075% (Axsain ♣, Zostrix-HP). Teach the patient to apply it four times daily for several weeks. The pain may worsen for several days after therapy is started before improving.

Unpleasant symptoms are noted with abrupt discontinuation of many of these drugs. A gradual reduction in the dose is recommended to prevent side effects.

Provide support and information on measures to reduce pain. Even having a bed cradle to lift bed clothes off hypersensitive skin can be beneficial. Help the patient maintain stable glucose control. *All patients with neuropathy are at increased risk for foot ulcers and require more frequent assessment and education in routine foot management.*

Preventing Injury From Reduced Vision

Planning: Expected Outcomes. The patient with DM is expected to be free of injury related to reduced SENSORY PERCEPTION for vision and to maintain current level of vision. Indicators include:

- No further reduction of visual fields
- No double vision

Interventions

Blood Glucose Control. Poor blood glucose control, proteinuria, hypertension, and long duration of DM are risk factors for vision loss among adults with diabetes. Surgical intervention for retinal hemorrhage or new retinal blood vessel growth can reduce vision loss.

Besides regular eye examinations to evaluate retinopathy, urge the patient with impaired vision to have an optometrist or ophthalmologist assess the remaining vision and prescribe appropriate vision support. A functional vision assessment, performed by a low-vision technician, rehabilitation teacher, or diabetes educator, determines the patient's use of lighting, contrast, nonoptical and low-vision devices, large-print options, and use of central or peripheral vision. Many low-vision reading aids are available as described in Chapter 47. The American Foundation for the Blind (AFB) maintains a list of services for visually impaired people that is organized by type of service and geographic area. More information is available at (800) 232-5463 and www.afb.org.

Environmental Management. Not all visually impaired patients need special devices. Adjustments in lighting, contrast, color, distance, type size of printed materials, and eye movement often improve visual abilities. Chapter 47 describes general methods of enhancing vision. For patients with DM and low vision, coding objects such as vials of insulin with bright colors or felt-tipped markers helps identify the correct bottle. Bringing the blood glucose lancet or insulin syringe close to the eye makes it easier to see.

Prefilled insulin pens are not approved for use by adults with severe visual impairment unless they are assisted by a person with good vision who is trained to use the pen correctly. Adaptive devices can help the patient self-administer insulin independently. Some syringes may have a magnifier attached to the syringe. Other devices include preset dose gauges (which measure the space between the end of the syringe barrel and the plunger) to help the patient draw up the correct amount of insulin by feeling this distance. The blind patient can accurately measure insulin by using products such as the Count-A-Dose Insulin Measuring Device. This device is designed to be used with the BD Lo-Dose syringe. It holds two insulin vials and has a slot to direct the syringe needle into the vials' rubber stoppers. The patient draws insulin into the syringe by turning a thumbwheel, which clicks for each unit (clicks can be both heard and felt). (See the Consumer Guide published yearly in the January edition of Diabetes Forecast [forecast.diabetes.org] for information to help patients determine which adaptive devices best meet their needs.) When teaching the patient to use an adaptive device, stress:

- Differentiating between bottles of fast-acting and slower-acting insulin by wrapping a rubber band around the fast-acting insulin bottle
- Ensuring proper placement of the device on the syringe
- Holding the insulin bottle upright when measuring insulin
- Avoiding air bubbles in the syringe by pulling a small amount of insulin into the syringe, moving the plunger in and out three times, and measuring insulin on the fourth draw

Help the patient determine how many doses can be drawn from a bottle so he or she does not inject air from an empty bottle instead of insulin.

Specialized adaptive equipment also is available to assist with blood glucose monitoring techniques. Help the patient select a blood glucose monitoring device best suited to his or her level of visual impairment. Some monitors have large display screens and easy-to-use features. Fully audio systems are available for patients who are visually impaired. Assess the ability of the patient to obtain an adequate blood sample and apply it to the test strip. Commercially made blood drop guides can help with this task.

Reducing the Risk for Kidney Disease

Planning: Expected Outcomes. The patient with diabetes is expected to maintain a normal urine elimination pattern. Indicators include:

- Urine protein levels within normal limits
- 24-hour intake and output balance
- Blood urea nitrogen (BUN) and serum creatinine within the normal ranges
- Serum electrolytes within the normal ranges

Interventions

Prevention. Diabetic kidney disease is more likely to develop in patients with poor blood glucose control. Progression to end-stage kidney disease can be delayed or prevented by normalizing blood pressure using drugs from either the angiotensin-converting enzyme inhibitor (ACEI) class or the angiotensin receptor blocker (ARB) class. Once used to "protect" the kidney, neither class of drug is recommended for patients with DM who have normal blood pressure and normal albumin excretion

(ADA, 2017c). Hypertension greatly accelerates the progression of diabetic kidney disease.

Stress the need for evaluation of kidney function according to the ADA Standards of Care. An annual test to quantify urine albumin is performed for patients who have had type 1 DM for over 5 years and in all those with type 2 DM starting at diagnosis and during pregnancy (ADA, 2017c). Persistent albuminuria in the range of 30 to 299 mg/24 hours (formerly called *microalbuminuria*) is the earliest stage of nephropathy in type 1 DM and a marker for the development of nephropathy in type 2 DM.

Aggressive control of blood glucose and hypertension in patients without albuminuria can avoid nephropathy. Once albuminuria develops, management focuses on controlling blood pressure and blood glucose and avoiding nephrotoxic agents.

Control of blood pressure and blood glucose levels requires the patient's participation and effort. Prescribed drugs must be taken according to schedules, and dietary restriction must be maintained. Teach patients about the roles of blood pressure and blood glucose levels in kidney disease. Help them maintain normal blood glucose levels and blood pressure levels below 140/80 mm Hg. Stress the need for yearly screening for albuminuria.

Smoking cessation is important in halting the progression of diabetic kidney disease. Teach the patient about the risks of smoking and refer him or her to appropriate resources for assistance in smoking cessation.

Drugs can affect kidney function either through toxic effects on the kidney or by an acute but reversible reduction in function. The most common nephrotoxic drugs are antifungal agents and aminoglycoside antibiotics. Outside the hospital, the leading nephrotoxic agents are NSAIDs such as ibuprofen (Advil) or naproxen (Aleve). Teach the patient to check with his or her primary health care provider or a pharmacist before taking over-the-counter drugs or herbal remedies.

Radiocontrast medium can also affect kidney function, especially in patients with pre-existing kidney problems. Monitor IV hydration before and after a contrast agent is used to prevent contrast-induced nephropathy in patients with DM.

Drug Therapy. Use of angiotensin-converting enzyme inhibitors (ACEIs) or angiotensin receptor blockers (ARBs) is recommended for all patients with persistent albuminuria or advanced stages of nephropathy (ADA, 2017c). ACE inhibitors reduce the level of albuminuria and the rate of progression of kidney disease, although they do not appear to prevent albuminuria. Monitor serum potassium levels for development of hyperkalemia (ADA, 2017c).

Dialysis for patients with DM and kidney failure is the same as for patients without diabetes (see Chapter 68). The dosage of insulin needs to be adjusted when dialysis starts.

Preventing Hypoglycemia.

Hypoglycemia is a low blood glucose level that induces specific symptoms and resolves when blood glucose concentration is raised. Once plasma glucose levels fall below 70 mg/dL (3.88 mmol/L), a sequence of events begins with release of counterregulatory hormones, stimulation of the autonomic nervous system, and production of *neurogenic* and *neuroglycopenic* symptoms. Peripheral autonomic symptoms, including sweating, irritability, tremors, anxiety, tachycardia, and hunger, serve as an early warning system and occur before the symptoms of confusion, paralysis, seizure, and coma occur from brain glucose deprivation. *Neuroglycopenic*

TABLE 64-11	Symptoms of Hypoglycemia
NEUROGLYCOPENIC SYMPTOMS	**NEUROGENIC SYMPTOMS**

• Weakness
• Fatigue
• Difficulty thinking
• Confusion
• Behavior changes
• Emotional instability
• Seizures
• Loss of consciousness
• Brain damage
• Death
	• Adrenergic:
	  • Shaky/tremulous
	  • Heart pounding
	  • Nervous/anxious
	• Cholinergic:
	  • Sweaty
	  • Hungry
	  • Tingling

TABLE 64-12	Differentiation of Hypoglycemia and Hyperglycemia	
FEATURE	**HYPOGLYCEMIA**	**HYPERGLYCEMIA**
Skin	Cool, clammy	Warm, moist
Dehydration	Absent	Present
Respirations	No particular or consistent change	Rapid, deep*; Kussmaul type; acetone odor ("fruity" odor) to breath
Mental status	Anxious, nervous*, irritable, mental confusion*, seizures, coma	Varies from alert to stuporous, obtunded, or frank coma
Symptoms	Weakness*, double vision, blurred vision, hunger, tachycardia, palpitations	None specific for DKA Acidosis; hypercapnia; abdominal cramps, nausea and vomiting Dehydration: decreased neck vein filling, orthostatic hypotension, tachycardia, poor skin turgor
Glucose	<70 mg/dL (3.9 mmol/L)	>250 mg/dL (13.8 mmol/L)
Urine or blood ketones	Negative	Positive

DKA, Diabetic ketoacidosis.
*Classic symptoms.

symptoms occur when brain glucose *gradually declines* to a low level. *Neurologic symptoms* result from autonomic nervous activity triggered by a *rapid decline* in blood glucose (Table 64-11).

Central nervous system (CNS) function depends on a continuous supply of glucose in the blood. The brain cannot make glucose and stores only a few minutes' supply as glycogen. This needed supply is not maintained when the blood glucose level falls below critical levels.

The first defense against falling blood glucose levels in the adult without DM is decreased insulin secretion, decreased glucose use, and increased glucose production. Normally, insulin secretion decreases when blood glucose levels drop to about 83 mg/dL (4.5 mmol/L). Counterregulatory hormones are activated at about 67 mg/dL (3.7 mmol/L), a level well above the threshold for symptoms of hypoglycemia. The main counterregulatory hormone is glucagon. Epinephrine also becomes important in patients with DM who are deficient in glucagon. Both glucagon and epinephrine raise blood glucose levels by stimulating liver glycogen breakdown and conversion of protein to glucose. Epinephrine also limits insulin secretion.

Type 1 DM disrupts the body's response to hypoglycemia, usually within 1 to 5 years of diagnosis. Regulation of circulating insulin levels is lost because insulin comes from an injection rather than from the pancreas. As blood glucose levels fall, insulin levels do not decrease. Over time, the pancreas loses its ability to secrete glucagon in response to hypoglycemia. After a few more years of type 1 DM, the response of epinephrine to falling blood glucose levels does not occur until the blood glucose level is very low. These problems greatly increase the risk for severe hypoglycemia.

A second problem with long-standing type 1 DM is *hypoglycemic unawareness*, in which patients no longer have the warning symptoms of impending hypoglycemia that should prompt them to take preventive action. This problem occurs most often in patients who have had type 1 DM for 30 years or longer.

The blood glucose level at which symptoms of hypoglycemia occur varies among patients. Thus clinical criteria used to categorize hypoglycemia are based on symptom severity rather than blood glucose levels. In mild hypoglycemia, the patient remains alert and able to self-manage symptoms. In severe hypoglycemia, neurologic function is so impaired that he or she needs another person's help to increase blood glucose levels.

Planning: Expected Outcomes. The patient is expected to have decreased episodes of hypoglycemia and remain oriented to person, place, and time, as indicated by a Glasgow Coma Scale score above 7.

Interventions. A blood glucose level below 70 mg/dL (3.9 mmol/L) alerts you to assess for symptoms of hypoglycemia. (see Table 64-11; Table 64-12).

Blood Glucose Management. Monitor blood glucose levels before giving antidiabetic drugs, before meals, before bedtime, and when the patient is symptomatic. All patients who take insulin, those taking long-acting insulin secretagogues (glyburide [glibenclamide]), and those taking metformin in combination with glyburide (Glucovance) are at risk for hypoglycemia. This risk is increased if they are older, have liver or kidney impairment, or are taking drugs that enhance the effects of antidiabetic drugs. Proper patient selection, drug dosage, and instructions are important factors in avoiding severe hypoglycemia. In the hospital setting it is important that mealtime insulin be coordinated with delivery of food for patient consumption to avoid episodes of hypoglycemia (see the Quality Improvement box).

Hypoglycemia may be difficult to recognize in those who take beta-blocking drugs. Symptoms are less intense and less obvious. Symptoms of hypoglycemia in older patients may be mistaken for other conditions.

The most common causes of hypoglycemia are:
• Too much insulin compared with food intake and physical activity
• Insulin injected at the wrong time relative to food intake and physical activity
• The wrong type of insulin injected at the wrong time
• Decreased food intake resulting from missed or delayed meals
• Delayed gastric emptying from gastroparesis
• Decreased liver glucose production after alcohol ingestion

QUALITY IMPROVEMENT (QSEN)

Increasing "Perfect Blood Glucose Control" Improved Insulin-Mealtime Match Among Inpatients With Diabetes

Engle, M., Fergusin, A., & Fields, W. (2016). A journey to improved inpatient glycemic control by redesigning meal delivery and insulin administration. *Clinical Nurse Specialist, 30*(2), 117–124.

Hypoglycemia is a common preventable occurrence in the acute care setting, most often caused by a lack of coordination between blood glucose testing, insulin administration, and meal delivery. This "never" event has the potential for serious adverse health outcomes and death and is the focus of the development of strategies for "perfect blood glucose (BG) control" in which BG does not fall below 70 mg/dL (3.68 mmol/L) nor elevates beyond 180 mg/dL (10 mmol/L).

The incidence of hyperglycemia and hypoglycemia in one large (540-bed) acute care community hospital was examined for a calendar year among all inpatients receiving insulin for diabetes. The rate of perfect blood glucose control was only 45%. This less-than-desirable rate was attributed primarily to issues relating to timing of premeal blood glucose checks, meal delivery, and administration of insulin. A major problem with inconsistent meal tray delivery through the dietary department was uncovered. This obstacle to perfect blood glucose control often resulted in patients having their point-of-care premeal blood glucose testing and insulin administration after, rather than before, consumption of a meal. The percentage of patients receiving mealtime insulin within 30 minutes of accurate blood glucose checks was only 35%.

A plan was developed in cooperation with the dietary department in which trays for patients receiving mealtime insulin were identified from a computer-generated list and were ticketed by dietary staff with a colored stamp stating "INSULIN" to differentiate them from trays for patients with diabetes who were not receiving insulin. Once the trays were prepared and ready to deliver to the nursing unit, dietary called the unit to inform nurses that a specific tray was en route. At that time, the nurse would perform point-of-care blood glucose testing. On arrival of the tray to the unit, the tray was delivered by the nurse who then administered the prescribed mealtime and correction insulin dose (based on the blood glucose level and the assessment by the nurse of the amount of carbohydrate the patient was expected to eat).

Examination of data after this policy was implemented hospital-wide revealed an increase of perfect blood glucose control rate to 53% and an improvement of the percentage of patients receiving mealtime insulin within 30 minutes of the blood glucose check from 35% to 73%. The incidence of both hyperglycemia and hypoglycemia decreased.

Commentary: Implications for Practice and Research

This quality improvement project demonstrated that barriers to best practice can be overcome for patient safety when interprofessional coordination is successful. The work flow for both nursing and dietary personnel required modification and coordination. Although improvement was significant, more research, especially in prevention of hypoglycemic episodes, is needed to achieve "perfect blood glucose control" in large acute care settings.

CHART 64-7 Patient and Family Education: Preparing for Self-Management

Management of Hypoglycemia at Home

For **mild** hypoglycemia (hungry, irritable, shaky, weak, headache, fully conscious; blood glucose usually less than 60 mg/dL [3.4 mmol/L]):
- Treat the symptoms of hypoglycemia with 10 to 15 g of carbohydrate. You may use one of these:
  - Glucose tablets or glucose gel (dosage is printed on the package)
  - ½ cup (120 mL) of fruit juice
  - ½ cup (120 mL) of regular (nondiet) soft drink
  - 8 ounces (240 mL) of skim milk
  - 6 to 10 hard candies
  - 4 cubes of sugar
  - 4 teaspoons of sugar
  - 6 saltines
  - 3 graham crackers
  - 1 tablespoon (15 mL) of honey or syrup
- Retest blood glucose in 15 minutes.
- Repeat this treatment if glucose remains less than 60 mg/dL (3 mmol/L). Symptoms may persist after blood glucose has normalized.
- Eat a small snack of carbohydrate and protein if your next meal is more than an hour away.

For **moderate** hypoglycemia (cold, clammy skin; pale; rapid pulse; rapid, shallow respirations; marked change in mood; drowsiness; blood glucose usually less than 40 mg/dL [2.2 mmol/L]):
- Treat the symptoms of hypoglycemia with 15 to 30 g of rapidly absorbed carbohydrate.
- Retest glucose in 15 minutes.
- Repeat treatment if glucose is less than 60 mg/dL (3 mmol/L).
- Eat additional food, such as low-fat milk or cheese, after 10 to 15 minutes.

For **severe** hypoglycemia (unable to swallow; unconsciousness or convulsions; blood glucose usually less than 20 mg/dL [1.0 mmol/L]):
- Treatment administered by family members:
  - Give 1 mg of glucagon as intramuscular or subcutaneous injection.
  - Give a second dose in 10 minutes if the person remains unconscious.
  - Notify the primary health care provider immediately and follow instructions.
  - If still unconscious, transport the person to the emergency department.
  - Give a small meal when the person wakes up and is no longer nauseated.

- Increased insulin sensitivity as a result of regular exercise and weight loss
- Decreased insulin clearance from progressive kidney failure

Nutrition Therapy. When the patient is hypoglycemic, start prescribed carbohydrate (CHO) replacement, usually ingestion of 15 to 20 g of glucose. If the patient can swallow, give a liquid form of CHO, although any CHO source can be used. Ingestion of 15 to 20 g of glucose is the preferred management for blood glucose levels less than 70 mg/dL (3.9 mmol/L),

repeated in about 15 minutes if symptoms have not improved or if blood glucose levels are still less than 70. The amount of CHO is increased to 30 g for glucose levels less than 50 mg/dL (2.8 mmol/L).

A 10-g amount of oral glucose raises plasma glucose levels by about 40 mg/dL over 30 minutes, and 20 g of oral glucose raises plasma glucose levels by about 60 mg/dL over 45 minutes. Specific recommendations are listed in Chart 64-7.

The blood glucose level determines the form and amount of glucose used. The response should be apparent in 10 to 20 minutes; however, test plasma glucose again in about 60 minutes because additional management may be needed. Fluid is absorbed much more quickly from the GI tract than are solids. Concentrated sweet fluids, such as juice with sugar added or a soft drink, may slow absorption.

Management of hypoglycemia requires ingestion of glucose or glucose-containing foods. The blood glucose response correlates better with the glucose content rather than the carbohydrate content of the food. Adding protein to CHO does not improve blood glucose response and does not prevent subsequent hypoglycemia. Adding fat may retard and then prolong the blood glucose response, resulting in post-treatment hyperglycemia. Commercially available products provide predictable glucose absorption.

Drug Therapy. Subcutaneous or IM glucagon and 50% IV dextrose are administered to patients who cannot swallow. Glucagon is the main counterregulatory hormone to insulin and is used as first-line therapy for severe hypoglycemia in DM. It converts liver glycogen to glucose but is not effective in severely starved patients. Take care to prevent aspiration in patients receiving glucagon, because it often causes vomiting. Give 50% dextrose carefully to avoid extravasation because it is hyperosmolar and can damage tissue. The effects of glucagon and dextrose are temporary. After the patient responds and is no longer nauseated, give a simple sugar followed by a small snack or meal. IV glucose is used to maintain mild hyperglycemia. Diazoxide (Proglycem) or octreotide (Sandostatin) may be required to treat sulfonylurea-induced hypoglycemia. Evaluate response by monitoring blood glucose levels for several hours because symptoms may persist. A target blood glucose level is 70 to 110 mg/dL (3.9 to 6.2 mmol/L).

⚠ NURSING SAFETY PRIORITY QSEN

Critical Rescue

Assess patients to recognize the presence and severity of hypoglycemia. For the patient with *severe* hypoglycemia (unable to swallow, unconscious or convulsing, blood glucose usually less than 20 mg/dL [1.0 mmol/L]), respond by:
1. Giving glucagon 1 mg subcutaneously or IM
2. Repeating the dose in 10 minutes if the patient remains unconscious
3. Notifying the primary health care provider immediately and following instructions

---

Prevention Strategies. Teach the patient how to prevent hypoglycemia by avoiding its four common causes: (1) excess insulin, (2) deficient intake or absorption of food, (3) exercise when insulin action is peaking, and (4) alcohol intake.

Insulin excess from variable absorption of insulin can cause hypoglycemia even when insulin is injected correctly. Increased insulin sensitivity can occur with weight loss, exercise programs, and resolution of an infection. Differences in insulin formulation can result in hypoglycemia. Teach the patient to not change insulin brands without medical supervision.

Deficient food intake from inadequate or incorrectly timed meals can result in hypoglycemia. Changes in gastric absorption may cause hypoglycemia in patients with delayed gastric emptying, which is more severe with solid meals and is made worse by illness or poor glucose control. Teach the patient the importance of regularity in timing and quantity of food eaten.

Exercise often causes blood glucose levels to fall in a patient with type 1 DM. Prolonged exercise increases muscle glucose uptake for several hours after exercise. Teach the patient about blood glucose monitoring and carbohydrate consumption before and during exercise. Also teach him or her to exercise at times when insulin activity is not peaking.

Alcohol inhibits liver glucose production and leads to hypoglycemia. It interferes with the counterregulatory response to hypoglycemia and impairs glycogen breakdown, making exercise-induced hypoglycemia more severe. Teach the patient to ingest alcohol only with or shortly *after* eating a meal with enough carbohydrate to prevent hypoglycemia. Warn patients to avoid excess alcohol at bedtime to prevent nighttime hypoglycemia.

Patient and Family Education. The cause of hypoglycemia may be subtle. At the onset of menses, a fall in hormone levels decreases insulin needs and contributes to hypoglycemia. When patients switch to a new bottle of insulin, hypoglycemia may occur because the fresh insulin has greater potency. Some patients have hypoglycemia when they change injection sites. Beta-blocking drugs mask warning signs and thus predispose patients to severe hypoglycemia. Some episodes of hypoglycemia occur without an obvious cause.

Many patients who have been treated in the emergency department for hypoglycemia do not receive adequate prevention instructions and are at continuing risk. Help each patient develop a personal treatment plan for hypoglycemia. The exact glucose rise from a set amount of carbohydrate (CHO) varies; however, using the estimate that each 5 g of CHO raises blood glucose about 20 mg/dL is a good starting plan. For example, the patient may be directed to take:

- 20 to 30 g of CHO if the blood glucose level is 50 mg/dL (2.8 mmol/L) or less
- 10 to 15 g of CHO if the blood glucose level is 51 to 70 mg/dL (2.9 to 3.9 mmol/L)

Use blood glucose monitoring results to revise or reinforce this plan.

Encourage the patient to wear a medical alert bracelet and help him or her obtain one. This bracelet is helpful if the patient becomes hypoglycemic and is unable to provide self-care.

Teach the patient and family about the symptoms of hypoglycemia. Stress that delaying a meal for more than 30 minutes raises the risk for hypoglycemia when using some insulin regimens. Instruct him or her to keep a CHO source nearby at all times. Teach the patient and family how to inject glucagon.

Hypoglycemia is a major risk for patients receiving intensive insulin protocols who engage in exercise programs. Explain that nightmares or headaches on days after prolonged or severe exercise may indicate hypoglycemia.

Establishing Treatment Plans. Blood glucose monitoring directs hypoglycemia management. Treatment continues until blood glucose levels reach and stay in the target range. Once blood glucose control is regained, the patient should identify the specific cause of the episode and take specific measures to prevent recurrence.

Preventing Diabetic Ketoacidosis. Diabetic ketoacidosis (DKA) is characterized by uncontrolled hyperglycemia, metabolic acidosis, and increased production of ketones. This condition results from the combination of insulin deficiency and an increase in hormone release that leads to increased liver and kidney glucose production and decreased glucose use in

CONSIDERATIONS FOR OLDER ADULTS
Patient-Centered Care (QSEN)

Older patients are especially vulnerable to hypoglycemia. Age-related declines in kidney function and liver enzyme activity may interfere with the metabolism of sulfonylureas and insulin, thereby potentiating their hypoglycemic effects. Older adults with DM have impaired epinephrine release and a reduced glucagon response to low blood glucose levels and often have hypoglycemic unawareness. Confusion and impairment in psychomotor skill when glucose is low prevent the older adult from taking steps to return glucose levels to normal.

Instruct the older patient's family to check blood glucose values when symptoms such as unsteadiness, light-headedness, poor concentration, trembling, or sweating occur (Touhy & Jett, 2016). Assess eating patterns to make sure that sufficient foods are eaten at appropriate times. Encourage a patient with a poor appetite to eat a small snack at bedtime to prevent hypoglycemia during the night.

The highest rates of severe and fatal episodes of hypoglycemia are associated with the use of glyburide in patients older than 70. Drug regimens that require that meals be eaten on time increase the potential for hypoglycemic reactions. Complex regimens that require multiple decision points should be simplified, especially for patients with decreased functional status (ADA, 2017h).

CLINICAL JUDGMENT CHALLENGE 64-2
Safety; Quality Improvement; Patient-Centered Care (QSEN)

The patient is a 67-year-old man with type 1 diabetes who is 2 days postoperative from a below-the-knee amputation. He is scheduled for an x-ray in an hour. His lunch has just arrived; and, after you check his blood glucose level, you administer the prescribed short-acting insulin. After updating the nurse who is covering for you, you go to lunch. When you return to the unit 45 minutes later, you receive a call from the radiology department that the patient is unconscious and his skin is cold and clammy. You check his room and find his lunch tray cold and untouched. It appears that transport services came early and did not notify anyone on the unit.

1. What is your first action? Provide a rationale.
2. What is the most likely cause leading to this problem?
3. What could be done to prevent such an incident from happening again?

peripheral tissues (Fig. 64-9). Laboratory diagnosis of DKA is shown in Table 64-13. All of these changes increase ketoacid production with resultant ketonemia and metabolic acidosis.

DKA occurs most often in patients with type 1 DM but also can occur in those with type 2 DM who are under severe stress (e.g., trauma, surgery, infection). Some adults with type 2 DM have a syndrome known as ketosis-prone diabetes or KPD. Regardless of whether the patient with DKA has type 1 or type

2 DM, management of the acute episode is the same. The most common precipitating factor for DKA is infection. *Death occurs in up to 10% of these cases even with appropriate treatment.*

Hyperglycemia leads to osmotic diuresis with dehydration and electrolyte loss. Classic symptoms of DKA include polyuria, polydipsia, polyphagia, a rotting citrus fruit odor to the breath, vomiting, abdominal pain, dehydration, weakness, confusion, shock, and coma. Mental status can vary from total alertness to profound coma. As ketone levels rise, the pH of the blood decreases, and acidosis occurs. **Kussmaul respirations** (very deep and rapid respirations) cause respiratory alkalosis in an attempt to correct metabolic acidosis by exhaling carbon dioxide. Initial serum sodium levels may be low or normal.

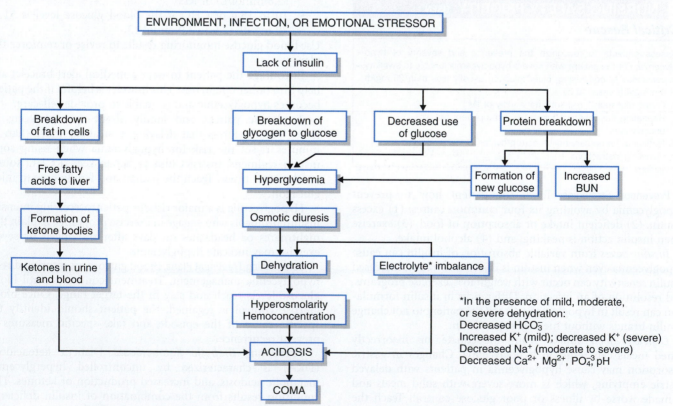

FIG. 64-9 Pathophysiologic mechanism of diabetic ketoacidosis (DKA). *BUN,* Blood urea nitrogen; *Ca²⁺,* calcium; *HCO₃⁻,* bicarbonate; *K⁺,* potassium; *Mg²⁺,* magnesium; *Na⁺,* sodium; *PO₄⁻³,* phosphate.

TABLE 64-13 Differences Between Diabetic Ketoacidosis and Hyperglycemic-Hyperosmolar State

	DIABETIC KETOACIDOSIS (DKA)	HYPERGLYCEMIC-HYPEROSMOLAR STATE (HHS)
Onset	Sudden	Gradual
Precipitating factors	Infection Other stressors Inadequate insulin dose	Infection Other stressors Poor fluid intake
Symptoms	Ketosis: Kussmaul respiration, "rotting fruit" breath, nausea, abdominal pain	Altered central nervous system function with neurologic symptoms
	Dehydration or electrolyte loss: polyuria, polydipsia, weight loss, dry skin, sunken eyes, soft eyeballs, lethargy, coma	Dehydration or electrolyte loss: same as for DKA
Laboratory Findings		
Serum glucose	>300 mg/dL (16.7 mmol/L)	>600 mg/dL (33.3 mmol/L)
Osmolarity/Osmolality	Variable	>320 mOsm/L (mOsm/kg)
Serum ketones	Positive at 1:2 dilutions	Negative
Serum pH	<7.35	>7.4
Serum HCO₃⁻	<15 mEq/L (mmol/L)	>20 mEq/L (mmol/L)
Serum Na⁺	Low, normal, or high	Normal or low
BUN	>30 mg/dL (10 mmol/L); elevated because of dehydration	Elevated
Creatinine	>1.5 mg/dL (60 mcmol/L); elevated because of dehydration	Elevated
Urine ketones	Positive	Negative

BUN, Blood urea nitrogen; *HCO₃⁻,* bicarbonate; *Na⁺,* sodium.

Initial potassium levels depend on how long DKA lasts before treatment. After therapy starts, serum potassium levels drop quickly.

Planning: Expected Outcomes. The patient is expected to have few episodes of hyperglycemia and avoid diabetic ketoacidosis. Indicators include that the patient consistently demonstrates these behaviors:

* Maintains blood glucose levels within the prescribed target range
* Adjusts insulin doses to match eating patterns and blood glucose levels during illness
* Maintains easily digestible liquid diet containing carbohydrate and salt when nauseated
* Describes correct procedure for urine ketone testing
* Describes when to seek help from health care professional

Interventions

Blood Glucose Management. Monitor for symptoms of DKA (see Table 64-13 and Fig. 64-9). Document and use these findings to determine therapy effectiveness. *First assess the airway, level of consciousness, hydration status, electrolytes, and blood glucose level.* Check the patient's blood pressure, pulse, and respirations every 15 minutes until stable. Record urine output, temperature, and mental status every hour. When a central venous catheter is present, assess central venous pressure every 30 minutes or as prescribed. After treatment starts and these values are stable, monitor and record vital signs every 4 hours. Use blood glucose values to assess therapy and determine when to switch from saline to dextrose-containing solutions.

Fluid and Electrolyte Management. *Closely assess the patient's FLUID AND ELECTROLYTE BALANCE.* Assess for acute weight loss, thirst, decreased skin turgor, dry mucous membranes, and oliguria with a high specific gravity. Assess for weak and rapid pulse; flat neck veins; increased temperature; decreased central venous pressure; muscle weakness; postural hypotension; and cool, clammy, and pale skin to determine if the patient is at risk for dehydration.

The first outcome of fluid therapy is to restore volume and maintain PERFUSION to vital organs. Typically initial infusion rates are 15 to 20 mL/kg/hr during the first hour.

The second outcome of replacing total body fluid losses is achieved more slowly. The choice for fluid replacement depends on blood pressure, hydration, serum electrolyte levels, and urinary output. In general, hypotonic fluids are infused at 4 to 14 ml/kg/hr after the initial fluid bolus. When blood glucose levels reach 250 mg/dL (13.8 mmol/L), give 5% dextrose in 0.45% saline. This solution helps prevent hypoglycemia and cerebral edema, which can occur when serum osmolarity declines too rapidly.

During the first 24 hours of treatment, the patient needs enough fluids to replace the actual volume lost and any ongoing losses. This may be as much as 6 to 10 L. Assess cardiac, kidney, and mental status to avoid fluid overload. Watch for symptoms of congestive heart failure and pulmonary edema. Central venous pressure may be monitored for older patients and those with cardiac disease. Assess the status of fluid replacement by monitoring blood pressure, intake and output, and changes in daily weight.

Drug Therapy. Insulin therapy is used to lower serum glucose by about 50 to 75 mg/dL/hr (2.8 to 4.2 mmol/L/hr) (Sanuth et al., 2014). Unless the episode of DKA is mild, regular insulin by continuous IV infusion is the usual management. Effective blood insulin levels are reached quickly when an IV bolus dose is given at the start of the infusion. An initial IV bolus dose of 0.1 unit/kg is followed by an IV infusion of 0.1 unit/kg/hr. Continuous insulin infusion is used because insulin half-life is short and subcutaneous insulin has a delayed onset of action. Subcutaneous insulin is started when the patient can take oral fluids and ketosis has stopped. DKA is considered resolved when blood glucose is less than 200 mg/mL (11.2 mmol/L) along with a serum bicarbonate level higher than 18 mEq/L (mmol/L), venous pH is higher than 7.3, and a calculated anion gap is less than 12 mEq/L (mmol/L). Assess therapy effectiveness by monitoring blood glucose levels and serial electrolyte levels.

Acidosis Management. The key feature of DKA is elevation in blood ketone concentration (measured as serum β-hydroxybutyrate). Accumulation of ketoacids results in an increased anion gap metabolic acidosis. A normal anion gap is between 7 and 9 mEq/L (mmol/L); an anion gap greater than 10 to 12 mEq/L (mmol/L) indicates metabolic acidosis.

Mild-to-moderate hyperkalemia is common in patients with hyperglycemia. Insulin therapy, correction of acidosis, and volume expansion decrease serum potassium concentration. To prevent hypokalemia, potassium replacement is initiated after serum levels fall below normal (5.0 mEq/L [mmol/L]). *Assess for signs of hypokalemia, including fatigue, malaise, confusion, muscle weakness, shallow respirations, abdominal distention or paralytic ileus, hypotension, and weak pulse.* An ECG shows conduction changes related to alterations in potassium. Hypokalemia is a common cause of death in the treatment of DKA.

! NURSING SAFETY PRIORITY QSEN

Action Alert

Before giving IV potassium-containing solutions, make sure that the urine output is at least 30 mL/hr.

Bicarbonate is used only for severe acidosis (Sanuth et al., 2014). Sodium bicarbonate, given by slow IV infusion over several hours, is indicated when the arterial pH is 7.0 or less or the serum bicarbonate level is less than 5 mEq/L (5 mmol/L).

Patient and Family Education. Exploring the factors leading to DKA helps in planning specific educational efforts. Teach the patient and family to check blood glucose levels every 4 to 6 hours as long as symptoms such as anorexia, nausea, and vomiting are present and as long as glucose levels exceed 250 mg/dL (13.8 mmol/L). Teach them to check urine ketone levels when blood glucose levels exceed 300 mg/dL (16.7 mmol/L).

Teach the patient to prevent dehydration by maintaining food and fluid intake. Unless another health problem is present that requires fluid restriction, suggest that he or she drink at least 2 L of fluid daily and increase this amount when infection is present. When nausea is present, instruct the patient to take liquids containing both glucose and electrolytes (e.g., regular sugar-sweetened soda pop, diluted fruit juice, and sports drinks [Gatorade]). Small amounts of fluid may be tolerated even when vomiting is present. When the blood glucose level is normal or elevated, the patient should take 8 to 12 ounces (240 to 360 mL) of calorie-free and caffeine-free liquids every hour while awake to prevent dehydration.

Liquids containing carbohydrate (CHO) can be taken if the patient cannot eat solid food. Ingesting at least 150 g of CHO daily reduces the risk for starvation ketosis. After consulting the primary health care provider, urge the patient to take additional rapid-acting (lispro) or short-acting (regular) insulin based on blood glucose levels.

Instruct the patient and family to consult the primary health care provider when these problems occur:

- Blood glucose exceeds 250 mg/dL (13.8 mmol/L) that does not respond to therapy.
- Ketonuria lasts for more than 24 hours.
- The patient cannot take food or fluids.
- Illness lasts more than 1 to 2 days.

Also instruct them to detect hyperglycemia by monitoring blood glucose whenever the patient is ill. Illness can result in dehydration with DKA, hyperglycemic-hyperosmolar state, or both. The sooner the patient seeks treatment, the less severe is the metabolic alteration. He or she should not omit insulin therapy during illness. Chart 64-8 lists guidelines for the ill patient.

Preventing Hyperglycemic-Hyperosmolar State (HHS). Hyperglycemic-hyperosmolar state (HHS) is a hyperosmolar (increased blood osmolarity) state caused by hyperglycemia.

👤 CHART 64-8 Patient and Family Education: Preparing for Self-Management

Sick-Day Rules

- Notify your primary health care provider that you are ill.
- Monitor your blood glucose at least every 4 hours.
- Test your urine for ketones when your blood glucose level is greater than 240 mg/dL (13.8 mmol/L).
- Continue to take insulin or other antidiabetic agents.
- To prevent dehydration, drink 8 to 12 ounces (240 to 360 mL) of sugar-free liquids every hour that you are awake. If your blood glucose level is below your target range, drink fluids that contain sugar.
- Continue to eat meals at regular times.
- If unable to tolerate solid food because of nausea, consume more easily tolerated foods or liquids equal to the carbohydrate content of your usual meal.
- Call your primary health care provider for any of these danger signals:
  - Persistent nausea and vomiting
  - Moderate or large ketones
  - Blood glucose elevation after two supplemental doses of insulin
  - High (101.5°F [38.6°C]) temperature or increasing fever; fever for more than 24 hours
- Treat symptoms (e.g., diarrhea, nausea, vomiting, fever) as directed by your primary health care provider.
- Get plenty of rest.

The processes of HHS are outlined in Fig. 64-10. Both HHS and diabetic ketoacidosis (DKA) are caused by hyperglycemia and dehydration. HHS differs from DKA in that ketone levels are absent or low and blood glucose levels are much higher. Blood glucose levels may exceed 600 mg/dL (33.3 mmol/L), and blood osmolarity may exceed 320 mOsm/L. Table 64-13 lists the differences between DKA and HHS.

HHS results from a sustained osmotic diuresis. Kidney impairment in HHS allows for extremely high blood glucose levels. As serum concentrations of glucose exceed the renal threshold, the kidney's capacity to reabsorb glucose is exceeded.

Decreased blood volume, caused by osmotic diuresis, or underlying kidney disease, common in many older patients with DM, results in further reduction of kidney function. The decreased volume further reduces glomerular filtration rate, causing the glucose level to increase. Decreased kidney PERFUSION from hypovolemia further impairs kidney function.

🧓 CONSIDERATIONS FOR OLDER ADULTS

Patient-Centered Care QSEN

HHS occurs most often in older patients with type 2 DM, many of whom are unaware they have the disease (Touhy & Jett, 2016). Mortality rates in older patients are high. The onset of HHS is slow and may not be recognized. The older patient often seeks medical attention later and is sicker than the younger patient. HHS does not occur in well-hydrated patients. Older patients are at greater risk for dehydration and HHS because of age-related changes in thirst perception, poor urine-concentrating abilities, and use of diuretics. Assess all older adults for dehydration, regardless of whether they are known to have DM.

Myocardial infarction, sepsis, pancreatitis, stroke, and some drugs (glucocorticoids, diuretics, phenytoin [Dilantin], beta blockers, and calcium channel blockers) also may cause or contribute to HHS. Central nervous system (CNS) changes range from confusion to complete coma. Unlike DKA, patients with HHS may have seizures and reversible paralysis. The

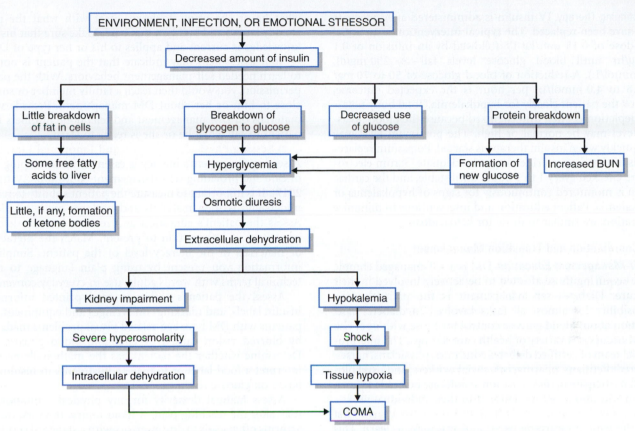

FIG. 64-10 Pathophysiologic mechanism of hyperglycemic-hyperosmolar state (HHS). *BUN,* Blood urea nitrogen.

degree of neurologic impairment is related to serum osmolarity, with coma occurring once serum osmolarity is greater than 350 mOsm/L (350 mmol/L).

The development of HHS rather than DKA is related to residual insulin secretion. In HHS, the patient secretes just enough insulin to prevent ketosis but not enough to prevent hyperglycemia. The hyperglycemia of HHS is more severe than that of DKA, greatly increasing blood osmolarity, leading to extreme diuresis with severe dehydration and electrolyte loss.

Planning: Expected Outcomes. The patient with DM is expected to have few episodes of hyperglycemia and avoid HHS. Indicators include that the patient consistently demonstrates these behaviors:

- Maintains blood glucose levels within the target range
- Uses antidiabetic drugs appropriately
- Remains well hydrated
- Describes when to seek help from health care professionals

Interventions

Monitoring. Assess for indications of HHS. (See Tables 64-11 and 64-12 for symptoms of hyperglycemia.) Continually assess fluid status.

Fluid Therapy. The expected outcomes of therapy are to rehydrate the patient and restore normal blood glucose levels within 36 to 72 hours. The choice of fluid replacement and the rate of infusion are critical in managing HHS. The severity of the CNS problems is related to the level of blood hyperosmolarity and cellular dehydration. Re-establishing fluid balance in brain cells is a difficult and slow process, and many patients do not recover baseline CNS function until hours after blood glucose levels have returned to normal.

The *first* priority for fluid replacement in HHS is to increase blood volume. In shock or severe hypotension, normal saline is used. Otherwise half-normal saline is used. Infuse fluids at 1 L/hr until central venous pressure or pulmonary capillary wedge pressure begins to rise or until blood pressure and urine output are adequate. The rate is then reduced to 100 to 200 mL/hr. Half of the estimated fluid deficit is replaced in the first 12 hours, and the rest is given over the next 36 hours. Body weight, urine output, kidney function, and the presence or absence of pulmonary congestion and jugular venous distention determine the rate of fluid infusion. In patients with heart failure, kidney disease, or acute kidney injury, monitor central venous pressure. *Assess the patient hourly for signs of cerebral edema (i.e., abrupt changes in mental status, abnormal neurologic signs, and coma).* Lack of improvement in level of consciousness may indicate inadequate rates of fluid replacement or reduction in plasma osmolarity. Regression after initial improvement may indicate a too-rapid reduction in plasma osmolarity. A slow but steady improvement in CNS function is the best evidence that fluid management is satisfactory.

❗ NURSING SAFETY PRIORITY (QSEN)

Critical Rescue

Continually monitor the patient being managed for hyperglycemic-hyperosmolar state to recognize status changes. When you notice changes in the level of consciousness; changes in pupil size, shape, or reaction; or seizures, respond by immediately notifying the primary health care provider.

Continuing Therapy. IV insulin is administered after adequate fluids have been replaced. The typical intervention is an initial bolus dose of 0.15 unit/kg IV followed by an infusion of 0.1 unit/kg/hr until blood glucose levels fall to 250 mg/dL (13.9 mmol/L). A reduction of blood glucose of 50 to 70 mg/dL (2.8 to 4.0 mmol/L) per hour is the expected outcome. Monitor the patient closely for hypokalemia. Total body potassium depletion is often unrecognized because the blood potassium level may be normal or high. The potassium level may drop quickly when insulin therapy is started. Potassium replacement is initiated once urine output is adequate. Serum electrolytes are checked every 1 to 2 hours until stable, and the cardiac rhythm is monitored continuously for signs of hypokalemia or hyperkalemia. Patient education and interventions to minimize dehydration are similar to those for ketoacidosis.

Care Coordination and Transition Management

Self-Management Education. DM is a self-managed chronic disease requiring those affected to be actively involved in their own care. Diabetes self-management is the patient's daily responsibility for almost all tasks involved in diabetes care. Education about blood glucose control for those with or at risk for DM occurs in a variety of health care settings. The interprofessional team of certified diabetes educators, physicians, nurses, registered dietitians, pharmacists, social workers, and psychologists all participate in the education. Adults are best able to learn through educational efforts tailored to their individual needs.

Assessing Learning Needs and Readiness to Learn. First assess the patient's learning needs and readiness to learn. This assessment establishes what the patient already knows and what he or she needs to know. It also helps you determine the patient's ability and desire to learn. Assess the needs of both the patient and family before teaching. Table 64-14 lists areas to include in this assessment.

Patients want information that applies directly to them. Find out what concerns the patient most about having DM, and ask what he or she wants to learn. Start with what the patient already knows and build on that base. Make sure that his or her knowledge is current and applies to his or her type of DM.

Your assessment may indicate that the patient is not ready to learn needed self-management behaviors. With the patient's permission, you would then teach a family member or someone close to him or her about DM management. Provide written materials on DM management and telephone numbers for the patient to call when he or she is ready to learn.

Assessing Physical, Cognitive, and Emotional Limitations. Assessing the patient's literacy is essential in developing a plan of care and providing self-management education (Watts et al., 2017). It is important to measure the patient's ability to read and understand written materials and perform math calculations. Assess the patient's education and reading level to determine what level of information to present. Match the literacy level of materials to the literacy level of the patient. Simplify the information you present by using plain language to replace technical terms with words adults use in everyday conversation.

Assess the patient's ability to read printed information, insulin labels, and markings on syringes and equipment. Many patients with DM have age-related visual problems made worse by blurred vision caused by changing blood glucose levels. Determine whether the patient has the math skills needed to interpret a food label or to make adjustments in insulin doses based on glucose readings.

Assess manual dexterity for any physical limitations that may alter the teaching plan. A hand injury, tremors, or severe arthritis often leads to dosing errors with a standard syringe and may require a change in insulin preparation.

Individual learning styles vary. Visual learners think in terms of pictures and remember things best by seeing something written or by seeing visual aids. Auditory learners learn best through hearing. Kinesthetic or tactile learners learn best through touching, feeling, and experiencing what they are trying to learn. Tactile learners remember best by writing or physically manipulating the equipment. Successful self-management education provides written handouts, discusses steps involved in a procedure such as insulin administration or self-monitoring of blood glucose (SMBG), and encourages the learner to touch and manipulate equipment. Confirm that the patient understands your instructions by using "teach-back" techniques.

Tailor educational sessions to the time available and to the condition of the patient. Hospitalized adults require only basic education when they are acutely ill. In these situations, it is appropriate to teach basic survival skills or focused problem-solving skills while reserving more detailed education for follow-up sessions.

Survival Skills Information. The initial phase of education involves teaching information necessary for the survival of any adult diagnosed with DM. Survival information includes:

- Simple information on pathophysiology of DM
- Learning how to prepare and administer insulin or how to take other antidiabetic drugs
- Recognition, treatment, and prevention of hypoglycemia and hyperglycemia
- Basic diet information
- Monitoring of blood glucose and urine ketones
- Sick-day management rules
- Where to buy DM supplies and how to store them
- When and how to notify the primary health care provider

TABLE 64-14   Assessment of Learning Needs for the Patient With Diabetes

- Health and medical history
- Nutrition history and practices
- Physical activity and exercise behaviors
- Prescription and over-the-counter medications and complementary and integrative therapies and practices
- Factors that influence learning such as education and literacy levels, perceived learning needs, motivation to learn, and health beliefs
- Diabetes self-management behaviors, including experience with self-adjusting the treatment plan
- Previous diabetes self-management training, actual knowledge, and skills
- Physical factors, including age, mobility, visual acuity, hearing, manual dexterity, alertness, attention span, and ability to concentrate or special needs or limitations requiring adaptive support and use of alternative skills
- Psychosocial concerns, factors, or issues, including family and social support
- Current mental health status
- History of substance use, including alcohol, tobacco, and recreational drugs
- Occupation, vocation, education level, financial status, and social, cultural, and religious practices
- Access to and use of health care resources

In-Depth Education. In-depth education and counseling involve teaching more detailed information about survival skills and actions for avoiding long-term complications. Educational sessions with patient and family are needed to "patientize" the DM regimen for their needs and abilities.

The adult with DM needs to understand the disease pathology. He or she must be able to discuss the action of insulin and the effects of insulin deficiency and to explain the effects of diet, drugs, and activity on blood glucose. The patient should be able to relate maintaining normal blood glucose levels to preventing complications. This includes relating changes in glucose level to the possible need for a change in insulin dosage.

Provide education about the symptoms of hypoglycemia along with the prescribed treatment options if the patient takes any drugs that will lower blood glucose levels. Educate patients and their families about common causes of hypoglycemia such as changes in drug regimen, increase in physical activity, and delayed or missed meals. Review indications of hypoglycemia at each visit. Advise patients to check their blood glucose levels before driving and to make sure they have easy-to-reach snacks and/or fast-acting sugars with them at all times. Encourage them to always wear a medical ID tag or bracelet and to contact their primary health care provider if they experience low blood glucose levels more than twice a week.

Many patients require combination drug therapy to achieve glucose control in addition to aspirin and drugs for lowering lipids and blood pressure. If the patient takes an antidiabetic drug, ask him or her to identify the drug and describe the prescribed schedule. Determine if the patient is able to administer insulin or other injectable antidiabetic drugs accurately by having him or her demonstrate injection techniques. Ask the patient to discuss the onset, peak, and duration of the insulin used. The patient must be able to state when insulin is to be injected, where it is injected, and how it is stored. Review formulas for self-adjustment in insulin (when supported by the primary health care provider), and explain blood glucose monitoring requirements needed to evaluate the effects of additional insulin. Stress the dangers of skipping doses. Review drug interactions, especially with older patients taking oral antidiabetic drugs.

Teach patients receiving diet therapy alone, glucose-lowering drugs, or fixed insulin doses to eat the consistent amounts of carbohydrate (CHO) at meals and snacks. Patients who adjust mealtime doses of insulin or those on insulin pump therapy can be taught to match their insulin dose to the CHO content of their diet. The patient needs to understand what to eat, how much to eat, and when to eat. Stress the importance of eating on time, the dangers of skipping meals, and how to maintain food intake during illness. Ask the patient to describe the meal plan and explain the adjustments needed to meet diabetic diet requirements. Include the family member usually responsible for buying groceries and preparing meals in this teaching.

Regular physical activity is important for physical fitness, weight management, and blood glucose control. Help all patients identify activities they can do to achieve the goal of moderate-intensity activity 3 or more days a week. For patients taking insulin and/or insulin secretagogues, physical activity can cause hypoglycemia if carbohydrate intake isn't increased. Review how to perform physical activities safely. Instruct the patient on blood glucose levels that are safe for exercise, the frequency of glucose monitoring during exercise, drug adjustments before exercise, food required before exercise, and what food to have available during exercise. He or she should be aware of the risk for injury during exercise and be able to explain the importance of protective footwear.

Self-monitoring of blood glucose (SMBG) provides immediate information on a patient's blood glucose level and provides feedback on the effects of recent activity, drugs, and meals. The nurse's role includes teaching skills of performing the test, educating how to interpret results, and problem solving to adjust behaviors and therapy based on the information. Teach patients how to recognize when blood glucose levels are out of range, how to adjust therapy and behaviors based on SMBG results, and how to verify the effects of these adjustments by performing subsequent glucose testing. In addition, show patients who use insulin how to use SMBG to adjust dosages to achieve glucose control while avoiding episodes of hypoglycemia.

Teach patients sick-day procedures when initially diagnosed with DM. Hyperglycemia often develops before infection symptoms and can serve as a warning sign that infection is developing. Provide guidelines for the frequency of glucose testing, ketone testing, and insulin adjustment for those patients able to self-adjust insulin doses.

Psychosocial Preparation. The diagnosis of DM may represent a loss of control and flexibility. Life becomes ordered, and routines must be followed. Some events surrounding DM are predictable. Injecting insulin and not eating for several hours causes hypoglycemia. Poorly controlled DM leads to complications and premature death. Tight control of blood glucose prevents complications.

The stress of DM is in addition to the demands of normal daily life. The patient must be able to integrate the demands of DM into daily schedules while keeping blood glucose stable.

Patients are more likely to adhere to disease management activities when the strategies make sense and seem effective. Other factors promoting adherence include the patient's belief that the activity is important, having confidence in himself or herself, and having support. Assist in healthy psychological adaptation to DM by providing successful educational experiences. Mastery of blood glucose monitoring helps the patient feel control over the disease. Knowing the effects of extra activities, extra food, or extra insulin is helpful in learning to adjust the regimen.

Feeling a sense of control over the condition promotes a positive attitude about DM. Success in injecting insulin provides concrete evidence that he or she can master the disease. Teach by breaking a task into small, achievable units to ensure mastery. For example, a patient may begin learning how to inject insulin by first obtaining an accurate dose.

Devote as much teaching time as possible to insulin injection and blood glucose monitoring. Patients with newly diagnosed DM may fear giving themselves injections. After this technique is mastered, he or she may be less anxious and more able to attend to other tasks.

Recognize that not everyone will adapt to DM. Some patients are unable to progress beyond the survival level. Major depression affects many patients, having an impact on quality of life and all aspects of functioning, including self-management behaviors. Refer those who have significant problems coping with the day-to-day demands of DM to mental health counseling for appropriate treatment.

Home Care Management. Patients with DM self-manage their disease. Each day they decide what to eat, whether to exercise, and whether to take prescribed drugs. Maintaining blood

CHART 64-9 Focused Assessment

The Insulin-Dependent Patient With Diabetes During a Home or Clinic Visit

- Assess overall mental status, wakefulness, ability to converse.
- Take vital signs and weight:
  - Fever could indicate infection.
  - Are blood pressure and weight within target range? If not, why?
- Question patient regarding any change in visual acuity; check current visual acuity.
- Inspect oral mucous membranes, gums, and teeth.
- Question patient about injection areas used; inspect areas being used; assess whether patient is using areas and sites appropriately.
- Inspect skin for intactness, wounds that have not healed, new sores, ulcers, bruises, or burns; assess any previously known wounds for infection, progression of healing.
- Question patient regarding foot care.
- Assess lower extremities and feet for peripheral pulses, lack of or decreased sensation, abnormal sensations, breaks in skin integrity, condition of toes and nails.
- Question patient regarding color and consistency of stools and frequency of bowel movements; assess abdomen for bowel sounds.
- Review patient's home health diary:
  - Is blood glucose within targeted range? If not, why?
  - Is glucose monitoring being recorded often enough?
  - Is the patient's food intake adequate and appropriate? If not, why?
  - Is exercise occurring regularly? If not, why?
- Assess patient's ability to perform self-monitoring of blood glucose.
- Assess patient's procedures for obtaining and storing insulin and syringes, cleaning equipment, disposing of syringes and needles.
- Assess patient's insulin preparation and injection technique.
- Assess patient's knowledge of antidiabetic drug regimen and for which side effects to look.

TABLE 64-15 Outcome Criteria for Diabetes Teaching

Before self-management begins to home, the patient with diabetes or the significant other should be able to:
- Tell why insulin or a noninsulin antidiabetic drug is being prescribed
- Name which insulin or noninsulin antidiabetic drug is being prescribed, and name the dosage and frequency of administration
- Discuss the relationship between mealtime and the action of insulin or the other antidiabetic agent
- Discuss plans to follow diabetic diet instructions
- Prepare and administer insulin accurately
- Test blood for glucose or state plans for having blood glucose levels monitored
- Test urine for ketones and state when this test should be done
- Describe how to store insulin
- List symptoms that indicate a hypoglycemic reaction
- Tell which carbohydrate sources are used to treat hypoglycemic reactions
- Tell which symptoms indicate hyperglycemia
- Tell which dietary changes are needed during illness
- State when to call the primary health care provider or the nurse (frequent episodes of hypoglycemia, symptoms of hyperglycemia)
- Describe the procedures for proper foot care

◆ *Evaluation: Reflection*

Evaluate the care of the patient with DM based on the identified priority patient problems. Outcome success for diabetes education is the ability of the patient to maintain blood glucose levels within their established target range. General outcome criteria are listed below and in Table 64-15. The expected outcomes include that the patient should:

- Achieve blood glucose control
- Avoid acute and chronic complications of diabetes
- Avoid injury
- Experience relief of pain
- Maintain optimal vision
- Maintain a urine output in the expected range
- Have an optimal level of mental status functioning
- Have decreased episodes of hypoglycemia
- Have decreased episodes of hyperglycemia

glucose control depends on the accuracy of self-management skills. The role of the nurse is to provide support and education and to empower the patient to make informed decisions. Self-management education allows patients to identify their problems and provides techniques to help them make decisions, take appropriate actions, and alter these actions as needed.

Provide information about resources. The patient must know whom to contact in case of emergency. Older adults who live alone need to have daily telephone contact with a friend or neighbor. The patient may also need help shopping and preparing meals. He or she may have limited access to transportation and may not have sufficient supplies of food, particularly in bad weather. Because of the likelihood of visual problems in older patients, they may need help in preparing insulin syringes for injection or in monitoring blood glucose. Make referrals to home care or public health agencies as needed. Chart 64-9 identifies areas for assessment during a home or clinic visit.

GET READY FOR THE NCLEX® EXAMINATION!

KEY POINTS

Review these key points for each NCLEX Examination Client Needs Category.

Safe and Effective Care Environment

- Use aseptic technique during any invasive procedure when caring for a patient with diabetes. **QSEN: Safety**

- Administer antidiabetic drugs and insulin in a safe manner. **QSEN: Safety**
- Ensure that meals are available with or immediately after the patient receives an antidiabetic drug or insulin. **QSEN: Safety**
- Use good handwashing techniques before providing any care to a patient with diabetes. **QSEN: Safety**

- Collaborate with the primary health care provider, diabetes nurse educator, registered dietitian, pharmacist, social worker, and case manager to individualize patient care for the adult with diabetes in any care setting. **QSEN: Patient-Centered Care**
- Never dilute or mix insulin glargine with any other insulin or solution. **QSEN: Safety**
- Avoid injecting insulin within a 2-inch radius of the umbilicus. **QSEN: Evidence-Based Practice**
- Reinforce to all patients with diabetes that tight control over blood glucose levels reduces the risk for the vascular complications of diabetes. **QSEN: Evidence-Based Practice**
- Instruct the patient and family about complications and when to seek assistance. **QSEN: Safety**
- Assess patients' visual acuity and peripheral tactile sensation to determine needed adjustments in teaching self-medication and self-monitoring of blood glucose levels. **QSEN: Safety**
- Teach patients with peripheral neuropathy to use a bath thermometer to test water for bathing, to avoid walking barefoot, and to inspect their feet daily. **QSEN: Safety**
- Teach the patient and family about the symptoms of infection and when to seek medical advice. **QSEN: Safety**
- Instruct patients with diabetes to wear a medical alert bracelet. **QSEN: Safety**
- Instruct patients to not share blood glucose monitoring equipment. **QSEN: Safety**
- Teach patients to rotate insulin injection sites within one area rather than to other areas, to prevent changes in absorption. **QSEN: Evidence-Based Practice**
- Teach patients who experience Somogyi phenomenon (early morning hyperglycemia) to ensure an adequate dietary intake at bedtime. **QSEN: Evidence-Based Practice**
- Instruct patients to always carry a glucose source. **QSEN: Safety**
- Teach patients who exercise to test urine for ketone bodies if blood glucose levels are greater than 250 mg/dL before engaging in strenuous exercise. **QSEN: Safety**

Health Promotion and Maintenance

- Encourage all patients to maintain weight within an appropriate range. **QSEN: Patient-Centered Care**
- Encourage patients with diabetes, to participate regularly in exercise or physical activity appropriate to their health status. **QSEN: Evidence-Based Practice**
- Instruct all patients with diabetes to avoid becoming dehydrated and to drink at least 2 L of water each day unless another medical condition requires fluid restriction. **QSEN: Patient-Centered Care**
- Refer patients newly diagnosed with diabetes to local resources and support groups. **QSEN: Patient-Centered Care**
- Remind patients with diabetes to have yearly eye examinations by an ophthalmologist. **QSEN: Evidence-Based Practice**
- Instruct patients in foot care as outlined in Chart 64-6.

Psychosocial Integrity

- Explore with the patient what the diagnosis of diabetes means to him or her. **QSEN: Patient-Centered Care**
- Allow the patient the opportunity to express concerns about the diagnosis of diabetes or the treatment regimen. **QSEN: Patient-Centered Care**
- Pace your education sessions to match the learning needs and style of the patient. **QSEN: Patient-Centered Care**
- Urge patients newly diagnosed with DM to attend diabetes education classes to become a fully engaged partner in management of the disease. **QSEN: Patient-Centered Care**

Physiological Integrity

- Help patients who have pain from peripheral neuropathy determine which pain-relieving drugs and techniques work best for them. **QSEN: Patient-Centered Care**
- Assess the patient's hemoglobin A1C for indications of adherence to prescribed regimens and their effectiveness. **QSEN: Evidence-Based Practice**
- Explain all procedures, restrictions, drugs, and follow-up care to the patient and family. **QSEN: Patient-Centered Care**
- Use return demonstration with "teach-back" strategies when teaching the patient about drug regimen, insulin injection, blood glucose monitoring, and foot assessment. **QSEN: Patient-Centered Care**
- Teach patients to administer an accurate dose of insulin using a prefilled or disposable insulin pen. **QSEN: Patient-Centered Care**
- Instruct patients who are taking sulfonylurea drugs about an increased risk for hypoglycemic reactions. **QSEN: Patient-Centered Care**
- Teach patients who are taking metformin the symptoms of lactic acidosis (fatigue, dizziness, difficulty breathing, stomach discomfort, irregular heartbeat). **QSEN: Patient-Centered Care**
- Warn patients to not take over-the-counter drugs with their oral antidiabetic drugs without consulting their primary care provider. **QSEN: Patient-Centered Care**
- Start carbohydrate replacement per the primary health care provider's prescription or standing protocols immediately on identifying a patient with hypoglycemia. **QSEN: Evidence-Based Practice**
- Give glucagon subcutaneously or IM and 50% dextrose IV to patients identified with hypoglycemia who cannot swallow. **QSEN: Evidence-Based Practice**
- First assess the airway, level of consciousness, hydration status, electrolytes, and blood glucose level of any patient with diabetic ketoacidosis. **QSEN: Evidence-Based Practice**
- Use blood glucose values to assess therapy effectiveness and determine when to switch from saline to dextrose-containing solutions in a patient with diabetic ketoacidosis. **QSEN: Evidence-Based Practice**
- Continually assess fluid status and level of consciousness in a patient with hyperglycemic-hyperosmolar state (HHS) during the resuscitation period. **QSEN: Evidence-Based Practice**
- Immediately report indications of cerebral edema (abrupt changes in mental status; changes in level of consciousness; changes in pupil size, shape, or reaction; seizures) in a patient with HHS to the primary health care provider. **QSEN: Patient-Centered Care**

SELECTED BIBLIOGRAPHY

Akindana, A., & Ogunedo, C. (2015). Managing type 2 diabetes in black patients. *The Nurse Practitioner, 40*(9), 20–27.

American Association of Diabetes Educators (AADE). (2015). *AADE position statement: Diabetes and physical activity*. www.diabetese-ducator.org/docs/default-source/default-document-library/dia-betes-and-physical-activity2f6fd636a05f68739c53ff0000b8561d.pdf?sfvrsn=0.

American Diabetes Association (ADA). (2014a). Diabetic retinopathy and other ocular findings in the Diabetes Control and Complications Trial/Epidemiology of Diabetes Interventions and Complications Study. *Diabetes Care, 37*(1), 17–23.

American Diabetes Association (ADA). (2014b). Kidney disease and related findings in the Diabetes Control and Complications Trial/Epidemiology of Diabetes Interventions and Complications Study. *Diabetes Care, 37*(1), 24–30.

American Diabetes Association (ADA). (2016). Intensive diabetes treatment and cardiovascular outcomes in type 1 diabetes: The DCCT/EDIC study 30-year follow-up. *Diabetes Care, 39*(5), 686–693.

American Diabetes Association (ADA). (2017a). Standards of medical care in diabetes—2017: Cardiac disease and risk management. *Diabetes Care, 40*(Suppl. 1), S75–S87.

American Diabetes Association (ADA). (2017b). Standards of medical care in diabetes—2017: Classification and diagnosis of diabetes. *Diabetes Care, 40*(Suppl. 1), S11–S24.

American Diabetes Association (ADA). (2017c). Standards of medical care in diabetes—-2017: Comprehensive medical evaluation and assessment of comorbidities. *Diabetes Care, 40*(Suppl. 1), S25–S32.

American Diabetes Association (ADA). (2017d). Standards of medical care in diabetes—2017: Glycemic targets. *Diabetes Care, 40*(Suppl. 1), S48–S56.

American Diabetes Association (ADA). (2017e). Standards of medical care in diabetes—2017: Management of diabetes in pregnancy. *Diabetes Care, 40*(Suppl. 1), S114–S119.

American Diabetes Association (ADA). (2017f). Standards of medical care in diabetes—2017: Microvascular complications and foot care. *Diabetes Care, 40*(Suppl. 1), S88–S98.

American Diabetes Association (ADA). (2017g). Standards of medical care in diabetes—2017: Obesity management for the treatment of type 2 diabetes. *Diabetes Care, 40*(Suppl. 1), S57–S63.

American Diabetes Association (ADA). (2017h). Standards of medical care in diabetes—2017: Older adults. *Diabetes Care, 40*(Suppl. 1), S99–S104.

American Diabetes Association (ADA). (2017i). Standards of medical care in diabetes—2017: Pharmacologic approaches to glycemic treatment. *Diabetes Care, 40*(Suppl. 1), S64–S74.

American Diabetes Association (ADA). (2017j). Standards of medical care in diabetes—2017: Prevention or delay of type 2 diabetes. *Diabetes Care, 40*(Suppl. 1), S44–S47.

Aschenbrenner, D. (2015). Ketoacidosis possible from some type 2 diabetes drugs. *American Journal of Nursing, 115*(9), 22–23.

Aschenbrenner, D. (2017). Diabetes drug receives new indication. *American Journal of Nursing, 117*(4), 24–25.

Burchum, J., & Rosenthal, L. (2016). *Lehne's pharmacology for nursing care* (9th ed.). St. Louis: Elsevier.

Centers for Disease Control and Prevention (CDC). (2015). *2014 National diabetes statistics report*. http://www.cdc.gov/diabetes/data/statistics/2014StatisticsReport.html.

Centers for Disease Control and Prevention (CDC). (2016). *Chronic disease prevention and health promotion: Diabetes at a glance*. http://www.cdc.gov/chronicdisease/resources/publications/aag/diabetes.htm.

Engle, M., Fergusin, A., & Fields, W. (2016). A journey to improved inpatient glycemic control by redesigning meal delivery and insulin administration. *Clinical Nurse Specialist, 30*(2), 117–124.

Frank, M., & Gerhardt, A. (2015). Treating dyslipidemia in patients with type 2 diabetes mellitus. *The Nurse Practitioner, 40*(8), 18–22.

Frazer, C. (2015). Metabolic syndrome. *Medsurg Nursing, 24*(2), 125–126.

Freeland, B., & Farber, M. (2015). Type 2 diabetes drugs: A review. *Home Healthcare Now, 33*(6), 304–310.

Giddens, J. F. (2017). *Concepts for nursing practice* (2nd ed.). St. Louis: Elsevier.

Greenwood, D. (2015). Better type 2 diabetes self-management using paired testing and remote monitoring. *American Journal of Nursing, 115*(2), 58–65.

Jarvis, C. (2016). *Physical examination & health assessment* (7th ed.). St. Louis: Elsevier.

Kidney Foundation of Canada. (2015). *Facing the facts 2015*. From: www.kidney.ca/file/Facing-the-Facts-2015-infographic-portrait.pdf.

Lampe, J. (2015). Boost your confidence in caring for patients with insulin pumps. *American Nurse Today, 10*(8), 1–8.

McCance, K., Huether, S., Brashers, V., & Rote, N. (2014). *Pathophysiology: The biologic basis for disease in adults and children* (7th ed.). St. Louis: Mosby.

Moran, K., & Burson, R. (2015). Exercise and diabetes. *Home Healthcare Now, 33*(4), 226–227.

National Institute of Diabetes and Digestive and Kidney Diseases (NIDDKD) of the National Institutes of Health. (2014). *National Diabetes Information Clearing House: National diabetes statistics, 2014*. http://www.cdc.gov/diabetes/pubs/statsreport14/national-diabetes-report-web.pdf.

Nwankwo, R., & Funnell, M. (2016). What's new in nutrition for adults with diabetes? *Nursing, 46*(3), 28–33.

Pagana, K., Pagana, T., & Pike-MacDonald, S. (2013). *Mosby's Canadian manual of diagnostic and laboratory tests*. St. Louis: Mosby.

Pagana, K., Pagana, T. J., & Pagana, T. N. (2017). *Mosby's diagnostic and laboratory test reference* (13th ed.). St. Louis: Mosby.

Paparella, S. (2015). Insulin pens: Single patient use is mandatory for safety. *Journal of Emergency Nursing, 41*(4), 340–342.

Sanuth, B., Bidlencik, A., & Volk, A. (2014). Management of acute hyperglycemic emergencies: Focus on diabetic ketoacidosis. *AACN Advanced Critical Care, 25*(3), 314–324.

Se, S., & Tucher, K. (2015). Hypoglycemia prevention: An innovative approach. *Nursing, 45*(6), 19–22.

Statistics Canada. (2015). *Health: All subtopics for health—Diabetes by age-group and sex*. http://www.statcan.gc.ca/tables-tableaux/sum-som/l01/cst01/health53a-eng.htm.

The Joint Commission (TJC). (2016). *Advanced certification in inpatient diabetes*. https://www.jointcommission.org/certification/inpatient_diabetes.aspx.

Touhy, T., & Jett, K. (2016). *Ebersole & Hess' Toward healthy aging* (9th ed.). St. Louis: Mosby.

U.S. Department of Health and Human Services (USDHHS). (2015). *Organ Procurement and Transplantation Network*. Retrieved from: http://optn.transplant.hrsa.gov/data/view-data-reports/.

United States Department of Veterans Affairs. (2016). *Diabetes type 2 and agent orange*. http://www.publichealth.va.gov/exposures/agentorange/conditions/diabetes.asp.

Watts, S., & Howard, J. (2016). Prediabetes: What nurses need to know. *American Journal of Nursing, 116*(7), 54–58.

Watts, S., Stevenson, C., & Adams, M. (2017). Improving health literacy in patients with diabetes. *Nursing, 47*(1), 25–31.

Zimmer, P., Braun, L., Fraser, R., Hecht, L., & Kelliher, F. (2015). Promoting success in self-injection: Listening to patients. *Medsurg Nursing, 24*(4), 279–285.

CHAPTER **65**

Assessment of the Renal/Urinary System

Chris Winkelman

 http://evolve.elsevier.com/Iggy/

PRIORITY AND INTERRELATED CONCEPTS

The priority concept for this chapter is ELIMINATION.

The interrelated concepts for this chapter are:
• FLUID AND ELECTROLYTE BALANCE
• ACID-BASE BALANCE

LEARNING OUTCOMES

Safe and Effective Care Environment

1. Collaborate with the interprofessional team to perform a complete urinary and renal system assessment, including ELIMINATION, FLUID AND ELECTROLYTE BALANCE, and ACID-BASE BALANCE.
2. Protect the patient, yourself, and others from injury and infection during assessment of the renal and urinary systems.

Health Promotion and Maintenance

3. Explain how physiologic changes of the urinary/renal system affect ELIMINATION and the associated care of older adults.

Psychosocial Integrity

4. Implement patient-centered nursing interventions to help patients and families cope with the psychosocial impact caused by a urinary ELIMINATION health problem.

Physiological Integrity

5. Apply knowledge of anatomy and physiology to perform an evidence-based assessment for the patient with a urinary ELIMINATION health problem.
6. Interpret assessment findings for the patient with a urinary or renal system health problem.
7. Teach the patient and caregivers about diagnostic procedures associated with assessment of kidney and urinary health problems.

The kidneys and urinary tract together make up the renal system, which is responsible for urine elimination. The concept of **ELIMINATION** is the excretion of waste from the body by the GI tract (as feces) and by the kidneys (as urine). See Chapter 2 for a summary overview of the concept of elimination and how it relates to the concepts of FLUID AND ELECTROLYTE BALANCE and ACID-BASE BALANCE.

The urinary tract includes the ureters, bladder, and urethra. It is the drainage route for the excretion of urine. The kidneys filter fluids and small compounds from the blood for elimination of waste. Structural or functional problems in the kidneys or urinary tract may alter FLUID AND ELECTROLYTE BALANCE and ACID-BASE BALANCE.

The kidneys help maintain health in many ways. *Most important, they maintain body fluid volume and composition and create urine for waste* ELIMINATION. The kidneys also help adjust blood pressure, regulate ACID-BASE BALANCE, produce erythropoietin for red blood cell (RBC) synthesis, and convert vitamin D to an active form.

Assessment of the patient at risk for or with actual problems of the kidneys or urinary system begins with a history and physical assessment. Understanding the anatomy, physiology, and diagnostic tests of the renal system helps you problem solve about kidney and urinary tract function in the clinical setting. It also helps you teach the patient about the purpose of procedures and physically and emotionally prepare the patient for assessment.

ANATOMY AND PHYSIOLOGY REVIEW

Kidneys

Structure

Gross Anatomy. The two kidneys are located behind the peritoneum, not in the abdominal cavity, one on either side of the spine (Fig. 65-1). The adult kidney is 4 to 5 inches (10 to 13 cm) long, 2 to 3 inches (5 to 7 cm) wide, and about 1 inch (2.5 to 3 cm) thick. The left kidney is slightly longer and narrower than the right kidney. Larger-than-usual kidneys may indicate obstruction or polycystic disease. Smaller-than-usual kidneys may indicate chronic kidney disease (CKD).

Variation in kidney shape and number is relatively common and does not always indicate a problem in kidney function. Some adults have more than two kidneys or may have only one large, horseshoe-shaped kidney. As long as tests of kidney function are normal, these variations are of no significance (Brenner, 2016).

Several layers of tissue surround the kidney, providing protection and support. The outer surface of the kidney is a layer of fibrous tissue called the *capsule* (Fig. 65-2). It covers most of the kidney except the *hilum*, which is the indented area where the kidney blood vessels and nerves enter and exit. It is also where the ureter exits. The capsule is surrounded by layers of fat and connective tissue.

Lying beneath the capsule are the two layers of functional kidney tissue: the cortex and the medulla. The *renal cortex* is the outer tissue layer. The *medulla* is the medullary tissue lying below the cortex in the shape of many fans. Each "fan" is called a pyramid. The *renal columns* are cortical tissue that dips down into the interior of the kidney and separates the pyramids.

The tip of each pyramid is called a *papilla*. The papillae drain urine into the collecting system. A cuplike structure called a *calyx* collects the urine at the end of each papilla. The calices join together to form the *renal pelvis,* which narrows to become the ureter.

The kidneys have a rich blood supply and receive a blood flow from 600 to 1300 mL/min. The blood supply to each kidney comes from the renal artery, which branches from the abdominal aorta. The renal artery divides into progressively smaller arteries, supplying all blood to areas of the kidney tissue and the nephrons. The smallest arteries *(afferent arterioles)* feed the nephrons directly to form urine.

Venous blood from the kidneys starts with the capillaries surrounding each nephron. These capillaries drain into

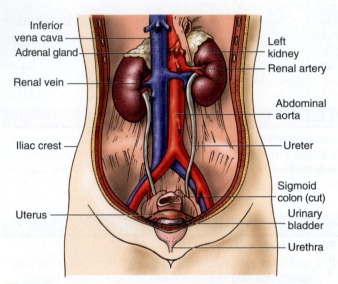

FIG. 65-1 Anatomic location of the kidneys and structures of the urinary system.

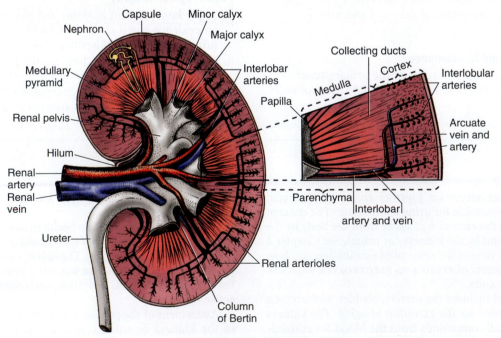

FIG. 65-2 Bisection of the kidney showing the major structures of the kidney.

progressively larger veins, with blood eventually returned to the inferior vena cava through the renal vein.

Microscopic Anatomy. The **nephron** is the functional unit of the kidney and forms urine by filtering waste products and water from the blood. There are about 1 million nephrons per kidney, and each nephron separately performs filtration and makes urine from blood.

There are two types of nephrons: *cortical nephrons* and *juxtamedullary nephrons.* The cortical nephrons are short and lie totally within the renal cortex. The juxtamedullary nephrons (about 20% of all nephrons) are longer, and their tubes and blood vessels dip deeply into the medulla. The purpose of these nephrons is to concentrate urine during times of low fluid intake to allow continued excretion of body waste with less fluid loss (McCance et al., 2014).

Blood supply to the nephron is delivered through the *afferent arteriole* (i.e., the smallest, most distal portion of the renal arterial system). From the afferent arteriole, blood flows into the *glomerulus,* which is a series of specialized capillary loops. It is through these capillaries that water and small particles are filtered from the blood to make urine. The remaining blood leaves the glomerulus through the *efferent arteriole,* which is the first vessel in the kidney's venous system. From the efferent arteriole, blood exits into either the *peritubular capillaries* around the tube of the cortical nephrons or the *vasa recta* around the tube of juxtamedullary nephrons.

Each nephron is a tubelike structure with distinct parts (Fig. 65-3). The tube begins with Bowman's capsule, a saclike structure that surrounds the glomerulus. The tubular tissue of Bowman's capsule narrows into the *proximal convoluted tubule (PCT).* The PCT twists and turns, finally straightening into the descending limb of the *loop of Henle.* The descending loop of Henle dips in the direction of the medulla but forms a hairpin

loop and comes back up into the cortex as the ascending loop of Henle.

The two segments of the ascending limb of the loop of Henle are the thin segment and the thick segment. The *distal convoluted tubule (DCT)* forms from the thick segment of the ascending limb of the loop of Henle. The DCT ends in one of many collecting ducts located in the kidney tissue. The urine in the collecting ducts passes through the papillae and empties into the renal pelvis.

Special cells in the afferent arteriole, efferent arteriole, and DCT are known as the *juxtaglomerular complex* (Fig. 65-4). These cells produce *renin,* which is a hormone that helps regulate blood flow, glomerular filtration rate (GFR), and blood pressure. Renin is secreted when sensing cells in the DCT (called the *macula densa*) sense changes in blood volume and pressure. The macula densa touches the renin-producing cells. Renin is produced when the macula densa cells sense that blood volume, blood pressure, or blood sodium level is low. Renin then converts renin substrate (angiotensinogen) into angiotensin I. This leads to a series of reactions that cause secretion of the hormone aldosterone (Fig. 65-5). Aldosterone increases kidney reabsorption of sodium and water, restoring blood pressure, blood volume, and blood sodium levels (McCance et al., 2014). It also promotes excretion of potassium (see Chapter 11).

The glomerular capillary wall has three layers (Fig. 65-6): the endothelium, the basement membrane, and the epithelium. The endothelial and epithelial cells lining these capillaries are separated by pores that filter water and small particles from the blood into Bowman's capsule. This fluid is called the *filtrate.*

Function

The kidneys have both regulatory and hormonal functions. The regulatory functions control FLUID AND ELECTROLYTE BALANCE and ACID-BASE BALANCE. The hormonal functions control red blood cell (RBC) formation, blood pressure, and vitamin D activation.

Regulatory Functions. The kidney processes that maintain FLUID AND ELECTROLYTE BALANCE and ACID-BASE BALANCE through urine ELIMINATION are glomerular filtration, tubular reabsorption, and tubular secretion. These processes use

FIG. 65-3 Anatomy of the nephron—the functional unit of the kidney. The differences in appearance in tubular cells seen in a cross section reflect the differing functions of each nephron segment. Note that the particular nephron labeled here is a juxtamedullary nephron. (From Patton, K.T., & Thibodeau, G.A. [2018]. *The human body in health & disease* [7th ed.]. St. Louis: Mosby.)

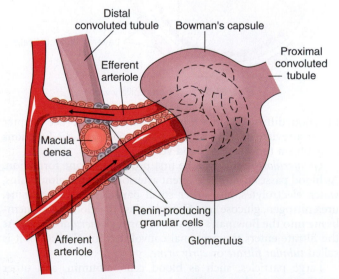

FIG. 65-4 Juxtaglomerular complex showing juxtaglomerular cells and the macula densa.

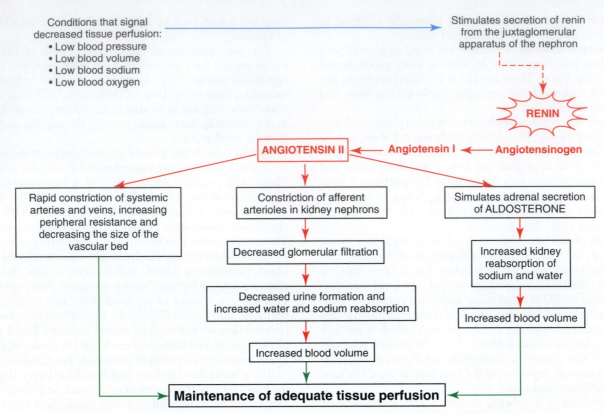

FIG. 65-5 Role of aldosterone, renin substrate (angiotensinogen), angiotensin I, and angiotensin II in the renal regulation of water and sodium.

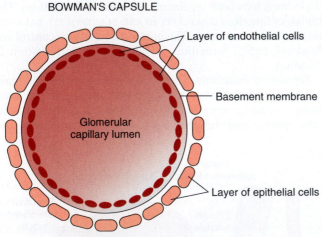

FIG. 65-6 Glomerular capillary wall.

filtration, diffusion, active transport, and osmosis. (See Chapter 11 for a review of these actions.) Table 65-1 lists the functions of nephron tubules and blood vessels.

Glomerular filtration is the first process in urine formation. As blood passes from the afferent arteriole into the glomerulus, water, electrolytes, and other small particles (e.g., creatinine, urea nitrogen, glucose) are filtered across the glomerular membrane into the Bowman's capsule to form *glomerular* filtrate. As the filtrate enters the proximal convoluted tubule (PCT), it is called *tubular filtrate* or *early urine.*

Large particles, such as blood cells, albumin, and other proteins, are too large to filter through the glomerular capillary walls. *Therefore these substances are not normally present in the excreted final urine.*

Filtration rate is expressed in milliliters per minute. Normal glomerular filtration rate (GFR) averages 125 mL/min, totaling about 180 L daily. If the entire amount of filtrate were excreted as urine, death would occur from dehydration. Actually, only about 1 to 3 L is excreted each day as urine. The rest is reabsorbed back into the blood (McCance et al., 2014).

GFR is controlled by blood pressure and blood flow. The kidneys self-regulate their own blood pressure and blood flow, which keeps GFR constant. GFR is controlled by selectively constricting and dilating the afferent and efferent arterioles. When the afferent arteriole is constricted or the efferent arteriole is dilated, pressure in the glomerular capillaries falls, and filtration decreases. When the afferent arteriole is dilated or the efferent arteriole is constricted, pressure in the glomerular capillaries rises, and filtration increases. This way the kidney maintains a constant GFR, even when systemic blood pressure changes. When systolic pressure drops below 65 to 70 mm Hg, these self-regulation processes do not maintain GFR.

Tubular reabsorption is the second process in urine formation. Tubular reabsorption of most of the filtrate (early urine) keeps normal urine output at 1 to 3 L/day and prevents dehydration. As the filtrate passes through the tubular parts of the nephron, water and electrolytes are reabsorbed from the tubular lumen of the nephron and into the peritubular capillaries. This process returns much of the water, electrolytes, and other particles to the blood.

The tubules return about 99% of filtered water back into the body (Fig. 65-7). Most water reabsorption occurs in the proximal convoluted tubule (PCT). Water reabsorption continues as the filtrate flows down the descending loop of Henle. The thin and thick segments of the ascending loop of Henle are *not* permeable to water, and no water reabsorption occurs here.

TABLE 65-1   Vascular and Tubular Components of the Nephron

STRUCTURE	ANATOMIC FEATURES	PHYSIOLOGIC ASPECTS
Vascular Components		
Afferent arteriole	Delivers arterial blood from the branches of the renal artery into the glomerulus	Autoregulation of renal blood flow via vasoconstriction or vasodilation Renin-producing granular cells
Glomerulus	Capillary loops with thin, semipermeable membrane	Site of glomerular filtration Glomerular filtration occurs when hydrostatic pressure (blood pressure) is greater than opposing forces (tubular filtrate and oncotic pressure)
Efferent arteriole	Delivers arterial blood from the glomerulus into the peritubular capillaries or the vasa recta	Autoregulation of renal blood flow via vasoconstriction or vasodilation Renin-producing granular cells
Peritubular capillaries (PTCs) and vasa recta (VR)	PTCs: surround tubular components of cortical nephrons VR: surround tubular components of juxtamedullary nephrons	Tubular reabsorption and tubular secretion allow movement of water and solutes to or from the tubules, interstitium, and blood
Tubular Components		
Bowman's capsule (BC)	Thin membranous sac surrounding $\frac{7}{8}$ of the glomerulus	Collects glomerular filtrate (GF) and funnels it into the tubule
Proximal convoluted tubule (PCT)	Evolves from and is continuous with Bowman's capsule Specialized cellular lining facilitates tubular reabsorption	Site for reabsorption of sodium, chloride, water, glucose, amino acids, potassium, calcium, bicarbonate, phosphate, and urea
Loop of Henle	Continues from PTC Juxtamedullary nephrons dip deep into the medulla Permeable to water, urea, and sodium chloride	Regulation of water balance
Descending limb (DL)	Continues from the loop of Henle Permeable to water, urea, and sodium chloride	Regulation of water balance
Ascending limb (AL)	Emerges from DL as it turns and is redirected up toward the renal cortex	Potassium and magnesium reabsorption in the thick segment Thin segment is impermeable to water
Distal convoluted tubule (DCT)	Evolves from AL and twists so the macula densa cells lie adjacent to the juxtaglomerular cells of afferent arteriole	Site of additional water and electrolyte reabsorption, including bicarbonate Potassium and hydrogen secretion
Collecting ducts	Collect formed urine from several tubules and deliver it into the renal pelvis	Receptor sites for antidiuretic hormone regulation of water balance

The distal convoluted tubule (DCT) can be permeable to water, and some water reabsorption occurs as the filtrate continues to flow through the tubule. The membrane of the DCT may be made more permeable to water when *vasopressin* (antidiuretic hormone [ADH]), and aldosterone are present. Vasopressin increases tubular permeability to water, allowing water to leave the tube and be reabsorbed into the capillaries. Vasopressin also increases arteriole constriction. Arteriole constriction alters blood pressure, which then affects the amounts of fluid and particles that exit glomerular capillaries. Aldosterone promotes the reabsorption of sodium in the DCT. Water reabsorption occurs as a result of the movement of sodium (where sodium goes, water follows).

The ability of the kidneys to vary the volume or concentration of urine helps regulate water balance regardless of fluid intake. In this way, the healthy kidney can prevent dehydration when fluid intake is low and can prevent circulatory overload when fluid intake is high.

In addition to water, electrolytes are reabsorbed as needed to maintain FLUID AND ELECTROLYTE BALANCE in the blood. Most sodium, chloride, and water reabsorption occurs in the proximal convoluted tubule (PCT). The collecting ducts are the other site of sodium, chloride, and water reabsorption.

Here reabsorption is caused by aldosterone. Potassium is mostly reabsorbed in the PCT and in the thick segment of the loop of Henle.

Bicarbonate, calcium, and phosphate are mostly reabsorbed in the PCT. Bicarbonate reabsorption helps ACID-BASE BALANCE and maintains a normal blood pH. Blood levels of calcitonin and parathyroid hormone (PTH) (see Chapters 11 and 63) control calcium balance.

Some types of particles in the tubular filtrate also are returned to the blood by *tubular reabsorption*. About 50% of all urea in the filtrate is reabsorbed; creatinine is not reabsorbed.

The kidney reabsorbs some of the glucose filtered from the blood. However, there is a limit to how much glucose the kidney can reabsorb. This limit is called the **renal threshold** or **transport maximum (tm)** for glucose reabsorption. The usual renal threshold for glucose is about 220 mg/dL (12 mmol/L). This means that at a blood glucose level of 220 mg/dL (12 mmol/L) or less, all glucose is reabsorbed and returned to the blood, with no glucose present in final urine. When blood glucose levels are greater than 220 mg/dL (12 mmol/L), some glucose stays in the filtrate and is present in the urine. Normally, almost all glucose and most proteins are reabsorbed and thus are not present in the urine.

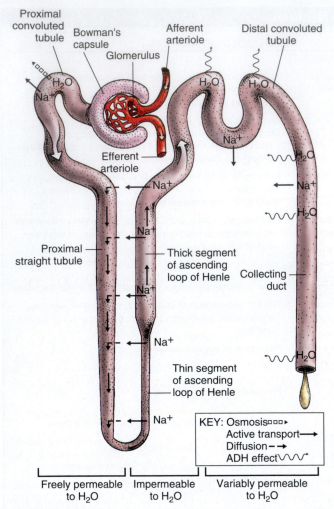

FIG. 65-7 Sodium and water reabsorption by the tubules of a cortical nephron. *ADH,* Antidiuretic hormone; *Na+,* sodium.

Tubular secretion is the third process of urine formation. It allows substances to move from the blood into the urine. During tubular secretion, substances move from the peritubular capillaries in reverse, across capillary membranes, and into the cells that line the tubules. From the cells, these substances are moved into the urine and excreted from the body. Potassium (K^+) and hydrogen (H^+) ions are some of the substances moved in this way to maintain FLUID AND ELECTROLYTE BALANCE and ACID-BASE BALANCE (pH).

Hormonal Functions. The kidneys produce renin, prostaglandins, erythropoietin, and activated vitamin D (Table 65-2). Other kidney products, such as the kinins, change kidney blood flow, regulate blood pressure, and influence capillary permeability. The kidneys also help break down and excrete insulin and many other drugs.

Renin, as discussed in the Microscopic Anatomy section, assists in blood pressure control. It is formed and released when there is a decrease in blood flow, blood volume, or blood pressure through the renal arterioles or when too little sodium is present in kidney blood. These conditions are detected through the receptors of the juxtaglomerular complex.

Renin release causes the production of *angiotensin II* through a series of steps (see Fig. 65-5). Angiotensin II increases systemic blood pressure with powerful blood vessel constricting effects and triggers the release of aldosterone from the adrenal glands. Aldosterone increases the reabsorption of sodium in the distal tubule of the nephron. Therefore more water is reabsorbed, which increases blood volume and blood pressure. When blood flow to the kidney is reduced, this system also prevents fluid loss and maintains circulating blood volume (see Chapter 11).

Prostaglandins are produced in the kidney and many other tissues. Those produced specifically in the kidney help regulate

TABLE 65-2	Kidney Hormones and Hormones Influencing Kidney Function	
	SITE	**ACTION**
Kidney Hormones		
Renin	Renin-producing granular cells	Raises blood pressure as result of angiotensin (local vasoconstriction) and aldosterone (volume expansion) secretion
Prostaglandins	Kidney tissues	Regulate intrarenal blood flow by vasodilation or vasoconstriction
Bradykinins	Juxtaglomerular cells of the arterioles	Increase blood flow (vasodilation) and vascular permeability
Erythropoietin	Kidney parenchyma	Stimulates bone marrow to make red blood cells
Activated vitamin D (1,25-dihydrocholecalciferol)	Kidney parenchyma	Promotes absorption of calcium in the GI tract
Hormones Influencing Kidney Function		
Vasopressin (Antidiuretic hormone [ADH])	Released from posterior pituitary	Makes DCT and CD permeable to water to maximize reabsorption and produce a concentrated urine
Aldosterone	Released from adrenal cortex	Promotes sodium reabsorption and potassium secretion in DCT and CD; water and chloride follow sodium movement
Natriuretic hormones	Cardiac atria, cardiac ventricles, brain	Cause tubular secretion of sodium

CD, Collecting duct; *DCT,* distal convoluted tubule.

glomerular filtration, kidney vascular resistance, and renin production. They also increase sodium and water excretion.

Erythropoietin is produced and released in response to decreased oxygen tension in the kidney's blood supply. It triggers red blood cell (RBC) production in the bone marrow. When kidney function is poor, erythropoietin production decreases, and anemia results.

Vitamin D activation occurs through a series of steps. Some of these steps take place in the skin when it is exposed to sunlight, and then more processing occurs in the liver. From there, vitamin D is converted to its active form in the kidney. Activated vitamin D is needed to absorb calcium in the intestinal tract and regulate calcium balance (McCance et al., 2014).

Ureters

Each kidney usually has a single ureter, which is a hollow tube that connects the renal pelvis with the urinary bladder. The ureter is about ½ inch (1.25 cm) in diameter and about 12 to 18 inches (30 to 45 cm) in length. The diameter of the ureter narrows in three areas:

- In the upper third of the ureter, at the point at which the renal pelvis becomes the ureter, is a narrowing known as the **ureteropelvic junction (UPJ)**.
- The ureter also narrows as it bends toward the abdominal wall (aortoiliac bend).
- Each ureter narrows at the point at which it enters the bladder; this point is called the **ureterovesical junction (UVJ)**.

The ureter tunnels through bladder tissue for a short distance and then opens into the bladder at the trigone (Fig. 65-8).

The ureter has three layers: an inner lining of mucous membrane *(urothelium)*, a middle layer of smooth muscle fibers, and an outer layer of fibrous tissue. The middle layer of muscle fibers is controlled by several nerve pathways from the lower spinal cord.

Contractions of the smooth muscle in the ureter move urine from the kidney pelvis to the bladder. Stretch receptors in the kidney pelvis regulate this movement. For example, a large volume of urine in the kidney pelvis triggers the stretch receptors, which respond by increasing ureteral contractions and ureter peristalsis.

Urinary Bladder

Structure

The urinary bladder is a muscular sac (see Fig. 65-8) that lies directly behind the pubic bone. In men, the bladder is in front of the rectum. In women, it is in front of the vagina.

The bladder is composed of the *body* (the rounded sac portion) and the *bladder neck* (posterior urethra), which connects to the bladder body. The bladder has three linings: an inner lining of epithelial cells *(urothelium)*, middle layers of smooth muscle *(detrusor muscle)*, and an outer lining. The *trigone* is an area on the posterior wall between the points of ureteral entry (ureterovesical junctions [UVJs]) and the urethra.

The **internal urethral sphincter** is the smooth detrusor muscle of the bladder neck and elastic tissue. The **external urethral sphincter** is skeletal muscle that surrounds the urethra. In men, the external sphincter surrounds the urethra at the base of the prostate gland. In women, the external sphincter is at the base of the bladder. The pudendal nerve from the spinal cord controls the external sphincter.

Function

The bladder stores urine, provides continence, and enables voiding. The secretions of the urothelium lining the bladder resist bacteria.

Continence is the ability to voluntarily control bladder emptying. It occurs during bladder filling through the combination of detrusor muscle relaxation, internal sphincter muscle tone, and external sphincter contraction. As the bladder fills with urine, stretch sensations are transmitted to spinal sacral nerves.

Maintaining continence occurs by the interaction of the nerves that control the muscles of the bladder, bladder neck, urethra, and pelvic floor, as well as by factors that close the urethra. In the continent person, the smooth muscle of the detrusor remains relaxed during a period of urine filling and storage. Sympathetic nervous system fibers prevent detrusor muscle contraction. These control centers for voiding are located in the cerebral cortex, the brainstem, and the lower spinal cord. For urethral closure to be adequate for continence, the mucosal surfaces must be in contact and must be adhesive. Contact depends on the presence and proper function of the involved nerves and muscles. Adhesion depends on the secretion of mucuslike substances.

Micturition (voiding, urination) is a reflex of autonomic control that triggers contraction of the detrusor muscle (closing the ureter at the UVJ to prevent backflow) at the same time as relaxation of the external sphincter and the muscles of the pelvic floor. Voluntary urine ELIMINATION (voiding) occurs as a learned response and is controlled by the cerebral cortex and the brainstem. Contraction of the external sphincter inhibits the micturition reflex and prevents voiding.

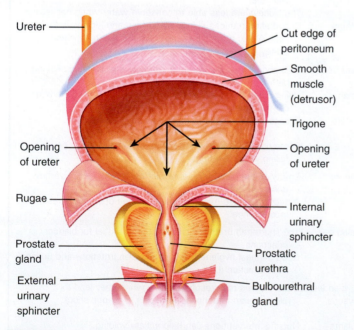

Ureter

Opening of ureter

Rugae

Prostate gland

External urinary sphincter

Cut edge of peritoneum

Smooth muscle (detrusor)

Trigone

Opening of ureter

Internal urinary sphincter

Prostatic urethra

Bulbourethral gland

FIG. 65-8 Gross anatomy of the urinary bladder. (Modified from Patton, K.T., & Thibodeau, G.A. [2013]. *Anatomy & physiology* (8th ed.). St. Louis: Mosby.)

Urethra

The urethra is a narrow tube lined with mucous membranes. Its purpose is to allow urine ELIMINATION from the bladder. The

urethral meatus, or opening, is the endpoint of the urethra. In men, the urethra is about 6 to 8 inches (15 to 20 cm) long, with the meatus located at the tip of the penis. The male urethra has three sections:

- The prostatic urethra, which extends from the bladder through the prostate gland
- The membranous urethra, which extends from the prostate to the wall of the pelvic floor
- The cavernous urethra, which is external and extends through the length of the penis

In women, the urethra is 1 to 1.5 inches (2.5 to 3.75 cm) long and exits through the pelvic floor. The meatus lies slightly below the clitoris and directly in front of the vagina and rectum.

Kidney and Urinary Changes Associated With Aging

Kidney Changes

Changes occur in the kidney as a result of the aging process that can affect urine ELIMINATION and health (Chart 65-1). The kidney loses cortical tissue and nephrons and gets smaller with age as a result of reduced blood flow to the kidney (Touhy & Jett, 2016). The medulla is not affected by aging, and the juxta-medullary nephron functions are preserved. The glomerular and tubular linings thicken. Both the number of glomeruli and their surface areas decrease with aging. Tubule length decreases. The changes reduce the older adult's ability to filter blood and excrete waste products.

Blood flow to the kidney declines by about 10% per decade as blood vessels thicken. This means that blood flow to the kidney is not as adaptive in older adults, leaving nephrons more vulnerable to damage during episodes of either hypotension or hypertension.

Glomerular filtration rate (GFR) decreases with age. By age 65 years, the GFR is about 65 mL/min (half the rate of a young adult) and increases the risk for fluid overload. This decline is more rapid in patients with diabetes, hypertension, or heart failure. The combination of reduced kidney mass, reduced blood flow, and decreased GFR contributes to reduced drug clearance and a greater risk for drug reactions and kidney damage from drugs and contrast media in older adults.

Tubular changes with aging decrease the ability to concentrate urine, resulting in **urgency** (a sense of a nearly uncontrollable need to urinate) and **nocturnal polyuria** (increased urination at night). The regulation of sodium, acids, and bicarbonate is less efficient. Along with an age-related impairment in the thirst mechanism, these changes increase the risk for disturbances of FLUID AND ELECTROLYTE BALANCE, such as dehydration and **hypernatremia** (increased blood sodium levels) in the older adult. Hormonal changes include a decrease in renin secretion, aldosterone levels, and activation of vitamin D.

Urinary Changes

Changes in detrusor muscle elasticity lead to decreased bladder capacity and reduced ability to retain urine (Touhy & Jett, 2016). The urge to void may cause immediate bladder emptying because the urinary sphincters lose tone and often become weaker with age. In women, weakened muscles in the pelvic floor shorten the urethra and promote incontinence. In men,

---

CHART 65-1   Nursing Focus on the Older Adult

Changes in the Renal System Related to Aging

PHYSIOLOGIC CHANGE	NURSING INTERVENTIONS	RATIONALES
Decreased glomerular filtration rate (GFR)	Monitor hydration status.	The ability of the kidneys to regulate water balance decreases with age.
	Ensure adequate fluid intake.	The kidneys are less able to conserve water when necessary.
	Administer potentially nephrotoxic agents or drugs carefully.	Dehydration reduces kidney blood flow and increases the nephrotoxic potential of many agents. Acute or chronic kidney failure may result.
Nocturia	Ensure adequate nighttime lighting and a hazard-free environment.	Falls and injuries are common among older patients seeking bathroom facilities.
	Ensure the availability of a bedside toilet, bedpan, or urinal.	Using these items instead of getting up to go the bathroom can help prevent falls.
	Discourage excessive fluid intake for 2-4 hr before the patient goes to bed.	Excessive fluid intake at night may increase nocturia.
	Evaluate drugs and timing.	Some drugs increase urine output and increase the risk for falling when toileting.
Decreased bladder capacity	Encourage the patient to use the toilet, bedpan, or urinal at least every 2 hr.	Emptying the bladder on a regular basis may avoid overflow urinary incontinence.
	Respond as soon as possible to the patient's indication of the need to void.	A quick response may alleviate episodes of urinary stress incontinence.
Weakened urinary sphincters and shortened urethra in women	Provide thorough perineal care after each voiding.	The shortened urethra increases the potential for bladder infections.
		Good perineal hygiene may prevent skin irritations and urinary tract infection (UTI).
Tendency to retain urine	Observe the patient for urinary retention (e.g., bladder distention) or urinary tract infection (e.g., dysuria, foul odor, confusion).	Urinary stasis may result in a UTI, which may lead to bloodstream infections, urosepsis, or septic shock.
	Provide privacy, assistance, and voiding stimulants such as warm water over the perineum as needed.	Nursing interventions can help initiate voiding.
	Evaluate drugs for possible contribution to retention.	Anticholinergic drugs promote urinary retention.

an enlarged prostate gland makes starting the urine stream difficult and may cause urinary retention.

CULTURAL/SPIRITUAL CONSIDERATIONS

Patient-Centered Care QSEN

African Americans have more rapid age-related decreases in GFR than do white adults. Kidney excretion of sodium is less effective in hypertensive African Americans who have high sodium intake, and the kidneys have about 20% less blood flow as a result of anatomic changes in small blood vessels and intrarenal responses to renin. Thus African-American patients are at greater risk for kidney failure than are white patients (Jarvis, 2016). Yearly health examinations should include urinalysis, checking for the presence of microalbuminuria, and evaluating serum creatinine.

ASSESSMENT: NOTICING AND INTERPRETING

Patient History

Demographic information, such as age, gender, race, and ethnicity, is important to consider as nonmodifiable risk factors in the patient with any kidney or urinary ELIMINATION problem. A sudden onset of hypertension in patients older than 50 years suggests possible kidney disease. Clinical changes in polycystic kidney disease typically occur in patients in their 40s or 50s. In men older than 50 years, altered urine patterns accompany prostate disease.

Anatomic gender differences make some disorders worse or more common. For example, men rarely have ascending urinary tract infections. Women have a shorter urethra and more commonly develop cystitis (bladder inflammation, most often with infection) because bacteria pass more readily into the bladder.

Ask the patient about any previous kidney or urologic problems, including tumors, infections, stones, or urologic surgery. A history of any chronic health problems, especially diabetes mellitus or hypertension, increases the risk for development of kidney disease because these disorders damage kidney blood vessels.

Exposure to certain contrast media during imaging can harm the kidneys. Iodinated contrast medium used for CT scans is associated with both acute and chronic kidney injury (Lambert et al., 2017). High-osmolarity contrast agents can also contribute to kidney function impairment. Exposure to gadolinium-enhanced MRI can result in nephrogenic systemic fibrosis.

Ask the patient about chemical exposures at the work place or with hobbies. Exposure to hydrocarbons (e.g., gasoline, oil), heavy metals (especially mercury and lead), and some gases (e.g., chlorine, toluene) can impair kidney function. Use this opportunity to teach patients who come into contact with chemicals at work or during leisure-time activities to avoid direct skin or mucous membrane contact with these chemicals. Use of heroin, cocaine, methamphetamine, ecstasy, and volatile solvents (inhalants) has also been associated with kidney damage.

Specifically ask the patient whether he or she has ever been told about the presence of protein or albumin in the urine. The question, "Have you ever been told that your blood pressure is high?" may prompt a response different from the one to the question, "Do you have high blood pressure?" Ask women about health problems during pregnancy (e.g., proteinuria, high blood pressure, gestational diabetes, urinary tract infections). Obtain information about:

- Chemical or environmental toxin exposure in occupational, diagnostic, or other settings
- Recent travel to geographic regions that pose infectious disease risks
- Recent trauma or injury, particularly to the abdomen or pelvic or genital areas
- A history of altered patterns of urinary ELIMINATION

Socioeconomic status may influence health care practices. Prevention, early detection, and treatment of kidney or urinary problems may be limited by lack of insurance or access to health care, lack of transportation, and reduced income. Low income may also result in difficulty following medical advice, having prescriptions filled, adhering to dietary instructions, and keeping follow-up appointments.

Educational level may affect health-seeking practices and the patient's understanding of a disease or its symptoms. Recurring urinary tract infections can result from not completing a course of antibiotic therapy or from not following up to ensure that the infection is cleared.

The patient's health beliefs affect the approach to health and illness. Cultural background or religious affiliation may influence the belief system, as well as comfort when discussing issues about ELIMINATION (Jackson et al., 2013).

The language used by patients may be different from that used by the health care professional. When obtaining a history, listen to and explore the terms used by the patient. By using the patient's own terms, you may help him or her provide a more complete description of the problem and may decrease the patient's discomfort when discussing bodily functions.

Nutrition History

Ask the patient with known or suspected kidney or urologic disorders about his or her usual diet and any recent changes in the diet. Note any excessive intake or omission of certain food categories. Ask about food and fluid intake. Assess how much and which types of fluids the patient drinks daily, especially fluids with a high calorie or caffeine content. Use this opportunity to teach the patient the importance of drinking sufficient fluid to cause urine to be dilute (clear or very light yellow). If another medical problem does not require fluid restriction, ingestion of about 2 liters of fluid daily is recommended to prevent dehydration and cystitis. If the patient has followed a diet for weight reduction, the details of the diet plan are important, and collaboration with a dietitian may be needed. A high-protein intake can result in temporary kidney problems. For example, a patient at risk for calculi (stone) formation who ingests large amounts of protein or has a poor fluid intake may form new stones.

Ask about any change in appetite or taste. These symptoms can occur with the buildup of nitrogenous waste products from kidney failure. Changes in thirst or fluid intake may also cause changes in the volume of urine ELIMINATION. Endocrine disorders may also cause changes in thirst, fluid intake, and urine output. (See Chapter 61 for a discussion of endocrine influences on fluid balance.)

Medication History

Identify all of the patient's prescription drugs because many can impair kidney function (Burchum & Rosenthal, 2016). Ask about the duration of drug use and whether there have been any recent changes in prescribed drugs. Drugs for diabetes mellitus, hypertension, cardiac disorders, hormonal disorders, cancer, arthritis, and psychiatric disorders are potential causes of kidney problems. Antibiotics, such as gentamicin (Garamycin, Cidomycin ✦), may also cause acute kidney injury. Drug-drug interactions and drug–contrast media interactions also may lead to kidney dysfunction (Lambert et al., 2017).

Explore the past and current use of over-the-counter (OTC) drugs or agents, including dietary supplements, vitamins and minerals, herbal agents, laxatives, analgesics, acetaminophen, and NSAIDs. Many of these agents affect kidney function and urine ELIMINATION. For example, dietary supplementation with synthetic creatine, used to increase muscle mass, has been associated with compromised kidney function. High-dose or long-term use of NSAIDs or acetaminophen can seriously reduce kidney function. Some agents are associated with hypertension, hematuria, or proteinuria, which may occur before kidney dysfunction.

Family History and Genetic Risk

The family history of the patient with a suspected kidney or urologic problem is important because some disorders have a familial pattern. Ask whether siblings, parents, or grandparents have had kidney problems. Past terms used for kidney disease include *Bright's disease, nephritis,* and *nephrosis.* Although nephritis is a current term for an inflammatory process in the kidney and nephrosis is a current term for a degenerative process in the kidney, these terms have been used by lay adults for years to describe any type of kidney problem. Polycystic kidney disease, which is a genetic disorder, can occur in either gender.

Current Health Problem

The effects of kidney failure are seen in all body systems. Document all of the patient's current health problems. Ask him or her to describe all health concerns, because some kidney disorders cause problems in other body systems. Recent upper respiratory problems, achy muscles or joints, heart disease, or GI conditions may be related to problems of kidney function.

Assess the kidney and urologic system by asking about any changes in the appearance (color, odor, clarity) of the urine, pattern of urine ELIMINATION, ability to initiate or control voiding, and other unusual symptoms. For example, urine that is reddish, rust-colored, brown or black, greenish, or different from the usual yellowish color may prompt the patient to seek health care assistance. Urine typically has a mild but distinct odor of ammonia. An increase in the intensity of color, a change in odor quality, or a decrease in urine clarity may suggest infection.

Ask about changes in urination patterns, such as **incontinence** (involuntary bladder emptying), **nocturia** (urination at night), **urgency** (unstoppable urge to urinate), frequency, or an increase or decrease in the amount of urine. The normal urine output for adults is about 1500 to 2000 mL/day or within 500 mL of the volume of fluid ingested daily. Ask about how closely the urine output is to the volume of fluid ingested. A bladder diary may be useful. Ask whether:

- Initiating urine flow is difficult
- A burning sensation or other discomfort occurs with urination
- The force of the urine stream is decreased (in men)
- Persistent dribbling of urine is present

The onset of pain in the flank, in the lower abdomen or pelvic region, or in the perineal area triggers concern and usually prompts the patient to seek assistance. Ask about the onset, intensity, and duration of the pain; its location; and its association with any activity or event.

Pain associated with kidney or ureteral irritation is often severe and spasmodic. Pain that radiates into the perineal area, groin, scrotum, or labia is described as *renal colic.* This pain occurs with distention or spasm of the ureter, such as in an obstruction or the passing of a stone. Renal colic pain may be intermittent or continuous and may occur with pallor, diaphoresis, and hypotension. These general symptoms occur because of the location of the nerve tracts near or in the kidneys and ureters (Brenner, 2016).

Because the kidneys are close to the GI organs and the nerve pathways are similar, GI symptoms may occur with kidney problems. These renointestinal reflexes often complicate the description of the kidney problem.

Uremia is the buildup of nitrogenous waste products in the blood from inadequate ELIMINATION as a result of kidney failure. Symptoms include anorexia, nausea and vomiting, muscle cramps, *pruritus* (itching), fatigue, and lethargy.

Physical Assessment

The physical assessment of the patient with a known or suspected kidney or urologic disorder includes general appearance, a review of body systems, and specific structure and functions of the kidney and urinary system.

Assess the patient's general appearance and check the skin for the presence of any rashes, bruising, or yellowish discoloration. The skin and tissues may show edema associated with kidney disease, especially in the *pedal* (foot), *pretibial* (shin), and sacral tissues and around the eyes. Use a stethoscope to listen to the lungs to determine whether fluid is present. Weigh the patient and measure blood pressure as a baseline for later comparisons.

Assess the levels of consciousness and alertness. Record any deficits in memory, concentration, or thought processes. Family members may report subtle changes. Cognitive changes may be the result of the buildup of waste products when kidney disease is present.

Assessment of the Kidneys, Ureters, and Bladder

Assess the kidneys, ureters, and bladder during an abdominal assessment (Jarvis, 2016). Auscultate before percussion and palpation because these activities can enhance bowel sounds and obscure abdominal vascular sounds.

Inspect the abdomen and the flank regions with the patient in both the supine and the sitting positions. Observe the patient for asymmetry (e.g., swelling) or discoloration (e.g., bruising or redness) in the flank region, especially in the area of the costovertebral angle (CVA). The CVA is located between the lower portion of the twelfth rib and the vertebral column.

Listen for a bruit by placing a stethoscope over each renal artery on the midclavicular line. A **bruit** is an audible swishing sound produced when the volume of blood or the diameter of the blood vessel changes. It often occurs with blood flow through a narrowed vessel, as in renal artery stenosis.

Kidney palpation is usually performed by a primary health care provider. It can help locate masses and areas of tenderness in or around the kidney. Lightly palpate the abdomen in all quadrants. Ask about areas of tenderness or pain, and examine nontender areas first. The outline of the bladder may be seen as high as the umbilicus in patients with severe bladder distention.

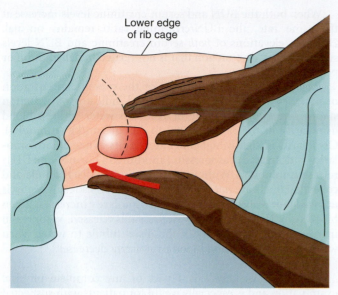

FIG. 65-9 Advanced technique for palpation of the kidney.

If tumor or aneurysm is suspected, palpation may harm the patient.

Because the kidneys are located deep and posterior, palpation is easier in thin patients who have little abdominal musculature. For palpation of the right kidney, the patient is in a supine position while the examiner places one hand under the right flank and the other hand over the abdomen below the lower right part of the rib cage. The lower hand is used to raise the flank, and the upper hand depresses the abdomen as the patient takes a deep breath (Fig. 65-9). The left kidney is deeper and often cannot be palpated. A transplanted kidney is readily palpated in either the lower right or left abdominal quadrant. The normal kidney is smooth, firm, and nontender.

A distended bladder sounds dull when percussed. After gently palpating to determine the outline of the distended bladder, begin percussion on the lower abdomen and continue in the direction of the umbilicus until dull sounds are no longer produced. If you suspect bladder distention, use a portable bladder scanner to determine the amount of retained urine.

If the patient reports flank pain or tenderness, percuss the nontender flank first. Have the patient assume a sitting, side-lying, or supine position, and then form one of your hands into a clenched fist. Place your other hand flat over the CVA of the patient. Quickly deliver a firm thump to your hand over the CVA area (Jarvis, 2016). Costovertebral tenderness often occurs with kidney infection or inflammation. Patients with inflammation or infection in the kidney or nearby structures may describe their pain as severe or as a constant, dull ache.

Assessment of the Urethra

Using a good light source and wearing gloves, inspect the urethra by examining the meatus and the tissues around it. Record any unusual discharge such as blood, mucus, or pus. Inspect the skin and mucous membranes of surrounding tissues. Record the presence of lesions, rashes, or other abnormalities of the penis or scrotum or of the labia or vaginal opening. Urethral irritation is suspected when the patient reports discomfort with urination. Use this opportunity to remind women to clean the perineum by wiping from front to back, never from back to front. Teach them that the front-to-back technique keeps organisms in stool from coming close to the urethra and decreases the risk for infection.

 ### CULTURAL/SPIRITUAL CONSIDERATIONS
Patient-Centered Care QSEN

Women from some cultures or religions may have undergone female circumcision. This procedure alters the appearance of the vulvar-perineal area and increases the risk for urinary tract infections. It also makes urethral inspection or catheterization difficult. Document any noted anatomic changes and ask the patient to describe her hygiene practices for this area.

Psychosocial Assessment

Concerns about the urologic system may evoke fear, anger, embarrassment, anxiety, guilt, or sadness in the patient. Childhood learning often includes the idea that toileting should take place in private and not be discussed with other people. Urologic disorders may bring up forgotten memories of difficult toilet training and bedwetting or of childhood experiences of exploring one's body. The patient may ignore symptoms or delay seeking health care because of emotional responses or cultural taboos about the urogenital area.

 ### NCLEX EXAMINATION CHALLENGE 65-1
Physiological Integrity

When obtaining a health history from a 22-year-old female client who has new-onset urinary incontinence, which findings or factors does the nurse consider significant? **Select all that apply.**
A. Chemical exposure in the workplace
B. A burning sensation occurring on urination
C. Urinating 10 times daily although fluid intake remains unchanged
D. A recent change in the client's oral contraceptive prescription
E. A new inability to hold urine (urgency)
F. A "stinky" odor from the urine

Diagnostic Assessment
Laboratory Assessment

Blood Tests. Serum creatinine is produced when muscle and other proteins are broken down. Because protein breakdown is usually constant, the serum creatinine level is a good indicator of kidney function. Serum creatinine levels are slightly higher in men than in women because men tend to have a larger muscle mass than do women. Similarly, adults with greater muscle mass or muscle mass turnover (e.g., athletes) may have a slightly higher-than-average serum creatinine level. Muscle mass and the amount of creatinine produced decrease with age. However, because of decreased rates of creatinine clearance, the serum creatinine level remains relatively constant in older adults unless kidney disease is present.

No common pathologic condition other than kidney disease increases the serum creatinine level. The serum creatinine level does not increase until at least 50% of the kidney function is lost; therefore *any* elevation of serum creatinine values is important and should be assessed further. Creatinine is excreted by the kidneys.

Blood urea nitrogen (BUN) measures the effectiveness of kidney excretion of urea nitrogen, a by-product of protein breakdown in the liver. Urea nitrogen is produced mostly from

Action Alert

A serum creatinine of 1.5 mg/dL (110 mcmol/L) or greater places a patient at risk for acute kidney injury (AKI) from iodinated contrast media and some drugs (Lambert et al., 2017). Monitor both baseline and trend values to recognize risk for and actual kidney damage, especially among patients exposed to agents that can cause kidney dysfunction. If indicated, respond by promptly informing the primary health care provider of increases in serum creatinine greater than 1.5 times the baseline and urine output values of less than 0.5 mL/kg/hr for 6 or more hours.

liver metabolism of food sources of protein. The kidneys filter urea nitrogen from the blood and excrete the waste as part of urine ELIMINATION.

Other factors influence the BUN level, and an elevation does not always mean that kidney disease is present (Chart 65-2). For example, rapid cell destruction from infection, cancer treatment, or steroid therapy may elevate BUN level. In addition, blood is a protein. Blood in the tissues rather than in the blood vessels is reabsorbed as if it were a general protein. Thus reabsorbed blood protein is processed by the liver and increases BUN levels. This means that injured tissues can result in increased BUN levels even when kidney function is normal. In addition, BUN is increased by protein turnover in exercising muscle and is elevated as a result of concentration during dehydration.

The liver must function properly to produce urea nitrogen. When liver and kidney dysfunction are present, urea nitrogen levels are actually *decreased* because the liver failure limits urea production. The BUN level is not always elevated with kidney disease and is not the best indicator of kidney function. However, an elevated BUN level suggests kidney dysfunction.

Blood urea nitrogen to serum creatinine ratio can help determine whether non–kidney-related factors, such as low cardiac output or red blood cell destruction, are causing the elevated BUN level. When blood volume is deficient (e.g., dehydration) or cardiac output is low, the BUN level rises more rapidly than the serum creatinine level. As a result, the ratio of BUN to creatinine is *increased*.

When both the BUN and serum creatinine levels increase at the same rate, the BUN/creatinine ratio remains normal. However, elevations of *both* serum creatinine and BUN levels suggest kidney dysfunction that is not related to dehydration or poor perfusion.

Blood osmolarity is a measure of the overall concentration of particles in the blood and is a good indicator of hydration status. The kidneys excrete or reabsorb water to keep blood osmolarity in the range of 280 to 300 mOsm/kg (mmol/kg). Osmolarity is slightly higher in older adults. When blood osmolarity is decreased, vasopressin (antidiuretic hormone [ADH]) release is inhibited. Without vasopressin, the distal tubule and collecting ducts are *not* permeable to water. As a result, water is *excreted*, not reabsorbed, and blood osmolarity increases. When blood osmolarity increases, vasopressin is released. Vasopressin increases the permeability of the distal tubule to water. Then water is reabsorbed, and blood osmolarity decreases.

Urine Tests

Urinalysis. Urinalysis is a part of any complete physical examination and is especially useful for patients with suspected kidney or urologic disorders (Chart 65-3). Ideally, the urine specimen is collected at the morning's first voiding. Specimens obtained at other times may be too dilute. The specimen may be collected by several techniques (Table 65-3).

Urine color comes from trichrome pigment. Color variations may result from increased levels of trichrome or other pigments, changes in the concentration or dilution of the urine, and the presence of drug metabolites in the urine. Urine smells faintly like ammonia and is normally clear without *turbidity* (cloudiness) or haziness.

Specific gravity is the concentration of particles (i.e., electrolytes, wastes) in urine. A high specific gravity indicates concentrated urine from dehydration, decreased kidney blood flow, or excess vasopressin associated with stress, surgery, anesthetic agents, and certain drugs (e.g., morphine, some oral antidiabetic drugs) or syndrome of inappropriate antidiuretic hormone (SIADH) (see Chapter 62). Low specific gravity indicates dilute urine that may occur from high fluid intake, diuretic drugs, or diabetes insipidus (DI) (see Chapter 62).

Specific gravity of urine is compared with distilled water, which has a specific gravity of 1.000. The normal specific gravity

---

⚑ CHART 65-2   **Laboratory Profile**

Kidney Function Blood Studies

TEST	NORMAL RANGE FOR ADULTS	CANADIAN NORMAL RANGE	SIGNIFICANCE OF ABNORMAL FINDINGS
Serum creatinine	*Males:* 0.6-1.2 mg/dL *Females:* 0.5-1.1 mg/dL *Older adults:* May be decreased	*Males:* 53-106 mcmol/L *Females:* 44-97 mcmol/L	An *increased level* indicates kidney impairment. A *decreased level* may be caused by a decreased muscle mass.
Blood urea nitrogen (BUN)	10-20 mg/dL *Older adults:* Slightly higher	3.6-7.1 mmol/L	An *increased level* may indicate liver or kidney disease, dehydration or decreased kidney perfusion, a high-protein diet, infection, stress, steroid use, GI bleeding, or other situations in which blood is in body tissues. A *decreased level* may indicate malnutrition, fluid volume excess, or severe hepatic damage.
BUN/creatinine ratio (BUN divided by creatinine)	6-25	6-25	An *increased ratio* may indicate fluid volume deficit, obstructive uropathy, catabolic state, or a high-protein diet. A *decreased ratio* may indicate fluid volume excess.

Data from Pagana, K., Pagana, T., & Pagana, T. (2017). *Mosby's diagnostic & laboratory test reference* (13th ed.). St. Louis: Mosby; and Pagana, K., Pagana, T., & Pike-McDonald, S. (2013). *Mosby's Canadian manual of diagnostic and laboratory tests*. St. Louis: Elsevier.

CHART 65-3 Laboratory Profile

Urinalysis

TEST	NORMAL RANGE FOR ADULTS	SIGNIFICANCE OF ABNORMAL FINDINGS
Color	Yellow	*Dark amber* indicates concentrated urine. *Very pale yellow* indicates dilute urine. *Dark red* or *brown* indicates blood in the urine. Brown may indicate increased bilirubin level. Red also may indicate the presence of myoglobin. *Other color* changes may result from diet or drugs.
Odor	Specific aroma, similar to ammonia	*Foul smell* indicates possible infection, dehydration, or ingestion of certain foods or drugs.
Turbidity	Clear	*Cloudy urine* indicates infection, sediment, or high levels of urine protein.
Specific gravity	Usually 1.005-1.030; possible range 1.000-1.040 *Older adult:* Decreased	*Increased* in decreased kidney perfusion, inappropriate ADH secretion, or heart failure. *Decreased* in chronic kidney disease, diabetes insipidus, malignant hypertension, diuretic administration, and lithium toxicity.
pH	Average: 6; possible range: 4.6-8	*Changes* are caused by diet, drugs, infection, age of specimen, acid-base imbalance, and kidney disease.
Glucose	Fresh specimen, negative 50-300 mg/day in a 24-hour specimen (<2.78 mmol/day in a 24-hour specimen)	*Presence* reflects hyperglycemia or a decrease in the kidney threshold for glucose.
Ketones	None	*Presence* occurs with diabetic ketoacidosis, prolonged fasting, anorexia nervosa.
Protein	0-0.8 mg/dL (0-0.08 g/L) 50-80 mg in a 24-hour specimen at rest <250 mg in a 24-hour specimen with exercise	*Increased* amounts may indicate stress, infection, recent strenuous exercise, or glomerular disorders.
Bilirubin (urobilinogen)	None	*Presence* suggests liver or biliary disease or obstruction.
Red blood cells (RBCs)	0-2 per high-power field	*Increased* is normal with catheterization or menses but may reflect tumor, stones, trauma, glomerular disorders, cystitis, or bleeding disorders.
White blood cells (WBCs)	0-4 per low-power field	*Increased* may indicate an infection or inflammation in the kidney and urinary tract, kidney transplant rejection, or exercise.
Casts	None	*Increased* indicates bacteria, protein, or urinary calculi.
Crystals	None	*Presence* may indicate that the specimen has been allowed to stand.
Bacteria	<1000 colonies/mL	*Increased* indicates the need for urine culture to determine the presence of urinary tract infection.
Parasites	None	*Presence* of *Trichomonas vaginalis* indicates infection, usually of the urethra, prostate, or vagina.
Leukocyte esterase	None	*Presence* suggests urinary tract infection.
Nitrites	None	*Presence* suggests urinary *Escherichia coli.*

Data from Pagana, K., Pagana, T., & Pagana, T. (2017). *Mosby's diagnostic & laboratory test reference* (13th ed.). St. Louis: Mosby; and Pagana, K., Pagana, T., & Pike-McDonald, S. (2013). *Mosby's Canadian manual of diagnostic and laboratory tests.* St. Louis: Elsevier.
ADH, Antidiuretic hormone.

of urine ranges from 1.005 to about 1.030. Kidney disease diminishes the concentrating ability of the kidney, and chronic kidney disease may be associated with a low (dilute) specific gravity.

pH is a measure of urine acidity or alkalinity. A pH value less than 7 is acidic, and a value greater than 7 is alkaline. Urine pH is affected by diet, drugs, systemic disturbances of ACID-BASE BALANCE, and kidney tubular function. For example, a high-protein diet produces acidic urine, whereas a high intake of citrus fruit produces alkaline urine.

Urine specimens become more alkaline when left standing unrefrigerated for more than 1 hour, when bacteria are present, or when a specimen is left uncovered. Alkaline urine increases cell breakdown; thus the presence of red blood cells may be missed on analysis. Ensure that urine specimens are covered and delivered to the laboratory promptly or refrigerated

(McGoldrick, 2015). During systemic acidosis or alkalosis, the kidneys, along with blood buffers and the lungs, normally respond to keep serum pH normal. Chapter 12 discusses ACID-BASE BALANCE and imbalance.

Protein is not normally present in the urine. Microalbumin levels greater than 80 mcg/24 hr (0.08 g/24 hr), are abnormal. Protein molecules are too large to pass through intact glomerular membranes. When glomerular membranes are not intact, protein molecules pass through and are excreted with urine ELIMINATION. Increased membrane permeability is caused by infection, inflammation, or immunologic problems. Some systemic problems cause production of abnormal proteins, such as globulin. Detection of abnormal protein types requires electrophoresis.

A random finding of proteinuria (usually albumin in the urine) followed by a series of negative (normal) findings

TABLE 65-3 Collection of Urine Specimens

NURSING INTERVENTIONS	RATIONALES
Voided Urine	
Collect the first specimen voided in the morning.	Urine is more concentrated in the early morning.
Send the specimen to the laboratory as soon as possible.	After urine is collected, cellular breakdown results in more alkaline urine.
Refrigerate the specimen if a delay is unavoidable.	Refrigeration delays the alkalinization of urine. Bacteria are more likely to multiply in an alkaline environment.
Clean-Catch Specimen	
Explain the purpose of the procedure to the patient.	Correct technique is needed to obtain a valid specimen.
Instruct the patient to self-clean before voiding:	Surface cleaning is necessary to remove secretions or bacteria from the urethral meatus.
Instruct the female patient to separate the labia and use the sponges and solution provided to wipe with three strokes over the urethra. The first two wiping strokes are over each side of the urethra; the third wiping stroke is centered over the urethra (from front to back).	
Instruct the male patient to retract the foreskin of the penis and to similarly clean the urethra, using three wiping strokes with the sponge and solution provided (from the head of the penis downward).	
Instruct the patient to initiate voiding after cleaning. The patient then stops and resumes voiding into the container.	A midstream collection further removes secretions and bacteria because urine flushes the distal portion of the internal urethra.
At no time should any part of the patient's anatomy touch the lip or inner aspect of the container.	
Only 1 ounce (30 mL) is needed; the remainder of the urine may be discarded into the commode.	
Ensure that the patient understands the procedure.	An improperly collected specimen may result in inappropriate or incomplete treatment.
Help the patient as needed.	The patient's understanding and the nurse's assistance ensure proper collection.
Catheterized Specimen	
For non-indwelling (straight) catheters:	The one-time passage of a urinary catheter may be necessary to obtain an uncontaminated specimen for analysis or to measure the volume of residual urine.
Follow facility procedures for urinary catheterization.	These procedures minimize bacterial entry.
For indwelling catheters:	Urine is collected from an indwelling catheter or tubing when patients have catheters for continence or long-term urinary drainage.
• Apply a clamp to the drainage tubing, distal to the injection port.	Clamping allows urine to collect in the tubing at the location where the specimen is obtained.
• Clean the injection port cap of the catheter drainage tubing with an appropriate antiseptic and allow to dry. Povidone-iodine solution or alcohol is acceptable.	Surface contamination is prevented by following the cleaning procedures.
• Attach a sterile 5-mL syringe into the port and aspirate the quantity of urine required.	A minimum of 5 mL is needed for culture and sensitivity (C&S) testing.
• Inject the urine sample into a sterile specimen container.	A sterile container is used for C&S specimens.
• Remove the clamp to resume drainage.	
• Properly dispose of the syringe.	
24-Hour Urine Collection	
Instruct the patient thoroughly.	A 24-hr collection of urine is necessary to quantify or calculate the rate of clearance of a particular substance.
Provide written materials to assist in instruction.	Instructional materials for patients, signs, etc. remind patients and staff to ensure that the total collection is completed.
Place signs appropriately.	
Inform all personnel or family caregivers of test in progress.	
Check laboratory or procedure manual on proper technique for maintaining the collection (e.g., on ice, in a refrigerator, or with a preservative).	Proper technique prevents breakdown of elements to be measured.
On initiation of the collection, ask the patient to void, discard the urine, and note the time. If a Foley catheter is in use, empty the tubing and drainage bag at the start time and discard the urine.	Proper techniques ensure that *all* urine formed within the 24-hr period is collected.
Collect all urine of the next 24 hr.	
Twenty-four hours after initiation, ask the patient to empty the bladder and add that urine to the container.	
Do not remove urine from the collection container for other specimens.	Urine in the container is not considered a "fresh" specimen and may be mixed with preservative.

does not imply kidney disease. If infection is the cause of the proteinuria, urinalyses after resolution of the infection should be negative for protein. Persistent proteinuria needs further investigation.

Microalbuminuria is the presence of albumin in the urine that is not measurable by a urine dipstick or usual urinalysis procedures. Specialized assays are used to quickly analyze a freshly voided urine specimen for microscopic levels of albumin. The normal microalbumin levels in a freshly voided specimen should be less than 2.0 mg/dL. Higher levels indicate microalbuminuria and could mean mild or early kidney disease, especially in patients with diabetes mellitus. In 24-hour urine specimens, levels greater than 80 mcg/24 hr (0.08 g/24 hr) indicate microalbuminuria.

Glucose in the urine may indicate a high level of glucose in the blood, typically greater than 220 mg/dL (12 mmol/L). Changes in the renal threshold for glucose may occur temporarily in patients who have infection or severe stress.

Ketone bodies are formed from the incomplete metabolism of fatty acids. Three types of ketone bodies are acetone, acetoacetic acid, and beta-hydroxybutyric acid. *Normally there are no ketones in urine.* Ketone bodies are produced when fat is used instead of glucose for cellular energy. Ketones present in the blood are partially excreted in the urine.

Leukoesterase is an enzyme found in some white blood cells, especially neutrophils. When the number of these cells increases in the urine or they are damaged (lysed), the urine then contains leukoesterase. A normal reading is no leukoesterase in the urine. A positive test (+ sign) is an indication of a urinary tract infection.

Nitrites are not usually present in urine. Many types of bacteria, when present in the urine, convert nitrates (normally found in urine) into nitrites. A positive test enhances the sensitivity of the leukoesterase test to detect urinary tract infection.

Sediment is precipitated particles in the urine. These particles include cells, casts, crystals, and bacteria. Normally, urine contains few, if any, cells. Types of cells abnormally present in the urine include tubular cells (from the tubule of the nephron), epithelial cells (from the lining of the urinary tract), red blood cells (RBCs), and white blood cells (WBCs). WBCs may indicate a urinary tract or kidney infection. RBCs may indicate *glomerulonephritis, acute tubular necrosis, pyelonephritis,* kidney trauma, or kidney cancer.

Casts are clumps of materials or cells. When cells, bacteria, or proteins are present in the urine, minerals and sticky materials clump around them and form a cast of the distal renal tubule and collecting duct. Casts are described by the type of particle they have surrounded (e.g., hyaline [protein-based] or cellular [from RBCs, WBCs, or epithelial cells]) or the stage of cast breakdown (whole cell or granular from cell breakdown). Although an isolated urinalysis with sediment from casts may be the result of strenuous exercise, repeated findings with sediment are more likely to be associated with disease.

Urine crystals come from mineral salts as a result of diet, drugs, or disease. Common salt crystals are formed from calcium, oxalate, urea, phosphate, magnesium, or other substances. Some drugs, such as the sulfates, can also form crystals.

Bacteria multiply quickly, so the urine specimen must be analyzed promptly to avoid falsely elevated counts of bacterial colonization. Normally urine is sterile, but it can be easily contaminated by perineal bacteria during collection.

Recent advances in technology and molecular biology have led to new diagnostic tests using urine, including identification of biomarkers of disease and profiling for specific proteins. For example, cystatin-C, produced by all nucleated cells, is formed at a constant rate and freely filtered by the kidneys. It is used to estimate glomerular filtration rate (GFR) and may predict progression of chronic kidney disease. Markers such as cystatin-C are being investigated to identify early-onset kidney dysfunction, target therapy, and predict responsiveness to intervention. Other markers for angiogenesis and kidney cell adhesion, regulation, and apoptosis (i.e., connective tissue growth factor [CTGF], neutrophil gelatinase-associated lipocalin [NGAL]) will likely contribute to clinical diagnostics in the future.

Urine for Culture and Sensitivity. Urine is analyzed for the number and types of organisms present. Symptoms of infection and unexplained bacteria in a urine specimen are indications for urine culture and sensitivity testing. Bacteria from urine are placed in a medium with different antibiotics. In this way we can know which antibiotics are effective in killing or stopping the growth of the organisms (organisms are "sensitive") and which are not effective (organisms are "resistant"). A clean-catch or catheter-derived specimen is best for culture and sensitivity testing.

Composite Urine Collections. Some urine collections are made for a specified number of hours (e.g., 24 hours) for precise analysis of urine levels of substances such as creatinine or urea nitrogen, sodium, chloride, calcium, catecholamines, or other components (Chart 65-4). For a composite urine specimen, *all* urine within the designated time frame must be collected (see Table 65-3). If other urine must be obtained while the collection is in progress, measure and record the amount collected but not added to the timed collection.

The urine collection may need to be refrigerated or stored on ice to prevent changes in the urine during the collection time. Follow the procedure from the laboratory for urine storage, including whether a preservative is to be added. The urine collection must be free from fecal contamination. Menstrual blood and toilet tissue also contaminate the specimen and can invalidate the results.

The collection of all urine for a 24-hour period is often challenging. With hospitalized patients, the cooperation of staff personnel, the patient, family members, and visitors is essential. Placing signs in the bathroom, instructing the patient and family, and emphasizing the need to save the urine are helpful.

Creatinine Clearance. Creatinine clearance is a measure of glomerular filtration rate (GFR) and kidney function. The patient's age, gender, height, weight, diet, and activity level influence the expected amount of excreted creatinine. Thus these factors are considered when interpreting creatinine clearance test results. Decreases in the creatinine clearance rate may require reducing drug doses and often signifies the need to further explore the cause of kidney deterioration.

Commonly, creatinine clearance is calculated from serum creatinine, age, weight, urine creatinine, gender, and race. Creatinine clearance can be based on the excretion of injected inulin or other substances that are not reabsorbed into the blood. Creatinine clearance to estimate GFR can also be based on a 24-hour urine collection, although urine can be collected for shorter periods (e.g., 8 or 12 hours). The analysis compares the urine creatinine level with the blood creatinine level; therefore a blood specimen for creatinine must also be collected. The range for normal creatinine clearance is 107 to 139 mL/minute

CHART 65-4 Laboratory Profile

24-Hour Urine Collections

COMPONENT	NORMAL RANGE FOR ADULTS	CANADIAN RANGE FOR ADULTS	SIGNIFICANCE OF ABNORMAL FINDINGS
Creatinine	*Males:* 1-2 g/24 hr or 14-26 mg/kg/24 hr *Females:* 0.6-1.8 g/24 hr *Older adults:* slightly lower	*Males:* 124-230 mcmol/kg/24 hr *Females:* 97-177 mcmol/kg/24 hr	*Decreased amounts* indicate deterioration in function caused by kidney disease. *Increased amounts* occur with infections, exercise, diabetes mellitus, and meat meals.
Urea nitrogen	12-20 g/24 hr	0.43-0.71 mmol/24 hr	*Decreased amounts* occur when kidney damage or liver disease is present. *Increased amounts* commonly result from a high-protein diet, dehydration, trauma, or sepsis.
Sodium	40-250 mEq/24 hr	40-250 mmol/day	*Decreased* in hemorrhage, shock, hyperaldosteronism, and prerenal acute kidney injury. *Increased* with diuretic therapy, excessive salt intake, hypokalemia, and acute tubular necrosis.
Chloride	110-250 mEq/24 hr *Older adults:* Lower	110-250 mmol/24 hr	*Decreased* in certain kidney diseases, malnutrition, pyloric obstruction, prolonged nasogastric tube drainage, diarrhea, diaphoresis, heart failure, and emphysema. *Increased* with hypokalemia, adrenal insufficiency, and massive diuresis.
Calcium	100-400 mg/24 hr	2.50-7.50 mmol/kg/24 hr	*Decreased* with hypocalcemia, hypoparathyroidism, nephrosis, and nephritis. *Increased* with calcium kidney stones, hyperparathyroidism, sarcoidosis, certain cancers, immobilization, and hypercalcemia.
*Total catecholamines	<100 mcg/24 hr	<591 mmol/24 hr	*Increased* with pheochromocytoma, neuroblastomas, stress, or heavy exercise.
Protein	<80 mg/24 hr	10-150 mg/24 hr	*Increased* in glomerular disease, nephrotic syndrome, diabetic nephropathy, urinary tract malignancies, and irritations.

Data from Pagana, K., Pagana, T., & Pagana, T. (2017). *Mosby's diagnostic & laboratory test reference* (13th ed.). St. Louis: Mosby; Pagana, K., Pagana, T., & Pike-McDonald, S. (2013). *Mosby's Canadian manual of diagnostic and laboratory tests.* St. Louis: Elsevier; and United States Library of Medicine. https://www.nlm.nih.gov/medlineplus/ency/srticle/003580.htm.
*Epinephrine and norepinephrine only; dopamine is not measured.

for men (1.78-2.32 mL/sec) and 87 to 107 mL/minute (1.45-1.78 mL/sec) for women tested with a 24-hour urine collection. Values decrease progressively per decade of life for adults older than 40 years because of age-related decline in GFR. However, these expensive and time-consuming methods are usually reserved for when a decision for starting renal replacement therapy (dialysis) is needed.

Current guidelines suggest that clinical laboratories report an estimate of GFR whenever a serum creatinine is ordered, based on the modified diet in renal disease (MDRD) study equation. The MDRD equation does not require urine to estimate GFR. The estimated GFR (eGFR) for the MDRD equation is >60 mL/min/1.73 m^2 (Pagana et al., 2017). An alternate approach for calculation is the Cockcroft-Gault equation, which has traditionally been used to determine drug dose adjustment when the eGFR is <50 mL/min/1.73 m^2.

Urine Electrolytes. Urine samples can be analyzed for electrolyte levels (e.g., sodium, chloride). Normally the amount of sodium excreted in the urine is nearly equal to that consumed. Urine sodium levels of less than 10 mEq/L (mmol/L) indicate that the tubules are able to conserve (reabsorb) sodium.

Urine Osmolarity. Osmolarity measures the concentration of particles in solution. The particles in urine contributing to osmolarity include electrolytes, glucose, urea, and creatinine. Urine osmolarity can vary from 50 to 1200 mOsm/kg or L (mmol/kg or L), depending on the patient's hydration status and kidney function. With average fluid intake, the range for urine osmolarity is 300 to 900 mOsm/kg or L (mmol/kg or L). Electrolytes, acids, and other normal metabolic wastes are continually produced. These particles are the solute load that must be excreted in the urine on a regular basis. This is referred to as *obligatory solute excretion.* If the patient loses excessive fluids, the kidney response is to save water while excreting wastes by excreting small amounts of highly concentrated urine. Diet, drugs, and activity can change urine osmolarity. Urine with an increased osmolarity is concentrated urine with less water and more solutes. Urine with a decreased osmolarity is dilute urine with more water and fewer solutes.

? NCLEX EXAMINATION CHALLENGE 65-2

Safe and Effective Care Environment

Which client being managed for dehydration does the nurse consider at **greatest** risk for possible reduced kidney function?
A. An 80-year-old man who has benign prostatic hyperplasia
B. A 62-year-old woman with a known allergy to contrast media
C. A 48-year-old woman with established urinary incontinence
D. A 45-year-old man receiving oral and IV fluid therapy

Bedside Sonography/Bladder Scanners. The use of portable ultrasound scanners in the hospital and rehabilitation setting by nurses is a noninvasive method of estimating bladder volume (Fig. 65-10). Bladder scanners are used to screen for post-void residual volumes and determine the need for intermittent

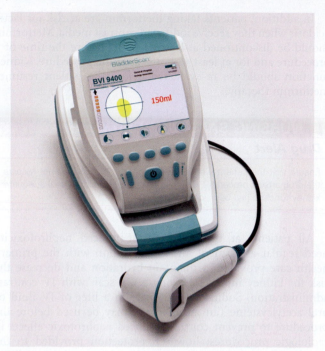

FIG. 65-10 "BladderScan" BVI 9400, a handheld portable bladder scanner. (Courtesy Verathon Corporation, Bothell, WA.)

catheterization based on the amount of urine in the bladder rather than the time between catheterizations. There is no discomfort with the scan, and no patient preparation beyond an explanation of what to expect is required.

Explain the reason the procedure is being done and what sensations the patient might experience during it. For example, "This test will measure the amount of urine in your bladder. I will place a gel pad just above your pubic area and then place the probe, which is a little bigger and heavier than a stethoscope, on the gel."

Before scanning, select the male or female icon on the bladder scanner. Using the female icon allows the scanner software to subtract the volume of the uterus from any measurement. Use the male icon on all men and on women who have undergone a hysterectomy.

Place an ultrasound gel pad right above the pubic bone or moisten the round dome of the scan head area with 5 mL of conducting gel to improve ultrasound conduction. Use gel on the scanner head for obese patients and those with heavy body hair in the area to be scanned. Place the probe midline over the abdomen about 1.5 inches (4 cm) above the pubic bone. Aim the scan head so the ultrasound is projected toward the expected location of the bladder, typically toward the patient's coccyx. Press and release the scan button. The scan is complete with the sound of a beep, and a volume is displayed. Two readings are recommended for best accuracy. An aiming icon on the portable bladder scanner indicates whether the bladder image is centered on the crosshairs of the scan head. If the crosshairs on the aiming icon are not centered on the bladder, the measured volume may not be accurate.

Imaging Assessment

Many imaging procedures are used to diagnose abnormalities within the renal-urinary system (Table 65-4). Explain the procedures to the patient, prepare him or her, and provide

TABLE 65-4 Radiologic and Special Diagnostic Tests for Patients With Disorders of the Kidney and Urinary System

TEST	PURPOSE
Radiography of kidneys, ureters, and bladder (KUB) (plain film of abdomen)	To screen for the presence of two kidneys To measure kidney size To detect gross obstruction in kidneys or urinary tract
Computed tomography (CT) with contrast, CT-arteriography or angiography	To measure kidney size To evaluate contour to assess for injury, masses, or obstruction in kidneys or the urinary tract To assess renal blood flow
Magnetic resonance imaging (MRI)	Similar to CT Useful for staging of cancers
Ultrasonography (US) Can be used with contrast media	To identify the urine volume in the bladder, size of the kidneys or obstruction (e.g., tumors, stones) in the kidneys or lower urinary tract Can also assess blood flow to and from the kidney
(Nuclear) renal scan	To evaluate renal perfusion To estimate glomerular filtration rate To provide functional information without exposing the patient to iodinated contrast medium
Cystoscopy	To identify abnormalities of the bladder wall and urethral and ureteral occlusions To treat small obstructions or lesions via fulguration, lithotripsy, or removal with a stone basket
Cystography and cystourethrography	To outline bladder's contour when full and examine structure during voiding To examine the structure of the urethra To detect backward urine flow
Metabolic imaging with positron emission tomography (PET)	To evaluate cysts, tumors, and other lesions, eliminating the need for biopsy in some patients

follow-up care. Patient education materials for many urologic tests have been developed by organizations such as the Society for Urologic Nurses and Associates and are freely available.

Kidney, Ureter, and Bladder X-rays. An x-ray of the kidneys, ureters, and bladder (KUB) is a plain film of the abdomen obtained without any specific patient preparation. The KUB study shows gross anatomic features and obvious stones, strictures, calcifications, or obstructions in the urinary tract. This test identifies the shape, size, and position of the organs in relation to other parts of the urinary tract. Other tests are needed to diagnose functional or structural problems.

There is no discomfort or risk from this procedure. Tell the patient that the x-ray will be taken while he or she is in a supine position. No specific follow-up care is needed.

Computed Tomography. Inform the patient that a CT scan provides three-dimensional information about the kidneys, ureters, bladder, and surrounding tissues. The CT scan is performed in a special room, usually in the radiology department. It can provide information about tumors, cysts, abscesses, other masses, and obstruction. CT can also be used to image the kidney's vascular system (i.e., CT angiography). Some hospitals require patients having CT scans to be NPO for some period before the scan, although there is no specific evidence guiding this practice.

Determine whether the scan requires contrast medium (often called *dye*). The most common contrast agents used for imaging of the kidney are radiopaque, contain iodine, are nonionic, and have varying osmolarity. These include Iohexol (Omnipaque), Iopromide (Ultravist), and Iodixanol (Visiopaque). Oral or injected contrast medium is usually given before starting the imaging procedure. Dye use may be omitted in patients at risk for contrast-induced acute kidney injury, but the images produced are less distinct.

When contrast is used, ensure that there is sufficient oral or IV intake to dilute and excrete the contrast media. Typically, the radiologist will specify a total fluid intake of 1 liter or a variable rate to maintain urine output at 1 to 2 mL/kg/hr for up to 6 hours. When no contrast is used, there is no special postprocedure care.

Contrast medium is potentially kidney-damaging (nephrotoxic). *Contrast-induced nephropathy* is the onset of *acute kidney failure* within 48 hours after the administration of iodinated contrast medium (Lambert et al., 2017; Wichmann et al., 2015). The risk for *contrast-induced nephropathy* is greatest in patients who are older or dehydrated, have pre-existing chronic kidney disease (CKD), or have comorbidities of diabetes, heart failure, or current hypotension (Silva et al., 2015). Patients who take nephrotoxic drugs also are at risk (Davenport et al., 2014). Chart 65-5 lists assessment questions to ask before a patient undergoes testing with contrast material.

CHART 65-5   Best Practice for Patient Safety & Quality Care QSEN

Assessing the Patient About to Undergo a Kidney Test or Procedure Using Contrast Medium

Before the procedure:
- Ask the patient if he or she has ever had a reaction to contrast media. (Such a patient has the highest risk for having another reaction.)
- Ask the patient about a history of asthma. (Patients with asthma have been shown to be at greater risk for contrast reactions than the general public. When reactions do occur, they are more likely to be severe.)
- Ask the patient about known hay fever or food or drug allergies, especially to seafood, eggs, milk, or chocolate. (Contrast reactions have been reported to be as high as 15% in these patients.)
- Ask the patient to describe any specific allergic reactions (e.g., hives, facial edema, difficulty breathing, bronchospasm).
- Assess for a history of renal impairment and for conditions that have been implicated in increasing the chance of developing kidney injury or impairment after contrast media (e.g., diabetic nephropathy, class IV heart failure, dehydration, concomitant use of potentially nephrotoxic drugs such as the aminoglycosides or NSAIDs, and cirrhosis).
- Ask the patient if he or she is taking metformin (Glucophage). (Metformin must be discontinued at least 24 hours before any study using contrast media because the life-threatening complication of lactic acidosis, although rare, could occur.)
- Assess hydration status by checking blood pressure, heart and respiratory rates, mucous membranes, skin turgor, and urine concentration.
- Ask the patient when he or she last ate or drank anything.

In addition, patients taking metformin are at risk for lactic acidosis when they receive iodinated contrast media. Metformin should be discontinued at least 24 hours before the time of a procedure and for at least 48 hours after the procedure. Kidney function should be re-evaluated before the patient resumes metformin therapy.

! NURSING SAFETY PRIORITY QSEN

Drug Alert

Ensure that the patient who is prescribed metformin does not receive the drug after a procedure requiring IV contrast material until adequate kidney function has been determined.

All patients at risk for contrast-induced nephrotoxicity need regular assessment and collaboration with the primary health care provider to maintain hydration and decrease the risk for kidney injury following a CT scan with IV contrast administration. Sodium bicarbonate in a liter of IV fluid or oral acetylcysteine (an antioxidant) may be used before the procedure to prevent contrast-induced nephrotoxic effects in radiologic procedures; however, protection provided to the kidneys is not consistent in clinical trials (Lameire & Kellum, 2013). Diuretics may be given immediately after the contrast is injected to enhance excretion in patients who are well hydrated.

Magnetic Resonance Imaging. MRI provides improved imaging between normal and abnormal tissue in the renal system compared with a CT scan. As with all MRIs, the patient with metal implants (pins, pacemaker, joint replacement, aneurysmal clips, or other cosmetic or medical devices) is not eligible for this test because the magnet can move the metal implant. Gadolinium-based contrast agents have been linked with nephrogenic systemic fibrosis (Pagana et al., 2017) and should not be used in patients with renal impairment, usually defined as a serum creatinine above 1.5 mg/dL (110 mcmol/L) or an estimated GFR less than 45 mL/minute. Adults older than 60 years should be carefully evaluated for renal impairment (see the Kidney and Urinary System Changes Associated with Aging section).

Kidney Ultrasonography. Inform the patient that ultrasonography does not cause discomfort and is without risk. This test usually requires a full bladder. Ask the patient to drink 500 to 1000 mL of water, if needed, about 2 to 3 hours before the test to help fill the bladder. The patient should not void after drinking the water until the test is complete. This test applies sound waves to structures of different densities to produce images of the kidneys, ureters, and bladder and surrounding tissues. Ultrasonography allows assessment of kidney size, cortical thickness, and status of the calices. The test can identify obstruction in the urinary tract, tumors, cysts, and other masses without the use of contrast. In addition, it can determine blood flow into and out from the kidney using Doppler color flow imaging.

The patient undergoing kidney ultrasound is usually placed in the prone position. Sonographic gel is applied to the skin over the back and flank areas to enhance sound wave conduction. A transducer in contact with and moving across the skin delivers sound waves and measures the echoes. Images of the internal structures are produced. Skin care to remove the gel is all that is needed after ultrasonography.

Renal Scan. This imaging test is used to examine the perfusion, function, and structure of the kidneys by the IV administration of a radioisotope. It does not use an iodinated contrast agent and thus may be used in preference to a CT scan when the patient is allergic to iodine or has impaired kidney function that places him or her at risk for kidney injury from IV contrast.

No fasting or sedation is used. A peripheral IV catheter is inserted to give the radioisotope contrast agent. While the patient lies in a prone or sitting position, a camera is passed over the kidney area and records the isotope uptake on film, minutes after the radioisotope is given. After initial images, the patient may be given furosemide or captopril to better visualize kidney function and blood flow. The isotope is eliminated 6 to 24 hours after the procedure. Encourage the patient to drink fluids to aid in excretion of the isotope. Because only tracer doses of radioisotopes are used, no precautions are needed related to radioactive exposure.

Renal Arteriography (Angiography). Renal arteriography allows the radiopaque contrast medium to enter the renal blood vessels and generates images to determine blood vessel size and abnormalities. This test has largely been replaced by other imaging techniques (e.g., nuclear renal scans, ultrasonography, computed tomography) and is seldom used as a stand-alone diagnostic procedure. The most common use of renal arteriography is at the time of a renal angioplasty or other intervention.

Cystoscopy and Cystourethroscopy

Patient Preparation. Cystoscopy and cystourethroscopy are endoscopic procedures and require completion of a preoperative checklist and a signed informed consent statement. The urologist provides a complete description of and reasons for the procedure, and the nurse reinforces this information. Cystoscopy may be performed for diagnosis or treatment. This test is used to examine for bladder trauma (cystoscopy) or urethral trauma (cystourethroscopy) and to identify causes of urinary tract obstruction. Cystoscopy also may be used to remove bladder tumors or plant radium seeds into a tumor, dilate the urethra and ureters with or without stent placement, stop areas of bleeding, or resect an enlarged prostate gland.

Cystoscopy may be performed under general anesthesia or under local anesthesia with sedation. The patient's age and general health and the expected duration of the procedure are considered in the decision about anesthesia. A light evening meal may be eaten. Usually the patient is NPO after midnight on the night before the cystoscopy. A bowel preparation with laxatives or enemas is performed the evening before the procedure so bowel contents do not interfere with the procedure.

Procedure. The cystoscopy is performed in a designated cystoscopic examination room. If the procedure is performed in a surgical suite under general anesthesia, the usual surgical support personnel are present (see Chapter 15). This procedure is often performed in clinics, ambulatory surgery or short-procedure units, or a urologist's office.

Assist the patient onto a table and, after sedation, place him or her in the lithotomy position. After the anesthesia is given and the area cleansed and draped, the urologist inserts a cystoscope through the urethra into the urinary bladder. This examination commonly includes the use of both the cystoscope and the urethroscope.

Follow-up Care. After this procedure with general anesthesia, the patient is returned to a postanesthesia care unit (PACU) or area. If local anesthesia and sedation were used, he or she may be returned directly to the hospital room. Patients undergoing cystoscopic examinations as outpatients are transferred to an area for monitoring before discharge to home. Monitor for airway patency and breathing, changes in vital signs (including temperature), and changes in urine output. Also observe for the complications of bladder puncture, excessive bleeding, and infection. Bladder puncture is accompanied by severe pain, including abdominal pain, nausea, and vomiting.

A catheter may or may not be present after cystoscopy. The patient without a catheter has urinary frequency as a result of irritation from the procedure. The urine may be pink tinged, but gross bleeding is not expected. Bleeding or the presence of clots may obstruct the catheter and decrease urine output. Monitor urine output and notify the urologist of obvious blood clots or a decreased or absent urine output. Irrigate the Foley catheter with sterile saline, if prescribed. Notify the urologist if the patient has a fever (with or without chills) or an elevated white blood cell (WBC) count, which suggests infection. Urge the patient to take oral fluids to increase urine output (which helps prevent clotting) and reduce the burning sensation on urination.

Cystography and Cystourethrography. These tests are a series of x-rays or a continuous radiographic visualization by fluoroscopy. During the imaging, radiopaque contrast medium fills the bladder, and the bladder is emptied. Images show structure and function of the bladder and urethra. Tumors, rupture or perforation of the bladder and urethra, abnormal backflow of urine, and distortion from trauma or other pelvic masses can be seen.

Patient Preparation and Procedure. Explain the procedure to the patient. A urinary catheter is temporarily needed to instill contrast medium directly into the bladder for both procedures. The contrast medium enhances x-ray visibility of the lower urinary tract and is not absorbed into the bloodstream, reducing the risk for contrast-induced kidney injury.

After bladder filling, x-rays are taken from the front, back, and side positions. For the voiding cystourethrogram (VCUG), the patient is requested to void, and x-rays are taken during the voiding. A VCUG can determine whether urine refluxes (flow backward) into the ureter. The cystogram is used in cases of trauma when urethral or bladder injury is suspected or for patients with recurrent *pyelonephritis* (kidney infection).

Follow-up Care. Monitor for infection as a result of catheter placement. In this test, the contrast medium is not nephrotoxic because it does not enter the bloodstream and does not reach the kidney. Encourage fluid intake to dilute the urine and reduce the burning sensation from catheter irritation after removal. Monitor for changes in urine output because pelvic or urethral trauma may be present.

Retrograde Procedures. Retrograde means going against the normal flow of urine. A retrograde examination of the ureters and pelvis (*pyelogram*), the bladder (*cystogram*), and the urethra (*urethrogram*) involves instilling radiopaque contrast medium into the lower urinary tract. Because the contrast agent is instilled directly to obtain an outline of the structures desired, the agent does not enter the bloodstream. Therefore the patient is not at risk for contrast-induced kidney injury.

The patient is prepared for retrograde procedures (retrograde pyelography, retrograde cystography, and retrograde urethrography) in the same way as for cystoscopy. Retrograde x-rays are obtained during the cystoscopy. After placement of the cystoscope by the urologist, catheters are placed into each ureter, and contrast is instilled into each ureter and renal pelvis. The catheters are removed by the urologist, and x-rays are taken to outline these structures as the agent is excreted. The procedure identifies obstruction or structural abnormalities.

For patients undergoing retrograde cystoscopy or urethrography, radiopaque contrast medium is instilled similarly into the bladder or urethra. Cystography and urethrography identify structural problems, such as fistulas, diverticula, and tumors.

After retrograde procedures, monitor the patient for infection caused by placing instruments in the urinary tract. Because these procedures are performed during cystoscopic examination, follow-up care is the same as that for cystoscopy, including monitoring for bladder puncture or perforation.

Other Diagnostic Assessments

Urodynamic Studies. Urodynamic studies examine the processes of voiding and include:

- Tests of bladder capacity, pressure, and tone
- Studies of urethral pressure and urine flow
- Tests of perineal voluntary muscle function

These tests are often used along with voiding urographic or cystoscopic procedures to evaluate problems with urine flow and disorders of the lower urinary tract.

Cystometrography (CMG) can determine how well the bladder wall (detrusor) muscle functions and how sensitive it is to stretching as the bladder fills. This test provides information about bladder capacity, bladder pressure, and voiding reflexes.

Explain the procedure and inform the patient that a urinary catheter will be needed temporarily during the procedure. Ask the patient to void normally. Record the amount and time of voiding. Insert a urinary catheter to measure the residual urine volume. The cystometer is attached to the catheter, and fluid is instilled via the catheter into the bladder. The point at which the patient first notes a feeling of the urge to void and the point at which he or she notes a strong urge to void are recorded. Bladder capacity and bladder pressure readings are recorded graphically. The patient is asked to void when the bladder instillation is complete (about 500 mL). The residual urine after voiding is recorded, and the catheter is removed. Electromyography of the perineal muscles may be performed during this examination.

For any procedure that involves inserting instruments into the urinary tract, monitor for infection. Record the patient's temperature, the character of the urine, and urine output volume.

Urethral pressure profile (also called a *urethral pressure profilometry [UPP]*) can provide information about the nature of urinary incontinence or urinary retention.

Explain the procedure and inform the patient that a urinary catheter will be needed temporarily during the procedure. A special catheter with pressure-sensing capabilities is inserted into the bladder. Variations in the pressure of the smooth muscle of the urethra are recorded as the catheter is slowly withdrawn.

As with any study involving inserting instruments into the urinary tract, monitor the patient for symptoms of infection.

Urine stream testing is used to evaluate pelvic muscle strength and the effectiveness of pelvic muscles in stopping the flow of urine. It is useful in assessing urinary incontinence.

Explain the procedure and reassure the patient that efforts will be made to ensure privacy. The patient is asked to begin urinating. Three to five seconds after urination begins, the

examiner gives the patient a signal to stop urine flow. The length of time required to stop the flow of urine is recorded.

Cleaning the perineal area, as after any voiding, is all that is necessary after the urine stream test.

Electromyography (EMG) of the perineal muscles tests the strength of the muscles used in voiding. This information may help identify methods of improving continence. Inform the patient that some mild, temporary discomfort may accompany placement of the electrodes.

In EMG of the perineal muscles, electrodes are placed in either the rectum or the urethra to measure muscle contraction and relaxation. After the completion of EMG, administer analgesics as prescribed to promote the patient's comfort.

🔍 NCLEX EXAMINATION CHALLENGE 65-3

Safe and Effective Care Environment

The nurse is admitting a client who has type 2 diabetes (T2D) and is scheduled for surgery. Which laboratory findings from this client's admission panel does the nurse report as indicating possible abnormal kidney function? **Select all that apply.**

A. Presence of ammonia in the urine
B. Urine microalbumin 240 mcg/24 hour (0.240 g/ 24 hour)
C. Urine specific gravity of 1.028
D. Blood urea nitrogen of 38 mg/dL (13.5 mmol/L)
E. Serum creatinine 2.2 mg/dL (294.3 mcmol/L)
F. Blood osmolarity 290 mOsm/kg (290 mmol/kg)

Kidney Biopsy

Patient Preparation. Explain that a kidney biopsy can help determine a cause of unexplained kidney problems and help direct or change therapy. Most kidney biopsies are performed **percutaneously** (through skin and other tissues) using ultrasound or CT guidance. The patient signs an informed consent. Patients are NPO for 4 to 6 hours before the procedure.

Because of the risk for bleeding after the biopsy, coagulation studies such as platelet count, activated partial thromboplastin time (aPTT), prothrombin time (PT), and bleeding time are performed before surgery. Hypertension is aggressively managed before and after the procedure because high blood pressure can make stopping the bleeding after the biopsy more difficult. Uremia also increases the risk for bleeding, and dialysis may be prescribed before a biopsy. A blood transfusion may be needed to correct anemia before biopsy.

Procedure. In a percutaneous biopsy, the nephrologist or radiologist obtains tissue samples without an incision. Patients receive sedation and are monitored throughout the procedure. The patient is placed in the prone position on the procedure table. The entry site is selected after taking preliminary images. The area is prepped and sterilely draped. A local anesthetic is injected, and the physician then inserts the biopsy device into the tissues toward the kidney. Needle depth and placement are confirmed by ultrasound or CT. While the patient holds his or her breath, the needle is advanced into the renal cortex. Samples are then taken with a spring-loaded coring biopsy needle and sent for pathologic study.

Follow-up Care. After a percutaneous biopsy, the major risk is bleeding into the kidney or into the tissues external from the kidney at the biopsy site. For 24 hours after the biopsy, monitor the dressing site, vital signs (especially fluctuations in blood pressure), urine output, hemoglobin level, and hematocrit. Even if the dressing is dry and there is no hematoma, the patient could be bleeding from the site. An internal bleed is not readily visible but is suspected with flank pain, decreasing blood pressure, decreasing urine output, or other signs of hypovolemia or shock. With severe bleeding, some patients develop bruising along the flank and back accompanied by pain.

The patient follows a plan of strict bedrest, lying in a supine position with a back roll for additional support for 2 to 6 hours after the biopsy. The head of the bed may be elevated, and the patient may resume oral intake of food and fluids. After bedrest, the patient may have limited bathroom privileges if there is no evidence of bleeding.

Monitor for hematuria, the most common complication of kidney biopsy. Hematuria occurs microscopically in most patients, but 5% to 9% have gross hematuria. This problem usually resolves without treatment 48 to 72 hours after the biopsy but can persist for 2 to 3 weeks. In rare cases, transfusions and surgery are required. There should be no obvious blood clots in the urine.

The patient may have some local pain after the biopsy. If aching originates at the biopsy site and begins to radiate to the flank, back, and around the front of the abdomen, bleeding may have started, or a hematoma is forming around the kidney. This pattern of pain with bleeding occurs because blood in the tissues around the kidney increases pressure on local nerve tracts.

If bleeding occurs, IV fluid, packed red blood cells, or both may be needed to prevent shock. In general, a small amount of bleeding creates enough pressure to compress bleeding sites. This is called a *tamponade effect*. If tamponade does not occur and bleeding is extensive, surgery for hemostasis or even nephrectomy may be needed. A hematoma in, on, or around the kidney may become infected, requiring treatment with antibiotics and surgical drainage.

If no bleeding occurs, the patient can resume general activities after 24 hours. Instruct him or her to avoid lifting heavy objects, exercising, or performing other strenuous activities for 1 to 2 weeks after the biopsy procedure. Driving may also be restricted. Refer to Chapter 16 for general postoperative care for the patient who has undergone an open kidney biopsy.

❓ NCLEX EXAMINATION CHALLENGE 65-4

Safe and Effective Care Environment

Which symptom(s) in a client during the first 12 hours after a kidney biopsy indicate(s) to the nurse a possible complication from the procedure?
A. The client experiences nausea and vomiting after drinking juice.
B. The biopsy site is tender to light palpation.
C. The abdomen is distended, and the client reports abdominal discomfort.
D. The heart rate is 118, blood pressure is 108/50, and peripheral pulses are thready.

❓ CLINICAL JUDGMENT CHALLENGE 65-1

Safety; Patient-Centered Care QSEN

You are assessing a 66-year-old patient who is scheduled for surgical repair of a hip fracture from a car crash 4 hours ago. The patient hit a telephone pole while traveling at 45-50 miles per hour and was wearing a seat belt at the time of the accident. When the patient voids, you notice that the urine is rust-colored. The patient reports a sensation of burning during this voiding but no other subjective urinary symptoms.
1. What assessment information will you document?
2. What additional information should you get from the patient and what else should you consider?
3. Organize your thoughts into a SBAR communication (see Chapter 1).
4. Which member(s) of the interprofessional team will you notify and why?

GET READY FOR THE NCLEX® EXAMINATION!

KEY POINTS

Review these Key Points for each NCLEX Examination Client Needs Category.

Safe and Effective Care Environment
- Use Contact Precautions with any patient who has drainage from the genitourinary tract. **QSEN: Safety**
- Wear gloves when testing or handling urine. **QSEN: Safety**
- Evaluate risk for injury from diagnostic testing by asking about adverse or allergic reactions to radiopaque contrast agents, iodine, or gadolinium. **QSEN: Safety**
- Ask the patient about the use of prescribed and over-the-counter drugs that increase risk for kidney dysfunction. **QSEN: Safety**
- Verify that informed consent has been obtained and that the patient has a clear understanding of the potential risks before he or she undergoes invasive procedures to assess the kidneys and urinary function. **QSEN: Safety**
- Assess the patient for bleeding, increased pain, and symptoms of perforation or infection after any invasive test of kidney/urinary function. **QSEN: Safety**
- Inform primary health care providers about any symptoms of complications following invasive or noninvasive tests of urinary and kidney structure or function. **QSEN: Safety**

Health Promotion and Maintenance
- Teach patients to clean the perineal area after voiding, after having a bowel movement, and after sexual intercourse. **QSEN: Evidence-Based Practice**
- Urge all patients to maintain an adequate fluid intake (sufficient to dilute urine to a light yellow color). A minimum of 2 L/day may be recommended unless another health problem requires fluid restriction. **QSEN: Evidence-Based Practice**
- Teach patients who come into contact with chemicals in their workplaces or for leisure-time activities to avoid direct skin or mucous membrane contact with these chemicals. **QSEN: Safety**

Psychosocial Integrity
- Allow the patient the opportunity to express fear or anxiety about tests of the kidneys and urinary tract or about a

potential change in kidney function. **QSEN: Patient-Centered Care**

- Assess the patient's level of comfort in discussing issues related to ELIMINATION and the urogenital area. **QSEN: Patient-Centered Care**
- Provide as much privacy as possible for patients undergoing examination or testing of the kidney/urinary tract. **QSEN: Patient-Centered Care**
- Use language and terminology that the patient can understand during discussions of kidney/urinary assessment. **QSEN: Patient-Centered Care**

Physiological Integrity

- Use sterile technique when inserting a urinary catheter. **QSEN: Evidence-Based Practice**
- Ask the patient about kidney problems in any other members of the family, because some problems have a genetic component. **QSEN: Patient-Centered Care**

- Ask the patient about current and past drug use (prescribed, over-the-counter, and illicit) and evaluate drug use for potential nephrotoxicity. **QSEN: Patient-Centered Care**
- Explain all diagnostic procedures, restrictions, and follow-up care to the patient scheduled for tests. **QSEN: Patient-Centered Care**
- Interpret laboratory data to distinguish between dehydration and kidney impairment. **QSEN: Evidence-Based Practice**
- Describe how to obtain a sterile urine specimen from a urinary catheter. **QSEN: Evidence-Based Practice**
- Describe which information regarding the urinary and renal system assessment should be documented in the patient's electronic health record. **QSEN: Patient-Centered Care**
- Assess urine output (compared with fluid intake) and serum tests of kidney function closely after any procedure in which IV radiopaque contrast agents are used. **QSEN: Evidence-Based Practice**

SELECTED BIBLIOGRAPHY

Brenner, B. M. (Ed.), (2016). *Brenner & Rector's the kidney* (10th ed.). Philadelphia: Saunders.

Burchum, J., & Rosenthal, L. (2016). *Lehne's pharmacology for nursing care* (9th ed.). St. Louis: Elsevier.

Davenport, M., Khalatbari, S., & Ellis, J. (2014). The challenges in assessing contrast-induced nephropathy: Where are we now? *American Journal of Roentgenology*, 202(4), 784–789.

Jackson, C., Botelho, E., Josepf, J., & Tennstedt, S. (2013). Accessing and evaluating urologic health information: Differences by race/ethnicity and gender. *Urologic Nursing*, 33(6), 282–287.

Jarvis, C. (2016). *Physical examination & health assessment* (7th ed.). St. Louis: Saunders.

Lambert, P., Chasson, K., Horton, S., Petrin, C., Marshall, E., Bowdon, S., et al. (2017). Reducing acute kidney injury due to contrast material: How nurses can improve patient safety. *Critical Care Nurse*, 37(1), 13–26.

Lameire, N., & Kellum, J. (2013). Contrast-induced acute kidney injury and renal support for acute kidney injury: A KDIGO summary (Part 2). *Critical Care: The Official Journal of the Critical Care Forum*, 17(1), 205.

McCance, K., Huether, S., Brashers, V., & Rote, N. (2014). *Pathophysiology: The biologic basis for disease in adults and children* (7th ed.). St. Louis: Mosby.

McGoldrick, M. (2015). Urine specimen collection and transport. *Home Healthcare Now*, 33(5), 285.

National Kidney Disease Education Program (NKDEP). (2015). *CKD and drug dosing: Information for providers.* http://www.niddk.nih.gov/health-information/health-communication-programs/nkdep/a-z/ckd-drug-dosing/Pages/CKD-drug-dosing.aspx.

Pagana, K., Pagana, T., & Pagana, T. (2017). *Mosby's diagnostic and laboratory test reference* (13th ed.). St. Louis: Mosby.

Pagana, K., Pagana, T., & Pike-McDonald, S. (2013). *Mosby's Canadian manual of diagnostic and laboratory tests*. St. Louis: Elsevier.

Puzantian, H., & Townsend, R. (2013). Understanding kidney function assessment: The basics and advances. *Journal of the American Association of Nurse Practitioners*, 25(7), 334–341.

Silva, S. A., Shah, P. M., Chertow, G. M., Harel, S., Wald, R., & Harel, Z. (2015). Risk prediction models for contrast-induced nephropathy: Systemic review. *British Medical Journal*, 351, h4395.

Society of Urologic Nurses and Associates. (2015). *Patient education*. https://www.suna.org/resource/patient-education.

Touhy, T., & Jett, K. (2016). *Ebersole & Hess' Toward healthy aging: Human needs & nursing response*. St. Louis: Elsevier.

U.S. Renal Data Systems. (2015). 2015 USRDS Annual Data Report. *Epidemiology of Kidney Disease in the United States. National Institutes of Health, National Institute of Diabetes and Digestive and Kidney Diseases*, Bethesda, MD. http://www.usrds.org/adr.aspx.

Wichmann, J. L., Katzberg, R. W., Litwin, S. E., Zwerner, P. L., De Cecco, C. N., Vogl, T. J., et al. (2015). Contrast-induced nephropathy. *Circulation*, 132(online), 1931–1936.

CHAPTER 66

Care of Patients With Urinary Problems

Chris Winkelman

PRIORITY AND INTERRELATED CONCEPTS

The priority concept for this chapter is ELIMINATION.

✳ The ELIMINATION concept exemplar for this chapter is Urinary Incontinence, below.

The interrelated concepts for this chapter are:
- COMFORT
- IMMUNITY
- TISSUE INTEGRITY

LEARNING OUTCOMES

Safe and Effective Care Environment

1. Collaborate with the interprofessional team to coordinate high-quality care and promote urinary ELIMINATION in patients who have problems in the urinary tract.
2. Teach the patient and caregiver(s) how home safety is affected by impaired ELIMINATION resulting from problems in the urinary tract.

Health Promotion and Maintenance

3. Identify community resources for patients requiring assistance with incontinence or any chronic urinary tract problem.
4. Teach adults how to decrease the risk for urinary tract infections.

Psychosocial Integrity

5. Implement nursing interventions to help patients and families cope with the psychosocial impact caused by urinary incontinence or any other chronic problem of the urinary tract.

Physiological Integrity

6. Apply knowledge of anatomy and physiology to assess patients with urinary problems affecting ELIMINATION.
7. Teach the patient and caregiver(s) about common drugs used for urinary tract problems, including pain control.

The urinary tract includes the ureters, bladder, and urethra. Although these structures play no role in the making of urine, their functions are essential for the urine made by the kidneys to be eliminated from the body. Both infectious and noninfectious problems in the urinary tract can disrupt urinary ELIMINATION and affect control of fluids, electrolytes, nitrogenous wastes, and blood pressure.

Any urinary problem can affect the storage or ELIMINATION of urine. Both acute and chronic urinary problems are common and costly. More than 20 million people in the United States are treated annually for urinary tract infections, cystitis, kidney and ureter stones, or urinary incontinence (U.S. Renal Data Systems, 2015). Although life-threatening complications are rare with urinary problems, patients may have functional, physical, and psychosocial changes that reduce quality of life. Nursing interventions are directed toward prevention, detection, and management of urologic disorders.

✳ ELIMINATION CONCEPT EXEMPLAR
Urinary Incontinence

❖ PATHOPHYSIOLOGY

Continence is the control over the time and place of urine ELIMINATION and is unique to humans and some domestic animals. It is a learned behavior in which a person can suppress the urge to urinate until a socially appropriate location is available (e.g., a toilet). Efficient bladder emptying (i.e., coordination between bladder contraction and urethral relaxation) is needed for continence.

Incontinence is an involuntary loss of urine severe enough to cause social or hygienic problems. It is *not* a normal consequence of aging or childbirth and often is a stigmatizing and an underreported health problem. Many adults suffer in silence, are socially isolated, and may be unaware that treatment is available. In addition, the cost of incontinence can be enormous.

Continence occurs when pressure in the urethra is greater than pressure in the bladder. For normal voiding to occur, the urethra must relax, and the bladder must contract with enough pressure and duration to empty completely. Voiding should occur in a smooth and coordinated manner under conscious control. Incontinence has several possible causes and can be either temporary or chronic (Table 66-1). Except for infection, temporary causes of incontinence usually do not involve a disorder of the urinary tract. The most common types of adult urinary incontinence are stress incontinence, urge incontinence, overflow incontinence, functional incontinence, and a mixed form.

Stress incontinence is the most common type. Its main feature is the inability to retain urine when laughing, coughing, sneezing, jogging, or lifting. In the continent adult, the urethra can be relaxed and tightened under conscious control because skeletal muscles of the pelvic floor surround it. When an adult feels the urge to urinate, the conscious contraction of the urethra can override a bladder contraction if the urethral contraction is strong enough.

Patients with *stress incontinence* cannot tighten the urethra enough to overcome the increased bladder pressure caused by contraction of the detrusor muscle. This is common after childbirth, when the pelvic muscles are stretched and weakened. The weakened pelvic floor allows the urethra to move during exertion. If the pelvic muscles are not strengthened, this condition continues. Low estrogen levels after menopause also contribute to stress incontinence. Vaginal, urethral, and pelvic floor muscles become thin and weak without estrogen.

Urge incontinence is the loss of urine for no apparent reason after suddenly feeling the need or urge to urinate. Normally when the bladder is full, contraction of the smooth muscle fibers of the bladder detrusor muscle signals the brain that it is time to urinate. Continent adults override that signal and relax the detrusor muscle for the time it takes to locate a toilet. Those who suffer from urge incontinence cannot suppress the signal and have a sudden strong urge to void and can leak large amounts of urine at this time. Urge incontinence is also known as an *overactive bladder (OAB)*. Overactivity may have no known cause or may be the result of abnormal detrusor contractions related to other problems. Such problems include stroke and other neurologic problems; other urinary tract problems; and irritation from concentrated urine, artificial sweeteners, caffeine, alcohol, and citric intake. Drugs, such as diuretics, and nicotine can also irritate the bladder. Often urine loss is related to both stress and urge incontinence, and symptoms mimic more than one subtype. This category is more common in older women.

Overflow incontinence occurs when the detrusor muscle fails to contract and the bladder becomes overdistended. This type of incontinence (*reflex incontinence* or *underactive bladder*) occurs when the bladder has reached its maximum capacity and some urine must leak out to prevent bladder rupture. Causes may include an underactive bladder muscle or a urethral obstruction. Causes for the underactive (acontractile) bladder may or may not be determined. A partially obstructed urethra can fail to relax enough to allow urine flow. Incomplete bladder emptying or urinary retention from urethral obstruction results in overflow incontinence.

Functional incontinence is incontinence occurring as a result of factors other than the abnormal function of the bladder and urethra. A common factor is the loss of cognitive function in patients affected by dementia. To maintain continence, an adult must be aware that urination occurs in a socially acceptable place. Patients with dementia may not have that awareness.

Etiology

Incontinence may have temporary or permanent causes. Evaluation of the incontinent patient means considering all possible causes, beginning with those that are temporary and correctable. Surgical and traumatic causes of urinary incontinence are related to procedures or surgery in the lower pelvic structures, which are areas that contain complex nerve pathways. Radical urologic, prostatic, and gynecologic procedures for treatment of pelvic cancers may result in urinary incontinence. Injury to segments S2 to S4 of the spinal cord may cause incontinence from impairment of normal nerve pathways.

Inappropriate bladder contraction may result from disorders of the brain and nervous system or from bladder irritation due to chronic infection, stones, chemotherapy, or radiation therapy. Other causes of bladder contraction failure include the neuropathies associated with diabetes mellitus, syphilis, and previous treatment with neurotoxic anticancer drugs. Constipation can lead to temporary urinary incontinence. Some drugs or drug-drug interactions from polypharmacy, such as anticholinergics, calcium channel blockers, diuretics, and sedatives, can cause or worsen urinary incontinence.

CONSIDERATIONS FOR OLDER ADULTS
Patient-Centered Care QSEN

Many factors contribute to urinary incontinence in older adults (Chart 66-1). An older adult may have decreased mobility from many causes. In inpatient settings, mobility is limited when the older patient is placed on bedrest. Vision and hearing impairments may also prevent the patient from locating a call light to notify the nurse or assistive personnel of the need to void. Assess for these factors and minimize them to prevent urinary incontinence. Getting out of bed to urinate is a common cause of falls among older adults in the home and other settings (Touhy & Jett, 2016).

Incidence and Prevalence

Incontinence is a major health problem. As many as 45% of woman over 65 years report some degree of urinary incontinence, with roughly half as many men reporting this condition (Gorina et al., 2014). As many as 75% of residents in long-term care facilities have urinary incontinence (Gorina et al., 2014).

Risk for urinary incontinence increases with chronic conditions such as diabetes mellitus, stroke, cognitive impairment, and impaired mobility. Urinary incontinence occurs not only with older age but with a history of vaginal delivery, particularly if the first child was delivered after age 30. Conditions of pelvic prolapse in women, prostate problems in men, diabetes, heart failure, spinal cord or nerve injury, and obesity also increase the risk for urinary incontinence (Cerruto et al., 2015; McCance et al., 2014). Both central nervous system diseases (i.e., dementia, multiple sclerosis, Parkinson disease) and musculoskeletal disorders (i.e., osteoporosis, osteoarthritis, paresthesia, pain or paralysis) contribute to cognitive and mobility impairment, resulting in the onset and severity of urinary incontinence (McCance et al., 2014). Many adults admitted to the hospital

TABLE 66-1	Types of Urinary Incontinence		
TYPE	**DEFINITION/DESCRIPTION**	**CAUSE**	**SYMPTOMS**
Stress incontinence	The involuntary loss of urine during activities that increase abdominal and detrusor pressure. Patients cannot tighten the urethra sufficiently to overcome the increased detrusor pressure; leakage of urine results.	Weakening of bladder neck supports; associated with childbirth. Intrinsic sphincter deficiency caused by such congenital conditions as epispadias (abnormal location of the urethra on the dorsum of the penis) or myelomeningocele. Acquired anatomic damage to the urethral sphincter (from repeated incontinence surgeries, prostatectomy, radiation therapy, and trauma). Vaginal prolapse from vaginal birth or aging.	Urine loss with physical exertion, cough, sneeze, or exercise. Usually only small amounts of urine are lost with each exertion. Normal voiding habits (≤8 times per day, ≤2 times per night). Post-void residual usually ≤50 mL. Pelvic examination shows hypermobility of the urethra or bladder neck with Valsalva maneuvers.
Urge incontinence	The involuntary loss of urine associated with a strong desire to urinate. Patients cannot suppress the signal from the bladder muscle to the brain that it is time to urinate.	Idiopathic. Brain and nerve disorders. Bladder inflammation or infection. Bladder cancer.	An abrupt and strong urge to void. May have loss of large amounts of urine with each occurrence.
Detrusor hyperreflexia (reflex incontinence)	The abnormal detrusor contractions result from neurologic abnormalities.	Central nervous system (CNS) lesions from stroke, multiple sclerosis, and parasacral spinal cord lesions. Local irritating factors such as caffeine, drugs, or bladder tumor.	Post-void residual ≤50 mL.
Overflow incontinence	The involuntary loss of urine associated with overdistention of the bladder when the bladder's capacity has reached its maximum. The urethra is obstructed, so it fails to relax sufficiently to allow urine to flow, resulting in incomplete bladder emptying or complete urinary retention, causing overflow incontinence.	Diabetic neuropathy; side effects of drugs; after radical pelvic surgery or spinal cord damage; outlet obstruction. Causes external to the mechanism of the urethra: an enlarged prostate (male patients) and large genital prolapse (female patients). When the cause is intrinsic to the urethra, abnormal contraction of the skeletal muscle occurs, causing obstruction. This condition, called *detrusor dyssynergia,* is seen in patients with spinal cord injuries and multiple sclerosis.	Bladder distention, often up to the level of the umbilicus. Constant dribbling of urine.
Mixed incontinence	A combination of stress, urge, and overflow incontinence.	As with each separate disorder.	As with each separate disorder.
Functional incontinence	Leakage of urine caused by factors other than disease of the lower urinary tract.	Decreased cognition such as with dementia, some central nervous system disorders; inability to walk to the toilet.	Quantity and timing of urine leakage vary; patterns are difficult to discern.
Transient causes	Transient causes improve with treatment of the underlying condition.	Reversible loss of cognitive functioning. Loss of awareness that urination is to occur in a socially acceptable place.	Altered mental state, as in sedation, delirium, confusion, depression, sepsis, mental illness, or severe psychological stress.
		Abnormal openings in the urinary tract, such as a fistula or diverticulum.	Urinary drainage noted from areas other than the urinary meatus.
		Drugs such as sedatives, hypnotics, diuretics, anticholinergics, decongestants, antihypertensives, and calcium channel blockers.	Some drugs cause altered mental state; others cause increased urine production.
		Diabetes insipidus or psychogenic polydipsia.	Increased urine output.
		Inability to get to toileting facilities.	Restraints, restricted mobility.
		Direct bladder pressure or urethral obstruction.	Constipation or fecal impaction.
Permanent causes	Permanent causes are organic but may be improved with treatment.	Cognitive impairment. Traumatic or surgical effects. Factors contributing to stress incontinence, urge incontinence, and overflow incontinence. Structural or functional defects of the bladder or the sphincters. Injuries or diseases of the spinal cord, brainstem, or cerebral cortex (neurogenic bladder). Congenital defects, including exstrophy of the bladder (bladder turned "inside out") and spina bifida.	Symptoms depend on the cause.

CHART 66-1 Nursing Focus on the Older Adult
Factors Contributing to Urinary Incontinence*

Drugs
- Central nervous system depressants, such as opioid analgesics, decrease the patient's level of consciousness and the urge to void and contribute to constipation.
- Diuretics cause frequent voiding, often of large amounts of urine.
- Multiple drugs can contribute to changes in mental status or mobility, and they can irritate the bladder.
- Anticholinergic drugs or drugs with anticholinergic side effects are especially challenging because they affect both cognition and the ability to void. Monitor patient responses to these drugs early in treatment.

Disease
- Stroke, Parkinson disease, dementia, and other neurologic disorders decrease mobility, sensation, or cognition.
- Arthritis decreases mobility and causes pain.

Depression
- Depression decreases the energy necessary to maintain continence.
- Decreased self-esteem and feelings of self-worth decrease the importance to the patient of maintaining continence.

Inadequate Resources
- Patients who need assistive devices (e.g., eyeglasses, cane, walker) may be afraid to ambulate without them or without personal assistance.
- Products that help patients manage incontinence of urine ELIMINATION are often costly.
- No one may be available to assist the patient to the bathroom or help with incontinence products.

*These factors are in addition to the physiologic changes of aging given in Chapter 3.

CHART 66-2 Focused Assessment
The Patient With Urinary Incontinence

Note the presence of risk factors for urinary incontinence:
- Age
- If female, menopausal status
- Central or peripheral neurologic disease with associated impairment in cognition or mobility
- Diabetes mellitus
- History of vaginal delivery; vaginal prolapse
- Urologic procedures
- Prescribed and over-the-counter drugs that affect cognition or mobility
- Bowel patterns; fecal impaction
- Stress/anxiety level

Detail the symptoms of urinary incontinence:
- Leakage
- Frequency
- Urgency
- Nocturia
- Sensation of full bladder before leakage

Obtain a 24-hour intake-and-output record or a voiding diary:
- Time and amount of oral intake and continent voiding
- Time and estimated amount of incontinent leakages
- Activity around the time of leakage

Assess the patient's:
- Mobility
- Self-care ability
- Cognitive ability
- Communication patterns

Assess the environment for barriers to toileting:
- Privacy
- Restrictive clothing
- Access to toilet

---

develop urinary incontinence. Because the problem is common among older adults, all adults older than 65 years are recommended to be screened for incontinence (Touhy & Jett, 2016).

❖ INTERPROFESSIONAL COLLABORATIVE CARE

Incontinence can occur in any setting and is very common in the community. Usually the adult with incontinence is treated using self-management strategies. Even when surgical intervention is used, hospitalization for incontinence is rare. Because urinary incontinence carries a burden of impaired COMFORT, activity disruption, shame or embarrassment, and loss of TISSUE INTEGRITY, it has a great impact on quality of life for most adults.

Assessment: Noticing

History. Incontinence may be underreported because health care professionals do not ask patients about urine loss. *Do not assume that patients will volunteer the information without specifically being asked* (Testa, 2015). Effective screening includes asking patients to respond "always," "sometimes," or "never" to these questions:
- Do you ever leak urine or water when you don't want to?
- Do you ever leak urine or water when you cough, sneeze, laugh, or exercise?
- Do you ever leak urine or water on the way to the bathroom?
- Do you ever use pads, tissue, or cloth in your underwear to catch urine?

If any answer is "always" or "sometimes," perform a focused assessment (Chart 66-2).

Physical Assessment/Signs and Symptoms. Assess the abdomen to estimate bladder fullness, rule out palpable hard stool, and evaluate bowel sounds. Urinary incontinence is confirmed by evaluating the force and character of the urine stream during voiding. Ask the patient to cough while wearing a perineal pad to assess for stress incontinence; a wet pad on forceful coughing indicates stress incontinence.

For women, inspect the external genitalia to determine whether there is apparent urethral or uterine prolapse, cystocele (herniation of the bladder into the vagina), or rectocele. These conditions occur with pelvic floor muscle weakness. A primary health care provider puts on an examination glove and inserts two fingers into the vagina to assess the strength of these muscles. Strength is described as *weak, adequate,* or *strong* based on the amount of pressure felt by the primary health care provider as the patient tightens her vaginal muscles. Describe and document the color, consistency, and odor of any secretions from the genitourinary orifices. The urine stream interruption test (i.e., asking a patient to voluntarily start and stop urine flow during a void at least twice) is another method of determining pelvic muscle strength. For men, inspect the urethral meatus for any discharge.

A digital rectal examination (DRE) is performed by the primary health care provider on both male and female patients. It provides information about the nerve integrity to the bladder. The examiner determines whether there is tactile sensation in the anal area by observing whether the rectal sphincter is relaxed or contracted on digital insertion. Because nerve supply to the bladder is similar to nerve supply to the rectum, the presence of tactile sensation and a rectal sphincter that contracts suggest that the nerve supply to the bladder is intact. Impaction of stool is a cause of transient urinary incontinence and can be detected during a rectal examination. The primary health care provider assesses for prostate enlargement in men as a possible cause of incontinence.

Laboratory Assessment. A urinalysis is useful to rule out urinary tract infection. This test is the first step in the assessment of incontinent patients of any age. The presence of red blood cells (RBCs), white blood cells (WBCs), leukocyte esterase, or nitrites is an indication for culturing the urine. Any infection is treated before further assessment of incontinence.

Imaging Assessment. Determine the amount of post-void residual urine (urine remaining in the bladder right after voiding) by portable ultrasound (bladder scanner). If prescribed, catheterizing the patient immediately after voiding can also be used to assess residual volume. Additional imaging is needed when surgery is being considered. CT is most useful for locating abnormalities in kidneys and ureters. A voiding cystourethrogram (VCUG) or urodynamic testing may be performed to assess the size, shape, support, and function of the urinary tract system. Urodynamic testing (see Chapter 65) may take several hours and more than one visit. Electromyography (EMG) of the pelvic muscles may be a part of the urodynamic studies.

◆ Analysis: Interpreting

The priority collaborative problems for patients with urinary incontinence include:

1. Stress incontinence due to weak pelvic muscles and structural supports
2. Urge incontinence due to decreased bladder capacity, bladder spasms, diet, and neurologic impairment
3. Reflex incontinence due to neurologic impairment
4. Functional incontinence due to impaired cognition or neuromuscular limitations
5. Total urinary incontinence (mixed) due to many causes

◆ Planning and Implementation: Responding

Several interventions are useful for each type of incontinence in addition to drugs, surgical repair, and nutrition therapy.

Reducing Stress Incontinence

Planning: Expected Outcomes. With appropriate therapy, the patient with stress incontinence is expected to develop continence of urine ELIMINATION. Indicators include that the patient rarely or never demonstrates these actions:

- Urine leakage between voidings
- Urine leakage with increased abdominal pressure (e.g., sneezing, laughing, lifting)

Interventions. Initial interventions for patients with stress incontinence include keeping a diary and pelvic muscle exercises (Kegel exercises) (Qaseem et al., 2014). Surgery also may be an option if other interventions are not effective (Testa, 2015). Explain the purpose of a detailed diary in which the patient records times of urine leakage, activities, and food eaten. The diary is then used by the primary health care provider to plan and evaluate interventions. Collection devices, absorbent pads, and undergarments may be used during the often lengthy process of assessment and treatment and by patients who elect not to pursue further interventions.

Nonsurgical Management. Changes to diet and regularly performing pelvic muscle exercises require the patient's active participation for success. Nursing interventions focus on teaching patients about the drugs and behavioral strategies and on providing ongoing encouragement, clarification, and support to maximize intervention effects.

Pelvic muscle (Kegel) exercise therapy for women with stress incontinence strengthens the muscles of the pelvic floor (circumvaginal muscles). These muscles become strengthened, as any other skeletal muscle does, by frequent, systematic, and repeated contractions. Pelvic floor muscle training improves not only continence but also quality of life in women with urinary incontinence (Wilde et al., 2014).

The most important step in teaching pelvic muscle exercises is to help the patient learn which muscles to exercise. During the pelvic examination in women and the rectal examination in men or women, instruct the patient to tighten the pelvic muscles around your fingers. Then provide feedback about the strength of the contraction. Starting and stopping the urine stream or stopping the passage of flatus indicates that the patient has correctly identified the pelvic muscles. Biofeedback devices, such as electromyography or perineometers, measure the strength of contraction. A perineometer is a tampon-shaped instrument inserted into the vagina to measure the strength of pelvic muscle contractions. The graph shows the amplitude of muscle contraction to the patient for biofeedback. Alternatively, retention of a vaginal weight also shows that the patient has identified the proper muscle (see discussion on vaginal cone therapy that follows).

Instructions for pelvic muscle exercises are given in Chart 66-3. Although improvement may take several months, most patients notice a positive change after 6 weeks. Teach patients

---

◘ CHART 66-3 Patient and Family Education: Preparing for Self-Management

Pelvic Muscle Exercises

- The pelvic muscles are composed of a sling of muscles that support your bladder, urethra, and vagina. Like any other muscles in your body, you can make your pelvic muscles stronger by alternately contracting (tightening) and relaxing them in regular exercise periods. By strengthening these muscles, you will be able to stop your urine flow more effectively.
- To identify your pelvic muscles, sit on the toilet with your feet flat on the floor about 12 inches apart. Begin to urinate, and then try to stop the urine flow. Do not strain down, lift your bottom off the seat, or squeeze your legs together. When you start and stop your urine stream, you are using your pelvic muscles.
- To perform pelvic muscle exercises, tighten your pelvic muscles for a slow count of 10 and then relax for a slow count of 10. Do this exercise 15 times while you are lying down, sitting up, and standing (a total of 45 exercises). Repeat—and this time rapidly contract and relax the pelvic muscles 10 times. This should take no more than 10 to 12 minutes for all three positions, or 3 to 4 minutes for each set of 15 exercises.
- Begin with 45 exercises a day in three sets of 15 exercises each. You will notice faster improvement if you can do this twice a day, or a total of 20 minutes each day. Remember to exercise in all three positions so your muscles learn to squeeze effectively despite your position. At first, it is helpful to have a designated time and place to do these exercises because you will have to concentrate to do them correctly. After you have been doing them for several weeks, you will notice improvement in your control of urine. However, many people report that improvement may take as long as 3 months.

to continue the exercises 10 times daily to improve and maintain pelvic muscle strength.

Nutrition therapy with weight reduction is helpful for obese patients because stress incontinence is made worse by increased abdominal pressure from obesity (Wilde et al., 2014). Teach the patient to avoid bladder irritants in the diet, such as caffeine, that can contribute to urgency and frequency. Stress the importance of maintaining an adequate fluid intake, especially water. Refer the patient to a registered dietitian as needed.

Drug therapy with topical estrogen to the perineal and vaginal orifice is used to treat postmenopausal women with stress incontinence. Estrogen may increase the blood flow and tone of the muscles around the vagina and urethra, thus improving the patient's ability to contract those muscles during times of increased intra-abdominal stress.

Vaginal cone weight therapy involves using a set of five small, cone-shaped weights (Touhy & Jett, 2016). They are of equal size but of varying weights and are used together with pelvic muscle exercise. The woman inserts the lightest cone, labeled *1*, into her vagina (Fig. 66-1A), with the string to the outside, for a 1-minute test period. If she can hold the first cone in place without its slipping out while she walks around, she proceeds to the second cone, labeled *2*, and repeats the procedure. The patient begins her treatment with the heaviest cone she can comfortably hold in her vagina for the 1-minute test period. Treatment periods are 15 minutes twice a day. When the patient can comfortably hold the cone in her vagina for 15-minutes, she progresses to the next heaviest weight. Treatment is completed with the cone labeled *5*.

Weighted vaginal cones can help strengthen the pelvic muscles and decrease stress incontinence but may not help pelvic prolapse. Vaginal cones do not require a prescription.

Other interventions for stress incontinence include behavior modification, psychotherapy, and electrical stimulation devices to strengthen urethral contraction. Intravaginal and intrarectal electrical stimulation devices have been used with varying degrees of success.

A *pessary* (plastic device, often ring shaped, that helps hold internal organs in place) inserted into the vagina may help with a prolapsed uterus or bladder when this condition is contributing to urinary incontinence. A prolapse occurs when the supportive tissue in the vagina weakens and stretches, allowing pelvic organs to protrude into the vaginal lumen. The pessary presses against the wall of the vagina to reposition pelvic organs. Generally, a pessary is removed and cleaned with soap and water on a monthly basis by the patient, but the nurse can do it for adults with cognitive or musculoskeletal impairment.

Urethral occlusion devices (urethral plugs) can be helpful for activity-induced incontinence. One device, the Reliance insert, is like a tiny tampon that the patient inserts into the urethra. After insertion, the patient inflates a tiny balloon, which rests at the bladder neck and prevents the flow of urine. To void, the patient pulls a string to deflate the balloon and removes the device. The applicator is reusable, although the tampon part is disposed of after each void.

Electrical stimulation with either an intravaginal or intrarectal electrical stimulation device is available to treat both urge and stress incontinence. Treatment consists of stimulating sensory nerves to decrease the sensation of urgency. It is done as an office-based procedure one to three times weekly for 6 to 8 weeks.

Magnetic resonance therapy involves targeted urinary tract nerves and muscles for depolarization. The patient sits on a chair containing a magnetic device that induces depolarization and helps reduce stress-induced incontinence similar to drug-induced relaxation of muscle and nerves.

Surgical Management. Stress incontinence may be treated by a surgical sling or bladder suspension procedure (Table 66-2). A sling procedure creates a sling around the bladder neck and urethra using strips of body tissue or synthetic mesh. Mid-urethral sling procedures are particularly effective for stress urinary incontinence (Cerruto et al., 2015). Bladder suspension procedures are more extensive than sling procedures, and the surgeon sutures tissue near the bladder neck to a pubic bone ligament to provide support and prevent sagging. A third surgical procedure is the injection of bulking agents into the urethral wall to provide resistance to urine outflow. Bulking agents include collagen, carbon-coated zirconium beads, and silicone implants.

Preoperative Care. Teach the patient about the procedure, and clarify the surgeon's explanation of events surrounding the surgery. Extensive urodynamic testing (see Chapter 65) has not been shown to be useful before surgical interventions for stress urinary incontinence (Cerruto et al., 2015).

Postoperative Care. After surgery, assess for and intervene to prevent or detect complications. For prevention of movement or traction on the bladder neck, secure the urethral catheter

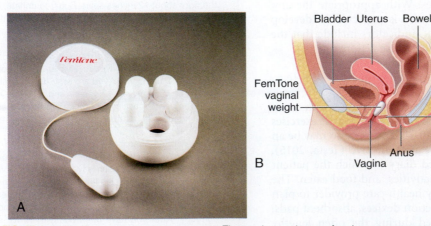

FIG. 66-1 A, FemTone vaginal weights, or cones. The number on the top of each cone represents increasing weight up to the heaviest cone, a *5*. **B,** Diagram showing the correct positioning of a vaginal weight, or cone, in place. (**A** Courtesy ConvaTec, A Bristol-Meyers Squibb Company, a Division of E.R. Squibb & Sons, Inc., Princeton, NJ.)

TABLE 66-2 Surgical Procedures for Stress Incontinence

PROCEDURE	PURPOSE	NURSING CONSIDERATIONS
Anterior vaginal repair (colporrhaphy)	Elevates the urethral position and repairs any cystocele.	Because the operation is performed by vaginal incision, it is often done in conjunction with a vaginal hysterectomy. Recovery is usually rapid, and a urethral catheter is in place for 24-48 hr.
Retropubic suspension (Marshall-Marchetti-Krantz or Burch colposuspension)	Elevates the urethral position and provides longer-lasting results.	The operation requires a low abdominal incision and a urethral or suprapubic catheter for several days after. Recovery takes longer, and urinary retention and detrusor instability are the most frequent complications.
Needle bladder neck suspension (Pereyra or Stamey procedure)	Elevates the urethral position and provides longer-lasting results without a long operative time.	The combined vaginal approach with a needle and a small suprapubic skin incision does not allow direct vision of the operative site; however, the high complication rates may be due to the selection of patients who, because of their medical condition, are not good candidates for longer retropubic procedures.
Pubovaginal sling procedures	A sling made of synthetic or fascial material is placed under the urethrovesical junction to elevate the bladder neck.	The operation uses an abdominal, vaginal, or combined approach to treat intrinsic sphincter deficiencies. Temporary or permanent urinary retention is common after surgery.
Midurethral sling procedures	A tensionless vaginal sling is made from polypropylene mesh (or other materials) and placed near the urethrovesical junction to increase the angle, which inhibits movement of urine into the urethra with lower intravesicular pressures.	This ambulatory surgery procedure uses a vaginal approach to improve symptoms of stress incontinence. Temporary or permanent urinary retention is common after surgery.
Artificial sphincters	A mechanical device to open and close the urethra is placed around the anatomic urethra.	The operation is done more frequently in men. The most common complications include mechanical failure of the device, erosion of tissue, and infection.
Periurethral injection of collagen or Siloxane	Implantation of small amounts of an inert substance through several small injections provides support around the bladder neck.	The procedure can be done in an ambulatory care setting and can be repeated as often as necessary. Certain compounds may migrate after injection; an allergy test to bovine collagen must be performed before implantation.

with tape or a tube holder. If a suprapubic catheter is used instead of a urethral catheter, monitor the dressing for urine leakage and other drainage. Catheters are usually in place until the patient can urinate easily and has residual urine volume of less than 50 mL after voiding. (See Chapters 14 and 16 for a discussion of general care before and after surgery.)

Reducing Urge Incontinence

Planning: Expected Outcomes. The patient with urge urinary incontinence is expected to use techniques to prevent or manage uncontrolled urine ELIMINATION. Indicators include that the patient often or consistently demonstrates these behaviors:

- Responds to urge in a timely manner
- Gets to toilet between urge and passage of urine
- Avoids substances that stimulate the bladder (e.g., caffeine, alcohol)

Interventions. Interventions for patients with urge incontinence or overactive bladder (OAB) are nonsurgical. These include bladder training and drug therapy if bladder training is not successful (Qaseem et al., 2014). *Neuromodulation* therapy, which involves stimulation of the nerves to the bladder, can be used to manage urge incontinence. Minor surgery is required to place the device. Most types of surgery are not the recommended treatment of this condition.

Drug Therapy. Because the hypertonic bladder contracts involuntarily in patients with urge incontinence, drugs that relax the smooth muscle and increase the bladder's capacity are prescribed (Chart 66-4). The most commonly prescribed drugs are anticholinergics (also known as antimuscarinics

because they target specific receptors in the cholinergic family of receptors), which include darifenacin (Enablex), fesoterodine (Toviaz), oxybutynin (Ditropan and Ditropan XL), propiverdine (Detrunorm), solifenacin (VESIcare), tolterodine (Detrol and Detrol LA), and trospium (Sanctura). Some of these drugs are available over-the-counter. This class of drugs has serious side effects, particularly for older adults, and is used along with behavioral interventions. These drugs inhibit the nerve fibers that stimulate bladder contraction. Tricyclic antidepressants with anticholinergic and alpha-adrenergic agonist activity, such as imipramine (Tofranil, Novopramine), have been used successfully in younger patients.

A beta-adrenergic agonist, mirabegron (Myrbetriq) has demonstrated effectiveness in reducing urge incontinence. The evidence comparing different drug categories for effectiveness in managing incontinence is limited, and no single drug or class is recommended over another.

Another drug therapy for urge incontinence is onabutulinumtoxinA (Botox). This drug is injected during cystoscopy into multiple areas of the detrusor muscle of the bladder. Usually 10 to 30 different sites are injected during one treatment session. This treatment relaxes the detrusor muscle and relieves the urge to urinate (Felicilda-Reynaldo & Backes, 2014). Some patients have had relief of incontinence for as long as 6 to 9 months after injection. Side effects may include urinary retention, painful urination, and an increased incidence of urinary tract infections. For most patients who experience urinary retention, the condition is temporary but does require intermittent self-catheterization.

CHART 66-4   Common Examples of Drug Therapy

Urinary Incontinence

DRUG CATEGORY	NURSING IMPLICATIONS
Hormones—Thought to enhance nerve conduction to the urinary tract, improve blood flow, and reduce tissue deterioration of the urinary tract	
Estrogen vaginal cream daily or an estrogen-containing ring inserted monthly	Teach patients to use only a thin application of the cream *to minimize excessive absorption and distribution and avoid systemic side effects.* Teach patients that it takes 4-6 weeks to achieve continence benefits and that benefits disappear after about 4 weeks after discontinuing regular use *because knowing the drug responses increases the likelihood of its correct use.*
Anticholinergics—Suppress involuntary bladder contraction and increase bladder capacity	
Darifenacin (Enablex) Fesoterodine (Toviaz) Oxybutynin (Ditropan) Propiverine (Detrunorm) Solifenacin (Vesicare) Tolterodine (Detrol) Trospium (Sanctura)	Ask whether the patient has glaucoma before starting any drugs from this class *because anticholinergics can increase intraocular pressure and make glaucoma worse.* Suggest that patients increase fluid intake and use hard candy to moisten the mouth *to reduce the dry mouth side effect.* Teach patients to increase fluid intake and the amount of dietary fiber *to prevent constipation associated with this drug category.* Teach patients to monitor urine output and to report an output significantly lower than intake to the primary health care provider *because all of these drugs can cause urinary retention, especially for men with an enlarged prostate.* Instruct patients taking the extended-release forms of these drugs not to chew or crush the tablet/capsule *to avoid both ruining the time-release feature and increasing the risk for a bolus dose with more side effects.*
Alpha-Adrenergic Agonists—Increase contractile force of the urethral sphincter, increasing resistance to urine outflow	
Midorine (ProAmatine, Orvaten)*	Teach the patient to monitor his or her blood pressure periodically when starting the *drug because these drugs can cause severe supine hypertension and should not be used in patients with severe cardiac disease.*
Beta₃ Blockers—Relax the detrusor smooth muscle to increase bladder capacity and urine storage	
Mirabegron (Myrbetriq)	Teach the patient to periodically obtain a blood pressure and to inform the health care provider if the systolic or diastolic values increase more than 10 mm Hg or above 180/110 *because this drug has the potential to increase blood pressure.* If the patient is taking warfarin, avoid this drug or schedule additional blood testing for potential increased risk for bleeding *because this drug uses the same metabolic pathway as warfarin and can potentiate warfarin's effects, leading to a prolonged international normalized ratio (INR) and increase the risk for bleeding.*
Antidepressants: Tricyclics and Serotonin-Norepinephrine Reuptake Inhibitors (SNRIs)—Increase norepinephrine and serotonin levels, which are thought to strengthen the urinary sphincters; also have anticholinergic actions	
Tricyclics Imipramine (Tofranil, Novo-Pramine) Amitriptyline (Elavil, Levate) *SNRI* Duloxetine (Cymbalta)*	Warn patients not to combine these drugs with other antidepressant drugs *to avoid a drug-drug interaction that can lead to a hypertensive crisis.* Instruct patients to inform their primary health care provider if they take drugs to manage hypertension. Teach patients to change positions slowly, especially in the morning *to avoid dizziness from orthostatic hypotension, which increases the risk for falls.* Teach patients the same interventions as for anticholinergic agents *because these drugs have anticholinergic activity and can produce the same side effects.*

*These drugs are used off label and do not have United States Food and Drug Administration (FDA) approval for use. However, they are commonly used to manage incontinence syndromes.

! NURSING SAFETY PRIORITY QSEN

Drug Alert

> Teach patients taking the extended-release forms of anticholinergic drugs to swallow the tablet or capsule whole without chewing or crushing it. Chewing or crushing the tablet/capsule ruins the extended-release feature, allowing the entire dose to be absorbed quickly, which increases adverse drug side effects.

Nutrition Therapy. Teach the patient to avoid foods that irritate the bladder such as caffeine and alcohol. Spacing fluids at regular intervals throughout the day (e.g., 120 mL every hour or 240 mL every 2 hours) and limiting fluids after the dinner hour (e.g., only 120 mL at bedtime) help avoid fluid overload on the bladder and allow urine to collect at a steady pace. Remind patients that maintaining an ideal body weight helps avoid the pressure that abdominal fat places on pelvic organs, thus reducing incontinence.

NCLEX EXAMINATION CHALLENGE 66-1

Safe and Effective Care Environment

> For which adverse drug effects does the nurse assess in a client who is hospitalized for an acute problem and is also prescribed an anticholinergic drug to manage incontinence? **Select all that apply.**
> A. Insomnia
> B. Blurred vision
> C. Constipation
> D. Dry mouth
> E. Loss of sphincter control
> F. Increased sweating
> G. Worsening mental function
> H. Hypotension

Bladder Training. Bladder training, sometimes called *behavioral training* for incontinence, includes the interventions listed in Chart 66-5 and electrical stimulation. Bladder training involves a great deal of patient participation. Provide ongoing

CHART 66-5 Best Practice for Patient Safety & Quality Care QSEN

Bladder Training and Habit Training to Reduce Urinary Incontinence

Bladder Training

- Assess the patient's awareness of bladder fullness and ability to cooperate with training regimen.
- Assess the patient's 24-hour urine ELIMINATION pattern for 2 to 3 consecutive days (bladder diary).
- Base the initial interval of toileting on the voiding pattern (e.g., 45 minutes).
- Teach the patient to void every 45 minutes on the first day and to ignore or suppress the urge to urinate between the 45-minute intervals.
- Take the patient to the toilet or remind him or her to urinate at the 45-minute intervals.
- Provide privacy for toileting and run water in the sink to promote the urge to urinate at this time.
- If the patient is not consistently able to resist the urge to urinate between the intervals, reduce the intervals by 15 minutes.
- Continue this regimen for at least 24 hours or for as many days as it takes for the patient to be comfortable with this schedule and not urinate between the intervals.
- When the patient remains continent between the intervals, increase the intervals by 15 minutes daily until a 3- to 4-hour interval is comfortable for the patient.
- Praise successes. If incontinence occurs, work with the patient to re-establish an acceptable toileting interval.

Habit Training

- Assess the patient's 24-hour voiding pattern for 2 to 3 days.
- Base the initial interval of toileting on the voiding pattern (e.g., 2 hours).
- Help the patient to the toilet or provide a bedpan/urinal every 2 hours (or whatever has been determined to be an appropriate toileting interval for the individual patient).
- During the toileting, remind the patient to void and provide cues such as running water.
- If the patient is incontinent between scheduled toileting, reduce the time interval by 30 minutes until the patient is continent between voidings.
- Help the patient to toilet and prompt to void at prescribed intervals.
- Do not leave the patient on the toilet or bedpan for longer than 5 minutes.
- Ensure that all nursing staff members comply with the established toileting schedule and do not apply briefs or encourage the patient to "just wet the bed."
- Reduce toileting interval by 30 minutes if there are more than two incontinence episodes in 24 hours.
- If the patient remains continent at the toileting interval, attempt to increase the interval by 30 minutes until a 3- to 4-hour continence interval is reached.
- Praise the patient for successes and spend extra time socializing with the patient.
- When incontinence occurs, ensure that the patient and bed are cleaned appropriately but do not spend extra time socializing with the patient.
- Discuss daily record of continence with staff to provide reinforcement and encourage compliance with toileting schedule.
- Include unlicensed assistive personnel in all aspects of the habit training.

encouragement, clarification, and support to increase the effectiveness of all interventions. This intervention may be combined with drug and diet therapy for weight loss.

Bladder training is an education program for the patient that begins with a thorough explanation of the problem of urge incontinence. Instead of the bladder being in control of the patient, the patient learns to control the bladder. For the program to succeed, he or she must be alert, aware, and able to resist the urge to urinate (Wilde et al., 2014).

Start a schedule for voiding, beginning with the longest interval that is comfortable for the patient, even if the interval is only 30 minutes. Instruct the patient to void every 30 minutes and to ignore any urge to urinate between the set intervals. Once he or she is comfortable with the starting schedule, increase the interval by 15 to 30 minutes. Instruct the patient to follow the new schedule until he or she achieves success again. As the interval increases, the bladder gradually tolerates more volume. Teach him or her relaxation and distraction techniques to maximize success in the retraining. Provide positive reinforcement for maintaining the prescribed schedule.

Habit training (scheduled toileting) is a type of bladder training that is successful in reducing incontinence in cognitively impaired patients. To use habit training, caregivers help the patient void at specific times (e.g., every 2 hours on the even hours). The goal is to get the patient to the toilet before incontinence occurs. The focus is on reducing incontinence. When that has been achieved, the focus may change to increasing bladder capacity by gradually lengthening the voiding intervals, but this is only secondary.

! NURSING SAFETY PRIORITY QSEN

Action Alert

Habit training is undermined when absorbent briefs are used in place of timed toileting. Do not tell patients to "just wet the bed." A common cause of falls in health care facilities is related to patient efforts to get out of bed unassisted to use the toilet. Work with all staff members, including unlicensed assistive personnel (UAP), to implement consistently the toileting schedule for habit training.

Prompted voiding, a supplement to habit training, attempts to increase the patient's awareness of the need to void and to prompt him or her to ask for toileting assistance. Habit training otherwise relies completely on a time schedule.

Pelvic muscle exercises for urge incontinence is helpful and is taught in the same way as for stress incontinence (see Chart 66-3). Improved urethral resistance helps the patient overcome abnormal detrusor contractions long enough to get to the toilet.

Surgical Management for Urge Incontinence. In contrast to stress urinary incontinence, urge urinary incontinence requires extensive preoperative testing for diagnosis and selection of surgery. The patient may need emotional support during this extensive diagnostic work-up. Surgical procedures and preoperative and postoperative management are the same as those described for stress urinary incontinence and in Table 66-2.

Reducing Reflex Incontinence

Planning: Expected Outcomes. With appropriate intervention, the patient with reflex incontinence is expected to achieve continence. Indicators include that the patient often or consistently demonstrates these behaviors:

- Recognizes the urge to void
- Maintains a predictable pattern of voiding
- Responds to urge in a timely manner
- Empties bladder completely
- Keeps urine volume in the bladder under 300 mL

Interventions. Interventions for the patient with reflex (overflow) incontinence caused by obstruction of the bladder outlet may include surgery to relieve the obstruction. The most common procedures are prostate removal (see Chapter 72) and repair of uterine prolapse (see Chapter 71).

Drug Therapy. Drugs are prescribed for short-term management of urinary retention, often after surgery. They are not used in long-term management of overflow incontinence caused by a hypotonic bladder. The most commonly used drug is bethanechol chloride (Urecholine), an agent that increases bladder pressure.

Behavioral Interventions. The most effective common behavioral interventions are bladder compression and intermittent self-catheterization.

Bladder compression uses techniques that promote bladder emptying and include the Credé method, the Valsalva maneuver, double-voiding, and splinting.

For the Credé method, teach the patient how to press over the bladder area, increasing the pressure, or to trigger nerve stimulation by tugging at pubic hair or massaging the genital area. These techniques manually help the bladder empty. In the Valsalva maneuver, breathing techniques increase chest and abdominal pressure. This increased pressure is then directed toward the bladder during exhalation. (The Valsalva maneuver is contraindicated in patients who have some cardiac problems because it can trigger a vagal response and cause bradycardia.) With the technique of double-voiding, the patient empties the bladder and then, within a few minutes, attempts a second bladder emptying.

For women who have a large *cystocele* (prolapse of the bladder into the vagina), a technique called *splinting* both compresses the bladder and moves it into a better position. The woman inserts her fingers into her vagina, gently lifts the cystocele, and begins to urinate. A *pessary,* described earlier, can also provide relief from cystocele-related incontinence.

Intermittent self-catheterization is often used to help patients with long-term problems of incomplete bladder emptying. It is effective, can be learned fairly easily, and remains the preferred method of bladder emptying in patients who have incontinence as a result of a neurogenic bladder (Prieto et al., 2015). These points are important in teaching the technique:

- Proper handwashing and cleaning of the catheter reduce the risk for infection.
- A small lumen and good lubrication of the catheter prevent urethral trauma.
- A regular schedule for bladder emptying prevents distention and mucosal trauma.

Patients must be able to understand instructions and have the manual dexterity to manipulate the catheter. Caregivers or family members in the home can also be taught to perform intermittent catheterization using clean (rather than sterile) technique with good outcomes (Bickhaus et al., 2015).

Reducing Functional Incontinence

Planning: Expected Outcomes. The patient with functional urinary incontinence is expected to remain dry and maintain skin TISSUE INTEGRITY. Indicators include that the patient often or consistently demonstrates these behaviors:

- Uses urine containment or collection measures to ensure dryness
- Manages clothing independently

Interventions. Causes of functional (or chronic intractable) incontinence vary greatly. Some are reversible, and others are not. The focus of intervention is treatment of reversible causes. When incontinence is not reversible, urinary habit training (see Chart 66-5) is used to establish a predictable pattern of bladder

emptying to prevent incontinence. A final strategy focuses on containment of the urine and protection of the patient's skin. Nonsurgical interventions include applied devices, containment, and catheterization.

Applied devices include intravaginal pessaries for women and penile clamps for men. The intravaginal pessary supports the uterus and vagina and helps maintain the correct position of the bladder. (See Chapter 71 for further discussion of pessaries.) The penile clamp is applied around the outside of the penis to compress the urethra and prevent urine leakage.

Adverse outcomes from pessaries and penile clamps include reduced TISSUE INTEGRITY with tissue damage from pressure and infection from colonization of damaged tissues. Both devices require that the patient have either manual dexterity or a caregiver to apply and remove the device. Instruct the patient or caregivers in the use of these devices. Male patients may use an external collecting device, such as a condom catheter. Design of an effective external collecting device for women has not been as successful.

Containment is achieved with absorbent pads and briefs designed to collect urine and keep the patient's skin and clothing dry. Many types and sizes of pads are available:

- Shields or liners inserted inside a panty
- Undergarments that are full-size pads with waist straps
- Plastic-lined protective underpants
- Combination pad and pant systems
- Absorbent bed pads

A major concern with the use of wearable protective pads is the risk for skin breakdown (loss of TISSUE INTEGRITY). Some patients develop incontinence-associated dermatitis (IAD) even when the skin is kept free of contact with urine (Gray et al., 2016). The wearable pads generate heat and sweat in the area that can cause dermatitis. Materials and costs of protective pads vary. Some are reusable; others are disposable. The disposal of these products raises ecologic concerns. Avoid use of the word "diaper" when discussing these adult pants, because of the association of diapers with a baby. More acceptable terms are "briefs" and "pads." See Chapter 25 for more information about IAD.

Catheterization for control of functional incontinence may be intermittent or involve a long-term catheter. Intermittent catheterization is preferred to a long-term catheter because of the reduced risk for infection. A long-term urinary catheter is appropriate for patients with disrupted TISSUE INTEGRITY who need a dry environment for healing, for those who are terminally ill and need COMFORT, and for those who are critically ill and require precise measurement of urine output.

Managing Total or Mixed Urinary Incontinence. Mixed or total urinary incontinence is a combination of two or more types of involuntary urine loss syndromes. For example, stress incontinence and urge incontinence often occur together in women during and after menopause. For the patient with mixed or total incontinence, combinations of assessment techniques (as discussed under each syndrome) are used. Interventions are also combined to promote continence. The problems and interventions for mixed incontinence are the same as for each specific type of incontinence separately. After identifying the specific types of incontinence that an individual patient has, apply the appropriate priority patient problems, interventions, and expected outcomes discussed earlier with each incontinence type.

CULTURAL/SPIRITUAL CONSIDERATIONS
Patient-Centered Care QSEN

Lower income is associated with fewer discussions between clinicians and patients about incontinence among women who have at least one episode of incontinence weekly (Duralde et al., 2016). Some evidence indicates that African-American women are less knowledgeable about risk factors associated with incontinence and its treatment options (Mandimika et al., 2015). Perform systematic screening of all women, including minority women, to overcome barriers to discussions and evaluation of incontinence and its treatment.

CLINICAL JUDGMENT CHALLENGE 66-1
Patient-Centered Care; Evidence-Based Practice QSEN

The patient is a 72-year-old woman who reports loss of a large volume of urine just as she enters the bathroom both at home and away from home. The problem started only recently and occurred about four times during the past week. She is an active church volunteer, lives independently with her husband, and recently passed a safe driving course to assure her that she is still safe to drive around town. The patient wants to continue to participate in her active lifestyle and wants to discuss options for preventing/managing this embarrassing condition.
1. What other information will you obtain from this patient?
2. What type or types of incontinence is she most likely to have from the information she has provided thus far?
3. What will you tell her regarding options for care?
4. She asks if there is anything she can do now to stop this problem of involuntary loss of urine. How do you respond?

Care Coordination and Transition Management

Community-based care for the patient with incontinence of urine ELIMINATION considers his or her personal, physical, emotional, and social resources. Important personal resources for self-care include mobility and manual dexterity. When planning care, consider who will be the primary caregiver and which factors may influence the effectiveness of the plan. A comparative effectiveness review from the Agency for Healthcare Research and Quality (AHRQ, 2013) reports that drugs for urinary incontinence can provide benefit but that adverse drug events, overall, lead to poor adherence. This report also provides information that nonpharmacologic and nonsurgical treatments provide significant clinical benefit with low risk for adverse effects but that these interventions are also associated with poor adherence. Ongoing relationships with primary health care providers may improve adherence.

Home Care Management. Assess the home environment for barriers that limit access to the bathroom. Eliminate hazards that might slow walking or lead to a fall. Such hazards include throw rugs, furniture with legs that extend into the walking area, slippery waxed or polished floors, and poor lighting.

If the patient must climb stairs to reach a bathroom, handrails should be installed and stairs kept free of obstacles. Toilet seat extenders may help provide the right level and height of seating so maximal abdominal pressure may be applied for voiding. Portable commodes may be obtained when ambulatory access to toilets is impractical. Physical and occupational therapists are valuable resources for assisting with home care management.

Self-Management Education. Teach the patient and family about the cause of the specific type of incontinence and discuss available treatment options for its management. The teaching plan addresses the prescribed drugs (purpose, dosage, method and route of administration, and expected and potential side effects). Instruct the patient and family about the importance of weight reduction and dietary modification to help control incontinence of urine ELIMINATION. Remind the patient who smokes that nicotine can contribute to bladder irritation and that coughing can cause urine leakage.

When external devices or protective pads are needed, describe the possible options and help the patient make a selection best for his or her lifestyle and resources. For patients who will use intermittent catheterization or those with artificial urinary sphincters, demonstrate the correct technique to the patient or caregiver. Evaluate return demonstrations for correct technique. Chart 66-6 also addresses teaching.

Psychosocial Preparation. The embarrassment of incontinence can be devastating to self-esteem, body image, and relationships. Sexual intimacy is adversely affected by it. Its unpredictable nature creates anxiety. Patients may be embarrassed to seek help and, even when resources are identified, they may need help to feel comfortable in using them. Buying supplies at a local store may threaten privacy.

Acknowledge the personal concerns of the patient and caregiver. Never make their concerns seem trivial. As he or she learns the specifics of the plan that will allow control of urinary incontinence, the confidence to resume social interactions should return. Many continence supplies can be purchased online and delivered to the home to maintain privacy.

Health Care Resources. Referral to home care agencies for help with personal care and to continence clinics that specialize in evaluation and treatment may be helpful. In many continence

CHART 66-6 Patient and Family Education: Preparing for Self-Management
Urinary Incontinence

- Maintain a normal body weight to reduce the pressure on your bladder.
- Do not try to control your incontinence by limiting your fluid intake. Adequate fluid intake is necessary for kidney function and health maintenance.
- If you have a catheter in your bladder, follow the instructions given to you about maintaining the sterile drainage system.
- If you are discharged with a suprapubic catheter in your bladder, inspect the entry site for the tube daily, clean the skin around the opening gently with warm soap and water, and place a sterile gauze dressing on the skin around the tube. Report any redness, swelling, drainage, or fever to your primary health care provider.
- Do not put anything into your vagina, such as tampons, drugs, hygiene products, or exercise weights, until you check with your primary health care provider at your 6-week checkup after surgery.
- Do not have sexual intercourse until after your 6-week postoperative checkup.
- Do not lift or carry anything heavier than 5 lb or participate in any strenuous exercise until your primary health care provider gives you postoperative clearance. In some cases, this could be as long as 3 months.
- Avoid exercises, such as running, jogging, step or dance aerobic classes, rowing, cross-country ski or stair-climber machines, and mountain biking. Brisk walking without any additional hand, leg, or body weights is allowed. Swimming is allowed after all drains and catheters have been removed and your incision is completely healed.
- If Kegel exercises are recommended, ask your nurse for specific instructions.

clinics, nurses collaborate with physicians and other health care professionals to evaluate and manage patients. The treatment plan is specific for each patient; supplies and products are custom selected.

Patients may benefit from education and from the support of others who experience similar concerns. The National Association for Continence (NAFC) (www.nafc.org), Access to Continence Care and Treatment (www.wellweb.com/INCONT/acct/contents.htm), and the Wound, Ostomy, and Continence Nurses (www.wocn.org) publish newsletters and educational materials written with easy-to-understand explanations. The American Foundation for Urologic Disease (www.afud.com) provides information on many areas of bladder dysfunction. Local hospitals often have local NAFC-approved support groups.

 NCLEX EXAMINATION CHALLENGE 66-2

Safe and Effective Care Environment

For which hospitalized client does the nurse recommend the ongoing use of a urinary catheter?

A. 35-year-old woman who was admitted with a splenic laceration and femur fracture (closed repair completed) following a car crash

B. 48-year-old man who has established paraplegia and is admitted for pneumonia

C. 61-year-old woman who is admitted following a fall at home and has new-onset dysrhythmia

D. 74-year-old man who has lung cancer with brain metastasis and is being transitioned to hospice for end-of-life care

---

◆ *Evaluation: Reflecting*

Evaluate the care of the patient with urinary incontinence based on the identified priority patient problems. The expected outcomes are that the patient will:

- Describe the type of urinary incontinence experienced
- Demonstrate knowledge of proper use of drugs and correct procedures for self-catheterization, use of the artificial sphincter, or care of an indwelling urinary catheter
- Demonstrate effective use of the selected exercise or bladder-training program
- Select and use incontinence interventions, devices, and products
- Have a reduction in the number of incontinence episodes
- Maintain TISSUE INTEGRITY of the skin and mucous membranes in the perineal area

CYSTITIS

❖ PATHOPHYSIOLOGY

Cystitis is an inflammatory condition of the bladder. Commonly, it refers to inflammation from an infection of the bladder. However, cystitis can be caused by inflammation without infection. For example, drugs, chemicals, or local radiation therapy cause bladder inflammation without an infecting organism. Irritants, such as feminine hygiene spray, spermicidal jellies, or long-term use of a catheter can cause cystitis without infection. Cystitis may sometimes occur as a complication of other disorders, such as gynecologic cancers, pelvic inflammatory disorders, endometriosis, Crohn's disease, diverticulitis, lupus,

or tuberculosis. Interstitial cystitis is a painful inflammatory bladder condition.

An infection can occur in any area of the urinary tract and the kidney. Such infections are known as *urinary tract infections* or *UTIs*. Risk factors associated with cystitis and other UTIs are listed in Table 66-3. An acute UTI is the invasion of a normal urinary tract by an infectious organism. A recurrent UTI occurs as more than two infections in 6 months or more than three infections in 1 year. These distinctions in UTIs are important because they have different approaches to management.

🧩 **GENDER HEALTH CONSIDERATIONS**

Patient-Centered Care QSEN

About 10% of young, sexually active women experience a UTI each year, and 60% of all women have one or more UTIs in their lifetime. Most UTIs are acute and uncomplicated in women. Acute, uncomplicated UTIs rarely occur in men.

A UTI is further categorized as *uncomplicated* or *complicated*. With an uncomplicated UTI, there is no anatomic or functional abnormality of the urinary tract or condition that increases the risk for infection or possibility of treatment failing to resolve the infection (such as the presence of a multi–drug-resistant organism or urologic dysfunction). Some factors and conditions that contribute to a diagnosis of complicated UTI are pregnancy, male gender, obstruction, diabetes, neurogenic bladder, chronic kidney disease, and reduced IMMUNITY (Nicolle, 2016). In men, a UTI is generally considered complicated even with normal structure and function because most UTIs occur in older men or in association with anal intercourse (resulting in exposure to potentially virulent pathogens). Complicated cystitis or other UTI requires greater vigilance to avoid or detect adverse events from the infection and a longer course of antimicrobial treatment. A diagnosis of complicated UTI may require additional testing to identify and manage other related health problems (comorbidities).

The presence of bacteria in the urine is bacteriuria and may occur with cystitis or any UTI. When the patient has bacteriuria but no symptoms of infection, it is called *colonization*, or *asymptomatic bacterial urinary tract infection* or *ABUTI*, and is more common in older adults. This problem may progress to acute infection or renal insufficiency when the patient has other conditions, and only then does it require treatment.

The urinary and genitourinary tracts are normally sterile, apart from the distal urethra. Several host defenses help protect against infection in the urinary tract. Mucin produced by cells lining the bladder helps maintain mucosal integrity and prevents cellular damage. Mucin prevents bacteria from adhering to urothelial cells. Urine pH and the concentration of organic acids also contribute to sustaining sterile urine. Polymorphonuclear (PMN) leukocytes (white blood cells [WBCs]) in the urinary tract are the IMMUNITY cells that engulf and destroy pathogens. Urine proteins, such as secreted antibodies, also are protective. In men, the prostate gland secretes additional protective proteins. Frequent voiding is another defense against bacterial growth and adherence by preventing urine stasis.

Etiology and Genetic Risk

UTIs, like other infections, result from interactions between a pathogen and the host. Usually a high bacterial *virulence*

TABLE 66-3 Factors Contributing to Urinary Tract Infections

FACTOR	MECHANISM
Obstruction	Incomplete bladder emptying creates a continuous pool of urine in which bacteria can grow, prevents flushing out of bacteria, and allows bacteria to ascend more easily to higher structures. Bacteria have a greater chance of multiplying the longer they remain in residual urine. Overdistention of the bladder damages the mucosa and allows bacteria to invade the bladder wall.
Stones (calculi)	Large stones can obstruct urine flow. The rough surface of a stone irritates mucosal surfaces and creates a spot where bacteria can establish and grow. Bacteria can live within stones and cause re-infection.
Vesicoureteral reflux	The urethra is colonized with bacteria. These bacteria are noninfectious until they move to upstream anatomy (bladder, ureters, kidneys) and colonize or form an infection with reflux (backward-flowing urine). Reflux of sterile urine can cause kidney scarring, which may promote kidney dysfunction.
Diabetes mellitus	Excess glucose in urine provides a rich medium for bacterial growth. Peripheral neuropathy affects bladder innervation and leads to a flaccid bladder and incomplete bladder emptying.
Characteristics of urine	Urine pH can promote different species of bacterial growth. Concentrated urine allows bacterial growth and adhesion to urinary tract anatomy.
Gender	**Women** Susceptibility to urethral colonization with coliform or pathogenic bacteria is increased, especially as estrogen levels fall during menopause. Use of douches, perfumed pads or toilet tissue, diaphragms, or spermicide (including spermicide-coated condoms) in women can inflame periurethral tissue and contribute to colonization. Bladder displacement during pregnancy predisposes women to cystitis and the development of pyelonephritis. A diaphragm or pessary that is too large can obstruct urine flow or traumatize the urethra. **Men** With increased age, the prostate enlarges and may obstruct the normal flow of urine, producing stasis. With increased age, prostatic secretions lose their antibacterial characteristics and predispose to bacterial proliferation in the urine. Sexually transmitted diseases may cause urethral strictures that obstruct the flow of urine and predispose to urinary stasis.
Age	Urinary stasis may be caused by incomplete bladder emptying as a result of an enlarged prostate in men and cystocele and vaginal prolapse in women. Neuromuscular conditions that cause incomplete bladder emptying, such as Parkinson disease and stroke, affect older adults more frequently. The use of drugs with intentional or unintentional anticholinergic properties in older adults contributes to delayed bladder emptying. Fecal incontinence contributes to urethral contamination. Low estrogen in menopausal women adversely affects the cells of the vagina and urethra, making them more susceptible to infections. Overall IMMUNITY declines with age, increasing the risk for uncomplicated infections to become complicated.
Sexual activity	Sexual intercourse is the strongest risk factor for uncomplicated cystitis, particularly in young women. Irritation of the perineum and urethra during intercourse can promote migration of bacteria from the perineal area to the urinary tract in some women. Inadequate vaginal lubrication may exacerbate potential urethral irritation. Bacteria may be introduced into the man's urethra during anal intercourse or during vaginal intercourse with a woman who has a bacterial vaginitis.
Recent use of antibiotics	Antibiotics change IMMUNITY and normal protective flora, providing opportunity for pathogenic bacterial overgrowth and colonization.

(ability to invade and infect) is needed to overcome normal host defenses and IMMUNITY. However, an adult with reduced immunity is more likely to become infected even with bacteria that have low virulence. With UTI, bacteria (and, infrequently, fungi), move up the urinary tract from the external urethra to the bladder to cause infectious cystitis. Less commonly, spread of infection through the blood and lymph fluid can occur, although this cause of UTI is not common. Invading bacteria with special adhesions are more likely to cause ascending UTIs that start in the urethra or bladder and move up into the ureter and kidney.

Infectious cystitis typically is caused by pathogens from the bowel or, in some cases, the vagina. About 90% of UTIs are caused by *Escherichia coli*. Less common organisms include *Staphylococcus saprophyticus*, *Klebsiella pneumoniae*, and organisms from the *Proteus* and *Enterobacter* species (Nicolle, 2016). Other infecting microbes causing infectious cystitis are viruses, mycobacteria, parasites, and yeast (fungus), especially *Candida* species. Reflux from the colonized distal urethra can also contribute to UTI in vulnerable patients. Irritation, trauma, or instrumentation of the urinary tract decreases host defenses and contributes to UTIs through the ascending migration of uropathogens.

Catheters are the most common factor associated with new-onset UTIs in the hospital and long-term care settings (Conway et al., 2017; Corley, 2015; Panchisin, 2016). Within 48 hours of catheter insertion, bacterial colonization along the urethra and the catheter itself begins. About half of patients with indwelling catheters become infected within 1 week of catheter insertion.

How a catheter-associated infection occurs varies between genders. Bacteria from a woman's perineal area are more likely to ascend to the bladder by moving along the urethra. The shorter urethra in women aids in the ascending organisms' migration. In men, bacteria tend to gain access to the bladder from the catheter itself (Conway et al., 2017). Any break in the closed urinary drainage system allows bacteria to move through the lumen of the catheter. The external catheter surface also provides route for migration. Best practices to reduce the risk for catheter contamination and catheter-associated UTIs are listed in Chart 66-7.

Organisms other than bacteria cause cystitis. Fungal infections, such as those caused by *Candida,* can occur during long-term antibiotic therapy, because antibiotics change normal protective flora that reduce the adherence and volume of pathogenic bacteria. Patients with reduced IMMUNITY (those who are severely immunosuppressed, are receiving corticosteroids or other immunosuppressive agents, or have diabetes mellitus or acquired immune deficiency syndrome) are at higher risk for fungal UTIs.

Viral and parasitic infections are rare and usually are transferred to the urinary tract from an infection at another body site. For example, *Trichomonas,* a parasite found in the vagina, can also be found in the urine. Treatment of the vaginal infection also resolves the UTI.

Noninfectious cystitis may result from chemical exposure, such as to drugs (e.g., cyclophosphamide [Cytoxan, Procytox]); from radiation therapy; and from IMMUNITY problems, as with systemic lupus erythematosus (SLE).

Interstitial cystitis is a rare, chronic inflammation of the entire lower urinary tract (bladder, urethra, and adjacent pelvic muscles) that is related to genetic and IMMUNITY dysfunction rather than infection (Martin et al., 2015). The condition affects women six to seven times more often than men, and the diagnosis is difficult to make. Symptoms are pain associated with bladder filling or voiding, usually accompanied by frequency, urgency, and nocturia (McCance et al., 2014). Pain occurs in suprapubic or pelvic areas, sometimes radiating to the groin, vulva, or rectum.

Although cystitis is not life threatening, infection of the urinary tract can lead to life-threatening complications, including pyelonephritis and sepsis. Severe kidney damage from an ascending UTI is a rare complication. Patients with predisposing factors, such as anatomic abnormalities, pregnancy, obstruction, reflux, calculi, or diabetes, are at greater risk for complications.

The urinary tract is the infection source of severe sepsis or septic shock in about 10% to 30% of cases (Wagenlehner et al., 2013). The spread of the infection from the urinary tract to the bloodstream is termed *bacteremia* or urosepsis. Urosepsis is associated with a mortality rate of 30% (Conway et al., 2015). Sepsis, regardless of the source, is a systemic reaction to infection that prolongs hospitalization and can lead to shock,

---

◎ **CHART 66-7   Best Practice for Patient Safety & Quality Care** QSEN

Minimizing Catheter-Associated Urinary Tract Infections (CAUTI)

- Maintain good hand hygiene during insertion and manipulation of the catheter system to avoid contamination.
- Insert urinary catheters for appropriate use only, including:
  - Acute urinary retention or bladder obstruction
  - Accurate measurement of urine volume in critically ill patients
  - Perioperative situations that involve urologic surgery, prolonged surgery, large-volume infusions or diuretics during surgery, or the need for monitoring intraoperative urine output
  - To assist in healing of open sacral or perineal wounds in incontinent patients
  - Potentially unstable spine conditions or multiple traumatic injuries, such as pelvic fractures, for which patient requires immobilization
  - To provide COMFORT at end of life
- Ensure that only properly trained personnel insert and maintain catheters.
- Use routine hygiene to clean periurethral area; antiseptic cleaning solutions are NOT recommended.
- Leave catheters in place only as long as needed. The strongest predictor of a CAUTI is the length of time the catheter dwells in a patient.
- Assess need for urinary catheter daily and document patient needs or indications.
  - For example, remove catheters in postanesthesia care or as soon as possible after surgery when intraoperative indications have resolved.
- Use aseptic technique and sterile equipment in the acute care setting when inserting a urinary catheter.
- Maintain a closed system by ensuring that catheter tubing connections are sealed securely; disconnections can introduce pathogens into the urinary tract.
- Obtain urine samples aseptically.
- If breaks in the system occur, replace the catheter and entire collecting system.

- Maintain unobstructed urine flow:
  - Keep the catheter and collecting tube free from kinking.
  - Keep the urine collection bag below the level of the bladder and do not rest the bag on the floor
- Empty the bag regularly, using a separate, clean container for each patient.
- Ensure that the drainage spigot does not come into contact with nonsterile surfaces.
- Secure the catheter to the patient's thigh (women) or lower abdomen (men); catheter movement can cause urethral friction and irritation.
- Consider the use of antiseptic or antimicrobial catheters for patients requiring urinary catheters for more than 3 to 5 days. These catheters reduce bacterial colonization (i.e., biofilm) along the catheter.
- Consider appropriate alternatives to an indwelling catheter:
  - External (condom) devices in cooperative men without obstruction or urinary retention
  - Intermittent catheterization in patients requiring drainage for neurogenic bladder or postoperative urinary retention
- Use portable ultrasound devices to assess urine volume to reduce unnecessary catheterization.
- Implement best practices in quality improvement to ensure that core recommendations for use, insertion, and maintenance are implemented. Examples of projects that improve patient care and reduce CAUTI include:
  - Nurse-initiated protocols for urinary catheter removal
  - Compliance with hand hygiene
  - Impact of educational programs on CAUTI occurrence
  - Compliance with documentation for catheter placement or maintenance
  - Number of CAUTI per 1000 catheter days or patient days on unit
  - Track number of catheters inserted

Adapted from www.cdc.gov/CAUTItoolkits;www.ihi.org/preventCAUTI.

multiple organ failure, and other profound complications (see Chapter 37).

Incidence and Prevalence

The incidence of UTI is second only to upper respiratory infections in primary care. Patients who have **frequency** (an urge to urinate frequently in small amounts), **dysuria** (pain or burning with urination), and **urgency** (feeling that urination will occur immediately) account for more than 8 million health care visits annually. Total direct and indirect costs for adult UTIs are estimated at $1.6 billion annually. In addition to a high prevalence in primary care, UTIs are the most common health care–associated infection (Conway et al., 2015).

CONSIDERATIONS FOR OLDER ADULTS

Patient-Centered Care QSEN

In men, the incidence of UTI greatly increases after 73 years of age. In women, the prevalence of UTIs increases from 20% among all women to 50% among those older than 80 years (U.S. Renal Data Systems, 2015). Skin and mucous membrane changes from a lack of estrogen appear to account for much of the increased risk in older women, together with overall decreased IMMUNITY. Prostate disease increases risk for UTIs in men. Often the older adult does not have the typical symptoms of UTI (i.e., flank pain, dysuria, fever). More common symptoms are grossly bloody, foul-smelling urine with increasing frequency of urination (Touhy & Jett, 2016). When UTI leads to urosepsis, mental status changes occur. Ask about these additional symptoms of UTI whenever you are assessing an older adult.

Health Promotion and Maintenance

Although infectious cystitis is common, in many cases it is preventable. **In the health care setting, using guidelines to prevent UTIs that are associated with catheter use is a National Patient Safety Goal (www.jointcommission.org, 2016).** When catheters must be used in institutional settings, strict attention to sterile technique during insertion is essential to reduce the risk for UTIs (see Chart 66-7). Long-term placement of urinary catheters requires aseptic technique for insertion. When *intermittent catheterization* was used in rehabilitation and other chronic settings, use of clean technique resulted in a similar rate of UTI compared with sterile technique as reported in a recent meta-analysis (Prieto et al., 2015). Clean technique for catheter insertion is used in home settings where multiple resistant organisms are less likely to be present.

! NURSING SAFETY PRIORITY QSEN

Action Alert

Ensuring that urinary catheters are used appropriately and discontinued as early as possible is everyone's responsibility (Panchisin, 2016). Do not allow catheters to remain in place for staff convenience.

Certain changes in fluid intake patterns, urinary ELIMINATION patterns, and hygiene patterns can help prevent or reduce cystitis in the general population. For example, a liberal water intake of 2.2 L for women and 3 L for men can promote general health. Another strategy to promote health is to have sufficient fluid intake to cause 1.5 L of clear or light yellow urine daily. Strategies to prevent cystitis and other UTIs are listed in Chart 66-8. Although these strategies do not have consistent or

CHART 66-8 Patient and Family Education: Preparing for Self-Management

Preventing a Urinary Tract Infection

- Drink fluid liberally, as much as 2 to 3 liters daily if not contraindicated by health conditions.
- Be sure to get enough sleep, rest, and nutrition daily to maintain immunologic health.
- If spermicides are used, consider changing to another method of contraception.
- [For women] Clean your perineum (the area between your legs) from front to back.
- [For women] Avoid using or wearing irritating substances such as douches, scented lubricants for intercourse, bubble bath, tight-fitting underwear, and scented toilet tissue. Wear loose-fitting cotton underwear.
- [For women] Empty your bladder before and after intercourse.
- [For both women and men] Gently wash the perineal area before intercourse.
- Do not routinely delay urination because the flow of urine can help remove bacteria that may be colonizing the urethra or bladder.
- If you experience burning when you urinate, if you have to urinate frequently, or if you find it difficult to begin urinating, notify your primary health care provider right away, especially if you have a chronic medical condition (e.g., diabetes) or are pregnant.
- Consider using one or more of these therapies to reduce the risk for developing a urinary tract infection:
  - Taking cranberry substances (juice, capsules, or tablets) daily. Avoid high fructose cranberry juice to minimize calories and high-glucose urine favorable to bacterial reproduction.
  - Applying topical estrogen to the perineal area, if postmenopausal. Topical estrogen normalizes vaginal flora. Oral estrogens are not effective.

high-quality evidence to support a reduced risk for UTI when followed, they are low risk and reasonable.

❖ INTERPROFESSIONAL COLLABORATIVE CARE

Cystitis and UTIs can occur in any setting and are very common in the community. Usually the adult with cystitis is treated at home using self-management strategies.

◆ Assessment: Noticing

Physical Assessment/Signs and Symptoms. Frequency, urgency, and dysuria are the common symptoms of a urinary tract infection (UTI), but other symptoms may be present (Chart 66-9). Urine may be cloudy, foul smelling, or blood tinged. Ask the patient about risk factors for UTI during the assessment (see Table 66-3). For noninfectious cystitis, the Pelvic Pain and Urgency/Frequency Patient Symptom Scale (PUF, 2011) can identify patients with interstitial cystitis.

For patients with a urinary catheter, in addition to common signs of UTI (e.g., fever with or without chills; leukocytosis; suprapubic or flank pain; urine with sediment, blood, or foul odor), new onset of hypotension or changes in mental status can indicate a UTI (Nelson & Good, 2015). If a catheter has been in place for more than 2 weeks, it may be necessary to first replace the catheter before obtaining a urine specimen for culture (McGoldrick, 2016).

Before performing the physical assessment, ask the patient to void so the urine can be examined and the bladder emptied before palpation. Assess vital signs to help identify the presence of infection (e.g., fever, tachycardia, and tachypnea). Inspect

CHART 66-9   Key Features

Urinary Tract Infection

Common Symptoms

- Frequency
- Urgency
- Dysuria
- Hesitancy or difficulty in initiating urine stream
- Low back pain
- Nocturia
- Incontinence
- Hematuria
- Pyuria
- Bacteriuria
- Retention
- Suprapubic tenderness or fullness
- Feeling of incomplete bladder emptying

Rare Symptoms

- Fever
- Chills
- Nausea or vomiting
- Malaise
- Flank pain

Symptoms That May Occur in the Older Adult

- The only symptom may be something as vague as increasing mental confusion or frequent, unexplained falls.
- A sudden onset of incontinence or a worsening of incontinence may be the only symptom of an early urinary tract infection (UTI).
- Fever, tachycardia, tachypnea, and hypotension, even without any urinary symptoms, may be signs of urosepsis.
- Loss of appetite, nocturia, and dysuria are common indications.

the lower abdomen and palpate the bladder. Distention after voiding indicates incomplete bladder emptying.

Using Standard Precautions, record any lesions around the urethral meatus and vaginal opening. To help differentiate between a vaginal and a urinary tract infection, note whether there is any vaginal discharge or irritation. Vaginal discharge and irritation are more indicative of vaginal infection. Women often report burning with urination when urine touches labial tissues that are inflamed or have lost TISSUE INTEGRITY with ulcerations by vaginal infections or sexually transmitted infections (STIs). Maintain privacy with drapes during the examination.

The prostate is palpated by digital rectal examination (DRE) by the primary health care provider for size, change in shape or consistency, and tenderness. A large prostate gland can obstruct urine outflow and contribute to urostasis and bacterial colonization of the urinary tract, contributing to the risk for a complicated UTI.

Laboratory Assessment. Laboratory assessment for a UTI begins with a clean-catch urine specimen that is divided into two containers. If the patient cannot produce a clean-catch specimen, you may need to obtain the specimen with a small-diameter (6 Fr) catheter. For a routine urinalysis, 10 mL of urine is needed; smaller quantities are sufficient for culture.

One container is used for a urinalysis. The combination of a positive leukocyte esterase and nitrate from a urinalysis is 68% to 88% sensitive in the diagnosis of a UTI. The presence of white blood cells (WBCs) (**pyuria**), red blood cells (RBCs)

(**hematuria**), or casts (clumps of material or cells) also may indicate UTI. The presence of more than 20 epithelial cells/high-power field (HPF) suggests contamination, and a new specimen should be collected for culture and sensitivity (if needed).

If the urinalysis suggests a UTI and there are no risk factors or conditions for complicated UTI in a woman, treatment can be started. If the UTI is complicated (described previously), the second specimen is analyzed as a urine culture. A culture also may be performed when a patient with a UTI does not respond to usual therapy, when the diagnosis is uncertain, to assess for sensitivity, or to determine resolution of UTI. Urinalysis is less specific in diagnosing a UTI in an older adult, especially one who has a urinary catheter (Nelson & Good, 2015).

A urine culture confirms the type of organism and the number of colonies. Urine culture is expensive, and initial results take at least 24 hours. A UTI is confirmed when more than 10^5 colony-forming units/mL are in the urine from any patient. In noncatheterized patients who have symptoms of UTI (e.g., fever, dysuria, new-onset frequency or urgency, suprapubic or flank pain, or hematuria), as few as 10^3 colony-forming units/mL in a voided specimen can confirm the infection. For patients with a catheter who are symptomatic, 10^2 colony-forming units/mL are diagnostic of a complicated UTI. The presence of many different types of organisms in low colony counts usually indicates that the specimen is contaminated. Sensitivity testing follows culture results when complicating factors are present (e.g., stones or recurrent infection), when the patient is older, or to ensure that appropriate antibiotics are prescribed.

Occasionally the serum WBC count may be elevated, with the differential WBC count showing a "left shift" (see Chapter 17). This shift indicates that the number of immature WBCs is increasing and the number of mature WBCs is decreasing in response to continued infection. Thus the number of "bands" or immature WBCs, is elevated, which indicates reduced IMMUNITY. Left shift most often occurs with urosepsis and rarely occurs with uncomplicated cystitis, because cystitis is a local rather than a systemic infection.

Other Diagnostic Assessment. The diagnosis of UTI and cystitis is based on history, physical examination, and laboratory data. If urinary retention and obstruction of urine outflow are suspected, pelvic ultrasound or CT may be needed to locate the site of obstruction or the presence of calculi. Voiding cystourethrography (see Chapter 65) is needed when urine reflux is suspected.

Cystoscopy (see Chapter 65) may be performed when the patient has recurrent UTIs (more than three or four a year). A urine culture is performed first to ensure that no infection is present. If infection is present, the urine is sterilized with antibiotic therapy before the procedure to reduce the risk for sepsis. Cystoscopy identifies abnormalities that increase the risk for cystitis. Such abnormalities include bladder calculi, bladder diverticula, urethral strictures, foreign bodies (e.g., sutures from previous surgery), and **trabeculation** (an abnormal thickening of the bladder wall caused by urinary retention and obstruction). Retrograde pyelography, along with the cystoscopic examination, shows outlines and images of the drainage tract.

Cystoscopy is needed to accurately diagnose interstitial (noninfectious) cystitis. A urinalysis usually shows WBCs and RBCs but no bacteria. Common findings in interstitial cystitis are a small-capacity bladder, the presence of Hunner's ulcers (a type of bladder lesion), and small hemorrhages after bladder distention.

◆ Interventions: Responding

Nonsurgical Management. The expected outcome is to maintain an optimal urine ELIMINATION pattern. Nursing interventions for the management of cystitis focus on COMFORT and teaching about drug therapy, fluid intake, and prevention measures. In a hospital setting, timely administration of antibiotics can prevent or reduce complications from urosepsis.

Drug Therapy. Drugs used to treat bacteriuria and promote patient COMFORT include urinary antiseptics or antibiotics, analgesics, and antispasmodics. Cure of a UTI depends on the antimicrobial levels achieved in the urine. Fluconazole is the drug of choice for treatment of *Candida* (fungal) infections. Antispasmodic drugs decrease bladder spasms and promote complete bladder emptying.

Antibiotic therapy is used for bacterial UTIs (Chart 66-10). Guidelines for uncomplicated cystitis recommend nitrofurantoin, trimethoprim/sulfamethoxazole, or fosfomycin as first-line therapy (Infectious Disease Society of America, 2013; Hopkins et al., 2014). Longer antibiotic treatment (7 to 21 days) and sometimes different agents are required for hospitalized patients and those with complicated UTIs (e.g., men, pregnant women, and patients with anatomic, functional or metabolic derangements that affect the urinary tract).

! NURSING SAFETY PRIORITY (QSEN)

Drug Alert

Sulfamethoxazole/trimethoprim (Bactrim DS, Septra DS) should be stopped at the first appearance of a skin rash. A rash may indicate the onset of Stevens-Johnson syndrome (aching joints and muscles; bilateral blistering skin) or toxic epidermal necrolysis (redness, blistering, and peeling skin and mucous membranes).

Antibiotics are one of the drug categories most frequently involved in the error of administration to patients who have documented allergies to these drugs.

Low-dose antibiotic therapy over 6 to 12 months is sometimes used for chronic, recurring infection caused by structural abnormalities or stones. Trimethoprim 100 mg daily may be used for long-term management of the older patient with frequent UTIs. For women who have recurrent UTIs after intercourse, antibiotics may be prescribed to be taken after intercourse. The three most common drug treatment regimens are (1) one low-dose tablet of trimethoprim (Proloprim, Trimpex), (2) sulfamethoxazole/trimethoprim (single-strength Bactrim, Cotrim), or (3) nitrofurantoin (Macrodantin, Nephronex ✸, Novo Furantoin ✦).

🚻 GENDER HEALTH CONSIDERATIONS

Patient-Centered Care (QSEN)

Pregnant women with a bacterial UTI require prompt and aggressive treatment because a UTI can lead to acute pyelonephritis during pregnancy. Pyelonephritis in pregnancy can cause preterm labor and adversely affect the fetus. Remind pregnant patients to contact their health care provider whenever symptoms of UTI are present.

Fluid Intake. Urge patients to drink enough fluid to maintain dilute urine throughout the day and night unless fluid restriction is needed for another health problem. Some urologists recommend sufficient fluid intake to result in at least 1.5 L of urine output or 7 to 12 voidings daily. Food can provide 20% or more of fluid intake, particularly the intake of fruits and vegetables.

Cranberry-containing products taken daily appear to decrease the ability of bacteria to adhere to the epithelial cells lining the urinary tract. In some patients, this may result in preventing UIT or decreasing the incidence of recurrent symptomatic UTIs, but the evidence is not high quality (Allan & Nicole, 2013). Cranberry juice, tablets, or capsules must be consumed for more than 4 weeks to affect the ability of *E. coli* to adhere to the urinary tract (Foxman et al., 2015). Cranberry juice can be an irritant to the bladder with interstitial cystitis and should be avoided by patients with this condition. Avoiding caffeine, carbonated beverages, and tomato products may decrease bladder irritation and promote COMFORT during cystitis.

Comfort Measures. A warm sitz bath two or three times a day for 20 minutes may provide COMFORT and some relief of local symptoms. If burning with urination is severe or urinary retention occurs, teach the patient to sit in the sitz bath and urinate into the warm water. Urinary tract analgesics or antispasmodics may also provide comfort (see Chart 66-10).

Surgical Management. Surgery for cystitis treats the conditions that increase the risk for recurrent UTIs (e.g., removal of obstructions and repair of vesicoureteral reflux). Procedures may include cystoscopy (see Chapter 65) to identify and remove calculi or obstructions.

Care Coordination and Transition Management

Assess the patient's level of understanding of the problem. Her or his knowledge about factors that promote the development of cystitis determines the teaching interventions planned.

Teach the patient how to take prescribed drugs. Stress the need for correct spacing of doses throughout the day and the need to complete all of the prescribed antibiotics. If the drug will change the color of the urine, as it does with phenazopyridine (Pyridium, Urogesic, Phenazo), inform the patient to expect this change.

Patients may associate discomfort with sexual activities and have feelings of guilt and embarrassment. Open and sensitive discussions with a woman who has recurrences of UTI after sexual intercourse can help her find techniques to handle the problem (see Chart 66-8). Explore with her the factors that contribute to her infections, such as sexual penetration when the bladder is full, diaphragm use, and her general IMMUNITY responses against infection. Some positions during intercourse may reduce urethral irritation and subsequent cystitis. Remind the patient that vigorous cleaning of the perineum with harsh soaps and vaginal douching may irritate the perineal tissues and *increase* the risk for UTI. At the patient's request, discuss the problem with her and her partner to help them find ways of maintaining their intimate relationship.

URETHRITIS

❖ PATHOPHYSIOLOGY

Urethritis is an inflammation of the urethra and can result from infectious and noninfectious conditions. The incidence is highest among adults ages 20 to 24 years. The most common

CHART 66-10 **Common Examples of Drug Therapy**

Urinary Tract Infections

DRUG	NURSING IMPLICATIONS
Trimethoprim*/ sulfamethoxazole (Bactrim DS, Septra DS, trimethoprim/ sulfamethoxazole orally)	Ask patients about drug allergies, especially to sulfa drugs, before beginning drug therapy *because allergies to sulfa drugs are common and require changing drug therapy.* Teach patients to drink a full glass of water with each dose and to have an overall fluid intake of 3 L daily *because these drugs can form crystals that precipitate in the kidney tubules. Fluids can prevent this complication.* Teach patients to keep out of the sun or to wear protective clothing outdoors and use a sunscreen *because these drugs increase sun sensitivity and can lead to severe sunburn.* Caution patients to complete the drug regimen even if the symptoms improve or disappear sooner *to prevent bacterial resistance and infection recurrence.*
Ciprofloxacin (Cipro, ProQuin) Levofloxacin (Levaquin) Ofloxacin (Floxin)	Teach patients taking the extended-release drugs to swallow them whole and not to crush or chew the tablets *because this action ruins the extended effect.* Warn patients not to take the drug within 2 hours of taking an antacid *to prevent interference with drug absorption.* Teach patients how to take their pulse, to monitor it twice daily while on this drug, and to notify the primary health care provider if new-onset irregular heartbeats occur *to identify serious drug-induced dysrhythmias.* Teach patients to keep out of the sun or to wear protective clothing outdoors and use a sunscreen *to avoid serious sunburns from increased sun sensitivity.* Caution patients to complete the drug regimen even if the symptoms improve or disappear sooner *to reduce bacterial resistance and infection recurrence.*
Amoxicillin (Amoxil) Amoxicillin/clavulanate (Augmentin, Clavulin)	Ask patients about drug allergies to penicillin before beginning drug therapy *because allergies to this drug category are common.* Teach patients to take the drug with food *to reduce the risk for GI upset.* Instruct patients to call the primary health care provider if severe or watery diarrhea develops *to recognize the complication of pseudomembranous colitis, which may require discontinuing the drug.* Suggest that women who take oral contraceptives use an additional method of birth control while taking this drug *because these drugs may reduce the effectiveness of estrogen-containing contraceptives.* Caution patients to complete the drug regimen even if the symptoms improve or disappear sooner *to prevent bacterial resistance and infection recurrence.*
Cefdinir, cefaclor, or cefpodoxime	Ask about drug allergies to penicillin or cephalosporins before beginning drug therapy *because these drugs are structurally similar to penicillin and anyone with allergies to penicillin is likely to be allergic to the cephalosporins.* Instruct patients to call the prescriber if severe or watery diarrhea develops *to recognize the complication of pseudomembranous colitis, which may require discontinuing the drug.* Caution patients to complete the drug regimen even if the symptoms improve or disappear sooner *to prevent bacterial resistance and infection recurrence.* Instruct patients to mix the contents of a package in about ½ cup of cold water, stir well, and drink all the liquid *to ensure that all granules are dissolved and the correct dose is taken.* Avoid taking this drug when also taking metoclopramide or any other drug that increases GI motility *to prevent interference with drug absorption.* Teach patients to shake the bottle well before measuring the drug *to thoroughly mix the suspension.* Suggest that patients obtain a calibrated spoon for liquid drugs and not to use household spoons *to ensure accurate dosing.* Teach patients to drink a full glass of water with each dose and to have an overall fluid intake of at least 3 L daily *to avoid having the drug precipitate in the kidneys and cause kidney damage.* Caution patients to complete the drug regimen even if the symptoms improve or disappear sooner *to prevent bacterial resistance and infection recurrence.*
Phenazopyridine (Azo-Dine, Prodium, Pyridiate, Pyridium, Uristat, Phenazo)	Remind patients that this drug will not treat an infection, only the symptoms *because these drugs have no antibacterial activity.* Teach patients to take the drug with or immediately after a meal *to reduce the risk for GI upset.* Warn patients that urine will turn red or orange *to reduce anxiety about this change.*
Hyoscyamine (Anaspaz, Cystospaz, many others)	Teach patients to notify the primary health care provider if blurred vision or other eye problems, confusion, dizziness or fainting spells, fast heartbeat, fever, or difficulty passing urine occurs *because these symptoms indicate drug toxicity.* Teach patients to wear dark glasses in sunlight or other bright-light areas *because these drugs dilate the pupil and increase eye sensitivity to light.*

*Trimethoprim can be given alone to patients with a sulfa allergy.

cause of infectious urethritis is sexually transmitted infections (STIs). These include gonorrhea or nonspecific urethritis caused by *Ureaplasma* (a gram-negative bacterium), *Chlamydia* (a sexually transmitted gram-negative bacterium), or *Trichomonas vaginalis* (a protozoan found in both the male and female genital tract). Urethritis is also known as *pyuria-dysuria syndrome, frequency-dysuria syndrome, trigonitis syndrome,* and *urethral syndrome.*

Many women with urethritis have symptoms similar to cystitis, vaginitis, or cervicitis. Men with urethritis may report symptoms of cystitis, as well as heaviness in the genitals *(orchalgia).* Noninfectious urethritis in postmenopausal women may be related to uretero-genital tissue changes resulting from low estrogen levels.

Symptoms of urethritis include discharge of mucopurulent or purulent material, dysuria, and itching or discomfort of the area (urethral pruritus). The discharge can be any color, depending on the infecting organism or source of irritation. Additional symptoms may include fever (with or without chills) and urgent or frequent urination.

❖ INTERPROFESSIONAL COLLABORATIVE CARE

Ask the patient about a history of STI, painful or difficult urination, discharge from the penis or vagina, and discomfort in the lower abdomen. Urinalysis may show **pyuria** (white blood cells [WBCs] in the urine) without a large number of bacteria. Similarly, a urethral smear may show WBCs. All patients with urethritis should be tested for *N. gonorrhoeae* and *C. trachoma* with an endourethral (in men) or endocervical (women) smear. Testing for *Chlamydia* may be done with the same sample. STI testing for VDRL serology and HIV is suggested by the Centers for Disease Control and Prevention (CDC, 2016a). A pregnancy test is performed for women who have had unprotected intercourse. In women, a pelvic examination may reveal tissue changes from low estrogen levels in the vagina. Urethroscopy may show low estrogen changes with inflammation of urethral tissues.

Noninfectious urethritis symptoms usually resolve spontaneously over time, regardless of treatment. Postmenopausal women often have improvement in urethral symptoms with the use of estrogen vaginal cream. Estrogen cream applied locally to the vagina increases the amount of estrogen in the urethra as well, reducing irritating symptoms. Urethritis from STIs is treated with antibiotic therapy. More information on STIs can be found in Chapter 74.

UROLITHIASIS

❖ PATHOPHYSIOLOGY

Urolithiasis is the presence of *calculi* (stones) in the urinary tract. Stones often do not cause symptoms until they pass into the lower urinary tract, where they can cause excruciating pain. **Nephrolithiasis** is the formation of stones in the kidney; formation of stones in the ureter is **ureterolithiasis**. Stones are particles in the urine that occur in amounts too high to stay dissolved (become supersaturated) in urine. As a result of

supersaturation, the particles precipitate and collect to form calculi.

The most common condition associated with stone formation is dehydration. Everyone excretes crystals in the urine at some time, but fewer than 10% of adults form stones. Most stones contain calcium as one part of the stone complex. Struvite (15%), uric acid (8%), and cystine (3%) are more rare compositions of stones. Formation of stones involves two conditions:

1. Supersaturation of the urine with the particular element (e.g., calcium, uric acid) that first becomes crystallized and later becomes the stone

2. Formation of a *nidus* (deposit of crystals that can be the point of infection) along the lining of the kidney and urinary tract

In addition, some patients may have decreased amounts of inhibitor substances in the urine that would otherwise prevent supersaturation with crystal aggregation. This type of metabolic risk factor can be inherited.

In addition to low urine volume, high urine acidity (as with uric acid and cystine stones) or alkalinity (as with calcium phosphate and struvite stones), as well as drugs (e.g., topiramate, corticosteroids, indinavir, acetazolamide), contribute to stone formation.

One example of a metabolic problem causing stone formation begins when excessive amounts of calcium are absorbed through the intestinal tract, leading to hypercalciuria. As blood circulates through the kidneys, the excess calcium is filtered into the urine, causing supersaturation of calcium in the urine. If fluid intake is poor, such as when a patient is dehydrated, supersaturation is more likely to occur.

Any stone may result in obstruction within the urinary tract, which can threaten both glomerular filtration rate (GFR) and kidney perfusion. When the stone occludes the ureter and blocks the flow of urine, the ureter dilates. Enlargement of the ureter is called **hydroureter**.

The pain associated with ureteral spasm is excruciating and may cause the patient to go into shock from stimulation of nearby nerves. **Hematuria** (bloody urine) may result from damage to the urothelial lining. If the obstruction is not removed, urinary stasis can lead to infection and impair kidney function on the side of the blockage. As the blockage persists, **hydronephrosis** (enlargement of the kidney caused by blockage of urine lower in the tract and filling of the kidney with urine) and permanent kidney damage may develop.

Etiology and Genetic Risk

The vast majority of adults who form stones have a metabolic risk factor. The cause of stone formation in a susceptible adult (e.g., one who has a metabolic risk factor) is dehydration. Table 66-4 lists some metabolic problems that cause stone formation. Patients who are white, are obese, or have diabetes or gout (hyperuricemia) have increased risk for initial stone formation (Rodgers, 2013). Other conditions associated with stone formation and recurrence are hyperparathyroidism, urinary tract obstruction, inflammatory bowel diseases, and a history of GI problems (Fink et al., 2013). Because a metabolic problem is so strongly associated with stone formation and is a nonmodifiable risk factor, an adult of any age who develops a stone is always at high risk for future stone development.

Diet is not considered a risk for stone formation. However, calcium (greater than 1000 mg daily) and vitamin D supplementation (greater than 800 IU daily) and high-dose ascorbic

TABLE 66-4 Metabolic Defects That Commonly Cause Kidney Stones

METABOLIC DEFICIT	ETIOLOGY
Hypercalcemia	
Primary	Absorptive: Increased intestinal calcium absorption Renal: Decreased kidney tubular excretion of calcium
Secondary	Resorptive: Hyperparathyroidism, vitamin D intoxication, kidney tubular acidosis, prolonged immobilization
Hyperoxaluria	
Primary	Genetic: Autosomal-recessive trait resulting in high oxalate production
Secondary	Dietary: Excess oxalate from foods such as spinach, rhubarb, Swiss chard, cocoa, beets, wheat germ, pecans, peanuts, okra, chocolate, and lime peel
Hyperuricemia	
Primary	Gout is an inherited disorder of purine metabolism (20% of patients with gout have uric acid calculi)
Secondary	Increased production or decreased clearance of purine from myeloproliferative disorders, thiazide diuretics, carcinoma
Struvite	Made of magnesium ammonium phosphate and carbonate apatite; formed by urea splitting by bacteria, most commonly, *Proteus mirabilis;* needs an alkaline urine to form
Cystinuria	Autosomal-recessive defect of amino acid metabolism that precipitates insoluble cystine crystals in the urine

acid (vitamin C) intake have been implicated in stone formation (Fletcher, 2013). Conversely, high intake of fluid, fruits, and vegetables; low consumption of protein; and a balanced intake of fats and carbohydrates are prescribed to prevent and treat recurrent urolithiasis (Fink et al., 2013).

GENETIC/GENOMIC CONSIDERATIONS
Patient-Centered Care QSEN

Family history has a strong association with stone formation and recurrence because of inherited metabolic variations. More than 30 genetic variations are associated with the formation of kidney stones, although single gene disorders are rare. More commonly, nephrolithiasis is a complex disease, with genetic variation in intestinal calcium absorption, kidney calcium transport, or kidney phosphate transport all associated with stone formation (Online Mendelian Inheritance in Man [OMIM], 2016). Always ask a patient with a renal stone whether other family members also have this problem.

Incidence and Prevalence

The incidence of stone disease is high and varies with geographic location, race, and family history. About 12% of adults will have at least one episode of renal stone disease (McCance et al., 2014). The incidence of most stone types is higher in men, although struvite stones are twice as common in women. This difference in struvite stone formation incidence is

thought to be related to the fact that women have more UTIs and struvite stones are associated with UTI. Recurrence rates vary depending on the type of treatment, although any adult who has had a stone is much more likely to have recurrence. Recurrence of stones occurs in patients with a family history of stone disease and in those who had their first occurrence by age 25 years.

🌐 CULTURAL/SPIRITUAL CONSIDERATIONS
Patient-Centered Care QSEN

The incidence of stone disease is most common in the southeastern United States, Japan, and western Europe. Calcium stone disease is more common in men than in women and tends to occur in young adults or during early middle adulthood. Initial onset of stone disease occurs more often in younger adults than older adults and more commonly among white adults (Rodgers, 2013). For patients in these higher-risk groups, nursing care includes teaching family members, as well as patients, to avoid dehydration. Collaborate with the interprofessional health care team about referring patients with recurrent stone formation to evaluate metabolic risk factors.

❖ INTERPROFESSIONAL COLLABORATIVE CARE
◆ Assessment: Noticing

Ask the patient about a personal or family history of urologic stones. Obtain a diet history, focusing on fluid intake patterns and supplemental vitamin or mineral intake. If he or she has a history of stone formation, ask about past treatment, whether chemical analysis of the stone was performed, and which preventive measures are followed.

The major symptom of stones is severe pain, commonly called **renal colic**. Flank pain suggests that the stone is in the kidney or upper ureter. Flank pain that extends toward the abdomen or to the scrotum and testes or the vulva suggests that stones are in the ureters or bladder. Pain is most intense when the stone is moving or the ureter is obstructed.

Renal colic begins suddenly and is often described as "unbearable." Nausea, vomiting, pallor, and diaphoresis often accompany the pain. However, a large stationary stone in the kidney (staghorn calculus) rarely causes much pain because it is not moving. Frequency and dysuria occur when a stone reaches the bladder. **Oliguria** (scant urine output) or **anuria** (absence of urine output) suggests obstruction, possibly at the bladder neck or urethra. *Urinary tract obstruction is an emergency and must be treated immediately to preserve kidney function.*

Assess the patient for bladder distention. He or she may appear pale, ashen, and diaphoretic and may have excruciating pain. Vital signs may be elevated with pain; body temperature and pulse are elevated with infection. Blood pressure may decrease if the severe pain causes shock.

Urinalysis is performed in patients with suspected stones. Measurement of urine specific gravity and osmolarity can provide a clue about the adequacy of fluid intake. Urine pH can help in the determination of stone type. (High urine acidity [low urine pH] is associated with uric acid and cystine stones; high urine alkalinity [high urine pH] is associated with calcium phosphate and struvite stones.) A 24-hour urine analysis can determine whether supersaturation of common stone particles is present. Hematuria during renal colic is common, and blood may make the urine appear smoky or rusty. RBCs are usually caused by stone-induced trauma to the lining of the ureter, bladder, or urethra. WBCs and bacteria may be present as a result of urinary stasis. Increased *turbidity* (cloudiness) and odor indicate that infection may also be present. Microscopic examination of the urine may identify possible stone-forming crystals.

The serum WBC count is elevated with infection. Increases in the serum levels of calcium, phosphate, or uric acid levels indicate that excess minerals are present that may contribute to stone formation.

The current standard for confirming urinary stones is an unenhanced helical CT scan of the abdomen and pelvis. Most stones are radiopaque; and the size, location, and surrounding anatomic structures are easily seen. In settings where a CT is not available, a plain abdominal x-ray (KUB) is useful (Fig. 66-2). Ultrasound may be used in pregnant women suspected to have stones, but it is not sensitive for ureteral stones and is not used for general screening.

◆ Interventions: Responding

Nursing interventions focus on promoting COMFORT and preventing infection and urinary obstruction. Most patients expel the stone without invasive procedures. Size (i.e., less than 5 mm) is the most important factor for whether a stone will pass on its own; its composition and location are also factors. The larger the stone and the higher up in the urinary tract it is, the less likely it is to pass. When the stone is passed, it should be captured and sent to the laboratory for analysis. Other interventions are needed when the stone does not pass spontaneously (Fig. 66-3).

Managing Pain. Nonsurgical and surgical approaches are used to help the patient with a kidney stone achieve an acceptable degree of pain relief and COMFORT.

Nonsurgical Management. Nonsurgical measures to relieve pain include strategies to enhance stone passing, as well as direct pain management.

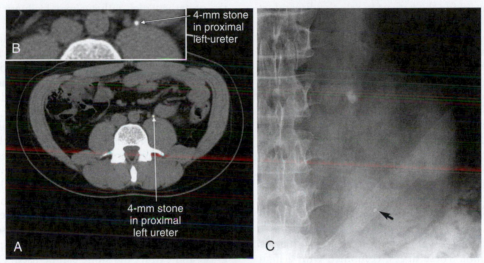

FIG. 66-2 **A** and **B,** Urinary stones on CT scan. **C,** Urinary stones on x-ray of the kidneys, ureters, and bladder (KUB). (**A** and **B** from Broder, J. K. [2011]. *Diagnostic imaging for the emergency physician.* Philadelphia: Saunders. **C** from Pollack, H.M. [2000]. *Clinical urography* [2nd ed.]. Philadelphia: Saunders.)

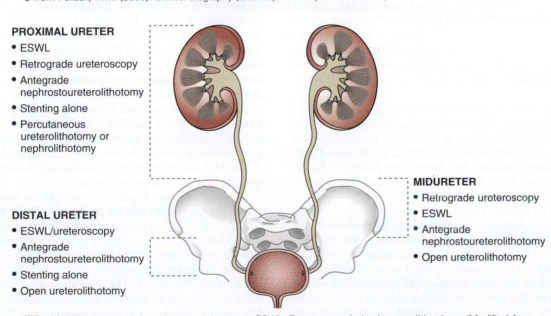

PROXIMAL URETER
- ESWL
- Retrograde ureteroscopy
- Antegrade nephrostoureterolithotomy
- Stenting alone
- Percutaneous ureterolithotomy or nephrolithotomy

DISTAL URETER
- ESWL/ureteroscopy
- Antegrade nephrostoureterolithotomy
- Stenting alone
- Open ureterolithotomy

MIDURETER
- Retrograde ureteroscopy
- ESWL
- Antegrade nephrostoureterolithotomy
- Open ureterolithotomy

FIG. 66-3 Treatment options for ureteral stones. *ESWL,* Extracorporeal shock wave lithotripsy. (Modified from Singal, R.K., & Denstedt, J.D. [1997]. Contemporary management of ureteral stones. *The Urologic Clinics of North America, 24*[1], 59-70.)

Drug therapy is needed in the first 24 to 36 hours when pain is most severe. Opioid analgesics are used to control the severe pain caused by stones in the urinary tract and may be given IV for rapid pain relief. NSAIDs such as ketorolac (Toradol) or ketoprofen (Nexcede) in the acute phase may be quite effective. When NSAIDs are used, there is an increased risk for kidney impairment from reduced perfusion. NSAIDs interfere with renal autoregulation, and the risk for impairment is greater among patients with pre-existing kidney dysfunction. Risk for bleeding also is increased from platelet inhibition when NSAIDs are used. Bleeding risk is particularly concerning when surgical intervention for stones is needed.

Control of pain and promotion of COMFORT are more effective when drugs are given at regularly scheduled intervals or by a constant delivery system (e.g., skin patch) instead of PRN. Spasmolytic drugs, such as oxybutynin chloride (Ditropan) and propantheline bromide (Pro-Banthine, Propanthel), are important for control of pain (see Chart 66-8). Give the drugs and assess the response by asking the patient to rate the discomfort on a pain-rating scale.

Other management techniques include avoiding overhydration and underhydration in the acute phase to help make the passage of a stone less painful. Strain the urine and teach the patient to strain it to monitor for stone passage. Send any stone passed to the laboratory for analysis because preventive therapy is based on stone composition.

Antibiotics may be used to manage struvite stones, because these are associated with urinary infections from urease-producing organisms such as *Proteus mirabilis, Klebsiella, Enterobacter,* or *Pseudomonas.* (*E. coli* does not produce urease.) When urease-producing bacteria remain in the urine and within the stone, urine becomes alkaline, causing phosphate to precipitate and allowing staghorn-shaped struvite stones to rapidly form.

Two drugs may be used to aid in stone expulsion: a thiazide diuretic and allopurinol. These drugs, combined with a high fluid intake, increase urine volume or decrease urine pH and help increase the excretion of stones or stone fragments. Alpha-adrenergic blockers and calcium channel blockers can shorten the time to stone passage by relaxing the smooth muscle within the ureters. Citrate may be used to alkalinize urine pH and dissolve uric acid stones. Implementing oral citrate treatment cannot be done until stone composition is known. It is typically reserved for prevention and treatment of recurrent stone formation.

A stone that has not passed within 1 to 2 months is unlikely to pass spontaneously. Other options for stone intervention are considered when infection occurs, when pain cannot be well managed, or when there is an actual or increased risk for reduced kidney function. An observation period of 1 to 2 weeks may be reasonable if the patient is comfortable or has few symptoms and stones are smaller than 5 mm.

Lithotripsy or extracorporeal *shock wave lithotripsy (SWL)* is the use of sound, laser, or dry shock waves to break the stone into small fragments. The patient receives moderate sedation and lies on a flat table with the lithotriptor aimed at the stone, which is located by fluoroscopy. A local anesthetic cream is applied to the skin site over the stone 45 minutes before the procedure. During the procedure, cardiac rhythm is monitored by ECG, and the shock waves are delivered in synchrony with the R wave. Shock waves at the rate of 60 to 120/min are applied over 30 to 45 minutes (Li et al., 2013). Continuous ECG monitoring for dysrhythmia and fluoroscopic observation for stone destruction are maintained.

After lithotripsy, strain the urine to monitor the passage of stone fragments. Bruising may occur on the flank of the affected side. Occasionally a stent is placed in the ureter before SWL to ease passage of the stone fragments.

Surgical Management. Minimally invasive surgical and open surgical procedures are used if urinary obstruction occurs or if the stone is too large to be passed.

Minimally Invasive Surgical Procedures. Minimally invasive surgical (MIS) procedures include stenting, ureteroscopy, percutaneous ureterolithotomy, and percutaneous nephrolithotomy.

Stenting is performed with a **stent**, a small tube that is placed in the ureter by ureteroscopy. The stent dilates the ureter and enlarges the passageway for the stone or stone fragments. This totally internal procedure prevents the passing stone from coming in contact with the ureteral mucosa, thereby reducing pain, bleeding, and infection risk, all of which could block the ureter. A Foley catheter may facilitate passage of the stone through the urethra.

Ureteroscopy is an endoscopic procedure. The ureteroscope is passed through the urethra and bladder into the ureter. Once the stone is seen, it is removed with grasping baskets, forceps, or loops. Lithotripsy also can be performed through the ureteroscope. A Foley catheter may be placed to facilitate passage of the stone fragments through the urethra.

Percutaneous ureterolithotomy or nephrolithotomy is the removal of a stone in the ureter or kidney through the skin. The patient lies prone or on the side and receives local or general anesthesia. The urologist or radiologist identifies the ideal entry point with fluoroscopy and passes a needle into the collecting system of the kidney. Once a tract has been made in the kidney, other equipment, such as an **intracorporeal** (inside the body) ultrasonic or laser lithotriptor, can be used to break up and remove the stone. An endoscope with a special attachment to grasp and extract the stone can be used. Often a nephrostomy tube is left in place at first to prevent the stone fragments from passing through the urinary tract.

Monitor the patient for complications after the procedure. Complications include bleeding at the site or through the tube, pneumothorax, and infection. Monitor nephrostomy tube drainage for volume and the presence of blood in the urine, which is normal for the first 24 to 48 hours after tube placement. Provide routine nephrostomy tube care, with sterile dressing changes and tube flushing (if ordered).

Open Surgical Procedures. When other stone removal attempts have failed or when risk for a lasting injury to the ureter or kidney is possible, an *open ureterolithotomy* (into the ureter), *pyelolithotomy* (into the kidney pelvis), or *nephrolithotomy* (into the kidney) procedure may be performed. These procedures are used for a large or impacted stone.

Preoperative Care. Explain to the patient how, when, and where the procedure will be performed. Describe what he or she can expect to see, hear, and feel before and after the procedure. The patient is given nothing by mouth and also receives a bowel preparation before the procedure. (See Chapter 14 for routine care before surgery.)

Operative Procedures. The retroperitoneal area is entered through a large flank incision, as for nephrectomy (see Chapter 67), pyelolithotomy, or nephrolithotomy and through a lower abdominal incision for ureterolithotomy. The urinary tract is entered surgically, and the stone is removed. Before closure, tubes and drains may be placed (e.g., nephrostomy tube, ureteral stent, Penrose or other wound drainage device, and Foley catheter).

Postoperative Care. Follow routine procedures for assessment of the patient who has received anesthesia. (See Chapter 16 for routine care after surgery.) Monitor the amount of bleeding from incisions and in the urine. Maintain adequate fluid intake. Strain the urine to monitor passage of stone fragments. Teach the patient how to prevent future stones with dietary changes, including consistent daily fluid intake to avoid dehydration and supersaturation.

❓ NCLEX EXAMINATION CHALLENGE 66-4

Safe and Effective Care Environment

A client with diabetes has all of the following changes after a percutaneous nephrolithotomy procedure. Which change is **most important** for the nurse need to immediately report to the health care provider?

A. Difficulty breathing and an oxygen saturation of 88% on 2 L of oxygen by nasal cannula

B. A point-of-care blood glucose of 150 mg/dL and client report of thirst

C. A decreased hematocrit by 1% (compared with preoperative values and hematuria

D. An oral temperature of 38° C (101° F) and cloudiness of urine draining from the nephrostomy tube right after IV administration of a broad-spectrum antibiotic

---

Preventing Infection. Infection control before invasive procedures is critical for preventing urosepsis. Interventions include giving antibiotics, either to eliminate an existing infection or to prevent new infections, and maintaining nutrition and fluid intake. Because infection always occurs with struvite stone formation, the health care team plans for long-term infection prevention.

Drug therapy involves the use of quinolones, ampicillin, or other broad-spectrum antibiotics. When urine culture and sensitivity (C&S) results are known, more specific antibiotics may be prescribed. C&S studies are often repeated 48 hours after completion of antibiotic therapy to evaluate whether urine sterility has returned.

Urine levels of antibiotics may be measured to ensure that adequate levels have been reached. If the antibiotic is not sufficiently concentrated in urine, organisms may not be completely eliminated. Evidence of a new infection (e.g., chills, fever, and altered mental status) warrants the collection of urine sample for new C&S tests.

For the patient with struvite stones, periodic and long-term monitoring of the urine for infection is needed. Urine cultures are checked monthly for as long as 1 year. Long-term use of antibiotics, while recommended, makes the development of resistant organisms more likely and antibiotic therapy less effective. Drugs that prevent bacteria from splitting urea, such as acetohydroxamic acid (Lithostat) and hydroxyurea (Hydrea), are often prescribed long term for patients with struvite stones. Serum creatinine levels are monitored in patients receiving acetohydroxamic acid, and the drug is stopped if creatinine levels are above 2 mg/dL. Review interventions aimed at preventing urinary tract infection (UTI). (See the Health Promotion discussion in the Cystitis section.)

Nutrition therapy ideally includes adequate calorie intake with a balance of all food groups. Encourage a fluid intake

sufficient to dilute urine to a light color throughout the 24-hour day (typically 2 to 3 L/day) unless another health problem requires fluid restriction.

Preventing Obstruction. Measures to prevent urinary obstruction by stones include a high intake of fluids (3 L/day or more) and accurate measures of intake and output. Fluid intake sufficient to provide diluted urine helps prevent dehydration, promotes urine flow, and decreases the chance of crystals forming a stone. Interventions also depend on the type of stone the patient has formed. Drugs, diet modification, and fluid intake are the major strategies used to prevent future stones.

Drug therapy to prevent obstruction depends on what is causing stone formation and the type of stone formed. Teach the patient the reason for the drug and assess for side effects or adverse drug reactions. Some drugs may need to be avoided because they may contribute to stone formation.

Drugs to treat *hypercalciuria* (high levels of calcium in the urine) include thiazide diuretics (e.g., chlorothiazide [Diuril] or hydrochlorothiazide [HydroDIURIL, Urozide ♣]). These drugs promote calcium reabsorption from the renal tubules back into the body, thereby reducing urine calcium loads. For patients with *hyperoxaluria* (high levels of oxalic acid in the urine), allopurinol (Zyloprim) or febuxostat (Uloric) is used.

For patients with hyperuricemia or chronic gout, both allopurinol and febuxostat help prevent the formation of urate (uric acid) stones. To alkalinize the urine, drugs such as potassium citrate, 50% sodium citrate, and sodium bicarbonate are used. Lemon or orange juice may also be ingested as a daily source of citrate. The desired urine pH is 6.0 to 6.5. Because the normal urine pH averages 5.0 to 6.0, the desired values are termed *alkaline.*

For patients with *cystinuria* (high levels of cystine in the urine), both alpha-mercaptopropionylglycine (AMPG) and captopril (Capoten) lower urine cystine levels. They are used when hydration and urine alkalization have not been successful.

Statins (i.e., drugs used to manage hypercholesterolemia) have also been found to reduce the incidence of stone recurrence in some patients (Sur et al., 2013). Usually patients with one stone are advised to increase fluid intake. With two or more stones, drug therapy is advised based on the type of stone as described previously (Fink et al., 2013).

Nutrition therapy depends on the type of stone formed (Table 66-5). Collaborate with the dietitian to plan for and teach the appropriate diet to the patient.

Other measures can help the stone pass more quickly. Urge the patient to walk as often as possible. Walking promotes passage of stones and reduces bone calcium resorption. Check the urine pH daily and strain all urine with filter paper or a special urine sieve/strainer to collect passed stones and fragments.

Self-management education includes the key points listed in Chart 66-11. Follow-up care to evaluate effects of intervention includes a 24-hour urine collection and serum chemical analysis. The patient often has great anxiety and fear that a stone and its pain may recur. In addition to anxiety about the pain, the risk for repeated surgical interventions or permanent and serious kidney damage may be present. Psychosocial preparation is enhanced when patients know what to expect and which actions to take if problems develop. Reassure the patient that preventive and health promotion activities help prevent recurrence.

TABLE 66-5 Dietary Treatment for Kidney and Urinary Stones

STONE TYPE	DIETARY INTERVENTIONS	RATIONALES
Calcium oxalate	Avoid oxalate sources, such as spinach, black tea, and rhubarb. Decrease sodium intake.	Reduction of urinary oxalate content may help prevent these stones from forming. Urinary pH is not a factor. High sodium intake reduces kidney tubular calcium reabsorption.
Calcium phosphate	Limit intake of foods high in animal protein to 5-7 servings per week and never more than 2 per day. Some patients may benefit from a reduced calcium intake (milk, other dairy products). Decrease sodium intake.	Reduction of protein intake reduces acidic urine and prevents calcium precipitation. Reduction of urine calcium concentration may prevent calcium precipitation and crystallization. High sodium intake reduces kidney tubular calcium reabsorption.
Struvite (magnesium ammonium phosphate)	Limit high-phosphate foods, such as dairy products, organ meats, and whole grains.	Reduction of urinary phosphate content may help prevent these stones from forming.
Uric acid (urate)	Decrease intake of purine sources, such as organ meats, poultry, fish, gravies, red wines, and sardines.	Reduction of urinary purine content may help prevent these stones from forming.
Cystine	Limit animal protein intake (as above). Encourage oral fluid intake (500 mL every 4 hours while awake and 750 mL at night).	Reduces urinary uric acid. Increased fluid helps dilute the urine and prevents the cystine crystals from forming.

CHART 66-11 Patient and Family Education: Preparing for Self-Management

Urinary Calculi

- Finish your entire prescription of antibiotics to ensure that you will not get a urinary tract infection.
- You may resume your usual daily activities.
- Remember to balance regular exercise with sleep and rest.
- You may return to work 2 days to 6 weeks after surgery, depending on the type of intervention, your personal tolerance, and your primary health care provider's directives.
- Depending on the type of stone you had, you may be advised to take medications or adjust your diet may to reduce the risk for further stone formation.
- Remember to drink at least 3 L of fluid a day to dilute potential stone-forming crystals, prevent dehydration, and promote urine flow.
- Monitor urine pH as directed (possibly up to three times per day).
- Expect bruising after lithotripsy. The bruising may be quite extensive and may take several weeks to resolve.
- Your urine may be bloody for several days after surgery.
- Pain in the region of the kidneys or bladder may signal the beginning of an infection or the formation of another stone. Report any pain, fever, chills, or difficulty with urination immediately to your primary health care provider or nurse.
- Keep follow-up appointments to check on infection and have repeat cultures done.

UROTHELIAL CANCER

❖ PATHOPHYSIOLOGY

Urothelial cancers are malignant tumors of the *urothelium*, which is the lining of transitional cells in the kidney, renal pelvis, ureters, urinary bladder, and urethra. Most urothelial cancers occur in the bladder, and the term *bladder cancer* describes this condition.

In North America, most urinary tract cancers are transitional cell carcinomas of the bladder (American Cancer Society [ACS], 2017; Canadian Cancer Society, 2016). The second most common site of urinary tract cancer is the kidney and renal pelvis. Urothelial cancers are usually low grade, have multiple points of origin (*multifocal*), and are recurrent. Once the cancer spreads beyond the transitional cell layer, it is highly invasive and can spread beyond the bladder. Because of the nature of

this cancer, patients may have recurrence up to 10 years after being cancer free (ACS, 2017).

Tumors confined to the bladder mucosa are treated by simple excision, whereas those that are deeper but not into the muscle layer are treated with excision plus **intravesical** (inside the bladder) chemotherapy. Cancer that has spread deeper into the bladder muscle layer is treated with more extensive surgery, often a **radical cystectomy** (removal of the bladder and surrounding tissue) with urinary diversion. Chemotherapy and radiation therapy are used in addition to surgery. If untreated, the tumor invades surrounding tissues, spreads to distant sites (liver, lung, and bone), and ultimately leads to death.

Exposure to toxins such as gasoline and diesel fuel, as well as to chemicals used in hair dyes and in the rubber, paint, electric cable, and textile industries, increases the risk for bladder cancer. The greatest risk factor for bladder cancer is tobacco use. Other risks include *Schistosoma haematobium* (a parasite) infection, excessive use of drugs containing phenacetin, and long-term use of cyclophosphamide (Cytoxan, Procytox).

In the United States and Canada, about 87,730 new cases of bladder cancer are diagnosed each year, and about 19,190 deaths occur each year from the disease (ACS, 2017; Canadian Cancer Society, 2016). This cancer is rare in adults younger than 40 years and is most common after 60 years of age.

As with many urologic conditions, sexual health is commonly affected by this diagnosis and treatment (Dunn, 2015). To manage sexual health concerns, encourage patients to discuss sexual health and ensure that the proper interprofessional care team member provides education to patients and their partners about:

- Potential implications of treatment on sexuality
- Treatment options
- Referrals to providers who specialize in sexual dysfunction

Health Promotion and Maintenance

Many adults believe that tobacco use is associated with cancers only of organs that come into direct contact with it, such as the lungs. However, many compounds in tobacco enter the bloodstream and affect other organs, such as the bladder. Therefore encourage everyone who smokes to quit and nonsmokers not to start (see the Health Promotion and Maintenance section of Chapter 27). Just as important, encourage anyone who comes in contact with dry, liquid, or gaseous chemicals to take precautions. Some adults work with chemicals, and others may come into contact with them while engaging in hobbies. Many chemicals and fumes can enter the body through contact with skin and with mucous membranes in the respiratory tract. Use of personal protective equipment, such as gloves and masks, can reduce this contact. Also encourage anyone who works with chemicals to shower or bathe and change clothing as soon as contact is completed.

❖ INTERPROFESSIONAL COLLABORATIVE CARE
◆ Assessment: Noticing

Physical Assessment/Signs and Symptoms. Ask about the patient's perception of his or her general health. Document the gender and age of the patient. Ask about active and passive exposure to cigarette smoke. To detect exposure to harmful environmental agents, ask the patient to describe his or her occupation and hobbies in detail. Also ask the patient to describe any change in the color, frequency, or volume of urine ELIMINATION and any abdominal discomfort.

Observe the patient's overall appearance, especially skin color and nutrition status. Inspect, percuss, and palpate the abdomen for asymmetry, tenderness, and bladder distention.

Examine the urine for color and clarity. Blood in the urine is often the first indication of bladder cancer. It may be gross or microscopic and is usually painless and intermittent. Dysuria, frequency, and urgency occur when infection or obstruction is also present.

Psychosocial Assessment. Assess the patient's emotions, including his or her response to a tentative diagnosis of bladder cancer, and note anxiety, fear, sadness, anger, or guilt. Early symptoms are painless, and many patients ignore the blood in the urine because it is intermittent. They also may be reluctant to seek treatment if they suspect a sexually transmitted infection (STI). As a result, they may have guilt or anger about their own delays in seeking medical attention.

Assess the patient's coping methods and available support from family members. Social support may provide motivation and improve coping during recovery from treatment.

Diagnostic Assessment. The only significant finding on a routine urinalysis is gross or microscopic hematuria. Cytologic testing on voided urine specimens usually is not helpful. Bladder-wash specimens and bladder biopsies are the most specific tests for cancer.

Cystoscopy is usually performed to evaluate painless hematuria. A biopsy of a visible bladder tumor can be performed during cystoscopy. This is essential for staging and is usually performed in an ambulatory care surgery center. Cystoureterography may be used to identify obstructions, especially where the ureter joins the bladder. CT scans show tumor invasion of surrounding tissues. Ultrasonography shows masses but is less valuable for tumor staging. MRI may help assess deep, invasive tumors.

◆ Interventions: Responding

Therapy for the patient with bladder cancer usually begins with surgical removal of the tumor for diagnosis and staging of disease. For tumors extending beyond the mucosa, surgery is followed by intravesical chemotherapy or immunotherapy. High-grade or recurrent tumors are treated with more radical surgery plus intravesical chemotherapy, radiotherapy, or both. Systemic chemotherapy is reserved for patients with distant metastases. (See Chapter 22 for general care of the patient receiving chemotherapy or radiation therapy.)

Nonsurgical Management. Prophylactic immunotherapy with intravesical instillation of bacille Calmette-Guérin (BCG), a live virus compound, is used to prevent tumor recurrence of superficial cancers. This procedure is more effective than single-agent chemotherapy. Usually the agent is instilled in an outpatient cancer clinic and allowed to dwell in the bladder for a specified length of time, usually 2 hours. When the patient urinates, live virus is excreted with the urine.

Teach patients receiving this treatment to prevent contact of the live virus with other members of the household by not sharing a toilet with others for at least 24 hours after instillation. Instruct men to urinate while sitting down to avoid splashing the urine. After 24 hours, the toilet should be completely cleaned using a solution of 10% liquid bleach. If only one toilet is available in the household, teach the patient to flush the toilet after use and follow this by adding one cup of undiluted bleach to the bowl water. The bowl is then flushed after 15 minutes, and the seat and flat surfaces of the toilet wiped with a cloth containing a solution of 10% liquid bleach. Instruct the patient to wear gloves during the cleaning and to dispose of the cloth after sealing it in a plastic bag.

Underwear or other clothing that has come in contact with the urine during the immediate 24 hours after instillation should be washed separately from other clothing in a solution of 10% liquid bleach. Sexual intercourse is avoided for 24 hours after the instillation.

Multi-agent chemotherapy is successful in prolonging life after distant metastasis has occurred but rarely results in a cure. Radiation therapy is also useful in prolonging life.

Surgical Management. The type of surgery for bladder cancer depends on the type and stage of the cancer and the patient's general health. Complete bladder removal (*cystectomy*) with additional removal of surrounding muscle and tissue offers the best chance of a cure for large, invasive bladder cancers. Four alternatives for urine ELIMINATION are used after cystectomy: ileal conduit; continent pouch; bladder reconstruction, also known as *neobladder*; and ureterosigmoidostomy.

Preoperative Care. Specific patient education depends on the type and extent of the planned surgical procedure. Coordinate education before surgery with the patient, surgeon, and enterostomal therapist (ET) or wound, ostomy, and continence nurse. Discuss the type of planned urinary diversion and the selection of a site for the stoma. Including the patient in this planning improves the chances for the patient to have a positive attitude about body image and a positive self-image. Use educational counseling to ensure understanding about self-care practices, methods of pouching, control of urine drainage, and management of odor.

The site selected for the stoma should be visible to the patient and avoid folds of skin, bones, and scar tissue. When possible, the waistline or belt area is avoided to reduce the risk for reducing TISSUE INTEGRITY. Prepare the patient for the number and type of drains that will be present after surgery. General care before surgery is discussed in Chapter 14.

Operative Procedures. Transurethral resection of the bladder tumor (TURBT) or partial cystectomy is performed for small, early, superficial tumors. In a partial (segmental) cystectomy, a portion of the bladder is removed when there is only a single isolated bladder tumor.

When the entire bladder must be removed (complete cystectomy), the ureters are diverted into a collecting reservoir. Techniques for urinary diversion are shown in Fig. 66-4. With an ileal conduit, the ureters are surgically placed in the ileum, and urine is collected in a pouch on the skin around the stoma. More often, a continent reservoir known as a "neobladder" is created from an intestinal graft to store urine and replace the surgically removed bladder. With cutaneous ureterostomy or ureteroureterostomy, the ureter opening is brought out onto the skin. The cutaneous ureterostomies may be located on either side of the abdomen or side by side.

Ureterostomies divert urine directly to the skin surface through a ureteral skin opening (stoma). After ureterostomy, the patient must wear a pouch.

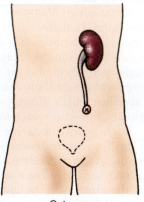

Cutaneous ureterostomy

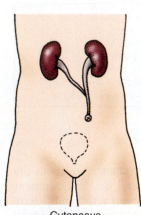

Cutaneous ureteroureterostomy

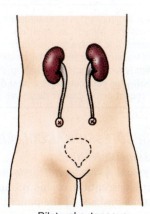

Bilateral cutaneous ureterostomy

Conduits collect urine in a portion of the intestine, which is then opened onto the skin surface as a stoma. After the creation of a conduit, the patient must wear a pouch.

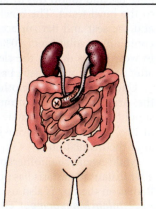

Ileal (Bricker's) conduit

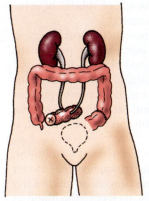

Colon conduit

Ileal reservoirs divert urine into a surgically created pouch, or pocket, that functions as a bladder. The stoma is continent, and the patient removes urine by regular self-catheterization.

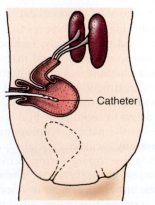

Catheter

Continent internal ileal reservoir (Kock's pouch)

Sigmoidostomies divert urine to the large intestine, so no stoma is required. The patient excretes urine with bowel movements, and bowel incontinence may result.

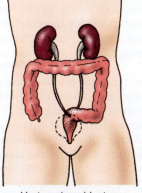

Ureterosigmoidostomy

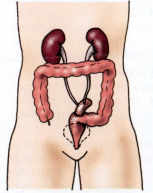

Ureteroiliosigmoidostomy

FIG. 66-4 Urinary diversion procedures used in the treatment of bladder cancer.

Postoperative Care. After cutaneous ureterostomy, an external pouch covers the ostomy to collect urine and maintain TISSUE INTEGRITY. Work with the ET to focus care on the wound, the skin, and urinary drainage. (See Chapter 56 for ostomy care.)

The patient with a Kock's pouch, a continent reservoir, may have a Penrose drain and a plastic Medena catheter in the stoma. The drain removes lymphatic fluid or other secretions; the catheter ensures urine drainage so incisions can heal. The patient with a neobladder usually requires 2 to 4 days in the ICU and will have a drain at first in the event the neobladder requires irrigation. Later, irrigation can be performed with intermittent catheterization. Irrigation is performed to ensure patency. There is no sensation of bladder fullness with a neobladder because sensory nerves are not attached. As a result, the patient will need to learn new cues to void, such as prescribed times or noticing a feeling of neobladder pressure. General care after surgery is discussed in Chapter 16.

Different types of drains and nephrostomy catheters are used, sometimes on a temporary basis, to drain urine from the kidney. Some are totally internal, with no drainage to the outside. Others may drain exclusively to the outside, and urine is collected in a pouch or bag. For this type of drainage system, urine output remains constant. Decreased or no drainage is cause for concern and must be reported to the surgeon or nephrologist, as is leakage around the catheter. Some nephrostomy tubes are connected both to the new bladder (internal drainage) and to an external drainage system. With this type of system, urine output from the external portion of the catheter varies. With any drainage system, intervention is needed if the external catheter is partially or completely pulled out accidentally. Immediately notify the surgeon or nephrologist. If the catheter remains partially in place, secure it from further movement. This action may result in a reinsertion process rather than a total replacement.

Care Coordination and Transition Management

Self-Management Education. Teach the patient and family about drugs, diet and fluid therapy, the use of external pouching systems, and the technique for catheterizing a continent reservoir.

With some procedures, the patient may need electrolyte replacement to prevent long-term deficits. Teach him or her to avoid foods that are known to produce gas if the urinary diversion uses the intestinal tract. When intestinal production of gas is excessive, flatus can induce incontinence.

Patients who have a neobladder created often have extreme weight loss during the first few weeks after surgery. Collaborate with a dietitian to develop a diet plan specific to the patient to meet his or her caloric needs.

Help the patient prepare for the impact of urinary diversion on self-image, body image, sexual functioning, and self-esteem. Counseling provides information and support to reduce feelings of powerlessness.

Through discussions with the patient about common social situations, help him or her gain control over new toileting practices. Men with a urinary diversion into the sigmoid colon need to learn the habit of sitting to urinate. For patients of either gender, promote confidence in social situations by encouraging frequent emptying of urinary collection devices before traveling or attending social functions. Resumption of sexual activity is a major concern for many, regardless of

age. Address this topic openly and with sensitivity. Cystectomy causes impotence in men, but treatment is available (see Chapter 72).

Health Care Resources. The United Ostomy Association and the ACS have educational materials that may be useful to patients. Refer patients and family members to local chapters or units of these organizations. In some areas, local support groups have meetings to help others and to send visitors to provide peer counseling and support. Home care personnel may help with follow-up, easing the transition from hospital to home. The Wound, Ostomy, and Continence Nurses Society has educational programs and a journal for the care of patients with ostomies.

BLADDER TRAUMA

❖ PATHOPHYSIOLOGY

Bladder trauma can be caused by penetrating or blunt injury to the lower abdomen. Penetrating injury may occur by stabbing, gunshot wound, or other trauma in which objects pierce the abdominal wall. A fractured pelvis with puncture of the bladder by bone fragments is the most common cause of bladder trauma. It also may result from sexual assault.

Blunt trauma compresses the abdominal wall and the bladder. A seat belt may compress the bladder hard enough to cause injury, especially when the bladder is full or distended.

❖ INTERPROFESSIONAL COLLABORATIVE CARE

Patients with a penetrating bladder wound often have anuria or hematuria. In the emergency department, initial assessment includes inspection of the urinary meatus for blood.

Bladder trauma, other than a simple contusion, requires surgical intervention. When bone fractures are present, they are stabilized before bladder repair to prevent further bladder damage. Surgical interventions include repairing the bladder wall and peritoneal membrane. Usually repairs of the bladder are procedures to close the abnormal opening(s) caused by the trauma.

Patients with an anterior bladder wall injury usually have a Penrose drain and a Foley catheter in place after surgery. Those with a posterior bladder wall injury have a Penrose drain and Foley or suprapubic catheter after surgery. In some instances, vaginal or rectal fistulas may also require repair.

Psychosocial support is critical for patients who have sustained traumatic injuries. Refer them to counseling resources to help them deal with psychosocial issues.

GET READY FOR THE NCLEX® EXAMINATION!

KEY POINTS

Review these Key Points for each NCLEX Examination Client Needs Category.

Safe and Effective Care Environment

- Use sterile technique when inserting a catheter or any other instrument into the urinary system. **QSEN: Safety**
- Use Contact Precautions with any drainage from the genitourinary tract. **QSEN: Safety**
- Assess daily to determine whether there is an ongoing need for an indwelling catheter. **QSEN: Evidence-Based Practice**
- Teach patients and families of patients with urge or stress incontinence to keep pathways to the bathroom well lighted and clear of obstacles to help prevent falls. **QSEN: Safety**

Health Promotion and Maintenance

- Teach patients to clean the perineal area daily, after voiding, after having a bowel movement, and after sexual intercourse. **QSEN: Patient-Centered Care**
- Encourage all patients to maintain an adequate fluid intake. **QSEN: Evidence-Based Practice**
- Teach women who have stress incontinence the proper way to perform pelvic floor–strengthening exercises. **QSEN: Patient-Centered Care**
- Urge adults who smoke to stop smoking. **QSEN: Evidence-Based Practice**
- Teach patients who come into contact with chemicals in their workplaces or with leisure-time activities to avoid direct skin and mucous membrane contact with these chemicals. **QSEN: Safety**

Psychosocial Integrity

- Allow the patient the opportunity to express feelings or concerns regarding a potential chronic urinary tract disorder or a cancer diagnosis. **QSEN: Patient-Centered Care**

- Use a nonjudgmental approach in caring for patients with urinary incontinence. **QSEN: Patient-Centered Care**
- Avoid referring to protective pads, briefs, or pants as "diapers." **QSEN: Patient-Centered Care**
- Recognize the need for the patient undergoing cystectomy and urinary diversion to grieve about the body image change. **QSEN: Patient-Centered Care**
- Assess the patient's level of COMFORT in discussing issues related to ELIMINATION and the urogenital area. **QSEN: Patient-Centered Care**
- Use language and terminology during kidney/urinary assessment that the patient is comfortable using. **QSEN: Patient-Centered Care**
- Refer patients to community resources and support groups. **QSEN: Patient-Centered Care**

Physiological Integrity

- Identify hospitalized patients at risk for bacteriuria and urosepsis. **QSEN: Evidence-Based Practice**.
- Report immediately any condition that obstructs urine flow. **QSEN: Safety**
- Instruct patients with UTI to complete all prescribed antibiotic therapy even when symptoms of infection are absent. **QSEN: Patient-Centered Care**
- Evaluate daily the indications for maintaining urinary catheters and discontinue their use as soon as possible. **QSEN: Evidence-Based Practice**
- Teach patients the expected side effects and any adverse reactions to prescribed drugs. **QSEN: Patient-Centered Care**
- Assess the patient's manual dexterity and cognitive awareness before teaching a regimen of intermittent self-catheterization. **QSEN: Patient-Centered Care**

SELECTED BIBLIOGRAPHY

Asterisk indicates a classic or definitive work on this subject.

Agency for Healthcare Research and Quality (AHRQ) (2012-reviewed for currency 2013). Non-surgical treatments for urinary incontinence in adult women: Diagnosis and comparative effectiveness. In *AHRQ Comparative Effectiveness Reviews*. Rockville, MD: Author. http://effectivehealthcare.ahrq.gov/index.cfm/search-for-guides-reviews-and-reports/?productid=1021&pageaction=displayproduct.

Allan, G. M., & Nicolle, L. (2013). Cranberry for preventing urinary tract infection. *Canadian Family Physician, 59*(4), 367.

American Cancer Society (ACS) (2017). *Cancer facts and figures 2017.* Report No. 01-300M—No. 500817. Atlanta: Author.

American Nurses Association (ANA) (2015), *Streamlined evidence-based RN tool: Catheter associated urinary tract infection (CAUTI) prevention*. http://nursingworld.org/ANA-CAUTI-Prevention-Tool.

Bates, F., & Porter, G. (2014). Inspiring confidence to overcome incontinence. *Canadian Nurse, 110*(7), 18–20.

Belizario, S. (2015). Preventing urinary tract infections with a two-person catheter insertion procedure. *Nursing, 45*(3), 67–69.

Bickhaus, J., Drobnis, E., Critchlow, W., Occhino, J., & Foster, R. (2015). The feasibility of clean intermittent self-catheterization teaching in an outpatient setting. *Female Pelvic Medicine and Reconstructive Surgery, 21*(4), 220–224.

Burchum, J., & Rosenthal, L. (2016). *Lehne's pharmacology for nursing care* (9th ed.). St. Louis: Elsevier.

Canadian Cancer Society, Statistics Canada (2016). *Canadian Cancer Statistics, 2016.* Toronto: Canadian Cancer Society.

Centers for Disease Control and Prevention (CDC). (2016a). *2015 Sexually transmitted disease treatment guidelines.* www.cdc.gov/std/tg2015.

Centers for Disease Control and Prevention (CDC). (2016b). *Urinary tract infection (catheter-associated urinary tract infection [CAUTI] and non–catheter-associated urinary tract infection [UTI]) and other urinary system infection (USI) events.* http://www.cdc.gov/nhsn/PDFs/pscManual/7pscCAUTIcurrent.pdf.

Cerruto, M., D'Elia, C., Balzarro, M., Porcaro, A., Sarti, A., & Artibani, W. (2015). Advances in female urology: A review of the 2013 literature. *Urologic Nursing, 35*(1), 32–38.

Conway, L., Carter, E., & Larson, E. (2015). Risk factors for nosocomial bacteremia secondary to urinary catheter-associated bacteriuria: A systematic review. *Urologic Nursing, 35*(4), 191–203.

Conway, L., Liu, J., Harris, A., & Larson, E. (2017). Risk factors for bacteremia in patients with urinary catheter-associated bacteriuria. *American Journal of Critical Care, 26*(1), 43–52.

Corley, L. (2015). CAUTI awakenings. *Nursing, 45*(1), 20–21.

Dunn, M. W. (2015). Bladder cancer: A focus on sexuality. *Clinical Journal of Oncology Nursing, 19*(1), 68–73.

Duralde, E., Walter, L., Van Den Eeden, S., Nakagawa, S., Subak, L., Brown, J., et al. (2016). Bridging the gap: Determinants of undiagnosed or untreated urinary incontinence in women. *American Journal of Obstetrics and Gynecology, 214*(2), 266.e1–266.e9.

Felicilda-Reynaldo, R., & Backes, K. (2014). Botox for overactive bladders: A look at the current state of the evidence. *Medsurg Nursing, 23*(1), 30–34.

Fink, H., Wilt, T., Eidman, K., Garimella, P., MacDonald, R., Rutks, I., et al. (2013). Medical management to prevent recurrent nephrolithiasis in adults: A systematic review for an American College of Physicians Clinical Guideline. *Annals of Internal Medicine, 158*(7), 535–543.

Fletcher, R. H. (2013). The risk of taking ascorbic acid. *JAMA Internal Medicine, 173*(5), 375–394.

Foxman, B., Cronenwett, A. E., Spino, C., Berger, M. B., & Morgan, D. M. (2015). Cranberry juice capsules and urinary tract infection after surgery: Results of a randomized trial. *American Journal of Obstetrics and Gynecology, 213*(2), 194 e191–194 e198.

Gorina, Y., Schappert, S., Bercovitz, A., Elgaddal, N., & Kramarow, E. (2014). Prevalence of incontinence among older Americans. *Vital and Health Statistics. Series 3, Analytical Studies, 36*, 1–33.

Gray, M., McNichol, L., & Nix, D. (2016). Incontinence-associated dermatitis: Progress, promises, and ongoing challenges. *Journal of Wound, Ostomy, and Continence Nursing, 43*(2), 188–192.

Hopkins, L., McCroskey, D., Reeves, G., & Tanabe, P. (2014). Implementing a urinary tract infection clinical practice guideline in an ambulatory urgent care practice. *The Nurse Practitioner, 39*(4), 50–54.

Infectious Disease Society of America (2013). *Guidelines for antimicrobial treatment of acute uncomplicated cystitis and pyelonephritis in women.* http://www.idsociety.org/Organ_System/#Genitourinary.

Li, K., Lin, T., Zhang, C., Fan, X., Xu, K., Bi, L., et al. (2013). Optimal frequency of shock wave lithotripsy in urolithiasis treatment: A systematic review and meta-analysis of randomized controlled trials. *Journal of Urology, 190*(4), 1260–1267.

Mandimika, C., Murk, W., McPencow, A., Lake, A., Miller, D., Connell, K., et al. (2015). Racial disparities in knowledge of pelvic floor disorders among community-dwelling women. *Female Pelvic Medicine and Reconstructive Surgery, 21*(5), 287–292.

Martin, E., Sheaves, C., & Childers, K. (2015). Underlying mechanisms and optimal treatment for interstitial cystitis: A brief overview. *Urological Nursing, 35*(3), 111–116.

McCance, K., Huether, S., Brashers, V., & Rote, N. (2014). *Pathophysiology: The biologic basis for disease in adults and children* (7th ed.). St. Louis: Mosby.

McGoldrick, M. (2016). Frequency for changing long-term indwelling urinary catheters. *Home Healthcare, Now, 34*(2), 105–106.

Nelson, J., & Good, E. (2015). Urinary tract infections and asymptomatic bacteremia in older adults. *The Nurse Practitioner, 40*(8), 43–48.

Nicolle, L. (2016). Urinary tract infections in adults. In K. Skorecki, G. Chertow, P. Marsden, M. Taal, & A. Yu (Eds.), *Brenner and Rector's the kidney* (10th ed.). Philadelphia: Elsevier.

Olson-Sitki, K., Kirkbride, G., & Forbes, G. (2015). Evaluation of a nurse-driven protocol to remove urinary catheters: Nurses' perceptions. *Urologic Nursing, 35*(2), 94–99.

Online Mendelian Inheritance in Man (OMIM). (2016). *Nephrolithiasis, Calcium oxalate; CAON.* www.omim.org/entry/167030.

Panchisin, T. (2016). Improving outcomes with the ANA CAUTI prevention tool. *Nursing, 46*(3), 55–59.

Pelvic Pain and Urinary Urgency/Frequency (PUF) Patient Symptom Scale. (2011). http://www.obgyn.net/urogynecology/pelvic-pain-and-urinary-urgency-frequency-puf-patient-symptom-scale#sthash.flECux6S.dpuf.

Prieto, J., Murphy, C., Moore, K., & Fader, M. (2015). Intermittent catheterization for long-term bladder management. *Neurology and Urodynamics Journal, 34*(7), 648–653.

Qaseem, A., Dallas, P., Forciea, M., Starkey, M., Denberg, T., Shekelle, P., et al. (2014). Nonsurgical management of urinary incontinence in women: A clinical practice guideline from the American College of Physicians. *Annals of Internal Medicine, 161*(6), 429–440.

Rodgers, A. L. (2013). Race, ethnicity and urolithiasis: A critical review. *Urolithiasis, 41*(2), 99–103.

Skorecki, K., Chertow, G., Marsden, P., Taal, M., & Yu, A. (Eds.), (2016). *Brenner & Rector's the kidney* (10th ed.). Philadelphia: Saunders.

Sur, R., Masterson, J., Palazzi, K., L'Esperance, J., Auge, B., Chang, D., et al. (2013). Impact of statins on nephrolithiasis in hyperlipidemic patients: A 10-year review of an equal access health care system. *Clinical Nephrology, 79*(5), 351–355.

Testa, A. (2015). Understanding adult urinary incontinence. *Urologic Nursing, 35*(2), 82–86.

Touhy, T., & Jett, K. (2016). *Ebersole & Hess' toward healthy aging: Human needs & nursing response.* St. Louis: Elsevier.

U.S. Renal Data Systems. (2015). *2015 USRDS Annual Data Report. Epidemiology of Kidney Disease in the United States.* National Institutes of Health, National Institute of Diabetes and Digestive and Kidney Diseases, Bethesda, MD, http://www.usrds.org/adr.aspx.

Wagenlehner, F., Lichtenstern, C., Rolfes, C., Mayer, K., Uhle, F., Weidner, W., et al. (2013). Diagnosis and management for urosepsis. *International Journal of Urology, 20*(10), 963–970.

Wilde, M., Bliss, D., Booth, J., Cheater, F., & Tannenbaum, C. (2014). Self-management of urinary and fecal incontinence. *American Journal of Nursing, 114*(1), 38–45.

Wilde, M., Fairbanks, E., Parshall, R., Zhang, F., Miner, S., Thayer, D., et al. (2015). A web-based self-management intervention for intermittent catheter users. *Urologic Nursing, 35*(3), 127–133.

Care of Patients With Kidney Disorders

Chris Winkelman

 http://evolve.elsevier.com/Iggy/

PRIORITY CONCEPTS AND INTERRELATED CONCEPTS

The priority concept in this chapter is ELIMINATION.

✳ The ELIMINATION concept exemplar for this chapter is Pyelonephritis, below.

The interrelated concepts for this chapter are:
- FLUID AND ELECTROLYTE BALANCE
- ACID-BASE BALANCE
- IMMUNITY
- CELLULAR REGULATION

LEARNING OUTCOMES

Safe and Effective Care Environment

1. Collaborate with the interprofessional team to coordinate high-quality care and promote urinary ELIMINATION in patients who have kidney disorders.
2. Teach the patient and caregiver(s) about home safety issues affected by impaired ELIMINATION and impairment of FLUID AND ELECTROLYTE BALANCE or ACID-BASE BALANCE resulting from kidney problems.
3. Prioritize evidence-based care for patients with kidney disorders that impair urinary ELIMINATION.

Health Promotion and Maintenance

4. Identify community resources for patients requiring assistance with any acute or chronic kidney problem.
5. Teach adults how to decrease the risk for kidney damage or kidney disease.

Psychosocial Integrity

6. Implement nursing interventions to help the patient and family cope with the psychosocial impact caused by acute or chronic kidney disorders.

Physiological Integrity

7. Apply knowledge of anatomy, physiology, pathophysiology, and genetics to assess patients with impaired kidney function affecting ELIMINATION, FLUID AND ELECTROLYTE BALANCE, or ACID-BASE BALANCE.
8. Teach the patient and caregiver(s) about common drugs and other management strategies used for kidney disease, including pain control.
9. Implement evidence-based nursing interventions to prevent complications of kidney disorders and their therapies.

Healthy kidneys are the major controllers of urinary ELIMINATION. They perform this function by filtering wastes from the blood and selectively determining which substances remain in the body and which are eliminated. Thus the kidneys maintain homeostasis by contributing to FLUID AND ELECTROLYTE BALANCE and ACID-BASE BALANCE. Any problem that disrupts kidney function has the potential to impair general homeostasis and all aspects of urinary elimination (Fig. 67-1). Interaction with other organs and systems is necessary for the kidneys to function effectively. In addition, when the kidneys are impaired, the buildup of toxic wastes affects all other body systems and can lead to life-threatening outcomes. This chapter describes a variety of infectious and noninfectious kidney disorders, kidney tumors, and kidney trauma. Acute kidney injury (AKI) and chronic kidney disease (CKD) are discussed in Chapter 68.

✳ ELIMINATION CONCEPT EXEMPLAR
Pyelonephritis

In the healthy adult, urine is normally sterile. Urinary tract infection (UTI) is an infection in any part of this normally sterile system. **Pyelonephritis** is a bacterial infection in the kidney and renal pelvis (McCance et al., 2014). It can be acute or chronic. Pyelonephritis interferes with urinary ELIMINATION, which is the excretion of waste from the body by the urinary system (as urine). Chapter 2 provides a summary of the concept of elimination in more detail.

❖ PATHOPHYSIOLOGY

Acute pyelonephritis is an active bacterial infection, whereas **chronic pyelonephritis** results from repeated or continued

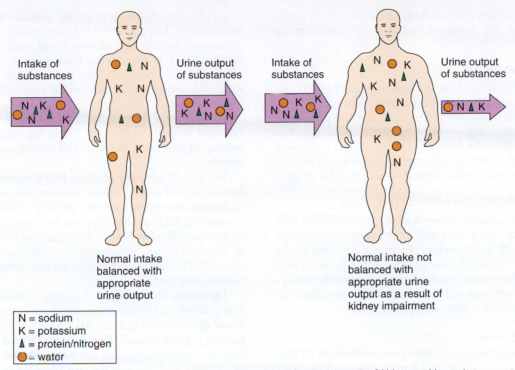

Intake of substances → Urine output of substances

Intake of substances → Urine output of substances

Normal intake balanced with appropriate urine output

Normal intake not balanced with appropriate urine output as a result of kidney impairment

N = sodium
K = potassium
▲ = protein/nitrogen
● = water

FIG. 67-1 Unbalanced body water, electrolytes, and waste products as a result of kidney problems that prevent adjustments in urinary elimination.

upper urinary tract infections that occur almost exclusively in patients who have anatomic abnormalities of the urinary tract. Bacterial infection causes local (e.g., kidney) and systemic (e.g., fever, aches, and malaise) inflammatory symptoms.

In pyelonephritis, organisms usually move up from the urinary tract into the kidney tissue. This is more likely to occur when urine refluxes from the bladder into the ureters and then to the kidney. **Reflux** is the reverse or upward flow of urine toward the renal pelvis and kidney. Infection also can be transmitted by organisms in the blood, but this cause of pyelonephritis is rare unless the patient has impaired IMMUNITY.

Acute pyelonephritis involves IMMUNITY responses leading to acute tissue inflammation, local edema, tubular cell necrosis, and possible abscess formation. **Abscesses**, which are pockets of infection, can occur anywhere in the kidney. The infection is scattered within the kidney; healthy tissues can lie next to infected areas. Fibrosis and scar tissue develop from chronic inflammation in the kidney glomerular and tubular structures. As a result, filtration, reabsorption, and secretion are impaired; and kidney function is reduced (Fig. 67-2).

Etiology and Genetic Risk

Single episodes of *acute pyelonephritis* result from bacterial infection, with or without obstruction or reflux. *Chronic pyelonephritis* usually occurs with structural deformities, urinary stasis, obstruction, or reflux. Conditions that lead to urinary stasis include prolonged bedrest and paralysis. Obstruction can be caused by stones, kidney cancer, scarring from pelvic radiation or surgery, recurrent infection, or injury. Reflux may occur from scarring or result from anatomic anomalies. Reflux also results from bladder tumors, prostate enlargement, or urinary stones. Reduced bladder tone from diabetic neuropathy, spinal cord injury, and neurodegenerative diseases (e.g., spina bifida, multiple sclerosis) contributes to stasis and reflux.

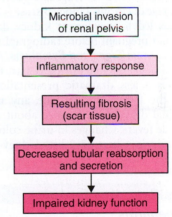

Microbial invasion of renal pelvis

↓

Inflammatory response

↓

Resulting fibrosis (scar tissue)

↓

Decreased tubular reabsorption and secretion

↓

Impaired kidney function

FIG. 67-2 Pathophysiology of pyelonephritis.

Pyelonephritis from an ascending infection may follow manipulation of the urinary tract (e.g., placement of a urinary catheter), particularly in patients who have reduced IMMUNITY or diabetes. In patients with chronic kidney stone disease, stones may retain organisms, resulting in ongoing infection and kidney scarring. Drugs, such as high-dose or prolonged use of NSAIDs, can lead to papillary necrosis and reflux.

The most common pyelonephritis-causing infecting organism among community-dwelling adults is *Escherichia coli*. *Enterococcus faecalis* is common in hospitalized patients. Both organisms are in the intestinal tract. Other organisms that cause pyelonephritis in hospitalized patients include *Proteus mirabilis*, *Klebsiella* species, and *Pseudomonas aeruginosa*. When the infection is bloodborne, common organisms include *Staphylococcus aureus* and the *Candida* and *Salmonella* species.

Other causes of kidney scarring contributing to increased risk for pyelonephritis are inflammatory responses resulting from IMMUNITY excesses with antibody reactions, cell-mediated immunity against the bacterial antigens, or autoimmune reactions.

Incidence and Prevalence

Acute pyelonephritis is most common in women 20 to 30 years of age (Nicolle, 2016). Because chronic pyelonephritis is rarely characterized by infection alone, the incidence and prevalence is linked to the underlying condition or conditions that lead to relapsing inflammatory damage of the kidney. These conditions include congenital structural abnormality, neurogenic bladder dysfunction, or primary vesicoureteral reflux (Nicolle, 2016).

❖ INTERPROFESSIONAL COLLABORATIVE CARE

Depending on the severity of the disease, pyelonephritis may be managed in any care setting and in the community. About 20% of women with acute pyelonephritis are admitted to the hospital (Nicolle, 2016). The focus of care for patients with chronic pyelonephritis requires continuing attention to managing the structural or functional abnormality that contributes to recurrent infection and inflammatory fibrosis.

◆ Assessment: Noticing

History. Ask about recurrent urinary tract infections (UTIs), diabetes mellitus, stone disease, and known defects of the genitourinary tract. Ask about disease or treatment that results in reduced IMMUNITY, which also increases risk for pyelonephritis. Ask about kidney function; knowledgeable patients may be able to describe their stage of chronic kidney disease (CKD) if chronic pyelonephritis has led to permanent kidney damage. Ensure that a woman is not pregnant before radiographic imaging.

Physical Assessment/Signs and Symptoms. Ask about specific symptoms of acute pyelonephritis (Chart 67-1). Chronic pyelonephritis has a less dramatic presentation but similar symptoms. Ask the patient to describe any urinary symptoms or abdominal discomfort. Inquire about any history of repeated low-grade fevers. Changes in urine color or odor may accompany bacteriuria. Chart 67-2 lists kidney-related effects of chronic pyelonephritis.

➤➤ CHART 67-1 Key Features

Acute Pyelonephritis

- Fever
- Chills
- Tachycardia and tachypnea
- Flank, back, or loin pain
- Tenderness at the costovertebral angle (CVA)
- Abdominal, often colicky, discomfort
- Nausea and vomiting
- General malaise or fatigue
- Burning, urgency, or frequency of urination
- Nocturia
- Recent cystitis or treatment for urinary tract infection (UTI)

➤➤ CHART 67-2 Key Features

Chronic Pyelonephritis

- Hypertension
- Inability to conserve sodium
- Decreased urine-concentrating ability, resulting in nocturia
- Tendency to develop hyperkalemia and acidosis

Inspect the flanks and gently palpate the costovertebral angle (CVA). Inspect both CVAs for enlargement, asymmetry, edema, or redness, all of which can indicate inflammation (Jarvis, 2016). If there is no tenderness to light palpation in either CVA, a primary health care provider firmly percusses each area. Tenderness or discomfort may indicate infection or inflammation.

Psychosocial Assessment. Any infection in an older adult can lead to acute confusion. Assess the older adult who has new-onset confusion for signs and symptoms of urinary/renal infection.

The patient with any problem in the genitourinary area may have feelings of anxiety, embarrassment, or guilt. Listen for signs of anxiety or specific fears and prevent embarrassment during assessment. Feelings of guilt, often associated with sexual habits or practices, may be masked through delay in seeking treatment or through vague, nonspecific responses to specific or direct questions. Encourage patients to tell their own story in familiar, comfortable language.

Laboratory Assessment. Urinalysis shows a positive leukocyte esterase and nitrite dipstick test and the presence of white blood cells (WBCs) and bacteria. Occasional red blood cells and protein may be present. The urine is cultured to determine the specific organisms causing the infection and the susceptibility or resistance of the specific organism to various antibiotics. The urine sample for culture and sensitivity testing is usually obtained by the clean-catch method. In patients with recurrent pyelonephritis, more specific testing of bacterial antigens and antibodies may help determine whether the same organism is responsible for the recurrent infections.

Blood cultures may be obtained to determine the source and spread of infectious organisms. Other blood tests include the WBC count and differential of the complete blood count, as well as C-reactive protein and erythrocyte sedimentation (ESR) rate to determine IMMUNITY responses and presence of inflammation. Serum tests of kidney function, such as blood urea nitrogen (BUN) and creatinine, are used as baseline and to trend recovery or deterioration. Estimate of glomerular filtration rate (GFR) also is used to trend kidney function.

Imaging Assessment. An x-ray of the kidneys, ureters, and bladder (KUB) or CT is performed to visualize anatomy, inflammation, fluid accumulation, abscess formation, and defects in kidneys and the urinary tract. These tests also identify stones, kidney tumors or cysts, or prostate enlargement. Urine reflux caused by incompetent bladder-ureter valve closure can be seen with a cystourethrogram. (See Chapter 65 for more information on imaging assessment.)

Other Diagnostic Assessment. Other diagnostic tests include examining antibody-coated bacteria in urine, testing for certain enzymes (e.g., lactate dehydrogenase isoenzyme 5), and radionuclide renal scan. Examining urine for antibody-coated bacteria helps identify patients who may need long-term antibiotic therapy. High-molecular-weight enzymes in urine, such as lactate dehydrogenase isoenzyme 5, are present with any kidney tissue deterioration problem and give trend data. The renal scan can identify active pyelonephritis or abscesses in or around the kidney. A kidney biopsy may be performed to rule out less obvious causes of inflammation.

◆ Analysis: Interpreting

The priority collaborative problems for the patient with pyelonephritis are:

1. Pain (flank and abdominal) due to inflammation and infection
2. Potential for chronic kidney disease (CKD) disease due to kidney tissue destruction

◆ Planning and Implementation: Responding

Managing Pain

Planning: Expected Outcomes. With proper intervention, the patient with pyelonephritis is expected to achieve an acceptable state of comfort. Indicators include that he or she often or consistently demonstrates these behaviors:

- Uses pharmacologic relief measures
- Uses NSAIDs appropriately
- Uses best practices for catheter replacement when chronic catheter use is indicated
- Reports pain controlled

Interventions. Interventions may be nonsurgical or surgical. Interventional radiologic techniques may be used to relieve obstruction or repair a stricture of the urinary tract.

Nonsurgical Management. Interventions include the use of drug therapy, nutrition and fluid therapy, and teaching to ensure the patient's understanding of the treatment.

Drug therapy can reduce pain. Acetaminophen is preferred over NSAIDs because it does not interfere with kidney autoregulation of blood flow. Reduction of fever will also reduce pain. Some patients may require the use of opioids in the short term for pain control.

Drug therapy with antibiotics is prescribed to treat the infection. At first the antibiotics are broad spectrum. After urine and blood culture and sensitivity results are known, more specific antibiotics may be prescribed. Antibiotics are given (usually IV in hospitalized patients; orally in community-dwelling patients) to achieve adequate blood levels or sterile blood culture results. A prophylactic antibiotic is not recommended for patients with impaired voiding or chronic catheter use because it does not limit recurrence or severity, of UTI (Nicolle, 2016).

Catheter replacement is supportive for a patient requiring a urinary catheter for 2 or more weeks (e.g., for neurogenic bladder or wound healing). This involves removal and replacement of the catheter and closed drainage system before starting antibiotic therapy. This intervention reduces bioburden by removing a device with a biofilm of concentrated organisms.

Nutrition therapy involves ensuring that the patient's nutrition intake has adequate calories from all food groups for healing to occur. A registered dietitian should be part of the interprofessional team. Fluid intake is recommended at 2 L/day, sufficient to result in dilute (pale yellow) urine, unless another health problem requires fluid restriction.

Surgical Management. Surgical interventions can correct structural problems causing urine reflux or obstruction of urine outflow or can remove the source of infection. Teach the patient the nature and purpose of the proposed surgery, the expected outcome, and how he or she can participate.

The surgical procedures may be one of these: **pyelolithotomy** (stone removal from the kidney), **nephrectomy** (removal of the kidney), ureteral diversion, or reimplantation of ureter(s) to restore proper bladder drainage.

A pyelolithotomy is needed for removal of a large stone in the kidney pelvis that blocks urine flow and causes infection. Nephrectomy is a last resort when all other measures to clear the infection have failed. For patients with poor ureter valve closure or dilated ureters, **ureteroplasty** (ureter repair or revision) or ureteral reimplantation (through another site in the bladder wall) preserves kidney function and eliminates infections.

Preventing Chronic Kidney Disease

Planning: Expected Outcomes. The patient is expected to conserve existing kidney function. Underlying genitourinary abnormalities must be identified, and appropriate interventions taken to manage a current infection and the risk for subsequent infections. The approach by the urologist or nephrologist depends on signs and symptoms as well as on patient history. Indicators include that he or she consistently demonstrates these behaviors:

- Describes the role of antibiotics and self-administration of drugs
- Explains and uses techniques to ensure adequate nutrition and hydration
- Describes the plan for post-treatment follow-up, including knowledge of recurrent symptoms
- Modifies prescribed regimen as directed by a health care professional

Interventions. Specific antibiotics are prescribed to treat the infection. Stress the importance of completing the drug therapy as directed. Discuss with the patient and family the importance of regular follow-up examinations and completing the recommended diagnostic tests.

Blood pressure control slows the progression of kidney dysfunction. Ensure that the patient is able to detect adverse changes in blood pressure using community resources such as free blood pressure readings at community settings or retail pharmacies. When pyelonephritis causes or worsens CKD, ensure a referral to a nephrologist for additional assessment and management (see CKD in Chapter 68). Encourage the patient to drink sufficient fluid during waking hours to prevent dehydration because dehydration could further reduce kidney function. When dietary protein is restricted, a registered dietitian can help the family select appropriate food and proportions. Collaborate with the dietitian and reinforce the prescribed interventions.

Care Coordination and Transition Management

Pyelonephritis may cause fear and anxiety in the patient and family. The severity of the acute process and its potential to develop into a chronic process are frightening. The patient and the family need reassurance that treatment and preventive measures can be successful.

Home Care Management. If no surgery is performed, the patient may need help with self-care, nutrition, and drug management at home. If surgery is performed, he or she may need help with incision care, self-care, and transportation for follow-up appointments.

Self-Management Education. After assessing the patient's and family's understanding of pyelonephritis and its therapy, explain:

- Drug regimen (purpose, timing, frequency, duration, and possible side effects)
- The role of nutrition and adequate fluid intake
- Best practices for chronic urinary catheter care, if needed
- The need for a balance between rest and activity, including any limitations after surgery
- The signs and symptoms of disease recurrence
- The use of previously successful coping mechanisms and community resources

Advise the patient to complete all prescribed antibiotic regimens and to report any side effects or unusual symptoms to the primary health care provider rather than stopping the drugs. Ensure that interprofessional care includes nutrition counseling, because many patients have special nutrition requirements, such as those for diabetes or pregnancy.

Health Care Resources. The patient may also briefly need a home health care nurse to help with drug or nutrition therapy at home. Housekeeping services may be helpful while he or she is regaining strength.

◆ *Evaluation: Reflecting*

Evaluate the care of the patient with pyelonephritis based on the identified priority patient problems. Expected outcomes may include that the patient will:

- Report that pain is controlled
- Be knowledgeable about the disease, its treatment, and interventions to prevent or reduce CKD progression

ACUTE GLOMERULONEPHRITIS

❖ *PATHOPHYSIOLOGY*

Glomerulonephritis is categorized into conditions that primarily involve the kidney (primary glomerular nephritis) and those in which kidney involvement is only part of a systemic disorder (secondary glomerulonephritis). It is a group of diseases that injure and inflame the glomerulus, the part of the kidney that filters blood. Inflamed glomeruli allow passage of protein and blood in the urine. Glomerulonephritis is associated with high blood pressure, progressive kidney damage (leading to CKD), and edema. Anemia from reduced production of erythropoietin and high cholesterol often co-occur. Glomerulonephritis can cause altered urinary ELIMINATION.

Acute glomerulonephritis (GN) develops suddenly from an excess IMMUNITY response within the kidney tissues. Usually an infection is noticed before kidney symptoms of acute GN are present. The onset of symptoms is about 10 days from the time of infection. Usually patients recover quickly and completely from acute GN.

Many causes of primary GN are infectious (Table 67-1). Secondary glomerulonephritis can be caused by multi-system diseases (Table 67-2) and can manifest as acute or chronic disease. However, the division of primary and secondary glomerulonephritis is complex because diagnostic findings, histologic changes, and other changes are the same in both kidney and systemic disease, with both demonstrating altered IMMUNITY. Drugs and inherited disorders are also implicated in glomerulonephritis with an acute or chronic presentation.

TABLE 67-1 Infectious Agents Associated With Glomerulonephritis
• Group A beta-hemolytic *Streptococcus*
• Staphylococcal or gram-negative bacteremia or sepsis
• Pneumococcal, *Mycoplasma*, or *Klebsiella* pneumonia
• Syphilis
• Tuberculosis
• Hepatitis B and C
• Herpes
• Infectious mononucleosis
• Malaria
• Rocky Mountain spotted fever
• Cytomegalovirus infection
• Histoplasmosis
• Toxoplasmosis
• Varicella
• *Chlamydia psittaci* infection
• Coxsackievirus infection
• Any systemic bacterial, parasitic, fungal, or viral infection (potentially). Prompt antimicrobial and anti-inflammatory treatment reduces the risk for acute glomerulonephritis becoming a chronic condition.

TABLE 67-2 Secondary Glomerular Diseases and Syndromes
• Systemic lupus erythematosus (SLE)
• Chronic pyelonephritis with vesicoureteral reflux
• Antiphospholipid antibody syndrome
• Small vessel vasculitis
• Allergic granulomatosis
• Henoch-Schönlein-Henoch purpura
• Goodpasture's syndrome and other basement membrane diseases
• Systemic necrotizing vasculitis
• Wegener's granulomatosis
• Periarteritis nodosa (also called *polyarteritis nodosa*)
• Fabry's disease
• Amyloidosis
• Diabetic glomerulopathy
• HIV-associated nephropathy
• Hereditary nephritis, including Alport's syndrome
• Multiple myeloma and other metastatic cancers
• Glomerular manifestations of sustained liver diseases (viral hepatitis B or C, autoimmune hepatitis, and cirrhosis)
• Sickle cell disease
• Hemolytic-uremic syndrome
• Thrombotic thrombocytopenia purpura

HIV, Human immune deficiency virus.

❖ *INTERPROFESSIONAL COLLABORATIVE CARE*

◆ *Assessment: Noticing*

History. Ask about recent infections, particularly of the skin or upper respiratory tract, and about recent travel or other possible exposures to viruses, bacteria, fungi, or parasites. Recent illnesses, surgery, or other invasive procedures may suggest infection. Ask about any systemic diseases that alter IMMUNITY, such as systemic lupus erythematosus (SLE), which could cause acute GN.

Physical Assessment/Signs and Symptoms. Inspect the patient's skin for lesions or recent incisions, including body piercings, because these may be the source of organisms causing GN. Assess the face, eyelids, hands, and other areas for edema because edema is present in most patients with acute GN. Assess for fluid overload and pulmonary edema that may result from fluid and sodium retention occurring with acute GN. Ask about any difficulty breathing or shortness of breath. Assess for crackles in the lung fields, an S_3 heart sound (gallop rhythm), and neck vein distention.

Ask about changes in urine ELIMINATION patterns and any change in urine color, volume, clarity, or odor. The patient may describe blood in the urine as smoky, reddish brown, rusty, or cola colored. Ask about dysuria or oliguria. Weigh him or her to assess for fluid retention.

Take the patient's blood pressure and compare it with the baseline blood pressure. Mild-to-moderate hypertension occurs with acute GN as a result of impaired FLUID AND ELECTROLYTE BALANCE with fluid and sodium retention. The patient may have fatigue, a lack of energy, anorexia, nausea, and/or vomiting if uremia from severe kidney impairment is present.

CONSIDERATIONS FOR OLDER ADULTS
Patient-Centered Care QSEN

The less common symptoms of acute GN are more likely to occur in older adults. Circulatory congestion and pulmonary edema often are present, causing acute GN to be easily confused with new onset of acute exacerbation of heart failure (AEHF) (Touhy & Jett, 2016). Ask any older adult with symptoms of circulatory overload mimicking heart failure about urine ELIMINATION patterns to determine whether the problem may be related to acute GN.

Laboratory Assessment. Urinalysis shows red blood cells (hematuria) and protein (proteinuria). An early morning specimen of urine is preferred for urinalysis because the urine is concentrated, most acidic, and filled with more intact formed elements at that time. Microscopic examination often shows red blood cell casts, as well as casts from other substances.

A 24-hour urine collection for total protein assay is obtained. The protein excretion rate for patients with acute GN may be increased from 500 mg/24 hr to 3 g/24 hr. Serum albumin levels are decreased because this protein is lost in the urine and fluid retention causes dilution.

Serum creatinine and BUN provide information about kidney function and may be elevated, indicating impairment of ELIMINATION. The glomerular filtration rate (GFR), either estimated from a single serum and urine creatinine value or measured by the 24-hour urine test for creatinine clearance, may be decreased to 50 mL/min. Recall that the older adult has a decline in GFR, which may make GFR results challenging to interpret.

Other tests for indicators of IMMUNITY problems include antistreptolysin-O titers, C3 complement levels, cryoglobulins, antinuclear antibodies (ANAs), and circulating immune complexes. Testing for human immune deficiency virus (HIV) is recommended. Blood, skin, or throat cultures may be obtained.

Antistreptolysin-O titers are increased after group A beta-hemolytic *Streptococcus* infections. Complement levels are decreased when the complement system is activated. Type III cryoglobulins may be found during acute illness. ANAs suggest an IMMUNITY excess (autoimmune response), and systemic lupus erythematosus (SLE) is just one possibility. Serum immune complexes containing IgG and C3 are often detected.

Other Diagnostic Assessment. A kidney biopsy provides a precise diagnosis of the condition, assists in determining the prognosis, and helps outline treatment (see Chapter 65). The specific tissue features are determined by light microscopy, immunofluorescent stains, and electron microscopy to identify cell type, the presence of immunoglobulins, or the type of tissue deposits.

◆ Interventions: Responding
Interventions focus on managing infection, preventing complications, and providing appropriate patient education.

Managing infection as a cause of acute GN begins with appropriate antibiotic therapy. Penicillin, erythromycin, or azithromycin is prescribed for GN caused by streptococcal infection. Check the patient's known allergies before giving any drug. Stress personal hygiene and basic infection control principles (e.g., handwashing) to prevent spread of the organism. Teach patients the importance of completing the entire course of the prescribed antibiotic.

Modifying immunity with drugs can also benefit patients with acute glomerulonephritis that is not due to acute infection but is related to excessive inflammation. Corticosteroids and cytotoxic drugs (e.g., cyclosporine, cyclophosphamide) to suppress IMMUNITY responses may be used. Patients receiving immunosuppressants need to take precautions to avoid exposure to new infections (see Chapters 19 and 20 for more information).

Preventing complications is an important nursing intervention, especially when FLUID AND ELECTROLYTE BALANCE is disrupted. For patients with fluid overload, hypertension, and edema, diuretics and sodium and water restrictions are prescribed. The usual fluid allowance is equal to the 24-hour urine output plus 500 to 600 mL. Patients with oliguria usually have increased serum levels of potassium and blood urea nitrogen (BUN). Potassium and protein intake may be restricted to prevent hyperkalemia and uremia as a result of the elevated BUN. Antihypertensive drugs may be needed to control hypertension (see Chapter 36).

Nausea, vomiting, or anorexia indicates that uremia is present. Dialysis is necessary if uremic symptoms or fluid volume excess cannot be controlled with nutrition therapy and fluid management (see Chapter 68). *Plasmapheresis* (removal and filtering of the plasma to eliminate antibodies) also may be used (see Chapter 40).

Coordinate care to conserve patient energy and balance activity with rest to maintain function. Relaxation techniques and diversional activities can reduce emotional stress.

Preparing for self-management includes teaching the patient and family members about the purpose of prescribed drugs, the dosage and schedule, and potential adverse effects. Ensure that they understand diet and fluid restrictions. Advise the patient to measure weight and blood pressure daily at the same time each day. Instruct him or her to notify the primary health care provider of any sudden increase in weight or blood pressure.

If short-term dialysis is required to control FLUID AND ELECTROLYTE BALANCE or uremic symptoms, explain vascular access care and dialysis schedules and routines (see Chapter 68).

Rapidly progressive glomerulonephritis (RPGN) is a primary glomerulonephritis also called *crescentic glomerulonephritis* because of the presence of crescent-shaped cells in the Bowman's capsule. RPGN develops acutely over several weeks or months. Patients become quite ill quickly and have symptoms of kidney impairment (fluid volume excess, hypertension, oliguria, electrolyte imbalances, and uremic symptoms).

Regardless of treatment, RPGN often progresses to end-stage kidney disease (ESKD).

CHRONIC GLOMERULONEPHRITIS

❖ PATHOPHYSIOLOGY

Chronic glomerulonephritis, or *chronic nephritic syndrome,* develops over years to decades. Mild proteinuria and hematuria, hypertension, fatigue, and occasional edema are often the only symptoms.

Although the exact cause is not known, changes in kidney tissue result from infection, hypertension, inflammation from IMMUNITY excess, or poor kidney blood flow. Kidney tissue atrophies, and functional nephrons are greatly reduced. Biopsy in the late stages of atrophy may show glomerular changes, cell loss, protein and collagen deposits, and fibrosis of the kidney tissue. Microscopic examination shows deposits of immune complexes and inflammation.

The loss of nephrons reduces glomerular filtration. Hypertension and renal arteriole sclerosis are often present. The glomerular damage allows proteins to enter the urine. Chronic glomerulonephritis always leads to end-stage kidney disease (ESKD) (see Chapter 68).

❖ INTERPROFESSIONAL COLLABORATIVE CARE

◆ Assessment: Noticing

History. Ask about other health problems, including systemic diseases, kidney or urologic disorders, infectious diseases (i.e., streptococcal infections), and recent exposures to infections. Ask about overall health status and whether increasing fatigue and lethargy have occurred.

Identify the patient's urine ELIMINATION pattern. Ask whether the frequency of voiding has increased or the quantity of urine has decreased. Ask about changes in urine color, odor, or clarity and whether dysuria or incontinence has occurred. Nocturia is a common symptom.

Assess the patient's general comfort and ask whether new-onset dyspnea has occurred because fluid overload can occur with decreased urine output. Ask about and observe for changes in cognition (i.e., irritability, an inability to read, or incapacity during job-related functions) or disturbed concentration. Changes in memory and the ability to concentrate occur as waste products collect in the blood.

Physical Assessment/Signs and Symptoms. Assess for systemic circulatory overload. Auscultate lung fields for crackles, observe the respiratory rate and depth, and measure blood pressure and weight. Assess the heart rate, rhythm, and presence of an S_3 heart sound. Inspect the neck veins for venous engorgement and check for edema of the feet and ankles, on the shins, and over the sacrum.

Assess for uremic symptoms, such as slurred speech, ataxia, tremors, or asterixis (flapping tremor of the fingers or the inability to maintain a fixed posture with the arms extended and wrists hyperextended). Inspect skin for a yellowish color, texture changes, bruises, rashes, or eruptions. Ask about itching and document areas of dryness or any excoriation from scratching.

Psychosocial Assessment. A diagnosis of chronic glomerulonephritis is associated with psychosocial responses of uncertainty, loss, and fear of the need for lifestyle changes as the disease progresses. While obtaining the history, listen carefully for spoken and unspoken feelings of anger, resentment, futility, sadness, or anxiety, all of which may need further exploration.

Diagnostic Assessment. Urine output decreases; and urinalysis shows protein, usually less than 2 g in a 24-hour collection. The specific gravity is fixed at a constant level of dilution (around 1.010) despite variable fluid intake. Red blood cells and casts may be in the urine.

The glomerular filtration rate (GFR) is low. The serum creatinine level is elevated, usually greater than 6 mg/dL (500 mcmol/L) but may be as high as 30 mg/dL (2500 mcmol/L) or more because of poor waste ELIMINATION. The BUN is increased, often as high as 100 to 200 mg/dL (35 to 70 mmol/L).

Decreased kidney function disturbs FLUID AND ELECTROLYTE BALANCE. Sodium retention is common, but dilution of the plasma from excess fluid can result in a falsely normal serum sodium level (135 to 145 mEq/L [mmol/L]) or a low sodium level (less than 135 mEq/L [mmol/L]). When oliguria develops, potassium is not excreted, and hyperkalemia occurs when levels exceed 5.4 mEq/L (mmol/L).

Hyperphosphatemia develops with serum levels greater than 4.7 mg/dL (1.73 mmol/L). Serum calcium levels are usually low normal or are slightly below normal.

Disturbances of ACID-BASE BALANCE with acidosis develop from hydrogen ion retention and loss of bicarbonate. However, there may be a decrease in serum carbon dioxide (CO_2) levels as patients breathe more rapidly to compensate for the acidosis. If respiratory compensation is present, the pH of arterial blood is between 7.35 and 7.45. A pH of less than 7.35 means that the patient's respiratory system is not completely compensating for the acidosis (see Chapter 12).

The kidneys are abnormally small on x-ray or CT in chronic glomerulonephritis.

◆ Interventions: Responding

Interventions focus on slowing the progression of the disease and preventing complications. Management is systemic and consists of diet changes, fluid intake sufficient to prevent reduced blood flow to the kidneys, and drug therapy to control the problems from uremia. Eventually ELIMINATION is so impaired that the patient requires dialysis or transplantation to prevent death. (Care for the patient requiring dialysis or transplantation is discussed in Chapter 68.)

NEPHROTIC SYNDROME

❖ PATHOPHYSIOLOGY

Nephrotic syndrome (NS) is an immunologic kidney disorder in which glomerular permeability increases so larger molecules

▶▶ CHART 67-3 Key Features

Nephrotic Syndrome

Sudden onset of these symptoms:
- Massive proteinuria
- Hypoalbuminemia
- Edema (especially facial and periorbital)
- Lipiduria
- Hyperlipidemia
- Delayed clotting or increased bleeding with higher-than-normal values for serum activated partial thromboplastin time (aPTT) coagulation or international normalized ratio for prothrombin (INR, PT)
- Reduced kidney function with elevated blood urea nitrogen (BUN) and serum creatinine and decreased glomerular filtration rate (GFR)

pass through the membrane into the urine and are then excreted. This process causes massive loss of protein into the urine, edema formation, and decreased plasma albumin levels. Many agents and disorders are possible causes of NS. All glomerulonephritis diseases have features of nephrosis (Pendergraft et al., 2016)

The most common cause of glomerular membrane changes is altered IMMUNITY with inflammation. Defects in glomerular filtration can also occur as a result of genetic defects of the glomerular filtering system, such as Fabry disease. Altered liver function may occur with NS, resulting in increased lipid production and hyperlipidemia.

❖ INTERPROFESSIONAL COLLABORATIVE CARE

The main feature of NS is increased protein ELIMINATION with severe proteinuria (with more than 3.5 g of protein in a 24-hour urine sample). Patients also have low serum albumin levels of less than 3 g/dL (30 g/L), high serum lipid levels, fats in the urine, edema, and hypertension (Chart 67-3). Renal vein thrombosis often occurs at the same time as NS, either as a cause of the problem or as an effect. NS may progress to end-stage kidney disease (ESKD), but treatment can prevent progression.

Management varies, depending on which process is causing the disorder (identified by kidney biopsy). Excess IMMUNITY may improve with suppressive therapy using steroids and cytotoxic or immunosuppressive agents. Angiotensin-converting enzyme inhibitors (ACEIs) can decrease protein loss in the urine, and cholesterol-lowering drugs can improve blood lipid levels. Heparin may reduce vascular defects and improve kidney function. Diet changes are often prescribed. If the glomerular filtration rate (GFR) is normal, dietary intake of proteins is needed. If the GFR is decreased, protein intake must be decreased. Mild diuretics and sodium restriction may be needed to control edema and hypertension. Assess the patient's hydration status because vascular dehydration is common. If plasma volume is depleted, kidney problems worsen. Acute kidney injury (AKI) may be avoided if adequate blood flow to the kidney is maintained.

NEPHROSCLEROSIS

❖ PATHOPHYSIOLOGY

Nephrosclerosis is a degenerative disorder resulting from changes in kidney blood vessels. Nephron blood vessels thicken,

resulting in narrowed lumens and decreased kidney blood flow. The tissue is chronically hypoxic, with ischemia and fibrosis developing over time.

Nephrosclerosis occurs with all types of hypertension, atherosclerosis, and diabetes mellitus. The more severe the hypertension, the greater the risk for severe kidney damage. Nephrosclerosis is rarely seen when blood pressure is consistently below 160/110 mm Hg. The changes caused by hypertension may be reversible or may progress to end-stage kidney disease (ESKD) within months or years.

Hypertension is the second leading cause of ESKD, with many patients requiring kidney replacement therapy (e.g., dialysis or transplantation).

🌐 CULTURAL/SPIRITUAL CONSIDERATIONS

Patient-Centered Care **QSEN**

Hypertension is more common in African Americans and American Indians, and the risks for ESKD from hypertension are also greater for these ethnic groups (U.S. Renal Data Systems, 2015). Between 25 and 45 years of age, the ratio of African Americans to Caucasians at risk for ESKD from hypertension is nearly 20:1. At any health care encounter with an African-American or American Indian patient, blood pressure should always be assessed. If hypertension is present, treatment and patient education can help reduce the risk for development of ESKD.

❖ INTERPROFESSIONAL COLLABORATIVE CARE

Management focuses on controlling high blood pressure and reducing albuminuria to preserve kidney function. Although many antihypertensive drugs may lower blood pressure, the patient's response is important in ensuring long-term adherence to the prescribed therapy. Factors that promote adherence include once-a-day dosing, low cost, and minimal side effects.

Lack of knowledge or misinformation about hypertension poses many challenges to health care professionals working with patients who have hypertension. When kidney disease occurs, adherence to therapy is even more important for preserving health.

Many drugs can control high blood pressure (see Chapter 36), and more than one agent may be needed for best control. Angiotensin-converting enzyme inhibitors (ACEIs) are very useful in reducing hypertension and preserving kidney function. Diuretics can maintain FLUID AND ELECTROLYTE BALANCE in the presence of kidney function insufficiency. Hyperkalemia needs to be prevented when potassium-sparing diuretics, alone or in combination with other diuretics, are used to treat hypertensive patients with known kidney disease.

POLYCYSTIC KIDNEY DISEASE

❖ PATHOPHYSIOLOGY

Polycystic kidney disease (PKD) is a genetic disorder in which fluid-filled cysts develop in the nephrons (Fig. 67-3). Relentless development and growth of cysts from loss of CELLULAR REGULATION and abnormal cell division result in progressive kidney enlargement. PKD is associated with hypertension, abdominal fullness and pain, episodes of cyst bleeding, hematuria, kidney stone formation, infections, and systemic disease (Chapman et al., 2015).

The cysts look like clusters of grapes (see Fig. 67-3). Over time, growing cysts damage the glomerular and tubular

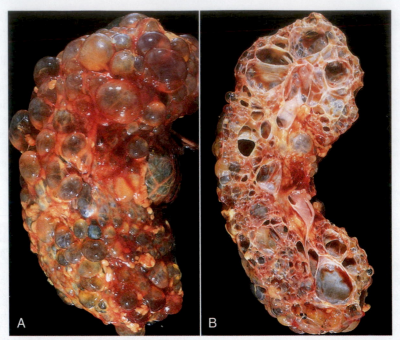

FIG. 67-3 External surface **(A)** and internal surface **(B)** of a polycystic kidney. (From Kumar, V., Abbas, A., Fausto, N., & Aster, J. (2010). *Robbins and Cotran pathologic basis of disease* (8th ed.). Philadelphia: Saunders.)

membranes. Each cystic kidney enlarges, becoming the size of a football, and may weigh 10 lb or more each. As cysts fill with fluid and become larger, kidney function becomes less effective, and urine formation and waste ELIMINATION are impaired.

Most patients with PKD have high blood pressure. The cause of hypertension is related to kidney ischemia from the enlarging cysts. As the vessels are compressed and blood flow to the kidneys decreases, the renin-angiotensin system is activated, raising blood pressure. Control of hypertension is a top priority because proper treatment can disrupt the process that leads to further kidney damage, as well as avoid complications such as stroke from hypertension.

Cysts may also occur in the liver and blood vessels. The incidence of cerebral *aneurysms* (outpouching and thinning of an artery wall) is higher in patients with PKD. Aneurysms may rupture, causing bleeding and sudden death. For unknown reasons, kidney stones occur in many patients with PKD. Heart valve problems (e.g., mitral valve prolapse), left ventricular hypertrophy, and colonic diverticula also are common in patients with PKD.

Etiology and Genetic Risk

Kidney cysts are genetically and clinically related to many symptoms and problems. PKD can be inherited as either an autosomal-dominant trait or, less often, as an autosomal-recessive trait. Autosomal-dominant PKD is the most common inherited kidney disease. People who inherit the recessive form of PKD usually die in early childhood. The 5% to 10% incidence of PKD in patients with no family history occurs as a result of a new gene mutation. The number of genes that influence PKD is challenging and requires that geneticists and genetic counselors be a part of the interprofessional team caring for patients with or at risk for the disease (Chapman et al., 2015). A clear genetic diagnosis can be made in about 90% of patients

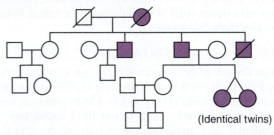

(Identical twins)

FIG. 67-4 Four-generation pedigree for autosomal-dominant polycystic kidney disease (ADPKD). *Colored-in symbols* indicate family members with ADPKD. *Slashes* indicate that the person has died.

undergoing genetic testing when kidney cysts occur (Ong et al., 2015).

🧬 GENETIC/GENOMIC CONSIDERATIONS
Patient-Centered Care QSEN

Autosomal-dominant PKD (ADPKD) is the most common form of the disease in adults, with a 50% risk of passing the mutated gene to their children. Fig. 67-4 shows a pedigree for a family with ADPKD. The onset, symptoms, and severity can vary; however, nearly 100% of people who inherit a PKD gene mutation will develop kidney cysts by age 30 (Online Mendelian Inheritance in Man [OMIM], 2016). ADPKD-1 is the most common and most severe form of the autosomal-dominant disease. ADPKD-2 has a slower rate of cyst formation, symptoms, and progression to end-stage kidney disease (ESKD) (OMIM, 2013).

There is no way to prevent PKD, although early detection and management of hypertension may slow the progression of kidney damage and impaired ELIMINATION. Genetic counseling may be useful for adults who have one parent with PKD. Family history analysis is used to help identify people at risk (see Fig. 67-4).

Incidence and Prevalence

PKD affects about 600,000 people of all ethnic groups in the United States (National Kidney Foundation, 2016). Men and women have an equal chance of inheriting the disease because the gene responsible for PKD is on an autosome (see Chapter 5).

❖ INTERPROFESSIONAL COLLABORATIVE CARE

◆ Assessment: Noticing

Because PDK is a chronic disease with periods of acute problems, most management occurs in the community rather than in an acute care hospital. With acute problems or when surgery is needed, initial care is in a hospital setting, and continuing care can occur in any setting.

History. Explore the family history of a patient with suspected or actual PKD and ask whether either parent was known to have PKD or whether there is any family history of kidney disease. Important information to obtain is the age at which the problem was diagnosed in the parent and any related complications. Ask about pain, abdominal discomfort, constipation, changes in urine color or frequency, hypertension, headaches, and a family history of stroke or sudden death.

Physical Assessment/Signs and Symptoms. Chart 67-4 lists key features of PKD. Pain is often the first symptom. Inspect the abdomen. A distended abdomen is common as the cystic kidneys swell and push the abdominal contents forward. Polycystic kidneys are easily palpated because of their increased size. Use *gentle* abdominal palpation because the cystic kidneys and nearby tissues may be tender and palpation is uncomfortable. The patient also may have flank pain as a dull ache or as a sharp and intermittent discomfort. Dull, aching pain is caused by increased kidney size with distention, abnormal stimulation of sensory neurons in the kidney, or infection within the cyst. Sharp, intermittent pain occurs when a cyst ruptures or a stone is present. When a cyst ruptures, the patient may have bright red or cola-colored urine. Infection is suspected if the urine is cloudy or foul smelling or if there is **dysuria** (pain on urination).

Nocturia (the need to urinate excessively at night) is an early symptom and occurs because of decreased urine concentrating ability. Patients with early PKD often have hyperfiltration leading to wasting of sodium and water, which disrupts FLUID AND ELECTROLYTE BALANCE. Later, as kidney function declines (i.e., reduced glomerular filtration rate [GFR]), the patient retains water and sodium, which causes hypertension, edema, and uremic symptoms such as anorexia, nausea, vomiting, pruritus, and fatigue (see Chapter 68). Because intracranial berry aneurysms often occur in patients with PKD, a severe headache with or without neurologic or vision changes requires attention.

▶▶ CHART 67-4 Key Features

Polycystic Kidney Disease

- Abdominal or flank pain
- Hypertension
- Nocturia
- Increased abdominal girth
- Constipation
- Bloody or cloudy urine
- Sodium wasting and inability to concentrate urine in early stage
- Progression to kidney failure with anuria

Psychosocial Assessment. A PKD diagnosis is associated with psychosocial responses of uncertainty, loss, and fear (Tong et al., 2015). The patient may have had a parent who died or relatives who required dialysis or transplantation. Listen for spoken and unspoken feelings of anger, resentment, futility, sadness, or anxiety. Such feelings may need further exploration. Feelings of guilt and concern for the patient's children may also complicate the issue.

Diagnostic Assessment. Ultrasonography is used to provide initial screening for PKD. The definitive diagnostic test is an MRI. CT scan with angiography may be used to assess kidney perfusion. A finding of five or more kidney cysts on MRI is diagnostic of PKD (Chapman et al., 2015). Estimation of kidney size by MRI or CT helps determine total kidney volume and disease progression.

Urinalysis may show **proteinuria** (protein in the urine), which indicates a decline in kidney function and impaired ELIMINATION. Hematuria may be gross or microscopic. Bacteria in the urine indicate infection, usually in the cysts. Obtain a urine sample for culture and sensitivity testing when there is evidence of infection. As kidney function declines, serum creatinine and blood urea nitrogen (BUN) levels rise. With further decline, creatinine clearance decreases, and the GFR is low. Changes in kidney handling of sodium may cause either sodium losses or sodium retention.

Genetic testing is not routinely performed for diagnostic assessment of PKD. It may be considered for patients who have atypical imaging findings or for those with symptoms who have no family history of PKD.

◆ Interventions: Responding

Currently no treatments are effective in extending kidney function in PKD. Drug therapies to interrupt the pathways that promote malignant cyst formation such as molecular signaling for cell division or endothelial growth are being evaluated. Supportive interventions for PKD include management of hypertension and pain, reducing complications from infection and constipation, and slowing disease progression. Be attentive to the psychosocial issues of uncertainty and fear related to an inherited disorder, as well as reproductive issues. Genetic counseling is part of comprehensive care of the patient and family experiencing PKD.

When the disease progresses and the kidneys no longer function for waste ELIMINATION, care becomes similar to that needed for the patient with end-stage kidney disease (see Chapter 68).

Managing Blood Pressure. Blood pressure control is necessary to reduce cardiovascular complications and slow the progression of kidney dysfunction. Nursing interventions include education for self-management. Initially patients with PKD may have salt-wasting and should **NOT** follow a sodium-restricted diet. As the disease progresses and *sodium retention* occurs, restricting sodium may then help control blood pressure. See Chapter 36 for hypertension management.

Drug therapy for blood pressure control is a mainstay of treatment when the disease progresses. Achieving a blood pressure goal of 120/80 slows kidney growth from cyst formation and sustains kidney function (Chapman et al., 2015). The most effective antihypertensive agents for PKD are angiotensin-converting enzyme inhibitors (ACEIs) (Ong et al., 2015). These drugs also help control the cell growth aspects of PKD and reduce microalbuminuria. ACEIs can cause birth defects and are contraindicated during pregnancy. Additional antihypertensive drugs, such as calcium channel blockers, beta blockers, and vasodilators, may be used (see Chapter 36).

Teach the patient and family how to measure and record blood pressure. Help the patient establish a schedule for self-administering drugs, monitoring daily weights, and keeping blood pressure records (Chart 67-5). Explain the potential side effects of the drugs. Make available written materials, such as drug teaching cards and booklets. Work with the patient and a dietitian to develop strategies to manage sodium and other dietary issues that contribute to hypertension.

Managing Pain. Because PKD-related pain is chronic, a multidisciplinary pain management approach is helpful. Drugs may include opioids along with acetaminophen. NSAIDs are used cautiously because they can reduce kidney blood flow. Aspirin-containing drugs are avoided to reduce bleeding risk.

Complementary therapy includes positioning and the application of dry heat to the abdomen or flank. Teach the patient methods of relaxation and comfort using deep breathing, guided imagery, or other strategies (see Chapter 4 for pain management). When pain is severe, cysts can be reduced by needle aspiration and drainage; however, they usually refill. When the quality or severity of pain abruptly increases, assess for infection.

Reducing Complications from Infection. Fever, abdominal pain, and either leukocytosis or serum markers of inflammation (e.g., elevated erythrocyte sedimentation rate [ESR] or C-reactive protein [CRP]) may be associated with cystic or systemic infection. Blood and urine cultures may or may not be positive with cyst infection. Early infection management can prevent or reduce complications and acute kidney injury. Monitor serum creatinine levels because some antibiotics are nephrotoxic.

Percutaneous or surgical drainage of the cyst may be indicated. Prepare the patients similarly to a kidney biopsy described in Chapter 65.

Preventing Constipation. Teach the patient who has adequate urine output to prevent constipation by maintaining adequate fluid intake (generally 2 to 3 L daily in food and beverages), maintaining dietary fiber intake, and exercising regularly. Explain that pressure on the large intestine may occur as the polycystic kidneys increase in size. These recommendations for bowel management might change, particularly when ESKD

develops. Advise the patient about the use of stool softeners and bulk agents, including careful use of laxatives, to prevent chronic constipation.

Slowing Progression of Chronic Kidney Disease. Early in the disease when patients have hyperfiltration with decreased urine concentration, nocturia, and low specific gravity, urge them to drink at least 2 L of fluid daily to prevent dehydration, which can further reduce kidney function. Hyperfiltration may persist for several years. Maintaining adequate fluid intake can reduce the vasopressin release that reduces kidney blood flow.

As the disease progresses, protein intake may be limited to slow the development of ESKD. Help the patient and family understand the diet plan and why it was prescribed. Work closely with the dietitian to foster the patient's understanding.

Strategies for kidney protection include the use of a vasopressin-suppressing agent such as tolvaptan (Samsca, Jinarc) to improve blood flow, slow kidney volume growth, and sustain kidney function. The use of "statin" drugs to reduce the growth of kidneys has not yet been proven effective in adults with PKD (Chapman et al., 2015).

Care Coordination and Transition Management

Health Care Resources. The Polycystic Kidney Research Foundation (www.pkdcure.org) and the National Kidney & Urologic Diseases Clearinghouse (NKUDIC) of the National Institute of Diabetes and Digestive and Kidney Diseases (www.niddk.nih.gov) conduct research and provide education about PKD. Many pamphlets are available; there is a fee for some materials. Chapters of the National Kidney Foundation (NKF) and the American Association of Kidney Patients (AAKP) also have resources for information and support.

💡 **NCLEX EXAMINATION CHALLENGE 67-3**

Health Promotion and Maintenance

Which statement made by a client newly diagnosed with polycystic kidney disease (PKD) in the hyperfiltration stage indicates to the nurse that additional teaching for self-management is needed?
A. "I'll need to decrease my daily water intake."
B. "I need to make certain my brothers and sisters know about this disease."
C. "Probably the best time of day to take my lisinopril each day is with breakfast."
D. "Regular low-impact exercise may help me feel better and help prevent constipation."

HYDRONEPHROSIS AND HYDROURETER

❖ PATHOPHYSIOLOGY

Hydronephrosis and hydroureter are problems of urinary ELIMINATION with outflow obstruction. Urethral strictures obstruct urine outflow and may contribute to bladder distention, hydroureter, and hydronephrosis. Prompt recognition and treatment are crucial to preventing permanent kidney damage.

In hydronephrosis, the kidney enlarges as urine collects in the renal pelvis and kidney tissue. Because the capacity of the renal pelvis is normally 5 to 8 mL, obstruction in the renal pelvis or at the point where the ureter joins the renal pelvis quickly distends the renal pelvis. Kidney pressure increases as the volume of urine increases. Over time, sometimes in only a matter of hours, the blood vessels and kidney tubules can be damaged extensively (Fig. 67-5).

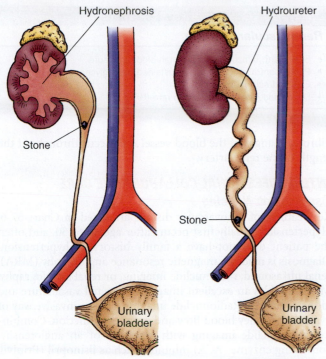

FIG. 67-5 Hydronephrosis is caused by obstruction in the upper part of the ureter. Hydroureter is caused by obstruction in the lower part of the ureter.

In patients with **hydroureter** (enlargement of the ureter), the effects are similar, but the obstruction is in the ureter rather than in the kidney. The ureter is most easily obstructed where the iliac vessels cross or where the ureters enter the bladder. Ureter dilation occurs above the obstruction and enlarges as urine collects (see Fig. 67-5).

Urinary obstruction causes damage when pressure builds up directly on kidney tissue. Tubular filtrate pressure also increases in the nephron as drainage through the collecting system is impaired and glomerular filtration decreases or ceases. Kidney necrosis can occur. Nitrogen waste products (urea, creatinine, and uric acid) and electrolytes (sodium, potassium, chloride, and phosphorus) are retained, and ACID-BASE BALANCE is impaired.

Causes of hydronephrosis or hydroureter include tumors, stones, trauma, structural defects, and fibrosis (McCance et al., 2014). With cancer, obstructed ureters may result from tumors pressing on the ureters, pelvic radiation, or surgical treatment. Early treatment of the causes can prevent ureteral problems and permanent kidney damage. The time needed to prevent permanent damage depends on the patient's kidney health. Permanent damage can occur in less than 48 hours in some patients and after several weeks in other patients.

❖ INTERPROFESSIONAL COLLABORATIVE CARE

◆ Assessment: Noticing

Obtain a history from the patient, focusing on known kidney or urologic disorders. A history of childhood urinary tract problems may indicate previously undiagnosed structural defects. Ask about his or her usual pattern of urinary ELIMINA-TION, especially amount, frequency, color, clarity, and odor. Ask about recent flank or abdominal pain. Chills, fever, and malaise may be present with a urinary tract infection (UTI).

Inspect each flank to identify asymmetry, which may occur with a kidney mass, and *gently* palpate the abdomen to locate areas of tenderness. Palpate and percuss the bladder to detect distention, or use a bedside bladder scanner (see Chapter 65). Gentle pressure on the abdomen may cause urine leakage, which reflects a full bladder and possible obstruction.

Urinalysis may show bacteria or white blood cells if infection is present. When urinary tract obstruction is prolonged, microscopic examination may show tubular epithelial cells. Blood chemistries are normal unless glomerular filtration has decreased and waste ELIMINATION is impaired. Blood creatinine and BUN levels increase with a reduced GFR. Serum electrolyte levels may be altered with elevated blood levels of potassium, phosphorus, and calcium along with a metabolic acidosis (bicarbonate deficit). Urinary outflow obstruction can be seen with ultrasound (US) or CT.

◆ Interventions: Responding

Urinary retention and potential for infection are the primary problems. Failure to treat the cause of obstruction leads to infection and acute kidney injury (AKI).

Urologic Interventions. If obstruction is caused by a kidney stone (calculus), it can be located and removed using cystoscopic or retrograde urogram procedures. See Chapter 66 for more information about kidney stone management. After stone removal, a plastic stent is usually left in the ureter for a few weeks to improve urine flow in the area irritated by the stone. The stent is later removed by another cystoscopic procedure.

Radiologic Interventions. When an abnormal narrowing of the urinary tract (**stricture**) causes hydronephrosis and cannot be corrected with urologic procedures, a **nephrostomy** is performed. Most nephrostomy drains provide only external drainage (diversion). Other styles of nephrostomy drains enter the kidney and extend to the bladder, draining urine out to a bag or past a ureteral obstruction and into the bladder. With these, there are both internal and external parts to the nephrostomy tubing. Externally, a fully external or an internal/external diversion drain appears the same. The urine output will fluctuate more if all urine goes to the bladder before external drainage.

Patient Preparation. If possible, the patient is kept NPO for 4 to 6 hours before the procedure. Clotting studies (e.g., international normalized ratio [INR], prothrombin time [PT], and partial thromboplastic time [PTT]) should be normal or corrected. Drugs are used to reduce hypertension. The patient receives moderate sedation for the procedure.

Procedure. The patient is placed in the prone position. The kidney is located under ultrasound or fluoroscopic guidance, and a local anesthetic is given. A needle is placed into the kidney, a soft-tipped guidewire is placed through the needle, and then a catheter is placed over the wire. The catheter tip remains in the renal pelvis, and the external end is connected to a drainage bag. The procedure immediately relieves the pressure and prevents further damage. The nephrostomy tube remains in place until the obstruction is resolved.

Follow-up Care. Assess the amount of drainage in the collection bag. The amount of drainage depends on whether a ureteral catheter is also being used (with a separate drainage bag). Patients with ureteral tubes may have all urine pass through to the bladder or may have it drain into the collection bags. The type of urine drainage system placed must be clearly communicated in the chart. If urine is expected to drain into the collection bag, assess the amount of drainage hourly for the first 24 hours. If the amount of drainage decreases and the patient has back pain, the tube may be clogged or dislodged.

Monitor the nephrostomy site for leaking urine or blood. Urine drainage may be bloody for the first 12 to 24 hours after the procedure and should gradually clear. If prescribed, the nephrostomy tube can be irrigated with 5 mL sterile saline to check patency and dislodge clots. It is common for diuresis to occur when a nephrostomy is placed for obstruction. Monitor intake and output hourly for the first several hours, and inform the surgeon if the patient begins to have symptoms of dehydration (i.e., hypotension, poor skin turgor, dry mucous membranes, increased thirst). Assess for indications of infection (i.e., fever, change in urine character).

> **! NURSING SAFETY PRIORITY** **QSEN**
>
> **Critical Rescue**
>
> After nephrostomy, monitor the patient to recognize indications of complications (i.e., decreased or absent drainage, cloudy or foul-smelling drainage, leakage of blood or urine from the nephrostomy site, back pain). If any indications are present, respond by notifying the surgeon immediately.

> **? NCLEX EXAMINATION CHALLENGE 67-4**
>
> **Physiological Integrity**
>
> When providing care to a client who has undergone a nephrotomy for hydronephrosis, which observation alerts the nurse to a possible complication? **Select all that apply.**
> A. Urine output of 15 mL for the first hour and then diminished
> B. Tenderness at the surgical site
> C. Pink-tinged urine draining from the nephrostomy
> D. A hematocrit value 3% lower than the preoperative value
> E. Sudden onset of abdominal pain that worsens after abdominal palpation
> F. Blood pressure of 180/90 that persists despite administration of pain medication
> G. The presence of a few small (less than 0.5 cm) clots with irrigation of the nephrostomy
> H. Bright red drainage through the nephrostomy tube 12 hours after the procedure

RENOVASCULAR DISEASE

❖ PATHOPHYSIOLOGY

Processes affecting the renal arteries may severely narrow the lumen and greatly reduce blood flow to the kidney tissues. Uncorrected renovascular disease, such as renal vein thrombosis or renal artery stenosis, atherosclerosis, or thrombosis, causes ischemia and atrophy of kidney tissue, leading to severe impairment of urinary ELIMINATION, FLUID AND ELECTROLYTE BALANCE, and ACID-BASE BALANCE.

Patients with renovascular disease, particularly those older than 50 years of age, often have a sudden onset of hypertension. Patients with high blood pressure but no family history of hypertension also may potentially have renal artery stenosis (RAS). RAS from atherosclerosis or blood vessel hyperplasia is the main cause of renovascular disease. Other causes include thrombosis and renal vessel aneurysms.

Atherosclerotic changes in the renal artery often occur along with sclerosis in the aorta and other major vessels. Renal artery changes are often located where the renal artery and aorta meet.

> **» CHART 67-6 Key Features**
>
> **Renovascular Disease**
>
> - Significant, difficult-to-control high blood pressure
> - Poorly controlled diabetes or sustained hyperglycemia
> - Elevated serum creatinine
> - Decreased glomerular filtration rate (GFR)

Fibrotic changes of the blood vessel wall occur throughout the length of the renal artery.

❖ INTERPROFESSIONAL COLLABORATIVE CARE

◆ Assessment: Noticing

Key features of renovascular disease are listed in Chart 67-6. Hypertension usually first occurs after age 40 to 50, and often the patient does not have a family history of hypertension. Diagnosis is made by magnetic resonance angiography (MRA), renal ultrasound, radionuclide imaging, or renal arteriography. MRA provides an excellent image of the renal vasculature and kidney anatomy. Radionuclide imaging is a noninvasive way of evaluating kidney blood flow and excretory function. Combining radionuclide imaging with ingestion of an angiotensin-converting enzyme (ACE) inhibitor such as lisinopril (Prinivil, Zestril) improves the accuracy of the test. A renal arteriogram makes the features of the renal blood vessels visible.

◆ Interventions: Responding

Identifying the type of defect, extent of narrowing, and condition of the surrounding blood vessels is critical for treatment choice as is the patient's overall health. Many patients with renovascular disease also have cardiovascular disease, and both conditions require treatment.

RAS may be managed by drugs to control high blood pressure and by procedures to restore the blood supply to the kidney. Drugs may control high blood pressure but may not lead to long-term preservation of kidney function. In younger adults, a lifetime of treatment with many drugs for high blood pressure makes treatment difficult and outcomes uncertain.

Endovascular techniques are nonsurgical approaches to repair RAS. Stent placement with or without balloon angioplasty is an example of an endovascular intervention (see Chapter 36). These techniques are less risky and require less time for recovery than does renal artery bypass surgery. After the procedure, the patient usually remains under close observation for 24 hours to monitor for sudden blood pressure fluctuations as the kidneys adjust to increased blood flow.

Renal artery bypass surgery is a major procedure and requires 2 or more months for recovery. A bypass may be performed for either one or both renal arteries. A synthetic blood vessel graft is inserted to redirect blood flow from the abdominal aorta into the renal artery, beyond the area of narrowing. A splenorenal bypass can also restore blood flow to the kidney. The process is similar to other arterial bypass procedures (see Chapter 38).

DIABETIC NEPHROPATHY

Diabetic nephropathy is a vascular complication of diabetes mellitus (DM) and the leading cause of end-stage kidney disease (ESKD) in North America (U.S. Renal Data Systems, 2015). It occurs with either type 1 or type 2 DM. Severity of diabetic kidney disease is related to the degree of hyperglycemia the patient generally experiences. With poor control of hyperglycemia, the complicating problems of atherosclerosis, hypertension, and neuropathy (which promotes loss of bladder tone, urinary stasis, and urinary tract infection) are more severe and more likely to cause kidney damage. Chapter 64 discusses diabetic nephropathy. Management of diabetic nephropathy is the same as for chronic kidney disease (see Chapter 68).

? NCLEX EXAMINATION CHALLENGE 67-5
Safe and Effective Care Environment

The charge nurse is preparing assignments on a busy medical unit. For this shift, there are two LPNs, two RNs, and one nursing assistant. Which client assignments are **most** appropriate? **Select all that apply.**

A. An LPN is assigned to a client who is receiving the first dose of an oral immunomodulating agent to manage acute glomerulonephritis.

B. An RN is assigned to the client who is receiving an IV corticosteroid twice daily to manage systemic lupus erythematous that has resulted in chronic glomerulonephritis.

C. An LPN is assigned to replace a urinary catheter (in place >2 weeks) in a client with a fever who requires a chronic urinary catheter to help healing from a genitourinary fistula.

D. An RN is assigned to administer IV antibiotics to a client admitted with pyelonephritis.

E. A nursing assistant is assigned to do all the morning baths.

F. LPNs are assigned to clients who have oral drugs prescribed and will do the vital signs for those clients.

G. An RN is assigned to the client who is being discharged with a new diagnosis of diabetic nephropathy that is serious (stage 3 CKD)

RENAL CELL CARCINOMA

❖ PATHOPHYSIOLOGY

Renal cell carcinoma (RCC) or adenocarcinoma of the kidney is the most common type of kidney cancer and occurs as a result of impaired CELLULAR REGULATION. Healthy kidney tissue is damaged and replaced by cancer cells, which impairs urine ELIMINATION for that kidney.

Systemic effects occurring with this cancer type are called *paraneoplastic syndromes* and include anemia, erythrocytosis, hypercalcemia, liver dysfunction with elevated liver enzymes, hormonal effects, increased sedimentation rate, and hypertension.

Anemia and erythrocytosis may seem confusing; however, most patients with this cancer have *either* anemia or erythrocytosis, not both at the same time. There is some blood loss from hematuria, but the small amount lost does not cause anemia. The cause of the anemia and the erythrocytosis is related to kidney cell production of erythropoietin. At times, the tumor cells produce large amounts of erythropoietin, causing erythrocytosis. At other times, the tumor cells destroy the erythropoietin-producing kidney cells and anemia results.

Parathyroid hormone produced by tumor cells can cause hypercalcemia. Other hormone changes include increased renin levels (causing hypertension) and increased human chorionic gonadotropin (hCG) levels, which decrease libido and change secondary sex features.

RCC has five distinct carcinoma cell types: clear cell, papillary cell, chromophobe cell, collecting duct carcinoma, and unclassified type (McCance et al., 2014). A few RCCs are hereditary.

TABLE 67-3	**Staging Kidney Tumors**

Stage I. Tumors up to 2.5 cm are situated within the capsule of the kidney. The renal vein, perinephric fat, and adjacent lymph nodes have no tumor.
Stage II. Tumors are larger than 2.5 cm and extend beyond the capsule but are within Gerota's fascia. The renal vein and lymph nodes are not involved.
Stage III. Tumors extend into the renal vein, lymph nodes, or both.
Stage IV. Tumors include invasion of adjacent organs beyond Gerota's fascia or metastasize to distant tissues.

Data from American Cancer Society. (2017). *Cancer facts and figures 2017.* Report No. 00-300M–No. 500817. Atlanta: Author.

The most well-known genetic syndrome that includes kidney cancer is von Hippel-Lindau syndrome. These cancers are highly vascular and may occur with cancers of the pancreas, central nervous system, and adrenal glands.

Kidney tumors are classified into four stages (Table 67-3). Complications include metastasis and urinary tract obstruction. The cancer usually spreads to the adrenal gland, liver, lungs, long bones, or the other kidney. When the cancer surrounds a ureter, hydroureter and obstruction may result.

The causes of nonhereditary RCC are unknown, but the risk is slightly higher for adults who use tobacco or are exposed to cadmium and other heavy metals, asbestos, benzene, and trichloroethylene. Men are slightly more likely to acquire RCC, as are obese, African-American, or hypertensive individuals. Regardless of cause or predisposing factor, RCC forms when CELLULAR REGULATION is disrupted.

Kidney cancers account for about 70,390 new cases of cancer and 16,260 deaths annually in the United States and Canada (American Cancer Society [ACS], 2017; Canadian Cancer Society, 2016). The 5-year survival rate is 60% in the United States. RCC occurs most often in adults between 55 and 60 years of age.

❖ INTERPROFESSIONAL COLLABORATIVE CARE

The most common treatment for RCC is a nephrectomy. When the cancer is local (i.e., only in the kidney), a nephrectomy can provide a cure. For patients with metastasis, nephrectomy is followed by targeted chemotherapy combined with cytokine treatment. Patients with RCC are at risk for CKD and cardiovascular complications. Patients need ongoing, interprofessional care with surveillance for best outcomes. Follow-up therapy is managed on an outpatient basis.

◆ Assessment: Noticing

History. Ask the patient about his or her age, known risk factors (e.g., smoking or chemical exposures), weight loss, changes in urine color, abdominal or flank discomfort, and fever. Also ask whether any other family member has ever been diagnosed with cancer of the kidney, bladder, ureter, prostate gland, uterus, or ovary.

Physical Assessment/Signs and Symptoms. Some patients with RCC have flank pain, obvious blood in the urine, and a kidney mass that can be palpated. Ask about the nature of the flank or abdominal discomfort. Patients often describe the pain as dull and aching. Pain may be more intense if bleeding into the tumor or kidney occurs. Inspect the flank area, checking for asymmetry or an obvious bulge. An abdominal mass may be felt with *gentle* palpation. A renal bruit may be heard on auscultation.

Bloody urine is a *late* common sign. Blood may be visible as bright red flecks or clots, or the urine may appear smoky or cola colored. Without gross hematuria, microscopic examination may or may not reveal red blood cells (RBCs).

Inspect the skin for pallor, darkening of the nipples, and, in men, breast enlargement *(gynecomastia)* caused by changing hormone levels. Other findings may include muscle wasting, weakness, and weight loss. All tend to occur late in the disease.

Diagnostic Assessment. Urinalysis may show RBCs. Hematologic studies show decreased hemoglobin and hematocrit values, hypercalcemia, increased erythrocyte sedimentation rate, and increased levels of adrenocorticotropic hormone, human chorionic gonadotropin (hCG), cortisol, renin, and parathyroid hormone. Elevated serum creatinine and blood urea nitrogen (BUN) levels indicate impaired kidney function.

Kidney masses may be detected by CT scan or MRI. Ultrasound is also used to detect masses or for initial screening. Kidney biopsy may be considered to help target therapy.

◆ **Interventions: Responding**

Interventions focus on controlling the cancer and preventing metastasis (ACS, 2017).

Nonsurgical Management. Microwave ablation (MWA) or cryoablation can slow tumor growth. It is a minimally invasive procedure carried out after MRI has precisely located the tumor. MWA is used most commonly for patients who have only one kidney or who are not surgical candidates.

Traditional chemotherapy has limited effectiveness against this cancer type. Use of biologic response modifiers (BRMs) such as interleukin-2 (IL-2), interferon (INF), and tumor necrosis factor (TNF) has increased survival time (see Chapters 17 and 22). Targeted therapy agents sorafenib (Nexavar), sunitinib (Sutent), and temsirolimus (Torisel) are approved as treatment for patients with advanced RCC. Sorafenib and sunitinib are oral drugs taken daily. They are multikinase inhibitors that slow cancer cell division and inhibit blood vessel growth in the tumor. Temsirolimus is a weekly IV infusion that blocks a protein that is needed for cell division, inhibiting cancer cell division. Other targeted drugs used to treat RCC are everolimus (Afinitor) and pazopanib (Votrient) (Burchum & Rosenthal, 2016).

Surgical Management. Renal cell carcinoma is usually treated surgically by *nephrectomy* (kidney removal). Renal cell tumors are highly vascular, and blood loss during surgery is a major concern. Before surgery, the arteries supplying the kidney may be occluded (embolized) by the interventional radiologist to reduce bleeding during nephrectomy.

Preoperative Care. Instruct the patient about surgical routines (see Chapters 14 to 16). Explain the probable site of incision and the presence of dressings, drains, or other equipment after surgery. Reassure the patient about pain relief. Care before surgery may include giving blood and fluids IV to prevent shock.

Operative Procedures. The patient is placed on his or her side with the kidney to be removed uppermost. The trunk area is flexed to increase exposure of the kidney area. The eleventh or twelfth rib may need to be removed to provide better access to the kidney. The surgeon removes either part or all of the kidney and all visible tumor. The renal artery, renal vein, and fascia also may be removed. A drain may be placed in the wound before closure. The adrenal gland may be removed when the tumor is near this organ.

When a *radical* nephrectomy is performed, local and regional lymph nodes are also removed. The surgical approach may be transthoracic (as discussed in the previous paragraph), lumbar, or through the abdomen, depending on the size and location of the tumor. Radiation therapy may follow a radical nephrectomy.

Postoperative Care. Refer to Chapter 16 for care of the patient after surgery. Nursing priorities are focused on assessing kidney function to determine effectiveness of the remaining kidney, pain management, and preventing complications.

Monitoring includes assessing for hemorrhage and adrenal insufficiency. Inspect the patient's abdomen for distention from bleeding. Check the bed linens under the patient because blood may pool there. Hemorrhage or adrenal insufficiency causes hypotension, decreased urine output, and an altered level of consciousness.

A decrease in blood pressure is an early sign of both hemorrhage and adrenal insufficiency. With hypotension, urine output also decreases immediately. Large water and sodium losses in the urine occur in patients with adrenal insufficiency, leading to impaired FLUID AND ELECTROLYTE BALANCE. As a result, a large urine output is followed by hypotension and oliguria (less than 400 mL/24 hr or less than 25 mL/hr). IV replacement of fluids and packed RBCs may be needed.

The second kidney is expected to provide adequate function, but this may take days or weeks. Assess urine output hourly for the first 24 hours after surgery (urine output of 0.5 mL/kg/hr or about 30 to 50 mL/hr is acceptable). A low urine output of less than 25 to 30 mL/hr suggests decreased blood flow to the remaining kidney and potential for acute kidney injury (AKI). The hemoglobin level, hematocrit values, and white blood cell count may be measured every 6 to 12 hours for the first day or two after surgery.

Monitor the patient's temperature, pulse rate, and respiratory rate at least every 4 hours. Accurately measure and record fluid intake and output. Weigh the patient daily.

The patient may be in a special care unit for 24 to 48 hours after surgery for monitoring of bleeding and adrenal insufficiency. A drain placed near the site of incision removes residual fluid. Because of the discomfort of deep breathing, the patient is at risk for atelectasis. Fever, chills, thick sputum, or decreased breath sounds suggest pneumonia.

Managing pain after surgery usually requires opioid analgesics (e.g., hydromorphone [Dilaudid] and morphine [Statex ♣]) given IV. The incision was made through major muscle groups used with breathing and movement. Liberal use of analgesics is needed for 3 to 5 days after surgery to manage pain. Oral agents may be tried when the patient can eat and drink.

Preventing complications focuses on infection and management of adrenal insufficiency. Antibiotics may be prescribed during and after surgery to prevent infection. The need for additional antibiotics is based on evidence of infection. Assess the patient at least every 8 hours for indications of systemic infection or local wound infection.

Adrenal insufficiency is possible as a complication of kidney and adrenal gland removal. Although only one adrenal gland may be affected, the remaining gland may not be able to secrete sufficient glucocorticoids immediately after surgery. Steroid replacements may be needed in some patients. Chapter 62 discusses the signs and symptoms of acute adrenal insufficiency in detail along with specific nursing interventions.

Patient-Centered Care; Teamwork and Collaboration; Evidence-Based Practice QSEN

You admit a 68-year-old woman who was diagnosed with renal cell carcinoma after experiencing a recurrent UTI with hematuria. When her UTI did not resolve with a second course of antibiotics, the cancer was discovered with a pelvic CT scan. She is on the surgical unit for exploratory surgery and possible nephrectomy. She asks, "Is it possible that the lump that was found on my CT is not cancer? Why not just do a biopsy? That is what happened when they found a lump in my breast, and it turned out not to be cancer. If it is cancer, could I walk out of here cured?"

1. What is the rationale for not using a biopsy to evaluate a kidney mass?
2. What are the characteristics of abnormal tissue that is cancer, distinctive from tissue that is not cancer? (You may need to refer to Chapter 21.)
3. Is nephrectomy a cure for renal cell cancer? Why or why not?
4. Following a nephrectomy, what are the concerns for this patient that require follow-up monitoring?

KIDNEY TRAUMA

❖ PATHOPHYSIOLOGY

Trauma to one or both kidneys may occur with penetrating wounds or blunt injuries to the back, flank, or abdomen. Another cause of kidney trauma is urologic procedures, such as extracorporeal shock wave lithotripsy, kidney biopsy, or percutaneous renal procedures. Blunt trauma accounts for most kidney injuries. Traumatic kidney injury is classified into five grades based on the severity of the injury. Grade one consists of low-grade injury in the form of kidney bruising, and grade five represents the most severe variety associated with shattering of the kidney and tearing of its blood supply. Adults of any age can suffer kidney trauma. Strategies to prevent trauma are reviewed in Chart 67-7.

❖ INTERPROFESSIONAL COLLABORATIVE CARE

◆ Assessment: Noticing

Obtain a history of the patient's usual health and the events involved in the trauma from the patient, a witness, or emergency personnel. Document the mechanism of injury to help determine the severity of the injury. For example, blunt trauma of the kidney from car crashes usually results in an injury of low severity. Critical information to acquire is a history of kidney or urologic disease, surgical intervention, or health problems such as diabetes or hypertension.

Ureteral or renal pelvic injury often causes diffuse abdominal pain. Urine outside of the urinary tract may be visible. Ask the patient about pain in the flank or abdomen. Is the pain dull? Sharp? Constant? Intermittent? Made worse by coughing?

Assess patients with kidney injuries carefully and thoroughly. Take the patient's blood pressure, apical and peripheral pulses, respiratory rate, and temperature. Inspect both flanks for bruising, asymmetry, or penetrating injuries. Also inspect the abdomen, chest, and lower back for bruising or wounds. Percuss the abdomen for distention. Inspect the urethra for blood.

Urinalysis shows hemoglobin or RBCs from tissue damage or kidney blood vessel rupture. Microscopic examination may also show red blood cell casts, which suggest tubular damage. Hemoglobin and hematocrit values decrease with blood loss (see Chapter 37).

Diagnostic procedures include ultrasound and CT. CT scan shows greater detail about blood vessel and tissue integrity. Hematomas within or through the kidney capsule can be seen, along with the integrity and patency of the urinary tract. If the patient is being taken to the operating room emergently, a high dose of ionic or nonionic IV contrast material can be given, followed by an abdominal x-ray (KUB) to visualize the traumatic injury and any organ damage.

◆ Interventions: Responding

Nonsurgical Management. *Drug therapy* is used for bleeding prevention or control. The need for clotting factors such as vitamin K and platelets is assessed, and they are given as needed.

Fluid therapy restores circulating blood volume and ensures adequate kidney blood flow. Crystalloid solutions replace water and some electrolytes and include 0.9% sodium chloride (normal saline solution [NSS]), 5% dextrose in 0.45% sodium chloride, and lactated Ringer's solution. When bleeding is extensive, packed RBC replacement restores hemoglobin and promotes oxygenation. Fresh frozen plasma or coagulation factors may help with uncontrolled bleeding. Plasma volume expanders, such as dextran or albumin, help restore plasma oncotic pressure and reduce the onset or severity of shock or fluid displacement to interstitial tissues.

During fluid restoration, give fluids at the prescribed rate and monitor the patient for signs of shock. Take vital signs as often as every 5 to 15 minutes. Measure and record urine output hourly. Output should be greater than 0.5 mL/kg/hr.

The interventional radiologist may use percutaneous or other instrumentation to drain collections of fluid or to embolize (clot) an artery or artery segment or place a stent to repair the urethra or ureters.

> ! **NURSING SAFETY PRIORITY** QSEN
>
> **Action Alert**
>
> If the urethral opening is bleeding, consult with the urologist or primary health care provider before attempting urinary catheterization to avoid making the injury worse.

Surgical Management. Most kidney injuries are managed without surgery. Many serious injuries can be treated with minimally invasive techniques such as angiographic embolization, which accesses the arteries of the kidneys through large blood vessels in the groin, similar to a cardiac catheterization. Surgery to explore the injured kidney occurs when the patient is in shock and may be losing a lot of blood from the kidney.

CHART 67-7 Patient and Family Education: Preparing for Self-Management

Preventing Kidney and Genitourinary Trauma

- Wear a seat belt.
- Practice safe walking habits.
- Use caution when riding bicycles and motorcycles.
- Wear appropriate protective clothing when participating in contact sports.
- Avoid all contact sports and high-risk activities if you have only one kidney.

Patients who have other significant abdominal injuries, such as injuries to the bowel, spleen, or liver, and require a laparotomy may also undergo inspection and repair of the injured kidney at the same time. The aim of surgical management is to repair the injured kidney and restore its ELIMINATION function. If the kidney is severely injured (Grade 5 injury), a nephrectomy is performed.

Care Coordination and Transition Management

Teach the patient and family how to assess for infection and other complications following kidney trauma. The most common complications are urine leakage and delayed bleeding.

Instruct the patient to check the pattern and frequency of urination and note whether the color, clarity, and amount appear normal. The development of an abscess surrounding the kidney also can occur. Instruct the patient to seek medical attention for worsening hematuria, any worrisome change, or pain with voiding. Chills, fever, lethargy, and cloudy, foul-smelling urine indicate a urinary tract infection or abscess formation. Traumatic kidney injury can also cause hypertension from changes in perfusion and activation of the renin-angiotensin-aldosterone system (see Chapter 65 and Fig. 65-5). Advise the patient to seek medical care promptly for all new and concerning signs or symptoms.

GET READY FOR THE NCLEX® EXAMINATION!

KEY POINTS

Review these Key Points for each NCLEX Examination Client Needs Category.

Safe and Effective Care Environment

- Report immediately any condition that obstructs urine flow. **QSEN: Safety**
- Check the blood pressure and urine output frequently in patients who have any type of kidney problem. **QSEN: Safety**
- Report immediately to the primary health care provider any sudden decrease of urine output in a patient with kidney disease or kidney trauma. In general, adult urine output expectations are 0.5-1 mL/kg/hr. **QSEN: Safety**
- Teach all patients with any kidney disorder strategies to prevent kidney damage from dehydration or trauma. **QSEN: Safety**
- Instruct patients with any type of kidney problem to weigh daily and to notify their primary health care provider if there is a sudden weight gain. **QSEN: Patient-Centered Care**

Health Promotion and Maintenance

- Refer patients with polycystic kidney disease to a geneticist or a genetic counselor. **QSEN: Patient-Centered Care**
- Refer patients to community resources, support groups, and information organizations such as the National Kidney Foundation, the Polycystic Kidney Disease Foundation, and the American Association of Kidney Patients. **QSEN: Patient-Centered Care**
- Encourage patients with diabetes to achieve tight glycemic control. **QSEN: Patient-Centered Care**
- Encourage patients with hypertension to follow their treatment regimens to maintain blood pressure within the target range. **QSEN: Evidence-Based Practice**
- Teach patients to match daily urine output with fluid intake, usually at least 2 L for kidney health unless another health

problem requires fluid restriction. **QSEN: Evidence-Based Practice**

Psychosocial Integrity

- Allow the patient the opportunity to express fear or anxiety regarding the potential for chronic kidney disease and end-stage kidney disease. **QSEN: Patient-Centered Care**
- Assess the patient's level of comfort in discussing issues related to ELIMINATION and the genitourinary area. **QSEN: Patient-Centered Care**
- Use language with which the patient is comfortable during assessment of the kidney and urinary system. **QSEN: Patient-Centered Care**
- Explain treatment procedures to patients and families. **QSEN: Patient-Centered Care**

Physiological Integrity

- Teach patients the expected side effects and any adverse reactions to prescribed drugs, especially as they relate to kidney function. **QSEN: Patient-Centered Care**
- Teach patients the indications of disease recurrence and when to seek medical help. **QSEN: Patient-Centered Care**
- Teach patients on antibiotic therapy for a UTI (pyelonephritis) to complete the drug regimen. **QSEN: Evidence-Based Practice**
- Explain the genetics of autosomal-dominant polycystic kidney disease.
- Use laboratory data and signs and symptoms to determine the effectiveness of therapy for pyelonephritis, polycystic kidney disease, glomerulonephritis, and renal cell carcinoma.
- Be aware of the signs and symptoms of hydronephrosis.
- Be aware of the relation between kidney disease and hypertension and the associated risk for cardiovascular events.

SELECTED BIBLIOGRAPHY

Asterisk indicates a classic or definitive work on this subject.

American Cancer Society (ACS). (2017). *Cancer facts and figures 2017.* Report No. 00-300M–No. 500817. Atlanta: Author.

Brookman-May, S., Langenhuijsen, J. F., Volpe, A., Minervini, A., Joniau, S., Salagierski, M., et al. (2013). Management of localized and locally advanced renal tumors. A contemporary review of current treatment options. *Minerva Medicine, 104*(3), 237–259.

Burchum, J., & Rosenthal, L. (2016). *Lehne's pharmacology for nursing care* (9th ed.). St. Louis: Elsevier.

Canadian Cancer Society, Statistics Canada (2016). *Canadian Cancer Statistics, 2016.* Toronto: Canadian Cancer Society.

Chapman, A., Devuyst, O., Eckardt, K., Gansevoort, R., Harris, T., Horie, S., et al. (2015). Autosomal-dominant polycystic kidney disease (ADPKD): Executive summary from a Kidney Disease:

Improving global outcomes (KDIGO) controversies conference. *Kidney International, 88*(1), 17–27.

Jarvis, C. (2016). *Physical examination & health assessment* (7th ed.). St. Louis: Elsevier.

McCance, K., Huether, S., Brashers, V., & Rote, N. (2014). *Pathophysiology: The biologic basis for disease in adults and children* (7th ed.). St. Louis: Mosby.

National Kidney Foundation. (2016). *Polycystic kidney disease.* https://www.kidney.org/atoz/content/polycystic.

Nicolle, L. (2016). Urinary tract infections in adults. Chapter 37. In K. Skorecki, G. Chertow, P. Marsden, M. Taal, & A. Yu (Eds.), *Brenner and Rector's the kidney* (10th ed., pp. 1231–1256). Philadelphia: Elsevier.

Ong, A. C., Devuyst, O., Knebelmann, B., Walz, G., & Era-Edta Working Group for Inherited Kidney Diseases. (2015). Autosomal-dominant polycystic kidney disease: The changing face of clinical management. *Lancet, 385*(9981), 1993–2002.

Online Mendelian Inheritance in Man (OMIM). (2013). *Polycystic kidney disease 2; PKD2.* www.omim.org/entry/613095.

Online Mendelian Inheritance in Man (OMIM). (2016). *Polycystic kidney disease 1; PKD1.* www.omim.org/entry/173900.

Pagana, K., Pagana, T. J., & Pagana, T. N. (2017). *Mosby's diagnostic and laboratory test reference* (13th ed.). St. Louis: Mosby.

Pendergraft, W., Nachman, P., Jennette, J., & Falk, R. (2016). Primary glomerular disease. Chapter 32. In K. Skorecki, G. Chertow, P. Marsden, M. Taal, & A. Yu (Eds.), *Brenner and Rector's the kidney* (10th ed., pp. 1012–1090). Philadelphia: Elsevier.

Pengo, M. F., Soloni, P., Cecchin, D., Maiolino, G., Rossi, G. P., & Caló, L. A. (2013). Pelvic-ureteric junction obstruction and hypertension with target organ damage: A case report and review of the literature. *Blood Pressure, 22*(5), 336–339.

Skorecki, K., Chertow, G., Marsden, P., Taal, M., & Yu, A. (Eds.), (2016). *Brenner & Rector's the kidney* (10th ed.). Philadelphia: Saunders.

Tong, A., Rangan, G. K., Ruospo, M., Saglimbene, V., Strippoli, G. F., Palmer, S. C., et al. (2015). A painful inheritance-patient perspectives on living with polycystic kidney disease: Thematic synthesis of qualitative research. *Nephrology Dialysis and Transplantation, 30*(5), 790–800.

Touhy, T., & Jett, K. (2016). *Ebersole & Hess' toward healthy aging: Human needs & nursing response.* St. Louis: Elsevier.

U.S. Renal Data Systems. (2015). *2015 USRDS Annual Data Report. Epidemiology of Kidney Disease in the United States.* National Institutes of Health, National Institute of Diabetes and Digestive and Kidney Diseases, Bethesda, MD. http://www.usrds.org/adr.aspx.

68 | CHAPTER

Care of Patients With Acute Kidney Injury and Chronic Kidney Disease

Chris Winkelman

 http://evolve.elsevier.com/Iggy/

PRIORITY AND INTERRELATED CONCEPTS

The priority concept for this chapter is ELIMINATION.

✳ The ELIMINATION concept exemplar for this chapter is Chronic Kidney Disease, p. 1398.

The interrelated concepts for this chapter are:
- ACID-BASE BALANCE
- FLUID AND ELECTROLYTE BALANCE
- IMMUNITY
- PERFUSION

LEARNING OUTCOMES

Safe and Effective Care Environment

1. Collaborate with the interprofessional team to coordinate high-quality care and promote urinary ELIMINATION in patients who have acute kidney injury or chronic kidney disease.
2. Teach the patient and caregiver(s) about home safety issues affected by impaired ELIMINATION and impairment of FLUID AND ELECTROLYTE BALANCE or ACID-BASE BALANCE resulting from acute kidney injury or chronic kidney disease.
3. Prioritize evidence-based care for patients with impaired urinary ELIMINATION from either acute kidney injury or chronic renal failure.

Health Promotion and Maintenance

4. Identify community resources for patients requiring assistance with management of altered ELIMINATION as a result of acute kidney injury or chronic kidney disease.
5. Teach adults how to decrease the risk for acute kidney injury or chronic kidney disease resulting in impaired urinary ELIMINATION.

Psychosocial Integrity

6. Implement nursing interventions to help patients and families cope with the psychosocial impact caused by acute kidney injury or chronic kidney disease.

Physiological Integrity

7. Apply knowledge of anatomy, physiology, and pathophysiology to assess patients with impaired kidney function from acute kidney injury or chronic kidney disease affecting ELIMINATION, FLUID AND ELECTROLYTE BALANCE, or ACID-BASE BALANCE.
8. Teach the patient and caregiver(s) about common drugs and other strategies used for acute kidney injury and chronic kidney disease, including pain control and depression management.
9. Implement evidence-based nursing interventions to prevent complications in patients undergoing kidney replacement therapy when urinary ELIMINATION is not effective in clearing waste or toxins.

The kidney function of urinary ELIMINATION includes excretion of waste, FLUID AND ELECTROLYTE BALANCE, regulation of ACID-BASE BALANCE, and hormone secretion. These processes are greatly impaired with kidney function loss, and every organ system is affected. Acute kidney injury (AKI) is most common in the acute care setting, whereas chronic kidney disease (CKD) is more likely to be seen in community settings or as a coexisting condition in acute care settings. The features of AKI and CKD are described in Table 68-1.

Both types of kidney problems can require kidney replacement therapy (e.g., dialysis). When kidney function is permanently or persistently impaired, as with end-stage kidney disease (ESKD), dialysis or kidney transplant is a lifesaving approach for urinary ELIMINATION to maintain homeostasis, FLUID AND ELECTROLYTE BALANCE, and ACID-BASE BALANCE. ESKD reduces independence, shortens life, and decreases quality of life. Many diseases and conditions are associated with the onset and severity of kidney function loss.

TABLE 68-1   Features of Acute Kidney Injury and Chronic Kidney Disease

CHARACTERISTIC	ACUTE KIDNEY INJURY	CHRONIC KIDNEY DISEASE
Onset	Sudden (hours to days)	Gradual (months to years)
% of nephron involvement	50%-95%	Varies by stage; generally symptomatic with 75% loss and dialysis with 90%-95% loss
Duration	May not progress; full recovery (return to baseline) possible ESKD occurs in 10%-20% with lifetime reliance on dialysis or kidney transplant	Progressive and permanent Treatment and lifestyle can slow progression and delay onset of ESKD
Prognosis	Good when kidney function is maintained or returns High mortality associated with renal replacement therapy requirements or prolonged illness	Progression of CKD depends on stage of GFR, stage of albuminuria, and specific conditions associated with the onset of the disorder ESKD fatal without a renal replacement therapy (dialysis or transplantation) Reduced life span and potential for complex medical regimen even with optimal treatment

CKD, Chronic kidney disease; *ESKD,* end-stage kidney disease; *GFR,* glomerular filtration rate.

TABLE 68-2   The KDIGO Classification System for Severity of Acute Kidney Injury

STAGE	SERUM CREATININE	URINE OUTPUT
Stage 1	Increased × 1.5-1.9 baseline or by ≥ 0.3 mg/dL (>26.2 mcmol/L)	<0.5 mL/kg/hr for 6-12 hr
Stage 2	Increased × 2-2.9 baseline	<0.5 mL/kg/hr for ≥12 hr
Stage 3	Increased × 3 baseline or by >4 mg/dL (≥354 mcmol/L) or initiation of renal replacement therapy	<0.3 mL/kg/hr for ≥24 hr or Anuria for ≥12 hr

KDIGO, **K**idney **D**isease: **I**mproving **G**lobal **O**utcomes (2013).

occurs over a few hours or days. The most current definition of AKI is an increase in serum creatinine by 0.3 mg/dL (26.2 mcmol/L) or more within 48 hours; or an increase in serum creatinine to 1.5 times or more from baseline, which is known or presumed to have occurred in the previous 7 days; or a urine volume of less than 0.5 mL/kg/hr for 6 hours (Dirkes, 2016; KDIGO, 2013). Criteria for staging the severity of AKI are in Table 68-2. These criteria are not applied universally but do provide the best evidence to date for early identification of AKI (Hain & Paixao, 2015). New biomarkers of tubular injury have great promise for improving the diagnosis and management of AKI (Dirkes, 2015).

Although glomerular filtration rate (GFR) is accepted as the best overall indicator of kidney function, it is not accurate during acute and critical illness (Puzantian & Townsend, 2013). Estimations of GFR from serum creatinine are affected by metabolic problems and treatments during critical illnesses. Urine output is altered when diuretics or IV fluids are used. AKI also causes systemic effects and complications described in Table 68-3. These complications increase discomfort and risk for death. Duration of oliguria or anuria closely correlates with lack of recovery of kidney function; the longer the duration of oliguria or anuria, the less likely it is that the patient will return to full or baseline kidney function.

Etiology

The causes of AKI are reduced PERFUSION to the kidneys, damage to kidney tissue, and obstruction of urine outflow. Diseases and conditions associated with reduced kidney PERFUSION, kidney damage, and urinary obstruction are listed in Table 68-4. (The diseases in Table 68-3 are described elsewhere in this text.)

Notice that several conditions resulting in AKI are listed more than once in Table 68-4. For example, coagulopathy (disorders of bleeding and clotting; see Chapter 40) reduces perfusion, causes inflammation and direct tissue damage, and creates obstruction of urinary flow.

Any patient with a pre-existing reduced GFR or elevated albumin-creatinine ratio is at increased risk for AKI during hospitalization (Grams et al., 2015). AKI is more likely to occur in hospitalized adults with advanced age or who have pre-existing conditions such as hypertension, diabetes, peripheral vascular disease, liver disease, or CKD (Thornburg & Gray-Vickery, 2016). Sepsis (see Chapter 37), cardiac surgery, hypotension, shock, or prolonged mechanical ventilation (see Chapter 32) also are independent risk factors for the development of AKI (Vrtis, 2013).

When kidney function declines gradually, it is diagnosed as CKD, formerly termed *chronic renal failure (CRF).* The patient may have many years of abnormal blood urea nitrogen and creatinine values, sometimes called *renal insufficiency,* before ESKD develops. When kidney function decline is sudden, acute kidney injury (AKI) is diagnosed. AKI can be a temporary condition that resolves, or it can progress to CKD. Even without progression to CKD, AKI is associated with high mortality in critically ill adults (Dirkes, 2015). AKI also can occur in a patient with established CKD. When these two conditions co-occur, the loss of kidney function and waste ELIMINATION is usually more severe and accelerated.

Acute kidney injury affects *many* body systems. Chronic kidney disease affects *every* body system. The problems that occur with kidney function loss are related to disturbances of FLUID AND ELECTROLYTE BALANCE, disturbances of ACID-BASE BALANCE, buildup of nitrogen-based wastes (uremia), and loss of kidney hormone function.

ACUTE KIDNEY INJURY

❖ *PATHOPHYSIOLOGY*

Acute kidney injury (AKI) is a rapid reduction in kidney function resulting in a failure to maintain waste ELIMINATION, FLUID AND ELECTROLYTE BALANCE, and ACID-BASE BALANCE. AKI

TABLE 68-3 Systemic Complications From Acute Kidney Injury

Metabolic
- Metabolic acidosis
- Hyperlipidemia
- Hyperkalemia
- Hyponatremia
- Hypocalcemia
- Hypophosphatemia

Cardiopulmonary
- Peripheral and pulmonary edema
- Heart failure
- Pulmonary embolism
- Pericarditis
- Pericardial effusion
- Hypertension
- Myocardial infarction

Neurologic
- Neuromuscular irritability or weakness
- Asterixis
- Seizures
- Mental status changes

Immune/Infectious
- Pneumonia
- Sepsis

Gastrointestinal
- Nausea
- Vomiting
- Decreased peristalsis
- Enteral nutrition intolerance
- Malnutrition
- Ulcer formation
- Bleeding

Hematologic
- Bleeding
- Thrombosis
- Anemia

Renal
- Chronic kidney disease (CKD)
- End-stage kidney disease (ESKD)

Other
- Hiccups
- Elevated parathyroid hormone
- Low thyroid hormone

TABLE 68-4 Diseases and Conditions That Contribute to Acute Kidney Injury

Perfusion Reduction (Prerenal Causes)
- Blood or fluid loss (e.g., surgery or trauma; severe sepsis, septic shock, or hypovolemic shock)
- Blood pressure drugs resulting in hypotension
- Heart attack or heart failure resulting in low ejection fraction and low cardiac output
- Infection (e.g., sepsis, septic shock)
- Liver failure
- Use of aspirin, ibuprofen (e.g., Advil, Motrin IB), naproxen (e.g., Aleve), or NSAIDs
- Severe allergic reaction (anaphylaxis)
- Severe burns
- Severe dehydration
- Renal artery stenosis
- Bleeding or clotting in the kidney blood vessels (coagulopathy)
- Atherosclerosis or cholesterol deposits that block blood flow in the kidneys

Kidney Damage (Intrinsic or Intrarenal Causes)
- Glomerulonephritis or inflammation of the glomeruli
- Bleeding in the kidney
- Thrombi or emboli in the kidney blood vessels
- Hemolytic uremic syndrome, a condition of premature destruction of red blood cells caused by infection
- Systemic infection (sepsis)
- Local infection (pyelonephritis)
- Lupus, an immune system disorder causing glomerulonephritis
- Drugs, such as certain chemotherapy agents, antibiotics, iodinated or hyperosmolar contrast media used during imaging tests (contrast-induced nephropathy), many antibiotics, and zoledronic acid (Reclast, Zometa), used to treat osteoporosis and high blood calcium levels (hypercalcemia)
- Multiple myeloma, a cancer of the plasma cells
- Scleroderma, a group of rare diseases affecting the skin and connective tissues
- Thrombotic thrombocytopenic purpura (TTP), a rare platelet disorder that increases clotting
- Ingested toxins, such as alcohol, heavy metals, and cocaine
- Vasculitis, an inflammation of blood vessels
- Ischemia in kidney tissue, including hypoxemia from respiratory and cardiac arrest

Urine Flow Obstruction (Postrenal Causes)
- Bladder cancer
- Cervical cancer
- Colon cancer
- Prostate cancer
- Enlarged prostate (prostate hypertrophy)
- Kidney stones (nephrolithiasis and ureterolithiasis)
- Nerve damage involving the nerves that control the bladder (neurogenic bladder)
- Blood clots in the urinary tract

Traditionally, AKI caused by reduced PERFUSION with a sustained mean arterial pressure (MAP) of less than 65 mm Hg is classed as prerenal failure. It is the most common cause of AKI in acute care. Damage to kidney tissue is classed as intrarenal or intrinsic renal failure and reflects injury to the glomeruli, nephrons, or tubules. Obstruction of urine flow is also called postrenal failure. Although this classification system is controversial, it provides a framework to guide care for prevention and treatment of AKI (Fournier, 2013). Any of these conditions can occur together. Coagulopathies can cause prerenal, intrarenal, and postrenal AKI.

With prerenal or postrenal pathology, the kidney compensates by the three responses of constricting kidney blood vessels, activating the renin-angiotensin-aldosterone pathway, and releasing antidiuretic hormone (ADH). These responses increase blood volume and improve kidney PERFUSION. However, these same responses reduce urine ELIMINATION, resulting in oliguria (urine output less than 400 mL/day) and azotemia (the retention and buildup of nitrogenous wastes in the blood). Toxins can also cause blood vessel constriction in the kidney, leading to reduced kidney blood flow, oliguria, and azotemia.

Activated IMMUNITY and damage from kidney toxins (nephrotoxins) (Table 68-5) cause intracellular changes of the tubular system in kidney tissue. Inflammatory proteins and immune-mediated complexes can damage cells and tissues in the kidney. With extensive damage, tubular cells slough and nephrons lose the ability to repair themselves. The presence of tubular debris and sediment in urine from kidney tissue damage (intrarenal failure or *acute tubular necrosis*) is related to systemic ischemia, reduced kidney PERFUSION, or nephrotoxin exposure.

Even with severe AKI (i.e., stage 2 or 3 in Table 68-2), some adults return to baseline kidney function during recovery from illness. It is the responsibility of all health care professionals to be alert to the possibility of AKI and implement prevention strategies when risk factors are present. *Timely interventions to remove the cause of AKI may prevent progression to ESKD and the need for lifelong renal replacement therapy or a renal transplant.*

Incidence and Prevalence

The reported prevalence of AKI from United States data ranges from 1% (community-acquired) up to 7.1% (hospital-acquired) among adults admitted to a hospital. As many as 30% of patients admitted to an ICU experience an episode of AKI (Fournier,

TABLE 68-5 Examples of Potentially Nephrotoxic Substances

Drugs

Antibiotics/Antimicrobials
- Amphotericin B
- Colistimethate
- Methicillin
- Polymyxin B
- Rifampin
- Sulfonamides
- Tetracycline hydrochloride
- Vancomycin

Aminoglycoside Antibiotics
- Gentamicin
- Kanamycin
- Neomycin
- Netilmicin sulfate
- Tobramycin

Chemotherapy Agents
- Cisplatin
- Cyclophosphamide
- Methotrexate

NSAIDs
- Celecoxib
- Flurbiprofen
- Ibuprofen
- Indomethacin
- Ketorolac
- Meclofenamate
- Meloxicam
- Nabumetone
- Naproxen
- Oxaprozin
- Rofecoxib
- Tolmetin

Other Drugs
- Acetaminophen
- Captopril
- Cyclosporine
- Fluorinate anesthetics
- Metformin
- D-Penicillamine
- Phenazopyridine hydrochloride
- Quinine

Other Substances

Organic Solvents
- Carbon tetrachloride
- Ethylene glycol

Nondrug Chemical Agents
- Radiographic contrast medium (e.g., iodinated media, hyperosmolar media, and gadolinium)
- Pesticides
- Fungicides
- Myoglobin (from breakdown of skeletal muscle)

Heavy Metals and Ions
- Arsenic
- Bismuth
- Copper sulfate
- Gold salts
- Lead
- Mercuric chloride

2013). Transient azotemia and oliguria are common among all inpatients. AKI is associated with an in-hospital and 1-year mortality rate of up to 60% (Ralib et al., 2013).

Health Promotion and Maintenance

Keep in mind that dehydration (severe blood volume depletion) reduces PERFUSION *and can lead to AKI even in adults who have no known kidney problems.* Urge all healthy adults to avoid dehydration by drinking 2 to 3 L of water daily. This is especially important for athletes or anyone who performs strenuous exercise or work and sweats heavily.

Nurses have an essential role in the prevention of AKI in hospitalized patients. Always be on the lookout for signs of impending kidney dysfunction through assessment and close monitoring of laboratory values. Early recognition and correction of problems causing reduced urinary ELIMINATION may avoid kidney tissue damage. Evaluate the patient's fluid status. Accurately measure intake and output and check body weight to identify changes in fluid balance. Note the characteristics of the urine and report new sediment, hematuria (smoky or red color), foul odor, or other worrisome changes. Immediately report a urine output of less than 0.5 mL/kg/hr that persists for more than 2 hours to the primary health care provider (Ralib et al., 2013). Waiting for 6 hours of oliguria to meet AKI criteria may allow progression of kidney damage—act early!

! NURSING SAFETY PRIORITY QSEN

Critical Rescue

In any acute care setting, preventing volume depletion and providing intervention early when volume depletion occurs are nursing priorities. Reduced PERFUSION from volume depletion is a common cause of AKI. Assess continually to recognize the signs and symptoms of volume depletion (low urine output, decreased systolic blood pressure, decreased pulse pressure, orthostatic hypotension, thirst, rising blood osmolarity). Respond by intervening early with oral fluids or, in the patient who is unable to take or tolerate oral fluid, requesting an increase in IV fluid rate from the primary health care provider to prevent permanent kidney damage.

Monitor laboratory values for any changes that reflect poor kidney function. A significant increase in creatinine, especially when the increase occurs over hours or a few days, is a concern and must be reported urgently to the primary health care provider. Other laboratory values that help monitor kidney function include serum blood urea nitrogen (BUN); serum potassium, sodium, and osmolarity; and urine specific gravity, albumin-creatinine ratio, and electrolytes. Know the baseline (steady-state) GFR because a reduced GFR makes the patient more vulnerable to AKI.

Be aware of nephrotoxic substances that the patient may ingest or be exposed to (see Table 68-5). Question any prescription for potentially nephrotoxic drugs, and validate the dose before the patient receives the drug. Many antibiotics have nephrotoxic effects. NSAIDs can cause or increase the risk for AKI. Combining two or more nephrotoxic drugs dramatically increases the risk for AKI. If a patient must receive a known nephrotoxic drug, closely monitor laboratory values, including BUN, creatinine, and drug peak and trough levels, for indications of reduced kidney function. When nephrotoxic agents are used, including contrast medium, nephrons may be protected by administering a pretreatment oral or IV bolus of fluid volume (Lambert et al., 2017).

❖ INTERPROFESSIONAL COLLABORATIVE CARE

AKI is managed initially in the hospital setting, most commonly in an ICU. During the acute phase of the problem, members of the interprofessional team include the nephrologist, nephrology nurse, registered dietitian, pharmacist, and dialysis technician. The responsibilities of each of these professionals are described within the interventions sections of this chapter. When the patient is discharged before urinary ELIMINATION returns to normal, continuing management is needed as part of the transition to community care.

◆ Assessment: Noticing

History. The accurate diagnosis of AKI, including its cause, depends on a detailed history. Know the risk factors for and criteria of AKI and chronic kidney disease (CKD). Ask about any change in urine appearance, frequency, or volume.

Ask about recent surgery or trauma, transfusions, allergic (hypersensitivity) reactions, or other factors that might lead to reduced kidney PERFUSION. Obtain a drug history, especially use of antibiotics and NSAIDs. Ask about recent imaging procedures requiring injection of a contrast medium. Coexisting conditions of advanced age, diabetes, long-term hypertension, major or systemic infection (sepsis), systemic inflammation, low cholesterol levels, and coagulopathy or treatment for bleeding or clotting disorders increase the risk for AKI (Dirkes, 2016).

To identify IMMUNITY-mediated AKI (i.e., acute glomerulonephritis), ask about acute illnesses such as influenza, colds, gastroenteritis, and sore throats. Allergic reactions from a drug or food allergy may result in AKI as late as 10 days after exposure. Ask about rashes, hives, or fever and evaluate the white blood cell differential for an increased eosinophil count.

Anticipate AKI following any episode of hypotension or shock. Any problem in which the blood volume is depleted can contribute to AKI by reducing PERFUSION. Such problems include cardiac bypass surgery, extensive bowel preparations, being NPO before surgery, or dehydration from exercise. Recent use of IV vasopressors (e.g., epinephrine or norepinephrine) may contribute to AKI when blood volume is reduced (hypovolemia).

Consider whether there is a history of urinary obstructive problems. Ask the patient about any difficulty in starting the urine stream, changes in the amount or appearance of the urine, narrowing of the urine stream, nocturia, urgency, or symptoms of kidney stones. Also ask about any cancer history that may cause urinary obstruction.

CONSIDERATIONS FOR OLDER ADULTS
Patient-Centered Care QSEN

Prevention of AKI in older adults first involves recognition of their increased vulnerability to kidney injury. There is a 20% greater rate of AKI among older adults in an ICU compared to younger adults (Hain & Paixao, 2015). Structural and functional changes in the aging kidney contribute to the risk for AKI. As kidneys age, there are fewer nephrons, more sclerotic glomeruli, and renal artery arteriosclerosis leading to reduced kidney PERFUSION and a decline in GFR. Age-related changes in tubular function decrease the ability to regulate sodium and potassium balance and to concentrate urine, increasing the risk for blood volume depletion (Touhy & Jett, 2016).

The use of multiple drugs is associated with drug-induced AKI, particularly in acute and critical care settings. Assess risk and take actions to reduce exposure to nephrotoxic agents, avoid hypotension and hypovolemia, evaluate drug-drug interactions for potential adverse kidney effects, and stop unnecessary drugs to maintain kidney function in older adults.

Physical Assessment/Signs and Symptoms. If a patient has a urinary catheter, assess urine output every hour after surgery until stable, during fluid resuscitation for shock or hypotension, and when the patient has a high risk for AKI following hospital admission. Even a brief period of oliguria, defined as less than 0.5 mL/kg/hour of urine output for 2 or more hours, can signal AKI.

Other symptoms of AKI are related to the buildup of nitrogenous wastes (azotemia) and decreased urine output (oliguria). As AKI progresses in severity, the patient may have symptoms of fluid overload because fluid is not eliminated. Indications of fluid overload include pulmonary crackles, dependent and generalized edema (anasarca), decreased oxygenation (low peripheral oxygenation or SpO2), confusion, increased respiratory rate, and dyspnea. See Chapter 11 for assessment of fluid overload.

Evaluate vital signs to recognize early hypoperfusion and hypoxemia. Symptoms of reduced blood volume such as mean arterial pressure (MAP) <65 mm Hg, tachycardia, thready peripheral pulses, or decreasing cognition may indicate risk for

AKI from poor PERFUSION; whereas an SpO2 <88% may indicate potential hypoxemic or ischemic damage to kidney tissue.

Laboratory Assessment. The many changes in laboratory values in the patient with AKI are similar to those occurring in chronic kidney disease (CKD) (Chart 68-1). Expect to see rising creatinine and BUN levels and abnormal blood electrolytes values. However, patients with AKI usually do *not* have the anemia associated with CKD unless there is blood loss from another condition (e.g., surgery, trauma) or when BUN levels are high enough to break (lyse) red blood cells.

In early AKI, urine tests provide important information. Urine sodium levels may reflect an inability to concentrate urine. Urine may be dilute with a specific gravity near 1.000 or concentrated with a specific gravity greater than 1.030. The presence of urine sediment (e.g., red blood cells, casts, and tubular cells), myoglobin, or hemoglobin may lead to nephron damage.

Imaging Assessment. Ultrasonography is useful in the diagnosis of kidney and urinary tract obstruction. Dilation of the renal calyces and collecting ducts, as well as stones, can be detected. Ultrasonography can show kidney size and patency of the ureters. Small kidney size may indicate an underlying CKD with loss of kidney tissue.

CT scans without contrast medium can determine adequacy of kidney PERFUSION and identify obstruction or tumors. Contrast medium is usually avoided to prevent further kidney damage (Lambert et al., 2017). An MRI may be used in place of CT scan.

X-rays of the pelvis or kidneys, ureters, and bladder (KUB) may provide an initial view of kidneys and the urinary tract to determine the cause of AKI. Enlarged kidneys with obstruction may show hydronephrosis. X-rays can show stones obstructing the renal pelvis, ureters, or bladder. More commonly, ultrasound is used to screen for hydronephrosis.

A nuclear medicine study called *MAG3* may be used to determine the nature of the kidney failure and measure GFR. A renal scan can determine whether PERFUSION of the kidneys is sufficient. Cystoscopy or retrograde pyelography may be needed to identify obstructions of the lower urinary tract (see Chapter 65).

Other Diagnostic Assessments. Kidney biopsy is performed if the cause of AKI is uncertain and symptoms persist or an immunologic disease is suspected. Prepare the patient before the test, particularly managing both hypotension and hypertension. Hypertension increases the risk for intrarenal hemorrhage following needle biopsy. Provide follow-up care. Be aware of all test results and understand how they might affect the treatment regimen. (See Chapter 65 for a detailed discussion of diagnostic tests related to the kidney.)

NCLEX EXAMINATION CHALLENGE 68-1
Safe and Effective Care Environment

The client is a 62-year-old admitted 2 days ago with traumatic injuries and hypovolemic shock from a car crash. The nurse reviewing the client's daily laboratory test results notices the following values. Which result is **most important** to report to the primary health care provider immediately?

A. Serum sodium 132 mEq/L (mmol/L)
B. Serum potassium 6.9 mEq/L (mmol/L)
C. Blood urea nitrogen 24 mg/dL (mmol/L)
D. Hematocrit 32% (0.32 volume fraction); hemoglobin 9.2 g/dL (92 g/L)

⚡ **CHART 68-1** **Laboratory Profile**

Kidney Disease

TEST	NORMAL RANGE FOR ADULTS	VALUES IN KIDNEY DISEASE
Serum creatinine	*Male:* 0.6-1.2 mg/dL (53-106 mcmol/L) *Female:* 0.5-1.1 mg/dL (44-97 mcmol/L) *Older adults:* Decreased *Older adults:* May be slightly increased	**In Chronic Kidney Disease** May increase by 0.5-1.0 mg/dL (50-100 mcmol/L) every 1-2 years May be as high as 15-30 mg/dL (500-1000 mcmol/L) *before symptoms* of severe CKD are present **In Acute Kidney Injury** Increase of 1-2 mg/dL (100-200 mcmol/L) every 24-48 hr May increase 1-6 mg/dL (100-600 mcmol/L) in 1 week or less
Serum sodium	136-145 mEq/L (136-145 mmol/L)	Normal, increased, or decreased
Serum potassium	3.5-5.0 mEq/L (3.5-5.0 mmol/L)	Increased
Serum phosphorus (phosphate)	3.0-4.5 mg/dL (0.97-1.45 mmol/L) *Older adults:* May be slightly decreased	Increased
Serum calcium	Total calcium: 9.0-10.5 mg/dL (2.25-2.75 mmol/L) Ionized calcium: 4.5-5.6 mg/dL (1.05-1.3 mmol/L) *Older adults:* Slightly decreased	Decreased
Serum magnesium	1.3-2.1 mEq/L (0.74-1.07 mmol/L)	Increased
Serum carbon dioxide combining power (bicarbonate) (venous)	23-30 mEq/L (23-30 mmol/L)	Decreased
Arterial blood pH	7.35-7.45	Decreased (in metabolic acidosis) or normal
Arterial blood bicarbonate (HCO_3^-)	21-28 mEq/L (21-28 mmol/L)	Decreased
Arterial blood $PaCO_2$	35-45 mm Hg	Decreased
Hemoglobin	*Female:* 12-16 g/dL (120-160 g/L) *Male:* 14-18 g/dL (140-180 g/L) *Older adults:* Slightly decreased	Decreased
Hematocrit	*Female:* 37%-47% (0.37–0.47 volume fraction) *Male:* 42%-52% (0.42-0.52 volume fraction) *Older adults:* May be slightly decreased	Decreased to 20%
Blood osmolarity	280-300 mOsm/L (mmol/L)	Elevated in volume-depleted states, increasing the risk for acute kidney injury
Blood osmolality	280-300 mOsm/kg (mmol/kg)	Elevated in volume-depleted states, increasing the risk for acute kidney injury

Data from Pagana, K., Pagana, T., & Pike-McDonald, S. (2013). *Mosby's Canadian manual of diagnostic and laboratory tests.* St. Louis: Elsevier; and Pagana, K., Pagana, T., & Pagana T. (2017). *Mosby's diagnostic and laboratory test reference* (13th ed.). St. Louis: Mosby.
CKD, Chronic kidney disease; *SI,* International System of Units.

◆ **Interventions: Responding**

Avoid hypotension and maintain normal fluid balance *(euvolemia)* to prevent and manage AKI. A reduction in kidney PERFUSION may initially not be recognized when there is no associated drop in systemic blood pressure. Autoregulation and the renin-angiotensin-aldosterone system (RAAS) effectively maintain normal kidney perfusion and glomerular filtration rate. However, these mechanisms may not be adequate in the critically ill patient, and some experts suggest maintaining a mean arterial pressure (MAP) of 80 mm Hg in high-risk or critically ill adults (Hain & Paixao, 2015). Ensure that the patient's MAP goal is shared with all interprofessional health team members.

Reduce exposure to nephrotoxic agents and drugs that alter kidney perfusion. When such substances cannot be avoided, monitor drug levels and communicate with the pharmacist to adjust doses to minimize harm. Contrast media can have serious toxic effects on tubular cells (Lambert et al., 2017). Ensure that kidney function is assessed before an imaging test that includes contrast media. A large volume of contrast, agents with high osmolarity (>2000 mOsm/L [mmol/L]), and frequent administration (given twice in 3 months or more often) of agents are more likely to cause contrast-induced nephropathy. Ensure that kidney function is assessed before an imaging test and that both the radiologist and the requesting primary health care provider are aware of reduced kidney function before contrast medium is given.

Communicate with the radiologist so the lowest dose of the contrast agent is used in high-risk adults. Adequate hydration is essential to prevent contrast-induced nephropathy (Honicker & Holt, 2016; Lambert et al., 2017). The patient may receive IV fluids at a rate of 1 mL/kg/hr for 12 hours before the imaging test or at 3 mL/kg/hour for 1 hour just before the procedure to ensure hydration and dilution of the contrast medium and to speed urinary ELIMINATION of the agent. A common desired outcome for patients undergoing a procedure with contrast medium is a urine output of 150 mL/hr for the first 6 hours after administration of the contrast agent.

Observations about new-onset or increased peripheral edema, increased daily weight, and reduced urine output can identify patients with a positive fluid balance from AKI who may require treatment with fluid restriction or diuretic therapy. Impairment of ACID-BASE BALANCE and electrolyte imbalance can occur and may require treatment, especially in older adults.

Blood sampling of patients at risk for AKI allows early recognition of elevated serum creatinine levels and trend data. Communicate observations about worsening kidney function early and often to the primary health care provider so interventions can promote kidney health and interrupt the progression of AKI when it occurs.

Not all patients with AKI experience oliguria. IMMUNITY and inflammatory causes of AKI may allow proteins to enter the glomerulus, and these proteins can hold fluid in the filtrate, causing a *polyuria* (excess urine output) that disrupts FLUID AND ELECTROLYTE BALANCE. During AKI with high-volume urine output, hypovolemia and electrolyte *loss* are the main problems. The patient in the diuretic phase of AKI needs a plan of care that focuses on fluid and electrolyte *replacement* and monitoring. Onset of polyuria can signal the start of recovery from AKI.

Surviving kidney tubule cells possess a remarkable ability to regenerate and proliferate, and early identification can stop progression of AKI, as well as aid in recovery of kidney function. Base the desired outcomes of care on collaboration and communication with interprofessional team members. Update the plan of care for either restriction (when fluid overload from new AKI is present) or liberal administration of fluid (to prevent AKI or promote elimination of contrast medium) based on timely and accurate team communication.

Frequent laboratory value monitoring, close surveillance of intake and output, drug therapy, nutrition, careful administration of fluids and minerals, and renal replacement therapy are commonly used to manage AKI.

💡 NCLEX EXAMINATION CHALLENGE 68-2

Safe and Effective Care Environment

Which actions/interventions are **most important** for the nurse to perform when caring for a 70-year-old client who is scheduled for a contrast-medium enhanced CT scan? **Select all that apply.**

A. Assess for coexisting conditions of pre-existing diabetes, heart failure, and established CKD.

B. Assess the hourly urine output for at least 6 hours before the procedure.

C. Assess creatinine clearance using a 24-hour urine collection test.

D. Alert the primary health care provider to a serum creatinine that has increased from 0.2 to 0.4 mg/dL (20-40 mcmol/L) in the previous 24 hours.

E. Alert the primary health care provider to a glomerular filtration rate (GFR) <60 mL/min/1.73 m^2.

F. Assess for hypovolemia, including evaluation of the mean arterial pressure (MAP).

G. Collaborate with the primary health care provider to determine whether isotonic IV fluids should be infused before the test.

H. Discuss with the primary health care provider about whether the client's prescribed diuretic should be held immediately before the test.

Drug Therapy. The interprofessional team consults the inpatient pharmacist for drug adjustment based on kidney function. As kidney function changes, drug dosages are changed. It is important to be knowledgeable about the site of drug metabolism and especially careful when giving drugs. Continuously monitor the patient with AKI for adverse drug events and interactions of the drugs that he or she is receiving. Diuretics may be used to increase urine output in AKI. Diuretic-induced urine output does not preserve kidney function or stop AKI, but diuretics do rid the body of retained fluid and electrolytes in the patient with AKI that has not progressed to end-stage kidney disease (ESKD).

Fluid challenges are often used to promote kidney PERFUSION. In patients without fluid overload, 500 to 1000 mL of normal saline may be infused over 1 hour. Patients with AKI often require central venous pressure (CVP) monitoring during a fluid challenge. When cardiac disease is also present and worsening, measurement of pulmonary arterial pressure by means of a pulmonary artery catheter for accurate evaluation of hemodynamic status may be needed. During fluid challenges, closely assess the response to fluid and slow the infusion if indications of fluid overload, particularly respiratory distress, occur.

Investigation is ongoing to identify biomarkers that can indicate kidney injury early. Neutrophil gelatinase-associated lipocalin (NGAL) and cystatin C appear to signal adverse changes in the kidney and may be useful to guide treatment (Dirkes, 2015).

Nutrition Therapy. Patients who have AKI often have a high rate of *catabolism* (protein breakdown). Increases in metabolism and protein breakdown may be related to the stress of illness and the increase in blood levels of catecholamines, cortisol, and glucagon. The rate of protein breakdown correlates with the severity of uremia and azotemia. Catabolism causes the breakdown of muscle protein and increases azotemia.

The interprofessional team's registered dietitian in the ICU setting calculates the patient's protein and caloric needs. A consultation may need to be requested for inpatients outside of the ICU or for those in the community settings. Work with the dietitian to establish a diet with specified amounts of protein, sodium, and fluids. For the patient who does not require dialysis, 0.6 g/kg of body weight or 40 g/day of protein is usually prescribed. For patients who require dialysis, the protein level needed ranges from 1 to 1.5 g/kg. The dietary sodium ranges from 60 to 90 mEq/kg (mmol/kg). If high blood potassium levels are present, dietary potassium is restricted to 60 to 70 mEq/kg (mmol/kg). The daily amount of fluid permitted is calculated to be equal to the urine volume plus 500 mL. Assess food intake every shift to ensure that caloric intake is adequate.

Many patients with AKI are too ill, or their appetite is too poor to meet caloric goals. For these patients, nutrition support with oral supplements, enteral nutrition, or parenteral nutrition (PN or hyperalimentation) is needed. Nutrition support in AKI aims to provide sufficient nutrients to maintain or improve nutrition status, preserve lean body mass, restore or maintain fluid balance, and preserve kidney function.

There are several kidney-specific formulations of oral supplements and enteral solutions (e.g., Nepro, Suplena Renalcal, and NovaSource Renal). Most specialty formulas for patients with kidney problems are lower in sodium, potassium, and phosphorus and higher in calories than are standard feedings. Enteral nutrition, delivered with a nasogastric or nasojejunal tube (these tubes can also be placed orally), can be used for nutrition support. If PN is used, the IV solutions are mixed to meet the patient's specific needs. Because kidney function is unstable in AKI, continuously monitor intake and output and serum electrolyte levels to determine how the supplementation affects FLUID AND ELECTROLYTE BALANCE. IV fat emulsion (Intralipid) infusions can provide a nonprotein source of calories. In uremic patients, fat emulsions are used in place of glucose to avoid the problems of excessive sugars.

Kidney Replacement Therapy. Kidney replacement therapy (KRT), also called renal replacement therapy (RRT), is used for patients with loss of kidney function and inadequate waste ELIMINATION. Indications for KRT include symptomatic uremia (e.g., pericarditis, neuropathy, decline in cognition), persistent or rapidly rising high potassium levels (i.e., greater than 6.5 mEq/L [mmol/L]), severe metabolic acidosis (pH less than 7.1), or fluid overload that inhibits tissue PERFUSION. When AKI occurs with drug or alcohol intoxication, KRT also can remove toxins.

Immediate vascular access for KRT in patients with AKI is made by placement of a catheter specific for dialysis (Fig. 68-1). The temporary catheter is placed in a central vein, most often the internal jugular (Schell-Chaple, 2017), using best practices to avoid catheter-associated bloodstream infections (see Chapter 13). Placement of the catheter requires informed consent and a "time-out" similar to other surgical procedures (see Chapter 14, Care of Preoperative Patients). This catheter is not used to acquire blood samples, give drugs or fluid, or monitor central venous pressure. Provide site care in accordance with agency

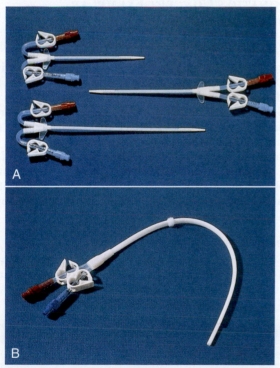

FIG. 68-1 Subclavian dialysis catheters. These catheters are radiopaque tubes that can be used for hemodialysis access. The Y-shaped tubing allows arterial outflow and venous return through a single catheter. **A,** Mahurkar catheters, made of polyurethane and used for short-term access. **B,** Perm-Cath catheter, made of silicone and used for long-term access. (Courtesy Kendall Company, Bothell, WA.)

policy and best practices to avoid catheter-related bloodstream infection (CRBSI).

A long-term dialysis catheter may be placed in the radiology department using a tunneling technique under moderate sedation. Under ultrasound or fluoroscopic guidance, the physician makes a small incision where the internal jugular vein passes behind the clavicle. A 6- to 8-cm tunnel is created away from the site of the incision. A long-term hemodialysis catheter is inserted through the tunnel and into the jugular vein. Keeping a segment of the catheter within the subcutaneous tissues before entering the jugular vein reduces the risk for infection. This central catheter is used only for dialysis and requires aseptic dressing changes.

Dialysis catheters have two lumens, one for outflow and one for inflow. This allows the patient's blood to flow out and, once dialyzed, to be returned through the inflow lumen. Some catheters have a third lumen to sample venous blood or give drugs and fluid during dialysis.

Intermittent Versus Continuous Kidney Replacement Therapy. Kidney replacement therapy (KRT) is a supportive strategy to purify blood, substituting for the normal function of the kidney. Particles are separated from blood based on the different ability of particles to pass through (diffuse) a membrane or across the peritoneal lining. KRT can be delivered intermittently, continuously, or as a hybrid of these approaches. Mortality is significant, regardless of modality, among patients who require KRT.

Intermittent KRT, sometimes called *hemodialysis*, is delivered over 3 to 6 hours. Generally a technician or dialysis nurse brings the dialysis machine to the bedside of a critically ill patient. Patients who do not need intensive care may be transported to an inpatient dialysis unit for the duration of the KRT treatment.

Intermittent KRT uses a dialysis machine to mix and monitor the *dialysate* (the fluid that helps remove the unwanted particles and waste products from blood). Dialysate is prescribed by the nephrology health care provider as an admixture to restore electrolytes and minerals to normal levels in the blood. The machine also monitors the flow of blood while it is outside of the body. Alarms are set and monitored by the dialysis technician or nurse to ensure safe and effective flow. This type of KRT is delivered three or four times weekly and requires anticoagulation in the dialysis circuit. However, dialysis creates shifts of fluid and electrolytes that may not be tolerated in critically ill patients. Another form of intermittent KRT is peritoneal dialysis, which is more commonly used for end-stage kidney disease. This therapy is discussed in detail in the Peritoneal Dialysis section of this chapter.

Continuous kidney replacement therapies (CKRTs), also known as *hemofiltration*, are alternative methods for removing wastes and restoring both ACID-BASE BALANCE and FLUID AND ELECTROLYTE BALANCE. They are used in hospitalized adults who are too unstable to tolerate the changes in blood pressure that occur with intermittent conventional hemodialysis. As with hemodialysis, blood is passed through a filter to remove waste and undesired particles. Unlike intermittent hemodialysis, CKRT removes and returns blood over 12 to 24 hours each day (Schell-Chaple, 2017). Another difference between CKRT and intermittent hemodialysis is the approach used to remove particles from blood. Hemofiltration uses ultrafiltration, whereas diffusion is used in intermittent dialysis to remove toxins and other particles. *Ultrafiltration* is the separation of particles from a suspension by passage through a filter with very fine pores. In ultrafiltration, the separation is performed by convective transport. During intermittent hemodialysis, separation depends on differential diffusion. Some approaches to CKRT combine ultrafiltration with diffusion (combined hemofiltration and hemodialysis).

CKRT occurs only in the ICU because of (1) the need for frequent monitoring and specialized skill set of the nurse to maintain safety during *extracorporeal circulation* (blood flow outside the body), and (2) the need for ongoing monitoring and replacement of fluid and electrolytes (Schell-Chaple, 2017). The American Nephrology Nurses Association provides resources for intermittent and continuous KRT policies and procedures.

Several strategies can be used to provide hemofiltration to critically ill patients. Continuous venovenous hemofiltration (CVVH) is more commonly used. CVVH is powered by a pump that drives blood from the patient catheter into the dialyzer (filter). The ultrafiltrate fluid is then collected into a bag for disposal. There may be a second pump that acts on the ultrafiltrate tubing to create negative pressure and increase fluid removal. Replacement fluid is infused via the inflow circuit in some systems. The pump increases the risk for an air embolus, and KRT systems have alarms that detect air. These systems also use anticoagulants but at lower doses than needed for systems using arterial access. CVVH can also be combined with dialysis (continuous venovenous hemofiltration and dialysis [CVVHD]). CVVHD is similar to intermittent KRT except that the rates of blood circulation and waste ELIMINATION are much slower with CVVHD, thus the need for continuous therapy (Dirkes, 2015).

Another modality for KRT is a hybrid of continuous and intermittent approaches. Slow continuous ultrafiltration (SCUF) provides slow removal of fluid over 12 to 24 hours and may be useful when azotemia or uremia is not a concern. Sustained low-efficiency dialysis (SLED) uses the dialysis machine to deliver prolonged dialysis for 12 to 24 hours. Lower blood flow and dialysate flow rates remove both particles and water and may be better tolerated by the unstable or critically ill patient, with fewer episodes of hypotension.

Continuous KRT is expensive and resource intensive. It requires consultation and collaboration with the nephrologist and close collaboration with a dialysis nurse. Conservative management of FLUID AND ELECTROLYTE BALANCE, ACID-BASE BALANCE, and drug therapy is an acceptable and reasonable approach to manage AKI.

Posthospital Care. Patients with AKI may have many outcomes. Some patients recover and return to baseline kidney function and general health. Others have partial recovery with mild or moderate chronic kidney disease (CKD). Still others may require permanent KRT. Some die from the acute illness.

The care for a patient with AKI after discharge from the hospital varies, depending on the status of the kidney function when the patient is discharged. Resolution of kidney injury may occur over several months, and follow-up care may be provided by a nephrologist or by the primary health care provider in consultation with the nephrologist. Frequent medical visits are necessary, as are scheduled laboratory blood and urine tests to monitor kidney function. A dietitian can plan modifications to the patient's diet according to the degree of kidney function and ongoing nutrition needs. Fluid restrictions and daily weights may be advised to avoid fluid overload while kidneys are recovering.

About 10% of patients who receive KRT for AKI in the hospital develop end-stage kidney disease (ESKD) and require intermittent dialysis or kidney transplantation (Dirkes, 2015). For patients who require dialysis at discharge following AKI, follow-up care is similar to that needed for patients with ESKD from CKD (see Care Coordination and Transition Management in the CKD section). Depending on their level of independence and family support, patients may need home care nursing or social work assistance.

❓ NCLEX EXAMINATION CHALLENGE 68-3
Health Promotion and Maintenance

The nurse is preparing a client for discharge who developed an acute kidney injury during coronary artery bypass graft surgery. The nurse notices that the client has a serum creatinine of 1.2 mg/dL (106 mcmol/L) and a glomerular filtration rate (GFR) of 75 mL/kg/1.73 m². Which is the **priority** nursing action?
A. Reminding the client to remain hydrated by drinking 500 mL of an electrolyte-based solution daily
B. Encouraging the client to reduce protein intake to reduce creatinine production until the follow-up visit with the nephrologist occurs
C. Checking the remaining values on the metabolic panel and informing the primary care provider of all results before the client is discharged
D. Educating the client about the need for follow-up, including re-evaluation of serum creatinine with the primary care provider or nephrologist in 8-12 weeks

---

❋ ELIMINATION CONCEPT EXEMPLAR
Chronic Kidney Disease

❖ PATHOPHYSIOLOGY

Unlike acute kidney injury (AKI), **chronic kidney disease (CKD)** is a progressive, irreversible disorder, and kidney function does *not* recover (Taal, 2016). It is defined as abnormalities in kidney structure or function that alter health and are present for longer than 3 months (KDIGO, 2013). When kidney function and waste ELIMINATION are too poor to sustain life, CKD becomes **end-stage kidney disease (ESKD)**. Terms used with CKD include **azotemia** (buildup of nitrogen-based wastes in the blood), **uremia** (azotemia with symptoms [Chart 68-2]), and **uremic syndrome**. See Table 68-1 for a comparison of AKI and CKD.

Stages of Chronic Kidney Disease

CKD is classified into five stages based on glomerular filtration rate (GFR) category. Direct measurement of urine creatinine (described in Chapter 65, using a 3-hour or 24-hour urine

---

▶▶ CHART 68-2   Key Features
Uremia

- Metallic taste in the mouth
- Anorexia
- Nausea
- Vomiting
- Muscle cramps
- Uremic "frost" on skin
- Itching
- Fatigue and lethargy
- Hiccups
- Edema
- Dyspnea
- Paresthesias

collection) is needed for most accurate GFR estimation. The five stages of CKD are described in Table 68-6. CKD starts with a normal GFR but increased risk for kidney damage. In the first stage, the patient may have a normal GFR (greater than 90 mL/min) but have abnormal urine findings, structural abnormalities, or genetic traits that point to kidney disease. The patient is at increased risk for kidney damage from infection, IMMUNITY responses with inflammation, pregnancy, dehydration, and hypotension. Careful management of conditions such as diabetes, hypertension, and heart failure can slow the onset and progression of CKD.

TABLE 68-6	**Stages of Chronic Kidney Disease**	
STAGE	**ESTIMATED GLOMERULAR FILTRATION RATE**	**INTERVENTION**
Stage 1 At risk; normal kidney function but urine findings, structural abnormalities, or genetic trait points to kidney disease	>90 mL/min	Screen for risk factors and manage care to reduce risk: • Uncontrolled hypertension • Diabetes with poor glycemic control • Congenital or acquired anatomic or urinary tract abnormalities • Family history of genetic kidney diseases • Exposure to nephrotoxic substances
Stage 2 Mild chronic kidney disease (CKD); reduced kidney function; laboratory values and other findings (e.g., structural changes) point to kidney disease	60-89 mL/min	Focus on reduction of risk factors.
Stage 3 Moderate CKD	30-59 mL/min	Implement strategies to slow disease progression.
Stage 4 Severe CKD	15-29 mL/min	Manage complications. Discuss patient preferences and values. Educate about options and prepare for renal replacement therapy.
Stage 5 End-stage kidney disease (ESKD)	<15 mL/min	Implement renal replacement therapy or kidney transplantation.

In Stage 2 CKD, GFR is reduced, ranging between 60 and 89 mL/min, and albuminuria may be present. Kidney nephron damage has occurred, and there may be slight elevations of metabolic wastes in the blood because of nephron loss. Levels of blood urea nitrogen (BUN), serum creatinine, uric acid, and phosphorus are not sensitive enough to define this stage. Increased output of dilute urine may occur at this stage of CKD and lead to severe dehydration.

> ⚠ **NURSING SAFETY PRIORITY** QSEN
> ### Action Alert
> Teach patients with mild chronic kidney disease (CKD) that carefully managing fluid volume, blood pressure, electrolytes, and other kidney-damaging diseases by following prescribed drug and nutrition therapies can slow progression to end-stage kidney disease (ESKD).

In Stage 3 CKD, GRF reduction continues and ranges between 30 and 59 mL/min, and albuminuria is usually present. Nephron damage is greater, and azotemia reflecting poor waste ELIMINATION is present. Ongoing management of the underlying conditions that cause nephron damage is essential, especially diabetes mellitus and blood pressure control. Restriction of fluids, proteins, and electrolytes is needed. Stage 3 is further divided into 3a and 3b to more accurately assess the risk for complications from CKD as GFR decreases below 45 mL/min/1.73 m².

Over time, patients progress to Stage 4 CKD and *end-stage kidney disease* (ESKD) (Stage 5). Waste ELIMINATION is poor with excessive amounts of urea and creatinine building up in the blood, and the kidneys cannot maintain homeostasis. Severe impairments of FLUID AND ELECTROLYTE BALANCE and ACID-BASE BALANCE occur. Without kidney replacement therapy, death results from ESKD.

Three albuminuria stages also are considered in evaluating CKD. These stages are defined by the albumin-to-creatinine ratio in urine. The first stage (A1) is none to mildly increased albumin, up to 29 mg/g creatinine (<3 mg/mmol) and is sometimes called *microalbuminuria*. The second (A2) stage has values of 30 to 300 mg/g creatinine (3 to 30 mg/mmol). The stage of greatest kidney damage (A3) has values >300 mg/g creatinine (>30 mg/mmol). The risk for progression of CKD, ESKD, and mortality is increased when urine albumin increases. Albumin in the urine is a marker of kidney damage, whereas GFR reflects kidney function. The combined values help identify adults at risk for progression of CKD and complications and guide interventions.

Kidney Changes

CKD with greatly reduced GFR causes many problems, including abnormal urine production, severe disruption of FLUID AND ELECTROLYTE BALANCE, and metabolic abnormalities. Because healthy nephrons become larger and work harder, urine production and water ELIMINATION are sufficient to maintain essential homeostasis until about three fourths of kidney function is lost. As the disease progresses, the ability to produce diluted urine is reduced, resulting in urine with a fixed osmolarity (isosthenuria). As kidney function continues to decline, the BUN increases, and urine output decreases. Patients with CKD can have a 10% to 20% increase in extracellular fluid volume, including blood volume (Scher et al., 2015). At this point, the patient is at risk for fluid overload with edema, pulmonary crackles, shortness of breath, and pleural or pericardial effusion (with symptoms of a friction rub on auscultation and/or decreased breath sounds or heart sounds).

Metabolic Changes

Urea and creatinine excretion are disrupted by CKD. Creatinine comes from proteins in skeletal muscle. The rate of creatinine excretion depends on muscle mass, physical activity, and diet. Without major changes in diet or physical activity, the serum creatinine level is constant. Creatinine is partially excreted by the kidney tubules, and a decrease in kidney function leads to a buildup of serum creatinine. Urea is made from protein metabolism and is excreted by the kidneys. The BUN level normally varies directly with protein intake.

Sodium excretion changes are common. Early in CKD, the patient is at risk for *hyponatremia* (sodium depletion) because there are fewer healthy nephrons to reabsorb sodium. Thus sodium is lost in the urine. Polyuria of mild-to-moderate CKD also causes sodium loss.

In the later stages of CKD, kidney excretion of sodium is reduced as urine production decreases. Then sodium retention and high serum sodium levels *(hypernatremia)* occur with only modest increases in dietary sodium intake. This problem leads to severe disruption of FLUID AND ELECTROLYTE BALANCE (see Chapter 11). Sodium retention causes hypertension and edema.

Even with sodium retention, the serum sodium level may appear normal because plasma water is retained at the same time. If fluid retention occurs at a greater rate than sodium retention, the serum sodium level is falsely low because of dilution (see Chart 68-1).

Potassium excretion occurs mainly through the kidney. Any increase in potassium load during the later stages of CKD can lead to hyperkalemia (high serum potassium levels). Normal serum potassium levels of 3.5 to 5 mEq/L (mmol/L) are maintained until the 24-hour urine output falls below 500 mL. High potassium levels then develop quickly, reaching 7 to 8 mEq/L (mmol/L) or greater. Life-threatening changes in cardiac rate and rhythm result from this elevation because of abnormal depolarization and repolarization. Other factors contribute to high potassium levels in CKD, including the ingestion of potassium in drugs, failure to restrict dietary potassium, tissue breakdown, blood transfusions, and bleeding or hemorrhage. (See Chapter 11 for discussion of potassium problems.)

ACID-BASE BALANCE is affected by CKD. In the early stages, blood pH changes little because the remaining healthy nephrons increase their rate of acid excretion. As more nephrons are lost, acid excretion is reduced and metabolic acidosis results (see Chapter 12).

Many factors lead to acidosis in CKD. First, the kidneys cannot excrete excessive hydrogen ions (acids). Normally, tubular cells move hydrogen ions into the urine for excretion, but ammonium and bicarbonate are needed for this movement to occur (Norton et al., 2017b). In patients with CKD, ammonium production is decreased and reabsorption of bicarbonate does not occur. This process leads to a buildup of hydrogen ions and reduced levels of bicarbonate *(base deficit)*. High potassium levels further reduce kidney ammonium production and excretion.

As CKD worsens and acid retention increases, increased respiratory action is needed to keep blood pH normal. The respiratory system adjusts or compensates for the increased blood

hydrogen ion levels (acidosis or decreased pH) by increasing the rate and depth of breathing to excrete carbon dioxide through the lungs. This breathing pattern, called Kussmaul respiration, increases with worsening kidney disease. Serum bicarbonate measures the extent of metabolic acidosis (bicarbonate deficit). Patients usually need alkali replacement to counteract acidosis.

Calcium and phosphorus balance is disrupted by CKD. A complex, balanced normal reciprocal relationship exists between calcium and phosphorus (used interchangeably with phosphate) and is influenced by vitamin D (see Chapter 11). The kidney produces a hormone needed to activate vitamin D, which then enhances intestinal absorption of calcium.

Normally, excess dietary phosphorus is excreted by the kidneys in the urine. In CKD, phosphorus overload leads to secretion of a phosphaturic hormone from bone (Fukagawa et al., 2013). This hormone, fibroblast growth factor 3 (FGFR3), contributes to mineral imbalance.

Parathyroid hormone (PTH) controls the amount of phosphorus in the blood by causing tubular excretion of phosphorus when there is an excess. An early effect of CKD is reduced phosphorus excretion (Fig. 68-2). As plasma phosphorus levels increase *(hyperphosphatemia)*, calcium levels decrease *(hypocalcemia)*. Chronic low blood calcium levels stimulate the parathyroid glands to release more PTH. With additional PTH, calcium is released from storage areas in bones *(bone resorption)*, which results in bone density loss. The extra calcium from the bone is needed to balance the excess plasma phosphorus level. The problem of low blood calcium levels is made worse with severe CKD because kidney cell damage also reduces production of active vitamin D. Thus less calcium is absorbed through the intestinal tract in the absence of sufficient vitamin D (Norton et al., 2017b).

The problems in bone metabolism and structure caused by CKD-induced low calcium levels and high phosphorus levels

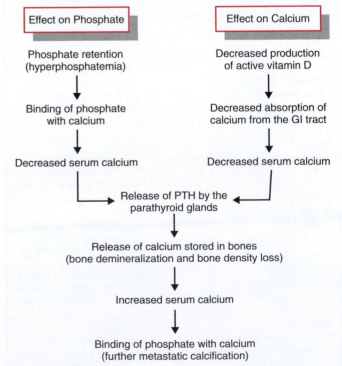

FIG. 68-2 Effects of kidney dysfunction on phosphorus and calcium balance. *PTH,* Parathyroid hormone.

are called **renal osteodystrophy**. Bone mineral loss causes bone pain, spinal sclerosis, fractures, bone density loss, osteomalacia, and tooth calcium loss.

Crystals formed from excessive calcium or phosphorus are called *metastatic calcifications* and may precipitate in many body areas. When the plasma level of the calcium-phosphorus product (serum calcium level multiplied by the serum phosphorus level) exceeds 70 mg/dL (6 mmol/L), the crystals may lodge in the kidneys, heart, lungs, blood vessels, joints, eyes (causing conjunctivitis), and brain. Itching increases with calcium-phosphorus imbalances.

Calcium is also deposited in atherosclerotic plaques in the lining of blood vessels. Vascular calcium deposits are a marker of significant risk for cardiovascular disease.

Cardiac Changes

Hypertension is common in most patients with CKD. It may be either the cause or the result of CKD. In patients who have other causes of hypertension such as atherosclerosis, the increased blood pressure damages the glomerular capillaries, and eventually ESKD results.

CKD itself elevates blood pressure by causing fluid and sodium overload and dysfunction of the renin-angiotensin-aldosterone system (RAAS). Hypertension alone can damage kidney arterioles, reducing PERFUSION. A decrease in kidney blood flow results in the production and release of a number of signaling chemicals, including renin, to improve blood flow to the kidney. The release of renin triggers the production of angiotensin and aldosterone. Angiotensin causes blood vessel constriction and increases blood pressure. Aldosterone stimulates kidney tubules to reabsorb sodium and water. These actions increase plasma volume and raise blood pressure. However, in the presence of CKD, an increase in blood pressure may not result in increased blood flow, and the production of renin continues, which creates a cycle of vasoconstriction in kidney arterioles and peripheral arterioles. The result is severe hypertension that is difficult to manage and worsens kidney function. Many patients with CKD have heart damage and enlargement from the long-term hypertension that results in coronary artery damage and poor coronary artery perfusion.

Hyperlipidemia occurs in CKD from changes in fat metabolism that increase triglyceride, total cholesterol, and low-density lipoprotein (LDL) levels. These changes increase the patient's risk for coronary artery disease and acute cardiac events. Problems with lipids and atherosclerosis are greatly increased for the patient with both CKD and diabetes mellitus.

Heart failure may occur in CKD because the workload on the heart is increased as a result of anemia, hypertension, and fluid overload. Left ventricular enlargement and heart failure are common in ESKD. Uremia may cause *uremic cardiomyopathy,* the uremic toxin effect on the myocardium. Heart failure also may occur in these patients because of hypertension and coronary artery disease. Cardiac disease is a leading cause of death in patients with ESKD.

Pericarditis also occurs in patients with CKD. The pericardial sac becomes inflamed by uremic toxins or infection. If it is not treated, this problem leads to pericardial effusion, cardiac tamponade, and death. Symptoms include shortness of breath from low cardiac output, severe chest pain, tachycardia, narrow *pulse pressure* (close values for systolic and diastolic blood pressure), low-grade fever, and a pericardial friction rub that can be heard with a stethoscope placed over the left sternal border. Dysrhythmias may occur with uremia and uremic pericarditis. Treatment of tamponade, which is a medical emergency, requires immediate removal of pericardial fluid by placement of a needle, catheter, or drainage tube into the pericardium.

Hematologic and Immunity Changes

Anemia is common in patients in the later stages of CKD and worsens CKD symptoms. The causes of anemia include a decreased erythropoietin level with reduced red blood cell (RBC) production, decreased RBC survival time from uremia, and iron and folic acid deficiencies (Norton et al., 2017b). The patient may have increased bleeding or bruising as a result of impaired platelet function.

CKD causes reduced IMMUNITY, which increases the risk for infection. Uremia disrupts white blood cell (WBC) production and function, decreasing host defenses. Protein, fluid, and electrolyte abnormalities contribute to inflammation and further immunity impairment.

Gastrointestinal Changes

Uremia affects the entire GI system. The flora of the mouth change with uremia. The mouth contains the enzyme *urease,* which breaks down urea into ammonia. The ammonia generated remains and then causes halitosis (uremic fetor) and *stomatitis* (mouth inflammation). Anorexia, nausea, vomiting, and hiccups are common in patients with uremia. The specific cause of these problems is unknown but may be related to high BUN and creatinine levels and acidosis.

Peptic ulcer disease is common in patients with uremia, but the exact cause is unclear. Uremic colitis with watery diarrhea or constipation may also be present with uremia. Ulcers may occur in the stomach or intestine, causing erosion of blood vessels. The blood loss caused by these erosions may lead to hemorrhagic shock from severe GI bleeding.

Cognitive and Functional Changes

Although CKD may be asymptomatic in the early stages, as it progresses complications include cognitive and physical impairment. There is also increased risk for systemic drug toxicity and adverse effects from interventions used to prevent or treat CKD.

Etiology and Genetic Risk

The causes of CKD are complex (Table 68-7). More than 100 different disease processes can result in progressive loss of kidney function (see also Chapter 67). Two main causes of CKD leading to dialysis or kidney transplantation are hypertension and diabetes mellitus. African-American patients are much more likely to develop ESKD and have hypertensive ESKD.

Incidence and Prevalence

The number of patients being treated for CKD is increasing, particularly among older adults. About 11% of adults in the United States have CKD, with more than half at stages 3 or 4 (Centers for Disease Control and Prevention [CDC], 2016). Over 800,000 people in the United States are being treated for ESKD (U.S. Renal Data Systems [USRDS], 2015). In Canada, more than 6000 adults have ESKD (Kidney Foundation of Canada, 2015). About 25% of patients receiving treatment for ESKD die in the first year of dialysis. Chart 68-3 addresses the prevention of kidney and urinary problems.

TABLE 68-7 Selected Causes of Chronic Kidney Disease

Glomerular Disease
- Glomerulonephritis
- Basement membrane disease
- Goodpasture's syndrome
- Intercapillary glomerulosclerosis

Tubular Disease
- Chronic hypercalcemia
- Chronic potassium depletion
- Fanconi's syndrome
- Heavy metal (lead) poisoning

Vascular Disease of the Kidney
- Ischemic disease of the kidney
- Bilateral renal artery stenosis
- Nephrosclerosis
- Hyperparathyroidism

Inherited or Genetic Conditions
- Hypoplastic kidneys
- Medullary cystic disease
- Polycystic kidney disease

Infection
- Pyelonephritis
- Tuberculosis

Systemic Vascular Disease
- Intrarenal renovascular hypertension
- Extrarenal renovascular hypertension

Metabolic Kidney Disease
- Diabetes
- Amyloidosis
- Gout (hyperuricemic nephropathy)
- Milk-alkali syndrome
- Sarcoidosis

Connective Tissue Disease
- Progressive systemic sclerosis
- Systemic lupus erythematosus
- Polyarteritis

Urinary Tract Disease
- Obstructive uropathy

NOTE: List is not all-inclusive.

CHART 68-3 Patient and Family Education: Preparing for Self-Management

Prevention of Kidney and Urinary Problems

- Be alert to the general appearance of your urine. Note any changes in its color, clarity, or odor.
- Changes in the frequency or volume of urine passage occur with changes in fluid intake. More frequent or infrequent voiding not associated with changes in fluid intake may signal health problems.
- Any discomfort or distress with the passage of urine is not normal. Pain, burning, urgency, aching, or difficulty with initiating urine flow or complete bladder emptying is of some concern. Report such symptoms to your primary health care provider.
- The kidneys need 1 to 2 liters of fluid a day to flush out your body wastes. Water is the ideal flushing agent.
- Avoid sugary, high-calorie drinks; they provide low-quality calories that contribute to weight gain and sugar-induced urination.
- Changes in kidney function are often silent for many years. Periodically ask your primary health care provider to measure your kidney function with a blood test (serum creatinine) and a urinalysis.
- If you have a history of kidney disease, diabetes mellitus, hypertension (high blood pressure), or a family history of kidney disease, you should know your serum creatinine level and your glomerular filtration rate (either estimated from serum creatinine or measured with a 24-hour creatinine urine collection). At least one checkup per year that includes laboratory blood and urine testing of kidney function is recommended.
- If you are identified as having decreased kidney function, ask about whether any prescribed drug, diagnostic test, or therapeutic procedure will present a risk to your current kidney function. Evaluate the contribution of diet to risk for kidney disease with your primary health care provider or a dietitian. Check out all nonprescription drugs with your primary health care provider or pharmacist before using them.

Health Promotion and Maintenance

Health promotion activities to prevent or delay the onset of CKD focus on controlling the diseases that lead to its development, such as diabetes and hypertension. Educating and encouraging the patient to accept lifestyle modifications and how to implement them are incorporated into the ongoing plan of care. Diet adjustments (e.g., sodium, protein, and cholesterol restriction), weight maintenance (i.e., achieve body mass index of 22 to 25 kg/m^2), smoking cessation, participation in 30 to 60 minutes of moderate-intensity exercise daily, and limitation of alcohol to 1 or 2 drinks daily are examples of lifestyle recommendations for the patient with CKD. Identifying patients who have diabetes or hypertension at an early stage is critical to CKD prevention (Norton et al., 2017a). Teach patients to adhere to drug and diet regimens and to engage in regular physical activity to prevent the blood vessel changes and kidney cell damage that lead to CKD. Instruct patients with diabetes to keep their blood glucose levels within the prescribed range. Teach patients with hypertension that drug therapy reduces vessel damage. Urge patients with diabetes or hypertension to have yearly testing for urine albumin-to-creatinine ratio (UACR) along with serum creatinine and BUN.

Teach adults treated for an infection anywhere in the kidney/urinary system to take all antibiotics as prescribed. Urge adults to drink at least 2 L of water daily unless a health problem requires fluid restriction. Caution adults who use NSAIDs to use the lowest dose for the briefest time period because these drugs interfere with blood flow to the kidney. High-dose and long-term NSAID use reduces kidney function.

NCLEX EXAMINATION CHALLENGE 68-4

Health Promotion and Maintenance

A 48-year-old African-American man is newly diagnosed with hypertension and Stage 1 chronic kidney disease (CKD). His primary health care provider has prescribed a thiazide diuretic. The client reports that he has increased his activity and changed his diet, which resulted in a 10-lb (4.5-kg) weight loss in the past 2 months. The client says he feels well and does not want to take any drugs. What is the nurse's **best** response?

A. "Reducing your blood pressure may slow or prevent progression of your chronic kidney disease."

B. "Your primary health care provider prescribed the diuretic because it will reverse the damage caused by kidney disease."

C. "Taking medications is a personal decision, and you have the right to decline this prescription."

D. "Because your lifestyle changes have resulted in weight loss, this intervention is all that is needed to reduce your risk for progression of kidney disease."

❖ INTERPROFESSIONAL COLLABORATIVE CARE

Although the patient with CKD may require hospitalization during exacerbation of imbalances or when other health problems require it, the vast majority of care occurs in the community. For best outcomes, the patient with CKD must be engaged in self-management. Because patients with CKD are at risk for so many adverse outcomes (not just ESKD), the interprofessional care team includes many specialists and health care professionals (e.g., nephrologists, nephrology nurses, pharmacists, registered dietitians, mental health therapists, physical therapists, case managers, social workers, clergy or pastoral care workers). The responsibilities of these interprofessional team members are described within the interventions sections for CKD. With so many professionals involved, care coordination is essential to positive outcomes in this population (Hain, 2015). The nurse coordinates the interprofessional team to support and counsel the patient and family, often over many years of treatment. The nurse has the most contact with the patient when he or she is hospitalized or undergoing in-center dialysis treatments.

◆ **Assessment: Noticing**

History. When taking a history from a patient with risk for or actual CKD, document the patient's age and gender. Accurately measure weight and height and ask about usual weight and recent weight gain or loss. Weight gain may indicate fluid retention from poor kidney function with disrupted FLUID AND ELECTROLYTE BALANCE. Weight loss may be the result of anorexia from uremia.

Ask about a history of kidney and urologic disorders, chronic health problems, and drug use. Chronic hypertension, diabetes, inflammatory diseases of systemic lupus erythematosus or arthritis, cancer, and tuberculosis can cause decreased kidney function. Ask the patient about family members' kidney disease that might indicate a genetic problem.

Document the use of current and past prescribed and over-the-counter drugs because many drugs are nephrotoxic and drug interactions can cause kidney damage (see Table 68-5) (Burchum & Rosenthal, 2016). Ask whether the patient has had x-rays or CT scan with contrast medium.

Examine the patient's dietary habits and discuss any GI problems. A change in the taste of foods often occurs with CKD. Patients may report that sweet foods are not as appealing or that meats have a metallic taste. Ask about the presence of nausea, vomiting, anorexia, hiccups, diarrhea, or constipation. These symptoms may be the result of excess wastes that the body cannot eliminate because of kidney disease.

Ask about the patient's energy level and any recent injuries or bleeding. Explore changes in his or her daily routine as a possible *result* of fatigue. Fatigue is a common and often profound problem among patients with CKD, particularly among patients receiving dialysis. Weakness, drowsiness, and shortness of breath suggest impending pulmonary edema or neurologic degeneration. Ask about bruising or bleeding caused by hematologic changes from uremia.

Discuss urine ELIMINATION in detail, including frequency of urination, appearance of the urine, and any difficulty starting or controlling urination. These data can help identify urologic problems that may influence kidney function.

Physical Assessment/Signs and Symptoms. CKD causes changes in all body systems (Chart 68-4). Most symptoms are related to changes in FLUID AND ELECTROLYTE BALANCE, ACID-BASE BALANCE, and buildup of nitrogenous wastes.

Neurologic symptoms of CKD and uremic syndrome vary (see Chart 68-4). Observe for problems ranging from lethargy to seizures or coma, which may indicate uremic encephalopathy. Fluid overload can cause changes in cognition. Assess for sensory changes that appear in a glove-and-stocking pattern over the hands and feet *(peripheral neuropathy).* Check for weakness in upper and lower extremities *(uremic neuropathy).* Fatigue can result in decreased activity.

If untreated, encephalopathy can lead to seizures and coma. Dialysis is used emergently when neurologic problems

---

▶▶ **CHART 68-4 Key Features**

Severe Chronic and End-Stage Kidney Disease

Neurologic Symptoms
- Lethargy and daytime drowsiness
- Inability to concentrate or decreased attention span
- Seizures
- Coma
- Slurred speech
- Asterixis (jerky movements or "flapping" of the hands)
- Tremors, twitching, or jerky movements
- Myoclonus
- Ataxia (alteration in gait)
- Paresthesias from peripheral neuropathy

Cardiovascular Symptoms
- Cardiomyopathy
- Hypertension
- Peripheral edema
- Heart failure
- Uremic pericarditis
- Pericardial effusion
- Pericardial friction rub
- Cardiac tamponade
- Cardiorenal syndrome

Respiratory Symptoms
- Uremic halitosis
- Tachypnea
- Deep sighing, yawning
- Kussmaul respirations
- Uremic pneumonitis
- Shortness of breath
- Pulmonary edema
- Pleural effusion
- Depressed cough reflex
- Crackles

Hematologic Symptoms
- Anemia
- Abnormal bleeding and bruising
- Reduced white blood cell count
- Increased risk for infection

Gastrointestinal Symptoms
- Anorexia
- Nausea
- Vomiting
- Metallic taste in the mouth
- Changes in taste acuity and sensation
- Uremic colitis (diarrhea)
- Constipation

- Uremic gastritis (possible GI bleeding)
- Uremic fetor (breath odor)
- Stomatitis

Urinary Symptoms
- Polyuria, nocturia (early)
- Oliguria, anuria (later)
- Proteinuria
- Hematuria
- Diluted, straw-colored urine appearance (early)
- Concentrated and cloudy urine appearance (later)

Integumentary Symptoms
- Decreased skin turgor
- Yellow-gray pallor
- Dry skin
- Pruritus
- Ecchymosis
- Purpura
- Soft-tissue calcifications
- Uremic frost (late, premorbid)

Musculoskeletal Symptoms
- Muscle weakness and cramping
- Bone pain
- Fractures
- Renal osteodystrophy

Reproductive Symptoms
- Decreased fertility
- Infrequent or absent menses
- Decreased libido
- Impotence
- Sexual dysfunction

Metabolic Symptoms
- Hyperparathyroidism
- Hyperlipidemia
- Alterations in vitamin D, calcium, and phosphorus adsorption and metabolism
- Metabolic acidosis
- Hyperkalemia

Psychosocial Symptoms
- Depression
- Fatigue
- Sleep disturbances
- Sexual dysfunction
- Cognitive impairment
- Unemployment

---

result from CKD. The symptoms of encephalopathy may resolve with dialysis. However, improvement in neuropathy can be limited by severe or recurrent episodes of brain dysfunction. Depression may compound cognitive and neurologic problems.

Cardiovascular symptoms of CKD result from fluid overload, hypertension, heart failure (HF), pericarditis, potassium-induced dysrhythmias, and cholesterol/calcium (plaque, atherosclerosis) deposits in blood vessels. Assess for indications of reduced sodium and water excretion. Blood volume overload, if untreated, leads to hypertension, pulmonary edema, peripheral edema, and HF.

Assess heart rate and rhythm, listening for extra sounds (particularly an S_3), irregular patterns, or a pericardial friction rub. Unless a dialysis vascular access has been created, measure blood pressure in each arm. Assess the jugular veins for distention, and assess for edema of the feet, shins, and sacrum and around the eyes. Crackles during lung auscultation and shortness of breath with exertion and at night suggest fluid overload.

Respiratory symptoms of CKD also vary (e.g., breath that smells like urine [*uremic fetor* or uremic halitosis], deep sighing, yawning, shortness of breath). Observe the rhythm, rate, and depth of breathing. Tachypnea and hyperpnea (increased depth of breathing) occur with metabolic acidosis.

With severe metabolic acidosis, extreme increases in rate and depth of ventilation (Kussmaul respirations) occur. A few patients have pneumonitis, or *uremic lung.* In these patients, assess for thick sputum, reduced coughing, tachypnea, and fever. A pleural friction rub may be heard with a stethoscope. Patients often have pleuritic pain with breathing. Auscultate the lungs for crackles, which indicate fluid overload.

Hematologic symptoms of CKD include anemia and abnormal bleeding. Check for indicators of anemia (e.g., fatigue, pallor, lethargy, weakness, shortness of breath, dizziness). Check for abnormal bleeding by observing for bruising, petechiae, purpura, mucous membrane bleeding in the nose or gums, or intestinal bleeding (black, tarry stools [melena]).

GI symptoms of CKD include foul breath (halitosis) and mouth inflammation or ulceration. Document any abdominal pain, cramping, or vomiting. Test all stools for occult blood.

Skeletal symptoms of CKD are related to osteodystrophy from poor absorption of calcium and continuous bone calcium loss. Adults with osteodystrophy have thin, fragile bones that are at risk for fractures with even slight trauma. Vertebrae become more compact and may bend forward, leading to an overall loss of height. Ask about changes in height and bone pain. Observe for spinal curvatures and any unusual bumps or protrusions in bone areas that may indicate fractures. Handle the patient carefully during examination and care.

Urine symptoms in CKD reflect the kidneys' decreasing function. Urine amount, frequency, and appearance change. Protein, sediment, or blood may be in the urine.

The amount and composition of the urine change as kidney function decreases and waste ELIMINATION is disrupted. With the onset of mild-to-moderate CKD, the urine may be more dilute and clearer because tubular reabsorption of water is reduced. The actual urine output in a patient with CKD varies with the amount of remaining kidney function. The patient with severe CKD or ESKD usually has oliguria, but some patients continue to produce 1 L or more daily. Daily urine volume usually changes again after dialysis is started. A long duration of oliguria is an indication that recovery of kidney function is not to be expected.

Skin symptoms of CKD occur as a result of uremia. Pigment is deposited in the skin, causing a yellowish coloration, or darkening when skin is brown or bronze. The anemia of CKD causes sallowness, appearing as a faded suntan on lighter-skinned patients.

Skin oils and turgor are decreased in patients with uremia. A distressing problem of uremia is severe *pruritus* (itching). Uremic frost, a layer of urea crystals from evaporated sweat, may appear on the face, eyebrows, axillae, and groin in patients with advanced uremic syndrome. Assess for bruises (*ecchymosis*), purple patches (*purpura*), and rashes.

Psychosocial Assessment. CKD and its treatment disrupt many aspects of a patient's life. Psychosocial assessment and support are part of the nurse's role from the time that CKD is first diagnosed. With ongoing issues, a mental health professional is an important member of the care team. Ask about the patient's understanding of the diagnosis and what the treatment regimen means to him or her (e.g., diet, drugs, dialysis). Assess for anxiety and fear and for coping styles used by the patient and family. CKD affects family relations, social activity, work patterns, body image, and sexual activity. The chronic nature of severe CKD and ESKD, the many treatment options, and the uncertainties about the disease and its treatment require ongoing psychosocial assessment, psychosocial interventions, and ongoing support. Support the recommendations of the mental health professional.

Laboratory Assessment. CKD causes extreme changes in many laboratory values (see Chart 68-1). Monitor these blood values: creatinine, blood urea nitrogen (BUN), sodium, potassium, calcium, phosphorus, bicarbonate, hemoglobin, and hematocrit. Also monitor GFR for trends.

A urinalysis is performed. In the early stages of CKD, urinalysis may show protein, glucose, red blood cells (RBCs) and white blood cells (WBCs), and decreased or fixed specific gravity. Urine osmolarity is usually decreased. As CKD progresses, urine output decreases dramatically, and osmolarity increases. A urine albumin-to-creatinine ratio (UACR) provides important information about kidney function and damage.

Glomerular filtration rate (GFR) can be estimated from serum creatinine levels, age, gender, race, and body size. But this type of estimation is generally used for screening rather than for staging of CKD. Estimation of GFR based on a formula that includes serum creatinine is also useful to calculate drug dose or drug frequency when reduced kidney function is a concern. However, to determine stage of CKD, a urine collection of 3 hours to 24 hours is usually done to assess creatinine clearance. A spot urine albumin-to-creatinine ratio also is completed.

In severe CKD, serum creatinine and BUN levels may be used to determine the presence and degree of uremia. Serum creatinine levels may increase gradually over a period of years, reaching levels of 15 to 30 mg/dL (500 to 1000 mcmol/L) or more, depending on the patient's muscle mass. BUN levels are directly related to dietary protein intake. Without protein restriction, BUN levels may rise to 10 to 20 times the value of the serum creatinine level. With dietary protein restriction, BUN levels are elevated but less than those of non–protein-restricted patients. Fluid balance also affects BUN.

Imaging Assessment. Few x-ray findings are abnormal with CKD. Bone x-rays of the hand can show renal osteodystrophy. With long-term ESKD, the kidneys shrink (except for ESKD caused by polycystic kidney disease) and may be 8 to 9 cm or smaller. This small size results from atrophy and fibrosis. If CKD progresses suddenly, a kidney ultrasound or CT scan without contrast medium may be used to rule out an obstruction. (See Chapter 65 for a complete description of diagnostic tests for kidney function.)

◆ Analysis: Interpreting

The patient with CKD usually has progressive reduction of kidney function. Management generally occurs in the community setting. In the acute or long-term care setting, the focus of care is to manage problems and prevent complications of CKD. The priority collaborative problems for patients with CKD include:

1. Fluid overload due to the inability of diseased kidneys to maintain body fluid balance
2. Potential for pulmonary edema due to fluid overload
3. Decreased cardiac function due to reduced stroke volume, dysrhythmias, fluid overload, and increased peripheral vascular resistance
4. Weight loss due to inability to ingest, digest, or absorb food and nutrients as a result of physiologic factors
5. Potential for infection due to skin breakdown, IMMUNITY-related kidney dysfunction, or malnutrition
6. Potential for injury due to effects of kidney disease on bone density, blood clotting, and drug elimination
7. Fatigue due to kidney disease, anemia, and reduced energy production
8. Anxiety due to change in health status, economic status, relationships, role function; threat of death; lack of knowledge about diagnostic tests, disease process, treatment; loss of control; or disrupted family life
9. Potential for depression due to chronic debilitating illness

◆ Planning and Implementation: Responding

The Concept Map discusses nursing care issues related to patients who have end-stage kidney disease (ESKD).

Managing Fluid Volume

Planning: Expected Outcomes. The patient with CKD is expected to achieve and maintain an acceptable FLUID AND ELECTROLYTE BALANCE. Indicators include that blood pressure, central venous pressure, and electrolytes are normal or nearly normal. Body weight is stable (±2 lb overnight and 5 lb weekly) and does not increase more than 3 lb between dialysis sessions.

Interventions. Management of the patient with CKD includes drug therapy, nutrition therapy, fluid restriction, and dialysis (when the patient reaches Stage 5). Hemodialysis is performed intermittently for 3 to 4 hours, typically 3 days per week. Alternatively, some patients with ESKD receive peritoneal dialysis. Peritoneal dialysis (PD) uses the peritoneum as the dialyzing membrane. The dialysate is infused through a catheter tunneled into the peritoneum. Dialysis for ESKD is described later in this chapter.

The purpose of fluid management is to attain fluid balance and prevent complications of fluid overload (Chart 68-5). Monitor the patient's intake and output and hydration status. Assess for indications of fluid overload (e.g., lung crackles, edema, distended neck veins).

Drug therapy with diuretics is prescribed for patients with mild-to-severe CKD to increase urinary ELIMINATION of fluid. The increased urine output with this therapy helps reduce fluid overload and hypertension in patients who still have some urine output. Diuretics are seldom used in ESKD after dialysis is started because, as kidney function is reduced, these drugs can accumulate and harm the remaining kidney cells and the patient's hearing.

Assess fluid status by obtaining daily weights and reviewing intake and output. Daily weight gain in these patients indicates fluid retention rather than true body weight gain. Estimate the amount of fluid retained: 1 kg of weight equals about 1 L of fluid retained. Weigh the patient daily at the same time each day, on the same scale, wearing the same amount of clothing, and after voiding (if the patient is not anuric). Monitor weight for changes before and after dialysis.

CHART 68-5   Best Practice for Patient Safety & Quality Care QSEN

Managing Fluid Volume

- Weigh the patient daily at the same time each day, using the same scale, with the patient wearing the same amount and type of clothing, and graph the results.
- Observe the weight graph for trends (1 L of water weighs 1 kg).
- Accurately measure all fluid intake and output.
- Teach the patient and family about the need to keep fluid intake within prescribed restricted amounts and to ensure that the prescribed daily amount is evenly distributed throughout the 24 hours.
- Monitor for these symptoms of fluid overload at least every 4 hours during critical illness:
  - Decreased urine output
  - Rapid, bounding pulse
  - Rapid, shallow respirations
  - Presence of dependent edema
  - Auscultation of crackles or wheezes
  - Presence of distended neck veins in a sitting position
  - Decreased oxygen saturation
  - Elevated blood pressure
  - Narrowed pulse pressure
- Assess level of consciousness and degree of cognition.
- Ask about the presence of headache or blurred vision.

Fluid restriction is often needed. Consider all forms of fluid intake, including oral, IV, and enteral sources, when calculating fluid intake. Help the patient spread oral fluid intake over a 24-hour period. Monitor his or her response to fluid restriction, and notify the primary health care provider if symptoms of fluid overload persist or worsen.

Preventing Pulmonary Edema

Planning: Expected Outcomes. The patient with CKD is expected to remain free of pulmonary edema by maintaining optimal fluid balance. Indicators include that the patient has no breathing difficulty and no adventitious lung sounds (e.g., crackles, wheezes) with auscultation and that oxygen saturation remains greater than 92%.

Interventions. Pulmonary edema can result from left-sided heart failure related to fluid overload or from blood vessel injury. In left-sided heart failure, the heart is unable to eject blood adequately from the left ventricle, leading to an increased pressure in the left atrium and in the pulmonary blood vessels. The increased pressure causes fluid to cross the capillaries into the pulmonary tissue, forming edema (McCance et al., 2014). Pulmonary edema can also occur from injury to the lung blood vessels as a result of uremia. This condition causes inflammation and capillary leak. Fluid then leaks from pulmonary circulation into the lung tissue and alveoli. It may also leak into the pleural space, causing a *pleural effusion*.

Assess the patient for early indicators of pulmonary edema, such as restlessness, anxiety, rapid heart rate, shortness of breath, and crackles that begin at the base of the lungs. As pulmonary edema worsens, the level of fluid in the lungs rises. Auscultation reveals increased crackles and decreased breath sounds. The patient may have frothy, blood-tinged sputum. As cardiac and pulmonary function decrease further, the patient becomes diaphoretic and cyanotic.

The patient with pulmonary edema usually is admitted to the hospital for aggressive treatment and continuous cardiac monitoring. Place the patient in a high-Fowler's position and give oxygen to improve gas exchange. Drug therapy with kidney failure and pulmonary edema is difficult because of potential

CONCEPT MAP

CHRONIC KIDNEY DISEASE

- ELIMINATION
- FLUID AND ELECTROLYTE BALANCE
- ACID-BASE BALANCE
- PERFUSION
- IMMUNITY

NOTICE IN THE HISTORY

Joe Brown is a 55-year-old African-American man who has a lengthy history of type 2 diabetes, coronary artery disease, and hyperlipidemia. He has had complete loss of kidney function for 4 months. His vital signs are T – 100° F; P – 104 and irregular; R – 32; BP – 160/100 mm Hg.

Noticing the details

- Age 55, male, height 5'9", 225 lbs, recent weight gain of 8 lbs.
- History of kidney stones, uncontrolled DM type 2, drug use, hypertension, and hyperlipidemia. Family history of polycystic kidney disease.
- Chronic use of NSAIDs for arthritis pain.
- Reports that desserts "don't taste sweet like before" and meat leaves a metallic taste. Some nausea and anorexia.
- Reports feeling weak and tired and is often short of breath. He has several bruises on his arms and legs at different stages.
- States he urinates dark-colored urine in small amounts a few times a day.

Interpreting the Data

PATIENT PROBLEMS

- Fluid Overload due to inability of kidneys to maintain body fluid balance
- Potential for pulmonary edema due to fluid overload
- Decreased PERFUSION due to reduced stroke volume, dysrhythmias, fluid overload, and increased peripheral vascular resistance
- Inadequate nutrition due to inability to ingest, digest, or absorb food and nutrients as a result of physiologic factors
- Potential for infection due to skin breakdown, IMMUNITY-related kidney dysfunction, or malnutrition
- Potential for injury due to effects of kidney disease on bone density, blood clotting, and drug elimination
- Fatigue due to kidney disease, anemia, and reduced energy production
- Anxiety due to threat to or change in health status, economic status, relationships, role function, systems, or self-concept; situational crisis; threat of death; lack of knowledge about diagnostic tests, disease process, treatment; loss of control; or disrupted family life

Planning Expected Outcomes

EXPECTED OUTCOMES

- Achieve and maintain acceptable FLUID AND ELECTROLYTE BALANCE
- Maintain a stable body weight
- No exhibiting signs of pulmonary edema
- Maintain adequate PERFUSION
- Maintain adequate nutrition
- Remain free of infection
- Remain free of injury
- Decreased fatigue

INTERVENTIONS—RESPONDING

1. Physical Assessment—Noticing

Assess for presence of S_3 or pericardial friction rub, chest pain, jugular vein distention, edema, fatigue, dyspnea, crackles, weight change, skin integrity, pruritus, skin discoloration, mental status, seizure activity, sensory changes, LE weakness, anorexia, nausea, vomiting, stomatitis, melena, urine amount/frequency/appearance, bone pain, presence of hyperglycemia secondary to diabetes, signs of bleeding disorders (petechiae, purpura, ecchymosis). *Guides patient care; assesses for signs of kidney failure.*

2. Fluid and Electrolyte Balance

Monitor vital signs, intake and output, weight, hydration status, treat hypertension with drug therapy. *Monitors for fluid overload; sodium retention causes hypertension and edema.*

3. Monitoring for Pulmonary Edema

- Assess for restlessness, anxiety, tachycardia, shortness of breath, crackles, decreased breath sounds, frothy, blood-tinged sputum, and diaphoresis. *Indicates pulmonary edema; uremic injury to lung blood vessels causes inflammation.*
- Position the patient in high Fowler's; give oxygen, loop diuretics, and measure urine output every 5-30 minutes. *Decreases fluid volume, improves gas exchange and PERFUSION.*
- Monitor vital signs and assess breath sounds at least every 2 hours. *Evaluates the patient's response to treatment.*

4. Maintaining Acid-Base Balance

Ensure participation in renal replacement therapies, either peritoneal dialysis (PD) or hemodialysis (HD). *Improves fluid, electrolyte, and acid-base balance; removes nitrogenous wastes.*

5. Interpreting Laboratory Values

Monitor these blood values: creatinine, blood urea nitrogen (BUN), sodium, potassium, calcium, phosphorus, bicarbonate, hemoglobin, and hematocrit. *Determines the effectiveness of therapy for kidney failure.*

6. Maintaining Adequate PERFUSION

- Assess for signs of heart failure. Administer calcium channel blockers, ACE inhibitors, alpha-adrenergic and beta-adrenergic blockers, vasodilators, and morphine. *Controls blood pressure, which is essential to preserve kidney function.*
- Monitor the patient's respiratory rate, O_2 saturation, and blood pressure hourly if given IV morphine. *Morphine reduces myocardial oxygen demand by triggering blood vessel dilation and to provide sedation. Avoid respiratory depression.*
- Monitor vital signs at least hourly when the patient is given a continuous infusion of nitroglycerin. *The combination of vasodilators causes severe hypotension. Nitroglycerin may be used to reduce pulmonary pressure from left heart failure.*

7. Enhancing Nutrition

Collaborate with the dietitian to determine calories; protein, fluid, potassium, sodium, and phosphorus restrictions; vitamin and mineral supplements. *Provides a balance of food and fluids to prevent malnutrition and avoid complications.*

8. Preventing Infection

Provide meticulous skin care; inspect vascular access site or peritoneal dialysis catheter site for redness, swelling, pain, and drainage. Monitor vital signs for fever and tachycardia. *Prevents and detects early signs of infection.*

9. Health Promotion and Maintenance

Teach the patient and family the importance of adhering to prescribed fluid and dietary restrictions, medications, and dialysis as scheduled. *Promotes health and reduces complications.*

10. Psychosocial Integrity

Encourage the expression of concerns about risks for death and lifestyle disruption; determine the presence of anxiety or maladaptive behavior. Refer to community health or support groups. *Minimizes the impact that depression, anxiety, and nonacceptance have on mental well-being.*

Concept Map by Deanne A. Blach, MSN, RN

adverse drug effects on the kidneys (Burchum & Rosenthal, 2016). Loop diuretics such as IV furosemide (Lasix) are used to manage pulmonary edema. Kidney impairment increases the risk for *ototoxicity* (ear damage with hearing loss) with furosemide; thus IV doses are given cautiously. Diuresis usually begins within 5 minutes of giving IV furosemide. Measure urine output hourly until the patient is stabilized. Monitor vital signs and assess breath sounds at least every 2 hours to evaluate the patient's response to this treatment.

IV morphine (1 to 2 mg) can be prescribed to reduce myocardial oxygen demand by triggering blood vessel dilation and to provide sedation. Dosage adjustments are needed to achieve the desired response and avoid respiratory depression. Monitor the patient's respiratory rate, oxygen saturation, and blood pressure hourly during this therapy. Other drugs that dilate blood vessels, such as nitroglycerin, may be given as a continuous infusion to reduce pulmonary pressure from left heart failure. Monitor vital signs at least hourly because this drug combination may cause severe hypotension.

Monitor serum electrolyte levels daily and report abnormalities to the primary health care provider so imbalances can be corrected quickly. If using ECG monitoring, identify dysrhythmias as they occur and report changes in rhythm that affect consciousness or blood pressure immediately to the provider. Monitor oxygen saturation levels by pulse oximetry and consult with the respiratory therapist for the optimal method to deliver oxygen (e.g., facemask, nasal cannula, or noninvasive mechanical support [see Chapter 28]). Monitor the patient for worsening of the condition with indications of increasing hypoxemia (decreasing Spo_2 values, restlessness, decreased cognition, or new-onset confusion). Temporary intubation and mechanical ventilation may be needed if respiratory failure occurs.

Patients with CKD who have existing cardiac problems, high blood pressure, or chronic fluid retention are at increased risk for developing pulmonary edema. They are less likely to respond quickly to treatment and are more likely to develop problems related to drug therapy. Kidney replacement therapy with ultrafiltration or dialysis may be used to reduce fluid volume.

Increasing Cardiac Function

Planning: Expected Outcomes. The patient with CKD is expected to attain and maintain adequate cardiac function. Indicators include that systolic and diastolic blood pressures, ejection fraction, peripheral pulses, and cognitive status are either normal or nearly normal.

Interventions. Many patients with long-standing hypertension are at risk for CKD and accelerated progression of kidney failure once CKD occurs. *Therefore blood pressure control is essential in preserving kidney function* (Norton et al., 2017a). To control blood pressure, diuretics (especially thiazides), calcium channel blockers, angiotensin-converting enzyme inhibitors (ACEIs), alpha-adrenergic and beta-adrenergic blockers, and vasodilators may be prescribed. ACEIs are the most effective drugs to decrease cardiovascular events when patients have CKD and hypertension. Calcium channel blockers can improve the GFR and blood flow within the kidney.

More information on the specific drugs for blood pressure control can be found in Chapter 36. Indications vary, depending on the patient, and these drugs are used carefully to avoid complications. Different dosages and combinations may be tried until blood pressure control is adequate and side effects are minimized. A common desired outcome of therapy for patients with CKD is to keep blood pressure below 135/85 (Scher et al., 2015).

Teach the patient and family to measure blood pressure daily. Evaluate their ability to measure and record blood pressure accurately using their own equipment. Recheck measurement accuracy on a regular basis. Teach the patient and family about the relationship of blood pressure control to diet and drug therapy. Instruct the patient to weigh daily and to bring records of blood pressure measurements and drug administration times and weights for discussion with the physician, nurse, or registered dietitian.

Assess the patient on an ongoing basis for signs and symptoms of reduced cardiac output, heart failure, and dysrhythmias. These topics are discussed in Chapters 34, 35, and 38.

Enhancing Nutrition

Planning: Expected Outcomes. The patient with CKD is expected to maintain adequate nutrition. He or she should have a protein-caloric intake appropriate for his or her weight-to-height ratio, muscle tone, and laboratory values (serum albumin, hematocrit, hemoglobin).

Interventions. The nutrition needs and diet restrictions for the patient with CKD vary according to the degree of kidney function and the type of kidney replacement therapy used (Table 68-8). The purpose of nutrition therapy is to provide the food and fluids needed to prevent malnutrition and avoid complications from CKD (Norton et al., 2017a).

The patient is referred to a dietitian for dietary teaching and planning. Work with the dietitian to teach the patient about diet changes that are needed as a result of CKD. Common changes include control of protein intake; fluid intake limitation; restriction of potassium, sodium, and phosphorus intake; taking vitamin and mineral supplements; and eating enough calories to meet metabolic need.

Protein restriction early in the course of the disease prevents some of the problems of CKD and may preserve kidney function (Norton et al., 2017b). Protein is restricted on the basis of the degree of kidney and waste ELIMINATION impairment

TABLE 68-8	Dietary Restrictions Needed for Severe Kidney Disease		
DIETARY COMPONENT	**WITH CHRONIC UREMIA**	**WITH HEMODIALYSIS**	**WITH PERITONEAL DIALYSIS**
Protein	0.55-0.60 g/kg/day	1.0-1.5 g/kg/day	1.2-1.5 g/kg/day
Fluid	Depends on urine output but may be as high as 1500-3000 mL/day	500-700 mL/day plus amount of urine output	Restriction based on fluid weight gain and blood pressure
Potassium	60-70 mEq or mmol daily	70 mEq or mmol daily	Usually no restriction
Sodium	1-3 g/day	2-4 g/day	Restriction based on fluid weight gain and blood pressure
Phosphorus	700 mg/day	700 mg/day	800 mg/day

(reduced glomerular filtration rate [GFR]) and the severity of the symptoms. Buildup of waste products from protein breakdown is the main cause of uremia.

The GFR and treatment of CKD are used to guide safe levels of protein intake. A patient with a severely reduced GFR who is *not* undergoing dialysis is usually permitted 0.55 to 0.60 g of protein per kilogram of body weight (e.g., 40 g of protein daily for a 150-lb [70-kg] adult). If protein is lost in the urine, it is added to the diet in amounts equal to that lost. Protein requirements are calculated by the registered dietitian based on actual body weight (corrected for edema), not ideal body weight.

The patient with ESKD receiving dialysis needs *more* protein because some protein is lost through dialysis. Protein requirements are tailored according to the patient's post-dialysis, or "dry," weight. Generally patients receiving hemodialysis are allowed about 1 to 1.5 g of protein/kg/day. Suggested protein-containing foods are meat and eggs. If protein intake is not adequate, muscle wasting can occur. BUN and serum prealbumin levels are used to monitor the adequacy of protein intake. Decreased serum prealbumin levels indicate poor protein intake.

Sodium restriction is needed in patients with little or no urine output to maintain FLUID AND ELECTROLYTE BALANCE. Both fluid and sodium retention cause edema, hypertension, and heart failure (HF). Most patients with CKD retain sodium; a few cannot conserve sodium.

Estimate fluid and sodium retention status by monitoring the patient's body weight and blood pressure. In uremic patients not receiving dialysis, sodium is limited to 1 to 3 g daily, and fluid intake depends on urine output. In patients receiving dialysis, the sodium restriction is 2 to 4 g daily, and fluid intake is limited to 500 to 700 mL plus the amount of any urine output. Instruct the patient not to add salt at the table or during cooking. Many foods are significant sources of sodium (e.g., processed food, fast food, potato chips, pretzels, pickles, ham, bacon, sausage) and difficult to moderate or remove from one's diet. Inattention to sodium intake can increase the duration or number of dialysis treatments and contribute to *disequilibrium syndrome* (feeling "zonked") following dialysis.

Potassium restriction may be needed because high blood potassium levels can cause dangerous cardiac dysrhythmias. Monitor the ECG for tall, peaked T waves caused by hyperkalemia. Document serum potassium levels. Instruct the patient with ESKD to limit potassium intake to 60 to 70 mEq (mmol) daily. Teach him or her to read labels of seasoning agents carefully for sodium and potassium content. Chart 11-6 lists common foods that are low in potassium and are permitted, along with foods that are high in potassium and should be avoided. Instruct patients to avoid salt substitutes composed of potassium chloride. Those receiving peritoneal dialysis or who are producing urine may not need potassium restriction.

Phosphorus restriction for control of phosphorus levels is started early in CKD to avoid renal osteodystrophy. Monitor serum phosphorus levels. Dietary phosphorus restrictions and drugs to assist with phosphorus control may be prescribed. Phosphate binders must be taken at mealtime. Most patients with CKD already restrict their protein intake; and, because high-protein foods are also high in phosphorus, this reduces phosphorus intake. Chapter 11 lists foods high in potassium, sodium, and phosphorus. Cinacalcet (Sensipar), a drug to control parathyroid hormone excess, is also used to manage hyperphosphatemia and hypocalcemia.

Vitamin and mineral supplementation is needed daily for most patients with CKD. Low-protein diets are also low in vitamins, and water-soluble vitamins are removed from the blood during dialysis. Anemia also is a problem in patients with CKD because of the limited iron content of low-protein diets and decreased kidney production of erythropoietin. Thus supplemental iron is needed. Calcium and vitamin D supplements may be needed, depending on the patient's serum calcium levels and bone status.

Nutrition needs for patients undergoing peritoneal dialysis (PD) are slightly different from those for patients undergoing dialysis. Because protein is lost with the dialysate in PD, protein replacement is needed. Often 1.2 to 1.5 g of protein per kilogram of body weight per day is recommended. Patients may have anorexia and have difficulty eating enough protein. High-calorie oral supplements may also be needed (e.g., Magnacal Renal, Ensure Plus). Sodium restriction varies with fluid weight gain and blood pressure. Usually dietary potassium does not need to be restricted because the dialysate is potassium free, causing excess potassium to be removed from the blood. Any potassium restriction is determined by serum potassium levels.

Collaborate with the dietitian to assess each patient's nutrition needs. Teach the patient the dietary regimen and evaluate his or her understanding of and adherence to it. Give the patient and family written examples of the diet to promote adherence. Help patients adapt diet restrictions to their budget, ethnic background, and food preferences.

🔎 NCLEX EXAMINATION CHALLENGE 68-5
Health Promotion and Maintenance

When the nurse caring for a client with severe chronic kidney disease asks what dietary modifications he has made for the disease, he reports the following actions. Which action indicates to the nurse that additional client education is needed?
A. Using a scale to measure protein weight
B. Taking calcium and vitamin D supplements daily
C. Eliminating bananas, citrus fruits, and avocados
D. Using a salt-substitute instead of ordinary table salt

Preventing Infection

Planning: Expected Outcomes. The patient with CKD is expected to remain free of infection. Indicators include that the patient will have mild or no fever, no lymph node enlargement, negative urine culture, negative dialysis access site culture, and white blood cell count either within the normal range or only slightly elevated.

Interventions. Provide meticulous care to nonintact skin areas (e.g., incisions, drain sites, puncture sites, cracked or excoriated skin, pressure injuries) and preventive skin care to intact areas. For patients undergoing dialysis, inspect the vascular access site or peritoneal dialysis catheter insertion site every shift for redness, swelling, pain, and drainage. Monitor vital signs for signs and symptoms of infection (e.g., fever, tachycardia).

Preventing Injury

Planning: Expected Outcomes. The patient with CKD is expected to remain free of injury. Indicators include that the patient is free of these problems:
- Pathologic fractures
- Toxic side effects from drug therapy
- Bleeding

Interventions. *Injury prevention strategies* are needed because the patient with long-standing CKD may have brittle, fragile bones that fracture easily and cause little pain. When lifting or moving a patient with fragile bones, use a lift sheet rather than pulling the patient. Teach unlicensed assistive personnel (UAP) the correct use of lift sheets. Observe for normal range of joint motion and for any unusual surface bumps or depressions over bony areas.

Managing drug therapy in patients with CKD is a complex clinical problem. Many over-the-counter drugs contain agents that alter kidney function. Therefore it is important to obtain a detailed drug history. Know the use of each drug, its side effects, and its site of metabolism.

Certain drugs must be avoided, and the dosages of others must be adjusted according to the degree of remaining kidney function (Gloe et al., 2016). As the patient's kidney function decreases, consult with the nephrologist and pharmacist to determine if further dosage adjustments are necessary. Assess for side effects and indications of drug toxicity and notify the prescriber as appropriate.

> **! NURSING SAFETY PRIORITY** **QSEN**
> *Drug Alert*
>
> Monitor the patient with severe CKD or ESKD closely for drug-related complications and ensure that dosages are adjusted as needed (Gloe et al., 2016). Consult with the pharmacist to determine safe effective doses.

Many drugs are routinely given to patients with CKD (Chart 68-6). Know the rationale for these drugs and the nursing interventions. Many patients also have cardiac disease and may require cardiac drugs such as digoxin. Patients with severe CKD and ESKD are particularly at risk for digoxin toxicity because the drug is excreted by the kidneys. When caring for patients with CKD who are receiving digoxin, monitor for indications of toxicity, such as nausea, vomiting, visual changes, restlessness, headache, confusion, bradycardia, and tachycardia. Monitor the serum drug levels to be certain they are in the therapeutic range (0.8 to 2 ng/mL). Closely monitor serum potassium levels of patients receiving digoxin because low potassium levels increase the risk for dysrhythmias and digoxin toxicity (Burchum & Rosenthal, 2016).

> **! NURSING SAFETY PRIORITY** **QSEN**
> *Drug Alert*
>
> Doses of digoxin are much lower than for most drugs. When digoxin is administered to older adults with kidney disease, the prescribed daily dose may be even lower (0.0625 mg). Check and recheck the dosage before administering digoxin to a patient with kidney disease.

Drugs to control an excessively high phosphorus level include phosphate-binding agents. These drugs help prevent renal osteodystrophy and related injuries. Stress the importance of taking these agents and all prescribed drugs.

Hypophosphatemia (low serum phosphorus levels) is a complication of phosphate binding, especially in patients who do not eat adequately but continue to take phosphate-binding drugs. *Hypercalcemia* (high serum calcium levels) can occur in patients taking calcium-containing compounds to control phosphorus excess. In patients taking aluminum-based phosphate binders for prolonged periods, aluminum deposits may cause bone disease or neurologic problems. Monitor the patient for muscle weakness, anorexia, malaise, tremors, and bone pain.

Teach patients with kidney disease to avoid antacids containing magnesium. These patients cannot excrete magnesium and thus should avoid additional intake.

Some drugs, in addition to those used to treat kidney failure, require special attention because they either are normally excreted by the kidney or can further damage the kidney. These drugs include antibiotics, opioids, antihypertensives, diuretics, insulin, and heparin.

Many antibiotics are safe for patients with CKD, but those excreted by the kidney and those that are nephrotoxic require dose adjustment (Gloe et al., 2016). To prevent complications of bloodstream infection from mouth bacteria, prophylactic antibiotics are given to patients with CKD before dental procedures.

Give opioid analgesics cautiously in patients with Stage 3 or 4 CKD or ESKD because the effects often last longer. Patients with uremia are sensitive to the respiratory depressant effects of these drugs. Because opioids are broken down by the liver and not the kidneys, the dosages are often the same, regardless of the level of kidney function. Monitor the patient's reactions closely after opioids are given to determine whether adjustments are needed.

As CKD progresses, the patient with diabetes often requires reduced doses of insulin or antidiabetic drugs because the failing kidneys do not excrete or metabolize these drugs well. Thus the drugs are effective longer, increasing the risk for hypoglycemia (Gloe et al., 2016). Monitor blood glucose levels at least four times daily to assess whether a dosage change is needed.

Poor platelet function and capillary fragility in CKD make anticoagulant therapy risky. Monitor patients receiving heparin, warfarin, or any anticoagulant every shift for bleeding. See Chapter 40 for more information on caring for patients at increased risk for bleeding.

Minimizing Fatigue

Planning: Expected Outcomes. The patient with CKD is expected to conserve energy by balancing activity and rest. Indicators include that the patient participates in self-care activities, has interest in surroundings, and demonstrates mental concentration.

Interventions. Some causes of fatigue in the patient with CKD include vitamin deficiency, anemia, and buildup of urea. All patients are given vitamin and mineral supplements because of diet restrictions and vitamin losses from dialysis. Avoid giving these supplements right before hemodialysis (HD) treatment because they will be dialyzed out of the body and the patient will receive no benefit.

The anemic patient with CKD is treated with agents to stimulate red blood cell production. The desired outcome of this therapy is to maintain a hemoglobin level around 10 g/dL (100 g/L). This therapy triggers bone marrow production of red blood cells if the patient has adequate iron stores. Iron supplements may be needed in patients who are iron deficient. Many who receive these drugs report improved appetite and sexual function along with decreased fatigue. The increased production of all blood cells from this therapy may increase blood pressure. The improved appetite challenges patients in

CHART 68-6 Common Examples of Drug Therapy

Chronic Kidney Disease

DRUG	NURSING IMPLICATIONS
Loop Diuretics—Increase urine output to manage volume overload when urinary elimination is still present	
• Furosemide (Lasix) • Bumetanide (Bumex, Burinex) • Dose varies with severity of kidney damage; not effective in ESKD	Monitor intake and output *to assess therapy effectiveness.* Generally the expected outcome is for output to be greater than intake by 500-1000/mL/24 hr. Monitor electrolytes *because these drugs result in loss of potassium*; this can be a desired effect in patients with hyperkalemia.
Vitamins and Minerals—Used to replace those lost through dialysis or poorly absorbed as a result of dietary restrictions and to lower vitamin or mineral excesses that could lead to more problems	
Phosphate binders form an insoluble calcium-phosphate complex to inhibit GI absorption to prevent hyperphosphatemia and renal osteodystrophy from hypocalcemia: • Calcium acetate (PhosLo) • Calcium carbonate (Caltrate, Oystercal, others) Noncalcium phosphate binders reduce blood phosphate levels without disturbing calcium levels: • Lanthanum carbonate • Sevelamer (Renagel, Renvela)	Teach patients to take drugs with meals *to increase the effectiveness in slowing or preventing the absorption of dietary phosphorus.* Teach patients not to take these drugs within 2 hours of other scheduled drugs *to prevent the inhibited absorption of other drugs, especially cardiac drugs and antibiotics.* Monitor both serum phosphorus and calcium levels because *these drugs lower phosphorus and can cause hypercalcemia.* Monitor for constipation *because these can cause significant constipation, leading to fecal impaction or ileus.* Teach patients to report muscle weakness, slow or irregular pulse, or confusion to the prescriber *because these are symptoms of hypophosphatemia, which require dosage adjustment.*
Multivitamins and vitamin B supplements: • Folic acid/folate (vitamin B$_6$, Folvite, Novo-Folacid ✦) cyanocobalamin (B$_{12}$)	Teach patients to take the drugs after dialysis *to prevent the supplement from being removed from the blood during dialysis.* Teach patients to take iron supplements (ferrous sulfate) with meals *to reduce nausea and abdominal discomfort.*
Oral iron salts: • Ferrous sulfate (Feosol, others) • Ferrous fumarate (Slow Fe, others) • Ferrous gluconate (Fergon, others)	Teach patients to take stool softeners daily while taking iron supplements, *which can cause constipation.* Remind patients that iron supplements change the color of the stool *because knowing the expected side effects decreases anxiety when they appear.*
Parenteral iron salts: • Iron dextran (IV) (INFeD) • Iron sucrose (IV) (Venofer)	A test dose of iron dextran is recommended *before IV administration because the incidence of allergic reactions is high.* Do not mix with drug with other parenteral drugs *because there are many incompatibilities.*
Vitamin D: • Calcitriol (Rocaltrol, Calcijex, Vectical) • Paricalcitol (Zemplar) • Doxercalciferol (Hectorol)	Monitor serum levels of calcium *because this active form of vitamin D suppresses parathyroid production and can lead to hypocalcemia.* Monitor serum levels of vitamin D *because this is a lipid-soluble vitamin that can be overingested and lead to toxicity.*
Erythropoietin-Stimulating Agents (ESAs)—Prevent or correct anemia caused by kidney disease through the stimulation of the bone marrow to increase red blood cell production and maturation	
• Epoetin alfa (Epogen, Procrit, generic) • Darbepoetin alfa (Aranesp)	Monitor hemoglobin values *because these drugs can overproduce blood cells, which increases blood viscosity and causes hypertension. This problem increases the risk for a myocardial infarction. The drug should not be given when hemoglobin levels are greater than 13 g/dL (130 g/L)* Teach patients to report any of these side effects to the prescriber as soon as possible: chest pain, difficulty breathing, high blood pressure, rapid weight gain, seizures, skin rash or hives, or swelling of feet or ankles *because these symptoms indicate possible serious cardiac complications.*
Parathyroid Hormone Modulator—Reduces parathyroid gland production of parathyroid hormone by decreasing the gland's sensitivity to calcium. This action helps maintain blood calcium and phosphorus levels closer to normal and can reduce renal osteodystrophy in patients with chronic kidney disease.	
• Cinacalcet (Sensipar)	Monitor blood levels of calcium and phosphorus *to assess drug therapy effectiveness and recognize imbalances of these important electrolytes.* Teach the patient to monitor for and report diarrhea and muscle pain (myalgia), *which are indications of calcium and/or phosphorus imbalance.*

ESKD, End-stage kidney disease.

their attempts to maintain protein, potassium, and fluid restrictions and requires additional education.

Reducing Anxiety

Planning: Expected Outcomes. The patient with CKD is expected to have reduced tension and apprehension. Indicators include that the patient consistently demonstrates these behaviors:

• Uses effective coping strategies
• Reports an absence of anxiety

Interventions. Perform an ongoing assessment of the patient's anxiety level. Observe behavior for cues indicating increasing anxiety (e.g., anxious facial expressions, clenching of hands, tapping of feet, withdrawn posture, absence of eye contact) and provide interventions to decrease the anxiety level.

Evaluate the support systems and the involvement of family and friends with the patient's care. Provide ongoing supportive interventions throughout therapy.

Unfamiliar settings and lack of knowledge about treatments and tests can increase the patient's anxiety level. Explain all procedures, tests, and treatments. Identify the patient's knowledge needs about kidney disease. Provide instruction at a level that he or she can understand using a variety of written and visual materials.

Provide continuity of care, whenever possible, by using a consistent and trusting nurse-patient relationship to decrease anxiety and encourage the patient to discuss his or her thoughts and feelings about any current problems or concerns.

Encourage the patient to ask questions and discuss fears about the diagnosis, treatment strategies, common outcomes. An open atmosphere that allows for discussion can decrease anxiety. Facilitate discussions with family members about the prognosis and the impact on lifestyle.

Recognizing and Managing Depression. In people with CKD the number and severity of symptoms and the presence of comorbidities may lead to depression (Tsai et al., 2015). Loss, such as loss of work or family roles may contribute to depression. Depressive symptoms have been associated with nonadherence to CKD treatments. Sleep disturbances, also interrelated with depression, are common among adults receiving dialysis for ESKD.

Planning: Expected Outcomes. The patient with CKD is expected to participate in self-care, have minimal social isolation, demonstrate effective coping, and have minimal spiritual distress related to CKD and its treatments. Indicators include that the patient consistently demonstrates these behaviors:

- Expresses feelings about performing self-care activities
- Initiates and assists with ADLs
- Sleeps and reports feeling refreshed from sleeping
- Discusses concerns about work and leisure involvement
- Maintains contact with family and friends
- Identifies resources such as self-help groups and religious communities for support

Interventions. Assess for indicators of despair and loneliness. Encourage involvement in decisions and community support groups. Identify community resources to maintain independence, including delivered meals, transportation, and financial or health care options. Ask about sleep patterns and quality. Assess the coping mechanisms and successful methods of dealing with problems.

In the general population, drugs are commonly used to manage depression. However, pharmacologic effects of drugs in adults with CKD or those receiving dialysis are altered and may need additional monitoring with alternative approaches for effective care. Care coordination for patients with CKD is essential because multiple health care professions may be involved in delivering care. Care coordination helps to avoid adverse drug effects (and drug-drug interactions), avoid hospitalizations, and decrease problems related to depression.

Kidney Replacement Therapies

Kidney replacement therapy (KRT) is needed when the pathologic changes of stage 4 and stage 5 CKD are life threatening or pose continuing discomfort. When the patient can no longer be managed with conservative therapies, such as diet, drugs, and fluid restriction, dialysis is indicated. Transplantation may be discussed at any time.

TABLE 68-9	Comparison of Hemodialysis and Peritoneal Dialysis
HEMODIALYSIS	**PERITONEAL DIALYSIS**
Advantages	
More efficient clearance of wastes	Flexible schedule for exchanges
Short time needed for treatment	Few hemodynamic changes during and following exchanges
	Fewer dietary and fluid restrictions
Complications	
Disequilibrium syndrome	Protein loss
Muscle cramps and back pain	Peritonitis
Headache	Hyperglycemia from dialysate
Itching	Respiratory distress
Hemodynamic and cardiac adverse events (hypotension, cell lysis contributing to anemia, cardiac dysrhythmias)	Bowel perforation
	Infection
Infection	Weight gain; discomfort from "carrying" 1-2 L in abdomen during dwell time; potential for back pain or development of hernia
Increased risk for subdural and intracranial hemorrhage from anticoagulation and changes in blood pressure during dialysis	
Contraindications	
Hemodynamic instability or severe cardiac disease	Extensive peritoneal adhesions, fibrosis, or active inflammatory GI disease (e.g., diverticulitis, inflammatory bowel conditions)
Severe vascular disease that prevents vascular access	
Serious bleeding disorders	Ascites or massive central obesity
Uncontrolled diabetes	Recent abdominal surgery
Access	
Vascular fistula, shunt, or catheter	Intra-abdominal catheter
Procedure	
Complex; requires a second person trained in the technique whether completed at home or at a dialysis unit/center	Simple, easier to complete at home compared with at-home hemodialysis
Special training for center personnel and in-home use	Less complex training; typically managed by patient; can be managed by one person

Hemodialysis. Intermittent hemodialysis (HD) is the most common KRT used with ESKD (Table 68-9). Dialysis removes excess fluids and waste products and restores FLUID AND ELECTROLYTE BALANCE and ACID-BASE BALANCE. HD involves passing the patient's blood through an artificial semipermeable membrane to perform the kidney's filtering and excretion functions. Safe HD therapy requires technicians to provide meticulous care to the machines delivering HD and nurses to implement and supervise direct care. Technical or human error can lead to avoidable complications (e.g., hemolysis, air embolism, dialysate error, contamination, exsanguination).

Patient Selection. Any patient may be considered for intermittent HD therapy. Starting HD depends on symptoms from disruptions of FLUID AND ELECTROLYTE BALANCE and waste and toxin accumulation, not the GFR alone. Dialysis is started immediately for patients who have:

- Acidosis that is severe (pH <7.2) or does not respond to therapy

- Fluid overload that does not respond to diuretics (including fluid overload with pulmonary edema or pericarditis)
- Symptomatic hyperkalemia with ECG changes
- Calciphylaxis (thrombosis and skin necrosis that can occur in stage 5 CKD)
- Toxin ingestion such as dialyzable drug overdose or poisoning (see Table 68-13)

Most commonly, hemodialysis for CKD is started when uremic symptoms (e.g., intractable nausea and vomiting, confusion, seizures, or severe bleed from platelet dysfunction) occur.

Many patients survive for years with HD therapy, and others may live only a few months. Length of survival with HD therapy depends on patient age, the cause of CKD, and the presence of other diseases, such as cardiovascular conditions or diabetes. Selection criteria include:

- Irreversible kidney failure when other therapies are unacceptable or ineffective
- No disorders that would seriously complicate HD
- Patient values and preferences
- Expected ability to continue or resume roles at home, work, or school

Dialysis Settings. Patients with CKD may receive HD treatments in many settings, depending on specific needs. Regardless of the setting for therapy, they need ongoing nursing support to maintain this complex and lifesaving treatment.

Patients may be dialyzed in a hospital-based center if they have recently started treatment or have complicated conditions that require close supervision. Stable patients not requiring intense supervision may be dialyzed in a community or free-standing dialysis center. Selected patients may participate in self-care in an ambulatory care center or with in-home HD.

In-home HD is the least disruptive treatment and allows the patient to adapt the regimen to his or her lifestyle. Newer technologies and HD equipment are making home dialysis an easier process to learn. It is growing in popularity and use. A water treatment system must be installed in the home to provide a safe, clean water supply for the dialysis process.

Procedure. Dialysis works using the passive transfer of toxins by diffusion. Diffusion is the movement of molecules from an area of higher concentration to an area of lower concentration. The rate of diffusion during dialysis is most dependent on the difference in the solute concentrations between the patient's blood and the dialysate. Large molecules, such as RBCs and most plasma proteins, cannot pass through the membrane.

When HD is started, blood and dialysate (dialyzing solution) flow in opposite directions across an enclosed semipermeable membrane. The dialysate contains a balanced mix of electrolytes and water that closely resembles human plasma. On the other side of the membrane is the patient's blood, which contains nitrogen waste products, excess water, and excess electrolytes. During HD, the waste products move from the blood into the dialysate because of the difference in their concentrations (diffusion). Some water is also removed from the blood into the dialysate by *osmosis.* Electrolytes can move in either direction, as needed, and take some fluid with them. Potassium and sodium typically move out of the plasma into the dialysate. Bicarbonate and calcium generally move from the dialysate into the plasma. This circulating process continues for a preset length of time, removing nitrogenous wastes, reestablishing FLUID AND ELECTROLYTE BALANCE, and restoring ACID-BASE BALANCE. Water

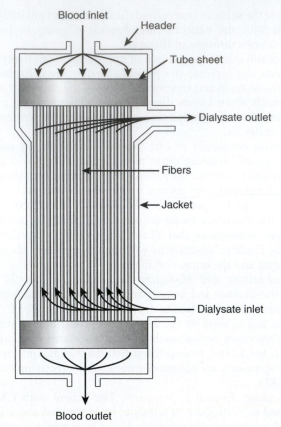

FIG. 68-3 Hollow fiber dialyzer (artificial kidney) used in hemodialysis. (From Feehally, J., Floege, J., & Johnson, R. [2007]. *Comprehensive clinical nephrology* [3rd ed.]. Philadelphia: Mosby.)

volume may be removed from the plasma by applying positive or negative pressure to the system.

The HD system includes a dialyzer, dialysate, vascular access routes, and an HD machine. The artificial kidney, or **dialyzer** (Fig. 68-3), has four parts: a blood compartment, a dialysate compartment, a semipermeable membrane, and an enclosed support structure.

Dialysate is made from water and chemicals and is free of any waste products or drugs. It is usually dispensed from the pharmacy in an acute care setting. The solution may be mixed in large or small batches by technicians in dialysis centers. Because bacteria and other organisms are too large to pass through the membrane, dialysate is not sterile. Water used in dialysate must meet specific standards and requires special treatment before mixing the dialysate. Dialysate composition may be altered for the patient's needs for management of electrolyte imbalances. During HD, the dialysate is warmed to 100° F (37.8° C) to increase the diffusion rate and prevent hypothermia.

The HD machine has built-in safety features such as the ability to record patient vital signs, blood and dialysate flows, arterial and venous pressures, delivered dialysis dose, plasma volume changes, and temperature changes. If any of these problems are detected, an alarm sounds to protect the patient from life-threatening complications.

All dialyzers function in a similar manner. Fig. 68-4 shows a comparison of fluid and particle movement across the dialyzer membranes, comparing intermittent HD with continuous kidney replacement circuits. For intermittent HD, the number and length of treatments depend on the amount of wastes and fluid to be removed, the clearance capacity of the dialyzer, and

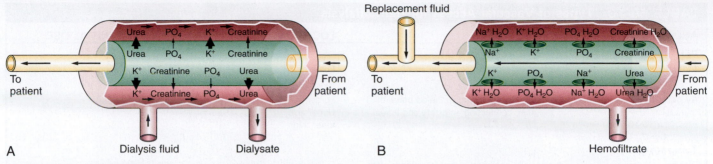

FIG. 68-4 Comparison of hemodialysis and hemofiltration fluid and solute movements across the membrane. Demonstrates this movement in hemodialysis **(A)** and hemofiltration **(B)**. The *arrows* that cross the membrane indicate the predominant direction of movement of each solute through the membrane; the relative size of the *arrows* indicates the net amounts of the solute transferred. Other *arrows* indicate the direction of flow. (From Feehally, J., Floege, J., & Johnson, R. [2007]. *Comprehensive clinical nephrology* [3rd ed.]. Philadelphia: Mosby.)

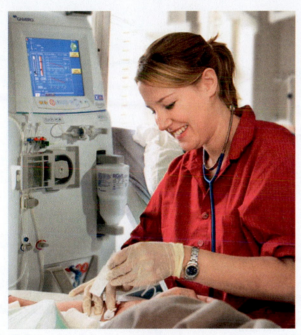

FIG. 68-5 Renal replacement therapy with an intermittent hemodialysis machine. (Courtesy Gambro Lundia AB, Lund, Sweden.)

the blood flow rate to and from the machine. Fig. 68-5 shows a typical intermittent dialysis machine. Most patients receive three 4-hour treatments over the course of a week. For those with some ongoing urine production, two 5- to 6-hour treatments a week may be adequate. If the patient gains large amounts of fluid, a longer HD treatment time may be needed to remove the fluid without hypotension or other severe side effects.

Anticoagulation. Blood clotting can occur during dialysis. Anticoagulation, usually with heparin, is delivered into the blood circuit via a pump. In patients with high risk for bleeding, a reduced dose, regional anticoagulation (using citrate rather than heparin for anticoagulation or reversing heparin actions by administering protamine before returning blood to the patient), or no anticoagulation may be used. Patient response to heparin varies, and the dose is adjusted on the basis of each patient's need.

Heparin remains active in the body for 4 to 6 hours after dialysis, increasing the patient's risk for hemorrhage during and immediately after HD treatments. Invasive procedures

must be avoided during that time. Monitor him or her closely for any signs of bleeding or hemorrhage. Protamine sulfate is an antidote to heparin and always should be available in the dialysis setting.

Vascular Access. Vascular access is required for hemodialysis (Table 68-10 and Fig. 68-6). The procedure requires the availability of a high blood flow: at least 250 to 300 mL/min, usually for a period of 3 to 4 hours (Norton et al., 2017b). Normal venous cannulation does not provide this high rate of blood flow.

Long-term vascular access is internal for most patients having long-term HD (see Table 68-10). The two common choices are an internal arteriovenous (AV) fistula or an AV graft (see Fig. 68-6A-C). *AV fistulas* are formed by surgically connecting an artery to a vein. The vessels used most often are the radial or brachial artery and the cephalic vein of the nondominant arm. Fistulas increase venous blood flow to the 250 to 400 mL/min needed for effective dialysis.

Time is needed after the surgeon creates the AV fistula for it to develop into a usable access site for HD. As the AV fistula "matures," the increased pressure of the arterial blood flow into the vein causes the vessel walls to thicken. This thickening increases their strength and durability for repeated cannulation. The amount of time needed for the fistula to mature varies. Some fistulas may not be ready for use for as long as 4 months after the surgery, and a temporary vascular access (AV shunt or HD catheter) is used during this time. Fig. 68-7 shows a mature fistula.

To access a fistula, cannulate it by inserting two needles: one toward the venous blood flow and one toward the arterial blood flow. This procedure allows the HD machine to draw the blood out through the arterial needle and return it through the venous needle.

Arteriovenous grafts are used when the AV fistula does not develop or when complications limit its use. The polytetrafluoroethylene (PTFE) graft is a synthetic material (GORE-TEX). This type of graft is commonly used for older patients using HD. Figs. 68-6A and 68-7 show a patient's fistula.

Precautions. Precautions are needed to ensure the functioning of an internal AV fistula or AV graft. First assess for adequate circulation in the fistula or graft and in the lower portion of the arm. Check distal pulses and capillary refill in the arm with the fistula or graft. Then check for a bruit or a thrill by auscultation or palpation over the access site. Chart 68-7 lists best practices for care of the patient with an HD access.

TABLE 68-10 Types of Vascular Access for Hemodialysis

ACCESS TYPE	DESCRIPTION	LOCATION	TIME TO INITIAL USE
Permanent			
AV fistula	An internal anastomosis of an artery to a vein	Forearm Upper arm	2-4 mo or longer
AV graft	Synthetic vessel tubing tunneled beneath the skin, connecting an artery and a vein	Forearm Upper arm Inner thigh	1-2 wk
Temporary			
Dialysis catheter	A specially designed catheter with separate lumens for blood outflow and inflow	Subclavian vein, internal jugular, or femoral vein	Immediately after insertion and x-ray confirmation of placement
Subcutaneous catheter	An internal device with two access ports and a cuff or dual-lumen catheter inserted into a large central vein	Subclavian vein, internal jugular, or femoral vein	Dedicated use; do not access for blood sampling or drug administration

AV, Arteriovenous.

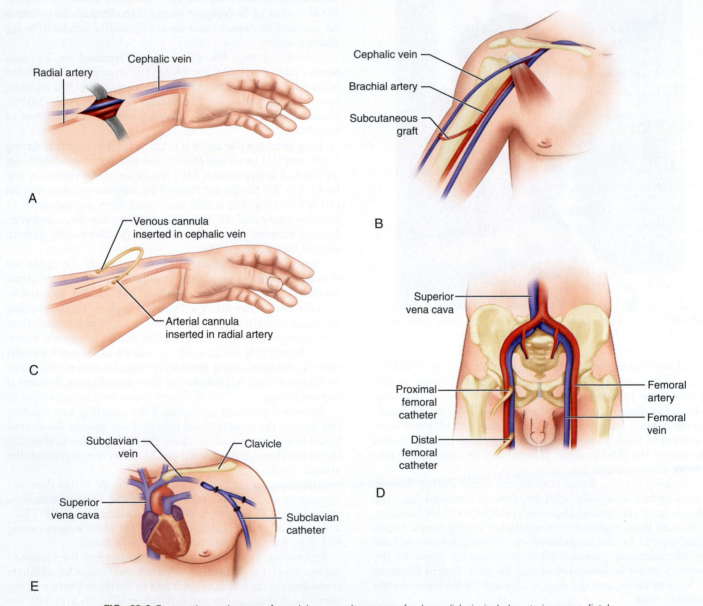

FIG. 68-6 Frequently used means for gaining vascular access for hemodialysis include arteriovenous fistula **(A)**, arteriovenous graft **(B)**, external arteriovenous shunt **(C)**, femoral vein catheterization **(D)**, and subclavian vein catheterization **(E)**. **A** and **B** are options for long-term vascular access for hemodialysis. **C**, **D**, and **E** are used for short-term access for intermittent hemodialysis or for continuous renal replacement therapy in acute care.

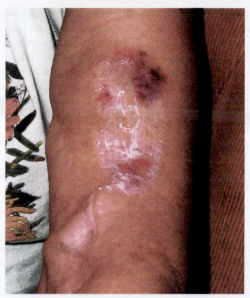

FIG. 68-7 A mature fistula for hemodialysis access. The increased pressure from the anastomosed artery forced blood into the vein. This process caused the vein to dilate enough for fistula needles to be placed for hemodialysis. When the vein is sufficiently dilated, a process that takes 8 to 12 weeks, the fistula is said to be *developed* or *mature.*

◎ CHART 68-7   Best Practice for Patient Safety & Quality Care QSEN

Caring for the Patient With an Arteriovenous Fistula or Arteriovenous Graft

- Do not take blood pressure readings using the extremity in which the vascular access is placed.
- Do not perform venipunctures or start an IV line in the extremity in which the vascular access is placed.
- Palpate for thrills and auscultate for bruits over the vascular access site every 4 hours while the patient is awake.
- Assess the patient's distal pulses and circulation in the arm with the access.
- Elevate the affected extremity after surgery.
- Encourage routine range-of-motion exercises.
- Check for bleeding at needle insertion sites.
- Assess for indications of infection at needle sites.
- Instruct the patient not to carry heavy objects or anything that compresses the extremity in which the vascular access is placed.
- Instruct the patient not to sleep with his or her body weight on top of the extremity in which the vascular access is placed.

⚠ NURSING SAFETY PRIORITY QSEN
Action Alert

Because repeated compression can result in the loss of the vascular access, avoid taking the blood pressure or performing venipunctures in the arm with the vascular access. Do not use an AV fistula or graft for general delivery of IV fluids or drugs.

Complications. Complications can occur with any type of access. Common problems include thrombosis or stenosis, infection, aneurysm formation, ischemia, and heart failure (Norton et al., 2017b). Table 68-11 lists strategies to prevent access complications.

Thrombosis, or clotting of the AV access, is the most frequent complication. Most grafts fail because of high-pressure arterial flow entering the venous system. The muscle layers of the veins react to this increased pressure by thickening. The venous thickening reduces or occludes blood flow. An interventional radiologist can re-open failing grafts with the injection of a thrombolytic drug (e.g., tPA) to dissolve the clot. The clot usually dissolves within minutes, and often a stricture is revealed at the point where the graft and the vein connect. The stricture can be corrected by balloon angioplasty.

Most infections of the vascular access are caused by *Staphylococcus aureus* introduced during cannulation. Prepare the skin with an antibacterial agent according to agency policy before cannulation to prevent infection. When using dialysis catheters, be sure to use only the cleansing agent recommended by the catheter manufacturer. Some disinfectants can damage the catheter (Stupak et al., 2016).

Aneurysms can form in the fistula and are caused by repeated needle punctures at the same site. Large aneurysms may cause loss of the fistula's function and require surgical repair.

Ischemia occurs in a few patients with vascular access when the fistula decreases arterial blood flow to areas below the fistula *(steal syndrome).* Symptoms vary from cold or numb fingers to gangrene. If the collateral circulation is poor, the fistula may need to be surgically tied off, and a new one created in another area to preserve extremity circulation.

Shunting of blood directly from the arterial system to the venous system through the fistula can cause heart failure in patients with limited cardiac function. This complication is rare; but, if it does occur, the fistula may need to be revised to reduce arterial blood flow.

TABLE 68-11	Interventions for Preventing Complications in Hemodialysis Vascular Access			
ACCESS TYPE	**BLEEDING**	**INFECTION**		**CLOTTING**
AV fistula or AV graft	Apply pressure to the needle puncture sites.	Prepare skin using best practices before cannulation. Typically 2% chlorhexidine is used, similar to central line skin preparation. Between hemodialysis sessions, the patient should wash the area with antibacterial soap and rinse with water.		Avoid constrictive devices such as blood pressure cuffs and tourniquets. Rotate needle insertion sites with each hemodialysis treatment. Assess for thrill and bruit.
Hemodialysis catheters (temporary and permanent)	Assess the access site every time you monitor vital signs.	Use aseptic technique to dress site and access catheter. Do not use catheters for blood sampling, IV fluids, or drug administration.		Place a heparin or heparin/saline dwell solution after hemodialysis treatment.

AV, Arteriovenous.

Temporary Vascular Access. Temporary access with special catheters can be used for patients requiring immediate HD. A catheter designed for HD may be inserted into the subclavian, internal jugular, or femoral vein. The lumens of these devices are much smaller than the permanent accesses, and more time (4 to 8 hours) is required to complete a dialysis session.

Subcutaneous devices may also be surgically inserted to provide temporary access for HD. Implanted beneath the skin, these devices are composed of two small metallic ports with attached catheters that are inserted into large central veins. The ports of subcutaneous devices have internal mechanisms that open when needles are inserted and close when needles are removed. Blood from one port flows from the body to the HD machine and returns to the body via the other port.

Hemodialysis Nursing Care. Many drugs are dialyzable (i.e., can be partially or completely removed from the blood during dialysis). Coordinate with the nephrology health care provider to assess the patient's drug regimen and determine which drugs should be held until after HD treatment. Table 68-12 lists common dialyzable drugs that should be given *after* rather than before HD. Consult the dialysis nurse or nephrologist to determine if antihypertensive drugs should be given before a scheduled dialysis treatment; some short-acting antihypertensives can contribute to hypotension during dialysis.

The time required to complete an HD treatment usually is at least 4 hours. During this time patients may use various distraction techniques to prevent boredom, such as reading, watching television or videos, visiting with friends or relatives, playing video games, or working puzzles. This time can be used also for brief health teaching opportunities.

Post-Dialysis Care. Closely monitor the patient immediately and for several hours after dialysis for any side effects from the treatment. Common problems include hypotension, headache, nausea, vomiting, dizziness, and muscle cramps.

Obtain vital signs and weight for comparison with pre-dialysis measurements. Blood pressure and weight are expected to be reduced as a result of fluid removal. Hypotension may require rehydration with IV fluids, such as normal saline. The patient's temperature may also be elevated because the dialysis machine warms the blood slightly. If he or she has a fever, sepsis may be present, and a blood sample is needed for culture and sensitivity.

The heparin or citrate required during HD increases the risk for excessive bleeding. All invasive procedures must be avoided for 4 to 6 hours after dialysis. Continually monitor the patient for hemorrhage during and for at least 1 hour after dialysis (Chart 68-8).

Complications of Hemodialysis. Few adverse events occur during a 3- to 4-hour HD treatment under current practice protocols. Improved water treatment, more physiologic solutions, and improvements in HD equipment and procedures have significantly improved safe care for patients receiving this treatment. Complications during HD include hypotension, dialysis disequilibrium syndrome, cardiac events, and reactions to dialyzers (Norton et al., 2017b).

! NURSING SAFETY PRIORITY **QSEN**

Critical Rescue

Monitor the patient closely during dialysis to recognize hypotension, which is common. Heat transfer from warm solutions can result in vasodilation and a drop in blood pressure. When this occurs, reduce the temperature of the dialysate to 35° C (95° F). Fluid shifts from the plasma volume related to differences in electrolyte concentrations between HD solutions and blood also reduce blood pressure. Respond to modest declines in blood pressure by adjusting the rate of dialyzer blood flow and placing the patient in a legs-up (Trendelenburg) position. Respond to sustained or symptomatic hypotension by giving a fluid bolus of 100 to 250 mL of normal saline, albumin, or mannitol (if prescribed). A second bolus may be needed. If hypotension persists, new-onset myocardial injury or pericardial disease may be a contributing factor; respond by applying oxygen, reducing the blood flow, and notifying the primary health care provider urgently. Discontinue HD when hypotension continues despite two bolus infusions.

◎ CHART 68-8 Best Practice for Patient Safety & Quality Care **QSEN**

Caring for the Patient Undergoing Hemodialysis

- Weigh the patient before and after dialysis.
- Know the patient's dry weight.
- Discuss with the nephrology health care provider or pharmacist whether any of the patient's drugs should be withheld until after dialysis.
- Be aware of events that occurred during previous dialysis treatments.
- Measure blood pressure, pulse, respirations, and temperature.
- Assess for indications of orthostatic hypotension.
- Assess the vascular access site when taking vital signs and follow agency policy for central line care and dressing changes.
- Observe for bleeding at the vascular access site and other sites where skin integrity is disrupted because anticoagulants given during dialysis and the presence of uremia increase bleeding risk.
- Assess the patient's level of consciousness.
- Assess for headache, nausea, and vomiting.
- Assess serum laboratory tests to evaluate effectiveness of treatment in removing wastes and achieving desired outcomes (e.g., FLUID AND ELECTROLYTE BALANCE, reduction of uremia).

TABLE 68-12 Examples of Dialyzable Drugs

Consult the pharmacist, nephrologist, or dialysis nurse to plan the best time to administer a drug based on the dialysis schedule.

Aminoglycosides
- Amikacin
- Gentamicin
- Tobramycin

Antituberculosis Agents
- Ethambutol
- Isoniazid

Antiviral and Antifungal Agents
- Acyclovir
- Ganciclovir
- Fluconazole

Cephalosporins
- Cefaclor
- Cefazolin
- Cefoxitin
- Ceftizoxime
- Ceftriaxone
- Cefuroxime
- Cefepime

Anticonvulsants
- Ethosuximide
- Gabapentin
- Phenobarbital

Penicillins
- Amoxicillin
- Ampicillin
- Cloxacillin
- Dicloxacillin
- Mezlocillin
- Penicillin G
- Ticarcillin

Miscellaneous
- Aztreonam
- Cimetidine
- Vitamins
- Clavulanic acid
- Allopurinol
- Enalapril
- Aspirin

Dialysis disequilibrium syndrome may develop during HD or after HD has been completed. It is characterized by mental status changes and can include seizures or coma, although this severity of disequilibrium syndrome is rare with today's HD practice. A mild form of disequilibrium syndrome includes symptoms of nausea, vomiting, headaches, fatigue, and restlessness. It is thought to be the result of a rapid reduction in electrolytes and other particles. Reducing blood flow at the onset of symptoms can prevent this syndrome.

Cardiac events during HD are associated with underlying cardiovascular disease, especially left ventricular hypertrophy, coronary vascular disease, and a history of cardiac dysrhythmias. These conditions are described in Chapters 34, 35, and 38. Although cardiac arrest is a rare event, the setting should be equipped with an automatic defibrillator and staff or family trained in cardiopulmonary resuscitation. Often cardiac arrest is related to new-onset cardiac ischemia. This problem is managed in an acute care setting in which the presence of myocardial disease can be evaluated and cardiac treatment optimized.

Pericardial disease is a complication of patients with ESKD. Assess the patient's heart sounds for the presence of a pericardial rub before starting dialysis. Intensification of dialysis may be used to treat this complication. Other treatment might include NSAID use or surgery.

Reactions to dialyzers still occur, although more biocompatible membranes and careful attention to rinsing the dialyzer before use (to eliminate sterilizing agents) have reduced this adverse event during HD. Reactions occur during a "first-time" use of the filter and resemble an anaphylactic episode early during HD, with profound hypotension. (Chapter 20 describes anaphylactic reactions.) With suspected dialyzer reactions, do not return the blood to the patient and discontinue HD. Corticosteroids may be used to treat the IMMUNITY reaction.

Other potential complications of HD require the nurse to monitor the level of consciousness and vital signs frequently during treatment and to slow or stop HD when symptoms occur. Hypoglycemia is a rare adverse HD event and more likely to occur when the patient has diabetes. It is managed by providing glucose and increasing dialysis glucose concentration in subsequent treatments. Hemorrhage can occur when needle dislodgment or circuit connections become loose and is amplified by anticoagulation used to maintain circuit patency. Some hemolysis occurs because of mechanical trauma to red blood cells, contributing to anemia in the patient with CKD and, perhaps, to sensations of dyspnea or chest tightness.

Infectious diseases transmitted by blood transfusion are a serious complication of long-term HD. Two of the most serious blood-transmitted infections are hepatitis and HIV infection. *Hepatitis B infection* and *hepatitis C infection* in patients with CKD have decreased because the use of erythropoietin-stimulating agents (ESAs) has reduced the need for blood transfusions to maintain red blood cell counts. Hepatitis is a problem because of the blood access and the risk for contamination during HD. The viruses can be transmitted through the use of contaminated needles or instruments, by entry of contaminated blood through open wounds in the skin or mucous membranes, or through transfusions with contaminated blood. Monitor all patients receiving HD for indications of hepatitis (see Chapter 58).

The risk for HIV transmission is reduced by the consistent practice of Standard Precautions, routine screening of donated blood for HIV, and decreased need for blood transfusions with CKD and ESKD. Patients who have been undergoing HD or who received frequent transfusions during the early to middle 1980s may have been infected at that time and are at risk for acquired immune deficiency syndrome (AIDS) (see Chapter 19).

CONSIDERATIONS FOR OLDER ADULTS
Patient-Centered Care QSEN

Between the years 2000 and 2010, a threefold increase in the number of older adults diagnosed with CKD occurred. In 2010, the number of patients ages 60 years and older increased to more than 25% of patients beginning ESKD therapy (USRDS, 2015). The overall mean age for new patients requiring dialysis is 64.6. Patients older than 65 years who are receiving HD are at greater risk for dialysis-induced hypotension. Older adults require more frequent monitoring during and after dialysis

Peritoneal Dialysis. Peritoneal dialysis (PD) allows exchanges of wastes, fluid, and electrolytes to occur in the peritoneal cavity. However, PD is slower than hemodialysis (HD), and more time is needed to achieve the same effect. Other disadvantages of PD are the protein loss in outflow fluid, risk for peritoneal injury, and potential discomfort from indwelling fluid. Advantages and complications are listed in Table 68-9. The use of PD has decreased and currently accounts for less than 10% of dialysis (USRDS, 2015).

Patient Selection. Most patients with CKD can select either HD or PD. For those who are unstable and those who cannot tolerate anticoagulation, PD is less hazardous than HD. For some patients, vascular access problems may eliminate HD as an option. At times a patient may use PD until a new arteriovenous (AV) fistula matures. PD is often the treatment of choice for older adults because it offers more flexibility if his or her status changes frequently.

Peritoneal dialysis *cannot* be performed if peritoneal adhesions are present or if extensive intra-abdominal surgery has been performed (Norton et al., 2017b). In these cases, the surface area of the peritoneal membrane is not sufficient for adequate dialysis exchange. Peritoneal membrane fibrosis may occur after repeated infection, which decreases membrane permeability.

Procedure. A siliconized rubber (Silastic) catheter is surgically placed into the abdominal cavity for infusion of dialysate (Fig. 68-8A-B). Usually 1 to 2 L of dialysate is infused by gravity *(fill)* into the peritoneal space over a 10- to 20-minute period, according to the patient's tolerance. The fluid stays *(dwells)* in the cavity for a specified time prescribed for each patient individually by the nephrologist. It then flows out of the body *(drains)* by gravity into a drainage bag. The peritoneal outflow contains the dialysate and the excess water, electrolytes, and nitrogen-based waste products. The dialyzing fluid is called peritoneal *effluent* on outflow. The three phases of the process (infusion, or "fill"; dwell; and outflow, or drain) make up one PD exchange. The number and frequency of PD exchanges are prescribed by the physician, depending on symptoms and laboratory data.

Process. Peritoneal dialysis occurs through diffusion and osmosis across the semipermeable peritoneal membrane and capillaries. The peritoneal membrane is large and porous. It allows particles and water to move from an area of higher

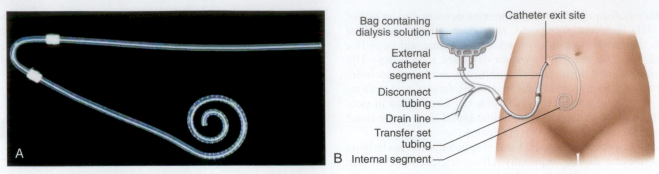

FIG. 68-8 Peritoneal dialysis catheter. **A,** The actual Silastic peritoneal dialysis catheter. **B,** Positioning of the Silastic catheter within the abdominal cavity. (**A** from Geary, D.F., & Schaefer, F. [2008]. *Comprehensive pediatric nephrology*. Philadelphia: Mosby.)

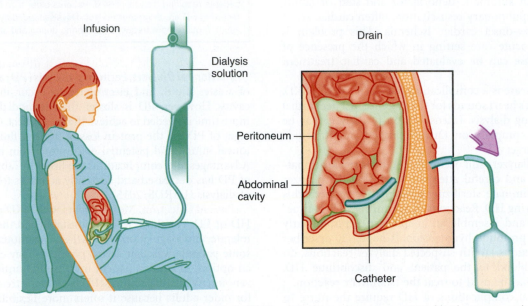

FIG. 68-9 Peritoneal dialysis exchange for control of fluids, electrolytes, nitrogenous wastes, blood pressure, and acid-base balance. The peritoneal membrane acts as the dialyzing membrane.

concentration in the blood to an area of lower concentration in the dialyzing fluid (diffusion).

The peritoneal cavity is rich in capillaries and is a ready access to the blood supply. The fluid and waste products dialyzed from the patient move through the blood vessel walls, the interstitial tissues, and the peritoneal membrane and are removed when the dialyzing fluid is drained from the body.

PD efficiency is affected by many factors. Infection can cause scarring and reduce capillary blood flow. Vascular disease and decreased PERFUSION of the peritoneum reduce PD diffusion. For PD, water removal depends on the concentration of the dialysate. PD efficiency can be altered by the *tonicity* (i.e., number of particles per liter of fluid) of the dialysate. Increasing the dialysate glucose concentration makes the solution more hypertonic (Schreiber, 2016). The more hypertonic the solution, the greater the osmotic pressure for water filtration and fluid removal from the patient during an exchange. The dialysate concentration is prescribed on the basis of the patient's fluid status.

Dialysate Additives. Heparin may be added to the dialysate to prevent clotting of the catheter or tubing. Usually intraperitoneal (IP) heparin is needed only after new catheter placement or if peritonitis occurs. IP heparin is not absorbed systemically and does not affect blood clotting.

Other agents that may be given in the dialysate include potassium and antibiotics. Commercially prepared dialysate does not contain potassium. Some patients need potassium added to the dialysate to prevent hypokalemia. Antibiotics may be given by the IP route when peritonitis is present or suspected. Potassium and antibiotics are not mixed in the same dialysate bag because interactions may reduce the antibiotic effect.

Types of Peritoneal Dialysis. Many types of PD are available, including continuous ambulatory PD, multiple-bag continuous ambulatory PD, automated PD, intermittent PD, and continuous-cycle PD. The type selected depends on the patient's ability and lifestyle. The two most commonly used types of PD are continuous ambulatory peritoneal dialysis and continuous cycling peritoneal dialysis.

Continuous ambulatory peritoneal dialysis (CAPD) is performed by the patient with the infusion of four 2-L exchanges of dialysate into the peritoneal cavity. Each time, the dialysate remains for 4 to 8 hours, and these exchanges occur 7 days a week (Figs. 68-9 to 68-11). During the dwell period, the patient can use a continuous connect system or disconnect and then reconnect at a later time. Most patients using PD long term prefer to complete exchanges overnight with an automated cycler (automatic peritoneal dialysis [APD], described in the following paragraphs).

With the continuous *connect* system (straight transfer set), the dialysate bag is attached to the catheter by 48-inch tubing. The empty bag and tubing are folded and worn beneath the clothing until they are used for outflow. After draining, the patient removes the bag and connects a new bag to repeat the process.

With the *disconnect system* (Y–transfer set), the patient removes the connecting tubing and empties the dialysate bag after inflow and attaches a cap to the PD catheter. The disconnect system eliminates the need to wear the tubing and bag but requires opening the system two extra times with each exchange. The extra opening of the system increases the risk for infection.

With CAPD, no machine is necessary, and no partner is required. However, it is best for a partner also trained in CAPD to be available as a support for the patient if illness occurs. Devices to assist in the safe, sterile connection of the tubing spike into the dialysate bag are available. These are useful for patients with poor vision, limited manual dexterity, or reduced hand and arm strength. CAPD allows constant removal of fluid and wastes and more closely resembles kidney action than HD. Some patients even perform their own exchanges while hospitalized.

Continuous-cycle peritoneal dialysis (CCPD) is a form of automated dialysis that uses an automated cycling machine. Exchanges occur at night while the patient sleeps. The final exchange of the night is left to dwell through the day and is drained the next evening as the process is repeated. CCPD offers the advantage of 24-hour dialysis, as in CAPD, but the sterile catheter system is opened less often.

Automated peritoneal dialysis (APD) may be used in the acute care setting, the ambulatory care dialysis center, or the patient's home. APD uses a cycling machine for dialysate inflow, dwell, and outflow according to preset times and volumes. A warming chamber for dialysate is part of the machine (Fig. 68-12). The functions are programmed for the patient's specific needs. A typical prescription calls for 30-minute exchanges (10/10/10 for inflow, dwell, and outflow) for a period of 8 to 10 hours. The machines have many safety monitors and alarms and are relatively simple to learn to use.

Automated peritoneal dialysis has advantages. It permits in-home dialysis during sleep, allowing the patient to be dialysis free during waking hours. The incidence of peritonitis is reduced with APD because fewer connections and disconnections are

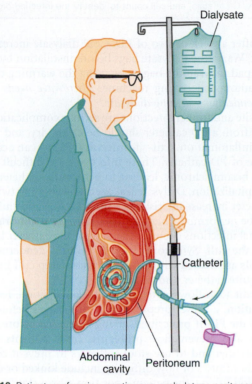

FIG. 68-10 Patient performing continuous ambulatory peritoneal dialysis (CAPD). Note that the patient can walk with this setup.

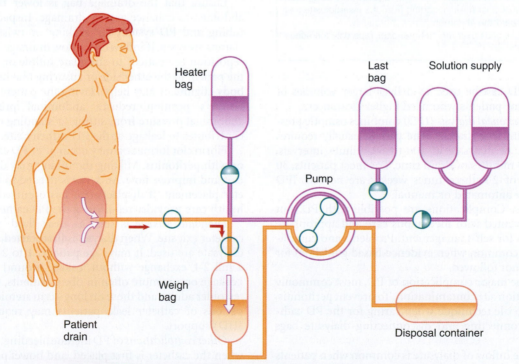

FIG. 68-11 Peritoneal dialysis machine circuit in automated peritoneal dialysis (APD).

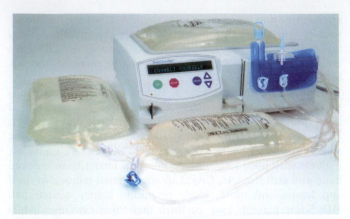

FIG. 68-12 Cycler machine for automated peritoneal dialysis at home. (Courtesy Baxter International, Inc., Deerfield, IL.)

CHART 68-9 Best Practice for Patient Safety & Quality Care QSEN

Caring for the Patient With a Peritoneal Dialysis Catheter

- Mask yourself and your patient. Wash your hands.
- Put on sterile gloves. Remove the old dressing. Remove the contaminated gloves.
- Assess the area for signs of infection, such as swelling, redness, or discharge around the catheter site.
- Use aseptic technique:
  - Open the sterile field on a flat surface and place two precut 4 × 4–inch gauze pads on the field.
  - Place three cotton swabs soaked in povidone-iodine or other solution prescribed by the nephrology health care provider on the field. Put on sterile gloves.
- Use cotton swabs to clean around the catheter site. Use a circular motion starting from the insertion site and moving away toward the abdomen. Repeat with all three swabs.
- As an alternative (if recommended by the nephrology health care provider or clinic), cleanse the area with sterile gauze pads using soap and water. Use a circular motion starting from the insertion site and moving away toward the abdomen. Rinse thoroughly.
- Apply precut gauze pads over the catheter site. Tape only the edges of the gauze pads.

needed. Also, APD can be used to deliver larger volumes of dialysis solution for patients who need higher clearances.

Intermittent peritoneal dialysis (IPD) combines osmotic pressure gradients with true dialysis. The patient usually requires exchanges of 2 L of dialysate at 30- to 60-minute intervals, allowing 15 to 20 minutes of drain time. For most patients, 30 to 40 exchanges of 2 L three times weekly are needed. IPD treatments can be automated or manual.

Complications. Complications are possible with PD, but many can be prevented with meticulous care and appropriate patient education for self-management. Problems and complications are more common when evidence-based guidelines for catheter care are not followed.

Peritonitis is the major complication of PD, most commonly caused by connection site contamination. To prevent peritonitis, use meticulous sterile technique when caring for the PD catheter and when connecting and disconnecting dialysate bags (Chart 68-9).

Pain during the inflow of dialysate is common when patients are first started on PD therapy. Usually this pain no longer

occurs after a week or two of PD. Cold dialysate increases discomfort. Warm the dialysate bags before instillation by using a heating pad to wrap the bag or by using the warming chamber of the automated cycling machine. *Microwave ovens are **not** recommended for warming dialysate.*

Exit site and tunnel infections are serious complications. The exit site from a PD catheter should be clean, dry, and without pain or inflammation. Exit-site infections (ESIs) can occur with any type of PD catheter. These infections are difficult to treat and can become chronic, leading to peritonitis, catheter failure, and hospitalization. Dialysate leakage and pulling or twisting of the catheter increase the risk for ESIs. A Gram stain and culture should be performed when exit sites have purulent drainage.

Tunnel infections occur in the path of the catheter from the skin to the cuff. Symptoms include redness, tenderness, and pain. ESIs are treated with antimicrobials. Deep cuff infections may require catheter removal.

Poor dialysate flow is often related to constipation. To prevent constipation, a bowel preparation is prescribed before placement of the PD. If prescribed, giving an enema before starting PD may also prevent flow problems. Teach patients to eat a high-fiber diet and to use stool softeners to prevent constipation. Other causes of flow difficulty include kinked or clamped connection tubing, the patient's position, fibrin clot formation, and catheter displacement.

Ensure that the drainage bag is lower than the patient's abdomen to enhance gravity drainage. Inspect the connection tubing and PD system for kinking or twisting. Ensure that clamps are open. If inflow or outflow drainage is still inadequate, reposition the patient to stimulate inflow or outflow. Turning the patient to the other side or ensuring that he or she is in good body alignment may help. Having the patient in a supine low-Fowler's position reduces abdominal pressure. Increased abdominal pressure from sitting or standing or from coughing contributes to leakage at the PD catheter site.

Fibrin clot formation may occur after PD catheter placement or with peritonitis. Milking the tubing may dislodge the fibrin clot and improve flow. An x-ray is needed to identify PD catheter placement. If displacement has occurred, the nephrology health care provider repositions the PD catheter.

Dialysate leakage is seen as clear fluid coming from the catheter exit site. When dialysis is first started, small volumes of dialysate are used. It may take patients 1 to 2 weeks to tolerate a full 2-L exchange without leakage around the catheter site. Leakage occurs more often in obese patients, those with diabetes, older adults, and those on long-term steroid therapy. During periods of catheter leak, patients may require hemodialysis (HD) support.

Other complications of PD include bleeding, which is expected when the catheter is first placed, and bowel perforation, which is serious. When PD is first started, the outflow may be bloody or blood tinged. This condition normally clears within a week or two. After PD is well established, the effluent should be clear and light yellow. Observe for and document any change in the color of the outflow. Brown-colored effluent occurs with a bowel perforation. If the outflow is the same color as urine and has the same glucose level, a bladder perforation is probable. Cloudy or opaque effluent indicates infection.

Nursing Care During In-Hospital Peritoneal Dialysis. In the hospital setting, PD is routinely started and monitored by the nurse. Before the treatment, assess baseline vital signs, including blood pressure, apical and radial pulse rates, temperature, quality of respirations, and breath sounds. Weigh the patient, always on the same scale, before the procedure and at least every 24 hours while receiving treatment. Weight should be checked after a drain and before the next fill to monitor the patient's "dry weight." Baseline laboratory tests, such as electrolyte and glucose levels, are obtained before starting PD and repeated at least daily during the PD treatment.

In the hospital setting, especially with a new access, continually monitor the patient receiving PD fluid exchanges. Take and record vital signs every 15 to 30 minutes. Assess for respiratory distress, pain, or discomfort. Check the dressing around the catheter exit site every 30 minutes for wetness during the procedure. Monitor the prescribed dwell time and initiate outflow. Assess blood glucose levels in patients who absorb glucose.

Observe the outflow pattern (outflow should be a continuous stream after the clamp is completely open). Measure and record the total amount of outflow after each exchange. Maintain accurate inflow and outflow records when hourly PD exchanges are performed. When outflow is less than inflow, the difference is retained by the patient during dialysis and is counted as fluid intake. Weigh the patient daily to monitor fluid status.

💡 NCLEX EXAMINATION CHALLENGE 68-6

Physiological Integrity

A client who performs home continuous ambulatory peritoneal dialysis reports that the drainage (effluent) has become cloudy in the past 24 hours. What is the nurse's **best first** action?
A. Remove the peritoneal catheter.
B. Notify the nephrology health care provider immediately.
C. Obtain a sample of effluent for culture and sensitivity.
D. Explain to the client the need to keep the dialysate in the refrigerator to prevent bacterial overgrowth.

Kidney Transplantation. Dialysis and kidney transplant are life-sustaining *treatments* for end-stage kidney disease (ESKD). Kidney transplant is not considered a "cure." Each patient, in consultation with a nephrologist, determines which type of therapy is best suited to his or her physical condition and lifestyle. About 17,000 to 18,000 kidney transplants are performed yearly in the United States, and about 1200 to 1400 are performed yearly in Canada (Kidney Foundation of Canada, 2015; Tran & Miniard, 2017). Currently about 165,000 people are awaiting kidney transplant in North America. The median time on the waiting list is 678 days (USRDS, 2015).

Candidate Selection Criteria. Candidates for transplantation must be free of medical problems that might increase the risks from the procedure. The usual age-range for kidney transplant is 2 to 70 years. Patients older than 70 years are considered for transplant on an individual basis.

The patient is thoroughly assessed before he or she is considered for a kidney transplant. Patients who have advanced, uncorrectable cardiac disease are excluded from the procedure because these problems are made worse by transplantation. Other conditions that preclude kidney transplant include metastatic cancer, chronic infection, and severe psychosocial problems such as alcoholism or chemical dependency. Longstanding pulmonary disease increases the risk for complications and death from respiratory infection. Patients with diseases of the GI system, such as peptic ulcers and diverticulosis, require treatment before transplantation because some diseases are made worse by the large doses of steroids used after surgery.

The urinary system is completely evaluated to ensure normal urine flow. Many patients with ESKD have not used their lower urinary tract for years, and ureteral or bladder problems may require surgical correction before a kidney is transplanted.

Patients with a recent history of cancer are treated with dialysis because of the shortage of donor organs and the uncertain life expectancy of these patients. In addition, the drugs used after the procedure increase the risk for cancer recurrence. If more than 2 to 5 years have passed since cancer eradication, the patient can be considered for a transplant.

Diabetes and other endocrine problems cause great risks. Patients with these problems can have a kidney transplant but require intense observation and management to limit complications. Other pre-existing conditions are considered on an individual basis, depending on the patient's health status. Kidney transplantation is considered for most patients with ESKD and is the optimal therapy for many adults.

Donors. Kidney donors may be living donors (related or unrelated to the patient), non–heart-beating donors (NHBDs), and cadaveric donors. The available kidneys are matched on the basis of tissue type similarity between the donor and the recipient. NHBDs are patients declared dead by cardiopulmonary criteria. Kidneys from NHBDs are removed (harvested) immediately after death in cases in which patients have previously given consent for organ donation. If immediate removal must be delayed, the organ is preserved by infusing a cool preservation solution into the abdominal aorta after death is declared and until surgery can be performed. Cadaveric donors are usually people who suffered irreversible brain injury, most often as a result of trauma. These donors are maintained with mechanical ventilation and must have sufficient PERFUSION for the kidneys to remain viable.

Organs from living *related* donors (LRDs) have the highest rates of kidney graft survival (90%). A living donor is one who is medically compatible with the recipient (Ficorelli et al., 2013). LRDs are usually at least 18 years old and are seldom older than 65 years, although there are donors over 70 years of age with good outcomes for both the donor and recipient (Medina-Polo et al., 2014). Physical criteria for donors include:

- Absence of systemic disease and infection
- No current active cancer
- No hypertension or kidney disease
- Adequate kidney function as determined by diagnostic studies

LRDs must express a clear understanding of the surgery and a willingness to give up a kidney. Some transplant centers require a psychiatric evaluation to assess the donor's motivation.

A paired or chain exchange donation can be done when two kidney donor/recipient pairs have blood types that are not compatible (Vazquez, 2015). The recipients trade donors so each recipient can receive a kidney with a compatible blood type and tissue type (Fig. 68-13). Once the evaluations of all donors and recipients are completed, the series of kidney transplant operations are scheduled to occur consecutively (www.paireddonation.org).

Because of advances in immunosuppressant therapy and medical management, the U.S. Department of Health and Human Services (USDHHS) and the Kidney Foundation of Canada report a 1-year kidney transplant graft survival to be almost 95% for all centers in the North America (Kidney Foundation of Canada, 2015; USDHHS, 2015).

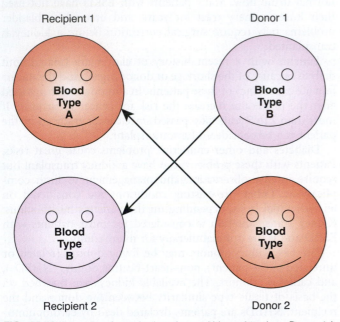

Recipient 1   Donor 1

Blood Type A   Blood Type B

Blood Type B   Blood Type A

Recipient 2   Donor 2

FIG. 68-13 Example of a paired exchange kidney donation. *Donor 1* is related to or acquainted with *recipient 1* and has agreed to donate a kidney but is not a blood type or tissue type match with *recipient 1*. *Donor 1* is compatible with *recipient 2* and agrees to donate a kidney to *recipient 2* if *donor 2* agrees to donate a kidney to *recipient 1* with confirmed compatibility to *recipient 1*.

Preoperative Care. Many issues related to patient health and the actual transplant procedure must be addressed before surgery. The *Clinical Pathway* on the *Evolve* website highlights care needs for the patient undergoing kidney transplantation.

Immunologic studies are needed because the major barrier to transplant success after a suitable donor kidney is available is the body's ability to reject "foreign" tissue. This immunologic process can attack the transplanted kidney and destroy it. For normal protective IMMUNITY to be overcome, tissue typing with human leukocyte antigen (HLA) studies and blood typing are performed on all candidates. A donated kidney *must* come from a donor who is the same blood type as the recipient. The HLAs are the main immunologic feature used to match transplant recipients with compatible donors. The more similar the antigens of the donor are to those of the recipient, the more likely the transplant will be successful, and rejection will be avoided (see Chapter 17).

Nursing actions before surgery include teaching about the procedure and care after surgery, in-depth patient assessment, coordination of diagnostic tests, and development of treatment plans. See Chapter 14 for more discussion of standard preoperative nursing care.

The patient usually requires dialysis within 24 hours of the surgery and often receives a blood transfusion before surgery. Usually blood from the kidney donor is transfused into the recipient. This procedure increases graft survival of organs from living related donors (LRDs).

Operative Procedures. The donor nephrectomy procedure varies depending on whether the donor is a non–heart-beating donor (NHBD), cadaveric donor, or living donor. The NHBD or cadaveric donor nephrectomy is a sterile autopsy procedure performed in the operating room. All arterial and venous vessels and a long piece of ureter are preserved. After removal, the kidneys are preserved until time for implantation into the recipient. The technique for kidney removal from living donors is a laparoscopic procedure. Donors need postoperative nursing care and support for the psychological adjustment to loss of a body part.

Transplantation surgery usually takes several hours. The new kidney is placed in the right or left anterior iliac fossa (Fig. 68-14) instead of the usual kidney position. This placement

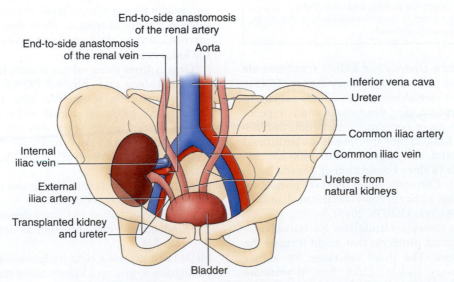

End-to-side anastomosis of the renal artery

End-to-side anastomosis of the renal vein

Aorta

Inferior vena cava

Ureter

Common iliac artery

Common iliac vein

Internal iliac vein

External iliac artery

Ureters from natural kidneys

Transplanted kidney and ureter

Bladder

FIG. 68-14 Placement of a transplanted kidney in the right iliac fossa.

allows easier connection of the ureter and the renal artery and vein. It also allows for easier kidney palpation. The recipient's own failed kidneys are not removed unless chronic kidney infection is present or, as in the case of polycystic kidney disease, the nonfunctioning, enlarged kidneys cause pain. After surgery, the patient is taken to the postanesthesia care unit and then, when stable, to a designated unit in the transplant center or to a critical care unit.

Postoperative Care. Care of the recipient after surgery requires nurses to be knowledgeable about the expected responses and potential complications. Nursing care includes ongoing physical assessment, especially evaluation of kidney function. The most common complications occurring in patients after kidney transplant are rejection and infection (Tran & Miniard, 2017). Drug therapy used to prevent tissue rejection reduces IMMUNITY, impairs healing, and increases the risk for infection.

Urologic management is essential to graft success. A urinary catheter is placed for accurate measurements of urine output and decompression of the bladder. Decompression prevents stretch on sutures and ureter attachment sites on the bladder.

Assess urine output at least hourly during the first 48 hours. An abrupt decrease in urine output (see Table 68-2) may indicate complications such as rejection, acute kidney injury (AKI), thrombosis, or obstruction. Examine the urine color. The urine is pink and bloody right after surgery and gradually returns to normal over several days to several weeks, depending on kidney function. Obtain daily urine specimens for urinalysis, glucose measurement, the presence of acetone, specific gravity measurement, and culture (if needed).

Occasionally, continuous bladder irrigation is prescribed to decrease blood clot formation, which could increase pressure in the bladder and endanger the graft. Perform routine catheter care, according to agency policy, to reduce catheter-associated urinary tract infection (CAUTI). The catheter is removed as soon as possible to avoid infection, usually 3 to 5 days after surgery. After surgery, the function of the transplanted kidney (graft) can result in either oliguria or diuresis. Oliguria may occur as a result of ischemia and acute kidney injury (AKI), rejection, or other complications. To increase urine output, the nephrology health care provider may prescribe diuretics and osmotic agents. Closely monitor the patient's fluid status because fluid overload can cause hypertension, heart failure, and pulmonary edema. Evaluate his or her fluid status by weighing daily, measuring blood pressure every 2 to 4 hours, and measuring intake and output.

Instead of oliguria, the patient may have diuresis, especially with a kidney from a living related donor (LRD). Monitor intake and output and observe for disruptions of FLUID AND ELECTROLYTE BALANCE, such as low potassium and sodium levels. Excessive diuresis may cause hypotension.

! NURSING SAFETY PRIORITY QSEN

Critical Rescue

Monitor the patient to recognize hypotension. If hypotension or excessive diuresis (e.g., unanticipated urine output 500 to 1000 mL greater than intake over 12 to 24 hours or other goal for intake and output) is present, respond by notifying the nephrology health care provider because hypotension reduces PERFUSION and oxygen to the new kidney, threatening graft survival.

Complications. Many complications are possible after kidney transplantation. Early detection and intervention improve the chances for graft survival.

Rejection is the most serious complication of transplantation and is the leading cause of graft loss. A reaction occurs between the tissues of the transplanted kidney and the antibodies and cytotoxic T-cells in the recipient's blood. These substances treat the new kidney as a foreign invader and cause tissue destruction, thrombosis, and eventual kidney necrosis.

The three types of rejection are hyperacute, acute, and chronic. Acute rejection is the most common type with kidney transplants. It is treated with increased immunosuppressive therapy and often can be reversed. Rejection is diagnosed by symptoms, a CT or renal scan, and kidney biopsy. Table 68-13 lists the features of the three types of rejection. Chapter 17 discusses their causes and treatment.

Ischemia from delayed transplantation following harvesting can contribute to acute kidney injury (AKI). Newly transplanted patients with AKI may need dialysis until adequate urine output returns and the blood urea nitrogen (BUN) and creatinine levels normalize. Biopsy can be used to determine if oliguria is the result of AKI or rejection.

Thrombosis of the major renal blood vessels may occur during the first 2 to 3 days after the transplant. A sudden decrease in urine output may signal impaired PERFUSION resulting from thrombosis. Ultrasound of the kidney may show decreased or absent blood supply. Emergency surgery is required to prevent ischemic damage or graft loss.

Renal artery stenosis may result in hypertension. Other signs include a bruit over the artery anastomosis site and decreased kidney function. A CT or renal scan can quantify the PERFUSION to the kidney. The involved artery may be repaired surgically or

---

TABLE 68-13 Comparison of Hyperacute, Acute, and Chronic Post-Transplant Rejection

HYPERACUTE REJECTION	ACUTE REJECTION	CHRONIC REJECTION
Onset		
Within 48 hours after surgery	1 week to any time after surgery; occurs over days to weeks	Occurs gradually during a period of months to years
Signs and Symptoms		
Increased temperature	Oliguria or anuria	Gradual increase in BUN and serum creatinine levels
Increased blood pressure	Temperature over 100° F (37.8° C)	
Pain at transplant site	Increased blood pressure	Fluid retention
	Enlarged, tender kidney	Changes in serum electrolyte levels
	Lethargy	Fatigue
	Elevated serum creatinine, BUN, potassium levels	
	Fluid retention	
Treatment		
Immediate removal of the transplanted kidney	Increased doses of immunosuppressive drugs	Conservative management until dialysis required

BUN, Blood urea nitrogen.

by balloon angioplasty in the radiology department. The decision to perform a balloon repair is determined by the amount of healing time after the surgery.

Other vascular problems include vascular leakage or thrombosis, both of which require an emergency transplant nephrectomy.

Other complications may involve the surgical wound or urinary tract. Wound problems, such as hematomas, abscesses, and lymphoceles (cysts containing lymph fluid), increase the risk for infection and exert pressure on the new kidney. Infection from reduced IMMUNITY is a major cause of death in the transplant recipient (Tran & Miniard, 2017). Prevention of infection is essential. Strict aseptic technique and handwashing must be rigorously enforced. Transplant recipients may not have the usual symptoms of infection because of the immunosuppressive therapy. Low-grade fevers, mental status changes, and vague reports of discomfort may be the only symptoms before sepsis. Always consider the possibility of infection with any patient after a kidney transplant. Urinary tract complications include ureteral leakage, fistula, or obstruction; stone formation; bladder neck contracture; and graft rupture. Surgical intervention may be required.

Immunosuppressive Drug Therapy. The success of kidney transplantation depends on changing the patient's IMMUNITY response so the new kidney is not rejected as a foreign organ. Immunosuppressive drugs protect the transplanted organ. These drugs include corticosteroids, inhibitors of T-cell proliferation and activity (azathioprine, mycophenolic acid, cyclosporine, and tacrolimus), mTOR inhibitors (to disrupt stimulatory T-cell signals), and monoclonal antibodies. Chapter 17 discusses the mechanisms of action for these agents and the associated patient responses. Patients taking these drugs are at an increased risk for death from infection. Usually, the patient receives a period of high-dose (induction) therapy followed by lower-dose maintenance immunosuppressive therapy.

Some patients do not follow the maintenance regimen correctly and are at high risk for losing the transplanted kidney. Work with the patient to ensure adherence to the drug regimen.

Despite the complexity of drug regimens following kidney transplantation, 85.5% of patients are living 5 years after transplantation compared with 35.8% of patients who receive dialysis for 5 years. The costs of hemodialysis (HD) are three times the cost of kidney transplantation over the same 5 years (Kidney Foundation of Canada, 2015; USRDS, 2015).

Although rejection is uncommon with immunosuppressive therapy, kidney transplant recipients are at risk for cardiovascular disease (the most common cause of death among kidney transplant recipients), diabetes, cancer, and infections. Prevention and management of these complications are important to maintaining the health of the transplanted kidney and prolonging patient survival. Be aware that some patient groups, including African Americans, Hispanic Americans, and Native Americans have a greater incidence of graft failure and systemic complications (especially cardiovascular disease) after transplantation.

Care Coordination and Transition Management

Home Care Management. Because of the complex nature of CKD, its progressive course, and many treatment options, a case manager is helpful in planning, coordinating, and evaluating care. As kidney disease progresses, the patient is seen by a nephrologist or nephrology nurse practitioner regularly. Together with the dietitian and social worker, evaluate the home environment and determine equipment needs before discharge. Once the patient is discharged, nephrology home care nurses direct care and monitor progress.

Provide health teaching about the diet in kidney disease and the progression of disease. As CKD approaches end-stage kidney disease (ESKD), treatment with hemodialysis (HD), peritoneal dialysis (PD), or transplantation is selected. For each form of treatment, the patient and partner must learn about the procedures and consider his or her personal lifestyle, support systems, and methods of coping. Decision making about treatment type or even whether to pursue treatment is difficult for patients and families. Provide information and emotional support to help patients with these decisions.

Teach patients who select hemodialysis (HD) about the machine and vascular access care. If in-home HD is selected, preparations are needed for the appropriate equipment, including a water-treatment system. A nephrology nurse is essential for a successful transition to at-home HD to teach the patient and monitor treatment and care. This nurse performs a home care visit before discharge to coordinate equipment setup. Family members must be available to respond to alarms during treatment. Nocturnal HD is a growing modality, and additional safety considerations must be addressed, including a plan for treatment discontinuation or generator backup during power outages. Regardless of whether the treatment occurs at home or in a center, promote independence through teaching and best practices in self-management.

The patient receiving PD needs extensive training in the procedure and help in obtaining equipment and the many supplies needed. A nephrology nurse assesses patients, monitors vital signs, assesses adherence with drug and diet regimens, and monitors for indications of peritonitis.

The nurse plays a vital role in the long-term care of the patient with a kidney transplant by facilitating acceptance and understanding of the antirejection drug regimen as a part of daily life. Carefully monitor patients for indications of graft rejection and for complications, such as infection. Chart 68-10 shows the focused assessment for the patient following kidney transplant.

Self-Management Education. Instruct patients and family members in all aspects of nutrition therapy, drug therapy, and complications. Teach them to report complications, such as fluid overload and infection. When a patient has a specific form of therapy, such as dialysis or transplantation, focus teaching on the chosen type of intervention. Assess the need for immunizations and request a prescription to administer needed ones before transplantation (Tran & Miniard, 2017).

Hemodialysis (HD) is the most complex form of therapy for the patient and family to understand. Even if patients receive HD in a dialysis center instead of at home, they are expected to have some knowledge of the process. Teach the patient or a

---

! NURSING SAFETY PRIORITY QSEN

Action Alert

Teach patients and families about the importance of adhering to the antirejection drug regimen to prevent transplant rejection.

CHART 68-10 **Focused Assessment**

The Patient Following Kidney Transplant

Assess cardiovascular and respiratory status, including:
- Vital signs, with special attention to blood pressure
- Presence of S_3 or pericardial friction rub
- Presence of chest pain
- Presence of edema (periorbital, pretibial, sacral)
- Jugular vein distention
- Presence of dyspnea
- Presence of crackles, beginning at the lung bases and extending upward

Assess nutritional status, including:
- Weight gain or loss
- Presence of anorexia, nausea, or vomiting

Assess kidney status, including:
- Amount, frequency, and appearance of urine (in nonanuric patients)
- Presence of bone pain
- Presence of hyperglycemia secondary to diabetes

Assess hematologic status, including:
- Presence of petechiae, purpura, ecchymosis
- Presence of fatigue or shortness of breath

Assess GI status, including:
- Presence of stomatitis
- Presence of melena

Assess integumentary status, including:
- Skin integrity
- Presence of pruritus
- Presence of skin discoloration

Assess neurologic status, including:
- Changes in mental status
- Presence of seizure activity
- Presence of sensory changes
- Presence of lower-extremity weakness

Assess laboratory data, including:
- BUN
- Serum creatinine
- Creatinine clearance
- CBC
- Electrolytes

Assess psychosocial status, including:
- Presence of anxiety
- Presence of maladaptive behavior

BUN, Blood urea nitrogen; *CBC,* complete blood count.

---

family member to care for the vascular access and to report signs of infection and clotting. Teaching also includes instructing the patient to assess daily for a bruit and thrill in the vascular access. Those who plan to have in-home HD will need a partner. Both the patient and the partner must be taught the entire process of HD and must be able to perform it independently before the patient is discharged.

Peritoneal dialysis (PD) involves extensive health teaching for the patient and family. Emphasize sterile technique because peritonitis is the most common complication of PD. Instruct patients to report any symptoms of peritonitis, especially cloudy effluent and abdominal pain. If peritonitis develops, teach patients how to give themselves antibiotics by the intra-peritoneal (IP) route. Stress the importance of completing the antibiotic regimen. Remind patients that repeated episodes of peritonitis can reduce the effectiveness of PD, which may require the transfer to HD.

The patient receiving a kidney transplant also needs extensive health teaching. Provide instruction about drug regimens,

home monitoring, immunosuppression, symptoms of rejection, infection, and prescribed changes in the diet and activity level.

Psychosocial Preparation. In collaboration with the patient's mental health professional or counselor, provide psychosocial support for the patient and family. Help the patient adjust to the diagnosis of kidney failure and eventually accept the treatment regimens.

Many patients view dialysis as a cure instead of lifelong management. For many patients, reduction of uremic symptoms and improved ELIMINATION in the first weeks after starting dialysis treatment create a sense of well-being (the "honeymoon" period). They feel better physically, and their mood may be happy and hopeful. At this time they tend to overlook the discomfort and inconvenience of dialysis. Use this time to begin health teaching. Stress that, although symptoms are reduced, not to expect a complete return to the previous state of well-being before ESKD.

Many patients become discouraged during the first year of treatment. This mood state may last a few months to a year or longer. The difficulties of incorporating dialysis into daily life are staggering, and patients may become depressed as problems occur. They may struggle with the idea of having to be permanently dependent on a disruptive therapy. Patients may feel helpless and dependent. Some patients may deny the need for dialysis or may not adhere to drug therapy and diet restrictions. Monitor any behaviors that may contribute to nonadherence and suggest psychiatric referrals. Help the patient and family focus on the positive aspects of the treatments. Continue health education with patients as active participants and decision makers.

Most patients with CKD eventually enter a phase of acceptance or resignation. Each patient reacts differently. To make this long-term adaptation, he or she must adjust to continuous change. Concerns depend on the patient's health and specific treatment method.

After patients have accepted or become resigned to the chronic aspect of their disease, they usually attempt to return to their previous activities. However, resuming the previous level of activity may not be possible. Help patients develop realistic expectations that allow them to lead active, productive lives.

Health Care Resources. Professionals from many disciplines are resources for the patient with ESKD. Home care nurses monitor the patient's status and evaluate maintenance of the prescribed treatment regimen (HD or PD). Social services are often involved because of the complex process of applying for financial aid to pay for the required medical care. A physical therapist may be beneficial in helping to improve the patient's functional health. A dietitian can help the patient and family members understand special dietary needs. A psychiatric evaluation may be needed if depressive symptoms are present. Pharmacists provide invaluable insight and teaching about drug therapy and adjustments to meet outcomes. Clergy and pastoral care specialists offer spiritual support.

Patients with CKD are routinely followed by a nephrologist. Organizations such as the National Kidney Foundation (NKF), the American Kidney Fund, and the National Association of Patients on Hemodialysis and Transplantation (NAPHT) may be helpful to patients and families.

◆ *Evaluation: Reflecting*

Evaluate the care of the patient with CKD based on the identified priority problems. The expected outcomes are that, with appropriate management, the patient should:

- Achieve and maintain appropriate FLUID AND ELECTROLYTE BALANCE
- Maintain an adequate nutrition status
- Avoid infection at the vascular access site
- Use effective coping strategies
- Prevent or slow systemic complications of CKD, including osteodystrophy
- Report an absence of physical signs of anxiety or depression

---

CLINICAL JUDGMENT CHALLENGE 68-1

Patient-Centered Care QSEN

Jamie is a 48-year-old woman who received a living related donor (LRD) kidney transplant 6 months ago. Today she learns that her blood sugar, which has been elevated since starting immunosuppressant therapy, is 180 mg/dL and her A1C is 8. You find her crying after her visit to the transplant surgeon, who advises that she start on an antidiabetic drug. The surgeon has left to consult with the nephrologist and primary health care provider to determine the best drug or drugs for glycemic control. Jamie states, "I can't take another med; I already take 10 tablets each day! Why is this happening to me?"

1. How will you respond to her feelings of anxiety or concern related to the number of tablets taken daily and feelings of "why me/why now"?
2. Which additional information would you gather to better understand the patient's emotional reaction to the new treatment plan?
3. Should you ask about who donated the kidney? Why or why not?
4. What possibility exists that some of Jamie's current emotional state is influenced by her antirejection drug therapy regimen? If a possibility does exist, which category of drugs is most likely to have a negative influence and why?
5. What are the next steps in communicating the patient concerns and emotional state to the interprofessional team members who are involved in Jamie's care?

GET READY FOR THE NCLEX® EXAMINATION!

KEY POINTS

Review these Key Points for each NCLEX Examination Client Needs Category.

Safe and Effective Care Environment

- Use sterile technique when initiating and providing kidney replacement therapy. **QSEN: Safety**
- Implement fall precautions and consider physical therapy referral for patients with CKD osteodystrophy to prevent fractures. **QSEN: Safety**
- Use skin protective measures to reduce injury and pressure injury in patients with CKD. **QSEN: Safety**
- Alert health care providers to patient assessments that indicate hypotension, dehydration, or hypovolemia to avoid inadequate kidney PERFUSION. **QSEN: Teamwork and Collaboration**
- Avoid taking blood pressure measurements or drawing blood from an arm with a vascular access (AV fistula or graft). **QSEN: Safety**
- Do not use a kidney replacement vascular access device (the AV fistula or graft site) to give IV fluids. **QSEN: Safety**

Health Promotion and Maintenance

- Encourage patients with AKI, CKD, or end-stage kidney disease (ESKD) to follow fluid and dietary restrictions regarding sodium, potassium, and protein. **QSEN: Evidence-Based Practice**
- Teach patients the expected side effects, any adverse reactions to prescribed drugs, and when to contact the prescriber. **QSEN: Safety**
- Teach patients using peritoneal dialysis the early signs and symptoms of peritonitis. **QSEN: Patient-Centered Care**

- Teach patients receiving immunosuppressive therapy for kidney transplantation to assess themselves daily for fever, general malaise, and nausea or vomiting, as well as changes in urine output and weight gain that indicate new fluid retention. **QSEN: Patient-Centered Care**

Psychosocial Integrity

- Allow patients the opportunity to express concerns about the disruption of lifestyle and considerations for end-of-life care as a result of kidney failure. **QSEN: Patient-Centered Care**
- Use language and terminology that are comfortable and understandable for the patient. **QSEN: Patient-Centered Care**
- Assess the patient for anxiety, depression, and nonacceptance of the diagnosis or treatment plan. **QSEN: Patient-Centered Care**
- Refer patients to community resources and support groups. **QSEN: Informatics**

Physiological Integrity

- Report immediately any condition that obstructs urine flow. **QSEN: Safety**
- Collaborate with the dietitian to teach patients about needed fluid, sodium, potassium, or dietary protein restriction to maintain FLUID AND ELECTROLYTE BALANCE. **QSEN: Teamwork and Collaboration**
- Inform the primary health care provider urgently or immediately about hemodynamic instability, change in cognition, signs of infection, newly abnormal serum electrolytes, and urine output less than 0.5 mL/kg/hr for more than 2 to 4 hours (unless the patient is oliguric or anuric from ESKD). **QSEN: Teamwork and Collaboration**

- Teach patients in the early stages of CKD the symptoms of dehydration. **QSEN: Patient-Centered Care**
- Evaluate the patient's laboratory values, especially the metabolic panel, trends in serum creatinine, GFR, and albumin-to-creatinine ratio to assess the status of kidney problems and communicate concerning changes to the interprofessional team. **QSEN: Teamwork and Collaboration**

- Teach patients in the later stages of CKD the indications of fluid overload and hyperkalemia. **QSEN: Patient-Centered Care**
- Avoid all invasive procedures in the 4 to 6 hours following hemodialysis. **QSEN: Evidence-Based Practice**

SELECTED BIBLIOGRAPHY

Burchum, J., & Rosenthal, L. (2016). *Lehne's pharmacology for nursing care* (9th ed.). St. Louis: Elsevier.

Centers for Disease Control and Prevention (CDC). (2016). *Chronic kidney disease surveillance system-United States.* http://www.cdc.gov/ckd.

Dirkes, S. (2015). Acute kidney injury: Causes, phases, and early detection. *American Nurse Today, 10*(7), 20–25.

Dirkes, S. (2016). Acute kidney injury. *Critical Care Nurse, 36*(6), 75–76.

Ficorelli, C. T., Edelman, M., & Weeks, B. H. (2013). Living donor renal transplant: A gift of life. *Nursing, 43*(1), 58–62.

Fournier, M. (2013). Stemming the rising tide of acute kidney injury. *American Nurse Today, 8*(1), 12–16.

Fukagawa, M., Komaba, H., & Kakuta, T. (2013). Hyperparathyroidism in chronic kidney disease patients: An update on current pharmacotherapy. *Expert Opinion on Pharmacotherapy, 14*(7), 863–871.

Gloe, D., Kenneally, M., & Felicilda-Reynaldo, R. F. D. (2016). Medication therapy adjustment in patients with chronic renal failure. *Medsurg Nursing, 25*(6), 325–328.

Grams, M., Sang, Y., Ballew, S., Gansevoort, R., Kimm, H., Kovesdy, C., et al. (2015). A meta-analysis of the association of estimated GFR, albuminuria, age, race, and sex with acute kidney injury. *American Journal of Kidney Disease, 66*(4), 591–601.

Hain, D. (2015). Where's the evidence? Care coordination for adults with chronic kidney disease. *Nephrology Nursing Journal, 42*(1), 77–82.

Hain, D., & Paixao, R. (2015). The perfect storm: Older adults and acute kidney injury. *Critical Care Nursing Quarterly, 38*(3), 271–279.

Honicker, T., & Holt, K. (2016). Contrast-induced acute kidney injury: Comparison of preventive therapies. (2016). *Nephrology Nursing Journal, 43*(2), 109–116.

KDIGO. (2013). *Kidney disease improving global outcomes. KDIGO 2012. Clinical practice guideline for the evaluation and management of chronic kidney disease.* http://www.kdigo.org/clinical_practice_guidelines/pdf/CKD/KDIGO_2012_CKD_GL.pdf.

Kidney Foundation of Canada. (2015). *Facing the facts 2015.* www.kidney.ca/file/Facing-the-Facts-2015-infographic-portrait.pdf.

Lambert, P., Chasson, K., Horton, S., Petrin, C., Marshall, E., Bowdon, S., et al. (2017). Reduing acute kidney injury due to contrast material: How nurses can improve patient safety. *Critical Care Nurse, 37*(1), 13–26.

McCance, K., Huether, S., Brashers, V., & Rote, N. (2014). *Pathophysiology: The biologic basis for disease in adults and children* (7th ed.). St. Louis: Mosby.

Medina-Polo, J., Pamplona-Casamayor, M., Miranda-Utrera, N., Gonzalez-Monte, E., Passas-Martinez, J., & Andres Belmonte, A. (2014). Dual kidney transplantation involving organs from expanded criteria donors: A review of our series and an update on current indications. *Transplant Proceedings, 46*(10), 3412–3415.

Norton, J., Newman, M., Romancito, G., Mahooty, S., Kuracina, T., & Narva, A. (2017a). Improving outcomes for patients with chronic kidney disease: Part 1. *American Journal of Nursing, 117*(2), 22–32.

Norton, J., Newman, M., Romancito, G., Mahooty, S., Kuracina, T., & Narva, A. (2017b). Improving outcomes for patients with chronic kidney disease: Part 2. *American Journal of Nursing, 117*(3), 26–35.

Pagana, K., Pagana, T., & Pike-McDonald, S. (2013). *Mosby's Canadian manual of diagnostic and laboratory tests.* St. Louis: Elsevier.

Pagana, K., Pagana, T., & Pagana, T. (2017). *Mosby's diagnostic and laboratory test reference* (13th ed.). St. Louis: Mosby.

Puzantian, H., & Townsend, R. (2013). Understanding kidney function assessment: The basics and advances. *Journal of the American Association of Nurse Practitioners, 25*(7), 334–341.

Ralib, A., Pickering, J., Shaw, G., & Endre, Z. (2013). The urine output definition of acute kidney injury is too liberal. *Critical Care : The Official Journal of the Critical Care Forum, 17*(3), R112.

Schell-Chaple, H. (2017). Continuous renal replacement therapy update: An emphasis on safe and high-quality care. *AACN Advanced Critical Care, 28*(1), 31–40.

Scher, H., Drew, M., & Cottrell, D. (2015). Treatment of resistant hypertension in the patient with chronic kidney disease. *The Journal for Nurse Practitioners, 11*(6), 587–604.

Schreiber, M. (2016). Peritoneal dialysis: Understanding, educating, and adhering to standards. *Medsurg Nursing, 25*(4), 270–274.

Stupak, D., Trubilla, J., & Groller, S. (2016). Hemodialysis catheter care: Identifying best cleansing agents. *Nephrology Nursing Journal, 43*(2), 153–155.

Taal, M. (2016). Risk factors and chronic kidney disease. Chapter 32. In K. Skorecki, G. Chertow, P. Marsden, M. Taal, & A. Yu (Eds.), *Brenner and Rector's The kidney* (10th ed., pp. 1012–1090). Philadelphia: Elsevier.

Thompson, A., Li, F., & Gross, A. K. (2017). Considerations for medication management and anticoagulation during continuous renal replacement therapy. *AACN Advanced Critical Care, 28*(1), 51–63.

Thornburg, B., & Gray-Vickery, P. (2016). Acute kidney injury: Limiting the damage. *Nursing, 46*(6), 24–34.

Touhy, T., & Jett, K. (2016). *Ebersole & Hess' toward healthy aging: Human needs & nursing response.* St. Louis: Elsevier.

Tran, A., & Miniard, J. (2017). Preventing infection after renal transplantation. *Nursing, 74*(1), 57–60.

Tsai, S., Wang, M., Miao, N., Chian, P., Chen, T., & Tsai, P. (2015). The efficacy of a nurse-led breathing training program in reducing depressive symptoms in patients on hemodialysis: A randomized controlled trial. *American Journal of Nursing, 115*(4), 24–32.

U.S. Department of Health and Human Services (USDHHS). (2015). *Organ Procurement and Transplantation Network.* http://optn.transplant.hrsa.gov/data/view-data-reports/.

U.S. Renal Data Systems (USRDS) (2015). *2015 USRDS Annual Data Report. Epidemiology of Kidney Disease in the United States.* Bethesda, MD: National Institutes of Health, National Institute of Diabetes and Digestive and Kidney Diseases. http://www.usrds.org/adr.aspx.

Vazquez, M. (2015). A nurse's journey through living kidney donation. *Nursing, 45*(10), 53–59.

Vrtis, M. (2013). Preventing and responding to acute kidney injury. *American Journal of Nursing, 113*(4), 38–47.

Wilson, B., & Lawrence, J. (2013). Implementation of a foot assessment program in a regional satellite hemodialysis setting. *Canadian Association of Nephrology Nurses and Technologists Journal, 23*(2), 41–47.

69 | CHAPTER

Assessment of the Reproductive System

Donna D. Ignatavicius

(e) http://evolve.elsevier.com/Iggy/

PRIORITY AND INTERRELATED CONCEPTS

The priority concept for this chapter is SEXUALITY.

The interrelated concept for this chapter is COMFORT.

LEARNING OUTCOMES

Health Promotion and Maintenance

1. Teach patients about evidence-based guidelines for selected reproductive screening tests.

Psychosocial Integrity

2. Identify general psychological responses to reproductive health problems that affect SEXUALITY.

Physiological Integrity

3. Briefly review the anatomy and physiology of the male and female reproductive systems.
4. Identify reproductive changes associated with aging and their implications for nursing care.

5. Perform a focused physical assessment of the patient with male or female reproductive system problems.
6. Explain the use of laboratory testing for patients with suspected or actual reproductive health problems.
7. Describe the postprocedure care and health teaching for a client undergoing a biopsy to determine the presence of cancer, including interventions for increasing COMFORT.
8. Develop an evidence-based teaching plan for a patient undergoing endoscopic studies for reproductive health problems.

The first health care professional to assess the patient with a reproductive system health problem or hear a patient's concern about a reproductive problem is often the nurse. These problems typically affect SEXUALITY, both its physical and psychosocial aspects, and are difficult for many people to discuss. Assessment of the male and the female reproductive systems should be part of every complete physical assessment. *Be aware of and sensitive to gender identity and differences in sexual orientation and practices.* A more detailed discussion of human SEXUALITY is found in Chapter 2.

ANATOMY AND PHYSIOLOGY REVIEW

Structure and Function of the Female Reproductive System

The female reproductive system is located both outside (external) and inside (internal) the body.

External Genitalia

The external female genitalia, or vulva, extend from the mons pubis to the anal opening. The mons pubis is a fat pad that covers the symphysis pubis and protects it during coitus (sexual intercourse).

The labia majora are two vertical folds of adipose tissue that extend posteriorly from the mons pubis to the perineum. The size of the labia majora varies, depending on the amount of fatty tissue present. The skin over the labia majora is usually darker than the surrounding skin and is highly vascular. It protects inner vulval structures and enhances sexual arousal.

The labia majora surround two thinner, vertical folds of reddish epithelium called the *labia minora*. The labia minora are highly vascular and have a rich nerve supply. Emotional or physical stimulation produces marked swelling and sensitivity. Numerous sebaceous glands in the labia minora lubricate the entrance to the vagina. The clitoris is a small, cylindric organ that is composed of erectile tissue with a high concentration of sensory nerve endings. During sexual arousal, the clitoris becomes larger and increases sexual sensation.

The vestibule is a longitudinal area between the labia minora, the clitoris, and the vagina that contains Bartholin glands and the openings of the urethra, Skene's glands (paraurethral glands), and vagina. The two Bartholin glands, located deeply toward the back on both sides of the vaginal opening, secrete lubrication fluid during sexual excitement. Their ductal openings are usually not visible.

The area between the vaginal opening and the anus is the perineum. The skin of the perineum covers the muscles, fascia, and ligaments that support the pelvic structures.

Internal Genitalia

The internal female genitalia are shown in Fig. 69-1. The vagina is a hollow tube that extends from the vestibule to the uterus. Ovarian hormones (primarily *estrogen*) influence the amounts of glycogen and lubricating fluid secreted by the vaginal cells. The normal vaginal bacteria (flora) interact with the secretions to produce lactic acid and maintain an acidic pH (3.5 to 5.0) in the vagina. This acidity helps prevent infection in the vagina.

At the upper end of the vagina, the uterine cervix projects into a cup-shaped vault of thin vaginal tissue. The recessed pockets around the cervix permit palpation of the internal pelvic organs. The posterior area provides access into the peritoneal cavity for diagnostic or surgical purposes.

The uterus (or "womb") is a thick-walled, muscular organ attached to the upper end of the vagina. This inverted pear-shaped organ is located within the true pelvis, between the bladder and the rectum. The uterus is made up of the body and the cervix.

The cervix is a short (1 inch [2.5 cm]), narrowed portion of the uterus and extends into the vagina. The surfaces of the cervix and the canal are the sites for Papanicolaou (Pap) testing. (See discussion later in this chapter.)

The fallopian tubes (uterine tubes) insert into the fundus of the uterus and extend laterally close to the ovaries. They provide a duct between the ovaries and the uterus for the passage of ova and sperm. In most cases, the ovum is fertilized in these tubes.

The ovaries are a pair of almond-shaped organs located near the lateral walls of the upper pelvic cavity. After menopause, they become smaller. These small organs develop and release ova and produce the sex steroid hormones (estrogen, progesterone, androgen, and relaxin). Adequate amounts of these hormones are needed for normal female growth and development and to maintain a pregnancy.

Breasts

The female breasts are a pair of mammary glands that develop in response to secretions from the hypothalamus, pituitary gland, and ovaries. The breasts are an accessory of the reproductive system that nourish the infant after birth.

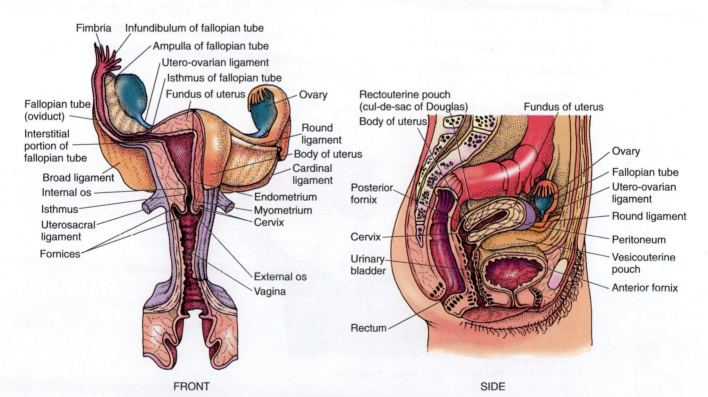

FIG. 69-1 Internal female genitalia.

Breast tissue is composed of a network of glandular and ductal tissue, fibrous tissue, and fat. The proportion of each component of breast tissue depends on genetic factors, nutrition, age, and obstetric history. The breasts are supported by ligaments that are attached to underlying muscles. They have abundant blood supply and lymph flow that drain from an extensive network toward the axillae (Fig. 69-2).

Structure and Function of the Male Reproductive System

The male reproductive system also consists of external and internal genitalia. The primary male hormone for sexual development and function is *testosterone*. Testosterone production is fairly constant in the adult male. Only a slight and gradual reduction of testosterone production occurs in the older adult male until he is in his 80s. Low testosterone levels decrease muscle mass, reduce skin elasticity, and lead to changes in sexual performance.

The penis is an organ for urination and intercourse consisting of the body or shaft and the glans penis (the distal end of the penis). The glans is the smooth end of the penis and contains the opening of the urethral meatus. The urethra is the pathway for the exit of both urine and semen. A continuation of skin covers the glans and folds to form the prepuce (foreskin). Surgical removal of the foreskin (**circumcision**) for religious or cultural reasons is a common procedure in the United States and other Western countries.

The scrotum is a thin-walled, fibromuscular pouch that is behind the penis and suspended below the pubic bone. This pouch protects the testes, epididymis, and vas deferens in a space that is slightly cooler than inside the abdominal cavity. The scrotal skin is darkly pigmented and contains sweat glands, sebaceous glands, and few hair follicles. It contracts with cold, exercise, tactile stimulation, and sexual excitement.

The internal male genitalia are shown in Fig. 69-3. The major organs are the testes and prostate gland. The testes are a pair of oval organs in the scrotum that produce sperm and testosterone. Each testis is suspended in the scrotum by the spermatic cord, which provides blood, lymphatic, and nerve supply to the testis. Sympathetic nerve fibers are located on the arteries in the cord, and sympathetic and parasympathetic fibers are on the vas deferens. When the testes are damaged, these autonomic nerve fibers transmit excruciating pain and a sensation of nausea.

The epididymis is the first portion of a ductal system that transports sperm from the testes to the urethra and is a site of sperm maturation. The vas deferens, or ductus deferens, is a firm, muscular tube that continues from the tail of each

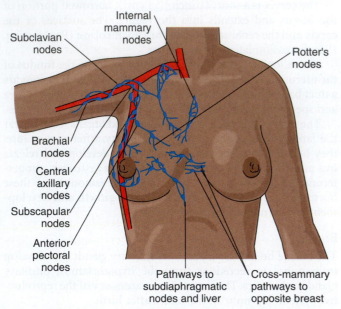

FIG. 69-2 Lymphatic drainage of the female breast.

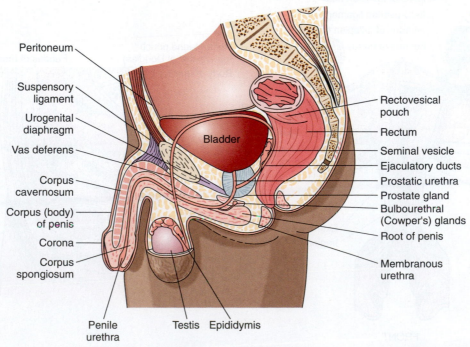

FIG. 69-3 Internal male genitalia.

epididymis. The end of each vas deferens is a reservoir for sperm and tubular fluids. They merge with ducts from the seminal vesicle to form the ejaculatory ducts at the base of the prostate gland. Sperm from the vas deferens and secretions from the seminal vesicles move through the ejaculatory duct to mix with prostatic fluids in the prostatic urethra.

The prostate gland is a large accessory gland of the male reproductive system that can be palpated via the rectum. The gland secretes a milky alkaline fluid that adds bulk to the semen, enhances sperm movement, and neutralizes acidic vaginal secretions. Men older than 50 years commonly have an enlarged prostate (benign prostatic hyperplasia [BPH]), which can cause problems such as overflow incontinence and nocturia (nighttime urination). Prostate function depends on adequate levels of testosterone.

Reproductive Changes Associated With Aging

Age affects the function of both the male and the female reproductive systems. Many changes in the reproductive system occur as people age (Chart 69-1).

Health Promotion and Maintenance

Many health problems of the reproductive system can be prevented through health promotion strategies and avoidance of risky lifestyle behaviors. For example, following recommended best practices for routine preventive screenings, such as mammography and Pap tests, can detect cancer early so it can be treated for a cure. Sexually transmitted infections (STIs) and other reproductive infections can be avoided using safe sex practices such as condoms or abstinence. Teach patients about these health promotion strategies and the rationale for practicing them. Additional health promotion interventions are

described under specific reproductive health problems within this unit.

ASSESSMENT: NOTICING AND INTERPRETING

Patient History

Establish a trusting relationship with the patient. Many patients are hesitant to share their reproductive history or concerns about SEXUALITY. Respect their choice to refuse to answer questions about their reproductive problems or sexual practices. Assess the patient's health habits, such as diet, sleep, and exercise patterns. Low levels of body fat may be related to ovarian dysfunction. Assess for alcohol, tobacco, and drug use (prescribed, over-the-counter [OTC], and illicit drugs), because **libido** (sex drive), sperm production, and the ability to have or sustain an erection can be affected by these substances.

Ask female patients about the date and result of their most recent Pap test, breast self-examination, and vulvar self-examination. Determine when male patients older than 50 years had their last prostate examination and prostate-specific antigen test.

Ask about childhood illnesses that could have an effect on the reproductive system. For example, mumps in men may cause **orchitis** (painful inflammation and swelling of the testes) and can lead to testicular atrophy and sterility. Also ask whether the patient has had any infections. Pelvic inflammatory disease or a ruptured appendix followed by peritonitis can cause pelvic scarring and strictures or adhesions in the fallopian tubes. **Salpingitis** (uterine tube infection) is often caused by chlamydia, a sexually transmitted infection (STI), and can result in female infertility. A history of infections or prolonged fever in males may have damaged sperm production or caused obstruction of the seminal tract, which can cause infertility.

CHART 69-1 Nursing Focus on the Older Adult

Changes in the Reproductive System Related to Aging

PHYSIOLOGIC CHANGE	NURSING INTERVENTIONS	RATIONALES
Women		
Graying and thinning of the pubic hair	Discuss changes with the patient (applies to all structures for both women and men).	Education helps prevent problems with body image (applies to all structures for both women and men).
Decreased size of the labia majora and clitoris		
Drying, smoothing, and thinning of the vaginal walls	Provide information about vaginal estrogen therapy and water-soluble lubricants.	Education enables the patient to make informed decisions about the treatment of vaginal dryness, which can cause painful intercourse.
Decreased size of the uterus	Provide information about Kegel exercises to strengthen pelvic muscles. Urinary incontinence can be a major problem.	Strengthening exercises may prevent or reduce pelvic relaxation and urinary incontinence.
Atrophy of the endometrium		
Decreased size and marked convolution of the ovaries		
Loss of tone and elasticity of the pelvic ligaments and connective tissue		
Increased flabbiness and fibrosis of the breasts, which hang lower on the chest wall; decreased erection of the nipples	Teach or reinforce the importance of breast self-awareness, clinical breast examinations, and mammography.	These methods can detect masses or other changes that may indicate the presence of cancer.
Men		
Graying and thinning of the pubic hair	Teach or reinforce the importance of testicular self-examination (TSE).	TSE may detect changes that may indicate cancer.
Increased drooping of the scrotum and loss of rugae		
Prostate enlargement, with an increased likelihood of urethral obstruction	Teach the patient the signs of urethral obstruction and the importance of prostate cancer screening.	Education helps the patient detect enlargement or obstruction, which may indicate the presence of cancer.

Assess for chronic illnesses or surgeries that could affect reproductive function. Disorders that affect a woman's metabolism or nutrition can depress ovarian function and cause amenorrhea (absence of menses). Patients with diabetes mellitus may experience physiologic changes such as vaginal dryness or impotence. Chronic disorders of the nervous system, respiratory system, or cardiovascular system can alter the sexual response.

Ask whether the patient has been treated with radiation therapy. Inquire about the prolonged use of corticosteroids, internal or external estrogen, testosterone, or chemotherapy drugs, which can lead to reproductive system dysfunction.

🧩 GENDER HEALTH CONSIDERATIONS
Patient-Centered Care (QSEN)

Data about sexual activity are vital parts of the patient's history. Sexual orientation and gender identity should not be assumed. Patients who are lesbian, gay, bisexual, transgender, and queer/questioning (LGBTQ) are often not fully assessed by health care professionals. These patients usually feel more comfortable sharing information about their reproductive health and sexual activity when approached in a caring, nonjudgmental way. Chapter 1 describes sensitive interviewing techniques that are appropriate for LGBTQ patients. Chapter 73 in this unit discusses assessment and care of transgender patients in detail.

🌐 CULTURAL/SPIRITUAL CONSIDERATIONS
Patient-Centered Care (QSEN)

Other cultural beliefs and practices influence lifestyle and SEXUALITY. A person's religious beliefs often influence specific sexual practices, the acceptable number of sexual partners, and contraceptive use. Be sensitive to these differences by being nonjudgmental and showing acceptance.

Nutrition History

A nutrition history is important when assessing the reproductive system. Fatigue and low libido may occur as a result of poor diet and anemia. The World Cancer Research Fund estimates that about one quarter to one third of the new *preventable* cancer cases in the United States in 2017 are related to overweight or obesity, physical inactivity, and poor nutrition (American Cancer Society [ACS], 2017a). Ask the patient to recall his or her dietary intake for a recent 24-hour period to assess nutritional quality.

Assess the patient's height, weight, and body mass index. The patient may be hesitant to discuss practices such as bingeing, purging, anorexic behaviors, or excessive exercise. A certain level of body fat and weight is necessary for the onset of menses and the maintenance of regular menstrual cycles. Decreased body fat results in insufficient estrogen levels.

🧩 GENDER HEALTH CONSIDERATIONS
Patient-Centered Care (QSEN)

Women have special nutrition needs. Heavy menstrual bleeding, particularly in women who have intrauterine devices, may require iron supplements. Teach all women about their body's need for calcium. Although adequate calcium intake throughout life is needed, it is especially important during and after menopause to help prevent osteoporosis caused by decreased estrogen production (see Chapter 50).

Family History and Genetic Risk

The family history helps determine the patient's risk for conditions that affect reproductive functioning. A delayed or early development of secondary sex characteristics may be a familial pattern.

The current age and health status of family members are important. Evidence of medical diseases or reproductive problems in family members (e.g., diabetes, endometriosis, reproductive cancer) provides a fuller understanding of the patient's current symptoms. For example, daughters of women who were given diethylstilbestrol (DES) to control bleeding during pregnancy are at increased risk for infertility and reproductive tract cancer.

Specific *BRCA1* and *BRCA2* gene mutations increase the overall risk for breast or ovarian cancer (ACS, 2017c). Men with first-degree relatives (e.g., father, brother) with prostate cancer are at greater risk for the disease than are men in the general population.

Current Health Problems

Patients often seek medical attention as a result of impaired COMFORT, bleeding, discharge, and masses (Chart 69-2). Pain related to reproductive system disorders may be confused with symptoms usually associated with GI or urinary health problems (e.g., urinary frequency). Ask the patient to describe the nature of the pain, including its type, intensity, timing and location, duration, and relationship to menstrual, sexual, urinary, or GI function. Assess the factors that exacerbate (worsen) or relieve the pain. Ask about sleeping patterns and if pain or other symptoms affect the ability to get adequate rest.

Heavy *bleeding* or a lack of bleeding may concern the patient. The possibility of pregnancy in any sexually active woman with amenorrhea must be considered. Postmenopausal bleeding needs to be evaluated. Ask the patient to describe

CHART 69-2 Best Practice for Patient Safety & Quality Care (QSEN)

Assessing the Patient With Reproductive Health Problems

PATIENT CONCERN	NURSING ASSESSMENT
Pain	Type and intensity of pain Location and duration of pain Factors that relieve or worsen pain Relationship to menstrual, sexual, urinary, or GI function Medications
Bleeding	Presence or absence of bleeding Character and amount of bleeding Relationship of bleeding to events or other factors (e.g., menstrual cycle) Onset and duration of bleeding Presence of associated symptoms, such as pain
Discharge	Amount and character of discharge Presence of genital lesions, bleeding, itching, or pain Presence of symptoms or discharge in sexual partner
Masses	Location and characteristics of mass Presence of associated symptoms, such as pain Relationship to menstrual cycle

the amount and characteristics of abnormal vaginal bleeding. Assess whether the bleeding occurs in relation to the menstrual cycle or menopause, intercourse, trauma, or strenuous exercise. For male patients, ask about the presence of penile bleeding. Ask any patient who has abnormal bleeding about associated symptoms, such as pain, cramping or abdominal fullness, a change in bowel habits, urinary difficulties, and weight changes.

Discharge from the male or female reproductive tract can cause irritation of the surrounding tissues, itching, altered COMFORT, embarrassment, and anxiety. Ask about the amount, color, consistency, odor, and chronicity of discharge that may be present from orifices used during sexual activity. Drugs (e.g., antibiotics) and clothing (e.g., tight jeans, synthetic underwear fabric) may cause or worsen genital discharge. Many types of discharge are caused by STIs or other infection (see Chapter 74).

Masses in the breasts, testes, or inguinal area are evaluated. Patients can sometimes relate changes in character or size of masses to menstrual cycles, heavy lifting, straining, or trauma. Ask about associated symptoms such as tenderness, heaviness, pain, dimpling, and tender lymph nodes.

Physical Assessment
Assessment of the Female Reproductive System
The clinical nurse generalist does not perform a comprehensive female or male reproductive examination. However, you should perform a focused assessment related to specific concerns of the patient. The primary health care provider conducts a more detailed gynecologic assessment as described in the following paragraphs; the clinical nurse often assists with the examination.

Immediately before the pelvic and breast examinations, ask the patient to empty her bladder and undress completely. Drape the patient adequately to provide modesty throughout the examination. Remove drapes only over the region being examined and replace them after that area has been assessed. Mirrors can be used to facilitate teaching if the patient so desires. The examination should be performed in a room that has adequate lighting for body inspection, has comfortable temperature, and ensures privacy.

The physical examination of the female reproductive system includes the breasts (see Chapter 70), abdomen, and pelvic examination. The patient's arms should be at her sides or over her chest to allow better relaxation of the abdominal muscles. During the gynecologic examination, the primary health care provider palpates for symptomatic and asymptomatic abdominopelvic masses, which can be of reproductive, intestinal, or urinary tract origin. Gynecologic masses, such as ovarian masses, may be further differentiated from lesions on the body of the uterus during the bimanual portion of the pelvic examination.

Inspection of the female genitalia and the pelvic examination are usually performed at the end of a head-to-toe physical assessment. The patient is often more apprehensive about these portions of the examination than about any other part. Impaired COMFORT or lack of privacy during previous pelvic or breast examinations may prevent the patient from relaxing.

Other than determining pregnancy or infertility, a pelvic examination is indicated to assess for:
- Menstrual irregularities
- Unexplained abdominal or vaginal pain
- Vaginal discharge, itching, sores, or infection
- Rape trauma or other pelvic injury
- Physical changes in the vagina, cervix, and uterus

Assessment of the Male Reproductive System
Unless a male patient seeks health care for a specific problem, the primary health care provider may not perform a reproductive assessment, depending on the setting and the age of the patient. Men are often embarrassed and anxious when the reproductive system is assessed. The patient may be concerned about impaired COMFORT, the developmental stage of his genitalia, or the possibility of an erection during the examination. If he does have an erection, the examiner should assure him that this is a normal response to a tactile stimulus (touch) and should continue the examination.

Explain each step of the assessment procedure before it is performed. The patient needs to be reassured that the health care provider will stop and change the assessment plan or technique if the patient experiences pain during the examination. Teach relaxation techniques and provide nonjudgmental support during the examination to increase COMFORT, especially during the rectal examination to palpate the prostate gland.

Psychosocial Assessment
The psychosocial assessment may provide information about factors that affect the patient's health status. During the social history, ask about sources of support, strengths, and coping reactions to illness or dysfunction.

⊕ CULTURAL/SPIRITUAL CONSIDERATIONS

Patient-Centered Care QSEN

A patient's personal experiences, culture, and/or spiritual beliefs may influence his or her SEXUALITY and ability to enjoy a satisfactory sex life. These factors may include:
- Sexual trauma or abuse inflicted during childhood or adulthood
- Punishment for masturbation
- Psychological trauma
- Cultural influences, such as the idea of female passivity during intercourse
- Concerns about sexual partners or sexual lifestyle
- Use of alcohol or street drugs

Fears may affect the patient's satisfaction with SEXUALITY or body image. He or she may also be concerned about the potential or actual reaction of family members to reproductive health problems (see Chart 69-2). Use nonjudgmental listening to continue development of trust between yourself and the patient, allowing the patient to openly express feelings or concerns.

Diagnostic Assessment
Laboratory Assessment
Chart 69-3 summarizes important laboratory tests associated with reproductive function. The **Papanicolaou test (Pap test)**, or **Pap smear**, is a cytologic study that is effective in detecting precancerous and cancerous cells within the female patient's cervix. It is done immediately before the pelvic examination. A speculum is inserted into the vagina, and several samples of cells from the cervix are obtained with a small brush or spatula. The specimens are placed on a glass slide and sent to the laboratory for examination.

The Pap test should be scheduled between the patient's menstrual periods so the menstrual flow does not interfere with laboratory analysis. Teach women not to douche, use vaginal medications or deodorants, or have sexual intercourse for at

CHART 69-3 Laboratory Profile

Reproductive Assessment

TEST	NORMAL RANGE FOR ADULTS	SIGNIFICANCE OF ABNORMAL FINDINGS
Serum Studies		
Follicle-stimulating hormone (FSH) (Follitropin)	*Men:* 1.42-15.4 IU/L *Women:* follicular phase, 1.37-9.9 units/L; midcycle, 6.17-17.2 units/L; luteal phase, 1.09-9.2 unis/L; postmenopause, 19.3-100.6 units/L	Decreased levels indicate possible infertility, anorexia nervosa, neoplasm. Elevations indicate possible Turner's syndrome.
Luteinizing hormone (LH) (Lutropin)	*Men:* 1.24-7.8 units/L *Women:* follicular phase, 1.68-15 units/L; midcycle, 21.9-56.6 units/L; luteal phase, 0.61-16.3 units/L; postmenopause, 14.2-52.3 unis/L	Decreased levels indicate possible infertility, anovulation. Elevations indicate possible ovarian failure, Turner's syndrome.
Prolactin	*Men:* 3-13 ng/mL *Women:* 3-27 ng/mL *Pregnant women:* 20-400 ng/mL	Elevations indicate possible galactorrhea (breast discharge), pituitary tumor, disease of hypothalamus or pituitary gland, hypothyroidism.
Estradiol	*Men:* 10-50 pg/mL *Women:* follicular phase, 20-350 pg/mL; midcycle, 150-750 pg/mL; luteal phase, 30-450 pg/mL; postmenopause, ≤20 pg/mL	Elevations of estradiol, total estrogens, and estriol in men indicate possible gynecomastia, decreased body hair, increased fat deposits, feminization, testicular tumor; in women, ovarian tumor.
Estriol	Men and nonpregnant women: N/A	Decreased levels of estradiol, total estrogens, and estriol in women indicate possible amenorrhea, climacteric, impending miscarriage, hypothalamic disorders.
Progesterone	*Men:* 10-50 ng/dL *Women:* follicular phase, <50 ng/dL; luteal phase, 300-2500 ng/dL; postmenopausal, <40 ng/dL	Decreased levels in women indicate possible inadequate luteal phase, amenorrhea. Elevations in women indicate possible ovarian luteal cysts. Decreased levels may indicate ovarian neoplasm, ovarian dysfunction.
Testosterone	*Men:* 280-1080 ng/dL *Women:* <70 ng/dL	Increased levels in men indicate possible testicular tumor, hyperthyroidism. Decreased levels in men indicate possible hypogonadism. Elevations in women indicate possible adrenal neoplasm, ovarian neoplasm, polycystic ovary syndrome.
Prostate-specific antigen	*Men:* 0-2.5 ng/mL	Increased levels may indicate prostatitis, benign prostatic hyperplasia, prostate cancer.
Urine Studies		
Total estrogens	*Men:* 4-25 mcg/24 hr *Women:* 4-60 mcg/24 hr	Elevations indicate possible testicular tumors. Decreased levels indicate possible ovarian dysfunction.
Pregnanediol	*Men:* 0-1.9 mg/24 hr *Women:* follicular phase, <2.6 mg/24 hr; luteal phase, 2.6-10.6 mg/24 hr	Elevations indicate possible luteal ovarian cysts, ovarian neoplasms, adrenal disorders. Decreased levels indicate possible amenorrhea.
17-Ketosteroids	Men (20-50 yr): 6-20 mg/24 hr Women (20-50 yr): 6-17 mg/24 hr Values decrease with age	Elevations indicate possible Cushing's syndrome, increased androgen or cortisol production, severe stress. Decreased levels indicate possible Addison's disease, hypopituitarism.

Data from Pagana, K.D., Pagana, T.J., & Pagana, T.N. (2017). *Mosby's diagnostic and laboratory test reference* (13th ed.). St. Louis: Mosby.
1 mcg, 1 microgram or 1 millionth of a gram; *1 ng,* 1 nanogram or 1 billionth of a gram; *1 pg,* 1 picogram or 1 trillionth of a gram.

least 24 hours before the test, because these may interfere with test interpretation.

The American Cancer Society (ACS) advises all women to begin having an annual Pap test at 21 years of age. Women younger than 21 years should not be tested (ACS, 2017a). Between ages 21 and 29 years, women should have a Pap test every 3 years; women between ages 30 and 65 years should have a Pap test plus a human papilloma virus (HPV) test ("co-testing") every 5 years. More information on the HPV test is found later in this chapter. According to the ACS, women older than 65 years who have had regular cervical cancer testing with normal results do not need Pap testing (ACS, 2017a). Recommended guidelines from other health care organizations suggest a Pap test every 3 years for women older than 60 years. Those who have had a history of a serious cervical precancerous lesion

should be tested annually for at least 20 years after that diagnosis, regardless of age (ACS, 2017a).

Canadian guidelines are similar and state that women should begin annual Pap testing at either 21 or 25 years of age, depending on the province. Between 30 and 69 years, women should have a Pap test every 3 years. After 70, Pap tests are not needed (Society of Obstetricians and Gynaecologists of Canada, 2013).

Other types of laboratory testing include cytologic vaginal *cultures,* which can detect bacterial, viral, fungal, and parasitic disorders. Examination of cells from the vaginal walls can evaluate estrogen balance.

The **human papilloma virus (HPV) test** can identify many high-risk types of HPV infection associated with the development of cervical cancer. This test can be done at the same time as the Pap test for women older than 30 years and for women of any age who have had an abnormal Pap test result (ACS, 2017a). It does not take the place of the Pap test because it tests for viruses that can cause cell changes in the cervix that, if not treated, could lead to cancer. Cells are collected from the cervix and sent to a laboratory for analysis. Women who have normal Pap test results and no HPV infection are at very low risk for developing cervical cancer. Conversely, women with an abnormal Pap test result and a positive HPV test are at higher risk if not treated.

Serum levels of follicle-stimulating hormone (FSH), luteinizing hormone (LH), and prolactin are helpful in the diagnosis of male and female reproductive tract disorders. No nutrition restrictions are necessary before the test. Serum testing can also detect estrogen, progesterone, and testosterone levels in men and women. See Chart 69-3 for normal values and the significance of abnormal findings.

Serologic studies detect antigen-antibody reactions that occur in response to foreign organisms. This form of diagnostic testing is helpful only after an infection has become well established. Serologic testing can be used in the evaluation of exposure to organisms causing syphilis, rubella, and herpes simplex virus type 2 (HSV2). Results may be read as *nonreactive, weakly reactive,* or *reactive.* A single titer is not as revealing as serial titers, which can detect the rise in antibody reactions as the body continues to fight the infection.

The *prostate-specific antigen (PSA)* test is used to screen for prostate cancer and to monitor the disease after treatment. PSA levels less than 2.5 ng/mL may be considered normal, although there is no agreement on that value and how it is affected by age. Elevated PSA levels may be associated with prostate cancer. Older men, particularly African-American men, often have a higher than normal PSA, especially as they age (Pagana et al., 2017). Chapter 72 discusses this test in more detail.

NCLEX EXAMINATION CHALLENGE 69-1

Health Promotion and Maintenance

A 70-year-old client asks the nurse if she needs a Pap smear. Her last Pap smear was 3 years ago, and it was normal. What is the correct nursing response?
A. "Yes, you need a Pap test this year."
B. "You aren't due for another Pap test until next year."
C. "A Pap smear is not needed unless you are sexually active."
D. "You may not need an annual Pap smear after 65 years of age."

Imaging Assessment

Computed Tomography. CT scans for reproductive system disorders involve the abdomen and the pelvis. Primary health care providers can detect and evaluate masses and identify lymphatic enlargement from metastasis. This scan can differentiate solid tissue masses from cystic or hemorrhagic structures.

Hysterosalpingography. A **hysterosalpingogram** is an x-ray that uses an injection of a contrast medium to visualize the cervix, uterus, and fallopian tubes. This test is used to evaluate tubal anatomy and patency and uterine problems such as fibroids, tumors, and fistulas. The study should not be attempted for at least 6 weeks after abortion, delivery, or dilation and curettage. Other contraindications include reproductive tract infection and uterine bleeding.

The examination is best performed in the first half (days 1 to 14) of the patient's menstrual cycle, which reduces the chance that the patient may be pregnant. Patients preparing to have a hysterosalpingogram should be instructed to follow the recommendations of their health care provider, which may include taking an over-the-counter pain reliever before the procedure.

On the day of the examination, confirm the date of the patient's last menstrual period. Ask about allergies to iodine dye or shellfish. The primary health care provider provides information about benefits and risks of the procedure with the patient. As the nurse, you may witness the signed informed consent. Be aware that the patient may experience some nausea and vomiting, abdominal cramping, or faintness during the procedure. Provide support and assistance with relaxation techniques as needed.

After the patient is placed in lithotomy position, the health care provider will insert a speculum to view the cervix. Dye is injected through the cervix to fill and highlight the interior of the cervix, uterus, and fallopian tubes. If the fallopian tubes are patent, the contrast material spills into the peritoneal cavity. Usually only two or three views are obtained to show the path and distribution of the contrast medium.

The patient may experience pelvic pain after the study and should receive analgesic medications as ordered. Inform her that she may also have referred pain to the shoulder because of irritation of the phrenic nerve. Provide a perineal pad after the test to prevent soiling of clothes as the dye drains from the cervix. Instruct the patient to contact her primary health care provider if bloody discharge continues for 4 days or longer and to immediately report any signs of infection, such as lower quadrant pain, fever, malodorous discharge, or tachycardia.

Mammography. **Mammography** is an x-ray of the soft tissue of the breast. Mammograms assess differences in the density of breast tissue. They are especially helpful in evaluating poorly defined masses, multiple masses or nodules, nipple changes or discharge, skin changes, and impaired COMFORT. Mammography can detect many cancers that are not palpable by physical examination. However, some actual cancers may not appear on mammography or may appear as benign (ACS, 2017b).

In young women's breasts, there is little difference in the density between normal glandular tissue and malignant tumors, which makes the mammogram less useful for evaluation of breast masses in these women. For this reason, annual screening mammograms are not recommended for women younger than 40 years (ACS, 2017b). In older women, the amount of fatty tissue is higher, and the fatty tissue appears lighter than cancers. Cancer and cysts may have the same density. Cysts usually have smooth borders, and cancers often have starburst-shaped margins.

No dietary restrictions are necessary before the mammogram. Remind the patient not to use creams, lotions, powders, or deodorant on the breasts or underarms before the study because these products may be visible on the mammogram and lead to misdiagnosis. If there is any possibility that the patient is pregnant, the test should be rescheduled. Explain the purpose of the study and its anticipated discomforts. The technician or assistant provides a gown and privacy for the woman to undress above the waist. Allow the patient to express concerns about the mammogram and the presence of any lumps.

When performing a standard mammogram, a technician positions the patient next to the x-ray machine with one breast exposed. A film plate and the platform of the machine are placed on opposite sides of the breast to be examined. The technician includes as much breast tissue as possible between the plates. The woman may experience some temporary discomfort when the breast is compressed (for about a minute for each of four positions). The entire test takes about 15 minutes. The patient usually is asked to wait until the films are reviewed in case a view needs to be repeated.

Most breast imaging centers offer digital 3D mammography, also known as digital breast tomosynthesis. This technology allows the radiologist to visualize through layers or "slices" of breast tissue, similar to a CT scan. If a digital mammogram is performed, the images are recorded and saved as computer files (ACS, 2017b). Medicare and most other health insurances pay for this newer and more expensive technology because it improves diagnosis accuracy.

Inform the patient when to expect the report of the results. Because this is a time when she is anxious about the health of her breasts, teach or reinforce the importance of breast self-awareness and provide instructions as needed.

Ultrasonography. Ultrasonography (US) is a technique that is used to assess fibroids, cysts, and masses. It can be used to monitor the progress of tumor regression after medical treatment. US is also helpful in differentiating solid tumors from cysts in breast examinations. In men, ultrasound can test for varicoceles, scrotal abnormalities, and problems of the ejaculatory ducts and seminal vesicles and the vas deferens (Pagana, et al., 2017).

For an abdominal, breast, or scrotal scan, the technician exposes the area and applies gel to the area to be scanned, which provides better transmission of sound waves from the transducer through the patient's skin. The transducer is moved in a linear pattern across the area being tested to outline and define soft-tissue masses and to differentiate tumor type, ascites, and encapsulated fluid.

For a *transvaginal* or *transrectal* scan, the transducer is covered with a condom onto which transmission gel has been placed. The transducer is then inserted into the vagina or rectum as indicated. Women should have an empty or only partially filled bladder if they are having a transvaginal ultrasound. For women who are incontinent, a urinary catheter may be inserted and filled with fluid to allow optimal visualization. Patients having an internal ultrasound should be informed that they might feel some mild impaired COMFORT associated with pressure of the probe.

Magnetic Resonance Imaging. MRI uses a magnetic field and radiofrequency energy to distinguish between normal and malignant tissues. MRIs are used in addition to mammograms to assess for breast cancer in women who have a genetic risk (ACS, 2017c). The use of MRI in evaluating patients with dense breast tissue may reduce the need for biopsy. MRI is also used to detect pelvic tumors.

Endoscopic Studies

Colposcopy. A colposcope allows three-dimensional magnification and intense illumination of epithelium with suspected disease. Colposcopy is suited for inspection of a female patient's cervical epithelium, vagina, and vulvar epithelium. Because it provides accurate site selection, this procedure can locate the exact site of premalignant and malignant lesions for biopsy.

Inform the patient that she should not douche or use vaginal preparations for 24 to 48 hours before the test. This nearly painless procedure is better tolerated if it is explained in advance and if the actual colposcope instrument is shown to the patient.

Explain that the primary health care provider may take a biopsy while performing colposcopy.

Provide the patient with a gown and privacy, and instruct her to undress from the waist down. Assist the patient to the lithotomy position. The primary health care provider locates the cervix or vaginal site through a speculum examination. Lubricants other than water should not be used. Cells in the area may be stained or left unstained to enhance visibility. The cervix will be cleaned and moistened with normal saline to increase the visibility of vascular patterns and the junction between the columnar epithelium and the squamous epithelium. Acetic acid is applied to the cervix to draw moisture from the tissue and to accentuate important features. The primary health care provider then uses a colposcope or colpomicroscope to inspect the area in question, and a biopsy specimen can be taken if abnormal cells are seen. (See Cervical Biopsy section later in this chapter.)

After the procedure, allow the patient to rest for a few minutes, especially if she had a biopsy performed. Provide privacy and supplies to clean the perineum and a perineal pad to absorb any dye or discharge. Inform the patient that she may wish to wear a sanitary pad because mild cramping, spotting, or dark or black-colored discharge (from medication applied to the cervix to reduce bleeding) may occur for several days. Remind the patient to take pain relievers as recommended by her primary health care provider but to avoid aspirin to decrease the chance of bleeding. The patient should be instructed to refrain from douching, using tampons, and having sexual intercourse for 1 week (or as instructed by the primary health care provider).

Laparoscopy. Laparoscopy is a direct examination of the pelvic cavity through an endoscope. This procedure can rule out an ectopic pregnancy, evaluate ovarian disorders and pelvic masses, and aid in the diagnosis of infertility and unexplained pelvic pain. Laparoscopy is also used during surgical procedures such as:

- Tubal sterilization
- Ovarian biopsy
- Cyst aspiration
- Removal of endometriosis tissue
- Lysis of adhesions around the fallopian tubes
- Retrieval of "lost" intrauterine devices

A laparoscopy may also be used instead of a laparotomy for minor surgical procedures because it uses small incisions, involves less discomfort, and typically does not require overnight hospitalization.

The surgeon describes benefits and risks of the procedure to the patient. Risks include complications associated with the use of anesthesia, postoperative shoulder pain from irritation of the phrenic nerve, effects of carbon dioxide gas and/or peritoneal stretching, irritation at the incision site, and the rare occurrence of infection or electrical burns. As the nurse, you may witness the patient signing the informed consent. A laparoscopy can be performed with a regional or general anesthetic.

After the patient is anesthetized and placed in the lithotomy position, a urinary catheter is inserted to drain the bladder. The operating table is placed in slight Trendelenburg position to allow the intestines to fall away from the pelvis. The cervix is held with a cannula to allow movement of the uterus during laparoscopy (Fig. 69-4). The surgeon inserts a needle below the umbilicus to infuse carbon dioxide (CO_2) into the pelvic cavity, which distends the abdomen and permits better visualization

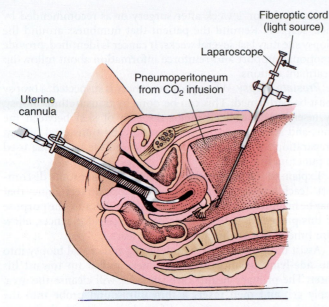

Uterine cannula

Pneumoperitoneum from CO_2 infusion

Laparoscope

Fiberoptic cord (light source)

FIG. 69-4 Laparoscopy. CO_2, Carbon dioxide.

The Patient Recovering From Cervical Biopsy

- Do not lift any heavy objects until the site is healed (about 2 weeks).
- Rest for 24 hours after the procedure.
- Report any excessive bleeding (more than that of a normal menstrual period) to your health care provider.
- Report signs of infection (fever, increased pain, foul-smelling drainage) to your health care provider.
- Do not douche, use tampons, or have vaginal intercourse until the site is healed (about 2 weeks).
- Keep the perineum clean and dry by using antiseptic solution rinses (as directed by your health care provider) and changing pads frequently.

of the organs. After the trocar and cannula are in place in the abdominal cavity, the surgeon removes the trocar and inserts the laparoscope. The surgeon can then visualize the pelvic cavity and reproductive organs. Further instrumentation is possible through one or more small incisions. The laparoscope is removed at the end of the procedure, and the abdomen is deflated. The small incision is closed with absorbable sutures and dressed with an adhesive bandage.

The patient is usually discharged on the day of the procedure. Discomfort from the incision is managed by oral analgesics. The greatest discomfort is caused by referred shoulder pain. Most of these sensations disappear within 48 hours depending on the extent of the procedure. Instruct the patient to change the small adhesive bandage as needed and to observe the incision for signs of infection or hematoma. Remind her also to avoid strenuous activity for the first week after the procedure.

Hysteroscopy. Hysteroscopy is a procedure that uses a fiberoptic camera to visualize the uterus to diagnose and treat causes of abnormal bleeding. The hysteroscope includes a fiberoptic camera that is inserted into the vagina to examine the cervix and uterus. Diagnostic hysteroscopy is used to diagnose new problems with the uterus or to confirm results from other tests. Hysteroscopy can also be used before or during other procedures (e.g., laparoscopy) for infertility and unexplained bleeding. The procedure is best performed 5 days after menses has ceased to reduce the possibility of pregnancy.

The physician informs the patient of benefits and risks associated with the procedure and obtains consent. You may witness the patient signing the informed consent. The preparation is the same as for a pelvic examination. After the patient is placed in lithotomy position, she is usually anesthetized with a paracervical or other regional block before the cervix is dilated. The physician inserts the hysteroscope through the cervix. Because this distends the uterus, cells can be pushed through the fallopian tubes and into the pelvic cavity. Therefore hysteroscopy is contraindicated in patients with suspected cervical or endometrial cancer, in those with infection of the reproductive tract, and in pregnant patients.

Care is the same as that after a pelvic examination. Analgesics may be prescribed if the patient has cramping or shoulder pain.

Biopsy Studies

Cervical Biopsy. In a cervical biopsy, cervical tissue is removed for cytologic study. A biopsy is indicated for an identifiable cervical lesion, regardless of the cytologic findings. The primary health care provider usually performs a biopsy in conjunction with colposcopy as a follow-up to a suspicious Pap test finding. The procedure may be performed in a clinic or office setting.

Several techniques can be used for a cervical biopsy. If a lesion is clearly visible, an endocervical curettage can be performed as an ambulatory care procedure and with little or no anesthetic. Conization (removal of a cone-shaped sample of tissue) and loop electrosurgical excision procedures (LEEPs) are usually not done unless the cervical biopsy findings are positive or the results of the colposcopy are unsatisfactory (Lowdermilk et al., 2016). Conization can be done as a cold-knife procedure, a laser excision, or an electrosurgical incision.

The biopsy is usually scheduled when the woman is in the early proliferative phase of the menstrual cycle, when the cervix is least vascular. Because a biopsy evaluates potentially cancerous cells, your patient may be anxious and need time to discuss her feelings and fears. The use of relaxation techniques may assist COMFORT. Assist her into the lithotomy position, recognizing that further preparation depends on the type of procedure to be performed.

The physician may anesthetize the patient according to the needs of the chosen procedure. He or she visualizes the cervix and obtains the tissue sample, which is immediately placed into a formalin solution. The type of anesthetic used for the procedure determines the type of immediate care that is needed after the procedure. Discharge instructions can be found in Chart 69-4.

Endometrial Biopsy. Both endometrial biopsy and aspiration are used to obtain cells directly from the lining of the uterus to assess for cancer of the endometrium. Biopsy helps assess menstrual disturbances (especially heavy bleeding) and infertility (corpus luteum dysfunction).

When menstrual disturbances are being evaluated, the biopsy is generally done in the immediate premenstrual period to provide an index of progesterone influence and ovulation. A biopsy performed in the second half of the menstrual cycle (about days 21 and 22) evaluates corpus luteum function and the presence or absence of a persistent secretory endometrium. Postmenopausal women may undergo biopsies at any time.

Menstrual data should be obtained from the patient and are included on the specimen request for the pathologist. Prepare the patient in the same way as you would for a pelvic examination. Advise her that she may experience some cramping when the cervix is dilated. Analgesia before the procedure and relaxation and breathing techniques during the procedure may be helpful to make her more comfortable.

An endometrial biopsy is usually done as an office procedure with or without anesthesia. After the uterus is measured and the cervix dilated, the primary health care provider inserts the curette or intrauterine cannula into the uterus. A portion of the endometrium is withdrawn using either the cuplike end of the curette or suction equipment and is placed into a formalin solution to be sent for histologic examination. The patient will likely have moderate cramping. Allow her to rest on the examining table until the cramping has subsided. Provide a perineal pad and a wipe to clean the perineum. Teach her that spotting may be present for 1 to 2 days but any signs of infection or excessive bleeding should be reported to the physician. Instruct the patient to avoid intercourse or douching until all discharge has ceased.

Breast Biopsy. All breast masses should be evaluated for the possibility of cancer. It is important to recognize that breast cancer can occur in both men and women; about 1% of breast cancers occur in men (National Cancer Institute, 2017). Fibrocystic lesions, fibroadenomas, and intraductal papillomas can be differentiated by biopsy. Any discharge from the breasts is examined histologically.

Provide instructions to the patient, depending on the type of biopsy performed and the type of anesthesia used. The patient usually receives a local anesthetic, and the tissue either is aspirated through a large-bore needle (core-needle biopsy) or is removed using a small incision to extract multiple samples of tissue.

Aspirated fluid from benign cysts may appear clear to dark green–brown. Bloody fluid suggests cancer. These specimens undergo histologic evaluation. If cancer is found, the tissue is evaluated for estrogen receptor analysis. Chapter 70 discusses types of breast cancer and their relationship to estrogen receptors.

Teach that discomfort after the procedure is usually mild and can be controlled with analgesics or the use of ice or heat, depending on the type and extent of the biopsy. Educate the patient about how to assess the area or incision for bleeding and edema. Tell women to wear a properly supportive bra

continuously for 1 week after surgery or as recommended by their surgeon. Remind the patient that numbness around the biopsy site may last several weeks. If cancer is identified, provide emotional support and reinforce information about follow-up treatment options.

Prostate Biopsy. When prostate cancer is suspected, a biopsy must be performed. This can be done by transurethral biopsy, by inserting a needle through the area of skin between the anus and scrotum, or, most commonly, by transrectal biopsy. Preparation for the procedure depends on the technique used to puncture the gland.

Explain to the patient that he may experience some discomfort. Teach him about breathing and relaxation techniques that may be helpful to use during the procedure. Because the purpose of this procedure is to evaluate prostate cells for cancer, allow him time to discuss his anxieties and fears.

Assist the patient who is undergoing transrectal biopsy into the side-lying position with his knees pulled up toward his chest. The primary health care provider will cleanse the area, apply gel, and then insert a thin ultrasound probe into the patient's rectum to anesthetize (if needed) and guide the biopsy needle into place. The biopsy is collected over a 5- to 10-minute period. The patient may experience a brief, uncomfortable feeling each time the needle collects a sample.

After prostate biopsy, educate the patient to take the entire prescribed antibiotic. Remind him that he may experience slight soreness, light rectal bleeding, and blood in the urine or stools for a few days. Semen may be red or rust colored for several weeks. Teach the patient to contact his primary health care provider if he has prolonged or heavy bleeding, worsening pain, swelling in the area of biopsy, and/or difficulty urinating. Rarely, sepsis can develop after a prostate biopsy. Teach the patient to contact his primary health care provider immediately if he experiences fever, pain when urinating, or penile discharge.

? NCLEX EXAMINATION CHALLENGE 69-2
Physiological Integrity

A client has undergone a breast biopsy. Which postprocedure symptoms will the nurse teach the client to report **immediately** to the primary health care provider?
A. Tenderness around the biopsy site
B. Numbness around the biopsy site
C. Heavy bleeding from the biopsy site
D. Slight edema near the biopsy site

GET READY FOR THE NCLEX® EXAMINATION!

KEY POINTS

Review these Key Points for each NCLEX Examination Client Needs Category.

Health Promotion and Maintenance
- Encourage women to follow recommended Pap screening guidelines for early detection of precancerous and cancerous cells from the cervix. **QSEN: Evidence-Based Practice**

- Assess and respect cultural preferences when identifying risks for certain reproductive problems and when evaluating health promotion practices. **QSEN: Patient-Centered Care**

Psychosocial Integrity
- Allow the patient to express fear or anxiety regarding potential changes in sexual or reproductive function.

- Assess the patient's level of COMFORT in discussing issues related to reproductive health and SEXUALITY. **QSEN: Patient-Centered Care**
- Encourage patients to express feelings of anxiety or impaired COMFORT related to genital examinations and testing of the reproductive system.

Physiological Integrity

- Urge patients with pain, bleeding, discharge, masses, or changes in reproductive function to see their health care provider. **QSEN: Safety**
- Provide privacy for patients undergoing examination or testing of the reproductive system.

- Recognize that reproductive changes occur with aging, as described in Chart 69-1.
- Recall the selected laboratory tests used for diagnosing reproductive health problems as outlined in Chart 69-3.
- Explain all diagnostic procedures, restrictions, and follow-up care to the patient scheduled for tests.
- Teach women to report symptoms of infection or bleeding to their health care provider after endoscopic procedures and biopsies of the breast, cervix, and endometrium. **QSEN: Safety**
- Instruct men to report symptoms of infection to their health care provider after a transrectal biopsy of the prostate. **QSEN: Safety**

SELECTED BIBLIOGRAPHY

American Cancer Society (ACS). (2017a). *Cancer facts and figures 2017.* www.cancer.org/acs/groups/content/@epidemiologysurveilance/documents/document/acspc-036845.pdf.

American Cancer Society (ACS). (2017b). *Mammograms.* www.cancer.org/cancer/breastcancer/moreinformation/breastcancerearlydetection/breast-cancer-early-detection-acs-recs-mammograms.

American Cancer Society (ACS). (2017c). *American Cancer Society recommendations for early breast cancer detection in women without breast symptoms.* www.cancer.org/cancer/breastcancer/moreinformation/breastcancerearlydetection/breast-cancer-early-detection-acs-recs.

Lowdermilk, D. L., Perry, S. E., Cashion, M. C., & Alden, K. R. (2016). *Maternity and women's health care* (11th ed.). St. Louis: Elsevier.

Mayo Clinic. (2017). *Prostate biopsy.* www.mayoclinic.com/health/prostate-biopsy/MY00182/DSECTION=what-you-can-expect.

National Cancer Institute at the National Institutes of Health. (2017). *General information about male breast cancer.* www.cancer.gov/cancertopics/pdq/treatment/malebreast/Patient/page1#Keypoint3.

Pagana, K. D., Pagana, T. J., & Pagana, T. N. (2017). *Mosby's diagnostic and laboratory test reference* (13th ed.). St. Louis: Mosby.

Society of Obstetricians and Gynaecologists of Canada. (2013). *Position Statement on Cervical Cancer Screening.* sogc.org/wp-content/uploads/2013/04/medCervicalCancerScreeningENG130220.pdf.

Care of Patients With Breast Disorders

Gail B. Johnson and Harriet Kumar

e http://evolve.elsevier.com/Iggy/

PRIORITY AND INTERRELATED CONCEPTS

The priority concepts for this chapter are:
- CELLULAR REGULATION
- COMFORT

※ The CELLULAR REGULATION concept exemplar for this chapter is Breast Cancer, below.

The interrelated concept for this chapter is SEXUALITY.

LEARNING OUTCOMES

Safe and Effective Care Environment

1. Collaborate with interprofessional health care team members to identify community resources for the patient with breast cancer.

Health Promotion and Maintenance

2. Describe the three-pronged approach to early detection of breast masses: mammography, clinical breast examination (CBE), and breast self-awareness.
3. Teach patients who choose breast self-examination (BSE) as an option to use correct technique.
4. Explain the options available to a person at high genetic risk for breast cancer.
5. Evaluate patient risk factors for impaired CELLULAR REGULATION in breast cancer.

Psychosocial Integrity

6. Discuss the psychosocial impact for the patient and family who have received a diagnosis of breast cancer.

7. Discuss SEXUALITY issues with the patient having breast surgery.
8. Describe body image changes that can result from breast cancer surgery.

Physiological Integrity

9. Compare assessment findings associated with benign breast lesions with those of malignant breast lesions.
10. Explain implications of breast reduction and breast augmentation.
11. Differentiate treatment options for breast cancer.
12. Use clinical judgment to prioritize nursing care for a patient with breast cancer, including managing impaired COMFORT.
13. Describe the role of radiation and drug therapy in the care of patients with breast cancer.
14. Identify the role of complementary and integrative therapy in breast cancer management.

Breast disorders may be benign or malignant. Changes in the breast tissue (CELLULAR REGULATION) can cause a great deal of anxiety and impaired COMFORT for women. Chapter 2 reviews these nursing concepts. Nurses are often in the position of assisting patients by providing accurate information about benign breast disorders and breast cancer.

※ CELLULAR REGULATION CONCEPT EXEMPLAR
Breast Cancer

❖ PATHOPHYSIOLOGY

Cancer is a common problem of impaired CELLULAR REGULATION. Cancer of the breast begins as a single transformed cell

that grows and multiplies in the epithelial cells lining one or more of the mammary ducts or lobules. It is a heterogeneous disease, having many forms with different clinical presentations and responses to therapy. Some breast cancers present as a palpable lump in the breast, whereas others show up only on a mammogram.

There are two broad categories of breast cancer: noninvasive and invasive. As long as the cancer remains within the mammary duct, it is referred to as *noninvasive*. The more common type of breast cancer is classified as *invasive*; this type grows into surrounding breast tissue. *Metastasis* occurs when cancer cells spread beyond the breast tissue and lymph nodes, via the blood and lymph systems, to distant sites. The most common sites of metastasis are bones, liver, lung, and brain, but breast cancer can spread to any organ. The course of metastatic breast cancer is related to the site affected and the level of functional impairment. The processes involved in cancer development are described in Chapter 21.

Noninvasive Breast Cancers

Ductal carcinoma in situ (DCIS) is an early *noninvasive* form of breast cancer. In DCIS, cancer cells are located within the duct and have not invaded the surrounding fatty breast tissue. Because of more precise mammography screening and earlier detection, the number of women diagnosed with DCIS has increased. Currently there is no way to determine which DCIS lesions will progress to invasive cancer and which ones will remain unchanged. This uncertainty causes anxiety and conflict regarding treatment decisions in many women diagnosed with DCIS. It is important to convey to patients the ways in which DCIS differs from invasive cancer and that DCIS cells lack the biologic capacity to metastasize.

Another type of noninvasive disease is lobular carcinoma in situ (LCIS). The cells look like cancer cells and are contained within the lobules (milk-producing glands) of the breast. LCIS is less common than DCIS and is not thought to be a precursor of invasive cancer. However, a diagnosis of LCIS is a marker for increased risk of developing invasive breast cancer (ACS, 2017a). It is usually diagnosed before menopause in women 40 to 50 years of age. Traditionally LCIS is treated with close observation only. Women with LCIS and other breast cancer risk factors may want to consider prophylactic treatment options such as tamoxifen, raloxifene, or prophylactic mastectomy (ACS, 2017a).

Invasive Breast Cancers

The most common type of invasive breast cancer is infiltrating ductal carcinoma. As the name implies, the disease originates in the mammary ducts and breaks through the walls of the ducts into the surrounding breast tissue. Once invasive, the cancer grows into the tissue around it in an irregular pattern. If a lump is present, it is felt as an irregular, poorly defined mass. As the tumor continues to grow, fibrosis (replacement of normal cells with connective tissue and collagen) develops around the cancer. This fibrosis may cause shortening of Cooper's ligaments and the resulting typical skin dimpling that is seen with more advanced disease (Fig. 70-1). Another sign, sometimes indicating late-stage breast cancer, is an edematous thickening and pitting of breast skin called *peau d'orange* (orange peel skin) (Fig. 70-2).

A rare but highly aggressive form of invasive breast cancer is inflammatory breast cancer (IBC). It is characterized by diffuse erythema and edema (peau d'orange). Patients typically complain of breast pain or a rapidly growing breast lump. Other common symptoms include a tender, firm, enlarged breast and breast itching. Because of its aggressive nature, IBC is usually diagnosed at a later stage than other types of breast cancer and is often harder to treat successfully (ACS, 2017a).

Breast Cancer in Men

Male breast cancer is rare and accounts for about 1% of all breast cancer cases in the United States and Canada. Similar to women, the incidence of male breast cancer increases with age; however, unlike women, the rates are similar among blacks and whites. Risk factors for male breast cancer include previous radiation, a family history of breast cancer (male or female), *BRCA 1/2* mutation, diabetes, gynecomastia (enlarged breasts), testicular disorders, and obesity (ACS, 2017b).

Men usually present with a hard, painless, subareolar mass; gynecomastia may be present. Other symptoms include nipple discharge (often blood stained), rash around the nipple, inverted nipple, ulceration or swelling of the chest, and possibly swollen lymph nodes. Because *men* usually do not suspect breast cancer, they often ignore the symptoms and postpone seeing their primary health care provider. As a result, many men are diagnosed at later stages than women. Treatment of breast cancer in men is the same as in women at a similar stage of disease.

Breast Cancer in Young Women

Genetic predisposition is a stronger risk factor for younger women than older women. Younger women frequently present with more aggressive forms of the disease; the number of cases of advanced breast cancer in younger women is increasing (Johnson et al., 2013). Screening tools can be less effective for this group because the breasts tend to be denser and mammographic recognition of breast cancer may be impaired in areas of dense tissue. Nurses should encourage women who have symptoms to seek evaluation and not watch and wait. Younger women with breast cancer face unique issues associated with treatment. These include earlier menopause, infertility after treatment, and impaired SEXUALITY (Kedde et al., 2013).

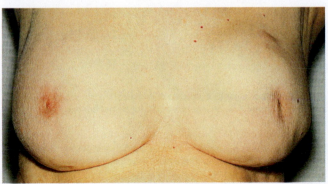

FIG. 70-1 Skin dimpling on a breast as a result of fibrosis or breast cancer. (From Mansel, R., & Bundred, N. (1995). *Color atlas of breast disease*. St. Louis: Mosby.)

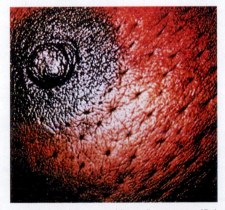

FIG. 70-2 Breast edema giving the skin an "orange peel" *(peau d'orange)* appearance. (From Gallager, H.S., Leis, H.P. Jr., Snyderman, R.K., & Urban, J.A. (1978). *The breast*. St. Louis: Mosby.)

Etiology and Genetic Risk

Increased age is the primary risk factor for developing breast cancer in both women and men. Several other factors are known to increase the risk of developing breast cancer; many are not modifiable, such as family history, early menarche, and late menopause. Modifiable risk factors include, but are not limited to, postmenopausal obesity, use of postmenopausal hormone replacement therapy (HRT), alcohol consumption, nulliparity, and lack of breast-feeding (ACS, 2017b).

According to the American Cancer Society (2017c), breast cancer is often diagnosed late in the disease process for lesbian and bisexual women because of their fear of discrimination, negative experiences with health care professionals, and lack of health insurance. In addition, many women in these groups have no children or have a child after they are 30 years of age or older. Having several risk factors for any woman increases one's risk more than having a single risk factor. Table 70-1 lists major breast cancer risk factors according to the varying degree of risk.

Incidence and Prevalence

One of every eight women in the United States will develop breast cancer by age 70 years (ACS, 2017b). Breast cancer is the

 GENETIC/GENOMIC CONSIDERATIONS

Patient-Centered Care OSEN

Mutations in several genes, such as *BRCA1* and *BRCA2*, are related to hereditary breast cancer. People who have specific mutations in either one of these genes are at an increased risk for developing breast cancer and ovarian cancer. However, these account for only 5% to 10% of all female breast cancers (ACS, 2017b). Only women with a strong family history and a reasonable suspicion that a mutation is present have genetic testing for *BRCA* and other mutations known to increase an individual's risk of developing breast cancer. Encourage women to talk with a genetics counselor to carefully consider the benefits and potential consequences of genetic testing before these tests are done.

second leading cause of cancer death in women, exceeded only by lung cancer (ACS, 2017b). Similar statistics can be found in Canada (Canadian Cancer Society, 2015). Early detection is the key to effective treatment and survival. The 5-year relative survival rate is lower for women who are diagnosed with an advanced stage of breast cancer. The 5-year relative survival rate for localized breast cancer is 99%, whereas the rate drops to 85% when the cancer has spread to the regional lymph nodes (ACS,

TABLE 70-1   Risk Factors for Breast Cancer

FACTORS	COMMENTS
Female gender	Ninety-nine percent of all breast cancers occur in women.
Age >65 years	Risk increases across all ages until age 80 years.
Genetic factors	Inherited mutations of *BRCA1* and/or *BRCA2* increase risk.
History of a previous breast cancer	The risk for developing a cancer in the opposite breast is five times greater than for the average population at risk.
Breast density	Dense breasts contain more glandular and connective tissue, which increases the risk for developing breast cancer.
Atypical hyperplasia	Biopsy-confirmed atypical hyperplasia is a high relative risk.
Family history	Two first-degree relatives with breast cancer increases risk.
Ionizing radiation	Women who received frequent low-level radiation exposure to the thorax had an increased risk, especially if the exposure occurred during periods of rapid breast formation.
High postmenopausal bone density	High estrogen levels over time both strengthen bone and increase breast cancer risk.
Reproductive history Nulliparity *or* First child born after age 30 years	Childless women have an increased risk, as do women who bear their first child near or after age 30.
Menstrual history Early menstruation *or* Late menopause *or* Both	The risk for breast cancer rises as the interval between menarche and menopause increases. Women who undergo bilateral oophorectomy before age 35 years have less risk for breast cancer than women who undergo natural menopause.
Recent oral contraceptive use	There is a slight increase in breast cancer risk in women taking oral contraceptives. The risk returns to normal after 10 years of stopping the pill.
Recent hormone replacement therapy (HRT)	Use of HRT containing both estrogen and progestin increases risk; risk diminishes after 5 years of discontinuation.
Obesity	Postmenopausal obesity (especially increased abdominal fat), increased body mass, insulin resistance, and hyperglycemia have been reported to be associated with an increased risk for breast cancer.
Other Risk Factors	
Alcohol consumption	Risk is dose dependent; consumption of 3 to 14 drinks per week is associated with a slight increase in risk; risk increases with increased consumption. This includes all forms of alcoholic beverages.
High socioeconomic status	Breast cancer incidence is greater in women of higher education and socioeconomic background. This relationship is possibly related to lifestyle differences, such as later age at first birth.
Jewish heritage	Women of Ashkenazi Jewish heritage have higher incidences of *BRCA1* and *BRCA2* genetic mutations.

Data from American Cancer Society. (2017). *Breast cancer facts & figures 2016-2017.* Atlanta: Author.

2017b). Survival drops dramatically when breast cancer is metastatic (spread to distant sites).

🌐 CULTURAL/SPIRITUAL CONSIDERATIONS
Patient-Centered Care QSEN

Overall, Euro-American women older than 40 years are at a greater risk for breast cancer than other racial/ethnic groups, but the rate of breast cancer in African-American women *younger than 40 years* is higher than for others in that age-group. African-American women also have a higher death rate at any age when compared with other women with the disease (ACS, 2017b). In their classic study, Ooi et al. (2011) found that American Indian, African-American, and Hispanic women are also likely to present with more aggressive breast cancer that is harder to treat, such as *triple-negative breast cancer*. In this type of breast cancer, cells lack receptors for estrogen, progesterone, and the protein *HER2*. African-American and Puerto Rican women have the highest risk for triple-negative breast cancer. These cultural disparities should be addressed with targeted interventions that are appropriate for specific cultural and ethnic groups. Nurses need to be culturally aware and competent to assist women to overcome barriers to care.

❓ NCLEX EXAMINATION CHALLENGE 70-1
Health Promotion and Maintenance

The nurse is caring for these clients. Which client does the nurse recognize as having the **highest** risk for development of breast cancer?
A. 55-year-old male with gynecomastia and obesity
B. 60-year-old female whose father died from colon cancer
C. 65-year-old male whose mother had ovarian cancer
D. 75-year-old female who was treated for breast cancer 5 years ago

Health Promotion and Maintenance

The American Cancer Society (ACS) and Canadian Cancer Society (CCS) establish evidence-based guidelines for breast cancer screening in women. Guidelines have not been recommended for screening men in the general population because breast cancer in men is so rare (ACS, 2017a). Encourage men with a strong family history or known genetic mutations to discuss screening with their primary health care provider.

Teach women that no single method for early detection of breast cancer is effective when used alone. The best approach for average-risk women is screening mammogram, clinical breast examination, and breast self-awareness.

Mammography

In 2015, the American Cancer Society (ACS) updated its breast cancer screening guidelines and recommends that women at average risk of breast cancer begin annual screening mammography at age 45. Women ages 40 to 45 should have the choice to start annual mammograms after the risks and potential benefits have been explained. Women age 55 and older may switch to mammograms every 2 years. Mammography should continue as long as a woman is in good health and has a life expectancy of at least 10 years (ACS, 2017a).

Canadian guidelines for mammography differ from those of the United States: no routine mammography screening is recommended until women reach 50 years of age. After 50, the recommended guidelines vary slightly across organizations but generally recommend that women after age 50 have mammography every 2 to 3 years until age 70 to 74 (Canadian Cancer Society, 2015).

Breast Self-Awareness/Self-Examination

Monthly breast self-examination (BSE) is less emphasized today than in the past several decades. Instead, it is recommended as an option that women increase breast self-awareness by becoming familiar with how their breasts look and feel.

Nurses working with women should teach them the importance of becoming familiar with the appearance and feel of their breasts. Any changes detected by the woman should be reported to her primary health care provider. Teach a woman that lumps are not necessarily abnormal. For premenopausal women, lumps can come and go with the menstrual cycle. Most lumps that are detected and tested are not malignant.

Some women may want to practice regular breast self-examination (BSE) as a method for breast self-awareness. Evidence shows that monthly BSE is no more beneficial than women simply being aware of what is normal for their own breasts and that women are just as likely to find a lump by chance (ACS, 2017a). However, BSE should be presented as an option to women beginning in their early 20s. In addition to breast self-awareness, place emphasis on mammography and clinical breast examination for early detection of breast cancer. The combined approach is better than any single test (ACS, 2017a). A woman who chooses to perform BSE should be taught the correct technique and have it reviewed by a health care professional during her clinical breast examination.

The BSE technique is similar for women and men. Use teaching models of normal and abnormal breasts when teaching BSE. Discuss the proper timing for BSE. Instruct premenopausal women to examine their breasts 1 week after the menstrual period. At this time, hormonal influence on breast tissue is decreased, so fluid retention and tenderness are reduced. Teach women whose breast tissue is no longer influenced by hormonal fluctuations, such as after a total hysterectomy or menopause, to pick a day each month to do BSE, such as the first day of the month. Chart 70-1 describes the procedure for breast self-examination and may be used as a patient resource.

Clinical Breast Examination

Clinical breast examination (CBE) is typically performed by advanced practice nurses and other health care providers. Clinicians who perform CBE ideally go through simulation training and exposure to patients to become proficient at the technique (Bryan & Snyder, 2013). It is recommended that the CBE be part of a periodic health assessment, at least every 3 years for women in their 20s and 30s and every year for asymptomatic women at least 40 years of age (ACS, 2017a). Teach patients what to expect during this examination. First, they will be asked to undress from the waist up. The examiner inspects the breasts for abnormalities in size and shape and for skin and nipple changes. Then, using the pads of the fingers, the examiner palpates the breasts for any lumps and, if present, whether such lumps are attached to the skin or deeper tissues. The area under both arms is also examined.

Options for High-Risk Women

Women with a personal history of breast cancer are at risk for developing a recurrence or a new breast cancer. Those with known *BRCA1* and/or *BRCA2* genetic mutation have a lifetime

◎ CHART 70-1   Best Practice for Patient Safety & Quality Care   QSEN

Performing Breast Self-Examination

1. Lie on your back and place your right arm behind your head. Lying down spreads the breast tissue evenly over the chest wall, making it easier to feel all the breast tissue.

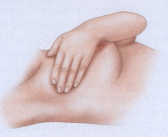

2. Use the finger pads of the three middle fingers on your left hand to feel for lumps in the right breast. Use overlapping dime-size circular motions of the finger pads to feel the breast tissue.

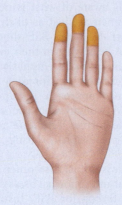

3. Use three different levels of pressure to feel all the breast tissue. Light pressure is needed to feel the tissue closest to the skin; medium pressure to feel a little deeper; and firm pressure to feel the tissue closest to the chest and ribs. It is normal to feel a firm ridge in the lower curve of each breast.

4. Move around the breast in an up-and-down pattern, starting at an imaginary line drawn straight down your side from the underarm and moving across the breast to the middle of the chest bone (sternum or breastbone). Be sure to check the entire breast area, going down until you feel only ribs and up to the neck.

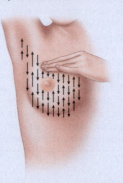

5. Repeat the examination on your left breast, putting your left arm behind your head and using the finger pads of your right hand to do the examination.

6. While standing in front of a mirror with your hands pressing firmly down on your hips, look at your breasts for any changes of size, shape, contour, or dimpling and look at your nipples and breast skin for redness or scaling. (The pressing down–on-the-hips position contracts the chest wall muscles and enhances any breast changes.)

7. Examine each underarm while sitting up or standing and with your arm only slightly raised so you can easily feel in this area. Raising your arm straight up tightens the tissue in this area and makes it harder to examine.

⚕ CONSIDERATIONS FOR OLDER ADULTS

Patient-Centered Care   QSEN

As women age, the breast tissue becomes flattened and elongated and is suspended loosely from the chest wall. On palpation, the breast tissue of the older woman has a finer, more granular feel than the lobular feel in a younger woman. The inframammary ridge may be more prominent as a result of atrophy of the breast tissue. Breast examination in older adults may be easier because of tissue atrophy and relaxation of the suspensory ligaments.

Women in nursing homes and other long-term care facilities often do not have clinical breast examinations and may not be deliberately aware of the normal appearance and feel of their breasts. Teach the importance of breast self-awareness and reporting any breast changes the woman may notice.

risk of breast cancer of about 20% to 25% or greater, according to risk assessment tools that are based mainly on family history or other high-risk factors. Women in this category usually practice *close surveillance* as a prevention option. It is referred to as *secondary prevention* and is used to detect cancer early in the initial stages. In addition to annual mammography and clinical breast examination, high-risk women are recommended to have an annual breast MRI screening (ACS, 2017b). Close surveillance may begin as early as age 30 years, but evidence is limited regarding the best age at which to start screening. *For women with a high risk for breast cancer development due to family history such as cancer in a mother or sister, it is recommended that cancer screening begin at the age that is 10 years younger than the age at which the affected cancer patient was initially diagnosed.* Encourage high-risk women to discuss their personal preferences for close surveillance with their primary health care providers.

Other options currently available for reducing a woman's breast cancer risk are **prophylactic mastectomy** (preventive surgical removal of one or both breasts), prophylactic **oophorectomy** (removal of the ovaries), and antiestrogen chemopreventive drugs. Although each option significantly reduces the risk for breast cancer, no option completely eliminates it. Each option has its own risks and potentially serious complications.

Even though a woman may decide to have a *prophylactic mastectomy*, there is a small risk that breast cancer will develop in residual breast glandular tissue because no mastectomy reliably removes all mammary tissue. Women must also understand that breast reconstruction after a prophylactic mastectomy is very different from breast augmentation. It is a more complex surgical procedure with a greater potential for complications. The decision to have this type of surgery can be a very difficult one to make. Women may find it helpful to reach out to a breast cancer support organization and talk to someone who has been through a prophylactic mastectomy.

Women undergoing *oophorectomy* will likely experience menopausal symptoms, although some estrogen remains in body fat tissue. *Antiestrogen drugs* reduce breast cancer recurrence but carry other risks such as blood clots and endometrial cancer. Encourage women to carefully consider the benefits and risks of breast cancer–risk-reducing options and discuss them with their health care provider.

❖ INTERPROFESSIONAL COLLABORATIVE CARE

◆ Assessment: Noticing

History. Often the history is taken after a mass has been discovered but before a diagnosis has been made for a woman or man with breast cancer. For some patients, the history may be obtained at the time they are seen for treatment of an identified

🌐 CULTURAL/SPIRITUAL CONSIDERATIONS
Patient-Centered Care QSEN

> Remember that some cultures do not allow the man to be part of a woman's care or only women are allowed to care for her, such as in the Arab Muslim culture. Other cultures are male predominant, and all decisions about female care are made by the man, such as in the Nigerian culture.

cancer. The interview should focus on three major areas: risk factors, the breast mass, and health maintenance practices.

Ask specific information on personal and family histories of breast cancer. In addition to increasing the woman's own risk, these factors also affect any sisters' or daughters' risk and should be part of later counseling.

Ask about the woman's gynecologic and obstetric (if any) history, including:

- Age at menarche
- Age at menopause
- Symptoms of menopause
- Age at first child's birth
- Number of children/pregnancies

Prolonged hormonal stimulation (e.g., early menses, late menopause) increases a woman's risk, as do birth of the first child after 30 years of age and nulliparity (having no children).

A history of the breast mass or lump reveals not only the course of the disease but also information related to health care–seeking practices and health-promoting behaviors. Ask the patient about how, when, and by whom the mass was discovered and the time between discovery and seeking care. If the patient found the mass, ask how it was discovered. The answer to this question reveals the need for discussion and teaching about health promotion practices, regardless of whether the mass proves to be cancerous. If there was a delay between discovery and seeing the health care provider, ask what caused the delay. These questions are linked to the psychosocial assessment but also reveal the length of time that the tumor has been present. Ask which procedures have been performed to diagnose the problem. Also ask patients if they have noticed any other changes in their body within the past year. This information can help determine whether there has been obvious cancer spread. Ask especially about the presence of joint or bone pain.

Ask about the use of alcohol intake because this is a factor that may increase breast cancer risk. Ask which prescribed and over-the-counter (OTC) drugs are used (specifically hormonal

◎ CHART 70-2 Best Practice for Patient Safety & Quality Care QSEN
Assessing a Breast Mass

- Identify the location of the mass by using the "face of the clock" method.
- Describe the shape, size, and consistency of the mass.
- Assess whether the mass is fixed or movable.
- Note any skin changes around the mass, such as dimpling of the skin, increased vascularity, nipple retraction, nipple inversion or skin ulceration.
- Assess the adjacent lymph nodes, both axillary and supraclavicular nodes.
- Ask patients if they experience pain or soreness in the area around the mass.

supplements such as estrogen and natural or herbal substances that stimulate hormones). Estrogen can be taken orally, intravaginally, or via a transdermal patch. Document the type and form of hormones (birth control pills or patches, supplements) and length of use.

Physical Assessment/Signs and Symptoms. Document in the electronic medical record any abnormal findings from the clinical breast examination. Describe specific information about a breast mass (Chart 70-2) such as location, using the "face of the clock" method; shape; size; consistency; and whether the mass is mobile or fixed to the surrounding tissue. Note any skin change, such as *peau d'orange* (dimpling, orange peel appearance), redness and warmth, nipple retraction, or ulceration, which can indicate advanced disease. Document the location of any enlargements of axillary and supraclavicular lymph nodes. Evaluate the presence of pain or tenderness in the affected breast.

Psychosocial Assessment. A breast cancer diagnosis is usually an unanticipated event in the life of a woman who feels physically well. It initiates a sudden and distressing transition into a potentially life-threatening illness. Feelings of fear, shock, and disbelief are predominant as a woman learns about her disease and faces numerous treatment decisions. Psychological distress is common at cancer diagnosis and at the end of treatment. A previous history of mental illness, age, and life circumstances can contribute to increased psychological distress. Encourage expression of feelings and determine if a referral to a breast cancer support group would be helpful. Talking with someone who has been through the experience is particularly helpful in dealing with the emotional aspects of the disease.

Assess the patient for problems related to SEXUALITY. Sexual dysfunction affects most breast cancer survivors in some way. Sometimes the sexual dysfunction is related to the loss of a breast and the threat to one's femininity, but many women also equate a breast cancer diagnosis and treatment effects with the aging process. Lack of libido (sexual desire) related to hormonal changes, psychological distress, and severe anxiety are commonly experienced by women with breast cancer. If the patient does not discuss sexual concerns voluntarily, ask about the frequency of and satisfaction with sexual relations with her partner. Use resources that provide education about alternative expressions of intimacy and a focus on pleasure rather than performance. Refer the patient and her partner to counseling if appropriate.

Laboratory Assessment. The diagnosis of breast cancer relies on pathologic examination of tissue from the breast mass. After

GENDER HEALTH CONSIDERATIONS
Patient-Centered Care QSEN

Research is limited about breast cancer and women who identify as lesbian or bisexual. Factors that are more likely to increase the risk of breast cancer in lesbian and bisexual women include nulliparity, increased age at birth of first child, and use of oral contraceptives (ACS, 2017a). Lesbian and bisexual women are less likely to have health insurance and get regular cancer screenings, possibly as a result of fear and distrust of culturally incompetent primary health care providers and/or health care access. They may also be less focused on their breasts and breast cancer risk. Nurses' awareness and sensitivity to these issues help establish trust. Emphasize the importance of screening and early detection. Assess the need for referrals to support organizations such as the National LGBT Cancer Network.

the diagnosis of cancer is established, laboratory tests, including pathologic study of the lymph nodes, help detect possible metastases. Elevated liver enzyme levels indicate possible liver metastases, and increased serum calcium and alkaline phosphatase levels suggest bone metastases.

Imaging Assessment. *Mammography* is a sensitive screening tool for breast cancer. The uniqueness of this test results from its ability to reveal preclinical lesions (masses too small to be palpated manually). Most breast centers now use *digital mammography,* a system that is able to read, file, and transmit mammograms electronically. Patient preparation and the procedure for mammography are discussed in Chapter 69. Some women may voice concern about radiation exposure with mammograms. Reassure them that the dose is very small and the risk for harm from radiation is minimal.

Digital breast *tomosynthesis* is a newer technology that is similar to mammography but uses three-dimensional images. It has the potential to improve detection of breast cancer by better differentiating suspicious from normal tissue (Alakhras et al., 2013). In the United States, currently it is covered by Medicare and most other major health insurances. This advanced technology is also available in Canada.

Ultrasonography of the breast is an additional diagnostic tool used to clarify findings on mammography. If the mammogram reveals a lesion, ultrasonography is helpful in differentiating a fluid-filled cyst from a solid mass. Mammography screening combined with ultrasound may be effective for detecting cancers in women with dense breasts, but currently it is not recommended for routine breast cancer screening (ACS, 2017b).

MRI is used for screening high-risk women and better examination of suspicious areas found by a mammogram (ACS, 2017b). It is more expensive than mammography. Most insurance companies will cover a portion of the cost if the woman is shown to be high risk. Although higher-quality images are produced, there is concern about high costs and access to quality breast MRI services for high-risk women (ACS, 2017b).

If the patient has an invasive breast cancer, other imaging tests may be done to rule out metastases. A chest x-ray is done to screen for lung metastases. Bone, liver, and brain scans and CT scans of the chest and abdomen can reveal distant metastases.

Other Diagnostic Assessment. Although imaging techniques serve as tools for screening and more precise visualization of potential breast cancers, *breast biopsy (pathologic examination of the breast tissue) is the only definitive way to diagnose breast cancer.* Breast tissue is obtained by one of several types of biopsies (see Chapter 69). Tissue samples are analyzed by a pathologist to determine the presence of breast cancer. If breast cancer is identified, it is classified according to the size and type of breast cancer, the histologic grade, and the type of receptors on the cells. These characteristics are used to guide treatment. For example, a small, noninvasive breast cancer may be treated only with lumpectomy and radiation; whereas a larger, aggressive tumor (one with a high histologic grade) may be treated with a mastectomy and chemotherapy, followed by radiation.

Cancer cells that contain estrogen receptors (*ER positive*) or progesterone receptors (*PR positive*) have a better prognosis and usually respond to hormonal therapy. If the type of breast cancer is *HER2,* or one in which the *neu* gene product is overexpressed, it may be treated successfully with trastuzumab (Herceptin), which is a breast cancer *targeted therapy* for this specific type.

Most women, even those with very small tumors, receive some sort of treatment in addition to surgery for breast cancer. Research has focused on ways to predict clinical outcomes so low-risk women may avoid unnecessary treatments. Gene expression profiling systems, such as Oncotype DX and MammaPrint, have been developed to help predict clinical outcomes by analyzing genes in breast cancer tissue. Some clinicians use this information in addition to the pathologic analysis for guiding treatment decisions. These multigene tests have been shown to be accurate predictors of patient prognosis and response to therapy in breast cancer (Jankowitz & Lee, 2013). Their role in clinical practice continues to evolve.

◆ Analysis: Interpreting

The priority collaborative problems for patients with breast cancer include:

1. Potential for metastasis of cancer to other parts of the body due to lack of treatment or inadequate treatment response
2. Potential for decreased ability to cope due to unanticipated breast cancer diagnosis and its treatment

◆ Planning and Implementation: Responding
Decreasing the Risk for Metastasis

Planning: Expected Outcomes. The patient who is treated for breast cancer is expected to remain free of metastases or recurrence of disease, if possible. If cancer recurs, the patient will experience optimal health outcomes, including potential palliation and end-of-life care.

Interventions. There are many surgical and nonsurgical options for breast cancer treatment. Because of the various options, the patient with breast cancer often faces difficult decisions. Although patients are living longer with metastatic disease, the 5-year survival rate remains low. Once cancer is diagnosed, the extent and location of metastases determine the overall therapeutic strategy. The emphasis of breast cancer treatment is on preventing or stopping the spread of tumor cells that leads to distant metastasis. Treatment is tailored specifically to each patient, taking into account other health problems and the patient's ability to tolerate a particular therapy.

Nonsurgical Management. For patients with breast cancer at a stage for which surgery is the main treatment, follow-up with adjuvant (in addition to surgery) radiation, chemotherapy, hormone therapy, or targeted therapy is commonly prescribed. For those who cannot have surgery or whose cancer is too advanced, these therapies are used to promote COMFORT (palliation). These options are discussed in the Adjuvant Therapy section later in this chapter.

Complementary and Integrative Health. Women with breast cancer often cope with distressing symptoms related to the

TABLE 70-2 Common Complementary and Integrative Therapies Used by Patients With Breast Cancer

SYMPTOM	COMPLEMENTARY AND INTEGRATIVE THERAPY
Physical	
Pain	Acupuncture, chiropractic therapy, hypnosis, massage, music, reiki, shiatsu
Nausea/vomiting	Acupuncture, aromatherapy, ginger, hypnosis, progressive muscle relaxation, shiatsu
Fatigue	Acupuncture, massage, meditation, reiki, tai chi, yoga
Hot flashes	Acupuncture, flaxseed
Muscle tension	Aromatherapy, massage, shiatsu
Emotional	
Anxiety/stress/fear	Aromatherapy, guided imagery, hypnosis, journaling, massage, meditation, music therapy, progressive muscle relaxation, prayer, support groups, tai chi, yoga
Depression	Aromatherapy, yoga, journaling, progressive muscle relaxation

disease itself or the side effects of treatment. Common symptoms associated with these therapies include pain, nausea, hot flashes, anxiety, depression, and fatigue. Physical and emotional symptoms associated with breast cancer may be eased with the use of complementary and integrative therapy. The most frequently used strategies are biologically based therapies such as vitamins, special cancer diets, and herbal therapy. Prayer is also widely used. Other types of therapies are mind-body or body based such as guided imagery and massage. Encourage women to seek a practitioner with a certification or license for the specific type of integrative therapy intervention. In some states, a certification or license is required for acupuncture, chiropractic therapy, massage, and shiatsu. Some types of complementary and integrative therapy can be self-taught or done alone after a few sessions of instruction. Table 70-2 lists complementary and integrative therapies for specific symptoms associated with breast cancer and its treatments.

Although the use of complementary and integrative therapy can improve quality of life, its use does not alter the outcome of breast cancer, and it should not be used in place of standard treatment. Encourage patients who are interested in trying these therapies to check with their health care provider before using them. The website breastcancer.org provides accurate information about complementary therapies and the extent to which they have been researched in breast cancer patients. Cost may be a factor in decision making since not all insurances provide coverage for complementary and integrative therapies. Teach the patient that all ingested complementary agents potentially risk interaction with conventional drugs.

Surgical Management. Although controversy exists concerning the best treatment for breast cancer, experts agree that the mass itself should be removed to reduce the risk for local recurrence. A large tumor is sometimes treated with chemotherapy, called *neoadjuvant therapy,* to shrink the tumor before it is surgically removed. An advantage of this therapy is that cancers can be removed by lumpectomy rather than mastectomy.

Axillary lymph nodes are analyzed for the presence of cancer and staging purposes. Axillary lymph node dissection (ALND) is usually done when there are palpable axillary lymph nodes or when cancer is suspected to be at a later stage. Sentinel lymph node biopsy (SLNB) is a much less invasive approach now preferred by most surgeons for analyzing lymph nodes in early-stage breast cancers with low-to-moderate risk for lymph node involvement. In this method, the sentinel lymph node is identified during breast surgery by injecting the breast with radioisotope and/or dye that travels via lymphatic pathways to the sentinel lymph node. The nodes that take up the dye (or give off a certain level of radiation picked up by a handheld counter) are removed and examined for the presence of cancer cells. It is believed that if cancer cells have traveled through the lymph channels, the cells will lodge in the sentinel nodes. Travel beyond these nodes to higher-level nodes may occur as a secondary event. Therefore the absence of cancer cells in the sentinel nodes is an indicator that no other nodes in the regional area are involved.

Preoperative Care. Care of the patient facing surgery for breast cancer focuses on psychological preparation and preoperative teaching. Priority nursing interventions are directed toward relieving anxiety and providing information to increase patient knowledge. *Include the spouse, partner, or other family member or significant other who may be experiencing similar stress and confusion, in the health teaching unless the patient's culture does not permit this approach.*

Review the type of procedure planned. Use open-ended questions (e.g., "What type of surgery are you having? Can you explain what will happen?") to assess the current level of knowledge. Provide postoperative information, including:

- The need for a drainage tube
- The location of the incision
- Mobility restrictions
- The length of the hospital stay (if any)
- The possibility of adjuvant therapy
- General preoperative and postoperative information needed by any surgical patient (see Chapters 14 and 16)

Supplement teaching with written or digital materials for the patient and family. This information should include whom to call in case there are any complications. Address body image issues before surgery to correct misconceptions about appearance after surgery. If available, suggest that patients and their caregivers attend classes before surgery in an ambulatory care setting, such as a breast cancer center, to promote successful early discharge from the hospital. Programs that provide emotional support, information, and opportunities for discussion related to SEXUALITY, body image, and preoperative and postoperative care enhance the recovery of the short-stay mastectomy patient.

Operative Procedures. Types of breast surgeries are shown in Fig. 70-3. During **breast-conserving surgery,** such as a *lumpectomy,* the surgeon removes the tumor and a small amount of tissue rather than the entire breast. A partial mastectomy is surgery to remove part of the breast that contains cancer and some normal tissue around it. *Margins* refer to the distance between the tumor and the edge of the surrounding tissue. The desired outcome of breast-conserving surgery is to obtain *negative margins* in which no cancer cells extend to the edge of the tissue. Typically, radiation therapy follows to kill any residual tumor cells.

Breast-conserving procedures are usually performed in same-day surgical settings. The cosmetic results of these surgeries are good to excellent, and the psychological benefits of avoiding breast removal are significant for patients who choose this option.

Breast-conserving Surgery

Lumpectomy

Partial Mastectomy

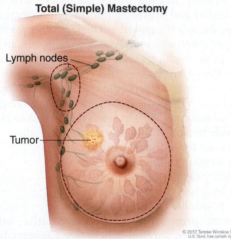

Breast-conserving surgery. Dotted lines show the area containing the tumor that is removed and some of the lymph nodes that may be removed.

Total (Simple) Mastectomy

Total (simple) mastectomy. The dotted line shows where the entire breast is removed. Some lymph nodes under the arm may also be removed.

Modified Radical Mastectomy

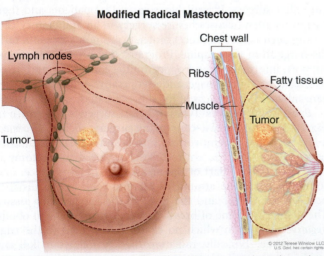

Modified radical mastectomy. The dotted line shows where the entire breast and some lymph nodes are removed. Part of the chest wall muscle may also be removed.

FIG. 70-3 Surgical treatment for breast cancer. (©2010 Terese Winslow. U.S. Govt. has certain rights.)

Despite advances in breast-conserving surgery, mastectomy remains a popular option for breast cancer treatment, and women are increasingly choosing it for prophylactic treatment (McLaughlin, 2013). Typically, indications for a mastectomy include multi-centric disease (tumor is present in different quadrants of the breast), inability to have radiation therapy, presence of a large tumor in a small breast, and patient preference. Mastectomy does not conserve the breast; the affected breast is completely removed. A total (simple) mastectomy is surgery to remove the whole breast that has cancer. A modified radical mastectomy removes the breast tissue, lymph nodes, and sometimes part of the underlying chest wall muscle. If reconstruction is to be performed at the same time as the mastectomy, less-invasive techniques, such as incising a ½-inch flap of skin around the nipple (excising the same amount of breast tissue as with conventional mastectomy), may be performed. Skin flaps or expanders may be used to create a breast mound at the time of the original procedure.

Postoperative Care. Before the patient returns from surgery, inform the staff to avoid using the affected arm for measuring blood pressure, giving injections, or drawing blood. He or she returns from the postanesthesia care unit (PACU) as soon as vital signs return to baseline levels and if no complications have occurred. Assess vital signs on a schedule of decreasing frequency, such as every 30 minutes for two times, every hour for two times, and then every 4 hours. During these checks, assess the dressing for bleeding.

During a *modified radical mastectomy*, the surgeon places one or two drainage tubes, usually Jackson-Pratt drains, under the skin flaps and attaches the tubes to a small collection chamber. Gentle suction is exerted, and fluid that would accumulate under the flaps and delay healing is collected. Various drains are available, but all allow the drainage to be seen and measured. When taking vital signs, monitor for the amount and color of drainage. Add this information to the intake and output record. Patients undergoing a *lumpectomy* may also have drainage tubes (usually Jackson-Pratt drains) placed if the lump is large or if axillary node dissection is performed.

! NURSING SAFETY PRIORITY QSEN

Action Alert

Per TJC National Patient Safety Goal recommendations, to decrease the chance of surgical site infection, carefully observe the surgical wound after breast surgery for signs of swelling and infection throughout recovery. Assess the incision and flap of the post-mastectomy patient for signs of bleeding, infection, and poor tissue perfusion. With short hospital stays, drainage tubes are usually removed about 1 to 3 weeks after hospital discharge when the patient returns for an office visit. The drainage amount should be less than 2 to 30 mL in a 24-hour period. Inform the patient that tube removal causes impaired COMFORT, although these tubes lie just under the skin. Provide or suggest analgesia before they are removed. Document all findings and report any abnormalities to the surgeon immediately.

Assess the patient's position to ensure that the drainage tubes or collection device is not pulled or kinked. The patient should have the head of the bed elevated at least 30 degrees, with the affected arm (the arm on the same side as the axillary dissection) elevated on a pillow while awake. Keeping the affected arm elevated promotes lymphatic fluid return after removal of lymph nodes and channels. Provide other basic COMFORT measures, such as repositioning and analgesics as prescribed on a regular basis until pain ceases. Patient-controlled analgesia may be used for some patients for a short time, depending on the type of surgery that was performed.

The hospital stay after breast surgery is short, often same day or just overnight, and recovery is usually not complicated. Because some managed care plans will not authorize an overnight stay in the hospital after a mastectomy, several states have enacted legislation mandating inpatient benefits. The patient who chooses an early discharge should have a home care visit within 24 hours of the discharge.

Ambulation and a regular diet are resumed by the day after surgery. While the patient is walking, the arm on the affected side may need to be supported at first. Gradually the arm should be allowed to hang straight by the side. Instruct the patient to avoid the hunched-back position with the arm flexed because of the risk for elbow contracture. Beginning exercises that do not stress the incision can usually be started on the first day after surgery. These exercises include squeezing the affected hand around a soft, round object (a ball or rolled washcloth) and flexion/extension of the elbow. The progression to more strenuous exercises depends on the subsequent procedures planned (e.g., reconstruction) and the surgeon's prescription.

As soon as the patient is ambulatory and surgical pain is under control, he or she is discharged to home. Common instructions for exercises after mastectomy are listed in Chart 70-3.

CHART 70-3 Patient and Family Education: Preparing for Self-Management

Post-Mastectomy Exercises

Hand Wall Climbing
- Face the wall and put the palms of your hands flat against the wall at shoulder level.
- Flex your fingers so your hands slowly "walk" up the wall.
- Stop when your arms are fully extended.
- Slowly "walk" your hands back down the wall until they return to shoulder level.

Pulley Exercise
- Drape a 6-foot-long rope over a shower curtain rod or over the top of a door. If you use a door for this exercise, have someone put a nail or hook at the top of the door so the rope does not slip off.
- Grab the ends of the rope, one in each hand, and extend your arms out to your sides until they are straight.
- Keeping your arms straight, pull down with your left arm to raise your right arm as high as you can.
- Pull down with your right arm to raise your left arm as high as you can.

Rope Turning
- Tie a rope to the knob of a closed door.
- Hold the other end of the rope and step back from the door until your arm is almost straight out in front of you.
- Swing the rope in a circle. Start with small circles and gradually increase to larger circles as you become more flexible.

NCLEX EXAMINATION CHALLENGE 70-2

Physiological Integrity

The nurse is assigned to care for a client who has undergone a modified radical right mastectomy for breast cancer. When delegating care, which statements by the nursing assistant would require **further** teaching by the nurse? **Select all that apply.**
A. "I'll irrigate the drainage tube after I empty it."
B. "If the client says she is in pain, I'll tell you right away."
C. "It's important for me to take blood pressure on the client's right arm."
D. "When helping the client walk, I'll remind her to stand straight."
E. "I'll let you know if her surgical dressing is intact and dry."

Breast Reconstruction. Breast reconstruction after or during mastectomy for women is common with few complications. Patients consult with the plastic surgeon to discuss the type of reconstruction, timing of the procedure, and technique desired. Many women prefer reconstruction immediately after mastectomy using their own tissue (autogenous reconstruction). Breast reconstruction at the time of mastectomy, both autogenous and prosthetic, may lessen the psychological strain associated with undergoing a mastectomy.

The surgeon should offer the option of breast reconstruction before surgery is performed. If the woman does not choose immediate reconstructive surgery, a temporary prosthesis can be used. Refer the patient to the American Cancer Society's *Reach to Recovery* program (www.cancer.org). In this program, a volunteer who has had breast cancer surgery visits the woman at home, offering information on breast forms, clothing, coping with breast cancer, and possible reconstructive options. For this intervention to be as helpful as possible, the volunteer should be about the same age as the patient and have experienced the same surgical procedure.

Evaluate the woman's level of satisfaction with her prosthesis several weeks after surgery. Assess her attitude by asking about future plans for restoring appearance. Although reconstruction is not appropriate for some women and others may not be interested in it, the surgeon should discuss the indications and contraindications, advantages and disadvantages, and typical recovery. If immediate reconstruction is chosen, the surgeon should be aware of this before surgery so plans can be coordinated with those of the plastic surgeon.

Several procedures are available for restoring the appearance of the breast (Table 70-3). Reconstruction may begin during the original operative procedure or later in one to several stages. Common types of breast reconstruction are:
- Breast expanders (saline or gel)
- Autologous reconstruction using the patient's own skin, fat, and muscle

Breast expanders are the most common method of breast reconstruction used today in the United States. A tissue expander is a balloon-like device with a resealable metal port that is placed under the pectoralis muscle. A small amount of normal saline is injected intraoperatively into the expander to partially inflate it. The patient then receives additional weekly saline injections for about 6 to 8 weeks until the expander is fully inflated. When full expansion is achieved, the tissue expander is then exchanged for a permanent implant during surgery in an ambulatory care center. The permanent implant is filled with either saline or silicone gel. Despite earlier claims that silicone gel caused autoimmune diseases such as lupus and arthritis, silicone implants have been used safely in most women who choose this type of breast implant.

Autologous reconstruction using the patient's own skin, fat, and muscle is advantageous because the donor site tissue is similar in consistency to that of the natural breast. Therefore

TABLE 70-3   Examples of Breast Reconstruction Procedures

PROCEDURE	DESCRIPTION	PROCEDURE	DESCRIPTION
Implantation	An implant matching the size of the other breast is placed under the muscle on the operative side to create a breast mound.	Myocutaneous flaps	A flap of skin, fat, and muscle is transferred from the donor site to the operative area. The flap contains an appropriate amount of fat to match the other breast and is similar in appearance to breast tissue. A blood supply is established by reanastomosis of vessels from the operative area to those with the flap when possible. A new nipple may be created with tissue from areas such as the labia or upper, inner thigh. Nipples can also be created by tattooing.

Latissimus dorsi musculocutaneous flap

Abdominal myocutaneous flap

PROCEDURE	DESCRIPTION
Tissue expansion (DIEP Reconstruction [Deep Inferior Epigastric Perforator Flap])	A tissue expander is placed under the muscle and gradually expanded with saline to stretch the overlying skin and create a pocket. After several weeks, the tissue expander is exchanged for an implant.

the results more closely resemble a real breast compared with implant reconstruction. Flap donor sites include the latissimus dorsi flap (back muscle); transverse rectus abdominis myocutaneous flap, known as the *TRAM flap* (abdominal muscle); and the gluteal flap (buttock muscle). Reconstruction of the nipple-areola complex is the last stage in the reconstruction of the breast. If necessary, a new nipple may be created with other body tissue, such as from the labia, abdomen, or inner thigh.

Women who have had a mastectomy and breast reconstruction in one breast should have close-surveillance breast cancer screening in the contralateral (opposite) breast, including imaging with mammography or mammography and MRI. Mammography and MRI are not recommended to be done routinely in reconstructed breasts because most local recurrences

of breast cancer in the residual tissue are palpable during clinical breast examination. Nursing care of the woman who has undergone breast reconstruction is outlined in Chart 70-4.

Adjuvant Therapy. The decision to follow the original surgical procedure with additional treatment to help keep the cancer from recurring is known as **adjuvant therapy**. This decision is based on several factors:

- The stage of the disease
- The patient's age and menopausal status
- Patient preferences
- Pathologic examination
- Hormone receptor status
- HER2/neu status
- Presence of a known genetic predisposition

CHART 70-4 Best Practice for Patient Safety & Quality Care QSEN

Postoperative Care of the Patient After Breast Reconstruction

- Assess the incision and flap for signs of infection (excessive redness, drainage, odor) during dressing changes.
- Assess the incision and flap for signs of poor tissue perfusion (duskiness, decreased capillary refill) during dressing changes.
- Avoid pressure on the flap and suture lines by positioning the patient on her nonoperative side and avoiding tight clothing.
- Monitor and measure drainage in collection devices, such as for Jackson-Pratt drains.
- Teach the patient to return to her usual activity level gradually and to avoid heavy lifting.
- Remind the patient to avoid sleeping in the prone position.
- Teach the patient to avoid participation in contact sports or other activities that could cause trauma to the chest.
- Teach the patient to minimize pressure on the breast during sexual activity.
- Remind the patient to refrain from driving until advised by the physician.
- Remind the patient to ask at the 6-week postoperative visit when full activity can be resumed.
- Reassure the patient that optimal appearance may not occur for 3 to 6 months after surgery.
- If implants have been inserted, teach the proper method of breast massage to enhance expansion and prevent capsule formation (consult with the physician).
- Emphasize breast self-awareness; if the patient performs breast self-examination (BSE), review her technique.
- Remind the patient of the importance of clinical breast examination and follow-up surveillance by her physician.

Adjuvant therapy for breast cancer consists of systemic chemotherapy, radiation therapy, or a combination of both. The purpose of radiation therapy is to reduce the risk for local recurrence of breast cancer. The goal of systemic therapy (with chemotherapy, hormone therapy, and targeted therapy) is to reduce the risk of recurrence (locally or at distant sites) and death. These drugs destroy breast cancer cells that may be present anywhere in the body. They are typically delivered after surgery for breast cancer, although neoadjuvant chemotherapy may be given to reduce the size of a tumor before surgery. Hormonal therapy may also be used as a chemoprevention option for high-risk women with a personal history of breast cancer.

Radiation Therapy. Radiation therapy is administered after breast-conserving surgery to kill breast cancer cells that may remain near the site of the original tumor. This therapy can be delivered to the whole breast or to only part of the breast. Whole-breast irradiation is delivered by external beam radiation over a period of 5 to 6 weeks. Partial breast irradiation (PBI) has become a newer option for women with early-stage breast cancer. PBI is a convenient alternative to whole breast radiation. Less time is needed for completion, and outcomes are comparable to those of whole breast radiation (Edwards et al., 2015). The advantage of this type of radiation is that it is delivered over a much shorter time interval, eliminating the need for daily trips for treatment. The types of methods available for delivering *partial-breast irradiation* include the following:

- Interstitial brachytherapy, in which several catheters loaded with a radioactive source are inserted at the lumpectomy cavity and surrounding margin, is given over a period of 4 to 5 days.
- Balloon brachytherapy, also known as *MammoSite*, involves the use of a single balloon-tipped catheter that is surgically placed near the tumor bed. The catheter is loaded with a radiation source and inflated to conform to the total cavity. Ten total treatments are given, with at least 6 hours between each treatment.
- Intraoperative radiation therapy is the most accelerated form of partial breast irradiation. It uses a high single dose of radiation delivered during the lumpectomy surgery.

Nursing care for the patient undergoing radiation therapy includes patient education and side effect management. Skin changes are a major side effect during this therapy (see Chapter 22). If brachytherapy is planned, instruct patients about the procedure. Assure them that they will be radioactive only while the radiation source is dwelling inside the breast tissue.

! NURSING SAFETY PRIORITY QSEN

Action Alert

Teach women undergoing brachytherapy for breast cancer that radiation is contained in the temporary implant. The risk for others to be exposed to radiation is very small. Body fluids and items contacted by patients with brachytherapy are not radioactive. However, during the time that radiation is delivered, it is recommended that visitors, including pregnant women and children, be limited.

Drug Therapy. Chemotherapy for breast cancer is delivered systemically via the central IV route, such as an implantable venous access device (e.g., Port-a-Cath). Its purpose is to kill undetected breast cancer cells that may have left the original tumor and moved to more distant sites. Chemotherapy is recommended for treatment of invasive breast cancer after surgery (adjuvant chemotherapy). It may also be given before surgery to reduce the size of the tumor (neoadjuvant chemotherapy) and is most effective when combinations of more than one drug are used. Chemotherapy drugs are usually delivered in four to six cycles, with each period of treatment followed by a rest period to give the body time to recover from the adverse effects of the drugs. Each cycle is 2 to 3 weeks long. The total treatment time is 3 to 6 months, although treatment may be longer for advanced breast cancer. Many combinations of drugs are used, and no one combination has been proven to be superior over others. A common chemotherapy regimen for breast cancer treatment is doxorubicin (Adriamycin, Caelyx ✦), cyclophosphamide (Cytoxan), and paclitaxel (Taxol), which, in the United States, is also known as AC-T (Burchum & Rosenthal, 2016). In early-stage breast cancer, chemotherapy regimens lower the risk for breast cancer recurrence and death. In metastatic breast cancer, chemotherapy regimens reduce cancer size and slow the progression of disease.

Nurses must be very proficient in the preparation and administration of chemotherapy drugs and knowledgeable about various venous access devices. They must also be able to manage the distressing symptoms associated with side effects of these drugs. Chapter 22 discusses chemotherapy in more detail and general nursing management of alopecia, nausea and vomiting, mucositis, and bone marrow suppression.

Chemotherapy is unpleasant and expensive and can have life-threatening short-term and long-term side effects. Because more women are living longer with breast cancer, more long-term effects are emerging. For example, ovarian suppression from chemotherapy drugs can result in infertility, a devastating effect for women of childbearing age.

> ! **NURSING SAFETY PRIORITY** QSEN
>
> **Action Alert**
>
> Teach patients undergoing chemotherapy with anthracyclines such as doxorubicin (Adriamycin) to be aware of cardiotoxic effects. Instruct them to report excessive fatigue, shortness of breath, chronic cough, and edema to the primary health care provider.

Targeted cancer therapies are drugs that target specific characteristics of cancer cells, such as a protein, an enzyme, or the formation of new blood vessels. The advantage of targeted therapy over traditional chemotherapy is that targeted therapy is less likely to harm normal, healthy cells and therefore it has fewer side effects. One of the first targeted therapies developed for breast cancer is the monoclonal antibody *trastuzumab* (Herceptin). This drug targets the *HER2/neu* gene product in breast cancer cells. Several other targeted therapies have been developed since Herceptin.

Hormonal drugs may also be used in breast cancer prevention and treatment. The purpose of hormonal therapy is to reduce the estrogen available to breast tumors to stop or prevent their growth. *Premenopausal* women whose main estrogen source is the ovaries may benefit from *LH-RH agonists* that inhibit estrogen synthesis. These drugs include leuprolide (Lupron) and goserelin (Zoladex), which suppress the hypothalamus from making luteinizing hormone–releasing hormone (LH-RH). When LH-RH is inhibited, the ovaries do not produce estrogen. Although the suppression of ovarian function decreases breast cancer risk, the drastic drop in estrogen causes significant menopausal symptoms. Therefore the decision to use these drugs is not made lightly.

Selective estrogen receptor modulators (SERMs), on the other hand, do not affect ovarian function. Rather, they block the effect of estrogen in women who have estrogen receptor (ER)–positive breast cancer (Burchum & Rosenthal, 2016). SERMs are also used as chemoprevention in women at high risk for breast cancer and in women with advanced breast cancer. For women with hormone receptor–positive breast cancer, tamoxifen reduces the chances of the cancer coming back by about half (ACS, 2017b). Common side effects of SERMs include hot flashes and weight gain. Rare but serious side effects of these drugs include endometrial cancer and thromboembolic events.

Aromatase inhibitors (AIs), such as letrozole (Femara) and anastrozole (Arimidex), are used in *postmenopausal* women whose main source of estrogen is not the ovaries but, rather, body fat (Burchum & Rosenthal, 2016). AIs reduce estrogen levels by inhibiting the conversion of androgen to estrogen through the action of the enzyme *aromatase.* They are beneficial when given to postmenopausal women for up to 5 years. Treatment with AIs usually follows treatment with tamoxifen. A side effect of AIs, not seen with tamoxifen, is loss of bone density. Women taking AIs are candidates for bone-strengthening drugs and must be closely monitored for osteoporosis. Fulvestrant (Faslodex), a second-line hormonal therapy for postmenopausal women with advanced breast cancer, is used after other hormonal treatments have stopped working.

Stem Cell Transplantation. Autologous or allogeneic stem cell transplantation is an option for patients with a high risk for recurrence or who have advanced disease. Autologous bone marrow transplantation (taken from the patient's bone marrow), peripheral blood stem cell transplantation (taken from circulating blood), or allogeneic bone marrow transplantation (taken from a healthy donor's bone marrow or peripheral blood) is performed as a means of rescue therapy after very high doses of chemotherapy. The general care of the patient undergoing bone marrow or stem cell transplantation is discussed in Chapter 22.

Developing Coping Strategies

Planning: Expected Outcomes. The patient with breast cancer is expected to report the use of methods to help increase coping ability and reduce anxiety. The patient will maintain relationships and participate as an active partner in management of the disease.

Interventions. The anxiety and uncertainty for the patient with breast cancer begin the moment a lump is discovered or when a mammogram reveals an abnormality. These feelings may be related to past experiences and personal associations with the disease. Assess the patient's perceptions of his or her own situation. Allow him or her to ventilate these feelings even if a diagnosis has not been established.

If the mass has been diagnosed as cancer, many people feel a partial sense of relief to be dealing with a known entity. A feeling of shock or disbelief usually occurs. It is difficult to accept a diagnosis of cancer when one feels basically well. Patients and their families or significant others deal in individual ways with the mix of feelings. Flexibility is the key to nursing care. Adjust your approach to care as the patient's emotional state changes. Those who have an interval between the diagnosis and treatment during which they actively participate in the choice of treatment cope more effectively after surgery, no matter which treatment is chosen.

An integral part of the plan to meet these emotional needs is the use of outside resources. Health care providers working with breast cancer may know other patients willing to make a preoperative visit. For example, the patient who is worried in particular about the side effects of radiation therapy may benefit more from talking to someone who has undergone radiation than from talking to the nurse or primary health care provider. Be sure to assess his or her preference.

Assess the patient's need for knowledge. Some may want to read and discuss any available information. Provide accurate information and clarify any misinformation the patient may have received by the media, on the Internet, or from family and friends.

Care Coordination and Transition Management

Home Care Management. In collaboration with the case manager and members of the interdisciplinary health care team, make the appropriate referrals for care after discharge. Preoperative teaching and arrangements for home care management and referrals (*Reach to Recovery,* social services, home care) can be started before surgery or other treatment.

The patient who has undergone breast surgery can be discharged to the home setting unless other physical disabilities exist. Some are discharged the day after surgery with Jackson-Pratt or other types of drains in place. Many patients are

CHART 70-5 Patient and Family Education: Preparing for Self-Management

Recovery From Breast Cancer Surgery

- There may be a dry gauze dressing over the incision when you leave the hospital. You may change this dressing if it becomes soiled.
- A small, dry dressing will be around the site where a drain is placed. Often there is some leakage of fluid around the drain. Check the gauze dressing for drainage and change it if it becomes soiled. Some leakage is normal; but, if the dressing becomes soaked more than once a day, call your primary health care provider.
- You have been taught how to empty the reservoir from your drain and how to measure the volume of drainage. You should empty the reservoir twice a day and record the measurements.
- Drains are generally removed when drainage is less than 30 mL/day for 3 consecutive days.
- You may take sponge baths or tub baths, making certain that the area of the drain and incision stays dry. You may shower after the stitches, staples, and drains are removed.
- You can begin using your arm for normal activities, such as eating or combing your hair. Exercises involving the wrist, hand, and elbow, such as flexing your fingers, circular wrist motions, and touching your hand to your shoulder, are very good. You can usually resume more strenuous exercises after the drains have been removed.
- You can expect some impaired COMFORT or mild pain after surgery; but within 4 to 5 days, most women have no need for pain medication or require medication only at bedtime.
- Numbness in the area of the surgery and along the inner side of the arm from the armpit to the elbow occurs in almost all women. It is the injury to the nerves that causes changes in sensation to the skin in those areas. Women have described sensations of heaviness, pain, tingling, burning, and "pins and needles." This is neuropathic pain, and short-acting analgesics may be given. These sensations may change over the next several months, becoming less and less noticeable, and may resolve entirely by the end of the first year following surgery.
- Pamphlets on exercises, hand and arm care, and general facts about breast cancer are available from your hospital or from a volunteer visitor of the local or national office on cancer or breast cancer. The American Cancer Society has volunteers who have had surgery similar to yours and are available to visit you.

CHART 70-6 Home Care Assessment

Patients Recovering From Breast Cancer Surgery

Assess cardiovascular, respiratory, and urinary status:
- Vital signs
- Lung sounds
- Urine output patterns

Assess for pain and effectiveness of analgesics.

Assess dressing and incision site:
- Excess drainage
- Symptoms of infection
- Wound healing
- Intact staples, sutures

Assess drain and site:
- Drainage around site and within drain reservoir
- Color and amount of drainage
- Symptoms of infection

Review patient's recordings of drainage.

Evaluate patient's ability to care for and empty drain reservoir.

Assess status of affected extremity:
- Range of motion
- Ability to perform exercise regimen
- Lymphedema

Assess nutritional status:
- Food and fluid intake
- Presence of nausea and vomiting
- Bowel sounds

Assess functional ability:
- ADLs
- Mobility and ambulation

Assess home environment:
- Safety
- Structural barriers

Assess patient's compliance and knowledge of illness and treatment plan:
- Follow-up appointment with surgeon
- Symptoms to report to health care provider
- Hand and arm care guidelines

Assess patient and caregiver coping skills:
- Whether patient and/or caregiver has looked at incision site
- Patient's and/or caregiver's reaction to incision site

---

discharged to home on the day of surgery. Older adults should not be sent home without a family member or friend who can stay with them for 1 to 2 days. These patients may need some assistance at home with drain care, dressings, and ADLs because of pain and impaired range of motion of the affected arm. Summaries of continuing care instructions are given in Charts 70-5 and 70-6.

Teach patients that activities involving stretching or reaching for heavy objects should be avoided temporarily. This restriction can be discussed with a family member or significant other who can perform these tasks or place the objects within easy reach.

Self-Management Education. The teaching plan for the patient after surgery includes:

- Care of the incision and drainage device
- Exercises to regain full range of motion
- Measures to avoid lymphedema
- Measures to improve body image, coping, and self-esteem
- Information about interpersonal relationships and roles
- **Measures to avoid injury, infection, and swelling of the affected arm (per The Joint Commission's National Patient Safety Goals)**

Postoperative Mastectomy Teaching. Teach incisional care to the patient, family, and/or other caregiver. The patient may wear a light dressing to prevent irritation. Explain that no lotions or ointments should be used on the area and that the use of deodorant under the affected arm should be avoided until healing is complete. Although swelling and redness of the scar itself are normal for the first few weeks, swelling, redness, increased heat, and tenderness of the surrounding area indicate infection and should be reported to the surgeon immediately. If a lymph node dissection was performed, instruct the patient to elevate the affected arm on a pillow for at least 30 minutes a day for the first 6 months. Ask the patient to have someone bring a loose-fitting, nonwire bra or camisole for her to try before discharge with a soft, cotton-filled or polyester fiber–filled form supplied by the hospital or by *Reach to Recovery*. The patient wears this form until the incision is completely healed and the health care provider approves the fitting of a more sophisticated prosthesis, usually 6 to 8 weeks after discharge. Encourage the patient to dress in loose-fitting street clothes at home, not pajamas, to further enhance a positive self-image.

Teach the patient to continue performing the exercises that began in the hospital. Active range-of-motion exercises should begin 1 week after surgery or when sutures and drains are removed. Emphasize that reaching and stretching exercises should continue only to the point of pain or pulling, never beyond that. Some YWCA locations have a free postmastectomy program that supports women and men following breast cancer surgery. The program includes exercise to music, exercise in water, and peer psychological support. Patients may participate as early as 3 weeks after surgery. Before discharge, the surgeon may prescribe precautions or limitations specific to plans for future procedures such as reconstruction.

Lymphedema, an abnormal accumulation of protein fluid in the subcutaneous tissue of the affected limb after a mastectomy, is a commonly overlooked topic in health teaching. Risk factors include injury or infection of the extremity, obesity, presence of extensive axillary disease, and radiation treatment. Once lymphedema develops, it can be very difficult to manage, and *lifelong measures must be taken to prevent it*. Nurses play a vital role in educating patients about this complication. Teach your patient to immediately report symptoms of lymphedema such as sensations of heaviness, aching, fatigue, numbness, tingling, and/or swelling in the affected arm, as well as swelling in the upper chest (Mohler & Mondry, 2013).

! NURSING SAFETY PRIORITY QSEN

Action Alert

Provide information needed to help the patient avoid infection and subsequent lymphedema of the affected arm after the mastectomy. Teach the importance of avoiding having blood pressure measurements taken on, having injections in, or having blood drawn from the arm on the side of the mastectomy. Instruct the patient to wear a mitt when using the oven, wear gloves when gardening, and treat cuts and scrapes appropriately. If lymphedema occurs, early intervention provides the best chance for control. Nurses should not assume that women with lymphedema are disabled; they are able to live full lives within this limitation. A referral to a lymphedema specialist may be necessary for the patient to be fitted for a compression sleeve and/or glove, to be taught exercises and manual lymph drainage, and to discuss ways to modify daily activities to avoid worsening the problem. Management is directed toward measures that promote drainage of the affected arm. Teach patients, especially those who have had axillary lymph nodes removed, that measures to prevent lymphedema are lifelong and include avoiding trauma to the arm on the side of the mastectomy.

Psychosocial Preparation. Concerns about appearance after surgery are common and are often a threat to the patient's self-concept as a woman. Before breast surgery, the woman and her partner can benefit from an explanation of the expected postoperative appearance. After a modified radical mastectomy, the chest wall is fairly smooth and has a horizontal incision from the axilla to the midchest area. After breast-conserving surgery, scars vary according to the amount of breast tissue removed. Women are sometimes shown pictures of post-mastectomy reconstruction but are disappointed with their own results. Emphasize that scars will fade and edema will lessen with time. Scars may be red and raised at first, but these features lessen in the first few months. After surgery, encourage the woman to look at her incision when she is ready. Do not push her to accept this body image change immediately.

Much of one's body image is a reflection of how others respond. Therefore the response of the patient's family or partner to the surgery is crucial in determining the effect on self-esteem. These people may also need the support of the nurse. They may have concerns about their ability to accept the changes and need to discuss these feelings with an objective listener. They may also need help with communicating their feelings, both negative and positive, to their loved one. Involving them in teaching may also help reinforce learning and increase retention.

Discuss sexual concerns before discharge. Most surgeons recommend avoiding sexual intercourse for 4 to 6 weeks. Patients may prefer to lay a pillow over the surgical site or to wear a bra, camisole, or T-shirt to prevent contact with the surgical site during intercourse. He or she may be embarrassed to discuss the topic of SEXUALITY. Be sensitive to possible concerns and approach the subject first.

For young women, issues related to childbearing may be a concern. Chemotherapy and radiation are considered serious teratogenic (birth defect–causing) agents. Advise sexually active patients receiving chemotherapy or radiotherapy to use birth control during therapy. The method and length of birth control should be discussed with the primary health care provider.

Health Care Resources. Resources available to the patient after discharge include personal support and community programs. After discharge, the spouse or partner may need help in planning support for home responsibilities. For example, a partner who may be assuming additional duties at home and work may feel stressed. Discussing the need for ongoing emotional support is also beneficial to both the patient and partner. Leaving the hospital and appearing normal do not end the anxiety and fear. Identifying a support person with whom the patient or couple can explore these feelings and discussing the need to ventilate feelings enhance personal and family recovery.

Numerous support and educational resources are available to those diagnosed with breast cancer. Nurses must provide accurate and current information to patients who may have obtained inaccurate information from various media. There are over 2 million breast cancer survivors in the United States, and many men and women are active in breast cancer support and advocacy organizations. National breast cancer organizations are accessible online, and many of them have local affiliates. Examples of such organizations are Susan G. Komen for the Cure, the National Breast Cancer Coalition, Y-Me, Sisters Network, Young Survival Coalition, and Pink Ribbon Girls. Local support organizations can be accessed through the health care provider, the local hospital, wellness centers, home care agencies, or by word of mouth.

The American Cancer Society (ACS) (www.cancer.org) is a comprehensive resource for information and support in the United States. Breast Cancer.Org (www.breastcancer.org) provides evidence-based information in language a lay person can understand.

The Canadian Breast Cancer Foundation (www.cbcf.org) offers information, resources, and support services for breast cancer patients and their families. The Breast Cancer Society of Canada (www.bcsa.ca) conducts research on breast cancer in Canada.

◆ Evaluation: Reflecting

Evaluate the care of the patient with breast cancer based on the identified priority patient problems. The expected outcomes include that the patient:

CLINICAL JUDGMENT CHALLENGE 70-1

Patient-Centered Care; Safety; Evidence-Based Practice QSEN

A 66-year-old woman is diagnosed with invasive breast cancer and scheduled for a modified right mastectomy and chemotherapy. She tells you that she has feared developing cancer because her mother and aunt "had the BRCA2 gene" and both were both diagnosed with breast cancer in their 40s. She says that she is worried and anxious because her older sister has ovarian cancer and has less than a year to live. The patient is married and has two female adult children who live with their families out of state. The patient tells you that she is very worried that her children may have the genetic predisposition to breast and/or ovarian cancer.

1. What evidence-based risk factors does this patient have for breast cancer?
2. What preoperative teaching will you provide for her and why?
3. What will you teach the patient about chemotherapy to maintain her safety?
4. In an effort to include a whole-person approach to her care, how might you help address the patient's emotional concerns?

- Has no recurrence or metastasis of breast cancer after completion of treatment; if metastasis occurs, have optimal palliative and end-of-life care
- States that she or he is coping with the uncertainty of having breast cancer and its treatment

BENIGN BREAST DISORDERS

Benign breast conditions are very common. Noncancerous changes to breast tissue can present as breast lumps, impaired COMFORT or pain, and nipple changes (Amin, et al., 2013). Most breast lumps are benign. Because the incidence of breast disease is related to age, breast disorders are described in the following paragraph in an age-related order (Table 70-4).

TABLE 70-4 Typical Presentation of Benign Breast Disorders

BREAST DISORDER	DESCRIPTION	INCIDENCE
Fibroadenoma	Most common benign lesion; solid mass of connective tissue that is unattached to the surrounding tissue	During teenage years into the 30s (most commonly)
Fibrocystic breast condition	Breast pain and tender lumps; the lumps are rubbery, ill defined, and commonly found in the upper outer quadrant of the breast	Onset late teens and 20s; usually subsides after menopause
Ductal ectasia	Hard, irregular mass or masses with nipple discharge, enlarged axillary nodes, redness, and edema; difficult to distinguish from cancer	Women approaching menopause
Intraductal papilloma	Mass in duct that results in nipple discharge; mass is usually not palpable	Women 40 to 55 years of age

FIBROADENOMA

Fibroadenomas are the most common benign tumor in women during the reproductive years. However, they also may occur in a few postmenopausal women. A fibroadenoma is a mass of connective tissue that is unattached to the surrounding breast tissue and is usually discovered by the woman herself or during mammography. Although the immediate fear is that of breast cancer, the risk for cancer occurring within a fibroadenoma is very small. On clinical examination, the tumors are oval, freely mobile, rubbery, and vary in size.

Fibroadenomas may occur anywhere in the breast. The primary health care provider may request a breast ultrasound examination or may perform a needle aspiration to establish whether the lump is cystic (fluid filled) or solid. If the lesion is solid, excision in an ambulatory care setting using local anesthesia is sometimes the treatment of choice.

FIBROCYSTIC BREAST CONDITION

❖ PATHOPHYSIOLOGY

Fibrocystic changes of the breast include a range of changes involving the lobules, ducts, and stromal tissues of the breast. Because these changes affect at least half of women over the life span, they are referred to as fibrocystic breast condition (FBC) rather than fibrocystic disease. This condition most often occurs in premenopausal women between 20 and 50 years of age and is thought to be caused by an imbalance in the normal estrogen-to-progesterone ratio. Typical symptoms include breast pain and tender lumps or swelling in the breasts. The symptoms are more noticeable before a woman's menstrual period (McCance et al., 2014).

The two main features of FBC are fibrosis and cysts. Areas of fibrosis are made up of fibrous connective tissue and are firm or hard. Cysts are spaces filled with fluid lined by breast glandular cells. Microcysts are small, nonpalpable cysts inside the breast glands. Macrocysts occur when fluid continues to build up. They often enlarge in response to monthly hormonal changes, stretching the surrounding breast tissue, and become painful. Symptoms usually resolve after menstruation and then recur before the next menstrual period in a cyclic fashion. Breast ultrasound is used to confirm the presence of a cyst.

Postmenopausal women taking hormone replacement therapy (HRT) may develop FBC or experience worsening of symptoms. Having cysts or fibrosis does not increase a woman's chance of developing breast cancer. However, if a lump is very firm or has other features raising the concern about cancer, mammography is indicated. A needle biopsy or surgical biopsy may be needed to make sure that cancer is not present. Biopsy may be indicated in these situations:

- No fluid is aspirated.
- The mammogram shows suspicious findings.
- A mass remains palpable after aspiration.
- The aspirated fluid reveals cancer cells.

Symptoms often resolve after menopause when estrogen decreases.

❖ INTERPROFESSIONAL COLLABORATIVE CARE

Management of FBC focuses on the symptoms of the condition. Suggest supportive measures for women with mild discomfort. The use of analgesics or limiting salt intake before menses to help decrease swelling may be helpful. Teach patients that wearing a supportive bra, even to bed, can reduce pain by decreasing tension on the ligaments. Local application of ice or heat may provide temporary relief of pain. For a small number of women, draining the cysts by needle aspiration can help relieve painful symptoms. Many women find relief with the reduction of dietary caffeine and other stimulants.

In women with severe symptoms of FBC, hormonal drugs such as oral contraceptives or selective estrogen receptor modulators (SERMs) may be prescribed to suppress oversecretion of estrogen and correct luteal insufficiency. Vitamin supplements have also been suggested to relieve symptoms, but research has not consistently shown these to be effective; some may have dangerous side effects if taken in large doses. Diuretics may be prescribed to decrease premenstrual breast engorgement.

> ### ! NURSING SAFETY PRIORITY QSEN
> #### *Drug Alert*
>
> Explain to women the benefits and risks associated with hormonal drug therapy for FBC, such as stroke, liver disease, and increased intracranial pressure. Teach them to seek medical attention immediately if any signs or symptoms of these complications occur.
> Encourage the patient to continue prescribed drug therapy and monitor the effectiveness of these interventions. Teach the patient to become familiar with the normal feel and texture of her breasts so she is aware of any changes.

ISSUES OF LARGE-BREASTED WOMEN

Although Western society emphasizes large breasts as a positive attribute, women with excessive breast tissue often have health problems and impaired COMFORT. For instance, a woman with large breasts may have difficulty finding clothes that fit well and in which she feels attractive. The breast size may be out of proportion to the rest of the body, which adds to the problem of finding clothes that fit. Larger bras are expensive and may need to be specially ordered. The woman may have large dents in the shoulders from bra straps. In addition, many large-breasted women develop fungal infections under the breasts, especially in hot weather, because it is difficult to keep this area dry and exposed to air.

Backaches from the added weight are also common. If well-fitting bras do not help and obesity is not part of the problem, the only alternative for this condition may be breast reduction surgery. The surgeon removes excess breast tissue and then repositions the nipple and remaining skin flaps to produce the best cosmetic effect. This operation is a major surgical procedure and is called a reduction mammoplasty.

The decision to have the procedure is usually made after years of living with the discomfort of excessive breast size. Listen to the woman verbalize her feelings and reinforce information as appropriate. The nursing care after surgery is similar to that for the woman having reconstructive surgery. (See discussion of Breast Reconstruction earlier in the Surgical Management section under Breast Cancer.)

ISSUES OF SMALL-BREASTED WOMEN

Some women choose to have breast augmentation surgery to increase or improve the size, shape, or symmetry of their breasts. Most health insurers do not pay for this procedure. Most surgeries involve the implantation of saline-filled or silicon prostheses. Some are constructed from the women's own tissue in much the same way as for reconstruction after mastectomy. *Saline* implants are filled with sterile saline and can be filled with the amount needed to get the shape and firmness the woman wants. If the implant shell leaks, the saline will be safely absorbed by the body. *Silicone* implants are filled with an elastic gel, which can leak into the breast and will not be absorbed. The plastic surgeon reviews the advantages and disadvantages of each implant or natural procedure.

Before breast augmentation surgery, teach the patient to stop smoking (to promote healing); avoid aspirin and other NSAID; and avoid herbs that can cause bleeding during the procedure, such as garlic, *Ginkgo biloba*, and ginseng. Tell her that the incisions will be hidden as much as possible, either under the pectoral muscle or directly behind the breast tissue as a submammary placement. One or more wound drains will be inserted during surgery, and she will need to know how to care for these drains at home. Review possible postoperative complications, including infection and implant leakage, which can cause severe pain and possible fever.

After surgery, the patient can be discharged to home the same day or the day after. Remind the family or significant other that someone should stay with her for at least 24 hours after surgery. The incisions may or may not have dressings, depending on the surgeon and type of surgery.

> ### ! NURSING SAFETY PRIORITY QSEN
> #### *Action Alert*
>
> Remind the patient after breast augmentation that for the first few days she should expect soreness in her chest and arms. Her breasts will feel tight and sensitive, and the skin over her breasts may feel warm or may itch. Teach the patient that she will have difficulty raising her arms over her head and should not lift, push, or pull anything until the surgeon permits. Teach her to also avoid strenuous activity or twisting above her waist. Remind the patient to walk every few hours to prevent deep vein thrombi. Tell her to expect some swelling of the breasts for 3 to 4 weeks after surgery.

An important issue for patients who have breast augmentation surgery is breast cancer surveillance. Breast self-examination (BSE) and clinical breast examination (CBE) can still be performed because the prosthesis is placed behind the woman's normal breast tissue, actually pushing it forward. However, screening mammography may not be as sensitive because the amount of visualized breast tissue is decreased. Additional x-rays, called *implant displacement views*, may be used to examine the breast tissue more completely. Although there is no conclusive evidence that breast augmentation increases breast cancer risk, further research is needed regarding diagnosis and prognosis of breast cancer among women with cosmetic breast implants (Lavigne et al., 2013). Teach women desiring cosmetic breast augmentation about the differences in breast cancer screening.

GET READY FOR THE NCLEX® EXAMINATION!

KEY POINTS

Review these Key Points for each NCLEX Examination Client Needs Category.

Safe and Effective Care Environment

- In collaboration with the health care team, identify community resources for patients with breast cancer, including *Reach to Recovery* of the American Cancer Society. **QSEN: Teamwork and Collaboration**

Health Promotion and Maintenance

- Identify patients at high risk for breast cancer, especially women with family history of breast cancer at a young age; those who have had early menarche, late menopause, or first pregnancy after 30 years of age; or those who are nulliparous (see Table 70-1).
- Discuss benefits and risks of options available to women who are high risk for breast cancer, including close surveillance, chemoprevention, and prophylactic surgery.
- Teach women to become self-aware of breasts and any breast changes; teach breast self-examination (BSE) to women who choose this method of breast self-awareness (see Chart 70-1). **QSEN: Patient-Centered Care**
- Encourage women to have a screening mammography according to recommended guidelines. Baseline screening should begin at 45 years of age and continue yearly. In high-risk women, screening should be started earlier. **QSEN: Evidence-Based Practice**
- Encourage women to have a clinical breast examination (CBE) according to recommended guidelines. **QSEN: Evidence-Based Practice; Informatics**

Psychosocial Integrity

- Assess and document patients' reactions to the diagnosis of breast cancer and the effect of breast cancer treatment on their body image and SEXUALITY. **QSEN: Patient-Centered Care; Informatics**
- Allow patients opportunities to express feelings of grief, fear, and anxiety.
- Teach women ways to minimize surgical area deformity and enhance body image, such as use of a breast implant (prosthesis) or the option of breast reconstruction.

- Address the reactions of family and significant others to the diagnosis of breast cancer; provide support and education. **QSEN: Patient-Centered Care**

Physiological Integrity

- Assess benign lumps as mobile and round or oval; assess possible malignant lumps as fixed and irregularly shaped, often in the upper outer breast quadrant (see Chart 70-2).
- A breast reduction is an option to promote COMFORT for women with very large, heavy breasts.
- A breast augmentation is an elective procedure for women with small breasts or for women who desire reconstruction after breast removal (see Table 70-3).
- After breast cancer surgery, assess vital signs, dressings, drainage tubes, and amount of drainage. **Clinical Judgment**
- Notify the health care team that the arm of the surgical mastectomy side should not be used for blood pressures, blood drawing, IV therapy, or injections. **QSEN: Safety**
- Assess the return of arm and shoulder mobility after breast surgery and axillary dissection.
- Assess for the presence of lymphedema and assist the patient to perform therapeutic measures to reduce lymphedema in the affected arm. **QSEN: Safety**
- Teach the patient measures to prevent lymphedema after axillary node dissection, including exercises as listed in Chart 70-3. **QSEN: Evidence-Based Practice**
- Observe for and report other complications of breast cancer surgery or breast reconstruction, especially infection and inadequate vascular perfusion (see Chart 70-4). **QSEN: Safety**
- After an axillary lymph node dissection, elevate the affected arm on a pillow.
- Teach self-management after breast surgery as listed in Chart 70-5.
- Radiation and drug therapy are used most often as adjuvant therapy after breast surgery but may be used before surgery to shrink the tumor.
- Benign problems of the breast may cause impaired COMFORT (see Table 70-4).

SELECTED BIBLIOGRAPHY

Asterisk indicates a classic or definitive work on this subject.

Alakhras, M. M., Bourne, R. R., Rickard, M. M., Ng, K. H., Pietrzyk, M. M., & Brennan, P. C. (2013). Digital tomosynthesis: A new future for breast imaging? *Clinical Radiology, 68*(5), e225–e236.

American Cancer Society (ACS) (2017a). *Breast cancer detailed guide*. Atlanta: Author.

American Cancer Society (ACS) (2017b). *Breast cancer facts & figures 2016-2017*. Atlanta: Author.

American Cancer Society (ACS) (2017c). *Cancer facts for lesbians and bisexual women*. www.cancer.org/healthy/findcancerearly/women-shealth/cancer-facts-for-lesbians-and-bisexual-women.htm.

Amin, A. L., Purdy, A. C., Mattingly, J. D., Kong, A. L., & Termuhlen, P. M. (2013). Multidisciplinary breast management benign breast disease. *Surgical Clinics of North America, 93*(2), 299–308.

*Beredjick, C. (2012). The lesbian breast cancer link. *Advocate (Boston, Mass.), 1062*, 16.

Bryan, T., & Snyder, E. (2013). The clinical breast exam: A skill that should not be abandoned. *JGIM: Journal of General Internal Medicine, 28*(5), 719–722.

Burchum, J. L. R., & Rosenthal, L. D. (2016). *Lehne's pharmacology for nursing care* (9th ed.). St. Louis: Elsevier.

Canadian Cancer Society. (2015). *Breast cancer*. www.cancer.ca/en/cancer-information/cancer-type/breast/statistics/?region-bc.

Edwards, J., Herzberg, S., Shook, J., Beirne, T., & Schomas, D. (2015). Breast conservation therapy utilizing partial breast brachytherapy for early-stage cancer of the breast: A retrospective review from the Saint Luke's Cancer Institute. *American Journal of Clinical Oncology*, 38(2), 174–178.

Jankowitz, R. C., & Lee, A. V. (2013). The evolving role of multi-gene tests in breast cancer management. *Oncology*, 27(3), 210–214.

Johnson, R. H., Chien, F. L., & Bleyer, A. (2013). Incidence of breast cancer with distant involvement among women in the United States, 1976-2009. *Journal of the American Medical Association*, 309(8), 800–805.

Kedde, H., Wiel, H. B., Weijmar Schultz, W. C., & Wijsen, C. (2013). Sexual dysfunction in young women with breast cancer. *Supportive Care in Cancer*, 21(1), 271–280.

Khatcheressian, J., Hurley, P., Bantug, E., Esserman, L., Grunfeld, E., Halberg, F., et al. (2013). Breast cancer follow-up and management after primary treatment: American Society of Clinical Oncology clinical practice guideline update. *Journal of Clinical Oncology*, 31(7), 961–965.

Lavigne, E., Holowaty, E. J., Pan, S. Y., Villeneuve, P. J., Johnson, K. C., Furgusson, D. A., et al. (2013). Breast cancer detection and survival among women with cosmetic breast implants: Systematic review and meta-analysis of observational studies. *British Medical Journal*, 346(f2399), 1–12.

McCance, K., Huether, S., Brashers, V., & Rote, N. (2014). *Pathophysiology: The biologic basis for disease in adults and children* (7th ed.). St. Louis: Mosby.

McLaughlin, S. (2013). Surgical management of the breast: Breast conservation therapy and mastectomy. *The Surgical Clinics of North America*, 93(2), 411–428.

Mohler, E., & Mondry, T. (2013). *Patient education: Lymphedema after breast cancer surgery (beyond the basics)*. www.uptodate.com.

*Ooi, S., Martinez, M., & Li, C. (2011). Disparities in breast cancer characteristics and outcomes by race/ethnicity. *Breast Cancer Research and Treatment*, 127(3), 729–738.

*Saquib, J., Parker, B., Natarajan, L., Madlensky, L., Saquib, N., Patterson, R., et al. (2012). Prognosis following the use of complementary and alternative medicine in women diagnosed with breast cancer. *Complementary Therapies in Medicine*, 20(5), 283–290.

CHAPTER 71

Care of Patients With Gynecologic Problems

Donna D. Ignatavicius

 http://evolve.elsevier.com/Iggy/

PRIORITY AND INTERRELATED CONCEPTS

The priority concepts for this chapter are:
- SEXUALITY
- COMFORT

❋ The SEXUALITY concept exemplar for this chapter is Uterine Leiomyoma, below.

The interrelated concepts for this chapter are:
- ELIMINATION
- REPRODUCTION

LEARNING OUTCOMES

Safe and Effective Care Environment
1. Collaborate with members of the health care team when providing safe quality care for patients with gynecologic cancers.

Health Promotion and Maintenance
2. Teach patients about community-based resources for patients with gynecologic health problems.
3. Identify risk factors for gynecologic cancers.
4. Teach women about evidence-based health promotion and maintenance measures to help prevent or early-detect gynecologic cancers.

Psychosocial Integrity
5. Identify interventions to help patients adapt to physical changes, including effects on SEXUALITY and REPRODUCTION, caused by gynecologic problems and their treatment.

Physiological Integrity
6. Develop a teaching plan for a patient to manage or prevent vaginal infections.
7. Prioritize care after surgery for the woman undergoing an anterior and/or posterior repair, including managing impaired COMFORT and ELIMINATION.
8. Develop an evidence-based plan of care for a patient undergoing a laparoscopic or traditional open hysterectomy.
9. Plan self-management education regarding radiation therapy for patients with gynecologic cancers.

Common gynecologic symptoms that women experience are pain or impaired COMFORT, vaginal discharge, and bleeding. Some patients also have urinary ELIMINATION symptoms associated with their gynecologic problem. Women are often hesitant to seek medical attention for these problems because of fear of a life-threatening disease diagnosis or concern about privacy and dignity. Be sensitive to the woman's concerns and encourage discussion about menstrual or other reproductive problems. Assess the effects of gynecologic disorders on SEXUALITY in any setting. These health problems often impair sexual function and therefore can affect the woman's relationship with her partner. Remember that sexuality affects a woman's sense of being,

self-esteem, and body image. See Chapter 2 for a brief review of the concept of SEXUALITY.

❋ SEXUALITY CONCEPT EXEMPLAR
Uterine Leiomyoma

❖ PATHOPHYSIOLOGY

Leiomyomas, also called **fibroids** or **myomas**, are benign, slow-growing solid tumors of the uterine myometrium (muscle layer). They are classified according to their position in the layers of the uterus: intramural, submucosal, and subserosal.

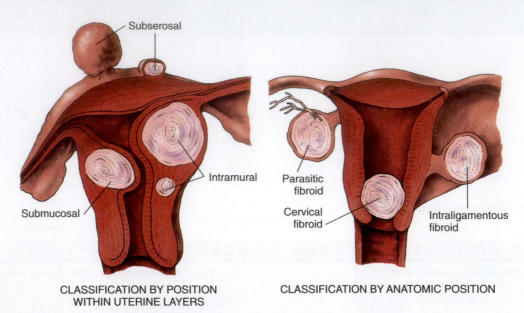

FIG. 71-1 Classification of uterine leiomyomas.

Intramural leiomyomas are contained in the uterine wall within the myometrium. *Submucosal* leiomyomas protrude into the cavity of the uterus and can cause bleeding and disrupt pregnancy. *Subserosal* leiomyomas protrude through the outer surface of the uterine wall and may extend to the broad ligament, pressing other organs (Fig. 71-1) (McCance et al., 2014).

Although most fibroids develop within the uterine wall, a few may appear in the cervix. Pedunculated leiomyomas are attached by a pedicle (stalk) to the outside of the uterus and occasionally break off and attach to other tissues (parasitic fibroids).

Etiology and Genetic Risk

Although the cause is not known, leiomyomas develop from excessive local growth of smooth muscle cells. This may be a genetic error causing a lack of ability to halt growth. The growth of leiomyomas may be related to stimulation by estrogen, progesterone, and growth hormone. This explains why fibroids sometimes enlarge during pregnancy and diminish in size after menopause (McCance et al., 2014).

Incidence and Prevalence

The incidence of leiomyomas increases as women get older. Women who have never been pregnant also are at a high risk. As many as 80% of women are likely to have fibroids (McCool et al., 2014). Many women have asymptomatic fibroids, whereas others have severe symptoms.

❖ INTERPROFESSIONAL COLLABORATIVE CARE

◆ Assessment: Noticing

Physical Assessment/Signs and Symptoms. Women with fibroids usually do not have impaired COMFORT, although acute pain may occur with twisting of the fibroid on its stalk. *The patient often seeks medical attention because of heavy vaginal bleeding.* Ask about how many tampons or menstrual pads she uses a day. Determine if she has a feeling of pelvic pressure and altered ELIMINATION patterns, including constipation and urinary frequency or retention. These symptoms result when the enlarged fibroid presses on other organs. The patient may notice that her abdomen has increased in size. Assess the woman's abdomen for distention or enlargement. Ask if she has **dyspareunia** (painful intercourse) and/or infertility (inability to become pregnant).

Abdominal, vaginal, and rectal examinations usually reveal the presence of a uterine enlargement. Further diagnostic procedures are needed to differentiate benign tumors from cancerous ones.

Psychosocial Assessment. Symptoms such as dyspareunia may significantly lower the patient's quality of life. A woman who is symptomatic may fear that she has cancer or may have anxiety about abnormal bleeding or her failure to conceive. She may also be concerned if surgery is recommended if she desires pregnancy. Assess the woman's feelings and concerns about her symptoms and fears of the unknown. If hysterectomy is recommended, explore the significance of the loss of the uterus for the woman and her partner, including effects on SEXUALITY and sexual function.

Diagnostic Assessment. A complete blood count may identify iron deficiency anemia (related to heavy or prolonged bleeding). A pregnancy test is done to determine whether pregnancy is the cause of the uterine enlargement. An endometrial biopsy may be performed to evaluate for endometrial cancer.

Transvaginal ultrasound (US) alone or with saline infusion (saline sonogram) provides a picture of a submucosal fibroid that may protrude into the uterine cavity. For this procedure, the US probe is placed into the woman's vagina to better visualize the uterine area. The primary health care provider may also choose to directly view a tumor and perform a biopsy using *laparoscopy* (for tumors on the outside of the uterus) or *hysteroscopy* (for tumors accessible inside the uterus). *MRI* can differentiate between benign and malignant lesions.

◆ Analysis: Interpreting

The priority collaborative problem for patients with uterine leiomyoma is *Potential for prolonged or heavy bleeding due to abnormal uterine growth.*

Planning and Implementation: Responding

Managing Bleeding

Planning: Expected Outcomes. The expected outcome for the patient who has one or more uterine leiomyomas is that she will not experience or continue to experience heavy (severe) or prolonged bleeding following treatment.

Interventions. Asymptomatic fibroids usually do not need treatment. Management depends on the size and location of the tumor and the woman's desire for future pregnancy. Women who want to become pregnant can take drug therapy or have magnetic resonance–guided focused ultrasound surgery or laparoscopic myomectomy to remove the tumor. Uterine artery embolization and hysterectomy are choices for women who no longer desire pregnancy.

Nonsurgical Management. If the woman is menopausal, the fibroids usually shrink, and surgery may not be necessary. Teach the patient who is receiving hormone replacement therapy for menopausal symptoms that the fibroids may continue to grow because of estrogen stimulation.

If the woman has few symptoms or desires childbearing, the primary health care provider may recommend intermittent observation and examination. As with dysfunctional uterine bleeding, mild leiomyoma symptoms can be managed with oral contraception.

Magnetic resonance–guided focused ultrasound is a noninvasive, painless technique for women with few smaller fibroids who wish to preserve their fertility. The woman lies prone on an MRI scanner, which provides a three-dimensional image of the pelvis. The radiologic clinician then guides a focused pulse of ultrasound to heat the tumor to destroy it.

An alternative to surgery for the woman who does not desire pregnancy is uterine artery embolization (also called *uterine fibroid embolization [UFE]*) under moderate sedation or short-term anesthesia. The interventional radiologist uses a percutaneous catheter inserted through the femoral artery to inject polyvinyl alcohol pellets into the uterine artery. The resulting blockage starves the tumor of circulation, allowing it (or them) to shrink.

! NURSING SAFETY PRIORITY QSEN

Action Alert

After uterine artery embolization, the woman may have severe cramping within the first 24 hours caused by decreased blood flow to the uterus. Cramping can last from a few days to 2 weeks. Assess the client's pain level and provide analgesics as needed. If a vascular closure device is used at the arterial insertion site (most commonly), raise the head of the bed. Help the patient ambulate about 2 hours after the procedure. If a closure device was not used, keep her on bedrest with the legs immobilized for 4 hours before ambulating to prevent bleeding. Patients generally recover quickly, returning to normal activities within 7 to 10 days after the procedure (Storck, 2012.)

Before discharge, tell the patient to observe for *postembolectomy syndrome*—a flulike illness that some women develop that lasts about 5 to 7 days. Teach her to resume usual activities slowly and avoid strenuous activity until the surgeon recommends it. Most patients can return to work or daily routine within a week.

Surgical Management. When possible, minimally invasive surgical (MIS) techniques are performed, such as a myomectomy, to prevent removing the uterus. If not, a hysterectomy is the procedure of choice.

Uterus-Sparing Surgeries. If the woman desires children, the surgeon may perform a laparoscopic or hysteroscopic myomectomy (the removal of leiomyomas from the uterus) (Bradley, 2013). During this procedure, a laser may be used to remove the tumors. This MIS procedure is usually performed in the early phase of the menstrual cycle to minimize blood loss and avoid the possibility of interrupting an unsuspected pregnancy. A small percentage of leiomyomas recur after surgery. Scarring makes the uterus more likely to rupture during labor, so future deliveries will be planned cesarean deliveries. Nursing care is similar to that for a woman undergoing a hysterectomy as discussed in the following paragraphs.

In selected cases (e.g., submucous fibroids, menorrhagia), a *transcervical endometrial resection (TCER)* is performed via hysteroscopy. A hysteroscope (endoscope) is inserted into the uterus, and the endometrium is destroyed using diathermy (heat) or radioablation.

! NURSING SAFETY PRIORITY QSEN

Critical Rescue

Monitor for rare but potential complications of hysteroscopic surgery, which include:

- Fluid overload (fluid used to distend the uterine cavity can be absorbed)
- Embolism
- Hemorrhage
- Perforation of the uterus, bowel, or bladder and ureter injury
- Persistent increased menstrual bleeding
- Incomplete suppression of menstruation

Monitor for any indications of these problems and report signs and symptoms, such as severe pain and heavy bleeding, to the surgeon or Rapid Response Team immediately.

Hysterectomy. Leiomyomas are the most common reason for hysterectomies. Hysterectomies may be performed abdominally, vaginally, or with laparoscopic or robotic assistance based on the patient's clinical reason for hysterectomy and the surgeon's area of technical expertise. Table 71-1 defines common terminology associated with gynecologic surgeries.

Preoperative Care. Preoperative teaching by the health care team typically begins in the surgeon's office or surgical clinic. Explain procedures that routinely take place before surgery, including laboratory tests and expected drugs such as a

---

TABLE 71-1 Common Gynecologic Surgeries

Total Hysterectomy

The entire uterus, including the cervix, is removed. The procedure may be vaginal or abdominal, with laparoscopic or robotic assistance.

Bilateral Salpingo-Oophorectomy (BSO)

Fallopian tubes and ovaries are removed.

Panhysterectomy

Total abdominal hysterectomy and BSO: The uterus, ovaries, and fallopian tubes are removed.

Radical Hysterectomy

The uterus, cervix, adjacent lymph nodes, upper third of the vagina, and surrounding tissues (parametrium) are removed.

prophylactic antibiotic. Depending on the type of surgical technique planned, teach about the need for turning, coughing, and deep-breathing exercises; incentive spirometry; early ambulation; and pain relief. (See Chapter 14 for a discussion of general patient care before surgery.)

Psychological assessment and support are essential. Assess the significance of the surgery for the woman and her partner related to SEXUALITY and REPRODUCTION. Many women relate their uterus to self-image and femininity or believe that their sexual function is related to their uterus. Although surgical menopause by hysterectomy can create loss of libido and vaginal changes if the ovaries are also removed, teach the patient that vaginal estrogen cream, lubricants, and gentle dilation can help with these issues (see the Evidence-Based Practice box). Reassure her regarding any misperceptions about the effects of hysterectomy, such as association with masculinization and weight gain. Assess the patient's support system and recognize that she may fear rejection by her sexual partner. To be patient centered, include the partner in all teaching sessions (if the patient prefers) *unless this practice is not culturally acceptable or the patient prefers not to do so for other reasons.*

Operative Procedures. A *total abdominal hysterectomy (TAH)* is usually performed for leiomyomas larger than the size of a 16-week pregnancy. The uterus and cervix are most often removed by laparoscopic-assisted minimally invasive surgery (MIS), which requires one or more very small umbilical incisions. Although not commonly done as often today, the traditional open surgery is performed through a horizontal "bikini" incision. A *total vaginal hysterectomy (TVH)* requires no skin incision because the uterus is removed through the vagina.

Some surgeons use robotic technology to assist in performing a TAH, although it is much more expensive than a traditional vaginal or laparoscopic approach (ACOG, 2013). Robotic surgery is helpful when performing hysterectomies on patients who are extremely obese. In both vaginal and abdominal hysterectomies, the surgeon removes the uterus from supporting ligaments, which are then attached to the vaginal cuff so normal depth of the vagina is maintained.

Postoperative Care. Nursing care of the woman who has undergone a *TAH* is similar to that of any patient who has had laparoscopic or traditional open abdominal surgery (see Chapter 16). Assess (Chart 71-1):

- Vaginal bleeding (there should be less than one saturated perineal pad in 4 hours)
- Abdominal bleeding at the incision site(s) (a small amount is normal)
- Intactness of the incision(s)
- Urine output per urinary catheter for 24 hours or less (for open surgery only)
- Incisional or abdominal pain

EVIDENCE-BASED PRACTICE QSEN

Does Having a Hysterectomy Affect a Woman's Sexuality?

Danesh, M., Hamzehgardeshi, Z., Moosazadeh, M., & Shabani-Asrami, F. (2015). The effect of hysterectomy on women's sexual function: A narrative review. *Medical Archives, 69*(6), 387-392.

The authors conducted a narrative systematic review of research using a five-step approach. An extensive literature review yielded 34 articles to include in the review. Five categories were examined to determine if having a hysterectomy had an effect on these areas summarized in the following points:

- *Sexual desire:* The research showed that most women had an increase in sexual desire after having a hysterectomy.
- *Sexual arousal:* The research showed mixed findings. Some women had an increase in sexual arousal and others had a decrease in arousal.
- *Orgasm:* The research again showed mixed results, with some women experiencing more orgasms and others experiencing fewer orgasms.
- *Dyspareunia:* The research showed little or no change in the incidence of dyspareunia. However, vaginal lubricants and dilators were used at times to prevent discomfort during sexual intercourse.
- *Sexual satisfaction:* The research showed an overall decrease in sexual satisfaction.

Level of Evidence: 1

The study was a systematic review, which is a strong source of evidence.

Implications for Research and Practice

Although more studies are needed to more specifically determine sexual function of women who had a hysterectomy, this study suggests that these patients need health teaching regarding sexuality after surgery. If culturally appropriate and if the patient agrees, the woman's sexual partner needs to be included in this health teaching.

📋 CHART 71-1 Focused Assessment

Postoperative Nursing Care of the Patient After Open Total Abdominal Hysterectomy

Assess cardiovascular, respiratory, renal, and gastrointestinal status, including:
- Vital signs
- Heart, lung, and bowel sounds
- Urine output
- Temperature and color of the skin
- Red blood cell, hemoglobin, and hematocrit levels
- Activity tolerance
- Dressing and drains for color and amount of drainage
- Perineal pads for vaginal bleeding and clots
- Fluid intake (IVs until peristalsis returns and patient is tolerating oral intake)

Teach the patient to use these interventions to prevent postoperative complications:
- Cough and deep-breathing exercises
- Incentive spirometry
- Sequential compression devices
- Ambulation
- Avoidance of heavy lifting or strenuous activity
- Adequate hydration

Assess the home care teaching needs of the patient related to the illness and surgery, including:
- Physiologic effects of the surgery
- Signs or symptoms to report
- Side or toxic effects of medications
- Activity limitations related to driving and use of stairs
- Follow-up care
- Postoperative restrictions related to sexual activity, use of tampons, and bathing
- Care of wound and/or drains

Assess the patient's coping skills and reaction to the diagnosis and surgical procedure.

Specific postoperative interventions for a *vaginal hysterectomy* include:

- Assessment of vaginal bleeding (there should be less than one saturated pad in 4 hours)
- Urinary catheter care
- Perineal care

❓ NCLEX EXAMINATION CHALLENGE 71-1
Physiological Integrity

A client returns from surgery after a laparoscopic total abdominal hysterectomy. On initial assessment, which finding by the nurse requires **immediate** intervention?

A. Decreased bowel sounds in all quadrants
B. Heavy vaginal bleeding with clots
C. Temperature of 99°F (37.2°C)
D. Client statement that pain is 4 on a scale of 0 to 10

Care Coordination and Transition Management

Discharge teaching, including activity restrictions, depends on the type of surgical procedure performed. Care coordination after discharge is also essential.

Home Care Management. Patients who have *uterus-sparing surgeries* usually go home the same day of surgery. They usually experience less postprocedural pain and fewer complications than patients who have their uterus and cervix removed. Teach patients that they should be able to return to usual daily activities in 2 weeks but sexual intercourse should be avoided for at least 6 weeks or as otherwise instructed by the primary health care provider.

If the patient had a *laparoscopic hysterectomy*, few limitations in activity are needed. For patients who had a *traditional open hysterectomy*, teach them to limit stair climbing for several weeks. If women live alone and are not permitted to drive for several weeks, they may need to arrange for transportation for follow-up surgical visits.

Self-Management Education. Teach the woman who has undergone an abdominal hysterectomy about the expected physical changes, any activity restrictions, diet, sexual activity, wound care (if any), complications, and the need for follow-up care. Some women experience impaired abdominal or shoulder COMFORT because of the introduction of carbon dioxide gas during a *laparoscopic* procedure. For patients who have a *vaginal* hysterectomy, teach them to promptly report excessive or increasing bleeding to their surgeon. Chart 71-2 lists areas to include for health teaching.

Generally, women are more accepting of surgery if they have completed childbearing, have interests outside the home, work, have no misconceptions about the effects of hysterectomy, and have support from the family, especially their sexual partner. Psychological reactions can occur months to years after surgery, particularly if sexual functioning and libido are diminished. Women identified as being at high risk for psychological problems may need long-term follow-up care or referral. They may need to be counseled about signs of depression. Intermittent sadness is normal, but continued feelings of low self-esteem or loss of interest or pleasure in usual activities and pastimes is not expected and should be evaluated. Provide written materials and focus on the positive aspects of the woman's life to help decrease adverse psychological reactions.

Health Care Resources. Loss of female reproductive organs causes many women to go through the grieving process. If

💠 CHART 71-2   Patient and Family Education: Preparing for Self-Management
Care After a Total Vaginal or Abdominal Hysterectomy

Expected Physical Changes

- You will no longer have a period, although you may have some vaginal discharge for a few days after you go home.
- It will not be possible for you to become pregnant, and birth control methods are no longer needed. (Condoms should still be used to decrease the chance of getting a sexually transmitted infection [STI].)
- If your ovaries were removed, you may have some menopause symptoms such as hot flushes, night sweats, and vaginal dryness.
- It is normal to tire more easily and require more sleep and rest during the first few weeks after surgery.

Activity (Typically for Vaginal and Traditional Open Surgeries)

- Limit stair climbing to fewer than five times per day.
- Do not lift anything heavier than 5 to 10 lb.
- Gradually increase walking as exercise, but stop before you become fatigued.
- Avoid the sitting position for any extended period. When you sit, do not cross your legs at the knees.
- Avoid jogging, aerobic exercise, participating in sports, and any strenuous activity for 2 to 6 weeks, depending on which type of surgical procedure was performed.
- Do not drive until your surgeon has told you that it's alright.

Sexual Activity

- Do not engage in sexual intercourse for 4 to 6 weeks or as prescribed by your surgeon.
- If you had a vaginal "repair" as part of your surgery, the first time you have intercourse you may have some tenderness or pain because the vaginal walls are tighter. Careful intercourse and the use of water-based lubricants can help reduce this discomfort. It usually goes away with time and stretching of the vagina.

Complications

- Take your temperature twice each day for the first 3 days after surgery. Report fevers of over 100°F (38°C).
- Check your incision, if you have any, daily for signs of infection (increasing redness, open areas, drainage that is thick or foul-smelling, incision pain).

Symptoms to Report to Your Surgeon

- Increased vaginal drainage or change in drainage (bloodier, thicker, foul-smelling)
- Temperature over 100°F (38°C)
- Pain, tenderness, redness, or swelling in your calves
- Pain or burning on urination

desired and culturally appropriate, refer the woman to a clergy member or spiritual counselor if needed to discuss feelings of sadness. Suggest that the patient consult with a mental health counselor or clinical psychologist as another option if needed.

◆ Evaluation: Reflecting

Evaluate the care of the patient with leiomyomas on the basis of the identified priority problem. The expected outcomes are that she:

- Has relief of bleeding from the fibroid tumor(s) after effective management
- Verbalizes positive perception of self and is satisfied with her own SEXUALITY

PELVIC ORGAN PROLAPSE

❖ PATHOPHYSIOLOGY

The pelvic organs are supported by a sling of muscles and tendons, which sometimes become weak and no longer able to hold an organ in place. Uterine prolapse, the most common type of pelvic organ prolapse (POP), can be caused by neuromuscular damage of childbirth; increased intra-abdominal pressure related to pregnancy, obesity, or physical exertion; or weakening of pelvic support caused by decreased estrogen. The stages of uterine prolapse are described by the degree of descent of the uterus through the pelvic floor.

Whenever the uterus is displaced, other structures such as the bladder, rectum, and small intestine can protrude through the vaginal walls (Fig. 71-2). A cystocele is a protrusion of the bladder through the vaginal wall (urinary bladder prolapse), which can lead to stress urinary incontinence (SUI) and urinary tract infections (UTIs). A rectocele is a protrusion of the rectum through a weakened vaginal wall (rectal prolapse).

❖ INTERPROFESSIONAL COLLABORATIVE CARE

◆ Assessment: Noticing

Patients with suspected uterine prolapse may report a feeling of "something falling out," dyspareunia (painful intercourse), backache, and heaviness or pressure in the pelvis. A pelvic examination may reveal a protrusion of the cervix or anterior vaginal wall when the woman is asked to bear down. Listen to her concerns and note signs of anxiety or depression from having long-term symptoms.

Ask the patient whether she has urinary ELIMINATION problems, such as difficulty emptying her bladder, urinary frequency and urgency, a urinary tract infection, or stress urinary incontinence (SUI) (loss of urine during activities that increase intra-abdominal pressure, such as laughing, coughing, sneezing, or lifting heavy objects). These symptoms may be associated with a *cystocele* (bladder prolapse).

Diagnostic tests include cystography (to show the presence of bladder herniation), measurement of residual urine by bladder ultrasound, and urine culture and sensitivity testing. Radiographic imaging of urinary anatomy and voiding function is useful in determining the degree of *cystocele* (prolapse).

Rectocele assessment usually includes symptoms of constipation, hemorrhoids, fecal impaction, and feelings of rectal or vaginal fullness. A vaginal and rectal examination may show a bulge of the posterior vaginal wall when the woman is asked to bear down.

◆ Interventions: Responding

Interventions are based on the degree of the POP. Conservative treatment is preferred over surgical treatment when possible.

Nonsurgical Management. Teach women to improve pelvic support and tone by doing pelvic floor muscle exercises (PFMEs, or Kegel exercises). Space-filling devices such as pessaries or spheres can be worn in the vagina to elevate the uterine prolapse. Intravaginal estrogen therapy may be prescribed for the postmenopausal woman to prevent atrophy and weakening of vaginal walls. Women with bladder symptoms may benefit from bladder training and attention to complete emptying. Management of a rectocele focuses on promoting bowel elimination. The primary health care provider usually prescribes a high-fiber diet, stool softeners, and laxatives.

Surgical Management. Surgery may be recommended for severe symptoms of POP, with preference given to the least invasive approach. Address the fears and concerns of the patient and her family.

Transvaginal repair for pelvic organ prolapse (POP) using surgical vaginal mesh or tape is a commonly performed minimally invasive technique. It is particularly useful for women who are very obese. Depending on the procedure that is planned, the patient has either local or general anesthesia. The surgeon creates a sling with the mesh or tape, and the woman is discharged the same day. Procedures done under local anesthesia can be done in the surgeon's office. Since 2008, patient report of complications associated with the use of transvaginal mesh has required the U.S. Food and Drug Administration (2011) to release a classic report and update advising about the safety and effectiveness of the use of this product for POP. Since that time, multiple legal cases have been filed because of continued problems and complications. Common complications associated with the use of transvaginal mesh for POP include mesh erosion, painful sexual intercourse (dyspareunia), infection, urinary ELIMINATION problems (e.g., stress urinary incontinence [SUI]), and organ perforation (e.g., bladder and bowel) (U.S. Food and Drug Administration [USFDA], 2011).

Teach patients who have had the mesh or tape procedure to avoid strenuous exercise, heavy lifting, and sexual intercourse

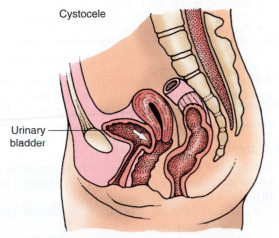
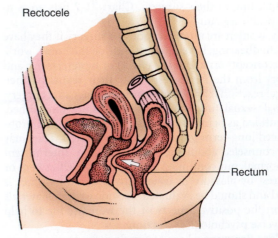

Cystocele — Urinary bladder

Rectocele — Rectum

FIG. 71-2 In cystocele, the urinary bladder is displaced downward, causing bulging of the anterior vaginal wall. In rectocele, the rectum is displaced, causing bulging of the posterior vaginal wall.

? **NCLEX EXAMINATION CHALLENGE 71-2**
Safe and Effective Care Environment

A client had an anterior and posterior colporrhaphy procedure this morning. What is the nurse's **current priority** assessment when caring for this client?
A. Monitoring for urinary incontinence
B. Determining pain level
C. Checking for bowel sounds
D. Inspecting the sternal incision

for 6 weeks. After 6 weeks, the patient may gradually begin to return to regular activities but must be educated about prevention of increasing intra-abdominal pressure (e.g., constipation, weight-lifting, cigarette smoking) for a minimum of 3 months to allow proper healing and prevent POP recurrence (Lazarou, 2012).

Alternatives to minimally invasive surgery are open surgical techniques. An **anterior colporrhaphy** (anterior repair) tightens the pelvic muscles for better *bladder* support. A vaginal surgical approach is used and may be done as a laparoscopic-assisted procedure. Nursing care for a woman undergoing an anterior repair is similar to that for a woman undergoing a vaginal hysterectomy.

After surgery, instruct the patient how to splint her abdomen to protect sutures and to limit her activities. Teach her to *avoid lifting anything heavier than 5 lb (2.27 kg), strenuous exercises, and sexual intercourse for 6 weeks.* For discomfort, she may use heat either as a moist heating pad or warm compresses applied to the abdomen. A hot bath may also be helpful. Sutures do not need to be removed because some are absorbable and others will fall out as healing occurs. Tell the woman to notify her health care provider if she has signs of infection, such as fever, persistent pain, or purulent, foul-smelling discharge. Encourage her to keep her follow-up appointment after surgery.

Posterior colporrhaphy (posterior repair) reduces *rectal* bulging. If both a cystocele and a rectocele are present, an *anterior and posterior colporrhaphy (A&P repair)* is performed. In this case, the woman may return from surgery with a urinary catheter in place to keep the surgical area clean and dry.

The nursing care after a posterior repair is similar to that after any rectal surgery. After surgery, a low-residue (low-fiber) diet is usually prescribed to decrease bowel movements and allow time for the incision to heal. Instruct the patient to avoid straining when she does have a bowel movement so she does not put pressure on the suture line. Bowel movements are often painful, and she may need pain medication before having a stool. Provide sitz baths or delegate this activity to unlicensed nursing personnel to relieve the woman's impaired COMFORT. Health teaching for the patient undergoing a posterior repair is similar to that for the patient undergoing an anterior repair. Vaginal hysterectomy may accompany any uterine prolapse repair surgery unless the woman wants to become pregnant. This procedure is described earlier in this chapter.

ENDOMETRIAL (UTERINE) CANCER

❖ *PATHOPHYSIOLOGY*

Endometrial cancer (cancer of the inner uterine lining) is the most common gynecologic malignancy (Nguyen et al., 2013). This chapter includes two other common gynecologic cancers, but the disease can affect any organ in the reproductive tract.

Endometrial cancer grows slowly in most cases, and early symptoms of vaginal bleeding generally lead to prompt evaluation and treatment. As a result, this type of cancer has a good prognosis. *Adenocarcinoma* is the most common type of tumor. It arises from the glandular part of the endometrium and usually follows endometrial hyperplasia (overgrowth).

The initial growth of the cancer is within the uterine cavity, followed by extension into the myometrium and the cervix. Stage I endometrial cancer is confined to the endometrium. Stage II cancer also involves the cervix, and stage III reaches the vagina or lymph nodes. Stage IV endometrial cancer has spread to the bowel or bladder mucosa and/or beyond the pelvis (McCance et al., 2014).

Metastasis outside the uterus occurs in these ways:
- Through lymphatic spread to the ovaries and parametrial, pelvic, inguinal, and para-aortic lymph nodes
- By blood to the lungs, liver, or bones
- By transtubal or intra-abdominal spread to the peritoneal cavity

Endometrial cancer is strongly associated with conditions causing prolonged exposure to estrogen without the protective effects of progesterone. Risk factors for endometrial cancer are listed in Table 71-2. Although most cases of endometrial cancer do not have a genetic predisposition, it is more common in

TABLE 71-2 Risk Factors for Endometrial (Uterine) Cancer and Cervical Cancer	
ENDOMETRIAL (UTERINE) CANCER	**CERVICAL CANCER**
• Women in reproductive years	• Girls and young women
• Family history of endometrial cancer or HNPCC	• Infection with HPV
• Diabetes mellitus	• Multiparity (multiple births)
• Hypertension	• Smoking
• Obesity	• Younger than 18 years at first intercourse
• Uterine polyps	• Multiple sex partners
• Late menopause	• African American
• Nulliparity (no childbirths)	• Oral contraceptive use
• Smoking	• History of STIs
• Tamoxifen (Nolvadex) given for breast cancer	• Obesity or poor diet
	• Family history of cervical cancer
	• HIV/AIDS
	• Lower socioeconomic status
	• Sexual partner had a previous partner who developed cervical cancer
	• Intrauterine exposure to DES

AIDS, Acquired immune deficiency syndrome; *DES,* diethylstilbestrol; *HIV,* human immune deficiency virus; *HNPCC,* hereditary nonpolyposis colon cancer; *HPV,* human papilloma virus; *STDs,* sexually transmitted diseases.

families who have gene mutations for hereditary nonpolyposis colon cancer (HNPCC) (National Cancer Institute [NCI], 2017).

White women get the disease more often than African-American women, but African-American women die more often from the disease. The causes for these differences are not known (NCI, 2017).

❖ INTERPROFESSIONAL COLLABORATIVE CARE

◆ Assessment: Noticing

The main symptom of endometrial cancer is postmenopausal bleeding. Ask the patient how many tampons or menstrual pads she uses each day. Some women also have a watery, bloody vaginal discharge, low back or abdominal pain, and low pelvic impaired COMFORT (caused by pressure of the enlarged uterus). Ask the patient to describe the exact location and intensity of her discomfort. A pelvic examination may reveal the presence of a palpable uterine mass or uterine polyp. The uterus is enlarged if the cancer is advanced.

Several laboratory tests are used to determine the overall condition of the woman with possible or confirmed endometrial cancer. For example, the complete blood count typically shows anemia because the patient has heavy bleeding. Serum tumor markers to assess for metastasis include CA-125 (cancer antigen–125) and alpha-fetoprotein (AFP), both of which may be elevated when ovarian cancer is present (Pagana et al., 2017). A human chorionic gonadotropin (hCG) level may be taken to rule out pregnancy before treatment for cancer begins.

Transvaginal ultrasound and *endometrial biopsy* are the gold standard diagnostic tests to determine the presence of endometrial thickening and cancer. Saline may be infused during the ultrasound to improve the image of the uterine cavity. The clinician then collects an endometrial biopsy from inside the uterus via a thin, flexible suction curette through the cervix (Pagana, et al., 2017).

Other diagnostic tests to determine the patient's overall health status and the presence of metastasis (cancer spread) include:

- Chest x-ray
- Intravenous pyelography (IVP) or excretory urography to assess renal function and to assess for renal metastasis
- Abdominal ultrasound
- CT of the pelvis
- MRI of the abdomen and pelvis
- Liver and bone scans to assess for distant metastasis

During the diagnostic phase, the woman may express fears and concerns about having the disease and the effect on her SEXUALITY and/or REPRODUCTION. After the diagnosis is confirmed, she may express disbelief, anger, depression, anxiety, or withdrawal behaviors. Assess these emotional reactions, and encourage the patient to discuss her feelings. Ask her about how she copes with other stressful events, and assess her support systems.

◆ Interventions: Responding

Surgical removal and cancer staging of the tumor with adjacent lymph nodes are the most important interventions for endometrial cancer. Cancer staging is often done using minimally invasive techniques, such as laparoscopic or robotic-assisted procedures.

Surgical Management. For stage I disease, the gynecology oncologist usually removes the uterus, fallopian tubes, and ovaries (total hysterectomy and bilateral salpingo-oophorectomy

[BSO]) and peritoneum fluid or washings for cytologic examination. Laparoscopic surgery has fewer complications, shorter hospital stay, and less cost. A *radical* hysterectomy with bilateral pelvic lymph node dissection and removal of the upper third of the vagina is performed for stage II cancer. Nursing care for a radical hysterectomy is the same as that for a simple hysterectomy except that the woman's hospitalization is usually longer and her convalescence may be extended. (See earlier discussion of Hysterectomy in this chapter.) Radical surgery and node dissection can also be done as a minimally invasive procedure using laparoscopic or robotic-assisted technology.

Nonsurgical Management. Nonsurgical interventions (radiation therapy and chemotherapy) are typically used after surgery and depend on the surgical staging.

Radiation Therapy. The oncologist may prescribe radiation therapy to be delivered by external beam and/or brachytherapy for stage II and stage III cancers. Women with stage II disease may use brachytherapy (internal) radiation to prevent recurrence of vaginal cancer and improve survival.

The purpose of *brachytherapy* is to prevent disease recurrence. The radiologist places an applicator within the woman's uterus through the vagina. After the correct position of the applicator is confirmed by x-ray, the radioactive isotope is placed in the applicator and remains for several minutes. This procedure may be repeated between two and five times once or twice a week. Some patients also have external beam radiation while having brachytherapy treatment sessions. There are no restrictions for the woman to stay away from her family or the public between treatments.

While the radioactive implant is in place, radiation is emitted that can affect other people. The amount of time needed for the therapy depends on the amount of radiation emitted from the source. The radiologist calculates the time needed for a specific dose of radiation.

Inform the patient that she is restricted to bedrest during the treatment session. Excessive movement in bed is restricted to prevent dislodgment of the radioactive source. Chart 71-3 lists the health teaching for the patient having brachytherapy for gynecologic cancer. Teach patients about when to call the primary health care provider after each treatment session.

External beam radiation therapy (EBRT or XRT) may be used to treat any stage of endometrial cancer in combination with surgery, brachytherapy, and/or chemotherapy. Depending on the extent of the tumor, the treatment is given on an ambulatory

---

◎ CHART 71-3 Best Practice for Patient Safety & Quality Care QSEN

Health Teaching for the Patient Having Brachytherapy for Gynecologic Cancer

- Teach the patient to report any of these signs and symptoms to the primary health care provider immediately:
  - Heavy vaginal bleeding
  - Urethral burning for more than 24 hours
  - Blood in the urine
  - Extreme fatigue
  - Severe diarrhea
  - Fever over 100°F (38°C)
  - Abdominal pain
- Teach the patient that she is not radioactive between treatments and there are no restrictions on her interactions with others.

care basis for 4 to 6 weeks. Tissue around the tumor and pelvic wall nodes also is treated. *Teach the patient to monitor for signs of skin breakdown, especially in the perineal area; to avoid sunbathing; and to avoid washing the markings outlining the treatment site.*

Reactions to radiation therapy vary. Some women feel "radioactive" or "unclean" after treatments and may exhibit withdrawal behaviors. Reassure them by correcting any misconceptions. Chapter 22 discusses nursing care of patients receiving radiation therapy in more detail.

Drug Therapy. *Chemotherapy* is used as palliative treatment in advanced and recurrent disease when it has spread to distant parts of the body, but it is not always effective. Although the combination can vary, three of the most common agents used for endometrial cancer are doxorubicin (Adriamycin), cisplatin (Platinol), and paclitaxel (Taxol).

Patients who have chemotherapy may be upset if alopecia (hair loss) occurs. Warn them of this possibility before treatment starts. Wigs, scarves, or turbans can be worn until the hair grows back. Many women select these replacements before they lose their hair. Others shave their head and begin wearing them immediately as the treatment begins. Tell women about these options so they can make decisions with which they are personally comfortable.

Chapter 22 describes chemotherapy and general nursing care during treatment.

Complementary and Integrative Health. Every woman experiences cancer differently. Many complementary and integrative therapies have evidence of benefit in decreasing the side effects of drug therapy and boosting the immune system. Provide your patient with information that will help her make informed, evidence-based decisions. Encourage her to check with her oncologist and/or pharmacist because some integrative therapies can be harmful or interfere with cancer treatment. Current evidence-based information is available at the American Cancer Society (www.cancer.org) and Canadian Cancer Society (www.cancer.ca) websites about mind-body therapies, healing touch, herbs, vitamins, nutrition, and biologic therapies.

Often patients experience emotional crises because of the physical effects of cancer treatments. Radical hysterectomy may be seen as mutilating. Both radiation and chemotherapy have side effects that change physical appearance and body image. Women may have a grief reaction to these changes. The feelings of loss depend on the visibility of the loss and the loss of function. Help the patient adapt to the body changes. Using a calm and accepting approach, encourage self-management as soon as her physical condition is stable.

Care Coordination and Transition Management

Home care after surgery for endometrial cancer is the same as that after a hysterectomy. (See discussion of Hysterectomy in the Uterine Leiomyoma section.) Patients who are receiving chemotherapy or radiation therapy are treated on an ambulatory care basis. Most women are surprised by the fatigue caused by radiation and chemotherapy. Help the patient and her family plan daily activities around trips to the clinic or the primary health care provider's office.

High doses of radiation cause sterility, and vaginal shrinkage can occur. Vaginal dilators can be used with water-soluble lubricants for 10 minutes each day until sexual activity resumes, generally within 4 weeks (ACS, 2017a). Reassure the woman

that she is not radioactive and that her partner will not "catch" cancer by engaging in sexual intercourse.

Death can occur with or without treatment. The patient and family want the woman to pass the 5-year survival mark without a recurrence of disease. If the tumor recurs and cure is not likely, the woman and her family need to think about hospice care and whether she can be cared for in the home. If there is a recurrence, they may be hostile and have signs of a grief reaction. Encourage patients and their families to discuss their feelings. Refer to support services such as a certified hospital chaplain or other spiritual leader, social worker, or counselor. Response to loss and grieving is discussed in Chapter 7.

In the United States, local American Cancer Society chapters provide written materials about endometrial cancer and information about local support groups. Each province in Canada also has a division of the Canadian Cancer Society (www.cancer.ca). If the patient is in the terminal stages of cancer, hospice care may be appropriate (see Chapter 7). If nursing care is needed at home, the hospital nurse or case manager makes referrals to a home health care agency. A referral to a social services agency may be needed if the patient cannot meet the financial demands of treatment and long-term follow-up.

OVARIAN CANCER

❖ PATHOPHYSIOLOGY

Ovarian cancer is the leading cause of death from female reproductive cancers, but it is not the most common type of cancer. Most ovarian cancers are epithelial tumors that grow on the surface of the ovaries. These tumors grow rapidly, spread quickly, and are often bilateral. Tumor cells spread by direct extension into nearby organs and through blood and lymph circulation to distant sites (McCance et al., 2014). Free-floating cancer cells also spread through the abdomen to seed new sites, usually accompanied by ascites (abdominal fluid).

Ovarian cancer seems to be disordered growth in response to excessive exposure to estrogen. This would explain the protective effects of pregnancies and oral contraceptive use, both of which interrupt the monthly estrogen exposure.

Women who have had tubal ligation, used oral contraception, and breast-fed their children have less risk for having the disease (ACS, 2017b). The incidence increases in women older than 50 years, and most are diagnosed after menopause. Family history accounts for a small percentage of cases. These women carry *BCRA1* or *BCRA2* genetic mutations. Of these, some choose to have an elective **bilateral salpingo-oophorectomy (BSO)** (removal of both ovaries and fallopian tubes) to prevent ovarian cancer. Table 71-3 lists known and suspected risk factors for ovarian cancer.

TABLE 71-3 **Risk Factors for Ovarian Cancer**	
• Older than 40 years	• Colorectal cancer
• Family history of ovarian or breast cancer or HNPCC	• Infertility
	• *BRCA1* or *BRCA2* gene mutations
• Diabetes mellitus	• Early menarche/late menopause
• Nulliparity	• Endometriosis
• Older than 30 years at first pregnancy	• Obesity/high-fat diet
• Breast cancer	

HNPCC, Hereditary nonpolyposis colon cancer.

Survival rates are low because ovarian cancer often is not detected until its late stages. It is important for nurses to teach women to *"think ovarian"* if they have vague abdominal and GI symptoms.

❖ INTERPROFESSIONAL COLLABORATIVE CARE

◆ Assessment: Noticing

Most women with ovarian cancer have had mild symptoms for several months but may have thought they were caused by normal perimenopausal changes or stress. They may report abdominal pain or swelling or have vague GI disturbances such as indigestion and gas. Ask the patient if she has had urinary frequency or incontinence, unexpected weight loss, and/or vaginal bleeding.

Complications of advanced metastatic cancer include:

- Pleural effusion
- Ascites
- Lymphedema
- Intestinal obstruction
- Malnutrition

On pelvic examination, an abdominal mass may not be palpable until it reaches a size of 4 to 6 inches (10 to 15 cm). Any enlarged ovary found after menopause should be evaluated as though it were malignant. A Pap smear is of limited value for detecting ovarian cancer.

A cancer antigen test, *CA-125,* measures the presence of damaged endometrial and uterine tissue in the blood. It may be elevated if ovarian cancer is present, but it can also be elevated in patients with endometriosis, fibroids, pelvic inflammatory disease, pregnancy, and even menses (Pagana, et al., 2017). It is also useful for monitoring a patient's progress during and after treatment. Transvaginal ultrasonography, chest radiography, and CT are part of a complete workup to evaluate for metastasis. Complete blood work includes a liver profile if there is ascites.

The woman with ovarian cancer has concerns similar to those described for the patient with endometrial cancer as described earlier in this chapter. Because the cancer is often diagnosed in an advanced stage, thoughts of death and dying, menopause, and loss of fertility come as a shock.

◆ Interventions: Responding

Nursing care of the patient with ovarian cancer is similar to that for endometrial or cervical cancer. The options for treatment depend on the extent of the cancer and usually include surgery first, followed by chemotherapy. Radiation is used for more widespread cancers.

Diagnosis depends on findings during surgical exploration. Exploratory laparotomy (abdominal surgery) is performed to diagnose, treat, and stage ovarian tumors. A total abdominal hysterectomy, bilateral salpingo-oophorectomy (removal of the ovaries and fallopian tubes), and pelvic and para-aortic lymph node dissection are usually performed. Very large tumors that cannot be removed are debulked (reduction). These procedures can be performed via laparoscopic technique to decrease recovery time, minimize pain, and reduce postoperative complications. Ovarian cancer is staged during surgery.

Nursing care of the patient is similar to that for any patient having abdominal surgery (see Chapter 16). As for any patient after abdominal surgery, assess vital signs and pain and maintain catheters and drains. Teach her the importance of antiembolism stockings, incentive spirometry, and early ambulation.

Infections after ovarian cancer surgery commonly affect the respiratory and urinary tracts. Assess vital signs and monitor the quantity and quality of urine output.

After removing and staging ovarian cancer, *chemotherapy* is the treatment that is used most often. Cisplatin (Platinol), carboplatin, and taxanes of all types are the most common postoperative *drugs* used for treating all stages of ovarian cancer. They may be given IV and/or intraperitoneally. Intraperitoneal (IP) therapy is described in Chapter 13. New drugs continue to be tested that use monoclonal antibodies, hormones, and agents that target cell growth and tumor blood supply. Chapter 22 describes chemotherapy in detail, including associated nursing care.

❓ CLINICAL JUDGMENT CHALLENGE 71-1

Clinical Judgment; Evidence-Based Practice; Informatics **QSEN**

A 48-year-old woman is scheduled to have a bilateral salpingo-oophorectomy (BSO) and total abdominal hysterectomy (TAH) using a traditional open procedure for ovarian cancer. Her oncologist told her that, after she recovers from surgery, she may need to have adjuvant chemotherapy to destroy any remaining cancer cells. She is married with a teenage daughter who is in the twelfth grade. The patient tells you as her nurse that she is devastated that she "may not live to see her daughter go to the prom and graduate from high school."

1. How will you respond to the patient at this time?
2. What preoperative teaching will you provide for this patient and why?
3. What will you tell her about chemotherapy that may be necessary after surgery?
4. Where would you search for evidence about her expected quality of life and prognosis?
5. To what community resources would you refer this patient after discharge?

Care Coordination and Transition Management

Patients having surgery usually return to their home. Teach them to avoid tampons, douches, and sexual intercourse for at least 6 weeks or as instructed by the primary health care provider. Remind them to keep their follow-up surgical appointment and talk with the primary health care provider about resuming usual activities. Refer patients and their families to Gilda's Club (www.gildasclub.org) and the National Ovarian Cancer Coalition (NOCC) (www.ovarian.org) for more information and support groups. In Canada, the National Ovarian Cancer Association (www.ovariancanada.org) is available for the same purpose.

For patients with advanced metastatic disease, collaborate with the case manager, patient, and family for possible referral to hospice. Chapter 7 discusses end-of-life care and hospice in detail. The woman who is faced with the diagnosis of advanced ovarian cancer understandably is very anxious about dying. Encourage her to discuss her feelings. Provide realistic assurance, as well as accurate information about treatments. Patients report that their most distressing moments in the hospital were when they thought they were not getting adequate information. Encourage them to use their support systems of family members, friends, and clergy, including the hospital chaplain. Grief counseling is very appropriate. A visit from another woman who has survived a similar disease or referral to a support group may decrease fears. Refer the patient who fears passing the *BRCA1* or *BRCA2* gene to her daughter for genetic counseling and testing.

Ovarian cancer has a high recurrence rate. After recurrence, the cancer is treatable but no longer curable. If this occurs, the patient may deny symptoms at first or express feelings of anger and grief. The family is often fearful of the outcome. Provide encouragement and support during this difficult time and help the patient and her family work through their grief and prepare for death.

CERVICAL CANCER

❖ PATHOPHYSIOLOGY

The uterine cervix is covered with squamous cells on the outer cervix and columnar (glandular) cells that line the endocervical canal. Papanicolaou (Pap) tests sample cells from both areas as a screening test for cervical cancer. The squamo-columnar junction is the *transformation zone* where most cell abnormalities occur. The adolescent has more columnar cells exposed on the outer cervix, which may be one reason that she is more vulnerable to sexually transmitted infections (STIs) and human immune deficiency virus (HIV). In contrast, in the menopausal woman, the squamo-columnar junction may be higher up in the endocervical canal, making it difficult to sample for a Pap test.

Premalignant changes are described on a continuum from *atypia* (suspicious) to *cervical intraepithelial neoplasia (CIN)* to *carcinoma in situ (CIS),* which is the most advanced premalignant change. It generally takes years for the cervical cells to transform from normal to premalignant to invasive cancer. CIN, sometimes called *dysplasia,* is graded on a scale of 1 to 3, depending on the appearance of the cervical tissue under a microscope (ACS, 2017c). Not much tissue appears abnormal in CIN1 (mild dysplasia), which is thought to be the least serious cervical precancer; more tissue appears abnormal in CIN2 (moderate dysplasia). Most tissue looks abnormal in CIN3 (severe dysplasia as well as carcinoma *in situ*), which is the most serious precancer (ACS, 2017c).

Most cervical cancers arise from the squamous cells on the outside of the cervix. The other cancers arise from the mucus-secreting glandular cells (adenocarcinoma) in the endocervical canal. The disease spreads by direct extension to the vaginal mucosa, lower uterine segment, parametrium, pelvic wall, bladder, and bowel. Metastasis is usually confined to the pelvis, but distant spread can occur through lymphatic spread and the circulation to the liver, lungs, or bones.

Human papilloma virus infection (HPV) is the most common type of sexually transmitted infection (STI) in the United States (Centers for Disease Control and Prevention [CDC], 2017). Almost all women will have HPV sometime in their life, but not all types lead to cancer. Most cases of cervical cancer are caused by certain types of HPV. The high-risk HPV types, especially strains 16 and 18, impair the tumor-suppressor gene and cause most of the cervical cancers. The unrestricted tissue growth can spread, becoming invasive and metastatic (McCance et al., 2014). Risk factors for cervical cancer are listed in Table 71-2. The number of cases of cervical cancer (and deaths from cervical cancer) has decreased significantly over the past 40 years because more women regularly get Pap tests and HPV vaccines are routinely given (CDC, 2017).

Health Promotion and Maintenance

Girls and young women (ages 9 through 26 years) should receive one of the two currently used HPV vaccines, *Gardasil* and *Cervarix,* ideally before their first sexual contact to receive protection against the highest-risk HPV types that are responsible for most cervical cancers. It is also given for boys and young men (ages 9 through 26 years) to prevent genital warts. Cervarix protects girls and women ages 9 through 25 years against HPV infection to prevent cervical cancer.

Teach all young adults and parents of minors about the importance of receiving the vaccine and the need to have the entire series (three injections over 6 months). Tell them that the most frequent side effects are related to local irritation from the injections (e.g., pain, redness). Other common side effects include nausea, vomiting, dizziness, headache, and diarrhea.

The American Cancer Society (ACS) recommends that women have periodic pelvic examinations and Pap tests to screen for cervical cancer early. Teach women that they should begin these screening precautions at the age of 21 years. Between ages 21 and 29 years, women should have a Pap test every 3 years; women between ages 30 and 65 years should have a Pap test plus a human papilloma virus (HPV) test ("co-testing") every 5 years. More information on the HPV test is found later in this chapter. In the absence of co-testing, this population should still have a Pap test every 3 years. According to the ACS, women older than 65 years who have had regular cervical cancer testing with normal results should not receive Pap tests. Recommended guidelines from other health care organizations suggest a Pap test every 3 years for women older than 60 years (ACS, 2017c).

Canadian guidelines have also changed as delineated by the Society of Obstetricians and Gynaecologists of Canada (www.sogc.org). The 2013 recommendations of this group recommend that Pap testing begin at the age of 25 years of age instead of the previous guideline of 21, with regular testing every 3 years until age 70.

❖ INTERPROFESSIONAL COLLABORATIVE CARE

◆ Assessment: Noticing

Physical Assessment/Signs and Symptoms. The patient who has pre-invasive cancer is often asymptomatic. *The classic symptom of invasive cancer is painless vaginal bleeding.* Ask the patient if she has had or now has bleeding. It may start as spotting between menstrual periods or after sexual intercourse or douching. As the cancer grows, bleeding increases in frequency, duration, and amount and may become continuous.

Ask the woman if she has a watery, blood-tinged vaginal discharge that becomes dark and foul smelling (occurs as the disease progresses). Leg pain (along the sciatic nerve) or swelling of one leg may be a late symptom or may indicate recurrent disease. Flank pain may be a late symptom of hydronephrosis, indicating advanced cancer pressing on the ureters, backing up the urine into the kidney. Ask the patient if she has had other signs of recurrence or metastasis such as:

- Unexplained weight loss
- Dysuria (painful urination)
- Pelvic pain (caused by pressure of the tumor on the bladder or the bowel)
- Hematuria (bloody urine)
- Rectal bleeding
- Chest pain

A physical examination may not reveal any abnormalities in early preinvasive cervical cancer. The internal pelvic examination may identify late-stage disease.

Diagnostic Assessment. If Pap results are abnormal, an *HPV-typing DNA test* of the cervical sample can determine the presence of one or more high-risk types. The primary health care provider may perform a colposcopic examination to view the transformation zone. **Colposcopy** is a procedure in which application of an acetic acid solution is applied to the cervix. The cervix is then examined under magnification with a bright filter light that enhances the visualization of the characteristics of dysplasia or cancer. If abnormal tissue is recognized, multiple biopsies of the cervical tissue are performed.

If atypical glandular cells are suspected, the health care provider may perform an *endocervical curettage* (scraping of the endocervix wall) as well. Inform her that a small amount of bleeding is expected for up to 2 weeks after the biopsies.

◆ **Interventions: Responding**

Interventions for the woman with cervical cancer are similar to those for endometrial cancer: surgery, which is possibly followed by radiation and chemotherapy for late-stage disease.

Surgical Management. Early stage I management focuses on one of several local *cervical ablation* procedures, including electrosurgical excision, laser therapy, or cryosurgery. Factors that influence the choice of localized treatment versus surgical intervention include patient overall health, desire for future childbearing, tumor size and stage, cancer cell type, degree of lymph node involvement, and patient preference.

The **loop electrosurgical excision procedure (LEEP)** is short (10 to 30 minutes) and is performed in a physician's office or an ambulatory care setting with a local anesthetic injected into the cervix. A thin loop-wire electrode that transmits a painless electrical current is used to cut away affected tissue. LEEP is both a diagnostic procedure and a treatment because it provides a specimen that can be examined by a pathologist to ensure that the lesion was completely removed. Minimal impaired COMFORT is associated with this procedure. Spotting (very scant bleeding) after the procedure is common. Teach patients to adhere for 3 weeks to the restrictions listed in Chart 71-4.

Laser therapy is also an office procedure used for early cancers. A laser beam is directed to the abnormal tissues, where energy from the beam is absorbed by the fluid in the tissues, causing them to vaporize. A small amount of bleeding occurs with the procedure, and the woman may have a slight vaginal discharge. Healing occurs in 6 to 12 weeks. A disadvantage of this procedure is that no specimen is available for study.

Cryotherapy involves freezing of the cancer, causing subsequent necrosis. The procedure is usually painless, although some women have slight cramping after it. The patient has a heavy watery discharge for several weeks after the procedure. Instruct her to follow the restrictions in Chart 71-4.

CHART 71-4 **Patient and Family Education: Preparing for Self-Management**

Care After Local Cervical Ablation Therapies

- Refrain from sexual intercourse.
- Do not use tampons.
- Do not douche.
- Take showers rather than tub baths.
- Avoid lifting heavy objects.
- Report any heavy vaginal bleeding, foul-smelling drainage, or fever.

The usual time period for these restrictions is 3 weeks. Your primary health care provider may prescribe a different (longer or shorter) time frame for you.

In cases of microinvasive cancer, a *conization* can remove the affected tissue while still preserving fertility. This procedure is done when the lesion cannot be visualized by colposcopic examination. A cone-shaped area of cervix is removed surgically and sent to the laboratory to determine the extent of the cancer. Potential complications from this procedure include hemorrhage and uterine perforation. Long-term follow-up care is needed because new cancers can develop.

A *total hysterectomy* may be performed as treatment of microinvasive cancer if the woman does not want children or more children. A laparoscopic approach is commonly used. A radical hysterectomy and bilateral pelvic lymph node dissection may be as effective as radiation is for treating cancer that has extended beyond the cervix but not to the pelvic wall. Care for patients undergoing hysterectomy is found in the Uterine Leiomyoma section earlier in this chapter.

Nonsurgical Management. Radiation therapy is reserved for invasive cervical cancer. Brachytherapy and external beam radiation therapy are used in combination, depending on the extent and location of the lesion. The procedure is similar to that described in the section on endometrial cancer.

A combination of chemotherapy with cisplatin (Platinol) and radiation may also be used. This treatment modality shows increased survival times but increased toxicity for many patients. Examples of other drugs used alone or in combination include paclitaxel (Taxol), carboplatin, fluorouracil (5-FU), and mitomycin. See Chapter 22 for more information about the general nursing care for the patient on chemotherapy and radiation.

VULVOVAGINITIS

❖ *PATHOPHYSIOLOGY*

Vaginal discharge and itching are two common problems experienced by most women at some time in their lives. Vaginal infections may be transmitted sexually and nonsexually. Gonorrhea, syphilis, chlamydia, and herpes simplex virus infections are sexually transmitted infections (STIs) discussed in Chapter 74.

Vulvovaginitis is inflammation of the lower genital tract resulting from a disturbance of the balance of hormones and flora in the vagina and vulva. It may be characterized by itching, change in vaginal discharge, odor, or lesions. The most common causes of *nonsexually* transmitted infections include:

- Fungus (yeast) *(Candida albicans)*
- Bacterial vaginosis
- Postmenopausal vaginal atrophy
- Changes in the normal flora or pH (from douching)
- Chemical irritant or allergens (vaginal spray, fabric dyes, detergent) or foreign body (tampon)
- Drugs, especially antibiotics
- Immunosuppression from diabetes or human immune deficiency virus (HIV)
- Atrophic vaginitis
- Lichen planus (thickened, leathery skin and possible lesions)
- Vulvar leukoplakia (postmenopausal atrophy and thickening of vulvar tissues)
- Vulvar cancer
- Urinary incontinence

Pediculosis pubis (crab lice, or "crabs") and scabies (itch mite) are common parasitic infestations of the skin of the vulva that can be *sexually* transmitted.

Some women may have an *itch-scratch-itch cycle,* in which the itching leads to scratching, which causes excoriation that then must heal. As healing takes place, itching occurs again. If the cycle is not interrupted, the chronic scratching may lead to the white, thickened skin of lichen planus. This dry, leathery skin cracks easily, increasing the risk for infection.

❖ **INTERPROFESSIONAL COLLABORATIVE CARE**

Assess for vulvovaginitis by asking questions about the symptoms, assisting with a pelvic examination, and obtaining vaginal smears for laboratory testing. Ask if the patient is experiencing an itching or burning sensation, erythema (redness), edema, and/or superficial skin ulcers. Use a nonjudgmental approach and provide reassurance during the assessment because the patient may be embarrassed or afraid to discuss her symptoms. Encourage her to talk about her problem and its effect on her sexual health.

Interventions for vulvovaginitis depend on the specific vaginal infection. Proper health habits can benefit treatment. Instruct the patient to get enough rest and sleep, observe good dietary habits, exercise regularly, and use good personal hygiene. Teach her about how to manage her infection and prevent further infections (Chart 71-5).

Wet compresses, warm or tepid sitz baths for 30 minutes several times a day, and topical drugs such as estrogens and lidocaine can help relieve itching. Encourage the patient to wear breathable fabrics such as cotton and to avoid irritants or allergens in products such as laundry detergents or bath products.

Treatment of pediculosis and scabies is used if needed and includes:

- Applying lindane (Kwell, Kwellada) lotion, shampoo, or cream to the affected area as directed
- Cleaning affected clothes, bedding, and towels
- Disinfecting the home environment (Lice cannot live for more than 24 hours away from the body.)

TOXIC SHOCK SYNDROME

Toxic shock syndrome (TSS) can result from menstruation and tampon use. Other conditions associated with TSS include gynecologic surgical wound infection, nonsurgical infections, and use of internal contraceptives. TSS can be fatal. Extensive public education has led to a dramatically decreased number of women developing the infection.

In infection related to menstruation, menstrual blood provides a growth medium for *Staphylococcus aureus* (or, less frequently, group A *Streptococcus* [GAS], also known as *Streptococcus pyogenes*). Exotoxins produced from the bacteria cross the vaginal mucosa to the bloodstream via microabrasions from tampon insertion or prolonged use.

TSS usually develops within 5 days after the onset of menstruation. Most common symptoms include fever, rash, myalgias, sore throat, edema, and hypotension (Low, 2013). The rash associated with TSS often looks like a sunburn, and patients often develop broken capillaries in the eyes and skin. Educate all women on prevention of TSS (Chart 71-6).

Treatment includes removal of the infection source, such as a tampon; restoring fluid and electrolyte balance; administering drugs to manage hypotension; and IV antibiotics. Other measures may include transfusions to reverse low platelet counts and corticosteroids to treat skin changes.

👤 CHART 71-5 Patient and Family Education: Preparing for Self-Management

Prevention of Vulvovaginitis

- Wear cotton underwear.
- Avoid wearing tight clothing, such as pantyhose or tight jeans, because it can cause chafing. You can also get hot and sweaty, which can increase the risk for infection.
- Always wipe front to back after having a bowel movement or urinating.
- During bath or shower, cleanse inner labial mucosa with water, not soap.
- Do not douche or use feminine hygiene sprays.
- If your sexual partner has an infection of the sex organs, do not have intercourse with him or her until he or she has been treated.
- You are more likely to get an infection if you are pregnant, have diabetes, take oral contraceptive drugs, or are menopausal.
- Practice vulvar self-examination monthly.

👤 CHART 71-6 Patient and Family Education: Preparing for Self-Management

Prevention of Toxic Shock Syndrome

- Wash your hands before inserting a tampon.
- Do not use a tampon if it is dirty.
- Insert the tampon carefully to avoid injuring the delicate tissue in your vagina.
- Change your tampon every 3 to 6 hours.
- Do not use superabsorbent tampons.
- Use perineal pads ("sanitary napkins") (instead of tampons) at night.
- Call your primary health care provider if you suddenly experience a high temperature, vomiting, or diarrhea.
- Do not use tampons at all if you have had toxic shock syndrome.
- Not using tampons almost guarantees that you will not get toxic shock syndrome.

GET READY FOR THE NCLEX® EXAMINATION!

▌KEY POINTS

Review these Key Points for each NCLEX Examination Client Needs Category.

Safe and Effective Care Environment

- Collaborate with the case manager when planning care for patients with gynecologic cancers. **QSEN: Teamwork and Collaboration**

Health Promotion and Maintenance

- Teach women to follow the American Cancer Society's screening guidelines to prevent and early-detect for gynecologic cancers. **QSEN: Evidence-Based Practice**
- Teach women to practice safe sex to prevent infection of the reproductive tract.
- Teach women about risk factors for gynecologic cancers as described in Tables 71-2 and 71-3.

- Teach women how to prevent toxic shock syndrome (TSS) as listed in Chart 71-6. **QSEN: Safety**
- Refer patients with gynecologic problems to appropriate community resources such as the American Cancer Society.

Psychosocial Integrity

- Explain all tests, procedures, and treatments, especially if they cause impaired COMFORT during or after the procedures.
- Assess the patient's anxiety before any gynecologic surgery and encourage her to discuss her feelings about self-esteem, SEXUALITY, and REPRODUCTION. **QSEN: Patient-Centered Care**
- Encourage women who are having procedures that may interfere with fertility and/or SEXUALITY to express feelings of fear or grief. **QSEN: Patient-Centered Care**
- Encourage women with chronic or serious health problems to consider using support groups or counseling.

Physiological Integrity

- Plan postoperative care for women having a laparoscopic or traditional open total abdominal hysterectomy (TAH) as outlined in Chart 71-1.

- Provide health teaching for the woman who had an open TAH or vaginal hysterectomy about self-care after discharge (see Chart 71-2). **Clinical Judgment**
- Teach patients about specific restrictions after local cervical ablation therapy (see Chart 71-4).
- When caring for a patient who has a radioactive implant, use best practices as described in Chart 71-3. **QSEN: Safety**
- Teach the patient who is going home after a hysterectomy how to monitor for infection and other complications. **QSEN: Safety**
- Instruct patients receiving external beam radiation to the abdomen to gently wash the area; to not apply creams or lotions (unless prescribed by the radiologist); to not wash off marking; to avoid exposing the area to sunlight or temperature extremes; and to wear soft, nonirritating clothing.
- Assess for symptoms associated with toxic shock syndrome.

SELECTED BIBLIOGRAPHY

Asterisk indicates a classic or definitive work on this subject.

American Cancer Society (ACS). (2017a). *Sex and pelvic radiation therapy*. www.cancer.org/treatment/treatmentsandsideeffects/physicalsideeffects/sexualsideeffectsinwomen/sexualityforthewoman/sexuality-for-women-with-cancer-pelvic-rad.

American Cancer Society (ACS). (2017b). *Ovarian cancer prevention*. www.cancer.gov/cancertopics/pdq/prevention/ovarian/Patient/page3.

American Cancer Society (ACS). (2017c). *Cervical cancer prevention and early detection*. http://www.cancer.org/acs/groups/cid/documents/webcontent/003167-pdf.pdf.

American Congress of Obstetricians and Gynecologists (ACOG). (2013). *Statement on robotic surgery by ACOG*. www.acog.org/About_ACOG/News_Room/News_Releases/2013/Statement_on_Robotic_Surgery.

Bradley, L. (2013). *Hysteroscopic myomectomy*. www.uptodate.com/contents/hysteroscopic-myomectomy.

Centers for Disease Control and Prevention (CDC). (2017). *Genital HPV infection: Fact sheet*. www.cdc.gov/std/hpv/stdfact-hpv.htm.

Danesh, M., Hamzehgardeshi, Z., Moosazadeh, M., & Shabani-Asrami, F. (2015). The effect of hysterectomy on women's sexual function: A narrative review. *Medical Archives, 69*(6), 387–392.

*Gallo, T., Kashani, S., Patel, D. A., Elsahwi, K., Silasi, D. A., & Azodi, M. (2012). Robotic-assisted laparoscopic hysterectomy: Outcomes in obese and morbidly obese patients. *Journal of the Society of Laparoendoscopic Surgeons, 16*(3), 421.

*Lazarou, G. (2012). *Pelvic organ prolapse treatment and management*. http://emedicine.medscape.com/article/276259-treatment#a1134.

Low, D. (2013). Toxic shock syndrome: Major advances in pathogenesis, but not treatment. *Critical Care Clinics, 29*, 651–675.

Lowdermilk, D. L., Perry, S. E., Cashion, M. C., & Alden, K. R. (2016). *Maternity and women's health care* (11th ed.). St. Louis: Elsevier.

Matzo, M., Graham, C., Troup, C. L., & Ferrell, B. (2014). Development of a patient education resource for women with gynecologic cancers: Cancer and sexual health. *Clinical Journal of Oncology Nursing, 18*(3), 343–348.

McCance, K., Huether, S., Brashers, V., & Rote, N. (2014). *Pathophysiology: The biologic basis for disease in adults and children* (7th ed.). St. Louis: Mosby.

McCool, W. F., Durain, D., & Davis, M. (2014). Overview of latest evidence of uterine fibroids. *Nursing for Women's Health, 18*(4), 314–332.

National Cancer Institute (NCI) (2017). *Endometrial cancer treatment: Endometrial cancer prevention*. www.cancer.gov/cancertopics/pdq/prevention/endometrial/Patient/page3.

Nguyen, M., LaFargue, C., Pua, T., & Tedjarati, S. (2013). Grade 1 endometrioid endometrial carcinoma presenting with pelvic bone metastasis: A case report and review of the literature. *Case Reports in Obstetrics and Gynecology*, 2013. doi:10.1155/2013/807205.

Pagana, K., Pagana, T. J., & Pagana, T. N. (2017). *Mosby's diagnostic and laboratory test reference* (13th ed.). St. Louis: Mosby.

Slatnik, C. L., & Duff, E. (2015). Ovarian cancer: Ensuring early diagnosis. *Nurse Practitioner, 40*(9), 47–54.

*Storck, S. (2012). *Uterine artery embolization*. www.nlm.nih.gov/medlineplus/ency/article/007384.htm.

*U.S. Food and Drug Administration (USFDA) (2011). *Urogynecologic surgical mesh: Update on the safety and effectiveness of transvaginal placement for pelvic organ prolapse*. www.fda.gov/downloads/MedicalDevices/Safety/AlertsandNotices/UCM262760.pdf.

CHAPTER 72

Care of Patients With Male Reproductive Problems

Donna D. Ignatavicius

 http://evolve.elsevier.com/Iggy/

PRIORITY AND INTERRELATED CONCEPTS

The priority concepts for this chapter are:
- ELIMINATION
- CELLULAR REGULATION

✳ The ELIMINATION concept exemplar for this chapter is Benign Prostatic Hyperplasia, p. 1474.

✳ The CELLULAR REGULATION concept exemplar for this chapter is Prostate Cancer, p. 1481.

The interrelated concepts for this chapter are:
- SEXUALITY
- REPRODUCTION

LEARNING OUTCOMES

Safe and Effective Care Environment
1. Collaborate with health care team members to provide care for patients with male reproductive health problems.

Health Promotion and Maintenance
2. Teach men and their partners about community resources for reproductive cancers.
3. Develop a health teaching plan for men to prevent or detect early male reproductive cancers.

Psychosocial Integrity
4. Explain the psychosocial needs of men who have male reproductive problems, including issues associated with SEXUALITY and REPRODUCTION.

Physiological Integrity
5. Identify the assessment findings of benign prostatic hyperplasia (BPH) as they affect urinary ELIMINATION.
6. Describe the nursing implications for safe pharmacologic management of BPH.

7. Develop an evidence-based postoperative plan of care for a patient undergoing surgery for benign prostatic hyperplasia.
8. Evaluate risk factors for impaired CELLULAR REGULATION that manifest as male reproductive cancers.
9. Identify complementary and integrative therapies to incorporate into the patient's plan of care.
10. Discuss treatment options for prostate cancer with patients, partners, and/or families.
11. Differentiate preoperative teaching for patients having an open or laparoscopic radical prostatectomy.
12. Identify adverse effects of radiation therapy for male reproductive cancers.
13. Describe common options for treating erectile dysfunction.
14. Identify cultural considerations related to male reproductive problems.
15. Develop a plan of care for a patient with testicular cancer, including fertility issues.

Male reproductive problems can range from short-term infections to long-term health care problems that require end-of-life care, such as cancers. Any health issue that affects the male reproductive system can affect the human need for SEXUALITY, ELIMINATION, and REPRODUCTION. For example, some patients have surgeries that damage essential nerves that are needed to have an erection. Others have disorders that psychologically prevent the patient from engaging in his usual sexual activity. Chapter 2 provides a review of the nursing concepts applied in this chapter.

The role of the nurse and other health care team members is to be open, supportive, and nonjudgmental when caring for men with reproductive problems. Respect the man's privacy at all times.

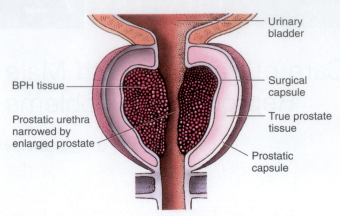

Urinary bladder

BPH tissue

Surgical capsule

Prostatic urethra narrowed by enlarged prostate

True prostate tissue

Prostatic capsule

FIG. 72-1 Benign prostatic hyperplasia (BPH) grows inward, causing narrowing of the urethra.

✳ ELIMINATION CONCEPT EXEMPLAR
Benign Prostatic Hyperplasia

❖ PATHOPHYSIOLOGY

With aging and increased dihydrotestosterone (DHT) levels, the glandular units in the prostate undergo nodular tissue **hyperplasia** (an increase in the number of cells). This altered tissue promotes local inflammation by attracting cytokines and other substances (McCance et al., 2014).

As the prostate gland enlarges, it extends upward into the bladder and inward, causing bladder outlet obstruction (BOO) (Fig. 72-1). In response, urinary ELIMINATION is affected in several ways, causing **lower urinary tract symptoms (LUTS)**. First, the detrusor (bladder) muscle thickens to help urine push past the enlarged prostate gland (McCance et al., 2014). In spite of the bladder muscle change, the patient has increased residual urine (stasis) and chronic urinary retention. The increased volume of residual urine often causes **overflow urinary incontinence**, in which the urine "leaks" around the enlarged prostate, causing dribbling. Urinary stasis can also result in urinary tract infections and bladder calculi (stones).

In a few patients, the prostate becomes very large, and the man cannot void (acute urinary retention [AUR]). The patient with this problem requires *emergent* care. In other patients, chronic urinary retention may result in a backup of urine and cause a gradual dilation of the ureters (**hydroureter**) and kidneys (**hydronephrosis**) if BPH is not treated. These urinary ELIMINATION problems can lead to chronic kidney disease as described in Chapter 68.

Etiology and Genetic Risk

Benign prostatic hyperplasia (BPH) is a very common health problem, but the exact cause is unclear. It is likely the result of a combination of aging and the influence of androgens that are present in prostate tissue, such as dihydrotestosterone (DHT) (McCance et al., 2014). A genetic or familial predisposition may contribute to the development of BPH in men younger than 60 years of age. Other risk factors for BPH development include (Patel & Parsons, 2014):

- Obesity
- Diabetes mellitus
- Testosterone and other androgen supplements
- Decreased physical activity

Incidence and Prevalence

Benign prostatic hypertrophy affects 8% of men under 40 years of age, 50% of those under 60 years of age, and 80% of men over 80 years of age. In 2020, 20 million men are expected to be over 60 years of age in the United States (Patel & Parsons, 2014).

❖ INTERPROFESSIONAL COLLABORATIVE CARE
◆ Assessment: Noticing

History. When taking a history, several standardized assessment tools are used to help the health care provider determine the severity of lower urinary tract symptoms (LUTS) associated with prostatic enlargement. One of the most commonly used assessments is the International Prostate Symptom Score (I-PSS), which incorporates the American Urological Association Symptom Index (AUA-SI) (Fig. 72-2) as questions 1 through 7. The additional question included on the I-PSS is the effect of the patient's urinary symptoms on quality of life. Most patients complete the questions as a self-administered tool because it is available in many languages. If the patient is illiterate (does not read) or does not feel like reading the questions, the nurse or health care provider can ask them. Be sure that older men wear their glasses or contact lenses if needed.

Physical Assessment/Signs and Symptoms. Ask about the patient's current urinary ELIMINATION pattern. Assess for urinary frequency and urgency. Determine the number of times the patient awakens during the night to void (**nocturia**). Other symptoms of LUTS include:

- Difficulty in starting (hesitancy) and continuing urination
- Reduced force and size of the urinary stream ("weak" stream)
- Sensation of incomplete bladder emptying
- Straining to begin urination
- Post-void (after voiding) dribbling or leaking

If frequency and nocturia do not occur with restricted urinary flow, the patient may develop an infection or other bladder problem. Ask whether the patient has had **hematuria** (blood in the urine) when starting the urine stream or at the end of voiding. BPH is a common cause of hematuria in older men due to infection.

The health care provider examines the patient for physical changes of the prostate gland. Remind him to void before the physical examination. Inspect and palpate the abdomen for a distended bladder. The primary health care provider may percuss the bladder. If the patient has a sense of urgency when gentle pressure is applied, the bladder may be distended. Obese patients are best assessed by percussion or bedside ultrasound bladder scanner rather than by inspection or palpation.

Prepare the patient for the prostate gland examination. Tell him that he may feel the urge to urinate as the prostate is palpated. Because the prostate is close to the rectal wall, it is easily examined by digital rectal examination (DRE). If needed, help the patient bend over the examination table or assume a side-lying fetal position, whichever is the easiest position for him. The primary health care provider examines the prostate for size and consistency. BPH presents as a uniform, elastic, nontender enlargement; whereas cancer of the prostate gland feels like a stony-hard nodule. Advise the patient that, after the prostate gland is palpated, it may be massaged to obtain a fluid sample for examination to rule out **prostatitis** (inflammation

International Prostate Symptom Score (I-PSS)

Patient Name:_____ Date of Birth:_____ Date Completed_____

In the past month:	Not at All	Less Than 1 in 5 Times	Less Than Half the Time	About Half the Time	More Than Half the Time	Almost Always	Your Score
1. Incomplete Emptying How often have you had the sensation of not emptying your bladder?	0	1	2	3	4	5	
2. Frequency How often have you had to urinate less than every 2 hours?	0	1	2	3	4	5	
3. Intermittency How often have you found you stopped and started again several times when you urinated?	0	1	2	3	4	5	
4. Urgency How often have you found it difficult to postpone urination?	0	1	2	3	4	5	
5. Weak Stream How often have you had a weak urinary stream?	0	1	2	3	4	5	
6. Straining How often have you had to strain to start urination?	0	1	2	3	4	5	
	None	**1 Time**	**2 Times**	**3 Times**	**4 Times**	**5 Times**	
7. Nocturia How many times do you typically get up at night to urinate?	0	1	2	3	4	5	
Total I-PSS Score							

Score: 1-7: Mild 8-19: Moderate 20-35: Severe

Quality of Life Due to Urinary Symptoms	Delighted	Pleased	Mostly Satisfied	Mixed	Mostly Dissatisfied	Unhappy	Terrible
If you were to spend the rest of your life with your urinary condition just the way it is now, how would you feel about that?	0	1	2	3	4	5	6

FIG. 72-2 The International Prostate Symptom Score (I-PSS). (Adapted from the American Urological Association Practice Guidelines Committee. [2003]. Guideline on the management of benign prostatic hyperplasia (BPH). *Journal of Urology, 170*[2 Pt 1], 530-547.)

Continued

About the I-PSS

The International Prostate Symptom Score (I-PSS) is based on the answers to seven questions concerning urinary symptoms and one question concerning quality of life. Each question concerning urinary symptoms allows the patient to choose one out of six answers indicating increasing severity of the particular symptom. The answers are assigned points from 0 to 5. The total score can therefore range from 0 to 35 (asymptomatic to very symptomatic).

The questions refer to the following urinary symptoms:

Questions	Symptom
1	Incomplete emptying
2	Frequency
3	Intermittency
4	Urgency
5	Weak Stream
6	Straining
7	Nocturia

Question 8 refers to the patient's perceived quality of life.

The first seven questions of the I-PSS are identical to the questions appearing on the American Urological Association (AUA) Symptom Index, which currently categorizes symptoms as follows:

Mild (symptom score less than or equal to 7)
Moderate (symptom score range 8 to 19)
Severe (symptom score range 20 to 35)

The International Scientific Committee (SCI), under the patronage of the World Health Organization (WHO) and the International Union Against Cancer (UICC), recommends the use of only a single question to assess the quality of life. The answers to this question range from "delighted" to "terrible," or 0 to 6. Although this single question may or may not capture the global impact of benign prostatic hyperplasia (BPH) symptoms or quality of life, it may serve as a valuable starting point for a doctor-patient conversation.

The SCI has agreed to use the symptom index for BPH, which has been developed by the AUA Measurement Committee, as the official worldwide symptoms assessment tool for patients suffering from prostatism.

The SCI recommends that physicians consider the following components for a basic diagnostic workup: history; physical examination; appropriate labs such as U/A, creatinine, etc.; and DRE or other evaluation to rule out prostate cancer.

FIG. 72-2, cont'd

and possible infection of the prostate), a common problem that can occur with BPH. If the patient has bacterial prostatitis, he is treated with broad-spectrum antibiotic therapy to prevent the spread of infection (McCance et al., 2014).

Psychosocial Assessment. Patients who have nocturia and other LUTS may be irritable or depressed as a result of interrupted sleep and annoying visits to the bathroom. Assess the effect of sleep interruptions on the patient's mood and mental status. Ask him about the impact of symptoms on SEXUALITY and libido (sexual desire).

Post-void dribbling and overflow incontinence may cause embarrassment and prevent the patient from socializing or leaving his home. For some patients, this social isolation can affect quality of life and lead to clinical depression and/or severe anxiety.

Laboratory Assessment. A *urinalysis* and urine *culture* are typically obtained to diagnose urinary tract infection and microscopic hematuria. If infection is present, the urinalysis measures the number of white blood cells (WBCs).

Other laboratory studies that may be performed include:
- A *complete blood count* (CBC) to evaluate any evidence of systemic infection (elevated WBCs) or anemia (decreased red blood cells [RBCs]) from hematuria
- *Blood urea nitrogen* (BUN) and serum creatinine levels to evaluate renal function (both are usually elevated with kidney disease)

- A *prostate-specific antigen* (PSA) and a serum acid phosphatase level if prostate cancer is suspected (both are typically elevated in patients who have prostate cancer)
- *Culture and sensitivity* of prostatic fluid (if expressed during the examination)

Other Diagnostic Assessment. Imaging studies that are typically performed are *transabdominal ultrasound* and/or *transrectal ultrasound (TRUS)* and an *MRI*. The patient having a TRUS lies on his side while the transducer is inserted into the rectum for viewing the prostate and surrounding structures. A tissue biopsy may also be done if the primary health care provider is uncertain whether the prostatic problem is benign or malignant.

In some cases, the physician uses a cystoscope to view the interior of the bladder, the bladder neck, and the urethra. This examination is used to study the presence and effect of bladder neck obstruction and is usually done in an ambulatory care setting. See Chapter 65 for a detailed description of *cystoscopy* and the nursing care needed for patients having this procedure.

Residual urine may be determined by *bladder ultrasound* immediately after the patient voids. As an alternative, because the patient voids before cystoscopy, residual urine may be measured when the cystoscope is inserted. *Urodynamic pressure-flow studies* may help diagnose and grade bladder outlet obstruction and detrusor muscle function.

◆ **Analysis: Interpreting**

The priority collaborative problems for the patient with benign prostatic hyperplasia (BPH) are:

1. Urinary retention due to bladder outlet obstruction
2. Decreased self-esteem due to overflow incontinence and possible sexual dysfunction with or without surgery

◆ **Planning and Implementation: Responding**

Improving Urinary Elimination

Planning: Expected Outcomes. The patient with BPH is expected to have a normal urinary ELIMINATION pattern without lower urinary tract symptoms (LUTS) or infection.

Interventions. Patients with symptomatic BPH are first treated with nonsurgical interventions, such as drug therapy. The Concept Map shows nursing assessment and collaborative interventions for the patient with BPH.

Nonsurgical Management. Drug therapy is a popular option for treating BPH. For patients with acute urinary retention (AUR) or those who do not respond to or cannot tolerate drug therapy, a noninvasive procedure or surgery is the treatment of choice for reducing bladder outlet obstruction.

Drug Therapy. Drugs from two major categories may be used alone, but most commonly they are given in combination. The health care provider usually prescribes a *5-alpha reductase inhibitor (5-ARI)* as first-line drug therapy. Examples of these drugs are finasteride (Proscar) and dutasteride (Avodart) (Burchum & Rosenthal, 2016). Normally, testosterone is converted to DHT in the prostate gland by the enzyme *5-alpha reductase*. By taking an enzyme-inhibiting agent, the patient's DHT levels decrease, which results in reducing the enlarged prostate.

The alpha-adrenergic receptors in prostatic smooth muscle enable the prostate gland to respond to *alpha-1 selective blocking agents,* such as tamsulosin (Flomax), alfuzosin (Uroxatral), doxazosin (Cardura, Cardura-1), and silodosin (Rapaflo). Tamsulosin is also available as an over-the-counter (OTC) drug (Burchum & Rosenthal, 2016). These drugs relax smooth

---

! NURSING SAFETY PRIORITY QSEN
Drug Alert

Remind patients who are being treated with a 5-ARI for BPH that they may need to take it for as long as 6 months before improvement is noticed. Teach them about possible side effects, which include erectile dysfunction (ED), decreased libido, and dizziness due to orthostatic hypotension. *Remind them to change positions carefully and slowly!*

---

muscles in the prostate gland, creating less urinary resistance and improved urinary flow. They also cause peripheral vasodilation and reduced peripheral vascular resistance.

! NURSING SAFETY PRIORITY QSEN
Drug Alert

If giving alpha blockers in an inpatient setting, assess for orthostatic (postural) hypotension, tachycardia, and syncope ("blackout"), especially after the first dose is given to older men. If the patient is taking the drug at home, teach him to be careful when changing position and to report any weakness, light-headedness, or dizziness to the health care provider immediately. Bedtime dosing may decrease the risk for problems related to hypotension. Teach patients taking a 5-ARI or an alpha-blocking drug to keep all appointments for follow-up laboratory testing because both drug classes can cause liver dysfunction.

The most effective drug therapy approach for many patients is a combination of a 5-ARI drug and an alpha-1 selective blocking agent. A commonly prescribed drug regimen is finasteride and doxazosin. Newer drugs, such as Jalyn, provide a combination of dutasteride and tamsulosin in a once-a-day capsule.

Other drugs may be helpful in managing specific urinary symptoms. For example, low-dose oral desmopressin, a synthetic antidiuretic analog, has been used successfully for nocturia (Burchum & Rosenthal, 2016). Tadalafil (Cialis), a drug usually given to treat erectile dysfunction, has also been approved for some men with BPH because it can improve lower urinary tract symptoms.

Complementary and Integrative Health. For many men with BPH, the U.S. Food and Drug Administration (FDA)–approved *Serenoa repens* (saw palmetto extract) helps manage the urinary symptoms associated with BPH and finasteride (Heidari et al., 2014). Results of studies to prove that this herb is effective are mixed. For patients who choose to take saw palmetto products (e.g., Permixon 160 mg twice a day), remind them to check with their health care provider before taking them because of potential interactions with prescribed drugs such as anticoagulants and NSAIDs. Side effects of saw palmetto are rare and mild (Burchum & Rosenthal, 2016).

Other Nonsurgical Interventions. Other interventions that may reduce obstructive symptoms include those that cause the release of prostatic fluid such as frequent sexual intercourse. This approach is helpful for the man whose obstructive symptoms result from an enlarged prostate with a large amount of retained prostatic fluid.

Teach patients with BPH to avoid drinking large amounts of fluid in a short time; to avoid alcohol, diuretics, and caffeine; and to void as soon as they feel the urge. These measures are aimed at preventing overdistention of the bladder, which may result in loss of detrusor muscle tone. Teach patients to avoid any drugs that can cause urinary retention, especially anticholinergics,

CONCEPT MAP

BENIGN PROSTATIC HYPERPLASIA (BPH)

PAIN — ELIMINATION — SEXUALITY

NOTICE IN THE HISTORY

Davey Smitt, a 64-year-old with BPH, is admitted with a urinary tract infection (UTI), hematuria, and hydronephrosis. His wife says their sexual relationship has been nonexistent due to her husband's BPH. He has used saw palmetto extract for his urinary symptoms with some relief.

Pathophysiology →

As the prostate gland enlarges, bladder outlet obstruction occurs and the patient develops urinary stasis and retention.
- Increased volume of residual → bladder outlet obstruction → urine stasis → urine "leaks" around enlarged prostate → dribbling
- Urinary stasis → UTI and bladder calculi
- Chronic retention → backup of urine causes gradual dilation of ureters, hydronephrosis if not treated

Data Synthesis →

PATIENT PROBLEMS

Urinary retention due to bladder outlet obstruction

Planning →

EXPECTED OUTCOMES

Normal urinary elimination pattern without urinary hesitancy, urgency, or infection

INTERVENTIONS—RESPONDING

1 Nonjudgment

Respect privacy at all times. *Being open, supportive, and nonjudgmental when caring for the patient with SEXUALITY issues facilitates trust.*

2 Physical Assessment of Elimination—Noticing

Perform focused assessment of urinary pattern: frequency, hesitancy, urgency, presence of weak stream, nocturia, sensation of incomplete emptying, straining, hematuria, and post-void dribbling. *Evaluates whether BPH is causing hematuria. If frequency and nocturia do not occur with this elimination problem of restricted urinary flow, it may be infection or other bladder problem.*

3 Drug Therapy

Explain the mechanisms of action, side effects, and implications for drug therapy for BPH. *Minimizes side effects and the potential for injury.*

4 Nursing Safety Priority: Drug Alert!

- Assess for orthostatic hypotension, tachycardia, and syncope from alpha blockers. *Minimizes potential for injury from falls from orthostatic hypotension.*
- Instruct the patient to report weakness, lightheadedness, or dizziness; monitor liver function, and side effects, including erectile dysfunction, and decreased libido. *Providing accurate discharge information prevents serious complications.*

5 Interpreting Laboratory Values

- Obtain urinalysis (U/A) and culture, and complete blood count. *U/A and culture detects UTI and hematuria; ↑ WBC is sign of infection, ↓ RBC indicates anemia from hematuria.*
- Obtain blood urea nitrogen (BUN) and serum creatinine, prostate-specific antigen (PSA), and serum acid phosphatase level. *BUN and serum creatinine increase detects renal dysfunction; increased PSA and serum phosphatase detects prostate cancer.*
- Obtain culture and sensitivity of prostatic fluid if expressed during the exam. *Rules out prostatitis.*

6 Reducing Obstructive Symptoms

- Instruct the patient to avoid large amounts of fluid, alcohol, diuretics, caffeine; void as soon as the urge is felt. *Promotes ELIMINATION and prevents bladder overdistention.*
- Inform the patient that frequent sexual intercourse can reduce obstructive symptoms. *Relieves symptoms in the patient who has a large amount of retained prostatic fluid.*
- Teach to avoid anticholinergics, antihistamines, and decongestants. *These medications cause urinary retention.*

7 Psychosocial Integrity and Sexuality

Assess the patient's acceptance of body image related to BPH and its impact on sleep and sexual function that affects mood and mental status. *Evaluates irritability or depression that may occur with nocturia. Evaluates embarrassment of postvoid incontinence that can prevent socialization. Evaluates effect on SEXUALITY.*

8 Herbal Remedies

Remind the patient to check with the provider before taking complementary therapies. *Teaches patients that scientific evidence is lacking. Some herbs such as saw palmetto used for urinary symptoms can interfere with prescription drugs.*

9 Treatment Options – TURP

If surgery is a chosen treatment option, consider the patient's general physical condition, size of prostate, patient preferences, anxiety, and misconceptions. *Assists with options for treatment of BPH and prevents postoperative complications.*

Concept Map by Deanne A. Blach, MSN, RN

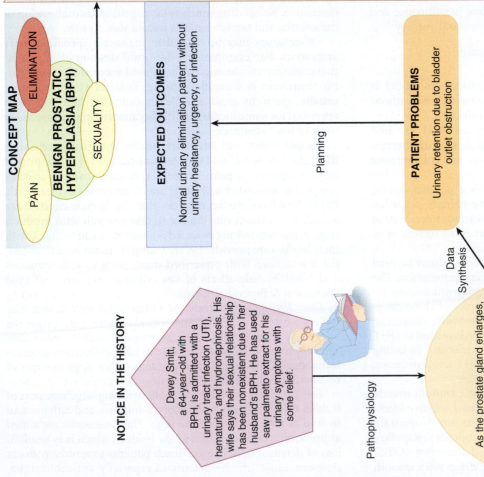

antihistamines, and decongestants. *Emphasize the importance of telling any health care provider about the diagnosis of BPH so these drugs are not prescribed.*

If drug therapy or other measures are not helpful in relieving urinary symptoms, several noninvasive techniques are available to shrink or destroy excess prostate tissue. For example, a new procedure called **prostate artery embolization** is performed by an interventional radiologist (IR) and is beginning to gain widespread acceptance in the United States. In this procedure, the IR threads a small vascular catheter into the prostate's arteries and injects particles blocking some of the blood flow to shrink the prostate gland. The patient is placed under moderate sedation rather than general anesthesia, which allows a typical discharge from the hospital in as few as 3 hours after the procedure. Most men report marked improvement in LUTS within the first month or so after the procedure.

Other procedures that destroy excess prostate tissue may be done in a primary health care provider's office or another ambulatory care setting. Examples include:

- *Transurethral needle ablation (TUNA)* (low radiofrequency energy shrinks the prostate)
- *Transurethral microwave therapy (TUMT)* (high temperatures heat and destroy excess tissue)
- *Interstitial laser coagulation (ILC)*, also called *contact laser prostatectomy (CLP)* (laser energy coagulates excess tissue)
- *Electrovaporization of the prostate (EVAP)* (high-frequency electrical current cuts and vaporizes excess tissue)

Prostatic stents may be placed into the urethra to maintain permanent patency after a procedure for destroying or removing prostatic tissue. All of these highly technical nonsurgical treatments use local or regional anesthesia and do not require an indwelling urinary catheter. They are also associated with less risk for complications such as intraoperative bleeding and erectile dysfunction when compared with traditional surgical approaches. Patients can return to their usual activities in a day or two.

Surgical Management. For patients who are not candidates for nonsurgical management or do not want to take drugs or have other treatment options, surgery may be performed. The gold standard surgery has been a **transurethral resection of the prostate (TURP),** in which the enlarged part of the prostate is removed through an endoscopic instrument. However, the holmium laser enucleation of the prostate (HoLEP) procedure, laparoscopic prostatic adenomectomy, and robotic-assisted simple prostatectomy (RASP) are safer minimally invasive surgeries (MISs) that may be performed for BPH. For a few men, an open prostatectomy (entire prostate removal) may be performed. (See discussion of Surgical Management in the Prostate Cancer section.) Some or all of these criteria indicate the need for surgery:

- Acute urinary retention (AUR)
- Chronic urinary tract infections secondary to residual urine in the bladder
- Hematuria
- Hydronephrosis

Preoperative Care. When planning surgical interventions, the patient's general physical condition, the size of the prostate gland, and the man's preferences are considered. The patient may have many fears and misconceptions about prostate surgery, such as believing that automatic loss of sexual functioning or permanent incontinence will occur. Assess the patient's anxiety, correct any misconceptions about the surgery, and

provide accurate information to him and his family. Regardless of the type of surgery to be performed, reinforce information about anesthesia (see Chapter 15). Remind patients taking anticoagulants that the drugs will be discontinued before a TURP or open prostate surgery to prevent postoperative bleeding. Other general preoperative care is described in Chapter 14.

The patient may have other medical problems that increase the risk for complications of general anesthesia and may be advised to have regional anesthesia. Epidural and spinal anesthesia are the most common types of anesthesia used for a TURP. Because the patient is awake, it is easier to assess for hyponatremia (low serum sodium), fluid overload, and water intoxication, which can result from large-volume bladder irrigations.

After a TURP, all patients have an indwelling urethral catheter. *Be sure that they know that they will feel the urge to void while the catheter is in place.* Tell the patient that he will likely have traction on the catheter that may cause discomfort. However, reassure him that analgesics will be prescribed to relieve his pain. Explain that it is normal for the urine to be blood tinged after surgery. Small blood clots and tissue debris may pass while the catheter is in place and immediately after it is removed. Some patients also have continuous bladder irrigation (CBI), depending on the procedure performed.

Operative Procedures. The traditional TURP is a "closed" surgery. To perform the procedure, the surgeon inserts a resectoscope (an instrument similar to a cystoscope, but with a cutting and cauterizing loop) through the urethra. The enlarged portion of the prostate gland is then removed in small pieces (prostate chips). A similar procedure is the transurethral incision of the prostate (TUIP) in which small cuts are made into the prostate to relieve pressure on the urethra. This alternate technique is used for smaller prostates. To prevent bleeding and excess clotting, a fibrinolytic inhibitor such as tranexamic acid (Cyklokapron) may be used during surgery.

The disadvantage of a TURP is that, because only small pieces of the gland are removed, remaining prostate tissue may continue to grow and cause urinary obstruction, requiring additional TURPs. Urethral trauma from the resectoscope with resulting urethral strictures is also possible.

In many large medical centers around the world, specialists can perform newer minimally invasive procedures, often using robotic-assisted techniques or laparoscopic procedures. Very little blood is lost during these procedures, and patient recovery is faster than that for the more traditional TURP.

Postoperative Care. During any surgical procedure for BPH, a urinary catheter is placed into the bladder. Traction is often applied on the catheter by pulling it taut and taping it to the patient's abdomen or thigh. If the catheter is taped to the patient's thigh, instruct him to keep his leg straight. The patient who had a TURP may have a catheter and continuous bladder irrigation (CBI) in place for several days. For the CBI, a three-way urinary catheter is used to allow drainage of urine and inflow of a bladder irrigating solution (Fig. 72-3). Be sure to maintain the flow of the irrigant to keep the urine clear. When measuring the fluid in the urinary drainage bag, be sure to subtract the amount of irrigating solution that was used to determine actual urinary output.

Patients having an MIS procedure do *not* typically have a CBI and are discharged within 24 hours after surgery. Most patients are discharged with the catheter in place.

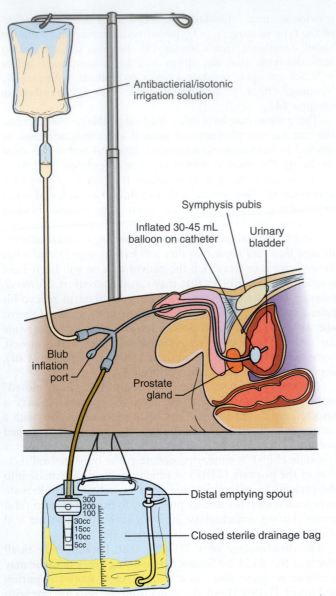

Antibactierial/isotonic irrigation solution

Symphysis pubis

Inflated 30-45 mL balloon on catheter

Urinary bladder

Blub inflation port

Prostate gland

Distal emptying spout

Closed sterile drainage bag

FIG. 72-3 Continuous bladder irrigation system after a TURP. *TURP,* Transurethral resection of the prostate.

❓ NCLEX EXAMINATION CHALLENGE 72-1

Physiological Integrity

A client has continuous bladder irrigation after surgery yesterday. The amount of bladder irrigating solution that has infused over the past 12 hours is 1050 mL. The amount of fluid in the urinary drainage bag is 1825 mL. The nurse records that the client had _____ mL urinary output in the past 12 hours. **Fill in the blank.**

⊛ CONSIDERATIONS FOR OLDER ADULTS

Patient-Centered Care QSEN

When caring for older men who may become confused after surgery, reorient them frequently and remind them not to pull on the catheter. If the patient is restless or "picks" at tubes, provide a familiar object such as a family picture for him to hold for distraction and a feeling of security. Do not restrain the patient unless all other alternatives have failed.

◎ CHART 72-1   Best Practice for Patient Safety & Quality Care QSEN

Care of the Patient After Transurethral Resection of the Prostate

- Monitor the patient closely for signs of infection. Older men undergoing prostate surgery often also have underlying chronic diseases (e.g., cardiovascular disease, chronic lung disease, diabetes).
- Help the patient out of the bed to the chair as soon as permitted to prevent complications of immobility. Older men may need assistance because of underlying changes in the musculoskeletal system (e.g., decreased range of motion, stiffness in joints). These patients are at *high risk* for falls.
- Assess the patient's pain every 2 to 4 hours and intervene as needed to control pain.
- Provide a safe environment for the patient. Anticipate a temporary change in mental status for the older patient in the immediate postoperative period as a result of anesthetics and unfamiliar surroundings. Reorient the patient frequently. Keep catheter tubes secure.
- Maintain the rate of the continuous bladder irrigation to ensure clear urine without clots and bleeding.
- Use normal saline solution for the intermittent bladder irrigant unless otherwise prescribed. Normal saline solution is isotonic.
- Monitor the color, consistency, and amount of urine output.
- Check the drainage tubing frequently for external obstructions (e.g., kinks) and internal obstructions (e.g., blood clots, decreased output).
- Assess the patient for reports of severe bladder spasms with decreased urinary output, which may indicate obstruction.
- If the urinary catheter is obstructed, irrigate it per agency or surgeon protocol.
- Notify the surgeon immediately if the obstruction does not resolve by hand irrigation or if the urinary return looks like ketchup.

Remind the patient that, because of the urinary catheter's large diameter and the pressure of the retention balloon on the internal sphincter of the bladder, he will feel the urge to void continuously. This is a normal sensation, not a surgical complication. Advise him not to try to void around the catheter, which causes the bladder muscles to contract and may result in painful spasms. Chart 72-1 summarizes the nursing care for patients having a TURP.

❗ NURSING SAFETY PRIORITY QSEN

Critical Rescue

After a TURP, monitor the patient's urine output every 2 to 4 hours and vital signs, including pain assessment, every 4 hours for the first postoperative day or according to agency or surgeon protocol. Assess for postoperative bleeding. *Patients who undergo a TURP are at risk for severe bleeding or hemorrhage after surgery. Although rare, bleeding is most likely within the first 24 hours.* Bladder spasms or movement may trigger fresh bleeding from previously controlled vessels. This bleeding may be arterial or venous, but venous bleeding is more common.

Observe for other possible but uncommon complications of TURP, such as infection and incontinence. Teach the patient that sexual function should not be affected after surgery but that retrograde ejaculation is possible. In this case, most of the semen flows backward into the bladder so only a small amount will be ejaculated from the penis.

Improving Self-Esteem

Planning: Expected Outcomes. The expected outcome is that the patient will experience improved self-esteem by managing incontinence through BPH treatment.

! NURSING SAFETY PRIORITY (QSEN)

Critical Rescue

If arterial bleeding occurs, the urinary drainage is bright red or ketchup-like with numerous clots. Notify the surgeon immediately and irrigate the catheter with normal saline solution per surgeon or hospital protocol. In rare instances the surgeon may prescribe aminocaproic acid (Amicar) to control bleeding. If this drug does not work, surgical intervention may be needed to clear the bladder of clots and stop bleeding.

If the bleeding is *venous,* the urine output is burgundy, with or without any change in vital signs. *Inform the surgeon of any bleeding.* Closely monitor the patient's hemoglobin (Hgb) and hematocrit (Hct) levels for anemia as a result of blood loss.

? NCLEX EXAMINATION CHALLENGE 72-2

Physiological Integrity

A client had a transurethral resection of the prostate (TURP) with continuous bladder irrigation yesterday. The staff nurse notes that the urinary drainage is pink tinged and clear. What is the nurse's **best** action?

A. Notify the charge nurse as soon as possible.
B. Increase the rate of the bladder irrigation.
C. Document the assessment in the medical record.
D. Prepare the patient for a blood transfusion.

Interventions. The patient with BPH typically has frequent urges to void and may have overflow incontinence at times because of urinary retention. Teach him to keep the surrounding area clean and dry to prevent skin breakdown. Remind him to toilet when he feels the urge and, if needed, to wear a small absorbent pad to prevent undergarment soiling. Involve the patient's sexual partner, if any, in teaching about the cause of the incontinence and any prescribed treatment. Once the patient is treated either with drug therapy or surgery, the incontinence subsides.

Care Coordination and Transition Management

The patient with benign prostatic hyperplasia (BPH) is typically managed at home. Patients who have nonsurgical interventions or surgery are also discharged to their home or other setting from where they were admitted.

Home Care Preparation. Patients having surgery typically are discharged with a urinary catheter in place for about a week or longer. Teach patients not to take a bath or swim to prevent a urinary tract infection while the catheter is in place. When the urinary catheter is removed, the patient may experience burning on urination and some urinary frequency, dribbling, and leakage. Reassure him that these symptoms are normal and will decrease. Instruct him to increase fluid intake to at least 2000 to 2500 mL daily, which helps decrease dysuria and keep the urine clear. *Be aware that an older patient who has renal disease or who is at risk for heart failure may not be able to tolerate this much fluid.*

Self-Management Education. Some patients, especially those who have had a TURP, may have temporary loss of control of urination or a dribbling of the urine. Reassure the patient that these symptoms are almost always temporary and will resolve. Also remind him that REPRODUCTION ability should not be affected by surgery.

Help the patient and his family find ways to keep his clothing dry until sphincter control returns. Instruct him to contract and relax his sphincter frequently to re-establish urinary ELIMINATION

EVIDENCE-BASED PRACTICE (QSEN)

What Is the Quality of Life for Patients Who Have Surgery for BPH?

Yim, P.W., Wang, W., Jiang, Y., Zakir, H.A., Toh, P.C., Lopez, V., et al. (2015). Health-related quality of life, physical well-being, and sexual function in patients with benign prostatic hyperplasia after prostatic surgery. *Applied Nursing Research, 28*(4), 274-280.

This research was a cross-sectional descriptive, correlational study using 94 volunteers from one hospital to examine quality of life for men who had previously had surgery for benign prostatic hyperplasia (BPH). The researchers asked these participants to complete five different tools to measure the study variables, including the International Index of Erectile Function and the Short-Form Health Survey. The findings revealed that many men who have surgery for BPH have poor physical health and continue to experience episodes of lower urinary tract symptoms (LUTS) and erective dysfunction (ED).

Level of Evidence: 4

This study used a nonexperimental, correlational research design.

Commentary: Implications for Practice and Research

Although the research design prevents generalizability, the implications for practice demonstrate the need for health teaching to ensure that patients who had surgery for BPH receive continued health care follow-up. Problems such as LUTS and ED can cause stress, depression, and a decreased quality of life. This study needs to be replicated using a larger sample across multiple settings and male demographic variables.

control (Kegel exercises). External urinary (condom) catheters are not used except in extreme cases because they may give the patient a false sense of security and delay urinary control.

Health Care Resources. Patients being managed for BPH usually do not require extensive follow-up care or health care resources. Men who are of advanced age may need one or two visits from a home health care agency to ensure that they are not experiencing complications and can provide self-care.

Teach patients to have follow-up care as recommended by the surgeon. After prostatic surgery, some men experience a return of LUTS and/or erectile dysfunction, which can decrease their quality of life (Yim et al., 2015) (see the Evidence-Based Practice box).

◆ Evaluation: Reflecting

Evaluate the care of the patient with BPH based on the identified priority patient problem. The primary expected outcome is that the patient will:

- Have improved urinary ELIMINATION as a result of appropriate and effective collaborative management
- Experience improved self-esteem as a result of effective BPH management

✳ CELLULAR REGULATION CONCEPT EXEMPLAR
Prostate Cancer

❖ PATHOPHYSIOLOGY

Testosterone and dihydrotestosterone (DHT) are the major androgens (male hormones) in the adult male. Testosterone is produced by the testis and circulates in the blood. DHT is a testosterone derivative in the prostate gland. In some patients, the prostate grows very rapidly, leading to noncancerous high-grade

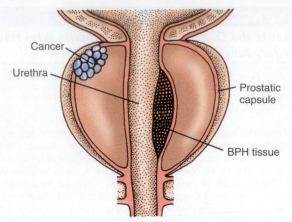

FIG. 72-4 Prostate gland with cancer and benign prostatic hyperplasia (BPH). Note that cancer normally arises in the periphery of the gland, whereas BPH occurs in the center of the gland.

prostatic intraepithelial neoplasia (PIN). This impairment of CELLULAR REGULATION causes men to be at a higher risk for developing prostate cancer than men who do not have that growth pattern.

Many prostate tumors are androgen sensitive (McCance et al., 2014). Most are adenocarcinomas and arise from epithelial cells located in the posterior lobe or outer portion of the gland (Fig. 72-4).

Of all malignancies, prostate cancer is one of the slowest growing, and it metastasizes (spreads) in a predictable pattern. Common sites of metastasis are the nearby lymph nodes, bones, lungs, and liver (McCance et al., 2014). The bones of the pelvis, sacrum, and lumbar spine are most often affected. Chapter 21 describes staging categories of localized and advanced cancers.

Etiology

Prostate cancer is caused by a number of factors. Advanced age is the leading risk factor. The risk increases for men who have a first-degree relative (brother, father) with the disease.

🌐 CULTURAL/SPIRITUAL CONSIDERATIONS
Patient-Centered Care **QSEN**

Race is the second most common risk factor for prostate cancer because the disease affects African Americans more often than other ethnic/racial groups, followed by Caucasians (Euro-Americans) and Hispanic-American men (McCance et al., 2014). The reasons for these differences are not known but may be related to socioeconomic factors, health care disparities, and lack of education (ACS, 2017).

Other risk factors that may play a role are eating a diet high in animal fat (e.g., red meat) and refined carbohydrates or having a low fiber intake. Men who have had a vasectomy or those who were exposed to environmental toxins, such as arsenic, may also be at increased risk for the disease (McCance et al., 2014).

Incidence and Prevalence

Prostate cancer is the second most common type of cancer in men in the world and, if found early, has a nearly 100% cure rate. Men older than 65 years have the greatest risk for the disease. In the United States, one in every six African-American

men and one in every eight Euro-American men have the disease (ACS, 2017).

Health Promotion and Maintenance

Teach men about the most recent American Cancer Society (ACS) guidelines for prostate cancer screening and early detection (ACS, 2017). The current recommendations are that men should make an informed decision about whether to have prostate cancer screening. Although not agreed on by all authoritative sources, starting at the age of 50 years, men should discuss the options of having prostate-specific antigen testing with their primary health care provider. Men at a higher risk for prostate cancer, including African Americans or men who have a first-degree relative with prostate cancer before the age of 65 years, should have this discussion at age 45 years. Men who have multiple first-degree relatives with prostate cancer at an early age should discuss screening at age 40 years (ACS, 2017).

Although a family history of prostate cancer cannot be changed, certain nutritional habits can be altered to possibly decrease the risk for the disease. First, teach men to eat a healthy, balanced diet, including decreasing animal fat (e.g., red meat). Instead of red meat, remind them to eat more fish and other foods high in *omega-3 fatty acids* because they are thought to be helpful in preventing cancer. Also reinforce the need to increase fruits, vegetables, and high-fiber foods.

❖ INTERPROFESSIONAL COLLABORATIVE CARE
◆ Assessment: Noticing

History. Assess the patient's age, race/ethnicity, and family history of prostate cancer. Ask about his nutritional habits, especially focusing on the intake of red meat, fish, and fruits and vegetables. Assess whether the patient has any problems with urinary ELIMINATION. Take a drug history to determine if he is taking any medication that could affect voiding. The first symptoms that the man may report are related to bladder outlet obstruction, such as difficulty in starting urination, frequent bladder infections, and urinary retention. Ask about urinary frequency, hematuria (blood in the urine), and nocturia (voiding during the night). Ask if he has had any pain during intercourse, especially when ejaculating. Inquire if he has had or currently has any other pain (particularly bone pain), a symptom associated with advanced prostate cancer. Ask him if he has had any recent unexpected weight loss.

Take a sexual history for recent changes in SEXUALITY, including libido or function. Ask about current or previous sexually transmitted infections, penile discharge, or scrotal pain or swelling.

Physical Assessment/Signs and Symptoms. Most *early* cancers are diagnosed while the patient is having a routine physical examination or is being treated for benign prostatic

---

🧬 GENETIC/GENOMIC CONSIDERATIONS
Patient-Centered Care **QSEN**

Many gene mutations play a role in various types of prostate cancer. Some men with the most aggressive prostate cancers have *BRCA2* mutations similar to those women who have *BRCA2*-associated breast and ovarian cancers. The most common genetic factor that increases the risk for prostate cancer is a mutation in the glutathione *S*-transferase (*GST P1*) gene. This gene is normally part of the pathway that helps prevent cancer (McCance et al., 2014).

hyperplasia (BPH). Gross blood in the urine (hematuria) is a common sign of *late* prostate cancer. Assess for pain in the pelvis, spine, hips, or ribs. Pain and swollen nodes indicate advanced disease that has spread. Take and record the patient's weight because unexpected weight loss is also common when the disease is advanced.

Prepare the patient for a digital rectal examination (DRE). On rectal examination, a prostate that is found to be stony hard and with palpable irregularities or indurations is suspected to be malignant.

Psychosocial Assessment. A diagnosis of any type of cancer causes fear and anxiety for most people. Some men, particularly African Americans, develop the disease in their 40s and 50s when they are perhaps planning their retirements, putting their children through college, and/or enjoying their middle years. Assess the reaction of the patient to the diagnosis and observe how his family reacts to the illness. Men may describe their feelings as shock, fear, anger, and "roller coaster." Expect that patients usually go through the grieving process and may be in denial or depressed. Determine what support systems they have, such as spiritual leaders or community group support, to help them through diagnosis, treatment, and recovery.

One of the biggest concerns for the man may be his ability for sexual function after cancer treatment. Tell him that function will depend on the type of treatment he has. Common surgical techniques used today do not involve cutting the perineal nerves that are needed for an erection. A dry climax may occur if the prostate is removed because it produces most of the fluid in the ejaculate. Refer the patient to his surgeon (urologist), sex therapist, or intimacy counselor if available.

Laboratory Assessment. **Prostate-specific antigen (PSA)** is a glycoprotein produced by the prostate. *PSA analysis is used as a screening test for prostate cancer.* If the test is performed, it should be drawn before the DRE because the examination can cause an increase in PSA caused by prostate irritation.

Most authoritative sources agree that the normal blood level of PSA in men younger than 50 years is less than 2.5 ng/mL. PSA levels increase to as high as 6.5 ng/mL when men reach their 70s. *African-American men have a slighter higher normal value, but the reason for this difference is not known. Because other prostate problems also increase the PSA level, it is not specifically diagnostic for cancer.* However, the level associated with prostate cancer is usually much higher than those occurring with problems such as prostatitis and benign prostatic hyperplasia (Pagana et al., 2017).

An elevated PSA level should decrease a few days after a prostatectomy for cancer. An increase in the PSA level several weeks after surgery may indicate that the disease has recurred.

Because PSA is not absolutely specific to prostate cancer, another test, *early prostate cancer antigen (EPCA-2),* may be a serum marker for prostate cancer. It can detect changes in the prostate gland early and is a very sensitive test. EPCA-2 may also eliminate the need to perform a biopsy of prostate tissue (Pagana et al., 2017).

Other Diagnostic Assessment. After assessments by DRE and PSA, most patients have a *transrectal ultrasound (TRUS)* of the prostate in an ambulatory care or imaging setting. The technician inserts a small probe into the rectum and obtains a view of the prostate using sound waves. If prostate cancer is suspected, a *biopsy* is usually performed in the physician's office to obtain an accurate diagnosis. Before the procedure, the physician uses lidocaine jelly on the ultrasound probe and/

or injects lidocaine into the prostate gland to promote patient comfort.

! NURSING SAFETY PRIORITY **QSEN**

Action Alert

After a transrectal ultrasound with biopsy, instruct the patient about possible complications, although rare, including hematuria with clots, signs of infection, and perineal pain. Teach him to report fever, chills, bloody urine, and any difficulty voiding. Advise him to avoid strenuous physical activity and to drink plenty of fluids, especially in the first 24 hours after the procedure. Teach him that a small amount of bleeding turning the urine pink is expected during this time. However, bright red bleeding should be reported to the health care provider immediately.

After prostate cancer is diagnosed, the patient has additional imaging and blood studies to determine the extent of the disease. Common tests include lymph node biopsy, CT of the pelvis and abdomen, and MRI to assess the status of the pelvic and para-aortic lymph nodes. A radionuclide bone scan may be performed to detect metastatic bone disease. An enlarged liver or abnormal liver function study results indicate possible liver metastasis.

Patients with advanced prostate cancer often have *elevated levels of serum acid phosphatase.* Most men with bone metastasis have *elevated serum alkaline phosphatase* levels and severe pain.

◆ Analysis: Interpreting

The priority collaborative problem for the patient with prostate cancer is *Potential for metastasis due to invasion of cancer cells in other parts of the body.*

◆ Planning and Implementation: Responding

Preventing Metastasis

Planning: Expected Outcomes. The expected outcome is that the patient will not experience metastasis as a result of prompt and effective collaborative management of prostate cancer.

Interventions. As with any cancer, accurate staging and grading of prostate tumors guide treatment planning and monitoring during the course of the disease. Patients are faced with several treatment options. A urologist and an oncologist usually collaborate to help patients make the best decision.

Active Surveillance. Because prostate cancer is slow growing with late metastasis, older men who are asymptomatic and have other illnesses may choose observation without immediate active treatment, especially if the cancer is early stage. This option is known as **active surveillance (AS)**. This form of treatment involves initial surveillance with active treatment only if the symptoms become bothersome. The average time from diagnosis to start of treatment is up to 10 years. During the AS period, men are monitored at regular intervals through DRE and PSA testing. Factors that are considered in choosing AS include potential side effects of treatment (e.g., urinary incontinence, erectile dysfunction), estimated life expectancy, and the risk for increased morbidity and mortality from not seeking active treatment.

Patients who have very early–stage cancer of the prostate who choose AS require close follow-up by their health care provider. If obstruction occurs, a transurethral resection of the prostate (TURP) may be done. The care of patients having this procedure is described in the discussion of Surgical Management in the Benign Prostatic Hyperplasia section.

Specific management is based on the extent of the disease and the patient's physical condition. The patient may undergo surgery for a biopsy, staging and removal of the tumor, or palliation to control the spread of disease or relieve distressing symptoms. As with AS, the health care provider and patient must weigh the benefits of treatment against potential adverse effects such as incontinence and erectile dysfunction (ED).

Surgical Management. *Surgery is the most common intervention for a cure.* Minimally invasive surgery (MIS) or, less commonly, an open surgical technique for radical prostatectomy (prostate removal) is usually performed. A **bilateral orchiectomy** (removal of both testicles) is another palliative surgery that slows the spread of cancer by removing the main source of testosterone.

Preoperative Care. Preoperative care depends on the type of surgery that will be done. Minimally invasive surgery (MIS) is most appropriate for localized prostate cancer and is used as a curative intervention. The most common procedure is the *laparoscopic radical prostatectomy (LRP),* most often with robotic assistance. Other newer procedures include transrectal high-intensity focused ultrasound (HIFU) and cryosurgery. Patients who qualify for LRP must have a PSA less than 10 ng/mL and have had no previous hormone therapy or abdominal surgeries. Remind the patient that the advantages of this procedure over open surgery include:

- Decreased hospital stay (1 to 2 days)
- Minimal bleeding
- Smaller or no incisions and less scarring
- Less postoperative discomfort
- Decreased time for urinary catheter placement
- Fewer complications
- Faster recovery and return to usual activities
- Nerve-sparing advantages

For the patient undergoing an *open* radical prostatectomy, provide preoperative care as for any patient having surgery (see Chapter 14).

Operative Procedures. For the *LRP procedure,* the patient is placed in lithotomy positioning with steep Trendelenburg. The urologist makes one or more small punctures or incisions into the abdomen. A laparoscope with a camera on the end is inserted through one of the incisions while other instruments are inserted into the other incisions. The robotic system may be used to control the movement of the instruments by a remote device. The prostate is removed along with nearby lymph nodes, but perineal nerves are not affected.

The *open* radical prostatectomy can be performed via several surgical approaches, depending on the patient's desired outcomes and the staging of the disease. The transperineal and retropubic (nerve-sparing) approaches are most commonly used. The surgeon removes the entire prostate gland along with the prostatic capsule, the cuff at the bladder neck, the seminal vesicles, and the regional lymph nodes. The remaining urethra is connected to the bladder neck. The removal of tissue at the bladder neck allows the seminal fluid to travel upward into the bladder rather than down the urethral tract, resulting in retrograde ejaculations.

Postoperative Care. Provide postoperative care of the patient after *open* radical prostatectomy as summarized in Chart 72-2. Nursing interventions include all the typical care for a patient undergoing major surgery. Maintaining hydration, caring for wound drains (open procedure), managing pain, and preventing pulmonary complications are important aspects of nursing care. (See general postoperative care in Chapter 16.)

 CHART 72-2 **Best Practice for Patient Safety & Quality Care** (QSEN)

Care of the Patient After an Open Radical Prostatectomy

- Encourage the patient to use patient-controlled analgesia (PCA) as needed.
- Help the patient get out of bed into a chair on the night of surgery and ambulate by the next day.
- Maintain the sequential compression device until the patient begins to ambulate.
- Monitor the patient for deep vein thrombosis and pulmonary embolus.
- Keep an accurate record of intake and output, including Jackson-Pratt or other drainage device drainage.
- Keep the urinary meatus clean using soap and water.
- Avoid rectal procedures or treatments.
- Teach the patient how to care for the urinary catheter because he may be discharged with the catheter in place.
- Teach the patient how to use a leg bag.
- Emphasize the importance of not straining during bowel movement. Advise the patient to avoid suppositories or enemas.
- Remind the patient about the importance of follow-up appointments with the surgeon and oncologist to monitor progress.

Assess the patient's pain level and monitor the effectiveness of pain management with opioids given as patient-controlled analgesia (PCA), a common method of delivery during the first 24 hours after surgery. Administer a stool softener if needed to prevent possible constipation from the drugs. Patients having the minimally invasive surgery have much less pain and fewer complications.

The patient has an indwelling urinary catheter to straight drainage to promote urinary ELIMINATION. Monitor intake and output every shift and record or delegate this activity to an supervise unlicensed assistive personnel (UAP). An antispasmodic may be prescribed to decrease bladder spasm induced by the indwelling urinary catheter. The time for catheter removal depends on the type of procedure that is performed and overall patient condition. Those with open surgical procedures use the catheter for 7 to 10 days or longer.

Ambulation should begin no later than the day after surgery. Provide assistance in walking the patient when he first gets out of bed. Assess for scrotal or penile swelling from the disrupted pelvic lymph flow. If this occurs, elevate the scrotum and penis and apply ice to the area intermittently for the first 24 to 48 hours.

Many patients who have the minimally invasive techniques are discharged 1 to 3 days after surgery and can resume usual activities in about a week or two. Those who have open procedures are discharged in 2 to 3 days or longer, depending on their progress.

Remind patients that common potential long-term complications of open radical prostatectomy are erectile dysfunction (ED) and urinary incontinence. For ED, drugs such as sildenafil (Viagra) may be effective. *Urge incontinence* may occur because the internal and external sphincters of the bladder lie close to the prostate gland and are often damaged during the surgery. Kegel perineal exercises may reduce the severity of urinary incontinence after radical prostatectomy. Teach the patient to contract and relax the perineal and gluteal muscles in several ways. For one of the exercises, teach him to:

1. Tighten the perineal muscles for 3 to 5 seconds as if to prevent voiding and then relax

2. Bear down as if having a bowel movement
3. Relax and repeat the exercise

Show him how to inhale through pursed lips while tightening the perineal muscles and how to exhale when he relaxes. To regain urinary control, teach the patient to practice holding an object, such as a pencil, in the fold between the buttock and the thigh. He may also sit on the toilet with the knees apart while voiding and start and stop the stream several times.

Nonsurgical Management. Nonsurgical management may be an adjunct to surgery or alternative intervention if the cancer is widespread or the patient's condition or age prevents surgery. Available modalities include radiation therapy, hormone therapy, and chemotherapy (less often).

Radiation Therapy. External or internal radiation therapy may be used in the treatment of prostate cancer or as "salvage" treatments when cancer recurs. It may also be done for palliation of the patient's symptoms.

External beam radiation therapy (EBRT or *XRT)* comes from a source outside the body. Patients are usually treated 5 days a week for 4 to 6 weeks. Three-dimensional conformal radiation therapy (3D-CRT) can more accurately target prostate tissue and reduce side effects such as damage to the rectum. An advanced type of this radiation called *intensity-modulated radiation therapy* provides very high doses to the prostate. EBRT can also be used to relieve pain from bone metastasis or be given following radical prostatectomy. Teach patients that external beam radiation causes ED in many men well after the treatment is completed.

Teach patients that other complications from EBRT include urinary frequency, diarrhea, and *acute radiation cystitis,* which causes persistent pain and hematuria. Symptoms are usually mild to moderate and subside 6 weeks after treatment. Drugs to prevent urinary urgency such as tolterodine (Detrol LA) may be prescribed. Teach the patient to avoid caffeine and continue drinking plenty of water and other fluids.

Radiation proctitis (rectal mucosa inflammation) may also develop but is less likely with 3D-CRT. The man reports rectal urgency and cramping and passes mucus and blood. Teach him to report these symptoms to the primary health care provider. Like cystitis, this problem usually resolves 4 to 6 weeks after the treatment stops. If proctitis occurs, teach patients to limit spicy or fatty foods, caffeine, and dairy products.

Low-dose brachytherapy (internal radiation) can be delivered by implanting low-dose radiation seeds, needles, or wires directly into and around the prostate gland. This treatment includes ultrasonically guided interstitial or radioactive implantation. These procedures are done on an ambulatory care basis and are the most cost-effective treatment for early-stage prostate cancer. Reassure the patient that the dose of radiation is low and that the radiation will not pose a hazard to him or others. Teach him that ED, urinary incontinence, and rectal problems do occur in a small percentage of cases. Fatigue is also common and may last for several months after the treatment stops. Chapter 22 describes general nursing care for patients having radiation therapy.

Drug Therapy. Drug therapy may consist of either hormone therapy (androgen deprivation therapy [ADT]) or chemotherapy. Because most prostate tumors are hormone dependent, patients with extensive tumors or those with metastatic disease may be managed by androgen deprivation. *Luteinizing hormone–releasing hormone (LH-RH) agonists* or anti-androgens can be used.

Examples of *LH-RH agonists* are leuprolide (Lupron), goserelin (Zoladex), and triptorelin (Trelstar). These drugs first stimulate the pituitary gland to release the luteinizing hormone (LH). After about 3 weeks, the pituitary gland "runs out" of LH, which reduces testosterone production by the testes (Burchum & Rosenthal, 2016).

> **! NURSING SAFETY PRIORITY** QSEN
>
> ### Drug Alert
>
> Teach patients taking LH-RH agonists that side effects include "hot flashes," erectile dysfunction, and decreased **libido** (desire to have sex). Some men also have **gynecomastia** (breast tenderness and growth). These drugs can also cause osteoporosis. Bisphosphonates such as pamidronate (Aredia) are prescribed to prevent bone fractures. They can also be used to slow the damage caused by bone metastasis.

Anti-androgen drugs, also known as *androgen deprivation therapy (ADT),* work differently in that they block the body's ability to use the available androgens (Burchum & Rosenthal, 2016). These drugs are the major treatment for metastatic disease. Examples include flutamide (Eulexin, Euflex), bicalutamide (Casodex), and nilutamide (Nilandron). They inhibit tumor progression by blocking the uptake of testicular and adrenal androgens at the prostate tumor site.

Anti-androgens may be used alone or in combination with LH-RH agonists for total or maximal androgen blockade (hormone ablation). Patients who have this drug combination often have "hot flashes" similar to those experienced by menopausal women, and they can decrease the patient's perceived quality of life. Ask the patient if he has been experiencing this problem. Megestrol acetate may be prescribed for this uncomfortable condition.

Systemic *chemotherapy* may be an option for patients whose cancer has spread and for whom other therapies have not worked. For example, small cell prostate cancer is rare and is more responsive to chemotherapy than to hormone therapy. Docetaxel (Taxotere) plus prednisone given every 3 weeks is the preferred treatment. A combination of cisplatin (Platinol) and etoposide (VP-16, VePesid) may also be effective for this type of cancer (Burchum & Rosenthal, 2016). Chapter 22 describes general nursing care for patients receiving chemotherapy.

Care Coordination and Transition Management

Interprofessional collaborative care of the man with prostate cancer should include his partner, if any, and family. The diagnosis and treatment of cancer greatly affect couples who survive the disease. Recognize that the patient and partner have specific physical and psychosocial needs that should be addressed before hospital discharge, and management should continue in the community setting.

Patients with prostate cancer may require care in a wide variety of settings: at the hospital, the radiation therapy department, the oncologist's office, or home at any stage of the disease process. Specific interventions depend on which treatment the patient had or if he had a combination of treatments. Regardless of treatment, care coordination to effectively manage transitions in care is essential. This section focuses on the needs of those who had a *radical prostatectomy.*

Home Care Management. Discharge planning and health teaching start early, even before surgery. A patient can better plan home care management when he knows what to expect.

Collaborate with the case manager to coordinate the efforts of various health care providers, surgical unit nursing staff, and possibly a home care nurse. As specified by The Joint Commission and other accrediting agencies, continuity of care is essential when caring for this patient because he may need weeks or months of therapies.

Self-Management Education. An important area of teaching for the patient going home after an *open* radical prostatectomy may be urinary catheter care. An indwelling urinary catheter may be in place for up to several weeks, depending on the surgical technique that was used. Teach him and his family how to care for the catheter, use a leg bag, and identify signs and symptoms of infection and other complications. See Chart 72-3 for patient and family education.

Encourage the patient to walk short distances. Lifting may be restricted to no more than 15 lb (6.8 kg) for up to 6 weeks if an open procedure was done. Remind him to maintain an upright position and not to walk bent or flexed. Vigorous exercise such as running or jumping should be avoided for at least 6 weeks and then gradually introduced. By contrast, patients having the minimally invasive laparoscopic surgery can usually return to work or usual activities in about a week.

Teach the patient not to strain to defecate. A stool softener may be prescribed to reduce the need for straining. If an opioid is prescribed for pain management, encourage the patient to drink adequate water to prevent constipation.

If the patient had an *open* radical prostatectomy, teach him to shower for the first 2 to 3 weeks rather than soak in a bathtub. Patients who had a *laparoscopic* procedure can usually shower in 1 to 2 days. Teach them to remove the small bandage but leave the Steri-Strips in place (they should fall off in about a week). Show patients how to inspect the incision or puncture site(s) daily for signs of infection. Remind them to keep all follow-up appointments. PSA blood tests are taken 6 weeks after surgery and then every 4 to 6 months to monitor progress.

Health Care Resources. Refer the patient and partner to agencies or support groups such as the American Cancer Society's *Man-to-Man* program to help cope with prostate cancer. This program provides one-on-one education, personal visits, educational presentations, and the opportunity to engage in open and candid discussions. Another prostate cancer support group is *Us TOO International* (www.ustoo.com) sponsored by the Prostate Cancer Education and Support Network. This group provides education and support with national and international chapters. Information can also be obtained from the Prostate Cancer Foundation (www.prostatecancerfoundation.org) or the National Prostate Cancer Coalition (www.fightprostatecancer.org). In Canada, the Prostate Cancer Canada organization (www.prostatecancer,ca) is dedicated to research and support for this disease. Other personal and community support services such as spiritual leaders or churches and synagogues are also important to many patients.

For same-sex couples surviving prostate cancer, *Malecare* (http://malecare.org) is an excellent resource. This nonprofit organization provides support groups for gay and bisexual men and their partners. Another resource is *A Gay Man's Guide to Prostate Cancer.*

Some men have erectile dysfunction (ED) for the first 3 to 18 months after a prostatectomy. Refer them to a specialist who can help with this problem. (ED is discussed later in this chapter.) Refer patients with urinary incontinence to a urologist who specializes in this area. Drug therapy and other strategies may be used. Chapter 66 discusses incontinence management in detail.

◆ Evaluation: Reflecting

Evaluate the care of the patient with prostate cancer based on the identified priority patient problem. The primary expected outcome is that the patient will not experience cancer metastasis as a result of appropriate and effective collaborative management.

TESTICULAR CANCER

❖ PATHOPHYSIOLOGY

Testicular cancer is a rare cancer that most often affects men between 20 and 35 years of age but can affect men of any age. It usually strikes men at a productive time of life and thus has significant economic, social, and psychological impact on the patient and his family and/or partner. With early detection by testicular self-examination (TSE) (Chart 72-4) and treatment, testicular cancer has a 95% cure rate (McCance et al., 2014). It can occur in one testicle or both.

Primary testicular cancers fall into two major groups:
- Germ cell tumors arising from the sperm-producing cells (account for most testicular cancers)

👤 CHART 72-3 Patient and Family Education: Preparing for Self-Management

Urinary Catheter Care at Home

- Once a day, gently wash the first few inches of the catheter starting at the penis and washing outward with mild soap and water.
- Rinse and dry the catheter well.
- If you have not been circumcised, push the foreskin back to clean the catheter site; when finished, push the foreskin forward.
- Change the drainage bag at least once a week as needed:
  - Hold the catheter with one hand and the tubing with the other hand and twist in opposite directions to disconnect.
  - Place the end of the catheter in a clean container to catch leakage of urine.
  - Remove the rubber cap from the tubing of the leg bag or clean drainage bag.
  - Clean the end of the new tubing with alcohol swabs.
  - Insert the end of the new tubing into the catheter and twist to connect securely.
  - Clean the drainage bag just removed by pouring a solution of one part vinegar to two parts water through the tubing and bag. Rinse well with water and allow the bag to dry.

👤 CHART 72-4 Patient and Family Education: Preparing for Self-Management

Testicular Self-Examination

- Examine your testicles monthly immediately after a bath or a shower, when your scrotal skin is relaxed.
- Examine each testicle by gently rolling it between your thumbs and fingers. Testicular tumors tend to appear deep in the center of the testicle.
- Look and feel for any lumps; smooth, rounded masses; or any change in the size, shape, or consistency of the testes.
- Report any lump or swelling to your primary health care provider as soon as possible.

TABLE 72-1 Classification of Testicular Tumors

GERM CELL (GERMINAL) TUMORS	NON–GERM CELL (NONGERMINAL) TUMORS

• Seminoma
• Nonseminoma:
  • Embryonal carcinoma
  • Teratoma
  • Choriocarcinoma
	• Interstitial cell tumor
	• Androblastoma

• Non–germ cell tumors arising from the stromal, interstitial, or Leydig cells that produce testosterone (account for a very small percentage of testicular cancers)

Testicular germ cell tumors are classified into two broad categories: seminomas and nonseminomas (Table 72-1). The most common type of testicular tumor is *seminoma*. Patients with seminomas have the most favorable prognoses because the tumors are usually localized, metastasize late, and respond to treatment. They often are diagnosed when they are still confined to the testicles and retroperitoneal lymph nodes.

Non–germ cell tumors are classified as either *interstitial cell tumors* or *androblastomas* (testicular adenomas). Most of these tumors do not metastasize. Interstitial cell tumors arise from the Leydig cells, which secrete testosterone into the bloodstream. Androblastomas sometimes secrete estrogen, which accounts for the feminization and **gynecomastia** (breast enlargement) occasionally seen in these men.

The risk for testicular tumors is higher in males who have an undescended testis (**cryptorchidism**) or human immune deficiency virus (HIV) infection (McCance et al., 2014).

GENETIC/GENOMIC CONSIDERATIONS
Patient-Centered Care QSEN

Men are at a higher risk for testicular cancer if they have a family history of the disease (Viatori, 2012). The incidence is higher among identical twins, brothers, and other close male relatives. Euro-American men are at a higher risk for testicular cancer than men of other races or ethnicities (Viatori, 2012). The reason for these differences is not known.

Primary testicular cancer is rarely bilateral. Other cancers such as leukemia, lymphoma, and metastatic carcinomas may invade the testes. A man with bilateral testicular tumors is more likely to have metastatic disease to the testes than primary cancer.

❖ INTERPROFESSIONAL COLLABORATIVE CARE
◆ Assessment: Noticing

Physical Assessment/Signs and Symptoms. When taking a history from a patient with a suspected testicular tumor, consider the risk factors. Assess for other risk factors, including a history or presence of an undescended testis and a family history of testicular cancer.

The most common report is a painless, hard swelling or enlargement of the testicle. Patients with discomfort such as heaviness or aching in the lower abdomen or scrotum may have metastatic disease. Determine how long any signs and symptoms have been present.

Assess the patient's family situation. Is the patient sexually active? If so, what is his sexual preference? Does he have children? Does he want children in the future? Depending on the

treatment plan chosen, would he be interested in sperm storage in a sperm bank?

If the man has one healthy testis, he can function sexually and may not have any problem with REPRODUCTION. If he has a retroperitoneal lymph node dissection or chemotherapy, he may become sterile because of treatment effects on the sperm-producing cells or surgical trauma to the sympathetic nervous system resulting in retrograde ejaculations.

The testes, lymph nodes, and abdomen should be examined thoroughly. Patients may feel embarrassed about having this examination. Provide privacy and explain the procedure to the patient. Inspect the testicles for swelling or a lump that the patient reports is painless. An advanced practice nurse or other health care provider palpates the testes for lumps and swelling that are not visible. The presence of any testicular pain, lymph node swelling, bone pain, abdominal masses, sudden hydrocele (fluid in the scrotum), or gynecomastia often indicates metastatic disease.

Psychosocial Assessment. Because testicular cancer and its treatment often lead to sexual dysfunction, pay close attention to the psychosocial aspects of the disease. SEXUALITY is an issue for men of any age, but it may be even more of an issue for younger men. Even if the cancer is detected at an early stage and the patient is cured after surgery, he may be afraid that he will be sexually deficient. He may also think of himself as "less than a whole person." These fears can disrupt the psychosocial and sexual development of young males and can threaten their identity. The patient may be afraid that he will be unable to perform sexually, will no longer be sexually attractive or desirable, and will face rejection. Feelings of sexual inadequacy may be denied, repressed, or displaced, causing increased stress on the man's personal and work relationships.

Assess the man's support systems, including his partner, family members, and friends. Ask him where he feels that he can be supported, such as a religious or spiritual group, community club, or social group. Friends are often very helpful during this difficult time.

Laboratory Assessment. Common serum tumor markers that confirm a diagnosis of testicular cancer are:
• Alpha-fetoprotein (AFP)
• Beta human chorionic gonadotropin (hCG)
• Lactate dehydrogenase (LDH)

Serum testosterone levels are increased when the tumor affects the Leydig cells, which produce this hormone. Drugs such as alcohol and antiepileptic drugs can also cause an increase in testosterone (Pagana et al., 2017).

Other Diagnostic Assessment. When a patient has a change in testis size, shape, or texture, *ultrasonography* can determine whether the mass is solid or fluid filled. It also can help differentiate benign masses from malignant ones.

After the diagnosis of testicular cancer, the patient should have a *CT scan* of the abdomen and the chest to identify small metastatic lesions. *Lymphangiography* shows a view of the body's lymph system to look for spread to other areas.

MRI is used to detect enlarged lymph nodes and abnormal nodules in certain organs that may indicate metastasis from the testicles. Chest x-rays and bone scans may also be performed if metastasis is suspected.

◆ Interventions: Responding.

At diagnosis, the incidence of **oligospermia** (low sperm count) and **azoospermia** (absence of living sperm) is common in patients with testicular cancer. This problem is thought to be related to higher testicular temperatures created by cancer cell metabolism. The man may not discover that he has reduced sperm count until he has a sperm count performed before surgery.

Health teaching about REPRODUCTION, fertility, and SEXUALITY is started in the pretreatment phase. Review the normal reproductive function and the possible effects of cancer and its treatment on reproductive function. Explore with the patient various reproductive options if desired (Chart 72-5). A sperm bank facility provides comprehensive information on semen collection, storage of semen, the storage contract, costs, and the insemination process.

When preparing the patient for the collection and storage of sperm, assume the role of patient advocate and keep in mind the effect of the cancer diagnosis. The psychological benefit of having stored sperm may be important for the man and may influence his response to treatment. For some men, knowing that the potential for being a father still exists may help them cope with other fears, such as alopecia or erectile dysfunction (ED).

Suggest that the patient arrange for semen storage, if desired, as soon as possible after diagnosis. Sperm collection should be completed before he begins radiation therapy or chemotherapy or undergoes a radical lymph node dissection. After radiation therapy or chemotherapy has been started, the patient is at increased risk for producing mutagenic sperm, which may not be viable or may result in fetal abnormalities.

The patient's diagnosis and his physical condition may not allow treatment to be postponed, thus making sperm storage impossible. Also, some men may have personal or religious beliefs that do not allow sperm storage. For those who are not candidates for sperm storage in a sperm bank and those who choose not to bank, discuss other options for REPRODUCTION such as donor insemination or adoption.

Surgical Management. Surgery is the main treatment for testicular cancer. For stage 0 or 1 (localized disease), the surgeon performs a unilateral orchiectomy to remove the affected testicle. Every effort is made to remove the cancerous testis as an intact organ to prevent releasing cancer cells into the surgical site. Depending on the type and stage of the cancer, radical retroperitoneal lymph node dissection (RPLND) may also be done.

Preoperative Care. Like most patients with cancer, the man with testicular cancer is very apprehensive. Offer support and reinforce the teaching provided by the surgeon. Teach the patient and his family or partner about what to expect after surgery. For patients with very early disease, minimally invasive surgery (MIS) using a laparoscope is performed rather than using an open incision. For patients having MIS, teach them that carbon dioxide may be used as part of the surgery. Carbon dioxide can cause chest or shoulder pain from diaphragmatic irritation after the procedure.

Operative Procedures. Most patients with seminoma have only one surgery to remove the diseased testicle through the groin (inguinal) for a cure. A frozen section of the tumor is examined to confirm the type and stage of the cancer. A gel-filled silicone prosthesis may be surgically implanted into the scrotum at the time of the orchiectomy or later if the patient desires. Reassure the patient that this procedure does not impair fertility or sexual function. He cosmetically appears to have two testes (reconstructive surgery).

Some men have more advanced disease or tumor types that are more aggressive. Two options are available for the lymph node dissection: a traditional open approach and minimally invasive surgery (MIS) using a laparoscope. To perform the *open* approach, the surgeon removes the retroperitoneal nodes in the iliac and lumbar regions. Because the blood supply and the lymphatic vessels of the testes and kidneys are directly related, an extensive midline incision from the xiphoid process to the pubis is necessary. Removal of the sympathetic ganglia eliminates peristalsis in the vas deferens and contractions of the seminal vesicles. This disruption results in sterility because the man's ejaculate no longer contains sperm. However, having a normal erection and experiencing orgasm usually are not affected.

The MIS procedure involves using a laparoscope through several small "keyhole" incisions through which the nodes are dissected for examination. This technique shortens the time the patient is in the operating suite, minimizes bleeding, and causes less pain after surgery. The patient has fewer postoperative complications and a shorter hospital stay.

Postoperative Care. Nursing care for the patient after surgery depends on the type of surgical procedure that was performed and the extent of the disease process.

⚠ NURSING SAFETY PRIORITY QSEN

Action Alert

Because of the length of the *open* orchiectomy and lymph node dissection approach, manipulation of the abdominal and retroperitoneal viscera, and the loss of lymphatic fluid, observe, assess, and report any complications of this major abdominal surgery (e.g., paralytic ileus) (see Chapter 16). Monitor vital signs (including pain), hydration, and pulmonary function carefully for the first 24 to 48 hours. Ambulate the patient as soon as possible and teach him how to use the incentive spirometer. Assess the patency of the urinary catheter. Be sure that the patient wears antiembolism stockings or devices and provide care for surgical incisions and wound drains.

The patient having the *laparoscopic* procedure may have a urinary catheter in place for 1 to 2 days. The other advantages of the MIS procedure are that patients have less pain and fewer complications than those who had the open surgery. Chapter 15 describes laparoscopic surgery in detail.

Nonsurgical Management. Combination *chemotherapy* may be used as adjuvant therapy for nonseminomatous testicular tumors or as primary treatment when there is evidence of metastatic disease. Many drug regimens are used, including varying combinations of bleomycin, etoposide, and cisplatin (BEP). The specific combination of drugs and the frequency, cycling, and duration of treatment vary from patient to patient, depending on the extent of the disease and the protocol being followed. Chapter 22 discusses the general nursing care for the patient receiving chemotherapy.

After orchiectomy for localized disease, *external beam radiation therapy* (EBRT) may be used. The remaining testis is shielded with a lead cup to preserve reproductive function. Even with these precautions, the patient may have a temporary decreased sperm count as a result of radiation scatter. Normally the sperm count returns to the pretreatment level within 24 to 30 months after the radiation treatment is completed. If metastases develop outside the lymphatic system, the man may still be cured with radiation therapy if the area of involvement is limited. If lymphatic involvement is extensive or if the visceral organs are involved, combination chemotherapy is used.

Care Coordination and Transition Management

The patient is usually hospitalized for multiple days after an *open* radical retroperitoneal lymph node dissection but for just 1 to 2 days for the *MIS* laparoscopic procedure.

After an open *orchiectomy,* unless the patient has a wound complication, he is discharged without a dressing on the inguinal incision. A scrotal support may be needed for several days. He may want to wear a dry dressing to prevent clothing from rubbing on the sutures and causing irritation. Tell him that the sutures will be removed in the physician's office 7 to 10 days after surgery. Patients who also had an *open retroperitoneal lymph node dissection* recover more slowly. They should not lift anything over 15 lb (6.8 kg), should avoid stair climbing, and should not drive a car for several weeks. Be sure that bathroom facilities are on the first floor of the house where he can easily access them.

NURSING SAFETY PRIORITY QSEN

Action Alert

For the patient who has undergone testicular surgery, emphasize the importance of scheduling a follow-up visit with the surgeon to examine the incision for healing and complications. Instruct him to notify the surgeon if chills, fever, increasing tenderness or pain around the incision, drainage, or dehiscence of the incision occurs. These signs and symptoms may indicate infection for which antibiotics are needed. Instruct the patient who had a laparoscopic orchiectomy that he will be able to resume most of his usual activities within 1 week after discharge. He can take a shower 1 or 2 days after surgery, but be sure that he does not remove the Steri-Strips. These strips will loosen and fall off about a week after surgery.

Explain the importance of performing monthly testicular self-examination (TSE) on the remaining testis and scheduling follow-up examinations with the physician. The patient who has had testicular cancer should schedule tests for urinary and serum levels of tumor markers and CT or MRI studies as part of his routine follow-up for at least 3 years.

The man who has testicular cancer needs emotional support. If permanent sterility occurs and sperm storage has not been feasible, he may desire counseling about other reproductive options. Refer the patient to agencies or support groups, such as the American Fertility Society (www.theafa.org) or RESOLVE: The National Infertility Association (www.resolve.org) (organizations for infertile couples).

ERECTILE DYSFUNCTION

❖ PATHOPHYSIOLOGY

Erectile dysfunction (ED), also known as *impotence,* is the inability to achieve or maintain an erection for sexual intercourse. It affects millions of men throughout the world. There are two major types of ED: organic and functional.

Organic ED is a gradual deterioration of function. The man first notices diminishing firmness and a decrease in frequency of erections. Causes include (McCance et al., 2014):

- Inflammation of the prostate, urethra, or seminal vesicles
- Surgical procedures such as prostatectomy
- Pelvic fractures
- Lumbosacral injuries
- Vascular disease, including hypertension
- Chronic neurologic conditions, such as Parkinson disease or multiple sclerosis
- Endocrine disorders, such as diabetes mellitus (a major cause) or thyroid disorders
- Smoking and alcohol consumption
- Drugs, such as antihypertensives
- Poor overall health that prevents sexual intercourse

If the patient has episodes of ED, it usually has a *functional* (psychological) cause. Men with functional ED usually have normal nocturnal (nighttime) and morning erections. Onset is usually sudden and follows a period of high stress.

❖ INTERPROFESSIONAL COLLABORATIVE CARE

If possible, the health care provider determines the cause of the ED through a variety of diagnostic testing, including measuring serum hormone levels and using Doppler ultrasonography to determine blood flow to the penis. The most common intervention for ED is drug therapy. Other interventions include vacuum devices, intracorporal injections, intraurethral applications, and prostheses (implants).

First-line oral drugs used to manage ED, phosphodiesterase-5 (PDE-5) inhibitors, work by relaxing the smooth muscles in the corpora cavernosa so blood flow to the penis is increased. The veins exiting the corpora are compressed, limiting outward blood flow and resulting in penile **tumescence** (swelling). Teach patients to take the pill 1 hour before sexual intercourse. For some drugs, such as sildenafil (Viagra) and vardenafil (Levitra), sexual stimulation is needed within $\frac{1}{2}$ to 1 hour to promote the erection. With other drugs, such as tadalafil (Cialis), erection can be stimulated over a longer period (Burchum & Rosenthal, 2016). Because the erection occurs more naturally compared with other treatment options, most men and their partners prefer this option.

Drug Alert

Instruct patients taking PDE-5 inhibitors to abstain from alcohol before sexual intercourse because it may impair the ability to have an erection. Common side effects of these drugs include dyspepsia (heartburn), headaches, facial flushing, and stuffy nose. If more than one pill a day is being taken, leg and back cramps, nausea, and vomiting also may occur. *Teach men who take nitrates to avoid PDE-5 inhibitors because the vasodilation effects can cause a profound hypotension and reduce blood flow to vital organs (Burchum & Rosenthal, 2016).* For patients who cannot take these drugs or do not respond to them, other methods are available to achieve an erection.

The basic design of a *vacuum constriction device (VCD)* is a cylinder that fits over the penis and sits firmly against the body. Using a pump, a vacuum is created to draw blood into the penis to maintain an erection. A rubber ring (tension band) is placed around the base of the penis to maintain the erection, and the cylinder is removed.

Injecting the penis with vasodilating drugs can make the penis erect by engorging it with blood. The most common agents used for this purpose include (Burchum & Rosenthal, 2016):

- Alprostadil (Caverject), a synthetic vasodilator identical to prostaglandin E_1 produced in the body
- Paverine, also a vasodilator
- Phentolamine (Regitine), an alpha-1, alpha-2 selective adrenergic receptor antagonist
- A combination of any or all of these drugs

Adverse drug effects include priapism (prolonged erection), penile scarring, fibrosis, bleeding, bruising at the injection site, pain, infection, and vasovagal responses.

Penile implants (prostheses) are used when other modalities fail. Devices include semirigid, flexible, or hydraulic inflatable and multi-component or one-piece instruments. The three-piece inflatable device is the most commonly implanted prosthesis. A reservoir is placed in the scrotum. Tubes carry the fluid into the inflatable pieces that are placed in the penis. To inflate the prosthesis, the man squeezes the pump located in the scrotum. To deflate the prosthesis, a release button is activated. Advantages include the man's ability to control his erections. The major disadvantages include device failure and infection. The device is implanted as an ambulatory care surgical procedure. *Teach the patient to observe the surgical site for bleeding and infection.*

? **NCLEX EXAMINATION CHALLENGE 72-4**

Health Promotion and Maintenance

The nurse is teaching a client about taking sildenafil (Viagra) for erectile dysfunction. Which statement by the client indicates a need for further teaching?
A. "I should have sex within an hour after taking the drug."
B. "I should avoid alcohol when on the drug or it might not work well."
C. "I can expect to maybe feel flushed or get a headache when I take the drug."
D. "If I have chest pain during sex, I should take a nitroglycerin tablet."

GET READY FOR THE NCLEX® EXAMINATION!

KEY POINTS

Review these Key Points for each NCLEX Examination Client Needs Category.

Safe and Effective Care Environment
- Teach patients with prostate cancer about American Cancer Society's *Man-to-Man* program and the American Foundation for Urologic Disease's *Us TOO International* program to help men and their partners cope with prostate cancer; contact the Prostate Cancer Canada organization for more research on prostate cancer in Canada.

Health Promotion and Maintenance
- Teach men at risk for prostate cancer to follow the current American Cancer Society's screening and early detection guidelines. **QSEN: Evidence-Based Practice**
- Teach men how to perform testicular self-examination as described in Chart 72-4.
- Teach uncircumcised men the importance of keeping the penis clean to prevent penile cancer.

Psychosocial Integrity
- Because most patients with testicular cancer are young and middle-age adults, assess their reaction to the possible loss of REPRODUCTION ability and SEXUALITY issues.

- Because of the high incidence of erectile dysfunction after radical prostatectomy, assess the patient's adjustment to these changes in body function. **QSEN: Patient-Centered Care**
- Assess the patient's anxiety before prostate surgery and allow him to express feelings of fear or grief. **QSEN: Patient-Centered Care**

Physiological Integrity
- Perform a focused physical assessment for patients reporting lumps or swelling in their genital area; inspect and palpate bladder and scrotum.
- Observe for and report complications after radical prostatectomy, including infection, severe pain, urinary infection, urinary ELIMINATION problems, and erectile dysfunction. **Clinical Judgment**
- Observe for and report bloody urine with clots after TURP; increase continuous bladder irrigation or irrigate the bladder per agency or surgeon protocol. **QSEN: Safety**
- Teach patients to report signs of infection when caring for a urinary catheter in the home. **Safety**
- Maintain traction on the urinary catheter and continuous bladder irrigation after a TURP. **Safety**
- Teach patients about drug therapies (5-ARIs and alpha blocking agents) used to treat BPH, including side effects such

as orthostatic hypotension, erectile dysfunction, decreased libido, dizziness, and liver dysfunction. **QSEN: Safety**
- Teach patients to avoid any drugs that can cause urinary retention, especially anticholinergics, antihistamines, and decongestants if BPH is present. **QSEN: Evidence-Based Practice**
- Remind patients wanting to use complementary and integrative therapies to check with their primary health care providers before using them.
- Eating a well-balanced diet with plenty of fish and fruits and vegetables may help prevent prostate cancer.
- Reinforce the man's option for managing prostate cancer; some procedures and drugs cause erectile dysfunction and incontinence either temporarily or permanently.

- Use the information listed in Chart 72-3 to teach patients urinary catheter care after prostate cancer surgery.
- Teach patients about not lifting more than 15 lb (6.8 kg) after open prostate surgery. **QSEN: Safety**
- Options for erectile dysfunction (ED) include drug therapy (most common), vacuum-assist devices, penile injections, transurethral suppositories, or penile implants.
- Be aware that African-American middle-age men are the most at risk for prostate cancer; Euro-American young men are the most at risk for testicular cancer.
- Teach patients and their partners about hormone therapy used to manage prostate cancer: LH-RH agonists and anti-androgen drugs.

SELECTED BIBLIOGRAPHY

Asterisk indicates a classic or definitive work on this subject.

American Cancer Society (ACS). (2017). *ACS Cancer facts and figures for African Americans* 2016-2018. www.cancer.org/groups/content/@editorial/documents/document/acspc-047403.pdf.

Burchum, J. L. R., & Rosenthal, L. D. (2016). *Lehne's pharmacology for nursing care* (9th ed.). St. Louis: Elsevier.

Dunn, M. W., & Kazer, M. W. (2011). Prostate cancer overview. *Seminars in Oncology Nursing, 27*(4), 244–250.

Heidari, M., Hosseinabadi, R., Anbari, K., Pournia, Y., & Tarverdian, A. (2014). Seidlitzia Rosmarinus for lower urinary tract symptoms associates with benign prostatic hyperplasia: A pilot randomized controlled clinical trial. *Complementary Therapies in Medicine, 22*(4), 607–613.

Jarvis, C. (2014). *Physical examination & health assessment* (7th ed.). St. Louis: Elsevier Saunders.

*King, D. (2012). Benign prostatic hyperplasia. *Nursing, 42*(5), 37.

McCance, K., Huether, S., Brashers, V., & Rote, N. (2014). *Pathophysiology: The biologic basis for disease in adults and children* (7th ed.). St. Louis: Mosby.

Pagana, K. D., Pagana, T. J., & Pagana, T. N. (2017). *Mosby's diagnostic and laboratory test reference* (13th ed.). St. Louis: Mosby.

Patel, N. D., & Parsons, J. K. (2014). Epidemiology and etiology of benign prostatic hyperplasia and bladder outlet obstruction. *Indian Journal of Urology, 30*(2), 170–176.

*Roehrborn, C. G. (2011). Male lower urinary tract symptoms (LUTS) and benign prostatic hyperplasia (BPH). *The Medical Clinics of North America, 95*(1), 87–100.

*Viatori, M. (2012). Testicular cancer. *Seminars in Oncology Nursing, 28*(3), 180–189.

Yim, P. W., Wang, W., Jiang, Y., Zakir, H. A., Toh, P. C., Lopez, V., et al. (2015). Health-related quality of life, physical well-being, and sexual function in patients with benign prostatic hyperplasia after prostatic surgery. *Applied Nursing Research, 28*(4), 274–280.

Care of Transgender Patients

Donna D. Ignatavicius and Stephanie M. Fox

ⓔ http://evolve.elsevier.com/Iggy/

PRIORITY AND INTERRELATED CONCEPTS

The priority concepts for this chapter are:
- PATIENT-CENTERED CARE
- HEALTH CARE DISPARITIES

The interrelated concepts for this chapter are:
- SEXUALITY
- REPRODUCTION

LEARNING OUTCOMES

Safe and Effective Care Environment

1. Describe the need to collaborate with members of the health care team to provide high-quality care for transgender patients.
2. Explain the role of the nurse as a leader in promoting advocacy for transgender people to provide quality care and minimize HEALTH CARE DISPARITIES.

Health Promotion and Maintenance

3. Develop a health teaching plan for transgender patients who take hormone therapy and/or have gender reassignment surgery.
4. Identify appropriate resources for accurate trans-health information and ongoing preventive health care.

Psychosocial Integrity

5. Discuss how to use culturally sensitive terminology when providing care for transgender patients.

6. Identify the major sources of stress that contribute to transgender health issues.
7. Explain the major challenges for transgender patients in obtaining health care.

Physiological Integrity

8. Describe the side effects and adverse effects of feminizing and masculinizing hormone therapy, including effects on SEXUALITY and REPRODUCTION.
9. Identify laboratory test values that require monitoring for patients taking hormone therapy.
10. Describe the preoperative care needed for male-to-female or female-to-male patients having genital surgery.
11. Prioritize PATIENT-CENTERED postoperative nursing CARE for patients having feminizing or masculinizing genital surgery.

The American Nurses Association (ANA) *Code of Ethics* states that the nurse practices with compassion and respect for the dignity and worth of every patient (ANA, 2015). The Institute of Medicine (now the National Academy of Medicine [NAM]) and the Quality and Safety Education for Nurses (QSEN) Institute further identified the need for nurses to be competent in PATIENT-CENTERED CARE (see Chapter 1 for review of this concept). This competency ensures that nurses provide care with sensitivity and respect for diverse patients, even if those patients have values and preferences different from their own (ANA, 2015). Diversity is often discussed as ethnicity and race, but other cultural aspects such as sexual orientation and gender identity are part of the diverse human experience.

People of minority sexual and gender identities are often grouped under one population category described by the acronym **LGBTQ**—lesbian, gay, bisexual, transgender, and queer/questioning (people who do not feel they belong in any other subgroup) (Table 73-1) (Eliason et al., 2013). Some literature includes only "LGBT." These evolving labels are misleading regarding people who identify as transgender. The grouping of SEXUALITY (sexual attraction and behavior) and *gender identity* (sense of maleness or femaleness) suggests that these two concepts are related or dependent on one another, but they are very different. *LGB* refers to specific sexual orientation. However, transgender people may identify as heterosexual, homosexual, both, or neither. Nurses and other health care professionals should not assume that transgender patients have the same

TABLE 73-1	Appropriate Terminology Associated With Transgender Health
TERM	**DEFINITION**
Coming out	A lesbian, gay, bisexual, transgender, and queer/questioning (LGBTQ) person's public disclosure regarding sexual orientation or gender identity
Female-to-male	An adjective to describe people who were identified as female at birth and are changing (or have changed) to a more masculine body or male
Gender dysphoria	Emotional or psychological distress caused by an incongruence between one's natal (birth) sex and gender identity
Gender identity	A person's inner sense of being a male, a female, or an alternative gender (e.g., genderqueer)
Genderqueer	An identity label used by some people whose gender identity does not conform to one of the two categories of male or female
Male-to-female	An adjective to describe people who were identified as male at birth and are changing (or have changed) to a more feminine body or female
Sex (also called *natal sex*)	The gender assigned at one's birth
Gender reassignment surgery (also called *sex reassignment surgery [SRS], gender-affirming surgery, or gender-confirming surgery*)	A group of surgical procedures that change primary and/or secondary sex characteristics to affirm a person's gender identity
Transgender	An adjective to describe a person who crosses or transcends culturally defined categories of gender
Transition	The period of time when transgender people change from the gender role associated with their sex to a different gender role
Transsexual	Term often used by health care professionals to describe people who want to change or have changed their primary and/or secondary sex characteristics

experiences or health care needs as those who identify as lesbian, gay, or bisexual.

PATIENT-CENTERED TERMINOLOGY

Commonly, gender is categorized as one of two terms: *male* and *female*. For the majority of people, these descriptors are accurate. However, some people do not clearly fit into either category and may define themselves as *transgender*. Identifying oneself as transgender is not a choice or lifestyle but, rather, an inner sense of being born in the wrong body. When transgender people pursue ways of affirming their physical body and appearance with their gender identity, their interaction with the health care system requires knowledge, respect, compassion, and specialized nursing care.

Using appropriate terminology is essential to demonstrating respect (see Table 73-1). Of utmost importance is the distinction between gender and sex. Gender, also known as **gender identity**, describes a person's inner sense of maleness or femaleness and is not related to REPRODUCTION anatomy. Gender identity describes one's social role as a man or a woman (American Psychiatric Association [APA], 2013). Sex, also known as *biological* or **natal sex**, refers to a person's genital anatomy present at birth (Edwards-Leeper & Spack, 2013).

When babies are born, the gender of the child is determined by the genitalia present, but there is no way of knowing the child's true sense of gender. The sense of gender and feelings toward maleness or femaleness can develop in children as early as age 2 years and is usually present in most children during the early elementary years. Transgender people feel a mismatch between their gender identity and natal sex, often extending back into early childhood. When this incongruence occurs, they can experience **gender dysphoria**, or discomfort with one's natal sex (APA, 2013; Edwards-Leeper & Spack, 2013). Some people who have gender dysphoria may seek interventions to transition to the identified gender.

The term *transgender* is often used as an umbrella description for all people whose gender identity and presentation do not conform to social expectations. In this text, **transgender** describes patients who self-identify as the opposite gender or a gender that does not match their natal sex (Merryfeather & Bruce, 2014). For proper usage, transgender should be used only in adjective form. For example, a patient "is transgender," "identifies as transgender," or "is a transgender patient." Note that "transgender" never ends in "-ed." The term *transgender* should not be used as a noun, and a patient should never be described as "*a* transgender."

According to *The Diagnostic and Statistical Manual of Mental Disorders* (APA, 2013), prevalence of gender dysphoria worldwide ranges from 5 to 14 in 1000 natal males and from 2 to 3 in 1000 natal females. However, these data describe the number of people who experience discontent with the gender they were assigned at birth and do not give an accurate estimate of the number of people who identify as transgender. Other data on the transgender population indicate that there are approximately 1.4 million adults in the United States who identify as transgender (Flores et al., 2016). Most scholars suggest that the prevalence is much higher, and more research is needed to collect accurate demographic data for this population. Statistical data for the number of adults who identify as transgender in Canada are not available.

Another common term is **transsexual**, which generally describes a person who has modified his or her natal body to match the appropriate gender identity, either through cosmetic, hormonal, or surgical means (Merryfeather & Bruce, 2014). "Transsexual" can be used as both an adjective and a noun, such that a patient can be described "as transsexual" or "as a transsexual." (*NOTE: As with other terms, use terminology only if the patient identifies as such*). People who were born with anatomically male parts but identify as and/or live as female are known as "male-to-female" or "MtF." Male-to-female people are also known as "transwomen," with the gender descriptor indicating the current-lived gender identity. Conversely, "transmen" are natal females who identify as and/or live as men. They are described as "female-to-male" or "FtM."

Transgender people are sometimes described as "transvestites" or "cross-dressers," often in a judgmental or negative manner. These terms should not be used unless the patient identifies as such. Other terms, such as *tranny, he-she,* or *shemale,* are offensive and hurtful. These terms and other negative comments should never be used.

A patient may self-identify with any of the above terms or choose not to be defined at all. Become familiar with appropriate terms and concepts, but do not force definitions on your patients. *Instead, if you are unsure how to address patients, during your nursing assessment ask them how they define their gender identity.*

TRANSGENDER HEALTH ISSUES

Transgender people (also referred to as *trans-people*) encounter frequent discrimination and are faced with numerous stressful situations related to their identity. Sources of stress such as job discrimination and bias-related harassment can have an impact on patients' physical and psychological health. In the most recent large-scale national survey on discrimination, the majority of transgender people had experienced mistreatment in the workplace. Also, almost half of transgender respondents reported loss of job or denial of promotion because of their transgender identity. As a result, they may be homeless, use alcohol or illicit drugs as coping mechanisms, and ignore their health needs (Grant et al., 2011). In some cases, they may turn to sex work (prostitution) as a mechanism for survival (Chestnut et al., 2013; Grant et al., 2011). Only a small subset of primarily MtF transgender people engage in sex work, which can expose them to human immune deficiency virus (HIV) and sexually transmitted infection (STI).

Transgender people are also vulnerable to bias-related violence and verbal harassment, including threats and intimidation. MtF people are more than two times more likely to experience physical violence and discrimination than nontranswomen; the likelihood of harassment is even greater for transwomen of color (Chestnut et al., 2013). A recent report indicated that half of LGBTQ-related hate-crime homicides in the United States were committed against transwomen (Chestnut et al., 2013). Factors that increase this risk for violence include poverty, homelessness, and sex work.

Having an identity that puts a person at risk for violence and mistreatment can lead to emotional distress, particularly if the person has been victimized directly. Transgender people who have experienced traumatic situations may demonstrate symptoms of posttraumatic stress disorder (PTSD) and/or depression. They may turn to a variety of coping strategies to deal with distress, some of which can negatively impact physical health. In a classic large-scale national survey, 26% of transgender people reported current or previous alcohol or illicit drug use to cope with discrimination and mistreatment; however, the number of people who use substances recreationally may be higher (Grant et al., 2010). Rates of smoking in the transgender community are higher than the rates in the LGB community and general population of U.S. adults. Most important, major life stressors, emotional distress, and lack of resources can lead to suicidal ideation or suicide attempt when all other methods of coping have failed. In a sample of over 7000 transgender adults, 41% reported at least one suicide attempt in their lifetime (Grant et al., 2010). Data support similar trends in Canada (Bauer & Scheim, 2015).

STRESS AND TRANSGENDER HEALTH

Transgender people have additional sources of stress when attempting to access health care, such as lack of health insurance due to unemployment and lack of health care–professional knowledge. This barrier to health care causes them to postpone both acute and preventive medical care. For people who are insured, coverage for health care related to gender transition, such as hormone use and surgery, is usually denied.

When transgender people gain access to health care, they are often fearful and anxious about the providers and setting. In particular, they may be hesitant to disclose their transgender status because of fear of discrimination or ridicule (Redfern & Sinclair, 2014). They may also fear that this information will be documented in health records and shared with family members. This reluctance is increased if they have had previous negative experiences with primary health care providers. One national survey found that 19% of transgender adults were refused health care services due to their gender identity, and 28% reported receiving verbal harassment in a health care setting. Male-to-female transgender people were more likely to encounter discrimination and avoid health care because of these experiences (Grant et al., 2010). Even with providers who seem tolerant and caring with transgender patients, there is still a risk for patients overhearing jokes in the hallway and defamatory comments (Rounds et al., 2013).

Another source of stress faced by many transgender people is lack of health care–professional knowledge regarding health care needs (Rounds et al., 2013). When this situation occurs, transgender patients are put in a position of acting as health care experts, which can limit the quality of their care. Although most transgender patients generally expect their providers to have some level of knowledge or know where to seek answers, at least half of them find that they have to teach their providers (Rounds et al., 2013). When they encounter primary health care providers who are unfamiliar with the specific health care needs of their population, patient confidence is likely to diminish drastically and affect desire for future health care.

Although transgender patients may encounter health care professionals who do not understand or who overlook their gender identity, some may encounter those who over-focus on it. Although it is important to be generally knowledgeable about a patient's gender status and understand how it may affect health care needs, this factor is not always relevant for every health problem. For example, transgender patients with fractures or influenza do not need to be questioned extensively about their gender identity. Although there are instances in which the presenting problems require transgender-specific care, many other instances require the same health care that all patients receive. At these times, most transgender patients prefer to be treated as any other patient (Rounds et al., 2013). Therefore use sound clinical judgment to decide if one's gender identity impacts patient assessment and care.

THE NEED TO IMPROVE TRANSGENDER HEALTH CARE

During the past few years, several national documents were published by the U.S. Department of Health and Human

Services and private health care organizations that call for improvement in LGBTQ health care. These important publications include:

- Healthy People 2020
- The Institute of Medicine's (IOM) (now NAM) report on LGBT health
- The Joint Commission field guide for care of LGBT patients
- World Professional Association for Transgender Health (WPATH) standards of care

The U.S. Department of Health and Human Services' *Healthy People 2010* publication did *not* include the need to improve health care for LGBT people. As a result of this omission, a companion document was developed by the Gay and Lesbian Medical Association (GLMA) to address special health care needs of this population across the life span. Ten common health problems affecting the LGBT group were identified, including cancer, nutrition and weight, and sexually transmitted infection.

The *Healthy People 2020* agenda added objectives for improving the health of LGBT people, including the need to recognize and address the special health needs of transgender patients of all ages. One major objective is to develop a system to identify patients who identify as LGBTQ. This objective is similar to the recommendation in the IOM's (now NAM's) publication entitled *The Health of LGBT People: Building a Foundation for Better Understanding* (IOM, 2011).

The IOM LGBT health report calls for the need for more research to identify the special health care concerns of LGBT people of all ages. To help meet this outcome, the document outlined the need to collect more demographic data to better identify this population. LGBTQ people need to feel safe when disclosing this very personal information.

In 2011, The Joint Commission (TJC) published a similar document that recommends ways for health care agencies to create a welcoming and safe environment for LGBT patients. In response to growing attention to the need for cultural competence for all health care professionals and to provide quality health care for sexual and gender minority patients, TJC published a field guide for health care agencies to improve LGBT patient care (TJC, 2011). Chart 73-1 lists the recommendations for health care agencies in designing a safe environment for LGBT patient care. Fig. 73-1 shows an example of a "safe zone" image that should be used to reassure these patients that they are in a safe place where they can receive respectful and knowledgeable quality care.

Also in 2011, the World Professional Association for Transgender Health (WPATH) updated its Standards of Care (Coleman et al., 2011). As of press time, this edition of the Standards of Care (SOC) remains the most current. The SOC document outlines core principles that nurses and other health care professionals should follow when caring for transgender patients (Table 73-2).

❖ INTERPROFESSIONAL COLLABORATIVE CARE

◆ Assessment: Noticing

As with any patient, it is best to ask during the nursing history and physical assessment how he or she prefers to be addressed. For example, for non-transgender patients, some people may go by a nickname or by their middle name and prefer to be addressed as such. For transgender patients, it is not uncommon for driver's licenses, insurance cards, and other forms of identification to retain their birth names (and by extension,

---

CHART 73-1 Best Practice for Patient Safety & Quality Care QSEN

The Joint Commission Recommendations for Creating a Safe, Welcoming Environment for LGBTQ Patients

- Post the *Patients' Bill of Rights* and nondiscrimination policies in a visible place.
- Make waiting rooms inclusive for LGBTQ patients and families, such as posting *Safe Zone*, rainbow, or pink triangle signs.
- Designate unisex or single-stall restrooms.
- Ensure that visitation policies are equitable for families of LGBTQ patients.
- Avoid assumptions about any patient's sexual orientation and gender identity.
- Include gender-neutral language on all medical forms and documents (e.g., "partnered" in addition to married, single, or divorced categories).
- Do not limit gender options on medical forms to "male" and "female."
- Reflect the patient's choice of terminology in communication and documentation.
- Provide information on special health concerns for LGBTQ patients.
- Become knowledgeable about LGBTQ health needs and care.
- Refer LGBTQ patients to qualified health care professionals as needed.
- Provide community resources for LGBTQ information and support as needed.

Adapted from The Joint Commission (TJC). (2011). *Advancing effective communication, cultural competence, and patient- and family-centered care for the lesbian, gay, bisexual, and transgender community.* www.jointcommission.org/lgbt.

---

birth sex) because it can be difficult to change this information, particularly if a person is in the process of transitioning. Therefore nurses may receive patient documentation with misleading patient data. For example, a nurse may receive a health care record listing a male name and birth sex yet encounter a patient presenting as female in appearance. It can be offensive and embarrassing for the patient who clearly identifies as female to be called "Mister," "sir," or the male birth name. Not only does it communicate disrespect, it also signals to the patient that she may receive inadequate care or that the environment is unsafe.

In addition to preferred names, correct pronoun usage is also important. Each patient has his or her own preference. For example, an MtF patient may visit a clinic during lunch hour at work. Because the patient has not disclosed the transgender identity at work, this patient maintains male dress and demeanor at the office. Although the patient may identify as female and live as female at home, the patient may request the nurse to use male pronouns (he, him, his) to match the patient's current presentation and may not disclose the transgender identity to the nurse. Conversely, even though the patient presents at the time as male, the patient may ask the nurse to use female pronouns (she, her, hers) because the patient identifies with a female gender identity.

In general, use pronouns that match the patient's physical presentation and dress unless the patient requests otherwise. Even though the biologic sex may not match, patients presenting as female should be addressed as female, and patients presenting as male should be addressed as male. With changing styles and trends, it can sometimes be difficult to assess by clothing alone. However, with a patient whose birth sex is listed as female yet presents in traditionally male attire, facial hair, and a men's hairstyle, it is most appropriate to address this patient as male.

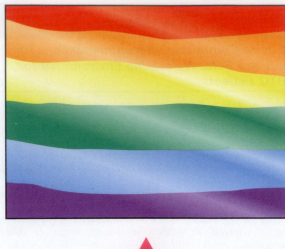

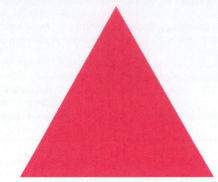

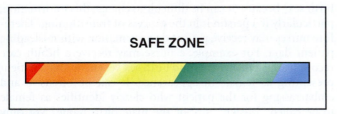

SAFE ZONE

FIG. 73-1 The Safe Zone—rainbow or pink triangle signs welcome LGBTQ patients in a health care agency.

Understandably, the clinical setting can be fast paced, and nurses may encounter multiple patients at a time; however, taking time to use clinical judgment is important. Appropriately interacting with a transgender patient can sometimes mean the difference between the patient continuing to seek health care or not.

In some cases, patients may not identify as male or female and prefer not to use male or female pronouns. These patients often feel that the binary gender system in which a person must fit clearly into one category or the other is too limiting. Although this is a small subset of the transgender population, it is important to be aware of this subculture in case you encounter a patient who refuses to identify with a specific gender. Some patients may request the use of gender-neutral pronouns, or they may use these pronouns in the nurse's presence. Some examples of gender neutral pronouns are "they/their/their" and "ze/hir/hir."

Getting used to using the correct name or pronoun can take some time. Occasionally, nurses know their patient's preferred name or pronoun but accidentally say the wrong one.

TABLE 73-2 **Core Principles for Health Care Professionals Who Care for Transgender Patients**

- Become knowledgeable about the health care needs of transgender and other gender-nonconforming people.
- Become knowledgeable about the treatment options for transgender patients and required follow-up care.
- Do not assume that all transgender patients are the same; treat each one as an individual and develop an individualized plan of care.
- Demonstrate respect for patients with nonconforming gender identities.
- Provide culturally sensitive care and use appropriate terminology that affirms the patient's gender identity.
- Facilitate patient access to appropriate and knowledgeable health care providers.
- Seek informed consent before providing treatment.
- Offer continuity of care or refer patients for ongoing quality health care.
- Advocate for patients within their families and communities.

Data from Coleman, E., Bockting, W., Botzer, M., Cohen-Kettenis, P., DeCuypere, G., Fladman, J., et al., (2011). Standards of care for the health of transsexual, transgender, and gender-nonconforming people (Version 7). *International Journal of Transgenderism, 13,* 165-232; and Rounds, K.E., McGrath, B.B., & Walsh, E. (2013). Perspectives on provider behaviors: A qualitative study of sexual and gender minorities regarding quality of care. *Contemporary Nurse, 44*(1), 99-110.

Transgender patients encounter this situation often and typically anticipate an error at times. When this error occurs, it is best to self-correct and continue with care rather than make a prolonged apology. Focusing too much on the error may make the patient more uncomfortable because more attention has been drawn to the situation. Most transgender patients, particularly those who live full time in their gender-affirming role, wish to be treated like any other patient.

History. Interventions for transgender people who experience gender dysphoria (discomfort with one's natal sex) include one or more of these options (Coleman et al., 2011):

- Changes in gender expression that may involve living part time or full time in another gender role
- Psychotherapy to explore gender identity and expression, improve body image, or strengthen coping mechanisms
- Hormone therapy to feminize or masculinize the body
- Surgery to change primary and/or secondary sex characteristics (e.g., the breasts/chest, facial features, internal and/or external genitalia)

During the health history, inquire about which interventions the patient has had, if any, or if there are plans to have them in the future. Ask about current use of *drug therapy,* including hormones, and other feminizing or masculinizing agents, including silicone injections. These medications are usually prescribed by endocrinologists or other specialists in transgender health care, but some patients may obtain them from nonmedical sources, including the Internet.

Exogenous hormone therapy can cause adverse health problems and requires careful patient monitoring, including laboratory testing. For example, estrogen therapy can cause increased health risks such as increased blood clotting causing venous thromboembolism (VTE), elevated blood glucose, hypertension, estrogen-dependent cancers, and fluid retention. Smoking and obesity increase these risks. The risks also increase with higher doses of the medication. Ask the patient about a history of these problems.

Inquire about the patient's *surgical history*. For the MtF patient, ask about breast surgery and any surgical changes to the genitalia, such as a penectomy (removal of the penis) and vaginoplasty (creation of a vagina). The MtF patient still has a prostate gland. For older patients, ask about any problems with prostate health problems, such as urinary dribbling and retention. For the FtM patient, ask whether a hysterectomy, bilateral salpingo-oophorectomy (BSO), mastectomy, phalloplasty (creation of a penis), and/or scrotoplasty (creation of a scrotum) was performed.

Keep in mind that health insurance usually does not cover the cost of the transition process and patients may seek alternative care. For example, hormones may be obtained illegally or from countries that do not have quality controls for medication. MtF patients may seek silicone for creating breasts from nonmedical people, causing a high risk for hepatitis C and silicone complications. Ask patients about the use of these alternatives as a part of their transition process.

Physical Assessment. Be sure to review the transgender patient's health record carefully before performing a physical assessment. Be culturally sensitive, nonjudgmental, and respectful during the assessment. Be aware that transgender patients may be young, middle-age, or older adults. To help increase the patient's comfort with examinations and the purpose of the assessment, explain why the information or examination is important to their health care (Redfern & Sinclair, 2014)

🕐 CONSIDERATIONS FOR OLDER ADULTS

Patient-Centered Care QSEN

Transgender patients who are older than 65 years lived in an era when most of them concealed their sexual orientation and true gender identity because of social stigma. These people have not been well studied as a group, but research indicates that those who lived with a partner have fewer mental health problems and better self-esteem than those who lived alone (Brennan et al., 2012).

When assessing transgender patients, be aware that they will be in varying stages of transition. Some patients present with no obvious physical signs that they are in the process of transitioning. Others have had gender reassignment surgery such that their new appearance matches their gender identity. Realize that a transgender patient's genitalia may not match his or her physical appearance.

Psychosocial Assessment. If gender and SEXUALITY are relevant to the patient's presenting health problem, ask specific questions to determine how these factors may impact care. Again, it is helpful to share with patients why this information is relevant to their treatment. Reassure patients that their responses are confidential and will not be shared with any family, friends, or significant others without the patient's permission. However, evidence of abuse must be reported as mandated by law. Appropriate screening questions about psychosocial functioning related to gender and sexuality include:

- Are you experiencing any challenges, concerns, or anxiety related to your sexuality?
- Related to your gender, how do you identify?
- Are you experiencing any sadness, depression, or thoughts of hurting yourself?
- Have you experienced any violence or discrimination in your personal or work life?

- Are you currently being seen by a counselor or psychologist related to your sexuality and gender identity? If so, why?

If the responses to these questions indicate that the patient has potential or actual mental health problems, consult with the health care provider for further evaluation by a qualified mental health care professional, such as a licensed counselor or clinical psychologist.

◆ Interventions: Responding

Nurses care for transgender patients who are transitioning or have completed gender reassignment. They may care for them for health problems related to their transition process or for problems that are unrelated to the patient's SEXUALITY or gender identity. In general, care for transgender patients with most health problems is the same as for any other patient. However, some interventions such as hormone therapy may affect nursing assessment and care. As a leader in health care, advocate for transgender patients and provide health teaching to promote their health. Encourage them to include their sexual partner, if any, in discussions about the transition process.

Nonsurgical Management. The primary nonsurgical interventions for transgender patients include drug (hormone) therapy, counseling about REPRODUCTION and reproductive health, and vocal therapy. The type of intervention depends on whether the patient is transitioning from MtF or FtM.

Drug Therapy. Drug therapy may be started after a psychosocial assessment by a qualified mental health care professional and informed consent has been obtained. According to WPATH's most recent standards of care, the criteria for hormone therapy include:

- Continuing and well-documented gender dysphoria
- Patient ability to make a fully informed decision and give consent to treatment
- Patient older than 18 years
- Well-controlled existing medical or mental health problems, if any

Drugs for MtF Patients. Patients transitioning from male to female (MtF) typically take a combination of estrogen therapy and androgen-reducing medications to achieve feminizing effects. Expected physical changes from *estrogen therapy* are breast enlargement, thinning hair, decreased testicular size, decreased erectile function, and increased body fat compared with muscle mass (Table 73-3). Because oral estrogen (ethinyl

TABLE 73-3 **Feminizing Drug Therapy for MtF Patients: Expected Changes and Monitoring**	
Expected Physical Changes	**Laboratory/Imaging Studies**
• Enlargement of breast tissue (gynecomastia)	• Chemistry panel (including glucose and electrolytes)
• Decreased testicular size	• Liver function tests
• Decreased erectile function	• Lipid profile
• Decreased libido (sex drive)	• Complete blood count
• Decreased body hair growth	• Prostate-specific antigen (PSA) if recommended for age-group
• Decreased male pattern baldness	• Mammogram (when breast tissue develops)
• Increased fat compared with muscle	• Papanicolaou (Pap) smear (if vagina present)
• Softening of skin	

estradiol) can increase the risk for venous thromboembolism, transdermal estrogen (Climara) or injectable estradiol is preferred for use in transgender patients. The typical dosing is two 0.1-mg patches changed twice weekly. Injectable estradiol is usually prescribed in a dose between 5 and 20 mg IM every 2 weeks. Progesterone may also be prescribed for 10 days each month (Burchum & Rosenthal, 2016).

> **! NURSING SAFETY PRIORITY** QSEN
>
> **Drug Alert**
>
> Before the first dose of transdermal estrogen, teach the patient to apply the patch to an area that is hairless to ensure good contact with the skin. When changing to a new patch, wash any excess drug from the skin where the previous patch was applied.

Teach patients taking any form of estrogen about side effects such as headache, breast tenderness, nausea/vomiting, and weight gain (often due to fluid retention) or loss. Tell them to report increased feelings of anxiety or depression to their primary health care provider. Estrogens can also cause estrogen-dependent cancers, hypertension (due to fluid retention), venous thromboembolism (VTE) such as deep vein thrombosis (DVT), and gallbladder disease. Teach patients to follow up with their primary health care provider to monitor for these potential adverse drug effects. Diagnostic testing is part of follow-up and monitoring, as listed in Table 73-3.

> **? NCLEX EXAMINATION CHALLENGE 73-1**
>
> **Physiological Integrity**
>
> The nurse provides health teaching for a client receiving estrogen therapy. Which statement by the client indicates that the teaching was effective? **Select all that apply.**
> A. "I need to check my blood pressure frequently when taking this drug."
> B. "I'll call my doctor if I have any redness or swelling in my legs."
> C. "I'll drink extra fluids because this drug will cause me to urinate a lot."
> D. "I know that the drug will cause my breast to feel tender."
> E. "I can get frequent headaches from taking this drug."

In addition to estrogen therapy, androgen-reducing agents (anti-androgens) are often given to block the effects of testosterone, including (Burchum & Rosenthal, 2016):
- Spironolactone (Aldactone), a low-cost diuretic that also inhibits testosterone secretion and androgen binding to androgen receptors
- 5-alpha reductase inhibitors (e.g., finasteride [Proscar]), drugs typically used to treat benign prostatic hyperplasia (BPH) (These drugs block the conversion of testosterone to a more active ingredient to decrease the hair loss associated with estrogen therapy and shrink prostate tissue.)
- GnRH agonists (e.g., goserelin [Zoladex]), neurohormones that block the gonadotropin-releasing hormone receptor, thus inhibiting the release of the follicle-stimulating hormone (FSH), and luteinizing hormone (LH) (These drugs are more expensive and are available only as implants and parenteral preparations.)

> **! NURSING SAFETY PRIORITY** QSEN
>
> **Drug Alert**
>
> Teach patients taking *spironolactone* to monitor their blood pressure and have periodic laboratory tests to assess for hyperkalemia if the health care provider determines them to be at risk for these drug effects. Remind them that increased serum potassium can cause cardiac dysrhythmias and skeletal muscle spasticity.

Common side effects of finasteride and other *5-alpha reductase inhibitors* include dizziness, cold sweats, and chills. These symptoms typically decrease over time. If patients continue to have them, instruct them to contact their primary health care provider.

Teach patients receiving *GnRH agonists* how to self-administer subcutaneous injections. Major side effects of these drugs are tachycardia and other cardiac dysrhythmias. Remind patients to follow up with their health care provider to monitor heart rate and rhythm. Teach them to call 911 if they experience chest pain (Burchum & Rosenthal, 2016).

Drugs for FtM Patients.   Testosterone is the major drug used for achieving masculinizing effects in transgender people transitioning from female to male; however, much of the available drug converts to estrogen in the body. This drug can be taken orally, transdermally, or parenterally (IM). Buccal and implantable forms of testosterone are also available. Oral testosterone (Andriol) is the least effective form of the drug. Depo-Testosterone, the most common IM preparation, is usually started in a low dose and increased to 100 to 200 mg every 1 to 2 weeks (Burchum & Rosenthal, 2016). Teach patients the importance of not sharing needles to prevent bloodborne diseases such as hepatitis C.

AndroGel and Androderm are topical forms that are more expensive than other testosterone preparations but may provide more consistent (although slower) results. A newer topical form of the drug, Axiron, can be applied to the armpits to increase serum testosterone levels. For all topical testosterone preparations, be sure that the patient washes his hands between applications and covers the area with clothing.

Expected effects of testosterone therapy include deepening of the voice, increased libido (sex drive), increased body hair growth, breast and ovarian atrophy, clitoral enlargement, and cessation of menses (Table 73-4). Teach the patient taking testosterone that some of these changes take up to a year to appear. If menses does not stop in the first few months of drug therapy, the patient is placed on Depo-Provera (progesterone) every 3 months until the testosterone becomes effective.

Common side effects of testosterone therapy include edema, acne, seborrhea (oily skin), headaches, weight gain, and possible psychotic symptoms. Before taking this medication, the patient is screened for a history of liver and heart disease. Testosterone therapy can cause increased liver enzymes, increased low-density lipoproteins (LDLs, or "bad" cholesterol), and decreased high-density lipoproteins (HDLs, or "good" cholesterol). Increased blood glucose and decreased clotting factors can also occur when taking the drug. Teach patients that these changes can lead to diabetes, heart disease, and stroke. Therefore remind patients that they need to follow up with their primary health care providers for careful monitoring for these complications, including having extensive diagnostic and laboratory testing (see Table 73-4).

TABLE 73-4 Masculinizing Drug Therapy for FtM Patients: Expected Changes and Monitoring

Expected Changes	Laboratory/Imaging Studies
• Voice deepening	• Lipid profile
• Body hair growth (hirsutism)	• Liver function tests
• Breast atrophy	• Complete blood count
• Increased libido	• Papanicolaou (Pap) smear (if
• Increased aggression	vagina present)
• Clitoral growth	• Mammogram (if breast tissue
• Redistribution of fat	present)
• Laryngeal prominence	

Reproductive Health Options. Using feminizing or masculinizing hormone therapy affects reproductive health, especially fertility. Therefore be sure that patients know their options for REPRODUCTION, if desired, *before* transition begins. MtF patients may want to consider sperm banking before drug therapy or gender reassignment surgery if they desire to have a biologic child. FtM patients may want to consider oocyte (egg) or embryo freezing. These frozen gametes or embryo could be implanted in a surrogate woman to become pregnant and carry to birth. Inform patients that these options are expensive, but be sure that all patients are informed. Be sure to include the patient's sexual partner, if any, in discussions related to reproductive options.

Voice and Communication Therapy. Communication is an essential aspect of human behavior and gender expression. Voice deepening for transgender people who are transitioning from female to male is accomplished by taking masculinizing hormones, such as testosterone. However, feminizing hormones have no effect on the adult MtF voice.

MtF patients may seek assistance from a voice and communication specialist to help them develop certain vocal characteristics, such as pitch and intonation. Vocal therapy can assist in management of gender dysphoria and be a positive step in the transition process. Specialists include speech-language pathologists and speech-voice clinicians. Remind patients to seek a specialist who is licensed, is knowledgeable in transgender health, and has specialized training in assessment and development of communication skills for transgender patients.

The purpose of vocal therapy is to help patients adapt their voice and communication such that it is authentic and reflects their gender identity. The voice therapist should take the patient's communication preferences and style into consideration as part of the assessment process to develop an individualized treatment plan. Some patients choose follow-up sessions for vocal therapy following voice feminization surgery, also called *feminization laryngoplasty*. This surgery is described in the next section.

Surgical Management. Many transgender people are satisfied with their gender identity, role, and self-expression without surgery. Surgery, particularly procedures that affect the external or internal genitalia, is usually the last and most carefully considered option for transitioning from one's natal sex to one's inner gender identity. These procedures are often referred to as **gender** or **sex reassignment surgery (SRS)** but are also known as gender-affirming surgery or gender-confirming surgery. The patient has a number of surgical options to achieve either feminizing or masculinizing effects. Regardless of the procedure performed, the nurse collaborates with the patient, family, and health care team to promote positive outcomes for the transition process.

Gender reassignment surgeries are procedures that alter anatomically healthy structures. Not all surgeons feel comfortable in performing procedures that could "harm" transgender patients. However, these procedures help treat gender dysphoria. Some patients elect to undergo the full range of surgeries, whereas others choose to have only some or none of them, typically because of the profound medical expense.

Genital surgeries "below the waist" are the most invasive procedures. The criteria for genital surgery depend on the type of surgery being requested. For example, most surgeons (usually urologists or plastic surgeons) require 12 months of hormone therapy plus one or two referrals from qualified psychotherapists for MtF patients who desire an orchiectomy (removal of testes). The same requirements are needed for FtM patients who desire a hysterectomy (uterus removal) and bilateral salpingo-oophorectomy (BSO), or removal of both fallopian tubes and ovaries.

The psychotherapist assesses the patient's readiness for genital surgery and hormone therapy, including a discussion of risks and out-of-pocket costs. The patient's support system is assessed to ensure that the patient makes the best possible decision and achieves the desired outcomes.

For MtF patients requesting a vaginoplasty (creation of a vagina) or FtM patients desiring a phalloplasty (creation of a penis), the required criteria include 12 continuous months of living in a gender role that is congruent with the patient's gender identity. It is also recommended that these patients have regular visits with a mental health care professional (Coleman et al., 2011).

Feminizing Surgeries for MtF Patients. Feminizing surgeries are performed for MtF patients to create a functional and/or aesthetic (cosmetic) female anatomy, including:

- Breast/chest surgeries, such as breast augmentation (mammoplasty to increase breast tissue)
- Genital surgeries, such as partial penectomy (removal of the penis), orchiectomy (removal of the testes), vaginoplasty and labiaplasty vulvoplasty (creation of a vagina and labia/vulva), and clitoroplasty (creation of a clitoris)
- Other surgeries, such as facial feminizing surgery (to achieve feminine facial contour); liposuction (fatty tissue removal), often from the waist or abdominal area; vocal feminizing surgery; and other body-contouring procedures.

Breast augmentation creates breast tissue for the MtF patient through the use of silicone or saline implants. Although not a prerequisite, it is recommended that MtF patients take feminizing hormones for 12 months before surgery for the best results (Coleman et al., 2011).

Voice surgery, such as reduction thyroid chondroplasty, is performed to decrease the size of the "Adam's apple." The procedure is done through a bronchoscope for cosmetic purposes. Nursing care of the patient having a bronchoscopy is discussed in Chapter 27.

The most common "below the waist" genital surgeries for MtF patients are bilateral *orchiectomy* to remove the testes and vaginoplasty with partial penectomy. Orchiectomy procedures and associated nursing care are the same for the transgender patient as they are for other natal males (see Chapter 72 for a detailed discussion).

A **vaginoplasty** is the construction of a neovagina (new vagina), usually with inverted penile tissue (obtained during a partial penectomy) or a colon graft. The procedure also includes creating a clitoris and labia using scrotal or penile tissue and skin grafts.

Preoperative Care. In addition to the required criteria to qualify for a vaginoplasty (also called *transvaginal surgery*), the transgender patient is medically evaluated like any other pre-surgical patient. Patients who have poorly controlled diabetes with vascular complications, coronary artery disease, or other systemic disease that limits functional ability are not candidates for gender reassignment surgery. Chapter 14 describes general preoperative care for any patient.

The surgeon explains the options for selected procedures, postoperative care expectations, and potential for complications after surgery. Postoperative recovery for transvaginal surgery takes a long time and has a high complication rate. Overweight patients have a higher incidence of wound infection and may have problems with adequate ventilation (breathing) and ambulation after surgery. Refer these patients for nutritional counseling as needed.

Written and verbal preoperative instructions are provided by the surgeon, including optional methods of body hair removal. A bowel preparation may be started 24 hours before surgery and includes a clear liquid diet, laxatives, and Fleet's enemas. Increased fluids are recommended until the patient goes to bed the night before surgery because the bowel "prep" can be very dehydrating. Antimicrobials such as neomycin sulfate and metronidazole (Flagyl) are typically given on the day of surgery to minimize the risk for infection.

Some surgeons require that the patient take supplements to prevent bruising and promote tissue healing, such as vitamin C. Patients who are very thin are encouraged to eat a high-protein diet. A powdered protein supplement with arginine (an amino acid) may also be prescribed to promote wound healing.

Patients have a number of laboratory tests to ensure that they are healthy before surgery. Adequate hemoglobin and hematocrit (H&H) levels are especially important because some blood is lost during surgery. For patients who have low H&H levels, an erythropoietin such as epoetin alfa (Procrit) or IM testosterone with iron is given. Most patients choose testosterone because it is a lower-cost drug.

Operative Procedures. Because surgery requires multiple procedures to create a female anatomy, the patient is on the operating table for many hours. The surgery may be performed in a hospital or specialized center for transgender surgeries. After general or epidural anesthesia is administered, the patient is placed in a lithotomy position (feet in stirrups) for the procedure. Epidural anesthesia is preferred for patients who are asthmatic or obese. The patient is transferred to the postanesthesia care unit (PACU) with a perineal dressing and packing, Jackson-Pratt drain, and indwelling urinary catheter.

Postoperative Care. Provide general postoperative care as described in Chapter 16. In addition, immediately after surgery, apply an ice pack to the perineum to decrease pain and bruising. Monitor the patient's pain level carefully and offer analgesia as needed. Genital surgery is painful because there is a high concentration of nerve endings in the perineum.

Although not a common postoperative complication, monitor the patient for bleeding. Observe the surgical dressing and surrounding area for oozing or bright red blood. Report and document any indication of bleeding immediately to the surgeon and keep the patient in bed.

Encourage the patient to drink liquids after surgery; discontinue the patient's IV line once oral fluids are tolerated. Evaluate the patient's intake and output every 8 to 12 hours.

> **! NURSING SAFETY PRIORITY** QSEN
>
> **Action Alert**
>
> Patients are in a lithotomy position for an extended period during surgery. Therefore, after surgery, monitor lower-extremity neurovascular status and encourage the patient to move the legs often during the first 24 hours after surgery. Report and document any unexpected findings, such as continued numbness or inability to move the lower legs or feet. Patients who had epidural anesthesia are not able to move their legs for several hours after surgery until the effect of the drug diminishes.

All patients stay in the hospital for at least one night after surgery, but some patients may stay longer, depending on the number and complexity of the surgical procedures. Some agencies transfer the patient the day after surgery to a local hotel for continued follow-up and monitoring by a health care professional (usually a nurse). Collaborate with the case manager for discharge planning and follow-up care.

The Jackson Pratt drain is removed typically 3 to 5 days after surgery when drainage is less than 15 to 20 mL in a 24-hour period. About a week after surgery, the surgical pressure dressing, packing, and external sutures are removed.

At this time, patients are taught how to douche and insert vaginal stents to dilate the vagina. Sexual intercourse also helps keep the vagina dilated. Remind patients that routine douching and douching after intercourse are needed to prevent infection in the new vagina. A solution of vinegar and water or a commercial product such as Massengill can be used. Vaginal stents (also called *dilators*) must be inserted several times a day for months after surgery. The stent should remain in the vagina for 30 to 45 minutes or as instructed by the surgeon. Teach patients the importance of using the stents with water-based lubrication. Collaborate with the surgeon to determine patient-specific instructions.

The urinary catheter is removed between postoperative day 7 and 12. Early removal can cause urinary retention, but prolonged placement can lead to catheter-associated urinary tract infection (CAUTI).

Patients should continue follow-up visits with their primary health care provider for signs and symptoms of complications. One of the worst complications is a vaginal-rectal fistula, which is caused by rectal perforation during surgery. Teach patients to report any leakage of stool into the vagina immediately to their surgeon. The treatment for this complication is a temporary colostomy and fistula wound management for many months. Other surgical complications of vaginoplasty are listed in Table 73-5.

In addition to physical complications after surgery, some MtF patients are not satisfied with the quality of the results. For example, the neovagina may not be functional for sexual intercourse. Some patients request another surgery to achieve more satisfying results.

Masculinizing Surgeries for FtM Patients. Masculinizing surgeries are performed for FtM patients to create a functional and/or aesthetic male anatomy, including:

TABLE 73-5 Postoperative Complications of Vaginoplasty Surgery

Most Serious Complications
- Vaginal-rectal fistula
- Rectal perforation
- Bleeding

Other Complications
- Surgical wound infection
- Urinary leakage/incontinence
- Chronic urinary tract infections
- Urinary meatus stenosis
- Vaginal stenosis
- Vaginal collapse
- Labial hematoma
- Inadequate vaginal length or width
- Lack of sensation
- Lack of sexual pleasure

? NCLEX EXAMINATION CHALLENGE 73-2

Physiological Integrity

A client is admitted to the postanesthesia care unit (PACU) following a vaginoplasty. For which surgical complications will the nurse monitor in the PACU? **Select all that apply.**
A. Bleeding
B. Rectal perforation
C. Urinary incontinence
D. Surgical site infection
E. Urinary retention

- Breast/chest surgeries, usually a bilateral mastectomy (removal of both breasts) and chest reconstruction
- Genital surgeries, such as a hysterectomy and bilateral BSO, vaginectomy (removal of the vagina), phalloplasty (creation of an average-size male penis) with uretero-plasty (creation of a urethra) or metoidioplasty (creation of a small penis using hormone-enhanced clitoral tissue), and scrotoplasty (creation of a scrotum) with insertion of testicular prostheses
- Other surgeries, such as liposuction, pectoral muscle implants, and other body-contouring procedures

Care of transgender patients having a mastectomy, hysterectomy, and bilateral salpingo-oophorectomy (BSO) is similar to care for any patient having these procedures as described elsewhere in this text. If the patient has not had previous abdominal surgery, a laparoscopic procedure is preferred for the hysterectomy and BSO surgery.

Procedures to create a male anatomy are not performed as often as MtF surgeries. Phalloplasties are the most difficult reconstructive genital surgeries to perform and usually require several stages. Skin flaps from the radial forearm, anterior lateral thigh, or back are used to create the penis. Fat grafts may be needed to increase penile girth, and buccal mucosal tissue may be used to create the urethra. A penile prosthesis or implant is not inserted until months after surgery when the initial surgical healing has occurred.

Complications from phalloplasty include urinary tract stenosis, donor graft site scarring, and occasionally necrosis of the neopenis (new penis). In addition to these physical problems, the patient may not be satisfied with the results of the surgery, such as an inadequate length of the penis. For these reasons, most FtM patients do not have this procedure and prefer to have only a laparoscopic hysterectomy and BSO.

? CLINICAL JUDGMENT CHALLENGE 73-1

Patient-Centered Care; Teamwork and Collaboration QSEN

A 58-year-old male-appearing patient visits the gender identity clinic to discuss the desire to have gender reassignment surgery. As the clinical nurse, you take the patient's history and find that the patient was married to a woman for 30 years and had three children. The couple divorced 3 months ago when the patient's wife discovered that her husband identified as a woman. The couple's children have had no contact with the patient since that time. The patient is employed as the vice-president of a large commercial construction company and has health insurance. The patient is interested in learning about options for male-to-female transitioning.

1. How would you address this patient?
2. What other data do you need to collect for the patient's history and why?
3. What options for transitioning to a female does this patient have?
4. After a physical examination, the clinic physician prescribed transdermal estrogen and spironolactone for the patient. What instructions will you provide for the patient before beginning drug therapy?

Care Coordination and Transition Management

Transgender patients often take hormone therapy for many years. Teach them that ongoing follow-up with a qualified health care professional is needed to maintain health and detect any complications, such as diabetes or cardiovascular problems, as early as possible.

Long-term follow-up with the surgeon after gender reassignment is essential to detect and treat the frequent complications that occur. Assess the patient's support systems and coping strategies, including financial status and health insurance benefits. Collaborate with the case manager to ensure a smooth transition into the community, including the possible need for any ongoing mental health counseling or therapy.

Urogenital care is also needed for patients who have gender reassignment surgery. FtM patients usually do not have a vaginectomy and therefore may experience vaginal atrophy causing itching and burning. Recommend that they seek gynecologic care to treat this problem, although the examination can be physically and emotionally painful.

MtF patients need counseling about SEXUALITY, genital hygiene, and prevention of sexually transmitted diseases. They are also at a high risk for frequent urinary tract infections as a result of a shortened urethra and urinary incontinence as a result of genital surgery. Teach patients the importance of having follow-up care for these problems.

Preventive health care screenings for transgender patients are also important. For example, the MtF patient requires prostate health care screenings that natal males need. Mammograms are also recommended to monitor for early signs of breast cancer.

A number of community resources and organizations are available for transgender support and information, such as:
- National Coalition for LGBT Health (http://lgbthealth.webolutionary.com/content/resources)
- Services and Advocacy for Gay, Lesbian, Bisexual, and Transgender Elders (www.sageusa.org)
- Transgender Health Information Program (www.transhealth.phsa.ca)
- University of San Francisco Center for Transgender Health (www.transhealth.ucsf.edu)
- World Professional Association for Transgender Health (www.wpath.org)

GET READY FOR THE NCLEX® EXAMINATION!

KEY POINTS

Review these Key Points for each NCLEX Examination Client Needs Category.

Safe and Effective Care Environment
- Depending on identified health care needs, collaborate with the primary health care provider, mental health professional, surgeon, pharmacist, and/or vocal/speech specialist when caring for the transgender patient. **QSEN: Teamwork and Interprofessional Collaboration**
- Advocate for the transgender patient who may be distrustful of health care professionals and fearful when seeking health care. **QSEN: Patient-Centered Care**

Health Promotion and Maintenance
- Teach patients taking hormone therapy about the need for ongoing health care monitoring for adverse drug events and health complications (see Tables 73-3 and 73-4). **QSEN: Safety**
- Refer the transgender patient and significant others, as appropriate, to community resources for information and support, such as the University of San Francisco Center for Transgender Health and the Transgender Health Information Program through Vancouver Coastal Health. Be knowledgeable about local resources and refer patients as needed.

Psychosocial Integrity
- Use culturally sensitive and accurate language when communicating with transgender patients; use pronouns that match the patient's physical appearance and dress unless the patient requests a specific term (see Tables 73-1 and 73-2). **QSEN: Patient-Centered Care**

- Provide PATIENT-CENTERED transgender CARE with dignity and respect for all patients. **Ethics**
- Be aware that transgender people may experience gender dysphoria, which presents an inner conflict between the person's natal (birth) sex and perceived gender identity.
- Assess transgender patients for sources of stress in the community that can lead to health issues, such as depression, anxiety, and substance use.
- Be aware that transgender patients may avoid health care settings because they are often unemployed, have no health insurance, and/or fear lack of respect and understanding based on previous experiences. These concerns contribute to HEALTH CARE DISPARITIES for this population. **QSEN: Patient-Centered Care**

Physiological Integrity
- Monitor for expected, side, and adverse effects of hormone therapy, including effects on SEXUALITY and REPRODUCTION, as described in Tables 73-3 and 73-4.
- Recognize that patients receiving hormone therapy need to have periodic laboratory testing to monitor for complications as listed in Tables 73-3 and Table 73-4. **QSEN: Evidence-Based Practice**
- Provide preoperative care for a patient having a vaginoplasty, including teaching about bowel preparation, food and fluid intake, hair-removal methods, and the need for informed consent.
- Monitor for potentially life-threatening complications of gender reassignment surgery, such as fistula development, bleeding, and wound infection (see Table 73-5).

SELECTED BIBLIOGRAPHY

Asterisk indicates a classic or definitive work on this subject.

American Nurses Association (ANA) (2015). *Code of ethics for nurses.* Washington, DC: Author.

American Psychiatric Association (APA) (2013). *Diagnostic and statistical manual of mental disorders* (5th ed.). Washington, DC: Author.

Bauer, G. R., & Scheim, A. I. (2015). *Transgender people in Ontario, Canada: Statistics from the Trans PULSE Project to inform human rights policy.* London, ON: Canadian Institute of Health Research.

Brennan, A. M. W., Barnsteiner, J., de Leon Siantz, M. L., Cotter, V. T., & Everett, J. (2012). Lesbian, gay, bisexual, transgendered, or intersexed content for nursing curricula. *Journal of Professional Nursing, 28*(2), 96–104.

Burchum, J. L. R., & Rosenthal, L. D. (2016). *Lehne's pharmacology for nursing care* (9th ed.). St. Louis: Elsevier.

Chestnut, S., Dixon, E., & Jindasurat, C. (2013). *Lesbian, gay, bisexual, transgender, queer, and HIV-affected hate violence in 2012.* National Coalition of Anti-Violence Programs. www.avp.org/storage/documents/ncavp_2012_hvreport_final.pdf.

*Coleman, E., Bockting, W., Botzer, M., Cohen-Kettenis, P., DeCuypere, G., Fladman, J., et al. (2011). Standards of care for the health of transsexual, transgender, and gender-nonconforming people (Version 7). *International Journal of Transgenderism, 13*, 165–232.

Edwards-Leeper, L., & Spack, N. P. (2013). Psychological evaluation and medical treatment of transgender youth in an interdisciplinary "Gender Management Services" (GeMS) in a major pediatric center. In J. Drescher & W. Byne (Eds.), *Treating transgender children and adolescents: An interdisciplinary discussion.* New York: Routledge.

Eliason, M. J., Chinn, P., Dibble, S. L., & DeJoseph, J. (2013). Open the door for LGBTQ patients. *Nursing, 43*(8), 44–50.

Flores, A. R., Herman, J. L., Gates, G. J., & Brown, T. N. T. (2016). *How many adults identify as transgender in the United States?* Los Angeles, CA: The Williams Institute.

*Grant, J. M., Mottet, L. A., & Tanis, J. (2010). *National transgender discrimination survey report on health and health care.* National Center for Transgender Equality and National Gay and Lesbian Task Force. http://transequality.org/PDFs/NTDSReportonHealth_final.pdf.

*Grant, J. M., Mottet, L. A., & Tanis, J. (2011). *Injustice at every turn: A report of the national transgender discrimination survey.* National Center for Transgender Equality and National Gay and Lesbian Task Force. http://www.thetaskforce.org/static_html/downloads/reports/reports/ntds_full.pdf.

*Institute of Medicine (IOM) (2011). *The health of LGBT people: Building a foundation for better understanding.* Washington, DC: National Academies Press.

Merryfeather, L., & Bruce, A. (2014). The invisibility of gender diversity: Understanding transgender and transsexuality in nursing literature. *Nursing Forum, 49*(2), 110–123.

Redfern, J. S., & Sinclair, B. (2014). Improving health care encounters and communication with transgender patients. *Journal of Communication in Healthcare, 7*(1), 25–40.

Rounds, K. E., McGrath, B. B., & Walsh, E. (2013). Perspectives on provider behaviors: A qualitative study of sexual and gender minorities regarding quality of care. *Contemporary Nurse, 44*(1), 99–110.

Spack, N. P. (2013). Management of transgenderism. *Journal of the American Medical Association, 309*, 478–484.

*The Joint Commission (TJC) (2011). *Advancing effective communication, cultural competence, and patient- and family-centered care for the lesbian, gay, bisexual, and transgender community.* www.jointcommission.org/lgbt.

74 | CHAPTER

Care of Patients With Sexually Transmitted Infections

Donna D. Ignatavicius

ⓔ http://evolve.elsevier.com/Iggy/

LEARNING OUTCOMES

Safe and Effective Care Environment
1. Maintain patient confidentiality and privacy related to sexually transmitted infection (STI).

Health Promotion and Maintenance
2. Educate patients with STIs and their partners on self-care measures.
3. Describe the role of expedited partner therapy in reducing STI recurrence.
4. Develop a teaching plan for young adults and other at-risk people about risk factors, prevention, and treatment for STIs.
5. Explain the importance of respect for patients' personal values and beliefs regarding practices associated with SEXUALITY.
6. Describe HEALTH CARE DISPARITIES associated with the incidence and management of STIs.

Psychosocial Integrity
7. Assess patients' and their partners' responses to a diagnosis of STI.
8. Reduce the psychological impact for the patient who has been diagnosed with STI.

Physiological Integrity
9. Develop a health teaching plan for patients on how to self-manage their STI, including antibiotic therapy.
10. Describe the assessment findings, including impaired COMFORT, that are typical in patients with STIs.
11. Determine typical assessment findings for women with pelvic inflammatory disease (PID).
12. Develop a patient-centered collaborative plan of care for a patient with PID, including its possible impact on REPRODUCTION.

OVERVIEW

Sexually transmitted infections (STIs) are caused by infectious organisms that have been passed from one person to another through intimate contact—usually oral, vaginal, or anal intercourse. Some organisms that cause these diseases are transmitted only through sexual contact. Others are transmitted also by parenteral exposure to infected blood, fecal-oral transmission, intrauterine transmission to the fetus, and perinatal transmission from mother to neonate. If the STI continues to recur and become chronic, the term sexually transmitted disease (STD) is used. STD continues to be the most acceptable term used by the Centers for Disease Control and Prevention (CDC).

Improved diagnostic techniques, increased knowledge about organisms that can be sexually transmitted, and changes in SEXUALITY (see Chapter 2 for a review) and sexual practices have led to an increasing number of reported cases of STIs. *Sexual issues are often sensitive, personal, and controversial, and nurses must respect the patients' lifestyle. Providing confidentiality is essential for patients to receive correct information, make informed decisions, and obtain appropriate care.*

The prevalence of STIs is a major public health concern worldwide. Populations at greatest risk for acquiring STIs and suffering from their complications are pregnant women, adolescents, and men who have sex with men (MSM). External factors such as an increasing population, cultural factors (e.g., earlier first intercourse), political and economic policies, incidences of sexual abuse and human trafficking, and international travel and migration affect the prevalence of STIs.

CONSIDERATIONS FOR OLDER ADULTS
Patient-Centered Care QSEN

Another factor contributing to STI prevalence is the increasing number of older adults that will continue as baby boomers age. People older than 50 years may not realize their risk for STIs or feel comfortable discussing their SEXUALITY with health care providers. Health care professionals may also lack awareness of the sexual activity of older adults. Be sure to teach older adults who are sexually active about their risk for developing STIs.

In the United States, one of the greatest factors associated with STI prevalence is the secrecy that surrounds SEXUALITY, sexual behavior, and intimacy in the American culture. The stigma of STIs in the United States has been associated with higher rates of these infections compared with rates in other developed countries. The prevalence of STIs is also affected by changing human physiology patterns such as earlier onset of menarche, comorbidities associated with human immune deficiency virus (HIV) and diabetes, treatments given for cancer or organ transplantation, and HEALTH CARE DISPARITIES (see Chapter 1 for a review of this concept). Substance use disorder has also been identified as a significant risk factor because of the effects that illicit drugs have on sexual risk-taking behavior.

STIs cause complications that can contribute to severe physical and emotional suffering, including infertility, ectopic pregnancy, cancer, and death. Some of the most common complications caused by sexually transmitted organisms are listed in Table 74-1.

Chlamydia infection, gonorrhea, syphilis, chancroid, human immune deficiency virus (HIV) infection, and acquired immune deficiency syndrome (AIDS) are reportable to local health authorities in every state (Centers for Disease Control and Prevention [CDC], 2017c). Other STIs such as genital herpes (GH) may or may not be reported, depending on local legal requirements. Positive results can be reported by clinicians and laboratories. Reports are kept strictly confidential.

Nurses in a variety of settings are responsible for identifying people at risk for STIs, caring for patients with diagnosed STIs, and preventing further cases through education and case finding. Nurses in primary care community settings and acute care settings have a responsibility to recognize patients who are at risk for or who have STIs, possibly while being treated for another unrelated health problem.

The CDC provides regularly updated guidelines for treatment of STIs. These best practice guidelines provide information, treatment standards, and counseling advice to help decrease the spread of these diseases and their complications (CDC, 2015).

HEALTH PROMOTION AND MAINTENANCE

One of the *Healthy People 2020* objectives is to completely eliminate syphilis in the United States (U.S. Department of Health and Human Services [USDHHS], 2017) (Table 74-2). One of the primary tools for prevention of sexually transmitted diseases (STIs), including syphilis, is education. All people, regardless of age, gender, ethnicity, socioeconomic status,

TABLE 74-1	Complications Caused by Sexually Transmitted Organisms
COMPLICATION	**CAUSATIVE ORGANISMS**
Salpingitis, infertility, and ectopic pregnancy	Neisseria gonorrhoeae Chlamydia trachomatis Mycoplasma hominis Ureaplasma urealyticum
Puerperal infection	N. gonorrhoeae C. trachomatis
Perinatal infection	Hepatitis B virus Human immune deficiency virus Human papilloma virus N. gonorrhoeae C. trachomatis Herpes simplex virus Treponema pallidum Cytomegalovirus Group B streptococcus
Cancer of genital area	Human papilloma virus
Male urethritis	M. hominis Herpes simplex virus N. gonorrhoeae C. trachomatis U. urealyticum
Vulvovaginitis	Herpes simplex virus Trichomonas vaginalis Bacterial vaginosis Candida albicans
Cervicitis	N. gonorrhoeae C. trachomatis Herpes simplex virus
Proctitis	N. gonorrhoeae C. trachomatis Herpes simplex virus Campylobacter jejuni Shigella species Entamoeba histolytica
Hepatitis	T. pallidum Hepatitis A, hepatitis B, and hepatitis C viruses
Dermatitis	Sarcoptes scabiei Phthirus pubis
Genital ulceration or warts	C. trachomatis Herpes simplex virus Human papilloma virus T. pallidum Haemophilus ducreyi Calymmatobacterium granulomatis

education level, gender identity, or sexual orientation, are susceptible to these diseases. Health literacy, motivation, and perceived risk can affect the health status of any patient. STIs are largely preventable through safer sex practices. Do not assume that a person is not sexually active because of his or her age, education, marital status, profession, or religion. Discuss prevention methods, including safer sex, with all patients who are or may become sexually active.

Safer sex practices are those that reduce the risk for nonintact skin or mucous membranes coming in contact with infected body fluids and blood. These practices include:
- Using a latex or polyurethane condom for genital and anal intercourse

TABLE 74-2 Meeting *Healthy People 2020* Objectives and Targets for Improvement: Sexually Transmitted Infections/Diseases

- Reduce the proportion of adolescents and young adults with *Chlamydia trachomatis* infections (by 10%).
- Reduce the proportion of females ages 15 to 44 years who have ever required treatment for pelvic inflammatory disease (by 10%).
- Reduce gonorrhea rates (by 10%).
- Reduce sustained domestic transmission of primary and secondary syphilis (by 10%).
- Reduce the proportion of females with human papilloma virus (HPV) infection (no specific target).
- Reduce the proportion of young adults with genital herpes due to herpes simplex type 2 (by 10%).

GENDER HEALTH CONSIDERATIONS

Patient-Centered Care QSEN

Because of the very vascular and large surface area of the mucous membranes of the vagina, women are more easily infected with STIs and are at greater risk for STI-related health problems than are men. Young women who are sexually active with men have the greatest risk for contracting an STI. Younger adults have greater rates of sexual activity, including more partners and more unprotected sex than older adults. Women are also more vulnerable to infections because of the exposure of cervical basal epithelium cells. Lesbian women have a *decreased* risk for STIs because of fewer partners, although many have or have had sex with men.

Some women may also be at high risk because they:
- Lack knowledge about the risk for disease
- Believe that they are not vulnerable to disease
- Mistakenly believe that contraceptives also protect them from STIs
- Drink alcohol in binges, which promotes risky sexual behavior

Postmenopausal women also may be at risk for STIs because many perceive that pregnancy is no longer likely and thus do not use barrier protection. Changing social relationships (e.g., divorce and widowhood in the middle years) have changed risk for exposure to STIs. Physiologic changes during menopause such as mucosal tears from vaginal atrophy may also place them at risk.

Women have more asymptomatic infections that may delay diagnosis and treatment. Many infectious organisms reside in the cervical os and cause little change in vaginal discharge or vulvar tissue, so women are not aware that they are infected. This delay increases the likelihood of complications, including ascending infections that may cause reproductive organ damage and illness. Embarrassment, denial, or fear about STIs may further delay treatment, increasing the potential for serious complications.

- Using a condom or latex barrier (dental dam) over the genitals or anus during oral-genital or oral-anal sexual contact
- Wearing gloves for finger or hand contact with the vagina or rectum
- Abstinence
- Mutual monogamy
- Decreasing the number of sexual partners

GENITAL HERPES

❖ PATHOPHYSIOLOGY

Genital herpes (GH) is an acute, recurring, incurable viral disease. It is the most common STI in the United States. The prevalence among African Americans is higher than for Euro-Americans, disproportionately affecting African-American women more than men (CDC, 2017c).

Two serotypes of herpes simplex virus (HSV) affect the genitalia: type 1 (HSV-1) and type 2 (HSV-2) (McCance et al., 2014). Most *nongenital* lesions such as cold sores are caused by HSV-1, transmitted via oral-oral contact. Historically HSV-2 caused most of the genital lesions. However, this distinction is academic because the transmission, symptoms, diagnosis, and treatment are nearly identical for the two types. Either type can produce oral or genital lesions through oral-genital or genital-genital contact with an infected person. HSV-2 recurs and sheds asymptomatically more often than HSV-1. Most people with GH have not been diagnosed because they have mild symptoms and shed virus intermittently.

The incubation period of genital herpes is 2 to 20 days, with the average period being 1 week. Many people do not have symptoms during the primary outbreak. Whether the patient is symptomatic or not, the virus remains dormant and recurs periodically. *Therefore, recurrences are not caused by re-infection. However, there is viral shedding, and the patient is infectious.* Long-term complications of GH include the risk for neonatal transmission and an increased risk for acquiring HIV infection (McCance et al., 2014).

❖ INTERPROFESSIONAL COLLABORATIVE CARE

◆ Assessment: Noticing

The diagnosis of GH is based on the patient's history and physical examination (Chart 74-1). Ask the patient if he or she felt itching or a tingling sensation in the skin 1 to 2 days before the outbreak, known as the *prodrome*. These sensations are usually followed by the appearance of **vesicles** (blisters) in a typical cluster on the penis, scrotum, vulva, vagina, cervix, or perianal region at the site of inoculation. The blisters rupture spontaneously in a day or two and leave painful ulcerations that can become extensive. Assess for other symptoms such as headaches, fever, general malaise, and swelling of inguinal lymph nodes. Ask if urination is painful. External dysuria is a painful symptom when urine passes over the eroded areas. Patients with urinary retention may need to be catheterized. Lesions resolve within 2 to 6 weeks.

After the lesions heal, the virus remains in a dormant state in the sacral nerve ganglia. Periodically the virus may activate, and symptoms recur. These recurrences may be triggered by many factors, including stress, fever, sunburn, poor nutrition, menses, and sexual activity. Assess the patient for these risk factors to provide anticipatory guidance for prevention of outbreaks.

GH is confirmed through a viral cell culture or polymerase chain reaction (PCR) assays of the lesions. PCR is the more sensitive test and is currently the gold standard; however, it is very expensive and usually not available. Fluid from inside the blister obtained within 48 hours of the first outbreak will yield the most reliable results because accuracy decreases as the blisters begin to heal. Serology testing, which is glycoprotein G antibody based, can identify the HSV type, either 1 or 2. Serologic tests are used to identify infection in high-risk groups such as HIV-positive patients, patients who have partners with HSV, or men who have sex with men (MSM) (CDC, 2017a). Antibodies may take up to 12 weeks to develop, so false-negative results can occur if tested too soon after the initial infection.

CHART 74-1 Focused Assessment

The Patient With a Sexually Transmitted Infection

Assess history of present illness:
- Chief concern
- Onset
- Symptoms by quality and quantity, precipitating and palliative factors
- Any treatments taken (self-prescribed or over-the-counter products)

Assess past medical history:
- Major health problems, including any history of STIs/PID or immunosuppression
- Surgeries: obstetric and gynecologic, circumcision

Assess current health status:
- Menstrual history for irregularities
- Sexual history:
- Type and frequency of sexual activity
- Number of lifetime and past 6 months sexual contacts/partners; monogamous
- Sexual orientation
- Contraception history
- Medications
- Allergies
- Lifestyle risks: drugs, alcohol, tobacco

Assess preventive health care practices:
- Papanicolaou (Pap) tests
- Regular STI screening
- Use of barrier contraceptives to prevent STIs and pregnancy

Assess physical examination findings:
- Vital signs
- Oropharyngeal findings
- Abdominal findings
- Genital or pelvic findings
- Anorectal findings

Assess laboratory data:
- Urinalysis
- Hematology
- ESR or CRP if PID is being considered
- Cervical, urethral, oral, rectal specimens
- Lesion samples for microbiology and virology
- Pregnancy testing

CRP, C-reactive protein; ESR, erythrocyte sedimentation rate; PID, pelvic inflammatory disease; STI, sexually transmitted infection.

CHART 74-2 Best Practice for Patient Safety & Quality Care QSEN

Care of or Self-Management for the Patient With Genital Herpes

- Administer oral analgesics as prescribed.
- Apply local anesthetic sprays or ointments as prescribed.
- Apply ice packs or warm compresses to the patient's lesions.
- Administer sitz baths three or four times a day.
- Urge an increase in fluid intake to replace fluid lost through open lesions.
- Encourage frequent urination.
- Pour water over the patient's genitalia while voiding or encourage voiding while the patient is sitting in a tub of water or standing in a shower.
- Catheterize the patient as necessary.
- Encourage genital hygiene, and encourage keeping the skin clean and dry.
- Wash hands thoroughly after contact with lesions and launder towels that have had direct contact with lesions.
- Wear gloves when applying ointments or making any direct contact with lesions.
- Advise the patient to avoid sexual activity when lesions are present.
- Advise the patient to use latex or polyurethane condoms during all sexual exposures.
- Instruct the patient in the use, side effects, and risks versus benefits of antiviral agents.
- Advise the patient to discuss the diagnosis of genital herpes (GH) with current and new partners.

prevent outbreaks, even for those with infrequent recurrent episodes (Burchum & Rosenthal, 2016).

Suppression reduces recurrences in most patients, but it does not prevent viral shedding, even when symptoms are absent. Patients receiving continuous therapy should periodically (possibly once a year) be reassessed for recurrences, usually by stopping the antiviral drug temporarily.

IV acyclovir and hospitalization may be indicated for patients with severe HSV infections, such as disseminated (systemic) disease or encephalitis (brain infection). These are severe complications of genital herpes and may be fatal.

Self-Management Education. Nursing interventions focus on patient education about the infection, sexual transmission, potential for recurrent episodes, and correct use and possible side effects of antiviral therapy. Frank discussion about sexual activity, including whether the patient has new or multiple partners, is an essential component of the nurse's intervention.

! NURSING SAFETY PRIORITY QSEN

Action Alert

Remind patients to abstain from sexual activity while GH lesions are present. Sexual activity can be painful, and likelihood of viral transmission is higher. Urge condom use during all sexual exposures because of the increased risk for HSV transmission from viral shedding, which can occur even when lesions are not present. Teach the patient about how to use condoms (Chart 74-3).

Assess the patient's and partner's emotional responses to the diagnosis of genital herpes. Many people are initially shocked and need reassurance that they can manage the disease. Infected patients may have feelings of disbelief, uncleanness, isolation, and loneliness. They may also be angry at their partner(s) for

◆ Interventions: Responding

The desired outcomes of treatment for HSV-infected patients are to decrease the impaired COMFORT from painful ulcerations, promote healing without secondary infection, decrease viral shedding, and prevent infection transmission (Chart 74-2).

Drug Therapy. Antiviral drugs are used to treat GH. The drugs decrease the severity, promote healing, and decrease the frequency of recurrent outbreaks but do not cure the infection.

Drug therapy should be offered to anyone with an initial outbreak of GH regardless of the severity of the symptoms. Topical therapy is not recommended. Acyclovir (Zovirax, Avirax), famciclovir (Famvir), or valacyclovir (Valtrex) may be prescribed. The main differences in these drugs are cost and frequency of use. Dosage and length of treatment differ for primary outbreaks (7 to 10 days) and recurrent outbreaks (1 to 5 days). Therapy for recurrent outbreaks is most beneficial if it is started within 1 day of the appearance of lesions or during the period of itching or tingling before lesions appear. Intermittent or continuous (daily) suppressive antiviral therapy is offered to patients to lessen the severity and frequency of or to

CHART 74-3 Patient and Family Education: Preparing for Self-Management

Use of Condoms

- Use latex or polyurethane condoms rather than natural membrane condoms.
- Use a condom with every sexual encounter (including oral, vaginal, and anal).
- Female condoms (Reality)—polyurethane or nitrile sheaths in the vagina—are effective in preventing transmission of viruses, including HIV.
- Condoms infrequently (2 per 100) break during sexual intercourse.
- Keep condoms (especially latex) in a cool, dry place, out of direct sunlight.
- Do not use condoms that are in damaged packages or are brittle or discolored.
- Always handle a condom with care to avoid damaging it with fingernails, teeth, or other sharp objects.
- Put condoms on before any genital contact. Hold the condom by the tip and unroll it on the penis. Leave a space at the tip to collect semen.
- If you use a lubricant with condoms, make sure that the lubricant is water based and washes away with water. Oil-based products damage latex condoms.
- Use of spermicide (nonoxynol-9) with condoms, either lubricated condoms or vaginal application, has *not* been proven to be more or less effective against STIs than use without spermicide. Spermicide-coated condoms have been associated with *Escherichia coli* urinary tract infections in women. *Nonoxynol-9 may increase risk for transmission of HIV during vaginal and anal intercourse. Its use is discouraged.*
- If a condom breaks, replace it immediately.
- After ejaculation, withdraw the erect penis carefully, holding the condom at the base of the penis to prevent the condom from slipping off.
- Never use a condom more than once.

Modified from Centers for Disease Control and Prevention (CDC). (2015). Sexually transmitted diseases treatment guidelines, 2015. *Morbidity and Mortality Weekly Report, 64*(RR-3), 1-137.
HIV, Human immune deficiency virus; *STI,* sexually transmitted infection.

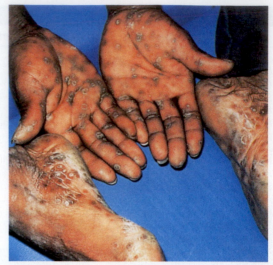

FIG. 74-1 Palmar and plantar secondary syphilis. (From Morse, S., Ballard, R., Holmes, K., & Moreland, A. (2003). *Atlas of sexually transmitted diseases and AIDS* (3rd ed.). Edinburgh: Mosby.)

transmitting the infection or fear rejection because they have it. Help patients cope with the diagnosis by being sensitive and supportive during assessments and interventions. Encourage social support and refer patients to support groups (e.g., local support groups of the National Herpes Resource Center [www.ashasexualhealth.org/std-sti/Herpes.html]) and therapists. Symptomatic care may include oral analgesics, topical anesthetics, sitz baths, and increased oral fluid intake. People who have tested serology positive to HSV-1 or HSV-2 but have never had GH symptoms should be counseled with the same information as those who have symptoms.

SYPHILIS

❖ PATHOPHYSIOLOGY

Syphilis is a complex sexually transmitted infection (STI) that can become systemic and cause serious complications, including death. The causative organism is a spirochete called *Treponema pallidum.* The infection is usually transmitted by sexual contact and blood exposure, but transmission can occur through close body contact such as kissing.

Syphilis progresses through four stages: primary, secondary, latent, and tertiary. The appearance of an ulcer called a **chancre** is the first sign of *primary* syphilis. It develops at the site of entry

(inoculation) of the organism from 10 to 90 days after exposure (3 weeks is average). Chancres may be found on any area of the skin or mucous membranes but occur most often on the genitalia, lips, nipples, and hands and in the mouth, anus, and rectum.

During this highly infectious stage, the chancre begins as a small papule. Within 3 to 7 days, it breaks down into its typical appearance: a painless, indurated, smooth, weeping lesion. Regional lymph nodes enlarge, feel firm, and are not painful. Without treatment, the chancre usually disappears within 6 weeks. However, the organism spreads throughout the body, and the patient is still infectious.

Secondary syphilis develops 6 weeks to 6 months after the onset of primary syphilis. During this stage, syphilis is a systemic disease because the spirochetes circulate throughout the bloodstream. Commonly mistaken for influenza, manifestations include flulike symptoms (malaise, low-grade fever, headache, muscular aches, sore throat) and a generalized rash. There is no typical appearance of this rash except for its presence on the palms and soles of the feet and on mucous membranes. It can appear as diffuse macules (reddish brown), papules (usually less than 5 mm) or pustules, scaly psoriasis-like lesions (Fig. 74-1), or gray-white wartlike lesions (condylomata lata). *All of these lesions are highly contagious and should not be touched without gloves.* Patchy alopecia on the scalp or facial hair (missing part of the eyebrow, "moth-eaten" appearance) is another symptom. The rash subsides without treatment in 4 to 12 weeks (McCance et al., 2014).

After the second stage of syphilis, there is a period of latency. *Early latent* syphilis occurs during the first year after infection, and infectious lesions can recur. *Late latent* syphilis is a disease of more than 1 year's duration after infection. This stage is not infectious except to the fetus of a pregnant woman. Patients with latent syphilis may or may not have reactive serologic test (e.g., Venereal Disease Research Laboratory [VDRL]) findings.

Tertiary, or late, syphilis occurs after a highly variable period, from 4 to 20 years. This stage develops in untreated cases and can mimic other conditions because any organ system can be affected. Signs and symptoms of late syphilis include (McCance et al., 2014):

- Benign lesions of the skin, mucous membranes, and bones
- Cardiovascular syphilis, usually in the form of aortic valvular disease and aortic aneurysms
- Neurosyphilis, causing central nervous system symptoms (e.g., meningitis, hearing loss, generalized paresis [weakness])

🌐 CULTURAL/SPIRITUAL CONSIDERATIONS

Patient-Centered Care (QSEN)

HEALTH CARE DISPARITIES exist between racial and ethnic groups in the incidence of primary and secondary syphilis. In the most recent report from the CDC (2017c), the rates increased among Hispanics, American Indians/Alaska Natives, Euro-Americans, and most dramatically among Asian/Pacific Islanders; rates have *decreased* among African Americans. Nevertheless, African Americans have a seven times greater rate of acquiring syphilis than whites. Compared with Euro-Americans, the 2014 rate for Hispanics was two times higher (CDC, 2017c). The reason for these differences is unclear, but status of health literacy and lack of access to health care may be factors.

👥 GENDER HEALTH CONSIDERATIONS

Patient-Centered Care (QSEN)

Unique needs regarding sexual health and prevention and treatment of STIs for lesbian, gay, bisexual, transgender, and questioning (LGBTQ) patients should be identified and addressed by the nurse. Because of discrimination, HEALTH CARE DISPARITIES, and health care provider lack of understanding, the overall health status of people in these populations may be poor. LGBTQ people may have difficulty finding health care that identifies and addresses their particular risks and concerns. Taking a health history that provides opportunity for the patient to identify his or her sexual orientation, gender identity, and sexual activity is crucial. Especially among transgender people, opportunities for physical examination are avoided or missed by both the patient and care provider because of fears of being misunderstood or inadequately prepared to give or receive appropriate care (CDC, 2017a). The CDC does not currently collect or report the incidence or prevalence of STIs among transgender people.

Men who have sex with men (MSM) are at greatest risk for contracting primary and secondary syphilis and made up 75% of cases of these diseases in 2012 (CDC, 2017a). These men are 17 times more likely to have anal cancer than heterosexual men, and those infected with HIV are at even greater risk. Infection with high-risk human papilloma virus (HPV) has been associated with greater risk for anal cancers among this population (CDC, 2017a).

Assuming that lesbian women or gay men have sex only with same-gender partners or similarly assuming that heterosexual patients never have sexual encounters with partners of their same sex may limit the accuracy of the nurse's risk assessment. Nurses must be aware that patients may not reveal that they are bisexual. Establish a trusting relationship and be culturally sensitive and nonjudgmental when working with LGBTQ patients. Chapter 1 describes recommendations for communicating with this population. Chapter 73 discusses the special health care needs of transgender patients.

❖ INTERPROFESSIONAL COLLABORATIVE CARE

◆ Assessment: Noticing

Assessment of the patient who has signs and symptoms of syphilis begins with a history to gather information about any ulcers or rash. Take a sexual history and conduct a risk assessment to include whether previous testing or treatment for syphilis or other STDs has ever been done (see Chart 74-1). Ask about allergic reactions to drugs, especially penicillin. A woman may report inguinal lymph node enlargement resulting from a chancre in the vagina or cervix that is not easily visible to her. She may state a history of sexual contact with a male partner who had an ulcer that she noticed during the encounter. Men usually discover the chancre on the penis or scrotum.

Conduct a physical examination, including inspection and palpation, to identify signs and symptoms of syphilis. *Wear gloves while palpating any lesions because of the highly contagious treponemes that are present.* Observe for and document rashes of any type because of the variable presentation of secondary syphilis.

After the physical examination, the health care provider obtains a *specimen of the chancre* for examination under a darkfield microscope. Diagnosis of primary or secondary syphilis is confirmed if *T. pallidum* is present.

Blood tests are also used to diagnose syphilis. The usual screening and/or diagnostic nontreponemal tests are the *Venereal Disease Research Laboratory (VDRL)* serum test and the more sensitive *rapid plasma reagin (RPR)*. These tests are based on an antibody-antigen reaction that determines the presence and amount of antibodies produced by the body in response to an infection by *T. pallidum*. They become reactive 2 to 6 weeks after infection. VDRL titers are also used to monitor treatment effectiveness. The antibodies are not specific to *T. pallidum;* and false-positive reactions often occur from conditions such as viral infections, hepatitis, and systemic lupus erythematosus (SLE) (Pagana et al., 2017).

If a VDRL result is positive, the primary health care provider requests or the laboratory may automatically perform a more specific treponemal test, such as the *fluorescent treponemal antibody absorption (FTA-ABS)* test or the *microhemagglutination assay for T. pallidum (MHA-TP)*, to confirm the infection. These tests are more sensitive for all stages of syphilis, although false-positive results may still occur. Patients who have a reactive test will have this positive result for their entire life, even after sufficient treatment. This poses a challenge when receiving a positive result for a patient who denies a history of or does not know that he or she had syphilis.

◆ Interventions: Responding

Interprofessional collaborative care includes drug therapy and health teaching to resolve the infection and prevent infection transmission to others. Benzathine penicillin G given IM as a single 2.4 million-unit dose is the evidence-based treatment for primary, secondary, and early latent syphilis (CDC, 2015). Patients in the late latent stage receive the same dose every week for 3 weeks (CDC, 2015). A different regimen, found in the CDC's *2015 STD Treatment Guidelines,* is recommended for patients who are HIV-infected or pregnant.

⚠ NURSING SAFETY PRIORITY (QSEN)

Drug Alert

Allergic reactions to benzathine penicillin G can occur. Monitor for allergic manifestations (e.g., rash, edema, shortness of breath, chest tightness, anxiety). Penicillin desensitization is recommended for penicillin-allergic patients. *Keep all patients at the health care agency for at least 30 minutes after they have received the antibiotic so manifestations of an allergic reaction can be detected and treated. The most severe reaction is anaphylaxis. Treatment should be available and implemented immediately if symptoms occur.* Chapter 20 describes the management of drug allergies in detail.

After treatment, the CDC recommends follow-up evaluation, including blood tests at 6, 12, and 24 months. Repeat treatment may be needed if the patient does not respond to the initial antibiotic.

The *Jarisch-Herxheimer reaction* may also follow antibiotic therapy for syphilis. This reaction is caused by the rapid release of products from the disruption of the cells of the organism. Symptoms include generalized aches, pain at the injection site, vasodilation, hypotension, and fever. They are usually benign and begin within 2 hours after therapy with a peak at 4 to 8 hours. This reaction may be treated symptomatically with analgesics and antipyretics (Burchum & Rosenthal, 2016).

Discuss with the patient with syphilis the importance of partner notification and treatment, including the risk for re-infection if the partner goes untreated. All sexual partners must be prophylactically treated as soon as possible, preferably within 90 days of the syphilis diagnosis.

Inform the patient that the disease will be reported to the local health authority and that all information will be held in strict confidence. Encourage him or her to provide accurate information for this follow-up to ensure that all at-risk partners are treated appropriately. Provide a setting that offers privacy and encourages open discussion. Urge the patient to keep follow-up appointments. For primary and secondary syphilis, drug therapy is provided at the first visit, which may suggest to the patient that no further visits are indicated or important. Remind the patient that follow-up for partners and assessment that symptoms have resolved are imperative and part of continuing care. Recommend sexual abstinence until the treatment of both the patient and partner(s) is completed.

The emotional responses to syphilis vary and may include feelings of fear, depression, guilt, and anxiety. Patients may experience guilt if they have infected others or anger if a partner has infected them. If further psychosocial interventions are needed, encourage the patient to discuss these feelings or refer him or her to other resources such as psychotherapy, self-help support groups, or STI/STD clinics.

? NCLEX EXAMINATION CHALLENGE 74-1

Physiological Integrity

The nurse gives a client an IM dose of penicillin G for primary syphilis. Which client statement indicates a need for further teaching?

A. "I'll wait in the clinic for 30 minutes to be sure I don't have a reaction."

B. "When I get home, I'll call my partner to tell them about my diagnosis."

C. "If I have sex with someone, I don't have to worry about spreading the disease."

D. "I plan to return to see my primary care provider for follow-up in 6, 12, and 24 months."

CONDYLOMATA ACUMINATA (GENITAL WARTS)

❖ PATHOPHYSIOLOGY

Condylomata acuminata (also known as *genital warts*) are caused by certain types of *human papilloma virus (HPV)*, most of which are types 6 and 11 or low-risk HPV. These types *rarely* result in invasive cancer of the genital tract such as cervical cancer. However, HPV types 16, 18, 31, 33, and 35, considered high-risk HPV, can be found on the skin of the genitalia and increase the risk for genital cancers, especially cervical cancer

(McCance et al., 2014). Infection with several HPV types can occur at the same time. The presence of one strain increases the risk for acquiring a higher-risk strain. Genital warts are the most common viral disease that is sexually transmitted and are often seen with other infections.

HPV infection has been established as the primary risk factor for development of cervical cancer. Sites commonly affected by infection include the urinary meatus, labia, vagina, cervix, penis, scrotum, anus, and perineal area. The incubation period is usually 2 to 3 months. There is growing evidence that HPV infection through oral and anal sex, especially in men who have sex with men (MSM), may be a risk factor for developing oral and anal cancers (CDC, 2017a).

❖ INTERPROFESSIONAL COLLABORATIVE CARE

◆ Assessment: Noticing

The diagnosis of condylomata acuminata is made by examination of the lesions. They are initially small, white or flesh-colored papillary growths that may grow into large cauliflower-like masses (Fig. 74-2). Multiple warts usually occur in the same area. Bleeding may occur if the wart is disturbed. Warts may disappear or resolve on their own without treatment. They may occur once or recur at the original site. Warts can occur on the external or internal surfaces of the genitalia, including the mucosal surfaces of the vagina and urethra.

Screening for HPV and dysplasia of the cervix is done by obtaining cervical specimens for Papanicolaou (Pap) and HPV DNA testing. Identifying high-risk strains of HPV and correlating with abnormal Pap smear findings are the standard of care (CDC, 2015). High-risk HPV may coexist with low-risk HPV, the likely cause of the warts. The diagnosis should include consideration of condyloma lata or secondary syphilis since STIs frequently coexist. A VDRL test, HIV test, and cultures for chlamydia and gonorrhea infections are done. Condylomata lata (secondary syphilis) can resemble condylomata acuminata (genital warts). If a wartlike lesion bleeds easily, appears infected, is atypical, or persists, a biopsy of the lesion is performed to rule

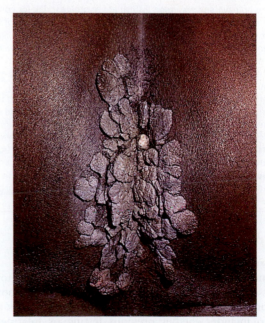

FIG. 74-2 Perianal condylomata acuminata. (From Morse, S., Ballard, R., Holmes, K., & Moreland, A. [2003]. *Atlas of sexually transmitted diseases and AIDS* [3rd ed.]. Edinburgh: Mosby.)

out other pathologic problems such as cancer. A biopsy of warts that are seen on the cervix should be performed before any treatment to eradicate them.

◆ Interventions: Responding

The outcome of treatment is to remove the warts. No current therapy eliminates the HPV infection, and recurrences after treatment are likely. It is not known whether removal of visible warts decreases the risk for disease transmission.

Drug Therapy. Patients may apply podofilox (Condylox) 0.5% cream or gel twice daily for 3 days with no treatment for the next 4 days. This regimen should be repeated for four cycles. Other options are imiquimod (Aldara) 5% cream applied topically at bedtime three times a week and sinecatechins 15% ointment (made from green tea extract) applied three times a day, both until the warts disappear or for up to 16 weeks. Imiquimod boosts the immune system rather than simply destroying the warts (Burchum & Rosenthal, 2016). These self-treatments are less expensive than those performed in the health care provider's office, but they take longer for healing. *Teach patients that over-the-counter (OTC) wart treatments should not be used on genital tissue.*

Cryotherapy, trichloroacetic acid (TCA) or bichloroacetic acid (BCA), and podophyllin (Pododerm) are provider-applied treatments. **Cryotherapy** (freezing), usually with liquid nitrogen, can be used every 1 to 2 weeks until lesions are resolved. TCA/BCA (80% to 90%) can be applied weekly. Podophyllin resin can be applied weekly but needs to be washed off 1 to 4 hours after application. Extensive warts have been treated with the carbon dioxide laser, intra-lesion interferon injections, and surgical removal (CDC, 2015).

Self-Management Education. The priority nursing intervention is patient and sexual partner education about the mode of transmission, incubation period, treatment, and complications, especially the association with cervical cancer. Reinforce instructions about local care of the lesions or patient-applied treatment for self-management.

> **! NURSING SAFETY PRIORITY** QSEN
>
> *Drug Alert*
>
> Teach patients that, after treatment with cryotherapy, podophyllin, or TCA, they may experience impaired COMFORT, bleeding, or discharge from the site or sloughing of parts of warts. Instruct them to keep the area clean (shower or bath) and dry. Teach them to be alert for any signs or symptoms of infection or side effects of the treatment.

Inform patients that recurrence is likely, especially in the first 3 months, and that repeated treatments may be needed. Urge all patients to have complete STI testing, since exposure to one STI may increase risk for contracting another. Sexual partners should also be evaluated and offered treatment if warts are present. Teach patients to avoid intimate sexual contact until external lesions are healed. Recommend condoms to help reduce transmission even after warts have been treated (see Chart 74-3). Encourage women to have a Pap test annually, starting at age 21 years; after they have had three normal smears, they should have a Pap test every 3 years if no new risk factors are present (e.g., new partner, other STIs). The presence of warts should increase suspicion that the patient may have had exposure to other STDs, which warrants additional testing.

Gardasil is used to provide immunity for HPV types 6 and 11 (predominantly types causing warts, low risk for cervical cancer) and 16 and 18 (high risk for cervical cancer). Initially approved for females, the vaccine is also recommended for males ages 9 to 26 years. Cervarix may be given to 9- to 25-year-old females and protects only against HPV types 16 and 18 (Burchum & Rosenthal, 2016). Both vaccines are recommended before onset of sexual activity (and before age 26 years) and possible exposure to HPV. Because exposure to HPV is likely for most sexually active young adults, vaccination protects them against the strains to which they have not yet been exposed. Vaccination is also especially encouraged for MSM and immunocompromised young adults up to the age of 26 years (CDC, 2015).

CHLAMYDIA INFECTION

❖ PATHOPHYSIOLOGY

Chlamydia trachomatis is an intracellular bacterium and the causative agent of genital chlamydia infections. It invades the epithelial tissues in the reproductive tract. The incubation period ranges from 1 to 3 weeks, but the pathogen may be present in the genital tract for months without producing symptoms.

C. trachomatis is reportable to local health departments in all states. Diagnosed cases continue to increase yearly, which reflects more sensitive screening tests and increased public health efforts to screen high-risk people. Because it is frequently asymptomatic, the estimated incidence is about double that reported. African-American women between 15 and 24 years of age are at the highest risk for the disease (CDC, 2017c). The exact reason for this health care disparity is not known.

❖ INTERPROFESSIONAL COLLABORATIVE CARE

◆ Assessment: Noticing

Obtain a complete history, including a genitourinary system review, psychosocial history, and sexual history (see Chart 74-1). In particular, ask about:

- Presence of symptoms, including vaginal or urethral discharge, dysuria (painful urination), pelvic pain, irregular bleeding
- Any history of sexually transmitted diseases (STIs)
- Whether sexual partners have had symptoms or a history of STIs
- Whether patient has had a new or multiple sexual partner(s)
- Whether patient or partner has had unprotected intercourse

About 70% of chlamydia infections are asymptomatic in women. For men and women, their history may reveal only risk factors associated with *C. trachomatis,* such as new or multiple sexual partners, age younger than 26 years and female, or a male having sex with a male (MSM). As with all interviews concerning sexual behavior, use a nonjudgmental approach and provide privacy and confidentiality.

> **GENDER HEALTH CONSIDERATIONS**
>
> *Patient-Centered Care* QSEN
>
> For men, ask about dysuria, frequent urination, and a mucoid discharge that is more watery and less copious than a gonorrheal discharge. These signs and symptoms indicate urethritis, the main symptom of chlamydia infection in men. Some men have the discharge only in the morning on arising. Complications include epididymitis, prostatitis, infertility, and Reiter's syndrome, a type of connective tissue disease.

In contrast, many women have no symptoms. Those with symptoms have mucopurulent vaginal discharge (typically yellow and more opaque), urinary frequency, and abdominal discomfort or pain. Cervical bleeding, from infected and therefore fragile tissue, may present as spotting or bleeding between menses and frequently after intercourse. Complications of infection with *C. trachomatis* include salpingitis (inflammation of the fallopian tubes), pelvic inflammatory disease (PID), and REPRODUCTION problems including ectopic pregnancy and infertility. These health problems are discussed in detail in maternal-child textbooks.

Diagnosis is made by sampling cells from the endocervix, urethra, or both, easily obtained with a swab. Because chlamydiae can reproduce only inside cells, cervical (or host) cells that harbor the organism (or parts of it) are required in the sample. Tissue culture (the gold standard) obtained from the cervical os during the female pelvic examination or from male urethral examination obtained by swabbing has been replaced by genetic tests. As with gonorrhea, the nucleic acid amplification tests (NAATs) and gene amplification tests (ligand chain reaction [LCR], and polymerase chain reaction [PCR] transcription-mediated amplification) are the newest methods of detecting *Chlamydia* in endocervical samples, urethral swabs, and urine. They are more sensitive than the tissue culture. Samples can be obtained by swab by the examining clinician or by a patient-collected urine specimen. This urine self-collection method has been found to be more acceptable and highly sensitive and specific. The acceptability of urine testing has resulted in increased identification of asymptomatic people.

All sexually active women 24 years old or younger and all women older than 25 years with new or multiple partners should be screened annually for *Chlamydia*. There is no recommendation for or against screening asymptomatic men, regardless of age or other risk, and low-risk asymptomatic women.

◆ *Interventions: Responding*

The treatment of choice for chlamydia infections is azithromycin (Zithromax) 1 g orally in a single dose or doxycycline (Monodox, Doxy-Caps, Doxycin) 100 mg orally twice daily for 7 days. The one-dose course, although more expensive, is preferred because of the ease in completing the treatment. Directly observing the patient taking the medication in the health care setting assures the nurse of compliance. Drugs that are prescribed for patients with allergies to these drugs include erythromycin, ofloxacin, and levofloxacin, all for 7 days (CDC, 2015).

Sexual partners should be treated and tested for other STDs. Expedited partner therapy, or patient-delivered partner therapy, shows signs of reducing chlamydia infection rates (CDC, 2015). **Expedited partner therapy (EPT)** is the practice of treating sexual partners of patients diagnosed with chlamydia infection or gonorrhea by providing prescriptions or medication to the patient, which they can take to their partner(s), without the primary health care provider examining the partner(s). When patients have been given the drug to give to their partner, rates of infection have decreased, and more partners have reported receiving treatment (CDC, 2015).

Patient and partner education is a crucial nursing intervention. Explain:
- The sexual mode of transmission
- The incubation period
- The high possibility of asymptomatic infections and the usual symptoms if present

- Treatment of infection with antibiotics and need for completion of course of treatment
- The need for abstinence from sexual intercourse until the patient and partner(s) have all completed treatment (7 days from the start of treatment, including a single-dose regimen)
- That women should be re-screened for re-infection 3 to 12 months after treatment because of the high risk for PID; also, that there is less evidence of the need for re-screening of treated men, but it should be considered
- The need to return for evaluation if symptoms recur or new symptoms develop (most recurrences are re-infections from a new or untreated partner)
- Complications of untreated or inadequately treated infection, which may include PID, ectopic pregnancy, or infertility

GONORRHEA

❖ *PATHOPHYSIOLOGY*

Gonorrhea is a sexually transmitted bacterial infection that occurs in both men and women. The causative organism is *Neisseria gonorrhoeae*, a gram-negative intracellular diplococcus. It is transmitted by direct sexual contact with mucosal surfaces (vaginal intercourse, orogenital contact, or anogenital contact) (McCance et al., 2014).

The first symptoms of gonorrhea may appear 3 to 10 days after sexual contact with an infected person. The disease can be present without symptoms and can be transmitted or progress without warning. In women, ascending spread of the organism can cause pelvic infection (pelvic inflammatory disease [PID]), **endometritis** (endometrial infection), **salpingitis** (fallopian tube infection), and pelvic peritonitis.

🌐 **CULTURAL/SPIRITUAL CONSIDERATIONS**

Patient-Centered Care QSEN

> Significant HEALTH CARE DISPARITIES exist between age and racial groups. Young (ages 15 to 24 years) African-American women have the highest gonorrhea rate, followed by young African-American men (CDC, 2017c). The reasons for these differences are not known, although lack of access to health care may be a factor.

❖ *INTERPROFESSIONAL COLLABORATIVE CARE*

◆ *Assessment: Noticing*

A complete history includes reviewing the genitourinary systems, including taking a sexual history that includes sexual orientation and sites of sexual exposure or intercourse. Assess for allergies to antibiotics (see Chart 74-1). Establish a trusting relationship and use a nonjudgmental approach to gather more complete information. This approach may decrease the patient's anxiety and fear about having an STI.

The infection can be asymptomatic in both men and women, but women have asymptomatic, or "silent," infections more often than do men. If symptoms are present, men usually notice dysuria and a penile discharge that can be either profuse, yellowish-green fluid, or scant, clear fluid. The urethra is most commonly affected, but infection can extend to the prostate, the seminal vesicles, and the epididymis. Men seek curative treatment sooner, usually because they have symptoms, and thereby avoid some of the serious complications.

Women may report a change in vaginal discharge (yellow, green, profuse, odorous), urinary frequency, or dysuria. The cervix and urethra are the most common sites of infection.

Anal signs and symptoms may include itching and irritation, rectal bleeding or diarrhea, and painful defecation. Assess the mouth for a reddened throat, ulcerated lips, tender gingivae, and lesions in the throat. Fig. 74-3 shows common sites of gonococcal infections.

If fever occurs, this may be a sign of an ascending (PID or epididymitis) or systemic infection (disseminated gonococcal infection). Symptoms could include joint or tendon pain, either

in a single joint or as migratory arthralgias, especially of the knees, elbows, fingers, or toes, and a rash usually on the palms and soles.

Clinical symptoms of gonorrhea can resemble those of chlamydia infection and need to be differentiated. *Molecular testing for* N. gonorrhoeae *is currently the most widely used standard and preferred over cultures or microscopic examinations.* These nucleic acid amplification tests (NAATs) are highly sensitive and specific. During examination, providers can swab the male urethra or female cervix to obtain specimens. These specimens can be placed in medium for molecular testing, cultured on chocolate agar (gold standard), or viewed microscopically after Gram staining (male urethral specimens only). Patient-collected urine or vaginal swabs can also be used to diagnose both gonorrhea and chlamydia infections, allowing for testing without a full examination.

In men, gonorrhea can be diagnosed by Gram staining smears of urethral discharge that has been swabbed onto a glass slide, dried, and stained. The presence of gram-negative diplococci is diagnostic for gonococcal urethritis in men. If the man has symptoms, Gram stains are very sensitive and specific for gonorrhea and allow for immediate diagnosis and treatment in the clinical setting. Without symptoms, Gram stains are less reliable. Smears do not confirm the diagnosis in women because the female genital tract normally harbors other *Neisseria* organisms that resemble *N. gonorrhoeae* (Pagana et al., 2017).

All patients with gonorrhea should be tested for syphilis, chlamydia, hepatitis B and hepatitis C, and HIV infection and, if possible, examined for HSV and HPV because they may have been exposed to these STIs as well. Sexual partners who have been exposed in the past 30 days should be examined, and specimens should be obtained.

◆ Interventions: Responding

Uncomplicated gonorrhea is treated with antibiotics. Chlamydia infection, which is four times more common, is frequently found in patients with gonorrhea. Because of this, patients treated for gonorrhea should also be managed with drugs that treat chlamydia infection.

Drug Therapy. Drug therapy recommended by the CDC is ceftriaxone (Rocephin) 250 mg IM *plus* azithromycin (Zithromax) 1 g orally in a single dose *or* doxycycline (Monodox, Doxy-Caps, Doxycin) 100 mg orally twice daily for 1 week to treat a presumed co-infection with *Chlamydia* (up to 40%), unless a negative *Chlamydia* result has been obtained. These combinations seem to be effective for all mucosal gonorrheal infections; treatment failure is rare (CDC, 2015). A test of cure is not required for treatment with ceftriaxone. Advise the patient to return for a follow-up examination if symptoms persist after treatment. Re-infection is usually the cause of these symptoms.

Sexual partners must be treated, not just evaluated, to prevent re-infection. Sexual partners also need to receive education about the infection.

Because the best treatment for gonorrhea is injected Rocephin (ceftriaxone), expedited partner therapy (EPT) is not ideal for treating it. If there is concern that the partner may not come to a health care facility for treatment, providing oral cefixime as an alternative has been recommended by the CDC (2015). Because of the potential for resistance of gonorrhea to cefixime, a test of cure is recommended after treatment is completed.

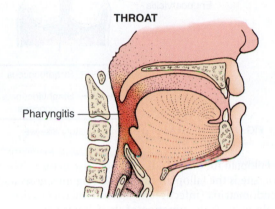

THROAT

Pharyngitis

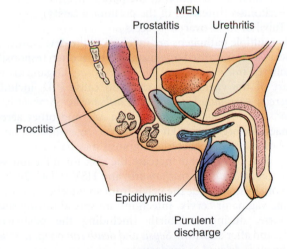

PELVIC/GENITAL

MEN

Prostatitis   Urethritis

Proctitis

Epididymitis

Purulent discharge

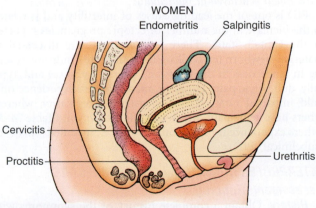

WOMEN

Endometritis   Salpingitis

Cervicitis

Proctitis

Urethritis

FIG. 74-3 Areas of involvement of gonorrhea in men and women.

Gonorrhea infection can become disseminated, requiring hospitalization and IV or IM ceftriaxone 1 g every 24 hours. If symptoms resolve within 24 to 48 hours, the patient may be discharged to home to continue oral antibiotic therapy (cefixime 400 mg twice a day) for at least a week (CDC, 2015).

Self-Management Education. Teach the patient about transmission and treatment of gonorrhea. The use of medication to treat chlamydia infection at the same time as treating gonorrhea should be explained to the patient since the likelihood of co-infection is high. Discuss the possibility of re-infection, including the risk for pelvic inflammatory disease (PID) (see discussion of PID later in this chapter). Instruct patients to cease sexual activity until the antibiotic therapy is completed and they no longer have symptoms; but, if abstinence is not possible, urge men and women to use condoms. Explain that gonorrhea is a *reportable disease.*

When a diagnosis of gonorrhea is made, patients may have feelings of fear or guilt. They may be concerned that they have contracted other STIs or consider the disease a punishment for promiscuity or "unnatural" sex acts. They may believe that acquiring gonorrhea (or any STI) is a risk that they must take to pursue their desired lifestyle. Such feelings can impair relationships with sexual partners. Encourage patients to express their feelings and offer other information and professional resources to help them have a correct understanding of their diagnosis and treatment. Ensuring privacy during your discussion with them and maintaining confidentiality of personal health information are essential in meeting psychosocial needs.

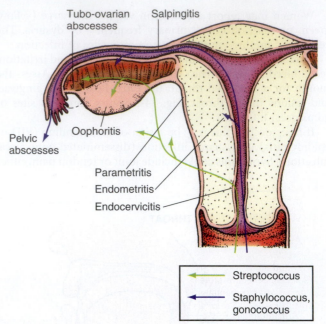

FIG. 74-4 The spread of pelvic inflammatory disease.

CLINICAL JUDGMENT CHALLENGE 74-1

Patient-Centered Care; Evidence-Based Practice QSEN

A 20-year-old man has been diagnosed with a chlamydial infection and provided with treatment for the infection. After learning how the infection is transmitted, he states that he is engaged to be married and realizes that his fiancée obviously had sex with someone else who gave her the infection, which he now has. He expresses his anger and states that he is breaking up with her immediately. As the nurse, you explain that medication treatment is available with expedited partner therapy (EPT) for his fiancée and the person with whom she had sexual intercourse. The patient becomes angry and says, "I don't ever want to speak to her again!"

1. What is the best therapeutic approach for working with this patient?
2. What emotional feelings is this patient experiencing? How will you respond to the patient's statement?
3. What is the value of EPT?
4. What health teaching is required about this infection for the patient, including drug therapy and sexual activity?

❊ SEXUALITY CONCEPT EXEMPLAR
Pelvic Inflammatory Disease

❖ PATHOPHYSIOLOGY

Pelvic inflammatory disease (PID) is a complex infectious process in which organisms from the lower genital tract migrate from the endocervix upward through the uterine cavity into the fallopian tubes. The spread of infection to other organs and tissues of the upper genital tract occurs from direct contact with mucosal surfaces or through the fimbriated ends of the tubes to the ovaries, parametrium, and peritoneal cavity (Fig. 74-4). This may involve one or more pelvic structures, including the uterus, fallopian tubes, and adjacent pelvic structures. The most common site is the fallopian tube. Resulting infections include:

- Endometritis (infection of the endometrial cavity)
- Salpingitis (inflammation of the fallopian tubes)
- Oophoritis (ovarian infection)
- Parametritis (infection of the parametrium)
- Peritonitis (infection of the peritoneal cavity)
- Tubal or tubo-ovarian abscess

Usually multiple pathogens are involved in the development of PID. Sexually transmitted organisms are most often responsible, especially *C. trachomatis* and *N. gonorrhoeae*. Organisms that are part of the vaginal flora can also cause PID, including *Gardnerella vaginalis, Haemophilus influenzae, Staphylococcus, Streptococcus, Mycoplasma, Escherichia coli,* and other aerobic and anaerobic organisms. There is increasing evidence that the anaerobes involved in bacterial vaginosis may have a role in the development of PID and increase the risk for infection with HIV, *N. gonorrhoeae, C. trachomatis,* and HSV (CDC, 2017b).

The organisms invade the pelvis from an infection ascending from the vagina or cervix. Infections are spread during sexual intercourse, during childbirth (including the postpartum period), and after abortion. *Sepsis and death can occur, especially if treatment is delayed or inadequate.*

PID is one of the leading causes of infertility and is related to the increase in the number of ectopic pregnancies reported in the United States. These complications are discussed in maternal-newborn textbooks. PID is an acute syndrome resulting in tenderness in the tubes and ovaries (adnexa) and, typically, dull pelvic pain. However, many women experience only mild impaired COMFORT or menstrual irregularity, whereas others have acute pain, which can affect their gait (Table 74-3). Others experience no symptoms at all (i.e., so-called "silent" or "subclinical" PID).

❖ INTERPROFESSIONAL COLLABORATIVE CARE
◆ Assessment: Noticing

History. Obtain a complete history of the symptoms with menstrual, obstetric, sexual, and family history and a history of

TABLE 74-3 **Diagnostic Criteria for Pelvic Inflammatory Disease**

Minimum Criteria for Initiating Empiric Treatment for Pelvic Inflammatory Disease

- Sexually active woman and at risk for STIs
- Pelvic or lower abdominal pain
- No other cause for illness can be found (e.g., appendicitis)

And

- Uterine tenderness *or*
- Adnexal tenderness *or*
- Cervical motion tenderness (chandelier sign)

Additional Criteria to Increase the Specificity of the Diagnosis of PID

- Oral temperature >101° F (>38.3° C)
- Abnormal cervical or vaginal mucopurulent discharge
- Presence of white blood cells on saline microscopy of vaginal secretions
- Elevated erythrocyte sedimentation rate
- Elevated C-reactive protein
- Laboratory documentation of cervical infection with *Neisseria gonorrhoeae* or *Chlamydia trachomatis*

Definitive Criteria for Diagnosing PID, Warranted in Selected Cases

- Histopathologic evidence of endometritis on endometrial biopsy
- Transvaginal sonography or MRI techniques showing thickened, fluid-filled tubes with or without free pelvic fluid or tubo-ovarian complex or Doppler studies suggesting pelvic infection
- Laparoscopic abnormalities consistent with PID

Modified from Centers for Disease Control and Prevention (CDC). (2015). Sexually transmitted diseases treatment guidelines, 2015. *Morbidity and Mortality Weekly Report, 64*(RR-3), 1-137.
PID, Pelvic inflammatory disease; *STDs,* sexually transmitted diseases.

previous episodes of pelvic inflammatory disease (PID) or other sexually transmitted infections (see Chart 74-1). Assess for contraceptive use, a history of reproductive surgery, and other risk factors previously discussed. Ask the patient if sexual abuse has occurred. If so, encourage her to discuss what happened and whether she was seen by a primary health care provider.

Many of the same factors that place women at risk for STIs also place them at risk for PID. Risk factors for sexually active women include:

- Age younger than 26 years
- Multiple sexual partners
- Intrauterine device (IUD) placed within the previous 3 weeks
- Smoking
- A history of PID
- Chlamydial or gonococcal infection; bacterial vaginosis
- A history of sexually transmitted diseases (STIs)

Physical Assessment/Signs and Symptoms. One of the most frequent symptoms of PID is lower abdominal or pelvic pain. Conduct a complete pain assessment. Other symptoms include irregular vaginal bleeding (spotting or bleeding between periods), dysuria (painful urination), an increase or change in vaginal discharge, dyspareunia (painful sexual intercourse), malaise, fever, and chills.

Observe whether the patient has impaired COMFORT with movement. Often she has a hunched-over gait to protect her abdomen. She may find it difficult to independently get on the examination table or stretcher. Assess for lower abdominal tenderness, possibly with rigidity or rebound tenderness. A pelvic examination by the primary health care provider may reveal yellow or green cervical discharge and a reddened or friable cervix (a cervix that bleeds easily). Criteria for accurate diagnosis of PID are listed in Table 74-3. The diagnosis of PID is usually based on health history, physical examination, and laboratory tests. Imaging studies and laparoscopy are not generally used to make the diagnosis.

Psychosocial Assessment. The woman who has symptoms of PID is usually anxious and fearful of the examination and unknown diagnosis. She may need much reassurance and support during the physical examination because her abdomen may be very tender or painful. Explain what is taking place to help promote comfort during the examination.

Because PID is often associated with an STI, the woman may feel embarrassed or uncomfortable discussing her symptoms or history. Use a nonjudgmental approach and encourage the patient to express her feelings and concerns. Determining her ability to follow through with the interprofessional collaborative plan of care is essential in deciding whether hospitalization should be considered.

Laboratory Assessment. The health care provider obtains specimens from the cervix, urethra, and rectum to determine the presence of *N. gonorrhoeae* or *C. trachomatis.* The white blood cell (WBC) count, erythrocyte sedimentation rate (ESR), and C-reactive protein may be elevated but are not specific for PID. A sensitive test that detects human chorionic gonadotropin (hCG) in urine or blood should be performed to determine whether the patient is pregnant (Pagana et al., 2017). Microscopic examination of vaginal discharge should be done to evaluate for the presence of WBCs.

Other Diagnostic Assessment. Abdominal *ultrasonography* may be used to determine the presence of appendicitis and tubo-ovarian abscesses that need to be ruled out when the diagnosis of PID is made. Transvaginal ultrasound and *MRI* are used in some cases to detect tubal wall thickening, fluid-filled tubes, and free pelvic fluid or a tubo-ovarian abscess, all associated with PID. *Endometrial biopsy* also has been used to increase the accuracy of the diagnosis.

◆ **Analysis: Interpreting**

The priority collaborative problem for patients with pelvic inflammatory disease (PID) is *Infection due to invasion of pelvic organs by sexually transmitted pathogens.*

◆ **Planning and Implementation: Responding**

Managing Infection

Planning: Expected Outcomes. The patient with PID is expected to have her infection resolved, be free of abdominal pain, and prevent re-infection.

Interventions. Interprofessional collaborative care includes antibiotic therapy and self-management measures.

Uncomplicated PID is usually treated on an ambulatory care basis. The CDC (2017b) recommends hospitalization for PID if the patient:

- Has appendicitis, ectopic pregnancy, or other surgical emergency that has not been excluded
- Is pregnant
- Does not respond to oral antibiotic therapy
- Is unable to follow or tolerate treatment on an ambulatory care basis

- Has severe illness, nausea and vomiting, or high fever
- Has a tubo-ovarian abscess

There are no recommendations about whether HIV-infected women should be hospitalized. Assess the ability of high-risk women for self-management at home. The patient's health status and availability of support systems are important considerations for home care. If the infection has not responded to treatment, the patient may need to be hospitalized for IV antibiotic therapy and further evaluation.

The CDC recommends oral and/or parenteral antibiotics for PID (CDC, 2017b). Drug therapy is required for 14 days. If the woman has not responded to oral antibiotics, she is hospitalized for IV antibiotic therapy and further evaluation. Inpatient therapy involves a combination of several IV antibiotics until the woman shows signs of improvement (e.g., decreased pelvic tenderness for at least 24 hours). Then oral antibiotics are continued at home until the course of treatment has lasted 14 days.

Antibiotic therapy relieves pain by destroying the pathogens and decreasing the inflammation caused by infection. Other pain-relief measures include taking mild analgesics and applying heat to the lower abdomen or back. As with any infection, encourage the patient to increase her intake of fluids and eat nutritious foods that can promote healing. *Teach the patient to rest in a semi-Fowler's position and encourage limited ambulation to promote gravity drainage of the infection that may help relieve pain.*

> ### ! NURSING SAFETY PRIORITY QSEN
> #### Action Alert
> Instruct women who are being treated for PID on an ambulatory care basis to avoid sexual intercourse for the full course of treatment and until their symptoms have resolved. Ask them to check their temperature twice a day. Teach them to report an increase in temperature to their health care provider. Remind them to be seen by the health care provider within 72 hours from starting antibiotic treatment and then 1 and 2 weeks from the time of the initial diagnosis.

In a small number of patients, the pain and tenderness may not be relieved by antibiotic therapy. The surgeon may perform a laparoscopy to remove an abscess through one or more subumbilical incisions to provide better access to the fallopian tubes. Before surgery, provide information about hospital routines and procedures. After surgery, the care of the woman with PID is similar to that of any patient after laparoscopic abdominal surgery. One difference is that she may have a wound drain for drainage of abscess fluid that may not have been completely removed during surgery. Observe, measure, and record wound drainage every 4 to 8 hours as requested.

Care Coordination and Transition Management.

If the woman is hospitalized, collaborate with the case manager or discharge planner before she is discharged to home. Teach the patient with PID to see her primary health care provider for follow-up to assess for complications and confirm that the infection has resolved. Establish an atmosphere of trust that encourages the woman to return frequently, if needed, for education or reassurance.

Home Care Management. Parenteral antibiotic therapy may be given at home, but usually the health care provider changes the treatment regimen to oral antibiotics before hospital

> ### CHART 74-4 Patient and Family Education: Preparing for Self-Management
> #### Oral Antibiotic Therapy for Sexually Transmitted Infections
> - Take your medicine for the number of times a day that it is prescribed and until it is completed.
> - Your sexual partner must be treated if you have a sexually transmitted infection (STI). Expedited partner therapy is one way to ensure that partners are treated.
> - Be sure to return for your follow-up appointment after completing your antibiotic treatment.
> - Call if you have any questions or concerns.
> - Do not have sex until after you and your partner complete your antibiotic therapy. This should be at least 7 days, even if treatment is one dose.
> - Drink at least 8 to 10 glasses of fluid a day to help heal your infection, while taking your antibiotics.
> - Do not take antacids containing calcium, magnesium, or aluminum, such as Tums, Maalox, or Mylanta, with your antibiotics. They may decrease the effectiveness of the antibiotic.
> - Take your antibiotics on an empty stomach unless your health care provider instructs you to take them with food.

discharge. Home care for the patient who had laparoscopic surgery is discussed in Chapter 16.

Self-Management Education. Patient teaching focuses on providing information about PID, identifying symptoms that suggest persistent or recurrent infection (persistent pelvic pain, dysmenorrhea, low backache, fever), and urging completion of antibiotic treatment, rest, and healthy nutrition to resolve the infection and prevent complications. Review information for oral antibiotic therapy (Chart 74-4).

Counsel the patient to contact her sexual partner(s) for examination and treatment. All sexual partners should be treated for gonorrhea and chlamydia infection regardless of whether they have symptoms. Remind the patient about follow-up care, and counsel her about the complications that can occur after an episode of PID. These problems include increased risk for recurrence, ectopic pregnancy, and infertility. Chronic pelvic pain may also develop.

Discuss contraception and the patient's need or desire for it. This discussion includes the use of condoms that can decrease the risk for future episodes of PID. Consider the likelihood that the patient had unprotected (from pregnancy and STIs) intercourse, which resulted in PID. Contraception that includes the use of condoms is an important health message to be communicated. Help the patient understand that having sexual intercourse with multiple partners increases the risk for recurrent episodes. Douching has also been suggested as a risky behavior for development of PID and/or infection with *Chlamydia* or *N. gonorrhoeae*.

Psychosocial concerns may require counseling. A patient who has PID may exhibit a variety of feelings (guilt, disgust, anger) about having a condition that may have been transmitted to her sexually. These feelings may affect her relationship with significant others and future sexual partners. She may also have concerns about future fertility if PID has damaged or scarred the fallopian tubes and other reproductive organs. Provide nonjudgmental emotional support and allow time for her to discuss her feelings. The primary provider of care may refer the patient to a mental health care provider as another appropriate option.

Physiological Integrity

Which assessment findings will the nurse expect for a client who is suspected of having pelvic inflammatory disease? **Select all that apply.**
A. Vaginal bleeding
B. Fever
C. Lower abdominal pain
D. Constipation
E. Rigid abdomen

Health Care Resources. The cost of antibiotics for patients with PID and other STIs may be a concern for those who are uninsured, underinsured, or impoverished. In collaboration with the case manager or social worker, help locate community resources for free or discounted drugs for women who cannot afford them. Ask the patient directly if she has the ability to pay for the drug and her follow-up visits, regardless of her apparent financial status.

If infertility is a result of PID, the patient may need referral to a clinic specializing in infertility treatment and counseling. She can also contact support groups for infertile couples, which exist in many local communities.

◆ *Evaluation: Reflecting*

Evaluate the care of the patient with PID based on the identified priority patient problem. The expected outcomes include that the patient should:
- Show evidence that the infection has resolved
- Report or demonstrate that pain is relieved or reduced and that she feels more comfortable
- Demonstrate a plan for ensuring treatment of her partner, obtaining antibiotics, and returning for follow-up care

GET READY FOR THE NCLEX® EXAMINATION!

KEY POINTS

Review these Key Points for each NCLEX Examination Client Needs Category.

Safe and Effective Care Environment
- Maintain patient and partner confidentiality and privacy at all times. **QSEN: Patient-Centered Care**
- Use gloves when examining the patient's genitalia or skin lesions. **QSEN: Safety**

Health Promotion and Maintenance
- Teach patients not to have sexual intercourse during their treatment for sexually transmitted infection (STI). **QSEN: Safety**
- Assume that all adult patients may be sexually active, regardless of age or stage of life. Sexually transmitted infections are still spread within the older-adult population because perception of risk is lower.
- Educate young women about increased vulnerability to STIs; women's vaginal mucous membranes place them at higher risk for contracting an STI, and young women statistically have more partners and more unprotected sex, which further increases their risk. **QSEN: Safety**
- Teach the patient about the availability of expedited partner therapy; be sure that both the patient and the partner take all doses of the drug.
- Encourage all patients who are sexually active to use condoms during sexual intimacy (see Chart 74-3).
- Urge sexually active people, especially those younger than 26 years (or those older than 26 years if at high risk), to have STI screenings at least annually.
- Treat all patients, regardless of diagnosis, gender identity, or sexual orientation, with respect. **QSEN: Patient-Centered Care**
- Respect the sexual choices and practices of all patients. **QSEN: Patient-Centered Care**

Psychosocial Integrity
- Provide privacy for patients undergoing examination or testing for STIs.
- Allow the patient to express fears and/or anxiety regarding a diagnosis of STI. **QSEN: Patient-Centered Care**
- Refer patients newly diagnosed with an STI to local resources and support groups as needed based on their response. **QSEN: Teamwork and Collaboration**
- Encourage all patients who have an STI to inform their sexual partner(s) of their health status.

Physiological Integrity
- Assess patients with STI using the guidelines in Chart 74-1. **QSEN: Evidence-Based Practice**
- Recognize that each stage of syphilis has unique symptoms and it is important not to overlook symptoms that resolve.
- Understand that patients without symptoms may still be infected with an STI.
- Encourage patients to adhere to their entire anti-infective drug regimen (see Chart 74-4), even after they begin to feel better.
- Teach patients the expected side effects and possible adverse reactions to prescribed drugs, particularly antibiotics. **QSEN: Safety**
- Teach patients about the short-term and long-term complications of STI using the information in Table 74-1.
- Be aware that PID is diagnosed based on the criteria in Table 74-3. **QSEN: Evidence-Based Practice**
- Place the hospitalized patient with PID in semi-Fowlers position. **QSEN: Safety**
- Teach patients with PID about possible complications, the importance of drug therapy adherence, and sexual activity restrictions.

SELECTED BIBLIOGRAPHY

Burchum, J. L. R., & Rosenthal, L. D. (2016). *Lehne's pharmacology for nursing care* (9th ed.). St. Louis: Elsevier.

Centers for Disease Control and Prevention (CDC). (2015). Sexually transmitted diseases treatment guidelines, 2015. *Morbidity and Mortality Weekly Report, 64*(RR–3), 1–137.

Centers for Disease Control and Prevention (CDC). (2017a). *Gay and bisexual men's health: Sexually transmitted diseases.* www.cdc.gov/msmhealth/STD.htm.

Centers for Disease Control and Prevention (CDC). (2017b). *Pelvic inflammatory disease (PID).* Retrieved from www.cdc.gov/std/tg2015/treatment.htm.

Centers for Disease Control and Prevention (CDC). (2017c). *Sexually transmitted diseases surveillance.* www.cdc.gov/std/stats14/default.htm.

Koester, K. A., Collins, S. P., Fuller, S. M., Galindo, G. R., Gibson, S., & Steward, W. T. (2013). Sexual healthcare preferences among gay and bisexual men: A qualitative study in San Francisco, California. *PLoS ONE, 8*(8), e71546.

Markowitz, L. E., Hariri, S., Lin, C., Dunne, E. F., Steinau, M., McQuillan, G., et al. (2013). Reduction in human papillomavirus (HPV) prevalence among young women following HPV vaccine introduction in the United States, National Health and Nutrition Examination Surveys, 2003-2010. *J Infect Dis, 208*(3), 385–393.

McCance, K., Huether, S., Brashers, V., & Rote, N. (2014). *Pathophysiology: The biologic basis for disease in adults and children* (7th ed.). St. Louis: Mosby.

Owusu-Edusei, K., Chesson, H. W., Gift, T. L., Tao, G., Mahajan, R., Ocfemia, M. C., et al. (2013). The estimated direct medical cost of selected sexually transmitted infections in the United States, 2008. *Sexually Transmitted Diseases, 40*(3), 197–201.

Pagana, K. D., Pagana, T. J., & Pagana, T. N. (2017). *Mosby's diagnostic and laboratory test reference* (13th ed.). St. Louis: Mosby.

Satterwhite, C. L., Torrone, E., Meites, E., Dunne, E. F., Mahajan, R., Banez Ocfemia, M. C., et al. (2013). Sexually transmitted infections among U.S. women and men: Prevalence and incidence estimates, 2008. *Sexually Transmitted Diseases, 40*(3), 187–193.

U.S. Department of Health and Human Services (USDHHS), Office of Disease Prevention and Health Promotion. (2017). *Healthy People 2020.* www.healthypeople.gov/hp2020/.

U.S. Preventive Services Task Force (USPSTF). (2014). *Guide to clinical preventive services, 2014: Recommendations of the U.S. Preventive Services Task Force.* Rockville, MD: Agency for Healthcare Research and Quality. http://www.ahrq.gov/professionals/clinicians-providers/guidelines-recommendations/guide/index.html.

U.S. Preventive Services Task Force (USPSTF). (2017b). *Sexually transmitted infections: Behavioral Counseling.* U.S. Preventive Services Task Force recommendation statement. AHRQ Publication 08-05123-EF-2. www.uspreventiveservicestaskforce.org/uspstf08/sti/stirs.htm.

A

abdominal acute compartment syndrome (AACS) A complication after abdominal trauma that occurs when the intraabdominal pressure is sustained at greater than 200 mm Hg.

abdominoperineal (AP) resection The surgical removal of the sigmoid colon, rectum, and anus through combined abdominal and perineal incisions. This resection is performed when rectal tumors are present.

ablative The process or act of removing.

abscess A localized collection of pus caused by an inflammatory response to bacteria in tissues or organs.

absolute neutrophil count (ANC) The percentage and actual number of mature circulating neutrophils; used to measure a patient's risk for infection. The higher the numbers, the greater the resistance to infection.

absorption The uptake from the intestinal lumen of nutrients produced by digestion.

acalculia Difficulty with math calculations; caused by brain injury or disease.

acalculous cholecystitis Inflammation of the gallbladder occurring in the absence of gallstones; typically associated with biliary stasis caused by any condition that affects the regular filling or emptying of the gallbladder.

acceleration-deceleration Types of forces that involve rapid or sudden movement forward and then backward.

acclimatization The process of adapting to a high altitude; involves physiologic changes that help the body compensate for less available oxygen in the atmosphere.

accommodation The process of maintaining a clear visual image when the gaze is shifted from a distant object to a near object. The eye adjusts its focus by changing the curvature of the lens.

achlorhydria The absence of hydrochloric acid from gastric secretions.

acid A substance that releases hydrogen ions when dissolved in water. The strength of an acid is measured by how easily it releases hydrogen ions in solution.

acid-base balance The maintenance of arterial blood pH between 7.35 and 7.45 through control of hydrogen ion production and elimination.

acidosis An acid-base imbalance in which blood pH is below normal.

acinus The structural unit of the lower respiratory tract consisting of a respiratory bronchiole, an alveolar duct, and an alveolar sac.

Acorn cardiac support device A polyester mesh jacket that is placed over the ventricles to provide support and to avoid overstretching the myocardial muscle in the patient with heart failure; reduces heart muscle hypertrophy and assists with improvement of ejection fraction.

acoustic neuroma A benign tumor of cranial nerve VIII; symptoms include damage to hearing, facial movements, and sensation. The tumor can enlarge into the brain, damaging structures in the cerebellum.

active euthanasia Purposeful action that directly causes death; not supported by most professional organizations, including the American Nurses Association.

active immunity Resistance to infection that occurs when the body responds to an invading antigen by making specific antibodies against the antigen. Immunity lasts for years and is natural by infection or artificial by stimulation (e.g., vaccine) of the body's immune defenses.

active surveillance (AS) Observation for cancer without immediate active treatment.

activities of daily living (ADLs) The activities performed in the course of a normal day, such as bathing, dressing, feeding, and ambulating.

activity therapist See *recreational therapist*.

acute Having relatively greater intensity; marked by a sudden onset and short duration.

acute adrenal insufficiency A life-threatening event in which the need for cortisol and aldosterone is greater than the available supply. Also called *addisonian crisis*.

acute arterial occlusion The sudden blockage of an artery, typically in the lower extremity, in the patient with chronic peripheral arterial disease.

acute compartment syndrome (ACS) A complication of a fracture characterized by increased pressure within one or more compartments and causing massive compromise of circulation to the area. Compartments are sheaths of inelastic fascia that support and partition muscles, blood vessels, and nerves in the body.

acute coronary syndrome (ACS) A disorder, including unstable angina and myocardial infarction, that results from obstruction of the coronary artery by ruptured atherosclerotic plaque and leads to platelet aggregation, thrombus formation, and vasoconstriction.

acute gastritis Inflammation of the gastric mucosa or submucosa after exposure to local irritants. Various degrees of mucosal necrosis and inflammatory reaction occur in acute disease. Complete regeneration and healing usually occur within a few days.

acute glomerulonephritis Inflammation of the glomerulus that develops suddenly from an excess immunity response within the kidney tissues.

acute hematogenous infection An infection resulting from bacteremia, disease, or nonpenetrating trauma that is disseminated by the blood through the circulation.

acute kidney injury (AKI) A rapid decrease in kidney function, leading to the collection of metabolic wastes in the body; formerly called *acute renal failure (ARF)*.

acute pain The unpleasant sensory and emotional experience associated with tissue damage that results from acute injury, disease, or surgery.

acute pancreatitis A serious inflammation of the pancreas characterized by a sudden onset of abdominal pain, nausea, and vomiting. It is caused by premature activation of pancreatic enzymes that destroy ductal tissue and pancreatic cells and results in autodigestion and fibrosis of the pancreas.

acute paronychia Inflammation of the skin around the nail, which usually occurs with a torn cuticle or an ingrown toenail.

acute pericarditis An inflammation or alteration of the pericardium, the membranous sac that encloses the heart; may be fibrous, serous, hemorrhagic, purulent, or neoplastic.

acute pyelonephritis Active bacterial infection in the kidney.

acute respiratory distress syndrome (ARDS) Respiratory failure marked by hypoxemia that persists even when 100% oxygen is given, as well as decreased pulmonary compliance, dyspnea, noncardiac-associated bilateral pulmonary edema, and dense pulmonary infiltrates on x-ray.

acute sialadenitis Inflammation of a salivary gland; can be caused by infectious agents, irradiation, or immunologic disorders.

acute-on-chronic kidney disease A condition in which acute kidney injury occurs in addition to chronic kidney disease.

adaptive immunity The immunity that a person's body makes (or can receive) as an adaptive response to invasion by organisms or foreign proteins; occurs either naturally or artificially through lymphocyte responses and can be either active or passive.

addisonian crisis Acute adrenal insufficiency; a life-threatening event in which the need for cortisol and aldosterone is greater than the available supply.

adenocarcinoma Tumor that arises from the glandular epithelial tissue.

adenohypophysis The anterior lobe of the pituitary gland, which makes up about 70% of the gland.

adiponectin An anti-inflammatory and insulin-sensitizing hormone.

adipose Fatty.

adjuvant therapy Chemotherapy that is used along with surgery or radiation.

adjuvant A substance that aids another substance, such as a cancer treatment that uses chemotherapy in addition to surgery.

adrenal crisis Acute adrenocortical insufficiency, which can be life threatening.

adrenal Cushing's disease An excess of glucocorticoids caused by a problem in the adrenal cortex, usually a benign tumor (adrenal adenoma). This usually occurs in only one adrenal gland.

advance directive (AD) A written document prepared by a competent person to specify what, if any, extraordinary actions he or she would want when no longer able to make decisions about personal health care.

adverse drug event (ADE) An unintended harmful reaction to an administered drug.

adverse events Variations in the standard of care that are usually below the standard.

aerosolization Transmission via fine airborne droplets.

aesthetic plastic surgery Plastic surgery that is cosmetic and aims to alter a person's physical appearance.

afferent arteriole The smallest, most distal portion of the renal arterial system that supplies blood to the nephron. From the afferent arteriole, blood flows into the glomerulus, a series of specialized capillary loops.

after-drop A continued decrease in core body temperature after a victim is removed from a cold environment; results from equilibration of core and peripheral blood temperature and countercurrent cooling of the blood perfusing cold tissue.

afterload The pressure or resistance that the ventricles must overcome to eject blood through the semilunar valves and into the peripheral blood vessels; the amount of resistance is directly related to arterial blood pressure and blood vessel diameter.

agglutination A clumping action that results during the antibody-binding process when antibodies link antigens together to form large and small immune complexes.

agnosia A general term for a loss of sensory comprehension; may include an inability to write, comprehend reading material, or use an object correctly.

agraphia Loss of the ability to write; caused by brain injury or disease.

Airborne Precautions Infection control guidelines from the U.S. Centers for Disease Control and Prevention; used for patients with infections spread by the airborne transmission route, such as tuberculosis. Negative airflow rooms are required to prevent the airborne spread of microbes.

akinesia Slow or no movement, as seen in a patient with Parkinson disease. Also called *bradykinesia*.

albuminuria The presence of albumin in the urine.

alcoholic hepatitis Liver inflammation caused by the toxic effect of alcohol on hepatocytes. The liver becomes enlarged, with cellular degeneration and infiltration by fat, leukocytes, and lymphocytes.

aldosterone The chief mineralocorticoid produced by the adrenal cortex. Aldosterone increases kidney reabsorption of sodium and water, thus restoring blood pressure, blood volume, and blood sodium levels. Aldosterone secretion is regulated by the renin-angiotensin system, serum potassium ion concentration, and adrenocorticotropic hormone.

alert Awake, engaged, and responsive.

alexia Complete inability to understand written language; caused by brain injury or disease.

alkaline reflux gastropathy A complication of gastric surgery in which the pylorus is bypassed or removed. Endoscopic examination reveals regurgitated bile in the stomach and mucosal hyperemia. Symptoms include early satiety, abdominal discomfort, and vomiting. Also called *bile reflux gastropathy*.

alkalosis An acid-base imbalance in which blood pH is above normal.

allele An alternate form (or variation) of a gene.

allergen A foreign protein that is capable of causing a hypersensitivity response, or allergy, that ranges from uncomfortable (itchy, watery eyes or sneezing) to life threatening (allergic asthma, anaphylaxis, bronchoconstriction, or circulatory collapse); causes a release of natural chemicals, such as histamine, in the body.

allergy An increased or excessive response to the presence of a foreign protein or allergen (antigen) to which the patient has been previously exposed.

allogeneic bone marrow transplantation The transplantation of bone marrow from a sibling.

allograft A graft of tissue or bone between individuals of the same species but a different genotype; the donor may be a cadaver or a living person, either related or unrelated. Also called *homograft*.

alopecia Hair loss.

alveolitis Inflammation of the alveoli.

amaurosis fugax A transient, brief episode of blindness in one eye.

ambulatory aid Assistive device such as a cane or a walker.

ambulatory pump Infusion therapy pump generally used with a home care patient to allow a return to his or her usual activities while receiving infusion therapy.

ambulatory A term that refers to a patient who goes to the hospital or physician's office for treatment and returns home on the same day.

amenorrhea The absence of menstrual periods in women.

amnesia Loss of memory.

amputation The removal of a limb or other appendage of the body.

amylase An enzyme that converts starch and glycogen into simple sugars; found most commonly in saliva and pancreatic fluids.

amyotrophic lateral sclerosis (ALS) A progressive and degenerative disease of the motor system that is characterized by atrophy of the hands, forearms, and legs and that results in paralysis and death. There is no known cause, no cure, no specific treatment, no standard pattern of progression, and no method of prevention. Also called *Lou Gehrig's disease*.

anaerobic cellular metabolism Metabolism without oxygen.

anaerobic Lacking adequate oxygen.

anal fissure A painful ulcer at the margin of the anus.

analgesia Pain relief or pain suppression.

anaphylaxis The widespread reaction that occurs in response to contact with a substance to which the person has a severe allergy (antigen); characterized by blood vessel and bronchiolar smooth muscle involvement causing widespread blood vessel dilation, decreased cardiac output, and bronchoconstriction; results in cell damage and the release of large amounts of histamine, severe hypovolemia, vascular collapse, decreased cardiac contraction, and dysrhythmias, and causes extreme whole-body hypoxia.

anasarca Generalized edema.

anastomosis Surgical reattachment. Also a general term meaning "a connection."

anatomic dead space Places in which air flows but the structures are too thick for gas exchange.

anemia A clinical sign of some abnormal condition related to a reduction in one of the following: number of red blood cells, amount of hemoglobin, or hematocrit (percentage of packed red blood cells per deciliter of blood).

anergy The inability to mount an immune response to an antigen.

anesthesia An induced state of partial or total loss of sensation with or without loss of consciousness.

aneuploid (aneuploidy) An abnormal karyotype with more or fewer than 23 pairs of chromosomes.

aneurysm A permanent localized dilation of an artery (to at least 2 times its normal diameter) that forms when the middle layer (media) of the artery is weakened, stretching the inner (intima) and outer (adventitia) layers. As the artery widens, tension in the wall increases and further widening occurs, thus enlarging the aneurysm.

aneurysmectomy A surgical procedure performed to excise an aneurysm.

angina pectoris Literally, "strangling of the chest"; a temporary imbalance between the ability of the coronary arteries to supply oxygen and the demand for oxygen by the cardiac muscle. As a result, the patient experiences chest discomfort.

angioedema Diffuse swelling resulting from a vascular reaction in the deep tissues; can occur in a patient having an anaphylactic reaction.

anion Ion that has a negative charge.

anisocoria A difference in the size of the pupils.

ankle-brachial index (ABI) A ratio derived by dividing the ankle blood pressure by the brachial blood pressure; this calculation is used to assess the vascular status of the lower extremities. To obtain the ABI, a blood pressure cuff is applied to the lower extremities just above the malleoli. The systolic pressure is measured by Doppler ultrasound at both the dorsalis pedis and posterior tibial pulses. The higher of these two pressures is then divided by the higher of the two brachial pulses.

anomia Inability to find words.

anorectal abscess A localized induration and fluctuance that is caused by inflammation of the soft tissue near the rectum or anus and is most often the result of obstruction of the ducts of glands in the anorectal region by feces, foreign bodies, or trauma.

anorectic drugs Drugs that suppress appetite, which reduces food intake and, over time, may result in weight loss; may be prescribed for obese patients in a comprehensive weight reduction program.

anorexia nervosa An eating disorder of self-induced starvation resulting from a fear of fatness, even though the patient is underweight.

anorexia The loss of appetite for food.

anorexin Neuropeptide that decreases appetite.

anoxic Completely lacking oxygen.

antalgic (gait) A term that refers to an abnormality in the stance phase of gait. When part of one leg is painful, the person shortens the stance phase on the affected side.

anterior colporrhaphy Surgery for severe symptoms of cystocele in which the pelvic muscles are tightened for better bladder support.

anterior nares The nostrils or external openings into the nasal cavities.

antibody-mediated immunity (AMI) or anti-body-mediated immune system The defense response that produces antibodies directed against certain pathogens. The antibodies inactivate the pathogens and protect against future infection from that microorganism.

antidepressants A group of drugs that help manage clinical depression.

antiepileptic drugs (AEDs) A class of drugs used to control seizures. Also called *anticonvulsants*.

antigen A foreign protein or allergen that is capable of causing an immune response; protein on the surface of a cell.

anuria Complete lack of urine output; usually defined as less than 100 mL/24 hr.

aortic regurgitation The flow of blood from the aorta back into the left ventricle during diastole; occurs when the aortic valve leaflets do not close properly during diastole and the annulus (the valve ring that attaches to the leaflets) is dilated or deformed.

aortic stenosis Narrowing of the aortic valve orifice and obstruction of left ventricular outflow during systole.

aphasia Inability to use or comprehend spoken or written language due to brain injury or disease.

apheresis A procedure in which whole blood is withdrawn from the patient, a blood component (e.g., stem cells) is filtered out, and the plasma is returned to the patient.

aphonia Inability to produce sound; complete but temporary loss of the voice.

aphthous stomatitis Noninfectious stomatitis.

apical impulse The pulse located at the left fifth intercostal space in the midclavicular line in the mitral area (the apex of the heart). Also called the *point of maximal impulse*.

apolipoprotein E One of several regulators of lipoprotein metabolism.

appendectomy Surgical removal of the inflamed appendix.

appendicitis Acute inflammation of the vermiform appendix, which is the blind pouch attached to the cecum of the colon, usually located in the right iliac region just below the ileocecal valve.

approximated In a clean laceration or a surgical incision to be closed with sutures or staples, the act of bringing together the wound edges with the skin layers lined up in correct anatomic position so they can be held in place until healing is complete.

apraxia The loss of the ability to carry out a purposeful motor activity.

aqueous humor The clear, watery fluid that is continually produced by the ciliary processes and fills the anterior and posterior chambers of the eye. This fluid drains through the canal of Schlemm into the blood to maintain balanced intraocular pressure (pressure within the eye).

arcus senilis An opaque ring within the outer edge of the cornea caused by fat deposits. Its presence does not affect vision.

areflexic bladder Urinary retention and overflow (dribbling) caused by injuries to the lower motor neuron at the spinal cord level of S2 to S4 (e.g., multiple sclerosis and spinal cord injury below

T12). Bladder emptying may be achieved by performing a Valsalva maneuver or tightening the abdominal muscles. The effectiveness of these maneuvers should be ascertained by catheterizing the patient for residual urine after voiding. Also called *flaccid bladder*.

arrhythmogenic right ventricular cardiomyopathy (dysplasia) A form of cardiomyopathy that results from the replacement of myocardial tissue with fibrous and fatty tissue.

arterial revascularization The surgical procedure most commonly used to increase arterial blood flow in the affected limb of a patient with peripheral arterial disease.

arterial ulcers A painful complication in the patient with peripheral arterial disease. Typically, the ulcer is small and round, with a "punched out" appearance and well-defined borders. Ulcers develop on the toes (often the great toe), between the toes, or on the upper aspect of the foot. With prolonged occlusion, the toes can become gangrenous.

arteriography Angiography of the arterial vessels; this invasive diagnostic procedure involves fluoroscopy and the use of a contrast medium and is performed when an arterial obstruction, narrowing, or aneurysm is suspected.

arteriosclerosis A thickening, or hardening, of the arterial wall.

arteriotomy A surgical opening into an artery.

arteriovenous malformation (AVM) An abnormality that occurs during embryonic development, resulting in a tangled mass of malformed, thin-walled, dilated vessels. The congenital absence of a capillary network in these vessels forms an abnormal communication between the arterial and venous systems and increases the risk that the vessels may rupture, causing bleeding, such as into the subarachnoid space or into the intracerebral tissue with brain AVMs. In the absence of the capillary network, the thin-walled veins are subjected to arterial pressure.

arthralgia Pain in a joint.

arthritis Inflammation of one or more joints.

arthrodesis The surgical fusion of a joint.

arthrogram An x-ray study of a joint after contrast medium (air or solution) has been injected to enhance its visualization.

arthroscopy Procedure in which a fiberoptic tube is inserted into a joint for direct visualization of the ligaments, menisci, and articular surfaces of the joint.

articulations Joint surfaces.

artifact In the electrocardiogram, interference that is seen on the monitor or rhythm strip and may look like a wandering or fuzzy baseline; can be caused by patient movement, loose or defective electrodes, improper grounding, or faulty equipment.

ASA Physical Status Classification System From the American Society of Anesthesiologists (ASA), a system that assesses the fitness of patients for surgery.

ascending tracts Groups of nerves that originate in the spinal cord and end in the brain.

ascites The accumulation of free fluid within the peritoneal cavity. Increased hydrostatic pressure

from portal hypertension causes this fluid to leak into the peritoneal cavity.

assistive technology Electronic equipment that increases the ability of disabled patients to care for themselves.

assistive/adaptive device Any item that enables the patient to perform all or part of an activity independently.

asterixis A coarse tremor characterized by rapid, nonrhythmic extensions and flexions in the wrists and fingers; a motor disturbance seen in portal-systemic encephalopathy. Also called a *liver flap* or *flapping tremor*.

asthma A chronic respiratory condition in which reversible airway obstruction occurs intermittently, reducing airflow.

asthma A chronic respiratory condition in which reversible airflow obstruction in the airways occurs intermittently.

astigmatism A refractive error caused by unevenly curved surfaces on or in the eye (especially of the cornea) that distort vision.

ataxia Gait disturbance or loss of balance.

atelectasis Collapse of alveoli.

atelectrauma Shear injury to alveoli from opening and closing.

atherectomy An invasive nonsurgical technique in which a high-speed, rotating metal burr uses fine abrasive bits to scrape plaque from inside an artery while minimizing damage to the vessel surface.

atherosclerosis A type of arteriosclerosis that involves the formation of plaque within the arterial wall; the leading contributor to coronary artery and cerebrovascular disease.

atrial fibrillation (AF) A cardiac dysrhythmia in which multiple rapid impulses from many atrial foci, at a rate of 350 to 600 times per minute, depolarize the atria in a totally disorganized manner, with no P waves, no atrial contractions, a loss of the atrial kick, and an irregular ventricular response.

atrial gallop An abnormal fourth heart sound that occurs as blood enters the ventricles during the active filling phase at the end of ventricular diastole; may be heard in patients with hypertension, anemia, ventricular hypertrophy, myocardial infarction, aortic or pulmonic stenosis, and pulmonary emboli.

atrioventricular (AV) junction In the cardiac conduction system, the area consisting of a transitional cell zone, the atrioventricular (AV) node itself, and the bundle of His. The AV node lies just beneath the right atrial endocardium, between the tricuspid valve and the ostium of the coronary sinus.

atrophic gastritis A type of gastritis that involves all layers of the stomach and includes diffuse inflammation and destruction of deeply located glands.

attenuated The quality of making a substance weaker; for example, antigens that are used to make vaccines are specially processed to make them less likely to grow in the body.

atypical angina Angina that manifests itself as indigestion, pain between the shoulders, an aching jaw, or a choking sensation that occurs with exertion. Many women experience atypical angina.

atypical migraine The least common of the three types of migraine headaches, after migraines with aura and migraines without aura; the atypical category includes menstrual and cluster migraines.

aura A sensation that signals the onset of a headache or seizure; the patient may experience visual changes, flashing lights, or double vision.

autoamputation of the distal digits A condition in which the tips of the digits fall off spontaneously; can occur in severe cases of Raynaud's phenomenon.

autoantibodies Antibodies directed against self tissues of cells.

autocontamination The occurrence of infection in which the patient's own normal flora overgrows and penetrates the internal environment.

autodigestion Self-digestion. Specifically, the process of the stomach digesting itself if there is a break in its protective mucosal barrier.

autogenous Belonging to the person, such as a person's vein being moved from one part of the body to another.

autoimmune pancreatitis A chronic inflammatory form of pancreatitis that can also affect the bile ducts, kidneys, and other major connective tissues.

autologous blood transfusion Reinfusing the patient's own blood during surgery.

autologous bone marrow transplantation A type of bone marrow transplant in which patients receive their own stem cells, which were collected before high-dose chemotherapy.

autologous donation The donation of a patient's own blood before scheduled surgery for use, if needed, during the surgery to eliminate transfusion reactions and reduce the risk of bloodborne disease.

autolysis The spontaneous disintegration of tissue by the action of the patient's own cellular enzymes.

automaticity The ability of a cell to initiate an impulse spontaneously and repetitively; in cardiac electrophysiology, the ability of primary pacemaker cells (SA node, AV junction) to generate an electrical impulse.

autonomic dysreflexia (AD) A syndrome that affects the patient with an upper spinal cord injury; characterized by severe hypertension and headache, bradycardia, nasal stuffiness, and flushing; caused by a noxious stimulus, usually a distended bladder or constipation. This is a neurologic emergency and must be promptly treated to prevent a hypertensive brain attack.

autonomic nervous system (ANS) The part of the nervous system that is not under conscious control; consists of the sympathetic nervous system and the parasympathetic nervous system.

autonomy Ethical principle that implies a person's self-determination and self-management.

autosome Any of the 22 pairs of human chromosomes containing genes that code for all the structures and regulatory proteins needed for normal function but do not code for the sexual differentiation of a person.

axial loading A mechanism of injury that involves vertical compression. An example is a diving accident, in which the blow to the top of the head causes the vertebrae to shatter and pieces of bone enter the spinal canal and damage the cord.

azoospermia The absence of living sperm in the semen.

azotemia An excess of nitrogenous wastes (urea) in the blood.

B

Babinski's sign Dorsiflexion of the great toe and fanning of the other toes, which is an abnormal reflex in response to testing the plantar reflex with a pointed (but not sharp) object; indicates the presence of central nervous system disease. The normal response is plantar flexion of all toes.

bacteremia The presence of bacteria in the bloodstream.

bacteriuria Bacteria in the urine.

bad death A death embodied by pain, not having one's wishes followed at the end of one's life, isolation, abandonment, and constant agonizing about losses associated with death.

Baker's cyst Enlarged popliteal bursa.

banding See *endoscopic variceal ligation*.

barbiturate coma The use of drugs such as pentobarbital sodium or sodium thiopental at dosages to maintain complete unresponsiveness; used for patients whose increased intracranial pressure cannot be controlled by other means. These drugs decrease the metabolic demands of the brain and cerebral blood flow, stabilize cell membranes, decrease the formation of vasogenic edema, and produce a more uniform blood supply. The patient in a barbiturate coma requires mechanical ventilation, sophisticated hemodynamic monitoring, and intracranial pressure monitoring.

bariatrics Branch of medicine that manages obesity and its related diseases.

baroreceptors Sensory receptors in the arch of the aorta and at the origin of the internal carotid arteries that are stimulated when the arterial walls are stretched by an increased blood pressure.

barotrauma Damage to the lungs by positive pressure.

Barrett's epithelium Columnar epithelium (instead of the normal squamous cell epithelium) that develops in the lower esophagus during the process of healing from gastroesophageal reflux disease. It is considered premalignant and is associated with an increased risk of cancer in patients with prolonged disease.

Barrett's esophagus Ulceration of the lower esophagus caused by exposure to acid and pepsin, leading to the replacement of normal distal squamous mucosa with columnar epithelium as a response to tissue injury.

base A substance that binds (reduces) free hydrogen ions in solution. Strong bases bind hydrogen ions easily; weak bases bind less readily.

Basic Cardiac Life Support (BCLS) Procedure that involves ventilating the patient who has stopped breathing, as well as giving chest compressions in the absence of a carotid pulse. Also known as *cardiopulmonary resuscitation (CPR)*.

Bell's palsy Acute paralysis of cranial nerve VII; characterized by a drawing sensation and paralysis of all facial muscles on the affected side. The patient cannot close the eye, wrinkle the forehead, smile, whistle, or grimace. The face appears masklike and sags. Also called *facial paralysis*.

beneficence The ethical principle of preventing harm and ensuring the patient's well-being.

benign tumor cells Normal cells growing in the wrong place or at the wrong time.

benign Altered cell growth that is harmless and does not require intervention.

bereavement Grief and mourning experienced by the survivor before and after a death.

bicaval technique Surgical technique in heart transplantation in which the intact right atrium of the donor heart is preserved by anastomoses at the recipient's superior and inferior vena cavae.

bifurcation The point of division of a single structure into two branches.

bigeminy A type of premature complex that exists when normal complexes and premature complexes occur alternately in a repetitive two-beat pattern, with a pause occurring after each premature complex so that complexes occur in pairs.

bilateral orchiectomy The surgical removal of both testes, typically performed as palliative surgery in patients with prostate cancer. It is not intended to cure the prostate cancer but to arrest its spread by removing testosterone.

bilateral salpingo-oophorectomy (BSO) Surgical removal of both fallopian tubes and both ovaries.

biliary colic Intense pain due to obstruction of the cystic duct of the gallbladder from a stone moving through or lodged within the duct. Tissue spasm occurs in an effort to mobilize the stone through the small duct.

biliary stent A plastic or metal device that is placed percutaneously to keep a duct of the biliary system open in patients experiencing biliary obstruction.

biofilm A complex group of microorganisms that functions within a "slimy" gel coating on medical devices.

biological response modifiers (BRMs) A class of immunomodulating drugs that attempt to modify the course of disease. Also called *biologics*.

biologics See *biological response modifiers*.

biomedical technician Member of the health care team who maintains the safety of adaptive and electronic devices by monitoring their function and making repairs as needed.

biotrauma Inflammatory response–mediated damage to alveoli.

bivalve To cut a cast lengthwise into two equal pieces.

black box warning A governmental designation indicating that a drug has at least one serious side effect and must be used with caution.

bladder ultrasound Less invasive test to determine postvoiding residual urine volumes for the patient with a reflex (upper motor neuron) or uninhibited bladder; often used to measure residual urine in the bladder of patients with spinal cord injury.

blanch To whiten or lighten.

blast effect The damage sustained by the force of an explosion.

blast phase cell Immature cell that divides.

blood pressure (BP) The force of blood exerted against the vessel walls.

blood stem cells Immature, unspecialized (undifferentiated) cells that are capable of becoming any type of blood cell, depending on the body's needs.

bloodborne metastasis The release of tumor cells into the blood; the most common cause of cancer spread.

Blumberg's sign Pain felt on abrupt release of steady pressure (rebound tenderness) over the site of abdominal pain.

blunt trauma A type of trauma resulting from impact forces (e.g., motor vehicle accident, fall, assault).

body mass index (BMI) A measure of nutritional status that does not depend on frame size; indirectly estimates total fat stores within the body by the relationship of weight to height.

bolus feeding A method of tube feeding that involves intermittent feeding of a specified amount of enteral product at specified times during a 24-hour period, typically every 4 hours.

bone biopsy Procedure in which the physician extracts a specimen of bone tissue for microscopic examination to confirm the presence of infection or neoplasm; not commonly done today.

bone mineral density (BMD) The quality of bone that determines bone strength. It peaks between 30 and 35 years of age, when both bone resorption activity and bone-building activity occur at a constant rate. When bone resorption activity exceeds bone-building activity, bone density decreases.

bone reduction Realignment of fractured bone ends for proper healing.

bone remodeling A process in which bone is constantly undergoing changes.

bone resorption Loss of bone density due to demineralization resulting from the release of calcium from storage areas in bones.

bone scan A radionuclide test in which radioactive material is injected for visualization of the entire skeleton; used to detect tumors, arthritis, osteomyelitis, osteoporosis, vertebral compression fractures, and unexplained bone pain.

borborygmus (borborygmi) Bowel sounds, especially loud gurgling sounds, resulting from hypermotility of the bowel.

boring In pain, the type of intense pain that feels as if it is going through the body.

Bouchard's nodes Swelling at the proximal interphalangeal joints in osteoarthritis involving the hands.

bowel retraining A program for patients with neurologic problems that is designed to include a combination of suppository use and a consistent toileting schedule.

bradycardia Slowness of the heart rate; characterized as a pulse rate less than 50 to 60 beats/min.

bradydysrhythmia An abnormal heart rhythm characterized by a heart rate less than 60 beats/min.

bradykinesia Slow or no movement, as seen in a patient with Parkinson disease. Also called *akinesia*.

brain abscess A collection of pus that forms in the extradural, subdural, or intracerebral area of the brain as a result of a purulent infection, usually due to bacteria invading the brain directly or indirectly.

brain attack Stroke; disruption in the normal blood supply to the brain, either as an interruption in blood flow (ischemic stroke) or as bleeding within or around the brain (hemorrhagic stroke). A medical emergency that occurs suddenly, a stroke should be treated immediately to prevent neurologic deficit and permanent disability. Formerly called *cerebrovascular accident,* the National Stroke Association now uses the term *brain attack* to describe stroke.

brain herniation syndrome In the patient with untreated increased intracranial pressure, protrusion (herniation) of the brain downward toward the brainstem or laterally from a unilateral lesion within one cerebral hemisphere, causing irreversible brain damage and possibly death.

breakthrough pain Additional pain that "breaks through" the pain that is being managed by mainstay analgesic drugs.

breast augmentation Cosmetic surgical procedure to enhance the size, shape, or symmetry of the breasts.

breast-conserving surgery Surgical method for breast cancer that removes the bulk of the tumor rather than the entire breast.

Broca's aphasia See *expressive aphasia.*

Broca's area An important speech area of the cerebrum. It is located in the frontal lobe and is composed of neurons responsible for the formation of words, or speech.

bronchoscopy Insertion of a tube in the airway, usually as far as the secondary bronchi, for the purpose of visualizing airway structures and obtaining tissue samples for biopsy or culture.

bruit Swishing sound in the larger arteries (carotid, aortic, femoral, and popliteal) that can be heard with a stethoscope or Doppler probe; may indicate narrowing of the artery and is usually associated with atherosclerotic disease.

B-type natriuretic peptide (BNP) A peptide produced and released by the ventricles when the patient has fluid overload as a result of heart failure (HF).

bulbar Pertaining to the muscles involved in facial expression, chewing, and speech.

bulimia nervosa An eating disorder that is characterized by episodes of binge eating in which the patient ingests a large amount of food in a short time, followed by purging behavior such as self-induced vomiting or excessive use of laxatives and diuretics.

bunion Hallux valgus deformity of the foot in which lateral deviation of the great toe causes the first metatarsal head to become enlarged.

bunionectomy Surgical removal of the hallux valgus deformity (bunion) of the foot.

butterfly rash A dry, scaly raised rash on the face; the major skin manifestation of systemic lupus erythematosus.

C

***C. difficile*–associated disease (CDAD)** Clinical manifestations that are caused by *Clostridium difficile* as a potential result of antibiotic therapy use, especially in older adults.

cachexia Extreme body wasting and malnutrition that develop from an imbalance between food intake and energy use.

calciphylaxis A condition of thrombosis and skin necrosis that can occur in stage 5 chronic kidney disease.

calculi Abnormal formations of a mass of mineral salts that can occur in the body; forms in the kidney when excess calcium precipitates out of solution. Also called *stones.*

calculous cholecystitis Inflammation of the gallbladder usually following and created by obstruction of the cystic duct by a stone (calculus).

callus The loose, fibrous vascular tissue that forms at the site of a fracture as the first phase of healing and is normally replaced by hard bone as healing continues.

calyx The anatomic term for a cuplike structure.

Canadian Triage Acuity Scale (CTAS) A standardized model for triage in which lists of descriptors are used to establish the triage level.

cancellous The softer tissue inside bones that contains large spaces, or trabeculae, that are filled with red and yellow marrow.

candidiasis An infection caused by the fungus *Candida albicans.*

canthus The place where the upper and lower eyelids meet at the corner of either side of the eye.

capillary closing pressure The amount of pressure needed to occlude skin capillary blood flow.

capillary leak syndrome The response of capillaries to the presence of biologic chemicals (mediators) that change blood vessel integrity and allow fluid to shift from the blood in the vascular space into the interstitial tissues.

Caplan's syndrome The presence of pneumoconiosis and rheumatoid nodules in the lungs; noted primarily in coal miners and asbestos workers.

capnography An end-tidal carbon dioxide ($EtCO_2$) monitor.

capsule The layer of fibrous tissue on the outer surface of the kidney, which provides protection and support. The renal capsule itself is surrounded by layers of fat and connective tissue.

carboxyhemoglobin Carbon monoxide on oxygen-binding sites of the hemoglobin molecule.

carcinoembryonic antigen (CEA) An oncofetal antigen that may be elevated in 70% of people with colorectal cancer. CEA is not specifically associated with the colorectal cancer and may be elevated in the presence of other benign or malignant diseases and in smokers. CEA is often used to monitor the effectiveness of treatment and to identify disease recurrence.

carcinogen Any substance that changes the activity of the genes in a cell so that the cell becomes a cancer cell.

carcinogenesis Cancer development.

cardiac axis In electrocardiography (ECG), the direction of electrical current flow in the heart. The relationship between the cardiac axis and the lead axis is responsible for the deflections seen on the ECG pattern.

cardiac catheterization The most definitive but most invasive test in the diagnosis of heart disease; involves passing a small catheter into the heart and injecting contrast medium.

cardiac index A calculation of cardiac output requirements to account for differences in body size; determined by dividing the cardiac output by the body surface area.

cardiac markers Serum studies that include troponin, creatine kinase–MB, and myoglobin.

cardiac output (CO) The volume of blood ejected by the heart each minute; normal range in adults is 4 to 7 L/min.

cardiac rehabilitation The process of actively assisting the patient with cardiac disease to achieve and maintain a productive life while remaining within the limits of the heart's ability to respond to increases in activity and stress. *Phase 1* begins with the acute illness and ends with discharge from the hospital. *Phase 2* begins after discharge and continues through convalescence at home. *Phase 3* refers to long-term conditioning.

cardiac resynchronization therapy (CRT) In patients with some types of heart failure, the use of a permanent pacemaker alone or in combination with an implantable cardioverter-defibrillator to provide biventricular pacing.

cardiac tamponade Compression of the myocardium by fluid that has accumulated around the heart; this compresses the atria and ventricles, prevents them from filling adequately, and reduces cardiac output.

cardiogenic shock Post–myocardial infarction heart failure in which necrosis of more than 40% of the left ventricle has occurred. Also called *class IV heart failure*.

cardiomegaly Enlarged heart.

cardiomyopathy A subacute or chronic disease of cardiac muscle; classified into four categories based on abnormalities in structure and function: dilated, hypertrophic, restrictive, and arrhythmogenic.

cardiopulmonary bypass (CPB) Diversion of the blood from the heart to a bypass machine, where it is heparinized, oxygenated, and returned to the circulation through a cannula placed in the ascending aortic arch or femoral artery to provide oxygenation, circulation, and hypothermia during induced cardiac arrest for coronary artery bypass surgery. This process ensures a motionless operative field and prevents myocardial ischemia.

cardioversion A synchronized countershock that may be performed in emergencies for hemodynamically unstable ventricular or supraventricular tachydysrhythmias or electively for stable tachydysrhythmias that are resistant to medical therapies. The shock depolarizes a critical mass of myocardium simultaneously during intrinsic depolarization and is intended to stop the re-entry circuit and allow the sinus node to regain control of the heart.

care coordination The deliberate organization of and communication about patient care activities among members of the health care team (including the patient) to facilitate continuous health care to meet patient needs.

carina The point at which the trachea branches into the right and left mainstem bronchi.

carpal tunnel syndrome (CTS) A common condition in which the median nerve in the wrist becomes compressed, causing pain and numbness.

carrier (1) A person who harbors an infectious agent without symptoms of active disease; (2) in genetics, a person who has one mutated allele for a recessive genetic disorder. A carrier does not usually have any manifestations of the disorder but can pass the mutated allele to his or her children.

case management The process of assessment, planning, implementation, evaluation, and interaction for patients who have complex health problems and incur a high cost to the health care system. Goals include promoting quality of life, decreasing fragmentation and duplication of care across health care settings, and maintaining cost-effectiveness.

caseation necrosis A type of necrosis in which tissue is turned into a granular mass.

cast A rigid device that immobilizes the affected body part while allowing other body parts to move. It is most commonly used for fractures but may also be applied to correct deformities (e.g., clubfoot) or to prevent deformities (e.g., those seen in some patients with rheumatoid arthritis).

cataract A lens opacity that distorts the image projected onto the retina.

catechol-*O*-methyltransferases (COMTs) Enzymes that inactivate dopamine.

catecholamines Hormones (dopamine, epinephrine, and norepinephrine) released by the adrenal medulla in response to stimulation of the sympathetic nervous system.

catheter-related bloodstream infection (CR-BSI) Health care–acquired bloodstream infection caused by the presence of any type of intravenous catheter.

catheter-related bloodstream infection (CRBSI) prevention bundle An nationally recognized set of evidence-based interventions to prevent CR-BSIs.

cation Ion that has a positive charge.

cell saver system A technique that allows for collection of the person's own red blood cells during surgery, which is then reinfused directly back to the patient via a closed system.

cell-mediated immunity Microbial resistance that is mediated by the action of specifically sensitized T-lymphocytes.

cellular regulation The physiologic processes used to control cellular growth, replication, and differentiation (maturation into a specific cell type) to maintain homeostasis.

cellulitis An acute, spreading, edematous inflammation of the deep subcutaneous tissues; usually caused by infection of a wound or burn.

central IV therapy IV therapy in which a vascular access device (VAD) is placed in a central blood vessel, such as the superior vena cava.

central line–associated bloodstream infection (CLA-BSI) Health care–acquired bloodstream infection caused by the presence of a central intravenous line.

cerebral angiography (arteriography) Visualization of the cerebral circulation (carotid and vertebral arteries) after injecting a contrast medium into an artery (usually the femoral).

cerebral blood flow (CBF) Useful in evaluating cerebral vasospasm; can be measured in many areas of the brain with the use of radioactive substances.

cerebral perfusion pressure (CPP) The pressure gradient over which the brain is perfused. It is influenced by oxygenation, cerebral blood volume, blood pressure, cerebral edema, and intracranial pressure (ICP) and is determined by subtracting the mean ICP from the mean arterial pressure. A cerebral perfusion pressure above 70 mm Hg is generally accepted as an appropriate goal of therapy.

cerebral salt wasting (CSW) The primary cause of hyponatremia in the neurosurgical population; characterized by hyponatremia, decreased serum osmolality, and decreased blood volume. It is thought to result from the extrarenal influence of atrial natriuretic factor.

cerumen The wax produced by glands within the external ear canal; helps protect and lubricate the ear canal.

cervical polyp Tumor that arises from the mucosa and extends to the opening of the cervical os. Polyps result from hyperplasia of the endocervical epithelium, inflammation, or an abnormal local response to hormonal stimulation or localized vascular congestion of the cervical blood vessels. Polyps are the most common benign growth of the cervix.

CHADS₂ scoring system Acronym for Congestive heart failure, Hypertension, Age ≥75 years, Diabetes mellitus, Stroke. Determines whether a patient with atrial fibrillation needs preventive anticoagulant therapy.

chalazion An inflammation of a sebaceous gland in the eyelid.

chancre The ulcer that is the first sign of syphilis. It develops at the site of entry (inoculation) of the organism, usually 3 weeks after exposure. The lesion may be found on any area of the skin or mucous membranes but occurs most often on the genitalia, lips, nipples, and hands and in the oral cavity, anus, and rectum.

chemotherapy The treatment of cancer with chemical agents that have systemic effects; used to cure and to increase survival time.

chemotherapy-induced peripheral neuropathy (CIPN) The loss of sensory or motor function of peripheral nerves associated with exposure to certain anticancer drugs.

chest tube A drain placed in the pleural space to allow closed–chest drainage, which restores intrapleural pressure and allows re-expansion of the lung after surgery in patients who have undergone thoracotomy (incision of the chest wall).

Cheyne-Stokes respirations Common sign of nearing death in which apnea alternates with periods of rapid breathing.

choked disc See *papilledema*.

cholecystectomy The surgical removal of the gallbladder.

cholecystitis Inflammation of the gallbladder.

cholecystokinin A hormone that stimulates digestive juices and that may work with leptin to increase or decrease appetite.

choledochojejunostomy Surgical anastomosis of the common bile duct with the jejunum.

cholelithiasis The presence of gallstones.

cholesteatoma A benign overgrowth of squamous cell epithelium.

cholesterol Serum lipid that includes high-density lipoproteins and low-density lipoproteins.

cholinergic crisis Overmedication with cholinesterase inhibitors.

cholinesterase inhibitors Drugs that improve cholinergic neurotransmission in the central nervous system by delaying the destruction of acetylcholine by acetylcholinesterase, thus delaying the onset of cognitive decline. These are approved for symptomatic treatment of Alzheimer's disease but do not affect the course of the disease.

chondroitin A supplement that may play a role in strengthening cartilage.

choreiform movement Rapid, jerky movement.

chronic Having a slow onset and symptoms that persist for an extended period.

chronic calcifying pancreatitis (CCP) Alcohol-induced chronic pancreatitis that is characterized by protein precipitates that plug the ducts and lead to ductal obstruction, atrophy, and dilation. The epithelium of the ducts undergoes histologic changes, resulting in metaplasia (cell replacement) and ulceration. This inflammatory process causes fibrosis of the pancreatic tissue.

chronic constrictive pericarditis A fibrous thickening of the pericardium that prevents adequate filling of the ventricles and eventually results in cardiac failure; caused by chronic pericardial inflammation due to tuberculosis, radiation therapy, trauma, kidney failure, or metastatic cancer.

chronic fatigue syndrome (CFS) A chronic illness characterized by severe fatigue for 6 months or longer, usually following flu-like symptoms. At least four of the following criteria are required for diagnosis: sore throat; substantial impairment in short-term memory or concentration; tender lymph nodes; muscle pain; multiple joint pain with redness or swelling; headaches of a new type, pattern, or severity; unrefreshing sleep; and postexertional malaise lasting more than 24 hours.

chronic gastritis A patchy, diffuse inflammation of the mucosal lining of the stomach. Chronic gastritis usually heals without scarring but can progress to hemorrhage and ulcer formation.

chronic health condition A condition that has existed for at least 3 months.

chronic hepatitis Chronic liver inflammation that usually occurs as a result of hepatitis B or C. Superimposed infection with hepatitis D virus (HDV) in patients with chronic hepatitis B may also result in chronic hepatitis. Can lead to cirrhosis and liver cancer.

chronic kidney disease (CKD) A condition characterized by loss of kidney function over time.

chronic obstructive pancreatitis Pancreatitis that develops from inflammation, spasm, and obstruction of the sphincter of Oddi. Inflammatory and sclerotic lesions occur in the head of the pancreas and around the ducts, causing obstruction and backflow of pancreatic secretions.

chronic osteomyelitis Bone infection that persists over a long time due to misdiagnosis or inadequate treatment. Also called *subchronic osteomyelitis*.

chronic pain Pain that persists or recurs for indefinite periods (usually more than 3 months), often involves deep body structures, is poorly localized, and is difficult to describe. Also called *persistent pain*.

chronic pancreatitis A progressive, destructive disease of the pancreas characterized by remissions and exacerbations. Inflammation and fibrosis of the tissue contribute to pancreatic insufficiency and diminished function of the organ.

chronic paronychia Inflammation of the skin around the nail that persists for months. People at risk for chronic paronychia are those with frequent exposure to water, such as homemakers, bartenders, and laundry workers.

chronic pyelonephritis A kidney disorder that results from repeated or continued upper urinary tract infections or the effects of such infections.

chronic stable angina (CSA) Type of angina characterized by chest discomfort that occurs with moderate to prolonged exertion and in a pattern that is familiar to the patient.

chyme The liquid formed when food is transformed during the digestion process in the gastrointestinal tract.

circle of Willis At the base of the brain, the ring formed by the anterior, middle, and posterior cerebral arteries where they are joined together by small communicating arteries.

circumcision The surgical removal of the prepuce or foreskin of the penis.

circumferential Referring to something that completely surrounds an extremity or the thorax.

cirrhosis Liver disease that is characterized by extensive scarring of the liver and that is usually caused by a chronic irreversible reaction to hepatic inflammation and necrosis; disease typically develops insidiously and has a prolonged, destructive course.

classic heat stroke A form of heat stroke in which the body's ability to dissipate heat is significantly impaired; occurs over time as a result of long-term exposure to a hot, humid environment such as a home without air-conditioning in the high heat of the summer.

clinical practice guideline An "official recommendation" based on evidence to diagnose and/or manage a health problem (e.g., pain management).

clinical psychologist Member of the health care team who counsels patients and families on their psychological problems and on strategies to cope with disability.

clinically competent The condition of being legally competent and having decisional capacity.

clonic (rhythmic) Pertaining to a state of alternating muscle stiffness followed by rhythmic jerking motions, as in a tonic-clonic seizure.

clonus The sudden, brief, jerking contraction of a muscle or muscle group often seen in seizures. Also called *myoclonus*.

closed fracture A fracture that does not extend through the skin and therefore has no visible wound. Also called *simple fracture*.

closed reduction A nonsurgical method for managing a simple fracture. While applying a manual pull, or traction, on the bone, the health care provider manipulates the bone ends so that they realign.

closed traumatic brain injury A type of traumatic primary brain injury that occurs as the result of blunt trauma; the integrity of the skull is not violated, and damage to brain tissue depends on the degree and mechanisms of injury.

clotting A complex, multi-step process by which blood forms a protein-based structure (clot) in an appropriate area of tissue injury to prevent excessive bleeding while maintaining whole-body blood flow (perfusion).

clubbing Changes in the tissue beds of the fingers and toes, with the base of the nail becoming spongy; results from chronic oxygen deprivation in the tissue beds.

cluster headache A type of oculotemporal or oculofrontal headache marked by unilateral, excruciating, nonthrobbing pain that is felt deep in and around the eye and may radiate to the forehead, temple, cheek, ear, occiput, or neck. Average duration is 10 to 45 minutes. Headaches occur every 8 to 12 hours and up to 24 hours daily at the same time for about 6 to 8 weeks (hence the term *cluster*), followed by remission for 9 months to a year. Cause and mechanism are unknown but have been attributed to vasoreactivity and oxyhemoglobin desaturation.

clysis See *hypodermoclysis*.

coagulopathy Clotting abnormalities.

cognition The ability of the brain to process, store, retrieve, and manipulate information.

cognitive rehabilitation A way of helping brain-injured patients regain function in areas that are essential for a return to independence and a reasonable quality of life.

cognitive therapist A member of the rehabilitative health care team, usually a neuropsychologist, who works primarily with patients who have experienced head injuries and have cognitive impairments.

cohorting The practice of grouping patients who are colonized or infected with the same pathogen.

cold antibody anemia A form of immunohemolytic anemia (in which the immune system attacks a person's own red blood cells for unknown reasons) that occurs with complement protein fixation on immunoglobulin M (IgM). In this condition, the arteries in the hands and feet constrict profoundly in response to cold temperatures or stress.

cold phase A phase after peripheral nerve trauma resulting in complete denervation in which the skin appears cyanotic, mottled, or reddish blue and feels cool compared with the contralateral unaffected extremity. The cold phase follows the warm phase, which lasts 2 to 3 weeks after injury.

colectomy Surgical removal of part or all of the colon.

collaboration The planning, implementing, and evaluation of patient care using an interdisciplinary (ID) plan of care.

collateral circulation Circulation that provides blood to an area with altered tissue perfusion through smaller vessels that develop and compensate for the occluded vessels.

colon interposition A surgical procedure that may be performed in patients with an esophageal tumor when the tumor involves the stomach or the stomach is otherwise unsuitable for anastomosis. In colon interposition, a section of right or left colon is removed and brought up into the thorax to substitute for the esophagus.

colon resection Surgery performed for colorectal cancer in which the tumor and regional lymph nodes are removed.

colonoscopy The endoscopic examination of the entire large bowel.

colostomy The surgical creation of an opening between the colon and the surface of the abdomen.

colposcopy Examination of the cervix and vagina using a colposcope, which allows three-dimensional magnification and intense illumination of epithelium with suspected disease. This procedure can locate the exact site of precancerous and malignant lesions for biopsy.

comatose Unconscious and cannot be aroused despite vigorous or noxious simulation.

comfort A state of physical well-being, pleasure, and absence of pain or stress.

command center See *emergency operations center*.

commando procedure Mnemonic for combined neck dissection, mandibulectomy, and oropharyngeal resection—a procedure in which the surgeon removes a segment of the mandible with the oral lesion and performs a radical neck dissection.

communicable The ability of an infection, such as influenza, to be transmitted from person to person.

communicating hydrocephalus Form of hydrocephalus that occurs when the flow of cerebrospinal fluid (CSF) is blocked after it exits the ventricles; this form is "communicating" because CSF can still flow between the ventricles, which remain open.

compartment syndrome A condition in which increased tissue pressure in a confined anatomic space causes decreased blood flow to the area, leading to hypoxia and pain.

compensated cirrhosis A form of cirrhosis in which the liver has significant scarring but is still able to perform essential functions without causing significant symptoms.

compensatory mechanism The means of producing compensation. Also called *adaptive mechanism.*

complement activation and fixation Actions triggered by some classes of antibodies that can remove or destroy antigen.

complete spinal cord injury An injury in which the spinal cord has been severed or damaged in a way that eliminates all innervation below the level of the injury.

complex regional pain syndrome (CRPS) A complex disorder that includes debilitating pain, atrophy, autonomic dysfunction (excessive sweating, vascular changes), and motor impairment (most notably muscle paresis), probably caused by an abnormally hyperactive sympathetic nervous system. This syndrome most often results from traumatic injury and commonly occurs in the feet and hands; formerly called *reflex sympathetic dystrophy (RSD)*.

compliance In respiratory physiology, a measure of elasticity within the lung. Also, a patient's fulfillment of a caregiver's prescribed course of treatment.

compound fracture See *open fracture*.

compression fracture A fracture that is produced by a loading force applied to the long axis of cancellous bone. These fractures commonly occur in the vertebrae of patients with osteoporosis.

computed tomography coronary angiography (CTCA) 64-slice diagnostic scan used to diagnose coronary artery disease in symptomatic patients.

conductive hearing loss Hearing loss that results from any physical obstruction of sound wave transmission (e.g., a foreign body in the external canal, a retracted or bulging tympanic membrane, or fused bony ossicles).

conductivity The ability of a cell to transmit an electrical stimulus from cell membrane to cell membrane.

congestive heart failure (CHF) Former term for *left-sided heart failure*. Categorized as either systolic heart failure or diastolic heart failure, which may be acute or chronic and mild to severe.

conization The removal of a cone-shaped sample of tissue from the cervix for cytologic study.

conjunctivae The mucous membranes of the eye that line the undersurface of the eyelids (palpebral conjunctiva) and cover the sclera (bulbar conjunctiva).

connective tissue disease (CTD) A group of diseases that are the major focus of rheumatology (the study of rheumatic diseases); most are musculoskeletal disorders.

consensual response In assessing pupillary reaction to light, a slight constriction of the pupil of the eye not being tested when a penlight is brought in from the side of the patient's head and shined into the eye being tested as soon as the patient opens his or her eyes.

consolidation Solidification; lack of air spaces in the lung, such as occurs in pneumonia.

constipation The passage of hard, dry stool fewer than 3 times a week (as defined by the Association of Rehabilitation Nurses).

contact laser prostatectomy (CLP) Procedure for treating benign prostatic hyperplasia that uses laser energy to coagulate excess tissue. Also called *interstitial laser coagulation (ILC)*.

Contact Precautions Infection control guidelines from the U.S. Centers for Disease Control and Prevention; used for patients with infections spread by direct contact or contact with items in the patient's environment, such as pediculosis.

contiguous Something in direct contact with, or adjacent to, another area or structure.

continence The ability to voluntarily control emptying the bladder and colon. Continence is a learned behavior whereby a person can suppress the urge to urinate until a socially appropriate location is available.

continuous feeding A method of tube feeding in which small amounts of enteral product are continuously infused (by gravity drip or by a pump or controller device) over a specified time.

continuous femoral nerve blockade A method used to administer anesthesia using an IV moderate sedation agent is used in addition to the neuraxial or PNB drug. PNB may be either a single injection or continuous infusion by a portable pump.

continuous positive airway pressure (CPAP) A respiratory treatment that improves obstructive sleep apnea in patients with heart failure.

contractility The ability of a cell to contract in response to an impulse. In cardiac electrophysiology, the ability of atrial and ventricular muscle cells to shorten their fiber length in response to electrical stimulation, generating sufficient pressure to propel blood forward. Contractility is the mechanical activity of the heart.

contraction The closure of a wound as new collagen replaces damaged tissue, pulling the wound edges inward along the path of least resistance.

contralateral Pertaining to the opposite side.

contrecoup injury Bruising of the brain tissue, with damage occurring on the side opposite the site of impact.

control therapy drugs Drugs used every day, regardless of symptoms, to reduce airway responsiveness to prevent asthma attacks from occurring.

contusion A bruise; when referring to closed head injury, a bruising of brain tissue usually found at the site of impact (coup injury). Compare with *contrecoup injury*.

cor pulmonale Right-sided heart failure caused by pulmonary disease.

cordectomy Excision of a vocal cord in surgery for laryngeal cancer.

cornea The clear layer that forms the external coat on the front of the eye.

corneal abrasion Scrape or scratch of the cornea that disrupts its integrity.

corneal ulceration Deep disruption of the corneal epithelium that extends into the stromal layer and is caused by bacteria, protozoa, or fungi.

coronary artery bypass graft (CABG) A surgical procedure in which occluded coronary arteries are bypassed with the patient's own venous or arterial blood vessels or synthetic grafts.

coronary artery disease (CAD) Disease affecting the arteries that provide blood, oxygen, and nutrients to the myocardium; partial or complete blockage of the blood flow through the coronary arteries, causing ischemia and infarction of the myocardium, angina pectoris, and acute coronary syndromes. Also known as *coronary heart disease* or simply *heart disease*.

coronary artery vasculopathy (CAV) A form of coronary artery disease that presents as diffuse plaque in the arteries of the donor heart in patients who have received a heart transplant.

cortisol The main glucocorticoid produced by the adrenal cortex.

coryza The common cold, or acute viral rhinitis.

cough assist A technique for assisting the tetraplegic patient to cough. Place his or her hands on either side of the rib cage or upper abdomen below the diaphragm; then, as the patient inhales, push upward to help expand the lungs and cough.

craniotomy Surgical incision into the cranium.

creatine kinase (CK) An enzyme specific to cells of the brain, myocardium, and skeletal muscle. Its appearance in the blood indicates tissue necrosis or injury, with levels following a predictable rise and fall during a specified period.

Credé maneuver A technique used to assist in urination in which a patient places his or her hand in a cupped position directly over the bladder area and pushes inward and downward gently as if massaging the bladder to empty.

crepitus A continuous grating sensation caused when irregular cartilage or bone fragments rub together and which may be felt or heard as a joint is put through passive range of motion; also, a crackling sensation that can be felt on a patient's chest, indicating that air is trapped within the tissues.

CREST syndrome In patients with systemic sclerosis, the combination of calcinosis (calcium deposits), Raynaud's phenomenon, esophageal dysmotility, sclerodactyly (scleroderma of the digits), and telangiectasia (spider-like hemangiomas).

cricothyroidotomy Surgical procedure in which an opening is made between the thyroid cartilage and cricoid cartilage ring and results in a tracheostomy. Also called *cricothyrotomy*. The procedure is used in an emergency for access to the lower airways.

crises In the patient with sickle cell disease, periodic episodes of extensive cellular sickling that have a sudden onset and can occur as often as weekly or as seldom as once a year.

critical access hospital A small rural facility of 15 or fewer inpatient beds that provides around-the-clock emergency care services 7 days per week. Considered a necessary provider of health care to community residents who are not close to other hospitals in a given region.

cross-contamination A type of contamination in which organisms from another person or from the environment are transmitted to the patient.

cryotherapy (1) A way of decreasing muscle pain by "cooling down" the area with a local, short-acting gel or cream, such as after physical therapy; (2) in ophthalmologic surgery, use of a freezing probe to repair retinal detachment.

cryptorchidism Failure of the testes to descend into the scrotum.

culture of safety A blame-free approach to improving care in high-risk, error-prone health care organizations using interprofessional collaboration. Patients and families are encouraged to become safety partners in protecting patients from harm.

culture A procedure for identifying a microorganism by cultivating and isolating it in tissue cultures or artificial media.

Curling's ulcer Acute ulcerative gastroduodenal disease, which may develop within 24 hours

of a severe burn injury because of reduced gastrointestinal blood flow and mucosal damage.

Cushing's disease (Cushing's syndrome) Hypercortisolism caused by oversecretion of hormones by the adrenal cortex.

Cushing's triad A classic yet late sign of increased intracranial pressure (ICP) manifested by severe hypertension with a widened pulse pressure and bradycardia. As ICP increases, the pulse becomes thready, irregular, and rapid. Cerebral blood flow increases in response to hypertension.

Cushing's ulcer Acute ulcerative gastroduodenal disease that may develop as a result of increased intracranial pressure.

cutaneous (superficial) reflexes Superficial reflexes. Usually the plantar and abdominal reflexes are tested.

cyanosis Bluish or darkened discoloration of the skin and mucous membranes; results from an increased amount of deoxygenated hemoglobin.

cyclic feeding A method of tube feeding similar to continuous feeding (see definition of *continuous feeding*) except the infusion is stopped for a specified time in each 24-hour period ("down time"); the down time typically occurs in the morning to allow bathing, treatments, and other activities.

cystitis Inflammation of the bladder.

cystocele Herniation of the bladder into the vagina.

cytokines Small protein hormones produced by white blood cells.

cytotoxic Having cell-damaging effects.

D

dandruff An accumulation of patchy or diffuse white or gray scales on the surface of the scalp.

death rattle Loud, wet respirations caused by secretions in the respiratory tract and oral cavity of a patient who is near death.

death When illness or trauma overwhelms the compensatory mechanisms of the body and the lungs and heart cease to function.

débridement The removal of infected tissue from a healing wound.

debriefing After a mass casualty incident or disaster, (1) the provision of sessions for small groups of staff in which teams are brought in to discuss effective coping strategies (critical incident stress debriefing), and (2) the administrative review of staff and system performance during the event to determine opportunities for improvement in the emergency management plan.

debris Dead cells and tissues in a wound.

decerebrate posturing Abnormal posturing and rigidity characterized by extension of the arms and legs, pronation of the arms, plantar flexion, and opisthotonos; usually associated with dysfunction in the brainstem area. Also called *decerebration*.

decerebration See *decerebrate posturing*.

decompensated cirrhosis A form of cirrhosis in which liver function is significantly impaired with obvious manifestations of liver failure.

decompressive craniectomy Removal of a section of the skull in the patient with uncontrolled intracranial pressure (ICP); allows for additional space for edema without increasing ICP.

decorticate posturing Abnormal posturing seen in the patient with lesions that interrupt the corticospinal pathways. The arms, wrists, and fingers are flexed with internal rotation and plantar flexion of the legs. Also called *decortication*.

decortication See *decorticate posturing*.

deep tendon reflexes Tested as part of the neurologic assessment. An intact reflex arc is indicated when the muscle contracts in response to the tendon being struck with a reflex hammer.

deep vein thrombophlebitis Presence of a thrombus associated with inflammation in the deep veins, usually in the legs. Compared with superficial thrombophlebitis, it presents a greater risk for pulmonary embolism. Also called *deep vein thrombosis*.

deep vein thrombosis (DVT) Common term for *deep vein thrombophlebitis*.

defibrillation An asynchronous countershock that depolarizes a critical mass of myocardium simultaneously to stop the re-entry circuit, allowing the sinus node to regain control of the heart.

dehiscence A partial or complete separation of the outer layers of a wound, sometimes described as a "splitting open" of the wound.

dehydration Fluid intake less than what is needed to meet the body's fluid needs.

delayed union Term describing a fracture that has not healed within 6 months of injury.

delegation The process of transferring to a competent person the authority to perform a selected nursing task or activity in a selected patient care situation.

delirium An acute state of confusion, usually short-term and reversible within 3 weeks. Often seen among older adults in a hospital or other unfamiliar setting.

dementia A syndrome of slowly progressive cognitive decline with global impairment of intellectual function. The most common type is Alzheimer's disease.

demyelination Destruction of myelin between the nodes of Ranvier; a major pathologic finding in multiple sclerosis or Guillain-Barré syndrome.

depolarization The ability of a cell to respond to a stimulus by initiating an impulse. Also called *excitability*.

depression A response to multiple life stresses, a single situation, a primary disorder, or a problem associated with dementia; this response can range from mild, transient feelings of sadness to a severe sense of helplessness and hopelessness.

dermal papillae Fingerlike projections of dermal tissue that anchor the epidermis to the dermis.

dermatomes Specific areas of the skin that receive sensory input from spinal nerves.

descending tracts Groups of nerves that begin in the brain and end in the spinal cord.

desquamation The shedding or peeling of skin.

diabetic nephropathy A vascular complication of diabetes mellitus that causes permanent damage to kidney tissue and is a leading cause of end-stage kidney disease.

diabetic peripheral neuropathy (DPN) A progressive deterioration of nerves that results in loss of nerve function (sensory perception). A common complication of diabetes, it often involves all parts of the body.

diagnostic peritoneal lavage (DPL) Test that determines the presence of internal bleeding following abdominal trauma.

dialysate The solution used in dialysis. It is composed of water, glucose, sodium chloride, potassium, magnesium, calcium, and bicarbonate; dialysate composition may be altered according to the patient's needs for treatment of electrolyte imbalances.

dialyzer The apparatus used to perform hemodialysis. Also known as the "artificial kidney," it has four parts: a blood compartment, a dialysate compartment, a semipermeable membrane, and an enclosed structure to support the membrane.

diaphragmatic pacing A pacemaker for the phrenic nerve to cause the diaphragm to contract (leading to inhalation). Also known as *phrenic nerve pacing*.

diarrhea A condition in which the stool can be watery and without solid form.

diastole The phase of the cardiac cycle that consists of relaxation and filling of the atria and ventricles; normally about two thirds of the cardiac cycle.

diastolic blood pressure The amount of pressure/force against the arterial walls during the relaxation phase of the heart.

diastolic heart failure Heart failure that occurs when the left ventricle is unable to relax adequately during diastole, which prevents the ventricle from filling with sufficient blood to ensure adequate cardiac output.

Dietary Guidelines for Americans Recommendations made by the USDA and U.S. Department of Health and Human Services to help people maintain nutritional health; updated every 5 years.

Dietary Reference Intakes (DRIs) Nutrition guide developed by the Institute of Medicine of the National Academies that provides a scientific basis for food guidelines in the United States and Canada.

diffuse axonal injury (DAI) A type of closed head injury that is usually related to high-speed acceleration/deceleration, as with motor vehicle crashes. There is significant damage to axons in the white matter, and there are lesions in the corpus callosum, midbrain, cerebellum, and upper brainstem. Patients with severe injury may present with immediate coma, and most survivors require long-term care.

diffuse cutaneous systemic sclerosis Skin thickening on the trunk, face, and proximal and distal extremities in patients with systemic sclerosis.

diffuse light reflex A description of a light reflex that is spotty or multiple because of a changed eardrum shape from either retraction or bulging.

diffusion The spontaneous, free movement of particles (solute) across a permeable membrane down a concentration gradient; that is, from an area of higher concentration to an area of lower concentration.

digestion The mechanical and chemical process in which complex foodstuffs are broken down into simpler forms that can be used by the body.

digital 3D mammography Breast imaging procedure that allows the radiologist to visualize through layers or "slices" of breast tissue, similar to a CT scan.

digoxin toxicity A reaction to therapy with digitalis derivatives (digoxin) that is identified by monitoring serum digoxin and potassium levels (hypokalemia potentiates digitalis toxicity). Signs of toxicity are nonspecific (anorexia, fatigue, changes in mental status). Toxicity may cause dysrhythmia, most commonly premature ventricular contractions.

dilated cardiomyopathy (DCM) A type of cardiomyopathy that involves extensive damage to the myofibrils and interference with myocardial metabolism. There is normal ventricular wall thickness but dilation of both ventricles and impairment of systolic function.

dilation Increase in the diameter of blood vessels.

diplopia Double vision.

direct current stimulation (DCS) The placement of an implantable device to promote bone fusion; used as an adjunct for patients for whom spinal fusion may be difficult.

direct inguinal hernia A sac formed from the peritoneum that contains a portion of the intestine and passes through a weak point in the abdominal wall.

direct response Pupil constriction in response to bringing a penlight in from the side of the patient's head and shining the light in the eye being tested as soon as the patient opens his or her eyes.

directly observed therapy (DOT) A technique in which a health care professional watches the patient swallow prescribed drugs.

disabling health condition Any physical or mental health problem that can cause disability.

disaster triage tag system A system that categorizes triage priority by colored and numbered tags.

disaster A mass casualty incident in which the number of casualties exceeds the resource capabilities of a particular community or hospital facility.

discoid lesion Round lesion in patients who have discoid lupus erythematosus; evident when exposed to sunlight or ultraviolet light.

disease-modifying antirheumatic drugs (DMARDs) Drugs prescribed to slow the progression of mild rheumatoid disease before it worsens, such as hydroxychloroquine, sulfasalazine, or minocycline.

disequilibrium A condition in which the hydrostatic pressure is not the same in the two fluid spaces on either side of a permeable membrane.

disinfection A method of infection control in which the level of disease-causing organisms is reduced but the organisms are not killed; adequate when an item is entering a body area that has resident bacteria or normal flora, such as the respiratory tract.

diskitis Disk inflammation.

dislocation of a joint Occurrence of the articulating surfaces of two or more bones moving away from each other.

dissociate The act of separating and releasing ions.

diverticula Sacs resulting from the herniation of the mucosa and submucosa of a tubular organ into surrounding tissue.

diverticulitis The inflammation of one or more diverticula.

diverticulosis The presence of many abnormal pouchlike herniations (diverticula) in the wall of the intestine.

dizziness A disturbed sense of a person's relationship to space.

DNR Do not resuscitate; order from a physician or other authorized health care provider who instructs that CPR not be attempted in the event of cardiac or respiratory arrest.

dopamine agonist A class of drugs that mimic dopamine. Dopamine agonists stimulate dopamine receptors and are typically the most effective during the first 3 to 5 years of use. Prescribed for the patient with Parkinson disease to reduce dyskinesias (problems with movement).

dose-dense chemotherapy Chemotherapy that uses higher doses more often for aggressive cancer treatment, especially breast cancer.

double-barrel stoma The least common type of colostomy, which is created by dividing the bowel and bringing both the proximal and distal portions to the abdominal surface to create two stomas.

double-contrast barium enema A type of contrast radiography (x-rays) in which the patient's colon and rectum are visualized after a liquid containing barium, and then air, is placed into the colon.

doubling time The amount of time it takes for a tumor to double in size.

Droplet Precautions Infection control guidelines from the U.S. Centers for Disease Control and Prevention; used for patients with infections spread by the droplet transmission route, such as influenza.

drug holiday Period of time lasting up to 10 days in which the patient with Parkinson disease receives no drug therapy.

dual x-ray absorptiometry (DXA or DEXA) A type of radiographic scan that measures bone mineral density in the hip, wrist, or vertebral column; used as a screening and diagnostic tool for diagnosis and for follow-up evaluation of treatment of osteoporosis.

ductal carcinoma in situ (DCIS) An early, noninvasive form of breast cancer in which cancer cells are located within the duct and have not invaded the surrounding fatty breast tissue.

ductal ectasia A benign breast disease caused by dilation and thickening of the collecting ducts in the subareolar area. The ducts become distended and filled with cellular debris, which activates an inflammatory response. It is usually seen in women approaching menopause.

dumping syndrome A constellation of vasomotor symptoms that typically occur within 30 minutes after eating; believed to occur as a result of the rapid emptying of gastric contents into the small intestine, which shifts fluid into the gut and causes abdominal distention. Early manifestations include vertigo, tachycardia, syncope, sweating, pallor, and palpitations.

Dupuytren's contracture A slowly progressive contracture of the palmar fascia that results in flexion of the fourth or fifth digit of the hand and occasionally affects the third digit. Although a fairly common problem, the cause is unknown. It usually occurs in older men, tends to occur in families, and can be bilateral.

durable power of attorney for health care (DPOAHC) A legal document in which a person appoints someone else to make health care decisions in the event he or she becomes incapable of making decisions.

dysarthria Slurred speech.

dysfunctional uterine bleeding (DUB) A nonspecific term to describe bleeding that is excessive or abnormal in amount or frequency without predisposing anatomic or systemic conditions. Such bleeding occurs most often at either end of the span of a woman's reproductive years, when ovulation is becoming established or when it is becoming irregular at menopause.

dyskinesia Difficulty with movement.

dyslexia Problems understanding written language; caused by brain injury or disease.

dysmetria The inability to direct or limit movement.

dyspareunia Painful sexual intercourse.

dyspepsia Indigestion or heartburn following meals.

dysphagia Difficulty in swallowing.

dysphasia Slurred speech.

dyspnea on exertion (DOE) Dyspnea that is associated with activity, such as climbing stairs.

dyspnea Difficulty in breathing or breathlessness.

dysrhythmia A disorder of the heartbeat involving a disturbance in cardiac rhythm; irregular heartbeat.

dystrophic Pertaining to or characterized by dystrophy; abnormal.

dystrophin A muscle protein that maintains muscle integrity by sending signals to coordinate smooth, synchronous muscle fiber contraction. Faulty action of this protein causes muscular dystrophy.

dysuria Painful urination.

E

Eaton-Lambert syndrome A form of myasthenia gravis that affects the muscles of the trunk and the pelvic and shoulder girdles; often observed in combination with small cell carcinoma of the lung. Although weakness increases after exertion, there may be a temporary increase in muscle strength during the first few contractions, followed by a rapid decline.

ecchymoses Large purple, blue, or yellow bruises of the skin resulting from small hemorrhages; these bruises are larger than petechiae.

ecchymotic Pertaining to a bruise.

ECG caliper A measurement tool used in analysis of an electrocardiographic (ECG) rhythm strip.

echocardiography In cardiovascular assessment, the use of ultrasound waves to assess cardiac structure and mobility, particularly of the valves; a noninvasive, risk-free test that is easily performed at the bedside or on an ambulatory care basis.

echolalia Automatic repetition of what another person says.

ectopic Out of place.

ectropion A turning outward and sagging of the eyelid, which is caused by relaxation of the orbicular muscle.

edema Tissue swelling as a result of the accumulation of excessive fluid in the interstitial spaces.

edentulous Without teeth.

efferent arterioles The extremely small blood vessels that carry the remaining blood out of the glomerulus (once the glomerulus has filtered the blood to make urine) and into one of two additional capillary systems (the peritubular capillaries or the vasa recta).

effluent Drainage.

effusion An accumulation of fluid, such as in a joint (where it may limit movement).

ejection fraction The percentage of blood ejected from the heart during systole.

electrical bone stimulation The use of an electronic device (e.g., magnetic coils applied on the skin or over a cast to deliver a pulsed magnetic field) to promote bone union after a fracture. The exact mechanism of action is unknown, but this procedure is based on research showing that bone has inherent electrical properties that are used in healing.

electrocardiogram (ECG) A graphic recording of the electrical current generated by the heart. The ECG provides information about cardiac dysrhythmias, myocardial ischemia, site and extent of myocardial infarction, cardiac hypertrophy, electrolyte imbalances, and effectiveness of cardiac drugs. It is a routine part of cardiovascular evaluation and is a valuable diagnostic test.

electroencephalography (EEG) A recording of the electrical activity of the cerebral hemispheres; it represents the voltage changes in various areas of the brain as determined by recording the difference between two electrodes.

electrolyte A substance in body fluids that carries an electrical charge. Also called an *ion.*

electromyography (EMG) A recording of the electrical activity of peripheral nerves by testing muscle activity.

electrophysiologic study (EPS) In cardiovascular assessment, an invasive procedure performed in a catheterization laboratory during which programmed electrical stimulation of the heart is used to induce and evaluate lethal dysrhythmias and conduction abnormalities to permit accurate diagnosis and effective treatment. The study is used in patients who have survived cardiac arrest, have recurrent tachydysrhythmias, or experience unexplained syncopal episodes.

electrovaporization of the prostate (EVAP) Procedure for treating benign prostatic hyperplasia with high-frequency electrical current to cut and vaporize excess tissue.

elimination The excretion of waste from the body by the GI tract (as feces) and by the kidneys (as urine).

embolectomy Removal of a blood clot.

embolic stroke Damage to the brain when a blood clot forms somewhere in the body (usually the heart) and travels through the bloodstream to block one or more of the arteries supplying the brain.

embolus The occurrence of inflammation and thickening of the vein wall around a clot (thrombus).

emergence Recovery from anesthesia.

emergency medical technician (EMT) Prehospital care provider who supplies basic life-support interventions such as oxygen, basic wound care, splinting, spinal immobilization, and monitoring of vital signs.

emergency medicine physician A member of the emergency health care team with education and training in the specialty of emergency patient management.

emergency operations center (EOC) A designated location in the Hospital Incident Command System (HICS) with accessible communication technology. Also called the *command center.*

emergency preparedness A goal or plan to meet an extraordinary need for hospital beds, staff, drugs, personal protective equipment, supplies, and medical devices such as mechanical ventilators.

Emergency Severity Index (ESI) A standardized model for triage that categorizes both patient acuity and resource utilization into five levels, from most urgent to least urgent.

emergent triage In a three-tiered triage scheme, the category that includes any condition or injury that poses an immediate threat to life or limb, such as crushing chest pain or active hemorrhage.

emetogenic A substance that induces nausea and vomiting.

emmetropia The state of perfect refraction of the eye; with the lens at rest, light rays from a distant source are focused into a sharp image on the retina.

emotional abuse The intentional use of threats, humiliation, intimidation, and isolation to another person.

emotional lability Having uncontrollable emotions; for example, the patient laughs and then cries unexpectedly for no apparent reason.

empyema A collection of pus in the pleural space.

encephalitis An inflammation of the brain parenchyma (brain tissue) and meninges that affects the cerebrum, brainstem, and cerebellum; usually caused by a virus.

endogenous An infection in which organisms are carried by the bloodstream from other areas of infection in the body.

endometrial ablation Procedure for dysfunctional uterine bleeding that removes a built-up uterine lining using a laser, roller ball, or balloon.

endometrial cancer Cancer of the inner uterine lining.

endometriosis The abnormal occurrence of endometrial tissue outside the uterine cavity.

endometritis An infection of the endometrium.

endoscope A tube that allows viewing and manipulation of internal body areas.

endoscopic retrograde cholangiopancreatography (ERCP) The visual and radiographic examination of the liver, gallbladder, bile ducts, and pancreas by means of an endoscope and the injection of radiopaque dye to identify the cause and location of obstruction.

endoscopic variceal ligation (EVL) The application of small "O" bands around the base of esophageal varices to cut off their blood supply. Also called *banding.*

endoscopy The direct visualization of the gastrointestinal tract by means of a flexible fiberoptic endoscope.

endothelin A secretion produced by the endothelial cells when they are stretched.

endovascular stent graft The repair of an abdominal aortic aneurysm using a stent made of flexible material; the stent is inserted through a skin incision into the femoral artery by way of a catheter-based system.

end-stage kidney disease (ESKD) Acute renal failure combined with chronic renal insufficiency, resulting in the inability of the kidney to excrete waste products normally. The patient may need hemodialysis or a kidney transplant.

energy conservation Strategies to reduce the fatigue associated with chronic and disabling conditions, such as allowing rest periods and setting priorities.

engraftment The successful transplantation of cells in the patient's bone marrow.

enophthalmos Backward displacement of the eyeball into the orbit so that the eye appears sunken.

enteroscopy Visualization of the small intestine.

enterostomal feeding tube A tube used for patients who need long-term enteral feeding; the physician directly accesses the gastrointestinal tract using surgical, endoscopic, or laparoscopic techniques.

entropion The turning inward of the eyelid, causing the eyelashes to rub against the eye.

enucleation The surgical removal of the entire eyeball.

envenomation Venom injection from a snakebite.

epididymitis Inflammation of the epididymis.

epidural hematoma An accumulation of clotted blood resulting from arterial bleeding into the space between the dura and the skull; a neurosurgical emergency.

epidural Term for the space between the dura mater and vertebrae; it consists of fat, connective tissue, and blood vessels.

epiglottis A leaf-shaped, elastic structure that is attached along one edge to the top of the larynx; it closes over the glottis during swallowing to prevent food from entering the trachea and opens during breathing and coughing.

epiglottitis Infection or inflammation of the epiglottis and supraglottic structures that results in swelling. If swelling is great enough, the airway can be obstructed.

epilepsy A chronic disorder characterized by recurrent, unprovoked seizure activity; may be caused by an abnormality in electrical neuronal activity, an imbalance of neurotransmitters, or a combination of both.

epistaxis Nosebleed.

erectile dysfunction (ED) The inability to achieve or maintain a penile erection sufficient for sexual intercourse.

ergonomics An applied science in which the workplace is designed to increase worker comfort (thus reducing injury) while increasing efficiency and productivity.

erosion Ulceration.

eructation The act of belching.

erythema migrans A round or oval flat or slightly raised rash.

erythema Redness of the skin.

erythrocyte A red blood cell (RBC). Red blood cells are the major cells in the blood and are responsible for tissue oxygenation.

erythroplakia A velvety red mucosal lesion, most often occurring in the oral cavity.

erythropoiesis The selective maturation of stem cells into mature erythrocytes.

eschar The crust of dead tissue that forms from coagulated particles of destroyed dermis in a patient with a full-thickness burn injury.

escharotomy Incision made through tight eschar to relieve pressure and allow normal blood flow and breathing.

esophageal stricture Narrowing of the esophageal opening.

esophageal varices The distention of fragile, thin-walled esophageal veins due to increased pressure; the increased pressure is a result of portal hypertension, in which the blood backs up from the liver and enters the esophageal and gastric vessels that carry it into the systemic circulation.

esophagectomy The surgical removal of all or part of the esophagus.

esophagitis Inflammation of the esophagus.

esophagogastroduodenoscopy (EGD) The visual examination of the esophagus, stomach, and duodenum by means of a fiberoptic endoscope.

esophagogastrostomy The surgical creation of a communication between the stomach and the esophagus; it involves the removal of part of the esophagus and proximal stomach.

essential hypertension Elevated blood pressure that is not caused by a specific disease. The major risk factor is a family history of hypertension. Also called *primary hypertension*.

euploid Having the correct number of chromosome pairs for the species.

euploidy The normal diploid number for a cell.

eustachian tube Tube that connects the nasopharynx with the middle ear and opens during swallowing to equalize pressure within the middle ear.

euthyroid Having normal thyroid function.

euvolemia A state of balanced fluid intake and output.

evidence-based practice (EBP) A QSEN competency in which the nurse integrates best current evidence with clinical expertise and patient/family preferences and values for delivery of optimal health care.

evisceration The total separation of all layers of a wound and the protrusion of internal organs through the open wound.

evoked potentials Tests to measure the electrical signals to the brain generated by hearing, touch, or sight. Also called *evoked response*.

exacerbation An increase in severity of a disease. Also called *flare-up*.

excitability The ability of a cell to respond to a stimulus by initiating an impulse. Also called *depolarization*. In cardiac electrophysiology, it is the ability of non-pacemaker myocardial cells to respond to an electrical impulse generated from pacemaker cells and to depolarize.

exemplars Selected health problems and issues that are associated with health and professional nursing concepts.

exercise electrocardiography In cardiovascular assessment, a test that assesses cardiovascular response to an increased workload. Also called *exercise tolerance* or a *stress test*. Exercise electrocardiography helps determine the functional capacity of the heart, screens for coronary artery disease, and identifies dysrhythmias that develop during exercise. It also aids in evaluating the effectiveness of antidysrhythmic drugs.

exercise tolerance See *exercise electrocardiography*.

exertional dyspnea Breathlessness or difficulty breathing that develops during activity or exertion.

exertional heat stroke A form of heat stroke with a sudden onset, typically due to strenuous physical activity in hot, humid conditions. Lack of acclimatization to hot weather and wearing clothing too heavy for the environment are common contributing factors.

exogenous hyperthyroidism Hyperthyroidism caused by excessive use of thyroid replacement hormones.

exogenous Originating outside the body.

exophthalmos Abnormal protrusion of the eyeball (proptosis).

expedited partner therapy (EPT) Therapy used to treat chlamydia in which patients are given a drug or prescription with specific instructions for administration to their partners without direct evaluation by a health care provider. Also called *patient-delivered partner therapy*.

exploratory laparotomy A surgical opening of the abdominal cavity to investigate the cause of an obstruction or peritonitis.

exposure (1) The final component of the primary survey that allows for thorough assessment of the trauma patient; (2) in radiation therapy, the amount of radiation that is delivered to a tissue.

expressed gene When a particular gene has been "turned on."

expressed Turned on or activated.

expressive aphasia A type of aphasia resulting from damage in Broca's area of the frontal lobe of the brain. A motor speech problem in which the patient understands what is said but is unable to communicate verbally and has difficulty writing; rote speech and automatic speech, such as responses to a greeting, are often intact. The patient is aware of the deficit and may become frustrated and angry. Also called *Broca's aphasia* or *motor aphasia*.

expressivity In genetics, the degree of expression a person has when a specific autosomal dominant gene is present. The gene is always expressed, but some people have more severe results.

external fixation A system in which pins or wires are passed through skin and bone and connected to a rigid external frame to immobilize a fracture during healing.

external fixator See *external fixation*.

external hemorrhoid A hemorrhoid that lies below the anal sphincter and can be seen on inspection of the anal region.

external otitis A painful irritation or infection of the skin of the external ear, with resulting allergic response or inflammation. When it occurs in patients who participate in water sports, external otitis is called *swimmer's ear*.

external urethral sphincter The sphincter composed of the skeletal muscle that surrounds the urethra.

extracapsular Located outside the joint capsule.

extracellular fluid (ECF) The portion of total body water (about one third) that is in the space outside the cells. This space also includes interstitial fluid, blood, lymph, bone, and connective tissue water, and the transcellular fluids.

extracranial-intracranial bypass A surgical procedure in which the surgeon performs a craniotomy and bypasses the blocked artery by making a graft (bypass) from the first artery to the second artery to establish blood flow around the blocked artery and re-establish blood flow to the involved areas.

extramedullary tumor A tumor found within the spinal dura but outside the cord.

extrapulmonary Involving nonpulmonary tissues.

extravasation Escape of fluids or drugs into the subcutaneous tissue; a complication of intravenous infusion.

extrinsic factor In hematology, an event (e.g., trauma) that occurs outside the blood to cause platelet plugs to form.

extubation The removal of an endotracheal tube.

F

facial paralysis See *Bell's palsy*.

facilitated diffusion Diffusion across a cell membrane that requires the assistance of a transport system or membrane-altering system. Also called *facilitated transport*.

facilitated transport See *facilitated diffusion*.

failed back surgery syndrome (FBSS) A combination of organic, psychological, and socioeconomic factors in patients for whom back surgery is not successful. Discouraged by repeated surgical procedures, these patients must continue long-term nonsurgical management of pain, including nerve blocks.

failure to rescue The inability of nurses or other interprofessional health team members to save a patient's life in a timely manner when a health care issue or medical complication occurs.

fall An unintentional change in body position that results in the patient's body coming to rest on the floor or ground.

fallophobia In some older adults, the fear of falling and sustaining a serious injury.

far point (of vision) The farthest point at which the eye can see an object.

fascia An inelastic tissue that surrounds groups of muscles, blood vessels, and nerves in the body.

fasciculation Abnormal, involuntary twitching of a muscle.

fasciotomy A surgical procedure in which an incision is made through the skin and subcutaneous tissues into the fascia of the affected compartment to relieve the pressure in and restore circulation to the affected area in the patient with acute compartment syndrome.

fat embolism syndrome (FES) A serious complication, usually resulting from a fracture, in which fat globules are released from the yellow bone marrow into the bloodstream. This syndrome usually occurs within 48 hours of the fracture and can result in respiratory failure or death, often from pulmonary edema.

fatigue (stress) fracture A fracture that results from excessive or repeated strain and stress on a bone.

fatty liver Caused by the accumulation of fats in and around the hepatic cells. It may be caused by alcohol abuse or other factors. Also known as *steatosis*.

fecal microbiota transplantation (FMT) A procedure in which healthy normal flora is placed into the lower GI system of the infected patient who does not respond to antibiotic therapy or has recurrent disease .

fecal occult blood test (FOBT) A diagnostic test that measures the presence of blood in the stool from gastrointestinal bleeding; this is a common finding associated with colorectal cancer.

Felty's syndrome The combination of rheumatoid arthritis, hepatosplenomegaly (enlarged liver and spleen), and leukopenia.

femoral hernia A hernia that protrudes through the femoral ring.

fetor hepaticus The distinctive fruity or musty breath odor of chronic liver disease and portal-systemic encephalopathy.

fibrinolysis The breakdown of a clot.

fibrinolytic Drug that targets the fibrin component of the coronary thrombosis; used to dissolve thrombi in the coronary arteries and restore myocardial blood flow; examples include tissue plasminogen activator, anisoylated plasminogen-streptokinase activator complex, and reteplase.

fibroadenoma A solid, slowly enlarging benign mass of connective tissue that is unattached to the surrounding breast tissue and is typically discovered by the patient herself. The mass is usually round, firm, easily movable, nontender, and clearly delineated from the surrounding tissue.

fibrocystic breast condition (FBC) Physiologic nodularity of the breast that is thought to be caused by an imbalance in the normal estrogen-to-progesterone ratio. It is the most common breast problem of women between 20 and 30 years of age.

fibroids See *leiomyomas*.

fibromyalgia syndrome (FMS) A chronic pain syndrome characterized by pain and tenderness at specific sites in the back of the neck, upper chest, trunk, low back, and extremities along with fatigue, sleep disturbances, and headache.

fibrosis Replacement of normal cells with connective tissue and collagen (scar tissue).

fidelity Ethical principle that refers to the agreement that nurses will keep their obligations or promises to patients to follow through with care.

filter The movement of fluid from the space with higher hydrostatic pressure through the membrane into the space with lower hydrostatic pressure.

filtration The movement of fluid through a cell or blood vessel membrane because of hydrostatic pressure differences on both sides of the membrane.

financial abuse Mismanagement or misuse of the patient's property or resources.

first heart sound (S_1) Sound created by the closure of the mitral and tricuspid valves (atrioventricular valves).

first intention Healing in which the wound can be easily closed and dead space eliminated without granulation, which thus shortens the phases of tissue repair. Inflammation resolves quickly, and connective tissue repair is minimal, resulting in a thin scar.

fistula An abnormal opening between two adjacent organs or structures.

five cardinal manifestations of inflammation Warmth, redness, swelling, pain, and decreased function.

fixed occlusion Wiring the jaws together in the mouth closed position.

flaccid bladder See *areflexic bladder*.

flaccid paralysis Paralysis of a part of the body that is characterized by loss of muscle tone due to hypotonia; may be seen in the patient who has experienced a brain attack.

flail chest Inward movement of the thorax during inspiration, with outward movement during expiration; results from multiple rib fractures caused by blunt chest trauma that leaves a segment of the chest wall loose.

flat bone Bone that protects vital organs and often contains blood-forming cells, such as the scapula.

flatulence The presence of an excessive amount of gas in the stomach or intestines.

fluid and electrolyte balance The regulation of body fluid, fluid osmolality, and electrolytes by processes such as filtration, diffusion, and osmosis.

fluid overload An excess of body fluid. Also called *overhydration*.

folliculitis A superficial bacterial infection involving only the upper portion of the hair follicle.

forensic nurse examiner (RN-FNE) Emergency department specialist who is trained to recognize evidence of abuse and to intervene on the patient's behalf and who obtains patient histories, collects forensic evidence, and offers counseling and follow-up care for victims of rape, child abuse, and domestic violence.

fracture A break or disruption in the continuity of a bone.

fremitus Vibrations felt on the chest or back when the patient talks.

fremitus Vibration.

frequency (1) The highness or lowness of tones (expressed in hertz). The greater the number of vibrations per second, the higher the frequency (pitch) of the sound; the fewer the number of vibrations per second, the lower the pitch; (2) an urge to urinate frequently in small amounts.

fresh frozen plasma (FFP) Plasma that is frozen immediately after donation so that the clotting factors are preserved.

friable Easily crumbled or damaged.

frostbite A cold injury characterized by the degree of tissue freezing and the resultant damage it produces. Frostbite injuries can be superficial, partial, or full thickness.

frostnip A form of superficial frostbite (typically on the face, fingers, or toes) that produces pain, numbness, and pallor but is easily remedied with the application of warmth and does not induce tissue injury.

Fulmer SPICES A framework that identifies six serious "marker conditions" that can lead to longer hospital stays for patients, higher medical costs, and deaths.

fulminant hepatitis A severe acute and often fatal form of hepatitis caused by failure of the liver cells to regenerate, with progression to necrosis.

furuncle A localized inflammation of the skin caused by bacterial infection, usually *Staphylococcus*, of a hair follicle. Also called a *boil*.

G

gallium scan A test that is similar to a bone scan but that uses the radioisotope *gallium citrate* and is more specific and sensitive in detecting bone problems. This substance also migrates to brain, liver, and breast tissue and therefore is used to examine these structures when disease is suspected.

gamma globulin See *immunoglobulin*.

ganglion A round, cystlike lesion, often overlying a wrist joint or tendon.

gas exchange The process of oxygen transport to the cells and carbon dioxide transport away from the cells through ventilation and diffusion.

gastrectomy The surgical removal of part or all of the stomach.

gastric bypass A type of gastric restriction surgery in which gastric resection is combined with malabsorption surgery. The patient's stomach, duodenum, and part of the jejunum are bypassed so that fewer calories can be absorbed. Also known as a *Roux-en-Y gastric bypass*, or *RNYGB*.

gastric lavage Procedure of irrigating the stomach in which a large-bore nasogastric tube is inserted into the stomach and room-temperature solution is instilled in volumes of 200 to 300 mL. The solution and blood are repeatedly withdrawn manually until returns are clear or light pink and without clots.

gastritis An inflammation of the gastric mucosa (stomach lining).

gastroenteritis An increase in the frequency and water content of stools or vomiting as a result of inflammation of the mucous membranes of the stomach and intestinal tract. It affects primarily the small bowel and can be of either viral or bacterial origin.

gastroesophageal reflux (GER) Condition that occurs as a result of backward flow of stomach contents into the esophagus.

gastroesophageal reflux disease (GERD) An upper gastrointestinal disease caused by the backward flow (reflux) of gastrointestinal contents into the esophagus.

gastrojejunostomy Surgical anastomosis of the stomach to the jejunum.

gastroparesis Delay in gastric emptying.

gastrostomy A stoma created from the abdominal wall into the stomach.

gel phenomenon In patients with rheumatoid arthritis, morning stiffness that lasts between 45 minutes and several hours after awakening.

gender dysphoria Discomfort with one's natal sex.

gender identity A person's inner sense of maleness or femaleness not related to reproductive anatomy.

gender reassignment surgery See *sex reassignment surgery*.

gene The deoxyribonucleic acid (DNA) in the form of chromosomes within the nucleus of each cell that contains the instructions for making all the different proteins any organism makes. Every human cell with a nucleus contains the entire set of human genes.

general anesthesia A reversible loss of consciousness induced by inhibiting neuronal impulses in the central nervous system.

generalized seizure One of the three broad categories of seizure disorders along with partial seizures and unclassified seizures. There are six types: tonic-clonic, tonic, clonic, absence, myoclonic, and atonic (akinetic).

genetics The science concerned with the general mechanisms of heredity and the variation of inherited traits.

genital herpes (GH) An acute, recurring incurable viral disease of the genitalia caused by the herpes simplex virus and transmitted through contact with an infected person. An outbreak typically is preceded by a tingling sensation of the skin followed by the appearance of vesicles (blisters) on the penis, scrotum, vulva, perineum, vagina, cervix, or perianal region. The blisters rupture spontaneously, leaving painful erosions. After the lesions heal, the virus remains dormant, periodically reactivating with a recurrence of symptoms.

genome The complete set of human genes. Each human cell with a nucleus contains the entire set of human genes. The human genome contains about 35,000 individual genes.

genomic health care The application of known genetic variation to enhance health care to individuals and their families.

genomics The science focusing on the function of all of the human DNA, including genes and noncoding DNA regions.

genotype The actual alleles for a genetic trait, not just what can be observed.

genu valgum A deformity in which the knees are abnormally close together and the space between the ankles is increased. Also called *knock-knee*.

genu varum A deformity in which the knees are abnormally separated and the lower extremities are bowed inward. Also called *bowleg*.

Geriatric Depression Scale—Short Form (GDS-SF) A valid and reliable screening tool to help determine if an older patient has clinical depression.

geriatric failure to thrive (GFTT) A complex syndrome including under-nutrition, impaired physical functioning, depression, and cognitive impairment.

geriatric syndromes Major health issues that are associated with late adulthood in community and inpatient settings.

ghrelin The "hunger hormone" that is secreted in the stomach; increases in a fasting state and decreases after a meal.

Glasgow Coma Scale (GCS) An objective and widely accepted tool for neurologic assessment and documentation of level of consciousness. It establishes baseline data for eye opening, motor response, and verbal response. The patient is assessed and assigned a numeric score for each of these areas. A score of 15 represents normal neurologic functioning, and a score of 3 represents a deep coma state.

glaucoma A group of ocular diseases resulting in increased intraocular pressure, causing reduced blood flow to the optic nerve and retina and followed by tissue damage.

glomerulus A series of specialized capillary loops that receive blood from the afferent arteriole and then filter water and small particles from the blood to make urine. The remaining blood leaves the glomerulus via the efferent arteriole.

glossectomy The partial or total surgical removal of the tongue.

glossitis A smooth, beefy red tongue.

glottis The opening between the true vocal cords inside the larynx.

glucagon A hormone secreted by the pancreas that increases blood glucose levels. It is a "counterregulatory" hormone that has actions opposite those of insulin. It causes the release of glucose from cell storage sites whenever blood glucose levels are low.

gluconeogenesis The conversion of proteins and amino acids to glucose in the body.

glucosamine A supplement that may decrease inflammation.

glycemic A term referring to blood glucose.

glycogenesis The production of glycogen in the body.

glycogenolysis The breakdown of glycogen into glucose.

glycoprotein (GP) IIb/IIIa inhibitors Drugs that target the platelet component of the thrombus. They are administered intravenously to prevent fibrinogen from attaching to activated platelets at the site of a thrombus and are given to patients with acute coronary syndromes (especially unstable angina and non–Q-wave myocardial infarction). Examples include abciximab, eptifibatide, and tirofiban.

glycosylated hemoglobin (A1C) A standardized test that measures how much glucose permanently attaches to the hemoglobin molecule. A1C levels greater than 6.5% are diagnostic of diabetes mellitus.

"go bag" See *personal readiness supplies*.

goiter Enlargement of the thyroid gland.

gonadotropins Hormones that stimulate the ovaries and testes to produce sex hormones.

gonads The male and female reproductive endocrine glands. Male gonads are the testes, and female gonads are the ovaries.

goniometer An instrument for measuring angles; also refers to a tool used to measure joint range of motion.

good death A death that is free from avoidable distress and suffering for patients, families, and caregivers; in agreement with patients' and families' wishes; and consistent with clinical practice standards.

gout A systemic disease in which urate crystals deposit in the joints and other body tissues, causing inflammation.

grading System of classifying cellular aspects of a cancer tumor.

granulation The formation of scar tissue for wound healing to occur.

granuloma Growth that develops in the lungs of patients with sarcoidosis and contains lymphocytes, macrophages, epithelioid cells, and giant cells; scar tissue.

Graves' disease Toxic diffuse goiter characterized by hyperthyroidism, enlargement of the thyroid gland, abnormal protrusion of the eyes, and dry, waxy swelling of the front surfaces of the lower legs.

gray (gy) Unit of measurement for an absorbed radiation dose.

gray matter In the spinal cord, neuron cell bodies.

grief The emotional feeling related to the perception of loss.

grommet A polyethylene tube that is surgically placed through the tympanic membrane to allow continuous drainage of middle-ear fluids in the patient with otitis media.

ground substance A lubricant composed of protein and sugar groups that surrounds the dermal cells and fibers and contributes to the skin's normal suppleness and turgor.

guardian A person appointed to make health care decisions for a patient who is determined to not be legally competent.

Guillain-Barré syndrome (GBS) An acute autoimmune disorder characterized by varying degrees of motor weakness and paralysis. It may be referred to by a variety of other names, such as *acute idiopathic polyneuritis* and *polyradiculoneuropathy*.

gynecomastia Abnormal enlargement of the breasts in men.

H

H₂-receptor antagonists A group of drugs that inhibit gastric acid secretion by blocking the effects of histamine on parietal cell receptors in the stomach.

half-life Time it takes for the amount of drug in the body to be reduced by 50%.

halitosis A foul odor of the mouth.

hallux valgus A common deformity of the foot that occurs when the great toe deviates laterally at the metatarsophalangeal joint; sometimes referred to as a *bunion*.

halo fixator A static traction device used for immobilization of the cervical spine. Four pins or screws are inserted into the skull, and a metal halo ring is attached to a plastic vest or cast when the spine is stable, allowing increased patient mobility.

"halo" sign A clear or yellowish ring surrounding a spot of blood.

hammertoe The dorsiflexion of any metatarsophalangeal joint with plantar flexion of the adjacent proximal interphalangeal joint. The second toe is most often affected.

hand hygiene Infection control protocol that refers to both handwashing and alcohol-based hand rubs.

hantavirus pulmonary syndrome A severe and potentially lethal respiratory disease that is a complication of hantavirus infection carried by mice and rats.

health care–associated infection (HAI) Infections associated with the provision of health care; for example, microorganisms can enter the body through the genitourinary tract in patients with indwelling urinary catheters.

heart failure A general term for the inadequacy of the heart to pump blood throughout the body, causing insufficient perfusion of body tissues with vital nutrients and oxygen. Also called *pump failure*.

heart rate (HR) Term referring to the number of times the ventricles contract each minute.

heart transplantation A surgical procedure in which a heart from a donor with a comparable body weight and ABO compatibility is transplanted into a recipient less than 6 hours after procurement. It is the treatment of choice for patients with severe dilated cardiomyopathy and may be considered for patients with restrictive cardiomyopathy.

heat exhaustion A syndrome primarily caused by dehydration from heavy perspiration and inadequate fluid and electrolyte consumption during heat exposure over hours to days; if left untreated, can be a precursor to heat stroke.

heat stroke A true medical emergency in which the victim's heat regulatory mechanisms fail and are unable to compensate for a critical elevation in body temperature; if uncorrected, organ dysfunction and death will ensue.

Heberden's nodes Swelling at the distal interphalangeal joints in osteoarthritis that involves the hands.

hematemesis The vomiting of blood.

hematochezia The passage of red blood via the rectum.

hematocrit The percentage of packed red blood cells per deciliter of blood.

hematogenous See *endogenous*.

hematogenous tuberculosis A form of tuberculosis that spreads throughout the body when a large number of organisms enter the blood. Also called *miliary tuberculosis*.

hematopoiesis The production of blood cells, which occurs in the red marrow of bones.

hematuria Blood in the urine.

hemianopsia Blindness in half of the visual field of one or both eyes. Also called *hemianopia*.

hemiarthroplasty Surgical replacement of part of the shoulder joint, typically the humeral component, as an alternative to total shoulder arthroplasty.

hemiparesis Weakness on one side of the body.

hemiplegia Paralysis on one side of the body.

hemoconcentration Elevated plasma levels of hemoglobin, hematocrit, serum osmolarity, glucose, protein, blood urea nitrogen, and electrolytes that occur when only the water is lost and other substances remain.

hemodilution Excessive water in the vascular space.

hemoglobin A (HbA) Normal adult hemoglobin. The molecule has two alpha chains and two beta chains of amino acids.

hemoglobin S (HbS) An abnormal beta chain of hemoglobin associated with sickle cell disease that is sensitive to low oxygen content of red blood cells.

hemolytic anemia Anemia caused by the destruction of red blood cells.

hemolytic The characteristic of destroying red blood cells.

hemoptysis Coughing up blood or blood-stained sputum.

hemorrhoid Unnaturally swollen or distended vein in the anorectal region.

hemorrhoidectomy The excision of a hemorrhoid.

hemostasis The multistep process of controlled blood clotting.

hemothorax Bleeding into the chest cavity.

heparin-induced thrombocytopenia (HIT) The aggregation of platelets into "white clots" that can cause thrombosis, usually in the form of an acute arterial occlusion; occurs with heparin administration. Also called *white clot syndrome*.

hepatic encephalopathy See *portal-systemic encephalopathy*.

hepatitis A Hepatitis that is caused by the hepatitis A virus (HAV) and is characterized by a mild course similar to that of a typical viral syndrome and often goes unrecognized. It is spread via the fecal-oral route by oral ingestion of fecal contaminants. Sources of infection include contaminated water, shellfish caught in contaminated water, and food contaminated by infected food handlers. The virus may also be spread by oral-anal sexual activity. The incubation period is usually 15 to 50 days. The disease is usually not life threatening but may be more severe in people older than 40 years. It can also complicate pre-existing liver disease.

hepatitis B A form of hepatitis that is caused by the hepatitis B virus (HBV), which is shed in the body fluids of infected people and asymptomatic carriers. It is spread through unprotected sexual intercourse with an infected partner, needle sharing, blood transfusions, and other modes. Symptoms usually occur within 25 to 180 days of exposure and include nausea, fever, fatigue, joint pain, and jaundice. Most adults who get hepatitis B recover, clear the virus from their bodies, and develop immunity; however, up to 10% of patients with the disease do not develop immunity and become carriers.

hepatitis C Hepatitis that is caused by the hepatitis C virus (HCV). Transmission is blood to blood, most commonly by needle sharing or needlestick injury with contaminated blood. The rate of sexual transmission is very low; it is not spread by casual contact and is rarely transmitted from mother to fetus. The average incubation period is 7 weeks. Most people are asymptomatic and are not diagnosed until long after the initial exposure when an abnormality is detected during a routine laboratory evaluation or when symptoms of liver impairment appear. Hepatitis C causes chronic inflammation in the liver that eventually causes the hepatocytes to scar and may progress to cirrhosis.

hepatitis carrier Person who has had hepatitis B but has not developed immunity. Hepatitis carriers can infect others even though they are not sick and demonstrate no obvious signs of disease. Chronic carriers are at high risk for cirrhosis and liver cancer.

hepatitis D The hepatitis D virus (HDV) co-infects with hepatitis B virus (HBV) and needs the presence of HBV for viral replication. HDV can co-infect a patient with HBV or can occur as a superinfection in a patient with chronic HBV. Superinfection usually develops into chronic HDV infection. The incubation period is 14 to 56 days. As with HBV, the disease is transmitted primarily by parenteral routes.

hepatitis E Hepatitis E virus (HEV) was originally identified by its association with waterborne epidemics of hepatitis in the Indian subcontinent. Since then, it has occurred in epidemics in Asia, Africa, the Middle East, Mexico, and Central and South America, typically after heavy rains and flooding. In the United States, hepatitis E has been found only in travelers returning from endemic areas. The virus is transmitted via the fecal-oral route, and the clinical course resembles that of hepatitis A. HEV has an incubation period of 15 to 64 days. There is no evidence at this time of a chronic form of hepatitis E.

hepatitis The widespread inflammation of liver cells.

hepatocyte Liver cell.

hepatomegaly Enlargement of the liver.

hepatorenal syndrome (HRS) A state of progressive oliguric renal failure associated with hepatic failure, resulting in functional impairment of kidneys with normal anatomic and morphologic features. It indicates a poor prognosis for the patient with hepatic failure and is often the cause of death in patients with cirrhosis.

hereditary chronic pancreatitis Pancreatitis that may be associated with *SPINK1* and *CFTR* gene mutations.

heritability The risk that a disorder can be transmitted to one's children in a recognizable pattern.

hernia A weakness in the abdominal muscle wall through which a segment of the bowel or other abdominal structure protrudes.

herniated nucleus pulposus (HNP) The protrusion (herniation) of the pulpy material from the center of a vertebral disk; herniated disks occur most often between the fourth and fifth lumbar vertebrae (L4-5) but may occur at other levels. A herniation in the lumbosacral area can press on the adjacent spinal nerve (usually the sciatic nerve), causing severe burning or stabbing pain into the leg or foot, or it may press on the spinal cord itself, causing leg weakness and bowel and bladder dysfunction. The specific area of pain depends on the level of herniation.

hernioplasty Surgical repair of a hernia in which the surgeon reinforces the weakened outside muscle wall with a mesh patch.

herniorrhaphy The surgical repair of a hernia.

heterotopic ossification Abnormal bony overgrowth, often into muscle; seen as a complication of prolonged immobility in patients with spinal cord injury.

hiatal hernia Protrusion of the stomach through the esophageal hiatus of the diaphragm and into the thorax. Also called *diaphragmatic hernia*.

high altitude disease (HAD) See *high altitude illnesses*.

high altitude illnesses Pathophysiologic responses in the body caused by exposure to low partial pressure of oxygen at high elevations.

high altitude pulmonary edema (HAPE) A form of acute mountain sickness often seen with high altitude cerebral edema. Clinical indicators include persistent dry cough, cyanosis of the lips and nail beds, tachycardia and tachypnea at rest, and rales auscultated in one or both lungs. Pink, frothy sputum is a late sign.

high-alert drug A drug that has an increased risk for causing patient harm if given in error.

high-density lipoproteins (HDLs) Part of the total cholesterol value that should be more than 45 mg/dL for men and more than 55 mg/dL for women; "good" cholesterol.

highly sensitive C-reactive protein (hsCRP) A serum marker of inflammation and a common and critical component to the development of atherothrombosis.

high-output heart failure Heart failure that occurs when cardiac output remains normal or above normal. It is usually caused by increased metabolic needs or hyperkinetic conditions such as septicemia (fever), anemia, and hyperthyroidism. This type of heart failure is different from left- and right-sided heart failure, which are typically low-output states, and is not as common as other types.

hilum The area of the kidney in which the renal artery and nerve plexus enter and the renal vein and ureter exit. This area is not covered by the renal capsule.

hirsutism Abnormal growth of body hair, especially on the face, chest, and the linea alba of the abdomen of women.

homeostasis The narrow range of normal conditions (e.g., body temperature, blood electrolyte values, blood pH, blood volume) in the human body; the tendency to maintain a constant balance in normal body states.

homeostatic mechanism A safeguard or control mechanism within the human body that prevents dangerous changes.

homocysteine An essential sulfur-containing amino acid that is produced when dietary protein breaks down; elevated values (greater than 15 mmol/L) may be a risk factor for the development of cardiovascular disease.

homonymous hemianopsia Condition in which there is blindness in the same side of both eyes.

hordeolum An infection of the sweat glands in the eyelid.

hormone Chemical produced in the body that exerts its effects on specific tissues known as *target tissues*.

hospice An interdisciplinary approach to facilitate quality of life and a "good" death for patients near the end of their lives, with care provided in a variety of settings.

Hospital Incident Command System (HICS) An organizational model for disaster management in which roles are formally structured under the hospital or long-term care facility incident commander, with clear lines of authority and accountability for specific resources.

hospital incident commander As defined in a hospital's emergency response plan, the person (either an emergency physician or administrator) who assumes overall leadership for implementing the institutional plan at the onset of a mass casualty incident. The hospital incident commander has a global view of the entire situation, facilitates patient movement through the system, and brings in resources to meet patient needs.

hospitalist Family practitioner or internist employed by a hospital.

human leukocyte antigen (HLA) Antigen that is present on the surfaces of nearly all body cells as a normal part of the person and acts as an antigen only if it enters another person's body.

human papilloma virus (HPV) test A test that can identify many high-risk types of HPV associated with the development of cervical cancer.

humoral immunity A type of immunity provided by antibodies circulating in body fluids.

Huntington disease (HD) A hereditary disorder transmitted as an autosomal dominant trait at the time of conception (formerly called *Huntington chorea*). Men and women between 35 and 50 years of age are affected; clinical onset is gradual. The two main symptoms are progressive mental status changes (leading to dementia) and choreiform movements (rapid, jerky movements) in the limbs, trunk, and facial muscles.

hydrocephalus The abnormal accumulation of cerebrospinal fluid within the skull.

hydronephrosis Abnormal enlargement of the kidney caused by a blockage of urine lower in the tract and filling of the kidney with urine.

hydrophilic Tending to absorb water readily.

hydrophobic Not readily absorbing water; waterproof.

hydrostatic pressure The force of the weight of water molecules pressing against the confining walls of a space.

hydrotherapy The application of water for treatment of injury or disease.

hydroureter Abnormal distention of the ureter.

hyperacusis An intolerance for sound levels that do not bother other people.

hyperaldosteronism Excessive mineralocorticoid production.

hypercalcemia A total serum calcium level above 10.5 mg/dL or 2.75 mmol/L, which can cause fatigue, anorexia, nausea and vomiting, constipation, polyuria, and serious damage to the urinary system.

hypercapnia Increased arterial carbon dioxide levels.

hypercarbia Increased partial pressure of arterial carbon dioxide ($PaCO_2$) levels.

hypercellularity An abnormal number of cells.

hypercoagulability Increased clotting ability.

hyperemia Increased blood flow to an area.

hyperesthesia Abnormally increased sensation.

hyperextension A mechanism of injury that occurs when a part of the body is suddenly accelerated and then decelerated, causing extreme extension.

hyperflexion A mechanism of injury that occurs when a part of the body is suddenly and forcefully accelerated forward, causing extreme flexion.

hyperglycemia Abnormally high levels of blood glucose.

hyperinsulinemia Chronic high blood insulin levels.

hyperkalemia An elevated level of potassium in the blood.

hyperlipidemia An elevation of serum lipid (fat) levels in the blood.

hypermagnesemia A serum magnesium level above 2.1 mEq/L.

hypernatremia An excessive amount of sodium in the blood.

hyperopia An error of refraction that occurs when the eye does not refract light enough, causing images to fall (converge) behind the retina and resulting in poor near vision. Also called *farsightedness.*

hyperosmotic Describes fluids with osmolarities (solute concentrations) greater than 300 mOsm/L; hyperosmotic fluids have a greater osmotic pressure than do isosmotic fluids and tend to pull water from the isosmotic fluid space into the hyperosmotic fluid space until an osmotic balance occurs. Also called *hypertonic.*

hyperpharmacy See *polypharmacy.*

hyperphosphatemia A serum phosphorus level above 4.5 mg/dL.

hyperpituitarism Hormone oversecretion that occurs with pituitary tumors or hyperplasia.

hyperplasia Growth that causes tissue to increase in size by increasing the number of cells; abnormal overgrowth of tissue.

hyperpnea An abnormal increase in the depth of respiratory movements.

hypersensitivity An overreaction to a foreign substance.

hypertension A cardiovascular condition pertaining to people who have a systolic blood pressure of 140 mm Hg or higher or a diastolic blood pressure of 90 mm Hg or higher or who take medication to control blood pressure; approximately 1 of every 5 Americans has hypertension.

hypertensive crisis A severe elevation in blood pressure (greater than 180/120 mm Hg) that can cause damage to organs such as the kidneys or heart.

hyperthermia Elevated body temperature; fever.

hyperthyroidism A condition caused by excessive production of thyroid hormone.

hypertonia A condition of excessive muscle tone, which tends to cause fixed positions or contractures of the involved extremities and restricted range of motion of the joints.

hypertonic See *hyperosmotic.*

hypertriglyceridemia Elevated levels (150 mg/dL or above) of triglyceride in the blood.

hypertrophic cardiomyopathy (HCM) A type of cardiomyopathy that involves disarray of the myocardial fibers and asymmetric ventricular hypertrophy; leads to a stiff left ventricle that results in diastolic filling abnormalities.

hypertrophy The enlargement or overgrowth of an organ; tissue increases in size by the enlargement of each cell.

hyperuricemia An excess of uric acid in the blood.

hyperventilation A state of increased rate and depth of breathing.

hyperviscous The quality of being thicker than normal.

hypervolemia Increased plasma volume; or fluid excess.

hypocalcemia A total serum calcium level below 9.0 mg/dL or 2.25 mmol/L.

hypocapnia Decreased arterial carbon dioxide levels.

hypocarbia $Paco_2$ less than 40 to 45 mm Hg or decreased partial pressure of carbon dioxide in arterial blood.

hypodermoclysis The slow infusion of isotonic fluids into subcutaneous tissue.

hypoesthesia Abnormally decreased sensation.

hypoglycemia Abnormally low levels of glucose in the blood.

hypokalemia A decreased serum potassium level; a common electrolyte imbalance.

hypomagnesemia A low serum magnesium level, usually lower than 1.8 mEq/L or 0.74 mmol/L.

hyponatremia A serum sodium level below 136 mEq/L (mmol/L).

hypo-osmotic Describes fluids with osmolarities of less than 270 mOsm/L. Hypo-osmolar fluids have a lower osmotic pressure than isosmotic fluids, and water tends to be pulled from the hypo-osmotic fluid space into the isosmotic fluid space until an osmotic balance occurs. Also called *hypotonic.*

hypophonia Soft voice.

hypophosphatemia Inadequate levels of phosphate in the blood (below 3.0 mg/dL).

hypophysectomy Surgical removal of the pituitary gland.

hypoproteinemia A decrease in serum proteins.

hypothalamic-hypophysial portal system The small, closed circulatory system that the hypothalamus shares with the anterior pituitary gland; it allows hormones produced in the hypothalamus to travel directly to the anterior pituitary gland.

hypothalamus A structure within the brain; an integral part of autonomic nervous system control (controlling temperature and other functions) that is essential in intellectual function.

hypothermia A core body temperature less than 95° F (35° C).

hypotonia An abnormal condition of inadequate muscle tone, with an inability to maintain balance.

hypotonic See *hypo-osmotic.*

hypoventilation A state in which gas exchange at the alveolar-capillary membrane is inadequate so that too little oxygen reaches the blood and carbon dioxide is retained.

hypovolemia Abnormally decreased volume of circulating fluid in the body; fluid deficit.

hypoxemia (hypoxemic) Decreased blood oxygen levels; hypoxia.

hypoxia A reduction of oxygen supply to the tissues.

hysterosalpingogram An x-ray of the cervix, uterus, and fallopian tubes that is performed after injection of a contrast medium. This test is used in infertility workups to evaluate tubal anatomy and patency and uterine problems such as fibroids, tumors, and fistulas.

hysteroscopy Examination of the interior of the uterus and cervical canal using an endoscope.

I

icterus Yellow discoloration of the sclerae.

idiopathic chronic pancreatitis Pancreatitis that may be associated with *SPINK1* and *CFTR* gene mutations.

idiopathic seizure See *unclassified seizure.*

ileostomy The surgical creation of an opening into the ileum, usually by bringing the end of the terminal ileum through the abdominal wall and forming a stoma, or ostomy.

immediate memory Short-term or new memory. Test by asking the patient to repeat two or three unrelated words to make sure they were heard; after about 5 minutes, while continuing the examination, ask the patient to repeat the words.

immunity Resistance to infection; usually associated with the presence of antibodies or cells that act on specific microorganisms.

immunocompetent Having proper functioning of the body's ability to maintain itself and defend against disease.

immunoglobulin Antibody. Also called *gamma globulin.*

impermeable Not porous.

implanted port A device used for long-term or frequent infusion therapy; consists of a portal body, a dense septum over a reservoir, and a catheter that is surgically implanted on the upper chest or upper extremity.

inactivation The process of binding an antibody to an antigen to cover the antigen's active site and to make the antigen harmless without destroying it. Also called *neutralization.*

incisional hernia Protrusion of the intestine at the site of a previous surgical incision resulting from inadequate healing. Most often caused by postoperative wound infections, inadequate nutrition, and obesity. Also called *ventral hernia.*

incomplete spinal cord injury An injury in which the spinal cord has been damaged in a way that allows some function or movement below the level of the injury.

incontinence Involuntary loss of urine or stool severe enough to cause social or hygienic problems.

independent living skills See *instrumental activities of daily living (IADLs).*

indirect inguinal hernia A sac formed from the peritoneum that contains a portion of the intestine or omentum. The hernia pushes downward at an angle into the inguinal canal. In males, indirect inguinal hernias can become large and often descend into the scrotum.

indolent Slow-growing.

induration Hardening.

infarction Necrosis, or cell death.

infective endocarditis A microbial infection (e.g., viruses, bacteria, fungi) involving the endocardium; previously called *bacterial endocarditis.*

inferior vena cava filtration Surgical procedure in which the surgeon inserts a filter device percutaneously into the inferior vena cava of a patient with recurrent deep vein thrombosis (to prevent pulmonary emboli) or pulmonary emboli that do not respond to medical treatment. The device is meant to trap emboli in the inferior vena cava before they progress to the lungs. Holes in the device allow blood to pass through, thus not significantly interfering with the return of blood to the heart.

inferior wall myocardial infarction A type of myocardial infarction that occurs in patients with obstruction of the right coronary artery, causing significant damage to the right ventricle.

infiltrating ductal carcinoma The most common type of breast cancer; it originates in the mammary ducts and grows in the epithelial cells lining these ducts.

infiltration The leakage of IV solution into the tissues around the vein.

inflammatory breast cancer A rare but highly aggressive form of invasive breast cancer. Symptoms include swelling, skin redness, and pain in the breasts.

inflammatory cytokines Proteins produced primarily by white blood cells that assist in the inflammatory and immune responses of the body (e.g., tumor necrosis factor, interleukins).

inflow disease Chronic peripheral arterial disease with obstruction at or above the common iliac artery, abdominal aorta, or profunda femoris artery. The patient experiences discomfort in the lower back, buttocks, or thighs after walking a certain distance. The pain usually subsides with rest.

informatics A QSEN competency in which the nurse uses information and technology to communicate, manage knowledge, mitigate error, and support decision making.

infratentorial Located below the tentorium of the cerebellum.

infusate A solution that is infused into the body.

infusion therapy The delivery of parenteral medications and fluids through a variety of catheter types and locations using multiple techniques and procedures, such as intravenous and intra-arterial therapy to deliver solutions into the vascular system.

inpatient rehabilitation facilities (IRFs) Free-standing rehabilitation hospitals, rehabilitation or skilled units within hospitals (e.g., transitional care units), and skilled nursing facilities to which the patient is typically admitted for 1 to 3 weeks or longer.

inpatient A patient who is admitted to a hospital.

insensible water loss Water loss from the skin, lungs, and stool that cannot be controlled.

instrumental activities of daily living (IADLs) Special activities performed in the course of a day such as using the telephone, shopping, preparing food, and housekeeping. Also called *independent living skills.*

insufflation The practice of injecting gas or air into a cavity before surgery to separate organs and improve visualization.

intensity A quality of sound that is expressed in decibels; generally, having a high degree of energy or activity.

intensivist A physician who specializes in critical care.

intention tremor A tremor that occurs when performing an activity.

interbody cage fusion Cagelike spinal device that is implanted into the space where a disk was removed. Bone graft tissue grows into and around the cage and creates a stable spine at that level.

intercostally Located between the ribs.

intermittent claudication A characteristic leg pain experienced by patients with chronic peripheral arterial disease. Typically, patients can walk only a certain distance before a cramping muscle pain forces them to stop. As the disease progresses, the patient can walk only shorter and shorter distances before pain recurs. Ultimately, pain may occur even at rest.

internal derangement A broad term for disturbances of an injured knee joint.

internal fixation The use of metal pins, screws, rods, plates, or prostheses to immobilize a fracture during healing. The surgeon makes an incision (open reduction) to gain access to the broken bone and implants one or more devices.

internal hemorrhoid A hemorrhoid that is located above the anal sphincter and cannot be seen on inspection of the perineal area.

internal urethral sphincter The smooth detrusor muscle that lines the interior of the bladder neck.

interstitial cystitis A bladder inflammation of unknown etiology that occurs predominantly in women and is characterized by urinary frequency and pain on bladder filling.

interstitial fluid A portion of the extracellular fluid that is between cells, sometimes called the *third space.*

interstitial laser coagulation (ILC) Procedure for treating benign prostatic hyperplasia that uses laser energy to coagulate excess tissue. Also called *contact laser prostatectomy (CLP).*

intra-abdominal hypertension (IAH) Condition of sustained or repeated intra-abdominal pressure of 12 mm Hg or higher.

intra-abdominal pressure Pressure contained within the abdominal cavity.

intra-aortic balloon pump (IABP) An intra-aortic counterpulsation device. It may be used as an invasive intervention to improve myocardial perfusion during an acute myocardial infarction, to reduce preload and afterload, and to facilitate left ventricular ejection. It is also used when patients do not respond to drug therapy with improved tissue perfusion, decreased workload of the heart, and increased cardiac contractility.

intra-arterial infusion therapy The use of catheters placed into arteries to obtain repeated arterial blood samples, to monitor various hemodynamic pressures continuously, and to infuse chemotherapy agents or fibrinolytics.

intracapsular Located within the joint capsule.

intracellular fluid (ICF) The portion of total body water (about two thirds) that is found inside the cells.

intracerebral hemorrhage Bleeding within the brain tissue caused by the tearing of small arteries and veins in the subcortical white matter.

intracorporeal Situated or occurring inside the body.

intramedullary tumor Tumor originating within the spinal cord in the central gray matter and anterior commissure. It is often malignant.

intraocular pressure (IOP) Pressure of the fluid within the eye; may be measured by methods that involve direct contact with the eye or by noncontact techniques.

intraoperative During surgery.

intraosseous (IO) therapy Infusion therapy that is delivered to the vascular network in the long bones.

intraperitoneal (IP) infusion therapy The administration of antineoplastic agents into the peritoneal cavity.

intrapulmonary Within the respiratory tract.

intrarenal/intrinsic renal failure Decreased renal function resulting from damage to the glomeruli, interstitial tissue, or tubules. It can contribute to acute renal failure.

intrathecal Referring to the spine.

intravascular ultrasonography (IVUS) In cardiac catheterization, the use of a flexible catheter with a miniature transducer that emits sound waves. Sound waves are reflected off the plaque and the arterial wall, creating an image of the blood vessel; used as an alternative to injecting a contrast medium into the coronary arteries.

intravenous (systemic) fibrinolytic therapy The intravenous administration of thrombolytic agents to dissolve a thrombus.

intravesical Situated inside the bladder.

intrinsic factor A substance normally secreted by the gastric mucosa and needed for intestinal absorption of vitamin B_{12}. A deficiency of intrinsic factor and the resulting failure to absorb vitamin B_{12} lead to pernicious anemia.

intussusception The telescoping of a segment of the intestine within itself.

invasive hemodynamic monitoring System used in critical care areas to provide quantitative information about vascular capacity, blood volume, pump effectiveness, and tissue perfusion. It directly measures pressures in the heart and great vessels.

ion A substance found in body fluids that carries an electrical charge. Also called *electrolyte.*

iontophoresis A treatment for lower back pain in which a small electrical current and dexamethasone are typically used.

ipsilateral Occurring on the same side.

iris The colored portion of the external eye; its center opening is the pupil. Muscles of the iris contract and relax to control pupil size and the amount of light entering the eye.

irreducible hernia A hernia that cannot be reduced or placed back into the abdominal cavity; requires immediate surgical evaluation.

irregular bone Bone that has a unique shape, such as the carpal bones of the wrist.

irritability An overresponse to stimuli.

irritable bowel syndrome (IBS) A chronic gastrointestinal disorder characterized by chronic or recurrent diarrhea, constipation, and/or abdominal pain and bloating. Also called *spastic colon, mucous colon,* or *nervous colon.*

ischemia Blockage of blood flow through a blood vessel resulting in a lack of oxygen. Prolonged severe ischemia can cause irreversible damage to tissue.

ischemic stroke A type of brain attack caused by occlusion of a cerebral artery by either a thrombus or an embolus. About 80% of all brain attacks are ischemic.

ischemic Cell dysfunction or death from a lack of oxygen resulting from decreased blood flow in a body part.

isoelectric Having equal electric potentials, such as in the heart.

isosmotic Having the same osmotic pressures. Also called *isotonic* or *normotonic*.

isotonic See *isosmotic*.

J

jaundice A syndrome characterized by excessive circulating bilirubin levels. Liver cells cannot effectively excrete bilirubin, and skin and mucous membranes become characterized by a yellow coloration.

jejunostomy The surgical creation of an opening between the jejunum and the surface of the abdominal wall.

joint The place at which two or more bones come together. Also referred to as "articulation" of the joint. The primary function is to provide movement and flexibility in the body.

jugular venous distention (JVD) Enlargement of the jugular vein of the neck; caused by an increase in jugular venous pressure.

juxtaglomerular complex Specialized cells that produce and store renin in the afferent arteriole, efferent arteriole, and distal collecting tubule; taken together, the juxtaglomerular cells and the macula densa.

K

karyotype Technique used to make an organized arrangement of all the chromosomes within one cell during the metaphase section of mitosis.

keratin The protein produced by keratinocytes; makes the outermost skin layer waterproof.

keratinocytes Basal skin cells attached to the basement membrane of the epidermis that undergo cell division and differentiation to continuously renew skin tissue integrity and maintain optimal barrier function. As basal cells divide, keratinocytes are pushed upward and flattened to form the stratified layers of the epithelium (Malpighian layers).

keratoconjunctivitis sicca A condition of the eyes that results from changes in tear composition, lacrimal gland malfunction, or altered tear distribution. Also called *dry eye syndrome*.

keratoconus The degeneration of the corneal tissue resulting in abnormal corneal shape.

keratoplasty Corneal transplant. The surgical removal of diseased corneal tissue and replacement with tissue from a human donor cornea.

ketogenesis The conversion of fats to acids in the body.

ketone bodies Substances, including acetone, that are produced as by-products of the incomplete metabolism of fatty acids. When insulin is not available (as in uncontrolled diabetes mellitus), they accumulate in the blood and cause metabolic acidosis. Also called *ketones*.

knee height caliper Device that uses the distance between the patella and heel to estimate height.

Kupffer cells Phagocytic cells that are part of the body's reticuloendothelial system and that are involved in the protective function of the liver. Kupffer cells engulf harmful bacteria and anemic red blood cells.

Kussmaul respiration A type of breathing that occurs when excess acids caused by the absence of insulin increase hydrogen ion and carbon dioxide levels in the blood. This state triggers an increase in the rate and depth of respiration in an attempt to excrete more carbon dioxide and acid.

kwashiorkor Lack of protein quantity and quality in the presence of adequate calories. Body weight is somewhat normal, and serum proteins are low.

kyphoplasty A minimally invasive surgery for managing vertebral fractures in patients with osteoporosis. Bone cement is injected into the fracture site to provide pain relief, and an inflated balloon is used to restore height to the vertebra.

L

labyrinthectomy Surgical removal of the labyrinth; used as a radical treatment of Ménière's disease when medical therapy is ineffective and the patient already has significant hearing loss.

labyrinthitis An infection of the labyrinth of the ear; may occur as a complication of acute or chronic otitis media.

laceration A type of wound characterized by tearing or mangling and usually caused by sharp objects and projectiles.

lacrimal gland A small gland that produces tears; located in the upper outer part of each ocular orbit.

lacto-ovo-vegetarian A vegetarian diet pattern in which milk, cheese, eggs, and dairy foods are eaten but meat, fish, and poultry are avoided.

lactose intolerance The inability to convert lactose (found in milk and dairy products) to glucose and galactose in the body.

lacto-vegetarian A vegetarian diet pattern in which milk, cheese, and dairy foods are eaten but meat, fish, poultry, and eggs are avoided.

laparoscopy A minimally invasive procedure in which the surgeon makes several small incisions near the umbilicus through which a small endoscope is placed to examine the abdomen; direct examination of the pelvic cavity through an endoscope.

laparotomy An open surgical approach in which a large abdominal incision is made.

laryngectomee A person who has had a laryngectomy.

laryngopharynx The area behind the larynx that extends from the base of the tongue to the esophagus. It is the critical dividing point at which solid foods and fluids are separated from air.

larynx The "voice box"; it is composed of several cartilages and is located above the trachea and just below the throat at the base of the tongue; part of the upper respiratory tract.

laser An acronym for light amplification by stimulated emission of radiation. As a surgical tool, a laser emits a high-powered beam of light that cuts tissue more cleanly than do scalpel blades. A laser creates intense heat, rapidly clots blood vessels or tissue, and turns target tissue (e.g., a tumor) into vapor.

latency period The time between the initiation of a cell and the development of an overt tumor.

latex allergy Reactions to exposure to latex in gloves and other medical products; reactions include rashes, nasal or eye symptoms, and asthma.

latrodectism A syndrome caused by the venom of a black widow spider bite in which neurotransmitter releases from nerve terminals to cause severe abdominal pain, muscle rigidity and spasm, hypertension, and nausea and vomiting.

lead axis In electrocardiography, the imaginary line that joins the positive and negative poles of the lead systems.

lead In an ECG, the provider of one view of the heart's electrical activity.

left shift An increase in the band cells (immature neutrophils) in the white blood cell differential count; an early indication of infection.

left-sided heart (ventricular) failure Inadequacy of the left ventricle of the heart to pump adequately; results in decreased tissue perfusion from poor cardiac output and pulmonary congestion from increased pressure in the pulmonary vessels; typical causes include hypertensive, coronary artery, or valvular disease involving the mitral or aortic valve. Most heart failure begins with failure of the left ventricle and progresses to failure of both ventricles.

legally competent A legal term used to describe a person 18 years of age or older, a pregnant or a married minor, a legally emancipated (free) minor who is self-supporting, or a person not declared incompetent by a court of law.

leiomyomas Benign, slow-growing solid tumors of the uterine myometrium (muscle layer). These are the most commonly occurring pelvic tumors. Also called *myomas* and *fibroids*.

lens The circular, convex structure of the eye that lies behind the iris and in front of the vitreous body. Normally transparent, the lens bends the rays of light entering through the pupil so that they focus on the retina. The curve of the lens changes to focus on near or distant objects.

leptin A hormone that is released by fat cells and possibly by gastric cells; it also acts on the hypothalamus to control appetite.

lethargic Drowsy but easily awakened.

leukemia A type of cancer with uncontrolled production of immature white blood cells in the bone marrow; the bone marrow becomes overcrowded with immature, nonfunctional cells, and the production of normal blood cells is greatly decreased.

leukocyte White blood cell (WBC); this immune system cell protects the body from the effects of invasion by organisms.

leukopenia A reduction in the number of white blood cells.

leukoplakia White, patchy lesions on a mucous membrane.

level of consciousness (LOC) The degree of alertness or the amount of stimulation needed to engage a patient's attention and can range from *alert* to *coma*.

levels of evidence Term used to refer to the status, rank, or strength of evidence.

LGBTQ Acronym for "lesbian, gay, bisexual, transgender, and queer/questioning" culture.

libido Sexual desire.

lichenified An abnormal thickening of the skin to a leathery appearance; can occur in patients with chronic dermatitis because of their continual rubbing of the area to relieve itching.

Lichtenberg figures Branching or ferning marks that appear on the skin as a result of a lightning strike. Also called *keraunographic markings* or *erythematous arborization*.

life review A structured process of reflecting on one's life that is often facilitated by an interviewer.

ligament Connective tissue that attaches bones to other bones at joints.

light reflex The reflection of the otoscope's light off the eardrum in the form of a clearly demarcated triangle of light in the normal ear.

limited cutaneous systemic sclerosis Thick skin that is usually limited to sites distal to the elbow and knee but also involves the face and neck.

lipid Fat, including cholesterol and triglycerides, that can be measured in the blood.

lipolysis The decomposition or splitting up of fat to provide fuel for energy when liver glucose is unavailable.

liposuction A cosmetic procedure to reduce the amount of adipose tissue in selected areas of the body.

literacy challenged An individual who has a low reading level ability.

lithotripsy The use of sound, laser, or dry shock wave energy to break a kidney stone into small fragments. Also called *extracorporeal shock wave lithotripsy*.

living will A legal document that instructs physicians and family members about what life-sustaining treatment is wanted (or not wanted) if the patient becomes unable to make decisions.

lobectomy Surgical removal of an entire lung lobe.

lobular carcinoma in situ (LCIS) A noninvasive form of breast cancer that does not show up as a calcified cluster on a mammogram and is therefore most often diagnosed incidentally during a biopsy for another problem.

local anesthesia Anesthesia that is delivered by applying it to the skin or mucous membranes of the area to be anesthetized or by injecting it directly into the tissue around an incision, wound, or lesion.

locus The specific chromosome location for a gene.

log rolling Turning technique in which the patient turns all at once while his or her back is kept as straight as possible.

long bone Bone that is cylindric with rounded ends and often bears weight, such as the femur.

loop electrosurgical excision procedure (LEEP) Diagnostic procedure/treatment in which a thin loop-wire electrode that transmits a painless electrical current is used to cut away affected cervical cancer tissue.

lordosis The anterior concavity in the curvature of the lumbar and cervical spine when viewed from the side; a common finding in pregnancy and abdominal obesity.

Lou Gehrig's disease See *amyotrophic lateral sclerosis (ALS)*.

low back pain (LBP) Pain in the lumbosacral region of the back caused by muscle strain or spasm, ligament sprain, disk degeneration, or herniation of the nucleus pulposus from the center of the disk. Herniated disks occur most often between the fourth and fifth lumbar vertebrae (L4-5) but may occur at other levels.

low-density lipoproteins (LDLs) Part of the total cholesterol value that should be less than 130 mg/dL; "bad" cholesterol.

lower esophageal sphincter (LES) The portion of the esophagus proximal to the gastroesophageal junction; when at rest, the sphincter is closed to prevent reflux of gastric contents into the esophagus.

lower urinary tract symptoms (LUTS) Symptoms that occur as a result from prostatic hyperplasia, such as urinary retention and overflow incontinence, or urinary leaking.

low-intensity pulsed ultrasound A method using ultrasonic waves to promote bone union in slow-healing fractures or for new fractures as an alternative to surgery.

low-profile gastrostomy device (LPGD) A gastrostomy device that uses a firm or balloon-style internal bumper or retention disk; an antireflux valve keeps gastric contents from leaking onto the skin.

loxoscelism Systemic effects from the injected toxin of a spider bite.

lumbar puncture (spinal tap) The insertion of a spinal needle into the subarachnoid space between the third and fourth (sometimes the fourth and fifth) lumbar vertebrae to withdraw spinal fluid for analysis.

lumen The inside cavity of a tube or tubular organ, such as a blood vessel or airway.

lung compliance The quality of elasticity of the lungs.

lunula The white crescent-shaped portion of the nail at the lower end of the nail plate.

lurch An abnormality in the swing phase of gait; occurs when the muscles in the buttocks or legs are too weak to allow the person to change weight from one foot to the other.

Lyme disease A systemic infectious disease that is caused by the spirochete *Borrelia burgdorferi* and results from the bite of an infected deer tick. Signs and symptoms include a large "bull's-eye" circular rash, malaise, fever, headache, and muscle or joint aches.

lymphadenopathy Persistently enlarged lymph nodes.

lymphedema Abnormal accumulation of protein fluid in the subcutaneous tissue of the affected limb after a mastectomy.

lymphoblastic Pertaining to abnormal leukemic cells that come from the lymphoid pathways and develop into lymphocytes.

lymphocytic Pertaining to abnormal leukemic cells that come from the lymphoid pathways.

lymphokine Cytokine produced by T-cells.

lysis Breakage, for example, of a cell membrane.

M

macrocytic anemia A form of vitamin B_{12} deficiency anemia characterized by abnormally large precursor cells.

macrovascular Referring to large blood vessels.

macular degeneration The deterioration of the macula, the area of central vision.

macular Referring to a macula, a discolored spot on the skin that is not raised above the surface.

magnesium (Mg^{2+}) A mineral that forms a cation when dissolved in water.

magnetoencephalography (MEG) A noninvasive imaging technique that measures the magnetic fields produced by electrical activity in the brain via extremely sensitive devices such as superconducting quantum interference devices (SQUIDs).

malabsorption A syndrome associated with a variety of disorders and intestinal surgical procedures and characterized by impaired intestinal absorption of nutrients.

malignant cell growth Altered cell growth that is serious and, without intervention, leads to death; cancer.

malignant hypertension A severe type of elevated blood pressure that rapidly progresses, with systolic blood pressure greater than 200 mm Hg and diastolic blood pressure greater than 150 mm Hg (greater than 130 mm Hg when there are pre-existing complications).

malignant transformation The process of changing a normal cell into a cancer cell.

malignant Referring to cancer.

mammography An x-ray of the soft tissue of the breast.

mandibulectomy Surgical removal of the jaw.

marasmic-kwashiorkor A combined protein and energy malnutrition that often presents clinically when metabolic stress is imposed on a chronically starved patient.

marasmus A calorie malnutrition in which body fat and protein are wasted but serum proteins are often preserved.

marsupialization Surgical formation of a pouch that is a new duct opening.

mass casualty event A situation affecting the public health that is defined based on the resource availability of a particular community or hospital facility. When the number of casualties exceeds the resource capabilities, a disaster situation is recognized to exist.

mastication The process of chewing.

mastoiditis An acute or chronic infection of the mastoid air cells caused by untreated or inadequately treated otitis media.

maze procedure An open chest surgical technique often performed with coronary artery bypass grafting for patients in atrial fibrillation with decompensation.

mean arterial pressure (MAP) The arterial blood pressure (between 60 and 70 mm Hg) necessary to maintain perfusion of major body organs, such as the kidneys and brain.

mechanical débridement Method of débriding a wound by mechanical entrapment and detachment of dead tissue.

mechanical obstruction The physical obstruction of the bowel by disorders outside the intestine (e.g., adhesions or hernias) or by blockages in the lumen of the intestine (e.g., tumors, inflammation, strictures, or fecal impactions).

mechanism of injury (MOI) The method by which a traumatic event occurred.

mediastinal shift A shift of central thoracic structures toward one side; seen on chest x-ray.

mediastinitis Infection of the mediastinum.

medical command physician As defined in a hospital's emergency response plan, the person responsible for determining the number, acuity, and medical resource needs of victims arriving from the incident scene and for organizing the emergency health care team response to injured or ill patients.

medical harm Physician incidents and all errors caused by members of the health care team or system that lead to patient injury or death.

medical nutrition supplements (MNSs) Enteral products taken by patients who cannot consume enough nutrients in their usual diet (e.g., Ensure, Boost).

medication overuse headache See *rebound headache*.

medication reconciliation A formal evaluative process in which the patient's actual current medications are compared with his or her prescribed medications at time of admission, transfer, or discharge to identify and resolve discrepancies.

medulla A general term for the most interior portion of an organ or structure.

melena Blood in the stool, with the appearance of black tarry stools.

memory cell A type of B-lymphocyte that remains sensitized but does not start to produce antibodies until the next exposure to the same antigen.

Ménière's disease Tinnitus, one-sided sensorineural hearing loss, and vertigo that is related to overproduction or decreased reabsorption of endolymphatic fluid and causes a distortion of the entire inner canal system.

meninges The immediate protective covering of the brain and the spinal cord.

meningioma A type of benign brain tumor that arises from the coverings of the brain (the meninges) and causes compression and displacement of adjacent brain tissue.

meningitis Inflammation, usually bacterial or viral, of the arachnoid and pia mater of the brain and spinal cord and the cerebrospinal fluid. May be caused by bacteria or viruses; symptoms are the same regardless of the causative organism.

meniscectomy Surgical excision of a meniscus, as in a knee joint.

menses The monthly flow of blood from the genital tract of women.

metabolic syndrome A collection of related health problems with insulin resistance as a main feature. Other features include obesity, low levels of physical activity, hypertension, high blood levels of cholesterol, and elevated triglyceride levels. Metabolic syndrome increases the risk for coronary heart disease. Also called *syndrome X*.

metastasis The growth and spread of cancer.

metastasize To spread cancer from the main tumor site to many other body sites.

metastatic Referring to disease, such as cancer, that transfers from one organ to another organ or part not directly connected; pertains to additional tumors that form after cancer cells move from the primary location by breaking off from the original group and establishing remote colonies.

methemoglobinemia The conversion of normal hemoglobin to methemoglobin.

microalbuminuria The presence of very small amounts of albumin in the urine that are not measurable by a urine dipstick or usual urinalysis procedures. Specialized assays are used to analyze a freshly voided urine specimen for microscopic levels of albumin.

microbiome The genomes of all the microorganisms that coexist in and on an adult and can affect cellular regulation.

microcytic Abnormally small in size, such as an abnormally small red blood cell.

microvascular decompression A surgical procedure to relieve the pain of trigeminal neuralgia by relocating a small artery that compresses the trigeminal nerve as it enters the pons. The surgeon carefully lifts the loop of the artery off the nerve and places a small silicone sponge between the vessel and the nerve.

microvascular Referring to small blood vessels.

midline catheter A type of catheter that is 6 to 8 inches long and inserted through the veins of the antecubital fossa; used in therapies lasting from 1 to 4 weeks.

migraine headache An episodic familial disorder manifested by a unilateral, frontotemporal, throbbing pain that is often worse behind one eye or ear. It is often accompanied by a sensitive scalp, anorexia, photophobia, and nausea with or without vomiting. Three categories of migraine headache are migraines with aura, migraines without aura, and atypical migraines.

migratory arthritis In the early stage of rheumatoid arthritis, symptoms that are migrating or involve more joints.

miliary tuberculosis See *hematogenous tuberculosis*.

minimally invasive direct coronary artery bypass (MIDCAB) Surgical procedure that does not require cardiopulmonary bypass and may be used for patients with a lesion of the left anterior descending artery. Also known as "keyhole" surgery.

minimally invasive esophagectomy (MIE) A laparoscopic surgical procedure to remove part of the esophagus; may be performed in patients with early-stage cancer.

minimally invasive inguinal hernia repair (MIIHR) Surgical repair of an inguinal hernia through a laparoscope, which is the treatment of choice.

minimally invasive surgery (MIS) A general term for any surgery performed using laparoscopic technique.

Minimum Data Set (MDS) 3.0 Interdisciplinary tool required by the U.S. Centers for Medicare and Medicaid Services (CMS) to assess patients (residents) in nursing homes.

miosis Constriction of the pupil of the eye.

mitosis Cell division.

mitotic index The percentage of actively dividing cells within a tumor.

mitral regurgitation Inability of the mitral valve to close completely during systole, which allows the backflow of blood into the left atrium when the left ventricle contracts; usually due to fibrosis and calcification caused by rheumatic disease. Also called *mitral insufficiency*.

mitral stenosis Thickening of the mitral valve due to fibrosis and calcification and usually caused by rheumatic fever. The valve leaflets fuse and become stiff, the chordae tendineae contract, and the valve opening narrows, preventing normal blood flow from the left atrium to the left ventricle. As a result, left atrial pressure rises, the left atrium dilates, pulmonary artery pressures increase, and the right ventricle hypertrophies.

mitral valve prolapse (MVP) Dysfunction of the mitral valve that occurs because the valvular leaflets enlarge and prolapse into the left atrium during systole; usually benign but may progress to pronounced mitral regurgitation.

mixed conductive-sensorineural hearing loss A profound hearing loss that results from a combination of both conductive and sensorineural types of hearing loss.

mobility The ability of an individual to perform purposeful physical movement of the body.

modifiable risk factor A factor in disease development that can be altered or controlled by the patient. Examples include elevated serum cholesterol levels, cigarette smoking, hypertension, impaired glucose tolerance, obesity, physical inactivity, and stress.

monokine Cytokine made by macrophages, neutrophils, eosinophils, and monocytes.

morbid obesity A weight that has a severely negative effect on health; usually more than 100% above ideal body weight or a body mass index greater than 40.

morbidity An illness or an abnormal condition or quality.

mortality Death.

Morton's neuroma Plantar digital neuritis, a condition in which a small tumor grows in a digital nerve of the foot. The patient usually describes the pain as an acute, burning sensation in the web space that involves the entire surface of the third and fourth toes.

motor aphasia See *expressive aphasia*.

motor cortex Area in the frontal lobe of the brain that controls voluntary movement.

motor end plate The junction of a peripheral motor nerve and the muscle cells that it supplies.

motor Facilitating movement.

mourning The outward social expression of loss.

MR elastography A noninvasive diagnostic procedure that provides information about tissue stiffness by assessing qualities of shear waves generated into the tissue.

mucositis Open sores on mucous membranes.

multi-casualty event A disaster event in which a limited number of victims or casualties are involved and can be managed by a hospital using local resources.

multigated blood pool scanning In nuclear cardiology, cardiac blood pool imaging is a noninvasive test to evaluate cardiac motion and calculate ejection fraction by using a computer to synchronize the patient's electrocardiogram with pictures obtained by a gamma-scintillation camera. In multigated blood pool scanning, the computer breaks the time between R waves into fractions of a second, called "gates." The camera records blood flow through the heart during each gate. By analyzing information from multiple gates, the computer can evaluate ventricular wall motion and calculate ejection fraction (percentage of the left ventricular volume that is ejected with each contraction) and ejection velocity.

multiple organ dysfunction syndrome (MODS) The sequence of inadequate blood flow to body tissues, which deprives cells of oxygen and leads to anaerobic metabolism with acidosis, hyperkalemia, and tissue ischemia; this is followed by dramatic changes in vital organs and leads to the release of toxic metabolites and destructive enzymes.

multiple sclerosis (MS) A chronic autoimmune disease that affects the myelin sheath and conduction pathway of the central nervous system. It is one of the leading causes of neurologic disability in persons 20 to 40 years of age.

murmur Abnormal heart sound that reflects turbulent blood flow through normal or abnormal valves; murmurs are classified according to their timing in the cardiac cycle (systolic or diastolic) and their intensity depending on their level of loudness.

muscle biopsy The extraction of a muscle specimen for the diagnosis of atrophy (as in muscular dystrophy) and inflammation (as in polymyositis).

muscular dystrophy (MD) A group of degenerative myopathies characterized by weakness and atrophy of muscle without nervous system involvement. At least nine types have been clinically identified and can be broadly categorized as slowly progressive or rapidly progressive.

mutation A change in deoxyribonucleic acid (DNA) that is passed from one generation to another.

myalgia Muscle aches/muscle pain.

myasthenia gravis (MG) A chronic autoimmune disease of the neuromuscular junction. It is characterized by remissions and exacerbations, with fatigue and weakness primarily in the muscles innervated by the cranial nerves and in the skeletal and respiratory muscles. It ranges from mild disturbances of the ocular muscles to a rapidly developing, generalized weakness that may lead to death from respiratory failure.

myasthenic crisis Undermedication with cholinesterase inhibitors.

mydriasis Dilation of the pupil of the eye.

myelin sheath A white, lipid covering of the axon.

myelocytic Pertaining to leukemias in which the abnormal cells come from the myeloid pathways.

myelogenous Pertaining to leukemias in which the abnormal cells come from the myeloid pathways.

myelography Radiography of the spine after injection of contrast medium into the subarachnoid space of the spine; used to visualize the vertebral column, intervertebral disks, spinal nerve roots, and blood vessels.

myocardial hypertrophy Enlargement of the myocardium.

myocardial infarction (MI) Injury and necrosis of myocardial tissue that occurs when the tissue is abruptly and severely deprived of oxygen; usually caused by atherosclerosis of a coronary artery, rupture of the plaque, subsequent thrombosis, and occlusion of blood flow.

myocardial nuclear perfusion imaging (MNPI) The use of radionuclide techniques in which radioactive tracer substances are used to view, record, and evaluate cardiovascular abnormalities; useful for detecting myocardial infarction

and decreased myocardial blood flow and for evaluating left ventricular ejection.

myocardium The heart muscle.

myoglobin A low–molecular-weight heme protein found in cardiac and skeletal muscle; an early marker of myocardial infarction.

myoglobinuria The release of muscle myoglobulin into the urine.

myomas See *leiomyomas.*

myomectomy The surgical removal of leiomyomas with preservation of the uterus.

myopathy A problem in muscle tissue.

myopia An error of refraction that occurs when the eye over-refracts or over-bends the light and focuses images in front of the retina; this results in normal near vision but poor distance vision. Also called *nearsightedness.*

myositis Inflammation of a muscle.

myosplint Electrical stimulation of tension splints in the heart to help the ventricle change to a more normal shape in the patient with heart failure; under investigation in Europe and the United States.

myringoplasty Surgical reconstruction of the eardrum.

myringotomy The surgical creation of a hole in the eardrum; performed to drain middle-ear fluids and relieve pain in the patient with otitis media (middle-ear infection).

myxedema coma A rare, serious complication of untreated or poorly treated hypothyroidism in which decreased metabolism causes the heart muscle to become flabby and the chamber size to increase, resulting in decreased cardiac output and decreased perfusion to the brain and other vital organs.

myxedema Dry, waxy swelling of the skin that is accompanied by nonpitting edema (especially around the eyes, in the hands and feet, and between the shoulder blades) and is associated with primary hypothyroidism.

N

nadir In cancer treatment therapy, the period of greatest bone marrow suppression, when the patient's platelet count may be very low.

nasoduodenal tube (NDT) A tube that is inserted through a nostril and into the small intestine.

nasoenteric tube (NET) Any feeding tube that is inserted nasally and then advanced into the gastrointestinal tract.

nasogastric (NG) tube A tube that is inserted through a nostril and into the stomach for liquid feeding or for withdrawing gastric contents.

nasotracheal The route for inserting a tube into the trachea via the nose.

natal sex A person's genital anatomy present at birth. Also known as *biological sex.*

National Patient Safety Goals (NPSGs) Goals published by The Joint Commission that require health care organizations to focus on specific priority safety practices.

natural chemical débridement Method of débriding a wound by creating an environment that promotes self-digestion of dead tissues by bacterial enzymes.

near point of vision The closest distance at which the eye can see an object clearly.

near-drowning Recovery after submersion in a liquid medium (usually water); this term is no longer used because language that describes drowning incidents has been standardized.

near-syncope Dizziness with an inability to remain in an upright position.

necrotizing hemorrhagic pancreatitis (NHP) Inflammation of the pancreas that is characterized by diffusely bleeding pancreatic tissue with fibrosis and tissue death. This form affects about 20% of patients with pancreatitis.

needle thoracostomy A quick, temporary method of chest decompression in which a large-bore needle is used to vent trapped air pending chest tube insertion.

negative deflection In electrocardiography, the flow of electrical current in the heart (cardiac axis) away from the positive pole and toward the negative pole.

negative feedback control mechanism The condition of maintaining a constant output of a system by exerting an inhibitory control on a key step by a product of that system. Used in a series of reactions that control hormone secretion and cellular activity based on responses to correct any movement away from normal function. An example of a simple negative feedback hormone response is the control of insulin secretion in which the action of insulin (decreasing blood glucose levels) is the opposite of the condition that stimulated insulin secretion (elevated blood glucose levels).

negative nitrogen balance A net loss of protein that occurs when the breakdown (degradation) of protein exceeds buildup (synthesis).

neglect In nursing, failure to provide for a patient's basic needs.

neoadjuvant therapy Treatment of a cancerous tumor with chemotherapy to shrink the tumor before it is surgically removed.

neoplasia Any new or continued cell growth not needed for normal development or replacement of dead and damaged tissues.

nephrectomy The surgical removal of the kidney.

nephrolithiasis The formation of stones in the kidney.

nephron The "working" unit of the kidney where urine is formed from blood. Each kidney consists of about 1 million nephrons, and each nephron separately makes urine. There are two types of nephrons: cortical and juxtamedullary.

nephropathy Pathologic change in the kidney that reduces kidney function and leads to renal failure.

nephrosclerosis Thickening in the nephron blood vessels that results in narrowing of the vessel lumen, with decreased renal blood flow and chronically hypoxic kidney tissue.

nephrostomy The surgical creation of an opening directly into the kidney; performed to divert urine externally and prevent further damage to the kidney when a stricture is causing hydronephrosis and cannot be corrected with urologic procedures.

nephrotic syndrome (NS) A condition of increased glomerular permeability that allows larger molecules to pass through the membrane into the urine and be removed from the blood.

This process causes massive loss of protein into the urine, edema formation, and decreased plasma albumin levels.

neuraxial Referring to the epidural or spinal area.

neuritic plaques Degenerating nerve terminals found particularly in the hippocampus, an important part of the limbic system, and marked by increased amounts of an abnormal protein called *beta amyloid*; a characteristic change of the brain found in patients with Alzheimer's disease.

neurofibrillary tangles Tangled masses of fibrous elements throughout the neurons; a classic finding at autopsy in the brains of patients with Alzheimer's disease.

neurogenic shock Hypotension and bradycardia associated with cervical spinal injuries and caused by a loss of autonomic function. The patient is at greatest risk in the first 24 hours after injury.

neuroglia cells Cells of varying size and shape that provide protection, structure, and nutrition for the neurons.

neurohypophysis The posterior lobe of the pituitary gland that stores hormones produced in the hypothalamus.

neuroma A sensitive tumor consisting of nerve cells and nerve fibers.

neuron Excitable nerve cell that processes and transmits information through electrical and chemical signals.

neuropathic pain A type of chronic noncancer pain that results from a nerve injury. Examples of causes include diabetic neuropathy, postherpetic neuralgia, radiculopathy (spinal nerve damage), and trigeminal neuralgia. Neuropathic pain is described as burning, shooting, stabbing, and the sensation of "pins and needles."

neuropathy A problem in nerve tissue that can cause muscle weakness.

neurotransmitter Regulatory chemical that exerts inhibitory (slowing down) or excitatory (speeding up) activity at postsynaptic nerve cell membranes. Acetylcholine, norepinephrine, epinephrine, dopamine, and serotonin are neurotransmitters.

neurovascular assessment Assessment of the neuromuscular system that includes inspection of skin color, temperature, and capillary refill distal to an injury, surgical procedure, or cast. Palpation of pulses in the extremities below level of injury and assessment of sensation, movement, and pain in the injured part give a complete assessment.

neutralization See *inactivation.*

neutropenia Decreased numbers of leukocytes, especially neutrophils, which causes immunosuppression.

neutrophilia Increased number of circulating neutrophils.

nevus A mole; a benign skin growth of the pigment-forming cells.

new-onset angina Cardiac chest pain that occurs for the first time.

nitroglycerin (NTG) A drug prescribed for patients with angina. It increases collateral blood flow, redistributes blood flow toward the subendocardium, and causes dilation of the coronary arteries.

nits Lice eggs.

N-methyl-D-aspartate (NMDA) receptor antagonist A group of drugs that block excess amounts of glutamate, which damages nerve cells in the brain; used to treat Alzheimer's disease.

nociception Term used to describe how pain becomes a conscious experience.

nociceptive pain Pain related to the skin, musculoskeletal structures, or body organs.

nociceptors Sensory neurons that respond to pain or other noxious stimuli.

nocturia The need to urinate excessively at night. Also called *nocturnal polyuria.*

nocturnal polyuria See *nocturia.*

nonadherence In health care, accidental failure by a patient to take medication.

noncompliance In health care, deliberate failure by a patient to take medication.

nonmaleficence Ethical principle that emphasizes the importance of preventing harm and ensuring the patient's well-being.

nonmechanical obstruction Intestinal obstruction that does not involve a physical obstruction in or outside the intestine. Instead, decreased or absent peristalsis results in a slowing of the movement or a backup of intestinal contents. This is also known as *paralytic ileus* or *adynamic ileus* because it is a result of neuromuscular disturbance.

nonmodifiable risk factor Factor in disease development that cannot be altered or controlled by the patient. Examples include age, gender, family history, and ethnic background.

non–ST-segment elevation myocardial infarction (NSTEMI) Myocardial infarction in which the patient typically has ST and T-wave changes on a 12-lead ECG; this indicates myocardial ischemia.

nonsustained ventricular tachycardia (NSVT) Occurrence of three or more successive premature ventricular complexes.

nontunneled percutaneous central venous catheter (CVC) A type of catheter, usually 15 to 20 cm long and with dual or triple lumens, that is inserted through the subclavian vein in the upper chest or through the jugular veins in the neck using sterile technique.

nonurgent In a three-tiered triage scheme, the category that includes patients who can generally tolerate waiting several hours for health care services without a significant risk of clinical deterioration, such as those with sprains, strains, or simple fractures.

normal flora The microorganisms living in or on the human host without causing disease; the bacteria that are characteristic of each body location. Normal flora often compete with and prevent infection from unfamiliar microorganisms attempting to invade a body site.

normal sinus rhythm (NSR) The rhythm originating from the sinoatrial node (dominant pacemaker), with atrial and ventricular rates of 60 to 100 beats/min and regular atrial and ventricular rhythms.

normotonic See *isosmotic.*

North American pit vipers The Crotalidae, one of two families of indigenous poisonous snakes in North America; named for the characteristic depression between each eye and nostril. They include rattlesnakes, copperheads, and water moccasins and account for most poisonous snakebites in the United States.

nosocomial (infection) Acquired in an inpatient health care setting; for example, infections that were not present at hospital admission. Also called *hospital-acquired infections* and *health care–associated infections.*

nothing by mouth (NPO) No eating, drinking (including water), or smoking.

nuchal rigidity Stiff neck, which can be a sign of cerebrospinal fluid leak; nuchal rigidity is not checked until a spinal cord injury has been ruled out.

nucleotide The final form of a base that actually gets put into the strand of deoxyribonucleic acid. A nucleoside becomes a complete nucleotide by the attachment of phosphate groups.

nursing assistant A member of the rehabilitative health care team who assists the registered nurse in the care of patients.

nursing technician See *nursing assistant.*

nutrition The process of ingesting and using food and fluids to grow, repair, and maintain optimal body functions.

nutritional screening A screening by the health care provider that includes visual inspection, measured height and weight, weight history, usual eating habits, ability to chew and swallow, and any recent changes in appetite or food intake. The screening is a way to determine which patients need more extensive nutritional assessment.

nutritional status Reflects the balance between nutrient requirements and intake.

nystagmus Involuntary rapid eye movements.

O

obesity An increase in body weight at least 20% above the upper limit of the normal range for ideal body weight, with an excess amount of body fat; in an adult, a body mass index greater than 30.

obligatory urine output The minimum amount of urine per day needed to dissolve and excrete toxic waste products.

obstipation The inability to pass stool; intractable constipation.

obstruction Blockage.

obstructive jaundice Jaundice caused by an impediment to the flow of bile from the liver to the duodenum; may be caused by edema of the ducts or gallstones.

obstructive sleep apnea A breathing disruption during sleep that lasts at least 10 seconds and occurs a minimum of 5 times in an hour.

Occupational Safety and Health Administration (OSHA) A federal agency that protects workers from injury or illness at their place of employment.

occupational therapist (OT, OTR) A member of the rehabilitation health care team who works to develop the patient's fine motor skills used for activities of daily living and the skills related to coordination and cognitive retraining.

odynophagia Pain on swallowing.

oligomenorrhea Scant or infrequent menses.

oligospermia Low sperm count.

oliguria Scant urine output. Usually less than 400 mL per day.

oliguria Decreased excretion of urine in relation to amount of fluid intake; usually defined as urine output less than 400 mL/day.

oncogene Proto-oncogene that has been "turned on" and can cause cells to change from normal cells to cancer cells.

oncogenesis Cancer development.

oncovirus Virus that causes cancer.

oophorectomy Surgical removal of the ovary.

open fracture A fracture in which the skin surface over the broken bone is disrupted, causing an external wound. Also called *compound fracture*.

open reduction The reduction of a fracture after surgical incision into the site to allow direct visualization of the fracture. See *internal fixation*.

open traumatic brain injury A type of traumatic primary brain injury that occurs with a skull fracture or when the skull is pierced by a penetrating object. The integrity of the brain and the dura is violated, and there is exposure to outside contaminants, with damage to the underlying vessels, dural sinus, brain, and cranial nerves.

opportunistic infection Infection caused by organisms that are present as part of the normal environment and would be kept in check by normal immune function.

optic disc The point at the inside back of the eye where the optic nerve enters the eyeball. It appears as a creamy pink to white depressed area in the retina and contains only nerve fibers and no photoreceptor cells.

optic fundus The area at the inside back of the eye that can be seen with an ophthalmoscope.

optic nerve The nerve of sight; connects the optic disc to the brain.

orbit The bony socket of the skull that surrounds and protects the eye along with the attached muscles, nerves, vessels, and tear-producing glands.

orchiectomy The surgical removal of one or both testes.

orchitis An acute testicular inflammation resulting from trauma or infection.

orexin Neuropeptide that is an appetite stimulant.

organ donor An individual who has consented to donating one or more organs when he or she dies.

orotracheal The route for inserting a tube into the trachea via the mouth.

orthopnea Shortness of breath that occurs when lying down but is relieved by sitting up.

orthostatic hypotension A decrease in blood pressure (20 mm Hg systolic and/or 10 mm Hg diastolic) that occurs during the first few seconds to minutes after changing from a sitting or lying position to a standing position. Also called *postural hypotension*.

orthostatic Pertaining to or caused by standing erect.

orthotopic The most common type of transplantation procedure in which a diseased organ is removed and a donor organ is grafted in its place. For example, during heart transplantation, the surgeon removes the diseased heart and leaves the posterior walls of the patient's atria, which serve as the anchor for the donor heart; anastomoses

are made between the recipient and donor atria, aorta, and pulmonary arteries.

osmolality The number of milliosmoles in a kilogram of solution.

osmolarity The number of milliosmoles in a liter of solution.

osmosis The movement of a solvent across a semipermeable membrane (a membrane that allows the solvent but not the solute to pass through) from a lesser to a greater concentration.

ossiculoplasty Replacement of the ossicles within the middle ear.

osteitis deformans See *Paget's disease*.

osteoarthritis Noninflammatory form of arthritis characterized by the progressive deterioration and loss of cartilage in one or more joints; most common form of arthritis.

osteoblast Cell associated with formation of bone.

osteoclast Cell associated with destruction or resorption of bone.

osteocyte Bone cell.

osteomalacia Abnormal softening of the bone tissue characterized by inadequate mineralization of osteoid. It is the adult equivalent of rickets (vitamin D deficiency) in children.

osteomyelitis An inflammation of bone tissue caused by pathogenic microorganisms; produces an increased vascularity and edema often involving the surrounding soft tissues.

osteonecrosis The death of bone tissue, usually because the blood supply to the bone is disrupted. Usually a complication of a hip fracture or any fracture in which there is displacement of bone.

osteopenia A condition of low bone mass that occurs when there is a disruption in the bone remodeling process.

osteophyte Bone spur.

osteoporosis A metabolic disease in which bone demineralization results in decreased density and subsequent fractures.

osteotomy Surgical resection of bone.

ostomate A patient with an ostomy.

ostomy The surgical creation of an opening, usually referring to an opening in the abdominal wall; stoma.

otorrhea Ear discharge.

otosclerosis Irregular bone growth around the ossicles.

otoscope An instrument used to examine the ear; consists of a light, a handle, a magnifying lens, and a pneumatic bulb for injecting air into the external canal to test mobility of the eardrum.

ototoxic Having a toxic effect on the inner ear structures.

outflow disease Chronic peripheral arterial disease with obstruction at or below the superficial femoral or popliteal artery. The patient experiences burning or cramping in the calves, ankles, feet, and toes after walking a certain distance; the pain usually subsides with rest.

outpatient A patient who goes to the hospital for treatment and returns home on the same day.

overflow urinary incontinence The involuntary loss of urine when the bladder is overdistended.

overweight An increase in body weight for height compared with a reference standard (e.g., the Metropolitan Life height and weight tables) or 10% greater than ideal body weight. However,

this weight may not reflect excess body fat, which in an adult is a body mass index of 25 to 30.

ovoid pupil In evaluating pupils for size and reaction to light, the midstage between a normal-size pupil and a dilated pupil; indicates the development of increased intracranial pressure.

oxygen concentrator A machine that removes nitrogen, water vapor, and hydrocarbons from room air. Also known as *oxygen extractor*.

oxygen dissociation The transfer of oxygen from hemoglobin to tissues.

P

P wave In the electrocardiogram, the deflection representing atrial depolarization.

pack-years The number of packs of cigarettes per day multiplied by the number of years the patient has smoked; used in recording a patient's smoking history.

Paget's disease A metabolic disorder of bone remodeling, or turnover, in which increased resorption or loss results in bone deposits that are weak, enlarged, and disorganized. Also known as *osteitis deformans*.

pain An unpleasant sensory and emotional experience associated with actual or potential tissue damage; the most reliable indication of pain is the patient's self-report.

palliation Relieving symptoms.

palliative care A compassionate and supportive approach to patients and families who are living with life-threatening illnesses; involves a holistic approach that provides relief of symptoms experienced by the dying patient.

palpitations A feeling of fluttering in the chest, an unpleasant awareness of the heartbeat, or an irregular heartbeat; may result from a change in heart rate or rhythm or from an increase in the force of heart contractions.

pancreatic abscess A collection of purulent material that results from extensive inflammatory necrosis of the pancreas after infection by organisms such as *Escherichia coli*; the most serious complication of pancreatitis. It is fatal if left untreated.

pancreatic pseudocyst A false cyst, so named because, unlike a true cyst, it does not have an epithelial lining. It is an encapsulated saclike structure that forms on or surrounds the pancreas and develops as a complication of acute or chronic pancreatitis. It may contain up to several liters of straw-colored or dark-brown viscous fluid, the enzymatic exudate of the pancreas.

pancreaticojejunostomy Surgical anastomosis of the pancreatic duct with the jejunum.

pancytopenia A deficiency of all three cell types (red blood cells, white blood cells, and platelets) of the blood.

pandemic A general epidemic spread over a wide geographic area and affecting a large proportion of the population.

panniculectomy The surgical removal of any panniculus, most often the abdominal apron; usually done as a follow-up to bariatric surgery in an obese patient.

panniculitis Infection of the panniculus.

panniculus A layer of membrane; also used to refer to skinfold areas in the obese patient.

pannus Vascular granulation tissue composed of inflammatory cells that forms in a joint space; erodes articular cartilage and eventually destroys bone.

Papanicolaou test (Pap smear) A cytologic study that is effective in detecting precancerous and cancerous cells obtained from the cervix.

papilla The anatomic term for a small, nipple-shaped projection or structure.

papilledema Edema and hyperemia of the optic disc; a sign of increased intracranial pressure found on ophthalmoscopic examination. Also called a *choked disc.*

papilloma A pedunculated outgrowth of tissue.

papillotomy An incision of a papilla, a small nipple-shaped projection or structure.

papular Referring to a papule, a small, solid elevation of the skin.

paracentesis A procedure in which the physician inserts a trocar catheter into the abdomen to remove and drain ascitic fluid from the peritoneal cavity.

paradoxical blood pressure An exaggerated decrease in systolic pressure by more than 10 mm Hg during the inspiratory phase of the respiratory cycle (normal is 3 to 10 mm Hg); clinical conditions that may produce a paradoxical blood pressure include pericardial tamponade, constrictive pericarditis, and pulmonary hypertension. Also known as *paradoxical pulse* and *pulsus paradoxus.*

paradoxical chest wall movement The "sucking inward" of the loose chest area during inspiration and a "puffing out" of the same area during expiration in a patient with a flail chest.

paradoxical pulse See *paradoxical blood pressure.*

paradoxical splitting Abnormal splitting of the S_2 heart sound heard in patients with severe myocardial depression; causes early closure of the pulmonic valve or a delay in aortic valve closure.

paralysis Absence of movement.

paralytic ileus Absence of peristalsis.

paramedic Prehospital care provider for patients who require care that exceeds basic life support resources. Advanced life support (ALS) may include cardiac monitoring, advanced airway management and intubation, establishing IV access, and administering drugs en route to the emergency department.

paranasal sinuses The air-filled cavities within the bones that surround the nasal passages. Lined with ciliated membrane, the sinuses provide resonance during speech and decrease the weight of the skull.

paraparesis Weakness that involves only the lower extremities, as seen in lower thoracic and lumbosacral injuries or lesions.

paraplegia Paralysis that involves only the lower extremities, as seen in lower thoracic and lumbosacral injuries or lesions.

paresis Weakness.

paresthesia Abnormal or unusual nerve sensations of touch, such as tingling and burning.

parietal cells Cells lining the wall of the stomach that secrete hydrochloric acid and produce intrinsic factor.

Parkinson disease (PD) A debilitating neurologic disease that affects motor ability and is characterized by four cardinal symptoms: tremor, rigidity, akinesia (slow movement), and postural instability. It is the third most common neurologic disorder of older adults. Also called *paralysis agitans.*

parotidectomy The surgical removal of the parotid glands.

paroxysmal nocturnal dyspnea (PND) In the patient with heart disease, difficulty breathing that develops after lying down for several hours and causes the patient to awaken abruptly with a feeling of suffocation and panic. Occurs because the heart is unable to compensate for the increased volume when blood from the lower extremities is redistributed to the venous system, which increases venous return to the heart. A diseased heart is ineffective in pumping the additional fluid into the circulatory system, and pulmonary congestion results.

paroxysmal supraventricular tachycardia (PSVT) A form of supraventricular tachycardia that occurs when the rhythm is intermittent; it is initiated suddenly by a premature complex, such as a premature atrial complex, and terminated suddenly with or without intervention.

partial left ventriculectomy (PLV) A ventricular reconstructive procedure that involves removing a triangle-shaped section of the weakened heart in the left lateral ventricle to reduce the ventricle's diameter and decrease wall tension. Also known as *heart reduction surgery* and *Batista procedure.*

partial seizure One of the three broad categories of seizure disorders along with generalized seizure and unclassified seizure. Partial seizures are of two types: complex and simple. Partial seizures begin in a part of one cerebral hemisphere; some can evolve into generalized tonic-clonic, tonic, or clonic seizures. They are most often seen in adults and in general are less responsive to medical treatment. Also called *focal seizures* or *local seizures.*

passive euthanasia See *withdrawing or withholding life-sustaining therapy.*

passive immunity Resistance to infection that is of short duration (days or months) and either natural by transplacental transfer from the mother or artificial by injection of antibodies (e.g., immunoglobulin).

patellofemoral pain syndrome (PFPS) A health problem that occurs most often in people who are runners or who overuse their knee joints. For that reason, it is sometimes referred to as "runner's knee." These patients describe pain as being behind or around their patella (knee cap) in one or both knees.

pathogen Any microorganism capable of producing disease.

pathogenicity The ability to cause disease.

pathologic (spontaneous) fracture A fracture that occurs after minimal trauma to a bone that has been weakened by a disease such as bone cancer or osteoporosis.

patient-centered care A QSEN competency in which the nurse recognizes the patient or designee as the source of control and full partner in providing compassionate and coordinated care based on respect for the patient's preferences, values, and needs.

patient-controlled analgesia A method that allows the patient to control the dosage of opioid analgesic received by using an infusion pump to deliver the desired amount of medication through a conventional IV route.

PDSA Acronym for plan, do, study, act, which is one of the steps of the evidence-based practice improvement (EBPI) model.

peaceful death A death that is free from avoidable distress and suffering for patients and families, is in agreement with patients' and families' wishes, and is consistent with clinical practice standards.

pedal Pertaining to the feet.

pediculosis An infestation by human lice.

pedigree A graph of a family history for a specific trait or health problem over several generations.

pelvic inflammatory disease (PID) Any infection of the pelvis involving the upper genital tract beyond the cervix in women. It occurs when organisms from the lower genital tract migrate from the endocervix upward through the uterine cavity into the fallopian tubes.

pelvic organ prolapse (POP) Condition in which the sling of muscles and tendons that support the pelvic organs becomes weak and is no longer able to hold them in place.

penetrance In genetics, how often or how well a gene is expressed when it is present within a population.

penetrating trauma Injuries caused by piercing; classified by the velocity of the vehicle (e.g., knife or bullet) causing the injury. Low-velocity injuries from knife wounds cause damage directly at the site; high-velocity injuries from gunshot wounds cause both direct and indirect damage. Also called *penetrating injury.*

peptic ulcer disease (PUD) The impairment of gastric mucosal defenses so that they no longer protect the epithelium from the effects of acid and pepsin.

peptic ulcer A mucosal lesion of the stomach or duodenum.

percutaneous alcohol septal ablation Surgical procedure for hypertrophic cardiomyopathy (HCM) in which alcohol is injected into a target septal branch of the left anterior descending coronary artery to produce a small septal infarction. This procedure also widens the left ventricular outflow tract.

percutaneous coronary intervention (PCI) See *percutaneous transluminal coronary angioplasty (PTCA).*

percutaneous endoscopic gastrostomy (PEG) A stoma created from the abdominal wall into the stomach for insertion of a short feeding tube.

percutaneous stereotactic rhizotomy (PSR) Procedure performed under general anesthesia to treat trigeminal neuralgia; a hollow needle is passed through the inside of the patient's cheek into the trigeminal nerve fibers, and a heating current (radiofrequency thermocoagulation) goes through the needle to destroy some of the fibers.

percutaneous transhepatic cholangiography (PTC) The radiographic study of the biliary duct system using an iodinated dye instilled via a percutaneous needle inserted through the liver into the intrahepatic ducts. It may be performed when a patient has jaundice or persistent upper abdominal pain, even after cholecystectomy, but it is rarely performed as a diagnostic procedure.

percutaneous transluminal coronary angioplasty (PTCA) A nonsurgical method of improving arterial flow by opening the vessel lumen and creating a smooth inner vessel surface. One or more arteries are dilated with a balloon catheter advanced through a cannula, which is inserted into or above an occluded or stenosed artery. Also called *percutaneous vascular intervention* and *percutaneous coronary intervention (PCI).*

percutaneous vascular intervention See *percutaneous transluminal coronary angioplasty.*

percutaneous Performed through the skin and other tissues.

perfusion Adequate arterial blood flow to the peripheral tissues (peripheral perfusion) and blood that is pumped by the heart to oxygenate major body organs (central perfusion).

pericardial effusion Complication of pericarditis that occurs when the space between the parietal and visceral layers of the pericardium fills with fluid.

pericardial friction rub An abnormal sound that originates from the pericardial sac and occurs with the movements of the heart during the cardiac cycle; usually transient and a sign of inflammation, infection, or infiltration; may be heard in patients with pericarditis resulting from myocardial infarction, cardiac tamponade, or post-thoracotomy.

pericardiectomy Surgical excision of the pericardium (the sac around the heart).

pericardiocentesis Withdrawal of pericardial fluid through a catheter inserted into the pericardial space to relieve the pressure on the heart.

pericarditis An inflammation of the tissue (pericardium) surrounding the heart.

perichondrium A tough, fibrous tissue layer that surrounds the ear cartilage and gives shape to the pinna.

periodontal disease Gum disease in which mandibular bone loss has occurred.

perioperative The operative experience consisting of the preoperative, intraoperative, and postoperative time periods.

peripheral blood stem cells (PBSCs) Stem cells that are collected from peripheral blood for transplantation into the patient.

peripheral chemoreceptors Several 1- to 2-mm collections of tissue identified in the carotid arteries and along the aortic arch.

peripheral IV therapy IV therapy in which a vascular access device (VAD) is placed in a peripheral vein, usually in the arm.

peripheral vascular disease (PVD) Any disorder that alters the natural flow of blood through the arteries and veins of the peripheral circulation.

peripherally inserted central catheter (PICC) A long catheter inserted through a vein of the antecubital fossa (inner aspect of the bend of the arm) or the middle of the upper arm.

peritonitis Acute inflammation of the visceral/parietal peritoneum and endothelial lining of the abdominal cavity, or peritoneum.

peritonsillar abscess (PTA) A complication of acute tonsillitis. The infection spreads from the tonsil to the surrounding tissue, which forms an abscess.

periungual lesion Skin lesion around the nail bed.

permeable The quality of being porous.

pernicious anemia A form of megaloblastic anemia caused by failure to absorb vitamin B_{12} because of a deficiency of intrinsic factor (normally secreted by the gastric mucosa) needed for intestinal absorption of vitamin B_{12}.

PERRLA An acronym that stands for the phrase "*P*upils should be *e*qual in size, *r*ound and *r*egular in shape, and react to *l*ight and *a*ccommodation."

personal emergency preparedness plan An individual plan that outlines specific arrangements in the event of disaster, such as childcare, pet care, and older adult care.

personal protective equipment (PPE) Infection control protocol that refers to the use of gloves, isolation gowns, face protection, and respirators with N95 or higher filtration.

personal readiness supplies A preassembled disaster supply kit for the home and/or automobile that contains clothing and basic survival supplies. Also called a "*go bag.*"

petechiae Pinpoint red spots on the mucous membranes, palate, conjunctivae, or skin.

pH monitoring examination The most accurate testing method of diagnosing GERD, accomplished by placing a small catheter into the distal esophagus or esophageal wall (depending on the specific technique). The patient then records a diary of activities and symptoms over a 24- to 48-hour period while pH is continuously monitored.

pH A measure of the free hydrogen ion level in body fluid.

phagocytosis The process of engulfing, ingesting, killing, and disposing of an invading organism by neutrophils and macrophages; a key process of inflammation.

Phalen's maneuver Test to determine the presence of carpal tunnel syndrome (CTS); a positive test for CTS causes paresthesia in the medial nerve distribution of the palm of the hand in 60 seconds.

phantom limb pain (PLP) A frequent complication of amputation in which the patient perceives sensation in the absent (amputated) foot or hand. This sensation usually diminishes over time.

pharmacist Member of the health care team who oversees the prescription and preparation of medications and provides the team with essential information regarding drug safety.

pharmacologic stress echocardiogram A form of echocardiography in which either dobutamine (increases heart's contractility) or adenosine (dilates coronary arteries) is given to the patient; usually used when patients cannot tolerate exercise.

phenotype Any genetic characteristic that can actually be observed or, in some cases, determined by laboratory test.

pheochromocytoma A tumor of the adrenal medulla, which can cause excessive secretion of catecholamines.

phlebitis Inflammation of a vein, which can predispose patients to thrombosis.

phlebothrombosis Presence of a thrombus in a vein without inflammation.

phonophobia Abnormal sensitivity to sound.

phonophoresis Treatment for back pain in which a topical drug (e.g., lidocaine, hydrocortisone) is applied followed by continuous ultrasound for 10 minutes.

photophobia Abnormal sensitivity to light.

photopsia The appearance of bright flashes of light due to the onset of retinal detachment.

physiatrist A physician who specializes in rehabilitative medicine.

physical abuse The use of a physical force, such as hitting, burning, pushing, and molesting the patient, that results in bodily injury.

physical therapist (PT, RPT) A member of the rehabilitation health care team who helps the patient achieve mobility and who teaches techniques for performing certain activities of daily living.

piggyback set See *secondary administration set.*

pitting Indentation of the skin; often occurs with edema.

pituitary Cushing's disease Oversecretion of ACTH by the anterior pituitary gland, which causes hyperplasia of the adrenal cortex in both adrenal glands and an excess of most hormones secreted by the adrenal cortex.

placebo Any medication or procedure, including surgery, that produces an effect in a patient because of its implicit or explicit intent and not because of its specific physical or chemical properties.

Plan-Do-Study-Act (PDSA) A specific systematic model of quality improvement.

plantar fasciitis An inflammation of the plantar fascia, which is located in the area of the arch of the foot. It is often seen in athletes, especially runners.

plasma cell A short-lived B-lymphocyte that begins to function immediately to produce antibodies against sensitizing antigens.

plasmapheresis The separation of plasma from whole blood, after which the blood cells are returned to the patient without the plasma to eliminate antibodies.

plethoric A flushed appearance of the skin.

pleura The continuous smooth membrane composed of two surfaces that totally enclose the lungs.

pleural effusion Fluid in the pleural space.

pleuritic chest pain A stabbing pain on taking a deep breath.

plexus Cluster of nerves.

ploidy The number and appearance of chromosomes; used to describe cancer cells.

pluripotent stem cell The precursor cell involved in the production of red blood cells.

pneumonectomy Removal of an entire lung, including all blood vessels.

pneumonia Excess fluid in the lungs resulting from an inflammatory process that can include infection.

pneumothorax Air in the pleural (chest) cavity.

podagra Inflammation of the metatarsophalangeal joint of the great toe.

point of maximal impulse (PMI) See *apical impulse.*

polycystic kidney disease (PKD) An inherited disorder in which fluid-filled cysts develop in the kidneys.

polycythemia vera (PV) A disease that involves massive production of red blood cells, leukocytes, and platelets.

polydipsia Excessive intake of water.

polymedicine The use of many drugs to treat multiple health problems for older adults.

polymorphism A variation in form.

polyp An abnormal outgrowth from a mucous membrane.

polyphagia Excessive eating.

polypharmacy The use of many drugs to treat multiple health problems for older adults. Also known as *hyperpharmacy.*

polyuria Frequent and excessive urination.

pores Openings or spaces.

portal hypertension An abnormal persistent increase in pressure within the portal vein; a major complication of cirrhosis.

portal hypertensive gastropathy A complication that can occur in patients with portal hypertension, with or without esophageal varices. Slow gastric mucosal bleeding may result in chronic slow blood loss, occult positive stools, and anemia.

portal-systemic encephalopathy (PSE) A clinical disorder seen in hepatic failure and cirrhosis; it is manifested by neurologic symptoms and is characterized by an altered level of consciousness, impaired thinking processes, and neuromuscular disturbances. Also called *hepatic encephalopathy* and *hepatic coma.*

positive deflection In electrocardiography, the flow of electrical current in the heart (cardiac axis) toward the positive pole.

positive inotropic agents Drugs that increase myocardial contractility; such drugs are prescribed to improve cardiac output.

postanesthesia care unit (PACU) Recovery room.

postcholecystectomy syndrome (PCS) The occurrence of the clinical manifestations of biliary tract disease following cholecystectomy; caused by residual or recurring calculi, inflammation, or stricture of the common bile duct.

post-concussion syndrome A group of clinical manifestations following a concussion that consist of personality changes, irritability, headaches, dizziness, restlessness, nervousness, insomnia, memory loss, and depression. The prolonged pattern is classified as post-trauma syndrome.

posterior colporrhaphy The surgical procedure to repair a rectocele by strengthening pelvic supports and reducing the bulging.

posteroanterior Back to front; position for standard chest x-rays.

postherpetic neuralgia Pain that persists after herpes zoster lesions have resolved.

postictal stage Referring to the time immediately after a seizure.

postoperative period After surgery.

postpericardiotomy syndrome Symptoms, including pericardial and pleural pain, pericarditis, friction rub, elevated temperature and white blood cell count, and dysrhythmias, that occur in patients after cardiac surgery; may occur days to weeks after surgery and seems to be associated with blood that remains in the pericardial sac.

postrenal failure Decrease in renal function related to an obstruction in the flow of urine. It can progress to acute renal failure.

postural hypotension See *orthostatic hypotension.*

posture A person's body build and alignment when standing and walking.

post-void residual (PVR) The amount of urine remaining in the bladder within 20 minutes after voiding.

power air purifying respirator (PAPR) Device with a high efficiency particulate air (HEPA) filter and battery to promote positive pressure air flow; more effective than an N95 respirator.

PQRST A mnemonic (memory device) that may help in the current problem assessment of patients with gastrointestinal tract disorders. The letters represent these areas: P, precipitating or palliative (What brings it on? What makes it better or worse?); Q, quality or quantity (How does it look, feel, or sound?); R, region or radiation (Where is it? Does it spread anywhere?); S, severity scale (How bad is it [on a scale of 0 to 10]? Is it getting better, worse, or staying the same?); T, timing (Onset, duration, and frequency?).

PR interval In the electrocardiogram, the interval measured from the beginning of the P wave to the end of the PR segment; represents the time required for atrial depolarization as well as impulse delay in the atrioventricular node and travel time to the Purkinje fibers.

PR segment In the electrocardiogram, the isoelectric line from the end of the P wave to the beginning of the QRS complex, when the electrical impulse is traveling through the atrioventricular node, where it is delayed.

Prader-Willi syndrome (PWS) A complex neurodevelopmental genetic disorder that results from a hypothalamic-pituitary dysfunction that prevents appetite control. Patients with this syndrome are typically morbidly obese.

prandial (insulin secretion) The increased levels of insulin that are secreted after eating. Within 10 minutes of eating, an early burst of insulin secretion occurs, which is followed by an increasing insulin release that lasts as long as hyperglycemia is present.

prealbumin (PAB) A protein secreted by the liver that binds thyroxine.

precipitation The formation of large, insoluble antigen-antibody complexes during the antibody-binding process.

prediabetes An impaired fasting glucose (IFG) or impaired glucose tolerance (IGT).

prehospital care provider Typically, any of the first caregivers encountered by the patient if he or she is transported to the emergency department by an ambulance or helicopter.

preictal phase Referring to events that a patient experiences before a seizure, such as the presence of an aura.

pre-infarction angina Chest pain that occurs in the days or weeks before a myocardial infarction.

preload The degree of myocardial fiber stretch at the end of diastole and just before contraction; determined by the amount of blood returning to the heart from both the venous system (right heart) and the pulmonary system (left heart).

premature atrial complex (contraction) (PAC) In the electrocardiogram, an early complex that occurs when atrial tissue becomes irritable. This ectopic focus fires an impulse before the next sinus impulse is due, thus usurping the sinus pacemaker. The premature P wave from the atrial focus is early and has a shape different from that of the P wave generated from the sinus node.

premature complex In the electrocardiogram, an early complex that occurs when a cardiac cell or cell group other than the sinoatrial node becomes irritable and fires an impulse before the next sinus impulse is generated. After the premature complex, there is a pause before the next normal complex, which creates an irregularity in the rhythm.

premature ventricular complex (PVC) In the electrocardiogram, an early ventricular complex is followed by a pause that results from increased irritability of ventricular cells. The QRS complexes may be unifocal or uniform (of the same shape), or multifocal or multiform (of different shapes).

preoperative Before surgery.

prerenal failure Condition that causes inadequate kidney perfusion; can progress to acute renal failure.

presbycusis The loss of hearing, especially for high-pitched sounds; occurs as a result of aging.

presbyopia An age-related impairment of vision characterized by a loss of lens elasticity and the ability of the eye to accommodate. The near point of vision increases, and near objects must be placed farther from the eye to be seen clearly.

presence A type of communication that consists of listening and acknowledging the legitimacy of the patient's and/or family's pain.

pressure ulcer Tissue damage caused when the skin and underlying soft tissue are compressed between a bony prominence and an external surface for an extended period; commonly occurs over the sacrum, hips, and ankles.

pretibial myxedema Dry, waxy swelling of the front surfaces of the lower legs.

pretibial Pertaining to the front of the leg below the knee.

primary angle-closure glaucoma A form of glaucoma characterized by a narrowed angle and forward displacement of the iris so that movement of the iris against the cornea narrows or closes the chamber angle, obstructing the outflow of aqueous humor. It can have a sudden onset and is an emergency. Also called *closed-angle glaucoma, narrow-angle glaucoma,* or *acute glaucoma.*

primary arthroplasty A total joint arthroplasty procedure that has been performed for the first time.

primary gout The most common type of gout; results from one of several inborn errors of purine metabolism.

primary lesions In describing skin disease, the initial reaction to a problem that alters one of the structural components of the skin.

primary open-angle glaucoma (POAG) The most common form of primary glaucoma; characterized by reduced outflow of aqueous humor through the chamber angle. Because the fluid cannot leave the eye at the same rate it is produced, intraocular pressure gradually increases.

primary prevention Strategies used to avoid or delay the actual occurrence of a specific disease.

primary progressive multiple sclerosis (PPMS) A type of multiple sclerosis (MS) that involves a steady and gradual neurologic deterioration without remission of symptoms. Patients with this type of MS are usually between 40 and 60 years of age at onset of the disease and experience progressive disability with no acute attacks.

primary survey Priorities of care addressed in order of immediate threats to life as part of the initial assessment in the emergency department. Survey is based on an "ABC" mnemonic with "D" and "E" added for trauma patients: airway/cervical spine (A), breathing (B), circulation (C), disability (D), and exposure (E).

primary tumor The original tumor, usually identified by the tissue from which it arose (parent tissue), such as in breast cancer or lung cancer.

progressive multifocal leukoencephalopathy (PML) Rare disease affecting the white matter of the brain caused by a virus that attacks the cells that make myelin; occurs most often in patients who are immunosuppressed.

progressive-relapsing multiple sclerosis (PRMS) A type of multiple sclerosis (MS) that occurs in only 5% of patients with MS. It is characterized by the absence of periods of remission, and the patient's condition does not return to baseline. Progressive cumulative symptoms and deterioration occur over several years.

proliferative diabetic retinopathy A form of retinopathy associated with diabetes mellitus in which a network of fragile new blood vessels develops, leaking blood and protein into surrounding tissue. The new blood vessels are stimulated by retinal hypoxia that results from poor capillary perfusion of the retinal tissues. New blood vessels grow in the retina, onto the iris, and into the back of the vitreous. The vitreous contracts and pulls away from the retina, causing blood vessels to break and bleed into the vitreous.

promoter In oncology, a substance that promotes or enhances growth of the initiated cancer cell; may be a hormone, drug, or chemical.

pronator drift Occurs in a patient with muscle weakness due to cerebral or brainstem reasons. The arm on the weak side tends to fall, or "drift," with the palm pronating (turning inward) after the patient has closed his or her eyes and held the arms perpendicular to the body with the palms up for 15 to 30 seconds; part of the neurologic assessment.

prophylactic mastectomy Highly controversial practice of surgically removing the breast in order to reduce the risk of breast cancer.

proportionate palliative sedation A care management approach involving the administration of drugs such as benzodiazepines for the purpose of lowering patient consciousness.

proprioception (proprioceptive) Awareness of body position and movement.

prosopagnosia The inability to recognize oneself and other familiar faces; occurs in patients in the later stages of Alzheimer's disease.

prostaglandins Chemicals that are produced in the cells and cause inflammation and swelling.

prostate artery embolization A procedure in which the interventional radiologist threads a small vascular catheter into the prostate's arteries and injects particles blocking some of the blood flow to shrink the prostate gland.

prostate-specific antigen (PSA) A glycoprotein produced solely by the prostate. The normal blood level of PSA is less than 4 ng/mL; levels are higher in patients with increased prostatic tissue as a result of benign prostatic hyperplasia, prostatic infarction, prostatitis, and prostate cancer. Levels associated with prostate cancer are usually much higher than those occurring with other prostate tissue enlargement.

prostatitis Inflammation of the prostate.

protein synthesis The process by which genes are used to make the proteins needed for physiologic function.

protein-calorie malnutrition (PCM) A disorder of nutrition that may present in three forms: marasmus, kwashiorkor, and marasmic-kwashiorkor. Also called *protein-energy malnutrition*.

protein-energy malnutrition (PEM) See *protein-calorie malnutrition*.

proteinuria The presence of protein in the urine.

proteolysis The breakdown of proteins to provide fuel for energy when liver glucose is unavailable.

proton pump inhibitor (PPI) A group of drugs that inhibit the proton pump in the stomach to decrease gastric acid production.

pruritus An unpleasant itching sensation.

psoriasis A chronic autoimmune disorder of the skin with exacerbations and remissions. It results from overstimulation of the immune system (Langerhans' cells) in the skin that activates T-lymphocytes. The features include increased skin cell division in patchy areas forming scaly plaques.

psoriatic arthritis (PsA) A syndrome of inflammatory arthritis associated with psoriasis, the skin condition characterized by a scaly, itchy rash.

psychiatric crisis nurse team An emergency department specialty team whose nurses interact with patients and families in crisis.

psychotropic drugs Antipsychotic and neuroleptic drugs. These are appropriately given to patients with emotional and behavioral health problems (e.g., hallucinations and delusions) that accompany dementia but are sometimes inappropriately used for agitation, combativeness, or restlessness. They are considered chemical restraints because they decrease mobility and patients' ability to care for themselves.

ptosis Drooping of the eyelid.

pulmonary artery occlusive pressure (PAOP) See *pulmonary artery wedge pressure*.

pulmonary artery wedge pressure (PAWP) Measurement of pressure in the left atrium using a balloon-tipped catheter introduced into the pulmonary artery. When the balloon at the catheter tip is inflated, the catheter advances and wedges in a branch of the pulmonary artery. The tip of the catheter is able to sense pressures transmitted from the left atrium, which reflect left ventricular end-diastolic pressure. Also called *pulmonary artery occlusive pressure*.

pulmonary autograph The relocation of the patient's own pulmonary valve to the aortic position for aortic valve replacement (Ross procedure).

pulmonary embolism (PE) A collection of particulate matter, most commonly a blood clot, that enters venous circulation and lodges in the pulmonary vessels, obstructing pulmonary blood flow and leading to decreased systemic oxygenation, pulmonary tissue hypoxia, and potential death.

pulmonary empyema A collection of pus in the pleural space most commonly caused by a pulmonary infection.

pulse deficit The difference between the apical and peripheral pulses.

pulse pressure The difference between the systolic and diastolic pressures.

pulse therapy Any therapy given at a high dose for a short duration.

pulsus alternans A type of pulse in which a weak pulse alternates with a strong pulse despite a regular heart rhythm; seen in patients with severely depressed cardiac function.

punctum The opening through which tears drain; located at the nasal side of the eyelid edges.

pupil The opening through which light enters the eye; located in the center of the iris of the eye.

Purkinje cells In the cardiac conduction system, the cells that make up the bundle of His, bundle branches, and terminal Purkinje fibers. These cells are responsible for the rapid conduction of electrical impulses throughout the ventricles, leading to ventricular depolarization and subsequent ventricular muscle contraction.

purpura Purple patches on the skin that may be caused by blood disorders, vascular abnormalities, or trauma.

pyelolithotomy The surgical removal of a stone from the kidney.

pyelonephritis A bacterial infection in the kidney and renal pelvis (the upper urinary tract).

pyloromyotomy An incision through the serosa and muscularis of the pylorus, down to the mucosa; created to prevent gastric motility disturbances in patients who have undergone esophagectomy.

pyuria The presence of white blood cells (pus) in the urine.

Q

QRS complex In the electrocardiogram, the portion consisting of the Q, R, and S waves, representing ventricular depolarization.

QRS duration In the electrocardiogram, the time required for depolarization of both ventricles; measured from the beginning of the QRS complex to the J point (the junction at which the QRS complex ends and the ST segment begins).

QT interval In the electrocardiogram, the time from the beginning of the QRS complex to the end of the T wave. It represents the total time required for ventricular depolarization and repolarization.

quadriceps-setting exercise Postoperative leg exercise performed by straightening the legs and pushing the back of the knees into the bed.

quadrigeminy A type of premature complex consisting of a repetitive four-beat pattern; usually occurs as three sequential normal complexes followed by a premature complex and a pause, with the same pattern repeating itself in a four-beat pattern.

quadriparesis Weakness that involves all four extremities; seen with cervical spinal cord injury.

qualitative question A clinical question that focuses on the meanings and interpretations of human phenomena or experience of people and usually analyzes the content of what a person says during an interview or what a researcher observes.

quality improvement A QSEN competency in which the nurse uses data to monitor the outcomes of care processes and uses improvement methods to design and test changes to continuously improve the quality and safety of health care systems.

quantitative question A clinical question that asks about the relationship between or among defined, measurable phenomena and includes statistical analysis of information that is collected to answer a question.

R

radiation dose The amount of radiation absorbed by the tissue.

radiation proctitis Rectal mucosa inflammation that results from external beam radiation therapy.

radical cystectomy Removal of the bladder and surrounding tissue with urinary diversion.

radicular Referring to a nerve root.

radiculopathy Referring to radicular pain; spinal nerve root involvement.

radiofrequency catheter ablation An invasive procedure that uses radiofrequency waves to abolish an irritable focus that is causing a supraventricular or ventricular tachydysrhythmia.

Rapid Response Team Team of critical care experts who save lives and decrease the risk for harm by providing care to patients before a respiratory or cardiac arrest occurs. Also called *Medical Emergency Team*.

rapidly progressive glomerulonephritis A primary inflammation of the glomeruli, nephrons, and kidney tissue that develops over several weeks to months.

RBC Red blood cell.

rebound headache Headache that occurs as a side effect of a drug that has relieved an initial migraine headache. Also called *medication overuse headache*.

recall memory Recent memory, which can be tested during the history taking by asking about items such as the dates of clinic or physician appointments.

receptive aphasia A type of aphasia caused by injury to Wernicke's area in the temporoparietal area of the brain and characterized by an inability to understand the spoken and written word; reading and writing ability are equally affected. Although the patient can talk, the language is often meaningless and neologisms (made-up words) are common parts of speech. Also called *Wernicke's aphasia* or *sensory aphasia*.

reconstructive plastic surgery Type of plastic surgery that corrects or improves functional defects that have occurred as a result of congenital problems, trauma and scarring, or other types of therapy.

recreational therapist A member of the health care team who works to help patients continue or develop hobbies or interests. Also called *activity therapist*.

rectocele A protrusion of the rectum through a weakened vaginal wall.

red reflex A reflection of light on the retina seen as a red glare during ophthalmoscopic examination. An absent red reflex may indicate a lens opacity or cloudiness of the vitreous.

redirection An intervention to help with communication problems in patients with dementia; consists of attracting the patient's attention before conversing, keeping the environment as free of distractions as possible, and speaking directly to the patient in a distinct manner using clear and short sentences.

reducible hernia A hernia that can be placed back into the abdominal cavity by gentle pressure.

reduction mammoplasty Breast reduction surgery in which the surgeon removes excess breast tissue and then repositions the nipple and remaining skin flaps to produce an optimal cosmetic effect.

Reed-Sternberg cell A specific cancer cell type, found in lymph nodes, that is a marker for Hodgkin's lymphoma.

re-epithelialization In partial-thickness (superficial) wounds involving damage to the epidermis and upper layers of the dermis, a form of healing by means of the production of new skin cells by undamaged epidermal cells in the basal layer of the dermis.

refeeding syndrome Life-threatening metabolic complication that can occur when nutrition is restarted for a patient who is in a starvation state.

reflex arc A closed circuit of spinal and peripheral nerves that requires no control by the brain.

reflex sympathetic dystrophy (RSD) See *complex regional pain syndrome*.

reflux esophagitis Damage to the esophageal mucosa, often with erosion and ulceration, in patients with gastroesophageal reflux disease.

reflux Reverse or backward flow.

refraction The bending of light rays.

refractory hypoxemia Low blood oxygen levels that persist even when 100% oxygen is given.

regional anesthesia A type of local anesthesia that blocks multiple peripheral nerves in a specific body region.

registered dietitian (RD) Member of the health care team who ensures that patients meet their nutritional needs. Also called *nutritionist*.

regurgitation Flowing in the opposite direction from normal, as the occurrence of warm fluid traveling up the throat, unaccompanied by nausea, in the patient with gastroesophageal reflux disease.

rehabilitation assistants Assistants to rehabilitation therapists.

rehabilitation case manager Nurse or other health care professional who coordinates health care for patients undergoing rehabilitation in home or acute care settings.

rehabilitation nurse Nurse who coordinates the efforts of health care team members for patients undergoing rehabilitation in the inpatient setting; may be designated as the patient's case manager.

rehabilitation therapists The collective group of physical therapists (PTs), occupational therapists (OTs), and speech-language pathologists (SLPs).

rehabilitation The process of learning to live with chronic and disabling conditions by returning the patient to the fullest possible physical, mental, social, vocational, and economic capacity.

reinfusion system A technique that allows for collection of red blood cells from a joint drain over a specific time frame, which then can be reinfused directly back into the patient's systemic circulation.

relapsing-remitting multiple sclerosis (RRMS) A type of multiple sclerosis that occurs in 85% of cases and is characterized by a mild or moderate course, depending on the degree of disability. Relapses develop over 1 to 2 weeks and resolve over 4 to 8 months, after which the patient returns to baseline.

reliever drugs Drugs used in asthma therapy to stop an asthma attack once it has started.

religions Formal belief systems that provide a framework for making sense of life, death, and suffering and responding to universal spiritual questions; a formal expression of spirituality.

relocation stress syndrome Physiologic or psychosocial distress following transfer from one environment to another, such as after admission to a hospital or nursing home. Also called *relocation trauma*.

reminiscence The process of randomly reflecting on memories of events in one's life.

remote memory Long-term memory of events; can be tested by asking patients about their birth date, schools attended, city of birth, or anything from the past that can be verified.

renal colic Severe pain associated with distention or spasm of the ureter, such as with an obstruction or the passing of a stone; the pain radiates into the perineal area, groin, scrotum, or labia. Pain may be intermittent or continuous and may be accompanied by pallor, diaphoresis, and hypotension.

renal columns Cortical tissue that dips into the interior of the kidney and separates the pyramids in the medulla. Also called *columns of Bertin*.

renal cortex The outermost layer of functional kidney tissue lying beneath the renal capsule.

renal osteodystrophy The problems in bone metabolism and structure caused by renal failure–induced hypocalcemia and hyperphosphatemia.

renal pelvis The expansion from the upper end of the ureter into which the calices of the kidney open.

renal threshold The limit to the amount of glucose that the kidney can reabsorb as glucose is filtered from the blood. Also called the *transport maximum*.

renin A hormone that is produced in the juxta-glomerular complex of the kidney and that helps regulate blood flow, glomerular filtration rate, and blood pressure. Renin is secreted when sensing cells (macula densa) in the distal convoluted tubule sense changes in blood volume and pressure.

repetitive stress injury (RSI) Injury caused by repeated movements of the same part of the body (e.g., carpal tunnel syndrome).

replication The reproduction of DNA that occurs each time a cell divides.

resident An individual who lives in an inpatient facility and has all the rights of anyone living in his or her home.

residuals Amount of feeding that remains in the stomach after enteral nutrition.

resistin A hormone produced by fat cells that creates resistance to insulin activity.

resorption In referring to bone, the loss of bone minerals and density; the release of free calcium from bone storage sites directly into the extracellular fluid.

restorative aide A member of the health care team, often with the nursing department, who assists the therapists, especially in the long-term care setting.

restraint Any device (physical restraint) or drug (chemical restraint) that prevents the patient from moving freely.

restrictive (lung disorder) Any lung disorder that prevents good expansion and recoil of the gas exchange unit.

restrictive cardiomyopathy A form of cardiomyopathy that restricts the filling of the ventricles; a type of lung disease that prevents good expansion and recoil of the gas exchange unit.

resurfacing Regrowth of new skin cells across the open area of a wound as it heals.

resuscitation phase The first phase of a burn injury, beginning at the onset of injury and continuing to about 48 hours.

rete pegs The fingers of epidermal tissue that project into the dermis.

reticular activating system (RAS) Special cells throughout the brainstem that constitute the system that controls awareness and alertness.

retina The innermost layer of the eye, made up of sensory receptors that transmit impulses to the optic nerve. It contains blood vessels and two types of photoreceptors called *rods* and *cones*. Rods work at low light levels and provide peripheral vision; cones are active at bright light levels and provide color and central vision.

retinal detachment Separation of the retina from the epithelium.

retinal hole A break in the retina; can be caused by trauma or can occur with aging.

retinal tear Jagged and irregularly shaped break in the retina resulting from traction on the retina.

retinopathy Inflammation of the retina. Also used as a general term for vision problems.

retrograde Going against the normal direction of flow.

retroviruses The family of viruses that includes the human immune deficiency virus.

revision arthroplasty Surgical replacement of a prosthesis that has loosened and is causing pain.

rhabdomyolysis The breakdown or disintegration of muscle tissue; associated with excretion of myoglobin in the urine.

rheumatic carditis Inflammatory lesions in the heart due to a sensitivity response that develops after an upper respiratory tract infection with group A beta-hemolytic streptococci, which occurs in about 40% of patients with rheumatic fever. Inflammation results in impaired contractile function of the myocardium, thickening of the pericardium, and valvular damage. Also called *rheumatic endocarditis*.

rheumatic disease Any disease or condition involving the musculoskeletal system.

rheumatoid arthritis (RA) A chronic, progressive, systemic, inflammatory autoimmune disease process that primarily affects the synovial joints; one of the most common connective tissue diseases and the most destructive to the joints.

rhinitis An inflammation of the nasal mucosa.

rhinoplasty A surgical reconstruction of the nose done for cosmetic purposes and improvement of airflow.

rhinorrhea Watery drainage from the nose; a "runny" nose.

rhinosinusitis An inflammation of the mucous membranes of one or more of the sinuses; usually seen with rhinitis, especially the common cold (coryza).

rickets Vitamin D deficiency in children.

right-sided heart (ventricular) failure The inability of the right ventricle to empty completely, resulting in increased volume and pressure in the systemic veins and systemic venous congestion with peripheral edema.

robotic technology Technology that provides mechanical parts for extremities when they are not functional or have been amputated.

Romberg sign Swaying or falling when the patient is standing with arms at the sides, feet and knees close together, and eyes closed; a test of equilibrium in neurologic assessment.

rotation A mechanism of injury in which the head is turned excessively beyond the normal range.

rubor Dusky red discoloration of the skin.

rugae Folds, as of a mucous membrane.

S

S₃ gallop The third heart sound; an early diastolic filling sound that indicates an increase in left ventricular pressure and may be heard on auscultation in patients with heart failure.

safer sex practices Interventions that reduce the risk of nonintact skin or mucous membranes coming in contact with infected body fluids and blood, such as using a condom.

safety A QSEN competency in which the nurse minimizes risk of harm to patients and providers through both system effectiveness and individual performance.

Salem sump tube Tube inserted through the nose and placed into the stomach that is attached to low continuous suction. It has a vent ("pigtail") that prevents the stomach mucosa from being pulled away during suctioning.

salpingitis Infection of the fallopian tube.

sanguineous Having a bloody appearance.

sarcoidosis A granulomatous disorder of unknown cause that can affect any organ but most often involves the lung.

SBAR Acronym for a formal method of communication between two or more members of the health care team. It is used most often when there is an unmet patient need or problem but can also be used to communicate continuing care issues when a patient is discharged from one agency to another. It consists of four steps: S̲ituation, B̲ackground, A̲ssessment, R̲ecommendation.

scabies A contagious skin disease caused by mite infestations.

sclera The external white layer of the eye.

scleroderma See *systemic sclerosis*.

sclerotherapy The injection of a sclerosing agent via a catheter, usually in an endoscopic procedure, to stop variceal bleeding.

sclerotic Hard, or hardening.

scoliosis An abnormal lateral curve in the spine, which normally should be a straight vertical line.

scotomas Changes in peripheral vision.

sebum A mildly bacteriostatic, fat-containing substance produced by the sebaceous glands. Sebum lubricates the skin and reduces water loss from the skin surface.

second intention Healing of deep tissue injuries or wounds with tissue loss in which a cavity-like defect requires gradual filling of the dead space with connective tissue, which prolongs the repair process.

secondary administration set A short conduit that is attached to the primary administration set at a Y-injection site and is used to deliver intermittent medications. Also called a *piggyback set*.

secondary gout Gout involving hyperuricemia.

secondary hypertension Elevated blood pressure that is related to a specific disease (e.g., kidney disease) or medication (e.g., estrogen).

secondary lesion Describing skin disease in terms of changes in the appearance of the primary lesion. These changes occur with progression of an underlying disease or in response to a topical or systemic therapeutic intervention.

secondary prevention Early detection of a disease or condition, sometimes before signs and symptoms are evident, to prevent or limit permanent disability or death.

secondary progressive multiple sclerosis (SPMS) A type of multiple sclerosis that begins with a relapsing-remitting course and later becomes steadily progressive. Attacks and partial recoveries may continue to occur.

secondary survey In the emergency department, a more comprehensive head-to-toe assessment performed to identify other injuries or medical issues that need to be managed or that might impact the course of treatment.

secondary tumor Additional tumor that is established when cancer cells move from the primary location to another area in the body. Also called *metastatic tumor*.

seizure An abnormal, sudden, excessive, uncontrolled electrical discharge of neurons within the brain that may result in an alteration in consciousness, motor or sensory ability, and/or behavior. A single seizure may occur for no known reason; however, seizures may be due to a pathologic condition of the brain, such as a tumor.

self-tolerance In immunology, the ability to recognize self cells versus non-self cells, which is necessary to prevent healthy body cells from being destroyed along with invading cells.

Sengstaken-Blakemore tube Tube similar to a nasogastric tube that is placed through the nose and into the stomach in which an attached balloon is inflated to apply pressure to bleeding variceal areas of the esophagus.

sensitivity The likelihood that infecting bacterial organisms will be killed or stopped by a particular antibiotic drug. Sensitivity is determined by testing different antibiotics against the organisms. Organisms are sensitive if the antibiotic is effective in stopping their growth; organisms are resistant if the antibiotic is not effective.

sensorineural hearing loss Hearing loss that results from a defect in the cochlea, the eighth cranial nerve, or the brain itself. Exposure to loud noises and music may cause this type of hearing loss as a result of damage to the cochlear hair cells.

sensory aphasia See *receptive aphasia*.

sensory perception The ability to perceive and interpret sensory input into one or more meaningful responses. Sensory input is usually received through the five major senses of vision, hearing, smell, taste, and touch.

sensory Facilitating sensation.

sentinel event As defined by The Joint Commission, an unexpected occurrence involving serious physical or psychological injury or the risk thereof and requiring an intense analysis of the contributing factors and corrective action.

sepsis Systemic infection.

septic shock The type of shock that occurs when large amounts of toxins and endotoxins produced by bacteria are released into the blood, causing a whole-body inflammatory reaction.

septicemia Systemic disease associated with sepsis; the presence of pathogens in the blood.

sequestrum A piece of necrotic bone that has separated from surrounding bone tissue; a common complication of osteomyelitis.

serologic testing Laboratory testing that is performed to identify pathogens by detecting antibodies to the organism.

serositis Inflammation of a serous membrane, such as the pleura or peritoneum.

serous Having a serum-like appearance, or yellow color.

serum sickness A type III hypersensitivity reaction that develops first as a skin rash and occurs within 3 to 21 days of the administration of antivenin (Crotalidae) polyvalent. This allergic response is often accompanied by other manifestations such as fever, arthralgias (joint pains), and pruritus (itching).

severe acute respiratory syndrome (SARS) An easily spread respiratory infection first identified in China in November 2002. At first appearing as an atypical pneumonia, it is caused by a new, more virulent form of coronavirus, and there is no known effective treatment.

severe sepsis The progression of sepsis with an amplified inflammatory response.

sex chromosomes The pair of chromosomes containing the genes for sexual differentiation in humans. In males, the sex chromosomes are an X and a Y; in females, the sex chromosomes are two Xs.

sex reassignment surgery (SRS) Surgery, particularly procedures that affect the external or internal genitalia, that transitions an individual from one's natal sex to one's inner gender identity. Also known as *gender reassignment surgery*.

sexuality An integration of the physiologic, emotional, and social aspects of well-being related to intimacy, self-concept, and role relationships.

sexually transmitted infections (STIs) Any of a group of diseases caused by infectious organisms that have been passed from one person to another through intimate contact. Some organisms that cause these diseases are transmitted only through sexual contact. Other organisms are transmitted by parenteral exposure to infected blood, fecal-oral transmission, intrauterine transmission to the fetus, and perinatal transmission from mother to neonate. Also known as *sexually transmitted diseases (STDs)*.

SHARE Acronym standing for Standardize critical content, Hardwire within your system, Allow opportunity to ask questions, Reinforce quality and measurement, Educate and coach.

shift to the left An increased number of immature neutrophils found on a differential count in patients with infections; can be characterized by changes in percentages of different types of leukocytes. Also known as *left shift*.

shock The whole-body response to poor tissue oxygenation. Any problem that impairs oxygen delivery to tissues and organs can start the syndrome of shock and lead to a life-threatening emergency.

short bone Bone that is small and bears little or no weight, such as the phalanges (fingers and toes).

short peripheral catheter A catheter that consists of a plastic cannula built around a sharp stylet for venipuncture, which extends slightly beyond the cannula and is advanced into the vein.

sialagogue An agent that stimulates the flow of saliva.

simple fracture See *closed fracture*.

single-photon emission computed tomography (SPECT) A diagnostic tool using a radiopharmaceutical (agent that enables radioisotopes to cross the blood-brain barrier) that is administered by IV injection, after which the patient is scanned.

sinoatrial (SA) node In the cardiac conduction system, the primary pacemaker of the heart; located close to the epicardial surface of the right atrium near its junction with the superior vena cava. It can spontaneously and rhythmically generate electrical impulses at a rate of 60 to 100 beats/min. Also called the *sinus node*.

sinus arrhythmia A variant of normal sinus rhythm that results from changes in intrathoracic pressure during breathing; heart rate increases slightly during inspiration and decreases slightly during exhalation. Atrial and ventricular rates are between 60 and 100 beats/min, and atrial and ventricular rhythms are irregular.

sinus bradycardia A cardiac dysrhythmia caused by a decreased rate of sinus node discharge, with a heart rate that is less than 60 beats/min.

sinus tachycardia A cardiac dysrhythmia caused by an increased rate of sinus node discharge, with a heart rate that is more than 100 beats/min.

sinusitis An inflammation of the mucous membranes of the sinuses.

SIRS Acronym for systemic inflammatory response syndrome, an inflammatory state affecting the whole body.

Sjögren's syndrome In patients with advanced rheumatoid arthritis, the triad of dry eyes, dry mouth, and dry vagina caused by the obstruction of secretory ducts and glands by inflammatory cells and immune complexes.

skilled nursing facility (SNF) Part of either a hospital or long-term care (nursing home) setting in which care is reimbursed through Medicare Part A for the first 21 days after admission.

skinfold measurement Measurement that estimates body fat.

smart pump An infusion pump with dosage calculation software.

social justice Ethical principle that refers to equality and fairness—that all patients should be treated equally and fairly, regardless of age, gender, religion, race, ethnicity, or education.

social worker Member of the health care team who helps patients identify support services and resources and who coordinates transfers to or discharges from the rehabilitation setting.

sodium (Na⁺) A mineral that is the major cation in the extracellular fluid and maintains extracellular fluid (ECF) osmolarity.

solute A particle dissolved or suspended in the water portion (solvent) of body fluids; a solution consists of a solute and a solvent.

solvent The water portion of fluids.

spastic bladder Incontinence characterized by sudden, gushing voids, usually without completely emptying the bladder; caused by neurologic problems affecting the upper motor neuron, such as with spinal cord injuries above the twelfth thoracic vertebra.

spastic paralysis Paralysis of a part of the body that is characterized by spasticity of muscles due to hypertonia; may be seen in the patient who has experienced a brain attack.

specialized nutrition support (SNS) Total nutritional intake orally or intravenously with commercially prepared products (either total enteral nutrition or total parenteral nutrition).

speech-language pathologist (SLP) A member of the rehabilitation health care team who evaluates and retrains patients with speech, language, or swallowing problems.

sphincter of Oddi The sheath of muscle fibers surrounding the papillary opening of the duodenum.

sphincterotomy A procedure for opening a sphincter.

spider angiomas See *telangiectasias.*

spinal cord stimulation An invasive stimulation technique that provides pain control by applying an electrical field over the spinal cord.

spinal fusion (arthrodesis) A surgical procedure to stabilize the spine after repeated laminectomies have been unsuccessful. Chips of bone are removed (typically from the iliac crest) or are obtained from donor bone; the chips are grafted between the vertebrae for support and to strengthen the back.

spinal shock syndrome Loss of reflex activity below the level of a spinal lesion; occurs immediately after injury as a result of disruption in the communication pathways between the upper motor neurons and the lower motor neurons. Also called *spinal shock.*

spinal shock See *spinal shock syndrome.*

spinal stenosis Narrowing of the spinal canal; typically seen in people older than 60 years.

spiritual counselor Counselor who specializes in spiritual assessments and care, usually a member of the clergy.

spirituality The connection to self, others, the environment, and a "higher power."

splenectomy Surgical removal of the spleen.

splenomegaly Enlargement of the spleen.

splint Any object or device that extends to the joints above and below a fracture to immobilize it.

splinter hemorrhage Black longitudinal line or small red streak on the distal third of the nail bed; seen in patients with infective endocarditis.

spondee Two-syllable words in which there is generally equal stress on each syllable, such as *airplane, railroad,* and *cowboy;* used in testing speech reception threshold.

spondylolisthesis Condition in which one vertebra slips forward on the one below it, often as a result of spondylolysis. This problem causes pressure on the nerve roots, leading to pain in the lower back and into the buttocks.

spondylolysis A defect in one of the vertebrae; usually found in the lumbar spine.

spontaneous bacterial peritonitis (SBP) Bacterial infection of the abdominal peritoneum caused by ascites; often seen in patients with cirrhosis of the liver.

spore An encapsulated inactive organism.

sprain Excessive stretching of a ligament.

ST segment In the electrocardiogram, the line (normally isoelectric) representing early ventricular repolarization. It occurs from the J point to the beginning of the T wave.

staging System of classifying clinical aspects of a cancer tumor.

Standard Precautions Infection control guidelines from the U.S. Centers for Disease Control and Prevention stating that all body excretions, secretions, and moist membranes and tissues are potentially infectious; combines protective measures from Universal Precautions and Body Substance Isolation.

stasis dermatitis In patients with venous insufficiency, discoloration of the skin along the ankles, which may extend up to the calf.

stasis ulcer In patients with long-term venous insufficiency, ulcer formed as a result of edema or minor injury to the limb; typically occurs over the malleolus.

status epilepticus Prolonged seizures lasting more than 5 minutes or repeated seizures over the course of 30 minutes; a potential complication of all types of seizures.

steatorrhea An excessive amount of fat in the stool.

ST-elevation myocardial infarction (STEMI) Myocardial infarction in which the patient typically has ST elevation in two contiguous leads on a 12-lead ECG; this indicates myocardial infarction/necrosis.

stem cell An immature, undifferentiated cell produced by the bone marrow.

stent A small tube that is placed in a tubular structure to dilate it; a wirelike device that may be used along with percutaneous transluminal angioplasty to help keep the vessel open.

stereotactic pallidotomy A surgical treatment for the patient with Parkinson disease when drugs are ineffective in symptom management. An electrode is used to create a lesion in a targeted area within the pallidum, with the goal of reducing tremor and rigidity.

sterilization A method of infection control in which all living organisms and bacterial spores are destroyed; used on items that invade human tissue where bacteria are not commonly found.

stoma The surgical creation of an opening; usually refers to an opening in the abdominal wall.

stomatitis Inflammation of the oral mucosa; characterized by painful single or multiple ulcerations that impair the protective lining of the mouth. The ulcerations are commonly referred to as "canker sores."

strain Excessive stretching of a muscle or tendon when it is weak or unstable; sometimes referred to as "muscle pulls."

strangulated hernia A tightly constricted hernia that compromises the blood supply to the herniated segment of the bowel as a result of pressure from the hernial ring (the band of muscle around the hernia); leads to ischemia and obstruction of the bowel loop, with necrosis of the bowel and possibly bowel perforation.

strangulated obstruction Intestinal obstruction with compromised blood flow.

stratum corneum The outermost layer of the skin.

stress test See *exercise electrocardiography.*

stress ulcers Multiple shallow erosions of the proximal stomach and occasionally the duodenum.

stress urinary incontinence (SUI) Loss of urine during activities that increase intra-abdominal pressure, such as laughing, coughing, sneezing, or lifting heavy objects.

striae Reddish purple streaks on the skin. Also called *stretch marks.*

stricture Narrowing.

stridor A high-pitched crowing sound caused by laryngospasm or edema above or below the glottis; heard during respiration.

stroke volume (SV) The amount of blood ejected by the left ventricle during each heartbeat.

stroke See *brain attack.*

stuporous Arousable only with vigorous or painful stimulation.

subarachnoid space Term for the space between the arachnoid mater and pia mater of the spinal cord. Also called *subarachnoid.*

subcutaneous emphysema The presence of bubbles under the skin because of air trapping; an uncommon late complication of fracture.

subcutaneous infusion therapy Infusion therapy that is delivered under the skin when patients cannot tolerate oral medications, when intramuscular injections are too painful, or when vascular access is not available.

subcutaneous nodule Characteristic round, movable, nontender swelling under the skin of the arm or fingers in patients with severe rheumatoid arthritis.

subdural hematoma (SDH) The collection of clotted blood that typically results from venous bleeding into the space beneath the dura and above the arachnoid.

subdural space Term for the space between the dura mater and the middle layer (arachnoid).

subluxation Partial joint dislocation.

submucous resection (SMR) Surgical procedure to straighten a deviated septum when chronic symptoms or discomfort occur. Also called *nasoseptoplasty.*

submucous resection Surgical procedure to straighten a deviated septum.

substernally Located below the ribs.

subtotal thyroidectomy The surgical removal of part of the thyroid tissue.

sundowning In patients with Alzheimer's disease, increased confusion at night or when excessively fatigued.

superinfection Reinfection or a second infection of the same type.

supervision Guidance or direction, evaluation, and follow-up by the nurse to ensure that the task or activity is performed appropriately.

supratentorial Located within the cerebral hemispheres, in the area above the tentorium of the cerebellum; the tentlike fold of dura that surrounds the cerebellar hemisphere and supports the occipital lobe.

supraventricular tachycardia (SVT) A form of tachycardia that involves the rapid stimulation of atrial tissue at a rate of 100 to 280 beats/min. It is most often due to a re-entry mechanism in which one impulse circulates repeatedly throughout the atrial pathway, re-stimulating the atrial tissue at a rapid rate.

surfactant A fatty protein secreted by type II pneumocytes to reduce surface tension in the alveoli.

surveillance Term used to describe the tracking of infections by health care agencies.

susceptibility The risk of the host to infection; may be increased by the breakdown of host defenses against pathogens.

swimmer's ear See *external otitis.*

sympathectomy Surgical cutting of the sympathetic nerve branches via endoscopy through a small axillary incision.

sympathetic tone A state of partial blood vessel constriction caused when nerves from the sympathetic division of the autonomic nervous system continuously stimulate vascular smooth muscle.

synapse The area through which impulses are transmitted to their eventual destination.

syncope Transient loss of consciousness (blackouts), most commonly caused by decreased perfusion to the brain.

syndrome of inappropriate antidiuretic hormone (SIADH) Persistent hyponatremia, hypovolemia, and inappropriately elevated urine osmolality that occurs when vasopressin (antidiuretic hormone) is secreted even when plasma osmolarity is low or normal.

synovectomy The surgical removal of synovium.

synovial joint Type of joint lined with synovium, a membrane that secretes synovial fluid for lubrication and shock absorption.

synovitis Inflammation of synovial membrane.

syphilis A complex sexually transmitted disease that can become systemic and cause serious complications and even death. It is caused by the spirochete *Treponema pallidum,* which is found in the mouth, intestinal tract, and genital areas of people and animals. The infection is usually transmitted by sexual contact, but transmission can occur through close body contact and kissing.

syringe pump Pump for infusion therapy that uses a battery-powered piston to push the plunger continuously at a selected mL/hr rate; limited to small-volume continuous or intermittent infusions.

systemic lupus erythematosus (SLE) A chronic, progressive inflammatory connective tissue disorder that can cause major body organs and systems to fail; characterized by spontaneous remissions and exacerbations.

systemic sclerosis (SSc) A chronic connective tissue disease characterized by inflammation, fibrosis, and sclerosis of the skin and vital organs. Also called *scleroderma* and formerly called *progressive systemic sclerosis.*

systemic Affecting the body system as a whole.

systole The phase of the cardiac cycle that consists of the contraction and emptying of the atria and ventricles.

systolic blood pressure The amount of pressure/force generated by the left ventricle to distribute blood into the aorta with each contraction of the heart.

systolic heart failure (systolic ventricular dysfunction) Heart failure that results when the heart is unable to contract forcefully enough during systole to eject adequate amounts of blood into the circulation.

T

T wave In the electrocardiogram, the deflection that follows the ST segment and represents ventricular repolarization.

tachycardia An excessively fast heart rate; characterized as a pulse rate greater than 100 beats/min.

tachydysrhythmia An abnormal heart rhythm with a rate greater than 100 beats/min.

tactile (vocal) fremitus A vibration of the chest wall produced when the patient speaks; can be palpated on the chest wall.

target tissues The tissues that respond specifically to a given hormone.

taut Tightly stretched.

teamwork and collaboration A QSEN competency in which the nurse functions effectively within nursing and interprofessional teams, fostering open communication, mutual respect, and shared decision making to achieve quality patient care.

telangiectasias Vascular lesions with a red center and radiating branches. Also called *spider angiomas, spider nevi,* or *vascular spiders.*

telemetry In electrocardiography (ECG), the use of a battery-powered transmitter system for monitoring an ambulatory patient; allows freedom of movement within a certain radius without losing transmission of the ECG.

temporal field blindness A decrease in lateral peripheral vision.

temporary pacing A nonsurgical intervention for cardiac dysrhythmia that provides a timed electrical stimulus to the heart when either the impulse initiation or the intrinsic conduction system of the heart is defective.

tendon transplant Removal of a tendon from one part of the body and transplantation into the affected area to replace a ruptured tendon that cannot be repaired surgically.

tendon Any one of many bands of tough, fibrous tissue that attach muscles to bones.

tenesmus Straining, especially painful straining to defecate.

tension pneumothorax A life-threatening complication of pneumothorax in which air continues to enter the pleural space during inspiration and does not exit during expiration.

teratogenic Tending to produce birth defects.

tetany Continuous contractions of muscle groups; hyperexcitability of nerves and muscles.

tetraplegia Another term for *quadriplegia* (paralysis that involves all four extremities).

thalamotomy An alternative to stereotactic pallidotomy as a surgical treatment for the patient with Parkinson disease; uses thermocoagulation of brain cells to reduce tremor. Usually only unilateral surgery is performed to benefit the side of the body most affected by the disease.

thalamus A structure within the brain; functions as the "central switchboard" for the central nervous system.

thallium scan A test that is similar to a bone scan but uses the radioisotope *thallium* and is more sensitive in diagnosing the extent of disease in patients with osteosarcoma.

The Joint Commission An organization that offers peer evaluation for accreditation every 3 years for all types of health care agencies that meet their standards. Formerly known as the *Joint Commission for Accreditation of Healthcare Organizations (JCAHO).*

therapeutic hypothermia Treatment that lowers the body core temperature to reduce the risk of cell, tissue, and organ damage from a low or absent blood flow. Usually follows cardiac arrest.

thermotherapy Technique for treating benign prostatic hyperplasia that uses a variety of heat methods to destroy excess prostate tissue.

third intention Delayed primary closure of a wound with a high risk for infection. The wound is intentionally left open for several days until inflammation has subsided and is then closed by first intention.

thoracentesis The aspiration of pleural fluid or air from the pleural space.

threshold In evaluating hearing, the lowest level of intensity at which pure tones and speech are heard by a patient; in general, the lowest level at which a stimulus is perceived.

thrombectomy Removal of a clot (thrombus) from a blood vessel.

thrombocytopenia A reduction in the number of blood platelets below the level needed for normal coagulation, resulting in an increased tendency to bleed.

thrombophlebitis The presence of a thrombus associated with inflammation; usually occurs in the deep veins of the lower extremities.

thrombosis The formation of a blood clot (thrombus) within a blood vessel.

thrombotic stroke Damage to the brain when blood flow is impaired from a clot, resulting in blockage to one or more of the arteries supplying blood to the brain.

thrombus A blood clot believed to result from an endothelial injury, venous stasis, or hypercoagulability.

thymectomy Removal of the thymus gland.

thymoma An encapsulated tumor of the thymus gland.

thyrocalcitonin (TCT) A hormone produced and secreted by the parafollicular cells of the thyroid gland to help regulate serum calcium levels; secreted in response to excess plasma calcium.

thyroid storm (thyroid crisis) A life-threatening event that occurs in patients with uncontrolled hyperthyroidism and is usually caused by Graves' disease. Key manifestations include fever, tachycardia, and systolic hypertension.

thyroiditis Inflammation of the thyroid gland.

thyrotoxicosis The condition caused by excessive amounts of thyroid hormones.

thyroxine (T_4) A hormone that is produced by the follicular cells of the thyroid gland and that increases metabolism.

Tinel's sign Test that confirms a diagnosis of carpal tunnel syndrome; a positive test causes palmar paresthesias when the area of the median nerve is tapped lightly.

tinnitus A continuous ringing or noise perception in the ears.

tissue integrity The intactness of the structure and function of the integument (skin and subcutaneous tissue) and mucous membranes.

titration Adjustment of IV fluid rate on the basis of the patient's urine output plus serum electrolyte values.

TNM (tumor, node, metastasis) System developed by the American Joint Committee on Cancer to describe the anatomic extent of cancers.

toe brachial pressure index (TBPI) Toe systolic pressure divided by brachial (arm) systolic pressure; may be performed instead of or in addition to ankle-brachial index to determine arterial perfusion in the feet and toes.

toll-like receptors (TLRs) Receptors on immune system cells of humans and other animals that interact with the surface of any invading organism and allow recognition of non-self so actions are taken to rid the body of this invader.

tonic phase Pertaining to a state of stiffening or rigidity of the muscles, particularly of the arms and legs, and immediate loss of consciousness of a tonic-clonic seizure.

tonsillitis An inflammation and infection of the tonsils and lymphatic tissues located on each side of the throat.

tophi A collection of uric acid crystals that form hard irregular, painless nodules on the ears, arms, and fingers of patients with gout.

topical chemical débridement Method of débriding a wound by applying topical enzyme preparations to loosen necrotic tissue.

torn meniscus Tear of the knee meniscus (medial or lateral) in which the patient typically has pain, swelling, and tenderness in the knee.

torsades de pointes A type of ventricular tachycardia that is related to a prolonged QT interval.

total hysterectomy Removal of the uterus and cervix; the procedure may be vaginal or abdominal.

total joint arthroplasty (TJA) Surgical creation of a joint, or total joint replacement; commonly performed in patients with osteoarthritis. Also called *total joint replacement (TJR)*.

total joint replacement (TJR) See *total joint arthroplasty*.

total parenteral nutrition (TPN) Provision of intensive nutritional support for an extended time; delivered to the patient through access to central veins, usually the subclavian or internal jugular veins.

total thyroidectomy The surgical removal of all of the thyroid tissue.

touch discrimination Part of the neurologic examination. The patient closes his or her eyes while the practitioner touches the patient with a finger and asks that the patient point to the area touched.

toxic and drug-induced hepatitis Liver inflammation resulting from exposure to hepatotoxins (e.g., industrial toxins, alcohol, and medications).

toxic epidermal necrolysis (TEN) A rare acute drug reaction of the skin that results in diffuse erythema and blister formation, with mucous membrane involvement and systemic toxicity.

toxic megacolon Acute enlargement of the colon along with fever, leukocytosis, and tachycardia; usually associated with ulcerative colitis.

toxic multinodular goiter Hyperthyroidism caused by multiple thyroid nodules, which may be enlarged thyroid tissues or adenomas, and a goiter that has been present for several years.

toxic shock syndrome (TSS) A severe illness caused by a toxin produced by certain strains of *Staphylococcus aureus*. It was first recognized in 1980 as related to menstruation and tampon use. It is characterized by abrupt onset of a high fever and headache, sore throat, vomiting, diarrhea, generalized rash, and hypotension. The most common manifestations are skin changes (initially a rash that resembles a severe sunburn and changes to a macular erythema similar to a drug-related rash).

toxidrome A syndrome related to drug toxicity.

toxin Protein molecule released by bacteria that affects host cell at a distant site. Continued multiplication of a pathogen is sometimes accompanied by toxin production.

trabeculation An abnormal thickening of the bladder wall caused by urinary retention and obstruction.

tracheostomy The (tracheal) stoma, or opening, that results from a tracheotomy.

tracheotomy The surgical incision into the trachea for the purpose of establishing an airway.

trachoma A chronic conjunctivitis caused by *Chlamydia trachomatis*.

traction The application of a pulling force to a part of the body to provide reduction, alignment, and rest.

transcellular fluid Any of the fluids in special body spaces, including cerebrospinal fluid, synovial fluid, peritoneal fluid, and pleural fluid.

transcutaneous electrical nerve stimulation (TENS) A battery-operated device capable of delivering small electrical currents through electrodes applied to an area of the body to relieve pain.

transcutaneous pacing Temporary pacing that is accomplished through the application of two large external electrodes.

transesophageal echocardiography (TEE) A form of echocardiography performed transesophageally (through the esophagus); an ultrasound transducer is placed immediately behind the heart in the esophagus or stomach to examine cardiac structure and function.

transferrin An iron-transport protein that can be measured directly or calculated as an indirect measurement of total iron-binding capacity.

transgender Patients who self-identify as the opposite gender or a gender that does not match their natal sex.

transient ischemic attack (TIA) A brief attack (lasting a few minutes to less than 24 hours) of focal neurologic dysfunction caused by a brief interruption in cerebral blood flow, possibly resulting from cerebral vasospasm or transient systemic arterial hypertension. Repeated attacks may damage brain tissue; multiple attacks indicate significant increased risk for brain attack.

transition manager A role of the professional nurse to facilitate continuity of care for patients as they transfer among health care settings and the community.

transmyocardial laser revascularization A new surgical procedure for patients with unstable angina and inoperable coronary artery disease with areas of reversible myocardial ischemia. After a single-lung intubation, a left anterior thoracotomy is performed and the heart is visualized. A laser is used to create 20 to 24 long, narrow channels through the left ventricular muscle to the left ventricle. The channels eventually allow oxygenated blood to flow from the left ventricle during diastole to nourish the muscle.

transport maximum See *renal threshold*.

transsexual A person who has modified his or her natal body to match the appropriate gender identity, either through cosmetic, hormonal, or surgical means.

transurethral microwave therapy (TUMT) Procedure for treating benign prostatic hyperplasia using high temperatures to heat and destroy excess tissue.

transurethral needle ablation (TUNA) Procedure for treating benign prostatic hyperplasia using low radiofrequency energy to shrink the prostate.

transurethral resection of the prostate (TURP) The traditional "closed" surgical procedure for removal of the prostate. In this procedure, the surgeon inserts a resectoscope (an instrument similar to a cystoscope, but with a cutting and cauterizing loop) through the urethra. The enlarged portion of the prostate gland is then resected in small pieces.

trauma center Specialty care facility that provides competent and timely trauma services to patients depending on its designated level of capability.

trauma system An organized and integrated approach to trauma care designed to ensure that all critical elements of trauma care delivery are aligned to meet the injured patient's needs.

trauma Bodily injury.

triage officer In a hospital's emergency response plan, the person who rapidly evaluates each patient who arrives at the hospital. In a large hospital, this person is generally a physician who is assisted by triage nurses; however, a nurse may assume this role when physician resources are limited.

triage In the emergency department, sorting or classifying patients into priority levels depending on illness or injury severity, with the highest acuity needs receiving the quickest evaluation and treatment.

trigeminy A type of premature complex consisting of a repetitive three-beat pattern; usually occurs as two sequential normal complexes followed by a premature complex and a pause, with the same pattern repeating itself in triplets.

trigger points In patients with fibromyalgia syndrome, tender areas that can typically be palpated to elicit pain in a predictable, reproducible pattern.

triglycerides Serum lipid profile that includes the measurement of cholesterol and lipoproteins.

triiodothyronine (T$_3$) A hormone produced by the follicular cells of the thyroid gland.

troponin A myocardial muscle protein released into the bloodstream after injury to myocardial muscle. Because it is not found in healthy patients, any rise in values indicates cardiac necrosis or acute myocardial infarction.

truss A device, usually a pad made with firm material, that is held in place over the hernia with a belt to keep the abdominal contents from protruding into the hernial sac.

tuberculosis (TB) A highly communicable disease caused by *Mycobacterium tuberculosis*. It is the most common bacterial infection worldwide.

tumescence The condition of being swollen.

tunneled central venous catheter A type of catheter used for long-term infusion therapy in which a portion of the catheter lies in a subcutaneous tunnel, separating the points where the catheter enters the vein from where it exits the skin.

turbidity Cloudiness of a solution.

turbinates Three bony projections that protrude into the nasal cavities from the walls of the internal portion of the nose.

turgor The condition of being swollen and congested; indicates the amount of skin elasticity; the normal resiliency of a pinched fold of skin.

type A gastritis A type of gastritis that refers to an inflammation of the glands, fundus, and body of the stomach.

type B gastritis A type of gastritis that affects the glands of the antrum and may involve the entire stomach.

tyrosine kinase inhibitors (TKIs) Drugs with the main action of inhibiting activation of tyrosine kinases. There are many different TKIs. Some are unique to the cell type; others may be present only in cancer cells that express a specific gene mutation. As a result, the different TKI drugs are effective in disrupting the growth of some cancer cell types and not others.

U

U wave In the electrocardiogram, the deflection that follows the T wave and may result from slow repolarization of ventricular Purkinje fibers. When present, it is of the same polarity as the T wave, although generally smaller. Abnormal prominence of the U wave suggests an electrolyte abnormality or other disturbance.

ulcerative colitis (UC) A chronic inflammatory process that affects the mucosal lining of the colon or rectum; one of a group of bowel diseases of unknown etiology characterized by remissions and exacerbations. It can result in loose stools containing blood and mucus, poor absorption of vital nutrients, and thickening of the colon wall.

umbilical hernia Protrusion of the intestine at the umbilicus; can be congenital or acquired. Congenital umbilical hernias appear in infancy. Acquired umbilical hernias directly result from increased intra-abdominal pressure and are most commonly seen in obese people.

unclassified seizure One of the three broad categories of seizure disorders along with *partial seizure* and *generalized seizure*. They occur for no known reason, do not fit into the generalized or partial classifications, and account for about half of all seizure activity. Also called *idiopathic seizure*.

uncus The inner part of the temporal lobe of the brain that can move downward and cause pressure on the brainstem; the vital sign center.

undermining Separation of the skin layers at the wound margins from the underlying granulation tissue.

unilateral body neglect syndrome In the patient who has had a brain attack, an unawareness of the existence of the paralyzed side. For example, the patient may believe he or she is sitting up straight when actually he or she is leaning to one side. Another typical example is the patient who washes or dresses only one side of the body.

Unna boot A wound dressing constructed of gauze moistened with zinc oxide; used to promote venous return in the ambulatory patient with a stasis ulcer and to form a sterile environment for the ulcer. The boot is applied to the affected limb, from the toes to the knee, after the ulcer has been cleaned with normal saline solution and covered with an elastic wrap. The dressing hardens like a cast.

upper endoscopy See *esophagogastroduodenoscopy*.

upper esophageal sphincter (UES) The ringlike band of muscle fibers at the upper end of the esophagus. When at rest, the sphincter is closed to prevent air from entering into the esophagus during respiration.

upper GI (gastrointestinal) radiographic series The radiographic visualization of the gastrointestinal tract from the oral part of the pharynx to the duodenojejunal junction; used to detect disorders of structure or function of the esophagus (barium swallow), stomach, or duodenum.

uremia The accumulation of nitrogenous wastes in the blood (azotemia); a result of renal failure, with clinical symptoms including nausea and vomiting.

uremic frost A layer of urea crystals from evaporated sweat; may appear on the face, eyebrows, axilla, and groin in patients with advanced uremic syndrome.

uremic syndrome The systemic clinical and laboratory manifestations of end-stage kidney disease.

ureterolithiasis Formation of stones in the ureter.

ureteropelvic junction (UPJ) The narrow area in the upper third of the ureter at the point at which the renal pelvis becomes the ureter.

ureteroplasty Surgical repair of the ureter.

ureterovesical junction (UVJ) The point at which each ureter becomes narrow as it enters the bladder.

urethral meatus The opening at the endpoint of the urethra.

urethral stricture An obstruction that occurs low in the urinary tract due to decreased diameter of the urethra, causing bladder distention before hydroureter and hydronephrosis.

urethritis An inflammation of the urethra that causes symptoms similar to urinary tract infection.

urethroplasty Surgical treatment of the urethral stricture to remove the affected area with or without grafting to create a larger opening.

urgency The feeling that urination will occur immediately.

urgent triage In a three-tiered triage scheme, the category that includes patients who should be treated quickly but in whom an immediate threat to life does not currently exist, such as those with abdominal pain or displaced fractures or dislocations.

urinary tract infection (UTI) An infection in the normally sterile urinary system. The unobstructed and complete passage of urine from the renal and urinary systems is critical in maintaining a sterile urinary tract. When any structural abnormality is present, the risk for damage as a result of infection is greatly increased.

urolithiasis The presence of calculi (stones) in the urinary tract.

urosepsis The spread of an infection from the urinary tract to the bloodstream, resulting in systemic infection accompanied by fever, chills, hypotension, and altered mental status.

urticaria A transient vascular reaction of the skin marked by the development of wheals (hives).

uterine artery embolization Treatment for leiomyomas in which a radiologist uses a percutaneous catheter inserted through the femoral artery to inject polyvinyl alcohol pellets into the uterine artery. The resulting blockage starves the tumor of circulation, allowing it (or them) to shrink.

uterine prolapse Downward displacement of the uterus into the vagina.

uvea The middle layer of the eye, which consists of the choroid, ciliary body, and iris. The choroid has many blood vessels that supply nutrients to the retina.

V

vagal maneuver Nonsurgical management of cardiac dysrhythmias that is intended to induce vagal stimulation of the cardiac conduction system, specifically the sinoatrial and atrioventricular nodes. Vagal maneuvers may be attempted to terminate supraventricular tachydysrhythmia.

vaginoplasty The construction of a new vagina in a male-to-female patient, usually with inverted penile tissue or a colon graft, and the creation of a clitoris and labia using scrotal or penile tissue and skin grafts.

validation therapy For the patient with moderate or severe Alzheimer's disease, the process of recognizing and acknowledging the patient's feelings and concerns without reinforcing an erroneous belief (e.g., if the patient is looking for his or her deceased mother).

Valsalva maneuver A form of vagal stimulation of the cardiac conduction system in which the health care provider instructs the patient to bear down as if straining to have a bowel movement.

valvular regurgitation Regurgitation of any heart valve. See also *mitral regurgitation*.

variant (Prinzmetal's) angina A type of angina caused by coronary vasospasm (vessel spasm); usually associated with elevation of the ST segment on an electrocardiogram obtained during anginal attacks.

varicose veins Distended, protruding veins that appear darkened and tortuous; common in patients older than 30 years whose occupations require prolonged standing. As the vein wall weakens and dilates, venous pressure increases and the valves become incompetent (defective). The incompetent valves enhance the vessel dilation, and the veins become tortuous and distended.

vascular access device (VAD) A catheter; a plastic tube placed in a blood vessel to deliver fluids and medications.

vasculitis Blood vessel inflammation.

vasoconstriction Decrease in diameter of blood vessels.

vasopressin Secretion of the posterior pituitary gland. Also known as *antidiuretic hormone* or *ADH*.

vasospasm A sudden and transient constriction of a blood vessel.

Vaughn-Williams classification System used to categorize antidysrhythmic agents according to their effects on the action potential of cardiac cells.

vegan A vegetarian diet pattern in which only foods of plant origin are eaten.

venous beading A complication of diabetes; the abnormal appearance of retinal veins in which areas of swelling and constriction along a segment of vein resemble links of sausage. Such bleeding occurs in areas of retinal ischemia and is a predictor of proliferative diabetic retinopathy.

venous insufficiency Alteration of venous efficiency by thrombosis or defective valves; caused by prolonged venous hypertension, which stretches the veins and damages the valves, resulting in further venous hypertension, edema, and, eventually, venous stasis ulcers, swelling, and cellulitis.

venous thromboembolism (VTE) A term that refers to both deep vein thrombosis and pulmonary embolism; obstruction by a thrombus.

ventilator-associated events (VAEs) Complications of ventilator therapy that result in a significant and sustained deterioration in oxygenation (greater than 20% increase in the daily minimum fraction of inspired oxygen or an increase of at least 3 cm H_2O in the daily minimum positive end-expiratory pressure [PEEP] to maintain oxygenation).

ventilator-associated lung injury (VALI) Damage from prolonged ventilation causing loss of surfactant, increased inflammation, fluid leakage, and noncardiac pulmonary edema. Also known as *ventilator-induced lung injury*.

ventilator-induced lung injury (VILI) See *ventilator-associated lung injury*.

ventral hernia See *incisional hernia*.

ventricular asystole The complete absence of any ventricular rhythm. There are no electrical impulses in the ventricles and therefore no ventricular depolarization, no QRS complex, no contraction, no cardiac output, and no pulse, respirations, or blood pressure. The patient is in full cardiac arrest.

ventricular fibrillation (VF) A cardiac dysrhythmia that results from electrical chaos in the ventricles; impulses from many irritable foci fire in a totally disorganized manner so that ventricular contraction cannot occur; there is no cardiac output or pulse and therefore no cerebral, myocardial, or systemic perfusion. This rhythm is rapidly fatal if not successfully terminated within 3 to 5 minutes.

ventricular gallop An abnormal third heart sound that arises from vibrations of the valves and supporting structures and is produced during the rapid passive filling phase of ventricular diastole when blood flows from the atrium to a noncompliant ventricle. In patients older than 35 years, it is an early sign of heart failure or ventricular septal defect.

ventricular remodeling (1) Progressive myocyte (myocardial cell) contractile dysfunction over time; results from activation of the renin-angiotensin system caused by reduced blood flow to the kidneys, a common occurrence in low-output states; (2) after a myocardial infarction, permanent changes in the size and shape of the left ventricle due to scar tissue; such remodeling may decrease left ventricular function, cause heart failure, and increase morbidity and mortality.

ventricular tachycardia (VT) An abnormal heart rhythm that occurs with repetitive firing of an irritable ventricular ectopic focus, usually at a rate of 140 to 180 beats/min or more.

ventriculomyomectomy The surgical excision of a portion of the hypertrophied ventricular septum to create a widened outflow tract in patients with obstructive hypertrophic cardiomyopathy. Also called *ventricular septal myectomy*.

veracity Ethical principle that requires that the nurse is obligated to tell the truth to the best of his or her knowledge.

vertebroplasty A minimally invasive surgery for managing vertebral fractures in patients with osteoporosis. Bone cement is injected directly into the fracture site to provide immediate pain relief.

vertigo A sense of spinning movement that may result from diseases of the inner ear.

vesicant medications Drugs that cause severe tissue damage if they escape into the subcutaneous tissue; also referred to as vesicants.

vesicants Chemicals or drugs that cause tissue damage on direct contact or extravasation.

vesicle In health care, a small bladder or blister.

vestibule A longitudinal area between the labia minora, the clitoris, and the vagina that contains Bartholin glands and the openings of the urethra, Skene's glands (paraurethral glands), and vagina.

viral hepatitis Inflammation of the liver that results from an infection caused by one of five major categories of viruses (hepatitis A, B, C, D, or E). Viral hepatitis is the most common type and can be either acute or chronic.

viral load testing Test that measures the presence of human immune deficiency virus genetic material (ribonucleic acid) or other viral proteins in the patient's blood.

Virchow's triad The occurrence of stasis of blood flow, endothelial injury, or hypercoagulability; often associated with thrombus formation.

viremia The presence of viruses in the blood.

virilization The presence of male secondary sex characteristics.

virtual colonoscopy A noninvasive alternative to the colonoscopy procedure. A scanner is used to view the colon.

virulence A term used to describe the frequency with which a pathogen causes disease (degree of communicability) and its ability to invade and damage a host. Virulence can also indicate the severity of the disease; often used as a synonym for *pathogenicity*.

visceral proteins Proteins such as albumin that circulate in the bloodstream and may be produced by the liver.

vitiligo An abnormality of the skin characterized by patchy areas of pigment loss with increased pigmentation at the edges. It is seen with primary hypofunction of the adrenal glands and is due to autoimmune destruction of melanocytes in the skin.

vitreous body The clear, thick gel that fills the vitreous chamber of the eye (the space between the lens and the retina). This gel transmits light and shapes the eye.

vocational counselor A member of the rehabilitative health care team who assists the patient with job placement, training, or further education.

volutrauma Damage to the lung by excess volume delivered to one lung over the other.

volvulus Obstruction of the bowel caused by twisting of the bowel.

vulva The external female genitalia.

vulvovaginitis Inflammation of the lower genital tract resulting from a disturbance of the balance of hormones and flora in the vagina and vulva.

W

warm antibody anemia A form of immunohemolytic anemia (in which the immune system attacks a person's own red blood cells for unknown reasons) that occurs with immunoglobulin G antibody excess and may be triggered by drugs, chemicals, or other autoimmune problems.

warm phase A phase lasting 2 to 3 weeks after peripheral nerve trauma resulting in complete denervation; the extremity is warm, and the skin appears flushed or rosy. The warm phase is gradually superseded by a cold phase.

water brash Reflex salivary hypersecretion that occurs in response to reflux in the patient with gastroesophageal reflux disease.

WBC White blood cell.

weaning The process of going from ventilatory dependence to spontaneous breathing.

wedge resection Removal of small, localized areas of disease.

Wernicke's aphasia See *receptive aphasia*.

Wernicke's area An important speech area of the cerebrum. It is located in the temporal lobe and plays a significant role in higher-level brain function. It enables the processing of words into coherent thought and recognition of the idea behind written or printed words (language).

Whipple procedure (radical pancreaticoduodenectomy) A surgical treatment for cancer of the head of the pancreas. The procedure entails removal of the proximal head of the pancreas, the duodenum, a portion of the jejunum, the stomach (partial or total gastrectomy), and the gallbladder, with anastomosis of the pancreatic duct (pancreaticojejunostomy), the common bile duct (choledochojejunostomy), and the stomach (gastrojejunostomy) to the jejunum.

white matter In the spinal cord, myelinated axons that surround the gray matter (neuron cell bodies).

Williams position A position in which the patient lies in the semi-Fowler's position and flexes the knees to relax the muscles of the lower back and relieve pressure on the spinal nerve root. This is typically more comfortable and therapeutic for the patient with low back pain.

withdrawing or withholding life-sustaining therapy The withdrawal or withholding of one or more therapies that might prolong the life of a person who cannot be cured by the therapy; the withdrawal of therapy does not directly cause death. Formerly called *passive euthanasia*.

work-related musculoskeletal disorders (MSDs) Disorders caused by heavy lifting and dependent transfers by staff members.

X

xenograft Tissue transplanted (grafted) from another species; for example, a heart valve transplanted from a pig to a human.

xerosis Abnormally dry skin.

xerostomia Abnormal dryness of the mouth caused by a severe reduction in the flow of saliva.

x-ray Radiation that is generated by machine.

Z

Zika virus A virus carried by mosquitoes that has affected people in over a dozen countries, including the United States, and can cause microcephaly (abnormally small heads) in newborns and Gullain-Barré syndrome in adults.

NCLEX® EXAMINATION CHALLENGES ANSWER KEY

Chapter 3
3-1   B
3-2   A, B, D, E, F
3-3   B
3-4   B

Chapter 4
4-1   A, B, D
4-2   A, C, D, E
4-3   0.2
4-4   A

Chapter 5
5-1   C
5-2   B
5-3   C, D, E

Chapter 6
6-1   B
6-2   B, C, D
6-3   D

Chapter 7
7-1   D
7-2   B

Chapter 8
8-1   D
8-2   A, C, D
8-3   B

Chapter 9
9-1   D
9-2   A, B, C, D, E, G
9-3   B, C, D, E

Chapter 10
10-1   D
10-2   A, C
10-3   A, B, C, D, F, G

Chapter 11
11-1   C
11-2   A
11-3   B, D, E, F
11-4   D
11-5   B

Chapter 12
12-1   D
12-2   B, D, E
12-3   B

Chapter 13
13-1   D
13-2   125

Chapter 14
14-1   C
14-2   B, C, F
14-3   C

Chapter 15
15-1   D
15-2   B, C, D, F
15-3   B
15-4   A

Chapter 16
16-1   A
16-2   D
16-3   C, D
16-4   C

Chapter 17
17-1   B, D, E
17-2   C

Chapter 18
18-1   A, C, E
18-2   A, D, E
18-3   A
18-4   A, B, C, D, E
18-5   A, C, D, E
18-6   C

Chapter 19
19-1   B
19-2   B, C, F
19-3   D

Chapter 20
20-1   A, D

Chapter 21
21-1   A, D, E
21-2   A
21-3   A, E, F

Chapter 22
22-1   A, D, E
22-2   B
22-3   A, C, D
22-4   C

Chapter 23
23-1   A, E
23-2   B, E

Chapter 24
24-1   B
24-2   B
24-3   A, B, D, E, F, G

Chapter 25
25-1   C
25-2   D
25-3   A, B, F
25-4   C

Chapter 26
26-1   D
26-2   D
26-3   A, C, D
26-4   B, D, E

Chapter 27
27-1   C
27-2   A, D
27-3   A, C, D, F
27-4   B

Chapter 28
28-1   C
28-2   A, C, D, F
28-3   C

Chapter 29
29-1   B, D, F
29-2   A, F
29-3   A

Chapter 30
30-1   C
30-2   A, B, D, G
30-3   A
30-4   B
30-5   D

Chapter 31
31-1   B, C, E
31-2   A, D, E
31-3   B
31-4   B

Chapter 32
32-1   A, E, F
32-2   C, D, E, G, H
32-3   C, E, G

Chapter 33
33-1   B, C, E, F
33-2   C
33-3   B

Chapter 34
34-1   B
34-2   C
34-3   D

Chapter 35
35-1   A, C, D, E
35-2   A
35-3   D
35-4   C

Chapter 36
36-1   A, B, C, E
36-2   A
36-3   D
36-4   A
36-5   A, D, E

Chapter 37
37-1   A
37-2   A, B, D, E, H
37-3   D
37-4   C

Chapter 38
38-1   B, D, F
38-2   C, E, F
38-3   B

Chapter 39
39-1   D
39-2   B, E
39-3   C

Chapter 40
40-1   A
40-2   A, B, H
40-3   C
40-4   B

Chapter 41
41-1   B, E
41-2   B
41-3   B
41-4   A

Chapter 42
42-1   B, D, E
42-2   B
42-3   C
42-4   B
42-5   C, D, E, F

Chapter 43
43-1   A
43-2   D
43-3   B
43-4   A, B, C, D, E

Chapter 44
44-1   A, C, D, E
44-2   A, B, D
44-3   D

Chapter 45
45-1 B, C, D, E
45-2 B
45-3 C
45-4 C
45-5 B

Chapter 46
46-1 A
46-2 A, B, C, F

Chapter 47
47-1 C
47-2 B
47-3 D
47-4 A, B, E
47-5 C

Chapter 48
48-1 D
48-2 C
48-3 C, E
48-4 C

Chapter 49
49-1 A, B, D, E
49-2 D

Chapter 50
50-1 A, B, C, D, E, F
50-2 D
50-3 C
50-4 B

Chapter 51
51-1 B
51-2 B, C, D, E
51-3 D
51-4 A

Chapter 52
52-1 B, D, E
52-2 B
52-3 A, C, D, E, F

Chapter 53
53-1 D
53-2 B
53-3 C
53-4 A, D, F
53-5 A

Chapter 54
54-1 B
54-2 C
54-3 A
54-4 B, E

Chapter 55
55-1 A, B, E
55-2 A
55-3 B
55-4 C

Chapter 56
56-1 D
56-2 B
56-3 B, C, E
56-4 A, B, C, E

Chapter 57
57-1 B, C, D
57-2 A, B, C
57-3 B
57-4 A
57-5 B, C

Chapter 58
58-1 B
58-2 B, D, E
58-3 C

Chapter 59
59-1 B, E
59-2 A, D, E
59-3 D
59-4 C
59-5 C

Chapter 60
60-1 41
60-2 A, B, C, D
60-3 B, C, D

Chapter 61
61-1 A
61-2 B, C, E, F

Chapter 62
62-1 A, C, D, E
62-2 C
62-3 D

Chapter 63
63-1 B
63-2 A
63-3 B, C, D, H
63-4 C

Chapter 64
64-1 A, C, G, H
64-2 C
64-3 D
64-4 B

Chapter 65
65-1 B, C, E, F
65-2 A
65-3 B, D, F
65-4 D

Chapter 66
66-1 B, C, D, G
66-2 D
66-3 C, E, F, G
66-4 A
66-5 C

Chapter 67
67-1 B
67-2 C
67-3 A
67-4 A, D, E, F, H
67-5 B, C, D, E, F, G

Chapter 68
68-1 B
68-2 A, E, F, G
68-3 D
68-4 A
68-5 D
68-6 C

Chapter 69
69-1 D
69-2 C

Chapter 70
70-1 D
70-2 A, C, E

Chapter 71
71-1 B
71-2 B

Chapter 72
72-1 775
72-2 C
72-3 A
72-4 D

Chapter 73
73-1 A, B, D, E
73-2 A, B

Chapter 74
74-1 C
74-2 A, B, C, E

A

Abatacept, 323b, 369, 370b
Abdomen
    assessment of, 803
    auscultation of, 1067, 1123,
        1128–1129
    chronic pancreatitis findings in,
        1203
    distention of, 1124, 1162–1163,
        1222
    inspection of, 1067
    palpation of, 1067–1068
    percussion of, 1067
    quadrants of, 1066–1068, 1066f,
        1067t
    sickle cell disease effects on, 810
    ultrasound of, 1123
Abdominal aortic aneurysms,
    739–740
Abdominal breathing, 578, 578b
Abdominal hernias, 1137–1138,
    1137f
Abdominal obesity, 1287
Abdominal pain
    acute pancreatitis as cause of,
        1199–1201
    appendicitis as cause of,
        1147–1148
    cholecystitis as cause of, 1193
    Crohn's disease as cause of, 1159
    in pancreatic cancer, 1206
Abdominal thrust maneuver, 561f
Abdominal ultrasonography, 1163,
    1515
Abdominal x-rays, for peritonitis
    evaluation, 1146
Abdominoperineal transition, 1130
Abducens nerve, 844t
Abduction, 1010f
ABI. See Ankle-brachial index
AbioCor Implantable Replacement
    Heart, 701f
Above-the-knee amputation, 1051,
    1054, 1055f
Abscess
    anorectal, 1164–1165
    definition of, 880–881
    pancreatic, 1205
    peritonsillar, 611
    renal, 1373
    in ulcerative colitis, 1151t
Absolute neutrophil count, 293
Absorbable sutures, 267
Absorption, 1062
Absorptive atelectasis, 530, 531b
A1C. See Glycosylated hemoglobin

Acalculia, 933
Acalculous cholecystitis, 1192
Acarbose, 1118, 1292b–1293b
Accelerated graft atherosclerosis,
    301
Acceleration-deceleration injury,
    941, 941f, 1035–1036
Accessory muscles of respiration,
    511
Accessory nerve, 844t
Accidents. See also Motor vehicle
        accidents
    chronic and disabling health
        conditions caused by, 87
    in older adults, 33–34
Acclimatization, 145
Accommodation, 960
AccuVein AV300, 203f
Acetaminophen
    dosing of, 307b
    hepatotoxicity caused by, 55
    osteoarthritis uses of, 307, 307b
    pain management uses of, 55, 307
Acetazolamide, for acute mountain
    sickness, 146
Acetic acid, 186
Acetylcholine, 868
Acetylcholine receptors, 917
Achlorhydria, 1115
Acid(s)
    definition of, 186
    formation of, 190
    sources of, 188
Acid deficit, 195–196
Acid-base assessment, 188b
Acid-base balance
    acids, 186
    assessment of, 14
    bases, 186
    buffers, 186–189, 186f–187f
    chemistry of, 186–187
    definition of, 13, 185
    importance of, 185
    maintenance of, 185–190
    postoperative, 276
    promotion of, 14
    regulatory actions and
        mechanisms, 188–190
        chemical, 188–189, 189t
        kidneys, 189t, 190
        respiratory, 189–190, 189f, 189t
    scope of, 14f
Acid-base imbalances
    acidosis. See Acidosis
    alkalosis. See Alkalosis
    arterial blood gas monitoring of,
        14
    compensatory mechanisms for, 14,
        190
    definition of, 13, 190

Acid-base imbalances (Continued)
    interventions for, 14
    kidney compensation for, 190
    physiologic consequences of, 14
    prevention of, 14
    respiratory compensation for, 190
    risk factors for, 13–14
Acidic pH, 186f
Acidosis
    assessment of, 192–194
    in chronic kidney disease, 1400
    complications of, 195
    definition of, 13
    laboratory assessment of, 193–194
    lactic, 191–192
    metabolic, 13, 191, 191t, 193–195,
        193b, 1122
    metabolic/respiratory, 192
    pathophysiology of, 190–192, 191t
    potassium levels in, 194
    psychosocial assessment of, 193
    respiratory, 13, 191t, 192,
        194–195
    signs and symptoms of, 192–193,
        193b
Acinus, 510, 511f
Acitretin, 333, 465b
ACLS. See Advanced cardiac life
    support
Acorn cardiac support device, 702
Acoustic neuroma, 951, 996
Acquired immunity, 295, 298
Acquired immunodeficiency
        syndrome. See also Human
        immunodeficiency virus
        infection
    assessments in, 356b
    defining conditions for, 340t
    diagnostic criteria for, 339
    diarrhea management in, 354
    features of, 346b
    health care resources for, 357
    high-risk populations for, 340
    human immunodeficiency virus
        infection versus, 338
    incidence of, 340
    infection control in, 357b
    Kaposi's sarcoma associated with,
        347, 348f, 354–355
    malignant lymphomas associated
        with, 347–348
    pathophysiology of, 337–340
    prevalence of, 340
    psychosocial preparation in,
        356–357
    seizures in, 355
Acromegaly, 1247, 1247f, 1248b
Actemra. See Tocilizumab
Acticoat, 501b
Actinic keratosis, 475, 475t

Actinic lentigo, 435f
Actiq. See Fentanyl
Activated partial thromboplastin
    time, 619–620
Active immunity, 21–22, 298, 414
Active listening, 158
Active range of motion, 1010
Activities of daily living
    in Alzheimer's disease patients,
        863
    assessment of, 1009–1010
    definition of, 23, 92, 96
    dyspnea and, 517t
    rehabilitation for, 96
    self-management education for
        performing, 100
Activity therapists, 89
Acupressure, 876
Acupuncture, 876
Acute abdomen series, 1070
Acute adrenal insufficiency, 1253,
    1253b
Acute arterial occlusion, 737
Acute chest syndrome, 810, 812
Acute compartment syndrome,
    1033–1034, 1034b, 1044–1045,
    1044b
Acute coronary syndromes
    angina pectoris. See Angina
        pectoris
    antiplatelet agents for, 777, 777b
    assessment of, 772–774
    cardiac rehabilitation for, 779, 792
    coping with, 779
    coronary artery disease. See
        Coronary artery disease
    definition of, 769–770
    description of, 655
    drug therapy for, 774–775, 776b
    dysrhythmias caused by, 779–780
    etiology of, 771
    functional ability promotion in,
        778–779
    genetic risks of, 771, 771b
    health care resources for, 792
    incidence of, 772
    medical assistance indications in,
        791–792
    myocardial infarction. See
        Myocardial infarction
    nitrates for, 776b
    pathophysiology of, 769–771
    percutaneous coronary
        intervention for, 778
    physical assessment of, 772–773
    prevalence of, 772
    signs and symptoms of, 772–773
Acute gastritis, 1104–1105, 1105b
Acute glomerulonephritis,
    1376–1378, 1376t

Page numbers followed by f indicate
figures; t, tables; b, boxes

Acute hematogenous infection, 1022–1023

Acute kidney injury
assessment of, 1393–1394
chronic kidney disease versus, 1391t
classification of, 1391t, 1392
complications from, 1392t
contributing factors, 1392t
definition of, 1391
diseases and conditions contributing to, 1392t
drug therapy for, 1396
end-stage renal disease secondary to, 1398
etiology of, 1391–1392
features of, 1391t
health promotion and maintenance, 1393
history-taking for, 1393–1394
imaging assessment of, 1394
incidence of, 1392–1393
interventions for, 1395–1398
KDIGO classification system for, 1391t
kidney biopsy of, 1394
kidney replacement therapy for, 1397–1398, 1397f
laboratory assessment of, 1394, 1395b
nephrotoxic substances that cause, 1393t
nutrition therapy for, 1396–1397
in older adults, 1394b
oliguria associated with, 1396, 1423
pathophysiology of, 1391–1393
physical assessment of, 1394
prevalence of, 1392–1393
renal replacement therapy for, 1397, 1397f
signs and symptoms of, 1394

Acute leukemia
consolidation therapy for, 820–821
description of, 817, 819b
drug therapy for, 820–821
induction therapy for, 820

Acute lung injury, 626
Acute lymphocytic leukemia, 814t
Acute mountain sickness, 145–146, 145b–146b
Acute myelogenous leukemia, 814t, 820
Acute osteomyelitis, 1023, 1023b
Acute otitis media, 991
Acute pain, 46–47, 46t, 52
Acute pain transfusion reaction, 836
Acute pancreatitis
abdominal pain associated with, 1199–1201
alcohol consumption as cause of, 1200
assessment of, 1199–1200
autodigestion in, 1198f

Acute pancreatitis (Continued)
care coordination for, 1202
complications of, 1197–1198, 1198t, 1201
death caused by, 1199
definition of, 1197
drug therapy for, 1200–1201
endoscopic retrograde cholangiopancreatography -related trauma as cause of, 1199
etiology of, 1199
gallstones as cause of, 1201
genetic risk of, 1199
history-taking for, 1199
home care management of, 1202
imaging assessment of, 1200
incidence of, 1199
interventions for, 1200–1201
laboratory assessment of, 1200, 1200t
multi-system organ failure caused by, 1198
nonsurgical management of, 1200–1201
nutrition promotion in, 1201
in older adults, 1199
paralytic ileus secondary to, 1201b
pathophysiology of, 1197–1199
physical assessment of, 1199
prevalence of, 1199
psychosocial assessment of, 1200
respiratory status monitoring in, 1201b
shock caused by, 1198, 1199b
signs and symptoms of, 1199
surgical management of, 1201
transition management for, 1202
ultrasonography of, 1200

Acute paronychia, 442
Acute peripheral arterial occlusion, 737–738
Acute promyelocytic leukemia, 814t
Acute radiation cystitis, 1485
Acute respiratory distress syndrome
acute lung injury in, 626
acute pancreatitis as risk factor for, 1198
assessment of, 627
in burn injury, 497
causes of, 626t
definition of, 626
diagnostic assessment of, 627
drug therapy for, 628
etiology of, 626, 626t
extracorporeal membrane oxygenation for, 628
fluid therapy for, 628
genetic risks for, 626, 627b
health promotion and maintenance for, 627
incidence of, 626
interventions for, 627–628

Acute respiratory distress syndrome (Continued)
nutrition therapy for, 628
pathophysiology of, 626
positive end-expiratory pressure for, 627
prevalence of, 626
in sepsis, 764
signs and symptoms of, 627

Acute respiratory failure, 624–626, 625t
Acute sialadenitis, 1084–1085
Acute stress disorder, 156, 156b, 158
Acute transfusion reaction, 835–836
Acute transplant rejection, 301
Acute tubular necrosis, 1392
Acyclovir
for encephalitis, 884
for genital herpes, 1507
Adalimumab, 323b, 466b, 1153
Adam's apple, 510
Addiction, opioid, 58
Addisonian crisis, 1253
Addison's disease, 1253–1254
Adduction, 1010f
Adefovir, 1185t
A-delta fibers, 47–48, 49f
Adenocarcinomas. See also Cancer
colorectal, 1127
endometrial, 1465
Adenohypophysis, 1236, 1237f
Adenomas, 1126
Adenomatous polyposis coli gene, 1127b
Adenosine, 677b–678b, 678
Adenosine triphosphate, 802
Adipokines, 1225
Adiponectin, 1225
Adjustable gastric band, laparoscopic, 1229, 1230f
Adjuvant analgesics, 55, 63–65
ADLs. See Activities of daily living
Administration sets, for infusion therapy
add-on devices, 209–210
definition of, 209
filters used with, 210
intermittent, 209
needleless connection devices, 210–211, 210f, 214
secondary, 209, 209f
slip lock, 210
Administrative review, 157
Adrenal cortex, 1235t, 1237–1238
Adrenal crisis, 1253
Adrenal gland(s)
anatomy of, 1237–1238
hypofunction of, 1253–1255, 1254b–1255b, 1254f
laboratory assessment of, 1255b
Adrenal gland disorders
Cushing's disease. See Cushing's disease
hyperaldosteronism, 1260–1261
pheochromocytoma, 1261–1262

Adrenal glucocorticoids, 1006
Adrenal insufficiency, 1386
acute, 1253, 1253b
features of, 1254b
primary, 1253t
secondary, 1253t
sepsis as cause of, 765
Adrenal medulla, 1238
Adrenalectomy, 1259
Adrenergic agonists, for glaucoma, 966b
Adrenocorticotropic hormone
deficiency of, 1246, 1246b
description of, 1235t, 1236, 1238, 1254
overproduction of, 1248b
Advance directives, 104–115, 241, 263, 705
Advanced cardiac life support
certifications in, 120t, 123
dysrhythmias treated with, 687
Advanced life support providers, 119
Advanced practice nurses
in rehabilitation settings, 88
trauma, 131
Adventitious breath sounds, 519, 521t
Adverse drug events, 42b, 111b
Adverse events
definition of, 4–5
as sentinel events, 4–5
Adynamic ileus, 1122
Aerobic exercise, 32
Aerophagia, 1095
Afatinib, 589t
Afferent arterioles, 1322–1323
Afferent neurons, 840
Affordable Care Act, 118
African Americans
Alzheimer's disease in, 859b, 864b
angioedema in, 362b
hypertension in, 722b
sickle cell disease in, 809
"Africanized" bees, 137
Afterload
definition of, 645
drugs that affect, 698
Age-related macular degeneration, 979
Agglutination, 297
Aging. See also Older adults
cancer risks associated with, 380
cardiovascular system affected by, 646, 647b
endocrine system changes associated with, 1240, 1241b
eye changes associated with, 961, 961b
fluid balance affected by, 165b
gastrointestinal system changes associated with, 1064, 1064b
hearing affected by, 986
hematologic system changes associated with, 800, 800b

Aging (Continued)
  immune system affected by, 291b
  immunity changes caused by, 290, 300
  musculoskeletal system affected by, 1007–1008, 1007b
  neurologic changes associated with, 234b, 844–845, 845b
  renal system changes associated with, 234b, 1328–1329, 1328b
  reproductive system changes associated with, 1431, 1431b
  respiratory changes associated with, 512, 513b
  skin changes associated with, 234b, 433, 652
  spinal cord injury and, 902b
  urinary system changes associated with, 234b, 1328–1329
Agitated delirium, 111
Agnosia, 860, 933
Agraphia, 933
AIDS. See Acquired immunodeficiency syndrome
AIDS dementia complex, 348
AIDS wasting syndrome, 348
Air embolism, 214–215
Air trapping, 572
Airborne infection isolation room, 416
Airborne precautions, 419, 420t, 609
Airborne transmission
  description of, 416
  precautions for, 419, 420t, 609
Air-fluidized beds, 97
Airway. See also Upper airway
  anatomy of, 510, 511f
  in angioedema patients, 363
  artificial
    description of, 273
    suctioning of, 541–542, 541b
  burn injury of, 489–490
  clearance of, in tuberculosis, 607–608
  narrowing of, 565f
  postoperative maintenance of, 280
  primary survey of, 129, 131t
  in spinal cord injury patients, 897–898
  in traumatic brain injury patients, 948–949
Airway obstruction
  burn injury as cause of, 490t, 494
  head and neck cancer as cause of, 549–553
  monitoring for, 629b
  pathophysiology of, 563
  in pneumonia, 604
  respiratory acidosis caused by, 192
  upper, 560–561, 561f
Airway pressure-release ventilation, 627
Airway secretions, 129
AKI. See Acute kidney injury
Akinesia, 868

Alanine aminotransferase, 1068, 1069b, 1174, 1200
Albiglutide, 1292b–1293b
Albumin
  functions of, 796
  laboratory testing for, 1069b
  in malnutrition assessments, 25
  serum, 1217
Albuminuria, 1283, 1399
Albuterol
  asthma treated with, 569b–570b
  bronchospasm treated with, 365
Alcohol consumption, 610
  blood glucose levels affected by, 1299
  cirrhosis caused by, 1172
  surgical risks associated with, 232–233
Aldosterone
  deficiency of, 1255
  description of, 485, 1237, 1323
  fluid balance regulation by, 165
  sodium reabsorption affected by, 1326
Aldosterone antagonists, for heart failure, 700
Alectinib, 589t
Alefacept, 333
Alendronate, 1021
Alexia, 933
Alirocumab, 730–731
Alkaline pH, 187f
Alkaline phosphatase, 1011, 1069b
Alkaline reflux gastropathy, 1118
Alkalis, 487
Alkalosis
  definition of, 13
  metabolic, 13, 193b, 196, 196t, 1122
  pathophysiology of, 195–196, 196t
  relative, 195
  respiratory, 13, 196, 196t
Alkylating agents, 391
Alleles, 74–75, 75f, 79
Allergens, 360–361, 364b
Allergic rhinosinusitis, 365–366
Allergy/allergies
  to anesthesia, 263
  atopic, 360–361
  breathing affected by, 516
  definition of, 360
  food, 234–235, 1212b
  history-taking, 1008
  latex, 234–235, 419
  preoperative evaluation for, 234–235
Allogeneic bone marrow transplantation, 822
Allogeneic stem cells, 822
Allografts, 499
Allopurinol, 331–332, 1364
Alopecia
  chemotherapy as cause of, 395, 400, 588, 1467
  drugs as cause of, 820

Alosetron, 1136–1137, 1137b
5-Alpha reductase inhibitors, 1477, 1498
Alpha₁-antitrypsin deficiency, 573, 573b, 573t
Alpha-fetoprotein, 1186–1187
Alpha-glucosidase inhibitors, 1292b–1293b, 1293
Alteplase, 935, 936b
Altitude-related illnesses, 145–146, 145b–146b
Aluminum hydroxide, 1091, 1106b–1107b
Alveolar ducts, 510
Alveolar edema, 486
Alveolar-capillary diffusion, 192
Alveoli
  age-related changes in, 513b
  anatomy of, 510
Alzheimer's disease
  abuse concerns in, 865–866
  accident prevention in, 864–865
  activities of daily living in, 863
  in African Americans, 859b, 864b
  antidepressants for, 864
  assessment of, 860–861
  behavior changes associated with
    description of, 861
    management of, 862–864, 865t
  care coordination for, 866–867
  caregivers for, 866, 866b–867b
  cholinesterase inhibitors for, 864
  cognitive changes associated with, 860–861
  cognitive stimulation training for, 862
  communication methods for, 863b, 865
  complementary and integrative health for, 863
  depression in, 864
  drug therapy for, 863–864
  elder abuse concerns, 865–866
  etiology of, 858
  family caregivers for, 866, 866b
  genetic risk of, 858, 859b
  genetic testing for, 861
  health care resources for, 867
  health promotion and maintenance for, 859
  in Hispanics, 866b
  history-taking for, 860
  imaging assessments for, 861
  incidence of, 859
  injury prevention in, 864–865
  laboratory assessments for, 861
  memory impairments associated with, 860, 862
  neuritic plaques associated with, 858, 859f
  neurofibrillary tangles associated with, 858, 859f
  neuropsychiatric symptoms associated with, 861

Alzheimer's disease (Continued)
  nonpharmacologic management of, 862–863
  pathophysiology of, 857–859
  personality changes associated with, 861
  physical assessment of, 860–861
  prevalence of, 859
  psychosocial assessment of, 861
  psychotropic drugs in, 864
  reminiscence therapy for, 862
  risk factors for, 858, 859b
  Safe Return Program for, 867
  screening for, 860–861
  self-management education for, 866–867
  self-management skills associated with, 861
  sexual disinhibition associated with, 861
  signs and symptoms of, 860–861
  stages of, 860, 860b
  transition management for, 866–867
  validation therapy for, 863
  vascular dementia versus, 858t
  in veterans, 859b, 867b
  wandering associated with, 864, 864b
Amantadine, 871
Ambulation
  assistive devices for, 95, 95f
  after burn injury, 503
  nurse-initiated protocol for, 24b
Ambulatory aids, 23
Ambulatory care rehabilitation, 88
Ambulatory pumps, 211
Ambulatory surgical centers, 228, 271
Amebiasis, 1165–1166
Amebic meningoencephalitis, 883
Amenorrhea, 1173, 1246
American Chronic Pain Association, 52–53
American Nurses Association
  Code of Ethics, 9t, 1492
  ethics as defined by, 8–9
American Nurses Credentialing Center's Magnet Recognition, 7
American Occupational Therapy Association, 93
American Physical Therapy Association, 93
American Sign Language, 1001
American Society of Anesthesiologists Physical Status Classification system, 230–232, 233t, 257
Americans with Disabilities Act, 92
Amevive. See Alefacept
AMI. See Antibody-mediated immunity
Amino acids, 76, 76f
Aminocaproic acid, 620
Aminosalicylates, 1152, 1153t

5-Aminosalicylates, 1152, 1153t
Amiodarone, 200b, 677b–678b, 708
Amitriptyline, 1137
Ammonia, 190, 1068, 1073b
Ammonium, 190
Amnesia, 257
Amoxicillin, 612b, 1359b
Amoxicillin/clavulanate, 1359b
Amphiarthrodial joints, 1006
Amputation
    above-the-knee, 1051, 1054,
        1055f
    assessment of, 1052–1053
    bandaging of stump, 1054, 1055f
    below-the-knee, 1051, 1051f, 1054,
        1055f
    care coordination for, 1055–1056,
        1056b
    complications of, 1051–1052
    contracture prevention in, 1054
    definition of, 1050
    diagnostic assessment of, 1052
    emergency care for, 1053
    health care resources for, 1056,
        1056t
    health promotion and
        maintenance for, 1052
    home care management of, 1055,
        1056b
    infection prevention after, 1054
    levels of, 1051, 1051f
    lower-extremity, 1051, 1051b,
        1051f
    mobility promotion after,
        1053–1054
    pain caused by, 1051, 1053
    physical assessment of, 1052
    psychosocial assessment of, 1052,
        1052b
    self-esteem promotion in,
        1054–1055
    self-management education for,
        1055–1056
    signs and symptoms of,
        1052–1056
    Syme, 1051, 1051f
    tissue perfusion monitoring after,
        1053
    transition management for,
        1055–1056, 1056b
    traumatic, 1050, 1053
    types of, 1050
AMS. See Acute mountain sickness
Amylase
    serum, 1062, 1068, 1069b
    urine, 1068
Amylin analogs, 1292b–1293b,
    1293–1294
Amyloid beta protein precursor, 861
Amyotrophic lateral sclerosis, 889t
Anaergy, 607
Anaerobic conditions, 188
Anaerobic metabolism, 191–192
Anakinra, 323b
Anal canal, 1064

Anal disorders
    anal fissure, 1165
    anal fistula, 1165
    anorectal abscess, 1164–1165
    parasitic infections, 1165–1166
Anal intercourse, 342
Analgesia. See also Opioid analgesics;
    specific analgesics
    definition of, 257
    intraspinal, 61–62
    intrathecal, 61–62, 62b
    multimodal, 54–55
    patient-controlled, 55, 283–284
    preemptive, 54
Analgesic trial, 59b
Anamnestic response, 298
Anaphylaxis
    antihistamines for, 365
    assessment of, 364
    definition of, 361, 753
    emergency care of, 365b
    epinephrine injectors for, 363f,
        364b, 365
    features of, 364b
    health promotion and
        maintenance for, 363–364
    interventions for, 364–365, 365b
    pathophysiology of, 363
Anaplasia, 374
Anaplastic carcinoma, 1275
Anasarca, 651, 1394
Anastomosis, 1131
Anatomic dead space, 531–532
Androblastomas, 1487
Androderm, 1498
AndroGel, 1498
Androgen deprivation therapy,
    1485
Androgens
    description of, 1006
    hypopituitarism treated with,
        1247
Anemia
    aplastic, 814t, 815–816
    autoimmune hemolytic, 815
    causes of, 814t
    chemotherapy as cause of, 397
    in chronic kidney disease, 1401
    cold antibody, 815
    in Crohn's disease, 1159
    definition of, 813
    fatigue associated with, 802
    folic acid deficiency, 814–816,
        814t
    glucose-6-phosphate
        dehydrogenase deficiency,
        814t, 815–816
    immunohemolytic, 815–816
    iron deficiency, 814–816, 814t,
        815b
    management of, 815–816
    megaloblastic, 814
    in older adults, 803
    pernicious, 814, 1104–1105
    sickle cell. See Sickle cell disease

Anemia (Continued)
    types of, 814
    vitamin B₁₂ deficiency, 814, 814t,
        815f, 816
    warm antibody, 815
Aneroid pressure manometer, 541f
Anesthesia
    allergies to, 263
    definition of, 256
    epidural, 261t, 262f, 275, 275b
    general, 257–260, 258t–259t, 260b,
        275
    local, 260–261
    moderate sedation, 261–262, 262t
    previous experiences with, 234
    providers of, 256–257
    regional, 260–261, 261f–262f, 261t
    selection criteria for, 256–257
    spinal, 261t, 262f, 275, 275b
    total hip arthroplasty, 310
Anesthesiologist, 253t, 256
Anesthesiologist assistant, 256
Aneuploid, 74
Aneuploidy, 374, 376–377
Aneurysm(s)
    abdominal aortic, 739–740
    arterial, 738–740, 739f
    arteriovenous fistula, 1415
    assessment of, 739
    atherosclerosis as cause of,
        738–739
    definition of, 738, 929
    dissecting, 738–739
    femoral, 740
    interventions for, 739–740
    nonsurgical management of, 739
    pathophysiology of, 738–739
    peripheral arteries, 740
    surgical management of, 739–740
    thoracic aortic, 738–739
Aneurysmectomy, 739
Angina pectoris, 650t
    atypical, 773b
    chronic stable, 768–769
    definition of, 768–769
    features of, 773b
    new-onset, 770
    nitroglycerin for, 774–775
    pre-infarction, 770
    Prinzmetal's, 770
    self-management education for,
        792b
    unstable, 769–770
    variant, 770, 774
Angioedema, 361–366, 362b, 362f
Angiogenesis inhibitors, 404t, 405
Angiography, 657
Angiotensin I, 1237
Angiotensin II, 167, 1237, 1326
Angiotensin receptor blockers
    afterload affected by, 698
    hypertension treated with, 167,
        725b, 726–727
Angiotensin receptor neprilysin
    inhibitor, 698

Angiotensin-converting enzyme
    inhibitors
    afterload affected by, 698
    albuminuria treated with, 1308
    hypertension managed with, 167,
        725b, 726
Angiotensinogen, 167, 1237, 1324f
Anions, 172
Anisocoria, 963
Ankle fracture, 1043, 1049
Ankle-brachial index, 653, 733, 1052
Ankylosing spondylitis, 334t
Anomia, 860
Anorectal abscess, 1164–1165
Anorexia, 1065
Anorexia nervosa, 1216
Anorexins, 1225
ANP. See Atrial natriuretic peptide
Antacids
    for gastroesophageal reflux
        disease, 1090–1091
    for peptic ulcer disease,
        1106b–1107b, 1112
Antalgic gait, 1009
Anterior cerebral artery
    anatomy of, 841
    stroke involving, 933b
Anterior cervical diskectomy and
    fusion, 909–910, 910b
Anterior colporrhaphy, 1349t, 1465
Anterior pituitary gland
    hormones produced by, 1235t,
        1237t, 1245–1246
    hyperfunction of, 1248b
Anterior wall myocardial infarction,
    771
Anthralin, 464
Anthrax
    bioterrorism uses of, 428, 466b
    cutaneous, 466–468, 467f
    inhalation, 611–612, 612b
Anthropometric measurements,
    1213–1215
Anti-androgen drugs, 1485
Antibiotics
    dyspnea treated with, 110
    gastroenteritis treated with, 1149
    nonabsorbable, 1178–1179
    pelvic inflammatory disease
        treated with, 1516, 1516b
    preoperative prophylaxis, 247
Antibody
    antigen and, interactions between,
        296–298
    classification of, 298, 298t
    monoclonal. See Monoclonal
        antibodies
    production of, 297
Antibody-antigen binding, 297, 297f
Antibody-mediated immune system,
    417
Antibody-mediated immunity
    acquiring of, 298–299
    antigen-antibody interactions in,
        296–298

Antibody-mediated immunity (Continued)
B-lymphocytes in, 295–296
cells involved in, 292t, 797t
definition of, 295
description of, 22, 290–291
sequence of, 296f
Anticholinergics
Parkinson disease treated with, 871
respiratory secretions during dying treated with, 110
urinary incontinence treated with, 1349
Anticoagulants. See also specific drug
best practices for, 744b
clotting inadequacies treated with, 16
direct thrombin inhibitors, 801
heparin-induced thrombocytopenia treated with, 832
indirect thrombin inhibitors, 801
injury prevention in patients using, 623b
mechanism of action, 801
Anticoagulation
blood tests for monitoring, 634t
during hemodialysis, 1413
Anticonvulsants
fibromyalgia treated with, 333
pain management uses of, 63–64
Anti-cyclic citrullinated peptide, 320
Antidepressants. See also specific antidepressants
in Alzheimer's disease patients, 864
pain management uses of, 63–64
Antidiuretic hormone
age-related changes in, 1241b
deficiency of, 1246b, 1250
fluid balance regulation by, 165–166
secretion of, 407
syndrome of inappropriate. See Syndrome of inappropriate antidiuretic hormone
Antidysrhythmics, 677b–678b, 685–686
Antiembolism stockings, 244
Antiemetics, 399
Antiepileptic drugs
dry mouth caused by, 26
migraine headaches treated with, 875
pain management uses of, 63–64
seizures treated with, 111, 877–878, 878b
Anti-factor Xa test, 805
Antigen
antibody and, interactions between, 296–298
inactivation of, 297
sensitization to, 297

Antigen recognition, 296
Antihemophilic factor, 798t
Antihistamines
anaphylaxis treated with, 365
pruritus treated with, 463
rhinosinusitis treated with, 611, 611b
Antimetabolites, 391, 391t
Antimicrobial-resistant infection, 421, 421b
Antimicrobials
fever treated with, 425
infective endocarditis treated with, 712
sensitivity testing for, 424
Antimitotic agents, 391, 391t
Antinuclear antibodies, 326
Antinuclear antibody test, 320
Antiplatelet agents
acute coronary syndromes treated with, 777, 777b
clotting inadequacies treated with, 16
injury prevention in patients using, 623b
mechanism of action, 801–802
peripheral arterial disease treated with, 734–737
Antipsychotic drugs
adverse drug events caused by, 42b, 111b
in Alzheimer's disease patients, 864
indications for, 41
in older adults, 41, 42b
Antipyretic drugs, 426
Antithymocyte globulin, 302b
α₁-Antitrypsin, 83
Anuria, 18, 1362
Anxiety
in angioedema patients, 363
in chronic kidney disease, 1410–1411
in chronic obstructive pulmonary disease, 580
in head and neck cancer, 553
in hearing loss patients, 1001
management of, 622–623, 1410–1411
postoperative, 280
preoperative, 237, 246
in pulmonary embolism, 622–623
signs and symptoms of, 280
surgery-related, 17
in tuberculosis patients, 609
Anzemet, 399
AORN. See Association of periOperative Registered Nurses
Aorta
blood flow in, 642
dissection of, 740–741
Aortic regurgitation, 706b, 707
Aortic stenosis, 706–707, 706b
Aortic valvuloplasty, 708

Aortofemoral bypass surgery, 735, 736f
APC gene, 382
Aphasia, 91, 860, 933, 938, 938t
Apheresis, for polycythemia vera, 816
Aphthous stomatitis, 1076
Aphthous ulcers, 1076
Apical impulse, 654
Aplastic anemia, 814t, 815–816
Apo-Acetazolamide. See Acetazolamide
Apocrine sweat glands, 433
Apolipoprotein E, 1225
Apolipoprotein E4, 861
Apoptosis, 373
Appendectomy, 1148
Appendicitis, 1147–1148, 1147b, 1148f
Appendix, 1064
Appetite, 1225
Apraxia, 860, 934
Apremilast, 369
aPTT. See Activated partial thromboplastin time
Aquacel Ag, 501b
Aqueous humor
creation of, 972
definition of, 958
flow of, 959f
Arachidonic acid, 295
Arachnoid, 840
Arava. See Leflunomide
Arboviruses, 883
Archiving, 350
Arcus senilis, 435f, 961
ARDS. See Acute respiratory distress syndrome
Areflexic bladder, 97–98, 98t
Aromatase inhibitors, 1452
Aromatherapy, 109, 111
Around-the-clock dosing, of analgesics, 54–55, 59b
Arrhythmogenic right ventricular cardiomyopathy, 715
Arterial aneurysms, 738–740, 739f
Arterial baroreceptors, 721
Arterial blood gas
analysis of, 521, 522b
monitoring of
acid-base imbalance, 14
gas exchange assessments, 21
postoperative, 280
Arterial embolization, 711
Arterial pulses, 653, 653f
Arterial system, 645–646
Arterial thrombosis, 16b
Arterial ulcers, 732–733, 734b
Arterial vasoconstriction, 694
Arteriography, 657
Arteriosclerosis
assessment of, 729–730
definition of, 728
pathophysiology of, 728–729
Arteriotomy, 738

Arteriovenous fistulas, 1413, 1414f–1415f, 1414t–1415t, 1415b
Arteriovenous grafts, 1413, 1414f, 1414t–1415t, 1415b
Arteriovenous malformation, 929, 935, 952
Arteriovenous shunt, 1414f
Arthritis
definition of, 305
disease-associated, 332–333, 333t
energy conservation in, 324b
osteoarthritis. See Osteoarthritis
psoriatic, 332–333
rheumatoid. See Rheumatoid arthritis
Arthritis Foundation, 317, 324, 328, 334
Arthrocentesis, for rheumatoid arthritis, 321
Arthrodesis, 906
Arthrogram, 1011
Arthropod bites, 136–137, 137b, 137f, 138t–140t
Arthroscope, 1013
Arthroscopy
complications of, 1014
follow-up care after, 1014, 1014b
musculoskeletal system applications of, 1013–1014, 1013f
patient preparation for, 1013
procedure for, 1014
Articular cartilage, 1006–1007
Artifacts, electrocardiogram, 670
Artificial airway
description of, 273
suctioning of, 541–542, 541b
Artificial skin, 499
Ascending colostomy, 1131f
Aschoff bodies, 714
Ascites, 1170, 1173, 1173f, 1202, 1206
Aseptic meningitis, 881
Aspartate aminotransferase, 1068, 1069b, 1174
Aspiration
during drowning, 147
in head and neck cancer, 553
nasogastric feeding tube as cause of, 553
precautions for, 1081b
during swallowing, 543b
Aspirin
mechanism of action, 801–802
myocardial infarction treated with, 776–777
stroke prophylaxis using, 937
Assist-control ventilation, 631
Assistive/adaptive devices
for ambulation, 95–96, 95f, 96t
for self-care, 96
types of, 96t
Association of periOperative Registered Nurses, 229, 251

Association of Rehabilitation Nurses, 93
Asterixis, 1173, 1378
Asthma
    action plan for, 567–568
    assessment of, 565–567
    barrel chest associated with, 566, 567f
    deaths caused by, 563
    definition of, 563
    drug therapy for
        anti-inflammatory agents, 569b–571b, 571
        bronchodilators, 568–571, 569b–570b
        cholinergic antagonists, 569b–570b, 571
        corticosteroids, 569b–570b, 571
        cromones, 569b–570b, 571
        leukotriene modifiers, 569b–570b, 571
        metered dose inhaler for, 568–570, 570b, 570f
        step system for, 566b
        xanthines, 571
    etiology of, 563–565
    exercise for, 571
    features of, 566b
    gas exchange affected by, 21
    gastroesophageal reflux disease as trigger of, 565
    genetic risk of, 563–565
    history-taking for, 565
    incidence of, 565, 565b
    inflammation as trigger of, 565
    laboratory assessment of, 567
    oxygen therapy for, 571
    pathophysiology of, 563–565, 564f
    physical assessment of, 566–567, 567f
    prevalence of, 565, 565b
    pulmonary function tests for, 567
    self-management education for, 567–568, 568b, 568f
    signs and symptoms of, 566–567, 567f
    status asthmaticus, 572
Astigmatism, 960, 980–981
Asymptomatic bacterial urinary tract infection, 1354
Ataxia, 145–146, 933–934, 946
Atelectasis, 233–234
    absorptive, 530, 531b
Atelectrauma, 635
Atherectomy
    for coronary artery disease, 784
    for peripheral arterial disease, 735
Atherosclerosis
    aneurysms caused by, 738–739
    assessment of, 729–730
    complementary and integrative health for, 731
    coronary artery disease caused by, 771
    cross-section of, 769f

Atherosclerosis (Continued)
    definition of, 728, 928
    drug therapy for, 730–731, 730t
    incidence of, 729
    interventions for, 730–731
    nutrition therapy for, 730
    pathophysiology of, 728–729, 729f
    physical activity for, 730
    plaque, 928
    risk factors for, 729t
    statins for, 731b
    triglycerides in, 729–730
Atopic allergy, 360–361
Atopic dermatitis, 462, 463b
Atrial dysrhythmias
    atrial fibrillation. See Atrial fibrillation
    description of, 675–676
    drug therapy for, 677b–678b
    premature atrial complexes, 676
    supraventricular tachycardia, 676–678
Atrial fibrillation
    assessment of, 679
    biventricular pacing for, 681
    clotting inadequacies associated with, 15
    definition of, 678
    drug therapy for, 679–680
    electrocardiographic findings, 679f
    etiology of, 679
    genetic risk of, 679
    heart failure in, 680–681
    incidence of, 679
    interventions for, 679–680
    pathophysiology of, 678–679
    permanent, 679
    persistent, 679
    prevalence of, 679
    pulmonary embolism risks in, 680b
    stroke risks in, 16
    valvular heart disease and, 708
Atrial gallop, 654–655
Atrial kick, 665
Atrial natriuretic peptide, 166
Atrioventricular junctional area, 665
Atrioventricular valves, 642–643
Atrophic gastritis, 1104, 1115
Atrophic glossitis, 1118
Atrophy, 438f
Atropine sulfate, 677b–678b, 898
Atypical angina, 773b
Atypical chest pain, 1089
Atypical migraines, 873–874
Audiometry, 990–991
Audioscopy, 989
Auditory brainstem-evoked response, 991
Auditory evoked potentials, 855
Auscultation
    of abdomen, 1067, 1123
    of cardiovascular system, 654–655
    of heart sounds, 654–655
    of lungs, 519, 520f

Autoamputation of the distal digits, 329–330
Autoantibodies, 367
Auto-contamination, 820
Autodigestion, 1104, 1198f
Autoimmune diseases
    antiproliferative drugs for, 368–369, 370b
    calcineurin inhibitors for, 369, 370b
    corticosteroids for, 368
    cytotoxic drugs for, 368
    description of, 368
    disease-modifying antirheumatic drugs for, 368–369, 370b
    immunosuppressive therapy for, 368–369, 370b
Autoimmune hemolytic anemia, 815
Autoimmune pancreatitis, 1202
Autoimmune thrombocytopenic purpura, 830–831
Autoimmunity
    disorders with, 367t
    incidence of, 367
    pathophysiology of, 367–368
    self-reactions, 368
Autologous blood donation
    intraoperative, 263, 264b
    preoperative, 235
Autologous blood transfusions, 836
Automated external defibrillator
    dysrhythmias treated with, 686–687, 687f
    illustration of, 687f
    ventricular fibrillation treated with, 685
Automated peritoneal dialysis, 1419–1420, 1419f–1420f
Automaticity, 665
Autonomic dysreflexia, 896, 896b, 898, 898b
Autonomic hyperreflexia, 896
Autonomic nervous system, 646, 842–844
Autonomic neuropathy, 1285, 1285t, 1305
Autonomy, 9
Autoregulation, 945
Autosomal dominant pattern of inheritance, 78–79, 78t
Autosomal recessive pattern of inheritance, 78t, 79, 79f
Autosomal-dominant polycystic kidney disease, 1380, 1380b, 1380f
Autosomes, 74
Avascular necrosis, 1021, 1035, 1047
Axial loading, 894, 895f
Axillary lymph node dissection, 1447
Axillofemoral bypass surgery, 735–736, 736f
Axon, 840, 840f
Azathioprine
    autoimmune diseases treated with, 368
    immunosuppression uses of, 302b

Azithromycin
    for chlamydia infection, 1512
    for gonorrhea, 1513
Azoospermia, 1487–1488
Azotemia, 1392, 1398

B
B cells
    in antibody-mediated immunity, 295–296, 797t
    differentiation of, 295f
    types of, 297
Babinski's sign, 848
Bacille Calmette- Guérin vaccine, 606–607
Bacillus anthracis, 611–612
Back pain
    acute, 903–904
    areas commonly affected by, 903
    assessment of, 904–905
    care coordination for, 908–909
    chronic, 903
    contributing factors for, 904b
    diskectomy for, 906
    exercises for, 906b
    health care resources for, 909
    health promotion and maintenance for, 904
    home care management of, 908
    imaging assessment of, 905
    laminectomy for, 906
    laser-assisted laparoscopic lumbar diskectomy for, 906
    microdiskectomy for, 906
    minimally invasive surgery for, 906
    nonsurgical management of, 905–906, 906b
    pathophysiology of, 903–904
    physical assessment of, 904–905
    prevalence of, 903
    prevention of, 904b, 908b
    self-management education for, 908–909
    subacute, 903–904
    surgical management of, 906–908, 907b
    transition management for, 908–909
Bacteremia
    catheter-acquired, 415–416
    description of, 1356–1357
Bacterial gastroenteritis, 1148t, 1149
Bacterial infections
    of skin, 466–468, 466f, 467b
    skin cultures for, 444
Bacterial overgrowth, of intestine, 1142
Bacterial peritonitis, 1122
Bacteriuria, 1354
Bad death, 103
Bag-valve-mask ventilation, 129
Baker's cysts, 319
Balance
    assessment of, 991
    testing of, 849–850

Ball-and-socket joints, 1007
Balloon brachytherapy, 1451
Balloon valvuloplasty, 708
Band neutrophils, 292–293
Bandemia, 280, 293
Bar code-point of care system, 833
Bar-code medication administration
   as best safety practice, 4
   description of, 8
   example of, 4f
Bariatric surgery, 1229–1231
Barium enema, 1152
Barium swallow study, 1089, 1093, 1096
Baroreceptors, 646, 754
Barotrauma, 635, 995
Barrel chest
   in asthma, 566, 567f
   in chronic obstructive pulmonary disease, 576
Barrett's epithelium, 1088
Barrett's esophagus, 1095, 1115
Bartholin glands, 1429
Basal cell carcinoma, 475t, 476, 476f, 1079
Basal ganglia, 868
Base, 73, 186
Base deficit, 191
Base excess, 191
Base pairs, 73
Basic cardiac life support, 686
Basic life support, 120t, 123
Basilar artery, 841
Basilar skull fracture, 880–881, 946
Basiliximab, 302b
Basophils, 293–294, 361, 565, 797t
Batista procedure, 702
Beau's grooves, 443t
Bedaquiline fumarate, 609
Bedbugs, 471
Bedside sonography, 1336–1337, 1337f
Bee stings, 137, 137b, 138t–140t
Beers criteria, 35, 36t
Behavior, Alzheimer's disease-related
   changes in
     description of, 861
     management of, 862–864, 865t
Belimumab, 328
Bell's palsy. See Facial paralysis
Below-the-knee amputations, 1051, 1051f, 1054, 1055f
Beneficence, 9
Benign cellular growth, 14
Benign prostatic hyperplasia
   assessment of, 1474–1477, 1475f–1476f
   care coordination for, 1481
   complementary and integrative health for, 1477
   concept map for, 1477f–1478f
   drug therapy for, 1477
   etiology of, 1474
   genetic risk of, 1474

Benign prostatic hyperplasia (Continued)
   health care resources for, 1481
   history-taking for, 1474
   home care management of, 1481
   incidence of, 1474
   International Prostate Symptom Score, 1474, 1475f–1476f
   interventions for, 1477–1480
   laboratory assessment of, 1476–1477
   lower urinary tract symptoms associated with, 1474, 1477
   nonsurgical management of, 1477–1479
   pathophysiology of, 1474, 1474f
   physical assessment of, 1474–1476
   prevalence of, 1474
   prostate artery embolization, 1479
   prostate cancer and, 1482f
   psychosocial assessment of, 1476
   quality of life after, 1481b
   self-management education for, 1481
   signs and symptoms of, 1474–1476
   surgical management of, 1479–1480, 1480b, 1480f
   transition management for, 1481
   transurethral resection of the prostate for, 1479–1480, 1480b, 1480f
   urinary retention caused by, 18
Benign tumor cells, 373–374
Benlysta. See Belimumab
Benzathine penicillin G, for syphilis, 1509, 1509b
Benzocaine spray, 525
Benzodiazepines
   chemotherapy-induced nausea and vomiting treated with, 399b
   overdose of, 281b
   shivering managed with, 135
Bereavement, 108
Beta amyloid, 858
Beta blockers
   acute coronary syndromes treated with, 776b
   atrial fibrillation treated with, 680
   glaucoma treated with, 966b
   heart failure treated with, 700
   hemorrhage treated with, 1177
   hypertension treated with, 725b, 727
   migraine headaches prophylaxis using, 875
   myocardial infarction treated with, 777
   types of, 677b–678b
Beta cells, 72
Beta particles, 387, 387f
Bevacizumab, 405, 589t, 1130

Bicarbonate
   absorption of, 1325
   description of, 187
   overelimination of, 192
   renal movement of, 190
   sources of, 188
   underproduction of, 192
Bichloroacetic acid, 1511
Bigeminy, 671
Biguanides, 1291, 1292b–1293b
Bilateral salpingo-oophorectomy, 1461t, 1466–1467
Bile, 1064
Bile acid breath test, 1141
Bile reflux gastropathy, 1118
Bile salt deficiencies, 1141
Bi-level positive airway pressure, 535, 631
Biliary cirrhosis, 1170
Biliary colic, 1193, 1193b
Biliary obstruction, 1170
Biliary stents, 1207
Biliary system
   components of, 1191
   gallbladder. See Gallbladder
   liver. See Liver
   obstruction of, 1191
   pancreas. See Pancreas
Bilirubin, 1068, 1069b
BIMS. See Brief Interview for Mental Status
Binge eating, 1216
Biofilm, 421, 991
Biologic dressings, 499
Biologic heart valve replacement, 709–710
Biological response modifiers
   bone marrow suppression treated with, 396
   cancer treated with, 401–402
   connective tissue diseases treated with, 323b
   Crohn's disease treated with, 1153, 1159
   interferons, 402, 402t
   interleukins, 402, 402t
   psoriatic arthritis treated with, 332–333
   renal cell carcinoma treated with, 1386
   rheumatoid arthritis treated with, 321–322, 323b
   self-management education for, 1156
   side effects of, 402
   ulcerative colitis treated with, 1153
Biopsy
   bone, 1013, 1013b
   bone marrow. See Bone marrow aspiration and biopsy
   breast, 1438, 1446
   cervical, 1437, 1437b
   endometrial, 1437–1438, 1466
   excisional, 445

Biopsy (Continued)
   hepatitis diagnosis using, 1184
   intraoral, 1080
   kidney, 1340–1341
   lung. See Lung biopsy
   muscle, 1013
   needle, 1243
   prostate, 1438
   punch, 445
   reproductive system assessments, 1437–1438, 1437b
   shave, 445
   skin, 445
Bioterrorism, 427–428, 466b
Biotherapy
   head and neck cancer treated with, 549–550
   non-Hodgkin's lymphoma treated with, 829
   skin cancer treated with, 477
Biotrauma, 635
BiPAP. See Bi-level positive airway pressure
Biphenotypic leukemia, 818
Bisacodyl, 99
Bismuth subsalicylate, 1112
Bisphosphonates
   bone tumors treated with, 1026
   osteoporosis treated with, 1021, 1021b
Bitemporal hemianopia, 934f
Bites
   arthropod, 136–137, 137b, 137f, 138t–140t
   snakebites, 135–137, 136b, 136f–137f, 136t, 138t–140t
   spider, 136–137, 137b, 137f, 138t–140t
Bivalirudin, 744, 784
Biventricular pacemaker, 675
Biventricular pacing, 681
Black box warnings, 1291
Black widow spider bite, 136–137, 137b, 137f, 138t–140t
Bladder
   anatomy of, 1327, 1327f
   capacity of, 98
   distention of, 1331
   function of, 1327
   neurogenic, 98t
   transitional cell carcinoma of, 1366
   trauma to, 1369
Bladder cancer, 380b
Bladder scanners, 1336–1337, 1337f
Bladder suspension procedure, 1348
Bladder training, for urinary incontinence, 1350–1351, 1351b
BladderScan, 98
Blanch, 483
Blast phase cells, 820
Bleeding. See also Hemorrhage
   in high-risk patients, 827b
   laboratory tests for, 805

Bleeding *(Continued)*
  in leukemia, 825, 825*b*
  management of, in pulmonary
      embolism, 622
  upper gastrointestinal. *See* Upper
      gastrointestinal bleeding
Blink reflex, 963
Blood
  accessory organs in formation of,
      797–798
  components of, 796–797
  infusion therapy of, 200
  spleen in formation of, 797
Blood administration set, 834*f*
Blood cells
  growth of, 797*f*
  laboratory assessment of, 803–805,
      804*b*
  types of, 796
Blood clot embolism, 1034*b*
Blood donation, autologous
  intraoperative, 263, 264*b*
  preoperative, 235
Blood glucose
  alcohol consumption effects on,
      1299
  continuous monitoring of,
      1298–1299
  exercise effects on, 1311
  fasting levels of, 1281*f*, 1282
  glycosylated hemoglobin and,
      1289*t*
  in hospitalized patients,
      1301–1302
  monitoring of, 1296*f*, 1298–1300,
      1311
  self-monitoring of, 1298, 1317
Blood osmolarity, 1332
Blood pH, 13–14, 188
Blood pressure
  ambulatory monitoring of, 728
  calculation of, 720–721
  definition of, 645
  determinants of, 645
  diastolic, 646
  elevated. *See* Hypertension
  as hydrostatic filtering force,
      161
  lifestyle modifications for,
      1284
  management of, 1284, 1381–1382
  measurement of, 652–653, 781,
      1284
  mechanisms that influence,
      720–721
  normal range for, 720
  paradoxical, 652–653
  in polycystic kidney disease,
      1381–1382
  regulation of, 646
  renal regulation of, 646
  screening of, 722*f*
  systolic, 646
Blood stem cells, 796, 796*f*
Blood thinners, 801

Blood transfusion. *See also*
      Transfusion
  allergies to, 263
  autologous, 836
  cell savers, 235, 310
  indications for, 832*t*
  infusion therapy for, 200
  in older adults, 834*b*
  reactions to, 835–836
  red blood cells, 834–835
    compatibility determinations
        for, 834, 834*t*
    indications for, 832*t*, 834–835
    sickle cell disease treated with,
        812
  reinfusion system, 310
  responsibilities in, 832–834
  safety in, 833*b*
  setup for, 832, 834*f*
  types of, 834–835
Blood urea nitrogen, 1331–1332,
      1332*b*
Blood urea nitrogen to serum
      creatinine ratio, 1332, 1332*b*
Bloodborne metastasis, 375
Bloodborne Pathogen Standards,
      202
Blood-brain barrier, 390–391, 841
Bloodstream infections, 416, 423
BLS. *See* Basic life support
Blumberg's sign, 1194
Blunt trauma, 129
BMI. *See* Body mass index
BNP. *See* Brain natriuretic peptide
Boceprevir, 1185*t*
Body fat, 1225
Body fluids. *See also* Fluid(s)
  chemistry of, 187–188, 188*b*
  electrolytes in, 173*f*
  pH of, 185–186
Body image, 92, 1019
Body mass index, 1215, 1215*b*, 1225
Body temperature
  in heat stroke victims, 134
  normal, 482
Body water
  insensible loss of, 165
  total, 160, 161*f*
Bolus feeding, 1221
Bone
  cancellous tissue of, 1005
  classification of, 1005
  flat, 1005
  function of, 1005–1006
  haversian system of, 1005, 1005*f*
  healing of, 1032, 1033*b*, 1033*f*
  irregular, 1005
  long, 1005, 1005*f*
  matrix of, 1005
  minerals and hormones associated
      with, 1006
  resorption of, 1006, 1239, 1276
  short, 1005
  structure of, 1005, 1005*f*
  vascularity of, 1005

Bone banking, 1043
Bone biopsy, 1013, 1013*b*
Bone marrow
  age-related changes in, 800
  blood stem cells produced by, 796,
      796*f*
  chemotherapy-induced
      suppression of, 396–398
  functions of, 795–796
  harvesting of, 823
  stem cell production in, 290,
      291*f*
  transplantation of, 822
Bone marrow adipose tissue, 1019
Bone marrow aspiration and biopsy
  description of, 806
  leukemia diagnosis using, 820,
      820*f*
Bone mineral density, 1016, 1019
Bone morphogenetic protein-2,
      1017*b*
Bone reduction, 1038
Bone scan, 1011
Bone tumors
  assessment of, 1025–1026
  benign, 1024–1025
  care coordination for, 1027–1028
  chondroma, 1024–1025
  chondrosarcoma, 1025
  drug therapy for, 1026
  Ewing's sarcoma, 1025
  fibrosarcoma, 1025
  giant cell tumor, 1025
  health care resources for, 1028
  home care management of, 1027
  interventional radiology for, 1026
  interventions for, 1026–1027
  malignant, 1025
  metastatic, 1028
  nonsurgical management of, 1026
  osteochondroma, 1024
  osteosarcoma, 1012, 1025
  pain management in, 1027–1028
  pathophysiology of, 1024–1025
  radiation therapy for, 1026
  radical resection of, 1026
  self-management education for,
      1027–1028
  surgical management of,
      1026–1027
  transition management for,
      1027–1028
Bone turnover markers, 1019, 1019*t*
Bony ossicles, 984, 985*f*–986*f*
Boots, for fractures, 1038, 1038*f*
Borborygmus, 1067, 1123
Bordetella pertussis, 613
Borrelia burgdorferi, 332
Bortezomib, 405
Bosentan, 330, 585
Bowel continence, 99
Bowel elimination
  assessment of, 90*t*, 91
  description of, 18, 18*f*
  rehabilitation for, 99

Bowel preparation, preoperative, 242
Bowel retraining programs, 99
Bowel sounds, 276, 1067, 1199
Bowel strictures, 1161
Bowman's capsule, 1323, 1324*f*
Brachial plexus injury, 267*b*
Brachytherapy
  balloon, 1451
  description of, 388
  endometrial cancer treated with,
      1466–1467, 1466*b*
  interstitial, 1451
  oral cancer treated with, 1081
  prostate cancer treated with, 1485
Braden Scale for Predicting Pressure
      Sore Risk, 42, 457*t*
Bradycardia
  heart rate in, 670
  sinus, 673*f*–674*f*, 674–675
Bradydysrhythmias, 671–672
BRAF gene, 477
Brain
  age-related changes in, 858
  anatomy of, 840–841, 840*f*
  cerebellum, 841
  cerebrum, 840–841
  circulation in, 841, 842*f*
  diencephalon, 840, 840*f*
  frontal lobe of, 841*t*
  occipital lobe of, 841*t*
  in older adults, 858
  parietal lobe of, 841*t*
  temporal lobe of, 841*t*
Brain cancer, 376*t*
Brain death, 947
Brain disorders
  Alzheimer's disease. *See*
      Alzheimer's disease
  encephalitis, 883–884, 884*b*
  meningitis. *See* Meningitis
  migraine headaches. *See* Migraine
      headaches
  Parkinson disease. *See* Parkinson
      disease
  seizures. *See* Seizures
Brain herniation syndromes,
      942–943, 943*f*
Brain injuries
  hypotension as cause of, 941
  secondary causes of, 941–943
  traumatic. *See* Traumatic brain
      injury
Brain natriuretic peptide, 166
Brain tumors
  assessment of, 951
  care coordination for, 955
  cerebral tumors, 950
  classification of, 950–951, 951*t*
  clinical features of, 951*b*
  craniotomy for, 952–953, 954*t*
  drug therapy for, 952
  etiology of, 951
  genetic risk of, 951
  increased intracranial pressure
      caused by, 954

Brain tumors (Continued)
infratentorial, 950, 953
interventions for, 951–954
meningiomas, 951
nonsurgical management of, 952
pathophysiology of, 950–951
pituitary, 951
stereotactic radiosurgery for, 952, 952f
supratentorial, 950
surgical management of, 952–954
transition management for, 955
Brainstem
anatomy of, 841, 841t
assessment of, 848
traumatic injuries to, 945
BRCA1 gene, 81, 83, 382, 1432
BRCA2 gene, 79, 382, 1432
Breakthrough pain, 54–55
Breast(s)
anatomy of, 1429–1430
biopsy of, 1438, 1446
clinical examination of, 1443, 1456
large-breasted women, 1456
lymphatic drainage of, 1430f
mammography of, 1435–1436
reduction mammoplasty of, 1456
small-breasted women, 1456
ultrasonography of, 1446
Breast augmentation
description of, 1456
in male-to-female transgender patients, 1499
Breast cancer, 376t
adjuvant therapy for, 1450–1451
aromatase inhibitors for, 1452
assessment of, 1445–1455
axillary lymph node dissection for, 1447
BRCA1 gene, 81, 83, 1442b
BRCA2 gene, 79, 1442b
breast-conserving surgery for, 1447, 1448f
care coordination for, 1452–1454
chemotherapy for, 1451–1452
complementary and integrative health for, 1446–1447, 1447t
coping strategies for, 1452
diagnostic assessment of, 1446
drug therapy for, 1451–1452
ductal carcinoma in situ, 1441
early detection of, 83
etiology of, 1442
genetic risk of, 1442, 1442b
health care resources for, 1454
health promotion and maintenance for, 1443–1445
in high-risk women, 1443–1445
history-taking for, 1445
home care management of, 1452–1453
imaging assessment of, 1446
incidence of, 1442–1443

Breast cancer (Continued)
infiltrating ductal carcinoma, 1441
inflammatory, 1441
interventions for, 1446–1454
invasive, 1440–1441, 1441f
laboratory assessment of, 1445–1446
in lesbian and bisexual women, 1446b
lobular carcinoma in situ, 1441
magnetic resonance imaging of, 1446
mammographic screening for, 1443, 1446
mastectomy for
adjuvant therapy after, 1450–1451
breast reconstruction after, 1449–1450, 1450t, 1451b
exercises after, 1451b
modified radical, 1448, 1448f
postoperative teaching for, 1453–1454
prophylactic, 1444
total, 1448f
in men, 1441
metastasis of, 1440–1441, 1446–1452
noninvasive, 1440–1441
nonsurgical management of, 1446–1447
pathophysiology of, 1440–1443
physical assessment of, 1445
prevalence of, 1442–1443
prophylactic mastectomy for, 1444
psychosocial assessment of, 1445
psychosocial preparation for, 1454
radiation therapy for, 1451
risk factors for, 1442, 1442t
screening for, 382, 1441, 1443
selective estrogen receptor modulators for, 1452
self-management education for, 1453–1454
sexuality issues, 1445
signs and symptoms of, 1445
stem cell transplantation for, 1452
surgical management of, 1447–1452, 1448b, 1448f, 1453b
survival rates for, 1442–1443
targeted therapy for, 1452
transition management for, 1452–1454
in young women, 1441
Breast disorders
benign, 1455–1456, 1455t
cancer. See Breast cancer
fibroadenoma, 1455, 1455t
fibrocystic breast condition, 1455–1456, 1455t
in large-breasted women, 1456
in small-breasted women, 1456

Breast implants, 1450t, 1456
Breast mass, 1445, 1445b
Breast reconstruction, 1449–1450, 1450t, 1451b
Breast self-examination, 1443, 1444b, 1456
Breast-conserving surgery, 1447, 1448f
Breath sounds, 519, 520t, 897b
Breathing
allergy effects on, 516
in lung cancer, 587
postoperative exercises, 281
primary survey of, 129, 131t
purpose of, 509
techniques in, for chronic obstructive pulmonary disease, 578, 578b
Brief Interview for Mental Status, 91, 861
BRMs. See Biological response modifiers
Broca's aphasia, 938
Bromocriptine, 870–871, 1248, 1248b
Bronchi, 510, 511f
Bronchial sounds, 520t
Bronchioles, 510, 511f
Bronchodilators
asthma treated with, 568–571, 569b–570b
bronchospasm treated with, 110, 604
Bronchogenic carcinomas, 586
Bronchopneumonia, 599
Bronchoscopy, 494, 525
Bronchospasm, 565
in artificial airway suctioning, 542
interventions for, 365
Bronchovesicular sounds, 520t
Brown recluse spider bite, 136–137, 137b, 137f, 138t–140t
Bruits, 653, 723, 729, 1067, 1330
B-type natriuretic peptide
description of, 694, 697
human, 698
Buerger's disease, 741t
Buffers, 186–189, 186f–187f
Bulimia nervosa, 1216
Bullae, 572
Bumetanide, 699
Bundle of His, 665
Bunion, 1028, 1028f
Bunionectomy, 1028–1029
Bupropion, for smoking cessation, 515, 515b
Burkholderia cepacia, 583
Burn injury
acute phase of, 497–504
acute respiratory distress syndrome in, 497
age-related complications that affect, 490b
airway maintenance in, 493–494

Burn injury (Continued)
airway obstruction caused by, 490t
ambulation after, 503
assessment of
cardiopulmonary, 497
cardiovascular, 491
gastrointestinal, 492
imaging, 493
immune, 497–498
kidney, 491–492
laboratory, 492, 493b
musculoskeletal, 498
neuroendocrine, 497
physical, 489–493
respiratory, 489–491
in resuscitation phase, 489–493
skin, 492
urinary, 491–492
capillary response to, 485, 485f
carbon monoxide poisoning secondary to, 490, 491t
cardiac changes caused by, 485–486
cardiovascular assessment of, 491
care coordination for, 505
chemical, 487
circumferential, 484
classification of, 482
compensatory responses for, 486
compression dressings in, 503–504, 504f
contact, 486
contracture prevention after, 503–504, 503b, 504f
deaths caused by, 488
deep full-thickness, 482t, 485, 485f
deep partial-thickness, 483–484
depth of, 482–485, 482t
direct airway injury caused by, 489–490
dry heat as cause of, 486
electrical, 487–488, 487f–488f
emergency management of, 489b
escharotomies for, 484, 494–496, 496f
etiology of, 486–488
fluid resuscitation for, 494–495, 495b
fluid shift after, 485, 485f
full-thickness, 482t, 484–485, 484f
gastrointestinal assessment of, 492
gastrointestinal changes caused by, 486
health care resources for, 505
health promotion and maintenance for, 488–489
history-taking for, 489
home care management of, 505
hypovolemic shock prevention in, 494–496
immunologic changes caused by, 486
incidence of, 488

Burn injury (Continued)
inhalation injury caused by, 490t
laboratory assessment of, 492, 493b
metabolic changes caused by, 486
minor, 483t
mobility after, 502–504
moderate, 483t
moist heat as cause of, 486
oxygen therapy for, 494
oxygenation support in, 493–497
pain management in, 491
partial-thickness, 482t, 483–484, 484f
pathophysiology of, 481–488
patient positioning, 503
prevalence of, 488
psychosocial preparation in rehabilitative phase of, 505
pulmonary changes caused by, 486
pulmonary fluid overload associated with, 491
radiation, 488
rehabilitative phase of, 504–506
respiratory assessment of, 489–491
resuscitation phase of assessment in, 489–493
overview of, 486, 489
rule of nines for, 492, 492f
scald, 486
self-esteem promotion in, 504
self-management education for, 505
skin changes caused by, 481–485, 484f, 492
smoke poisoning caused by, 491
superficial-thickness, 482–483, 482t, 484f
thermal, 488, 490
tissues involved in, 483f
total body surface area of, 489, 492
transition management for, 505
vascular changes caused by, 485
weight loss minimization after, 502
wound care management in
biosynthetic dressings for, 499
dressings for, 499
enzymatic débridement, 499
excision, 500
hydrotherapy, 498–499
mechanical debridement, 498–499
nonsurgical, 498–499
skin grafts, 500–501
surgical, 499–501
wound infections secondary to
drug therapy for, 501–502, 501b
indicators of, 498t
nonsurgical management of, 501–502
potential for, 501–502
surgical management of, 502
wound sepsis, 497–498, 498t

Burnout, 124
Butorphanol tartrate, 284b
Butterfly needles, 203–204
"Butterfly" rash, 326–327, 327f

C
C fibers, 47–48, 49f
CA-125, 1468
CA19-9, 1068, 1069b
CABG. See Coronary artery bypass graft
Cachexia, 1216
Café au lait spots, 79
CAHs. See Critical care access hospitals
Calcineurin inhibitors
autoimmune diseases treated with, 369, 370b
immunosuppression uses of, 302b
Calcipotriene, 464–465
Calcitonin, 1006
Calcitriol, 1277
Calcium
absorption of, 179
in bone, 1006
bound, 179
chronic kidney disease effects on, 1400, 1400f
description of, 179–181
free, 179
imbalances of
hypercalcemia, 181, 181t
hypocalcemia, 179–181, 180f, 180t, 196
in postmenopausal women, 180b
laboratory testing for, 1069b
in older adults, 165b
osteoporosis prevention with, 1020–1021, 1021b
parathyroid hormone effects on, 179, 1239, 1275
serum levels of, 164t
Calcium carbonate, 1020, 1112
Calcium channel blockers
chronic stable angina treated with, 777
coronary spasm prevention using, 717
high-altitude pulmonary edema treated with, 146
hypertension treated with, 725b, 726
migraine headaches prophylaxis using, 875
types of, 677b–678b
Calculous cholecystitis, 1192
Calf circumference, 1215
Callus, 1029t
Caloric testing, 991
CAM. See Confusion Assessment Method
Campylobacter enteritis, 1148t
Canada Food Guide, 1212

Canadian Hospice Care Association, 113–114
Canadian Triage Acuity Scale, 124
Canagliflozin, 1292b–1293b
Canal of Schlemm, 958
Cancellous tissue, 1005
Cancer. See also Adenocarcinomas; Oncologic emergencies; Tumor(s)
cardiac function affected by, 386
cervical, 1469–1470, 1470b
chemoprevention of, 382
classification of, 375–376, 377t
clotting affected by, 385
colorectal. See Colorectal cancer
development of, 375–382
dietary factors associated with, 379, 379b
emergencies caused by. See Oncologic emergencies
endometrial, 1465–1467, 1465t, 1466b
etiology of, 377–381
external factors that cause, 378t, 379
gastric. See Gastric cancer
gastrointestinal function affected by, 385
gene mutations associated with, 382
genetic risk of, 377–381, 380b
genetic testing for, 380–382
grading of, 376–377, 377t
head and neck. See Head and neck cancer
immunity affected by, 385
incidence of, 378f, 380, 381b
liver, 1186–1187
lung. See Lung cancer
management of. See Cancer management
metastasis of. See Metastasis
motor deficits caused by, 385
nasal, 556
nutrition support for, 385
in older adults, 380b
oral. See Oral cancer
ovarian, 1467–1469, 1467t
pain caused by, 385–386
pancreatic. See Pancreatic cancer
pathophysiology of, 372–374
peripheral nerve function affected by, 385
personal factors associated with, 380–381
physical function affected by, 384–386
prevalence of, 372
prevention of, 381–382
primary prevention of, 381–382
prostate. See Prostate cancer
race-based incidence of, 381b
radiation exposure as cause of, 379
respiratory function affected by, 386

Cancer (Continued)
risk factors for, 380–381
screening for, 382
secondary prevention of, 382
sensory deficits caused by, 385
skin. See Skin cancer
staging of, 376–377, 378t
testicular. See Testicular cancer
thyroid, 1275
TNM staging of, 377, 378t
tobacco use as cause of, 379
urothelial. See Urothelial cancer
vaccinations for prevention of, 382
warning signs of, 380t
Cancer cells, 387
Cancer management
angiogenesis inhibitors, 404t, 405
biological response modifiers, 401–402
brachytherapy. See Brachytherapy
chemotherapy. See Chemotherapy
cytotoxic systemic therapy. See Chemotherapy
epidermal growth factor/receptor inhibitors, 404t, 405
hormonal manipulation, 406–407, 406t
immunotherapy, 401–403, 402t
monoclonal antibodies, 402–403
multikinase inhibitors, 404t, 405
photodynamic therapy, 405–406
proteasome inhibitors, 404t, 405
radiation therapy. See Radiation therapy
small molecule inhibitor targeted therapy, 403–405, 403f–404f, 404t
surgery, 386–387
tyrosine kinase inhibitors, 404t, 405
vascular endothelial growth factor/receptor inhibitors, 404t, 405
Cancer pain
chronic, 47
intrathecal pump for, 62b
self-management education for, 68
Cancer therapy symptom distress, 395
Candida albicans, 346–347, 468, 1076
Candidiasis, 346–347, 347f, 467b, 468, 1076–1077, 1076b, 1077f
Cane, 1044
Cangrelor, 783–784
Canker sores, 1076
Canthus, 958
Capillaries
hydrostatic pressure in, 162
structure of, 162f
Capillary closing pressure, 451
Capillary leak syndrome, 485, 753
Capnography, 523, 523f, 524b
Capnometry, 523, 1222

Capsaicin, 308, 1307
Capsule endoscopy, 1071–1072
Carbapenem-resistant
    Enterobacteriaceae, 422–423
Carbohydrate counting, 1300
Carbohydrate metabolism, 188
Carbon dioxide
    blood pH determined by, 188
    definition of, 187
    description of, 508–509
    hydrogen ions and, 187–188
    metabolism effects on, 189
Carbon monoxide poisoning, 490,
    491*t*
Carbonic acid, 187, 187*f*
Carbonic anhydrase equation, 187*f*
Carbonic anhydrase inhibitors,
    974–975
Carboxyhemoglobin, 233–234
Carcinoembryonic antigen, 1068,
    1069*b*, 1129
Carcinogenesis. *See also* Cancer
    chemical, 379
    definition of, 375, 377–378
    physical, 379
    viral, 378*t*, 379
Carcinogens, 375, 378, 381
Cardiac arrest
    hypothermic, 143–144
    lightning injury as cause of, 141
    spinal anesthesia as cause of, 261
Cardiac axis, 666, 666*f*
Cardiac blood pool imaging, 661
Cardiac catheterization, 657–659,
    657*t*–658*t*, 658*f*
Cardiac conduction system, 664–665,
    665*f*
Cardiac cycle, 644–645, 644*f*
Cardiac muscle, 1007
Cardiac output
    burn injury effects on, 485–486
    calculation of, 645
    decreased, 25
    definition of, 645
    determinants of, 720–721
    diuretics effect on, 495
    in valvular heart disease, 708
Cardiac rehabilitation, 779, 790, 792
Cardiac resynchronization therapy,
    701
Cardiac tamponade, 713–714, 788
Cardiac valves, 642, 643*f*
Cardinal positions of gaze, 964, 964*f*
Cardiogenic shock
    acute coronary syndrome as cause
        of, 782
    etiology of, 753
    risk factors for, 752*t*, 756*b*
CardioMEMS implantable
    monitoring system, 701
Cardiomyopathy
    arrhythmogenic right ventricular,
        715
    assessment of, 715
    dilated, 714, 715*t*

Cardiomyopathy (*Continued*)
    heart transplantation for, 716–717,
        717*f*
    hypertrophic, 714–716, 715*t*
    interventions for, 715–717
    myomectomy and ablation for,
        716
    nonsurgical management of,
        715–716
    pathophysiology of, 714–715, 715*t*
    percutaneous alcohol septal
        ablation for, 716
    restrictive, 714–715, 715*t*
    signs and symptoms of, 715*t*
    surgical management of, 716–717
    treatment of, 715*t*
    uremic, 1401
Cardiopulmonary bypass, 143, 785,
    786*f*
Cardiopulmonary resuscitation, 129,
    686–687
Cardiovascular autonomic
    neuropathy, 1285
Cardiovascular disease
    contributory factors for, 649*b*
    description of, 642
    diabetes mellitus as risk factor for,
        1283–1284
    orthopnea associated with,
        649–650
    risk factors for, 646–648,
        1283–1284
    sedentary lifestyle as risk factor
        for, 647–648
    smoking as cause of, 647
Cardiovascular system. *See also*
    Heart
    acidosis effects on, 192, 193*b*
    age-related changes in, 646, 647*b*
    alkalosis effects on, 196, 196*b*
    arterial system, 645–646
    assessment of, 90, 90*t*, 802–803
        angiography, 657
        cardiac catheterization,
            657–659, 657*t*–658*t*, 658*f*
        computed tomography, 661
        current health problems,
            649–651
        diagnostic, 655–661
        echocardiography, 660
        electrocardiography, 659
        exercise electrocardiography,
            659–660, 660*f*
        extremities, 652
        family history, 649
        functional history, 651
        general appearance, 651
        genetic risk, 649
        history-taking, 646–651
        laboratory, 655–661, 656*b*
        magnetic resonance imaging,
            661
        myocardial nuclear perfusion
            imaging, 661
        nutrition history, 648–649

Cardiovascular system (*Continued*)
        physical, 651–655
        positron emission tomography,
            661
        psychosocial, 655
        serum lipids, 656
        skin, 651–652
        in spinal cord injury, 896
        in stroke patients, 934
        transesophageal
            echocardiography, 660
    auscultation of, 654–655
    burn injury effects on, 485–486,
        491
    dehydration effects on, 168
    emotional behaviors' effect on,
        646
    fluid overload effects on, 171*f*
    functions of, 641
    hypercalcemia effects on, 181
    hyperkalemia effects on, 178
    hypernatremia effects on, 175
    hypocalcemia effects on, 180
    hypokalemia effects on, 176
    hypomagnesemia effects on, 182
    hyponatremia effects on, 174
    inspection of, 653, 654*f*
    leukemia effects on, 819
    lightning injury effects on, 141
    nutrition assessments, 1213*b*
    in older adults, 222–223, 234*b*,
        647*b*
    postoperative assessments of, 274
    postoperative procedures and
        exercises for, 244–246
    preoperative assessment of, 236
    sickle cell disease effects on, 810
    venous system, 646
Cardioversion, 680–681
Care coordination, 3. *See also specific*
    disorder, care coordination for
Carotenoids, 979
Carotid artery angioplasty with
    stenting, 936
Carotid sinus massage, 678
Carpal tunnel syndrome, 1057–1059,
    1058*b*
Carrier, 79, 414
Case management
    of emergency department
        patients, 125
    purpose of, 3
Case manager
    care coordination by, 3
    in emergency departments,
        119–120, 125
    functions of, 3
    rehabilitation, 88
Caseation necrosis, 605
Cast (orthopedic)
    bivalving of, 1039
    circulation impairment caused by,
        1040
    definition of, 1039
    fiberglass, 1039, 1039*f*

Cast (orthopedic) (*Continued*)
    fractures treated with, 1039–1040,
        1039*f*
    infection concerns with,
        1039–1040
    removal of, 1045*b*
Cast (urine), 1335
Catabolism, 486, 1396
Cataracts
    assessment of, 969
    care coordination for, 971
    definition of, 958, 968
    etiology of, 960*t*, 968
    eye injury as risk factor for, 961
    genetic risks of, 968
    health care resources for, 971
    health promotion and
        maintenance for, 960*t*
    history-taking for, 969
    home care management of, 962*b*,
        971, 971*f*
    incidence of, 968
    interventions for, 969–971, 970*f*
    pathophysiology of, 968
    phacoemulsification for, 970, 970*f*
    physical assessment of, 969
    prevalence of, 968
    psychosocial assessment of, 969
    self-management education for,
        971
    signs and symptoms of, 969*f*
    surgery for, 969–971, 970*f*
    transition management for, 971
    ultraviolet light exposure and, 961
    visual impairment caused by,
        969*f*
Catechol O-methyltransferase
    inhibitors, 870
Catecholamines, 770
    adrenal medulla secretion of, 1238
    stress response activated by, 486
Catheter(s)
    central venous. *See* Central venous
        catheters
    complications of, 226
    dialysis, 1397, 1397*f*, 1414*t*
    dressings with, 212–214
    embolism caused by, 219*t*–220*t*
    epidural, 226
    flushing of, 214–215
    hemodialysis, 208
    intraperitoneal infusion therapy,
        225
    intraspinal, 226
    midline, 204–205, 204*f*, 213
    peripherally inserted central,
        205–206, 205*f*, 206*b*, 212–213
    peritoneal dialysis, 1418*f*, 1420*b*
    securing of, 212–214, 213*f*, 222*b*
    short peripheral, 202–204,
        202*f*–203*f*, 202*t*, 203*b*,
        214–215
    subclavian dialysis, 1397*f*
    urinary tract infections caused by,
        415, 415*b*, 421, 1355–1356

Catheter-acquired bacteremia, 415–416
Catheter-associated urinary tract infection, 415, 415b, 421, 1356b, 1423, 1500
Catheter-related bloodstream infection, 204–206, 211–212, 216, 216t, 220t–221t
Cations, 172
CAUTIs. See Catheter-associated urinary tract infection
Caval-atrial junction, 205
CBT. See Cognitive-behavioral therapy
CCR5 antagonists, 351b–352b
CD16+ cells, 299
CD4+ T-cells, 337–339
Cecum, 1064
Cefaclor, 1359b
Cefdinir, 1359b
Cefpodoxime, 1359b
Ceftriaxone, 1513–1514
Celecoxib, 321
Celiac disease, 1164, 1164b
Cell(s)
    abnormal, 373–374, 374t
    biology of, 372–373, 373f
    cancer, 373–374, 374t
    features of, 374t
    malignant transformation of, 375
    mitosis of, 373
    plasma membrane of, 290f
    specific morphology of, 373, 373f
Cell cycle, 373, 373f
Cell differentiation, 14
Cell replication, 14
Cell salvage, 235
Cell savers, 235, 310
Cell-mediated immunity
    cells involved in, 292t, 299–300, 797t
    cytokines in, 299–300, 300t
    description of, 22, 290–291, 299
    protection provided by, 300
    tuberculosis and, 605
Cellular growth
    benign, 14
    definition of, 14
Cellular regulation
    definition of, 14, 71, 372
    impaired, 14–15
    orderly and well-regulated growth of, 373
    promotion of, 15
    proteins involved in, 373
Cellulitis, 28, 453, 466, 467b
Center for Epidemiological Studies Depression-Revised, 850–851
Centers for Disease Control and Prevention, 414
Central cyanosis, 651

Central intravenous therapy
    hemodialysis catheters, 208
    implanted ports, 207–208, 207f–208f
    peripherally inserted central catheters, 205–206, 205f, 206b, 212–213
    tunneled central venous catheters, 207, 207f, 213, 226
    vascular access devices for, 205
Central line-associated bloodstream infections, 205, 762
Central nervous system
    acidosis effects on, 193, 193b
    alkalosis effects on, 196, 196b
    assessment of, 803
    brain. See Brain
    components of, 840–842
    function of, 840–842
    hypernatremia effects on, 175
    hypokalemia effects on, 176
    hypomagnesemia effects on, 182
    leukemia effects on, 819
    lightning injury effects on, 142
    sickle cell disease effects on, 810
    spinal cord, 842
    structure of, 840–842
Central nervous system disorders
    Alzheimer's disease. See Alzheimer's disease
    encephalitis, 883–884, 884b
    meningitis. See Meningitis
    migraine headaches. See Migraine headaches
    multiple sclerosis. See Multiple sclerosis
    Parkinson disease. See Parkinson disease
    seizures. See Seizures
Central perfusion, 25
Central venous catheters
    blood samples obtained from, 215
    central line-associated bloodstream infection with, 205
    complications of, 220t–221t
    dislodgement of, 220t–221t
    home care of, 826b
    migration of, 220t–221t
    nontunneled percutaneous, 206–207, 206f, 215
    rupture of, 220t–221t
    tunneled, 207, 207f, 213, 226
Central venous pressure, 653, 1396
Cerebellar pontine angle tumors, 951
Cerebellum
    anatomy of, 841
    function assessments, 849–850
Cerebral aneurysms, 1380
Cerebral angiography, 852–853, 852b
Cerebral cortex, 841, 841t

Cerebral edema
    high-altitude, 145–146, 145b–146b
    pathophysiology of, 950
Cerebral functioning, 274–275
Cerebral hemispheres, 840–841
Cerebral hypoxia, 758
Cerebral perfusion, 935–938
Cerebral vasospasm, 937
Cerebrospinal fluid
    functions of, 841
    leakage of, 907b, 946
    lumbar puncture examination of, 855
Cerebrovascular disease, 1284
Cerebrum
    anatomy of, 840–841
    assessment of, 848
    hyponatremia-related changes, 174
    tumors of, 950
Certifications, for emergency nursing, 120t, 123
Certified registered nurse anesthetist, 253t, 256
Certified wound, ostomy, continence nurse, 1130, 1131t, 1153, 1156–1157
Certolizumab, 1160b
Cerumen
    definition of, 984
    impaction of, 995b
    pathophysiology of, 994
    removal of, 987b, 994–995, 994b, 994f
Cervarix, 1469, 1511
Cervical ablation, 1470, 1470b
Cervical biopsy, 1437, 1437b
Cervical cancer, 1469–1470, 1470b
Cervical collar, 899, 899f, 945
Cervical intraepithelial neoplasia, 1469
Cervical lymph nodes
    anatomy of, 1080, 1080f
    metastasis to, 1082
Cervical neck pain, 909–910, 910b
Cervical spinal cord injury, 896–897
Cervical spine, 319b
Cervix, 1429. See also specific cervical entries
Cetuximab, 1130
Chagas disease, 1166
Charcot foot, 1304, 1305f
Checklist of Nonverbal Pain Indicators, 54
CHEK2 gene, 382
Chemical burns, 487
Chemical carcinogenesis, 379
Chemical débridement, 457, 457t
Chemoprevention, 382
Chemoradiation, for head and neck cancer, 549
Chemotherapy
    breast cancer treated with, 1451–1452
    cardiac function affected by, 386

Chemotherapy (Continued)
    cervical cancer treated with, 1470
    colorectal cancer treated with, 1130
    combination, 392
    drugs used in
        administration of, 392
        categories of, 391–392, 391t
        disposal of, 394
        dose-dense, 392
        intra-arterial infusion of, 225
        oral, 393–394, 393t, 394b
    endometrial cancer treated with, 1467
    esophageal tumors treated with, 1097
    gastric cancer treated with, 1116
    head and neck cancer treated with, 549
    intra-arterial infusion of, 392
    intrathecal administration of, 392
    intravenous administration of, 392
    intraventricular administration of, 392
    intravesicular administration of, 392
    liver cancer treated with, 1187
    lung cancer treated with, 588
    oral cancer treated with, 1080–1081
    pancreatic cancer treated with, 1206–1207
    polycythemia vera treated with, 816–817
    prostate cancer treated with, 1485
    protections during administration of, 392
    psychosocial issues during, 395–396
    side effects of, 395–396, 1119
        alopecia, 395, 400
        anemia, 397
        bone marrow suppression, 396–398
        cognitive function changes, 400–401
        extravasation, 392–393
        mucositis, 395, 399–400, 400b
        myelosuppression, 396–398, 397b
        nausea and vomiting, 398–399, 399b
        neutropenia, 395, 396b
        peripheral neuropathy, 385, 401, 401b
        short-term, 395
        thrombocytopenia, 397–398
    testicular cancer treated with, 1488–1489
    urothelial cancer treated with, 1366
Cherry angiomas, 439, 439f

Chest
  auscultation of, 1242
  landmarks of, 518f
  palpation of, 518–519
Chest expansion
  assessment of, 518
  inadequate, 192
  postoperative exercises for, 243, 244b
  semi-Fowlers position for, 21
Chest pain, 517. *See also* Angina pectoris
  atypical, 1089
Chest physiotherapy, 583
Chest trauma
  flail chest, 637, 637f
  fractures caused by, 1049–1050
  pulmonary contusion, 636
  rib fracture, 636–637
Chest tubes
  drainage systems for, 590–592, 591f, 592b
  placement of, 590–592, 590f
Chest x-rays
  acute respiratory distress syndrome evaluations, 627
  chronic obstructive pulmonary disease evaluations using, 577
  pneumonia evaluations using, 603
  preoperative, 237
  respiratory system assessment using, 521
Cheyne-Stokes respirations, 107
Chimerism, 824
Chlamydia infection, 1511–1512
Chlamydia trachomatis, 1511–1512
Chlorhexidine, 216–222
Chloride
  in older adults, 165b
  serum levels of, 164t
Cholecystectomy
  cholecystitis treated with, 1195–1197
  laparoscopic, 1195–1196
  postcholecystectomy syndrome, 1196, 1196t
  traditional, 1196–1197
Cholecystitis
  acalculous, 1192
  acute, 1192
  acute pancreatitis caused by, 1201
  assessment of, 1193–1194
  calculous, 1192
  care coordination for, 1197
  cholecystectomy for, 1195–1197
  chronic, 1192, 1194
  definition of, 1191
  diagnostic assessment of, 1194
  drug therapy for, 1195
  etiology of, 1192
  extracorporeal shock wave lithotripsy for, 1195
  features of, 1193b

Cholecystitis (*Continued*)
  genetic risk of, 1192
  hepatobiliary scan for, 1194
  icterus as cause of, 1192
  illustration of, 1192f
  incidence of, 1193
  jaundice associated with, 1192
  nonsurgical management of, 1195
  nutrition promotion in, 1194
  pain management in, 1194–1197
  pathophysiology of, 1191–1193
  percutaneous transhepatic biliary catheter for, 1195
  physical assessment of, 1193–1194
  prevalence of, 1193
  risk factors for, 1193t
  signs and symptoms of, 1193–1194
  surgical management of, 1195–1197
  transition management for, 1197
  ultrasonography of, 1194
Cholecystokinin, 1225
Cholecystotomy, 1195
Choledochojejunostomy, 1207
Cholelithiasis, 1192, 1195
Cholesterol, 656, 1069b
Cholesterol stones, 1192
Cholinergic agonists, 966b
Cholinergic antagonists, 569b–570b, 571
Cholinergic crisis, 918–920, 920t
Cholinesterase inhibitors
  Alzheimer's disease treated with, 864
  myasthenia gravis treated with, 919–920
  Parkinson disease treated with, 871
Chondroitin, 309
Chondroma, 1024–1025
Chondrosarcoma, 1025
Choreiform movements, 868
Choroid, 957
Christianity, 112t
Christmas disease, 831
Christmas factor, 798t
Chromatographic assays, 1243
Chromosomes
  formation of, 73, 73f
  genes in, 72
  locus of, 72
  number of, 72, 74
  sex, 74, 75f
  structure of, 74
Chronic airflow limitation, 564f, 572f, 635
Chronic back pain, 903
Chronic bacteriuria, 98
Chronic bronchitis, 573, 576
Chronic calcifying pancreatitis, 1202
Chronic cholecystitis, 1192, 1194
Chronic constrictive pericarditis, 712–713

Chronic gastritis, 1104–1105, 1105b
Chronic glomerulonephritis, 1378
Chronic health conditions, 86–87
Chronic hepatitis, 1182
Chronic kidney disease
  acidosis in, 1400
  acute kidney injury versus, 1391t
  albuminuria secondary to, 1399
  anxiety management in, 1410–1411
  assessment of, 1403–1404
  cardiac changes caused by, 1401, 1403–1404
  cardiac function in, 1407
  care coordination for, 1424–1425, 1425b
  causes of, 1401, 1402t
  cognitive changes associated with, 1401
  concept map for, 1405f–1406f
  definition of, 1398
  depression secondary to, 1411
  dietary restriction for, 1407t
  end-stage kidney disease progression of, 1398–1399
  etiology of, 1401, 1402t
  fatigue associated with, 1409–1410
  features of, 1391t
  fluid restriction for, 1405
  fluid volume management in, 1405, 1405b
  gastrointestinal changes associated with, 1401, 1404
  genetic risk of, 1401
  health care resources for, 1425
  health promotion and maintenance of, 1402, 1402b
  heart failure in, 1401
  hematologic changes associated with, 1401, 1404
  hemodialysis for
    anticoagulation during, 1413
    arteriovenous fistulas, 1413, 1414f–1415f, 1414t–1415t, 1415b
    arteriovenous grafts, 1413, 1414f, 1414t–1415t, 1415b
    cardiac events during, 1417
    care after, 1416, 1416b
    complications of, 1416–1417
    description of, 1411
    dialyzers, 1412–1413, 1412f, 1417
    hemofiltration versus, 1413f
    home care management of, 1424
    infectious disease transmission during, 1417
    nursing care during, 1416
    patient selection, 1411–1412
    peritoneal dialysis versus, 1411t
    procedure, 1412–1413, 1412f–1413f

Chronic kidney disease (*Continued*)
  self-management education for, 1424–1425
  settings, 1412
  temporary vascular access, 1416
  vascular access, 1413–1416, 1414f, 1414t–1415t
  history-taking for, 1403
  home care management of, 1424
  hospitalization for, 1402–1403
  hyperkalemia risks, 1400
  hyperlipidemia in, 1401
  hypertension in, 1401, 1407
  hyponatremia risks, 1400
  imaging assessment of, 1404
  immunity changes associated with, 1401
  incidence of, 1401
  infection prevention in, 1408
  injury prevention in, 1408–1409
  kidney changes caused by, 1399–1400
  kidney replacement therapies for, 1411–1424, 1411t, 1412f–1415f
  indications for, 1411
  kidney transplantation for
    acute rejection, 1423–1424, 1423t
    assessments after, 1425b
    candidate selection criteria, 1421
    chronic rejection, 1423–1424, 1423t
    complications of, 1423–1424, 1423t
    donors, 1421–1422, 1422f
    hyperacute rejection, 1423–1424, 1423t
    immunosuppressive drug therapy in, 1424
    incidence of, 1421
    living related donors, 1421, 1423
    operative procedures, 1422–1423, 1422f
    postoperative care, 1423
    preoperative care, 1422
    rejection, 1423–1424, 1423t
    self-management education after, 1425
  laboratory assessment of, 1404
  metabolic changes caused by, 1400–1401, 1400f
  nutrition in, 1407–1408, 1407t
  opioid analgesic dosing in, 1409
  pathophysiology of, 1398–1401
  patient and family education about, 1402b
  pericarditis in, 1401
  peritoneal dialysis for
    automated, 1419–1420, 1419f–1420f
    catheters, 1418f, 1420b

Chronic kidney disease (Continued)
  complications of, 1420–1421
  continuous ambulatory, 1418, 1419f
  continuous-cycle, 1419
  description of, 1408, 1417
  dialysate additives, 1418
  dialysate leakage during, 1420
  hemodialysis versus, 1411t
  home care management of, 1424
  intermittent, 1420
  nursing care during, 1421
  patient selection, 1417
  peritonitis caused by, 1420, 1420b
  procedure, 1417–1418, 1418f
  self-management education for, 1425
  types of, 1418–1420, 1418f–1419f
  phosphorus restriction in, 1408
  physical assessment of, 1403–1404
  polycystic kidney disease progression to, 1382
  potassium restriction in, 1408
  prevalence of, 1401
  prevention of, 1375
  priority problems for, 1404–1405
  protein restriction in, 1407–1408
  psychosocial preparation in, 1425
  pulmonary edema prevention in, 1405–1407
  respiratory symptoms of, 1404
  self-management education for, 1424–1425
  signs and symptoms of, 1403–1404, 1403b
  skeletal symptoms of, 1404
  sodium restriction in, 1408
  stages of, 1398–1399, 1399t
  transition management for, 1424–1425, 1425b
  uremic encephalopathy associated with, 1403
  urinary output affected by, 18
  vitamin supplementation for, 1408, 1410b
Chronic lymphocytic leukemia, 814t, 821
Chronic myelogenous leukemia, 814t
Chronic obstructive pancreatitis, 1202
Chronic obstructive pulmonary disease
  acid-base imbalances caused by, 13–14
  activity improvements in, 580
  alpha₁-antitrypsin deficiency as risk factor for, 573, 573b, 573t
  anxiety management in, 580
  assessment of, 574–577
  barrel chest associated with, 576

Chronic obstructive pulmonary disease (Continued)
  breathing techniques for, 578, 578b
  cardiac changes associated with, 576
  care coordination for, 581, 581b
  chronic bronchitis, 573, 576
  complications of, 573–574
  diagnostic assessments, 577, 577t
  digital clubbing associated with, 576, 576f
  drug therapy for, 578–579
  dry powder inhalers for, 579
  dyspnea in, 576, 580
  effective coughing for, 578
  emphysema, 572–573, 572f
  etiology of, 573
  exercise for, 579
  gas exchange affected by, 21, 21f
  genetic risks, 573
  health care resources for, 581, 581b
  health promotion and maintenance for, 574
  history-taking for, 574
  home care management of, 581, 581b
  hydration for, 579
  imaging assessment of, 577
  incidence of, 573
  laboratory assessment of, 576–577
  monitoring of, 578
  nonsurgical management of, 577–579
  oxygen therapy for, 578
  pathophysiology of, 572–574
  patient positioning with, 574, 576f, 578
  physical assessment of, 574–576
  prevalence of, 573
  psychosocial assessment of, 576
  pulmonary rehabilitation for, 579
  respiratory acidosis associated with, 195
  respiratory infections in, 573, 581
  self-care management of, 581
  severity assessments, 577t
  signs and symptoms of, 574–576
  smoking as cause of, 14, 21, 573
  stepped therapy for, 579
  suctioning in, 579
  surgical management of, 579–580
  transition management for, 581, 581b
  vibratory positive expiratory pressure device for, 579, 579f
  weight loss prevention in, 580
Chronic osteomyelitis, 1023–1024, 1023b
Chronic otitis media, 991

Chronic pain
  description of, 46–47
  epidural infusion for, 225
  in older adults, 56b
  psychosocial factors that affect, 52
  self-management education for, 68
Chronic pancreatitis, 1202–1204, 1203b–1204b
Chronic paronychia, 442
Chronic renal failure. See Chronic kidney disease
Chronic stable angina pectoris, 768–769
Chronic tophaceous gout, 331
Chronic transplant rejection, 301
Chronic venous insufficiency, 746–747
Chvostek's sign, 180, 180f, 182, 1201, 1277
Chyme, 1062–1063
Cigarette smoking. See Smoking
Ciliary body, 957
Cimex lectularius, 471
Cinacalcet, 1276–1277, 1408, 1410b
Ciprofloxacin, 612b, 1359b
Circle of Willis, 841, 842f
Circulation, 129–130, 131t
Circulator, 253t
Circumcision, 1430
Circumduction, 1010f
Cirrhosis
  abdominal assessment of, 1173
  advanced, 1173
  alcohol use as cause of, 1172
  ascites caused by, 1170, 1173, 1173f
  assessment of, 1172–1175
  biliary, 1170
  biliary obstruction caused by, 1170
  care coordination for, 1179–1180
  causes of, 1170t
  clotting factors affected by, 15
  compensated, 1170, 1173
  complications of, 1170–1172
  concept map for, 1175f–1176f
  decompensated, 1170
  definition of, 1169
  diagnostic assessment of, 1174–1175
  drug therapy for, 1175
  esophageal varices caused by, 1170
  esophagogastroduodenoscopy evaluations, 1175
  etiology of, 1172
  fluid volume management in, 1175–1177
  gastroesophageal varices caused by, 1170
  genetic risk of, 1172
  health care resources for, 1180
  hemorrhage management in, 1177–1178

Cirrhosis (Continued)
  hepatic encephalopathy caused by, 1170–1171, 1171t, 1178–1179
  hepatitis B as cause of, 1172
  hepatitis C as cause of, 1172
  hepatitis D as cause of, 1172
  hepatorenal syndrome caused by, 1171
  history-taking for, 1172
  home care management of, 1179, 1179b
  imaging assessment of, 1174
  jaundice secondary to, 1170
  laboratory assessment of, 1174, 1174t
  Laennec's, 1170
  magnetic resonance elastography of, 1174
  magnetic resonance imaging of, 1174
  nutrition therapy for, 1175
  paracentesis for, 1175–1177, 1177b
  physical assessment of, 1173
  portal hypertension caused by, 1170
  postnecrotic, 1170
  primary biliary, 1170
  psychosocial assessment of, 1173–1174
  respiratory support in, 1177
  self-management education for, 1179–1180, 1179b
  signs and symptoms of, 1173
  transition management for, 1179–1180
  transjugular intrahepatic portal-systemic shunt for, 1177–1178
  types of, 1170
CKD. See Chronic kidney disease
CLASBI. See Central line-associated bloodstream infection
Clean-catch urine specimen, 1334t
Clinical breast examination, 382, 1443, 1456
Clinical competence, 36
Clinical judgment, 8
Clinical psychologists, 89
Clitoris, 1429
Clock Drawing Test, 861
Clonus, 849
Closed fracture, 1032, 1032f
Closed reduction and immobilization, of fractures, 1038–1040
Closed-loop obstruction, 1122
Clostridium difficile
  microbiome changes and, 77
  stool tests for, 1068–1070
Clostridium difficile-associated disease, 428
Clostridium tetani, 501
Clot lysis, 15
Clothing, 142

Clotting
anti-clotting forces, 799–800
assessment of, 16
cancer effects on, 385
definition of, 15, 795, 798
drugs that affect, 801t
inadequate, 15–16
laboratory testing for, 16
nutrition effects on, 802
promotion of, 16
scope of, 15, 15f
Clotting cascade, 15, 798, 799f, 800
Clotting factors, 798–799, 798t
Clubbing, of nails, 443t, 652
CNPI. See Checklist of Nonverbal
   Pain Indicators
Coagulation, 805. See also Clotting
Co-analgesics, 55, 63
Co-carcinogens, 379
Coccidioidomycosis, 613
Cochlea, 986
Cochlear implantation, 999
Code of Ethics, American Nurses
   Association, 9, 9t, 1492
Codeine, 61, 77, 284b
Co-dominant, 75
Coercion, 81–82
Cognition
acidosis effects on, 193
age-related changes in, 844
Alzheimer's disease-related
   changes in, 860–861
assessment of, 847, 847b
   before rehabilitation, 91
   description of, 17
chemotherapy effects on,
   400–401
chronic kidney disease effects on,
   1401
definition of, 16, 860
diabetes mellitus effects on,
   1286
in human immunodeficiency
   virus infection, 355
in hypothyroidism, 1273
inadequate
   description of, 17
   in older adults, 35–38
   pain assessment challenges
      caused by, 53–54, 53t
promotion of, 17
scope of, 16
sleep deprivation effects on, 846
stroke effects on, 932–933
Cognitive impairment
in multiple sclerosis, 892b
pain management for, 59b
safe environment for, 17b
Cognitive rehabilitation, 948
Cognitive retraining, 1043
Cognitive therapists, 89
Cognitive-behavioral therapy,
   66–67
Cogwheel rigidity, 869
Cohorting, 421

Cold antibody anemia, 815
Cold-related injuries
frostbite, 144–145, 144b, 144f
health promotion and
   maintenance for, 142
hypothermia, 142–144, 143b
Colectomy, 1130
Collagen
in dermis, 431–432
in wound dressings, 499
Collagenase, 501b
Collateral circulation, 733
Colles' fracture, 1046, 1046f, 1057
Colloids, 170
Colon interposition, 1098–1099
Colon resection, 1130
Colon tumors, 1130t
Colonization, 455
Colonoscopy
American Cancer Society
   recommendations for, 1072
colorectal cancer diagnosis using,
   1128b, 1129
description of, 382
follow-up care for, 1072, 1073b
gastrointestinal system
   assessments using, 1072–1073
patient preparation for, 1072
procedure for, 1072
ulcerative colitis evaluations using,
   1152
virtual, 1073
Colony-stimulating factor, 294–295,
   826
Color vision
age-related changes in, 961b
testing of, 964
Colorectal cancer
adenocarcinomas, 1127
assessment of, 380b, 1128–1129
care coordination for, 1133–1135
chemotherapy for, 1130
colonoscopy of, 1128b, 1129
colostomy for, 1130, 1131f–1132f,
   1131t, 1132, 1134–1135,
   1134b
etiology of, 1127–1128
fecal occult blood test for,
   1128–1129, 1128b
genetic risk of, 1127–1128, 1133b
grief management in, 1132–1133
health care resources for, 1135
health promotion and
   maintenance for, 1128
hereditary nonpolyposis, 1126,
   1127b, 1466
history-taking for, 1128
home care management of,
   1133
imaging assessment of, 1129
incidence of, 1128
interventions for, 1129–1132
laboratory assessment of, 1129
metastasis of, 376t, 1127,
   1129–1132

Colorectal cancer (Continued)
minimally invasive surgery for,
   1130, 1132
nonsurgical management of,
   1129–1130
pathophysiology of, 1126–1128
physical assessment of, 1128–1129,
   1129f
prevalence of, 1128
psychosocial assessment of, 1129
psychosocial concerns in patients
   with, 1134–1135
radiation therapy for, 1129–1130
risk factors for, 1127–1128
screening for, 1070, 1128, 1128b
self-management education for,
   1133–1135
sigmoidoscopy of, 1128b, 1129
signs and symptoms of,
   1128–1129, 1129f
sites of, 1127f
staging of, 1129
surgical management of,
   1130–1132
transition management for,
   1133–1135
ulcerative colitis and, 1151t
vascular endothelial growth factor
   inhibitors for, 1130
Colostomy, for colorectal cancer,
   1130, 1131f–1132f, 1131t, 1132,
   1134–1135, 1134b
Colporrhaphy, 1465
Colposcopy, 1436, 1469–1470
Comatose, 846
Combination antiretroviral therapy,
   342–343, 350–353
Combination chemotherapy, 392
Comfort
decreased, 17–18
definition of, 17
in pericarditis patients, 713
scope of, 17
for urinary tract infections, 1359
Coming out, 1493t
Commando procedure, 1082
Common bile duct, 1064
Communicable infections, 414
Communicating hydrocephalus,
   943
Communication
with Alzheimer's disease patients,
   863b, 865
by emergency nurse, 123
hand-off, 119–120
with hearing-impaired patients,
   998b, 1001–1002
in patient unable to speak, 550b
with stroke patients, 938
in tracheostomy patients, 543–544
Community-acquired pneumonia,
   599t–600t
Community-associated
   methicillin-resistant
   Staphylococcus aureus, 422

Compartment syndrome
acute, 1033–1034, 1034b,
   1044–1045, 1044b
definition of, 224
description of, 738
fasciotomy for, 1044–1045
fractures as cause of, 1033–1034,
   1034b, 1044–1045, 1044b
frostbite as cause of, 144–145
in intraosseous therapy, 224
Compassion fatigue, 124
Compensated cirrhosis, 1170, 1173
Competence, 36
Competencies
core. See Core competencies
genetic, 72, 72t
Complement activation and fixation,
   297
Complement system, 294
Complementary and integrative
   health
agitation treated with, 111
Alzheimer's disease managed with,
   863
atherosclerosis treated with, 731
benign prostatic hyperplasia
   managed with, 1477
breast cancer managed with,
   1446–1447, 1447t
endometrial cancer treated with,
   1467
gastritis managed with, 1107t
human immunodeficiency virus
   infection treated with,
   353–354
hypertension managed with, 723
irritable bowel syndrome
   managed with, 1137
migraine headaches managed
   with, 875–876
multiple sclerosis managed with,
   892
after myocardial infarction, 791
nausea and vomiting treated with,
   111
obesity managed with, 1229
osteoarthritis managed with,
   308–309
pain management use of, 109, 285,
   308–309, 496
peptic ulcer disease managed with,
   1107t, 1112–1113
rheumatoid arthritis managed
   with, 324
sickle cell disease treated with,
   811–812
ulcerative colitis managed with,
   1153
Complete blood count, 803, 1068
Complete fracture, 1032
Complex patterns of inheritance,
   78t, 80
Complex regional pain syndrome,
   1035, 1041–1042
Compound fracture, 1032

Compression dressings, 503–504, 504f
Compression fracture, 1032, 1033f
Computed tomography
  cardiovascular system evaluations using, 661
  contrast-enhanced, 1338
  ear assessments using, 990
  gastrointestinal system assessments using, 1070
  musculoskeletal system assessments using, 1011
  neurologic system evaluations using, 853
  renal system assessments, 1337–1338, 1337t, 1338b
  reproductive system assessments, 1435
  respiratory system assessment using, 521–522
  urinary stones on, 1363f
  vision assessments, 965
Computed tomography angiography, 661, 853
Computed tomography colonography, 1073
Computed tomography coronary angiography, 774
Computed tomography perfusion study, 853
Computed tomography-based absorptiometry, 1019
Computed tomography–magnetic resonance imaging, 853–854
Concussion, 949b. See also Traumatic brain injury
Condoms, 1508b
Conductive hearing loss, 989, 996–997, 997t
Conductivity, 665
Condylomata acuminata, 1510–1511, 1510f
Cones, 957–958
Confidentiality, 81, 83
Confrontation test, 964
Confusion, 40–42
Confusion Assessment Method, 17, 38, 38t, 91
Congestive heart failure, 692
Conivaptan, 954, 1252b
Conization, 1437
Conjunctivae, 958
Connective tissue diseases
  ankylosing spondylitis, 334t
  biological response modifiers for, 323b
  characteristics of, 304–305
  dermatomyositis, 334t
  fibromyalgia syndrome, 333–334
  gout, 330–332, 331f
  laboratory assessments, 320–321, 320b
  lupus erythematosus. See Lupus erythematosus; Systemic lupus erythematosus

Connective tissue diseases (Continued)
  Lyme disease, 332, 333b
  Marfan syndrome, 334t
  osteoarthritis. See Osteoarthritis
  polymyalgia rheumatica, 334t
  polymyositis, 334t
  psoriatic arthritis, 332–333
  Reiter's syndrome, 334t
  rheumatoid arthritis. See Rheumatoid arthritis
  systemic necrotizing vasculitis, 334t
  systemic sclerosis, 326b, 329–330, 330b
  temporal arteritis, 334t
Conn's syndrome, 1260–1261
Consciousness
  definition of, 846
  level of. See Level of consciousness
Consensual response, 848, 963
Consent, informed, 239–241, 240f
Consolidation, 599
Constipation
  definition of, 18
  diabetes mellitus as cause of, 1285
  interventions for, 19
  nausea and vomiting caused by, 111
  in older adults, 31
  opioid analgesics as cause of, 63t
  in polycystic kidney disease, 1382
  postoperative, 277
  prevention of, 19, 1382
  risk factors for, 18, 31
Contact burns, 486
Contact dermatitis, 462, 463b
Contact transmission
  description of, 416
  precautions for, 419, 420t
Contiguous osteomyelitis, 1023
Continence, 18, 1327, 1343
Continuous ambulatory peritoneal dialysis, 1418, 1419f
Continuous bladder irrigation system, 1479, 1480f
Continuous blood glucose monitoring, 1298–1299
Continuous femoral nerve blockade, 315
Continuous kidney replacement therapies, 1397–1398
Continuous passive motion machine, 315, 315f, 316b, 1027
Continuous peripheral nerve block, 65
Continuous positive airway pressure
  heart failure treated with, 701
  indications for, 535, 536f, 559, 632
Continuous quality improvement, 7
Continuous sutures, 268f
Continuous tube feeding, 1221
Continuous venovenous hemofiltration, 1398

Continuous venovenous hemofiltration and dialysis, 1398
Continuous-cycle peritoneal dialysis, 1419
Contractility
  definition of, 665
  drugs that enhance, 699–700
Contractures
  after amputation, 1054
  prevention of, in burn injury patients, 503–504, 503b, 504f
  in spinal cord injury patients, 900–901
  Volkmann's, 1034
Contrast agents, 1338, 1338b
Contrast-induced nephropathy, 1338
Convergence, 960
Coombs' tests, 805
COPD. See Chronic obstructive pulmonary disease
Coping, 32–33, 655, 779, 1452
Copperhead snake bite, 136, 136f, 138t–140t
Cor pulmonale, 573–574, 574b, 584
Coral snakes, 136, 137f, 138t–140t
Cordectomy, 550, 551t
Core competencies
  clinical judgment, 8
  emergency nursing, 122–123
  ethics. See Ethics
  evidence-based practice, 7
  health care disparities, 10–11, 11t
  health care organizations. See Health care organizations
  informatics, 7–8
  patient-centered care, 2–3
  quality and safety education for, 2
  quality improvement, 7
  safety, 3–5
  teamwork, 5–6, 5t
  technology, 7–8
Core Measures, 7
Corn, 1029t
Cornea
  abrasion of, 977
  age-related changes in, 961b
  anatomy of, 958, 958f
  assessment of, 963
  infection of, 977
  lacerations of, 982
  opacities of, 977–979, 978f
  staining of, 965
  transplantation of, 978f
  ulceration of, 977
Corneal light reflex, 964
Corneal ring placement, 981
Coronary arteries
  anatomy of, 643, 643f
  atherosclerotic, 769f
Coronary arteriography, 658

Coronary artery bypass grafting
  bleeding after, 788b
  candidates for, 785
  cardiopulmonary bypass, 785, 786f
  complications of, 787–788
  description of, 784
  electrolyte imbalance after, 787
  endovascular vessel harvesting for, 789
  fluid imbalance after, 787
  health care resources for, 792
  home care management after, 789–790
  hypertension after, 787–788
  hypothermia after, 787
  indications for, 785
  internal mammary artery used in, 784–786
  mechanical ventilation after, 788
  mediastinitis after, 788–789
  methods of, 787f
  minimally invasive, 789
  off-pump, 789
  in older adults, 790b
  operative procedures, 785–786
  pain management after, 788
  postoperative care for, 786–789
  postpericardiotomy syndrome after, 789
  preoperative care for, 785
  self-management education for, 790–791
  special care unit transfer after, 788–789
  sternal wound infection as cause of, 785, 788–789
  sternotomy pain after, 788
  surgical site infections after, 786b
Coronary artery calcification, 661
Coronary artery disease
  atherosclerosis as risk factor for, 771. See also Atherosclerosis
  coronary artery bypass graft for. See Coronary artery bypass graft
  definition of, 768
  health promotion and maintenance for, 772
  home care management of, 789–790
  incidence of, 647
  percutaneous coronary intervention for, 783–784, 784f
  physical activity recommendations for, 791b
  prevention of, 771b
  risk factors for, 771–772, 772b, 790–791
  stents for, 783
  waist circumference and, 1225
  in women, 772b
Coronary artery vasculopathy, 717

Coronary heart disease. *See* Coronary artery disease
Coronary sinus, 642
Corpus callosum, 840–841
Cortical nephrons, 1323
Corticosteroids
asthma treated with, 569*b*–570*b*, 571
autoimmune diseases treated with, 368
chemotherapy-induced nausea and vomiting treated with, 399*b*
idiopathic pulmonary fibrosis treated with, 586
immunosuppression uses of, 302*b*
inflammation treated with, 462
psoriasis treated with, 464
side effects of, 324
Corticotropin-releasing hormone, 1236, 1238, 1260
Cortisol, 1237–1238, 1255, 1260*b*
Cosentyx. *See* Secukinumab
Costovertebral angle, 1330
Cough/coughing
for chronic obstructive pulmonary disease, 578
description of, 516
in spinal cord injury patients, 897–898, 898*f*
Counterimmunoelectrophoresis, 882
CPAP. *See* Continuous positive airway pressure
CPB. *See* Cardiopulmonary bypass
C-peptide, 1289
Crackles, 521*t*, 601, 696, 1089
Cranberry juice, 1359
Cranial nerves
assessment of, 847–848, 934
description of, 842, 844*t*
Guillain-Barré syndrome involvement of, 914
stroke-related effects to, 934
Cranial polyneuritis, 924
Craniotomy, for brain tumors, 952–953, 954*t*
CRBSI. *See* Catheter-related bloodstream infection
C-reactive protein, 1283
Creatinine, serum, 1331
Creatinine clearance, 1335–1336
chronic kidney disease effects on, 1400
gender differences in, 57*b*
test for, 34
Credé maneuver/method, 98, 1352
Crepitus, 305–306, 518
CREST syndrome, 329
Cricoid cartilage, 510
Cricothyroid membrane, 510
Cricothyroidotomy, 510, 558, 560–561
Critical access hospitals, 117
Critical care access hospitals, 9

Critical incident stress debriefing, 156–157
Crizotinib, 589*t*
Crohn's disease
abdominal assessments in, 1159
abdominal pain associated with, 1159
anemia associated with, 1159
assessment of, 1159
biologic response modifiers for, 1153, 1159
care coordination for, 1161–1162
clinical presentation of, 1158
complications of, 1151*t*, 1158
definition of, 1157–1158
drug therapy for, 1159, 1160*b*
family history of, 1158*b*
fistulas associated with, 1158, 1158*f*, 1160, 1160*b*, 1162
glucocorticoids for, 1160
health teaching plan for, 1161–1162
home care assessment for, 1158*b*
incidence of, 1158
interventions for, 1159–1161
magnetic resonance enterography of, 1159
nonsurgical management of, 1159–1160
nutrition therapy for, 1159–1160
pathophysiology of, 1157–1158
psychosocial assessment of, 1159
risk factors for, 1158*b*
signs and symptoms of, 1159
skip lesions associated with, 1157–1158
surgical management of, 1161
transition management for, 1161–1162
ulcerative colitis versus, 1150*t*
Cromones, 569*b*–570*b*, 571
Cross-bridges, 644
Cross-contamination, 820–822
CRPS. *See* Complex regional pain syndrome
Crusts, 438*f*
Crutches, 1043–1044, 1044*f*
Cryopexy, 979
Cryosurgery, 477
Cryotherapy, 66, 315
cervical cancer treated with, 1470
condylomata acuminata treated with, 1511
mucositis treated with, 400
oral cancer treated with, 1081
Cryptococcosis, 347
Cryptococcus neoformans
description of, 347
meningitis caused by, 881
Cryptorchidism, 1487
Cryptosporidium, 1166
Cryptosporidiosis, 346
Crystalloids
dehydration treated with, 170
hypovolemic shock treated with, 758–759

CSF. *See* Colony-stimulating factor
CTAS. *See* Canadian Triage Acuity Scale
CTD. *See* Connective tissue diseases
CTS. *See* Carpal tunnel syndrome
Cultural safety, 2
Culturally competent care, 152*b*
Culture (microorganism), 424, 444
Culture of safety, 4–5
Curative surgery, 386
Curettage and electrodesiccation, 477
Curling's ulcer, 486, 1108
Cushing's disease
adrenal, 1256
assessment of, 1256–1257
care coordination for, 1260
conditions that cause, 1256*t*
cortisol replacement therapy for, 1260*b*
description of, 1247, 1248*b*
dexamethasone suppression testing for, 1257
etiology of, 1256
features of, 1256, 1257*b*
fluid retention in, 1258
gastrointestinal bleeding in, 1259
health care resources for, 1260
home care management of, 1260
imaging assessment of, 1257
incidence of, 1256
infection prevention in, 1259–1260
injury prevention in, 1259
interventions for, 1258–1260
laboratory assessment of, 1257
nonsurgical management of, 1258
nutrition therapy for, 1258
pathologic fractures in, 1259
pathophysiology of, 1255–1256
physical assessment of, 1256–1257
pituitary, 1256
prevalence of, 1256
psychosocial assessment of, 1257
self-management education for, 1260
signs and symptoms of, 1256–1257
surgical management of, 1258–1259
transition management for, 1260
Cushing's syndrome, 721
Cushing's triad, 945
Cushing's ulcer, 1108
Cutaneous anthrax, 466–468, 467*f*
Cutaneous reflexes, 848
Cuticle, 432*f*, 433
Cyanosis, 443, 802*b*
central, 651
definition of, 651
CyberKnife, 952
Cyclic tube feeding, 1221
Cyclin D1, 1095*b*

Cyclooxygenase, 295
Cyclosporine, 302*b*, 1303
CYP450 enzymes, 57*b*
CYP2C9, 77
CYP2C19, 77
CYP2D6, 77, 77*b*
Cyst(s)
in fibrocystic breast condition, 1455
illustration of, 438*f*
Cystic fibrosis
assessment of, 582
chest physiotherapy for, 583
exacerbation therapy for, 583
gene therapy for, 583
genetics of, 582*b*
high-frequency chest wall oscillation for, 583, 583*f*
lung transplantation for, 583
nonsurgical management of, 582–583
pathophysiology of, 581–582
surgical management of, 583–584
sweat chloride test for, 582
Cystinuria, 1362*t*, 1365
Cystitis. *See also* Urinary tract infections
acute radiation, 1485
assessment of, 1357–1359
definition of, 1354
description of, 1329
diagnostic assessment of, 1358–1359
etiology of, 1354–1357
fungal infections as cause of, 1356
genetic risk of, 1354–1357
infectious, 1355
interstitial, 1354, 1356
noninfectious, 1356
pathophysiology of, 1354–1357
signs and symptoms of, 1358
surgical management of, 1359
Cystocele, 1352, 1464, 1464*f*
Cystogram, 1339
Cystography, 1337*t*, 1339
Cystometrography, 1340
Cystoscopy, 1339, 1358–1359, 1367
Cystourethrography, 1337*t*, 1339
Cystourethroscopy, 1339
Cytokines
in cell-mediated immunity, 299–300, 300*t*
definition of, 299
types of, 300*t*
Cytomegalovirus, 347
Cytoreductive surgery, 386
Cytotoxic drugs, 368
Cytotoxic edema, 942
Cytotoxic systemic therapy, 390–391. *See also* Chemotherapy
Cytotoxic T lymphocyte-associated protein 4, 367, 369, 477
Cytotoxic T-cells, 299, 797*t*

D

Dabigatran, 680, 801
Dacarbazine, 399
Daclizumab, 302b
Dalfampridine, 891
Dandruff, 441
Dantrolene sodium, 258–259
Dapagliflozin, 1292b–1293b
Darbepoetin alfa, 397, 402t
Dark-skin patients
    cyanosis in, 651, 802b
    jaundice in, 444
    oxygen saturation in, 516b
    pallor in, 802b
Dawn phenomenon, 1296
D-dimer test, 743
Death
    approaching, 107–108, 107b–108b
    definition of, 104
    direct causes of, 104
    in emergency department, 126–127
    leading causes of, 104t
    overview of, 103–104
    peaceful, 103
    physical manifestations of, 113b
    postmortem care after, 114, 114b
    pronouncement of, 114b
    without dignity, 103
Death rattle, 110
Débridement, of wound, 457, 457t
Debriefing, 156–157
Decadron. See Dexamethasone
Decerebrate posturing, 848, 848f, 946
Decerebration, 848, 848f
Decibel scale, 990
Decisional capacity, 36
Decompensated cirrhosis, 1170
Decorticate posturing, 848, 848f, 946
Decortication, 848, 848f
Deep brain stimulation, for Parkinson disease, 872
Deep breathing, 244b
Deep tendon reflexes, 848
Deep vein thrombophlebitis, 742
Deep vein thrombosis
    anticoagulants for, 743–745
    care coordination for, 746
    D-dimer test for, 743
    definition of, 742
    diagnostic assessment of, 743
    drug therapy for, 743–745
    fractures as risk factor for, 1034–1035
    health care resources for, 746
    home care management of, 746
    impedance plethysmography for, 743
    incidence of, 742
    low-molecular-weight heparin for, 744–745
    nonsurgical management of, 743–745
    novel oral anticoagulants for, 745

Deep vein thrombosis (Continued)
    pneumatic compression devices for prevention of, 245, 245f
    postoperative, 281
    prevalence of, 742
    prevention of, 23, 281, 744
    pulmonary embolism caused by, 617
    self-management education for, 746, 746b
    signs and symptoms of, 742–743
    surgical management of, 745–746
    thrombolytic therapy for, 745
    transition management for, 746
    unfractionated heparin for, 744
    venous duplex ultrasonography for, 743
    warfarin for, 745
Defecation, 1064, 1204
Defense mechanisms, 92
Defibrillation
    automated external defibrillator
        dysrhythmias treated with, 686–687, 687f
        illustration of, 687f
        ventricular fibrillation treated with, 685
    definition of, 686
    implantable cardioverter/ defibrillator, 686, 688b
Dehiscence, wound, 277, 278f, 282–283
Dehydration
    assessment of, 168–169, 1084
    care coordination for, 170
    in diabetes mellitus, 1283
    drug therapy for, 170
    fluid compartments affected by, 168f
    fluid replacement for, 169–170, 170t
    gender differences, 164b
    health promotion and maintenance of, 168
    injury prevention in patients with, 170
    interventions for, 169–170, 169b
    intravenous solutions for, 170, 170t
    isotonic, 167–168
    laboratory assessment of, 169
    in older adults, 167b, 1194b
    oral rehydration solutions for, 170
    pathophysiology of, 167–168, 167t
    prevention of, 1314
    relative, 167
    safety considerations in, 170
    signs and symptoms of, 168–169
    systemic changes associated with, 168–169
    transition management for, 170
    weight loss as sign of, 168
Delayed gastric emptying, 1118

Delayed union, of fracture, 1035
Delegation, 6
Delirium
    definition of, 16
    dementia versus, 20t
    in older adults, 38
    pain assessment challenges associated with, 53–54, 53t
    types of, 38
Delirium tremens, 232–233
Delta hepatitis, 1181
Dementia
    Alzheimer's disease, 857–858. See also Alzheimer's disease
    clinical features of, 858t
    definition of, 16, 857–858
    delirium versus, 20t
    emergency department visits for, 126b
    multi-infarct, 37
    in older adults, 37
    pain assessment challenges associated with, 53–54, 53t
    vascular, 857–858, 858t
    in veterans, 126b
Demerol. See Meperidine
Demyelination, 912–913
Dendrites, 839–840, 840f
Denial, 655
Denosumab, 1021, 1026
Deoxyribonucleic acid. See DNA
Depression, 1010f
    in Alzheimer's disease, 864
    in chronic kidney disease patients, 1411
    cognitive changes caused by, 850–851
    in older adults, 36–37, 37f
    post-stroke, 939
    screening tool for, 850–851
    selective serotonin reuptake inhibitors for, 37
    situational, 36
    after stroke, 939
Dermal appendages, 481–482
Dermal papillae, 432
Dermatitis
    atopic, 462, 463b
    contact, 462, 463b
    incontinence-associated, 1352
    radiation, 389
Dermatomes, 842, 843f, 896
Dermatomyositis, 334t
Dermatophytosis, 467b, 468
Dermis
    age-related changes, 434b
    anatomy of, 432
    definition of, 431
    functions of, 433t
Descending colostomy, 1131f
Desmopressin acetate, 1251, 1477
Detrusor hyperreflexia, 1345t
Dexamethasone, 146
Dexamethasone suppression testing, 1257

Dextran, 898
Diabetes insipidus, 1246b, 1250–1251, 1250b
Diabetes mellitus
    assessment of, 1288–1289
    blood glucose in
        continuous monitoring of, 1298–1299
        decreases of, 1309
        exercise effects on, 1311
        in hospitalized patients, 1301–1302
        levels of, 1281f
        monitoring of, 1296f, 1298–1300, 1311
        self-monitoring of, 1298, 1317
        therapy target goals for, 1298
    care coordination for, 1316–1318, 1316t, 1318b, 1318t
    Charcot foot deformity in, 1304, 1305f
    classification of, 1281–1282, 1281t
    complications of
        acute, 1283
        cardiovascular disease, 1283–1284
        cerebrovascular disease, 1284
        chronic, 1283–1286
        cognitive dysfunction, 1286
        constipation, 1285
        description of, 1280
        diabetic autonomic neuropathy, 1285, 1285t, 1305
        diabetic nephropathy, 1286, 1384–1385
        diabetic retinopathy, 1284, 1284b
        exercise adjustments for, 1301
        hyperglycemia, 1281
        hyperglycemic-hyperosmolar state, 1300b, 1313t, 1314–1316, 1314b, 1315f
        hyperlipidemia, 1280
        hypoglycemia. See Diabetes mellitus, hypoglycemia in
        immunity reductions, 1284
        ketoacidosis. See Diabetic ketoacidosis
        kidney disease, 1308
        macrovascular, 1283–1284
        microvascular, 1283–1286
        peripheral neuropathy, 1284–1285, 1285t, 1304–1307, 1305f
        sexual dysfunction, 1286
        stroke, 1284
        surgical complications secondary to, 1303
    concept map for, 1289f–1290f
    definition of, 1280
    dehydration associated with, 1283
    diagnosis of, 1288–1289, 1288t
    drug therapy for
        alpha-glucosidase inhibitors, 1292b–1293b, 1293

Diabetes mellitus (Continued)
amylin analogs, 1292b–1293b, 1293–1294
biguanides, 1291, 1292b–1293b
DPP-4 inhibitors, 1292b–1293b, 1293
examples of, 1292b–1293b
incretin mimetics, 1292b–1293b, 1293
insulin. See Diabetes mellitus, insulin for
metformin, 1291, 1291b
overview of, 1291–1299
patient education regarding, 1297–1298
selection of, 1291
sodium-glucose cotransport inhibitors, 1292b–1293b, 1294
thiazolidinediones, 1291, 1292b–1293b
in ethnic minorities, 1292b–1293b
etiology of, 1286–1287
exercise therapy for, 1300–1301, 1301b
foot care in, 1304–1307, 1305f–1306f, 1306b–1307b
foot deformities in, 1304–1307, 1305f–1306f, 1306b
foot ulcers associated with, 1305–1306
genetic risk of, 1286–1287, 1286b
gestational, 1281t, 1288
glycosylated hemoglobin in, 1289, 1289t
health promotion and maintenance for, 1287–1288
history-taking for, 1288
home care management of, 1317–1318, 1318b
hypoglycemia in
definition of, 1308–1309
drug therapy for, 1311
home care management of, 1310b
interventions for, 1309–1311
nutrition therapy for, 1310–1311
in older adults, 1312b
patient and family education about, 1311
patient education about, 1317
prevention of, 1308–1311
signs and symptoms of, 1308–1309, 1309t
incidence of, 1287
insulin for. See also Insulin
absorption of, 1295–1296
alternative administration methods for, 1296–1297
complications of, 1296, 1296f
continuous subcutaneous infusion of, 1294, 1296, 1296f
injection areas and sites, 1295f

Diabetes mellitus (Continued)
injection devices for, 1297
Lispro, 1294
long-acting, 1295t
mixing of, 1296
pen-type injectors for, 1297–1298
rapid-acting, 1295t, 1296
regimens, 1294–1295
short-acting, 1295t
stimulators of, 1291–1294, 1292b–1293b
storage of, 1297
subcutaneous administration of, 1297b
syringes for, 1297
types of, 1294
islet cell transplantation for, 1303
laboratory assessment of, 1288–1289, 1288b
learning needs assessments in, 1316, 1316t
lifestyle considerations for, 1288
meal planning for, 1300
medical nutrition therapy for, 1299–1300
nonsurgical management of, 1291–1302
nutrition therapy for, 1299–1301, 1299t
in older adults, 1300b
oral glucose tolerance testing for, 1289
pain management in, 1307
pancreatic transplantation for, 1302–1303
patient education about, 1317
polydipsia associated with, 1283
polyphagia associated with, 1283
polyuria associated with, 1283
prevalence of, 1287, 1292b–1293b
psychosocial preparation of, 1317
screening for, 1289
self-management education about, 1318t
signs and symptoms of, 1283
surgical management of, 1302–1304
survival skills information for patients with, 1316
testing for, 1287t
transition management for, 1316–1318, 1316t, 1318b, 1318t
type 1
etiology of, 1286
exercise therapy for, 1300–1301, 1301b
features of, 1281t, 1286t
genetic risk of, 1286b
hypoglycemic unawareness associated with, 1309
type 2 versus, 1286t

Diabetes mellitus (Continued)
type 2
etiology of, 1286–1287
features of, 1281t, 1286t
meal planning for, 1300
metabolic syndrome as risk factor for, 1287
prevalence of, 1287
testing for, 1287t
type 1 versus, 1286t
in veterans, 1291b
ulcers associated with, 732–733, 734b, 1305–1306
vision loss secondary to, 1307–1308
Diabetic autonomic neuropathy, 1285, 1285t
Diabetic ketoacidosis
acidosis management in, 1313–1314
characteristics of, 1311–1312
drug therapy for, 1313
hyperglycemic-hyperosmolar state versus, 1313t, 1314
interventions for, 1313–1314
pathophysiology of, 1312f
patient and family education about, 1314
signs and symptoms of, 1312–1313
Diabetic nephropathy, 1286, 1384–1385
Diabetic peripheral neuropathy, 1284–1285, 1285t, 1304–1307, 1305f
Diabetic retinopathy, 1284, 1284b
Diagnostic surgery, 386
Dialysate, 1412
Dialysis. See Hemodialysis; Peritoneal dialysis
Dialysis catheters, 1397, 1397f, 1414t
Dialysis disequilibrium syndrome, 1417
Dialyzer, 1412–1413, 1412f, 1417
Diamox. See Acetazolamide
Diaphragmatic breathing, 244b, 578, 578b
Diaphragmatic hernias. See Hiatal hernias
Diarrhea
antidiarrheal drugs for, 1153
best practices for, 19b
definition of, 18
Escherichia coli, 1148t
fluid and electrolyte imbalances caused by, 18
in human immunodeficiency virus infection, 354
interventions for, 19, 19b
skin care in, 1142b
in total enteral nutrition patients, 1223
in ulcerative colitis, 1152–1155
Diarthrodial joints, 1006–1007
Diascopy, 445

Diastole, 644, 706
Diastolic blood pressure, 646
Diastolic heart failure, 692
Diastolic murmurs, 655
Diazoxide, 1311
DIC. See Disseminated intravascular coagulation
Diencephalon, 840, 840f
Diet. See also Nutrition
chronic kidney disease managed with, 1407t
dumping syndrome managed with, 1118t
gastritis managed with, 1104–1105
gluten-free, 1164
hemorrhoids managed with, 1140
irritable bowel syndrome managed with, 1136
liquid formula, 1227
low-energy, 1228
novelty, 1228
nutritionally balanced, 1228
obesity managed with, 1227–1228
peptic ulcer disease managed with, 1112, 1112b
preoperative restrictions for, 241
urolithiasis treated with, 1365, 1366t
very-low-calorie, 1227
Dietary Guidelines for Americans, 1211, 1212t
Dietary Reference Intakes, 1211
Di-2-ethylhexylphthalate, 209
Diffusion, 162–163, 162f, 1412
Diffusion imaging, 853
Digestion, 1062
Digital breast tomosynthesis, 1446
Digital clubbing, 576, 576f
Digital 3D mammography, 1436, 1446
Digital rectal examination, 382, 1346–1347, 1474, 1483
Digoxin, 677b–678b
in chronic kidney disease patients, 1409b
heart failure treated with, 700, 700b
hypokalemia caused by, 176
toxicity caused by, 700b
Dihydroergotamine, 875
Dihydrotestosterone, 1481–1482
Dilated cardiomyopathy, 714, 715t
Dilation, 752
Dilaudid. See Hydromorphone
Dilutional hyponatremia, 1251
"Dinner fork" deformity, 1046, 1046f
Diphosphoglycerate, 512
Diplopia, 892, 917, 1246–1247
Direct commissurotomy, 709
Direct inguinal hernia, 1137, 1137f
Direct ophthalmoscopy, 966t
Direct response, 848
Direct thrombin inhibitors, 16, 617–618, 620, 801

Directed blood donation, 235
Directly observed therapy, 423, 610
Disability examination, 130, 131t
Disabling health conditions, 86–87
Disaster
    definition of, 149
    external, 149–151
    internal, 149
    nursing roles in, 155
    types of, 149–150
Disaster Medical Assistance Team, 153
Disaster triage tag system, 152, 152b
Discharge planning, 235
Discoid lesions, 327
Discoid lupus erythematosus, 326–328, 328b
Discomfort, 17
Disease-modifying antirheumatic drugs, 322, 368–369, 370b
Disequilibrium, 161
Disinfection, 418
Diskectomy
    back pain treated with, 906
    cervical neck pain treated with, 909–910, 910b
Dissecting aneurysms, 738–739
Disseminated intravascular coagulation
    assessment of, 763–764
    definition of, 761
    as oncologic emergency, 407
Distal convoluted tubule, 1323, 1325
Distal interphalangeal joint, 1009, 1009f
Distal radius fracture, 1046–1047, 1046f
Distal symmetric polyneuropathy, 1285t
Distraction, 66–67
Distress
    at end of life, 107–108
    refractory symptoms of, 111
    symptoms of, 108–111
Distributive shock
    chemical-induced, 753
    etiology of, 753
    risk factors for, 752t, 756b
Diuretics
    cardiac output affected by, 495
    fluid overload treated with, 20
    heart failure treated with, 699
    hypertension treated with, 725b, 726
    loop, 699b, 701
    potassium excretion caused by, 177
    potassium-sparing, 177, 699, 701
    syndrome of inappropriate antidiuretic hormone treated with, 1252
    thiazide, 699, 725b

Diverticula
    esophageal, 1101
    intestinal, 1162–1164, 1162f, 1163b
Diverticular disease, 1162–1164, 1162f, 1163b
Diverticulitis, 1162, 1164
Diverticulosis, 1162–1163
Diving reflex, 147
DLE. See Discoid lupus erythematosus
DMAIC model, 7
DMARDs. See Disease-modifying antirheumatic drugs
DMAT. See Disaster Medical Assistance Team
DNA
    base pairs of, 73
    bases of, 73
    complementary strands of, 73, 73f
    double-stranded, 73, 73f
    forms of, 73f
    replication of, 73–74, 74f
    structure of, 72–73, 73f
DNR order. See Do-not-resuscitate order
Dobutamine, 700, 783b
Docusate sodium, 1140
Dofetilide, 677b–678b
Dolophine. See Methadone
Do-not-attempt-to-resuscitate order, 104–106
Do-not-resuscitate order, 104–106, 263
Dopamine
    for myocardial infarction, 783b
    in Parkinson disease, 868
Dopamine agonists
    adverse effects of, 870b
    Parkinson disease treated with, 870–871, 870b
    restless legs syndrome treated with, 923
Dose-dense chemotherapy, 392
Double-barrel colostomy, 1131f
Double-barrel stoma, 1132
Double-contrast barium enema, 1070
Doubling time, 377
Douching, 1500
Dowager's hump, 1018, 1018f
Down syndrome, 988
Doxycycline, 612b
DPOAHC. See Durable power of attorney for health care
DPP-4 inhibitors, 1292b–1293b, 1293
Drain(s)
    postoperative, 277–278, 279f
    preoperative preparation for, 242
    types of, 279f
Drainage systems, for chest tubes, 590–592, 591f, 592b

Dressings
    biologic, 499
    biosynthetic, 499
    burn wound, 499
    with catheters, 212–214
    postoperative, 277–278, 278f, 281–282
    pressure, 267, 457–458
    synthetic, 499, 500f
    tracheostomy, 543, 543f
    transparent film, 499, 500f
    for venous stasis ulcers, 747
DRIs. See Dietary Reference Intakes
Driving safety, for older adults, 34, 34b
Dronedarone, 677b–678b
Droplet transmission
    description of, 416
    precautions for, 419, 420t
Drowning, 147, 147b
Drug(s). See also specific drug
    absorption of, 34
    acute pancreatitis treated with, 1200–1201
    age-related changes in metabolism of, 34
    allergic rhinosinusitis treated with, 365
    Alzheimer's disease treated with, 863–864
    angioedema treated with, 363
    assessment of, 35
    Beers criteria for, 35, 36t
    benign prostatic hyperplasia treated with, 1477
    bone tumors treated with, 1026
    brain tumors treated with, 952
    breast cancer treated with, 1451–1452
    cholecystitis treated with, 1195
    cirrhosis treated with, 1175, 1178–1179
    copayments for, 10
    Crohn's disease treated with, 1159, 1160b
    dehydration treated with, 170
    diabetes insipidus caused by, 1250
    diabetes mellitus treated with. See Diabetes mellitus, drug therapy for
    dialyzable, 1416t
    discoid lupus erythematosus managed with, 327–328
    distribution of, 34
    excretion of, 34
    fluid overload treated with, 172
    genital herpes treated with, 1507
    gout treated with, 331–332
    half-life of, 58–59
    hemorrhage treated with, 1177
    hepatitis B treated with, 1185t
    hepatitis C treated with, 1185t
    hepatitis treated with, 1184
    hypercalcemia treated with, 181

Drug(s) (Continued)
    hyperkalemia treated with, 178
    hypernatremia treated with, 175
    hyperpituitarism treated with, 1248
    hyperthyroidism treated with, 1267–1268, 1268b
    hypocalcemia treated with, 180
    hypokalemia treated with, 176
    hyponatremia treated with, 174
    infusion therapy, 201
    malabsorption treated with, 1142
    malnutrition treated with, 1219
    metabolism of, 34
    migraine headaches treated with, 874–875
    obesity caused by, 1226
    obesity treated with, 1228–1229
    osteoporosis treated with, 1020–1022
    ototoxicity caused by, 26
    peptic ulcer disease treated with, 1106b–1107b, 1111–1112
    peristalsis promotion using, 286
    preoperative, 241–242, 247, 257
    respiratory acidosis treated with, 195
    self-administration of, by older adults, 35, 35f
    stomatitis treated with, 1077–1078
    syndrome of inappropriate antidiuretic hormone treated with, 1252
    systemic lupus erythematosus managed with, 327–328
    transplant rejection treated with, 302b
    trigeminal neuralgia treated with, 924
    ulcerative colitis treated with, 1152–1153
    wound infection treated with, 282
Drug eruption, 463b
Drug holiday, 871
Drug reconciliation, 287
Drug-eluting stents, 783
Drug-induced hepatitis, 1180
Dry age-related macular degeneration, 979
Dry heat, 486
Dry powder inhalers
    asthma managed with, 570, 571b
    chronic obstructive pulmonary disease treated with, 579
Dual x-ray absorptiometry, 1019
Ductal carcinoma in situ, 1441
Ductal ectasia, 1455t
Dulaglutide, 1292b–1293b
Dulcolax. See Bisacodyl
Dumping syndrome, 1117–1119, 1118t
Duodenum
    anatomy of, 1064
    ulcers of, 1107–1108, 1108f, 1110

Dupuytren's contracture, 1028, 1028f
Dura mater, 840
Durable power of attorney for health
    care, 104, 105f
Duragesic. See Fentanyl
Dwarfism, 1006
Dying. See also End of life
    comfort during, 107, 107b
    dyspnea during, 109–111, 110b
    ethics and, 114–115
    grieving during, 112–114
    life review during, 112
    overview of, 103–104
    pain management during,
        108–109
    pathophysiology of, 104
    as process, 112
    psychosocial assessment of, 108b
    reminiscence during, 112
    signs and symptoms of, 107–108,
        107b
    storytelling during, 112
    weakness during, 109
Dysarthria, 938
Dyskinesias, 870, 872
Dyslexia, 933
Dyspareunia, 1165, 1246, 1515
Dyspepsia, 1065, 1088–1089, 1105,
    1110, 1193
Dysphagia, 109, 917, 934, 1077, 1089,
    1096, 1217b, 1275
Dysphasia, 91
Dyspnea, 517, 517t
    in asthma, 566
    in chronic obstructive pulmonary
        disease, 576, 580
    during dying, 109–111, 110b
    exertional, 695
    in follicular carcinoma, 1275
    in heart failure, 695
    in lung cancer, 593
    paroxysmal nocturnal, 517, 650,
        695
    pathophysiology of, 110
    visual analog scale for, 576, 576f
Dyspnea on exertion, 649
Dysrhythmias
    acute coronary syndromes as
        cause of, 779–780
    atrial. See Atrial dysrhythmias
    bradydysrhythmias, 671–672
    care coordination for, 681–684
    in chronic obstructive pulmonary
        disease, 574
    definition of, 671
    etiology of, 672
    home care management of,
        681–682
    in older adults, 682b
    pathophysiology of, 671–672
    patient care for, 672b
    premature complexes, 671
    prevention of, 682b
    self-management education for,
        682

Dysrhythmias (Continued)
    sinus, 672–675
    sinus tachycardia, 673, 673f
    tachydysrhythmias, 668b, 672
    transition management for,
        681–684
    ventricular. See Ventricular
        dysrhythmias
Dystrophic nails, 441
Dysuria, 236, 1381

E
Ear(s). See also Hearing
    age-related changes, 986, 987b
    anatomy of, 984–986, 985f
    assessment of, 988–989, 989f
    diagnostic assessment of, 990–991
    external, 984, 985f, 988
    foreign bodies in, 994–995, 994b,
        994f
    imaging assessment of, 990
    inner, 985–986
    irrigation of, 994b, 994f
    middle, 984–985, 985f
    otoscopic assessment of, 988–989,
        989f
    physical assessment of, 988–989,
        989f
Ear disorders
    acoustic neuroma, 951, 996
    external otitis, 993–994, 993b, 994f
    mastoiditis, 995
    Ménière's disease, 986–987,
        995–996
    otitis media, 991–993, 992f, 1023b
    tinnitus, 987, 995
    trauma, 995, 1000b
Ear infection, 1000b
Ear surgery, 993b
Eardrops, 993b
Eardrum
    anatomy of, 984–985, 986f
    otoscopic examination of,
        988–989, 989f
Earwax. See Cerumen
Eating disorders, 1216
Eaton-Lambert syndrome, 918
Ebola virus, 151, 427, 427t
EBP. See Evidence-based practice
EBPI. See Evidence-based practice
    improvement
Ecchymoses, 439, 802, 830, 1036,
    1173
Eccrine sweat glands, 433
Echocardiography
    description of, 660
    valvular heart disease evaluations,
        707
Edema
    assessment of, 652
    cerebral. See Cerebral edema
    formation of, 162
    in heart failure, 696b
    increased intracranial pressure
        caused by, 942

Edema (Continued)
    pitting, 171f, 652f
    pulmonary. See Pulmonary
        edema
    skin effects of, 437
Edentulous, 1218
Edrophonium chloride, 918–919,
    919b
Efferent arterioles, 1323
Efferent neurons, 840
EGD. See
    Esophagogastroduodenoscopy
EHR. See Electronic health record
Ejection fraction, 692
Elastase, 1197
Elder abuse and neglect. See also
        Older adults
    in Alzheimer's disease patients,
        865–866
    description of, 39, 39t
Elective surgery, 232t
Electrical bone stimulation, 1043
Electrical burn injuries, 487–488,
    487f–488f
Electrical cardioversion, 680–681
Electrical safety, 252
Electrical stimulation, 458–459
Electrocardiogram
    artifacts on, 670
    burn injury evaluations, 491
    graph paper for, 667, 668f
    normal sinus rhythm, 671, 671f
    P wave of, 665
    preoperative, 238
    rhythm analysis, 670–671
Electrocardiogram caliper, 670–671
Electrocardiography
    complexes, 667–670, 669f
    continuous monitoring using, 667
    description of, 659, 665–666
    electrode positioning for, 666,
        666f, 668b
    lead systems for, 666–667, 666f
    premature ventricular
        contractions on, 683f
Electroencephalography, 854
Electrolarynx, 552, 552f
Electrolyte(s). See also specific
        electrolyte
    abnormal levels of, 164t
    in body fluids, 173f
    deficit of, 20
    definition of, 19, 172
    excess of, 20
    in gastrointestinal tract
        dysfunction, 1068
    levels of, 164t, 165b, 173f
    in older adults, 165b
    plasma levels of, 165b
    serum levels of, 164t
    in urine, 1336
Electrolyte balance
    anatomy of, 160–164
    assessment of, 20
    definition of, 19

Electrolyte balance (Continued)
    homeostatic mechanisms in, 160
    laboratory testing for, 20
    physiology of, 160–164
    postoperative, 276
    promotion of, 20
    renin-angiotensin II pathway in,
        166–167, 166f
    scope of, 19
Electrolyte imbalances
    after coronary artery bypass
        grafting, 787
    diarrhea caused by, 18
    hypercalcemia, 181, 181t
    hyperkalemia, 178–179, 178t,
        179b, 192, 237
    hypermagnesemia, 182, 182t
    hypernatremia, 174–175, 175t
    hypocalcemia, 179–181, 180f, 180t,
        196
    hypokalemia, 175–177, 177b, 196,
        237
    hypomagnesemia, 181–182, 182t
    hyponatremia, 173–174, 174t
    interventions for, 20
    in older adults, 173b
    physiologic consequences of, 20
    preoperative assessment of, 237
    prevention of, 20
    risk factors for, 19
    severe, 172
    total enteral nutrition as cause of,
        1222–1223
    transfusion as cause of, 833
    types of, 20t, 164t
Electromyography
    description of, 854
    musculoskeletal system
        evaluations using, 1013
    myasthenia gravis evaluations
        using, 918
    renal system evaluations, 1340
Electromyoneurography, 918
Electronic health record
    description of, 8
    intraoperative review of, 263–264
    preoperative review of, 246–247
Electronic infusion devices, 211
Electronic infusion pumps, 211
Electronic medical record, 8
Electronic nicotine delivery systems,
    514
Electronic patient record, 8
Electronystagmography, 991
Electroretinography, 967
Elevation, 1010f
Elimination
    assessment of, 19
    bowel, 18, 18f
    changes in, 18–19
    definition of, 18
    interventions for, 19
    scope of, 18, 18f
    urinary, 18
E-mail, 5

Embolectomy, 621, 738, 936
Embolic stroke, 928–929, 929t, 934
Embolism
    blood clot, 1034b
    definition of, 15–16, 737
    fat, 1034, 1034b
    pulmonary. See Pulmonary
        embolism
Emergency care
    for amputation, 1053
    for drowning, 147
    for fractures, 1037–1038, 1038b
Emergency departments
    adverse events in, 121
    care environment of, 118–120,
        119f
    case management after, 125
    death in, 126–127
    dementia care in, 126b
    demographic data, 118
    disposition from, 124–127,
        130–131
    environment safety in, 120–121
    fall prevention in, 121
    family education in, 125–126
    forensic nurse examiners in, 118
    health care role of, 117–118
    health education, 125
    homelessness and, 127
    hospital-based, 117
    injury management in, 127
    interprofessional team in, 118–120
    language barriers in, 123b
    medical errors in, 121
    older adults in, 118b
    patient education in, 125–126
    patient identification in, 121
    patient safety in, 120b, 121–122
    physicians in, 119
    procedures commonly performed
        in, 122–123
    psychiatric crisis nurse team in,
        118–119
    skin integrity protection in, 121
    specialized nursing teams in,
        118–119
    staff in
        ancillary, 119–120
        professional, 119–120
        safety of, 120–121, 120b
    The Joint Commission metrics
        for, 117–118
    triage in, 123–124, 124t
    triage reception area in, 120–121
    vulnerable populations in, 118
Emergency management plan, 149
Emergency medical technicians, 119
Emergency medicine physician, 119
Emergency nurse
    communication by, 123
    core competencies of, 122–123
    description of, 119–120
    health teaching by, 125
    priority setting by, 122
Emergency Nurses Association, 124

Emergency nursing
    certifications for, 120t, 123
    core competencies of, 122–123
    principles of, 123–127
    scope of, 122–123
    training for, 120t, 123
Emergency operations center, 154
Emergency preparedness and
        response
    goal of, 151
    mass casualty triage, 151–153
    nursing's role in, 157
Emergency preparedness plan
    activation of, 153
    notification of, 153
    personal, 155
    The Joint Commission mandate
        for, 150
Emergency Severity Index, 124
Emergent surgery, 232t
Emergent triage, 124
Emetogenic, 398
EMLA, 65
Emmetropia, 960, 960f
Emotional abuse, of older adults, 39
Emotional lability, 934
Empagliflozin, 1292b–1293b
Emphysema, 83
    incidence of, 573
    pathophysiology of, 572–573,
        572f
    prevalence of, 573
Empyema, 604
EMR. See Electronic medical record
EMTs. See Emergency medical
        technicians
Enbrel. See Etanercept
Encephalitis, 883–884, 884b
End of life. See also Death; Dying
    advance directives for, 104–115
    agitation at, 111
    delirium at, 111
    grieving at, 112–114
    nausea and vomiting at, 111
    overview of, 103–104
    pain management during,
        108–109
    planning for, 104–115
    in prisoners, 106b
    psychosocial needs at, 111–112
    religious beliefs, 112t
    respiratory distress at, 110
    seizure management at, 111
    spiritual assessment at, 112–113
    spirituality during, 108
    symptom management at, 109
End stoma, 1132
Endocervical curettage, 1470
Endocrine disorders
    diabetes insipidus, 1250–1251,
        1250b
    hyperpituitarism, 1247–1250,
        1247f, 1248b
    hypopituitarism, 1245–1247,
        1246b

Endocrine disorders (Continued)
    psychosocial assessment of, 1242
    syndrome of inappropriate
        antidiuretic hormone,
        1251–1253, 1252t
Endocrine system
    adrenal glands, 1237–1238
    age-related changes in, 1240,
        1241b
    assays of, 1243
    assessment of, 1240–1243
    description of, 1234–1235
    diagnostic assessment of,
        1242–1243
    elimination affected by, 1241
    functions of, 1235
    genetic testing of, 1243
    glands of, 1234–1235, 1235f
    history-taking, 1240–1241
    hormones of, 1235t
    hypothalamus. See Hypothalamus
    imaging assessment of, 1243
    inspection of, 1241–1242
    laboratory assessment of,
        1242–1243, 1243b
    needle biopsy of, 1243
    in older adults, 1240, 1241b
    pancreas. See Pancreas
    parathyroid glands. See
        Parathyroid glands
    physical assessment of, 1241–1242
    pituitary gland. See Pituitary
        gland
    provocative testing of, 1243
    psychosocial assessment of, 1242
    suppression testing of, 1243
    thyroid gland. See Thyroid gland
    urine tests, 1243, 1243b
Endogenous osteomyelitis, 1022
Endolymph, 986
Endometrial biopsy, 1437–1438,
        1466
Endometrial cancer, 1465–1467,
        1465t, 1466b
Endorphins, 48
Endoscopes, 254, 255f
Endoscopic retrograde
        cholangiopancreatography
    acute pancreatitis diagnosis using,
        1194, 1199, 1201
    chronic pancreatitis diagnosis
        using, 1203
    description of, 1071, 1175
    pancreatic cancer evaluations,
        1206
Endoscopic sclerotherapy, 1177
Endoscopic ultrasound, for gastric
        cancer, 1116
Endoscopic variceal ligation, 1177
Endoscopy
    carpal tunnel release, 1058–1059
    definition of, 1070
    follow-up care for, 526
    gastroesophageal reflux disease
        treated with, 1091

Endoscopy (Continued)
    gastrointestinal system
        assessments using, 1070
    hemorrhage treated with, 1177
    pancreatic necrosectomy, 1204
    patient preparation for, 525
    procedure for, 525
    reproductive system assessments,
        1436–1437
    respiratory system assessment
        using, 524–526
    small bowel capsule, 1071–1072
    upper, 1089
    upper gastrointestinal bleeding
        treated with, 1113
Endothelin, 694
Endothelin-receptor agonists, 585
Endotoxins, 414
Endotracheal intubation
    description of, 561
    nursing care for, 629–630
    preparation for, 629
Endotracheal tube, 273
    complications of, 630
    description of, 628–629
    dislodgement of, 538, 629–630
    extubation of, 635–636
    obstruction of, 537–538
    placement of, 537, 628, 629f
    stabilization of, 629
Endovascular stent grafts, 739
Endoventricular circular patch
        cardioplasty, 702
ENDS. See Electronic nicotine
        delivery systems
End-stage kidney disease
    acute kidney injury progression
        to, 1398
    chronic kidney disease progression
        to, 1398–1399
    description of, 1286, 1379
    features of, 1403b
    treatment of, 1390
End-tidal carbon monoxide
        monitoring, 625
Enema, preoperative, 242
Energy balance, 1211
Enophthalmos, 963
Entacapone, 870
Entamoeba histolytica, 1165
Entecavir, 1185t
Enterostomal feeding tubes,
        1220–1221
Enteroviruses, 883
Enucleation, 982
Environmental emergencies
    altitude-related illnesses, 145–146,
        145b–146b
    drowning, 147, 147b
    frostbite, 144–145, 144b, 144f
    heat exhaustion, 133–134
    heat stroke, 133–135, 134b–135b
    hypothermia, 142–144, 143b
    lightning injuries, 141–142,
        141b

Environmental emergencies (*Continued*)
snakebites, 135–137, 136*b*, 136*f*–137*f*, 136*t*, 138*t*–140*t*
spider bites, 136–137, 137*b*, 137*f*, 138*t*–140*t*
stings, 137, 137*b*, 137*f*, 138*t*–140*t*, 141*b*
EOC. *See* Emergency operations center
Eosinophils
function of, 797*t*
in inflammation, 294
Epidermal growth factor, 1081
Epidermal growth factor/receptor inhibitors, 404*t*, 405, 549–550, 1130
Epidermis
age-related changes, 434*b*
anatomy of, 432, 432*f*
blood supply to, 432
functions of, 433*t*
Epidural analgesia
delivery of, 61, 61*f*
patient-controlled, 55, 61
Epidural anesthesia, 261*t*, 262*f*, 275, 275*b*
Epidural catheters, 226
Epidural hematoma, 226, 942, 942*f*, 954
Epidural space, 225, 840
Epiglottis, 510, 510*f*
Epiglottitis, 491*b*
Epilepsy
antiepileptic drugs for, 880
definition of, 876
health teaching for, 880*b*
Epinephrine, 1238
Epinephrine injectors, 363*f*, 364*b*, 365
EpiPen, 363*f*
EpiPen Jr., 363*f*
Epistaxis, 557–558, 557*b*, 558*f*
Epithalamus, 840, 840*f*
Epitympanum, 984
Epoetin alfa, 310, 397, 402*t*
Epoprostenol, 585
EPR. *See* Electronic patient record
Epstein-Barr virus
cancers associated with, 379*t*
leukoplakia caused by, 1078–1079
Eptifibatide, 736–737
Equianalgesia, 58, 60*t*
Equilibrium testing, 849–850
ERCP. *See* Endoscopic retrograde cholangiopancreatography
Erectile dysfunction, 27, 1286, 1484–1485, 1489–1490
Ergocalciferol, 1277–1278
Erlotinib, 589*t*
Eructation, 1089, 1193
Erythema migrans, 332
Erythrocyte(s), 290
description of, 796
growth pathway of, 797*f*

Erythrocyte count, 657
Erythrocyte sedimentation rate, 320–321, 425
Erythrocyte-stimulating agents, 797
Erythroplakia, 548, 1079
Erythropoiesis, 797
Erythropoiesis-stimulating agents, 397, 826
Erythropoietin, 290, 300*t*, 310, 1327
Erythropoietin-stimulating agents, 1410*b*
Eschar, 453, 466, 496*f*
Escharotomies, 484, 494–496, 496*f*
Escherichia coli
diarrhea caused by, 1148*t*
O157:H7, 427–428
Esophageal cancer
description of, 1095
physical assessment of, 1096
risk factors for, 1095–1096
Esophageal disorders
gastroesophageal reflux disease. *See* Gastroesophageal reflux disease
tumors. *See* Esophageal tumors
Esophageal manometry, 1089
Esophageal speech, 552
Esophageal stricture, 1088, 1096
Esophageal tumors
assessment of, 1096
care coordination for, 1100–1101
chemoradiation for, 1097
chemotherapy for, 1097
diagnostic assessment of, 1096
features of, 1096*b*
health care resources for, 1100–1101
history-taking for, 1096
home care management for, 1100
interventions for, 1097–1100, 1099*f*
nonsurgical management of, 1097–1098
nutrition therapy for, 1097
pathophysiology of, 1095
photodynamic therapy for, 1098
physical assessment of, 1096
psychosocial assessment of, 1096
radiation therapy for, 1097
self-management education for, 1100
squamous cell carcinoma, 1095
surgical management of, 1098–1100, 1099*f*
swallowing therapy for, 1097
targeted therapy for, 1097–1098
transition management for, 1100–1101
wound management of, 1099
Esophageal ultrasound, 1096
Esophageal varices, 1170
Esophagectomy, 1098

Esophagitis, 347*f*
reflux, 1087
Esophagogastroduodenoscopy
cirrhosis evaluations using, 1175
description of, 1089
esophageal diverticula evaluations using, 1101
esophageal tumor evaluations using, 1096
gastric cancer diagnosed using, 1116
gastritis diagnosed using, 1105
gastrointestinal uses of, 1070–1071, 1071*b*, 1071*f*
peptic ulcer disease diagnosed using, 1111
sliding hernia evaluations using, 1093
upper gastrointestinal bleeding treated with, 1113
Esophagogastrostomy, 1098, 1099*f*
Esophagus
anatomy of, 1062–1063, 1062*f*
chemical injury to, 1101
dilation of, 1098
diverticula of, 1101
functions of, 1087
perforation of, 1101*t*
trauma to, 1101–1102, 1101*t*
ESR. *See* Erythrocyte sedimentation rate
Essential hypertension, 721, 721*t*
Estrogen
for male-to-female transgender patients, 1493–1494, 1493*t*, 1497–1498, 1497*t*
osteoblast stimulation by, 1006
Estrogen agonists/antagonists, 1021, 1021*b*
ESWL. *See* Extracorporeal shock wave lithotripsy
Etanercept, 323*b*, 466*b*
Ethics
attributes of, 9
Code of, 9, 9*t*
context of, 9
definition of, 8–9
in genetic testing, 81–82
organizational, 9
professional, 9
Ethmoid sinus, 509*f*
Ethnic minorities
diabetes mellitus in, 1292*b*–1293*b*
special needs of, 10
Euploid, 74
Euploidy, 373, 376–377
Eustachian tube, 509, 509*f*, 985, 985*f*
Euthanasia, 114
Everolimus
autoimmune diseases treated with, 368–369
immunosuppression uses of, 302*b*
Eversion, 1010*f*

Evidence-based practice
attributes of, 7
context of, 7
definition of, 6
levels of evidence, 6, 6*f*
scope of, 6–7
Evidence-based practice improvement, 7
Evisceration, wound, 277, 278*f*, 283, 283*b*
Evoked potentials, 854–855
Ewing's sarcoma, 1025
Excisional biopsy, 445, 477
Excitability, 665
Exenatide, 1292*b*–1293*b*
Exercise
aerobic, 32
asthma managed with, 571
by older adults, 31–32, 32*f*
chronic obstructive pulmonary disease managed with, 579
diabetes mellitus managed with, 1300–1301, 1301*b*
obesity treated with, 1228
in osteoporosis prevention, 1020
peripheral arterial disease managed with, 740
swimming, 32
Exercise electrocardiography, 659–660, 660*f*
Exercise testing
for myocardial infarction, 774
for peripheral arterial disease, 733
for respiratory system assessment, 524
for valvular heart disease, 707
Exertional dyspnea, 695
Exertional heat stroke, 134, 135*b*
Exfoliative psoriasis, 464
Existential distress, 113
Exogenous osteomyelitis, 1022
Exophthalmos, 963, 1265, 1266*f*
Exotoxins, 414
Expedited partner therapy
for chlamydia infection, 1512
for gonorrhea, 1513
Exploratory laparotomy, 1125, 1146
Expressive aphasia, 938
Extended-care environment, 271
Extension, 1010*f*
External beam radiation therapy, 388. *See also* Radiation therapy
endometrial cancer treated with, 1466–1467
prostate cancer treated with, 1485
testicular cancer treated with, 1489
External disasters, 149–151
External ear, 984, 985*f*, 988
External fixator, 1043
External genitalia, 1428–1429
External hemorrhoids, 1139, 1140*f*
External otitis, 993–994, 993*b*, 994*f*
External trigeminal nerve stimulator, 875

External urethral sphincter, 1327, 1327f

Extracellular fluid, 19, 160, 162, 164, 173, 188

Extracorporeal membrane oxygenation, 628

Extracorporeal shock wave lithotripsy, 1195, 1364

Extraocular muscles, 959, 959f, 960t, 964, 964f

Extravasation, 200b, 204, 217t–219t, 392–393

Extremity assessment, 652

Extremity pain, 651

Extrinsic factors, 798

Extubation, of endotracheal tube, 635–636

Eye(s). See also Vision
   age-related changes in, 961, 961b
   anatomy of, 957–959, 958f–959f
   blood vessels of, 959
   donation of, for corneal transplantation, 979
   electroretinography of, 967
   external structures of, 958–959, 959f
   extraocular muscles of, 959, 959f, 960t, 964, 964f
   fluorescein angiography of, 966–967
   foreign bodies in, 981
   function of, 960
   gonioscopy of, 967
   innervation of, 959
   lacerations to, 981–982
   layers of, 957–958, 958f
   muscles of, 959, 959f, 960t
   ophthalmoscopy evaluations, 966, 966f, 966t
   penetrating injuries to, 982
   refractive structures and media of, 958
   slit-lamp examination of, 965, 965f
   structure of, 957–959, 958f
   trauma to, 981–982

Eye disorders
   cataracts. See Cataract
   cornea
      abrasion of, 977
      infection of, 977
      opacities, 977–979, 978f
      ulceration of, 977
   glaucoma. See Glaucoma
   keratoconus, 977–979, 978f
   refractive errors, 960, 960f, 980–981
   retinal detachment, 979–980
   retinal holes, 979–980
   retinal tears, 979–980

Eye infections, 961–962, 962b

Eyedrops, 961–962, 962b, 966b, 971f

Eyelids
   anatomy of, 958, 959f
   eversion of, 435f
   laceration of, 981

Ezetimibe, 730

F

Face tent, 534–535, 534t

Facemasks
   nonrebreather, 532t, 533, 533f
   partial rebreather, 532–533, 532t, 533f
   simple, 532, 532t, 533f

FACES pain scale—revised, 50–52

Facial expression
   in myasthenia gravis, 917–918, 918f
   in Parkinson disease, 869, 869f

Facial nerve, 844t

Facial paralysis, 924–925

Facial trauma, 558–559

Facilitated diffusion, 162–163

Factor V Leiden, 619b

Factor VIII replacement, 831

Failed back surgery syndrome, 909

Failure to rescue, 8

Fall(s)
   definition of, 40–41
   home modifications for prevention of, 33, 33b
   in older adults, 33, 33b, 40–42
   preoperative assessment of, 236
   prevention of
      in alkalosis patients, 197
      description of, 33, 33b
      in emergency departments, 121
   risk factors for, 41b
   toileting-related, 41

Fallophobia, 33

Fallopian tubes, 1429

Familial adenomatous polyposis, 1065, 1126, 1127b, 1128

Familial clustering, 80

Family caregivers, 866, 866b

Family-centered care, 2

Fanconi's anemia, 815

Fasciculations, 919

Fasciotomies, 484, 738, 1044–1045

Fasting blood glucose, 1281f

Fasting plasma glucose, 1289

Fat emboli, 617

Fat embolism syndrome, 1034, 1034b

Fat malabsorption, 1202–1203

Fatigue
   in anemia, 802
   assessment of, 90
   in chronic kidney disease, 1409–1410
   definition of, 650
   in heart failure, 702
   hepatitis as cause of, 1184
   in leukemia, 825–826
   in pancreatic cancer, 1206
   in systemic lupus erythematosus, 327
   in tuberculosis, 610

Fatigue fracture, 1032

Fatty liver, 1185–1186

Fc fragment, 297, 297f

Fear, preoperative, 237

Febrile transfusion reaction, 835

Febuxostat, 331–332

Fecal fats, 1068–1070, 1141

Fecal immunochemical test, 1068

Fecal impaction, 1125, 1126b

Fecal incontinence, 18

Fecal microbiota transplantation, 428

Fecal occult blood test, 1068, 1128–1129, 1128b

Federal Emergency Management Agency, 153

Feeding tubes, 552–553. See also Endotracheal tube

Felty's syndrome, 321

FEMA. See Federal Emergency Management Agency

Female reproductive system
   anatomy of, 1428–1430, 1429f–1430f
   breasts, 1429–1430
   external genitalia, 1428–1429
   internal genitalia, 1429, 1429f
   in older adults, 1431b
   pelvic examination, 1433
   physical assessment of, 1433
   structure of, 1428–1430

Female-to-male transgender patients
   definition of, 1493–1494, 1493t
   drug therapy for, 1498
   masculinizing surgeries for, 1500–1501
   phalloplasty for, 1501

Femoral aneurysms, 740

Femoral fractures, 1048

Femoral hernia, 1137, 1137f

Fenoldopam, 783b

Fentanyl (Fentora)
   equianalgesic dosing of, 60t
   transdermal delivery of, 60, 60b

Ferumoxytol, 815–816

Fetal hemoglobin, 808, 811

Fetor hepaticus, 1173

Fever
   antipyretic drugs for, 426
   cooling methods for, 426
   dehydration and, 168–169
   as infection sign, 424b, 425–426
   interventions for, 425–426

Fiberglass cast, 1039, 1039f

Fibrin clot, 798–799

Fibrinogen, 796, 798t

Fibrinolysis, 800f

Fibrinolytic system, 15

Fibrinolytics, 777–778, 778t
   acute arterial occlusions treated with, 738
   anticoagulant action of, 801
   injury prevention in patients using, 623b
   mechanism of action, 801
   pulmonary embolism treated with, 621b
   stroke treated with, 935

Fibrin-stabilizing factor, 798t

Fibroadenoma, 1455, 1455t

Fibrocystic breast condition, 1455–1456, 1455t

Fibroids, 1459–1460

Fibromyalgia syndrome, 333–334

Fibrosarcoma, 1025

Fibrosis, 1441

Fibular fracture, 1048–1049

Fidelity, 9

Field block, 261f, 261t

"Fight or flight" mechanism, 18, 46–47, 1238

Filgrastim, 402t

Filtration
   definition of, 161
   diagram of, 161f
   in fluid balance, 161–162, 161f–162f

FIM. See Functional Independence Measure

Financial abuse, of older adults, 39

Finasteride, 1498

Fingolimod, 891

Fire, 150b

Fire safety, 252

Fire triangle, 252, 254f

First aid
   for drowning, 147
   for frostbite, 144
   for heat stroke, 134
   for hypothermia, 143
   for lightning injury, 142

First heart sound, 654

First-degree frostbite, 144

Fissures, 438f

Fistulae
   anal, 1165
   in Crohn's disease, 1158, 1158f, 1160, 1160b
   skin barriers around, 1161f
   in ulcerative colitis, 1151t, 1158
   after Whipple procedure, 1208

Flaccid bladder, 97–98, 98t

Flaccid paralysis, 933, 938

Flail chest, 637, 637f

Flash burns, 488

Flat bones, 1005

Flatulence, 1089, 1193

Flexion, 1010f

Fludrocortisone, 1255b

Fluid(s)
   composition of, 161
   description of, 19, 160
   electrolyte composition of, 173f
   extracellular, 19, 160, 162, 164
   functions of, 160–161
   intake regulation, 164, 165t
   interstitial, 160
   intracellular, 19, 160, 162, 164
   loss of, 164–165, 165t
   pH, 185–186

Fluid balance
   age-related changes in, 165b
   aldosterone regulation of, 165

Fluid balance (*Continued*)
anatomy of, 160–164
antidiuretic hormone regulation of, 165–166
assessment of, 20
definition of, 19
diffusion in, 162–163, 162*f*
filtration in, 161–162, 161*f*–162*f*
homeostatic mechanisms in, 160
hormonal regulation of, 165–166
laboratory testing for, 20
natriuretic peptide regulation by, 166
osmosis in, 163–164, 163*f*
physiology of, 160–164
postoperative, 276
promotion of, 20
renin-angiotensin II pathway in, 166–167, 166*f*
scope of, 19
Fluid compartments
dehydration effects on, 168*f*
fluid overload effects on, 171*f*
Fluid deficit, 20
Fluid excess, 20
Fluid imbalances
after coronary artery bypass grafting, 787
dehydration. *See* Dehydration
diarrhea caused by, 18
fluid shift as cause of, 485
interventions for, 20
parenteral nutrition as cause of, 1224
physiologic consequences of, 20
prevention of, 20
risk factors for, 19
total enteral nutrition as cause of, 1222–1223
types of, 20*t*
Fluid overload
assessment of, 171
cardiac complications during, 171*f*
description of, 20
drug therapy for, 172
features of, 172*b*
fluid compartment changes associated with, 171*f*
hypervolemia, 171
interventions for, 171–172
nutrition therapy for, 172
pathophysiology of, 167*t*, 171
in pulmonary edema, 172*b*
respiratory complications during, 171*f*
safety considerations in, 172
in syndrome of inappropriate antidiuretic hormone, 1252
total enteral nutrition as cause of, 1222
Fluid remobilization, 485
Fluid replacement
dehydration treated with, 169–170, 170*t*

Fluid replacement (*Continued*)
hyperglycemic-hyperosmolar state treated with, 1315
kidney trauma treated with, 1387
Fluid restriction
by older adults, 31*b*
in chronic kidney disease, 1405
syndrome of inappropriate antidiuretic hormone treated with, 1252
Fluid resuscitation
burn injury treated with, 494–495, 495*b*
intravenous therapy for, 758–759
Fluid retention
in Cushing's disease, 1258
weight gain as sign of, 172
Fluid volume management
in chronic kidney disease, 1405, 1405*b*
in cirrhosis, 1175–1177
Fluorescein angiography, 966–967
Fluorescent antinuclear antibody test, 320
Fluorescent treponemal antibody absorption test, 1509
Fluoroscopy, 527
5-Fluorouracil
pancreatic cancer treated with, 1206–1207
skin cancer treated with, 477
Flushing of catheters, 214–215
Fluticasone, 569*b*–570*b*
Focal brain injury, 941
FOCUS-Plan-Do-Study-Act model, 7
Folic acid deficiency anemia, 814–816, 814*t*
Follicle-stimulating hormone
deficiency of, 1246, 1246*b*
description of, 1237*t*, 1435
overproduction of, 1248*b*
Follicular carcinoma, 1275
Folliculitis, 466, 467*b*
Food allergy, 234–235, 1212*b*
Foot care
in diabetes mellitus, 1304–1307, 1305*f*–1306*f*, 1306*b*–1307*b*
in peripheral vascular disease, 737*b*
Foot disorders
description of, 1028–1029, 1028*f*, 1029*t*
diabetes mellitus-related, 1304–1307, 1305*f*–1306*f*, 1306*b*
Foot drop, 267*b*
Foot fracture, 1038
Footwear, for diabetic patients, 1306
Forebrain, 840
Foreign bodies
in ear, 994–995, 994*b*, 994*f*
in eye, 981
Forensic nurse examiners, 118
Fosphenytoin, 879

Fourth-degree frostbite, 144
Fovea centralis, 958
Fraction of inspired oxygen, 529, 532–533, 618, 632
Fractional flow reserve, 659
Fractures
ankle, 1043, 1049
assessment of, 1035–1037
bone reduction for, 1038
care coordination for, 1045–1046
casts for, 1039–1040, 1039*f*, 1045*b*
chest, 1049–1050
classification of, 1032
closed, 1032, 1032*f*
closed reduction and immobilization of, 1038–1040
Colles', 1046, 1046*f*, 1057
complete, 1032
complications of, 1032–1035
acute compartment syndrome, 1033–1034, 1034*b*, 1044–1045, 1044*b*
avascular necrosis, 1035
chronic, 1035
complex regional pain syndrome, 1035, 1041–1042
delayed union, 1035
fat embolism syndrome, 1034, 1034*b*
hemorrhagic shock, 1034
hypovolemic shock, 1034
infection, 1035, 1045
venous thromboembolism, 1034–1035
compound, 1032
compression, 1032
definition of, 1032
delayed union of, 1035
distal radius, 1046–1047, 1046*f*
drug therapy for, 1041
emergency care for, 1037–1038, 1038*b*
etiology of, 1035
fatigue, 1032
femoral, 1048
fibular, 1048–1049
fragility, 1032
genetic risks of, 1035
healing stages for, 1032, 1033*f*
health care resources for, 1045–1046
health promotion and maintenance for, 1035
hip, 1035*b*, 1047–1049, 1047*f*–1048*f*, 1049*b*
history-taking for, 1035–1036
home care management of, 1045
humeral shaft, 1046
imaging assessment of, 1037
incidence of, 1035
incomplete, 1032
laboratory assessment of, 1037

Fractures (*Continued*)
lower-extremity, 1047–1049, 1047*f*–1048*f*
mandibular, 558
metacarpal, 1047
mobility promotion in, 1043–1044
nasal, 556–557, 556*f*
neurovascular compromise caused by
interventions for, 1044–1045
status assessments for prevention of, 1036*b*–1037*b*, 1044
nonsurgical management of, 1038–1042
nonunion of, 1035, 1043
open, 1032, 1032*f*
open reduction and internal fixation of, 1042–1043, 1042*f*, 1048
orthopedic boots/shoes for, 1038, 1038*f*
osteoporosis as risk factor for, 1016, 1018
pain management of, 1037–1043
pathologic, 1032
pathophysiology of, 1032–1035
pelvic, 1036, 1049–1050
phalangeal, 1047, 1049
physical assessment of, 1036
physical therapy for, 1041
prevalence of, 1035
proximal femur, 1035*b*
proximal humerus, 1046
psychosocial assessment of, 1036–1037
rib, 636–637
self-management education for, 1045
signs and symptoms of, 1036
simple, 1032
splints for, 1038
stress, 1032
surgical management of, 1042–1043, 1042*f*
swelling associated with, 1036*b*
tibial, 1048–1049
traction for, 1040–1041, 1040*t*, 1041*b*, 1041*f*
transition management for, 1045–1046
types of, 1032, 1032*f*
upper-extremity, 1046–1047, 1046*f*
vertebral compression, 1036, 1050
weight-bearing, 1050
Fragility fracture, 1032
Fremitus, 518–519, 587
Frequency (hearing), 990
Fresh frozen plasma, 832*t*, 835
Frontal lobe, 841*t*, 860
Frontal sinus, 509*f*
Frostbite, 144–145, 144*b*, 144*f*
Fructosamine, 1289

FSH. *See* Follicle-stimulating hormone
Full-body lift, 93, 95*f*
Full-thickness wound
    definition of, 27
    physiologic consequences of, 28
Fulmer SPICES framework, 40
Fulminant hepatitis, 1182
Functional ability, 23
    assessment of, 92
    definition of, 92
    rehabilitation for improving, 96
Functional electrical stimulation, for spinal cord injury, 902
Functional incontinence, 1344
Functional Independence Measure, 92
Functional magnetic resonance imaging, 853
Fungal infections
    antifungal agents for, 470
    cystitis caused by, 1356
    in HIV-infected patients, 346–347
    of skin, 467*b*, 468
    skin cultures for, 444
    treatment of, 1078
Furanocoumarins, 731*b*
Furosemide, 699, 1276
Furuncles, 466, 466*f*, 467*b*

G
Gabapentin, 63–64, 925
Gabapentinoids, 63–64
Gadolinium contrast, 852*b*
GAGs. *See* Glycosaminoglycans
Gait
    assessment of, 1009
    for crutches, 1044
    in Parkinson disease, 871
    testing of, 849–850
Gait training, 95–96, 95*b*, 95*f*
Galactorrhea, 1247–1248
Gallbladder
    anatomy of, 1063–1064, 1063*f*
    cholecystitis of. *See* Cholecystitis
Gallium scan, 1011
Gallops, 654
Gallstones
    acute pancreatitis caused by, 1201
    description of, 1191. *See also* Cholecystitis
    extracorporeal shock wave lithotripsy for, 1195
    sites of, 1192*f*
Gamma globulins, 298
Gamma knife, for brain tumors, 952, 952*f*
Gamma rays, 387, 387*f*
Gamma-glutamyl transpeptidase, 1174
Ganglion, 1028
Gardasil, 1469, 1511
Gas bloat syndrome, 1094–1095

Gas exchange
    assessment of, 21, 364–365
    breathing for, 509
    chronic obstructive pulmonary disease effects on, 21, 21*f*
    decreased, 21, 22*f*
    definition of, 20–21
    failure of, 625
    hematologic system in, 796*f*
    in human immunodeficiency virus infection, 353
    in hypothyroidism, 1272–1273
    improvement of, 195
    interventions for, 21
    patient positioning for, 1080
    in pneumonia, 604
    postoperative, 280–281, 1082*b*
    scope of, 21
Gastrectomy
    dumping syndrome secondary to, 1117–1119, 1118*t*
    gastric cancer treated with, 1117, 1117*f*
    in Whipple procedure, 1207, 1207*f*
Gastric bypass, 1229, 1230*f*
Gastric cancer
    advanced, 1116, 1116*b*
    assessment of, 1116
    care coordination for, 1118–1119
    chemotherapy for, 1116
    early, 1116, 1116*b*
    esophagogastroduodenoscopy diagnosis of, 1116
    etiology of, 1115
    gastrectomy for, 1117, 1117*f*
    genetic risk of, 1115
    health care resources for, 1119
    health promotion and maintenance for, 1116
    home care management of, 1119
    incidence of, 1115–1116
    interventions for, 1116–1118
    nonsurgical management of, 1116
    pathophysiology of, 1115–1116
    prevalence of, 1115–1116
    radiation therapy for, 1116
    self-management education for, 1119
    surgical management of, 1116–1118, 1117*f*
    transition management for, 1118–1119
Gastric distention, 1088
Gastric emptying, 1089, 1107
Gastric outlet obstruction, 1109
Gastric ulcers, 1107–1110, 1108*f*
Gastritis
    acute, 1104–1105, 1105*b*
    assessment of, 1105
    atrophic, 1104, 1115
    chronic, 1104–1105, 1105*b*
    complementary and integrative health for, 1107*t*
    definition of, 1103
    dietary prevention of, 1104–1105

Gastritis (*Continued*)
    esophagogastroduodenoscopy of, 1105
    etiology of, 1104
    features of, 1105*b*
    genetic risk of, 1104
    health promotion and maintenance of, 1104–1105
    Helicobacter pylori as cause of, 1104
    H$_2$-receptor antagonists for, 1105
    interventions for, 1105–1107, 1106*b*–1107*b*
    nonsteroidal anti-inflammatory drugs as cause of, 1104–1105
    pathophysiology of, 1103–1104
    prevention of, 1104*b*
    types of, 1104
Gastroenteritis, 1148–1150, 1148*t*, 1149*b*–1150*b*
Gastroesophageal reflux, 1087
Gastroesophageal reflux disease
    antacids for, 1090–1091
    assessment of, 1088–1089
    asthma triggered by, 565
    care coordination for, 1091–1092
    definition of, 1087
    diagnostic assessment of, 1089
    drug therapy for, 1090–1091
    dysphagia caused by, 1089
    endoscopic therapy for, 1091
    features of, 1088*b*
    health promotion and maintenance, 1088
    hiatal hernia and, 1088
    histamine receptor antagonists for, 1091
    interventions for, 1090–1091
    laparoscopic Nissen fundoplication for, 1091
    lifestyle changes for, 1090, 1090*b*
    lower esophageal sphincter in, 1088, 1088*t*
    nonsurgical management of, 1090–1091
    nutrition therapy for, 1090
    obesity and, 1090
    in older adults, 1089*b*
    pathophysiology of, 1087–1088
    physical assessment of, 1088–1089
    proton pump inhibitors for, 1090*b*, 1091
    reflux esophagitis secondary to, 1087
    risk factors for, 1088
    signs and symptoms of, 1088–1089
    Stretta procedure for, 1091, 1091*b*
    surgical management of, 1091
    transition management for, 1091–1092
Gastrointestinal bleeding
    in Cushing's disease, 1259
    lower, 1156, 1156*b*
    upper. *See* Upper gastrointestinal bleeding

Gastrointestinal system
    age-related changes in, 1064, 1064*b*
    anatomy of, 1061–1064
    assessment of, 90–91, 90*t*, 1065–1073
    burn injury effects on, 486, 492
    colonoscopy of, 1072–1073
    computed tomography of, 1070
    current health problems assessments, 1066
    diagnostic assessment of, 1068–1073, 1069*b*
    endoscopic retrograde cholangiopancreatography of, 1071
    endoscopy of, 1070
    esophagogastroduodenoscopy of, 1070–1071, 1071*b*, 1071*f*
    esophagus. *See* Esophagus
    family history assessments, 1066
    functions of, 1062–1064
    gallbladder, 1063–1064, 1063*f*
    history-taking, 1065–1066, 1065*b*
    imaging assessment of, 1070
    inspection of, 1067
    laboratory assessment of, 1068–1070, 1069*b*
    large intestine, 1064
    liver, 1063–1064, 1063*f*
    liver-spleen scan, 1073
    magnetic resonance imaging of, 1070
    nutrition assessments, 1213*b*
    nutrition history, 1065–1066
    oral cavity. *See* Oral cavity
    palpation of, 1067–1068
    pancreas. *See* Pancreas
    percussion of, 1067
    physical assessment of, 1066–1068
    postoperative assessment of, 276–277
    psychosocial assessment of, 1068
    radiographic assessments of, 1070
    sigmoidoscopy of, 1073
    small bowel capsule endoscopy of, 1071–1072
    small intestine, 1064
    stomach. *See* Stomach
    stool tests, 1068–1070
    structure of, 1061–1062, 1062*f*
    ultrasonography of, 1073
    urine tests, 1068
Gastrointestinal tract
    anatomy of, 1061
    functions of, 1061–1062
    infection transmission, 415
    lumen of, 1061–1062
    tumors of, 385
Gastrojejunostomy, 1207
Gastroparesis, 1285
Gastrostomy, 1221
Gaviscon, 1091

GCS. See Glasgow Coma Scale

G-CSF. See Granulocyte colony-stimulating factor

Gel phenomenon, 319

Gender dysphoria, 1493, 1493t

Gender identity, 11t, 123b, 1492–1493, 1493t

Gender reassignment surgery
  definition of, 1493t, 1499
  for male-to-female patients, 1499–1500

Genderqueer, 1493t

Gene(s)
  alleles, 74–75, 75f, 79
  in chromosomes, 72
  composition of, 72
  definition of, 72
  function of, 74–76
  genotype of, 76
  penetrance of, 79
  phenotype of, 75–76
  protein synthesis, 76
  purpose of, 71–72
  structure of, 74–76
  susceptibility, 76
  variations in, 76–77

Gene expression, 76

Gene mutations, 76–77

Gene products, 76

Gene sequences, 76

Gene therapy
  cystic fibrosis treated with, 583
  heart failure treated with, 701

General anesthesia, 257–260, 258t–259t, 260b, 275

General appearance, 651

Generalized osteoporosis, 1016

Generalized peritonitis, 1145

Generalized seizures, 876

Genetic counseling
  communication during, 82–83
  confidentiality of, 81, 83
  description of, 81
  medical-surgical nurse's role in, 82–83
  patient advocacy and support during, 83
  privacy of, 83
  steps for, 82b

Genetic disorders, 72

Genetic testing
  benefits of, 80–81
  for cancer, 380–382
  ethical issues in, 81–82
  purpose of, 80, 81t
  risks of, 80–81
  steps for, 82b

Genetics
  competencies in, 72, 72t
  genes. See Gene(s)
  genomics versus, 71
  inheritance patterns
    autosomal dominant, 78–79, 78t
    autosomal recessive, 78t, 79, 79f

Genetics (Continued)
  complex, 78t, 80
  overview of, 77–80
  pedigree, 77–78, 78f–79f
  sex-linked recessive, 78t, 79–80, 80f
  purpose of, 71

Genital herpes, 1506–1508, 1507b

Genital warts. See Condylomata acuminata

Genitourinary system
  nutrition assessments, 1213b
  trauma to, 1387b

Genome, 72

Genomics, 71

Genotype, 76

Gentamicin sulfate, 501b

Genu valgum, 1010

Genu varum, 1010

GER. See Gastroesophageal reflux

GERD. See Gastroesophageal reflux disease

Geriatric Depression Scale, 850–851

Geriatric Depression Scale—Short form, 36–37, 37f

Geriatric failure to thrive, 31

Geriatric syndromes
  decreased mobility, 31–32
  decreased nutrition and hydration, 30–31
  definition of, 29–30

Germline mutations, 76

GFTT. See Geriatric failure to thrive

Ghrelin, 1225

Giant cell tumor, 1025

Giardia lamblia, 1165

Giardiasis, 1165–1166

Gigantism, 1006

Ginkgo biloba, 801–802

Glans penis, 1430

Glasgow Coma Scale
  decreases in, 851b
  description of, 130, 850
  illustration of, 850f

Glass bottles, for infusion therapy, 208

Glatiramer acetate, 891, 891b

Glaucoma
  assessment of, 972–974
  carbonic anhydrase inhibitors for, 974–975
  care coordination for, 975–976
  concept map for, 972f–973f
  definition of, 972
  drug therapy for, 26, 974–975
  etiology of, 972
  eye injury as risk factor for, 961
  eyedrops for, 966b, 975f
  genetic risks of, 972
  health care resources for, 976
  health promotion and maintenance for, 972
  home care management of, 975

Glaucoma (Continued)
  incidence of, 972
  laser trabeculoplasty for, 975
  nonsurgical management of, 974–975
  pathophysiology of, 958, 962t, 972
  physical assessment of, 972–974
  prevalence of, 972
  primary angle-closure, 972
  primary open-angle, 972
  self-management education for, 975–976
  signs and symptoms of, 972–974
  surgical management of, 975
  trabeculectomy for, 975
  transition management for, 975–976
  types of, 962t, 972

Glimepiride, 1292b–1293b

Glipizide, 1292b–1293b

Global aphasia, 938

Globulins, 796

Glomerular filtration, 1324

Glomerular filtration rate
  in acute kidney injury, 1391
  age-related declines in, 1328, 1328b
  creatinine clearance used to estimate, 1335–1336
  description of, 1324
  in nephrotic syndrome, 1379

Glomerulonephritis
  acute, 1376–1378, 1376t
  chronic, 1378
  rapidly progressive, 1377–1378

Glomerulus
  anatomy of, 1323, 1323f
  capillary wall, 1324f

Glossectomy, 1082

Glossitis, 814, 815f

Glossopharyngeal nerve, 844t

Glottis, 510, 510f

Gloves, 418b, 419t

Gloving, 256, 257f

Glucagon, 1240, 1281

Glucagon-like peptide-1, 1293

Glucocorticoids
  Crohn's disease treated with, 1160
  Cushing's disease treated with, 1258–1259
  endogenous, 1237–1238, 1238t
  functions of, 1238t
  production of, 1237–1238
  release of, 1238
  rheumatoid arthritis treated with, 322–323
  ulcerative colitis treated with, 1152–1153

Gluconeogenesis, 1282

Glucosamine, 308–309, 309b

Glucose
  blood. See Blood glucose
  counterregulatory hormone effects on, 1282
  fasting blood, 1281f, 1282
  fasting plasma, 1289

Glucose (Continued)
  function of, 1281
  incomplete breakdown of, 188

Glucose regulation
  definition of, 1280–1281
  insulin for, 1282
  poor, 1283

Glucose-6-phosphate dehydrogenase deficiency anemia, 814t, 815–816

Glutamate, 864

Gluten-free diet, 1164

Glyburide, 1292b–1293b

Glycocalyx, 421

Glycogenesis, 1282

Glycogenolysis, 1282

Glycoprotein IIb/IIIa inhibitors, 776

Glycosaminoglycans, 1271

Glycosylated hemoglobin, 1243, 1289, 1289t, 1291

GM-CSF. See Granulocyte-macrophage colony-stimulating factor

Goiter, 1265, 1266f, 1266t, 1271

Goldmann applanation tonometer, 965, 965f

Golimumab, 323b, 333

Gonadotropin-releasing hormone agonists, 1498

Gonadotropins
  deficiency of, 1246b
  description of, 1246
  overproduction of, 1248b

Gonads, 1237

Goniometer, 1010

Gonorrhea, 1512–1514, 1513f

Good death, 103, 113

Gout, 330–332, 331f

Gowning, 256, 257f

gp120, 338

Graduated compression stockings
  varicose veins treated with, 748
  venous insufficiency treated with, 747b

Graft occlusion, 736b

Graft-versus-host-disease
  after hematopoietic stem cell transplantation, 824–825, 825f
  transfusion-associated, 836

Granulocyte colony-stimulating factor, 293, 300t

Granulocyte-macrophage colony-stimulating factor, 293, 300t

Granulocytes, 292–293

Granulomatous thyroiditis, 1275

Graves' disease, 1265, 1267, 1270

Gray, 387–388

Gray matter, 840

Grief/grieving
  in colorectal cancer patients, 1132–1133
  definition of, 112
  at end of life, 112–114

Grommet, 992, 992f
Groshong valve, 205
Ground substance, 431–432
Group homes, 88
Growth factors
    definition of, 1081
    in oral cancer treatment, 1081
    types of, 300t
Growth hormone
    deficiency of, 1246, 1246b
    description of, 1006, 1237t
    overproduction of, 1247, 1247f,
        1248b
Guaiac fecal occult blood test, 1068
Guanylate cyclase stimulators, for
        pulmonary arterial
        hypertension, 585
Guardian, 36
Guillain-Barré syndrome
    assessment of, 914
    care coordination for, 916–917
    clinical features of, 914b
    cranial nerve involvement in, 914
    definition of, 912
    description of, 849
    diagnostic assessment of, 914
    electrophysiologic studies of, 914
    etiology of, 913–914
    health care resources for, 917
    home care management of,
        916–917
    incidence of, 914
    interventions for, 914–916
    intravenous immunoglobulin for,
        915
    mobility manifestations of, 914,
        914b, 916
    pathophysiology of, 912–914
    physical assessment of, 914
    plasmapheresis for, 914–915, 915b
    prevalence of, 914
    signs and symptoms of, 914
    stages of, 913, 916b
    transition management of,
        916–917
Gum chewing, in postoperative
        period, 286
Gynecologic disorders
    cervical cancer, 1469–1470, 1470b
    endometrial cancer, 1465–1467,
        1465t, 1466b
    ovarian cancer, 1467–1469, 1467t
    overview of, 1459
    pelvic organ prolapse, 1464–1465,
        1464f
    toxic shock syndrome, 1471, 1471b
    uterine leiomyoma. See Uterine
        leiomyoma
    vulvovaginitis, 1470–1471, 1471b
Gynecomastia, 407, 1173, 1247, 1386,
        1441

H
Habit training, for urinary
        incontinence, 1351, 1351b

HACE. See High-altitude cerebral
        edema
HAD. See High-altitude disease
Hageman factor, 798t
Hair
    age-related changes, 434b
    anatomy of, 432
    assessment of, 441
    growth of, 432
    preoperative removal of, 242,
        243f
Half-life, 58–59
Halitosis, 1096
Hallux valgus, 1028, 1028f, 1304
Halo fixator device, 899, 899b
"Halo" sign, 946
Hammertoe, 1029, 1029f
Hand
    disorders of, 1028, 1028f
    Dupuytren's contracture of, 1028,
        1028f
    ganglion of, 1028
    joints of, 1009, 1009f
Hand hygiene, 418, 418b
Hand strength, 848, 848f
Hand-off communication, 119–120,
        317
Hand-off report, 271b
Handrails, 325, 325f
Hantavirus, 423
Hantavirus pulmonary syndrome,
        423
HAPE. See High-altitude pulmonary
        edema
Hashimoto's disease, 1275
Hashimoto's thyroiditis, 1265
Haversian system, 1005, 1005f
Hazardous materials (HAZMAT)
        training, 150, 151f
HCOs. See Health care organizations
Head
    assessment of, 802
    cancer of. See Head and neck
        cancer
Head and neck cancer
    airway obstruction caused by,
        549–553
    anxiety management in, 553
    aspiration prevention in, 553
    assessment of, 548–549
    biotherapy for, 549–550
    care coordination for, 554–555
    chemotherapy for, 549
    communication issues in, 550b,
        555
    composite resections for, 552–553
    etiology of, 548
    health care resources for, 555
    history-taking for, 548
    home care management of, 554,
        554b
    imaging assessment of, 548
    incidence of, 548
    interventions for, 549–553
    laboratory assessment of, 548

Head and neck cancer (Continued)
    metastasis of, 548
    neck dissection for, 550
    nonsurgical management of,
        549–550
    nutrition alterations in, 552
    pain management in, 551–552
    pathophysiology of, 547–548
    prevalence of, 548
    psychosocial assessment of, 548
    psychosocial preparation for, 555
    radiation therapy for, 549
    salivary glands, 549
    self-esteem support in, 553–554
    self-management education of,
        554–555
    signs and symptoms of, 548, 548t
    speech and language rehabilitation
        in, 552
    staging of, 548
    surgical management of, 550–553
    transition management for,
        554–555
Headache
    medication overuse, 874
    migraine. See Migraine headaches
    rebound, 874
Health Canada, 1212
Health care disparities, 10–11, 11t
Health care organizations
    attributes of, 10
    context of, 10
    critical care access hospitals, 9
    definition of, 9
    scope of, 9–10
Health care workers, HIV
        transmission to, 343, 344f,
        345b
Health care-associated infection
    biofilms and, 421
    definition of, 417
    in long-term care settings, 417
    risks for, 421
Health care-associated
        methicillin-resistant
        Staphylococcus aureus, 422, 422b
Health care-associated pneumonia,
        599t–600t
Health Professions Education: A
        Bridge to Quality, 2
Health-enhancing behaviors, 30b
Health-protecting behaviors, 30b
Healthy People 2020
    description of, 694b, 695t
    health care disparities, 10, 11t
    heart disease, 722t
    lesbian, gay, bisexual, transgender,
        and queer population, 10,
        1495
    medication assessments, 35
    nutrition, 1226t
    sexually transmitted infection
        objectives of, 1505, 1506t
    stroke, 722t
    syphilis objectives, 1505, 1506t

Hearing. See also Ear(s)
    age-related changes, 986, 987b
    assessment of, 986, 989–991, 1002
    audiometry assessments of,
        990–991
    diagnostic assessment of, 990–991
    history-taking, 986–988
    psychosocial assessment of, 990
    voice test for, 989
Hearing aids
    assessment of, 987–988
    care of, 999b
    definition of, 999
    description of, 26, 27f
Hearing loss
    anxiety associated with, 1001
    assessment of, 997–998, 998b
    assistive devices for, 999
    care coordination for, 1001–1002
    causes of, 26
    clinical manifestations of, 998,
        998b
    cochlear implantation for, 999
    communication in, 998b, 1001
    conductive, 989, 996–997, 997t
    family history of, 988
    genetic risk of, 988, 988b
    health care resources for, 1002
    health promotion and
        maintenance for, 997
    history-taking for, 997–998
    home care management of, 1001
    imaging assessment of, 998–1001
    incidence of, 997
    interventions for, 999–1001
    laboratory assessment of, 998
    in Ménière's disease, 996
    mixed conductive-sensorineural,
        989, 996
    nonsurgical management of,
        999–1001
    pathophysiology of, 996–997
    physical assessment of, 998
    prevalence of, 997
    psychosocial assessment of, 998
    self-management education for,
        1002
    sensorineural, 989, 997, 997t
    stapedectomy for, 1000–1001,
        1000f
    surgical management of, 999–1001
    totally implanted devices for, 1001
    transition management for,
        1001–1002
    tuning fork tests for, 989–990, 998
    tympanoplasty for, 999–1000,
        1000f
Heart. See also Cardiovascular
        system
    anatomy of, 642–644, 642f–643f
    blood flow in, 642
    conduction system of, 664–665,
        665f
    coronary arterial system of, 643,
        643f

Heart (*Continued*)
function of, 644–645
mechanical properties of, 645
structure of, 642–644, 642*f*–643*f*
valves of, 642, 643*f*
Heart attack. *See* Cardiac arrest
Heart failure
activity schedule for, 704–705
advance directives in, 705
aldosterone antagonists for, 700
assessment of, 695–697
beta-blockers for, 700
cardiac resynchronization therapy
for, 701
care coordination for, 703–705
in chronic kidney disease, 1401
in chronic obstructive pulmonary
disease, 573–574
classification of, 692, 781–782,
782*t*
compensatory mechanisms for,
692–694, 693*f*
congestive, 692
continuous positive airway
pressure for, 701
definition of, 691
diagnostic assessment of, 697
diastolic, 692, 701
digoxin for, 700
diuretics for, 699
drug therapy for, 697–701, 698*t*,
704–705, 705*b*
dyspnea in, 695
edema in, 696*b*
electrical cardioversion for,
680–681
etiology of, 694, 694*t*
fatigue in, 702
gas exchange in, 697
gene therapy for, 701
health care resources for, 705
heart transplantation for, 705
home care management of,
703
hyperpolarization-activated cyclic
nucleotide-gated channel
blocker for, 701
imaging assessment of, 697
incidence of, 694
infective endocarditis as cause of,
711
inotropic drugs for, 700
interventions for, 680–681
intra-aortic balloon pump for,
782
laboratory assessment of,
696–697
left-sided, 651, 692, 695–696,
780–782
nitrates for, 699
nonsurgical management of,
697–701, 698*t*
nutrition therapy for, 698–699,
705
in older adults, 694*b*

Heart failure (*Continued*)
partial left ventriculectomy for,
702
pathophysiology of, 691–694
prevalence of, 694
psychosocial assessment of, 696
pulmonary edema in, 702–703,
702*b*
re-hospitalization for, 704
right-sided, 651, 692, 694–695,
782
self-management education for,
703–705, 704*t*
staging of, 692
surgical management of, 701–702
sympathetic nervous system
stimulation from, 692
systolic, 692
transition management for,
703–705
types of, 692
ventricular assist devices for,
701–702, 701*f*
Heart rate, 645, 670
Heart sounds, 654–655, 696, 773
Heart transplantation
cardiomyopathy treated with,
716–717, 717*f*
discharge planning for, 717
heart failure treated with, 705
operative procedures for, 716,
717*f*
postoperative care for, 716–717
preoperative care for, 716
rejection of, 716*b*
survival rates after, 717
Heart valve replacement, 709–710,
709*f*
Heat exhaustion, 133–134
Heat stroke, 133–135, 134*b*–135*b*
Heat-related illnesses
environmental factors, 133
heat exhaustion, 133–134
heat stroke, 133–135, 134*b*–135*b*
prevention of, 134*b*
risk factors for, 133
Heberden's nodes, 306, 306*f*
Height measurements, 1213–1215
Heimlich maneuver. *See* Abdominal
thrust maneuver
Helicobacter pylori
drug therapy for, 1111–1112
gastric cancer risks associated
with, 1115
gastritis caused by, 1104
in older adults, 1111*b*
peptic ulcers caused by, 1107,
1109, 1111–1112
Helicopters, 119*f*
Helper/inducer T-cells, 299, 797*t*
Hematemesis, 1105, 1108, 1170
Hematochezia, 1128
Hematocrit, 803, 810–811, 813
Hematogenous tuberculosis,
605–606

Hematologic disorders
anemia. *See* Anemia
autoimmune thrombocytopenic
purpura, 830–831
hemophilia, 831, 832*t*
heparin-induced
thrombocytopenia, 832
hereditary hemochromatosis, 817
idiopathic thrombocytopenic
purpura, 830–831
leukemia. *See* Leukemia
lymphomas, 828–829, 829*t*
multiple myeloma, 829–830
polycythemia vera, 816–817, 817*b*
sickle cell disease. *See* Sickle cell
disease
thrombotic thrombocytopenic
purpura, 831
Hematologic system
age-related changes in, 800, 800*b*
anatomy of, 795–800
assessment of, 800–806
bone marrow, 795–796, 796*f*
current health problems that
affect, 802
diagnostic assessment of, 803–806,
804*b*
drugs that affect, 801*t*
functions of, 808
in gas exchange, 796*f*
imaging assessment of, 806
laboratory assessment of, 803–806,
804*b*
in older adults, 800*b*
physical assessment of, 802–803
psychosocial assessment of, 803
Hematoma
epidural, 226, 942, 942*f*
subdural, 942–943, 942*f*
Hematopoiesis, 1005
Hematopoietic stem cell
transplantation
aplastic anemia treated with, 816
bone marrow harvesting for, 823
chronic lymphoblastic leukemia
treated with, 821
complications of, 824–825
conditioning regimen for,
823–824, 823*f*
cord blood harvesting, 823
engraftment of, 824
graft-versus-host-disease
secondary to, 824–825, 825*f*
leukemia treated with, 822–825, 822*t*
myelodysplastic syndromes treated
with, 817
peripheral blood stem cell
harvesting, 823
sickle cell disease treated with, 812
stem cells for, 822–823
steps of, 823*f*
transplantation procedure for, 824
transplants, 822*t*
veno-occlusive disease secondary
to, 825

Hematuria, 16, 803, 1303, 1341,
1358, 1361, 1482
Hemianopsia, 934, 934*f*
Hemiarthroplasty, 316, 1047, 1048*b*
Hemilaryngectomy, 551*t*
Hemiparesis, 933–934
Hemiplegia, 933–934
Hemoconcentration, 485, 1283
Hemodialysis
anticoagulation during, 1413
arteriovenous fistulas, 1413,
1414*f*–1415*f*, 1414*t*–1415*t*,
1415*b*
arteriovenous grafts, 1413, 1414*f*,
1414*t*–1415*t*, 1415*b*
arteriovenous shunt for, 1414*f*
cardiac events during, 1417
care after, 1416, 1416*b*
catheters for, 208, 1414*t*
complications of, 1416–1417
description of, 1397, 1411
dialyzers, 1412–1413, 1412*f*,
1417
hemofiltration versus, 1413*f*
home care management of, 1424
infectious disease transmission
during, 1417
nursing care during, 1416
patient selection, 1411–1412
peritoneal dialysis versus, 1411*t*
procedure, 1412–1413,
1412*f*–1413*f*
self-management education for,
1424–1425
settings, 1412
subclavian vein catheterization for,
1414*f*
temporary vascular access, 1416
vascular access, 1413–1416, 1414*f*,
1414*t*–1415*t*
Hemofiltration
description of, 1397–1398
hemodialysis versus, 1413*f*
Hemoglobin
definition of, 796
fetal, 808, 811
formation of, 797
glycosylated, 1243, 1289, 1289*t*
in malnutrition, 1217
oxygen delivery to tissue by, 512
Hemoglobin A, 808, 809*f*
Hemoglobin electrophoresis, 805
Hemoglobin S, 809–810, 809*f*
Hemolytic transfusion reaction,
835
Hemophilia, 831, 832*t*
Hemoptysis, 559–560, 618
Hemorrhage. *See also* Bleeding
in cirrhosis, 1177–1178
drug therapy for, 1177
external, 129–130
intracerebral, 943
postpartum, 1246
postsurgical, 551
spinal cord, 894

Hemorrhage (Continued)
  subarachnoid
    cerebral vasospasm after, 937
    description of, 929, 931
    traumatic brain injury as cause of, 944–950
Hemorrhagic shock, 1034
Hemorrhagic stroke, 16, 929, 929t
Hemorrhoidectomy, 1140
Hemorrhoids, 1139–1140, 1140f
Hemostasis, 798
Hemothorax, 637–638
Hemovac drain, 278, 279f, 282
Hendrich II Fall Risk Model, 41
Heparin
  with hemodialysis catheters, 208, 1413
  low-molecular-weight, 744–745
  pulmonary embolism treated with, 617–618, 620, 621b
  unfractionated, 744
Heparin-induced thrombocytopenia, 744, 832
Hepatic arterial infusion, for liver cancer, 1187
Hepatic artery embolization, 1187
Hepatic encephalopathy, 1170–1171, 1171t, 1178–1179
Hepatitis
  assessment of, 1183–1184
  care coordination for, 1185
  carriers of, 1181
  chronic, 1182
  classification of, 1180–1181
  complications of, 1182
  delta, 1181
  drug therapy for, 1185t
  drug-induced, 1180
  etiology of, 1180–1181
  fatigue caused by, 1184
  fulminant, 1182
  health promotion and maintenance for, 1182
  incidence of, 1182
  jaundice in, 1183
  liver biopsy for, 1184
  nutrition promotion in, 1184
  pathophysiology of, 1180–1182
  prevalence of, 1182
  self-management education for, 1185b
  toxic, 1180
  transition management for, 1185
  viral, 1180, 1182b, 1185b
Hepatitis A, 1180–1182, 1184
Hepatitis B
  cancers associated with, 379t
  carriers of, 1181
  in chronic kidney disease patients, 1417
  cirrhosis caused by, 1172
  drug therapy for, 1185t
  symptoms of, 1181
  transmission of, 1181
  vaccines for, 1182

Hepatitis C
  cancers associated with, 379t
  in chronic kidney disease patients, 1417
  cirrhosis caused by, 1172
  diagnosis of, 1184
  drug therapy for, 1185t
  transmission of, 1181
  in veterans, 1183b
Hepatitis D, 1181, 1184
Hepatitis E, 1181, 1184
Hepatobiliary scan, 1194
Hepatocellular carcinoma, 1186
Hepatomegaly, 1067, 1173, 1205
Hepatopulmonary syndrome, 1177
Hepatorenal syndrome, 1171
Herbs, 232–233
Hereditary angioedema, 362
Hereditary chronic pancreatitis, 1202
Hereditary hemochromatosis, 817
Hereditary nonpolyposis colorectal cancer, 1126, 1127b, 1466
Heritability, 72
Hernia
  abdominal, 1137–1138, 1137f
  assessment of, 1138
  direct inguinal, 1137, 1137f
  examination for, 1138
  femoral, 1137, 1137f
  hiatal. See Hiatal hernias
  incisional, 1137f, 1138
  indirect inguinal, 1137–1138, 1137f
  interventions for, 1138–1139
  irreducible, 1138
  minimally invasive repair of, 1138–1139, 1139b
  nonsurgical management of, 1138
  pathophysiology of, 1137–1138
  reducible, 1138
  strangulated, 1138
  surgical management of, 1138–1139
  types of, 1137–1138, 1137f
  umbilical, 1137, 1137f
Herniated nucleus pulposus, 903, 903f
Hernioplasty, 1138
Herniorrhaphy, 1138
Herpes simplex virus
  in AIDS-infected patients, 347, 355
  assessment of, 1506
  description of, 467b, 468, 881
  drug therapy for, 1507
  encephalitis caused by, 883
  genital, 1506–1508, 1507b
  HSV-1, 1506
  HSV-2, 1506
  pathophysiology of, 1506
  self-management of, 1507b
Herpes zoster, 467b, 468, 468f
Herpetic whitlow, 468
Heterografts, 499, 499f
Heterotopic ossification, 897, 900
Heterozygous, 75

Hiatal hernias
  assessment of, 1093
  care coordination for, 1095
  definition of, 1092
  features of, 1093b
  gastroesophageal reflux disease risks, 1088
  nonsurgical management of, 1093
  paraesophageal, 1092, 1093b
  pathophysiology of, 1092, 1092f
  rolling, 1092–1093, 1092f
  sliding, 1092, 1092f
  surgical management of, 1093–1095
  transition management for, 1095
Hiccups, 1123
HICS. See Hospital Incident Command System
Hierarchy of Pain Measures, 53, 53t
High-altitude cerebral edema, 145–146, 145b–146b
High-altitude disease, 145–146, 145b–146b
High-altitude pulmonary edema, 145–146, 145b–146b
High-density lipoprotein cholesterol, 730
High-density lipoproteins, 656
High-flow nasal cannula, 534–535
High-frequency chest wall oscillation, 583, 583f
High-frequency oscillatory ventilation, 627
Highly sensitive C-reactive protein
  description of, 656
  in rheumatoid arthritis, 321
Hinge joints, 1007
Hip(s)
  arthroplasty of. See Total hip arthroplasty
  dislocation of, after total hip arthroplasty, 311–312
  flexion contractures of, 1052
  fracture of, 1047–1049, 1047f–1048f, 1049b
  mobility evaluations, 1010
Hip resurfacing, 310
Hirsutism, 441, 1242, 1256
Hispanics
  Alzheimer's disease in, 866b
  older adults, 39b
Histamine, 293–294, 361, 361f, 364
Histamine receptor antagonists
  gastritis treated with, 1105
  gastroesophageal reflux disease treated with, 1091
  peptic ulcer disease treated with, 1112
Histoplasmosis, 347
HIT. See Heparin-induced thrombocytopenia
HIV infection. See Human immunodeficiency virus infection

HIV-associated nephropathy, 348
HIV-associated neurocognitive disorder, 348
HLAs. See Human leukocyte antigens
HMG-CoA reductase inhibitors, 730
H1N1, 597
H5N1, 597–598
H7N9, 597
H1N1 virus, 151
Hodgkin's lymphoma, 828
Homans' sign, 742–743
Home care management
  for acute pancreatitis, 1202
  for amputation, 1055, 1056b
  for benign prostatic hyperplasia, 1481
  for bone tumors, 1027
  for breast cancer, 1452–1453
  for breast cancer surgery, 1453b
  for burn injury, 505
  for cataract, 962b, 971, 971f
  for central venous catheter, 826b
  for chronic obstructive pulmonary disease, 581, 581b
  for cirrhosis, 1179, 1179b
  for colorectal cancer, 1133
  for Cushing's disease, 1260
  for diabetes mellitus, 1317–1318, 1318b
  for esophageal tumors, 1100
  for fractures, 1045
  for gastric cancer, 1119
  for glaucoma, 975
  for head and neck cancer, 554, 554b
  health care resources in, 101
  for hearing loss, 1001
  for heart failure, 703
  for hypertension, 727
  for hypoglycemia, 1310b
  for hypothyroidism, 1273–1274
  for infection, 426
  for intestinal obstructions, 1125
  for laryngectomy, 554b
  leave-of-absence visit, 100–101
  for leukemia, 826
  for malnutrition, 1224
  for myasthenia gravis, 921–922
  for myocardial infarction, 789–790, 790b
  for obesity, 1231
  for oral cancer, 1083, 1083b
  for osteoarthritis, 317
  for osteoporosis, 1022
  for otitis media, 993
  for oxygen therapy, 536
  for pain, 67
  for pancreatic cancer, 1209
  for pelvic inflammatory disease, 1516
  for peptic ulcer disease, 1114, 1115b
  for peritonitis, 1146

Home care management (Continued)
  for pneumonia, 605
  postoperative, 286
  for pressure injuries, 459–460
  for prostate cancer, 1485–1486
  for pulmonary embolism, 623, 624b
  for pyelonephritis, 1375
  in rehabilitation, 100
  for rheumatoid arthritis, 325
  for stomatitis, 1078
  for stroke, 939
  for tracheostomy, 544
  for tuberculosis, 610
  for ulcerative colitis, 1156
  for urinary incontinence, 1353
  for uterine leiomyomas, 1463
  for valvular heart disease, 710
Home infusion therapy, 67
Homelessness
  emergency department care and, 127
  impact of, 127
  in older adults, 30
Homeostasis, 1235
Homocysteine, 656
Homografts, 499
Homonymous hemianopsia, 934, 934f
Homozygous, 75
Honeybee stings, 137
Hookah smoking, 514
Hormonal manipulation, for cancer, 406–407, 406t
Hormones. See also specific hormone
  appetite regulation by, 1225
  definition of, 1234–1235
  endocrine, 1235t
  "lock and key" model of, 1235, 1235f
  male reproductive, 1430
  positive and negative feedback control of, 1236f
  receptor binding by, 1235, 1235f
  thyroid gland, 1235t, 1239t
Hospice care, 106, 106b, 107t, 113–114, 593
Hospital(s)
  critical access, 117
  emergency preparedness in
    infrastructure of, 152–153
    nurse's role in, 154–156
    personnel roles and responsibilities, 153–156, 154t
  older adults in, 39–42
  restraints used by, 41, 42b
Hospital care
  drowning, 147
  frostbite, 144–145
  heat stroke, 134–135
  hypothermia, 143
  lightning injury, 142
Hospital Elder Life Program, 38

Hospital Incident Command System, 153–154
Hospital incident commander, 154, 154t
Hospital-acquired infection, 122, 216
Hospitalist, 8
Hostile patients, 121b
Hot packs, 323–324
Huber noncoring needle, 208
Human B-type natriuretic peptides, 698
Human immunodeficiency virus infection. See also Acquired immunodeficiency syndrome
  acquired immunodeficiency syndrome and, 338, 340
  in African-American women, 345b
  anal intercourse as risk factor for, 342
  antibody-antigen tests, 349
  archiving in, 350
  care coordination for, 356–357
  classification of, 339–340
  cognition enhancements in, 355
  complementary and integrative health for, 353–354
  counseling about, 341–342
  course of, 344–345
  diarrhea management in, 354
  "docking" proteins of, 338f
  drug therapy for
    antiretroviral drugs, 350–353
    CCR5 antagonists, 351b–352b
    combination antiretroviral therapy, 342–343, 350–353
    integrase inhibitors, 351b–352b
    non-nucleoside reverse transcriptase inhibitors, 338, 351b–352b
    nucleoside reverse transcriptase inhibitors, 338, 351b–352b
    protease inhibitors, 338, 348, 351b–352b
  effects of, 338
  endocrine complications of, 348
  etiology of, 337–340
  gas exchange in, 353
  gender differences, 342
  genetic risk for, 337–340
  health care resources for, 357
  health care worker exposure to, 343, 344f, 345b
  health promotion and maintenance for, 340–343
  history-taking, 345–346
  home care management of, 356
  home testing kits for, 350
  incidence of, 340
  increased intracranial pressure in, 355
  infectious process of, 337–339
  in injection drug users, 343
  laboratory assessments in, 349
  long-term nonprogressors, 338b

Human immunodeficiency virus infection (Continued)
  lymphocyte count in, 349
  malignancies associated with, 347–348, 348f
  mouth care in, 354
  nutrition promotion in, 354
  occupational exposure to, 343
  opportunistic infections associated with
    description of, 339, 346–347, 347f
    prevention of, 350–353
  pain management in, 353–354
  parenteral transmission of, 341, 343
  particle features of, 337–338, 338f
  pathophysiology of, 337–340
  perinatal transmission of, 341, 343
  postexposure prophylaxis for, 342–343, 344f
  pre-exposure prophylaxis for, 342
  in pregnancy
    outcomes affected by, 340
    perinatal transmission, 341, 343
  prevalence of, 340
  progression of, 340
  psychosocial assessment, 348
  psychosocial distress caused by, 355–356
  as retrovirus, 338
  schematic diagram of, 338f
  screening for, 341, 341b
  self-management education for, 356, 357b
  sexual transmission of, 341–343
  signs and symptoms of, 339
  skin integrity in, 354–355
  stages of, 339–340
  testing for, 341–342, 341b, 349
  transition management for, 356–357
  transmission of
    needlestick injuries as cause of, 343
    parenteral, 341, 343
    perinatal, 341, 343
    sexual, 341–343
  in veterans, 341b
  viral load, 342, 349
  virus-host interactions, 338
  in women, 340b, 345b
Human immunodeficiency virus protease, 338
Human leukocyte antigens
  B5701 allele test, 350b
  description of, 290, 294
  rheumatoid arthritis and, 318b
Human lymphotrophic virus type I, 379t
Human lymphotrophic virus type II, 379t

Human papilloma virus, 348
  cancers associated with, 379t
  cervical cancer risks, 1469
  condylomata acuminata caused by, 1510–1511, 1510f
  oral cancer associated with, 1079
  test for, 1434–1435
  vaccinations for, 382, 1469, 1511
Human trafficking, 131
Human waste management, 157
Humeral shaft fracture, 1046
Humidified oxygen, 531, 531f
Humira. See Adalimumab
Humoral immunity, 295. See also Antibody-mediated immunity
Huntington disease, 72, 79–81
  clinical features of, 868t
  definition of, 868
  Parkinson disease versus, 868t
Hurricane Katrina, 151
Hyaluronic acid, 308
Hyaluronidase, 223
Hydration
  in chronic obstructive pulmonary disease, 579
  peristalsis and, 286
  postoperative assessment of, 276
Hydrocephalus
  brain tumors as cause of, 954
  description of, 882, 937, 943
Hydrocodone
  equianalgesic dosing of, 60t
  pain management uses of, 60, 60t
Hydrocortisone, 1255b
Hydrogen breath test, 1136
Hydrogen ions
  bicarbonate effects on, 187
  carbon dioxide and, 187–188
  description of, 186
  overproduction of, 191
  underelimination of, 192
Hydromorphone
  equianalgesic dosing of, 60t
  pain management uses of, 60, 60t
  postoperative pain management using, 284b
Hydronephrosis, 1361, 1382–1384, 1383f, 1474
Hydrophilic dressing, 457
Hydrophobic dressing, 457
Hydrostatic pressure, 161
Hydrotherapy, 498–499
Hydroureter, 1361, 1382–1384, 1474
Hydroxychloroquine, 322, 327–328
17-Hydroxycorticosteroids, 1254, 1257
Hydroxyurea, 811
Hygiene
  hand, 418, 418b
  oral. See Oral hygiene
  of surgical team, 255
Hyoscyamine, 110, 1359b
Hyperactive reflexes, 849
Hyperacusis, 988
Hyperacute rejection, 301

Hyperaldosteronism, 1260–1261
Hyperbaric oxygen therapy
    description of, 458
    osteomyelitis treated with, 1024
Hypercalcemia
    cancer-induced, 408
    characteristics of, 181, 181t
    in chronic kidney disease, 1409
Hypercalciuria, 1365
Hypercapnia, 177, 646
Hypercarbia, 530, 576, 944–945
Hypercoagulability, 15
Hypercortisolism. See Cushing's
    disease
Hyperemia, 144, 294
Hyperextension spinal cord injury,
    894, 895f
Hyperflexion spinal cord injury, 894,
    894f
Hyperglycemia
    description of, 1265
    in hospitalized patients, 1301
    hypoglycemia versus, 1309t
    injury from, 1291–1303
    insulin absence as cause of,
        1282–1283
    metabolic syndrome risks, 1287
    vision complications of, 1284
Hyperglycemic-hyperosmolar state,
    1300b, 1313t, 1314–1316, 1314b,
    1315f
Hyperinsulinemia, 1300
Hyperkalemia
    burn injury as cause of, 485
    in chronic kidney disease, 1400
    definition of, 1254
    description of, 178–179, 178t,
        179b, 192, 237
    management of, 1253b
    potassium-sparing diuretic as
        cause of, 1261
Hyperkinetic pulse, 653
Hyperleptinemia, 1225
Hyperlipidemia, 729
    in chronic kidney disease, 1401
    metabolic syndrome risks, 1287
Hypermagnesemia, 182, 182t
Hypernatremia, 174–175, 175t, 953
Hyperopia, 960, 960f, 980–981
Hyperosmotic fluid, 163
Hyperoxaluria, 1362t
Hyperparathyroidism, 1275–1277,
    1276b, 1276t
Hyperperfusion syndrome, 936
Hyperphosphatemia, 1378, 1400,
    1409
Hyperpituitarism, 1247–1250, 1247f,
    1248b
Hyperpolarization-activated cyclic
    nucleotide-gated channel
    blocker, 701
Hypersensitivity reactions, 23.
        See also Allergy
    definition of, 360
    histamine in, 361, 361f

Hypersensitivity reactions
    (Continued)
    type I
        allergic rhinosinusitis,
            365–366
        anaphylaxis as. See Anaphylaxis
        angioedema as, 361–366, 362b,
            362f
        description of, 360–361
        examples of, 361t
        mechanism of action, 361t
    type II
        description of, 366
        examples of, 361t
        mechanism of action, 361t
    type III
        description of, 366
        examples of, 361t
        immune complex in, 366,
            366f
        mechanism of action, 361t
    type IV
        description of, 367
        examples of, 361t
        mechanism of action, 361t
Hypertension. See also Blood
        pressure
    adrenal-mediated, 721
    in African Americans, 722b
    assessment of, 722–728
    care coordination for, 727–728
    in chronic kidney disease, 1401,
        1407
    classification of, 721
    complementary and integrative
        health for, 723
    concept map for, 724f
    after coronary artery bypass
        grafting, 787–788
    definition of, 652, 720
    diagnostic assessment of, 723
    drug therapy for, 723–727, 725b
        angiotensin II receptor blockers,
            725b, 726–727
        angiotensin-converting enzyme
            inhibitors, 725b, 726
        beta blockers, 725b, 727
        calcium channel blockers, 725b,
            726
        diuretics, 725b, 726
    end-stage kidney disease caused
        by, 1379
    essential, 721, 721t
    etiology of, 721, 721t
    gender differences in, 722b
    health care resources for, 728
    health promotion and
        maintenance for, 722, 722t
    home care management of, 727
    incidence of, 722
    interventions for, 723–727,
        725b–726b, 726t, 916
    ischemic heart disease with, 727
    lifestyle changes for, 723
    malignant, 721

Hypertension (Continued)
    management of
        angiotensin receptor blockers
            for, 167
        angiotensin-converting enzyme
            inhibitors for, 167
        renin-angiotensin II pathway in,
            167
    metabolic syndrome risks, 1287
    pathophysiology of, 720–722
    in pheochromocytoma,
        1261–1262
    in polycystic kidney disease, 1380
    portal, 1170
    prevalence of, 722, 722b
    psychosocial assessment of, 723
    pulmonary arterial, 584–585, 585t
    renovascular, 721
    secondary, 721, 721t
    self-management education for,
        727
    signs and symptoms of, 722–723
    transition management for,
        727–728
Hypertensive crisis, 727, 727b
Hypertensive urgency, 727
Hyperthermia, 425
    malignant, 258–259, 259b–260b
Hyperthyroidism
    assessment of, 1265–1267
    drug therapy for, 1267–1268,
        1268b
    etiology of, 1265
    exogenous, 1265
    exophthalmos in, 1265, 1266f
    eye problems associated with,
        1266
    features of, 1265, 1265b
    genetic risk of, 1265
    goiter associated with, 1265, 1266f,
        1266t
    history-taking for, 1265–1266
    incidence of, 1265
    interventions for, 1267–1270
    iodine preparations for,
        1267–1268
    laboratory assessment of, 1266,
        1267b
    nonsurgical management of,
        1267–1268
    pathophysiology of, 1264–1265
    physical assessment of, 1266
    prevalence of, 1265
    psychosocial assessment of, 1266
    radioactive iodine therapy for,
        1266–1269, 1269b
    signs and symptoms of, 1266
    surgical management of,
        1269–1270
Hypertonia, 933
Hypertonic fluid, 163
Hypertonic saline, 1252
Hypertonic solution, 200
Hypertrophic cardiomyopathy,
    714–716, 715t

Hypertrophic ungual labium, 1029t
Hyperuricemia, 331, 1362t
Hyperventilation, 189, 196, 854
Hypervolemia, 171, 174
Hypnotics, 258
Hypoactive delirium, 111
Hypoactive reflexes, 849
Hypocalcemia, 179–181, 180f, 180t,
    196, 657, 1269, 1400
Hypocapnia, 145
Hypocarbia, 944–945
Hypochromic, 803–804
Hypodermoclysis, 223
Hypoglossal nerve, 844t
Hypoglycemia
    drug therapy for, 1311
    glucagon effects on, 1281
    hyperglycemia versus, 1309t
    management of, 1253b
    nutrition therapy for, 1310–1311
    in older adults, 1309, 1312b
    patient and family education
        about, 1311
    prevention of, 1302, 1308–1311
    signs and symptoms of, 1309
Hypoglycemic unawareness, 1309
Hypokalemia
    burn injury as cause of, 485
    characteristics of, 175–177, 177b
    description of, 18, 196, 237
Hypokinetic pulse, 653
Hypomagnesemia, 181–182, 182t,
    1277
Hyponatremia
    burn injury as cause of, 485
    in chronic kidney disease, 1400
    definition of, 1254
    description of, 173–174, 174t
    dilutional, 1252
Hypo-osmotic fluid, 163
Hypoparathyroidism, 1277–1278
Hypophysectomy, 1249–1250, 1249b,
    1258
Hypopituitarism, 1245–1247, 1246b
Hypotension
    brain injury caused by, 941
    description of, 20
    drug therapy for, 621–622
    monitoring for, 1423b
    orthostatic, 121, 134b, 168,
        174–175, 652, 723, 726b, 901,
        1285
    postural, 652
    in pulmonary embolism, 621–622
Hypothalamic-hypophysial portal
    system, 1236
Hypothalamus
    anatomy of, 840, 840f, 1236–1237
    function of, 1236
    hormones produced by, 1235t
Hypothermia, 142–144, 143b
    after coronary artery bypass
        grafting, 787
    shivering caused by, 280
    in trauma patients, 130

Hypothyroid crisis, 1271
Hypothyroidism
    assessment of, 1272
    care coordination for, 1273–1274
    cognition support in, 1273
    etiology of, 1271, 1272t
    features of, 1271b
    gas exchange in, 1272–1273
    health care resources for, 1274
    home care management of,
        1273–1274
    hypotension prevention in, 1273
    incidence of, 1271
    interventions for, 1273
    laboratory assessment of, 1272
    levothyroxine sodium for, 1273
    myxedema coma in, 1271, 1273,
        1273b–1274b
    pathophysiology of, 1270–1271
    physical assessment of, 1272
    prevalence of, 1271
    psychosocial assessment of, 1272
    self-management education of,
        1274
    signs and symptoms of, 1271b, 1272
    transition management for,
        1273–1274
Hypotonia, 933
Hypotonic fluid, 163
Hypotonic solution, 200
Hypoventilation
    description of, 189–190, 625
    intraoperative, 267–268
    oxygen-induced, 530
Hypovolemia, 167–168, 174, 1113,
    1283
Hypovolemic shock
    adaptive responses and events
        during, 754t
    assessment of, 756–758
    in burn injury, 494–496
    care coordination for, 760
    concept map for, 756f–757f
    drug therapy for, 495, 759b
    etiology of, 752–753, 755
    in fractures, 1034
    health promotion and
        maintenance for, 756
    incidence of, 755
    laboratory assessment of, 758,
        758b
    nonsurgical management of,
        758–760, 759b
    pathophysiology of, 754–755
    peritonitis as cause of, 1145
    physical assessment of, 756–758
    prevalence of, 755
    risk factors for, 752t, 756b
    signs and symptoms of, 756–758
    surgical management of, 760
    transition management for, 760
Hypoxemia, 177
    in asthma, 566–567
    in chronic obstructive pulmonary
        disease, 573, 576

Hypoxemia (Continued)
    definition of, 529, 617
    home care management of, 581
    management of, 619–621
    oxygen therapy for, 626, 775
    in pulmonary embolism,
        619–621
    pulse oximetry for, 603
    severe, 536
    traumatic brain injury as cause of,
        947
Hypoxia, 1283
    brain injury caused by, 941
    definition of, 529, 797, 809
    in drowning, 147
    prevention of, 541
    in tracheostomy, 541
Hypoxic-ventilatory response, 145
Hysterectomy, 1461–1463, 1461t,
    1462b–1463b, 1466
Hysterosalpingography, 1435
Hysteroscopy, 1437

I
IADLs. See Instrumental activities of
    daily living
Iatrogenic hypoparathyroidism,
    1277
Ibandronate, 1021
IBS. See Irritable bowel syndrome
Ibuprofen, 284b
Ibutilide, 677b–678b
Icterus, 1192
Idarucizumab, 745, 801
Ideal body weight, 1215, 1225
Idiopathic chronic pancreatitis,
    1202
Idiopathic hypoparathyroidism,
    1277
Idiopathic pulmonary fibrosis,
    585–586
Idiopathic thrombocytopenic
    purpura, 830–831
Ileo pouch-anal anastomosis,
    restorative proctocolectomy
    with, 1154–1155, 1154f
Ileostomy
    dietary considerations in, 1156
    health care resources for, 1157
    self-management education for,
        1157b
    stoma for, 1153, 1154b
    total proctocolectomy with
        permanent ileostomy, 1154,
        1155f
    ulcerative colitis treated with,
        1153–1154
Ilizarov technique, 1043
Iloprost, 585
Imagery, 67
Imatinib mesylate, 821
Immobility, 1044
Immune complexes, 297f, 366, 366f
Immune reconstitution
    inflammatory syndrome, 353

Immune status
    environmental factors that affect,
        414–415
    infection risks and, 414
Immune system
    age-related changes in, 291b
    antibody-mediated, 417
    burn injury effects on, 486
    leukocytes, 290–291, 292t
    organization of, 290–291
Immunity
    acquired, 295, 298
    active, 21–22, 298, 414
    age-related changes in, 290, 300
    antibody-mediated, 22, 290–291
    assessment of, 22–23
    cancer effects on, 385
    cell-mediated, 22, 290–291
    changes in, 22–23
    chronic kidney disease effects on,
        1401
    definition of, 21–23, 289, 414,
        605
    development of, 367
    divisions of, 290–291, 292f
    functions of, 379
    in hospitalized patients, 351b
    human leukocyte antigens,
        290
    inflammation. See Inflammation
    innate-naive, 291–292
    natural, 291–292
    non-self proteins, 289–290,
        290f
    passive, 21–22, 298–299, 414
    promotion of, 23
    risk factors for, 22
    scope of, 22
    self cells, 289–290, 290f
    specific, 295–300
    sustained, 298
Immunocompetent, 289–291
Immunoglobulin A, 298t
Immunoglobulin D, 298t
Immunoglobulin E, 298t
Immunoglobulin G, 298, 298t
Immunoglobulin M, 298, 298t
Immunoglobulins, 298, 298t
Immunohemolytic anemia,
    815–816
Immunologic assays, 1243
Immunomodulators, 1153
Immunosuppressants/
    immunosuppressive therapy
    autoimmune diseases treated with,
        368–369, 370b
    idiopathic pulmonary fibrosis
        treated with, 586
    in kidney transplantation patients,
        1424
    myasthenia gravis treated with,
        920
    systemic lupus erythematosus
        treated with, 328, 328b
    after transplantation, 302b

Immunotherapy
    allergic rhinosinusitis treated with,
        365–366
    cancer treated with, 401–403,
        402t
Impact of Event Scale—Revised, 158,
    158b
Impaired cellular regulation, 14–15
Impedance, 645
Impedance plethysmography, 743
Impermeable membrane, 162
Implantable cardioverter/
    defibrillator, 687–688, 688b
Implanted ports, 207–208, 207f–208f
IMRT. See Intensity-modulated
    radiation therapy
Incentive spirometry, 243–244, 244f,
    604, 1094
Incisional hernia, 1137f, 1138
Incomplete fracture, 1032
Incontinence
    age-related, 18
    definition of, 18, 1330, 1343–1344
    fecal, 18
    in older adults, 31
    pressure injuries and, 451
    urinary. See Urinary incontinence
Incontinence-associated dermatitis,
    1352
Increased intracranial pressure
    brain tumors as cause of, 954
    edema as cause of, 942
    in human immunodeficiency
        virus infection, 355
    management of, 937
    stroke as cause of, 936–937, 936b
    traumatic brain injury as cause of,
        941–942, 946
Incretin, 1282
Incretin mimetics, 1292b–1293b,
    1293
Incus, 984, 985f–986f
Indacaterol, 569b–570b
Indirect contact transmission, 416
Indirect Coombs' test, 805
Indirect inguinal hernia, 1137–1138,
    1137f
Indirect thrombin inhibitors, 801
Induration, 607
Infarction
    definition of, 928
    myocardial. See Myocardial
        infarction
Infection(s)
    airborne transmission of, 416
    antimicrobial therapy inadequacy
        for, 423–427
    antimicrobial-resistant, 421,
        421b
    assessment of, 423–425
    bloodstream, 416, 423
    care coordination for, 426
    CDC information about, 414
    communicable, 414
    contact transmission of, 416

Infection(s) (Continued)
corneal, 977
in Cushing's disease, 1259–1260
directly observed therapy for, 423
droplet transmission of, 416
ear, 1000b
emerging types of, 427–428, 427t
environmental exposure to, 423
fever associated with, 424b, 425–426
food contamination as source of, 427–428
fractures as risk factor for, 1035, 1045
fungal. See Fungal infections
gastrointestinal tract transmission of, 415
health care resources for, 426
health promotion and maintenance for, 417–421
history-taking for, 423–424
home care management for, 426
hospital-acquired, 122
host factors in development of, 414t
imaging assessment of, 425
immune status and, 414
inflammation and, 292
intraoperative, 267, 268f
laboratory assessment of, 424–425
in leukemia, 821–822, 821b
lymphadenopathy associated with, 424
mechanical ventilation-related, 635
multidrug-resistant organism
carbapenem-resistant Enterobacteriaceae, 422–423
contact precautions for, 419
methicillin-resistant Staphylococcus aureus, 422
types of, 421–422
vancomycin-resistant Enterococcus, 422
occupational exposure to, 423
opportunistic
description of, 339, 346–347, 347f
prevention of, 350–353
oxygen therapy as cause of, 531
pandemic, 427
physical assessment of, 424
physiologic defenses for, 416–417
portal of exit for, 416
prevention of. See Infection prevention
psychosocial assessment of, 424
reservoirs of, 414
respiratory tract transmission of, 415
risks of, 414, 415b, 417b
self-management education for, 426
sepsis caused by, 760–761

Infection(s) (Continued)
sexually transmitted. See Sexually transmitted infections
signs and symptoms of, 424
skin. See Skin infections
skin barrier against, 415
surgical site. See Surgical site infections
tracheostomy as cause of, 539
transition management for, 426
transmission of
description of, 414–416
precautions based on, 419, 420t
routes of, 415–416
urinary tract. See Urinary tract infections
Infection control
disinfection for, 418
hand hygiene for, 418, 418b
in health care settings, 417
methods of, 417–421
patient placement for, 421
for patient transfer, 421
staff considerations, 421
Standard Precautions for, 418–419, 419t
sterilization for, 418
transmission-based precautions for, 419, 420t
Infection prevention
after amputation, 1054
description of, 397b
disinfection for, 418
methods of, 417–421, 827b
patient placement for, 421
in pressure injuries, 459
staff considerations, 421
Standard Precautions for, 418–419, 419t
transmission-based precautions for, 419, 420t
Infectious cystitis, 1355
Infective endocarditis, 711–712, 711b
Inferior oblique muscle, 960t
Inferior rectus muscle, 960t
Inferior vena cava filter, 618, 621, 745
Inferior wall myocardial infarction, 771
Infertility, 1517
Infiltrating ductal carcinoma, 1441
Infiltration, 200, 217t–219t, 221t
Infiltration Scale, 221t
Inflammation
asthma caused by, 565
basophils in, 293–294
cells involved in, 292–294, 292t
complement system in, 294
as defense mechanism, 417
eosinophils in, 294
five cardinal symptoms of, 294
infection and, 292
leukocytes in, 292, 292t
leukocytes involved in, 797t

Inflammation (Continued)
macrophages in, 293–295
neutrophils in, 292–293, 292t
phagocytosis in, 294
pneumonia caused by, 599
sequence of, 294–295
stages of, 294–295
tissue mast cells in, 294
Inflammatory bowel disease. See Crohn's disease; Ulcerative colitis
Inflammatory breast cancer, 1441
Inflammatory cytokines, 1225
Infliximab, 323b, 466b, 1160b
Influenza
pandemic, 597–598
pandemic outbreaks of, 151
seasonal, 596–597
Informatics
attributes of, 8
context of, 8
definition of, 7
scope of, 8
Informed consent
for cardiac catheterization, 658
preoperative, 239–241, 240f
Infratentorial lesion, 840
Infratentorial tumors, 950
Infusate, 200
Infusion nurses, 199–200
Infusion Nurses Society, 200
Infusion pressure, 214
Infusion therapy. See also Intravenous therapy
administration sets for
add-on devices, 209–210
definition of, 209
filters used with, 210
intermittent, 209
needleless connection devices, 210–211, 210f, 214
secondary, 209, 209f
slip lock, 210
ambulatory pumps, 211
blood and blood components, 200
containers used in, 208–209
definition of, 199
dose-track technology for, 211
drugs, 201
electronic infusion devices for, 211
electronic infusion pumps, 211
fluids used in, 200
indications for, 199
intra-arterial, 224–225
intraosseous, 223–224, 224f
intraperitoneal, 225
intraspinal, 225–226
intrathecal, 225–226
intravenous. See Intravenous therapy
intravenous solutions, 200
mechanically regulated devices for, 211, 212f
overview of, 199–202
prescribing of, 201

Infusion therapy (Continued)
rate-controlling devices, 211
smart pumps for, 211
subcutaneous, 223
syringe pumps, 211
vascular access devices for, 201–202
Ingrown nail, 1029t
Inguinal hernia, 1137, 1137f
Inhalant irritants, 515
Inhalation anthrax, 611–612, 612b
Inheritance patterns
autosomal dominant, 78–79, 78t
autosomal recessive, 78t, 79, 79f
complex, 78t, 80
overview of, 77–80
pedigree, 77–78, 78f–79f
sex-linked recessive, 78t, 79–80, 80f
Inherited mutation, 76
Injection drug users, 343
Injection sclerotherapy, 1177
In-line filter, for intraspinal infusions, 226
Inner ear, 985–986
Inner maxillary fixation, 558–559
Inpatient rehabilitation facility, 87
Inpatient rehabilitation facility patient assessment instrument, 92
Inpatient surgery, 229–230
INR. See International normalized ratio
Insensible water loss, 165
Inspection
of abdomen, 1067
of endocrine system, 1241–1242
of myocardium, 653, 654f
of skeletal system, 1009–1010, 1009f
of skin, 436–439
Institute for Safe Medication Practices, 1297–1298
Institute of Medicine Health Professions Education: A Bridge to Quality, 2
Instrumental activities of daily living, 1217
definition of, 92
self-management education for performing, 100
Insufflation, 254
Insulin
absence of, 1282–1283, 1283t
absorption of, 1295–1296
complications of, 1296, 1296f
continuous subcutaneous infusion of, 1294, 1296, 1296f, 1313
functions of, 1236, 1240
gene for, 72
injection areas and sites for, 1295f
injection devices for, 1297
Lispro, 1294
long-acting, 1295t
metabolic effects of, 1282

Insulin (Continued)
mixing of, 1296
pen-type injectors for, 1297–1298
preoperative administration of, 242
rapid-acting, 1295t, 1296
regimens, 1294–1295
secretion of, 1281
sensitizers of, 1291, 1292b–1293b
short-acting, 1295t
stimulators of, 1291–1294, 1292b–1293b
storage of, 1297
structure of, 76, 1281, 1282f
subcutaneous administration of, 1297b
syringes for, 1297
Insulin pump, 1296f
Insulin resistance, 1286–1287
Insulin-dependent diabetes mellitus. See Diabetes mellitus, type 1
Integrase, 337–340
Integrase inhibitors, 351b–352b
Integrative care, 3
Integrative therapies, 3t
Integumentary system
assessment of, before rehabilitation, 90t, 91
components of, 431
hair, 432–433
nails, 432–433, 432f
nutrition assessments, 1213b
skin. See Skin
Intensity, of sound, 990
Intensity-modulated radiation therapy, 388, 549, 556
Intensivist, 8
Intention tremors, 848, 889
Interbody cage fusion surgery, 906
Intercostal space, 518
Interferons
cancer treated with, 402, 402t
multiple sclerosis treated with, 891b
Interleukins
-1, 300t
-2, 300t
-6, 300t
cancer treated with, 402, 402t
Intermittent catheterization, 98
Intermittent claudication, 651, 732, 735
Intermittent hemodialysis. See Hemodialysis
Intermittent self-catheterization, 1352
Internal carotid artery, 841
Internal cerebral artery, 933b
Internal derangement, 1056
Internal hemorrhoids, 1139, 1140f
Internal mammary artery, 784–786
Internal urethral sphincter, 1327, 1327f
International Critical Incident Stress Foundation, 156

International normalized ratio, 16, 622b, 657, 805, 1174
International Prostate Symptom Score, 1474, 1475f–1476f
International Society of Blood Transfusion, 200, 201f
Interprofessional collaboration
attributes of, 5
definition of, 5
scope of, 5
Interprofessional communication, 5–6
competencies for, 5t
e-mail for, 5
goals of, 5
SBAR process for, 5–6
Interprofessional Education Collaborative Expert Panel, 5
Interprofessional team
in emergency departments, 118–120
members of, 5
in rehabilitation settings, 88–89, 88t, 89f
Interrupted sutures, 268f
Interstitial brachytherapy, 1451
Interstitial cystitis, 1354, 1356
Interstitial edema, 942
Interstitial fluid, 160
Intestinal disorders
appendicitis, 1147–1148, 1147b, 1148f
bacterial overgrowth, 1142
celiac disease, 1164, 1164b
colorectal cancer. See Colorectal cancer
Crohn's disease. See Crohn's disease
diverticular disease, 1162–1164, 1162f, 1163b
gastroenteritis, 1148–1150, 1148t, 1149b–1150b
hemorrhoids, 1139–1140, 1140f
hernia, 1137–1139, 1137f
inflammatory, 1144–1168
irritable bowel syndrome, 1135–1137
malabsorption syndrome, 1141–1142
noninflammatory, 1121–1143
obstruction. See Intestinal obstructions
peritonitis. See Peritonitis
polyps, 1126
ulcerative colitis. See Ulcerative colitis
Intestinal ischemia, 1122
Intestinal obstructions
assessment of, 1123
care coordination for, 1125–1126
closed-loop, 1122
complications of, 1122
diagnostic assessment of, 1123
exploratory laparotomy for, 1125
features of, 1123b

Intestinal obstructions (Continued)
fecal impaction as cause of, 1125, 1126b
fluid replacement and maintenance for, 1124
health care resources for, 1126
history-taking for, 1123
home care management for, 1125
imaging assessment of, 1123
interventions for, 1123–1125
intussusception, 1122, 1122f
laboratory assessment of, 1123
large-bowel, 1123b
mechanical, 1122–1123, 1122f
minimally invasive surgery for, 1125
nasogastric tubes for, 1124, 1134b
nonmechanical, 1122–1123
nonsurgical management of, 1124–1125
nursing care for, 1124b
pain associated with, 1123
pathophysiology of, 1121–1122
physical assessment of, 1123
postoperative ileus, 1122, 1124
self-management education for, 1126
signs and symptoms of, 1123
small-bowel, 1123b
strangulated, 1122, 1125
surgical management of, 1125
transition management for, 1125–1126
types of, 1122
volvulus, 1122, 1122f
Intestinal tract, 1144
Intestinal villi, 1064
Intestine. See also Large intestine; Small intestine
contents of, 1122
obstruction of. See Intestinal obstruction
preoperative preparation of, 242
Intimate partner violence, 118
Intra-aortic balloon pump, 782
Intra-arterial infusion therapy, 224–225
Intra-arterial thrombolytic therapy, 736
Intracellular fluid, 19, 160, 162, 164
Intracerebral hemorrhage, 929, 943
Intracranial pressure
in encephalitis, 884b
after hypophysectomy, 1249
increased. See Increased intracranial pressure
normal level of, 941
Intraductal papilloma, 1455t
Intrahepatic obstructive jaundice, 1170
Intraocular pressure
activities that increase, 961t
definition of, 958

Intraocular pressure (Continued)
in glaucoma, 972
normal, 972
tonometry of, 965, 965f–966f
Intraoperative period
advance directives, 263
anesthesia
allergies to, 263
definition of, 256
general, 257–260, 258t–259t, 260b
local, 260–261
moderate sedation, 261–262, 262t
providers of, 256–257
regional, 260–261, 261f–262f, 261t
selection criteria for, 256–257
description of, 228
diagnostic tests, 263–264
electronic health record review in, 263–264
history-taking in, 262–263
hypoventilation prevention, 267–268
infection prevention, 267, 268f
laboratory testing, 263–264
moderate sedation, 261–262, 262t
nursing interventions, 264b
onset of, 251–252
overview of, 251–268
patient positioning, 264–267, 265f, 267b
retained surgical items, 267
surgical attire, 256, 256f
surgical scrub, 256, 257f
surgical team, 252, 253t. See also Surgical team
Intraosseous infusion therapy, 223–224, 224f
Intraperitoneal infusion therapy, 225
Intraspinal analgesia, 61–62
Intraspinal infusion therapy, 225–226
Intrathecal analgesia, 61–62, 62b
Intrathecal baclofen, 891, 900
Intrathecal contrast-enhanced computed tomography scan, 853
Intrathecal infusion, 225–226
Intravascular ultrasonography, 659
Intravenous immunoglobulin, 915
Intravenous pumps, 211
Intravenous solutions, 170, 170t, 200
Intravenous therapy
administration sets for
add-on devices, 209–210
changing of, 214
definition of, 209
filters used with, 210
intermittent, 209
needleless connection devices, 210–211, 210f, 214
secondary, 209, 209f
slip lock, 210

Intravenous therapy (Continued)
catheters used in
blood samples obtained from, 215
dressings with, 212–214
flushing of, 214–215
hemodialysis, 208
peripherally inserted central, 205–206, 205f, 206b, 212–213
securing of, 212–214, 213f, 222b
short peripheral, 202–204, 202f–203f, 202t, 203b, 214–215
central
hemodialysis catheters, 208
implanted ports, 207–208, 207f–208f
peripherally inserted central catheters, 205–206, 205f, 206b, 212–213
tunneled central venous catheters, 207, 207f, 213, 226
vascular access devices for, 205
complications of
catheter embolism, 219t–220t
catheter-related bloodstream infection, 204–206, 211–212, 216, 216t, 220t–221t
circulatory overload, 219t–220t
ecchymosis, 217t–219t
extravasation, 217t–219t
hematoma, 217t–219t
infiltration, 217t–219t, 221t
local, 216, 217t–219t
nerve damage, 217t–219t
phlebitis, 217t–219t
site infection, 217t–219t
speed shock, 219t–220t
systemic, 216, 219t–220t
thrombophlebitis, 217t–219t
thrombosis, 217t–219t
venous spasm, 217t–219t
documentation of, 216
drug delivery using, 201
nursing assessment for, 212
nursing care for, 211–216
in older adults
cardiac changes, 222–223
catheter selection for, 222
renal changes, 222–223
skin care, 216–222
vein selection for, 222
venous distention, 222
patient education about, 211–212
peripheral
midline catheters for, 204–205, 204f, 213
short peripheral catheters for, 202–204, 202f–203f, 202t, 203b, 214–215
site selection for, 203–204, 203f, 204b
skin preparation for, 203–204

Intravenous therapy (Continued)
ultrasound applications in, 202–203
vein selection for, 203–204, 203f, 204b
skin care in, 216–222
in trauma patients, 130
Intrinsic factor, 798, 814, 1063
Intrinsic renal failure, 1392
Intubation
complications of, 260
endotracheal. See Endotracheal intubation
Intussusception, 1122, 1122f
Inversion, 1010f
Iodine, 1239
Iodoform gauze, 1000
Iontophoresis, 1041
IPEC Expert Panel. See Interprofessional Education Collaborative Expert Panel
Ipratropium, 569b–570b, 571
IPV. See Intimate partner violence
IRF. See Inpatient rehabilitation facility
IRF-PAI. See Inpatient rehabilitation facility patient assessment instrument
Iris
age-related changes in, 961b
anatomy of, 957, 958f
Iron, 796
Iron deficiency anemia, 814–816, 814t, 815b
Irreducible hernia, 1138
Irregular bones, 1005
Irrigation
external ear canal, 994b, 994f
Irritability, 174–175
Irritable bowel syndrome, 1068, 1135–1137
I-SBAR, 5
I-SBAR-R, 5
ISBT. See International Society of Blood Transfusion
Ischemia-edema cycle, 1033
Ischemic heart disease, 727
Ischemic stroke, 927–929, 929t, 935
Ishihara chart, 964
Islam, 112t
Islet cell transplantation, 1303
Islets of Langerhans, 1063, 1239, 1240f, 1281
Isoelectric line, 666
Isosmotic fluids, 163
Isosthenuria, 1399–1400
Isotonic dehydration, 167–168
Isotonic fluids, 163
Isotonic solution, 200
Ivabradine, 701

J
Jacknife position, 265f
Jackson-Pratt drain, 278, 279f, 282, 1500
Jaeger card, 964

Janus kinases, 367, 369
Jarisch-Herxheimer reaction, 1510
Jaundice
cholecystitis as cause of, 1192
cirrhosis as cause of, 1170, 1171f
in dark-skin patients, 444
definition of, 1170
in hepatitis, 1183
intrahepatic obstructive, 1170
obstructive, 1192
in sickle cell disease, 810
Jaw osteonecrosis, bisphosphonate-related, 1021
Jehovah's Witnesses, 123b
Jejunostomy, 1221
Jejunum, 1064
Jitter, 918
Job analysis, 92
Joint(s)
anatomy of, 1006–1007
ball-and-socket, 1007
definition of, 1006
dislocation of, 1057t
hand, 1009, 1009f
hinge, 1007
pivot, 1007
synovial, 1006–1007
types of, 1006
Joint effusions
mobility affected by, 1010
in osteoarthritis, 306–307
in rheumatoid arthritis, 319
J-pouch, 1154, 1154f
Judaism, 112t
Jugular venous distention, 653
Juxtaglomerular complex, 1323, 1323f
Juxtamedullary nephrons, 1323
JVD. See Jugular venous distention

K
Kallidin, 1197
Kaposi's sarcoma, 347, 348f, 354–355
Karyotype, 74, 75f, 1079
Keratin, 432
Keratinocytes, 432
Keratoconus, 977–979, 978f
Keratoplasty, 978
Keraunographic markings, 142
Keraunoparalysis, 142
Ketoacids, 191
Ketogenesis, 1282
Ketone bodies, 1283, 1301, 1335
Ketorolac tromethamine, 284b, 1195
Kidney(s). See also Renal system
in acid-base balance, 189t, 190
acute injury of. See Acute kidney injury
age-related changes in, 234b, 1328
anatomy of, 1322–1323, 1322f–1323f
assessment of, 803, 1330–1331, 1331f
bicarbonate movement by, 190
biopsy of, 1340–1341, 1394
in blood pressure regulation, 646

Kidney(s) (Continued)
blood supply to, 1322, 1328
burn injury-related assessment of, 491–492
capsule of, 1322, 1322f
dehydration effects on, 169
functions of, 1321, 1323–1327, 1372, 1390
gross anatomy of, 1322–1323, 1322f–1323f
hormonal functions of, 1326–1327, 1326t
microscopic anatomy of, 1323, 1323f–1324f
nephrons, 1323, 1323f, 1325t
nephrotoxic substances for, 1393t
in older adults, 222–223, 1328b
palpation of, 1330–1331, 1331f
postoperative assessment of, 276
preoperative assessment of, 236
regulatory functions of, 1323–1326
scarring of, 1373–1374
sickle cell disease effects on, 810
structure of, 1322–1323, 1322f–1323f
trauma to, 1387–1388, 1387b
tubular reabsorption, 1325
tubular secretion, 1326
tumors of, 1385, 1385t
Kidney, ureter, and bladder x-rays, 1337, 1337t
Kidney disease
chronic. See Chronic kidney disease
diabetes mellitus as cause of, 1308
polycystic. See Polycystic kidney disease
terms used for, 1330
Kidney disorders
acute glomerulonephritis, 1376–1378, 1376t
chronic glomerulonephritis, 1378
diabetic nephropathy, 1286, 1384–1385
hydronephrosis, 1361, 1382–1384, 1383f
hydroureter, 1361, 1382–1384
nephrosclerosis, 1379
nephrotic syndrome, 1378–1379, 1379b
polycystic kidney disease. See Polycystic kidney disease
pyelonephritis. See Pyelonephritis
renal cell carcinoma, 1385–1386
renovascular disease, 1384
Kidney replacement therapies
acute kidney injury treated with, 1397–1398, 1397f
chronic kidney disease treated with, 1411–1424, 1411t, 1412f–1415f
Kidney stones, 1362t
Kidney transplantation
acute rejection, 1423–1424, 1423t
assessments after, 1425b

Kidney transplantation (Continued)
  candidate selection criteria, 1421
  chronic rejection, 1423–1424, 1423t
  complications of, 1423–1424, 1423t
  donors, 1421–1422, 1422f
  hyperacute rejection, 1423–1424, 1423t
  immunosuppressive drug therapy in, 1424
  incidence of, 1421
  living related donors, 1421, 1423
  operative procedures, 1422–1423, 1422f
  postoperative care, 1423
  preoperative care, 1422
  rejection, 1423–1424, 1423t
  self-management education after, 1425
Killip Classification, 651, 781, 782t
Kineret. See Anakinra
Kinins, 293–294
Klebsiella pneumoniae, 422
Knee
  arthroplasty of. See Total knee arthroplasty
  effusion of, 1010
  internal derangement of, 1056
  sports-related injuries of, 1056, 1056b, 1057f, 1057t
Knee height caliper, 1213
Knee immobilizer, 1057f
Knowledge, skills, attitudes, and abilities, 2
Kock's pouch, 1369
Koilonychia, 443t
Kupffer cells, 1063–1064
Kussmaul respiration, 193, 1283, 1312–1313, 1400, 1404
Kwashiorkor, 1215
Kyphoplasty, 1050
Kyphosis, 1009f

L
Labia majora, 1429
Labia minora, 1429
Laboratory technicians, 119–120
Labyrinthectomy, 996
Lacerations
  corneal, 982
  ocular, 981–982
Lacrimal gland, 959, 959f
Lactase deficiency, 1141
Lactate dehydrogenase, 1174
Lactic acidosis, 191–192
Lacto-ovo-vegetarian, 1212
Lactose intolerance, 1212b
Lactose tolerance test, 1141
Lacto-vegetarian, 1212
Lactulose, 1178
Laennec's cirrhosis, 1170
Lamellar keratoplasty, 978
Laminectomy, 906
Lamivudine, 1185t
Language assessment, 847

Lanreotide, 1248–1249
Laparoscopes, 254, 255f
Laparoscopic adjustable gastric band, 1229, 1230f
Laparoscopic Nissen fundoplication, 1091, 1093, 1093f, 1094b
Laparoscopic sleeve gastrectomy, 1229
Laparoscopy
  appendectomy through, 1148
  cholecystectomy, 1195–1196
  radical prostatectomy, 1484
  reproductive system assessments using, 1436–1437, 1437f
  Whipple procedure via, 1207
Laparotomy, 1148
Large intestine
  anatomy of, 1064
  cecum, 1064
  functions of, 1064
  obstruction of, 1123b
Large-volume parenteral infusions, 224
Laryngeal cancer
  description of, 549
  surgical management of, 550, 551t
Laryngeal edema, 363
Laryngeal stridor, 1269–1270
Laryngectomee, 552
Laryngectomy, 550, 554b
Laryngofissure, 551t
Laryngopharynx, 510
Laryngoscopy, 524–525
Larynx
  age-related changes in, 513b
  anatomy of, 509f, 510
  trauma to, 559–560
Laser in-situ keratomileusis, 981
Laser trabeculoplasty, 975
Laser-assisted laparoscopic lumbar diskectomy, 906
LASIK. See Laser in-situ keratomileusis
Late adulthood, 30
Latency period, 375
Latent syphilis, 1508
Latent tuberculosis, 606
Lateral position, 265f
Lateral rectus muscle, 960t
Latex allergy, 234–235, 419
Laxatives, 1136
Lead axis, 666, 666f
Leave-of-absence visit, 100–101
LEEP. See Loop electrosurgical excision procedure
Leflunomide, 322
Left atrial appendage, 681
Left hemisphere stroke, 932–933, 933b
Left main coronary artery, 643, 643f
Left shift, 280, 293
Left ventricular failure
  description of, 695b
  after myocardial infarction, 780–782

Left-sided cardiac catheterization, 658, 658f
Left-sided heart failure, 651, 692, 695–696, 780–782
Legal competence, 36
Leiomyomas, uterine
  assessment of, 1460
  bleeding in, 1461–1463
  care coordination for, 1463
  classification of, 1460f
  etiology of, 1460
  genetic risk of, 1460
  health care resources for, 1463
  home care management of, 1463
  hysterectomy for, 1461–1463, 1461t, 1462b–1463b
  incidence of, 1460
  interventions for, 1461–1463
  pathophysiology of, 1459–1460
  physical assessment of, 1460
  prevalence of, 1460
  psychosocial assessment of, 1460
  self-management education for, 1463
  signs and symptoms of, 1460
  submucosal, 1459–1460, 1460f
  subserosal, 1459–1460, 1460f
  surgical management of, 1461–1463
  transcervical endometrial resection for, 1461
  transition management for, 1463
  transvaginal ultrasound of, 1460
  uterine artery embolization for, 1461, 1461b
Lens
  age-related changes in, 961b
  anatomy of, 958, 958f
Leptin, 1225, 1226b
Leptin resistance, 1225
LES. See Lower esophageal sphincter
Lesbian, gay, bisexual, transgender, and queer population, 1492–1493. See also Transgender patients/health
  description of, 10–11, 11t, 1495
  environment for, 1495b
  sexually transmitted infections in, 1509b
  smoking in, 514b
  The Joint Commission recommendations for, 1495, 1495b
Lethargic, 846
Leukemia, 380b
  acute
    consolidation therapy for, 820–821
    description of, 817, 819b
    drug therapy for, 820–821
    induction therapy for, 820
  acute lymphocytic, 814t
  acute myelogenous, 814t, 820
  acute promyelocytic, 814t
  assessment of, 818–820
  biphenotypic, 818

Leukemia (Continued)
  bleeding precautions in, 825, 825b
  bone marrow aspiration and biopsy for, 820, 820f
  care coordination for, 826–827, 827b
  chronic lymphocytic, 814t, 821
  chronic myelogenous, 814t
  classification of, 818
  drug therapy for, 820–821
  energy conservation in, 826, 826b
  etiology of, 818
  fatigue in, 825–826
  genetic risks of, 818
  genetic syndromes associated with, 818
  health care resources for, 827
  hematopoietic stem cell transplantation for
    bone marrow harvesting for, 823
    complications of, 824–825
    conditioning regimen for, 823–824, 823f
    cord blood harvesting, 823
    engraftment of, 824
    graft-versus-host-disease secondary to, 824–825, 825f
    leukemia treated with, 822–825, 822t
    peripheral blood stem cell harvesting, 823
    stem cells for, 822–823
    steps of, 823f
    transplantation procedure for, 824
    transplants, 822t
    veno-occlusive disease secondary to, 825
  history-taking for, 818–819
  home care management of, 826
  imaging assessment of, 820
  incidence of, 818
  infection protection in, 821–822, 821b
  injury minimization in, 825
  interventions for, 820–825
  laboratory assessment of, 819
  lymphoblastic, 818, 818t
  lymphocytic, 818, 818t
  myelocytic, 818, 818t
  myelogenous, 818, 818t
  nutrition therapy in, 825–826
  pathophysiology of, 817–818
  physical assessment of, 819
  platelet function in, 819
  prevalence of, 818
  psychosocial assessment of, 819
  psychosocial preparation for, 827
  risk factors for, 818
  self-management education for, 826–827, 826b–827b
  transition management for, 826–827, 827b

Leukocyte alkaline phosphatase, 805
Leukocytes
    definition of, 290–291
    functions of, 797t
    in inflammation, 292, 292t
Leukoesterase, 1335
Leukopenia, 815
Leukoplakia, 548, 1078–1079
Leukotriene modifiers, 569b–570b, 571
Level I trauma center, 127, 128t
Level II trauma center, 127–128, 128t
Level III trauma center, 128, 128t
Level IV trauma center, 128, 128t
Level of consciousness
    assessment of, 130, 896
    definition of, 846
    during dying, 107
    postoperative assessment of, 274–275
    in stroke patients, 931–932
    in traumatic brain injury patients, 946
Levels of evidence, 6, 6f
Levodopa/carbidopa, 870
Levosimendan, 700
Levothyroxine sodium, 1273
LGBTQ population. See Lesbian, gay, bisexual, transgender, and queer population
LH. See Luteinizing hormone
Libido, 1265
Lichenifications, 438f
Lichtenberg figures, 142
Lidocaine patch, 65
Life planning, 100
Life review, 112
Life Safety Code, 150
Ligament tear, 1057t
Light therapy, 465
Lightning injuries, 141–142, 141b
Linagliptin, 1292b–1293b
Linear scleroderma, 329
Lipase, 1068, 1197, 1200
Lipids, 728–729
Lipoatrophy, 348
Lipodystrophy, 348
Lipophilicity, 60
Lipoprotein-a, 656
Liposomal bupivacaine, 65
Lip-reading, 1001
Liquid formula diet, 1227
Liquid oxygen, 536–537, 537f
Liraglutide, 1228, 1292b–1293b
Lispro insulin, 1294
Lithotomy position, 265f
Liver
    anatomy of, 1063–1064, 1063f
    cancer of, 1186–1187
    functions of, 1063
    palpation of, 803
    transplantation of, 1187–1189, 1188t, 1189b
    trauma to, 1186, 1186b
    in vitamin K formation, 798

Liver disorders
    cancer, 1186–1187
    cirrhosis. See Cirrhosis
    fatty liver, 1185–1186
    hepatitis. See Hepatitis
Liver-spleen scan, 1073
Living will, 104–106
Lixisenatide, 1292b–1293b
LMX-4, 65
Lobar pneumonia, 599
Lobectomy, 589
Lobular carcinoma in situ, 1441
Local anesthesia, 260–261
Local anesthetics, 64–65
Localized pain, 50
Localized peritonitis, 1145
"Lock and key" model, 1235, 1235f
Locus, 72
Loneliness, 31
Long bones, 1005, 1005f
Long-acting beta₂ agonists, 569b–571b, 570–571
Long-term care settings
    description of, 30
    health care-associated infections in, 417
    older adults in
        care coordination and transition management for, 42
        health issues for, 39–42
        restorative aids in, 89
Long-term nonprogressors, 338b
Loop diuretics, 699b, 701
Loop electrosurgical excision procedure, 1470
Loop of Henle, 1323
Lorazepam, 110, 879
Lorcaserin, 1228
Lordosis, 1009, 1009f
Lovaza, 731
Low back pain. See also Back pain
    assessment of, 904–905
    care coordination for, 908–909
    contributing factors for, 904b
    exercises for, 906b
    health care resources for, 909
    health promotion and maintenance for, 904
    herniated nucleus pulposus as cause of, 903, 903f
    imaging assessment of, 905
    nonsurgical management of, 905–906, 906b
    pathophysiology of, 903–904
    physical assessment of, 904–905
    prevention of, 904b, 908b
    signs and symptoms of, 904–905
    surgical management of, 906–908, 907b
    transition management for, 908–909
    weight reduction for, 905–906
Low-density lipoprotein, 656

Low-density lipoprotein cholesterol, 730
Low-energy diets, 1228
Lower esophageal sphincter, 1062–1063, 1087–1088, 1092
Lower extremity
    amputation of, 1051, 1051b, 1051f
    arterial disease of, 731
    fractures of, 1047–1049, 1047f–1048f
    traction for, 1040t
Lower gastrointestinal bleeding, 1156, 1156b
Lower motor neuron, 842
Lower motor neuron disease, 99
Lower respiratory tract, 510–511, 511f
Lower urinary tract symptoms, 1474, 1477
Low-intensity pulsed ultrasound, 1043
Low-molecular-weight heparin, 744–745
Low-profile gastrostomy device, 1220f, 1221
Lubiprostone, 1136
Luer-Lok connection, 210
Lukens tube, 601f–602f
Lumacaftor/ivacaftor, 583
Lumbar puncture, 855
Lung(s)
    age-related changes in, 513b
    anatomy of, 510–511, 511f
    assessment of, 518–521
    auscultation of, 519, 520f
    inspection of, 518, 518f
    percussion of, 519, 519f–520f, 519t
Lung biopsy
    follow-up care for, 527
    patient preparation for, 526–527
    percutaneous, 527
    procedure for, 527
    respiratory system assessments using, 526–527
Lung cancer
    assessment of, 380b, 587–588
    chemotherapy for, 588
    deaths caused by, 586
    diagnostic assessment of, 588
    dyspnea management in, 593
    etiology of, 587
    genetic risk of, 587
    history-taking for, 587
    hospice care for, 593
    incidence of, 587
    interventions for, 588–593
    metastasis of, 586
    metastatic sites of, 376t
    nonsurgical management of, 588–593
    pain management in, 593
    palliative interventions for, 593
    paraneoplastic syndromes associated with, 586, 586t

Lung cancer (Continued)
    pathophysiology of, 586–587
    photodynamic therapy for, 589
    physical assessment of, 587–588
    prevalence of, 587
    primary prevention of, 587
    psychosocial assessment of, 588
    radiation therapy for, 588–589, 593
    signs and symptoms of, 587–588, 587t
    staging of, 586–587
    surgical management of, 589–593
    targeted therapy for, 588, 589t
Lung transplantation
    cystic fibrosis treated with, 583–584
    pulmonary arterial hypertension treated with, 585
Lunula, 432–433, 432f
Lupus erythematosus
    discoid, 326–328, 328b
    pathophysiology of, 326
    systemic. See Systemic lupus erythematosus
Lupus nephritis, 326
Lurch, 1009
Lutein, 979
Luteinizing hormone
    deficiency of, 1246, 1246b
    description of, 1237t
    overproduction of, 1248b
Luteinizing hormone-releasing hormone agonists, 1485
Lyme disease, 332, 333b
Lymph nodes, cervical, 1080, 1080f
Lymphadenopathy, 424
Lymphangiography, 1487
Lymphedema, 652, 1454, 1454b
Lymphokines, 299
Lymphomas
    in AIDS-infected patients, 347–348
    assessment of, 828–829
    classification of, 827, 829t
    Hodgkin's, 828
    indolent, 828
    interventions for, 829
    mucosa-associated lymphoid tissue, 1115
    non-Hodgkin's, 828–829
    pathophysiology of, 828
    staging of, 828, 829t
    treatment of, 829
Lynch syndrome, 1127b, 1128
Lyrica. See Pregabalin
Lysis, 297

M
Macitentan, 585
Macrocytic, 803–804
Macrophages
    function of, 797t
    in inflammation, 293–295

Macula densa, 1323, 1323f
Macula lutea, 958
Macular degeneration, 979
Macular rash, 440
Macules, 438f
Maculopapular rash, 881
Mafenide acetate, 501b
MAG3, 1394
Magnesium
    description of, 181–182
    hypermagnesemia, 182, 182t
    hypomagnesemia, 181–182,
        182t
    in older adults, 165b
    serum levels of, 164t
Magnesium hydroxide, 1091,
    1106b–1107b
Magnesium sulfate, 182, 686, 1277
Magnetic resonance angiography
    description of, 853
    renovascular disease evaluations,
        1384
    stroke assessments using, 935
Magnetic resonance arthrography,
    1013
Magnetic resonance
    cholangiopancreatography,
    1070, 1194
Magnetic resonance enterography
    Crohn's disease assessments using,
        1159
    ulcerative colitis assessments
        using, 1152
Magnetic resonance imaging
    cardiovascular system evaluations
        using, 661
    cognition assessments with, 17
    contraindications for, 853
    ear assessments using, 990
    functional, 853
    gastrointestinal system
        assessments, 1070
    hyperpituitarism evaluations,
        1248
    multiple sclerosis evaluations, 890,
        890f
    musculoskeletal system
        evaluations using, 1012–1013,
        1013b
    neurologic system evaluations
        using, 853
    osteoporosis evaluations, 1019
    patient preparation for, 1013b
    renal system assessments using,
        1337t, 1338
    reproductive system assessments,
        1436
    traumatic brain injury
        evaluations, 946
    vision assessments, 965
Magnetic resonance spectroscopy
    description of, 853
    osteoporosis evaluations, 1019
Magnetoencephalography, 854
Malabsorption syndrome, 1141–1142

Male reproductive disorders
    benign prostatic hyperplasia. See
        Benign prostatic hyperplasia
    erectile dysfunction, 27, 1286,
        1484–1485, 1489–1490
    overview of, 1473
    testicular cancer. See Testicular
        cancer
Male reproductive system
    function of, 1430–1431
    genitalia, 1430f
    hormones of, 1430
    in older adults, 1431b
    physical assessment of, 1433
    structure of, 1430–1431
Male-to-female transgender patients
    definition of, 1493–1494, 1493t
    drug therapy for, 1497–1499, 1497t
    gender reassignment surgery for,
        1499–1500
    vaginoplasty for, 1499–1500
Malignant hypertension, 721
Malignant hyperthermia, 258–259,
    259b–260b
Malignant otitis, 993
Malleus, 984, 985f–986f
Malnutrition
    assessment of, 25, 1217
    care coordination for, 1224–1225
    complications of, 1215–1216
    description of, 24
    drug therapy for, 1219
    dysphagia as cause of, 1217b
    eating disorders as cause of, 1216
    health care resources for,
        1224–1225
    health promotion and
        maintenance for, 1216
    history-taking for, 1217
    home care management of, 1224
    inadequate nutrient intake as
        cause of, 1216
    incidence of, 1216
    infection risks associated with,
        414–415
    interventions for, 1217–1224
    laboratory assessment of, 1217
    manifestations of, 1218t
    meal management for, 1218
    nutrition supplements for,
        1218–1219
    in older adults, 40, 1216b
    partial parenteral nutrition for,
        1223–1224
    pathophysiology of, 1215–1216
    physical assessment of, 1217
    prevalence of, 1216
    protein-calorie, 1215
    protein-energy, 1215
    psychosocial assessment of, 1217
    risk assessment for, 1216b
    self-management education for,
        1224
    signs and symptoms of,
        1215–1217

Malnutrition (Continued)
    total enteral nutrition for
        abdominal distention caused by,
            1222
        administration of, 1220–1221,
            1220f
        complications of, 1221–1223
        description of, 1219–1223
        diarrhea secondary to, 1223
        electrolyte imbalances caused
            by, 1222–1223
        enterostomal feeding tubes used
            in, 1220–1221
        fluid imbalances caused by,
            1222–1223
        gastrostomy for, 1221
        jejunostomy for, 1221
        nasoduodenal tube delivery of,
            1220
        nasoenteric tube delivery of,
            1220, 1220f
        nasogastric tube delivery of,
            1220
        nausea and vomiting caused by,
            1222
        refeeding syndrome caused by,
            1221–1222
        tube misplacement and
            dislodgement, 1222
    total parenteral nutrition for,
        1224
    transition management for,
        1224–1225
Malunion, of fracture, 1035
Mammalian target of rapamycin, 405
Mammography, 382, 1435–1436,
    1443, 1446
MammoSite, 1451
Mandibular fractures, 558
Mandibulectomy, 1082
Mannitol, for traumatic brain injury,
    948, 948b
Marasmic-kwashiorkor, 1215
Marasmus, 1215
Marfan syndrome, 334t, 740
Mass casualty event
    acute stress disorder after, 156,
        156b, 158
    definition of, 149–150
    nurse's role in, 155
    post-traumatic stress disorder
        after, 156b
    resolution of, 156–157
    survivors to, psychosocial response
        of, 157–158
    triage for, 151–153, 152t
Massage, 109
Massive hemothorax, 637
Mast cells, 294, 361, 361f, 565
Mastectomy
    breast reconstruction after,
        1449–1450, 1450t, 1451b
    exercises after, 1451b
    lymphedema after, 1454
    modified radical, 1448, 1448f

Mastectomy (Continued)
    postoperative teaching for,
        1453–1454
    prophylactic, 1443–1444
    total, 1448f
Mastication, 1062
Mastoid process, 984, 988
Mastoiditis, 995
Mattress overlays, 97
Maxillary sinus, 509f
Maze procedure, 681
McBurney's point, 1147–1148, 1148f
McGill-Melzack Pain Questionnaire,
    50–52, 51f
MCH. See Mean corpuscular
    hemoglobin
MCV. See Mean corpuscular volume
Meal planning, for diabetes mellitus,
    1300
Mean arterial pressure, 643–644, 752,
    753f, 754, 756
Mean corpuscular hemoglobin,
    803–804
Mean corpuscular volume, 803–804
Mechanical débridement, 457, 457t
Mechanical obstruction, 1122–1123,
    1122f
Mechanical ventilation
    care for patient receiving, 630b
    complications of, 634–635
    dependence on, 635
    indications for, 628
    infections caused by, 635
    modes of, 631
    nursing management of, 632–635
    pain assessments in patients
        receiving, 54
    patient's response to, monitoring
        of, 632–633
    purposes of, 630
    respiratory acidosis and, 192, 195
    upper airway obstruction treated
        with, 561
    ventilators
        controls and settings for, 631–633
        types of, 631, 633
        ventilator-associated events,
            634, 634t
    weaning from, 635, 636t
Mechanically regulated devices, for
    infusion therapy, 211, 212f
Mechanism of injury, 128–129
Medial rectus muscle, 960t
Median nerve, 1057
Mediastinitis, 788–789, 1099
Mediastinoscopy, 524–525
Medical command physician, 154, 154t
Medical emergency team, 8
Medical history, 233–234
Medical nutrition supplements,
    1218–1219
Medical nutrition therapy, for
    diabetes mellitus, 1299–1300
Medical Reserve Corps, 153
Medical-surgical nursing, 1–2

Medicare, 32
Medicare Hospice Benefit, 106
Medication administration records, 201
Medication errors
    in emergency departments, 121
    in older adults, 35
Medication overuse headache, 874
Medication reconciliation
    definition of, 3
    information used for, 3
    nurse-led protocol for, 4b
Medicine wheel, 113f
Medullary carcinoma, 1275
Megaloblastic anemia, 814
Meglitinide analogs, 1291, 1292b–1293b
Melanin, 432
Melanocytes, 432
Melanocyte-stimulating hormone, 1237t, 1254
Melanoma, 376t, 475t, 476, 476f
Melatonin, 923
Melena, 1105, 1108, 1170
Memantine, 864
Memory, 16
    Alzheimer's disease-related impairments in, 860
    assessment of, 847
Memory cells, 297–298, 797t
Ménière's disease, 986–987, 995–996
Meniett device, 996
Meninges, 840
Meningiomas, 951
Meningitis
    aseptic, 881
    care for, 882b
    Cryptococcus neoformans, 881
    definition of, 954
    interventions for, 882–883
    meningococcal, 881
    pathophysiology of, 880–881
    viral, 881
Meningococcal meningitis, 881
Meniscus tear, 1057t
Menopause, 27
Mental status
    age-related changes in, 845
    assessment of, 846–847
    in heat stroke victims, 134
Meperidine, 59b, 61, 1047
Mepilex Ag, 501b
MERS. *See* Middle East respiratory syndrome
Mesalamine, 1152b
Mesenteric artery thrombosis, 16b
MET. *See* Medical emergency team
Metabolic acidosis, 13, 191, 191t, 193–195, 193b, 1122
Metabolic alkalosis, 13, 193b, 196, 196t, 1122
Metabolic syndrome
    clinical features of, 1287
    description of, 771, 772t
    type 2 diabetes mellitus risks, 1287

Metabolic/respiratory acidosis, 192
Metabolism
    burn injury effects on, 486
    chronic kidney disease effects on, 1400–1401, 1400f
    insulin effects on, 1282
    liver's function in, 1064
Metacarpal fractures, 1047
Metacarpophalangeal joint, 1009, 1009f
Metaproterenol, 365
Metastasis. *See also* Cancer
    bloodborne, 375
    brain tumors caused by, 951
    breast cancer, 1440–1441, 1446–1452
    cervical lymph node, 1082
    colorectal cancer, 1127, 1129–1132
    definition of, 375, 384–385
    esophageal cancer, 1095
    head and neck cancer, 548
    lung cancer, 586
    lymphatic spread for, 375
    prostate cancer, 1483–1485
    sites of, 376t, 1440–1441
    steps of, 376f
Metastatic calcifications, 1401
Metered dose inhaler, 568–570, 570b, 570f
Metformin, 1291, 1291b, 1338
Methacholine, 567
Methadone, 61
Methemoglobinemia, 525
Methicillin-resistant *Staphylococcus aureus*
    community-associated, 422
    contact precautions for, 419
    description of, 422
    health care-associated, 422, 422b
    in osteomyelitis, 1023
    prevention of, 468–469, 469b
    skin infections caused by, 466
    stool culture and sensitivity for, 19
Methimazole, 1268b
Methotrexate
    pregnancy contraindications with, 322
    for rheumatoid arthritis, 322
Metronidazole, 1166, 1179
Metyrapone, 1258
Microalbuminuria, 656, 697, 1308, 1335, 1399
Microbiome, 77, 414b
Microcytic, 803–804, 814
Microdiskectomy, for back pain, 906
Microhemagglutination assay, 1509
Microorganisms
    antimicrobial sensitivity testing of, 424
    culture of, 424
Microprocessor ventilators, 631, 631f
Microvascular bone transfers, 1024
Microvascular decompression, 924
Microwave ablation, 1026, 1386
Micturition, 1327

Midarm circumference, 1215
Midarm muscle mass, 1215
MIDCAB. *See* Minimally invasive coronary artery bypass grafting
Mid-clavicular catheter, 205
Middle cerebral artery
    anatomy of, 841
    stroke involving, 933b
Middle ear, 984–985, 985f
Middle East respiratory syndrome, 598
Midline catheters, 204–205, 204f, 213
Midrin, 875
Mifepristone, 1258, 1258b
Miglitol, 1292b–1293b
Migraine headaches
    abortive therapy for, 874–875
    assessment of, 873–874
    atypical, 873–874, 874b
    with aura, 873–874, 874b
    categories of, 873–874
    complementary and integrative health for, 875–876
    definition of, 873
    diagnosis of, 874
    drug therapy for, 874–875
    ergotamine preparations for, 875
    external trigeminal nerve stimulator for, 875
    neuroimaging of, 874
    nortriptyline for, 875
    pathophysiology of, 873
    preventive therapy for, 875
    triggers for, 873, 875, 876b
    triptans for, 874–875, 875b
    without aura, 873–874, 874b
Migratory arthritis, 318–319
Miliary tuberculosis, 605–606
Milrinone, 700, 783b
Mindfulness, 67
Mineralocorticoids, 1237
Mini Nutritional Assessment, 1213, 1214f
Minimally invasive coronary artery bypass grafting, 789
Minimally invasive esophagectomy, 1098
Minimally invasive inguinal hernia repair, 1138–1139, 1139b
Minimally invasive surgery
    back pain treated with, 906, 910
    bariatric surgery using, 1229
    benefits of, 252–254
    brain tumors treated with, 953
    colorectal cancer treated with, 1130, 1132
    description of, 232t, 235, 252–254
    endoscopes used in, 254, 255f
    gastroesophageal reflux disease treated with, 1091
    home care management of, 908
    injuries during, 255
    insufflation in, 254
    intestinal obstruction managed with, 1125

Minimally invasive surgery (Continued)
    nasogastric tubes in, 1125
    pancreatic cancer treated with, 1207
    peptic ulcer disease treated with, 1114
    prostate cancer treated with, 1484
    testicular cancer treated with, 1488
    thymomas treated with, 921
    total hip arthroplasty, 310
    total knee arthroplasty, 314
    urolithiasis treated with, 1364
    Whipple procedure, 1207
Mini-Mental State Examination, 860–861
Miosis, 960, 960f
Mirabegron, 1349
Mistriage, 124
Mitosis, 73–74
Mitoxantrone, 891
Mitraclip, 709
Mitral regurgitation, 706, 706b
Mitral stenosis, 705–706, 706b, 710b
Mitral valve
    anatomy of, 642–643, 643f
    annuloplasty of, 709
    prolapse of, 706
Mitral valvuloplasty, 708
Mixed agonists/antagonists, 57
Mixed aphasia, 938
Mixed conductive-sensorineural hearing loss, 989
Mixed incontinence, 1345t
Mixed urinary incontinence, 1345t, 1352
MMSE. *See* Mini-Mental State Examination
MNA. *See* Mini Nutritional Assessment
Mobility
    assessment of, 23, 94f, 1009–1010
    cane for, 1044
    crutches for, 1043–1044, 1044f
    decreased
        description of, 23–24, 23t
        in older adults, 31–32
        rehabilitation for, 93–96
    definition of, 23
    Guillain-Barré syndrome effects on, 914, 914b, 916
    in multiple sclerosis, 891–892
    musculoskeletal trauma effects on, 1032
    postoperative, 245
    promotion of
        after amputation, 1053–1054
        in burn injury patients, 502–504
        description of, 23–24
        in fracture patients, 1043–1044
        in myasthenia gravis patients, 919

Mobility (Continued)
in osteoarthritis patients, 316
in rheumatoid arthritis patients, 324
scope of, 23
spinal cord injury effects on, 23, 896, 900–901
stroke-related changes in, 933–934, 938
walker for, 1044
Moderate sedation, 261–262, 262t
Modified radical mastectomy, 1448, 1448f
Modified-release opioids, 58–59, 59b
MODS. See Multiple organ dysfunction score
Mohs' surgery, 477
Moist heat, 486
Moniliasis, 1076
Monoamine oxidase type B inhibitors, 870
Monoclonal antibodies
cancer treated with, 402–403
immunosuppression uses of, 302b
mechanism of action, 402–403
skin cancer treated with, 477
ulcerative colitis treated with, 1153
Monoclonal gammopathy of undetermined significance, 830
Monocytes, 797t
Monogenic traits, 74
Monokines, 299
Monounsaturated fatty acids, 1299
Montelukast, 569b–570b
Montgomery straps, 278, 278f, 282
Morbid obesity, 1225
Morbidity, 235
Morphine sulfate
acute coronary syndrome applications of, 775
description of, 59–60
dyspnea treated with, 110
equianalgesic dosing of, 60t
heart failure applications of, 699
postoperative pain management using, 284b
Mortality, 235
Motor aphasia, 938
Motor end plate, 1007
Motor function assessments, 848
Motor neurons, 839–840
Motor vehicle accidents
by older adults, 34, 34b
spinal cord injury caused by, 895
traumatic brain injury caused by, 943. See also Traumatic brain injury
Mourning, 112
MRSA. See Methicillin-resistant Staphylococcus aureus
MSH2 gene, 382

mTOR. See Mammalian target of rapamycin
Mu agonists, 56–57
Mucosa-associated lymphoid tissue lymphoma, 1115
Mucosal barrier fortifiers, 1105, 1106b–1107b, 1112
Mucositis, chemotherapy-related, 399–400, 400b, 588
Mucous fistula, 1132
Mucous membranes, 520, 530–531
Multi-casualty event, 149–152
Multidrug-resistant organism infections
carbapenem-resistant Enterobacteriaceae, 422–423
contact precautions for, 419
methicillin-resistant Staphylococcus aureus, 422
in osteomyelitis, 1023
types of, 421–422
vancomycin-resistant Enterococcus, 422
Multidrug-resistant tuberculosis, 609
Multigated blood pool scanning, 661, 697
Multi-infarct dementia, 37
Multikinase inhibitors, 404t, 405
Multimodal analgesia
continuous, 54
pain managed with, 54–55
Multimodal therapy, for oral cancer, 1080
Multiple endocrine neoplasia, 1246b
Multiple myeloma, 829–830
Multiple organ dysfunction score, 104
Multiple organ dysfunction syndrome, 754–755, 755b, 762
Multiple sclerosis
amyotrophic lateral sclerosis versus, 889t
assessment of, 888–890
care coordination for, 892–894
clinical features of, 889b
cognitive impairment in, 892b
complementary and integrative health for, 892
concept map for, 892f–893f
definition of, 888
diagnostic assessment of, 890, 890f
etiology of, 888
familial patterns of, 888b
health care resources for, 894
history-taking for, 888
home care management of, 892
incidence of, 888
infection prevention in, 890–891
intention tremor associated with, 889
interventions for, 890–891
laboratory assessment of, 890
magnetic resonance imaging of, 890, 890f
mobility interventions in, 891–892

Multiple sclerosis (Continued)
muscle spasticity in, 891
pathophysiology of, 888
plaques associated with, 890, 890f
prevalence of, 888
primary progressive, 888
progressive-relapsing, 888
psychosocial assessment of, 889–890
relapsing-remitting, 888, 890–891
secondary progressive, 888
self-management education for, 892
sexuality affected by, 890, 892
transition management for, 892–894
visual system manifestations of, 889, 892
Murmurs, 654–655
Muromonab-CD3, 302b
Muscarinic-receptor antagonists, 1137
Muscle biopsy, 1013
Muscle enzymes, 1011
Muscle fibers, 1007
Muscle spasticity, 891
Muscle strength, 1011, 1011t
Muscle-specific kinase, 918
Muscular system
anatomy of, 1007
assessment of, 1011
Musculoskeletal disorders
bone tumors. See Bone tumors
foot disorders, 1028–1029, 1028f, 1029t
hand disorders, 1028, 1028f
osteomyelitis, 1022–1024, 1023b, 1023f, 1035
osteoporosis. See Osteoporosis
overview of, 1015
Musculoskeletal system
age-related changes in, 234b, 1007–1008, 1007b
arthroscopy applications for, 1013–1014, 1013f
assessment of, 90t, 91, 803, 1008–1014
biopsies of, 1013, 1013b
bone. See Bone
computed tomography of, 1011
current health problems that affect, 1008–1009
diagnostic assessment of, 1011–1014
electromyography of, 1013
ethnic differences in, 1005t
functional assessments of, 1009–1010
gait assessments, 1009
health promotion and maintenance of, 1007–1008
history-taking, 1008–1009
hypernatremia effects on, 175
hypocalcemia effects on, 180
hypokalemia effects on, 176

Musculoskeletal system (Continued)
imaging assessment of, 1011–1013
inspection of, 1009–1010, 1009f
joints, 1006–1007
laboratory assessment of, 1011, 1012b
magnetic resonance imaging of, 1012–1013, 1013b
mobility assessments, 1009–1010
muscular system
anatomy of, 1007
assessment of, 1011
strength grading, 1011, 1011t
neurovascular assessment of, 1010, 1010b
nuclear scans of, 1011–1012
nutrition history, 1008
overview of, 1004–1005
posture assessments, 1009, 1009f
preoperative assessment of, 236
psychosocial assessment of, 1011
radiography of, 1011
range of motion assessments of, 1010, 1010f
sickle cell disease effects on, 810
skeletal system
anatomy of, 1005–1007, 1005f
assessment of, 1009–1010
bone. See Bone
ultrasonography of, 1013
Musculoskeletal trauma
amputation. See Amputation
carpal tunnel syndrome, 1057–1059, 1058b
description of, 1032
fractures. See Fractures
knee injuries, 1056, 1056b, 1057f, 1057t
mobility affected by, 1032
rotator cuff injuries, 1059
Music therapy, 109, 111
Mutations
gene, 76–77
somatic, 76
Myasthenia gravis
acetylcholine receptors in, 917
assessment of, 917–919
care coordination for, 921–922
cholinesterase inhibitors for, 919–920
clinical features of, 917b
definition of, 917
diagnostic assessment of, 918–919
drug therapy for, 919–921
Eaton-Lambert syndrome, 918
electromyography for, 918
facial expression in, 917–918, 918f
factors that worsen or precipitate, 922t
health care resources for, 922
home care management of, 921–922
immunosuppressants for, 920
interventions for, 919–921

Myasthenia gravis (Continued)
  mobility promotion in, 919
  nonsurgical management of, 919–921
  nutrition in, 921b
  pathophysiology of, 917
  plasmapheresis for, 920–921
  repetitive nerve stimulation for, 918
  respiratory support in, 919
  self-management education of, 922, 922b
  single-fiber electromyography for, 918
  surgical management of, 921
  thymoma associated with, 918
  transition management for, 921–922
Myasthenic crisis, 918–920, 920t
Mycobacterium avium complex, 347
Mycobacterium tuberculosis, 605–606
Mycophenolate
  autoimmune diseases treated with, 368
  immunosuppression uses of, 302b
Mydriasis, 960, 960f
Myelin sheath, 840
Myeloablation, 824
Myelodysplastic syndromes
  hematopoietic stem cell transplantation for, 817
  leukemia. See Leukemia
  in older adults, 817
  pathophysiology of, 817
  risk factors for, 817
Myelosuppression, chemotherapy-induced, 396–398
Myocardial contractility, 645
Myocardial hypertrophy, 694
Myocardial infarction
  anterior wall, 771
  aspirin for, 776–777
  beta blockers for, 777
  cardiac rehabilitation for, 790
  care coordination for, 789–792
  chest discomfort associated with, 650t
  complementary and integrative health after, 791
  coronary artery bypass graft for. See Coronary artery bypass graft
  drug therapy for, 774–778, 776b, 791
  electrocardiographic changes and patterns associated with, 770f
  emergency care for, 774–775
  features of, 773b
  gender and, 772b
  glycoprotein IIb/IIIa inhibitors for, 776
  heart failure after
    classification of, 781–782, 782t
    drug therapy for, 782

Myocardial infarction (Continued)
  hemodynamic monitoring of, 780
    left ventricular, 780–782
    right-ventricular, 782
  home care management of, 789–790, 790b
  imaging assessment of, 773–774
  incidence of, 772
  inferior wall, 771
  interventions for, 774–778
  laboratory assessment of, 773
  lateral wall, 771
  medical assistance indications in, 791–792
  nitroglycerin for, 774
  non–ST-segment elevation, 770
  pathophysiology of, 770
  percutaneous coronary intervention for, 783–784, 784f
  posterior wall, 771
  prevalence of, 772
  psychosocial assessment of, 773
  reperfusion therapy for, 777–778
  risk factor modification for, 790–791
  serum markers of, 655
  sexual activity after, 791
  ST-elevation, 770
  surgical complications caused by, 233
  thrombolytic therapy for, 777–778, 778t
  transition management for, 789–792
Myocardial nuclear perfusion imaging, 661
Myocardium
  coronary artery blood flow to, 643–644
  functions of, 641
Myoclonic seizures, 876
Myoglobin, 492
Myoglobinuria, 258–259
Myomas, 1459–1460
Myopathy, 1008–1009
Myopia, 960, 960f, 980–981
Myosplint, 702
Myotomes, 896
MyPlate, 1211–1212, 1212f
Myringoplasty, 999
Myringotomy, 992–993, 992f
Myxedema, 1265, 1271, 1271f
Myxedema coma, 1271, 1273, 1273b–1274b

N

NAFLD. See Nonalcoholic fatty liver disease
Nails
  age-related changes, 435f
  anatomy of, 432–433, 432f
  assessment of, 441–442, 442f, 442t
  clubbing of, 443t, 652

Nails (Continued)
  consistency of, 441
  dystrophic, 441
  ingrown, 1029t
  lesions of, 441–442
  pigmentation of, 441, 442f
  shape of, 441, 443t
Naloxone, 64b, 284
Naltrexone SR/bupropion SR, 1228
Narcan. See Naloxone
Nasal cannula, 531–532, 532f, 532t, 604
Nasal polyps, 517
Nasoduodenal tube, 1220
Nasoenteric tube, 1220, 1220f
Nasogastric tube
  aspiration risks associated with, 553
  in bariatric surgery patients, 1230b
  complications of, 277
  in esophageal surgery patients, 1100, 1100b
  intestinal obstruction managed with, 1124, 1134b
  postoperative monitoring of, 277
  total enteral nutrition delivery using, 1220
  upper gastrointestinal bleeding managed with, 1113
Nasopharyngeal secretions, 560
Nasopharynx, 509, 509f
Nasoseptoplasty, 557
Natal sex, 1493, 1493t
Natalizumab, 891
Nateglinide, 1292b–1293b
National Comprehensive Cancer Network Distress Thermometer, 395, 395f
National Fire Protection Association, 150
National Institute for Occupational Safety and Health safe patient handling guidelines, 93
National Institute on Aging, 38
National Institutes of Health Stroke Scale, 931, 931t–932t
National Patient Safety Goals
  blood components, 200, 833
  blood donation, 235
  description of, 4–5, 8
  drug safety, 201
  for falls, 40–41, 1018, 1020
  hand-off communication, 120, 317
  hand-off report, 271
  handwashing, 882, 1100
  infection control, 417
  influenza vaccine, 596–597
  informed consent, 658
  nutrition screening, 1212
  patient identification, 247, 262–263, 262b
  preoperative requirements, 238–239

National Patient Safety Goals (Continued)
  pressure injuries, 448–449
  for pressure injuries, 42
  surgical communication, 229
  tracheostomy communication, 544
  transfusion therapy, 833
  warfarin monitoring, 745
Natriuresis, 698
Natriuretic peptides
  B-type, 694, 697
  definition of, 694
  fluid balance regulation by, 166
Natural immunity, 291–292
Natural killer cells, 299, 797t
Natural orifice transluminal endoscopic surgery, 1148, 1153, 1196, 1204
Nausea and vomiting
  chemotherapy-induced, 398–399, 399b
  at end of life, 111
  opioid analgesics as cause of, 63t
  postoperative, 276
  total enteral nutrition as cause of, 1222
Near point of vision, 961
Near vision, 964
Near-drowning, 147
Near-syncope, 650–651
Necitumumab, 589t
Neck
  assessment of, 802
  cancer of. See Head and neck cancer
Neck dissection, 550
Neck veins, 168
Necrotic tissue
  debridement of, in frostbite patients, 145
  description of, 28
Necrotizing hemorrhagic pancreatitis, 1197–1198
Necrotizing otitis, 993
Nedocromil, 569b–570b
Needle biopsy, 1243
Needle thoracostomy, 638
Needleless connection devices, 210–211, 210f, 214
Needlestick injuries, 343
Needlestick Safety and Prevention Act, 210
Negative feedback, 1235–1236, 1236f
Negative nitrogen balance, 1265
Negative-pressure wound therapy, 278, 458, 1160
Neisseria gonorrhoeae, 1512
Neisseria meningitidis, 414
Neobladder, 1368, 1369b
Neodermis, 499
Neovascularization, 1284
Nephrectomy, 1375, 1386

Nephrogenic diabetes insipidus, 1250, 1250b
Nephrolithiasis, 1361
Nephrolithotomy, 1364
Nephrons, 1323, 1323f, 1325t
Nephrosclerosis, 1379
Nephrostomy, 1383
Nephrotic syndrome, 1378–1379, 1379b
Nerve block, 261f, 261t
Nervous system. See also Brain; Neurologic system; Spinal cord
  assessment of, 846–855
  autonomic, 842–844
  cells of, 839–840
  central. See Central nervous system
  complete assessment of, 846–850
  computed tomography–magnetic resonance imaging of, 853–854
  divisions of, 839
  history-taking for, 846
  imaging assessment of, 851–855
  laboratory assessment of, 851
  magnetic resonance imaging of, 853
  peripheral, 842
  physical assessment of, 846–850
  psychosocial assessment of, 850–851
  rapid/focused assessment of, 850
Nesiritide, 698, 698b
Neuritic plaques, 858, 859f
Neurofibrillary tangles, 858, 859f
Neurogenic bladder, 98t
Neurogenic bowel, 99t
Neurogenic diabetes insipidus, 1250
Neurogenic pulmonary edema, 954
Neurogenic shock, 898
Neuroglia cells, 840
Neurohypophysis, 1236, 1237f
Neurokinin receptor antagonists, for chemotherapy-induced nausea and vomiting, 399b
Neurologic disorders
  Alzheimer's disease. See Alzheimer's disease
  encephalitis, 883–884, 884b
  meningitis. See Meningitis
  migraine headaches. See Migraine headaches
  Parkinson disease. See Parkinson disease
  seizures. See Seizures
Neurologic system. See also Nervous system
  age-related changes in, 234b, 844–845, 845b
  assessment of, 90t, 91, 846–855
  auditory evoked potentials of, 855
  cerebral angiography evaluations of, 852–853, 852b
  complete assessment of, 846–850
  computed tomography of, 853

Neurologic system (Continued)
  computed tomography–magnetic resonance imaging of, 853–854
  dehydration effects on, 168–169
  electroencephalography of, 854
  electromyography of, 854
  evoked potentials of, 854–855
  health promotion and maintenance of, 845–846
  imaging assessment of, 851–855
  laboratory assessment of, 851
  lumbar puncture of, 855
  magnetic resonance imaging of, 853
  magnetoencephalography of, 854
  postoperative assessment of, 274–275, 274t
  psychosocial assessment of, 850–851
  rapid/focused assessment of, 850
  single-photon emission computed tomography of, 854
  somatosensory evoked potentials of, 855
  transcranial Doppler ultrasonography of, 855
  visual evoked potentials of, 855
  x-rays of, 851
Neuroma
  acoustic, 951, 996
  definition of, 1050
Neuromodulation therapy, 1349
Neuromuscular blocking agents, 258
Neuromuscular system
  acidosis effects on, 193, 193b
  alkalosis effects on, 196, 196b
  hypercalcemia effects on, 181
  hyperkalemia effects on, 178
  hypocalcemia effects on, 180
  hypomagnesemia effects on, 182
  hyponatremia-related changes, 174
Neuron
  afferent, 840
  efferent, 840
  functions of, 839–840
  motor, 839–840
  sensory, 839–840
  structure of, 839–840, 840f
  synapse in, 840
Neurontin. See Gabapentin
Neuropathic pain, 48, 48t, 1307
Neuropathy, 1008–1009
Neurotransmitters
  definition of, 840
  in Parkinson disease, 868
Neutropenia
  chemotherapy-induced, 395, 396b
  definition of, 817
Neutrophilia, 295
Neutrophils
  functions of, 293, 797t
  in inflammation, 292–293, 292t

New York Heart Association Functional Classification, 651, 651t
New-onset angina, 770
Nicotine replacement therapies, 514–515
Nifedipine, 146
NIOSH. See National Institute for Occupational Safety and Health
Nitrates
  acute coronary syndromes treated with, 776b, 783b
  heart failure treated with, 699
Nitrites, 1335
Nitrofurazone, 501b
Nitroglycerin
  for angina pectoris, 774–775
  drug interactions for, 775b
  for myocardial infarction, 783b
  sublingual, 791b
Nitroprusside sodium, 783b
Nivolumab, 477, 589t
NMDA receptor antagonists, 864
NNRTIs. See Non-nucleoside reverse transcriptase inhibitors
Nociception
  processes of, 47–48, 49f
  schematic diagram of, 49f
Nociceptive pain, 47–48, 48t
Nociceptors, 47, 873
Nocturia, 41, 91, 236, 1328b, 1330, 1381, 1474, 1482
Nocturnal polyuria, 1328
Nodes of Ranvier, 840
Nodules, 438f
Nonabsorbable sutures, 267
Nonalcoholic fatty liver disease, 1172, 1185–1186
Nonalcoholic steatohepatitis, 1185
Noncommunicating hydrocephalus, 943
Noncompliance, 423
Non-Hodgkin's lymphoma, 828–829
Noninfectious cystitis, 1356
Noninsulin-dependent diabetes mellitus. See Diabetes mellitus, type 2
Noninvasive positive-pressure ventilation
  description of, 535, 535b, 536f
  obstructive sleep apnea treated with, 535, 559
Nonmaleficence, 9
Nonmechanical obstruction, 1122–1123
Non-nucleoside reverse transcriptase inhibitors
  mechanism of action, 338
  types of, 351b–352b
Nonrebreather masks, 532t, 533, 533f
Non-self cells, 380
Non-self proteins, 289–290, 290f
Nonseminomas, 1487

Nonsteroidal anti-inflammatory drugs
  adverse effects of, 56, 56b
  cardiovascular risks, 791b
  carpal tunnel syndrome managed with, 1058
  fibromyalgia managed with, 334
  gastritis caused by, 1104–1105
  in older adults, 56b
  pain management uses of, 55–56, 56b, 284b, 307–308, 1364
  peptic ulcer disease caused by, 1109
  postoperative pain management using, 284b
  rheumatoid arthritis managed with, 321
  topical, 308
Non–ST-segment elevation myocardial infarction, 770
Nonsustained ventricular tachycardia, 683
Nontunneled percutaneous central venous catheters, 206–207, 206f, 215
Nonunion, of fracture, 1035, 1043
Nonurgent triage, 124
Norco. See Hydrocodone
Norepinephrine, 1238
Normal sinus rhythm, 671, 671f
Normotonic fluids, 163
Norovirus, 1148t, 1149
Nortriptyline, for migraine headaches, 875
Nose
  anatomy of, 509, 509f
  assessment of, 517
  cancer of, 556
  epistaxis of, 557–558, 557b, 558f
  fractures of, 556–557, 556f
Novel oral anticoagulants
  clinical uses of, 680, 708, 710
  deep vein thrombosis treated with, 745
Novelty diets, 1228
NPO status, 241
NPPV. See Noninvasive positive-pressure ventilation
NPSGs. See National Patient Safety Goals
NPWT. See Negative-pressure wound therapy
NRS. See Numeric rating scale
NRTIs. see Nucleoside reverse transcriptase inhibitors
Nuclear, biologic, and chemical threats, 150
Nuclear scans
  gastrointestinal bleeding evaluations using, 1111
  musculoskeletal system evaluations using, 1011–1012
Nuclear-to-cytoplasmic ratio, 373–374

Nucleic acid amplification test, 347, 1513

Nucleoside reverse transcriptase inhibitors
  mechanism of action, 338
  types of, 351*b*–352*b*

Nucynta. *See* Tapentadol

Numeric rating scale, 50

Nurse
  emergency. *See* Emergency
  health care facility emergency preparedness role of, 154–156
  perioperative, 229
  postanesthesia care unit, 271
  registered, 123–124, 253*t*
  rehabilitation, 88, 88*t*

Nursing assistants, 88

Nursing technicians, 88

Nutrition. *See also* Diet
  in acute pancreatitis, 1201
  for acute respiratory distress syndrome, 628
  age-related changes in, 31
  in cholecystitis, 1194
  in chronic kidney disease, 1407–1408, 1407*t*
  clotting affected by, 802
  decreased
    description of, 23*t*, 24–25
    in older adults, 30–31
  definition of, 24
  ethnic preferences, 1212*b*
  gastrectomy effects on, 1118
  gout treated with, 332
  head and neck cancer effects on, 552
  for health promotion and maintenance, 1211–1212
  Healthy People 2020 objectives for, 1226*t*
  in hepatitis, 1184
  in human immunodeficiency virus infection, 354
  laboratory testing for, 25
  malabsorption managed with, 1142
  in myasthenia gravis, 921*b*
  in older adults, 1219*b*
  preoperative assessment of, 236–237
  promotion of, 25, 1219*b*
  scope of, 24
  socioeconomic influences on, 1065–1066
  in tracheostomy, 543
  in tuberculosis, 610
  in wound healing, 97, 287

Nutrition assessment
  anthropometric measurements, 1213–1215
  before rehabilitation, 90–91, 90*t*
  body mass index, 1215, 1215*b*
  description of, 25
  nutrition screening, 1212–1213
  nutrition status, 1212, 1213*b*

Nutrition history
  cardiovascular system, 648–649
  description of, 1227, 1240
  gastrointestinal system, 1065–1066
  musculoskeletal system, 1008
  renal system, 1329
  reproductive system, 1432
  vision, 962–963

Nutrition screening
  description of, 1212–1213, 1213*b*
  for older adults, 31*b*

Nutrition status
  definition of, 1212
  evaluation of, 1212
  pressure injuries and, 449–451

Nutrition supplements, 1218–1219

Nutrition therapy. *See also* Total enteral nutrition; Total parenteral nutrition
  acute kidney injury treated with, 1396–1397
  atherosclerosis treated with, 730
  cirrhosis managed with, 1175, 1178
  Crohn's disease treated with, 1159–1160
  Cushing's disease treated with, 1258
  esophageal tumors treated with, 1097
  fluid overload treated with, 172
  gastroesophageal reflux disease treated with, 1090
  heart failure treated with, 698–699, 705
  hyperkalemia treated with, 179*b*
  hypernatremia treated with, 175
  hypocalcemia treated with, 181
  hypoglycemia treated with, 1310–1311
  hypokalemia treated with, 177
  hyponatremia treated with, 174
  leukemia treated with, 825–826
  obesity treated with, 1228
  osteoporosis treated with, 1020
  peptic ulcer disease managed with, 1112
  pressure injury wound healing through, 458
  ulcerative colitis managed with, 1153
  urinary incontinence treated with, 1348

Nutritionally balanced diet, 1228

Nystagmus
  description of, 934, 964, 996
  electronystagmography of, 991

O

Obesity
  assessment of, 1227
  bariatric surgery for, 1229–1231
  behavioral management of, 1229
  body fat distribution in, 1225
  care coordination for, 1231

Obesity (*Continued*)
  complementary and integrative health for, 1229
  complications of, 1225, 1225*t*
  definition of, 648, 1225
  diet programs for, 1227–1228
  dietary causes of, 1225–1226
  drug therapy for, 1228–1229
  drugs that cause, 1226
  etiology of, 1225–1226
  exercise for, 1228
  familial factors, 1226*b*
  gastric bypass for, 1229, 1230*f*
  gastroesophageal reflux disease risks, 1090
  genetic risk of, 1225–1226, 1226*b*
  health care resources for, 1231
  history-taking, 1227
  home care management of, 1231
  insulin resistance caused by, 1286–1287
  interventions for, 25
  laparoscopic adjustable gastric band for, 1229, 1230*f*
  malnutrition associated with, 236–237
  morbid, 1225
  nonsurgical management of, 1227–1229
  nutrition history for, 1227
  nutrition therapy for, 1228
  obstructive sleep apnea risks, 236
  overweight versus, 1225
  pathophysiology of, 1225–1226
  physical assessment of, 1227
  physical inactivity as cause of, 1226
  prevalence of, 1225
  Roux-en-Y gastric bypass for, 1229, 1230*f*
  self-management education for, 1231
  signs and symptoms of, 1227
  surgical management of, 1229–1231, 1230*f*, 1231*b*
  sympathomimetic drugs for, 1228–1229
  transition management for, 1231
  wound healing affected by, 236–237

Obligatory solute excretion, 1336

Obligatory urine output, 165

Obstipation, 18, 1123

Obstructive jaundice, 1192

Obstructive sleep apnea
  assessment of, 559
  interventions for, 559
  noninvasive positive-pressure ventilation for, 535, 559
  in obese patients, 236
  pathophysiology of, 559

Occipital lobe, 841*t*

Occupational Safety and Health Administration, 423

Occupational therapists, 89, 93

Occupational therapy assistants, 89

Octreotide, 1118, 1177, 1248–1249, 1311

Ocular trauma, 981–982

Oculomotor nerve, 844*t*, 847–848

Odynophagia, 1089, 1096

Off-pump coronary artery bypass, 789

OGTT. *See* Oral glucose tolerance testing

Older adults. *See also* Aging
  abuse of, 39, 39*t*
  acute kidney injury in, 1394*b*
  acute pancreatitis in, 1199
  adjuvant analgesics in, 64*b*
  adverse drug events in, 35*t*
  anemia in, 803
  brain in, 858
  burn injury in, 490*b*
  cancer in, 380*b*
  candidiasis in, 1076*b*
  cardiac changes in, 222–223
  cardiovascular system in, 647*b*
  cerumen impaction in, 995*b*
  chronic respiratory disorder in, 564*b*
  in community-based settings, 30–39
  constipation in, 31
  coping by, 32–33
  coronary artery bypass grafting in, 790*b*
  dehydration in, 167*b*, 1194*b*
  diabetic retinopathy in, 1284*b*
  diverticulitis in, 1164*b*
  driving safety for, 34, 34*b*
  drugs in
    adverse drug events, 35*t*
    age-related changes, 34
    assessment of, 35, 36*b*
    self-administration of, 35, 35*f*
    use and misuse of, 34–35, 35*f*, 35*t*
  dysrhythmias in, 682*b*
  electrolyte imbalances in, 173*b*
  electrolyte levels in, 165*b*
  emergency department care for, 118*b*
  endocrine system in, 1240, 1241*b*
  exercise for, 31–32, 32*f*
  fecal impaction in, 1126*b*
  fluid restriction by, 31*b*
  fractures in, 1047–1048, 1047*b*
  gastroesophageal reflux disease in, 1089*b*
  gastrointestinal system in, 1064*b*
  glomerular filtration rate in, 1328*b*
  health care for, 32
  health care-associated methicillin-resistant *Staphylococcus aureus* in, 422*b*
  health issues for
    abuse, 39, 39*t*
    accidents, 33–34
    alcoholism, 38

Older adults (*Continued*)
  cognition-related, 35–38
  in community-based settings, 30–39
  confusion, 40–42
  delirium, 38
  dementia, 37
  depression, 36–37, 37*f*
  drug use and misuse, 34–35, 35*f*, 35*t*
  falls, 33, 33*b*, 40–42
  in hospitals, 39–42
  hydration-related, 30–31
  in long-term care settings, 39–42
  loss, 32–33
  malnutrition, 40
  mobility-related, 31–32
  neglect, 39, 39*t*
  nutrition-related, 30–31
  pressure injuries, 42
  sleep disorders, 40
  stress, 32–33
  substance use, 38–39
  heart failure in, 694*b*
  Helicobacter pylori in, 1111*b*
  hematologic system in, 800*b*
  hip fractures in, 1047–1048, 1047*b*
  Hispanic, 39*b*
  history-taking in, 122*b*
  homelessness in, 30
  in hospitals, 39–42
  hydration in, 30–31
  hyperglycemic-hyperosmolar state in, 1300*b*, 1314*b*
  hypoglycemia in, 1309, 1312*b*
  incontinence in, 31
  iron deficiency anemia in, 815*b*
  kidneys in, 1328*b*
  living arrangements for, 30
  loneliness in, 31
  in long-term care settings
    care coordination and transition management for, 42
    health issues for, 39–42
  malnutrition in, 1216*b*
  meal management in, 1219*b*
  motor vehicle accidents by, 34, 34*b*
  musculoskeletal system in, 1007*b*
  myelodysplastic syndromes in, 817
  neglect of, 39, 39*t*
  nutrition in, 30–31, 1219*b*
  nutritional screening for, 31*b*
  opioid analgesics in, 64*b*, 279*b*
  oral cancer in, 1082*b*
  oral candidiasis in, 1076*b*
  orthostatic hypotension in, 134*b*
  overview of, 30
  pain in, 52*b*, 56*b*, 59*b*
  patient-controlled analgesia in, 284*b*
  peritonitis in, 1163*b*
  physical activity by, 31–32, 32*f*
  pneumonia in, 603*b*
  population growth of, 29
  preoperative care of, 236*b*

Older adults (*Continued*)
  protein-energy malnutrition in, 1216*b*
  in rehabilitation settings, 90*b*
  relocation stress syndrome in, 30–31, 33*b*
  renal changes in, 222–223
  renal system in, 1328*b*
  reproductive system in, 1431*b*
  sensory changes in, 844
  sexually transmitted infections in, 1505*b*
  special needs of, 10
  subgroups of, 30
  surgery in, 232
  thyroid disorders in, 1274*b*
  transfusion in, 834*b*
  transgender, 1497*b*
  traumatic brain injury in, 944*b*
  tricyclic antidepressants in, 37*b*
  urinary incontinence in, 1344*b*
  urinary tract infections in, 91
  vision impairments in, 963*b*
  water intake by, 1212*b*
  wellness promotion in, 30*b*
  wound infection in, 954
Olfactory nerve, 844*t*
Oligomenorrhea, 1256
Oligospermia, 1487–1488
Oliguria, 18, 236, 1362, 1392, 1423
Onabotulinumtoxin A, 875, 1349
Oncofetal antigens, 1068
Oncogenes, 378–379, 380*b*
Oncogenesis, 375
Oncologic emergencies
  description of, 385, 407–410
  disseminated intravascular coagulation, 407
  hypercalcemia, 408
  sepsis, 407
  spinal cord compression, 408
  superior vena cava syndrome, 408–409, 409*f*
  syndrome of inappropriate antidiuretic hormone, 407–408
  tumor lysis syndrome, 409–410, 409*f*
Oncoviruses, 379
On-Q PainBuster, 211, 212*f*
Onycholysis, 441–442
Oophorectomy, 1444–1445
Open fracture, 1032, 1032*f*
Open reduction and internal fixation, 1042–1043, 1042*f*, 1047–1048
Open reduction with internal fixation, 558
Open thoracotomy, 638
Operating rooms
  fire safety in, 252
  layout of, 252
  occupational hazards in, 252
  safety in, 252
  surgical attire in, 256, 256*f*

Ophthalmic artery, 959
Ophthalmic ointment, 961*b*, 970
Ophthalmoscopy, 966, 966*f*
Opioid analgesics
  addiction to, 58
  administration of, 57–58
  adverse effects of, 62–63, 63*t*
  age considerations in dosing of, 58*b*
  in chronic kidney disease patients, 1409
  chronic pain managed with, 225
  classification of, 56–57
  complications of, 284
  constipation caused by, 1147
  controlled release, 58–59
  description of, 55–56
  dosing of, 57, 59
  drug formulation terminology for, 58–59
  dual mechanism, 61
  dyspnea treated with, 110
  in end-of-life patients, 108–109
  epidural delivery of, 61, 61*f*, 225
  equianalgesia for, 58, 60*t*
  fast acting, 58
  fentanyl, 60, 60*t*
  general anesthesia use of, 258
  in human immunodeficiency virus infection, 354
  hydrocodone, 60, 60*t*
  hydromorphone, 60, 60*t*
  immediate release, 58
  intraspinal delivery of, 61–62
  intrathecal delivery of, 61–62, 62*b*
  lipophilicity of, 60
  mechanism of action, 56–57
  methadone, 61
  mixed agonists/antagonists, 57
  modified release, 58–59, 59*b*
  morphine, 59–60, 60*t*
  mu agonists, 56–57
  in older adults, 279*b*
  overdose of, 285*b*
  oxycodone, 60, 60*t*
  partial agonists, 57
  phantom limb pain managed with, 1053
  physical dependence on, 58
  postoperative ileus caused by, 286
  postoperative pain management using, 283–284, 284*b*
  respiratory depression caused by, 62–63, 63*t*, 64*b*, 524*b*
  sedation caused by, 62–63, 63*t*–64*t*
  short acting, 58
  side effects of, 63*t*, 64*b*
  sustained release, 58–59
  tapentadol, 61
  titration of, 57
  tolerance to, 58
  tramadol, 61
  types to avoid, 61
Opioid antagonists, 57, 64*b*, 284
Opioid naïve, 58

Opioid tolerant, 58
Opportunistic infections
  description of, 339, 346–347, 347*f*
  prevention of, 350–353
Oprelvekin, 398, 402*t*
Opsonins, 294
Optic disc, 958
Optic fundus, 958
Optic nerve
  description of, 844*t*
  ultrasonic imaging of, 967
Oral cancer
  assessment of, 1079–1080
  basal cell carcinoma, 1079
  brachytherapy for, 1081
  care coordination for, 1083–1084
  chemotherapy for, 1080–1081
  cryotherapy for, 1081
  features of, 1080*b*
  genetic mutations in, 1079*b*
  health care resources for, 1084
  home care management of, 1083, 1083*b*
  interventions for, 1080–1083
  multimodal therapy for, 1080
  nonsurgical management of, 1080–1081
  in older adults, 1082*b*
  pathophysiology of, 1079
  prevention of, 1079
  radiation therapy for, 1081
  self-management education for, 1083, 1083*b*
  squamous cell carcinomas, 1079
  surgical management of, 1081–1083
  targeted therapy for, 1081
  taste changes after, 1083
  transition management for, 1083–1084
Oral candidiasis, 1076–1077, 1076*b*
Oral cavity
  anatomy of, 1062, 1075–1076
  examination of, 1080
  health of, 1076*b*
  masticatory function of, 1062
  teeth, 1062
Oral cavity disorders
  erythroplakia, 1079
  high-risk patients for, 1075–1076
  leukoplakia, 1078–1079
  oral cancer. *See* Oral cancer
  oral tumors, 1078–1084
  stomatitis, 1076–1078
Oral glucose tolerance testing, 1289
Oral hairy leukoplakia, 1078
Oral hygiene
  mucositis managed with, 400
  in oral cancer patients, 1080–1081
  routine for, 1080–1081
  in tracheostomy, 543
Oral rehydration solutions
  dehydration treated with, 170
  gastroenteritis treated with, 1149
Oral tumors, 1078–1084

OralCDx, 1080
Orbit, 957
Orchiectomy
    in male-to-female gender
        reassignment surgery, 1499
    testicular cancer treated with,
        1488–1489
Orchitis, 1431
Orencia. *See* Abatacept
Orexins, 1225
Organ of Corti, 986
Organizational ethics, 9
Orientation, assessment of, 846–847
ORIF. *See* Open reduction and
    internal fixation
Orlistat, 1228
Oropharynx, 509, 509f
Ortho checks, 168
Orthopedic boots/shoes, 1038,
    1038f
Orthopnea, 517, 574, 576f, 625,
    649–650, 695
Orthostatic hypotension, 121, 134b,
    168, 174–175, 652, 723, 726b,
    901, 1285
Oseltamivir, 597–598
OSHA. *See* Occupational Safety and
    Health Administration
Osmolality, 163
Osmolarity
    blood, 1332
    description of, 163, 1222–1223
    urine, 1336
Osmoreceptors, 164
Osmosis, 163–164, 163f, 1412
Ossiculoplasty, 999
Osteoarthritis
    care coordination for, 316–317
    clinical features of, 306t
    definition of, 305
    etiology of, 305
    exercises for, 317b
    gender differences in, 305b
    genetic risk of, 305
    health care resources for, 317
    health promotion and
        maintenance for, 305–306
    history-taking, 306
    home care management of, 317
    incidence of, 305
    joint changes in, 305f
    joint effusions associated with,
        306–307
    laboratory assessment of, 307
    mobility improvements in, 316
    pain management in
        complementary and integrative
            health for, 308–309
        drugs for, 307–308
        hyaluronic acid for, 308
        nonpharmacologic
            interventions, 308
        nonsteroidal anti-inflammatory
            drugs, 307–308
    surgical options for, 309–316

Osteoarthritis (*Continued*)
    pathophysiology of, 305–306,
        1007
    physical assessment of, 306–307,
        306f
    physical therapy for, 316
    prevalence of, 305
    primary, 305
    psychosocial assessment of, 307
    rheumatoid arthritis versus, 306t
    secondary, 305
    self-management education for,
        317, 317b
    signs and symptoms of, 306–307,
        306f
    spinal involvement by, 307
    total hip arthroplasty for
        anesthesia used in, 310
        complications of, 311t, 312–313
        components of, 310–311, 310f
        hip dislocation after, 311–312
        hip resurfacing versus, 310
        low-molecular-weight heparin
            uses, 312
        minimally invasive, 310
        mobility after, 313–314, 313f
        operative procedures, 310–311
        pain management after, 312b,
            313
        patient positioning after, 311,
            313f
        postoperative care, 311–314,
            311b
        preoperative care, 309–310
        primary, 309
        quadriceps-setting exercises
            after, 312–313
        rehabilitation, 314
        revision, 309
        self-management education,
            312b, 314
        venous thromboembolism risks
            after, 310, 312–313
        weight-bearing restrictions,
            313–314
    total joint arthroplasty for, 309
    total knee arthroplasty for
        complications of, 316
        continuous passive motion
            machine, 315, 315f, 316b
        cryotherapy after, 315
        description of, 314–316
        discharge instructions, 316
        minimally invasive, 314
        operative procedures, 315
        pain management after,
            315–316
        postoperative care, 315–316,
            315f
        preoperative care, 314–315
        rehabilitation after, 316
    total shoulder arthroplasty for,
        316
    transition management for,
        316–317

Osteoblasts, 1005
Osteochondroma, 1024
Osteoclasts, 1005
Osteocytes, 1005
Osteomalacia
    definition of, 1016
    osteoporosis versus, 1016t
Osteomyelitis, 1022–1024, 1023b,
    1023f, 1035
Osteonecrosis
    bone healing affected by, 1032
    of jaw, bisphosphonate-related,
        1021
    in systemic lupus erythematosus,
        327
Osteopenia, 1007, 1016
Osteoporosis
    assessment of, 1018–1020
    bisphosphonates for, 1021, 1021b
    bone turnover markers in, 1019,
        1019t
    calcium intake for, 1020–1021,
        1021b
    care coordination for, 1022
    computed tomography-based
        absorptiometry of, 1019
    in Crohn's disease patients, 1151t
    definition of, 1007, 1015–1016
    denosumab for, 1021
    description of, 24–25
    dietary supplements for,
        1020–1021, 1021b
    dowager's hump associated with,
        1018, 1018f
    drug therapy for, 1020–1022
    dual x-ray absorptiometry of,
        1019
    estrogen agonists/antagonists for,
        1021, 1021b
    etiology of, 1016–1017
    fallophobia risks, 33
    falls secondary to, 1020
    fractures caused by, 1016, 1018,
        1047
    generalized, 1016
    genetic risk of, 1016–1017, 1017b
    growth hormone deficiency as
        cause of, 1246
    health care resources for, 1022
    health promotion and
        maintenance for, 1017–1018
    hip fracture risks associated with,
        1047
    home care management of, 1022
    imaging assessment of, 1019–1020
    immune factors in, 1017b
    incidence of, 1017
    interventions for, 1020–1022
    laboratory assessment of, 1019,
        1019t
    lifestyle changes for, 1020
    magnetic resonance imaging of,
        1019
    magnetic resonance spectroscopy
        of, 1019

Osteoporosis (*Continued*)
    nutrition therapy for, 1020
    osteomalacia versus, 1016t
    pathophysiology of, 1016–1017
    physical assessment of, 1018–1019,
        1018f
    prevalence of, 1017
    prevention of, 1018
    primary, 1017b
    psychosocial assessment of, 1019
    regional, 1016
    risk factors for, 1017b
    salmon calcitonin for, 1022
    secondary, 1016
    self-management education for,
        1022
    teriparatide for, 1022
    transition management for, 1022
    vertebral imaging of, 1019
    vitamin D$_3$ for, 1020–1021
Osteosarcoma, 1012, 1025
Osteotomy, 1028–1029
Ostomate, 1153
Ostomy, 1154
Otezla. *See* Apremilast
Otitis media, 991–993, 992f, 1023b
Otorrhea, 880–881
Otosclerosis, 986–987, 996–997
Otoscope, 988, 989f
Otoscopic examination
    description of, 988–989, 989f,
        998
    otitis media on, 992f
    tympanic membrane perforation
        on, 992f
Outpatient surgery, 229–230
Ova and parasites testing, 1068–1070
Ovarian cancer, 1467–1469, 1467t
Ovaries
    anatomy of, 1429, 1429f
    hormones produced by, 1235t
Overactive bladder, 97–98, 1344,
    1349
Overflow incontinence, 1344, 1345t,
    1351–1352
Overhydration. *See* Fluid overload
Overweight, 648, 1225
Ovoid pupil, 946
Oxybutynin, 98
Oxycodone
    equianalgesic dosing of, 60t
    pain management uses of, 60, 60t
    postoperative pain management
        using, 284b
Oxygen
    humidified, 531, 531f
    liquid, 536–537, 537f
    tissue delivery of, 512
Oxygen concentrator, 537
Oxygen tanks, 536, 536f
Oxygen therapy
    absorptive atelectasis caused by,
        530, 531b
    acute respiratory failure treated
        with, 626

Oxygen therapy (Continued)
  asthma treated with, 571
  burn injury treated with, 494
  care coordination for, 536–537
  chronic obstructive pulmonary
      disease treated with, 578
  combustion caused by, 530
  complications of, 530–531
  delivery systems for
      description of, 531–536
      face tent, 534–535, 534t
      facemasks, 532–533, 532t, 533f,
          604
      high-flow, 533–535, 534t
      low-flow, 531–533, 532f, 532t
      nasal cannula, 531–532, 532f,
          532t, 604
      T-piece, 534–535, 534t, 535f
      Venturi masks, 533–534, 534f,
          534t
  dyspnea treated with, 110
  hazards of, 530–531
  home care management of, 536
  home care preparation for,
      536–537, 536f
  humidified oxygen, 531, 531f
  hypoventilation caused by, 530
  hypoxemia treated with, 626, 775
  indications for, 529
  infection risks, 531
  mucous membrane drying caused
      by, 530–531
  noninvasive positive-pressure
      ventilation, 535, 535b, 536f
  overview of, 529
  patient safety in, 530b
  in pneumonia, 604
  postoperative, 280–281
  purpose of, 529
  respiratory acidosis treated with,
      195
  safety in, 530b
  self-management education for,
      536
  septic shock managed with,
      765
  toxicity caused by, 530
  transition management for,
      536–537
  transtracheal, 536
Oxygen toxicity, 530
Oxygenation, in burn injury
    patients, 493–497
Oxygen-hemoglobin dissociation
    curve, 512, 512f
Oxymorphone, 60t
Oxytocin, 1237t

P
P wave, 667
Pacemaker, permanent, 675, 675f,
    676b
Pacing
  asynchronous, 675
  biventricular, 681

Pacing (Continued)
  sinus bradycardia treated with,
      674–675
  synchronous, 675
  temporary, 674–675
  transcutaneous, 674, 674f
Packed red blood cells, 200
Pack-years, 514
PACU. See Postanesthesia care unit
Pain
  abdominal. See Abdominal pain
  acute, 46–47, 46t, 52
  amputation-related, 1051, 1053
  back. See Back pain
  breakthrough, 54–55
  cancer
      chronic, 47
      intrathecal pump for, 62b
      self-management education for,
          68
  categorization of, 46–48
  chronic
      description of, 46–47
      epidural infusion for, 225
      in older adults, 56b
      psychosocial factors that affect,
          52
      self-management education for,
          68
  definition of, 46
  drug therapy for. See Pain
      management
  duodenal ulcers as cause of, 1110
  duration-based categorization of,
      46–47
  extremity, 651
  gastric ulcers as cause of, 1110
  inadequate management of, 46
  intestinal obstruction-related,
      1123
  irritable bowel syndrome as cause
      of, 1136
  localized, 50
  low back. See Back pain
  mechanism-based categorization
      of, 46–48
  modulation of, 48, 49f
  neuropathic, 48, 48t, 1307
  nociceptive, 47–48, 48t
  in older adults, 52b, 59b
  overview of, 45–68
  perception of, 48, 49f
  persistent, 46–47
  phantom limb, 1051, 1053
  professional organizations for, 46
  projected, 50
  psychosocial factors, 52–53
  radiating, 50
  rectal, 1164
  referred, 50
  scope of problem, 45–46
  self-reports of, 48
  somatic, 48
  surgery-related, 47
  transduction of, 47, 49f

Pain (Continued)
  transmission of, 47–48, 49f
  treatment of. See Pain
      management
  unrelieved, impact of, 46, 46t
  visceral, 48
Pain assessment
  challenges for, 53–54
  components of, 50–52
  in delirium, 53–54, 53t
  in dementia, 53–54, 53t
  description of, 1008
  Hierarchy of Pain Measures, 53,
      53t
  locations of pain, 50–52, 51f
  McGill-Melzack Pain
      Questionnaire for, 50–52, 51f
  in mechanically ventilated
      patients, 54
  in older adults, 59b
  overview of, 49–50
  postoperative, 278
  psychosocial assessments as part
      of, 52–53
Pain Assessment in Advanced
    Dementia scale, 54
Pain management
  in acute pancreatitis, 1199–1201
  analgesics for
      acetaminophen, 55
      adjuvant, 55, 63–65
      anticonvulsants as, 63–64
      antidepressants as, 63–64
      around-the-clock dosing of,
          54–55, 59b
      local anesthetics as, 64–65
      nonopioid, 55–56
      nonsteroidal anti-inflammatory
          drugs, 55–56, 56b, 284b,
          1364
      opioid. See Opioid analgesics
      routes of administration, 54
  in bone tumors, 1027–1028
  in burn injury, 491
  care coordination and transition
      management, 67–68
  in cholecystitis, 1194–1197
  after coronary artery bypass
      grafting, 788
  during dying, 108–109
  in fractures, 1037–1043
  in head and neck cancer, 551–552
  health care resources for, 68
  home care management in, 67
  in human immunodeficiency
      virus infection, 353–354
  in lung cancer, 593
  multimodal analgesia, 54–55
  nonpharmacologic
      cognitive-behavioral therapy,
          66–67
      complementary and alternative
          therapies, 109, 285, 496
      cryotherapy, 66
      description of, 65

Pain management (Continued)
  interventions for, 65
  physical modalities, 65–66
  spinal cord stimulation, 66
  tactile stimulation, 496
  transcutaneous electrical nerve
      stimulation, 66, 66f
  in older adults, 59b
  after oral cancer surgery, 1083
  patient-controlled analgesia, 55, 497
  in peritonitis, 1146
  placebos for, 65, 65b
  in polycystic kidney disease, 1382
  postoperative, 283–285,
      284b–285b
  preemptive analgesia, 54
  in pyelonephritis, 1375
  referrals in, 68
  regional anesthesia for, 65
  in rheumatoid arthritis, 321–324
  self-management education as
      part of, 68
  in sickle cell disease, 811–812
  total hip arthroplasty-related,
      312b, 313
  total knee arthroplasty-related,
      315–316
  in ulcerative colitis, 1155–1156,
      1156b
  in urolithiasis, 1363–1365
Pain perception assessments, 849
Pain rating scales, 50–52, 50t, 52f
Pain resource nurse programs, 45
PAINAD scale. See Pain Assessment
    in Advanced Dementia scale
Palatine tonsils, 509
Palliation, 106
Palliative care
  description of, 106, 107t, 113
  in lung cancer, 593
  for Parkinson disease, 873
Palliative surgery, 386
Pallor, 443, 651, 802b
Palmoplantar pustulosis, 464
Palpation
  of chest, 518–519
  of gastrointestinal system,
      1067–1068
  of kidneys, 1330–1331, 1331f
  of skin, 440–441, 440t
  of testes, 1242
  of thyroid gland, 1242, 1242b
Palpitations, 650, 671
Pamidronate, 1021, 1026
Pancreas
  abscess of, 1205
  alpha cells of, 1281
  anatomy of, 1063, 1063f
  beta cells of, 1281
  cancer of. See Pancreatic cancer
  endocrine, 1197, 1202, 1239, 1281
  exocrine, 1197, 1239, 1281
  functions of, 1197
  hormones produced by, 1235t
  insulin production by, 1281

Pancreas (Continued)
islets of Langerhans, 1063, 1239, 1240f
necrosis of, 1197
pseudocyst of, 1205
tumors of, 1205
Pancreatectomy, 1207
Pancreatic cancer
abdominal pain associated with, 1206
assessment of, 1206
care coordination for, 1208–1209
chemotherapy for, 1206–1207
endoscopic retrograde cholangiopancreatography of, 1206
features of, 1206b
genetic risk for, 1205b
health care resources for, 1209
home care management of, 1209
laboratory assessment of, 1206
nonsurgical management of, 1206–1207
pathophysiology of, 1205–1206
radiation therapy for, 1207
risk factors for, 1206
self-management education for, 1209
signs and symptoms of, 1205–1206
surgical management of, 1207–1208, 1207f
transition management for, 1208–1209
venous thromboembolism secondary to, 1205
Whipple procedure for, 1207, 1207f, 1208t
Pancreatic insufficiency, 1202
Pancreatic transplantation
complications of, 1303
description of, 1204
diabetes mellitus treated with, 1302–1303
rejection of, 1302–1303
Pancreatic-enzyme replacement therapy, 1203
Pancreaticojejunostomy, 1207
Pancreatitis
acute
abdominal pain associated with, 1199–1201
alcohol consumption as cause of, 1200
assessment of, 1199–1200
autodigestion in, 1198f
care coordination for, 1202
complications of, 1197–1198, 1198t, 1201
death caused by, 1199
definition of, 1197
drug therapy for, 1200–1201
endoscopic retrograde cholangiopancreatography -related trauma as cause of, 1199

Pancreatitis (Continued)
etiology of, 1199
gallstones as cause of, 1201
genetic risk of, 1199
history-taking for, 1199
home care management of, 1202
imaging assessment of, 1200
incidence of, 1199
interventions for, 1200–1201
laboratory assessment of, 1200, 1200t
multi-system organ failure caused by, 1198
nonsurgical management of, 1200–1201
nutrition promotion in, 1201
in older adults, 1199
paralytic ileus secondary to, 1201b
pathophysiology of, 1197–1199
physical assessment of, 1199
prevalence of, 1199
psychosocial assessment of, 1200
respiratory status monitoring in, 1201b
shock caused by, 1198, 1199b
signs and symptoms of, 1199
surgical management of, 1201
transition management for, 1202
ultrasonography of, 1200
chronic, 1202–1204, 1203b–1204b
necrotizing hemorrhagic, 1197–1198
Pancytopenia, 327, 815
Pandemic, 151, 427, 597
Pandemic influenza, 597–598
Panendoscopy, 549
Panhysterectomy, 1461t
Panitumumab, 1130
Panniculitis, 1227
Panniculus, 1227
Pao₂. See Partial pressure of arterial oxygen
Papanicolaou test, 1433–1434, 1469
Papillae, 1062
Papillary carcinoma, 1275
Papilledema, 946, 951
Papillotomy, 1071
Papular rash, 440
Papules, 438f
Paracentesis, 1175–1177, 1177b
Paradoxical blood pressure, 652–653
Paradoxical chest wall movement, 637, 637f
Paradoxical pulse, 713
Paradoxical splitting, 654
Paraesophageal hiatal hernias, 1092, 1093b
Paraffin dips, 323
Paralysis, 91
Paralytic ileus, 176, 277, 1122, 1201b
Paranasal sinuses
anatomy of, 509, 509f
cancer of, 556
Paraneoplastic syndromes, 1385
Paraprotein, 830

Parasitic disorders/infections
bedbugs, 471
description of, 1165–1166
pediculosis, 470–471
scabies, 470–471, 471f
Parasympathetic nervous system, 842
Parathyroid disorders
hyperparathyroidism, 1275–1277, 1276b, 1276t
hypoparathyroidism, 1277–1278
Parathyroid glands
anatomy of, 1239
hormones produced by, 1235t
Parathyroid hormone
calcium levels affected by, 179, 1239
description of, 1006
functions of, 1239, 1239f
phosphorus levels regulated by, 1400, 1400f
Parathyroid hormone modulator, 1410b
Parathyroidectomy, 1277
Parent cells, 372
Parenteral nutrition, 204–205. See also Total parenteral nutrition
Paresis, 91
Paresthesia, 178, 904–905, 914, 934, 1261
Paresthesias, 319
Parietal cells, 1063
Parietal lobe, 841t
Parkinson disease
anticholinergics for, 871
assessment of, 869–870
care coordination for, 872–873
care for, 870b
catechol O-methyltransferase inhibitors for, 870
clinical features of, 868t
deep brain stimulation for, 872
dietary considerations for, 871
dopamine agonists for, 870–871, 870b
drug therapy for, 870–871
dyskinesias associated with, 870, 872
etiology of, 869
facial expression changes associated with, 869, 869f
fetal tissue transplantation for, 872
gait in, 871
genetic risk of, 869
health care resources for, 872–873
home care preparation for, 872
Huntington disease versus, 868t
imaging assessment of, 869–870
incidence of, 869
laboratory assessment of, 869–870
monoamine oxidase type B inhibitors for, 870
neurotransmitters in, 868
nonsurgical management of, 870–872
palliative care for, 873

Parkinson disease (Continued)
pathophysiology of, 868–869
physical assessment of, 869
postural instability associated with, 871
prevalence of, 869
rigidity associated with, 869
self-esteem promotion in, 872
self-management education for, 872
signs and symptoms of, 868–869, 869f, 871
speech difficulties associated with, 871–872
stages of, 868–869, 869t
stereotactic pallidotomy for, 872
substantia nigra degeneration in, 868
surgical management of, 872
transition management for, 872–873
Parkland formula, 494–495
Paromomycin, 1166
Paronychia, 442
Parotidectomy, 1085
Paroxysmal nocturnal dyspnea, 517, 650, 695
Paroxysmal supraventricular tachycardia, 676
Partial agonists, 57
Partial breast irradiation, 1451
Partial corpus callosotomy, 880
Partial left ventriculectomy, 702
Partial pancreatectomy, 1207
Partial parenteral nutrition, 1223–1224
Partial pressure of arterial oxygen, 194, 624, 646
Partial pressure of carbon dioxide, 14, 624
Partial pressure of end-tidal carbon dioxide, 523
Partial rebreather mask, 532–533, 532t, 533f
Partial seizures, 876–877, 878b
Partial thromboplastin time, 619–620, 622b, 657, 805
Partial-thickness wound, 473
definition of, 27
physiologic consequences of, 28
PAS. See Physician-assisted suicide
Pasero Opioid-Induced Sedation Scale, 64t
Pasireotide, 1258
Passive immunity, 21–22, 298–299, 414
Passive range of motion, 1010
Passive smoking, 514
Patches, 438f
Patellofemoral pain syndrome, 1057t
Pathogen
definition of, 414
transmission methods for, 416

Pathogenicity, 414

Pathologic fracture, 1032

Patient harm and error, 3–4

Patient identification
  in emergency departments, 121
  intraoperative, 262–263
  preoperative, 241, 247

Patient safety, 4

Patient Self-Determination Act, 104, 241

Patient transfer, 421

Patient-centered care
  attributes of, 2
  context of, 3
  definition of, 2
  for older veterans, 36b
  scope of, 2

Patient-controlled analgesia, 55, 283–284, 497, 592

Patient-controlled epidural analgesia, 55, 61

Patient-controlled regional anesthesia, 65

Patterns of inheritance. See Inheritance patterns

PAWP. See Pulmonary artery wedge pressure

PCA. See Patient-controlled analgesia

PCEA. See Patient-controlled epidural analgesia

PCRA. See Patient-controlled regional anesthesia

PCSK9 inhibitors, 730–731

Peaceful death, 103

Peak airway (inspiratory) pressure, 632

Peak expiratory flow, 567–568

Peak expiratory flow rate, 567

Peak flow meter, 568b, 568f, 577

Peau d'orange, 1441, 1441f, 1445

Pediatric advanced life support, 120t, 123

Pediculosis, 470–471

Pediculosis capitis, 470

Pediculosis corporis, 470

Pediculosis pubis, 470, 1470

Pedigree, 77–78, 78f–79f

PEEP. See Positive end-expiratory pressure

Pegfilgrastim, 402t

PEG-INF/RBV, 1185t

Pegloticase, 332

Pegvisomant, 1248–1249

Pelvic examination, 1433

Pelvic fractures, 1036, 1049–1050

Pelvic inflammatory disease
  abdominal ultrasonography of, 1515
  antibiotics for, 1516, 1516b
  assessment of, 1514–1515
  care coordination for, 1516–1517
  diagnostic criteria for, 1515t
  health care resources for, 1517
  home care management of, 1516
  infertility caused by, 1514, 1517

Pelvic inflammatory disease (Continued)
  interventions for, 1515–1516, 1516b
  laboratory assessment of, 1515
  pathogens that cause, 1514
  pathophysiology of, 1514, 1514f
  physical assessment of, 1515
  psychosocial assessment of, 1515
  risk factors for, 1515
  self-management education for, 1516–1517
  signs and symptoms of, 1515
  transition management for, 1516–1517

Pelvic muscle exercises, 1347, 1347b, 1351, 1464

Pelvic organ prolapse, 1464–1465, 1464f

Pelvic pouch, 1154, 1154f

PEM. See Protein-energy malnutrition

Pembrolizumab, 477

Penetrance, 79

Penetrating keratoplasty, 978, 978f

Penetrating trauma
  description of, 129
  ocular, 982
  osteomyelitis secondary to, 1023
  spinal cord injury caused by, 894

Penile implants, 1490

Penis, 1430, 1430f

Penrose drain, 278, 279f, 282

Pentamidine isethionate, 353

Pentoxifylline, 734

Peptic ulcer(s)
  complications of, 1108–1109
  definition of, 1107
  duodenal ulcers, 1107–1108, 1108f, 1110
  gastric ulcers, 1107–1110, 1108f
  Helicobacter pylori as cause of, 1107, 1109
  perforation of, 1108–1109
  stress ulcers, 1108
  types of, 1107–1108

Peptic ulcer disease
  antacids for, 1112
  assessment of, 1109–1111
  care coordination for, 1114–1115
  complementary and integrative health for, 1107t, 1112–1113
  complications of, 1108–1109
  definition of, 1107
  dietary considerations in, 1112, 1112b
  drug therapy for, 1106b–1107b, 1111–1112
  dyspepsia associated with, 1110
  esophagogastroduodenoscopy for, 1111
  etiology of, 1109
  genetic risk of, 1109
  health care resources for, 1115

Peptic ulcer disease (Continued)
  Helicobacter pylori as cause of, 1107, 1109
  histamine receptor antagonists for, 1112
  home care management of, 1114, 1115b
  imaging assessment of, 1111
  incidence of, 1109
  interventions for, 1111–1113
  laboratory assessment of, 1111
  minimally invasive surgery for, 1114
  nonsteroidal anti-inflammatory drugs as cause of, 1109
  nutrition therapy for, 1112
  pain caused by, 1111–1113
  pathophysiology of, 1107–1109, 1108f
  physical assessment of, 1110
  prevalence of, 1109
  psychosocial assessment of, 1111
  self-management education for, 1114–1115
  signs and symptoms of, 1110
  surgical management of, 1114
  transition management for, 1114–1115
  upper gastrointestinal bleeding caused by
    acid suppression for rebleeding prevention, 1114
    description of, 1108, 1109b
    endoscopic therapy for, 1113
    fluid replacement for, 1113
    hypovolemia concerns secondary to, 1113
    interventional radiologic procedures for, 1113–1114
    interventions for, 1113–1114
    nasogastric tube for, 1113
    nonsurgical management of, 1113–1114
  in uremia, 1401

Percussion
  of chest, 519, 519f–520f, 519t
  of gastrointestinal system, 1067

Percutaneous alcohol septal ablation, 716

Percutaneous cervical diskectomy, 910

Percutaneous coronary intervention
  acute coronary syndromes treated with, 778
  myocardial infarction treated with, 783–784, 784f

Percutaneous endoscopic gastrostomy, 1221

Percutaneous lung biopsy, 527

Percutaneous stereotactic rhizotomy, for trigeminal neuralgia, 924

Percutaneous transhepatic biliary catheter, 1195

Percutaneous transhepatic biliary drain, 1206

Percutaneous ureterolithotomy, 1364

Percutaneous vascular intervention, for peripheral arterial disease, 735, 735b

Perfusion
  central, 25
  decreased, 25–26
  definition of, 25, 795
  inadequate, 104
  peripheral, 25
  sickle cell disease effects on, 809

Perfusionist, 253t

Pericardial friction rub, 655, 713

Pericardiectomy, 713

Pericardiocentesis, 713–714

Pericarditis, 650t, 712–714, 712b, 1401

Pericardium, 642

Perilymph, 986

Perimetry, 964

Perineal wound, 1133b

Perineometer, 1347

Periodontal disease, 1079

Perioperative nurse, 229

Perioperative nursing data set, 229

Perioperative period
  definition of, 228
  patient safety in, 228–229
  patient-focused model, 229, 229f

Peripheral arterial disease
  aortofemoral bypass surgery for, 735, 736f
  assessment of, 731–733
  axillofemoral bypass surgery for, 735–736, 736f
  chronic, 732b
  drug therapy for, 734–735
  exercise for, 740
  exercise tolerance testing for, 733
  features of, 732b, 733f
  home care management of, 737b
  inflow disease, 732
  intermittent claudication associated with, 732
  interventions for, 733–737
  magnetic resonance angiography for, 733
  nonsurgical management of, 733–737
  obstructions associated with, 731, 732f
  outflow disease, 732
  pathophysiology of, 731
  patient positioning for, 740
  percutaneous vascular intervention for, 735, 735b
  surgical management of, 735–737
  ulcers associated with, 732–733, 734b
  vasodilation promotion in, 740–741

Peripheral artery aneurysms, 740

Peripheral blood smear, 803

Peripheral blood stem cell harvesting, 823

Peripheral chemoreceptors, 646
Peripheral cyanosis, 652
Peripheral intravenous therapy
    midline catheters for, 204–205,
        204f, 213
    short peripheral catheters for,
        202–204, 202f–203f, 202t,
        203b, 214–215
    site selection for, 203–204, 203f,
        204b
    skin preparation for, 203–204
    ultrasound applications in,
        202–203
    vein selection for, 203–204, 203f,
        204b
Peripheral nerves
    cancer effects on, 385
    distribution of, 913f
Peripheral nervous system
    description of, 842
    facial paralysis, 924–925
    Guillain-Barré syndrome. See
        Guillain-Barré syndrome
    myasthenia gravis. See Myasthenia
        gravis
    restless legs syndrome, 922–923
    trigeminal neuralgia, 923–924,
        923f
Peripheral neuropathy
    chemotherapy-induced, 385
    definition of, 912
    diabetic, 1284–1285, 1285t,
        1304–1307, 1305f
Peripheral perfusion, 25
Peripheral vascular disease
    description of, 731
    foot care in, 737b
Peripheral venous disease
    description of, 741–748
    venous thromboembolism. See
        Venous thromboembolism
Peripherally inserted central
        catheters, 205–206, 205f, 206b,
        212–213
Peristalsis
    peritonitis effects on, 1145
    in postoperative period, 285–286
Peristaltic contractions, 1064
Peritoneal dialysis
    automated, 1419–1420,
        1419f–1420f
    catheters, 1418f, 1420b
    chronic kidney disease treated
        with, 1408
    complications of, 1420–1421
    continuous ambulatory, 1418,
        1419f
    continuous-cycle, 1419
    description of, 1408, 1417
    dialysate additives, 1418
    dialysate leakage during, 1420
    hemodialysis versus, 1411t
    home care management of, 1424
    intermittent, 1420
    nursing care during, 1421

Peritoneal dialysis (Continued)
    nutrition needs for, 1408
    patient selection, 1417
    peritonitis caused by, 1420,
        1420b
    procedure, 1417–1418, 1418f
    self-management education for,
        1425
    types of, 1418–1420, 1418f–
        1419f
Peritonitis
    abdominal x-rays of, 1146
    assessment of, 1145–1146
    care coordination for, 1146–1147
    cholecystitis as cause of, 1192
    definition of, 1144
    etiology of, 1145, 1420
    features of, 1145b
    fluid volume restoration in, 1146
    generalized, 1145
    home care management of, 1146
    imaging assessment of, 1146
    incidence of, 1145
    interventions for, 1146
    laboratory assessment of, 1146
    localized, 1145
    nonsurgical management of, 1146
    in older adults, 1163b
    pain management in, 1146
    pathophysiology of, 1144–1145
    peptic ulcers as cause of,
        1108–1109
    peristalsis affected by, 1145
    peritoneal dialysis as cause of,
        1420, 1420b
    physical assessment of, 1145,
        1145b
    prevalence of, 1145
    psychosocial assessment of, 1145
    signs and symptoms of, 1145,
        1145b
    spontaneous bacterial, 1171, 1175
    surgical management of, 1146
    transition management for,
        1146–1147
Peritonsillar abscess, 611
Periungual lesions, 319
Permeable membrane, 161
Pernicious anemia, 814, 1104–1105
PERRLA, 847–848, 963
Persistent pain, 46–47
Personal emergency preparedness
    plan, 155
Personal protective equipment
    definition of, 418
    illustration of, 420f
    recommendation for, 419t
Personal readiness supplies, 155b,
    156t
Personality
    Alzheimer's disease-related
        changes in, 861
    description of, 16
Pertussis, 613
Pessary, 1348, 1352

Petechiae
    definition of, 802
    description of, 439, 440f, 1173
    infective endocarditis as cause of,
        711
PFPS. See Patellofemoral pain
    syndrome
pH
    acidic, 186f
    alkaline, 187f
    blood, 13–14, 188
    body fluids, 185–186
    gastric contents, 1222
    urine, 1333
pH monitoring examination, 1089
Phacoemulsification, 970, 970f
Phagocytosis, 293–294, 294f, 417
Phalangeal fractures, 1047, 1049
Phalen's maneuver, 1058
Phalloplasty, 1501
Phantom limb pain, 1051, 1053
Pharmacists, 89
Pharmacokinetics, 57b
Pharmacologic stress
    echocardiogram, 660
Pharynx
    age-related changes in, 513b
    anatomy of, 509–510
Phenazopyridine, 1359, 1359b
Phenotype, 75–76
Phenoxybenzamine, 1262
Phentermine-topiramate, 1228
Phenytoin, 952
Pheochromocytomas, 721, 1261–1262
"Philadelphia" chromosome,
    376–377, 820
Phlebitis, 200, 217t–219t, 742
Phlebitis Scale, 221t
Phlebostatic axis, 780b
Phlebothrombosis, 742
Phonophobia, 874, 881
Phosphodiesterase inhibitors, 700
    high-altitude pulmonary edema
        treated with, 146
    nitroglycerin and, interactions
        between, 775b
Phosphodiesterase-5 inhibitors, 1489
Phosphorus
    in bone, 1006
    chronic kidney disease effects on,
        1400, 1400f
Photodynamic therapy
    description of, 405–406
    esophageal tumors treated with,
        1098
    lung cancer treated with, 589
Photophobia, 874, 881, 1266, 1270
Photopsia, 979
Photoreceptors, 957–958
Physiatrists, 88
Physical abuse, of older adults, 39
Physical activity, 31–32, 32f. See also
    Exercise
Physical dependence, 58
Physical inactivity, 1226

Physical therapists, 88–89, 89f, 93
Physical therapy
    fractures treated with, 1041
    osteoarthritis uses of, 316
    wound care applications of, 458
Physical therapy assistants, 88–89
Physician assistants, 88
Physician-assisted suicide, 114
Physicians
    emergency medicine, 119
    medical command, 154, 154t
    in rehabilitation settings, 88
Physiotherapists, 88–89
Pia mater, 840
PICC. See Peripherally inserted
    central catheters
Pick's disease, 857–858
Piggyback set, 209, 209f
Pill boxes, 34
Pinna, 984, 985f, 988
Pioglitazone, 1291, 1292b–1293b
Pit vipers, 136, 136f, 136t, 138t–140t
Pitting edema, 171f, 652f
Pituitary adenoma, 1247
Pituitary gland
    anatomy of, 1236–1237
    anterior. See Anterior pituitary
        gland
    hormones produced by, 1235t
    magnetic resonance imaging of,
        1243
    posterior. See Posterior pituitary
        gland
Pituitary gland disorders
    hyperpituitarism, 1247–1250,
        1247f, 1248b
    hypopituitarism, 1245–1247, 1246b
Pituitary tumors, 951
Pivot joints, 1007
Placebos, 65, 65b
Plague, 428
Plan-Do-Study-Act model, 7
Plantar fasciitis, 1029
Plaques, 438f, 928
Plasma
    electrolyte levels in, 165b
    transfusion of, 835
Plasma cells, 297, 797t, 829
Plasma thromboplastin, 798t
Plasmapheresis, 366
    complications of, 915b
    Guillain-Barré syndrome treated
        with, 914–915, 915b
    myasthenia gravis treated with,
        920–921
Plasmin, 801
Plasminogen, 801
Plastic containers, for infusion
    therapy, 208–209
Platelet(s)
    activation of, 798
    aggregation of, 798, 805
    in clotting, 15
    definition of, 797
    leukemia effects on, 819

Platelet count, 805, 825
Platelet plugs, 798
Platelet transfusions
   idiopathic thrombocytopenic
        purpura treated with, 831
   indications for, 832t, 835
   reaction to, 835
Platelet-derived growth factor, 458
Plethysmography, 733
Pleura, 510
Pleural effusion, 1405
   description of, 518–519
   in lung cancer patients, 593
   thoracentesis for, 593
Pleural friction rub, 521t
Pleur-evac system, 590, 591f
Plexuses, 842
PMI. *See* Point of maximal impulse
PNDS. *See* Perioperative nursing
        data set
Pneumatic compression devices, 245,
        245f
Pneumocystis jiroveci pneumonia,
        346, 353
Pneumonectomy
   complications of, 593
   definition of, 589
   incisions for, 589f
   pain management after, 592
   postoperative care for, 590–593
   preoperative care for, 589
   respiratory management after,
        592–593
Pneumonia
   airway obstruction in, 604
   assessment of, 601–603
   care coordination for, 604–605
   chest x-rays for, 603
   community-acquired, 599t–600t
   empyema management in, 604
   etiology of, 599
   gas exchange in, 604
   health care resources for, 605
   health care-associated, 599t–600t
   health promotion and
        maintenance for, 599–601
   history-taking for, 601
   home care management of, 605
   hospital-acquired, 599t–600t
   imaging assessment of, 603
   incentive spirometry in, 604
   incidence of, 599
   inflammation as cause of, 599
   laboratory assessment of, 603,
        603f
   lobar, 599
   in older adults, 603b
   oxygen therapy in, 604
   pathophysiology of, 598–599,
        603t
   physical assessment of, 601–603
   prevalence of, 599
   prevention of, 600b
   psychosocial assessment of, 603
   risk factors for, 599, 599t

Pneumonia (Continued)
   self-management education for,
        605
   sepsis prevention in, 604
   signs and symptoms of, 601–603,
        603t
   transition management for,
        604–605
   vaccines/vaccination for, 599, 601
   ventilator-associated, 600t, 601,
        633
Pneumonia Severity Index, 603
Pneumothorax, 539, 637–638
Pneumovax, 599
PNS. *See* Parasympathetic nervous
        system
Podagra, 331
Podofilox, 1511
Point of maximal impulse, 654
Point-of-care testing, 656
Polyclonal antibodies, 302b
Polycystic kidney disease
   assessment of, 1381–1382
   autosomal-dominant, 1380, 1380b,
        1380f
   blood pressure management in,
        1381–1382
   care coordination for, 1382
   chronic kidney disease progression
        of, 1382
   constipation in, 1382
   definition of, 1379
   etiology of, 1380
   features of, 1379–1380, 1380f,
        1381b
   genetic risk of, 1380, 1380f
   health care resources for, 1382
   history-taking for, 1381
   incidence of, 1381
   interventions for, 1381–1382
   pain management in, 1382
   pathophysiology of, 1379–1381
   physical assessment of, 1381
   prevalence of, 1381
   self-management education for,
        1382b
   signs and symptoms of, 1381
   transition management for, 1382
Polycythemia vera, 15, 576–577,
        816–817, 817b
Polydipsia, 1261, 1283
PolyMem, 501b
Polymorphisms, 76–77
Polymorphonuclear cells, 292–293
Polymorphonuclear leukocytes, 417
Polymyalgia rheumatica, 334t
Polymyositis, 334t
Polymyxin B-bacitracin, 501b
Polypectomy, 1072, 1126
Polyphagia, 1283
Polyps
   hyperplastic, 1126
   intestinal, 1126
   nasal, 517
   screening for, 1070

Polyuria, 1261, 1283
PONV. *See* Postoperative nausea and
        vomiting
Pores, 162
Porfimer sodium, 1098
Portal hypertension, 1170
Portal hypertensive gastropathy,
        1170
Portal-systemic encephalopathy,
        1170–1171
Positive end-expiratory pressure,
        627, 632
Positive end-expiratory volume, 497
Positive inotropic agents, 622,
        699–700, 782
Positive-pressure valve, 210
Positive-pressure ventilation, 535,
        535b, 536f
Positron emission tomography
   cardiovascular system evaluations
        using, 661
   metastatic disease evaluations,
        1096
Post-acute care, 87, 92
Postanesthesia care unit
   description of, 270
   discharge from, 272, 272b
   pain assessment in, 278
Postanesthesia care unit nurse, 271
Postanesthesia care unit record, 273f
Postcholecystectomy syndrome,
        1196, 1196t
Postembolectomy syndrome, 1461b
Posterior cerebral artery
   anatomy of, 841
   stroke involving, 933b
Posterior colporrhaphy, 1465
Posterior nasal bleeding, 557
Posterior pituitary gland
   diabetes insipidus, 1250–1251,
        1250b
   hormones produced by, 1235t,
        1236–1237, 1237t
   syndrome of inappropriate
        antidiuretic hormone,
        1251–1253, 1252t
Posterior vitreous detachment, 979
Postherpetic neuralgia, 468
Post-irradiation sialadenitis, 1085
Postmenopausal women, 180b
Postmortem care, 114, 114b
Postnecrotic cirrhosis, 1170
Postoperative ileus, 285–286, 1122,
        1124
Postoperative nausea and vomiting,
        276
Postoperative period
   acid-base balance in, 276
   airway maintenance in, 280
   arterial blood gas tests in, 280
   breathing exercises in, 281
   cardiac monitoring in, 274
   cardiovascular system in
        assessment of, 274
        complications involving, 244–246

Postoperative period (Continued)
   care coordination in, 286–287
   comfort alterations in, 278
   complications in, 272t
   constipation in, 277
   definition of, 270
   description of, 228
   drains used in, 277–278, 279f,
        282
   dressings used in, 277–278,
        281–282
   drug reconciliation in, 287
   electrolyte balance in, 276
   fluid balance in, 276
   gas exchange in, 280–281
   gastrointestinal system, 276–277
   gum chewing in, 286
   hand-off report, 271b
   health care resources, 287
   history-taking, 271
   home care management, 286
   hydration status assessments, 276
   incentive spirometry in, 243–244,
        244f
   intake and output measurements,
        276
   kidneys in, 276
   laboratory assessment in, 280
   leg exercises in, 245, 245b
   mobility in, 245
   movement in, 281
   nasogastric tube monitoring, 277
   neurologic system, 274–275, 274t
   oxygen saturation monitoring in,
        280
   oxygen therapy in, 280–281
   pain in
        assessment of, 278
        management of, 283–285,
           284b–285b
   peripheral vascular assessment in,
        274
   peristalsis in, 285–286
   phases of, 270–271
   physical assessments, 272–278
   pressure injuries in, 283
   psychosocial assessment in,
        278–280
   renal system in, 276
   respiratory system in
        assessment of, 273–274
        complications involving,
           242–244
   self-management education in,
        286–287
   skin assessments, 277–278, 278f
   skin care, 281b
   total knee arthroplasty, 315–316,
        315f
   transition management in,
        286–287
   urinary system, 276
   venous thromboembolism
        prevention, 274, 281
   vital signs, 274

Postoperative period (Continued)
wound
dehiscence of, 277, 278f, 282–283
drains, 277–278, 279f, 282
dressings for, 277–278, 281–282
evisceration of, 277, 278f, 283, 283b
healing of, 277, 278f
nonsurgical management of, 281–282
staple closure of, 282
suture closure of, 282
wound infection prevention in, 281–283
Postpartum hemorrhage, 1246
Postpericardiotomy syndrome, 789
Postrenal failure, 1392
Posttraumatic stress disorder
after mass casualty event, 156b
in transgender patients, 1494
Postural hypotension, 121, 168, 652
Posture
assessments of, 1009, 1009f
instability, in Parkinson disease, 871
Post-void residual, 98
Potassium
in acidosis, 194
bicarbonate ion and, 194f
dietary sources of, 175
extracellular fluid, 175
laboratory testing for, 1069b
in older adults, 165b
replacement of, for hypokalemia, 176
restriction of, in chronic kidney disease, 1408
serum levels of, 164t, 175
Potassium imbalances
hyperkalemia, 178–179, 178t, 179b, 192, 237
hypokalemia, 175–177, 177b, 196, 237
Potassium-sparing diuretics, 177, 699, 701
Povidone-iodine allergy, 234–235
Powered air-purifying respirator, 120, 416
PPE. See Personal protective equipment
PQRST, 1066
PR interval, 669–670, 669f
PR segment, 667–669, 669f
Pramlintide, 1292b–1293b
Prasugrel, 783–784
Prealbumin, 25, 1217
Precipitation, 297
Precordium, 653–654, 654f
Prediabetes, 1287
Prednisolone, 302b
Prednisone, 1255b
asthma treated with, 569b–570b
immunosuppression uses of, 302b
rheumatoid arthritis treated with, 322–323

Prednisone (Continued)
ulcerative colitis treated with, 1152–1153
Preemptive analgesia, 54
Pregabalin, 63–64
Pregnancy
human immunodeficiency virus infection effects on, 340
methotrexate contraindications for, 322
in sickle cell disease patients, 813b
Prehospital care providers, 119, 119f
Pre-infarction angina, 770
Preload
definition of, 645
drugs that affect, 699–701
interventions that reduce, 698
Premature atrial complexes, 676
Premature complexes, 671
Premature ventricular complexes, 683–684, 683f, 779
Premature ventricular contractions, 683
Preoperative period
administering regularly scheduled drugs, 241–242
antibiotic prophylaxis in, 247
anxiety in, 237, 246
bowel preparation, 242
checklist for, 247–249, 248f
definition of, 229
description of, 228
dietary restrictions in, 241
discharge planning in, 235
drains, 242
drugs in, 241–242, 247, 257
electrocardiogram in, 238
electronic health record review in, 246–247
expected outcomes in, 238
family members, 246
fear in, 237
focused assessment in, 238b
hair removal, 242, 243f
history-taking in, 230–235
imaging assessments in, 237
informed consent, 239–241, 240f
interventions in, 238–246
intestinal preparation, 242
laboratory assessments in, 237
medical history, 233–234
National Patient Safety Goal requirements, 238–239
older adults, 236b
patient preparation in, 247
patient self-determination, 241
patient transfer to surgical suite, 247–249
physical assessments in, 235–237
postoperative procedures and exercises
antiembolism stockings, 244
for cardiovascular complications, 244–246
coughing and splinting, 244

Preoperative period (Continued)
incentive spirometry, 243–244, 244f
leg exercises, 245, 245b
overview of, 244
pneumatic compression devices, 245, 245f
for respiratory complications, 242–244
psychosocial assessments, 237
rest in, 246
skin preparation, 242, 243f
studies of, 239b
teaching in, 239t, 246
total hip arthroplasty, 309–310
total knee arthroplasty, 314–315
tubes, 242
urinalysis, 237
vascular access preparations, 242
Prerenal failure, 1392
Presbycusis, 26, 997
Presbyopia, 26, 33, 980–981
Presence, 112
Pressure dressings, 267
Pressure injuries
assessment of, 91
Braden scale for, 457t
care coordination for, 459–461
Concept Map for, 455f–456f
definition of, 447
description of, 27
features of, 452b
friction in, 448
health care resources for, 461
health promotion and maintenance for, 448–452
high-risk patients for, 448–451, 461b
home care management of, 459–460
incidence of, 448
incontinence and, 451
infection prevention in, 459
laboratory assessment of, 455
mechanical forces that cause, 448
nutrition status and, 449–451
in older adults, 42
pathophysiology of, 447–448
patient positioning for, 452
physical assessment of, 453
postoperative, 283
pressure-redistribution techniques for, 451–452
prevalence of, 448
prevention of, 96–97, 449, 449b, 900
psychosocial assessment of, 455
self-care management of, 460–461
shearing forces as cause of, 448, 448f
signs and symptoms of, 453
skin integrity care bundle for, 449b
in spinal cord injury patients, 901–903
stages of, 452b, 454f

Pressure injuries (Continued)
support surfaces and devices for, 451
transition management for, 459–461
wound caused by
assessment of, 453–455
best practices for, 460b
dressings for, 457–458
drug therapy for, 458
electrical stimulation for, 458–459
hyperbaric oxygen therapy for, 458
management of, 455–459, 457b
negative-pressure wound therapy for, 458
nonsurgical management of, 457–459
nutrition therapy for, 458
physical therapy for, 458
skin substitutes for, 458
surgical management of, 459
ultrasound-assisted wound therapy for, 458–459
Pressure support ventilation, 636t
Pressure-activated safety valve, 205
Pressure-cycled ventilators, 631
Pressure-reducing devices, 97
Pressure-relieving devices, 97
Pretibial myxedema, 1265, 1271f
Priapism, 810
Primary aldosteronism, 721
Primary angle-closure glaucoma, 972
Primary biliary cirrhosis, 1170
Primary gout, 330–331
Primary lesions, 436, 438f
Primary open-angle glaucoma, 972
Primary prevention
of cancer, 381–382
of impaired cellular regulation, 15
of sensory perception changes, 26
Primary progressive multiple sclerosis, 888
Primary survey and resuscitation interventions, 129–130, 131t
Primary syphilis, 1508
Primary tumor, 375
Prinzmetal's angina, 770
Priority setting, 122
Privacy, of genetic counseling, 83
Proaccelerin, 798t
Probenecid, 332
Probiotics, for irritable bowel syndrome, 1137
Procainamide hydrochloride, 685
Proctocolectomy
with ileo pouch-anal anastomosis, 1154–1155, 1154f
total proctocolectomy with permanent ileostomy, 1154, 1155f
Professional ethics, 9

Progressive multifocal leukoencephalopathy, 891
Progressive-relapsing multiple sclerosis, 888
Proinsulin, 1281, 1282f
Projected pain, 50
Prokinetic agents, for chemotherapy-induced nausea and vomiting, 399b
Prolactin, 1237t, 1248b
Prolactin-secreting tumors, 1247
Proliferative diabetic retinopathy, 1284
Pronation, 1010f
Pronator drift, 848
Prone position, 265f
Prophylactic mastectomy, 1443–1444
Prophylactic surgery, for cancer, 386
Proportionate palliative sedation, 111
Proprioception, 850, 932–933
Propylthiouracil, 1267, 1268b
Prostacyclin agents, 585
Prostaglandin agonists, for glaucoma, 966b
Prostaglandin analogs, 1106b–1107b
Prostaglandin-5 inhibitors, 892
Prostaglandins, 873, 1103, 1326–1327
Prostate artery embolization, 1479
Prostate cancer
    active surveillance of, 1483–1484
    anti-androgen drugs for, 1485
    assessment of, 380b, 1482–1483
    benign prostatic hyperplasia and, 1482f
    care coordination for, 1485–1486
    chemotherapy for, 1485
    etiology of, 1482
    health care resources for, 1486
    health promotion and maintenance for, 1482
    history-taking for, 1482
    home care management of, 1485–1486
    incidence of, 1482
    interventions for, 1483–1485
    laboratory assessment of, 1483
    laparoscopic radical prostatectomy for, 1484
    metastasis of, 376t, 1483–1485
    nonsurgical management of, 1485
    pathophysiology of, 1481–1482, 1482f
    physical assessment of, 1482–1483
    prevalence of, 1482
    psychosocial assessment of, 1483
    radiation therapy for, 1485
    risk factors for, 1482
    self-management education for, 1486, 1486b
    signs and symptoms of, 1482–1483

Prostate cancer (Continued)
    surgical management of, 1484–1485, 1484b
    transition management for, 1485–1486
    transrectal ultrasound for, 1483, 1483b
Prostate gland
    anatomy of, 1431
    benign hyperplasia of. See Benign prostatic hyperplasia
    biopsy of, 1438
    digital rectal examination of, 382, 1346–1347, 1474
Prostate-specific antigen, 1435, 1477, 1483
Prostatic intraepithelial neoplasia, 1481–1482
Prostatic stents, 1479
Prostatitis, 1474–1476
Prosthetic heart valves, 709–710
Protamine sulfate, 744
Protease inhibitors, 338, 348, 351b–352b
Proteases, 572
Proteasome inhibitors, 404t, 405
Protein
    restriction of, in chronic kidney disease, 1407–1408
    in urine, 1333
Protein buffers, 188–189
Protein C, 764
Protein malabsorption, 1202–1203
Protein synthesis, 76
Protein-calorie malnutrition, 414–415, 1215
Protein-energy malnutrition, 1215
Proteinuria, 1333–1335, 1377, 1381
Proteolysis, 1197
Prothrombin, 798t
Prothrombin time, 622b, 657, 805, 1068, 1174
Proton pump inhibitors
    gastritis treated with, 1105
    gastroesophageal reflux disease treated with, 1090b, 1091
    peptic ulcer disease treated with, 1106b–1107b, 1111–1112
Proto-oncogenes, 375
Proximal convoluted tubule, 1323–1324
Proximal femur fractures, 1035b
Proximal humerus fractures, 1046
Proximal interphalangeal joint, 1009, 1009f
Pruritus, 436, 461–462, 1192
PSDA. See Patient Self-determination Act
Pseudoaddiction, 58
Pseudocyst, pancreatic, 1205
Pseudomonas aeruginosa, 1023, 1135–1136
Psoralen and ultraviolet A therapy, 465

Psoriasis
    assessment of, 464
    collaborative care for, 463–465
    corticosteroids for, 464
    definition of, 463
    drug therapy for, 466b
    emotional support for, 465
    exfoliative, 464
    history-taking for, 464
    light therapy for, 465
    pathophysiology of, 463
    systemic therapy for, 465
    tar preparations for, 464
    topical therapy for, 464–465
Psoriasis vulgaris, 464, 464f
Psoriatic arthritis, 332–333, 463
PSVT. See Paroxysmal supraventricular tachycardia
Psychiatric crisis nurse team, 118–119
Ptosis, 917, 934, 963
Ptyalin, 1062
Pubovaginal sling procedure, 1349t
Pulmonary arterial hypertension, 584–585, 585t
Pulmonary artery, 511, 511f
Pulmonary artery occlusive pressure, 780
Pulmonary artery pressure, 697
Pulmonary artery wedge pressure, 697, 780–782
Pulmonary autographs, 709
Pulmonary circulation, 511
Pulmonary contusion, 636
Pulmonary edema
    in chronic kidney disease, 1405–1407
    fluid overload in, 172b
    in heart failure, 702–703, 702b
    high-altitude, 145–146, 145b–146b
    neurogenic, 954
    prevention of, 1405–1407
Pulmonary embolism
    anxiety management in, 622–623
    assessment of, 618–619
    in atrial fibrillation, 680b
    bleeding management in, 622
    care coordination for, 623–624
    collaborative care for, 618–624
    definition of, 616–617
    drug therapy for, 619–620, 620b
    fractures as risk factor for, 1034–1035
    health care resources for, 623–624
    health promotion and maintenance for, 617–618
    heparin for, 617–618, 620, 621b
    home care management of, 623, 624b
    hypotension, 621–622
    hypoxemia in, 619–621
    imaging assessment of, 619
    laboratory assessment of, 618–619
    lifestyle changes for prevention of, 617

Pulmonary embolism (Continued)
    nonsurgical management of, 619–621, 619b
    pathophysiology of, 616–617
    physical assessment of, 618
    prevention of, 617b
    psychosocial assessment of, 618
    risk factors for, 617
    self-management education for, 623, 623b
    severity of, 620t
    signs and symptoms of, 618, 618b
    surgical management of, 620–621
    transition management for, 623–624
    venous thromboembolism as cause of, 617, 716
Pulmonary fibrosis, idiopathic, 585–586
Pulmonary fluid overload, 491
Pulmonary function tests
    for asthma, 567
    description of, 523–524, 525t
Pulmonary rehabilitation, 579
Pulmonary tuberculosis. See Tuberculosis
Pulmonary vein isolation, 681
Pulmonic valve, 643
Pulse
    description of, 653
    palpation of, 729
Pulse antibiotic therapy, for urinary tract infections, 98
Pulse deficit, 672
Pulse oximetry
    description of, 247, 273
    respiratory system assessment using, 523, 523f
Pulse pressure, 652–653
Pulse therapy, 322
Pulsus alternans, 696
Pulsus paradoxus, 713
Punch biopsy, 445
Punctal occlusion, 975, 975f
Pupil(s)
    age-related changes in, 961b
    assessment of, 963
    constriction of, 847–848, 960
    definition of, 957
    dilation of, 960
Pupil testing
    description of, 847–848
    in traumatic brain injury patients, 946
Pure-tone air-conduction testing, 990
Pure-tone audiometry, 990–991
Pure-tone bone-conduction testing, 991
Purified protein derivative test, 322, 347, 367
Purkinje cells, 665
Purpura, 439
Pursed-lip breathing, 578, 578b
Pustules, 438f

PVCs. *See* Premature ventricular complexes
Pyelogram, 1339
Pyelolithotomy, 1375
Pyelonephritis, 1359*b*
  acute, 1372–1373, 1374*b*
  assessment of, 1374
  care coordination for, 1375–1376
  chronic, 1372–1373, 1374*b*
  definition of, 1372
  diagnostic assessment of, 1374
  health care resources for, 1376
  history-taking for, 1374
  home care management for, 1375
  imaging assessment of, 1374
  interventions for, 1375
  laboratory assessment of, 1374
  nonsurgical management of, 1375
  pain management in, 1375
  pathophysiology of, 1372–1374, 1373*f*
  physical assessment of, 1374
  psychosocial assessment of, 1374
  self-management education for, 1376
  signs and symptoms of, 1374
  surgical management of, 1375
  transition management for, 1375–1376
Pyloric obstruction, 1109, 1114
Pyloromyotomy, 1098
Pyuria, 1358

Q
QRS complex, 669–670
QRS duration, 669–670
QSEN initiative, 2
QSEN Institute, 2
QT interval, 669*f*, 670–671
Quadriceps-setting exercises, 312–313
Quadrigeminy, 671
Quadriparesis, 933–934
Quality and safety education, 2
Quality improvement
  attributes of, 7
  continuous, 7
  definition of, 7
  scope of, 7
QuantiFERON-TB Gold In-Tube test, 607

R
Radial nerve compression, 267*b*
Radiating pain, 50
Radiation dermatitis, 389
Radiation dose, 387–388
Radiation exposure, 379
Radiation injuries, 488
Radiation proctitis, 1485
Radiation therapy. *See also* Brachytherapy; External beam radiation therapy
  bone tumors treated with, 1026
  brachytherapy, 388

Radiation therapy (*Continued*)
  breast cancer treated with, 1451
  cervical cancer treated with, 1470
  colorectal cancer treated with, 1129–1130
  delivery methods and devices for, 388–389
  endometrial cancer treated with, 1466–1467
  esophageal tumors treated with, 1097
  external beam, 388
  gastric cancer treated with, 1116
  head and neck cancer treated with, 549
  high-dose rate implants, 388–389, 389*b*
  hoarseness secondary to, 549
  hyperpituitarism treated with, 1249
  intensity of, 388
  intensity-modulated, 388
  low-dose rate implants, 388–389, 389*b*
  lung cancer treated with, 588–589, 593
  oral cancer treated with, 1081
  overview of, 387–388
  prostate cancer treated with, 1485
  side effects of, 389–390, 389*t*, 1116, 1119
  skin cancer treated with, 477
  skin protection during, 390*b*
  stereotactic body, 388
  tissue effects of, 387
  xerostomia caused by, 1084–1085
Radical cystectomy, 1366
Radical hysterectomy, 1461*t*, 1466
Radical prostatectomy
  laparoscopic, 1484
  open, 1484*b*
Radical surgery, 232*t*
Radiculopathies, 905
Radioactive iodine therapy
  hyperthyroidism treated with, 1266–1269, 1269*b*
  thyroid cancer treated with, 1275
Radiofrequency ablation
  description of, 681
  liver cancer treated with, 1187
  supraventricular tachycardia treated with, 676–678
Radiofrequency identification, 8
Radiographs
  chest. *See* Chest x-rays
  gastrointestinal system assessments, 1070
  skeletal system assessments using, 1011
Radioisotope scanning, 965
Radiosurgery, for trigeminal neuralgia, 924
Rales, 521*t*
Raloxifene, 1021

Ramsay Sedation Scale, 261, 262*t*
Ramucirumab, 589*t*
Range of motion
  active, 1010
  assessments of, 1010, 1010*f*
  mobility rehabilitation exercises, 96, 503
  passive, 1010
Ranibizumab, 1284
Rapid influenza diagnostic test, 597
Rapid plasma reagin, 1509
Rapid response teams, 8
Rapid urease testing, 1105
Rapidly progressive glomerulonephritis, 1377–1378
Rattlesnake bites, 136, 138*t*–140*t*
Raynaud's disease, 741*t*
Raynaud's phenomenon, 329–330, 741*t*
Reasoning, 16
Rebound headache, 874
Rebound phenomenon, 146
Receptive aphasia, 938
Recombinant human bone morphogenetic protein-2, 1045
Reconstructive surgery, 386
Recreational therapists, 89
Rectal pain, 1164
Rectal tumors, 1130*t*
Rectocele, 1464, 1464*f*
Recurrent aphthous ulcers, 1076–1078
Red blood cells
  description of, 796
  gender differences, 800*b*
  production of, 797
  transfusion of
    compatibility determinations for, 834, 834*t*
    indications for, 832*t*, 834–835
    sickle cell disease treated with, 812
Red reflex, 966
Reducible hernia, 1138
Reduction mammoplasty, 1456
Reed-Sternberg cells, 828
Re-epithelialization, 473–474, 474*f*
Refeeding syndrome, 1221–1222
Referred pain, 50
Reflex arc, 842, 843*f*
Reflex incontinence, 1344, 1345*t*
Reflex sympathetic dystrophy, 1035
Reflexes
  assessment of, 848–849
  asymmetry of, 849, 849*f*
  components of, 842
  cutaneous, 848
  deep tendon, 848
  hyperactive, 849
  hypoactive, 849
Reflux, 1373
Reflux esophagitis, 1087
Refraction
  definition of, 960, 980
  errors of, 960, 960*f*, 980–981

Regional anesthesia, 65, 260–261, 261*f*–262*f*, 261*t*
Regional osteoporosis, 1016
Registered dietitians, 89
Registered nurse, 123–124, 253*t*
Regurgitation, 1089
Rehabilitation
  ambulatory care, 88
  for bowel continence, 99
  after cancer surgery, 387
  cognitive assessments before, 91
  continuum of care, 87
  definition of, 86
  desired outcome of, 88
  for functional abilities, 96
  functional ability assessments before, 92
  history-taking, 89–90
  home care preparation after, 100
  inpatient, 87
  interprofessional team for, 88–89, 88*t*, 89*f*
  for mobility issues, 93–96
  for pressure injury prevention, 96–97
  safe patient handling and mobility practices during, 93–95, 93*b*
  for spinal cord injury, 901–902
  telerehabilitation, 101
  for urinary continence, 97–98
Rehabilitation assistants, 89
Rehabilitation case manager, 88
Rehabilitation nurses, 88, 88*t*
Rehabilitation settings
  care coordination and transition management in, 99–101
  description of, 87–88
  gait training in, 95–96, 95*b*, 95*f*
  interprofessional team in, 88–89, 88*t*, 89*f*
  leave-of-absence visit, 100
  older adults in, 90*b*
  physical assessments in
    bowel elimination, 90*t*, 91
    cardiovascular system, 90, 90*t*
    gastrointestinal system, 90–91, 90*t*
    integumentary system, 90*t*, 91
    musculoskeletal system, 90*t*, 91
    neurologic system, 90*t*, 91
    nutrition, 90–91, 90*t*
    overview of, 90*t*
    renal system, 90*t*, 91
    respiratory system, 90, 90*t*
    skin, 90*t*, 91
    tissue integrity, 90*t*, 91
    urinary system, 90*t*, 91
  predischarge assessments, 100
  psychosocial assessments in, 92
  safe patient handling and mobility practices in, 93–95, 93*b*
  staff members in, work-related musculoskeletal disorders to, 93
  vocational assessments in, 92

Rehabilitation therapists, 89
Rehabilitative surgery, 386
Rehydration, 170
Reiter's syndrome, 334t
Relapsing-remitting multiple sclerosis, 888, 890–891
Relative alkalosis, 195
Relative dehydration, 167
Relative potency, 58
Relaxation techniques, 67, 285
Religion
  death rituals based on, 112t
  emergency department care affected by, 123b
Relocation stress syndrome, 30–31, 33b
Remicade. See Infliximab
Reminiscence/reminiscence therapy, 112, 862
Renal arteriography, 1339
Renal artery bypass surgery, 1384
Renal artery stenosis, 721, 1384, 1423–1424
Renal cell carcinoma, 1385–1386
Renal colic, 1330, 1362
Renal columns, 1322
Renal cortex, 1322
Renal medulla, 1322
Renal osteodystrophy, 1400–1401, 1404
Renal replacement therapies
  acute kidney injury treated with, 1397–1398, 1397f
  chronic kidney disease treated with, 1411–1424, 1411t, 1412f–1415f
Renal scan, 1339
Renal system. See also Kidney(s)
  age-related changes in, 234b, 1328–1329, 1328b
  assessment of
    blood tests, 1331–1332
    computed tomography, 1337–1338, 1337t, 1338b
    current health problems, 1330
    cystography, 1337t, 1339
    cystometrography, 1340
    cystoscopy, 1337t, 1339
    cystourethrography, 1337t, 1339
    cystourethroscopy, 1339
    description of, 90t, 91
    diagnostic, 1331–1341
    electromyography, 1340
    family history, 1330
    genetic risks, 1330
    history-taking, 1329–1330
    imaging, 1337–1341
    kidney, ureter, and bladder x-rays, 1337, 1337t
    kidney biopsy, 1340–1341
    laboratory, 1331–1341
    magnetic resonance imaging, 1337t, 1338
    medication history, 1329–1330
    nutrition history, 1329

Renal system (Continued)
    physical, 1330–1331
    positron emission tomography, 1337t
    psychosocial, 1331
    renal arteriography, 1339
    renal scan, 1339
    retrograde procedures, 1339–1340
    ultrasonography, 1337t, 1338
    urine tests. See Urine tests
    urodynamic studies, 1340
  dehydration effects on, 169
  description of, 1321
  kidneys. See Kidney(s)
  physical assessment of, 1330–1331
  postoperative assessment of, 276
  preoperative assessment of, 236
  ureters, 1327, 1327f
  urethra, 1327–1328
  urinary bladder, 1327, 1327f
Renal threshold, 1325
Renal transplantation. See Kidney transplantation
Renin, 166–167, 721, 1237, 1323, 1326
Renin-angiotensin II pathway
  in fluid balance, 166–167, 166f
  in hypertension management, 167
Renin-angiotensin system
  activation of, 694
  angiotensin receptor blockers effect on, 698
  angiotensin-converting enzyme inhibitors effect on, 698
  description of, 166
Renin-angiotension-aldosterone system
  activation of, 692
  blood pressure regulation by, 721
  chronic kidney disease effects on, 1401
Renovascular disease, 1384
Renovascular hypertension, 721
Repaglinide, 1292b–1293b
Reperfusion therapy, for myocardial infarction, 777–778
Repetitive nerve stimulation, for myasthenia gravis, 918
Repetitive stress injury, 1057
Replication, of DNA, 73–74, 74f
Reproductive system
  age-related changes in, 1431, 1431b
  assessment of, 1431–1438
  biopsy studies of, 1437–1438, 1437b
  colposcopy of, 1436
  current health problems in, 1432–1433
  diagnostic assessment of, 1433–1438
  endoscopic studies of, 1436–1437
  family history of, 1432

Reproductive system (Continued)
  female. See Female reproductive system
  genetic risk of, 1432
  health promotion and maintenance for, 1431
  history-taking for, 1431–1433
  hysteroscopy of, 1437
  imaging assessment of, 1435–1436
  laboratory assessment of, 1433–1435, 1434b
  laparoscopy of, 1436–1437, 1437f
  magnetic resonance imaging of, 1436
  male. See Male reproductive system
  nutrition history for, 1432
  in older adults, 1431b
  physical assessment of, 1433
  psychosocial assessment of, 1433
  ultrasonography of, 1436
Residents, of skilled nursing facilities, 87, 87f
Resistin, 1225
Respect, 2, 9
Respiration
  accessory muscles of, 511
  assessment of, 63b
  neural regulation of, 189f
Respiratory acidosis, 13, 191t, 192, 194–195
Respiratory alkalosis, 13, 196, 196t
Respiratory bronchioles, 511f
Respiratory depression
  opioid analgesics as cause of, 62–63, 63t, 64b, 524b
  respiratory acidosis as cause of, 192
Respiratory hygiene/cough etiquette, 419, 419t
Respiratory infections, 573, 581
Respiratory system. See also Lung(s)
  in acid-base balance, 189–190, 189f, 189t
  acidosis effects on, 193, 193b
  age-related changes in, 234b, 512, 513b
  alkalosis effects on, 196, 196b
  anatomy of
    airways, 510, 511f
    alveolar ducts, 510
    bronchi, 510, 511f
    bronchioles, 510, 511f
    description of, 508–512
    larynx, 509f, 510, 517–518
    lungs, 510–511, 511f, 518–521
    nose, 509, 509f, 517, 556
    paranasal sinuses, 509, 509f, 517, 556
    pharynx, 509–510, 517–518
    sinuses, 509, 509f, 517, 556
    thorax, 518–521
    trachea, 510, 511f, 517–518
  assessment of
    capnography, 523, 523f, 524b
    capnometry, 523

Respiratory system (Continued)
    chest pain, 517
    chest x-rays, 521
    computed tomography, 521–522
    current health problems, 516–517
    description of, 90, 90t, 802
    diagnostic, 521–527
    dyspnea, 517, 517t
    endoscopy, 524–526
    exercise testing, 524
    family history, 516
    genetic risks, 516
    history-taking, 515–517
    imaging, 521–524
    laboratory, 521, 522b
    lung biopsy, 526–527
    orthopnea, 517
    physical, 517–521
    psychosocial, 521
    pulmonary function tests, 523–524, 525t
    pulse oximetry, 523, 523f
    in spinal cord injury, 896
    thoracentesis, 526, 526f
  dehydration effects on, 168
  description of, 508
  drug use effects on, 516
  fluid overload effects on, 171f
  health promotion and maintenance of, 512–515
  hypokalemia effects on, 176
  inhalant irritants that affect, 515
  leukemia effects on, 819
  nutrition assessments, 1213b
  oxygen delivery by, 512
  oxygen-hemoglobin dissociation curve, 512, 512f
  postoperative assessments of, 273–274
  postoperative procedures and exercises
    coughing and splinting, 244
    incentive spirometry, 243–244, 244f
  preoperative assessment of, 236
  respiratory adequacy indicators, 520–521
  sickle cell disease effects on, 810
  smoking effects on, 514
Respiratory system disorders
  acute respiratory distress syndrome. See Acute respiratory distress syndrome
  acute respiratory failure, 624–626, 625t
  asthma. See Asthma
  chronic obstructive pulmonary disease. See Chronic obstructive pulmonary disease
  coccidioidomycosis, 613
  cystic fibrosis. See Cystic fibrosis

Respiratory system disorders
    (Continued)
  idiopathic pulmonary fibrosis,
      585–586
  influenza. See Influenza
  inhalation anthrax, 611–612,
      612b
  Middle East respiratory syndrome,
      598
  peritonsillar abscess, 611
  pertussis, 613
  pulmonary arterial hypertension,
      584–585, 585t
  pulmonary embolism. See
      Pulmonary embolism
  rhinosinusitis, 610–611
  tuberculosis. See Tuberculosis
Respiratory tract
  infection transmission, 415
  lower, 510–511, 511f
  upper, 509–510, 509f
Respite care, 866, 949
Resting metabolic rate, 1228
Restless legs syndrome, 922–923
Restorative aides, 89
Restorative nursing programs, 96
Restorative proctocolectomy with
      ileo pouch-anal anastomosis,
      1154–1155, 1154f
Restraints
  alternatives to, 42b
  chemical, 41
  definition of, 41
  hospital use of, 41
Restrictive cardiomyopathy, 714–715,
      715t
Retained surgical items, 267
Rete pegs, 432, 432f
Retention sutures, 267
Reticular activating system, 841
Reticulocyte count, 804–805
Retina
  anatomy of, 957–958
  detachment of, 979–980
  holes of, 979–980
  macular degeneration of, 979
  tears of, 979–980
  ultrasonic imaging of, 967
Retinitis pigmentosa, 980
Retrograde pyelography, 1358
Retroperitoneal lymph node
      dissection, 1489
Retropubic suspension, 1349t
Retrovirus, 338
Reverse transcriptase, 337–340
Rewarming
  frostbite treated with, 144–145
  hypothermia treated with, 143
RFID. See Radiofrequency
      identification
Rh antigen system, 835
Rheumatic carditis, 714
Rheumatic disease, 304
Rheumatic endocarditis, 714
Rheumatic fever, 714

Rheumatoid arthritis
  arthrocentesis for, 321
  care coordination for, 325
  cervical, 319b
  clinical features of, 306t
  complementary and integrative
      health interventions for, 324
  coping strategies for patients with,
      325
  definition of, 318
  diagnostic assessments for, 321, 321b
  drug therapy for
    biological response modifiers,
        321–322, 323b
    disease-modifying
        antirheumatic drugs, 322
    nonsteroidal anti-inflammatory
        drugs, 321
  early stage of, 318–319
  etiology of, 318
  exercises for, 317b
  extra-articular manifestations of,
      319
  features of, 318b
  genetic risk of, 318
  health care resources for, 325
  home care management of, 325
  human leukocyte antigens and,
      318b
  incidence of, 318
  joint deformities associated with,
      319, 319f
  laboratory assessment of, 320–321,
      320b
  mobility interventions in, 324
  nonpharmacologic interventions
      for, 323–324
  osteoarthritis versus, 306t
  pain management in, 321–324
  pathophysiology of, 318
  prevalence of, 318
  psychosocial assessment of,
      319–320
  referrals for, 319
  self-esteem promotion in, 324–325
  self-management education for,
      325
  signs and symptoms of, 318–319,
      319f
  subcutaneous nodules associated
      with, 319
  transition management of, 325
  vasculitis associated with, 319
Rheumatoid factor, 320
Rheumatology, 304
Rhinoplasty, 556–557, 556f
Rhinorrhea, 880–881
Rhinosinusitis, 610–611
Rhonchi, 521t
Rib fracture, 636–637
Rifater, 608
Rifaximin, 1137
Right atrial pressure, 780
Right atrium, 642
Right coronary artery, 643–644, 643f

Right hemisphere stroke, 932–933,
      933b
Right ventricle, 642
Right ventricular failure, 696, 696b,
      782
Right-sided heart failure, 651, 692,
      694–695
Rigidity, 869
Rinne tuning fork test, 989–990
Risedronate, 1021
Rituximab (Rituxan), 323b
Rivastigmine, 871
Robotic surgery, 254–255, 789
Rods, 957–958
Rollator, 95
Rolling hiatal hernias, 1092–1093,
      1092f
Romberg sign, 850
Rosenbaum Pocket Vision Screener,
      964
Rosiglitazone, 1291, 1292b–1293b
Rotation, 1010f
Rotator cuff injuries, 1059
Rotigotine, 870
Roux-en-Y gastric bypass, 1229,
      1230f
RRTs. See Rapid response teams
Rubor, 652
Rule of nines, 492, 492f

S
Sacubitril/valsartan, 698, 704–705
Safe patient handling and mobility,
      93–95, 93b
Safer sex practices, 1505–1506
SAFEs. See Sexual assault forensic
      examiners
Safety
  attributes of, 4
  context of, 4–5
  culture of, 4–5
  definition of, 3
  in dehydration patients, 170
  emergency department staff,
      120–121, 120b
  in fluid overload, 172
  oxygen therapy, 530b
  scope of, 3–4
  surgical checklist for, 228–229,
      230f
Safety promotion, 2
Salem sump tube, 1124
Saline lock, 203
Salivary glands
  acute sialadenitis of, 1084–1085
  disorders involving, 1084–1085
  radiation therapy effects on,
      549
  tumors of, 1085
Salmeterol, 569b–570b, 570–571
Salmon calcitonin, 1022
Salpingitis, 1431, 1512
Salt tablets, 134
Salt water drowning, 147
Same-day admission, 229–230

SANE. See Sexual assault nurse
      examiners
Sarcoma
  Ewing's, 1025
  fibrosarcoma, 1025
  Kaposi's, 347, 348f, 354–355
  osteosarcoma, 1012, 1025
Sargramostim, 402t
SARS. See Severe acute respiratory
      syndrome
Saxagliptin, 1292b–1293b
SBAR, 5–6, 895
SBRT. See Stereotactic body
      radiotherapy
Scabies, 470–471, 471f, 1470
Scald injuries, 486
Scales, 438f
Schilling test, 1141
Schwartz-Bartter syndrome, 1251
SCIP. See Surgical Care Improvement
      Project
Sclera
  anatomy of, 957
  assessment of, 963
Scleral buckling, 980
Scleroderma, 329
Scoliosis, 1009, 1009f
Scorpion stings, 136–137, 137b, 137f,
      138t–140t
Scrotum, 1430
Seasonal influenza, 596–597
Sebaceous glands, 433
Sebum, 433
Second heart sound, 654
Secondary administration set, 209,
      209f
Secondary gout, 331
Secondary hypertension, 721, 721t
Secondary lesions, 436, 438f
Secondary prevention
  of cancer, 382
  of impaired cellular regulation, 15
  of sensory perception changes, 26
Secondary progressive multiple
      sclerosis, 888
Secondary survey and resuscitation
      interventions, 130
Secondary syphilis, 1508
Secondary tuberculosis, 606
Secondary tumors, 375
Second-degree frostbite, 144
Secondhand smoke, 514
Secukinumab, 369, 370b, 466b
Sedation
  moderate, 261–262, 262t
  opioid analgesics as cause of,
      62–63, 63t–64t
Segmented neutrophils, 292–293,
      293f
Seizures
  in acquired immunodeficiency
      syndrome, 355
  antiepileptic drugs for, 877–878,
      878b
  assessment of, 877

Seizures (Continued)
care coordination for, 880
definition of, 876
drug therapy for, 877–878
emergency care for, 879
at end of life, 111
etiology of, 877
generalized, 876
genetic risk for, 877
management of, 878
myoclonic, 876
nonsurgical management of, 877–879
partial, 876–877, 878b
partial corpus callosotomy for, 880
pathophysiology of, 876
precautions for, 878
prevention of, 877t
surgical management of, 879–880
tonic-clonic, 876, 878b–879b
transition management for, 880
types of, 876–877
unclassified, 877
vagal nerve stimulation for, 879
Selective estrogen receptor modulators, 1452, 1456. See also Estrogen agonists/antagonists
Selective internal radiation therapy, 1187
Selective serotonin reuptake inhibitors
depression treated with, 37
tramadol interactions with, 61
Self cells, 289–290, 290f
Self-determination, 9
Self-esteem
in amputation patients, 1054–1055
in burn injury patients, 504
in head and neck cancer patients, 553–554
in Parkinson disease patients, 872
in rheumatoid arthritis patients, 324–325
Self-management, 9
Self-management education
for activities of daily living, 100
for Alzheimer's disease, 866–867
for amputation, 1055–1056
for asthma, 567–568, 568b, 568f
for back pain, 908–909
for benign prostatic hyperplasia, 1481
for bone tumors, 1027–1028
for burn injury, 505
for cataracts, 971
for chronic kidney disease, 1424–1425
for chronic obstructive pulmonary disease, 581
for cirrhosis, 1179–1180, 1179b
for colorectal cancer, 1133–1135
for deep vein thrombosis, 746, 746b

Self-management education (Continued)
for dysrhythmias, 682
for esophageal tumors, 1100
for fractures, 1045
for gastric cancer, 1119
for glaucoma, 975–976
for gonorrhea, 1514
for head and neck cancer, 554–555
for hearing loss, 1002
for heart failure, 703–705, 704t
for hepatitis, 1185b
for human immunodeficiency virus infection, 356, 357b
for hypothyroidism, 1274
for ileostomy, 1157b
for infection, 426
for instrumental activities of daily living, 100
for intestinal obstructions, 1126
for leukemia, 826–827, 826b–827b
for low back pain, 908–909
for malnutrition, 1224
for multiple sclerosis, 892
for myasthenia gravis, 922, 922b
for obesity, 1231
for oral cancer, 1083, 1083b
for osteoarthritis, 317, 317b
for osteoporosis, 1022
for otitis media, 993
for oxygen therapy, 536
for pain, 68
for pancreatic cancer, 1209
for Parkinson disease, 872
for pelvic inflammatory disease, 1516–1517
for peptic ulcer disease, 1114–1115
for pneumonia, 605
in postoperative period, 286–287
for prostate cancer, 1486, 1486b
for pulmonary embolism, 623, 623b
for pyelonephritis, 1376
for rheumatoid arthritis, 325
for sepsis, 766
for spinal cord injury, 902
for stomatitis, 1078
for stroke, 939–940, 940f
for systemic lupus erythematosus, 328
for total hip arthroplasty, 312b
for tracheostomy, 544
for traumatic brain injury, 949, 949b
for tuberculosis, 610
for ulcerative colitis, 1156–1157
for urinary incontinence, 1353, 1353b
for urolithiasis, 1366b
for uterine leiomyomas, 1463
for valvular heart disease, 710, 710b
Self-monitoring of blood glucose, 1298, 1317

Self-tolerance, 289–290
Sella turcica, 1243
Semicircular canals, 985–986
Semi-Fowlers position, 21
Semilunar valves, 643, 643f
Seminoma, 1487, 1487t
Semipermeable membrane, 163
Semmes-Weinstein monofilaments, 1305–1306, 1306f
Senile angiomas, 439f
Sensorineural hearing loss, 989, 997, 997t
Sensory function assessments, 849
Sensory neurons, 839–840
Sensory perception
auditory. See Ear(s); Hearing
cancer effects on, 385
definition of, 957
description of, 26–27, 27f
fall risks caused by changes in, 33
in spinal cord injury, 896, 896b
stroke-related changes in, 934, 939
after traumatic brain injury, 948–949
visual. See Eye(s); Vision
Sensory receptors, 842
Sentinel events, 4–5
Sepsis
assessment of, 763–764
burn wound, 497–498, 498t
care coordination for, 765–766
definition of, 407, 753, 760–761
description of, 28
diagnostic criteria for, 762t
etiology of, 762
health promotion and maintenance for, 763
home care management of, 766, 766b
inadequate antimicrobial therapy as cause of, 423
incidence of, 762
indicators of, 498t
infection as cause of, 760–761
interventions for, 765, 765t
laboratory assessment of, 764
as oncologic emergency, 407
pathophysiology of, 760–762
in pneumonia, 604
predisposing factors for, 762t
prevalence of, 762
prevention of, 604, 812, 1101
psychosocial assessment of, 764
self-management education for, 766
in sickle cell disease, 812
signs and symptoms of, 763–764
Surviving Sepsis Campaign for, 765
transition management for, 765–766
September 11, 2001, 150
Septic shock
assessment of, 763–764
definition of, 753, 762
description of, 423

Septic shock (Continued)
health promotion and maintenance for, 763
interventions for, 765
predisposing factors for, 762t
progression of, 760, 760f
signs and symptoms of, 763–764
Septicemia, 407
Sequestrectomy, 1024
Sequestrum, 1022
Serologic testing, 425
Serosanguineous drainage, 277
Serotonin antagonists, for chemotherapy-induced nausea and vomiting, 399b
Serous drainage, 277
Serum creatinine, 1331, 1332b
Serum ferritin test, 805
Serum protein electrophoresis, 918
Serum sickness, 366
Severe acute respiratory syndrome, 598
Sex, 1493, 1493t
Sex chromosomes, 74, 75f
Sex hormones, 1238
Sex-linked recessive pattern of inheritance, 78t, 79–80, 80f
Sexual assault forensic examiners, 118
Sexual assault nurse examiners, 118
Sexual disinhibition, 861
Sexual dysfunction, 1286
Sexual orientation, 11t
Sexual transmission, of HIV infection, 341–343
Sexuality
assessment of, 90
breast cancer and, 1445
description of, 27–28
hysterectomy effects on, 1462b
multiple sclerosis effects on, 890, 892
spinal cord injury effects on, 901–902
Sexually transmitted infections
assessment of, 1507b
chlamydia infection, 1511–1512
complications caused by, 1505t
condylomata acuminata, 1510–1511, 1510f
genital herpes, 1506–1508, 1507b
gonorrhea, 1512–1514, 1513f
health promotion and maintenance for, 1505–1506, 1506t
Healthy People 2020 objectives for, 1505, 1506t
interventions for, 27
in lesbian, gay, bisexual, transgender, and queer population, 1509b
in older adults, 1505b
overview of, 1504–1505
pelvic inflammatory disease secondary to. See Pelvic inflammatory disease

Sexually transmitted infections
(Continued)
prevalence of, 1504–1505, 1505b
safer sex practices for prevention
of, 1505–1506
screening for, 27
syphilis, 1508–1510, 1508f
Shave biopsy, 445
Shearing forces, 448, 448f
Sheehan's syndrome, 1246
Shigellosis, 1148t, 1149
Shingles. See Herpes zoster
Shivering, 135, 280
Shock
acute pancreatitis as cause of,
1198, 1199b
cardiogenic
acute coronary syndrome as
cause of, 782
etiology of, 753
risk factors for, 752t, 756b
classification of, 751
clinical features of, 752b
definition of, 751
distributive
chemical-induced, 753
etiology of, 753
risk factors for, 752t, 756b
hypovolemic
adaptive responses and events
during, 754t
assessment of, 756–758
care coordination for, 760
concept map for, 756f–757f
drug therapy for, 759b
etiology of, 752–753, 755
in fractures, 1034
health promotion and
maintenance for, 756
incidence of, 755
laboratory assessment of, 758,
758b
nonsurgical management of,
758–760, 759b
pathophysiology of, 754–755
physical assessment of, 756–758
prevalence of, 755
risk factors for, 752t, 756b
signs and symptoms of,
756–758
surgical management of, 760
transition management for, 760
multiple organ dysfunction
syndrome secondary to,
754–755, 755b
obstructive
etiology of, 753
risk factors for, 752t
overview of, 751–754
risk factors for, 756b
septic. See Septic shock
signs and symptoms of, 752, 752b
stages of, 754–755
types of, 752–754
Short bones, 1005

Short Michigan Alcoholism
Screening Test—Geriatric
Version, 38
Short peripheral catheters, 202–204,
202f–203f, 202t, 203b, 214–215
Short-acting beta₂ agonists, 568–570,
569b–570b
SIADH. See Syndrome of
inappropriate antidiuretic
hormone
Sialadenitis
acute, 1084–1085
post-irradiation, 1085
Sickle cell anemia. See Sickle cell
disease
Sickle cell disease
acute chest syndrome in, 810,
812
assessment of, 809–811
care coordination for, 812–813
crises in, 809, 811, 812b
definition of, 808
etiology of, 809
genetic risk of, 809
hematopoietic stem cell
transplantation for, 812
history-taking for, 809–810
hydroxyurea in, 811
imaging assessment of, 811
incidence of, 809
jaundice associated with, 810
laboratory assessment of, 810–811
pain management in, 811–812
pathophysiology of, 808–809
perfusion affected by, 809
physical assessment of, 810
pregnancy in, 813b
prevalence of, 809
priapism in, 810
psychosocial assessment of, 810
red blood cell transfusion for, 812
self-management education for,
812–813, 813b
sepsis prevention in, 812
signs and symptoms of, 810
transition management for,
812–813
ulcers associated with, 810
vaso-occlusive events, 809
Sickle cell trait, 79, 809
Sigmoid colon, 1064
Sigmoid colostomy, 1131f, 1134
Sigmoidoscopy
colorectal cancer diagnosis using,
1128b, 1129
description of, 1073
Sigmoidostomy, 1368f
Sign language, 1001
Sildenafil, 146, 1489
Silver sulfadiazine, 501b
Simple facemask, 532, 532t, 533f
Simple fracture, 1032
Simple hemothorax, 637
Simple surgery, 232t
Simponi. See Golimumab

SIMV. See Synchronized intermittent
mandatory ventilation
Sinemet, 870, 923
Single gene traits, 74
Single nucleotide polymorphisms,
76–77
Single-fiber electromyography, for
myasthenia gravis, 918
Single-incision laparoscopic
cholecystectomy, 1195
Single-photon emission computed
tomography, 854
Singultus, 1123
Sinoatrial node, 664, 672–673
Sinus(es)
anatomy of, 509, 509f
assessment of, 517
cancer of, 556
Sinus arrhythmia, 671
Sinus dysrhythmias, 672–675
Sinus tachycardia, 673, 673f
Sipuleucel-T, 402t
Sirolimus
autoimmune diseases treated with,
368
immunosuppression uses of, 302b
SIRS. See Systemic inflammatory
response syndrome
Sitagliptin, 1292b–1293b
Situational awareness, 157
Situational depression, 36
Sjögren's syndrome, 319–320
Skeletal system. See also
Musculoskeletal system
anatomy of, 1005–1007, 1005f
assessment of, 1009–1010
bone. See Bone
imaging assessment of, 1011–1013
radiography of, 1011
Skeletal traction, 1040
Skene's glands, 1429
Skilled nursing facilities
rehabilitation in, 87
residents of, 87, 87f
Skin
age-related changes in, 234b, 433,
652, 800b
anatomy of, 431–432, 432f
assessment of, 90t, 91, 433–445,
651–652, 802
barrier functions of, 415
burn injury-related changes to,
481–485, 484f, 491
cleanliness of, 439
in dark-skin patients, 443–444,
444b
dehydration effects on, 168
diagnostic assessment of, 444–445
edema effects on, 437
functions of, 433, 433t, 482
history-taking for, 433–436, 435b
hydration effects on, 436
inflammation of, 443
inspection of, 436–439
laboratory testing of, 444–445

Skin (Continued)
leukemia effects on, 819
nutrition assessments, 1213b
palpation of, 440–441, 440t
postoperative assessments of,
277–278, 278f
preoperative assessment of, 237
psychosocial assessment of, 444
radiation therapy effects on,
1084
sebaceous glands of, 433
self-examination of, 476
sepsis manifestations of, 764
sickle cell disease effects on, 810
structure of, 431–432, 432f
sweat glands of, 433
systemic lupus erythematosus
manifestations of, 326–328,
327f
temperature of, 652
trauma to
collaborative management of,
474
pathophysiology of, 471–474
turgor of, 441
Wood's light examination of, 445
Skin biopsy, 445
Skin cancer, 380b
assessment of, 436–437, 477
basal cell carcinoma, 475t, 476,
476f
collaborative care for, 476–477
drug therapy for, 477
etiology of, 475–476
genetic risk of, 475–476
health promotion and
maintenance for, 476
incidence of, 476
melanoma, 475t, 476, 476f
nonsurgical management of,
477
pathophysiology of, 474–476
prevalence of, 476
prevention of, 476b
radiation therapy for, 477
squamous cell carcinoma,
475–476, 475f, 475t
surgical management of, 477
types of, 475f, 475t
Skin care
in diarrhea patients, 1142b
infection spread prevention
through, 469
in older adults, 216–222
postoperative, 281b
for pressure injury prevention, 97
in systemic lupus erythematosus
patients, 328
for ulcerative colitis, 1156b
Skin color, 436, 437t
Skin disorders
inflammatory, 458–459, 462–463,
463b
pressure injuries. See Pressure
injuries

Skin disorders (Continued)
  pruritus, 461–462
  psoriasis. See Psoriasis
  Stevens-Johnson syndrome, 478, 478f
  toxic epidermal necrolysis, 478
  urticaria, 462
Skin grafts, for burn wound management, 500–501
Skin infections
  assessment of, 469
  bacterial, 466–468, 466f, 467b
  cutaneous anthrax, 466, 467f
  drug therapy for, 470
  folliculitis, 466, 467b
  fungal, 467b, 468
  furuncles, 466, 466f, 467b
  health promotion and maintenance for, 468–469
  history-taking for, 469
  methicillin-resistant Staphylococcus aureus as cause of, 466
  pathophysiology of, 466–470
  transmission-based precautions for, 469–470
  viral, 467b, 468
Skin lesions
  configuration of, 439t
  primary, 436, 438f
  secondary, 436, 438f
Skin substitutes, 458
Skin traction, 1040, 1041f
Skin turgor, 168, 169f
Skinfold measurements, 1215
Sleep deprivation, 845–846
Sleep disorders, 40
Sliding board, 901
Sliding hiatal hernias, 1092, 1092f
Slip lock, 210
Slit-lamp examination, 965, 965f
Slow continuous ultrafiltration, 1398
SLPs. See Speech-language pathologists
Small bowel capsule endoscopy, 1071–1072
Small intestine
  anatomy of, 1064
  functions of, 1064
  obstruction of, 1123b
Small molecule inhibitor targeted therapy, 403–405, 403f–404f, 404t
Smart pumps, for infusion therapy, 211
SMAST-G. See Short Michigan Alcoholism Screening Test—Geriatric Version
Smoke detectors, 488–489
Smoke poisoning, 491
Smoking
  assessment of, 514
  carboxyhemoglobin levels, 233–234

Smoking (Continued)
  cardiovascular disease risks, 512–514, 647
  cessation of, 514–515, 515b, 555, 1308
  chronic obstructive pulmonary disease caused by, 14, 21, 573
  hookah, 514
  pack-years for, 514
  passive, 514
  pneumonia risks secondary to, 605
  prevalence of, 514b
  secondhand smoke, 514
  social, 514
  surgical risks associated with, 232–233
  in transgender community, 1494
Smooth muscle, 1007
Snakebites, 135–137, 136b, 136f–137f, 136t, 138t–140t
Snellen eye chart, 963–964
SNFs. See Skilled nursing facilities
SNP. See Single nucleotide polymorphism
SNS. See Sympathetic nervous system
Social justice, 9
Social smokers, 514
Social workers
  in emergency departments, 119–120
  in rehabilitation settings, 89
Sodium
  description of, 173–175
  in older adults, 165b
  restriction of
    in chronic kidney disease, 1408
    cirrhosis managed with, 1175
  serum levels of, 164t
Sodium channel blockers, 677b–678b
Sodium imbalances
  hypernatremia, 174–175, 175t
  hyponatremia, 173–174, 174t
Sodium lauryl sulfate, 1077
Sodium polystyrene sulfonate, for hyperkalemia, 20
Sodium-glucose cotransport inhibitors, 1292b–1293b, 1294
Solar keratosis, 475, 475t
Solifenacin, 98
Solutes, 161
Solvent, 161
Somatic mutations, 76
Somatic pain, 48
Somatomedins, 1246
Somatosensory evoked potentials, 855
Somatostatin, 1239–1240
Somogyi phenomenon, 1296
Soriatane. See Acitretin
Sotalol, 677b–678b, 685
Sound
  decibel scale for, 990
  intensity of, 990

Sound judgment, 8
Spastic paralysis, 933, 938
Specific gravity, 1332–1333
Specific morphology, 373
SPECT. See Single-photon emission computed tomography
Speech
  assessment of, 847
  in Parkinson disease patients, 871–872
Speech and language rehabilitation, 552
Speech audiometry, 991
Speech discrimination testing, 991
Speech reception threshold, 991
Speech-language pathologist, 89
Speech-language pathologist assistants, 89
Sphenoid sinus, 509f
Sphincter of Oddi, 1064, 1192
Sphincterotomy, 1201
Spider angiomas, 1173
Spider bites, 136–137, 137b, 137f, 138t–140t
Spinal anesthesia, 261t, 262f, 275, 275b
Spinal column, 225
Spinal cord
  functions of, 842, 887
  hemorrhage of, 894
  multiple sclerosis. See Multiple sclerosis
Spinal cord compression, 408
Spinal cord injury
  aging and, 902b
  airway management in, 897–898
  assessment of, 895–897
  autonomic dysreflexia in, 896, 896b, 898, 898b
  axial loading as cause of, 894, 895f
  cardiovascular assessment in, 896
  care coordination for, 901–903, 901f
  cervical, 896–897
  cervical collar for, 899, 899f
  complete, 894
  complications of, 897
  contractures secondary to, 900–901
  "cough assist" technique in, 897–898, 898f
  drug therapy for, 900
  etiology of, 895
  functional electrical stimulation for, 902
  gastrointestinal assessment in, 896–897
  genitourinary assessment in, 896–897
  halo fixator device for, 899, 899b
  health care resources for, 903
  history-taking for, 895
  home care management of, 901–902
  hydration for, 898

Spinal cord injury (Continued)
  hyperextension as cause of, 894, 895f
  hyperflexion as cause of, 894, 894f
  imaging assessment of, 897
  incidence of, 895
  incomplete, 894
  laboratory assessment of, 897
  mechanism of injury, 894–895, 894f–895f
  mobility affected by, 23, 896, 900–901
  neurogenic shock after, 898
  pathophysiology of, 894–895
  penetrating trauma as cause of, 894
  physical assessment of, 896–897
  pressure injury risks secondary to, 901–903
  prevalence of, 895
  psychosocial adaptation for, 901
  psychosocial assessment of, 897
  rehabilitation for, 901–902
  respiratory assessment in, 896
  respiratory secretion management in, 897
  secondary, 894, 899–900, 899b, 899f
  self-management education for, 902
  sensory perception assessments in, 896, 896b
  sexuality affected by, 901–902
  signs and symptoms of, 896–897
  spinal immobilization and stabilization after, 899–900, 899b, 899f–900f
  surgical management of, 900
  traction for, 899
  transition management for, 901–903, 901f
  venous thromboembolism risks secondary to, 897
  vertical compression as cause of, 894, 895f
  in veterans, 903b
Spinal cord stimulation, 66, 909, 909b
Spinal fusion, 906, 908
Spinal nerves, 842
Spinal osteoarthritis, 307
Spinal shock, 896
Spine board, 945
Spine stabilization, 147
SPINK1 gene, 1202
Spiritual counselors, 89
Spiritual distress, 113
Spirituality, 108
Spironolactone, 1261, 1498
Spleen
  in blood formation, 797
  liver-spleen scan, 1073
  red pulp of, 797
  white pulp of, 797
Splenectomy, 797, 831, 1207

Splenic infarction, 711
Splenomegaly, 1067, 1170
Splint(s), 1038
Splinter hemorrhages, 711
Spondee, 991
Spontaneous bacterial peritonitis, 1171, 1175
Spores, 612
Sports-related injuries, 1056, 1056b, 1057f, 1057t
S-pouch, 1154, 1154f
Sprain, 1057t
Sputum, 516
Squamous cell carcinoma
    description of, 475–476, 475f, 475t
    esophageal, 1095
    oral, 1079
Squamous metaplasia, 548
St. John's wort, 701, 801–802
ST segment, 669, 669f
Staff nurses, 155
Staff safety, 4
Staffing, infection control through, 421
Standard Precautions, 418–419, 419t, 1358
Stapedectomy, 1000–1001, 1000f
Stapes, 984, 985f
Staphylococcal endotoxin, 1105
Staples, 268f
Starling's law, 645, 692–694
Starvation, 1221–1222
Statins
    for atherosclerosis, 731b
    myocardial infarction treated with, 777
Status asthmaticus, 572
Status epilepticus, 879
Stay sutures, 268f
Steal syndrome, 1415
Steatorrhea, 1068–1070, 1141, 1159, 1194, 1203
Steatosis, 1185–1186
Stelara. See Ustekinumab
ST-elevation myocardial infarction, 770
Stem cell transplantation, for breast cancer, 1452
Stem cells. See also Hematopoietic stem cell transplantation
    bone marrow production of, 290, 291f
    differentiation and maturation of, 290, 291f, 293
Stents, 783
Stereotactic body radiotherapy, 388
Stereotactic pallidotomy, for Parkinson disease, 872
Stereotactic radiosurgery, 952, 952f
Sterilization, 418
Sternal split procedure, 921
Sternal wound infection, 785, 788–789
Stevens-Johnson syndrome, 478, 478f, 1359b

Stings, 137, 137b, 137f, 138t–140t, 141b
Stoma
    colostomy, 1131–1132, 1132f
    home care management of, 1134b
    ileostomy, 1153, 1154b
    measurement of, 1134
    after total laryngectomy, 551, 554–555
Stomach
    anatomy of, 1063
    description of, 1103
    ulcers of, 1107–1109, 1108f
Stomach disorders
    cancer. See Gastric cancer
    gastritis. See Gastritis
    peptic ulcer disease. See Peptic ulcer(s); Peptic ulcer disease
Stomatitis, 399–400, 820, 1076–1078, 1401
Stool tests, 1068–1070, 1111
STOP-Bang Sleep Apnea Questionnaire, 559
Storytelling, during dying, 112
Strain, 1057t
Strangulated hernia, 1138
Strangulated obstruction, 1122, 1125
Stratum corneum, 432, 432f
Stratum germinativum, 432, 432f
Stratum granulosum, 432, 432f
Stratum lucidum, 432
Stress
    coping with, 32–33
    family caregiver, 866b
    management of, 1137
    in older adults, 32–33
    in transgender patients, 1494
Stress debriefing, 157
Stress fracture, 1032
Stress incontinence, 1344, 1348, 1349t, 1464
Stress testing, 659–660, 660f
Stress ulcers, 1108
Stretta procedure, 1091, 1091b
Striae, 1242, 1257
Striated muscle, 1007
Strictures
    bowel, 1161
    esophageal, 1088, 1096
    urinary tract, 1383
Stricturoplasty, 1161
Stridor, 274, 364, 636
Stroke. See also Transient ischemic attack
    anterior cerebral artery, 933b
    antithrombotics for, 937
    aphasia after, 938, 938t
    assessment of, 930–935
    in atrial fibrillation, 16
    cardiovascular assessment in, 934
    care coordination for, 939–940
    carotid artery angioplasty with stenting for, 936
    cerebral perfusion in, 935–938

Stroke (Continued)
    cognitive changes associated with, 932–933
    communication promotion after, 938
    complications of, 937
    cranial nerve function assessments after, 934
    definition of, 928
    depression after, 939
    diabetes mellitus as risk factor for, 1284
    drug therapy for, 937–938
    embolectomy for, 936
    embolic, 928–929, 929t, 934
    emotional lability assessments in, 934
    endovascular interventions for, 936
    etiology of, 929
    fibrinolytic therapy for, 935
    genetic risk of, 929
    health care resources for, 940
    health promotion and maintenance for, 930
    hemorrhagic, 929, 929t
    history-taking for, 930–931
    home care management of, 939
    imaging assessment of, 935
    incidence of, 929–930
    increased intracranial pressure monitoring after, 936–937, 936b
    internal cerebral artery, 933b
    interventions for, 935–938
    intracranial bleeding-induced, 831
    ischemic, 927–929, 929t, 935
    laboratory assessment of, 934–935
    left hemisphere, 932–933, 933b
    level of consciousness assessments in, 931–932
    magnetic resonance angiography of, 935
    middle cerebral artery, 933b
    mobility after, 933–934, 938
    National Institutes of Health Stroke Scale, 931, 931t–932t
    nonsurgical management of, 935–938
    pathophysiology of, 928–930
    physical assessment of, 931–935
    posterior cerebral artery, 933b
    prevalence of, 929–930
    psychosocial assessment of, 934
    racial predilection for, 930b
    recurrence of, 940
    right hemisphere, 932–933, 933b
    risk factors for, 930b
    self-management education for, 939–940, 940f
    sensory changes caused by, 934
    sensory perception changes after, 934, 939
    signs and symptoms of, 931–935
    thrombotic, 928, 929t

Stroke (Continued)
    transition management for, 939–940
    types of, 928–929, 928f, 929t
    vertebrobasilar artery, 933b
    visual loss secondary to, 934, 934f
    in women, 935b
Stroke center, 930, 939
Stroke syndromes, 933b
Stroke volume, 645, 692–694
Stromelysin, 305
Strong acid, 186
Strong bases, 186
Struvite stones, 1364
Stuart-Prower factor, 798t
Stuporous, 846
Subacute thyroiditis, 1275
Subarachnoid hemorrhage
    cerebral vasospasm after, 937
    description of, 929, 931
Subarachnoid space, 225, 840
Subclavian dialysis catheters, 1397f
Subclavian steal, 741t
Subcutaneous emphysema, 518
    definition of, 1036
    in fracture patients, 1036
    laryngeal trauma as cause of, 559–560
    tracheostomy as cause of, 539
Subcutaneous fat, 431, 432f
Subcutaneous infusion therapy, 223
Subcutaneous nodules, in rheumatoid arthritis, 319
Subdural hematoma, 942–943, 942f, 954
Subdural space, 840
Sublimaze. See Fentanyl
Submucous resection, 557
Substance P, 56–57
Substance use, 38–39
Substantia nigra, 868
Subsys. See Fentanyl
Subtotal thyroidectomy, 1269
Sucralfate, 1112
Suctioning
    of artificial airway, 541–542, 541b
    in chronic obstructive pulmonary disease, 579
Sulfamethoxazole/trimethoprim, 1359b–1360b
Sulfasalazine, 1152, 1152b
Sulfonylureas, 1291, 1292b–1293b
Sundowning, 861
Superior oblique muscle, 960t
Superior rectus muscle, 960t
Superior vena cava, 408–409
Superior vena cava syndrome, 408–409, 409f
Superstorm Sandy, 151
Supervision
    definition of, 6
    of unlicensed assistive personnel, 6
Supination, 1010f
Supine position, 265, 265f
Support systems, 92b

Suppressor genes, 378
Suppressor T-cells, 299
Suppurative cholangitis, 1192
Supraglottic partial laryngectomy, 551t
Supratentorial lesion, 840
Supratentorial tumors, 950
Supraventricular tachycardia, 676–678
Surfactant, 147, 510
Surgeon, 253t
Surgery
    administering regularly scheduled drugs before, 241–242
    American Society of Anesthesiologists Physical Status Classification system, 230–232, 233t, 257
    antibiotic prophylaxis before, 247
    appendicitis treated with, 1148
    back pain treated with, 906–908, 907b
    benign prostatic hyperplasia treated with, 1479–1480, 1480b, 1480f
    blood donation for, 235
    brain tumors treated with, 952–954
    breast cancer treated with, 1447–1452, 1448f, 1453b
    breast-conserving, 1447, 1448f
    cancer treated with, 386–387
    cataracts treated with, 969–971, 970f
    categories of, 232t
    cholecystitis treated with, 1195–1197
    chronic obstructive pulmonary disease managed with, 579–580
    complications of, 272t
        pulmonary, 233–234
        risk factors for, 233t
    consent for, 239–241, 240f
    cost reduction in, 228
    Crohn's disease treated with, 1161
    Cushing's disease treated with, 1258–1259
    cystic fibrosis treated with, 583–584
    discharge planning before, 235
    elective, 232t
    emergent, 232t
    esophageal tumors treated with, 1098–1100, 1099f
    fractures managed with, 1042–1043, 1042f
    gastric cancer treated with, 1116–1118, 1117f
    gastroesophageal reflux disease treated with, 1091
    glaucoma treated with, 975
    head and neck cancer treated with, 550–553

Surgery (Continued)
    hearing loss treated with, 999–1001
    hernia treated with, 1138–1139
    hiatal hernias treated with, 1093–1095
    history-taking before, 230–235
    hyperpituitarism treated with, 1249–1250
    informed consent for, 239–241, 240f
    low back pain treated with, 906–908, 907b
    lung cancer treated with, 589–593
    medical history before, 233–234
    minimally invasive. See Minimally invasive surgery
    myasthenia gravis treated with, 921
    NPO status before, 241
    obesity treated with, 1229–1231, 1230f, 1231b
    in older adults, 232
    oral cancer treated with, 1081–1083
    overview of, 229–249
    pain caused by, 47
    pancreatic cancer treated with, 1207–1208, 1207f
    patient identification before, 241
    patient positioning for, 264–267, 265f, 267b
    pelvic organ prolapse treated with, 1464–1465
    peritonitis treated with, 1146
    postoperative period. See Postoperative period
    preoperative period. See Preoperative period
    previous procedures, 234
    radical, 232t
    readiness for, 229
    reasons for, 232t
    robotic, 254–255
    safety checklist for, 228–229, 230f
    same-day admission, 229–230
    simple, 232t
    skin cancer treated with, 477
    skin preparation before, 242, 243f
    Surgical Care Improvement Project measures, 229, 231t, 244, 282
    trigeminal neuralgia treated with, 924
    types of, 232t
    ulcerative colitis treated with, 1153–1155, 1155f
    urgency of, 232t
    urgent, 232t
    urinary incontinence treated with, 1348–1349, 1349t
    urolithiasis treated with, 1364–1365
Surgical assistant, 253t

Surgical attire, 256, 256f
Surgical Care Improvement Project, 229, 231t, 244, 282
Surgical scrub, 256, 257f
Surgical settings
    inpatient, 229–230
    outpatient, 229–230
Surgical site infections
    after coronary artery bypass grafting, 786b
    definition of, 267
    after oral cancer surgery, 1083
    predisposing factors for, 242
    Surgical Care Improvement Project measures for, 229
Surgical suite
    fire safety in, 252
    layout of, 252
    occupational hazards in, 252
    patient transfer to, 247–249
    safety in, 252–256
    surgical attire in, 256, 256f
Surgical team
    gloving of, 256, 257f
    gowning of, 256, 257f
    health and hygiene of, 255
    members of, 252, 253t
    safety of, 252–256
    surgical attire worn by, 256, 256f
    surgical scrub by, 256, 257f
Surviving Sepsis Campaign, 765
Susceptibility genes, 76
Sustained immunity, 298
Sutures
    absorbable, 267
    nonabsorbable, 267
SVT. See Supraventricular tachycardia
Swallowing, 1062
    aspiration prevention during, 543b, 553
    evaluation of, 553
    supraglottic method of, 553, 553b
Swallowing therapy, 1097
Swimmer's ear. See External otitis
Swimming, 32
Syme amputation, 1051, 1051f
Sympathectomy, 1042
Sympathetic nervous system, 842
    burn injury compensation, 486, 487f
    heart failure stimulation of, 692
Sympathetic tone, 752
Sympathomimetics
    acute coronary syndromes treated with, 783b
    description of, 1228–1229
Synapse, 840
Synaptic cleft, 840
Synaptic knob, 840
Synarthrodial joints, 1006
Synchronized intermittent mandatory ventilation, 631, 636t
Syncope
    definition of, 650–651, 1285
    description of, 618, 706

Syndrome of inappropriate antidiuretic hormone
    characteristics of, 1251–1253, 1252t
    as oncologic emergency, 407–408
    signs and symptoms of, 954
Syndrome X, 771
Syngeneic stem cells, 822
Synovial joint, 1006–1007
Synovitis, 1006–1007, 1057
Syphilis, 1508–1510, 1508f
Syringe pumps, 211
Systemic inflammatory response syndrome, 761–762, 761f, 762t, 763b, 881
Systemic lupus erythematosus
    care coordination of, 328
    definition of, 326
    drug therapy for, 327–328
    features of, 326b
    laboratory assessment of, 327
    pathophysiology of, 326
    psychosocial assessment of, 327
    self-management education for, 328
    signs and symptoms of, 326–327, 327f
    skin manifestations of, 326–327, 327f
    skin protection in, 328, 328b
    transition management of, 328
Systemic necrotizing vasculitis, 334t
Systemic sclerosis, 326b, 329–330, 330b
Systole, 644, 706
Systolic blood pressure, 646
Systolic heart failure, 692
Systolic murmurs, 655

T
T3. See Triiodothyronine
T4. See Thyroxine
T cells
    differentiation of, 295f
    subsets of, 299
T wave, 669, 669f, 671
Tachycardia
    heart rate in, 670
    paroxysmal supraventricular, 676
    sinus, 673, 673f
    supraventricular, 676–678
    ventricular, 684, 684f
Tachydysrhythmias, 668b, 672
Tacrolimus, 302b, 1303
Tactile fremitus, 518–519
Tactile stimulation, for pain management, 496
Tadalafil, 146
Tamponade effect, 1341
Tapentadol, 61
Tar preparations, 464
Target tissues, 1234–1235
Targeted therapy
    breast cancer treated with, 1452
    esophageal tumors treated with, 1097–1098

Targeted therapy (Continued)
    oral cancer treated with, 1081
    pancreatic cancer treated with, 1207
    renal cell carcinoma treated with, 1386
Taste sense
    age-related changes in, 31
    oral cancer effects on, 1083
Tattoos, 439
Tbo-filgrastim, 402t
TBPI. See Toe brachial pressure index
TBSA. See Total body surface area
TeamSTEPPS, 6
Teamwork
    attributes of, 5
    definition of, 5
    scope of, 5
Technetium scan, 661
Technology
    attributes of, 8
    context of, 8
    definition of, 7
    scope of, 8
Telangiectasias, 748
Telaprevir, 1185t
Telehealth, 101
Telemetry, 667
Teleneurology, 935
Telerehabilitation, 101
Teletherapy, 388
Temporal arteritis, 334t
Temporal lobe, 841t
Temporary pacing, 674–675
Tendons
    definition of, 1007
    rupture of, 1057t
Tenesmus, 1150, 1166
Tenofovir, 1185t
TENS. See Transcutaneous electrical nerve stimulation
Tension pneumothorax, 637–638
Tentorium, 840
Teriparatide, 1022
Terminal dehydration, 115
Terminal delirium, 111
Terminal knob, 840
Terminally ill patients, withholding food in, 1219
Tertiary syphilis, 1508–1509
Testes
    anatomy of, 1430, 1430f
    hormones produced by, 1235t
    palpation of, 1242
    self-examination of, 1486b
Testicular cancer
    assessment of, 1487
    chemotherapy for, 1488–1489
    classification of, 1486–1487, 1487t
    laboratory assessment of, 1487
    pathophysiology of, 1486–1487
    psychosocial assessment of, 1487
    surgical management of, 1488
Testicular self-examination, 1486b

Testicular tumors, 1486–1487, 1487t
Testosterone, 1430, 1481–1482, 1498
Tetanus, 145
Tetany, 1269
Thalamus, 840, 840f
Thalidomide, 369
Thallium imaging, 661
Thallium scan, 1011–1012
The Joint Commission
    care coordination recommendations, 3
    emergency department metrics, 117–118
    emergency preparedness plan, 150
    family-centered care, 2
    interprofessional communication strategies, 5
    lesbian, gay, bisexual, transgender, and queer population, 1495, 1495b
    medication reconciliation requirements, 4b
    National Patient Safety Goals
        blood components, 200, 833
        blood donation, 235
        description of, 4–5, 8
        drug safety, 201
        for falls, 40–41, 1018, 1020
        hand-off communication, 120, 317
        hand-off report, 271
        handwashing, 882, 1100
        infection control, 417
        influenza vaccine, 596–597
        informed consent, 658
        nutrition screening, 1212
        patient identification, 247, 262–263, 262b
        preoperative requirements, 238–239
        pressure injuries, 448–449
        surgical communication, 229
        tracheostomy communication, 544
        transfusion therapy, 833
        warfarin monitoring, 745
    restraints used by hospitals, 41
    sentinel event reporting requirements, 4–5
    tobacco use screening, 514–515
Therapeutic hypothermia, 947
Therapeutic Touch, 109
Thermal burns, 488, 491
Thermoregulation, 135b
Thiazide diuretics, 699, 725b
Thiazolidinediones, 1291, 1292b–1293b
Third space fluid, 19
Third spacing, 485, 1145, 1170
Third-degree frostbite, 144
Thirst, 164
Thoracentesis, 526, 526f, 593

Thoracic aortic aneurysms, 738–739
Thoracic outlet syndrome, 741t
Thoracotomy, 638
Thorax assessments, 518–521
Threshold (hearing), 990
Thrombectomy, 736, 738, 745
Thrombocytopenia
    chemotherapy as cause of, 395, 397–398, 588
    definition of, 815, 817
    description of, 15
    heparin-induced, 832
    injury prevention in patients with, 398b
    management of, 825b
    platelet count in, 805
Thrombocytosis, 321
Thrombolytic therapy
    contraindications for, 778t
    deep vein thrombosis treated with, 745
    myocardial infarction treated with, 777–778, 778t
Thrombophlebitis
    definition of, 742
    intravenous therapy as cause of, 217t–219t
    management of, 743
Thrombopoietin, 300t, 797
Thrombosis
    arterial, 16b
    deep vein. See Deep vein thrombosis
    definition of, 15–16
    intravenous therapy as cause of, 217t–219t
    mesenteric artery, 16b
    vascular stasis as cause of, 816
    venous, 15–16
Thrombotic stroke, 928, 929t
Thrombotic thrombocytopenic purpura, 831
Thromboxane A$_2$, 798
Thrombus. See also Thrombosis
    definition of, 742
    etiology of, 742
    stroke caused by, 928
Thrush, 347f, 468
Thymoma, 918
Thyrocalcitonin, 179, 1239
Thyroid cancer, 1275
Thyroid cartilage, 510
Thyroid crisis, 1270
Thyroid disorders
    hyperthyroidism. See Hyperthyroidism
    hypothyroidism. See Hypothyroidism
    in older adults, 1274b
    thyroiditis, 1275
Thyroid gland
    anatomy of, 1238–1239, 1239f
    hormones produced by, 1235t, 1239t, 1264–1265
    palpation of, 1242, 1242b

Thyroid storm, 1267, 1270, 1270b
Thyroidectomy, 1269, 1275
Thyroiditis, 1275
Thyroid-stimulating hormone
    deficiency of, 1246, 1246b
    description of, 1237t, 1239, 1271
    overproduction of, 1248b
Thyroid-stimulating hormone receptors, 1265
Thyroid-stimulating immunoglobulins, 1265
Thyrotoxic periodic paralysis, 1268b
Thyrotoxicosis, 918, 1264–1265, 1268b
Thyrotropin-releasing hormone, 1239
Thyroxine, 697b, 1006, 1238, 1247, 1266, 1272
TIBC. See Total iron-binding capacity
Tibial fracture, 1048–1049
Tibial nerve, 267b
Tic douloureux. See Trigeminal neuralgia
Tidal volume, 631
Time-cycled ventilators, 631
Time-out, 265, 266f
Tinea capitis, 468
Tinea corporis, 468
Tinea cruris, 468
Tinea manus, 468
Tinea pedis, 468
Tinel's sign, 1058
Tinnitus, 987, 995
TIPS. See Transjugular intrahepatic portal-systemic shunt
Tirofiban, 736–737
Tissue integrity
    assessment of, before rehabilitation, 90t, 91
    description of, 27–28
Tissue mast cells, 294
Tissue perfusion
    after amputation, 1053
    hematologic system in, 796f
Tissue plasminogen activator, 736–738
Tissue thromboplastin, 798t
TJC. See The Joint Commission
TLS. See Tumor lysis syndrome
Tobacco, 379. See also Smoking
Tocilizumab, 323b, 369, 370b
Toe brachial pressure index, 653
Toe fracture, 1038
Tofacitinib, 369
Toileting-related falls, 41
Tolerance, 58
Toll-like receptors, 290, 300
Tolterodine, 98
Tolvaptan, 954, 1252, 1252b
Tongue, 1062
Tonic-clonic seizures, 876, 878b–879b
Tonometry, 965
Tono-Pen, 965, 966f

Tooth loss, 31
Topiramate, 875
Topoisomerase inhibitors, 391, 391t
Torsade de pointes, 657
Total abdominal hysterectomy, 1462, 1462b–1463b
Total body irradiation, 387
Total body surface area, 489, 492
Total body water, 160, 161f
Total enteral nutrition
  abdominal distention caused by, 1222
  administration of, 1220–1221, 1220f
  complications of, 1221–1223
  description of, 1219–1223
  diarrhea secondary to, 1223
  electrolyte imbalances caused by, 1222–1223
  enterostomal feeding tubes used in, 1220–1221
  fluid imbalances caused by, 1222–1223
  gastrostomy for, 1221
  jejunostomy for, 1221
  nasoduodenal tube delivery of, 1220
  nasoenteric tube delivery of, 1220, 1220f
  nasogastric tube delivery of, 1220
  nausea and vomiting caused by, 1222
  refeeding syndrome caused by, 1221–1222
  tube misplacement and dislodgement, 1222
Total hip arthroplasty
  anesthesia used in, 310
  complications of, 311t, 312–313
  components of, 310–311, 310f
  hip dislocation after, 311–312
  hip resurfacing versus, 310
  low-molecular-weight heparin uses, 312
  minimally invasive, 310
  mobility after, 313–314, 313f
  operative procedures, 310–311
  pain management after, 312b, 313
  patient positioning after, 311, 313f
  postoperative care, 311–314, 311b
  preoperative care, 309–310
  primary, 309
  quadriceps-setting exercises after, 312–313
  rehabilitation, 314
  revision, 309
  self-management education, 312b, 314
  venous thromboembolism risks after, 310, 312–313
  weight-bearing restrictions, 313–314
Total iron-binding capacity, 805

Total joint arthroplasty
  hip. See Total hip arthroplasty
  hospital length of stay after, 314b
  osteoarthritis treated with, 309
Total knee arthroplasty
  complications of, 316
  continuous passive motion machine, 315, 315f, 316b
  cryotherapy after, 315
  description of, 314–316
  discharge instructions, 316
  minimally invasive, 314
  operative procedures, 315
  pain management after, 315–316
  postoperative care, 315–316, 315f
  preoperative care, 314–315
  rehabilitation after, 316
Total laryngectomy, 551, 551t, 555
Total lymphocyte count, 1217
Total parenteral nutrition
  complications of, 1224
  fluid imbalance risks, 1224
  malnutrition treated with, 1224
  solutions for, 200
Total proctocolectomy with permanent ileostomy for, 1154, 1155f
Total shoulder arthroplasty, 316
Total thyroidectomy, 1269
Total vaginal hysterectomy, 1462, 1463b
Touch discrimination assessments, 849
Touch sense, 33
Tourniquets, 129–130, 222
Toxic diffuse goiter, 1265
Toxic epidermal necrolysis, 478
Toxic hepatitis, 1180
Toxic megacolon, 1151t, 1153
Toxic multinodular goiter, 1265
Toxic shock syndrome, 1471, 1471b
Toxicity
  digoxin, 700b
  oxygen, 530
Toxins, 414
Toxoplasma gondii, 346
Toxoplasmosis encephalitis, 346
T-piece, 534–535, 534t, 535f, 636t
Trabeculation, 1358
Trabeculectomy, 975
Trachea, 510, 511f
Trachea–innominate artery fistula, 538t
Tracheal stenosis, 538t
Tracheobronchial tree, 510
Tracheoesophageal fistula, 538t
Tracheoesophageal puncture, 552
Tracheomalacia, 538t
Tracheostomy
  air warming in, 540–541
  aspiration prevention during swallowing, 543b
  assessments in, 542b
  bronchial hygiene in, 543
  care coordination for, 544

Tracheostomy (Continued)
  care issues for patients with, 539–544
  care of, 542–543, 542b
  caregiver anxiety in, 555b
  communication issues during, 543–544
  complications of, 537–539, 538t
  definition of, 537
  dressings for, 543, 543f
  health care resources for, 544
  home care management of, 544
  humidification in, 540–541
  in laryngeal cancer, 550
  minimal leak technique in, 540
  nutrition in, 543
  operative procedures for, 537, 538f
  oral hygiene in, 543
  overview of, 537
  psychosocial needs in, 544
  self-concept needs in, 544
  self-management education for, 544
  suctioning of, 541–542, 541b
  tissue damage in, 539–540, 541f
  transition management for, 544
  tubes used in, 539, 540f, 543
  weaning from, 544
Tracheostomy button, 544
Tracheotomy, 494, 553, 561
Traction
  fractures treated with, 1040–1041, 1040t, 1041b, 1041f
  lower-extremity, 1040t
  skeletal, 1040
  skin, 1040, 1041f
  spinal cord injury treated with, 899
  upper-extremity, 1040t
Trafficking, human See Human trafficking
Training
  bladder, 1350–1351, 1351b
  for emergency nursing, 120t, 123
  gait, 95–96, 95b, 95f
  habit, 1351, 1351b
TRALI. See Transfusion-related acute lung injury
TRAM flap, 1449–1450
Tramadol, 61
Transarterial chemoembolization, for liver cancer, 1187
Transbronchial biopsy, 526
Transbronchial needle aspiration, 526
Transcatheter aortic valve replacement, 708–709, 708f
Transcervical endometrial resection, 1461
Transcranial Doppler ultrasonography, 855
Transcutaneous electrical nerve stimulation, 66, 66f
Transcutaneous oxygen pressure, 1052
Transcutaneous pacing, 674, 674f

Transesophageal echocardiography
  description of, 660
  valvular heart disease evaluations, 707
Transfer belts, 95
Transferrin, 805, 1217
Transfusion
  acute reactions to, 835–836
  allergies to, 263, 836
  autologous blood, 836
  bacterial reactions to, 836
  cell savers, 235, 310
  febrile reactions to, 835
  hemolytic reactions to, 835
  indications for, 832t
  infusion therapy for, 200
  in older adults, 834b
  plasma, 835
  platelet
    idiopathic thrombocytopenic purpura treated with, 831
    indications for, 832t, 835
    reaction to, 835
  reactions to, 835–836
  red blood cells, 834–835
    compatibility determinations for, 834, 834t
    indications for, 832t, 834–835
    sickle cell disease treated with, 812
  reinfusion system, 310
  responsibilities in, 832–834
  safety in, 833b
  setup for, 832, 834f
  types of, 834–835
  white blood cells, 832t, 835
Transfusion-associated circulatory overload, 836
Transfusion-associated graft-versus-host-disease, 836
Transfusion-related acute lung injury, 626, 836
Transgender patients/health
  assessment of, 1495–1497
  care coordination for, 1501
  communication therapy for, 1499
  definition of, 1493
  drug therapy for, 1497–1498
  environment for, 1495b
  estrogen for, 1497–1498
  female-to-male
    definition of, 1493–1494, 1493t
    drug therapy for, 1498
    masculinizing surgeries for, 1500–1501
    phalloplasty for, 1501
  gonadotropin-releasing hormone agonists, 1498
  health care for, 1494–1501, 1496t
  history-taking of, 1496–1497
  issues in, 1494
  male-to-female
    definition of, 1493–1494, 1493t
    drug therapy for, 1497–1499, 1497t

Transgender patients/health
  (Continued)
    gender reassignment surgery
      for, 1499–1500
    vaginoplasty for, 1499–1500
    nonsurgical management of,
      1497–1499
    older adults as, 1497b
    physical assessment of, 1497
    pronoun usage for, 1495–1496
    psychosocial assessment of, 1497
    reproductive health options in,
      1499
    stress experienced by, 1494
    surgical management of,
      1499–1501
    terminology associated with,
      1493–1494, 1493t
    transition management for, 1501
    violence and verbal harassment of,
      1494
    voice therapy for, 1499
Transient ischemic attack, 927–928,
  928b. See also Stroke
Transition management, 3. See also
  specific disorder, transition
  management for
Transition (transgender), 1493t
Transjugular intrahepatic
  portal-systemic shunt,
  1177–1178
Transmission-based precautions
  for infection control, 419, 420t
  for skin infections, 469–470
Transmyocardial laser
  revascularization, 789
Transparent film dressings, 499, 500f
Transplantation
  bone marrow, 822
  heart
    cardiomyopathy treated with,
      716–717, 717f
    discharge planning for, 717
    heart failure treated with, 705
    operative procedures for, 716,
      717f
    postoperative care for, 716–717
    preoperative care for, 716
    rejection of, 716b
    survival rates after, 717
  hematopoietic stem cell. See
    Hematopoietic stem cell
    transplantation
  immunosuppression after, 302b
  islet cell, 1303
  kidney. See Kidney transplantation
  liver, 1187–1189, 1188t, 1189b
  lung
    cystic fibrosis treated with,
      583–584
    pulmonary arterial
      hypertension treated with,
      585
  pancreatic
    complications of, 1303

Transplantation (Continued)
  description of, 1204
  diabetes mellitus treated with,
    1302–1303
  rejection of, 1302–1303
  rejection of
    acute, 301
    causes of, 300–301
    chronic, 301
    drugs for, 302b
    hyperacute, 301
    management of, 301, 302b
    renal. See Kidney transplantation
Transport maximum, 1325
Transrectal ultrasonography, 1436,
  1483, 1483b
Transsexual, 1493–1494, 1493t
Transtracheal oxygen therapy, 536
Transurethral resection of the
  bladder tumor, 1368
Transurethral resection of the
  prostate, 1479–1480, 1480b,
  1480f, 1483
Transvaginal ultrasonography
  description of, 1436
  uterine leiomyoma evaluations,
    1460
Transverse colostomy, 1131f
Trastuzumab, 405, 1097–1098
Trauma. See also Accidents; Motor
  vehicle accidents
  amputations caused by, 1050, 1053
  bladder, 1369
  blunt, 129
  chest
    flail chest, 637, 637f
    fractures caused by, 1049–1050
    pulmonary contusion, 636
    rib fracture, 636–637
  definition of, 127
  ear, 995, 1000b
  esophageal, 1101–1102, 1101t
  eye, 981–982
  facial, 558–559
  kidney, 1387–1388, 1387b
  laryngeal, 559–560
  liver, 1186, 1186b
  mechanism of injury, 128–129
  ocular, 981–982
  penetrating
    description of, 129
    ocular, 982
    osteomyelitis secondary to, 1023
    spinal cord injury caused by,
      894
Trauma centers, 127–128, 128f, 128t,
  130–131
Trauma nursing
  mechanism of injury, 128–129
  primary survey and resuscitation
    interventions, 129–130, 131t
  principles of, 127–131
  secondary survey and
    resuscitation interventions,
    130

Trauma systems, 128
Traumatic brain injury
  acceleration-deceleration
    mechanism of, 941, 941f
  airway assessments in, 948–949
  Alzheimer's disease risks, 858–859
  assessment of, 944–946
  brain death after, 947
  breathing pattern assessments in,
    948–949
  care coordination for, 949–950,
    949b
  cognitive rehabilitation for, 948
  death after, 947
  definition of, 940
  drug therapy for, 948, 948b
  epidural hematoma secondary to,
    942, 942f
  etiology of, 943
  features of, 945b
  health care resources for, 950
  health promotion and
    maintenance for, 943–944
  hemorrhage caused by, 944–950
  home care management of, 949
  hydrocephalus caused by, 943
  hypotension secondary to, 941
  hypoxemia after, 947
  hypoxia secondary to, 941
  imaging assessment of, 946
  incidence of, 943
  increased intracranial pressure
    after, 941–942, 946
  interventions for, 947–950
  laboratory assessment of, 946
  level of consciousness assessments
    in, 946
  magnetic resonance imaging of,
    946
  mannitol for, 948, 948b
  mild, 944t, 945b
  moderate, 944t, 949
  neurogenic pulmonary edema
    caused by, 954
  neurologic assessment of, 945–946
  nonsurgical management of,
    947–948
  in older adults, 944b
  pathophysiology of, 940–943
  patient positioning in, 947b
  physical assessment of, 944–946
  prevalence of, 943
  primary, 941
  psychosocial assessment of, 946
  secondary brain injuries caused
    by, 941–943, 947
  self-management education for,
    949, 949b
  sensory perception after, 948–949
  severe, 941, 944t, 947, 949
  severity of, 941, 944t, 947
  signs and symptoms of, 944–946
  spine precautions with, 945
  subdural hematoma secondary to,
    942–943, 942f

Traumatic brain injury (Continued)
  therapeutic hypothermia for, 947
  transition management for,
    949–950, 949b
  in veterans, 845–846, 950b
  vital signs assessment in, 945
Traumatic relocation syndrome,
  861
Trendelenburg position, 265f
Treponema pallidum, 415–416, 1508
Treprostinil, 585
TRH. See Thyrotropin-releasing
  hormone
Triage
  automated tracking systems for,
    152–153
  "civilian", 151–153
  in culturally competent care, 152b
  disaster triage tag system, 152,
    152b
  in emergency departments,
    123–124, 124t
  green-tagged patients, 152
  mass casualty event, 151–153, 152t
  radiofrequency technology for,
    152–153
  red-tagged patients, 152
  yellow-tagged patients, 152
Triage officer, 154, 154t
Trichloroacetic acid, 1511
Trichomonas, 1356
Tricuspid valve, 642–643, 643f
Tricyclic antidepressants
  in Alzheimer's disease, 864
  fibromyalgia treated with, 334
  in older adults, 37b
  pain management uses of, 64
  side effects of, 64
Trigeminal nerve
  description of, 844t
  external stimulator for, 875
Trigeminal neuralgia, 923–924, 923f
Trigeminy, 671
Trigger points, 333
Triglycerides, 656
Triiodothyronine, 1238, 1247, 1266,
  1272
Trimethoprim/sulfamethoxazole,
  1359b–1360b
Triptans, for migraine headaches,
  874–875, 875b
Trochlear nerve, 844t
Troponin, 656
Trousseau's sign, 180, 180f, 182,
  1201, 1277
Truss, 1138
Truvada, 342
Trypanosoma cruzi, 1166
Trypsin, 1197
TSH. See Thyroid-stimulating
  hormone
T-SPOT TB test, 607
TTP. See Thrombotic
  thrombocytopenic purpura
T-tube drain, 278, 279f

Tube feedings
administration of, 1221
bolus feeding, 1221
care and maintenance in,
1221b–1222b
continuous, 1221
cyclic, 1221
enterostomal, 1220–1221
tube misplacement and
dislodgement, 1222
Tuberculin skin test, 607, 607f
Tuberculosis
in AIDS-infected patients, 347
airborne precautions for, 609
airway clearance in, 607–608
anxiety management in, 609
assessment of, 606–607
care coordination for, 610
diagnostic assessment of, 607
drug therapy for, 608–609
etiology of, 606
fatigue management in, 610
health care resources for, 610
health promotion and
maintenance for, 606
hematogenous, 605–606
history-taking for, 606–607
home care management of, 610
imaging assessment of, 607
latent, 606
miliary, 605–606
multidrug-resistant, 609
nutrition in, 610
pathophysiology of, 605–606
physical assessment of, 607
psychosocial assessment of, 607
screening for, 607
secondary, 606
self-management education for,
610
signs and symptoms of, 607
sputum culture for, 607
transition management for, 610
tuberculin skin test for, 607, 607f
Tumor(s). See also Cancer
bone. See Bone tumors
brain. See Brain tumors
doubling time of, 377
esophageal. See Esophageal tumors
grading of, 377t
growth assessments, 377
kidney, 1385, 1385t
oral, 1078–1084
pancreatic, 1205
primary, 375
rectal, 1130t
salivary glands, 1085
secondary, 375
testicular, 1486–1487, 1487t
Tumor, node, metastasis system, 377,
378t
Tumor cells, 373–374
Tumor lysis syndrome, 409–410,
409f
Tumor necrosis factor, 300t

Tuning fork tests, 989–990, 998
Tunneled central venous catheters,
207, 207f, 213, 226
Turbinates, 509, 509f
Turgor, 441
24-hour urine collection, 1334t,
1336b
Two-point discrimination, 849
Tympanic membrane
anatomy of, 984, 985f–986f
perforation of, 992f
Tympanometry, 991
Tympanoplasty, 999–1000, 1000f
Tympany, 519t
Type 1 diabetes mellitus. See
Diabetes mellitus, type 1
Type 2 diabetes mellitus. See
Diabetes mellitus, type 2
Type A chronic gastritis, 1104
Type B chronic gastritis, 1104
Type II pneumocytes, 510, 626
Tyrosine, 1239
Tyrosine kinase inhibitors, 330, 404t,
405, 1207
Tyrosine kinases, 403
Tzanck smear, 445

U
U wave, 669–670, 669f
UAP. See Unlicensed assistive
personnel
UC. See Ulcerative colitis
UES. See Upper esophageal sphincter
Ulcer(s)
description of, 438f, 448
duodenal, 1107–1108, 1108f
foot, 1305
gastric, 1107, 1108f, 1110
peptic. See Peptic ulcer(s)
stress, 1108
Ulcerative colitis
activity restrictions for, 1153
American College of
Gastroenterologists
classification of, 1150t
assessment of, 1151–1152
blood loss monitoring in, 1156b
care coordination for, 1156–1157
colonoscopy of, 1152
complementary and integrative
health for, 1153
complications of, 1151t
Crohn's disease versus, 1150t
cultural considerations for, 1151b
definition of, 1150
diagnostic assessment of,
1151–1152
diarrhea management in,
1152–1155
drug therapy for, 1152–1153
etiology of, 1150–1151
genetic risk of, 1150–1151
health care resources for, 1157
history-taking for, 1151
home care management of, 1156

Ulcerative colitis (Continued)
ileostomy for, 1153–1154
immunomodulators for, 1153
incidence of, 1151
interventions for, 1152–1155
laboratory assessment of,
1151–1152
lower gastrointestinal bleeding in,
1156, 1156b
magnetic resonance enterography
for, 1152
nonsurgical management of,
1152–1153
nutrition therapy for, 1153
pain management in, 1155–1156,
1156b
pathophysiology of, 1150–1151
physical assessment of, 1151
prevalence of, 1151
psychosocial assessment of, 1151
restorative proctocolectomy with
ileo pouch-anal anastomosis,
1154, 1154f
self-management education for,
1156–1157
severity of, 1150, 1150t
signs and symptoms of, 1151
skin care for, 1156b
surgical management of,
1153–1155, 1155f
total proctocolectomy with
permanent ileostomy for,
1154, 1155f
transition management for,
1156–1157
Ultrafiltration, 1397–1398
Ultram. See Tramadol
Ultrasonography
abdominal, 1123
acute pancreatitis evaluations, 1200
breast evaluations, 1446
cholecystitis evaluations, 1194
gastrointestinal system
assessments using, 1073
malabsorption evaluations, 1141
musculoskeletal system
evaluations using, 1013
peripheral intravenous therapy
applications of, 202–203
renal system assessments, 1337t,
1338
reproductive system assessments,
1436
transrectal, 1436
transvaginal, 1436
vision assessments, 965
Ultrasound-assisted wound therapy,
458–459
Ultraviolet light therapy, 465
Ultraviolet radiation, 379
Umbilical hernia, 1137, 1137f
Umbo, 985f
Uncal herniation, 943, 943f
Undernutrition. See Malnutrition
Unfractionated heparin, 744

Unilateral inattention syndrome,
934, 939
Unintentional injury, 127
Unlicensed assistive personnel
delegation of tasks to, 6
fluid replacement therapy by,
169
pressure injury prevention by, 42b
skin care by, 97
supervision of, 6
Unna boot, 747–748
Unstable angina pectoris, 769–770
Upper airway
edema of, 490, 491b
obstruction of, 560–561, 561f
structures of, 547
Upper endoscopy, 1089
Upper esophageal sphincter,
1062–1063, 1087–1088
Upper extremity
amputations of, 1050
fractures of, 1046–1047, 1046f
traction for, 1040t
Upper gastrointestinal bleeding
acid suppression for rebleeding
prevention, 1114
description of, 1108, 1109b
endoscopic therapy for, 1113
fluid replacement for, 1113
hypovolemia concerns secondary
to, 1113
interventional radiologic
procedures for, 1113–1114
interventions for, 1113–1114
nasogastric tube for, 1113
nonsurgical management of,
1113–1114
Upper gastrointestinal radiographic
series, 1070
Upper respiratory tract, 509–510,
509f
Urea breath test, 1111
Urease, 1401
Uremia, 1330, 1398b
Uremic cardiomyopathy, 1401
Uremic encephalopathy, 1403
Uremic frost, 1404
Uremic syndrome, 1398
Ureter(s)
anatomy of, 1327, 1327f
assessment of, 1330–1331
Ureterolithiasis, 1361
Ureterolithotomy, 1364
Ureteropelvic junction, 1338
Ureteroplasty, 1375
Ureteroscopy, 1364
Ureterostomy, 1368f
Urethra
anatomy of, 1327–1328, 1430
assessment of, 1331
Urethral occlusion devices, 1348
Urethral pressure profile, 1340
Urethral sphincter, 1327, 1327f
Urethritis, 1359–1361
Urethrogram, 1339

Urge incontinence, 1344, 1345t, 1349–1351, 1350b, 1484–1485
Urgency, 1328, 1330
Urgent surgery, 232t
Urgent triage, 124
Urinalysis, 1332–1335, 1333b
    preoperative, 237
    urolithiasis evaluations, 1362–1363
Urinary bladder. See Bladder
Urinary diversion, 1368, 1368f
Urinary elimination, 18
Urinary incontinence
    areflexic bladder as cause of, 97–98, 98t
    assessment of, 1346–1347, 1346b
    behavioral interventions for, 1352
    bladder training for, 1350–1351, 1351b
    care coordination for, 1353–1354, 1353b
    contributing factors, 1346b
    description of, 19
    drug therapy for, 98, 1348, 1350b, 1352
    electrical stimulation for, 1348
    etiology of, 1344
    flaccid bladder as cause of, 97–98, 98t
    functional, 1352
    habit training for, 1351, 1351b
    health care resources for, 1353–1354
    history-taking for, 1346
    home care management of, 1353
    incidence of, 1344–1346
    intermittent catheterization for, 98, 1352
    interventions for, 1347–1349, 1347b
    magnetic resonance therapy for, 1348
    mixed, 1345t, 1352
    nonpharmacologic management of, 97–98
    nonsurgical management of, 1347–1348
    nutrition therapy for, 1348, 1350
    in older adults, 1344b
    overactive spastic bladder as cause of, 97
    overflow, 1344, 1345t, 1351–1352
    pathophysiology of, 1343
    pelvic muscle exercises for, 1347, 1347b, 1351
    pessary for, 1348, 1352
    physical assessment of, 1346–1347
    prevalence of, 1344–1346
    psychosocial preparation for, 1353
    rehabilitation for, 97–98
    risk factors for, 1344–1346
    self-management education for, 1353, 1353b
    signs and symptoms of, 1346–1347
    stress, 1344, 1348, 1349t, 1464

Urinary incontinence (Continued)
    surgical management of, 1348–1349, 1349t
    transition management for, 1353–1354, 1353b
    types of, 1345t
    urge, 1344, 1345t, 1349–1351, 1350b, 1484–1485
    vaginal cone weight therapy for, 1348, 1348f
Urinary retention, 18
Urinary stones. See Urolithiasis
Urinary system
    age-related changes in, 234b, 1328–1329
    assessment of, 90t, 91, 803
    burn injury-related assessment of, 491–492
    postoperative assessment of, 276
    sickle cell disease effects on, 810
    ureters, 1327
Urinary system disorders
    urethritis, 1359–1361
    urinary tract infection. See Urinary tract infections
    urolithiasis. See Urolithiasis
Urinary tract
    anatomy of, 1321, 1322f, 1343
    obstruction of, 1365
Urinary tract infections. See also Cystitis
    assessment of, 1357–1359
    asymptomatic bacterial, 1354
    care coordination for, 1359
    catheter-associated, 415, 415b, 1355–1356, 1356b, 1423, 1500
    comfort measures for, 1359
    complicated, 1354
    contributing factors for, 1355t
    definition of, 1354
    diagnostic assessment of, 1358–1359
    drug therapy for, 98, 1359, 1360b
    etiology of, 1354–1357
    features of, 1358b
    fluid intake for, 1359
    genetic risk of, 1354–1357
    nonsurgical management of, 1359
    in older adults, 91
    risk factors for, 1354
    signs and symptoms of, 98, 1358
    surgical management of, 1359
    transition management for, 1359
    uncomplicated, 1354
Urine
    casts in, 1335
    color of, 1332
    composition of, 18
    culture and sensitivity of, 1335
    early, 1324
    electrolytes in, 1336
    glucose in, 1335
    nitrites in, 1335
    osmolarity of, 1336

Urine (Continued)
    pH, 1333
    post-void residual, 98
    protein in, 1333
    sediment in, 1335
    specific gravity of, 1332–1333
Urine collections, 1335
Urine output, obligatory, 165
Urine specimens, 1334t
Urine stream testing, 1340
Urine tests
    description of, 1068, 1243, 1243b
    urinalysis, 1332–1335, 1333b
Urobilinogen, 1068, 1192
Urodynamic studies, 1340
Urolithiasis
    assessment of, 1362–1363
    computed tomography of, 1363f
    definition of, 1361
    dietary treatment of, 1365, 1366t
    etiology of, 1361–1362
    extracorporeal shock wave lithotripsy for, 1364
    genetic risk of, 1361–1362, 1362b
    incidence of, 1362
    infection prevention in, 1365
    interventions for, 1363–1365, 1363f
    minimally invasive surgery for, 1364
    nonsurgical management of, 1363–1364
    pain management in, 1363–1365
    pathophysiology of, 1361–1362
    prevalence of, 1362
    self-management education for, 1366b
    surgical management of, 1364–1365
    urinary obstruction caused by, 1365
Urosepsis, 1356–1357
Urothelial cancer
    assessment of, 1367–1369
    health promotion and maintenance of, 1366–1367
    interventions for, 1367–1369, 1368f
    pathophysiology of, 1366
Urothelium, 1327
Urticaria, 462, 1261
Ustekinumab, 333, 369, 370b, 466b
USWT. See Ultrasound-assisted wound therapy
Uterine artery embolization, 1461, 1461b
Uterine leiomyomas
    assessment of, 1460
    bleeding in, 1461–1463
    care coordination for, 1463
    classification of, 1460f
    etiology of, 1460
    genetic risk of, 1460
    health care resources for, 1463
    home care management of, 1463

Uterine leiomyomas (Continued)
    hysterectomy for, 1461–1463, 1461t, 1462b–1463b
    incidence of, 1460
    interventions for, 1461–1463
    pathophysiology of, 1459–1460
    physical assessment of, 1460
    prevalence of, 1460
    psychosocial assessment of, 1460
    self-management education for, 1463
    signs and symptoms of, 1460
    submucosal, 1459–1460, 1460f
    subserosal, 1459–1460, 1460f
    surgical management of, 1461–1463
    transcervical endometrial resection for, 1461
    transition management for, 1463
    transvaginal ultrasound of, 1460
    uterine artery embolization for, 1461, 1461b
Uterus
    anatomy of, 1429
    prolapse of, 1464
Uvea, 957
Uvulopalatopharyngoplasty, 559

V
Vaccines, influenza, 596–597
Vacutainer needle holder, 215, 215f
Vacuum constriction device, 1490
VAD. See Vascular access devices
Vagal maneuvers, 678
Vagal nerve stimulation, 542, 879
Vagina
    anatomy of, 1429
    bleeding from, 1469
Vaginal cone weight therapy, 1348, 1348f
Vaginoplasty, 1499–1500, 1501t
Vagus nerve, 844t
Validation therapy, 863
Valsalva maneuver, 98, 634, 1301, 1352
Valvular heart disease
    antibiotic prophylaxis for, 707b
    aortic regurgitation, 706b, 707
    aortic stenosis, 706–707, 706b
    assessment of, 707
    atrial fibrillation and, 708
    balloon valvuloplasty for, 708
    cardiac output in, 708
    care coordination for, 710–711
    direct commissurotomy for, 709
    drug therapy for, 707–708
    echocardiography of, 707
    health care resources for, 711–712
    heart valve replacement procedures for, 709–710, 709f
    home care management of, 710
    interventions for, 707–710
    mitral regurgitation, 706, 706b
    mitral stenosis, 705–706, 706b, 710b
    mitral valve annuloplasty for, 709

Valvular heart disease (Continued)
  mitral valve prolapse, 706
  noninvasive reparative procedures
      for, 708–709, 708f
  nonsurgical management of,
      707–709
  pathophysiology of, 705–707
  self-management education for,
      710, 710b
  surgical management of, 709–710
  transcatheter aortic valve
      replacement for, 708–709,
      708f
  transition management for,
      710–711
Vancomycin, 200b
Vancomycin-intermediate
    Staphylococcus aureus, 421–422
Vancomycin-resistant Enterococcus
  contact precautions for, 419
  description of, 422
Vancomycin-resistant Staphylococcus
    aureus, 421–422
Vaping, 514
Vardenafil, 1489
Varenicline, for smoking cessation,
    515, 515b
Variant angina, 770, 774
Varicella-zoster virus infection, 347
Varicose veins, 748
Vas deferens, 1430–1431
Vascular access
  hemodialysis, 1413–1416, 1414f,
      1414t–1415t
  preoperative preparation for, 242
Vascular access devices
  central intravenous therapy, 205,
      212
  definition of, 201–202
  removing of, 215
  securing of, 213b
  tunneled central venous catheters,
      207, 207f, 213
Vascular dementia
  Alzheimer's disease versus, 858t
  pathophysiology of, 857–858
Vascular endothelial growth factor,
    375, 784
Vascular endothelial growth factor/
    receptor inhibitors
  colorectal cancer treated with,
      1130
  description of, 404t, 405
  macular degeneration treated
      with, 979
Vascular leak syndrome, 293–294
Vascular system
  arterial system, 645–646
  purposes of, 645–646
Vasculitis
  in rheumatoid arthritis, 318–319
  systemic necrotizing, 334t
Vasoconstriction, 752
Vasodilators, for acute coronary
    syndromes, 783b

Vasogenic edema, 942
Vaso-occlusive events, 809
Vasopressin, 1237t, 1245, 1246b,
    1332. See also Antidiuretic
    hormone
VATS. See Video-assisted
    thoracoscopic surgery
Vaughn-Williams classification, 685
Vedolizumab, 1153
Vegetarians, 1212
Veins, 646
Venereal Disease Research
    Laboratory serum test, 1509
Veno-occlusive disease, 825
Venous beading, 1284
Venous distention, 222
Venous duplex ultrasonography, 743
Venous insufficiency
  assessment of, 747
  chronic, 746–747
  description of, 716
  graduated compression stockings
      for, 747b
  interventions for, 747–748, 747b
  pathophysiology of, 746–747
Venous pulse, 653
Venous system, 646
Venous thromboembolism. See also
    Deep vein thrombosis;
    Pulmonary embolism
  assessment of, 742–743
  Core Measure Set for, 742, 742t,
      746, 938
  diagnostic assessment of, 743
  etiology of, 742
  fractures as risk factor for,
      1034–1035
  heparin prophylaxis for, 617–618
  history-taking for, 742
  inadequate clotting secondary to, 15
  incidence of, 742
  pancreatic cancer as cause of, 1205
  pathophysiology of, 742
  physical assessment of, 742–743
  postoperative, 244, 274, 281
  preoperative prophylactic
      interventions for, 274
  prevalence of, 742
  prevention of, 23, 281, 312–313
  pulmonary embolism caused by,
      617, 716
  risk factors for, 244, 617
  signs and symptoms of, 742–743
  in spinal cord injury patients, 897
  thrombus in, 742
  after total hip arthroplasty, 310,
      312–313
Venous thrombosis, 15–16
Venous ulcers, 732–733, 734b, 747
Venous vasodilators, 699
Ventilation
  mechanical. See Mechanical
      ventilation
  noninvasive positive-pressure, 535,
      535b, 536f

Ventilation/perfusion mismatch, 625
Ventilator(s), 631–633
Ventilator-associated events, 634,
    634t
Ventilator-associated lung injury, 635
Ventilator-associated pneumonia
  description of, 600t, 601
  noninvasive positive-pressure
      ventilation for prevention of,
      535
  prevention of, 897
Ventilator-induced lung injury, 635
Ventilatory failure, 624–625, 625t
Ventricular assist devices, for heart
    failure, 701–702, 701f
Ventricular asystole, 686–688
Ventricular dysrhythmias
  description of, 683–688
  premature ventricular complexes,
      683–684, 683f
  ventricular asystole, 686–688
  ventricular fibrillation, 684–686,
      685f
  ventricular tachycardia, 684, 684f
Ventricular fibrillation, 684–686, 685f
Ventricular gallop, 654–655
Ventricular remodeling, 694, 771
Ventricular tachycardia, 684, 684f
Ventriculomyomectomy, 716
Venturi masks, 533–534, 534f, 534t
Veracity, 9
Vermiform appendix, 1064
Vertebral compression fractures,
    1036, 1050
Vertebrobasilar artery stroke, 933b
Vertebroplasty, 1050, 1050b
Vertical compression, of spine, 894,
    895f
Vertigo, 987, 995–996, 1001
Very-low-calorie diets, 1227
Vesicants, 204, 392
Vesicles, 438f
Vesicoureteral reflux, 1355t
Vesicular sounds, 520t
Vestibulocochlear nerve, 844t
Veterans
  Alzheimer's disease in, 859b, 867b
  chronic pain in, 36b, 47b
  cognitive-behavioral therapy for,
      67b
  dementia in, 126b
  depression in, 36b
  diabetes mellitus in, 1291b
  hepatitis C in, 1183b
  lower-extremity amputation in,
      1051b
  smoking in, 515b
  spinal cord injury in, 903b
  traumatic brain injury in,
      845–846, 950b
  type 2 diabetes mellitus in, 1291b
Veterans Administration
  description of, 9–10
  safe patient handling and mobility
      practices, 93, 95f

Vibratory positive expiratory
    pressure device, for chronic
    obstructive pulmonary disease,
    579, 579f
Vicodin. See Hydrocodone
Video-assisted thoracoscopic surgery,
    589
Viral carcinogenesis, 378t, 379
Viral gastroenteritis, 1148t, 1149
Viral hepatitis, 1180, 1185b
Viral infections
  of skin, 467b, 468
  skin cultures for, 444–445
Viral meningitis, 881
Virchow's triad, 742
Virtual colonoscopy, 1073
Virulence, 414
Visceral pain, 48
Visceral proteins, 1217
Vision. See also Eye(s)
  acuity of, 26
  assessment of, 962–967
  diagnostic assessment of, 965–967
  health promotion and
      maintenance of, 961–962
  imaging assessment of, 965
  impairment of, in older adults, 963b
  laboratory assessment of, 965
  loss of, 26, 934f
  near, 964
  near point of, 961
  psychosocial assessment of,
      964–965
  testing of, 963–964, 964f
Vision loss
  diabetes mellitus as cause of,
      1307–1308
  environmental management of,
      1307–1308
Visual acuity tests, 963–964
Visual analog dyspnea scale, 576, 576f
Visual evoked potentials, 855
Visual field testing, 964
Vital signs
  postoperative assessment of, 274
  in traumatic brain injury, 945
Vitamin B$_{12}$
  absorption of, 1141
  deficiency of
    anemia caused by, 814, 814t,
        815f, 816
    central nervous system affected
        by, 803
    in vegetarians, 1212
  pernicious anemia and, 1105
Vitamin D
  activation of, 1327
  deficiency of, 1277–1278
  description of, 432, 482, 1006
Vitamin D$_3$, 1020–1021
Vitamin K, 745b, 798
Vitamin K antagonists
  mechanism of action, 801
  pulmonary embolism treated
      with, 621b

Vitiligo, 1242
Vitreous body, 958, 958f
Vocal fremitus, 518–519
Vocational assessments, 92
Vocational counselors, 89
Voice sounds, 519
Voided urine, 1334t
Voiding
    facilitating techniques for, 98
    post-void residual urine after, 98
    toileting routines to re-establish, 98
Volkmann's contractures, 1034
Volume fraction, 803
Volume-cycled ventilators, 631
Voluntary stopping of eating and drinking, 115
Volutrauma, 635
Volvulus, 1092, 1122, 1122f
Vomiting. See Nausea and vomiting
VSED. See Voluntary stopping of eating and drinking
VTE. See Venous thromboembolism
Vulnerable populations, 118
Vulva, 1428–1429
Vulvovaginitis, 1470–1471, 1471b

W
Waist circumference, 1225
Waist-to-hip ratio, 1225
Walker, 1044
Wandering, 864, 864b
Warfarin
    antidote for, 745b
    deep vein thrombosis treated with, 745
    drug interactions with, 746b
    food interactions with, 746b
    genetic testing before using, 620b
    in mechanical valve patients, 710
Warm antibody anemia, 815
Wasp stings, 137, 137b, 138t–140t
Water brash, 1089
Water pressure, 161
Water-seal chest drainage system, 590–591, 590b
Weak acid, 186, 186f
Weak bases, 186
Weakness
    assessment of, 1008–1009
    during dying, 109
    in systemic lupus erythematosus, 327

Weaning
    from mechanical ventilation, 635, 636t
    from tracheostomy, 544
Weapons of mass destruction, 153
Wearable cardioverter/defibrillator, 688
Weber tuning fork test, 989–990
Wedge resection, 589
Weight
    assessment of, 1213b
    ideal body, 1215, 1225
    measurement of, 1213–1215
Weight gain
    fluid retention as cause of, 172
    mobility affected by, 93–95
Weight loss
    in burn injury patients, 502
    in chronic obstructive pulmonary disease, 580
    dehydration and, 168
    unintentional, 1215
Weight-bearing fractures, 1050
Wellness promotion, 30b
Wernicke's aphasia, 938
West Nile virus, 883, 884b
Wet age-related macular degeneration, 979
Wheelchair, 95
Wheelchair pushups, 97
Wheezes, 521t, 601
Whipple procedure, 1207, 1207f, 1208t
White blood cell(s)
    description of, 290–291
    formation of, 797
    transfusion of, 832t, 835
White blood cell count, 657
White blood cell count with differential, 424–425
White blood cell differential, 293, 293t
"White clot syndrome", 744
White matter, 840
Wild-type gene sequence, 76
Williams position, 905
Winged needles, 203–204
Withdrawing or withholding life-sustaining therapy, 114–115
Women
    carpal tunnel syndrome in, 1057b
    coronary artery disease in, 772b
    dehydration in, 164b

Women (Continued)
    human immunodeficiency virus infection in, 340b, 345b
    stroke in, 935b
Wong-Baker FACES pain rating scale, 50, 52f
Wood's light examination, 445
Work-arounds, 4
Work-related musculoskeletal disorders, 93
Wound
    breakdown of, 551
    chemical débridement of, 457, 457t
    closure of, 267, 268f
    colostomy, 1132
    contraction of, 474f
    débridement of, 457, 457t
    dehiscence of, 277, 278f, 282–283, 1099
    drains, 277–278, 279f, 282
    dressings for. See Dressings
    enzymatic débridement of, 499
    evisceration of, 277, 278f, 283, 283b
    full-thickness, 473–474
    mechanical débridement of, 457, 457t, 498–499
    partial-thickness, 473
    perineal, 1133b
    pressure injury
        assessment of, 453–455
        best practices for, 460b
        dressings for, 457–458
        drug therapy for, 458
        electrical stimulation for, 458–459
        hyperbaric oxygen therapy for, 458
        management of, 455–459, 457b
        negative-pressure wound therapy for, 458
        nonsurgical management of, 457–459
        nutrition therapy for, 458
        physical therapy for, 458
        skin substitutes for, 458
        surgical management of, 459
        ultrasound-assisted wound therapy for, 458–459
    staple closure of, 282
    suture closure of, 282

Wound exudate, 453t
Wound healing
    delayed primary intention, 278
    impaired, 277, 278f, 474t
    mechanisms of, 473–474
    normal, 471t
    nutrition for, 97, 287
    obesity effects on, 236–237
    phases of, 466f, 471–473, 471t
    postoperative, 277, 278f
    promotion of, 28
Wound infection
    drug therapy for, 282
    in older adults, 954
    postoperative prevention of, 281–283
Wrist
    carpal tunnel syndrome of, 1057–1059, 1058b
    Colles' fracture of, 1046, 1046f, 1057
Wrist drop, 267b

X
X chromosome, 74
Xanthine oxidase inhibitors, 331–332
Xanthines, 571
Xeljanz. See Tofacitinib
Xenografts, 499, 499f, 709
Xerosis, 449b, 461
Xerostomia, 319, 549, 1084–1085
Xylose absorption, 1069b

Y
Y chromosome, 72, 74
Y-tubing, 832

Z
Zanamivir, 597–598
Zeaxanthin, 979
Zegerid, 1091
Zenker's diverticula, 1101
Ziconotide, 905, 905b
Zika virus, 416
Zohydro. See Hydrocodone
Zoledronic acid, 1026
Zostavax, 469